Rehabilitation of the hand
SURGERY AND THERAPY

Rehabilitation of the hand
SURGERY AND THERAPY

Editors

JAMES M. HUNTER, M.D.

Professor of Orthopaedic Surgery,
Jefferson Medical College of Thomas Jefferson University;
Chief, Hand Surgery Services, Department of Orthopaedics,
Thomas Jefferson University Hospital,
Philadelphia, Pennsylvania

LAWRENCE H. SCHNEIDER, M.D.

Clinical Professor of Orthopaedic Surgery,
Jefferson Medical College of Thomas Jefferson University,
Philadelphia, Pennsylvania

EVELYN J. MACKIN, P.T.

Director of Hand Therapy, Hand Rehabilitation Center,
Philadelphia, Pennsylvania

ANNE D. CALLAHAN, M.S., O.T.R./L.

Hand Therapy Consultant; Former Assistant Director of Hand Therapy,
Hand Rehabilitation Center,
Philadelphia, Pennsylvania

THIRD EDITION

*With **2216** illustrations, including **25** in color*

The C. V. Mosby Company

ST. LOUIS · BALTIMORE · PHILADELPHIA · TORONTO   1990

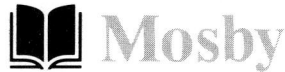

Editor: Eugenia A. Klein
Developmental Editor: Kathryn H. Falk
Assistant Editor: Ellen Baker Geisel
Project Manager: Teri Merchant
Production Editors: Betty Hazelwood, Gail Brower
Book and Cover Design: Gail Morey Hudson

THIRD EDITION

The C.V. Mosby Company
11830 Westline Industrial Drive, St. Louis, Missouri 63146

Library of Congress Cataloging-in-Publication Data

Rehabilitation of the hand: surgery and therapy/editors, James M.
  Hunter . . . [et al.].—3rd ed.
      p. cm.
    Includes bibliographical references.
    ISBN 0-8016-2472-X
    1. Hand—Wounds and injuries. 2. Hand—Surgery, 3. Hand—
Surgery—Patients—Rehabilitation.   I. Hunter, James M.
      [DNLM: 1. Hand. 2. Hand Injuries—rehabilitation.   WE 830 R345]
    RD559.R43   1990
    617.5'7506—dc20
                                                  89.12938

GW/MV/MV   9 8 7 6 5 4 3 2 1

Contributors

URSULA ALBION, P.T., O.T.

chapter 67

Victoria Hospital, University of Western Ontario,
London, Ontario, Canada

PETER C. AMADIO, M.D.

chapter 28

Consultant in Orthopaedics, Mayo Clinic;
Assistant Professor of Orthopaedics, Mayo Medical School,
Rochester, Minnesota

THOMAS J. ARMSTRONG, Ph.D.

chapter 97

Associate Professor, Department of Environmental
and Industrial Health, Department of Industrial
and Operations Engineering, The University of Michigan,
Ann Arbor, Michigan

PAT L. AULICINO, M.D.

chapter 4

Associate Professor of Orthopaedic Surgery, Eastern Virginia
Medical School, Norfolk, Virginia

LOIS M. BARBER, O.T.R., F.A.O.T.A.

chapter 56

Vice-President, LMB Hand Rehab Products, Inc., Product
Development, San Luis Obispo, California

JOHN BARBIS, M.A., P.T.

chapters 40 and 41

Assistant Professor, Thomas Jefferson University, College of
Allied Health Services, Philadelphia, Pennsylvania

**JOHN V. BASMAJIAN, M.D., F.R.C.P.(C.),
F.A.C.R.M. (Australia), F.S.B.M., F.A.B.M.R.**

chapter 78

Professor Emeritus of Medicine and Anatomy, McMaster
University, Hamilton, Ontario, Canada

PATRICIA L. BAXTER-PETRALIA, M.S., O.T.R./L.

chapters 7, 48, and 95

Clinical Director of Work Therapy, Hand Rehabilitation Center;
Adjunct Instructor of Orthopaedic Surgery, Thomas Jefferson
University, Jefferson Medical College, Philadelphia,
Pennsylvania

ROBERT B. BEACH, M.A., P.T.

chapter 9

Chief, Physical Therapy Department, Federal Correctional
Institution, Fort Worth, Texas; Former Chief of Rehabilitation
Research Department, U.S. Public Health Service Hospital,
Gillis W. Long Hansen's Disease Center, Carville, Louisiana

JANE BEAR-LEHMAN, M.S., O.T.R.

chapter 102

Adjunct Associate Professor, Department of Occupational
Therapy, New York University, New York, New York

DEBRA BEAULIEU, O.T.R./L.

chapter 98

Penn Therapy Associates, Broomall, Pennsylvania

JUDITH A. BELL-KROTOSKI, O.T.R., F.A.O.T.A.

chapters 9, 42, 43, 52, and 91

Clinical Research Therapist; Chief of Hand and Occupational
Therapy, Rehabilitation Research Department, U.S. Public
Health Service Hospital, Gillis W. Long Hansen's Disease
Center, Carville, Louisiana

STANLEY BERLIN, M.Ed., C.V.E., C.W.E.

chapter 101

Chief, Work Adjustment Services, The Raymond M. Curtis
Hand Center, Union Memorial Hospital, Baltimore, Maryland

JOHN N. BILLOCK, C.P.O.

chapter 85

Director of Orthotics, Prosthetics, and Rehabilitation
Engineering, Hillside Rehabilitation, Warren, Ohio

SUSAN M. BLACKMORE, M.S., O.T.R./L.

chapters 7, 79, and 95

Hand Rehabilitation Center, Instructor, Department of Occupational Therapy; College of Allied Health Services, Adjunct Instructor, Department of Orthopaedic Surgery, Thomas Jefferson University, Philadelphia, Pennsylvania

SIDNEY J. BLAIR, M.D., F.A.C.S.

chapter 102

Dr. William N. Scholl Professor and Chairman, Department of Orthopaedics and Rehabilitation, Loyola University Medical Center, Maywood, Illinois

JEANINE BOOZER, O.T.R.

chapter 73

Hand Therapy Unit, Blodgett Memorial Medical Center, Grand Rapids, Michigan

PAUL W. BRAND, M.D.

chapters 1, 50, and 87

Clinical Professor Emeritus, University of Washington, School of Medicine, Seattle, Washington; Former Chief, Rehabilitation Branch, National Hansen's Disease Center, Carville, Louisiana; Former Clinical Professor of Orthopaedics and Surgery, Louisiana State University Medical School, New Orleans, Louisiana

DONNA E. BREGER, M.A., O.T.R.

chapter 9

Deputy Chief and Clinical Director, Hand and Occupational Therapy, Rehabilitation Research Department, U.S. Public Health Service Hospital, Gillis W. Long Hansen's Disease Center, Carville, Louisiana

FORST E. BROWN, M.D.

chapter 66

Chairman, Section of Plastic Surgery, Dartmouth-Hitchcock Medical Center, Dartmouth College, Hanover, New Hampshire

LAURA A. BRUENING, O.T.R./L.

chapters 7, 95, and 98

Senior Therapist, Hand Rehabilitation Center, Philadelphia, Pennsylvania

†STERLING BUNNELL, M.D.

chapter 80

WILLIAM E. BURKHALTER, M.D.

chapters 10 and 15

Professor of Orthopaedics, Department of Orthopaedics and Rehabilitation; Associate Chairman for Clinical Affairs, University of Miami School of Medicine; Chief, Division of Hand Surgery, Jackson Memorial Hospital, Miami, Florida

PATRICIA M. BYRON, M.A., O.T.R./L.

chapters 17, 83, and 94

Clinical Director, Primary Care, Hand Rehabilitation Center, Philadelphia, Pennsylvania

ANNE D. CALLAHAN, M.S., O.T.R./L.

chapters 44 and 45

Hand Therapy Consultant, Philadelphia, Pennsylvania

CATHERINE A. CAMBRIDGE, M.S., P.T.

chapter 6

Director, Hand Therapy of Delaware, Wilmington, Delaware

MARGARET S. CARTER, O.T.R.

chapters 19 and 20

Director, Hand Rehabilitation Unit, Hand Surgery Associates, Phoenix, Arizona

STEPHEN L. CASH, M.D.

chapter 29

Clinical Assistant Professor of Orthopaedic 5urgery, Division of Hand Surgery, Thomas Jefferson University Hospital, Hand Rehabilitation Center, Philadelphia, Pennsylvania

ROBERT A. CHASE, M.D.

chapter 3

Emile Holman Professor of Surgery, Department of Surgery, Stanford University School of Medicine, Stanford, California

GAYLORD L. CLARK, M.D.

chapters 100 and 104

Assistant Professor of Orthopaedic Surgery, Department of Orthopaedic Surgery, Johns Hopkins University School of Medicine; Attending Hand Surgeon, Raymond M. Curtis Hand Center, The Union Memorial Hospital, Baltimore, Maryland

JUDY C. COLDITZ, O.T.R./L.

chapters 25, 26, 49, and 89

Administrator, Hand & Orthopaedic Rehabilitation Associates; Director, Hand Rehabilitation Center, Raleigh, North Carolina

CARL R. COLEMAN, M.D.

chapter 31

Clinical Professor and Codirector, Hand Service, Department of Surgery, Division of Orthopaedic Surgery, Ohio State University College of Medicine; Director of Orthopaedic Education, Riverside Methodist Hospital, Columbus, Ohio

KAY COLELLO-ABRAHAM, O.T.R

chapter 92

Director, Hand Therapy, Orange Rehabilitation Therapy, Orange, California

---

† Deceased.

JONATHAN K. COOPER, B.S.

chapter 100

Industrial Specialist, Work Adjustment Service, Union
Memorial Hospital, Baltimore, Maryland

RAYMOND M. CURTIS, M.D.

chapter 23

Associate Professor of Orthopaedic Surgery (Retired); Associate
Professor of Plastic Surgery (Retired), Johns Hopkins University
School of Medicine; Director, Hand Surgery (Retired), Union
Memorial Hospital, Baltimore, Maryland

GLORIA L. DeVORE, O.T.R.

chapter 75

Director, Hand Therapy Associates, Department of Surgery,
University of Arizona College of Medicine, Tucson, Arizona

MARY P. DIMICK, O.T.R.

chapter 93

Director, Rehabilitation Center; Director, Work Evaluation
Center; University of California, San Diego Medical Center,
San Diego, California

ADOLPH DIODA

chapter 96

Instructor in Sculpture, Pennsylvania Academy of Fine Arts,
Philadelphia, Pennsylvania

THEODORE E. DuPUY, M.D.

chapter 4

Associate Professor of Orthopaedic Surgery, Eastern Virginia
Medical School, Norfolk, Virginia

ROBERT J. DURAN, M.D.

chapter 31

Clinical Professor and Codirector, Hand Service, Department of
Surgery, Division of Plastic Surgery, Ohio State University
College of Medicine, Columbus, Ohio

ROSLYN BROWN EVANS, O.T.R.

chapter 36

Director, Indian River Hand Rehabilitation, Vero Beach, Florida

ELAINE EWING FESS, M.S., O.T.R., F.A.O.T.A.

chapters 5 and 88

Consultant in Private Practice, Hand Research,
Zionsville, Indiana

VINCENT G. FIETTI, Jr., M.D.

chapter 68

Associate Clinical Professor, Department of Orthopaedic
Surgery, Columbia University College of Physicians
and Surgeons; Assistant Attending Orthopaedic Surgeon,
St. Luke's-Roosevelt Hospital, New York, New York

VICTORIA M. FRAMPTON, M.C.S.P., S.R.P.

chapter 47

Superintendent Physiotherapist, Thanet District General Unit,
Margate, Kent, England

GARY K. FRYKMAN, M.D.

chapter 18

Professor, Department of Orthopaedic Surgery, Loma Linda
University Medical Center; Medical Director, Hand
Rehabilitation Center, Loma Linda, California

CARL GÖRAN-HAGERT, M.D.

chapter 8

Associate Professor of Surgery, Kuwait University, Kuwait

CHARLOTTE GOWLAND, O.T.R.

chapter 76

Director, Occupational Therapy, Rancho Los Amigos Medical
Center, Downey, California

LAURIE GRIGSBY, O.T.R./L.

chapter 65

Occupational Therapy Department, St. Christopher's Hospital
for Children, Philadelphia, Pennsylvania

MURRAY P. HAMLET, D.V.M.

chapter 66

Director, Cold Research Division, U.S. Army Research Institute
of Environmental Medicine, Natick, Massachusetts

FRED H. HOCHBERG, M.D.

chapter 99

Associate Professor of Neurology, Massachusetts General
Hospital, Boston, Massachusetts

JAMES M. HUNTER, M.D.

chapters 13, 28, 34, and 39

Professor of Orthopaedic Surgery, Jefferson Medical College of
Thomas Jefferson University; Chief, Hand Surgery Services,
Department of Orthopaedics, Thomas Jefferson University
Hospital, Philadelphia, Pennsylvania

KIMBERLY HUNTER, B.F.A.

chapter 96

Instructor in Ceramics, Hand Rehabilitation Center,
Philadelphia, Pennsylvania

RICHARD S. IDLER, M.D.

chapter 62

Hand Surgery Associates of Indiana, Inc., Indianapolis, Indiana

SCOTT H. JAEGER, M.D.

chapters 28 and 39

Penn Diagnostic Center, Philadelphia, Pennyslvania

PAULA BREME KADER, P.T.

chapter 63

Hand Rehabilitation Center, Philadelphia, Pennsylvania

MARY C. KASCH, O.T.R., C.V.E.

chapter 103

Director, Hand Rehabilitation Center of Sacramento, Sacramento, California

WILLIAM H. KIRKPATRICK, M.D.

chapter 21

Assistant Clinical Professor of Orthopaedic Surgery, Thomas Jefferson University Hospital, Philadelphia, Pennsylvania

LORI A. KLEREKOPER, O.T.R./L.

chapter 31

Senior Staff Therapist, Ohio State University Hospital, Columbus, Ohio

L. LEE LANKFORD, M.D.

chapter 59

Clinical Professor, Department of Orthopaedic Surgery, The University of Texas Health Science Center at Dallas, Texas, Dallas, Texas

GEORGIANN F. LASETER, O.T.R., F.A.O.T.A.

chapter 27

Director, Hand Rehabilitation Services, Dallas, Texas

VALERIE HOLDEMAN LEE, P.T.

chapter 61

Director, Hand Rehabilitation Associates, Phoenix, Arizona

ROBERT D. LEFFERT, M.D.

chapter 46

Associate Professor of Orthopaedic Surgery, Harvard Medical School, Boston, Massachusetts

JUDY LEONARD, O.T.R.

chapters 72 and 73

Regional Hand Rehabilitation Service, Grand Rapids, Michigan

EVELYN J. MACKIN, P.T.

chapters 13, 33, 34, 68, and 82

Director of Hand Therapy, Hand Rehabilitation Center, Philadelphia, Pennsylvania

JOHN W. MADDEN, M.D., F.A.C.S.

chapter 12

Clinical Professor of Orthopaedics, University of New Mexico, Albuquerque, New Mexico; Director, Tucson Hand Rehabilitation Program, Tucson, Arizona

LORETTA M. MAIORANO, O.T.R./L.

chapter 83

Director, Tri County Hand Therapy Center, Pottstown, Pennsylvania

EVA McCORMICK, O.T.R.

chapter 102

Director, Occupational Therapy Department, Foster G. McGaw Hospital of Loyola University, Maywood, Illinois

PAMELA M. McENTEE, M.S., O.T.R./L.

chapters 7 and 24

Director of Hand Therapy, PA Rehab, Inc., Swarthmore, Pennsylvania

ROBERT M. McFARLANE, M.D.

chapter 67

Professor and Chairman, Division of Plastic Surgery, Department of Surgery, University of Western Ontario, London, Ontario, Canada

WANDRA K. MILES, O.T.R.

chapter 65

Pennsylvania Hand Center, Bryn Mawr, Pennsylvania

ERIK MOBERG, M.D., Ph.D.

chapter 77

Emeritus Professor, Department of Orthopedics and Hand Surgery, Sahlgren University Hospital, Göteborg, Sweden

JOHN H. MOORE, Jr., M.D.

chapter 17

Assistant Professor of Surgery, Division of Plastic Surgery, Thomas Jefferson University Hospital, Philadelphia, Pennsylvania

CHRISTINE A. MORAN, M.S., P.T.

chapter 57

Adjunct Assistant Clinical Professor, Department of Physical Therapy, Old Dominion University, Norfolk, Virginia; Assistant Clinical Professor, Graduate Studies in Physical Therapy, Medical College of Virginia; Director, The Richmond Upper Extremity Center, Richmond, Virginia

PATRICIA A. TAYLOR MULLINS, P.T.

chapter 14

Director, Hand Rehabilitation Services of Oklahoma, Baptist Medical Center, Oklahoma Health Care Corporation, Oklahoma City, Oklahoma

EDWARD A. NALEBUFF, M.D.

chapter 74

Clinical Professor or Orthopaedic Surgery, Tufts University School of Medicine; Chief of Hand Surgery, New England Baptist Hospital, Boston, Massachusetts

JAMES F. NAPPI, M.D.

chapter 31

Hand and Microsurgery Center, Riverside Hospital; Clinical Assistant Professor of Surgery, Division of Plastic Surgery, Ohio State University College of Medicine, Columbus, Ohio

ARTHUR J. NELSON, Ph.D., P.T.

chapter 55

Professor, Department of Physical Therapy, School of Education, Health, Nursing and Arts Profession, New York University, New York, New York

ELVERT F. NELSON, M.D.

chapter 18

North Pacific Orthopaedic Associates, Portland, Oregon

BONNIE L. OLIVETT, O.T.R.

chapter 84

Director, Upper Extremity Rehabilitation; Clinical Instructor, University of Colorado Health Sciences and Research Center, Denver, Colorado

GEORGE E. OMER, Jr., M.D., M.S. (Orthop Surg)

chapters 37 and 58

Professor of Orthopaedics and Chairman, Department of Orthopaedics and Rehabilitation; Cochief, Division of Hand Surgery; Professor of Anatomy and Surgery; Chief, Division of Hand Surgery; Medical Director, Physical Therapy Program, The University of New Mexico School of Medicine, Albuquerque, New Mexico

KATRINA JONES PENDERGRAFT, M.A., C.V.E.

chapter 100

Program Manager, Workways, Inc., Joliet, Illinois

†RICHARD L. PETZOLDT, M.D.

chapter 103

CYNTHIA A. PHILIPS, O.T.R./L.

chapters 71 and 74

Director of Occupational Therapy, Newton Wellseley Hospital, Newton, Massachusetts

JEAN PILLET, M.D.

chapter 82

Director, Centre de Prosthese Plastique, Paris, France

†R. GUY PULVERTAFT, C.B.E., M.D., M. CHIR., F.R.C.S.

chapters 2 and 32

RICHARD L. READ, P.T.

chapter 39

Hand Rehabilitation Center, Philadelphia, Pennsylvania

SANDRA UTLEY REEVES, O.T.R.

chapter 64

Senior Therapist, Occupational Therapy Department, Shands Teaching Hospital, Gainesville, Florida

C. CHRISTOPHER REYNOLDS, P.T.

chapters 53 and 61

Co–clinical Director, Hand Rehabilitation Unit, Hand Surgery Associates, Phoenix, Arizona

ERIK A. ROSENTHAL, M.D.

chapter 35

Private Practice of Hand Surgery, Springfield, Massachusetts; Associate Clinical Professor of Orthopaedic Surgery, Tufts University School of Medicine, Boston, Massachusetts; Assistant Clinical Professor of Orthopaedic Surgery, University of Connecticut School of Medicine, Farmington, Connecticut

ROGER E. SALISBURY, M.D.

chapter 64

Professor of Surgery; Chief of Plastic and Reconstructive Surgery, New York Medical College; Director, Burn Unit, Westchester County Medical Center, Valhalla, New York

---

† Deceased

SANDRA RICHARDS SAUNDERS, M.S., P.T.

chapter 57

The Richmond Upper Extremity Center, Richmond, Virginia

RODNEY W. SCHLEGEL, P.T.

chapter 104

Private Practice; Consultant to Raymond M. Curtis Hand Center, Baltimore, Maryland

LAWRENCE H. SCHNEIDER, M.D.

chapters 33 and 51

Clinical Professor of Orthopaedic Surgery, Jefferson Medical College of Thomas Jefferson University, Philadelphia, Pennsylvania

DANIEL I. SINGER, M.D.

chapters 17 and 34

Assistant Clinical Professor of Orthopaedic Surgery, Division of Orthopaedics, Department of Surgery, John A. Burns School of Medicine, University of Hawaii, Honolulu, Hawaii

KEVIN L. SMITH, M.D., MSc

chapter 11

Assistant Professor of Plastic Surgery, University of North Carolina, Chapel Hill (Charlotte Division); Attending Surgeon, Charlotte Memorial Hospital and Medical Center, Charlotte, North Carolina

MORTON SPINNER, M.D.

chapter 38

Clinical Professor of Orthopaedic Surgery, Albert Einstein College of Medicine, Yeshiva University, New York, New York

BARBARA GOODWYN STANLEY, P.T.

chapter 54

Capital District Hand Therapy Center, Schenectady, New York

JAMES B. STEICHEN, M.D.

chapter 62

Clinical Professor of Orthopaedic Surgery, Department of Orthopaedic Surgery, Indiana University School of Medicine; Attending Hand Surgeon, St. Vincent Hospital and Health Care Center, Indianapolis, Indiana

KAREN M. STEWART, M.S., O.T.R.

chapter 16

Clinical Coordinator, Stewart Hand Therapy Group, Springfield, Massachusetts; Former Director, Upper Extremity Rehabilitation Service, Hesperia Hospital, Modena, Italy

JAMES W. STRICKLAND, M.D.

chapter 81

Chief, Section of Hand Surgery, St. Vincent Hospital and Health Care Center, Indianapolis; Clinical Professor, Department of Orthopaedic Surgery, Indiana University School of Medicine, Indianapolis, Indiana

ALFRED B. SWANSON, M.D.

chapters 8, 69, 70, and 73

Professor of Surgery, Michigan State University, Lansing, Michigan; Chief of Orthopaedic and Hand Surgery Training Program, Blodgett and Butterworth Hospitals; Chief and Director, Orthopaedic Research and Hand Surgery Fellowship, Blodgett Memorial Hospital, Grand Rapids, Michigan

GENEVIEVE de GROOT SWANSON, M.D.

chapters 8 and 73

Assistant Clinical Professor of Surgery, Michigan State University, Lansing, Michigan

DENNIS G. TOBIN, O.T.R.

chapter 66

Administrative Director, Department of Rehabilitation Medicine, Mary Hitchock Memorial Hospital, Hanover, New Hampshire

PATRICIA A. TOTTEN, O.T.R./L.

chapter 22

Hand Rehabilitation Center, Philadelphia, Pennsylvania

SUSAN M. TRIBUZI, O.T.R.

chapters 57 and 90

Director, Hand Rehabilitation Specialists, Division of Orthopaedic Specialists, Ltd., Richmond, Virginia

GWENDOLYN van STRIEN, M.S., P.T.

chapter 30

Hand Therapist and Consultant, Rotterdam Dijkzicht Hospital; Instructor, National Organization for Postgraduate Education for Physical Therapists (S.W.S.F.), Den Haag, The Netherlands

ROBERT L. WATERS, M.D.

chapter 76

Medical Director, Rancho Los Amigos Hospital, Downey, California; Clinical Professor of Orthopaedics, University of Southern California School of Medicine, Los Angeles, California

JANET WAYLETT-RENDALL, O.T.R.

chapter 60

Supervisor/Program Coordinator, Hand Rehabilitation Center, Loma Linda University Medical Center; Clinical Instructor, Department of Occupational Therapy, Loma Linda University, Loma Linda, California

STEVEN M. WENNER, M.D.

chapter 86

Clinical Associate Professor of Orthopaedic Surgery, Boston University; Staff Surgeon, Bayside Medical Center; Shriners Hospital for Crippled Children, Springfield, Massachusetts

STEPHAN H. WHITENACK, M.D., Ph.D., F.A.C.S.

chapter 39

Director, Vascular Laboratory; Chief, Thoracic Surgery; Director, Residency Affiliation; Chestnut Hill Hospital; Assistant Professor of Surgery, Jefferson Medical College, Philadelphia, Pennsylvania

DIANA A. WILLIAMS, O.T.R./L.

chapter 79

Supervisor, Hand Therapy Department, Hand Rehabilitation Service, Geisinger Medical Center, Danville, Pennsylvania

DOROTHY J. WILSON, O.T.R., F.A.O.T.A.

chapter 76

Clinical Assistant Professor, University of Southern California, School of Medicine, Los Angeles, California

ROBERT LEE WILSON, M.D.

chapters 19 and 20

Assistant Chief, Hand Surgery Service, Maricopa Medical Center, Phoenix, Arizona; Instructor in Surgery, University of Arizona, Tucson, Arizona

PHYLLIS WRIGHT, P.T.

chapter 64

Physical Therapy Department, North Carolina Memorial Hospital, Chapel Hill, North Carolina

To Erik Moberg, M.D., Ph.D.

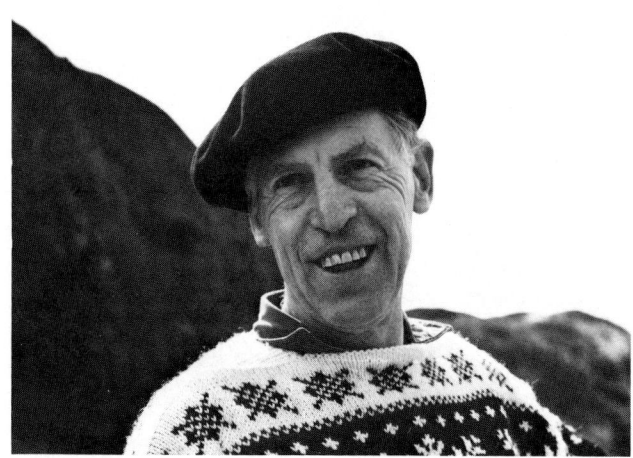

Erik Moberg was born on January 5, 1905, in Lund, a university city in the south of Sweden founded about 1000 AD. As a boy he developed an intense interest in zoology and had, as he says, "quite a fine collection of insects." He feels that he profited much from the preparation of their tiny structures for study under the microscope. Eventually this interest led him to study comparative anatomy at the early age of 16 years.

He earned his medical degree in 1932. Except for 14 months in Iran, all of his early studies were in Lund. In medical school Erik Moberg's attention was drawn to the surgical care of the disabled hand. He disliked the coarse way that hands were treated and believed that the tissues were not given the gentle handling essential to the care of such an intricate structure. Determined to "do it better," he began to use a bloodless field without having seen or read about it.

In 1945 Erik Moberg established a ward for the hand disabled patients at Sahlgren Hospital in Gothenberg. In 1947 he visited and was influenced by Bunnell, Koch, and others who had developed a deep interest in hand surgery as a specialty and who shared his belief in more refined hand surgical techniques.

Dr. Moberg was the first to correlate clinical sensory tests with hand function by defining hand function in terms of "what the hand can do." Vigorous and persuasive "in retirement," he continues to emphasize that none of the known methods for testing nerve recovery are reliable and repeatable and that to find such a test "will take decades." His never-ending emphasis for more than 2 decades on the evaluation of functional sensibility deserves our appreciation and thanks.

Many honors have been bestowed upon Erik Moberg. On May 14, 1962, he presented the first Annual Sterling Bunnell Lecture to the American Society for Surgery of the Hand on "Aspects of Sensation in Reconstructive Surgery of the Upper Extremity." He was elected the first president of the International Federation of Societies for Surgery of the Hand (IFSSH) and is a member of 13 international hand societies. He served as president of the Swedish Surgical Society in 1970. He was recognized as a "Pioneer in Hand Surgery" at the Third Congress of the IFSSH in Tokyo, Japan, in 1986. He has contributed 60 years of medical publications since his first publication in 1926.

Erik Moberg is an enthusiastic sailor. At the age of 70, he gathered with family and friends in a Swedish fishing village to celebrate his retirement. Unbeknown to him, his 46-foot yawl was brought up the coast for a surprise reunion. Those fortunate to be at his retirement watched this rare man "shimmy up" the 70-foot mast of his yawl and give a wave to his friends.

Dr. Moberg prides himself for having swum in almost all the seas of the world—"only missed one"—the Arctic Ocean.

Erik Moberg's legacy is that he has given us an exciting springboard to the challenge that is sensibility evaluation. He has also shown us by example, a love of life, profession, and family to be emulated. It is with great admiration and warm affection that we dedicate the third edition of *Rehabilitation of the Hand* to Erik Moberg.

DEDICATION TO THE SECOND EDITION

To Raymond M. Curtis, M.D.

The second edition of *Rehabilitation of the Hand* will reach an ever-expanding worldwide team of hand surgeons and therapists. The book has a definite personality that blends teamwork, scholarship, imagination, and compassion. It is with great pleasure that we dedicate this volume to a man we hold in high esteem, Dr. Raymond M. Curtis, because to enumerate those qualities is to describe Dr. Curtis—the surgeon and the man. We are grateful for his countless contributions to hand surgery and rehabilitation. This dedication is our way of thanking him for the contribution he has made to the professional lives of hand surgeons and hand therapists.

DEDICATION TO THE FIRST EDITION

To Paul W. Brand, M.D.

It is with great pride that we dedicate our book to Dr. Paul W. Brand. This devout man has unselfishly used his extraordinary skills and high standards of medicine in his service and devotion to God.

Therapists and surgeons who seek to know the origin and philosophy of hand rehabilitation centers should know that the idea began in the mind and heart of this humble, gentle man.

Born in India, the son of missionaries, Paul Brand was aware at an early age of the frustration that beset those stricken with Hansen's disease. With no hope of help, these persons merely existed as outcasts in the dark corners of their little world. Dr. Brand's efforts through reconstructive surgery restored useless hands and gave persons with Hansen's disease the opportunity to be educated and to work and live with dignity.

When Dr. Brand began his work in India, there were no hand centers or hand therapists. He trained young Indian men in specific phases of treatment, such as sensory evaluation or muscle training. After years of performing their specialties, they developed amazing expertise, and when physical therapy schools were established, these young men were the first to be admitted and graduated as physical therapists.

The first hand center was an old shack, but it was the birthplace of the hand rehabilitation team—surgeons, therapists, and patients working together. The center provided an environment where patients could have surgery, treatment, and training in a workshop. Having been a carpenter during his early years of life, Dr. Brand recognized the value of woodworking and other purposeful activities in treatment of the hand. Thus he employed concepts of occupational therapy to help restore crippled fingers to useful function.

We shall be forever indebted to the fates that led this quiet man to his great work in India with patients with Hansen's disease and later at the U.S. Public Health Service Hospital in Carville, Louisiana. Their good fortune has become ours because he has given us a precious charge. Surgeons and therapists together in hand centers throughout the world can build upon the work he started. As we try to emulate the high standards he has set for us, we offer this book in honor of Dr. Paul W. Brand.

Foreword to the *Third Edition*

It is a privilege to be invited to write the foreword for the third edition of this classic *Rehabilitation of the Hand*.

The first edition in 1978 was a direct result of the conference organized 2 years previously in Philadelphia. The continuing annual meetings run by the Hand Rehabilitation Center have attracted an ever-widening and increasingly enthusiastic, knowledgeable audience.

The success of the book is obvious. Any medical book that is in a third edition after only 10 years has attracted great interest. We know that this book has stimulated the close working association between hand surgeons and therapists that is now accepted throughout the world as necessary for the best results and has been one of the most significant developments in hand surgery over the past decade. This close relationship is reflected in the third edition, where the authorship is divided almost equally between doctors and therapists.

Many hand societies have invited therapist colleagues to participate at their meetings, and in 1989 the recently formed International Federation of Societies of Hand Therapists met in Israel at the same time as the Fourth Congress of the International Federation of Societies for Surgery of the Hand.

This remarkable progress over the past decade is commendable, and the principles of correct care of the injured or diseased hand, which are described so clearly in this book, have led to such marked improvement in the results of treatment.

The principles are simple and easily applied but are equally easily neglected and forgotten and must be constantly stressed. This is particularly important in a specialty where the other major advance of the past 15 years has been the application of surgery under the microscope. The outstanding technical achievements that have become commonplace in restoring circulation and performing complex reconstructions make it easy for the surgical team to neglect these basic principles, which prevent stiffness and contractures and retain a functional hand.

This consistent reminder is required for all of us who practice the art of hand surgery and will ensure the continuing success of and need for *Rehabilitation of the Hand*.

Douglas W. Lamb

Foreword *to the Second Edition*

Over the past few decades, advances in the treatment of lesions of the hand and upper extremity have been tremendous. This is the result of many factors, including the development of hand surgery as a specialty; the growth of knowledge of the functional anatomy of the hand, wound healing, and nerve physiology; new concepts in the treatment of tendon, nerve, bone, and joint problems; and the development of microsurgery.

However, the growth of the concept of centers combining hand surgeons and hand therapists in the same unit is perhaps the most significant advance of all. In these centers all the ingredients contributing to functional recovery after a hand lesion are synthesized.

The hand serves as both a receiver of information and an executor of the response. These two functions are closely intertwined and influence each other. The mobility of the fingers is indispensable for tactile identification of objects. The way the hand grips an object is directly influenced by the sensory input of the individual, and especially by the sensibility of the hand.

Thus the treatment of hand lesions cannot be accomplished without the combination of repair of the involved tissues and sensory and motor reeducation. A perfect anatomical repair without a functional recovery is useless.

I believe that this new philosophy of a "global approach" to the treatment of hand problems has not been better presented than in *Rehabilitation of the Hand*. The four editors have formed a hand rehabilitation center, consisting of both surgeons and therapists, that has served as a model around the world. Their experience, devotion, and contagious enthusiasm are evident in all their symposia and writings. In this work they have gathered together the most prestigious authors in all areas involving problems of the hand.

The first edition of this book immediately enjoyed a huge success. This new edition has been considerably revised and expanded. There are 25 more chapters than in the first edition, and the book covers all aspects of rehabilitation, from the evaluation of function and impairment to the management of replanted parts and the use of the new limb prostheses and orthoses. This book will be invaluable for those who read the previous edition, physicians and therapists alike, and for anyone, from student to specialist, who is interested in hand rehabilitation.

Raoul Tubiana

Foreword *to the First Edition*

The successful management of the crippled hand depends on accurate preoperative assessment, skilled surgery, and devoted aftercare. This trinity is the rock on which modern hand surgery is built. As surgeons, we look to physical therapists to assist us in the assessment and preparation of the patient as well as in the aftercare. It matters not whether we are engaged in the reconstruction of the mutilated hand or concerned with the palsy of leprosy, the stiff hand, or the tetraplegic patient. All require the coordinated effort of the team.

It was this concept that led to the Symposium on Rehabilitation of the Hand held in Philadelphia, in March, 1976. This, the first combined meeting of its kind, set a pattern for the future and a standard that will be difficult to surpass. From this union has arisen a new body, the American Society of Hand Therapists, which had its first meeting in February, 1978.

During the closing session of the symposium, the thought came of presenting the work to a wider audience. All will be grateful to the editors, on whom the burden of publication has fallen. The table of contents speaks for itself. In these pages is gathered the wisdom of a galaxy of talents, for all who contributed are leaders in their respective fields. The subjects range from basic principles and techniques, which need to be stated again and again, to the latest thoughts on some difficult problems. Pervading the entire volume is the personal experience of hand therapists in the widest sense of the word who have given years of practice to their subject. It is fitting that the words of Sterling Bunnell should be included, for no one has done more to raise surgery of the hand from the unknown to the position it holds today, and his words are still relevant. We welcome, also, the tribute to Paul Brand, who has shown that the same principles apply when the material is unpromising and the odds are long, provided there is the determination and the compassion to win through.

There is no need to wish success to this work, for it is assured a special place in the libraries of all who aspire to care for the wounded hand.

R. Guy Pulvertaft

Preface

Rehabilitation of the Hand: Surgery and Therapy is a publication for the nineties that acknowledges the growth of hand surgery as a specialty and the developing strengths of hand therapy as a support specialty. This third edition of *Rehabilitation of the Hand: Surgery and Therapy* represents the combined insight and expertise of both the hand surgeon and the therapist. There are 104 chapters dealing with surgery and therapy. Thirty-four chapters are new and 15 chapters are completely revised, so that actually 49 new chapters are presented as well as a revision of 55 chapters.

In the third edition, the surgical aspects are expanded, dealing with the anatomy of the hand, management of hand trauma, tendon inflammations and reconstructions, arthritis and burns, and fractures and dislocations. A major expansion in this text is in the field of nerve injury and disability, especially peripheral nerve disorders stemming from the brachial plexus and neurologic thoracic outlet syndromes. Rehabilitation subjects introduced in the text are upper extremity problems of the musician, prosthetic management of the limb-deficient child and adult, ergonomics, biomechanics and disability and return to work evaluation. Splinting has been expanded in the child and adult. We have also retained certain classic chapters unfaded by time by Bunnell, Pulvertaft, Swanson, Madden, and Bell-Krotoski.

The earlier dedications of *Rehabilitation of the Hand* were to Drs. Paul Brand and Raymond Curtis. This edition is dedicated to Dr. Erik Moberg. These three hand surgeons project a common empathy: to give the patient a surgical plan based on factual knowledge and a projected result based on a mutual apprenticeship. The coauthors of *Rehabilitation*

of the Hand: Surgery and Therapy, in a way shared this cognitive apprenticeship as they prepared this text for the reader.

Certain groups of persons have helped make the third edition of *Rehabilitation of the Hand: Surgery and Therapy* a more significant contribution than ever before. For consistent support of the goals of the Hand Rehabilitation Foundation, we sincerely thank Dorothy B. Kaufmann for her continuing efforts. Also, we wish to remember Commander Judith Bell-Krotoski, who helped launch the first edition of *Rehabilitation of the Hand.*

We wish to thank Teri Stahller, staff photographer at the Hand Rehabilitation Center, for her assistance and Christine Jackson for manuscript preparations. It has been a pleasure to work with Kathy Falk, senior developmental editor; Ellen Baker Geisel, assistant editor; and Betty Hazelwood and Gail Brower, production editors at The C.V. Mosby Company.

The editors feel that they have accomplished their mission in the third edition of *Rehabilitation of the Hand: Surgery and Therapy,* presenting a broad, in-depth text for the hand surgeon and therapist. We wish especially to thank the contributing authors. We feel that this edition has surpassed the high standard set by previous editions and look forward to seeing it serve as a valuable source to clinicians at all levels of experience.

James M. Hunter
Lawrence H. Schneider
Evelyn J. Mackin
Anne D. Callahan

Contents

I

BASIC CONSIDERATIONS
management by objectives, psychological aspects, and anatomy

1

Hand rehabilitation: management by objectives

Paul W. Brand

Hand surgery has been around a long time. The American Society for Surgery of the Hand has worked for 35 years "to improve and develop surgery of the hand" in response to the energy and foresight of Sterling Bunnell and with the purpose of promoting better understanding and better professional standards in surgery of the hand. This society and other similar societies around the world have influenced more and more surgeons to devote themselves wholly or mainly to this one specialization—surgery of the hand. Specialization gets results. By the time one surgeon has operated on a thousand cases of flexor tendon injury in the finger and has listened and discussed the techniques and problems with a dozen others who have done the same, he or she is able to do a far better job than the finest general surgeon who does one hand case a month and one flexor tendon case a year.

However, specialization also has its dangers. It tends to narrow our vision and to magnify the significance of small factors that are of statistical significance in those overall results we publish from time to time, which tend to become an index of our professional success. We may see a patient simply as our six-hundredth flexor tendon case with our eighty-fifth use of primary repair in the proximal segment and our fifth use of the newest suture material or prophylactic antibiotic.

If asked about our objective for the case, we might say that we want to assess the effect of wide excision of the tendon sheath at the suture site. The patient probably also has an objective, and this may affect the outcome even more than our objective. He may want to get back to work as fast as he can, or he may want to penalize his employer and maximize his financial compensation. I recently had a patient with the late results of a high nerve injury, and my objective was to use a new pattern of tendon transfers. This would require careful postoperative reeducation. The patient was an inmate of the state penitentiary, and he had his own overriding objective, which was to use his period of postoperative hospitalization to escape from prison. His success depended in part on his ability to remove his splints and use his operated hand to manipulate and remove his shackles and then to keep one jump ahead of the police. The strong motivation he had to use his hand and the fact that I had used synergistic tendon transfers and strong tendon suture techniques allowed our apparently diverse objectives to reinforce each other, so that when we met many months later, he had an almost perfect result.

Hand rehabilitation has a broader scope than hand surgery. It takes into account all factors that are important to the patient, as well as those local factors that are amenable to the surgeon's knife and the therapist's skill. It recognizes that the surgeon in his proper preoccupation with his art may miss or underrate the most significant elements of the case and that good teamwork must include not only the skilled and experienced allied health personnel but also the owner of the hand himself—that previously uninformed, fearful, and apprehensive person on whose faith, courage, and determination the success of the whole operation depends.

Because we are discussing management by objectives, we should start at the beginning to determine priorities. What are the first objectives for a hand surgeon who is developing a hand surgery unit into a hand rehabilitation program? I will mention two that concern patterns of staff and space and two that refer to patient care.

STAFF AND SPACE
The team

Therapists as team members. From my experience and from what I have observed, the first objective is to have a team, and the first step in attaining that objective is to have one designated therapist work with the surgeon. This objective is not attained by having therapists available in some other department or organization unless some very special understanding and commitment are reached. Physical therapy formerly had a bad image among the older hand surgeons. The reason was that standardized methods of therapy, suitable perhaps for backs and hips, have sometimes been disastrous for fingers. A few hands, moving slowly toward mobility, have become stiff again as a result of the treatment of an enthusiastic therapist who was unfamiliar with the case and probably unfamiliar with the stern disciplines that are second nature to a therapist who works mainly with hands.

In large medical centers, where all physical and occupational therapists are in a separate department directed by a physiatrist, and in private practice, where a number of therapists work out of their joint office, it may be difficult for a surgeon to know who is to be assigned to any given case. It may even be that different therapists handle the same case on different days. Such an arrangement does not fulfill the objective of a team and may sometimes cause real problems. The right thing for the surgeon to do in these circumstances is to take the time to achieve full understanding and cooperation with the physiatrist or chief therapist so that a certain therapist or two may be assigned to the hand cases and may be given the time and freedom to consult fully with the surgeon at every preoperative and postoperative stage. If a physiatrist has the time and interest to sit in on these discussions and to accept responsibility as a member of the team, this is even better, but continuity of the physiatrist is still not as significant as continuity of the therapist. It is the *touch* of the therapist's hands that helps a patient to relax and to make progress. At every fresh pair of hands, he tightens up again until further experience allows him to relax, develop confidence, and start to progress again. For the same reason, I like the concept of the "hand therapist" rather than simply physical therapists and occupational therapists. A hand therapist may start his or her professional life as either a physical therapist or an occupational therapist and then learn by experience the aspects of the skills of the other discipline that are applicable to hands. There is no need for a therapist to confine himself or herself to hands; it is just a matter of special interest and special skills. In a unit that is large enough to employ several therapists, there may be room for retention of some special distinctions. For example, one occupational therapist may make and adapt most of the splints. Even so, I think a patient does better with continuity of responsibility with one individual therapist.

Team interaction. After the identification of a therapist as a member of the team, the next step is to develop a working relationship in which there is true team interaction. It is sometimes difficult for a surgeon, or any physician, to discount the feeling that he or she is the sole source of all wisdom. Some knowledge comes from books; more comes from experience. In the case of the hand, most comes by touch—by skin-to-skin, eye-to-eye dynamic interaction, whereby a good therapist comes to know just how a patient feels and reacts. Many times I have planned an operation and then have been told firmly by the therapist who was working on the preoperative hand that in this particular case the planned procedure would be a waste of time or that it would be better if it were postponed or modified. More often than not the therapist has been right. I am indebted to a succession of therapists whose insights have contributed at least as much to my education as I have been able to contribute to theirs. It is good for hand therapists to come into the operating room and observe the actual placement of transferred tendons and to see the kinds of problems that may contribute to scar formation. This need not be a routine, but it is helpful in the training stages and for difficult cases.

There are probably therapists who work in situations in which they have little or no access to the surgeon and in which teamwork does not exist. My advice to them is to keep good records, especially graphs of range of motion, swelling, and the temperature of joints. When such graphs show a plateau that suggests a change of treatment is needed, the therapist should go to the prescribing surgeon armed with the graphs and ask for advice. The chances are the surgeon will be impressed that the therapist can contribute clear, pertinent, factual information about the patient, and he or she will probably begin asking for this kind of help with other patients. Teamwork can develop in many ways.

Time and space

The next objective concerns time and space. I believe that many hands become stiff from a dangerous mixture:

$$\left. \begin{array}{l} \text{Overtreatment—30 minutes} \\ \text{Disuse—23½ hours} \end{array} \right\} \text{daily}$$

This situation stems from hospital and clinic routines, in which therapists have a timetable and in which charges are made per session. A therapist knows that he or she has just 20 minutes or so to *do* something to improve range of motion or get a tendon gliding. He or she is likely to work too fast or push too hard. The patient also feels that those minutes are critical, and when they are over, he will relax his hand into immobile disuse. Human tissue cells, however, have no consciousness of timetables. They respond to sudden intense stress by inflammation and an outpouring of fibrinogen. Then they occupy the idle hours of disuse by knitting the strands of fibrin into a fabric that will resist further joint movement.

Some of the new generation of hand rehabilitation centers are being organized in a different way. They do not need more staff, but they use more space. The idea is that patients pay by the day or the week rather than by the minute or hour. Then they are free to come to the center in the morning and stay all day if they like. This may fit in with family programs, because a family member can drop the patient off on the way to work or school and pick him up on the way home. The therapists do not attempt to work with the patient all the time; rather they set him up with an exercise program or some therapeutic job or form of recreation. The therapists move around checking on progress and keeping activity going. New patients may be paired with older ones, and rheumatoid arthritics can exchange ideas on how to handle the activities of daily living without causing painful stress on their joints. This sort of program requires more room than the older type of program. There should be space for straight exercise programs and electronic, diagnostic, and stimulation apparatus. There must be room for a splint workshop or bench. A variety of benches and tables is needed for different types of manual tasks and a few games. There should be a rest area and, if I had my choice, a garden. In almost any condition of sickness and disability, it is therapeutic to mind and body to be part of a living system where seeds are sprouting and worms and bees are about their business. Life and growth are infectious.

PATIENT OBJECTIVES

If staff and space are available, what about objectives for the individual patient? This book will suggest many objectives related to surgery, therapy, and splinting. Two should be mentioned in relation to the patient as a whole—the person to whom the hand is attached and who must live with it when we have finished.

Responsibility and competence

The first objective is to establish responsibility and competence. We all know that the most successful results occur when the patient is determined to do well and believes that he can do well. He accepts advice, but he does things himself. Yet we all have a tendency to build up the importance and significance of what we as professionals can do for the patient, thereby downplaying the patient's contribution. We would like the patient to leave his hand with us in the morning and pick it up in the evening. We take credit for the improvements and blame the patient for poor results.

For real rehabilitation, from the very start we need to make the patient feel that he is doing it all himself. Only the surgery is done while he is asleep. Even that is something he has understood, asked for, and agreed to. Now as he starts to move his postoperative hand, he must understand what makes his hand swell, what makes it heal, and how tendons move. Above all, we must teach him the significance of pain. It is not an enemy. It is his own living cells keeping him informed about the limits within which he must stay. Each patient must see his own graph of changing range of motion at each joint, and he must be encouraged to feel responsible for improvement or to wonder why it got worse. He must see his hand volume measurements and perhaps measure the volume himself. This process is like biofeedback, because he quickly recognizes that when he hangs his hand down, his volume graph goes up; when the volume level comes down, his range of motion improves. He should see how the temperature of his joints is assessed by a touch of the thermistor probe—how it goes up and down with good activity but goes up and stays up if he pushes his exercises too hard. He may check the tension of the rubber bands of his splint and make sure they do not slip. He must see the dial of his dynamometer as he tests his improving strength. When the time comes for the therapist to use some passive motion, there must be such close rapport that the patient knows that he is not going to be subjected to a force against his will. As I hold and stroke a hand with my eyes on the face of the patient, I can soon feel that his nerve endings cross the interface of his hand and mine and that I feel his pain as soon as he does. As we talk together and I respond to his fear and build up his confidence, we soon get the feeling that he is in control of his own hand and I am acting only in place of his damaged or paralyzed muscle tendon units. Each time we sit together and hold hands, the symbiotic synergistic feeling increases until there is ideally an absolute mutual confidence and respect that is quite an exhilarating experience. I have become a new strength for the patient, but it is his strength now, not mine, and he can pick up from there and do things himself.

This is the value of a rehabilitation center as compared with a hospital ward. When I had my gallbladder removed several years ago, I was exposed for the first time to the full impact of the system of hospital medical care in this country. My overwhelming impression was that of being reduced to a cog in a remorseless machine—an incompetent cog at that. My sterile prison cell was visited by an assembly line of technicians who entered and left, each with his own competence and superiority: "Roll up your sleeve," "Pull down your pants," "I'm doing this again because your first blood clotted"—with a frown that implied it was poor-quality blood. The cumulative effect of a long succession of total strangers gathering data that were never shared with me produced the feeling that I was the only totally incompetent person on the ward. My bowels were one person's responsibility and my blood another's responsibility, whereas a third person took care of my mind by keeping up the proper level of pain medication. If I as a doctor could be given that feeling, what is the hope for a nonmedical person? So let's minimize hospitalization and maximize the patient's sense of personal competence. "It's my hand—I can do it!"

Patient's overall goals

We should always be ready to reevaluate and modify our minor and technical objectives in a flexible response to our understanding of the patient's overall goals for life. It is good to set ourselves measurable objectives. The tip of the finger should reach the distal crease of the palm after tendon grafting. Pinch strength in this hand should reach 2 kilograms. Metacarpophalangeal range of motion should be 80 degrees after Silastic joint replacement. These measurements are good, because they set targets for the patient and we can plot the progress on a graph for all to see. However, the danger of narrow objectives is that we forget the overall view. I recently had to stop and reevaluate the situation as I found myself prescribing more therapy to perfect the opposition of the thumb in a 68-year-old retired patient who could already use his hand for all ordinary activities. My objective of perfection was a matter of my professional pride. How long was this patient's expectation of life? What percentage of his remaining months should he spend undergoing treatment of his thumb? What did he ask of the function of his thumb?

CONCLUSION

The real trouble with management by objectives is that the most important goals in life and health are not amenable to measurement at all. We tend to fasten on things that we can measure and feed into a computer. We glorify technical progress and let the spirit languish. In agriculture, we maximize the harvest but lose the soil that is the basis of future harvests. In medicine we kill germs and mend bones, but we need to learn to combat fear and build confidence. A good surgeon will mend a lacerated hand, choosing what can be saved and what cannot. A good rehabilitation team will mobilize it as far as it can be mobilized, and then will convince the patient that life is still good and achievement still possible in spite of what has been lost.

It is here that teamwork has its greatest value. Not all of us inspire the kind of confidence that encourages a patient to speak his fears and shyly expose the inner ambitions or resentments that make up the very essence of who he is and where he is aimed. It may be the therapist or the social worker who gets the best insights, but he or she can help the other group members to adjust their sights and match their tempo to a new rhythm.

Like Thoreau, we all march better if we sense the beat of our own drum. However, we must learn to subdue our own rhythm and listen for the drummer who is real to the patient.

2

Psychological aspects of hand injuries

R. Guy Pulvertaft

Our President has asked me to undertake a task for which I feel inadequately equipped. Psychology is defined in the Oxford Dictionary as "The science of the nature, function and phenomenon of the human mind and conduct." It would not be fitting for me to attempt a description of the physiological and pathological patterns of behaviour. To those of you who wish to study the subject from a psychiatric viewpoint, I commend an Article written by Cone and Hueston[2] which appeared in the Medical Journal of Australia last January. What I have to say to you comes not from a knowledge of psychology but from a lifetime of surgical practice with its failures and its successes. I can do no more than draw your attention to some of the conditions which may be initiated or influenced by the patient's and the doctor's mental attitude. Human relationship is a matter of fundamental importance in the care of the patient, whether he be a child or an adult. You have all been through a long and arduous training designed to fit you for the many decisions and actions you are called upon to make. Few, if any, of you will have had formal instruction in the art of rapport. This has been left to your own personality and the attitudes you have observed in your teachers. I know that I feel deep gratitude to the men and women I served as student, house surgeon and registrar and to the many others whom I have been privileged to know throughout my life. Albert Schweitzer said, "One other thing strikes me when I look back on my youthful days. The fact that so many people gave me something, or were something to me, without knowing it. Much that I would otherwise not have felt so clearly or done so effectively was felt or done as it was, because I stood under the sway of these people. If we had before us those who have thus been a blessing to us and could tell them how it came about, they would be amazed to learn what had passed over from their life to ours."

It is often said that rehabilitation commences at the moment of injury. It is also true that the words spoken by the emergency surgeon can engender a feeling of confidence and trust, particularly for the patient who has suffered a mutilating injury of the hand; who sees his skills destroyed, his career ruined and his family's future placed in jeopardy. The same feeling of despair must enter the minds of parents when their child is born with a severe malformation. I do not mean to infer that it is right to be unduly optimistic and give promises which cannot be honoured. There are ways in which we can combine sympathy with truth.

The best service that we can give is to get on with the job as effectively as we can and see the patient through the ensuing weeks and months personally, with the assistance of the Social Worker and the Department of Physical Medicine. In Orthopaedic and Plastic Surgery there is a tradition of continuing personal care and the same is seen in those who practise Hand Surgery. The Resettlement Service for the Disabled is doing a most valuable work. I quote the words of George Cochrane, Director of Physical Medicine in Derby, with whom I have worked for many years. "Rehabilitation begins with the appraisal of clinical problems at the outset and the defining for all, and this includes the patient and his relatives, the problem and the expected outcome and what we should aim to achieve in various stages on the way to this. Well before the end of treatment, the District Resettlement Officer is advised of his abilities, limitations, interests and past skills and charged to seek out work for him."

I need hardly remind you that in the animal world a weak or wounded animal may be deserted or attacked by other members of the herd. The same may be seen in a more subtle form in the human race. It is our duty to see that the infirm are supported spiritually as well as physically. A man may react to a physical disaster by a determination to overcome or he may fold up and withdraw into himself. The response, no doubt, depends primarily upon the patient but it can be influenced by the personality of the doctor. As Cone put it "an unresponsive surgeon will find that he has an unresponsive patient." We may take encouragement from the knowledge that few give up whilst we can remember many who have been victorious.

This lad of 16 years (Fig. 2-1), whom Douglas Reid will remember, never lost heart and despite his disability qualified as a surveyor and now holds a responsible post. I recall the day when he demonstrated to us how he could lift the ash from a cigarette with his double hook without breaking it; a trick which none of us could do with our normal hands. This man (Fig. 2-2) suffered gross damage from the same cause—fireworks—at the age of 13. He, also, lost the other hand. In the surviving hand two stumps provided his sole grip. He has steady employment as a clerk.

One of the most remarkable stories of physical handicap overcome is that of Howard Blackburn,[5] who while fishing from a dory on the Newfoundland Banks was caught in a blizzard and was unable to rejoin his schooner. He rowed for two days through the intense cold and reached Newfoundland but frostbite destroyed all fingers and part of his thumbs. Some years later, Blackburn made a solo voyage

Reprinted with permission from *The Hand; 1975 Journal of the British Society for Surgery of the Hand,* Longman Group, Ltd., **7**:93-103.

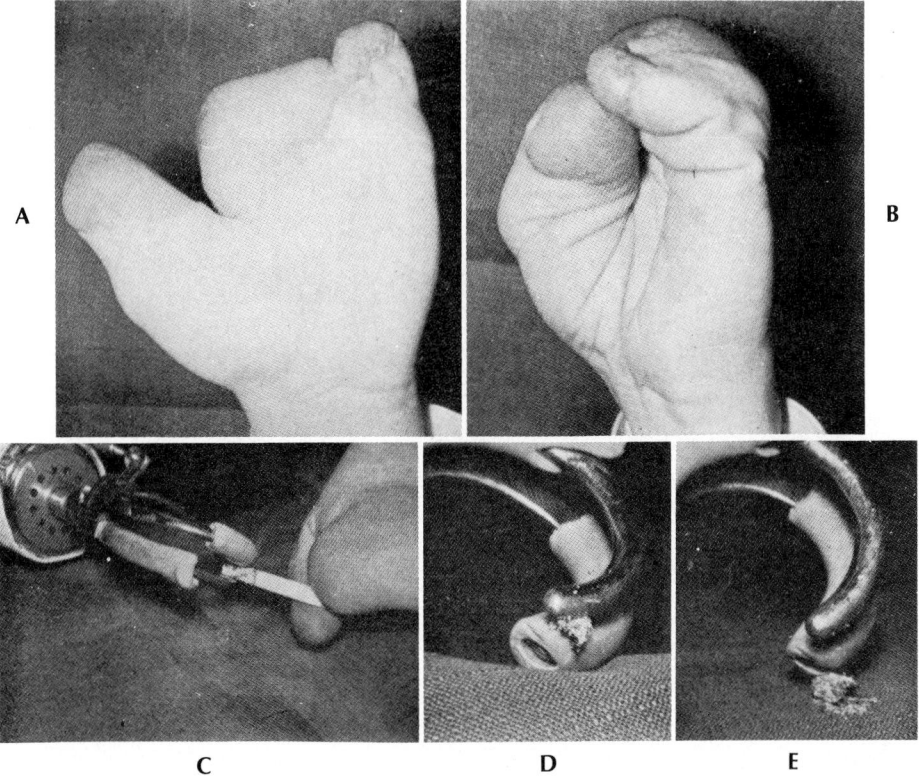

Fig. 2-1   Explosive injury at age of 16 years. **A** and **B,** Mutilated left hand (reconstruction by D.A.C. Reid). **C, D,** and **E,** Precision control of prosthesis, right hand.

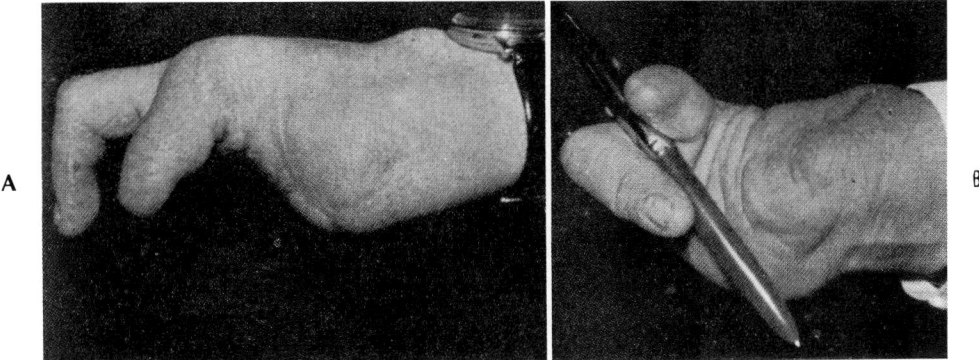

Fig. 2-2   Explosive injury at age of 13 years. **A** and **B,** Mutilated right hand. Left hand amputated. Reproduced from British Journal of Bone and Joint Surgery by permission of the Editor.

from Goucester, Massachusetts, to Gloucester, England, in a 30 foot open boat under sail. Two years later, he made another Atlantic crossing to Lisbon in a smaller boat.

While working in a Leprosy Hospital last year I was much struck by a patient who had lost one foot and numerous fingers. I came across him on my night rounds, when I found him surrounded by the other men in the ward playing rummy with great merriment. He was an inspiration to his friends and, though little did he know it, to the Staff as well. It was only later that I learned he read to the ward from the Bible every day.

The spirit in man can rise above the evils that can harm the body.

Although our prime objective is to restore function, the appearance of the hands may be of greater psychological significance for some persons. The hand is not only the symbol of man's power and the instrument of his perception; it is also the mirror of his emotion. Indeed, some of the operations we perform are governed by this thought, particularly in the field of congenital deformity. Correction of syndactyly, removal of supernumerary digits and straightening of the club hand are examples where surgery is designed to improve appearance as well as function.

Robert Jones[6] tells of a young woman "who was a housekeeper and applied for relief, not because a severe club hand was not useful in her work, but because of its unsightliness

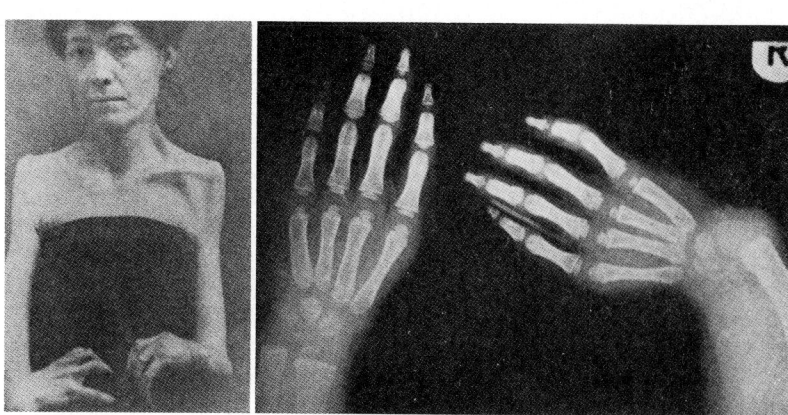

Fig. 2-3 Untreated club hands. *Right,* X-ray at age of 4 years. Reproduced from Orthopaedic Surgery by Jones and Lovett by permission of the Editor.

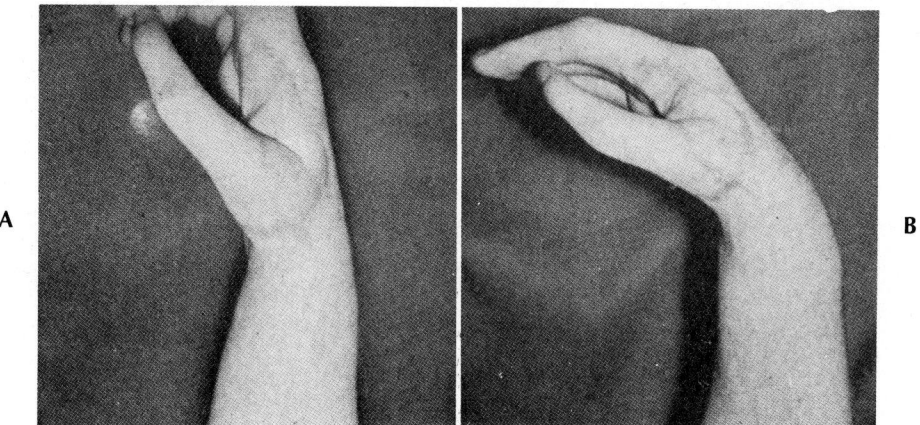

Fig. 2-4 Club hand. **A** and **B,** 11 years after centralisation at age of 5 years. Reproduced from British Journal of Bone and Joint Surgery by permission of the Editor.

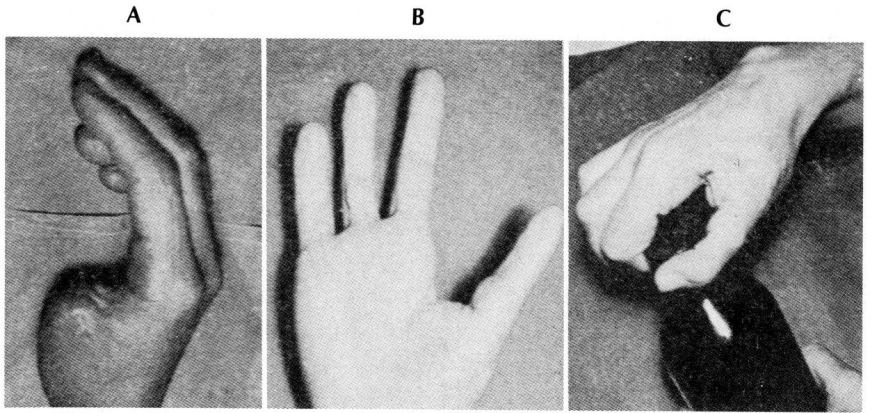

Fig. 2-5 Sub-total amputation of right thumb. **A,** Before reconstruction. **B** and **C,** 16 months after pollicisation of index finger.

and shortening which led her always to conceal it in public." Here is a similar case and we can understand her concern (Fig. 2-3). Here is a young patient in whom the appearance has been improved with functional benefit also (Fig. 2-4).

This woman came to us in great distress (Fig. 2-5). She was told that the thumb could be reconstructed and it was a matter of agreeing with her on the most suitable method. She chose, and I think rightly, to accept loss of the index finger to obtain a hand of reasonable appearance and good function. I have heard it argued that the ideal time to perform a pollicisation, when circumstances permit, is at the emergency operation. I believe this advice to be wrong for it ignores the psychological aspect of the injury. The patient is in no fit state to make a decision and the desire to accomplish a technical success must not override other considerations.

Beware of false pride! As news gets round that you can perform operations that were not possible in the past, an aura will surround you and your ego may be subconsciously influenced. Self-criticism is a quality which every surgeon should possess if he is to steer clear of avoidable disaster. I do not mean to denigrate self-confidence, for without this a surgeon would be a poor thing; nor do I wish to cry down enthusiasm for a cause. My remark is directed at the "enthusiastic" surgeon, a phrase which has a different shade of meaning.

Now let us consider some of the specific problems which you will encounter.

Pain arising from nerve injury

1. Causalgia. Recently, I had the opportunity of reading Weir Mitchell's classic description[9] of a case of causalgia written 100 years ago. Miss T. at the age of 2½ years ran a splinter into her right palm where the median nerve divides into its branches. The wood was not removed but the wound healed uneventfully. At the age of 22, Miss T. accidently struck her palm and experienced acute local pain which settled in a few days. Three months later, pain developed in the shoulder for which she was seen in Paris and a diagnosis of rheumatism was made. The pain spread down the arm and into the hand and became severe. She was seen in Milan by Dr. Sapolini, Surgeon to the King of Italy, who removed the fragment of wood found lying between the filaments of the median nerve. On waking from the anaesthetic, she felt intense pain in the index finger and thumb. Within a few days the pain became exquisite and was of a burning nature. The skin of the median territory became red and smooth "upon which the fall of a bit of lace or of a veil edge was simply anguish." Morphia was required. After she had endured this for two months, Dr. Sapolini, finding that pressure upon the *radial* nerve gave relief, resected one inch of this nerve at the elbow. Absolute ease followed but ten days later the pain suddenly returned with the same intensity.

After consulting many more surgeons of distinction without benefit, Miss T. was seen by Sir James Paget in London who advised her to return home to America. There she came under the care of Dr. Mitchell and I quote part of his very full description. "Miss T. was thin and pale. She slept with the hand supported upon its ulnar side, and wakened when the hand slipped over and was touched by the bed clothes, while all day she devoted herself to shield the hand from any foreign contact. This anxiety to avoid having the hand

touched, and the constant influence of pain, gave to her physiognomy a singular expression of vigilance, such as I have rarely seen since the terrible traumatic neuralgias of the late war." Mitchell was referring to the American Civil War, after which he had written his celebrated work on nerve injuries. Then follows a detailed account of his findings, which time does not permit me to relate. Let it suffice to say that not only was the median territory affected, but tenderness was present throughout the major nerve trunks of the arm and the plexus and the front of the chest. Mitchell removed ¾ inch of the median nerve in the lower forearm. Complete relief was experienced and at follow-up ten months later, the condition remained stable.

Although we would treat this case differently today, I have related the history in some detail to remind you of this distressing and mysterious complaint. I have little doubt that this young woman was thought by many to be suffering from an hysterical disorder.

Barnes[1] gives this description of the characteristic pain of causalgia:

1. It is severe, spontaneous and persistent.
2. It usually has a burning quality.
3. It may spread beyond the territory of the injured nerve.
4. It is invariably aggravated by both physical and emotional stimuli.

Doupe et al.[4] have postulated that the syndrome arises from a short circuit between the autonomic and the sensory fibres of the injured nerve. Efferent impulses in the autonomic fibres arising from various stimuli, including the emotions, leak across the artificial synapse and excite the sensory axons giving rise to pain and other effects (Fig. 2-6).

Sunderland[14] gives this warning:—"Some physicians and surgeons, finding it difficult to appreciate the fact that these patients suffer intensely, are ever on the alert for evidence that they are dramatising or exaggerating their symptoms . . . though the behavior of the patient may suggest that the disorder is psychogenic in origin, many have failed to find evidence of a constitutional psychic factor, and we are left with the conclusion that, in by far the majority of patients, the personality changes are the result and not the cause of the pain."

2. Irritative lesions. There is a group of painful nerve injuries which must be distinguished from causalgia; "the painful syndromes that lack the distinctive features of causalgia" as Seddon[12] put it, such as are seen after amputations, digital nerve divisions and some plexus injuries. These syndromes may arise from a variety of causes, whereas causalgia is most commonly a result of high velocity missile wounds. The nerve interruption is often complete in irritative lesions, but in causalgia it is usually incomplete. Irritative lesions may occur in any nerve, whilst causalgia as a rule arises from injuries to the median and tibial nerves and the brachial plexus.

This is not the occasion to discuss the management of these conditions, except to stress that the temptation to lose patience with those who suffer from them must be resisted. The subject is fully reviewed by Seddon, and Cullen's work on causalgia[3] should also be studied.

Hysteria

Hysteria is a functional disturbance in which symptoms are assumed for a personal advantage without the patient

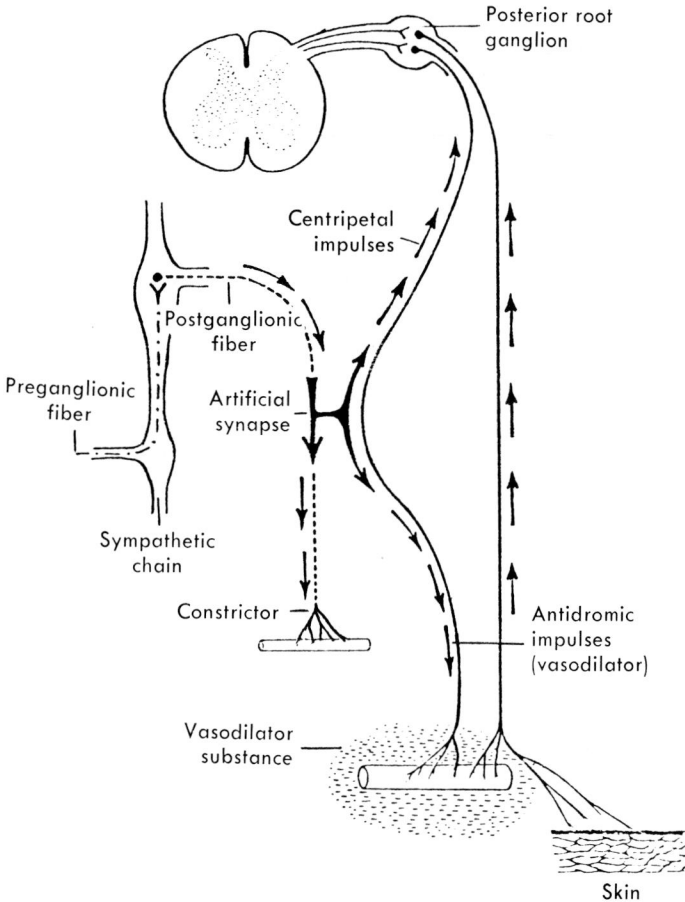

Fig. 2-6 The pain pathways in causalgia as postulated by Doupe. Reproduced from Barnes R, in Peripheral Nerve Injuries, M.R.C. Special Report Series No. 282, by permission of the Author and the Controller of H.M. Stationery Office.

being fully conscious of this motive. In making this diagnosis, it is essential to exclude organic disease and this may be difficult when hysteria is superimposed upon an organic disorder. In a limb the presenting features are usually an anaesthetic area and alternatively paralysis which do not accord with anatomy, unless the patient has a knowledge of anatomy. In a case of long standing there may be secondary trophic changes such as oedema, shiny skin and joint stiffening. The diagnosis is made after a thorough neurological examination including electrodiagnosis. A reasoned explanation to the patient may be sufficient to direct thought in the right direction and avoid prolonged incapacity. Aubrey Lewis[8] has said that common sense on the part of the physician is as important as psychological understanding and that too much treatment is as harmful as too little treatment. In a resistant case, there should be no hesitation in seeking psychiatric advice.

Malingering

There are those who deliberately set out to deceive, and the border line between true hysteria and malingering is sometimes difficult to determine. I have avoided the term when composing a medical report and have used a phrase such as "I am unable to find a satisfactory explanation for this man's complaints." When a remark of this kind follows an examination which clearly has been thoroughly performed, the reader of the report or the Judge may safely be left to draw his own conclusions. In my experience, no useful purpose is served by arguing with the patient about symptoms and signs which are manifestly not genuine. Repeat the examination quietly and without undue comment until you are convinced of the sincerity or otherwise of the patient and the unreality of the physical signs. Many years ago I came across the expression "Profitable Humbug." Francis Walshe,[15] in discussing these situations pointed out that we do not see this phenomenon arising after injuries sustained at sport. The sportsman, when injured, is expected to resume the game with the least possible delay and is not well regarded if he does not do so. No such code applies to the victim of an accident upon the roads or in industry, nor does he lose face if he behaves in the most extravagant fashion after the most trifling of injuries and claims disability for months or years. Sir Francis recalls that he was once asked by the Judge in a High Court action:—"Doctor, when these people kid themselves that they are ill, do they know that they are kidding themselves?" I give his reply verbatim:—"This is a difficult question to answer without qualification, but my view is that at some time in his 'illness,' if perhaps not all the time, the subject is aware that he is exploiting the situation for a known end. Possibly, as the months go by, the still small voice of conscience becomes less frequent and more still and finally falls silent. By this time the story of the accident has been rehearsed so many times in the circle of relatives and friends and to solicitor and doctors that the patient does not clearly know what is fact and what is legend. That the entire illness is determined and maintained by factors in the unconscious of the patient, I am not able to believe; willing as I am to credit these patients with a high capacity for self-deception."

The self-inflicted injury

You will meet these puzzling and worrying problems in many forms. For those of you who are not familiar with the life of Baron Munchausen I suggest you read "Singular Travels and Adventures of Baron Munchausen" published by the Cresset Press. To illustrate his remarkable initiative, I will relate one of his unpublished experiences. While riding alone through a Polish forest, Munchausen was thrown from his horse and was obliged to spend the night in that wolf infested place. Aware that wolves attack in single file, he stationed himself with his back to a tree and awaited the onslaught. It was not long before Munchausen observed their eyes gleaming in a long line and he braced himself for the attack. As the leading wolf sprang he, with great presence of mind, thrust his right arm through the jaws of the beast and seized its anus; then leaning back he withdrew his arm, thus turning the animal inside out. Naturally, the wolf made off in the opposite direction closely followed by the rest of the pack.

Sometimes, it seems that the symptoms to which we are obliged to listen rival these tales in their imaginative content. I think of a young lass of eight who presented with a weeping finger. The slightly frothy fluid appeared to ooze from a fault in the nail. We were mystified until it occurred to us that the simplest explanation should not be overlooked— placing the finger in the mouth. Mother found it difficult to

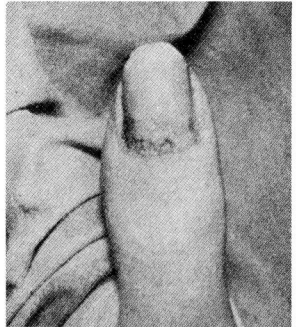

Fig. 2-7   Self-inflicted paronychia.

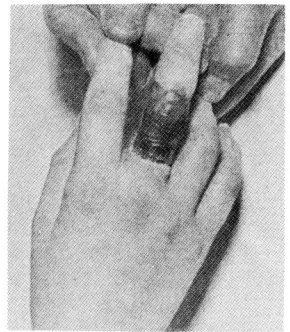

Fig. 2-8   Self-inflicted burn.

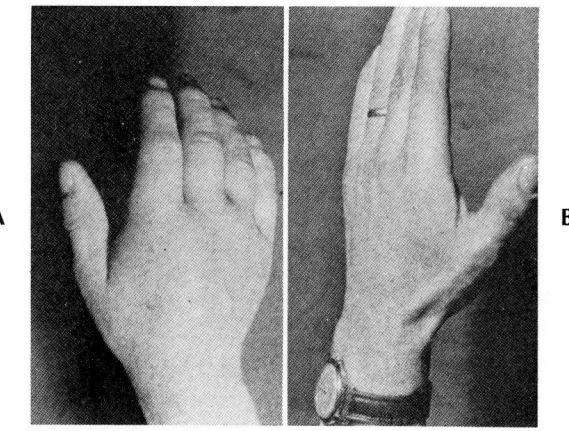

Fig. 2-9   Secretan's syndrome. **A,** Right hand. **B,** Normal left hand.

believe that her daughter could behave in this manner, even when the finger remained dry if it was protected by a covering. Another child came with a persistently swollen hand for no reason that her parents nor her doctor could detect. We could find no evidence that a constriction band had been used. However, admission to hospital and elevation of the limb allowed the oedema to disperse and a plaster cast prevented its recurrence. The parents accepted the evidence and it remained to cure the habit without causing the child to lose face. This was done to everyone's satisfaction and the trouble did not return. I believe that we should endeavour to resolve these situations in an understanding way. This may try our patience in a busy Clinic, but an early redirection of a young person may avoid worse trouble later.

Here is a case of chronic paronychia (Fig. 2-7) caused by deliberate insertion of thorns. Nineteen were removed. This unusual burn (Fig. 2-8) was caused by an encircling bandage soaked in some corrosive fluid. The physical defect was cured but, undefeated, this woman continued to haunt the out-patient department for years with a variety of self-inflicted injuries. Psychiatric treatment has failed to relieve her of these strange tendencies.

Peritendinous fibrosis of the dorsum of the hand (Fig. 2-9) which Secretan described in 1911[11] is a curious condition in which the extensor tendons become surrounded by a mass of organising fibrous tissue containing macrophages and haemosiderin. It probably results from repeated minor contusions of the hand and the suspicions of self-infliction should enter your mind. It is interesting to note that Secretan states that he had not seen a patient suffering from this condition who did not have some possible claim for occupational injury.

Attempted suicides demand the immediate help of the Psychiatrist and, indeed, this is a standing requirement in the National Health Service.

Sudeck's atrophy

Sudeck in 1900 described a syndrome of osteoporosis of the bones of the hand accompanied by oedema in the early stages, stiffness, pain, muscle atrophy and skin changes.[13] The cause remains unknown, but it appears to be an acute autonomic dystrophy occurring after injury, usually of a minor nature, surgery or inflammation. It is said to be more commonly seen in women than in men although a recent report by Kleinert[7] indicates otherwise. It tends to occur more often in persons who are introspective and apprehensive. Symptoms usually develop within a few weeks of the exciting cause, but the onset may be delayed for several months.

I have nothing to add to what is already known except to emphasize two lessons which experience has taught me; the importance of early recognition and the imperative need for immediate and determined treatment before the condition progresses to a state from which the hand may never fully recover. The early danger signs are oedema and pain, and when either of these present in the absence of a simple explanation action should be taken. The temptation is to compromise by advising physical treatment in the hope of seeing an improvement at the next visit. The patient should be admitted to hospital for elevation of the limb and for a full programme of physical treatment which can only be given effectively as an inpatient. It may be difficult to convince the patient that this action be necessary for to him the early signs do not appear to warrant this inconvenience. He must be told that a week's delay at this stage may mean a month's delay in final recovery. I have never had cause to regret insisting upon this course, but have regretted it when I have been complacent. I need hardly add that the psychological management of these situations is not unimportant. Strict observance of these rules may avoid the need for sympathetic block or sympathectomy later.

• • •

We commenced the day with "Evolution of the Hand." We have moved on through anatomy and treatment to the forefront of progress in the accomplishments of micro-surgery. We have been warned of the complications of surgery and I have spoken of psychological complications. I will conclude with some sound advice which you will find in the Book of Proverbs. "Wisdom is the principle thing; therefore get wisdom; and with all thy getting get understanding."[10]

ACKNOWLEDGMENTS

My thanks are due to Barry Wilks and his staff of the Department of Medical Illustration at the Derbyshire Royal Infirmary for their assistance.

REFERENCES

1. Barnes R Causalgia: a review of 48 Cases. Peripheral nerve injuries. Medical Research Council Special Report Series 282. London, 1954, H.M. Stationery Office.
2. Cone J and Hueston JT: Psychological aspects of hand injury. Med J Australia 1:104, 1974.
3. Cullen CH: Causalgia: Diagnosis and treatment, J Bone Joint Surg 30-B:467, 1948.
4. Doupe J Cullen CH and Chance GQ: Post-traumatic pain and the causalgic syndrome, J Neurol Neurosurg Psychiatry 7:33-48, 1944.
5. Garland JE: Lone voyager. Boston, 1963, Little, Brown & Co.
6. Jones R and Lovett RW: Orthopaedic surgery, London, 1923, Oxford University Press.
7. Kleinert HE, and others: Post-traumatic sympathetic dystrophy. J Bone Joint Surg 54A:899, 1972.
8. Lewis A: Price's textbook of the practice of medicine. Hunter D, editor, London, 1956, Oxford University Press, p. 1975.
9. Mitchell SW: Traumatic neuralgia: section of median nerve, Am J Med Sci 135:2-29, 1894.
10. Proverbs, chapter 4, verse 7.
11. Secretan H: Oedeme dur et Hyperplasie Traumatique du Metacarpe Dorsal. Revue Médicale de la Suisse Romande 21:409-416, 1901.
12. Seddon HJ: Surgical disorders of the peripheral nerves. Edinburgh and London, 1972, Churchill Livingstone, Inc.
13. Sudeck P: Uber die acute entzündliche Knochenatrophie. Archiv. Fur Klinische Chirurgie 62:147-156, 1900.
14. Sunderland S: Nerves and nerve injuries, Edinburgh and London, 1968, E & S Livingstone, Ltd.
15. Walshe FMR: The role of injury, of the law and of the doctor in the aetiology of the so-called traumatic neurosis, The Medical Press, 239:493, 1958.

3

Anatomy and kinesiology of the hand*

Robert A. Chase

The hand skeleton and associated ligaments constitute an architectural framework to allow the latitude of motion of the digits characteristic of human hand function. Some generalizations concerning allowable ranges of motion make up the patterns described by many observers through the centuries. The architectural units are divided into those functioning fixed and those with a sweep of motion in multiple planes. The mobile elements may be divided conveniently into three parts, each described below and illustrated in a manner described by J. William Littler.[7-9,11,13,34]

THE FIXED UNIT OF THE HAND

The fixed unit of the hand (Fig. 3-1, *4*), consisting of metacarpals 2 and 3 and the distal row of carpals, has very limited motion at the intermetacarpal joints and the second and third carpometacarpal joints. The distal row of carpal bones forms a stable, unchanging, transverse arch. It is fixed by virtue of the tough intercarpal ligaments and the arch configuration of the carpal bones with the capitate as the keystone. The volar carpal ligament attaching to the hook of the hamate and the palmar ridges of the trapezium further prevent the collapse of the fixed transverse carpal arch. Articulating with the distal carpal row and projecting distally from it are the five metacarpals. The index and long finger metacarpals are fixed quite intimately to the distal carpal row, and together with it they form the fixed unit of the hand skeleton. This central fixed unit forms a supporting base for the remaining mobile units of the hand. The fixed unit projects distally from the wrist under the influence of the major wrist extensors (extensor carpi radialis longus and extensor carpi radialis brevis) and the prime wrist flexor, the flexor carpi radialis. This central beam of the hand is then positioned for motion around it of the adaptive elements.

MOBILE ADAPTIVE HAND UNITS

The adaptive units of the hand which move about the central I-beam consist of three elements which are in descending order of specialization, the thumb ray, the index finger, and the fourth and fifth rays together with the long finger.

The thumb ray

The thumb with its metacarpal and two phalanges (Fig. 3-1, *1*) has the greatest latitude and sweep of any of the digits. The metacarpotrapezial joint is a biconcave, saddle joint allowing a wide range of motion in many planes, since

---

*From Flynn JE and Jupiter J: Hand surgery, ed 4, Baltimore, 1989, Williams & Wilkins.

the joint capsule, though tough and unyielding, is loose enough to allow substantial movement.* Five intrinsic muscles and four extrinsic muscles influence thumb positioning and activity.

The index finger

The index finger phalanges (Fig. 3-1, *2*) project from the fixed second metacarpal under the influence of three intrinsic and four extrinsic muscles. These muscles account for the relative independence of function of the index finger as compared with the long, ring, and little fingers. The interphalangeal joints move as hinge joints in flexion and extension, while the metacarpophalangeal (MP) joint has sub-

---

*References 2, 7, 13, 17, 23, 25, 28, 38, 39, 47.

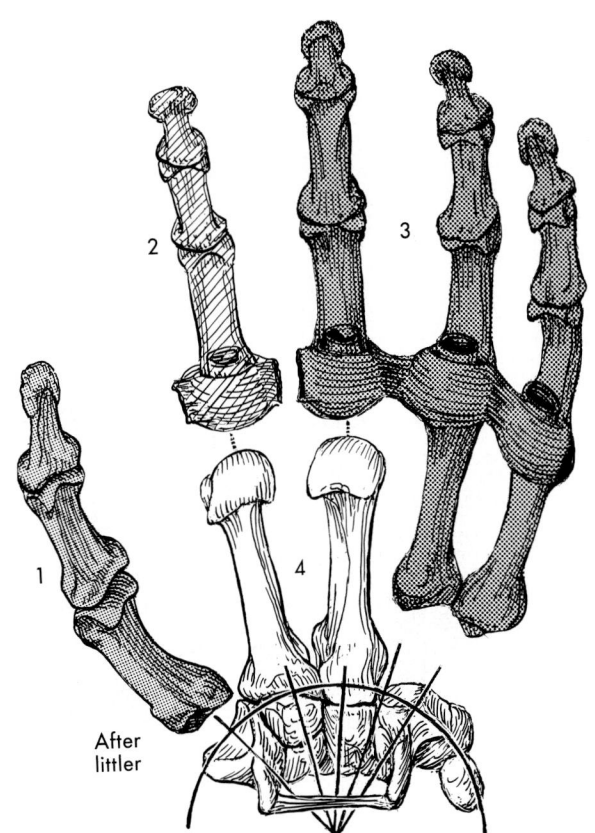

Fig. 3-1 The architectural components of the hand are divided into four separate units. Note the central fixed unit *(4)* and the mobile units *(1, 2* and *3)*—See text. (After Littler, as shown in Chase RA: Atlas of hand surgery, Philadelphia, 1973, WB Saunders Co.)

stantial medial and lateral range of motion when the joint is in extension.

Long, ring, and little fingers together with the fourth and fifth metacarpals

This unit on the ulnar side of the hand functions as a stabilizing vise to grasp objects for manipulation by the thumb and index finger (Fig. 3-1, *3*). There is a range of motion of approximately 30 degrees of flexion and extension at the fifth metacarpal hamate joint and approximately half this range of motion at the fourth metacarpal hamate joint. This motion together with flexion capabilities at the MP joints and interphalangeal joints of the ulnar fingers allows adaptation of the part to work in concert with other hand units in powerful grasp. The units of the hand are illustrated after Littler (Fig. 3-1): the fixed unit being designated number 4; the mobile first ray as number 1; the index digit with its independence as number 2; and the long, ring, and little fingers coupled with the 4th and 5th metacarpals as unit number 3.

Armed with an understanding of the degrees of motion in the various joints, it is possible to understand the arch principles in hand architecture (Fig. 3-2). For example, the fixed transverse arch of the hand occurs at the level of the distal carpal row. It is fixed by virtue of the fitted arch of carpals with the capitate as the keystone and the tough intercarpal ligaments together with the flexor retinaculum or volar carpal ligament, which bridges between the extreme

ends of the arch, taking attachment laterally on the hook of the hamate and pisiform and medially on the tubercle of the trapezium and tubercle of the scaphoid.

At the level of the metacarpal heads, the arch becomes adaptive by virtue of the wide range of motion of the first metacarpal at the metacarpotrapezial joint and the limited but definite range of motion at the fourth and fifth carpometacarpal joints. When the fixed transverse arch at the metacarpal heads is pulled into a half circle under the influence of the thenar and hypothenar muscles, the thumb is positioned to oppose the remaining digits as in pulp-to-pulp pinching. The fourth and fifth metacarpal heads are tethered to the central stable two metacarpals by the so-called intermetacarpal ligaments, which in fact attach to the volar plates of the MP joints. When the mobile metacarpal heads 1, 4, and 5 are pulled dorsally by the extrinsic extensor tendons with the thenar and hypothenar muscles relaxed, the transverse metacarpal arch is flattened or even reversed. Combined median and ulnar nerve palsy will produce this picture.

The MP joints of each of the four fingers move medially and laterally with the joint in extension but lose this capability when the joint is flexed. The reinlike collateral ligaments are loose and redundant with the MP joints in extension and hyperextension, allowing maximum medial and lateral deviation. As the MP joint is flexed, the cam effect of the eccentrically placed ligaments and the epicondylar bowing of the collateral ligaments results in tightening

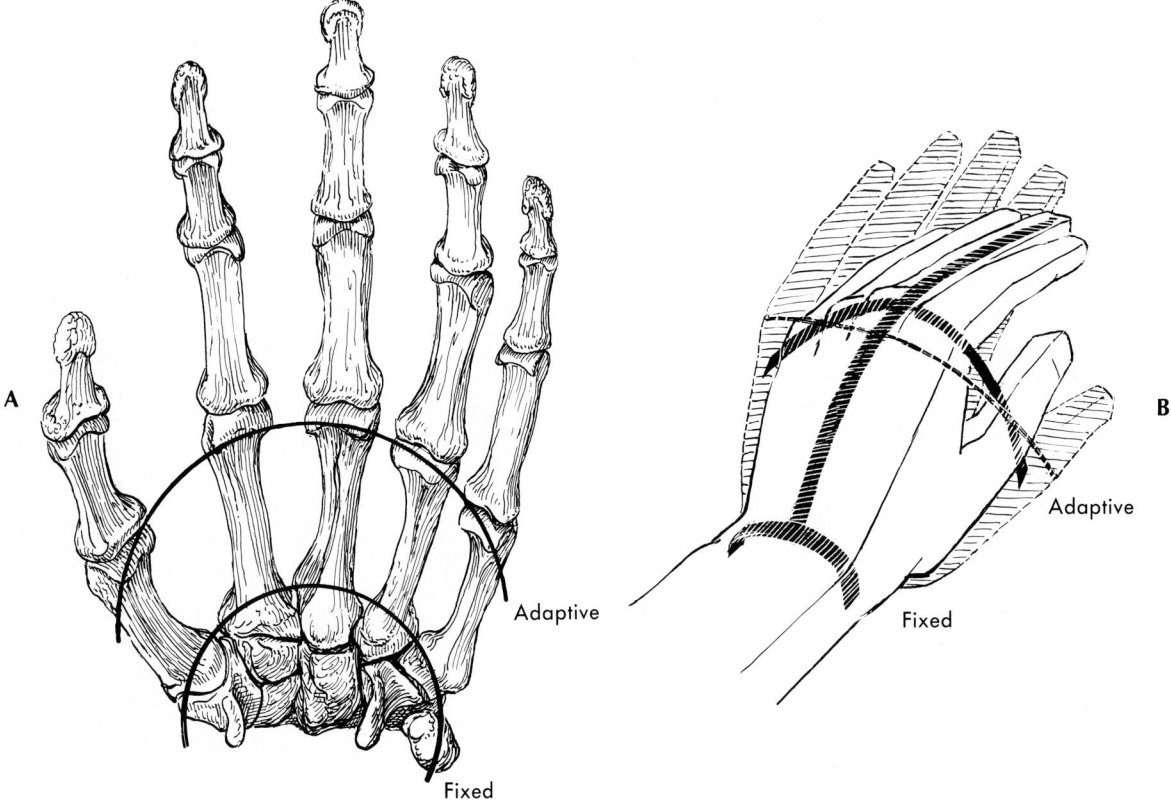

Fig. 3-2   A, The fixed and mobile transverse arches of the hand. **B,** Adaptive mobility at the level of the metacarpal heads, locus of the mobile transverse arch. This arch forms a semicircle with maximum action of the thenar and hypothenar positioning muscles. (From Flynn JE and Jupiter JB: Hand surgery, ed 4, Philadelphia, Williams & Wilkins [in press].)

and strict limitation of lateral mobility[33,47] (Fig. 3-3).

Lateral mobility of the MP joints is stabilized somewhat by the interosseous muscles. The selected variable contraction of the interossei normally influences lateral motion to the extent allowed by the unyielding collateral ligaments. Should the collateral ligaments be destroyed or purposefully sacrificed, the interossei remain the sole source of lateral stability of the MP joints. Thus when ulnar paralysis exists, caution must be exercised in MP joint capsulotomies, since all lateral stability is lost and disastrous ulnar deviation may occur.[50]

The proximal interphalangeal (PIP) joints of the fingers act like hinge joints, because the medial and lateral collateral ligaments are radially fixed in a manner which allows no medial or lateral deviation of the joint in either flexion or extension. The PIP joints flex beyond the right angle to approximately 120 degrees. Generally, hyperextension is limited because of the ligamentous volar plate, an inseparable part of the joint capsule. A loose volar plate allows a variable amount of hyperextension beyond the usual 5 degrees. The distal interphalangeal (DIP) joints flex to about 90 degrees and usually extend to nearly 30 degrees of hyperextension.

FASCIA AND COMPARTMENTS OF THE HAND AND FOREARM

The deep fascia of the forearm invests the forearm musculature and divides it into flexor and extensor compartments separated by the interosseous membrane, the radius and ulna, and intermuscular septa. The anterior compartment is subdivided into three compartments, a deep and superficial compartment medially, and a lateral compartment containing the brachioradialis, extensor carpi radialis longus, and extensor carpi radialis brevis. The closed dorsal and ventral compartments are subject to compartment pressure syndromes when the deep fascia remains intact.

In the hand, the fascia on the dorsum is quite different from that on the palm. Dorsally, the subcutaneous fascia is thin, loose, and areolar. The dorsal skin, therefore, is mobile and subject to avulsion injury and subcutaneous edema with swelling. A deep layer of fascia continuous with the extensor retinaculum at the wrist is present but thin. The extensor tendons are interlinked by membranous fascia which forms a distinct fascia layer.

The palmar fascia[4,20,35,36] is heavily fibrous and is arranged in longitudinal, transverse, oblique, and vertical fibers (Fig. 3-4). The longitudinally oriented fibers concentrate at the proximal origin from the palmaris longus at the wrist. If the palmaris longus is absent, which it is in about 15% to 20% of cases, the fascia terminates at the wrist crease. The fascia at the wrist level is separable from the underlying flexor retinaculum, the fibers of which are transverse in orientation in contrast to the longitudinal orientation of the palmar fascial fibers. From the proximal palm, the longitudinal fibers of the palmar fascia fan out, concentrating in flat bundles coursing toward each of the digits. These longitudinal fibers spread at the base of each digit and send minor fibers to the skin and the bulk of fibers distal into the fingers, where they attach to tissues making up the fibrous flexor sheath of the digits (Fig. 3-4, *A*). These fibers often extend well beyond the PIP joint and rarely as far as the DIP joint. There are some attachments of the fascia to the palmar plate and the intermetacarpal ligaments on each side of the flexor tendon sheath at the level of the MP joints. A bundle of variable thickness courses toward the thumb. These fibers are sometimes difficult to identify and are customarily less concentrated and numerous than the fibrous bands to the four fingers. The thumb fibers blend into the deep fascia overlying the thenar muscles. On the ulnar extreme side of the longitudinal fibers there is a blending of the fibers with the hypothenar fascia. The proximal portion of this ulnar border is the attachment site of the palmaris brevis muscle. Laterally, the muscle arises from hypothenar skin and fascia.

The transverse fibers of the palmar fascia are concentrated in the midpalm and the web spaces. The midpalmar transverse fibers lie deep to the longitudinal fibers, but they are inseparable from the deep vertical fibers that concentrate into the septa between the longitudinally oriented structures coursing to the digits. These transverse midpalmar fibers are called the transverse palmar ligament after the description by Skoog.[40] These transverse fibers form the roof of tunnels which act as palmar pulleys for the long flexors to the digits.

The vertical fibers of the palmar fascia, which lie superficial to the tough triangular membrane made up of the longitudinal and transverse fibers, consist of abundant vertical fibers attaching to the palm skin dermis (see Fig. 3-4, *B*). These fibers stabilize the palm skin and account for the palmar creases (Fig. 3-5). The vertical fibers on the deep side of the palmar fascial plate coalesce into a septa, forming compartments for the flexor tendons to each digit and separate compartments for the neurovascular bundles and lumbrical muscles (Fig. 3-4).

These eight compartments extend proximally to about the midpalm. Proximal to this there is a common central compartment. The medial and lateral marginal vertical septa extend more proximal than the seven intermediate septa closing the central compartment laterally and medially. The presence of the adductor pollicis, which crosses the palmar

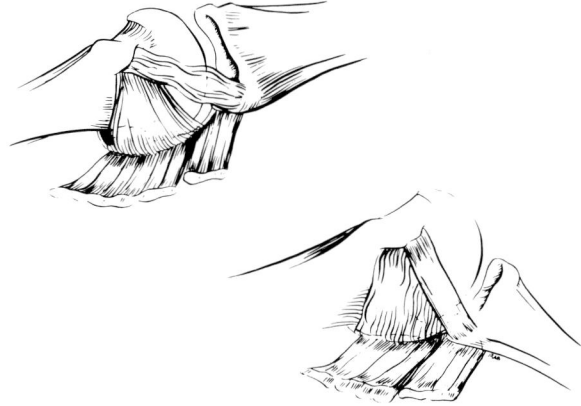

Fig. 3-3 Metacarpophalangeal Joint Collateral Ligaments. With the joint extended, the metacarpophalangeal joint component of the collateral ligament is loose and the component from the metacarpal to the palmar plate is taut. Lateral movement is possible in extension. In flexion, the metacarpophalangeal joint collateral ligament is taut and the part attached to the palmar plate is loose. Thus no lateral movement is possible in metacarpophalangeal flexion. (From Flynn JE and Jupiter JB: Hand surgery, ed 4, Philadelphia, Williams & Wilkins [in press].)

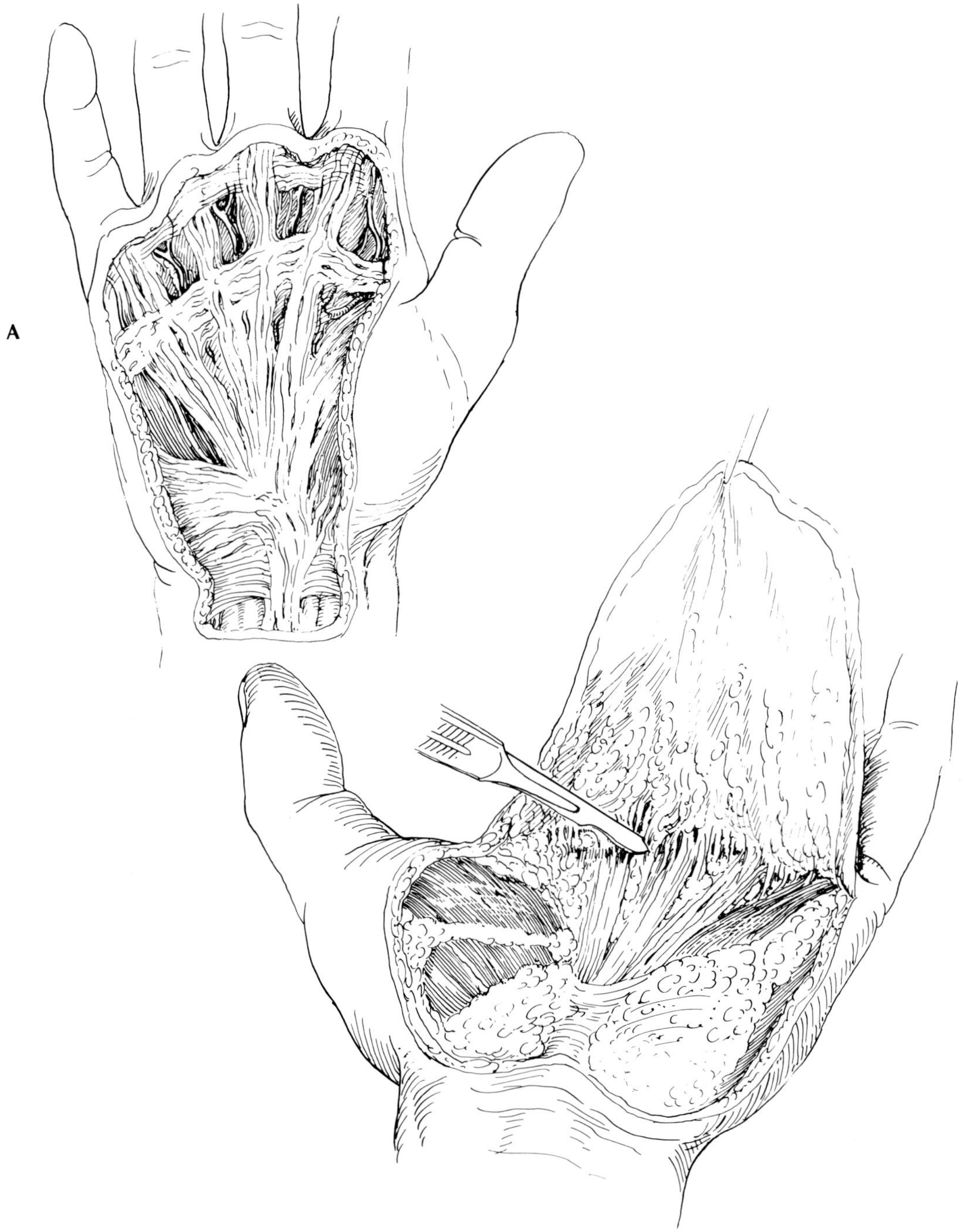

Fig. 3-4 The palmar fascia with its longitudinal, transverse, and vertical fibers. **A,** The longitudinal fibers originate in the palmaris longus (when present). Transverse fibers are concentrated in the distal palm supporting the web skin and in the midpalm, are deep to the longitudinal fibers as the transverse palmar ligament. **B,** Vertical fibers extend superficially as multiple tiny tethering strands to stabilize the thick palmar skin. The deep vertical components concentrate in septa between the longitudinally oriented structures to the fingers. (From Chase RA: Atlas of hand surgery, Philadelphia, 1973, WB Saunders Co.)

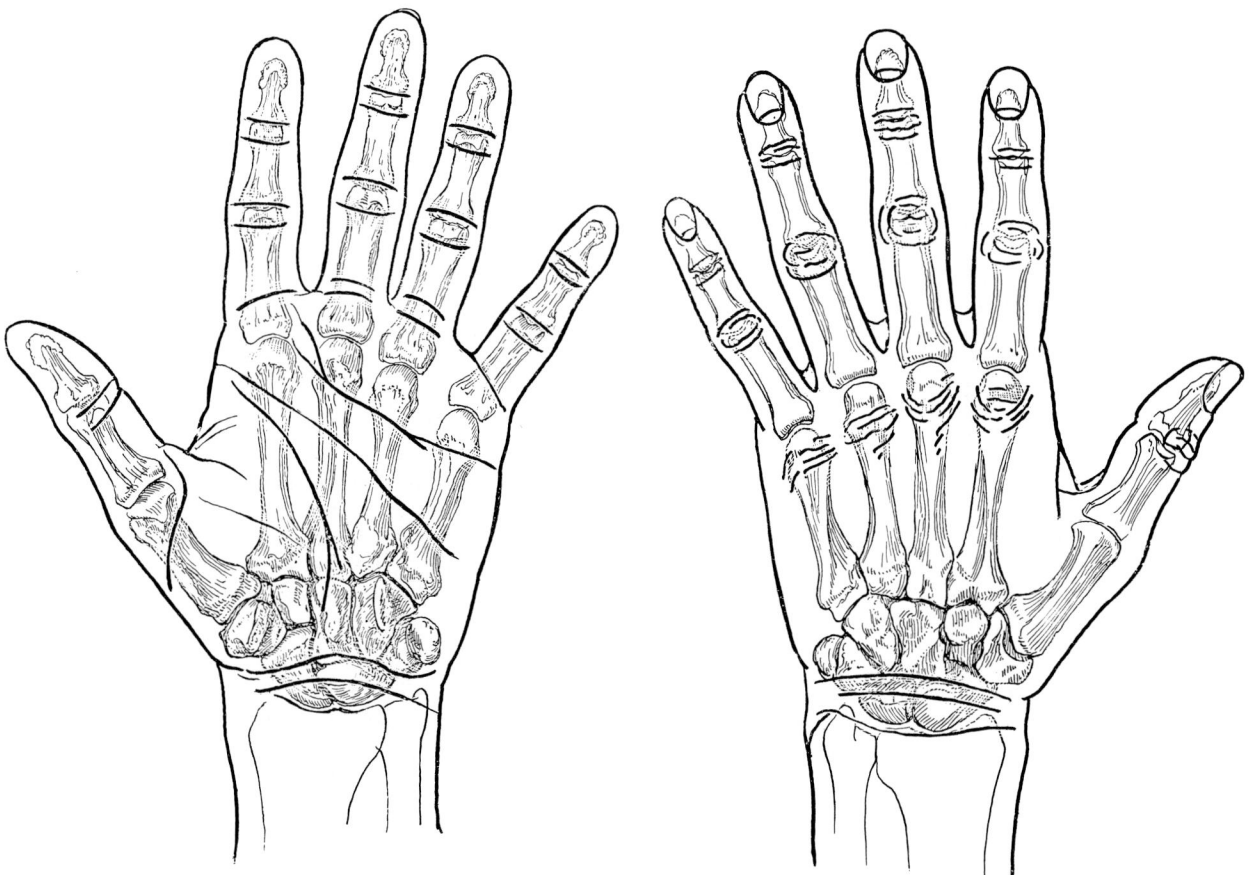

Fig. 3-5 Palmar and dorsal skin creases and their relationship to underlying joints. Note the fixed palmar creases resulting from skin fixation to the underlying palmar fascial plate by numerous vertical fibers. (From Flynn JE and Jupiter JB: Hand surgery, ed 4, Philadelphia, Williams & Wilkens [in press].)

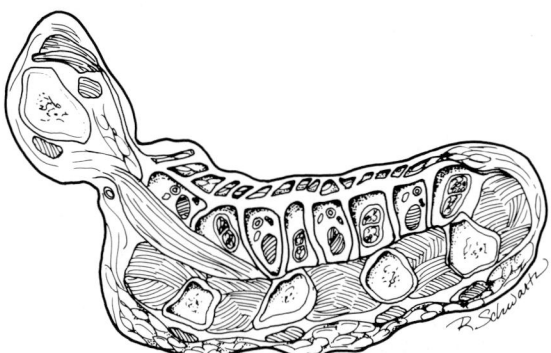

Fig. 3-6 Cross section at midpalm shows the white plaque of palmar fascia with vertical fibers extending upward to the dermis of the overlying skin. These tiny tethering strands stabilize the thick palmar skin. The deep vertical components of the fascia concentrate in septa between the longitudinally oriented structures to the fingers. Note the large fascial partition to the third metacarpal that separates the midpalmar space from the thenar space. (From Flynn JE and Jupiter JB: Hand surgery, ed 4, Philadelphia, Williams & Wilkens [in press].)

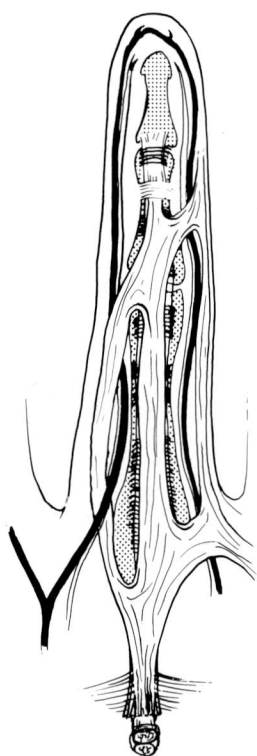

Fig. 3-7 Longitudinal fibers of the palmar fascia frequently extend down on each side of the flexor tendon sheath as spiral bands, often curling around the neurovascular bundles. (After Murray).

aspect of the second metacarpal, results in the appearance of a major septum between the index flexor tendons and the neurovascular and lumbrical space to the third interspace. This thick septum attaches to the third metacarpal, dividing the palmar space into a thenar or adductor space and a midpalmar space (Fig. 3-6).[24]

At the level of the MP joint some of the longitudinal fibers extend down each side of the flexor tendon sheath as spiral bands passing superficial or deep to the proper digital artery and nerve. Not infrequently these bands extend dorsal to the neurovascular bundle at the base of the finger, then curl back around the bundle prior to crossing the PIP joint (Fig. 3-7). These spiral cords sometimes make dissection of the neurovascular bundle at this level in Dupuytren's contracture quite tedious.[35,36,43]

MUSCLES AND TENDONS
Extrinsic extensors

The extensor digitorum is a series of tendons with a common muscle belly (Fig. 3-8, A). The tendon itself enters into the central extensor of each of the fingers and terminates in its insertion into the middle phalanx at the central slip of the extensor mechanism. Its primary action in each finger is to extend the MP joint through the shroudlike fibers that pass around the proximal phalanx medially and laterally, just distal to the MP joint.

The interplay between the long extrinsic extensors and intrinsic muscles at the interphalangeal joint is the source of extension power to the phalanges of the fingers and thumb. The extrinsic extensors with muscle bellies in the forearm consist of a group of extensors, which work in unison with one another, and two independent long extensors, one for the index finger and another for the little finger (Figs. 3-8, B and C). Extrinsic extensors of the thumb consist of the extensor pollicis longus and the extensor pollicis brevis. The latter accompanies the abductor pollicis brevis as one of the "outcropping" muscles emerging from beneath the long digital extensors and coursing superficial to the extensor carpi radialis longus and brevis to enter the first dorsal compartment at the wrist.[25]

On the dorsum of the hand there are intertendinous bridges between the separate tendons of the extensor digitorum. The extensor indicis is an independent long extensor to the index finger, and the extensor digiti minimi, usually represented by two separate tendons at the metacarpal level, acts as an independent extensor of the little finger. In each case the independent extensor lies on the ulnar side of the extensor digitorum contribution to each of these two fingers. The extensor pollicis longus, like the independent extensors of the index and little fingers, has its own separate muscle belly, which lies deep to the extensor digitorum muscle bellies. Extensor pollicis longus inserts on the distal phalanx of the thumb and is the primary extensor of the interphalangeal joint, acting secondarily to extend the MP joint and the wrist (Fig. 3-9, A). The oblique muscles to the thumb, the tendons of which occupy the first dorsal fibrous compartment, consist of the tendons of the abductor pollicis longus and the extensor pollicis brevis. The extensor pollicis brevis inserts on the proximal phalanx, acting primarily as an extensor of the MP joint (Fig. 3-9, B). The abductor pollicis longus inserts on the base of the first metacarpal, and it often sends tendon fibers to the proximal portion of the abductor pollicis brevis (Fig. 3-9, C). The abductor pollicis longus radially abducts the first metacarpal, but in bridging the wrist it, together with the extensor pollicis brevis, acts to aid in radial deviation of the wrist.

Extrinsic flexors

There are three layers of muscles in the flexor pronator group of the volar side of the forearm. The superficial group of muscles may be outlined by placing the hand on the palmar aspect of the opposite forearm with the thenar eminence at the medial epicondylar area and the ring finger along the ulnar border (Fig. 3-10). The thumb, index, long, and ring fingers then fall directly over the muscle tendon units, representing the superficial group of muscles on the flexor surface of the forearm. The thumb overlies the pronator teres; the index lies over the flexor carpi radialis; the long finger, over the palmaris longus; and the ring finger, over the flexor carpi ulnaris. The superficialis muscles make up the middle layer, and the deep layer consists of the flexor digitorum profundi, the flexor pollicis longus, and the pronator quadratus.

Each finger has a flexor digitorum profundus tendon inserting on the distal phalanx. The counterpart to the thumb is the flexor pollicis longus. The muscle bellies of the flexor profundi to the long, ring, and little fingers are often common and interdependent in the forearm, while the muscle belly of the flexor digitorum profundus to the index finger and the flexor pollicis longus each has a separate, identifiable independent muscle belly. Occasionally there is some interdependence between the flexor profundus to the index

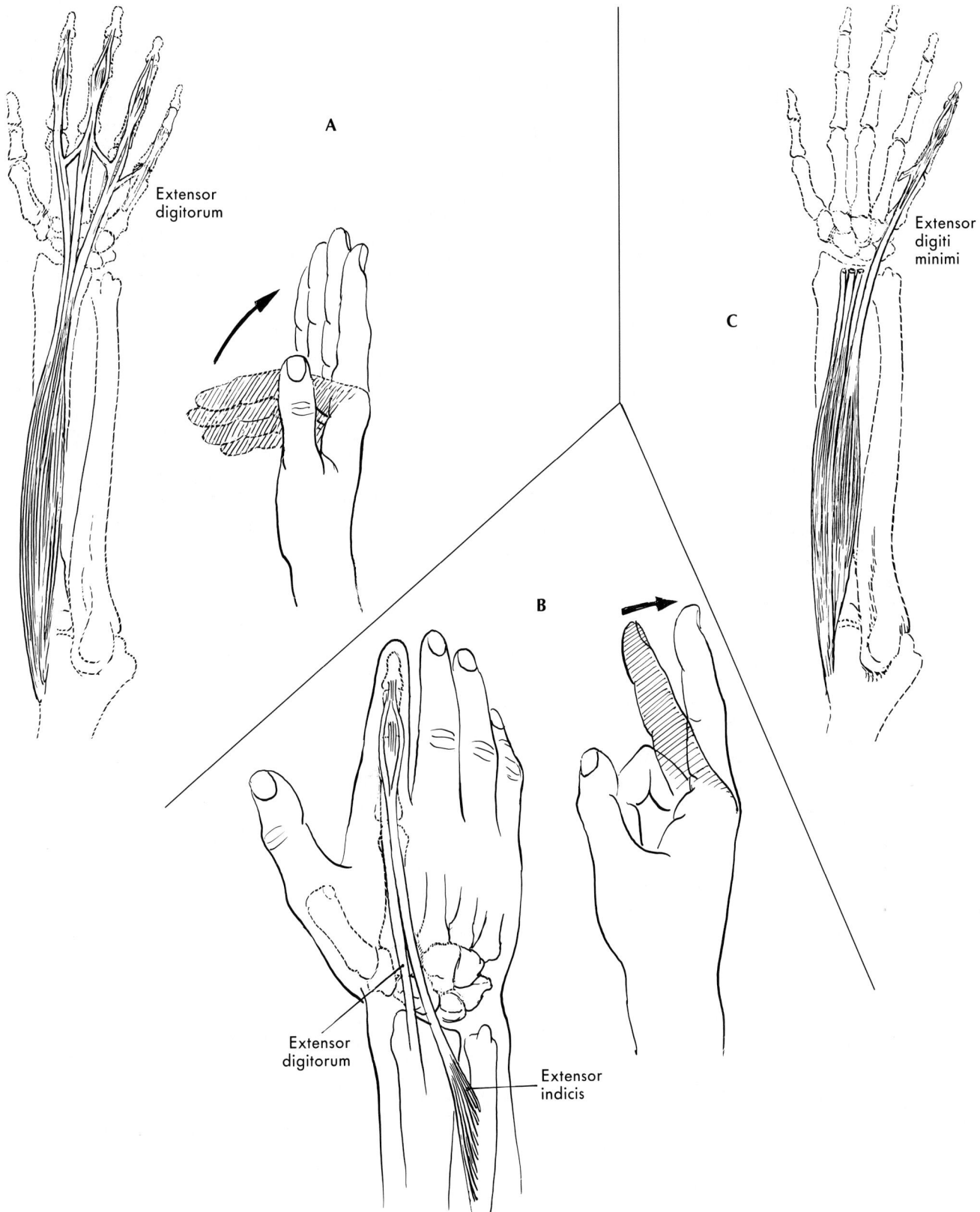

Fig. 3-8   **A,** Extensor digitorum has a common muscle belly and tendons extending to the four fingers. Note the intertendinous bridges at the level of the distal metacarpals. **B,** Extensor indicis to the index finger parallels the tendon to that finger from the extensor digitorum. **C,** Extensor digiti minimi allows independent extrinsic extension of the little finger. Tendons of the independent extensors of the index and little fingers lie on the ulnar side of the contribution to those fingers from the extensor digitorum. (From Chase RA: Atlas of hand surgery, Philadelphia, 1973, WB Saunders Co.)

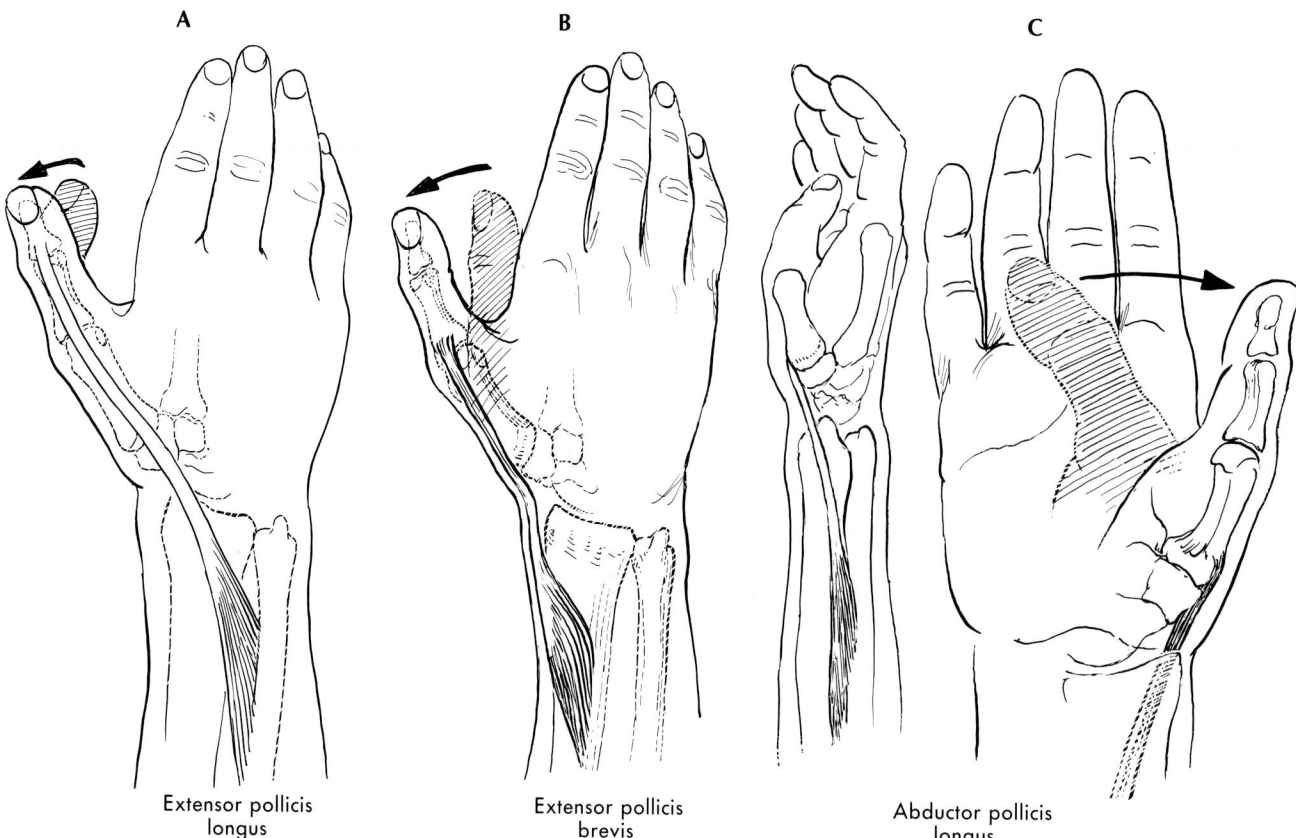

A

B

C

Extensor pollicis
longus

Extensor pollicis
brevis

Abductor pollicis
longus

Fig. 3-9 **A,** Extensor pollicis longus is the independent extensor of the distal phalanx of the thumb. **B,** Extensor pollicis brevis with attachment to the proximal phalanx extends to the metcarpophalangeal joint and aids in dorsal abduction of the thumb and radial deviation of the wrist. **C,** The abductor pollicis longus acts at the base of the first metacarpal to dorsally abduct the thumb and radially deviate the wrist. The extensor pollicis brevis and abductor pollicis longus, outcropping muscles to the thumb, occupy the first dorsal compartment at the wrist. (From Chase RA: Atlas of hand surgery, Philadelphia, 1973, WB Saunders Co.)

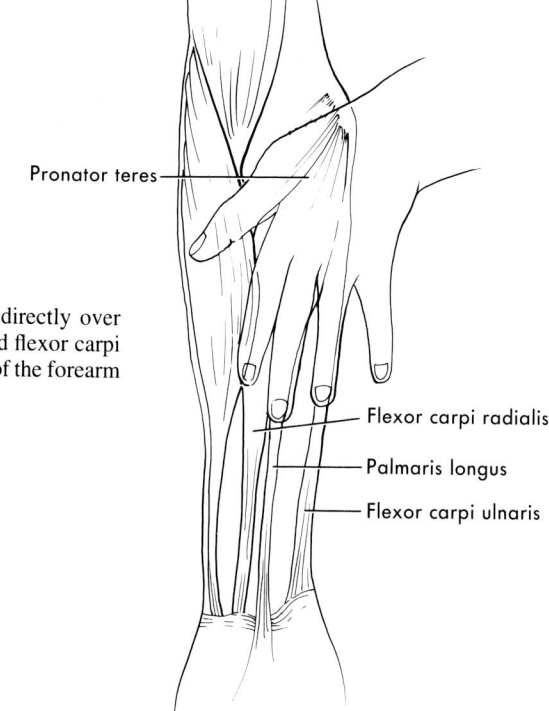

Pronator teres

Flexor carpi radialis

Palmaris longus

Flexor carpi ulnaris

Fig. 3-10 The thumb, index, long, and ring fingers lie directly over the pronator teres, flexor carpi radialis, palmaris longus, and flexor carpi ulnaris if the contralateral hand is placed on the volar aspect of the forearm as shown. (After Henry—Extensile Exposure).

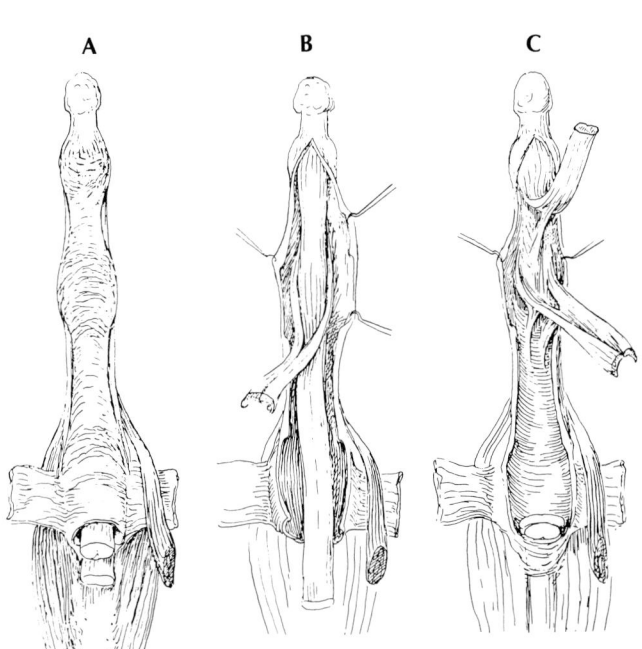

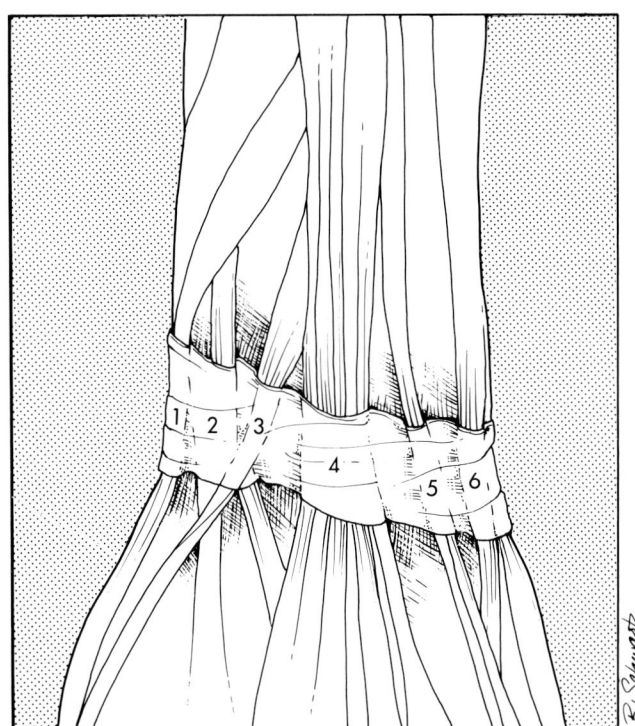

Fig. 3-11 **A,** Flexor tendons in the digit are surrounded by fibrous and synovial sheaths. **B,** The superficialis tendons split to allow the passage of the profundus tendon between its two tails to insert on the distal phalanx. **C,** The superficialis decussates behind the profundus tendon before inserting on the middle phalanx. (From Chase RA: Atlas of hand surgery, Philadelphia, 1973, WB Saunders Co.)

Fig. 3-12 The extensor retinaculum at the wrist forms a roof over the six extensor compartments. Each compartment has a synovial compartment that extends both proximally and distally to the retinaculum itself. (From Flynn JE and Jupiter JB: Hand surgery, ed 4, Philadelphia, Williams & Wilkens [in press].)

finger and the flexor pollicis longus. Each of the four fingers also has a flexor digitorum superficialis tendon, which lies superficial to the profundus tendon in the palm. As it passes into the finger, it flattens, then splits at the level of the proximal phalanx, and its two flat tails surround the profundus, decussate behind it to insert at the level of the middle phalanx (Fig. 3-11). The muscle bellies of the flexor digitorum superficialis tendons lie superficial on the palmar aspect of the forearm and are independent from one another. All of the extrinsic digital flexors pass through the carpal tunnel, where the flexor retinaculum acts as a major proximal pulley at the wrist.

THE RETINACULAR SYSTEM
Extensor retinaculum (Fig. 3-12)

The dorsal annular ligament of the wrist forms the roof over six separate extensor compartments at the level of the wrist. This dorsal transverse carpal ligament is essentially an area of thickening and specialization within the deep fascia of the forearm and hand. The compartments are separated by vertical, longitudinal septa. The retinaculum itself is continuous across the dorsum of the tendons, then deep to the extensors, generating a floor for the compartments, particularly on the ulnar side of the hand.[45]

The first radial compartment may be subdivided into several compartments for the tendons of the abductor pollicis longus and the extensor pollicis brevis. The next compartment contains the two major wrist extensors, extensor carpi

radialis longus and brevis. The third compartment forms a tunnel for the extensor pollicis longus just ulnar to Lister's tubercle. The fourth compartment houses the tendons of the extensor digitorum and the extensor indicis. The fifth compartment forms a pulley for the extensor digiti minimi. The sixth compartment houses the extensor carpi ulnaris.

THE FLEXOR RETINACULAR SYSTEM
(Fig. 3-13, *A* and *C*)
Wrist pulley

The transverse carpal liagment forms a broad restraining pulley at the wrist level. It attaches on the radial side to the tubercle of the trapezium and scaphoid. On the ulnar side it attaches to the hook of the hamate and the pisiform. The ligament confines the long flexor tendons and the median nerve within the carpal tunnel to prevent bowstringing of the long flexor tendons at the wrist.

Finger pulleys (Fig. 3-13, *B* and *C*)[14,15,21,42]

There are four or five discrete annular pulleys for the flexor tendons in each finger. Between the annular pulleys one finds variable cruciate bands, which act as minor pulleys. The A_1 annular pulley begins 0.5 cm proximal to the MP joint and is anchored to the volar plate and the proximal phalanx. Immediately distal to it is the A_2 pulley, the largest of the annular pulleys, which extends about half the length of the proximal phalanx. The third annular pulley, A_3, lies over the PIP joint arising from its volar plate. The fourth

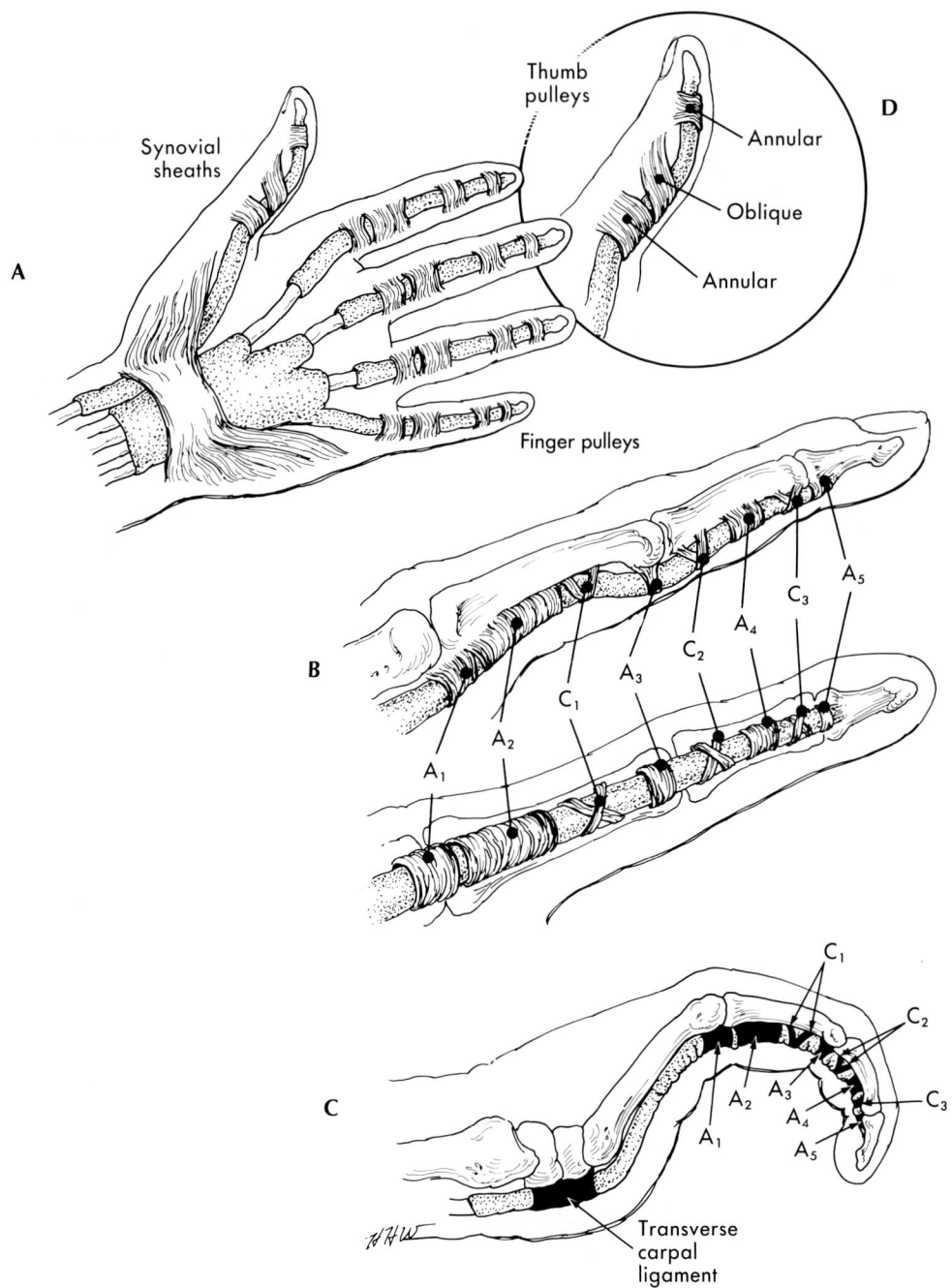

Fig. 3-13 **A,** Synovial and retinacular pulleys at the wrist and digit levels. **B,** The annular and cruciate pulleys within each of the fingers. **C,** The major retinacula occur where the longitudinal arches are adaptive at the wrist and within the digits. **D,** The thumb pulley. (From Chase RA: Atlas of hand surgery, vol 2, Philadelphia, 1984, WB Saunders Co.)

annular pulley is found over the middle one third of the middle phalanx, and a thickening of the sheath over the DIP joint is commonly designated as the fifth annular pulley, A_5. Between the A_2 and A_3 pulley, between the A_3 and A_4 pulley, and distal to the A_4 pulley, one commonly finds the more delicate cruciate ligaments, C_1, C_2, and C_3. The pulleys within the finger are placed to maintain the relationship of the flexor tendon to the long axis of each finger joint, and they prevent bowstringing of the tendon across the joints in flexion. The gaps between pulleys allow unrestrained

flexion of the joints by allowing folding and pleating of the thin synovial sheath, which remains as the sole covering of the flexor tendons beneath the overlying finger fascia between the pulleys. Pulleys for the thumb consist of annular pulleys at the MP joints and an oblique pulley between (Fig. 3-13, *D*).

FLEXOR TENDON ZONES (Fig. 3-14)[9]

Based on the anatomy of the fibrous sheaths and the insertion of the flexor digitorum profundus and superficialis,

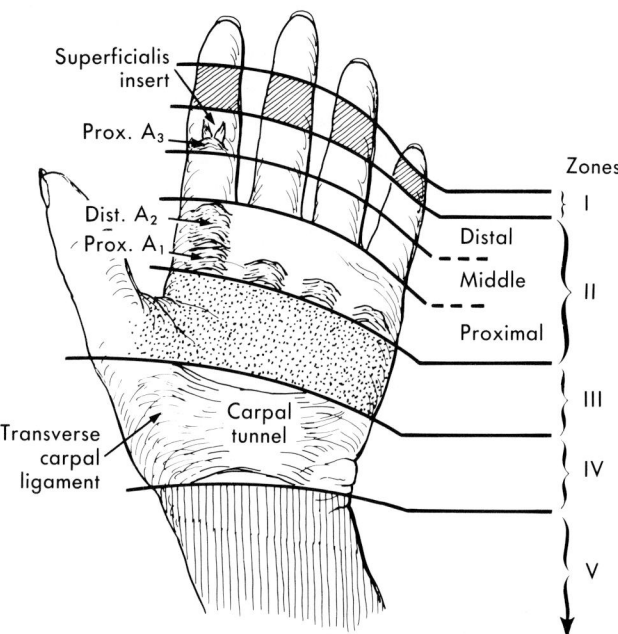

Fig. 3-14 Flexor tendon zones chosen for their relevance to flexor tendon injuries. (See text) (From Chase RA: Atlas of hand surgery, vol 2, Philadelphia, 1984, WB Saunders Co.)

the palmar aspect of the digits and hand are divided into specific zones.

Zone 1—Zone 1 is the area traversed by the flexor digitorum profundus distal to the insertion of the flexor digitorum superficialis on the middle phalanx.

Zone 2—Zone 2 extends from the proximal end of Zone 1 to the proximal end of the digital fibrous sheath. It is subdivided into distal, middle, and proximal components.

    Distal— The distal portion extends from the insertion of the superficialis on the middle phalanx deep to the profundus to the proximal end of the A_3 pulley.

    Middle— The middle component extends from the insertion of the A_3 pulley to the distal end of A_2. The roof of the sheath in this zone consists only of synovial sheath and the C_1 cruciate ligament.

    Proximal—The proximal portion extends from the distal end of A_2 to the proximal end of A_1, a tunnel covered by the tough A_1 and A_2 pulley system.

Zone 3—Zone 3 is the area traversed by the flexor tendons in the palm and is free of fibrous pulleys. It extends, therefore, from the proximal end of the finger pulley system (A_1) to the distal end of the wrist retinaculum, the transverse carpal ligament.

Zone 4—Zone 4 is the carpal tunnel. It extends from the

distal to the proximal borders of the transverse carpal ligament.

Zone 5—Zone 5 extends from the proximal border of the transverse carpal ligament to the musculotendinous junctions of the flexor tendon.

These tendon zones are particularly important to the hand surgeon treating tendon injuries. The management technique, the postoperative rehabilitation, and the prognosis vary according to the zone in which the flexor tendon injury occurs.

FUNCTION OF THE EXTRINSIC FLEXORS AND EXTENSORS[5]

In reviewing the function of muscles and their tendons, it is important to recall that a muscle-tendon unit affects every joint between its origin and insertion; that is, the flexor digitorum profundus crossing multiple joint linkages will primarily flex the DIP joint. However, secondarily, it will flex the PIP joint, followed by the MP joint, and, finally, the wrist. The complexity of its function multiplies when one takes into account the other antagonists and protagonists at each of the joints in the linkage of skeletal elements between the muscle's proximal and distal attachments. For example, flexion of the DIP and PIP joints by the profundus tendon is augmented by active extension of the MP joint by the long extensor tendon. Thus a principle is established that in a multiple linkage system, a tendon's function is, in fact, augmented at some joints by action of its antagonist at other joints in the system. It is certainly clear that wrist extensors which are antagonist to the profundus tendon at the wrist significantly augment profundus function at the MP and interphalangeal joints. This combination of wrist extension and finger flexion, in fact, is a synergistic function. The flexor digitorum profundus muscles which operate the ulnar three fingers are interdependent. Thus if one restrains any of those three fingers in extension, there is markedly diminished function of the profundus tendon in the other two fingers. This forms the basis for a test for superficialis tendon function. Muscle bellies of the flexor digitorum superficialis muscles are separate and independent. If one checkreins the function of the profundus tendons by holding the long finger or little finger in extension passively, the only effective flexor of the PIP joint is the superficialis tendon muscle unit. This is the basis for testing for superficialis function (Fig. 3-15).

The flexor pollicis longus is the only flexor of the interphalangeal joint of the thumb. Testing for its function, therefore, is simple. The extrinsic extensor muscles act primarily to extend the MP joints. Secondarily, they act as wrist extensors. Because of the nature of the extensor mechanism in the finger, if the MP joint is held passively in flexion, the long extensor tendon through its central slip and lateral bands acts to extend the interphalangeal joints. Thus when the interossei and lumbricals act to flex or stabilize the MP joint, the long extensor mechanism will augment the extension of the interphalangeal joints. Absence of such intrinsic support of the MP joints in neutral position or flexion results in extension and hyperextension of the MP joints and in loss of influence of the extrinsic extensors at the interphalangeal joints, which are then at the mercy of the long flexors to the fingers. The result is the classical claw or intrinsic minus position.[48]

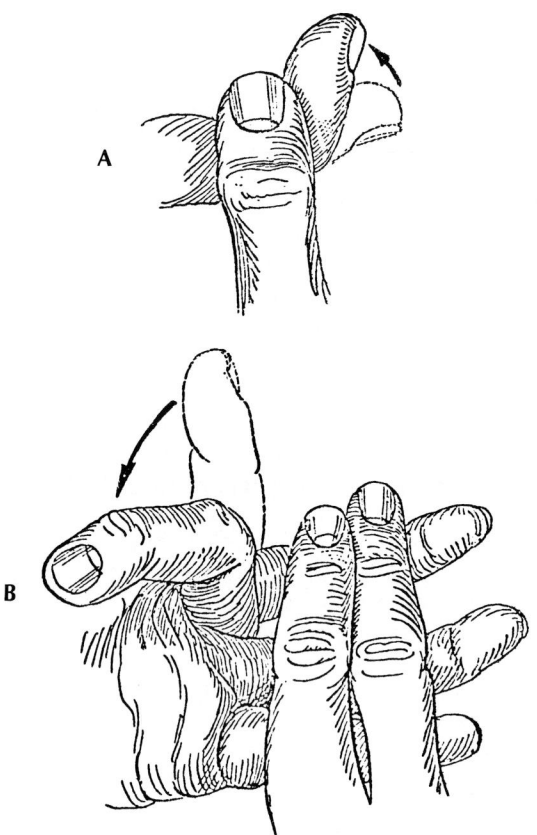

Fig. 3-15 **A,** The only flexor of the distal interphalangeal joint is flexor digitorum profundus. **B,** By checkreining the profundi, holding the fingers in extension, function of the superficialis muscle to the free finger may be tested. (From Chase RA: Atlas of hand surgery, vol 2, Philadelphia, 1984, WB Saunders Co.)

THE INTRINSIC MUSCLES OF THE HAND
Thenar muscles

The two and one-half muscles lying lateral to the flexor pollicis longus on the palmar aspect of the thumb represent the median-innervated positioning muscles of that member. They are the abductor pollicis brevis, the opponens pollicis, and the superficial head of the flexor pollicis brevis. The abductor pollicis brevis originates from the fascia and flexor retinaculum on the palmar aspect of the wrist and extends to insert in part on the proximal phalanx and in part into the extensor mechanism of the thumb at and just beyond the MP joint. The fleshy opponens pollicis lies just deep to the abductor pollicis brevis and inserts all along the body of the metacarpal. The flexor pollicis brevis consists of two heads, one lateral to and one medial to the flexor pollicis longus. The lateral or superficial head quite regularly inserts into the proximal phalanx after surrounding the sesamoid at the radial side of the MP joint. The medial or deep head varies greatly in its insertion, inserting on the proximal phalanx sometimes through the sesamoid on the medial aspect of the MP joint, sometimes through the lateral sesamoid, and sometimes through both. The adductor pollicis muscle consists of a transverse and oblique heads. It originates along the line of the palmar aspect of the third metacarpal and deep fascia of the hand. It inserts into the proximal phalanx by enshrouding the sesamoid on the ulnar side

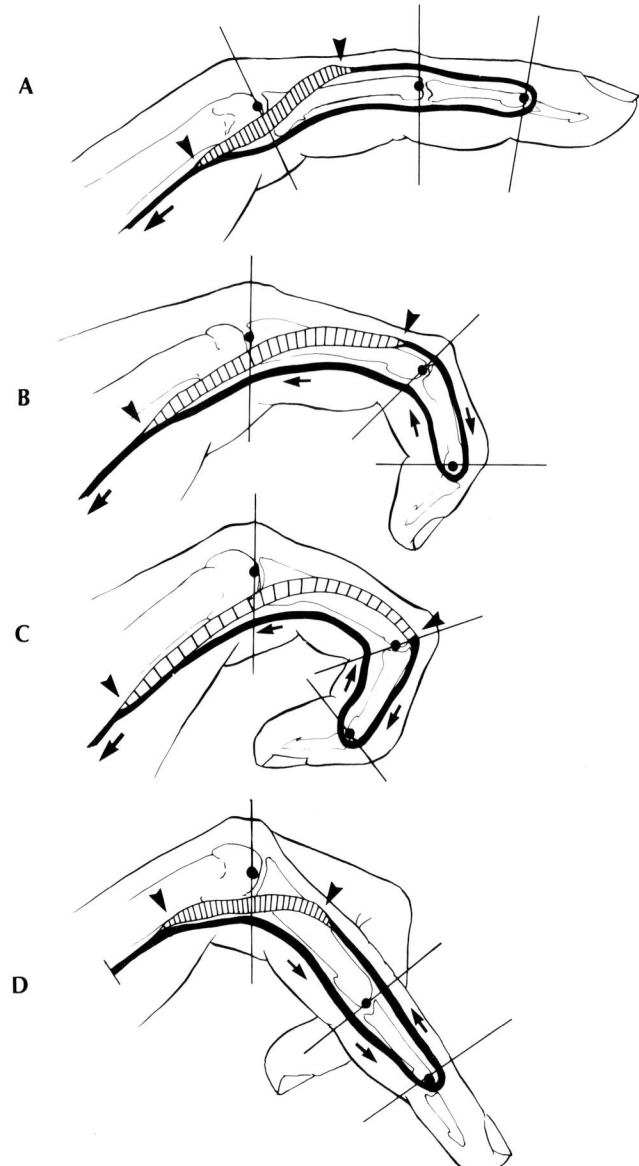

Fig. 3-16 The lumbrical muscle acts as a moderator band between the extensor and flexor mechanism in the finger. It has a moving origin from the profundus tendon and a moving insertion into the extensor mechanism through the lateral band. **A,** As the profundus tendon is pulled, the origin of the lumbrical moves proximal. **B,** Action of the profundus flexes the interphalangeal joints and moves the extensor mechanism distally, further separating the origin and insertion of the lumbrical. **C,** This becomes more exaggerated as the finger is pulled into flexion with the lumbrical relaxed. **D,** If the lumbrical muscle then contracts, its effect on the finger is to flex the metacarpophalangeal joint and extend the interphalangeal joints. This is the primary function of the lumbrical. (From Flynn JE and Jupiter JB: Hand surgery, ed 4, Philadelphia, Williams & Wilkens [in press].)

of the MP joint, often together with the deep head of the flexor pollicis brevis.

The hypothenar muscles are essentially mirror images of the thenar muscles except that there is an absence of the adductor. The muscles are abductor digiti minimi, flexor digiti minimi brevis, and opponens digiti minimi. The dorsal palmar interossei lie in the interosseous intervals taking origin from the opposing surfaces of the metacarpals. There are four dorsal interossei and three palmar. The interosseous tendons insert on the medial or lateral aspects of the proximal phalanx and have slips into the lateral band of the extensor mechanism. With the long finger as a central axis of the hand, the dorsal interossei are abductors, while the palmar interossei are adductors of the fingers. The lumbrical muscle has a moving site of origin from the profundus tendon or tendons in the palm of the hand. It extends palmar to the ligaments between the volar plates of the MP joints and inserts into the lateral band of the extensor mechanism. Diagrammatically, one sees that the relaxed lumbrical muscle is stretched by a separation of its origin and insertion as the finger is flexed by a pull on the profundus tendon. As the finger flexes, the extensor mechanism moves distally at the level of the interphalangeal joints, and thus the origin and insertion of the muscle are spread apart. If the muscle contracts, it produces flexion at the MP joint and extension at the PIP and DIP joints (Fig. 3-16).

The extensor mechanism in the finger[18,29-32,41,46]

There is a complex interdigitation of tendons of the extrinsic extensor mechanism and the intrinsic tendons within the digit. The extrinsic extensor tendon is linked to shroud fibers at the level of the MP joint called the sagittal bands. It is through this sagittal band mechanism that the long extensors create extension at the MP joint as their primary function. The extensor, however, continues as a central slip inserting beyond the PIP joint into the middle phalanx. Prior to its insertion it subdivides, giving off lateral slips, which

join the lateral conjoint tendon or band through which the long extensor may influence the DIP joint. The tendinous extension of the interossei extends into the finger, forming a lateral tendon palmar to the joint axis of the MP joint. This extends distally, coursing dorsal to the PIP joint where it is joined by the lateral slips of the common extensor mechanism. These lateral tendons of the interossei also give slips to the central slip for insertion into the proximal dorsal lip of the middle phalanx. The lumbrical muscle whose tendon lies just palmar to the intermetacarpal ligament extends as tendon to join the dorsal mechanism in passing dorsal to the axis of the PIP joint (Fig. 3-16). In addition to these active structures, there is a passive oblique retinacular ligament, which inserts together with the distal insertion of the extensor mechanism on the distal phalanx. It therefore passes dorsal to the joint axis of the DIP joint, then obliquely palmar to take its origin from the fibrous tissues surrounding the flexor tendons just proximal to the PIP joint. It acts to extend the DIP joint when the PIP joint is extended.[10] The extensor mechanism is held centrally at the level of the PIP joint by the transverse retinacular ligaments.

The complex interplay of the extrinsic and intrinsic muscles within the finger allows wide variation of postures within the range allowed by the collateral ligaments and the capsular ligaments of the MP joint and the PIP and DIP joints.

BLOOD SUPPLY[1,12,37]

Arterial blood supply to the hand and forearm is furnished by branches from the brachial artery, including the superior and inferior ulnar collateral arteries and the profunda bra-

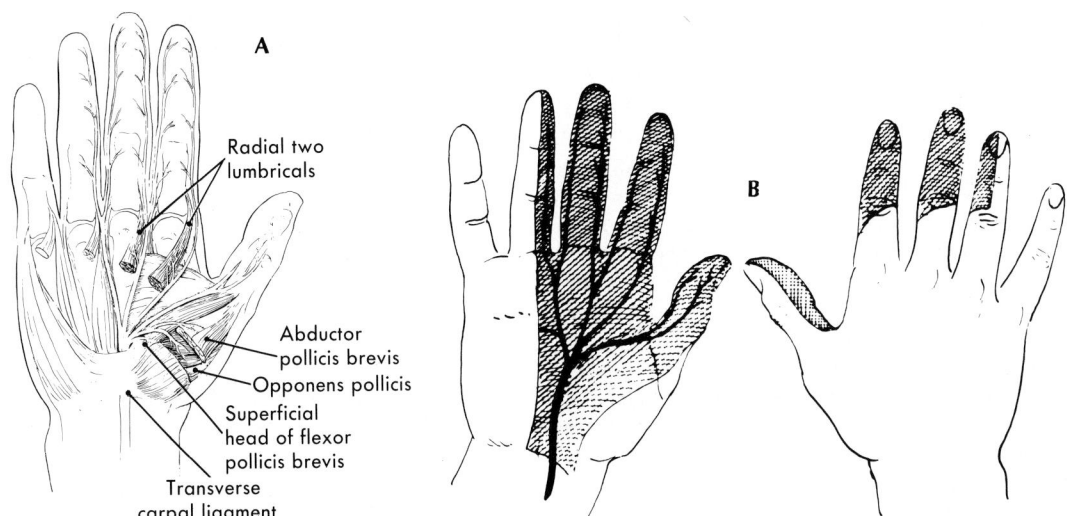

Fig. 3-17 **A,** The median nerve, the most superficial structure in the carpal tunnel, generally arborizes as it passes through the carpal tunnel into its terminal motor and sensory branches. The recurrent motor branches, which may actually pass through the flexor retinaculum rather than distal to it; generally innervate the two and one-half thenar muscles on the radial side of the long flexor to the thumb, the abductor pollicis brevis, the opponens pollicis, and the superficial head of the flexor pollicis brevis. In addition, there are motor branches to the two radial lumbricals from the nerve branches coursing towards the index and long fingers. **B,** Sensory branches course to the thumb, index, and long fingers and to the radial side of the ring finger. The median nerve classically lends sensibility to the palmar aspect and the distal dorsum of the thumb, index, and long fingers and the radial one half of the ring finger. Intrinsic muscles radial to the flexor pollicis longus and the two radial lumbricals receive motor innervation from the median nerve. (From Chase RA: Atlas of hand surgery, vol 2, Philadelphia, 1984, WB Saunders Co.)

chial artery, which contribute to the collateral anastomoses around the elbow. The terminal branches of the brachial artery, the radial and ulnar, are the major contributors of blood supply to the forearm and the hand. An early branch of the ulnar artery as it courses deep across the proximal forearm is the common interosseous artery, which gives rise to the anterior posterior interosseous arteries deep within the forearm. The radial and ulnar arteries continue through the forearm, contributing multiple muscular and osseous branches. At the wrist level interarterial arches between the two major vessels furnish blood supply to the carpal bones. At the wrist level the radial artery courses dorsally at the level of the radiocarpal joint to pass across the depression between the long and short extensors to the thumb, often referred to as the anatomical snuffbox. Before doing so, it generally gives off a superficial branch, which crosses the thenar eminence at various depths superficial to and deep within the thenar muscles to contribute to the superficial vascular arch. The branch crossing dorsally represents the major radial arterial contribution to the hand, particularly on its radial aspect. There are multiple variations in the nature of branching of the radial artery after it passes through the first web space between the second metacarpal and the first dorsal interosseous attachments to it. After giving off arterial branches to the thumb and index finger, it becomes the major contributor to the deep palmar vascular arch. The ulnar artery courses distally adjacent to the ulnar nerve lying just deep to the flexor carpi ulnaris. As it approaches the wrist, it contributes to the vascular arches at the wrist level, then turns superficial to lie just deep to the palmaris brevis muscles within Guyon's tunnel. After giving off a deep branch which anastomoses deep within the palm with the contribution to the deep vascular arch from the radial artery, the ulnar artery continues across the palm just deep to the palmar fascia as the superficial palmar arch. Arteries radiate distally from the superficial arch as common digital arteries which divide into proper digital arteries to the adjacent sides of the index, long, ring, and little fingers. Proper digital arteries arise from the superficial arch to the ulnar side of the little finger and from either the deep or superficial arch to the radial side of the index finger.

Blood supply to the thumb comes variably from the deep branch of the radial artery as a princeps pollicis or as branches directly from the deep arch. A discussion of the multiple variations of the blood supply within the hand is beyond the scope of this chapter, and the author suggests that a more complete review is available in the classic studies by Coleman and Anson[12] (1961) and the detailed studies by Murakami[37] (1969) and Adachi[1] (1928). Venous return from the hand is found both as classical venae comitantes from each of the arteries and the networks of veins which drain toward the dorsum of the fingers and hand into the cephalic and basilic venous systems. A detailed knowledge of vascular anatomy has become much more important with the advent of microvascular surgery with prospects for replantation and transfer of composite parts from one place to another.

NERVE SUPPLY[16,44,49]

Sensory nerve supply to the forearm and hand comes from the medial, lateral, and posterior antebrachial cutaneous nerves and the radial, ulnar, and median nerves within

the hand. The radial aspect of the dorsum of the hand is innervated by the superficial sensory branch of the radial nerve. The dorsal branch of the ulnar nerve supplies the ulnar aspect of the dorsum of the hand as well as the palmar aspect of the little finger and ulnar half of the ring finger. The remaining portion of the palm, which includes the palmar aspect of the thumb, index, long, and half of the ring fingers, is supplied by the median nerve.

The median nerve

The median nerve enters the forearm lying adjacent to the brachial artery at the elbow and beneath the lacertus fibrosus or bicipital fascia. After giving off motor branches to the pronator teres muscle, the nerve passes between its deep and superficial heads. It gives off the anterior interosseous nerve in varying relationships to the pronator teres. The anterior interosseous nerve courses deep and distally along the interosseous membrane, giving motor branches to the flexor pollicis longus, the flexor digitorum profundus to the index finger, and to the pronator quadratus in which the nerve terminates. The main trunk of the median nerve passes through a second muscular arcade at the origins of the superficialis muscles of the forearm. It then lies on the deep surface of the superficialis muscles and tendons to the distal quarter of the forearm. In this position it gives off motor branches to the flexor digitorum superficialis and the flexor carpi radialis. The nerve emerges to become superficial by coursing around the radial aspect of the superficialis tendons just above the wrist. It then becomes the most superficial structure within the carpal tunnel (Fig. 3-17, A). After passing through the carpal tunnel, the nerve arborizes into its sensory branches and the recurrent motor branch to the thenar muscles. The recurrent motor branch may come off at various levels, including a point within the carpal tunnel where it may penetrate the volar carpal ligament to pass to the thenar muscles. The sensory nerves consist of a proper digital nerve to the thumb, which divides into a medial and lateral proper digital nerve, a proper digital nerve to the radial side of the index finger, and common digital nerves, which divide into proper digital nerves to the adjacent sides of the index, long, and ring fingers (Fig. 3-17, B). Tiny motor branches to the radial two lumbricals originate from the proper digital nerve to the radial side of the index finger and the common digital nerve to the adjacent sides of the index and long fingers.

Ulnar nerve

The ulnar nerve enters the forearm by passing through the cubital tunnel at the medial epicondylar groove of the humerus. It penetrates between the two heads of origin of the flexor carpi ulnaris. It lies on the deep side of that muscle throughout the forearm. It gives off motor branches to the flexor carpi ulnaris and the ulnar two or three flexor digitorum profundus muscles. At the wrist the nerve courses superficial to enter the hand beneath the palmaris brevis muscle and fascia in Guyon's tunnel (Fig. 3-18, A). At this point it gives off a deep motor branch and superficial branches, including a proper digital nerve to the ulnar side of the little finger and a common digital nerve to the adjacent sides of the little and ring fingers (Fig. 3-18, B). Other branches go to the palmaris brevis muscle and the abductor digiti minimi muscle. The deep motor branch of the ulnar

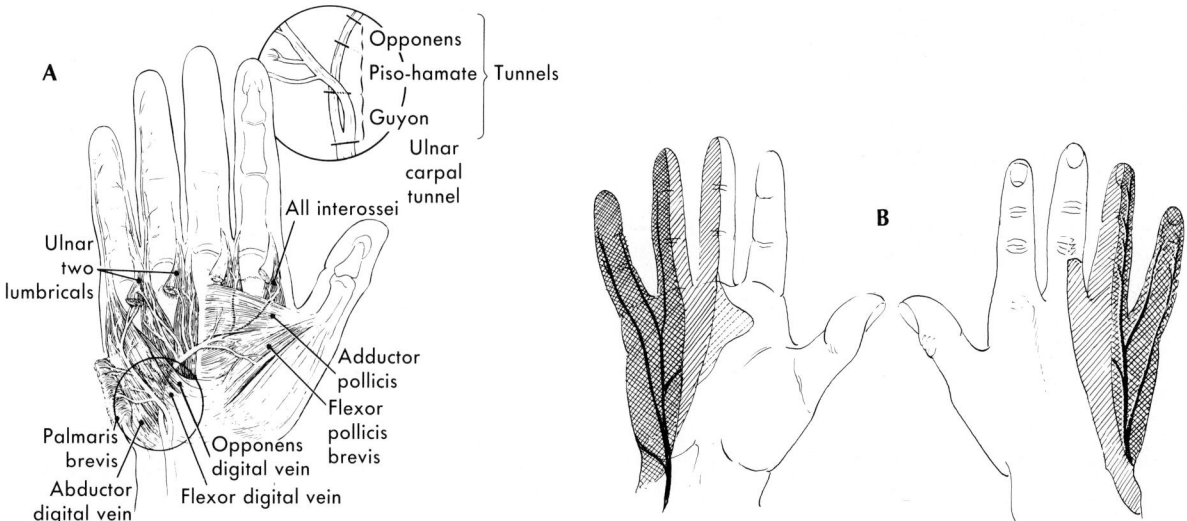

Fig. 3-18 **A,** The ulnar nerve arrives at the hand just medial to the flexor carpi ulnaris, where it becomes superficial coursing just beneath the palmaris brevis within Guyon's tunnel. The deep motor branch continues by coursing through the pisohamate tunnel and the opponens tunnel between the superficial and deep head of the opponens digiti minimi muscle. It courses across the deep palm in company with the deep vascular arch to give innervation to all of the interossei, the two ulnar lumbricals, the adductor pollicis, and generally the deep head of the flexor pollicis brevis. **B,** The superficial branch gives motor twigs to the palmaris brevis and the abductor digiti minimi before it continues to give sensory innervation to the little finger and ulnar side of the ring finger. (From Chase RA: Atlas of hand surgery, vol 2, Philadelphia, 1984, WB Saunders Co.)

nerve then passes through two more components of the ulnar tunnel at the wrist/hand level.[26] The first portion is that which lies between the hook of the hamate and the pisiform called the pisohamate tunnel, and the second is a tunnel between the two heads of the opponens digiti minimi called the opponens tunnel. The nerve then courses with the deep vascular arch and gives off tiny motor branches to the remaining hypothenar muscles, all of the interossei, the ulnar two lumbricals, the adductor pollicis, and the deep head of the flexor pollicis brevis. Variation in nerve supply to the intrinsic muscles between median and ulnar nerves occurs at the flexor pollicis brevis level.[49] The two heads of the muscle are often separately innervated by the median and ulnar nerve respectively, but quite often the superficial head may be innervated by the ulnar nerve or by both nerves.

Radial nerve

The radial nerve enters the forearm just deep to the brachioradiali muscle. It courses across the radial aspect of the elbow region close to the head of the radius, where it penetrates between the two heads of the supinator muscle at an arcade of fibers called the Arcade of Frohse. Prior to entering the arcade, the radial nerve gives motor branches to the brachioradialis, the flexor carpi, radialis longus and brevis, and a sensory branch which courses deep to the brachioradialis throughout the forearm to emerge as the dorsal sensory branch on the radial aspect of the dorsum of the hand (Fig. 3-19). The radial nerve passes through the Arcade of Frohse to become the posterior interosseous nerve. It innervates the supinator, and after passing between the two heads of the supinator, the nerve arborizes to give off motor branches to the extensor digitorum, the extensor carpi ulnaris, the

extensor indicis, the extensor digiti minimi, the extensor pollicis longus, the extensor pollicis brevis, and the abductor pollicis longus.

HAND KINESIOLOGY—SOME PRINCIPLES[3,5,6]

Movements in the hand represent a complex series of muscular actions around multiple joint linkages. Muscle protagonists, antagonists, and modifiers all work in centrally controlled coordination based on movement commands voluntarily generated cerebrally, modified by reflex interactions

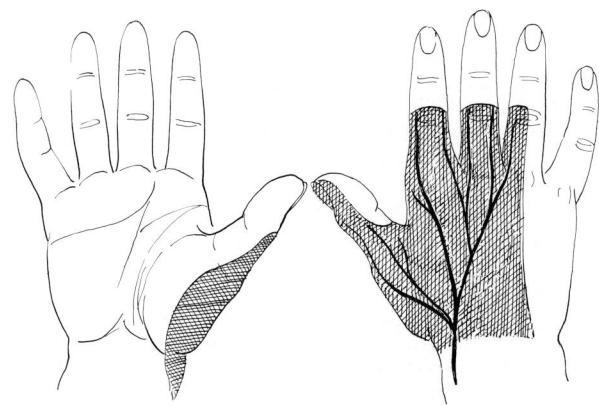

Fig. 3-19 The dorsal or sensory branch of the radial nerve courses over the radial dorsal aspect of the wrist to supply sensory innervation to the radial aspect of the dorsum of the hand and the proximal dorsal aspect of the thumb, index, and long fingers and variably the ring finger.

at various levels in the central nervous system. A muscle rarely acts independently to create movement. For each muscle tendon unit, however, there are some principles worth noting:

1. A muscle tendon unit acts on every joint between its origin and insertion (see section on Function of Extrinsic Flexors and Extensors).
2. Afferent fibers from stretch sensors within muscles serve as one arm of a reflex servo-mechanism to help control muscular contraction.
3. Reflexes may be conditioned through a complex learned reflexive response in such examples as those automatically demonstrated by complex movements done by conditioned athletes.
4. The arrangement of muscles and tendons in relationship to a specific joint determines their effect on joint action within the range allowed by the joint configuration and ligamentous limitations.
5. The forces on a joint by a muscle depend not alone upon muscle power but upon the combination of vectors affecting the joint at a given axis of motion.
6. The torque generated for rotary movement around a joint axis depends not only on the force generated by the muscle but by the lever arm or perpendicular distance from the axis or center of rotation. This is popularly known as the moment arm.
7. The function of a muscle tendon unit which crosses several joints has its function augmented at any given joint by action of its antagonists at any or all other joints in the linkage. For example, the profundus flexors have their function at the MP and interphalangeal joints augmented by the wrist extensors which are antagonists of the profundi at the wrist. This is the practical explanation of muscle synergism.

For an up-to-date, nicely presented, comprehensive discussion of upper limb kinesiology, see Brand.[5]

REFERENCES

1. Adachi B: Das Arterie System der Japaner, vol 1, p 382, Maruzan Co, Kyoto, 1928.
2. Aubriot JH: The metacarpophalangeal joint of the thumb. In Tubiana R, editor: The hand, Philadelphia, 1985, WB Saunders Co.
3. Bell C: The hand—its mechanism and vital endowments as Evincing Design, London, 1834, The Pickering Press.
4. Bojsen-Moller F and Schmidt L: The palmar aponeurosis and the central spaces of the hand, J Anat 117:55, 1974.
5. Brand PW: Clinical mechanics of the hand, St. Louis, 1985, The CV Mosby Co.
6. Bunnell S: Surgery of the hand, Philadelphia, 1944, JB Lippincott Co.
7. Chase RA: Atlas of hand surgery, vol 1, Philadelphia, 1973, WB Saunders Co.
8. Chase RA: Atlas of hand surgery, vol 2, Philadelphia, 1984, WB Saunders Co.
9. Chase RA: Surgical anatomy of the hand, Surg Clin North Am 44:1349, 1964.
10. Chase RA: Muscle tendon kinetics, Am J Surg 109:277, 1965.
11. Chase RA: Anatomy and examination of the hand. In May JW and Littler JW, editors: Converse textbook of plastic surgery (in preparation).
12. Coleman SS and Anson BJ: Arterial patterns in the hand based upon a study of 650 specimens, Surg Gynecol Obstet 113:408, 1961.
13. Dahhan P, Fischer L, and Alliey Y: The trapeziometacarpal articulation, Anatomia Clinica 2:43, 1980.
14. Doyle JR and Blythe WF: The finger flexor tendon sheath and pulleys: anatomy and reconstruction, AAOS symposium on tendon surgery in the hand, St. Louis, 1975, The CV Mosby Co.
15. Doyle JR and Blythe WF: Anatomy of the flexor tendon sheath pulleys of the thumb, J Hand Surg 2:149, 1977.
16. Duchenne GBA: Physiologie des Mouvements, Paris, 1867, Bailliere (Translation by Kaplan EB, Philadelphia, 1959, JB Lippincott Co.).
17. Eaton RG and Littler JW: A study of the basal joint of the thumb, J Bone Joint Surg 51A:661, 1969.
18. Eyler DL and Markee JE: The anatomy of the intrinsic musculature of the fingers, J Bone Joint Surg 36A:1, 1954.
19. Henry AK: Extensile exposure, Baltimore, 1945, Williams & Wilkins.
20. Hueston JT: Dupuytren's contracture, Baltimore, 1963, Williams & Wilkins.
21. Hunter JM and others: The pulley system, Proceedings of the American Society for Surgery of the Hand: orthopedic transactions 4:4, 1980.
22. Jones FW: Principles of anatomy as seen in the hand, Philadelphia, 1920, Blakistons' Son.
23. Joseph J: Further studies of the metacarpo-phalangeal and interphalangeal joints of the thumb, J Anat 85:221, 1951.
24. Kanavel AB: Infections of the hand, Philadelphia, 1925, Lea & Febiger.
25. Kaplan EB: Functional and Surgical Anatomy of the Hand, Philadelphia, 1953, JB Lippincott Co.
26. Kim S: The ulnar tunnel at the wrist, Personal communication, 1986.
27. Kuczynski K: Carpometacarpal joint of the human thumb, J Anat 118:119, 1974.
28. Kuczynski K: The thumb and the saddle, The Hand 7:120, 1975.
29. Landsmeer JMF: Anatomy of the dorsal aponeurosis of the human finger and its functional significance, Anat Rec 104:31, 1949.
30. Landsmeer JMF: Anatomical and functional investigations on the articulation of the human fingers, Acta Anat 25:1, 1955.
31. Landsmeer JMF: A report on the coordination of the interphalangeal joints of the human finger and its disturbances, Acta Morphol Neerl Scand 2:59, 1958.
32. Landsmeer JMF: The coordination of finger-joint motion, J Bone Joint Surg 45A:1654, 1963.
33. Littler JW: Architectural principles of reconstructive hand surgery, Surg Clin North Am 31:463, 1951.
34. Littler JW: On the adaptability of man's hand (with reference to the equiangular curve), The Hand 5:187, 1973.
35. McFarlane RM: Patterns of the diseased fascia in the fingers in Dupuytren's contracture, Plast Reconstr Surg 54:31, 1974.
36. McFarlane RM: Dupuytren's contracture. In Green DP: Operative hand surgery, New York, 1982, Churchill Livingstone, Inc.
37. Murakami T, Takaya K, and Outi H: The origin, course and distribution of arteries to the thumb, with special reference to the so-called A. princeps pollicis, Okajimas folica anatomica japonica 46:123, 1969.
38. Ou CJA: The biomechanics of the carpometacarpal joint of the thumb, doctoral dissertation, Department of Mechanical Engineering, Louisiana State University and Agricultural and Mechanical College. Ann Arbor, 1980, University Microfilms International.
39. Pagalidis T, Kuczynski K, and Lamb DW: Ligamentous stability of the base of the thumb, The Hand 13:29, 1981.
40. Skoog T: The transverse elements of the palmar aponeurosis in Dupuytren's contracture, Scand J Plast Reconstr Surg 1:51, 1967.
41. Stack HG: A study of muscle function in the fingers, Ann Royal Coll Surg Engl 33:307, 1963.
42. Strauch B and Maura W: Digital flexor tendon sheath: an anatomic study, J Hand Surg 10A:785, 1985.
43. Strickland JW and Bassett RL: The isolated digital cord in Dupuytren's contracture: anatomy and clinical significance, J Hand Surg 10A:118, 1985.
44. Sunderland S: Nerves and nerve injuries, New York, 1978, Churchill Livingstone, Inc.
45. Taleisnik J and others: Extensor retinaculum of the wrist, J Hand Surg 9A:495, 1984.
46. Tubiana R and Valentine P: L'extension des doigts, Rev Chir Orthop 49:543, 1963.
47. Tubiana R: The Hand, vol 2, Philadelphia, 1985, WB Saunders Co.
48. White WL: Restoration of function and balance of the wrist and hand by tendon transfers, Surg Clin North Am 40:427, 1960.
49. Woodhall B and Beebe GW, editors: Peripheral nerve regeneration: A follow-up study of 3656 World War II injuries, Veterans Administration Medical Monograph, 1956.
50. Zancolli E: Structural and dynamic bases of hand surgery, Philadelphia, 1979, JB Lippincott Co.

II
EVALUATION

4

Clinical examination of the hand

Pat L. Aulicino and Theodore E. DuPuy

Clinical examination of the hand is a basic skill that should be mastered by both the surgeon and the therapist. To master this skill, it is necessary to have an understanding of the functional anatomy of the hand. A thorough history, a systematic examination, and knowledge of disease processes that affect the hand will leave the examiner with few diagnostic dilemmas. Radiographs, electrodiagnostics, and specialized laboratory tests are ancillary tools that only confirm a diagnosis that has been made on a clinical basis.

An organized approach and clear and concise records are of paramount importance. Either line drawings of the deformities or clinical photographs should be prepared for each new patient evaluated. Range of motion of the affected parts should be recorded and dated in a table format. If there is a discrepancy between active and passive motion, this should also be noted. A good hand examination is useless if the results are not recorded accurately.

This chapter will outline one approach to examination of the hand. The most important points have already been made: perform a systematic, organized clinical examination, and record the results accurately and clearly.

HISTORY

Before examination of a patient's hand, an accurate history must be taken. The patient's age, hand dominance, occupation, and avocations are elicited. If the patient has had an injury, the exact mechanism as well as the time and date of the injury and prior treatment are recorded. Prior surgical procedures, infections, medications, and prior therapy are also noted. Once this background data is obtained, the patient is questioned specifically regarding his involved extremity. Does he have pain? What is the character of the pain? When does it occur? Is it work related, or constant? Does it occur at night or during the day? What relieves the pain, and what exacerbates it? What is the patient not able to do now that he could do before his injury? What does the patient desire from you? This last question is extremely important. The patient's reply will assist you in determining whether the patient has a realistic understanding of the true nature of his injury. Unrealistic expectations can never be fulfilled. They result in both an unhappy patient and an unhappy surgeon. During this interview it is also important to assess the impact that the injury or disease process has upon the patient's family, economic, and social life. Patients who have litigation pending or significant secondary gain are usually poorly motivated and are not optimum candidates for elective hand surgery. Successful hand surgery requires precise surgical techniques followed by expert hand therapy in conjunction with a well-motivated, compliant patient.

The patient's pertinent medical history is now obtained. Does he have rheumatoid arthritis or some other progressive collagen-vascular disease? Is the patient taking systemic steroids or some other medication? Does the patient have any other chronic systemic illness that would make him a poor surgical risk? The history is completed only after the surgeon or therapist has a complete understanding of the patient's problem and how this affects the patient physically, psychologically, and economically.

PHYSICAL EXAMINATION
General inspection

When examining a patient's upper extremity, one must be able to observe the shoulder, arm, forearm, and hand. Therefore the patient should be disrobed. The gross appearance of the entire extremity is noted. Are the shoulder muscles atrophied? Does the patient have a normal-appearing upper extremity or is there a traumatic or congenital anomaly? Are there any scars? How does the patient carry this limb? Can he move his shoulder and arm without pain? Is the patient able to place his hand? If the hand cannot be placed in a functional position, a brilliantly reconstructed hand is useless.

After the general appearance of the limb has been noted, the attention is directed to the integument. The color, tone, and moisture of the skin are noted. Are the normal skin creases present (Fig. 4-1)? Is there any edema of the hand? Are the nails ridged, pitted, or deformed? Is there correct rotational alignment of the nail plates (Fig. 4-2)? Are there any obvious deformities of the hand? Do the thenar or hypothenar muscles appear atrophied? Are there any contractures? When the patient's injured extremity is being inspected, the uninjured extremity should also be inspected for comparison. The attitude of the hand is then noted. Normally with the hand resting and the wrist in neutral, the fingers are progressively more flexed from the radial to the ulnar side of the hand. A loss of the normal attitude of the hand can indicate a tendon laceration, a contracture, or possibly a peripheral nerve injury (Fig. 4-3).

Part of the general inspection is noting how the patient treats his injured limb. Does he cradle his injured hand and stare at it as if it did not belong to him, or does he appear relatively unhampered by his injury? All observations are, of course, assiduously recorded.

Range of motion

The motion of the entire extremity should be measured and compared with the opposite side. As previously stated, discrepancies between active and passive motion should be noted. Fixed deformities are also noted.

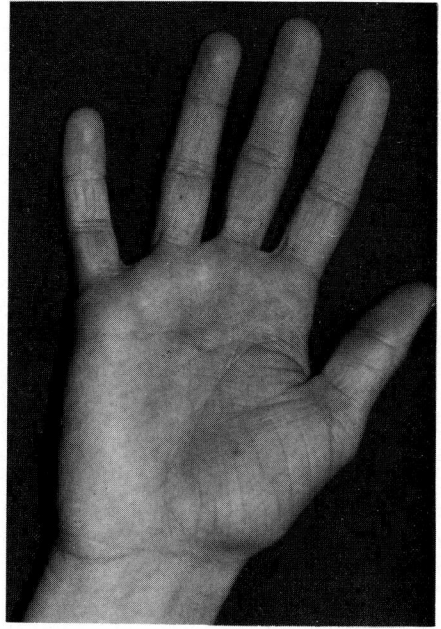

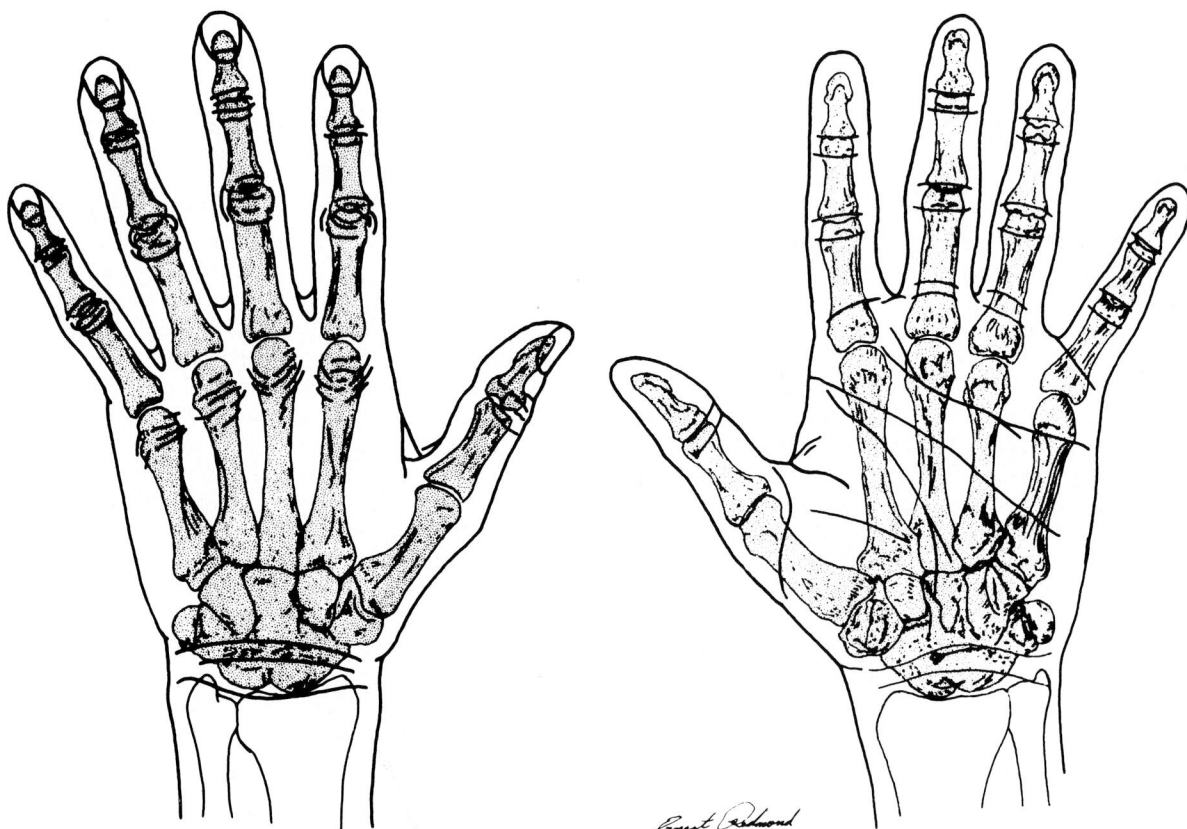

Fig. 4-1 Clinical photograph and diagrammatic illustrations of the relationship of the volar and dorsal skin creases to the underlying joints. The absence of a volar skin crease may indicate the presence of an underlying joint anomaly and thus the inability of the patient to flex that digit, as is seen in congenital symphalangism. The absence of both volar and dorsal skin creases is seen in conditions that cause edema, or as a result of the atrophic phase of a reflex sympathetic dystrophy. (Redrawn from Chase RA: Atlas of hand surgery, Philadelphia, 1973, WB Saunders Co.)

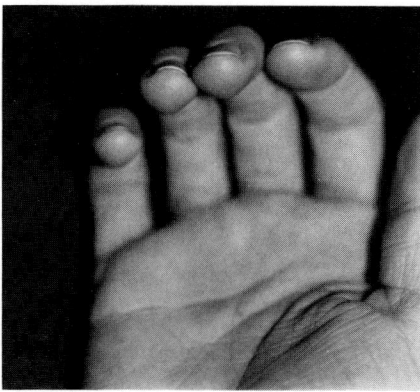

Fig. 4-2 Normal rotational alignment of nail plates.

The shoulder should be tested for forward flexion, extension, abduction, and internal and external rotation. Elbow extension and flexion and forearm supination and pronation are also checked and recorded. Wrist dorsiflexion, volar flexion, and ulnar and radial deviation are recorded. Thumb extension, flexion, opposition, adduction, carpometacarpal extension, and carpometacarpal abduction are measured and recorded. A finger goniometer should be used to make each of these measurements.[35] If motion is lacking, the distance from the tip of the finger to the distal palmar crease is measured. If the finger touches the palm but does

not reach the crease, as in the profundus tendon disruption, this should be noted and the distance from the tip of the finger to the distal palmar crease should be recorded; however, it should be stated that the finger did touch the palm but did not reach the distal palmar crease (Fig. 4-4).

Once all active and passive motions have been examined, the wrist is flexed and extended to see of the normal tenodesis effect is present. In an uninjured hand, when the wrist is flexed, the fingers and the thumb will extend, and as the wrist is extended, the fingers will assume an attitude of flexion and the thumb will oppose the fifth digit (Fig. 4-5). The alignment of the digits is then inspected. As stated, the nail plates should all be parallel to one another, and their alignment should be similar to that of the other hand. Each finger should point individually to the tuberosity of the scaphoid, and the longitudinal axis of all fingers when flexed should point in the direction of the scaphoid (Fig. 4-6).

Muscle testing

The hand is powered by intrinsic and extrinsic muscles. The extrinsic muscles have their origin in the forearm and the tendinous insertions in the hand. The extrinsic flexors are on the volar side of the forearm and flex the digits and the wrist. The extrinsic extensors originate on the dorsal aspect of the forearm and extend the fingers, thumb, and wrist. The intrinsic muscles originate and insert in the hand. These include the thenar and hypothenar muscles as well as the lumbricals and the interossei. The thenar and hy-

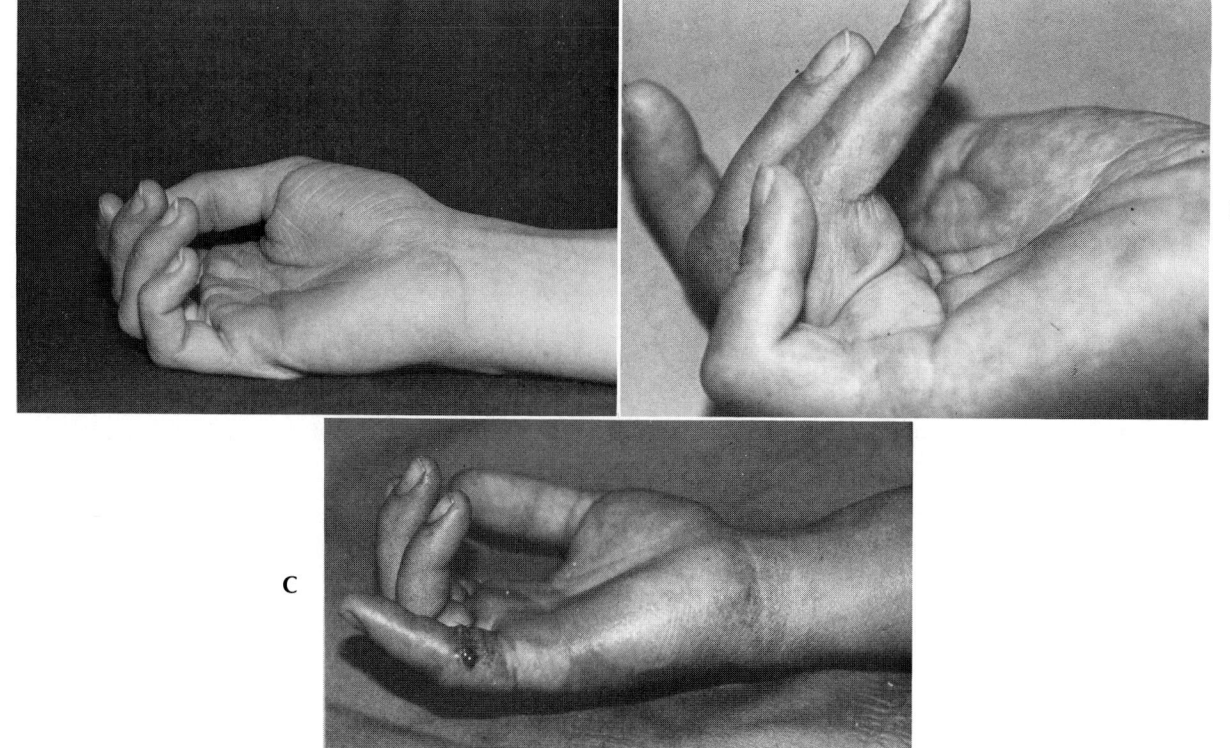

Fig. 4-3 **A,** Normal attitude of the hand in a resting position. Notice that the fingers are progressively more flexed from the radial aspect to the ulnar aspect of the hand. In **B** this normal attitude is lost because of flexion contractures of the digits as a result of Dupuytren's disease. **C,** Loss of the normal attitude as a result of a laceration of the flexor tendons to the fifth digit.

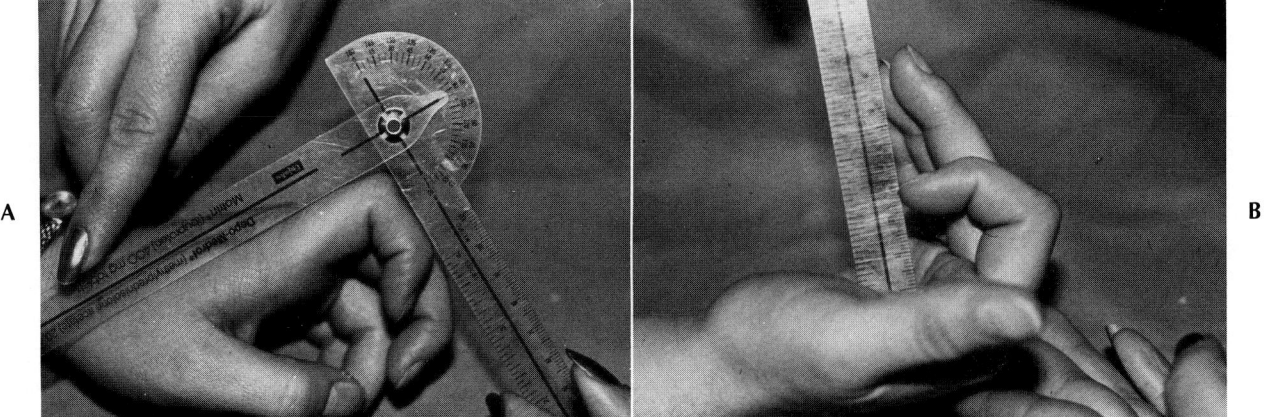

Fig. 4-4   A, A finger goniometer is used to measure the range of motion of the proximal interphalangeal joint of the index finger. **B,** A ruler is then used to measure the distance of the pulp of the finger from the distal palmar crease. Active and passive motions should be noted and recorded.

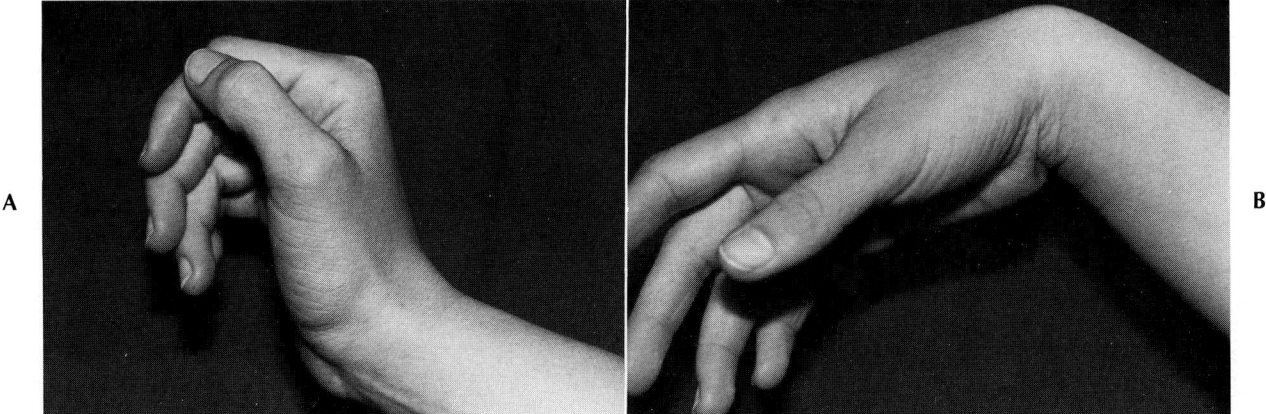

Fig. 4-5   Tenodesis of the hand. In an uninjured hand, **A,** on wrist dorsiflexion the fingers and thumb will flex and **B,** on flexion of the wrist the thumb and fingers will extend. In the presence of a tendon laceration, contractures of the joints, or adhesions of the flexor or extensor systems, the normal tenodesis effect will be lost. This test can be performed actively by the patient or passively by the examiner.

pothenar muscles help to position the thumb and the fifth finger and also aid in opposition of the thumb and in pinch. The interossei assist in abduction and adduction of the digits. The lumbricals flex the metacarpophalangeal (MP) joints and extend the interphalangeal joints. The interossei also have the function of flexing the MP joints and, by and large, are much stronger than the lumbricals. The function and testing of the intrinsic muscles will be discussed later in this chapter.

Extrinsic muscle testing—the extrinsic flexors. As each specific extrinsic muscle-tendon unit is tested, its strength should be graded and recorded. Strength should be graded from 0 to 5, with 5 being normal. In grade 0, there is no evidence of contractility. In grade 1 (trace), there is slight evidence of contractility and no joint motion. In grade 2 (poor), there is complete range of motion with gravity eliminated. In grade 3 (fair), there is complete range of motion against gravity. In grade 4 (good), there is complete range of motion against gravity with some resistance. In

grade 5 (normal), there is complete range of motion against gravity with full resistance.

The flexor pollicis longus (long flexor of the thumb) flexes the interphalangeal joint of the thumb. This muscle is tested by asking the patient to actively flex the last joint of his thumb (Fig. 4-7).

The flexor digitorum profundus of each finger is then tested, in sequence, by having the patient flex the distal interphalangeal (DIP) joint of the finger being tested while the examiner holds the digit in full extension and blocks motion at the proximal interphalangeal (PIP) joint and the MP joint. During the testing of each profundus tendon, the other fingers are maintained in a slightly flexed position (Fig. 4-8).

The flexor digitorum superficialis of each finger is then tested. The examiner must hold the adjacent fingers in full extension. The PIP joint of the finger being tested is not blocked (Fig. 4-9). If the flexor system is functioning properly, the PIP will flex, and the DIP joint will remain in

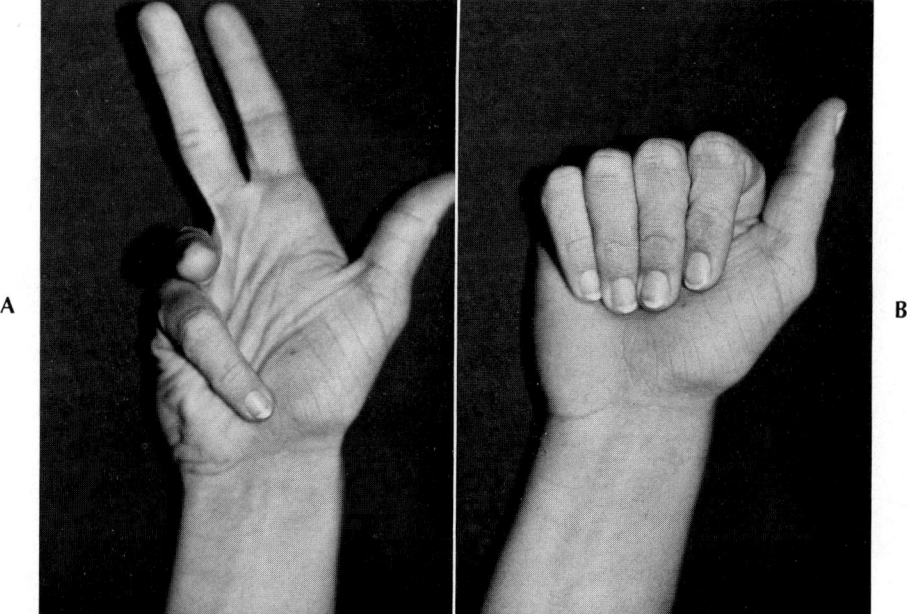

Fig. 4-6   **A,** On flexion the tip of the fifth finger will point directly to the tuberosity of the scaphoid, as will all the fingers when individually flexed. **B,** When all the digits are flexed simultaneously, the longitudinal axes of all fingers converge at an area proximal to the tuberosity of the scaphoid, because of crowding of the adjacent digits. If there is a malunited fracture, the rotational alignment will be off and often there will be crossover of the digits.

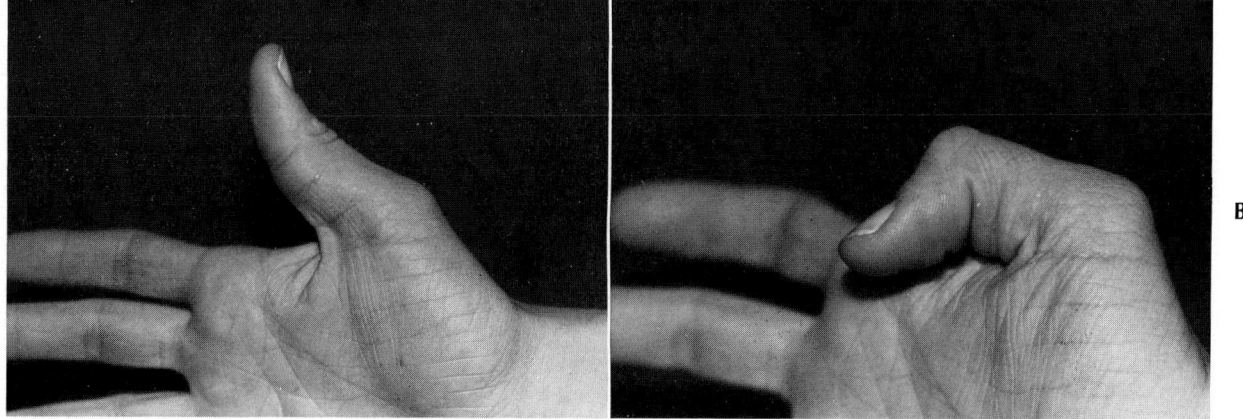

Fig. 4-7   Testing the flexor pollicis longus. With the thumb in a position of full extension at the interphalangeal joint, **A,** the patient is asked to actively flex this joint, **B.** The range of motion and grade of strength are recorded. It is also important to note whether the motion is obtained with or without blocking of the preceding joint by the examiner. This applies not only to testing the flexor pollicis longus, but to testing all other flexor systems, since more power and motion can be obtained when blocking is used.

extension. The fifth finger often has a deficient superficialis.[3] That is, it is not strong enough to flex the interphalangeal joint: on testing, the MP joint will flex and the DIP joint and the PIP joint will remain in extension.

The flexors of the wrist can be tested by having the patient flex the wrist against resistance in a radial and then in an ulnar direction, while the examiner palpates each tendon. The flexor carpi radialis is palpated on the radial side of the wrist, and the flexor carpi ulnaris is palpated on the ulnar side of the wrist. The palmaris longus tendon can be palpated just ulnar to the flexor carpi radialis tendon.

Extrinsic muscle testing—the extensors. As was previously stated, the extensors of the digits and the wrist originate on the dorsal aspect of the forearm and pass through six discrete retinacular compartments at the dorsum of the wrist before their insertions in the hand.

The first dorsal compartment contains the abductor pollicis longus and the extensor pollicis brevis tendons. The abductor pollicis longus usually has multiple tendon slips and inserts on the base of the first metacarpal, and often has insertions on the trapezium. The extensor pollicis brevis and abductor pollicis longus function in unison and are

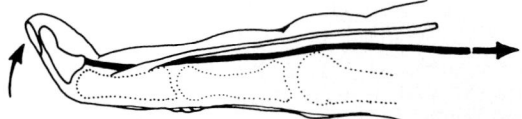

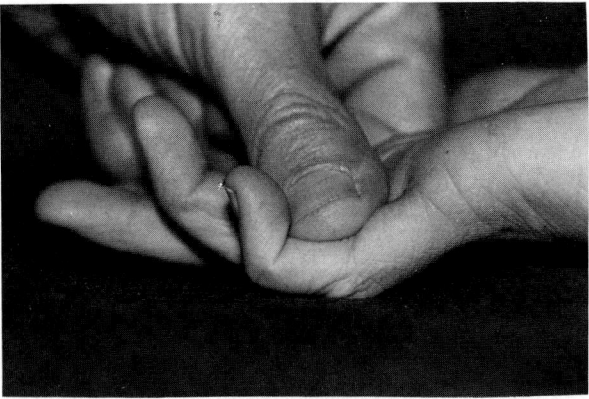

Fig. 4-8 Profundus test. The flexor digitorum profundus tendon flexes the distal interphalangeal joint. With the metacarpophalangeal joint and the proximal interphalangeal joint held in extension by the examiner, the patient is asked to flex the distal interphalangeal joint. (Redrawn from Hoppenfeld S: Physical examination of the spine and extremities, New York, 1976, Appleton-Century-Crofts.)

Fig. 4-9 Superficialis test. The flexor digitorum superficialis tendon flexes the proximal interphalangeal joint. The examiner must hold the adjacent fingers in full extension while asking the patient to flex the finger being tested. If the flexor system is functioning normally, the proximal interphalangeal joint will flex, while the distal interphalangeal joint remains in extension. (Redrawn by permission from Hoppenfeld S: Physical examination of the spine and extremities, New York, 1976, Appleton-Century-Crofts.)

responsible for abduction of the first metacarpal and extension into the plane of the metacarpals. These musculotendinous units are tested by asking the patient to bring the thumb "out to the side and the back." Pain in the area of the first dorsal compartment and radial styloid is common and often a result of stenosing tenovaginitis of these tendons. This was first described by de Quervain in 1895 and now is a well-established clinical entity, which bears his name. Finkelstein, in 1930, stated that acute flexion of the thumb and deviation of the wrist in an ulnar direction would produce excruciating pain at the first dorsal compartment, near the radial styloid, in patients who had stenosing tenovaginitis. This examination is now universally known as Finkelstein's test (Fig. 4-10).[13]

The extensor carpi radialis longus and brevis run in the second dorsal compartment. The longus inserts on the base of the second metacarpal and the brevis on the third. These

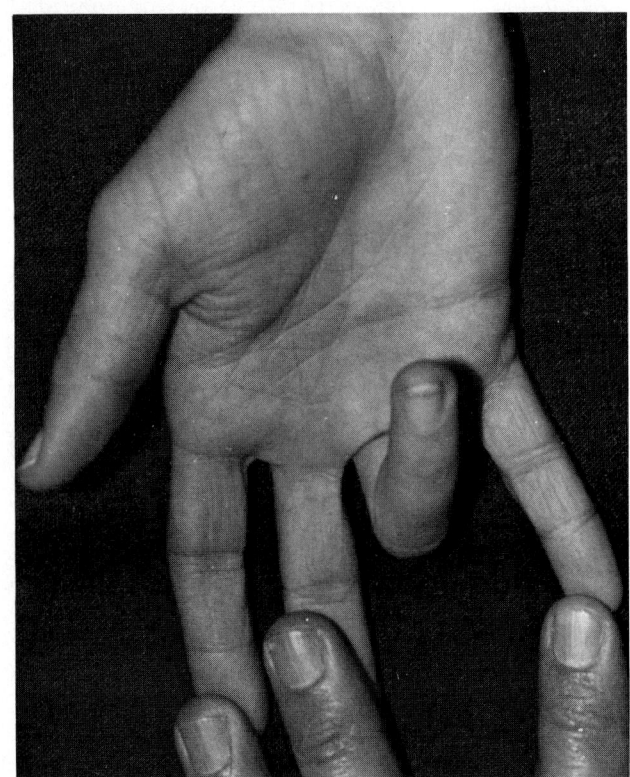

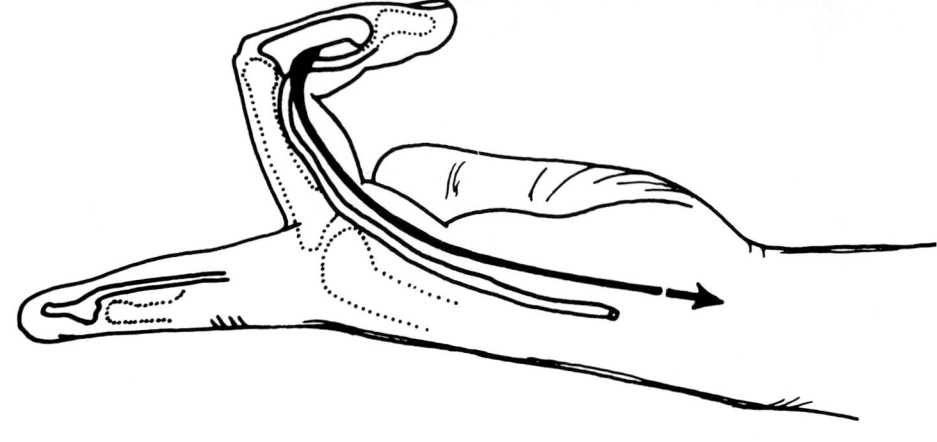

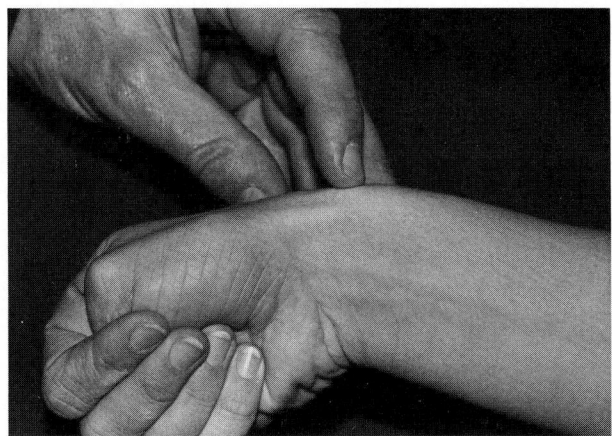

Fig. 4-10 Finkelstein's test for de Quervain's stenosing tenovaginitis of the first dorsal compartment. Acute flexion of the thumb and deviation of the wrist in an ulnar direction will produce excruciating pain at the first dorsal compartment, near the radial styloid, in patients who have this pathologic entity.

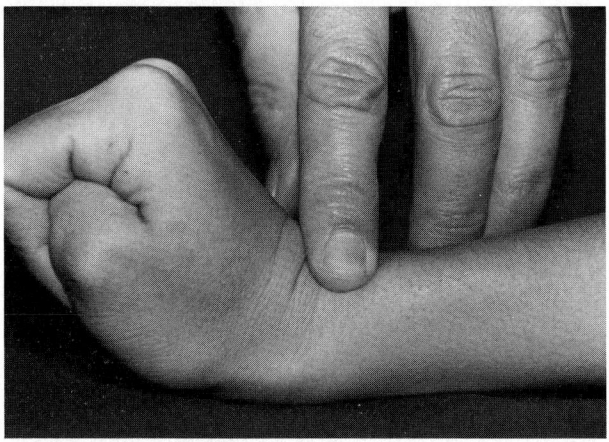

Fig. 4-11 On dorsiflexion of the wrist, the examiner can palpate the extensor carpi radialis longus, inserting on the base of the second metacarpal, and the extensor carpi radialis brevis, inserting on the base of the third metacarpal.

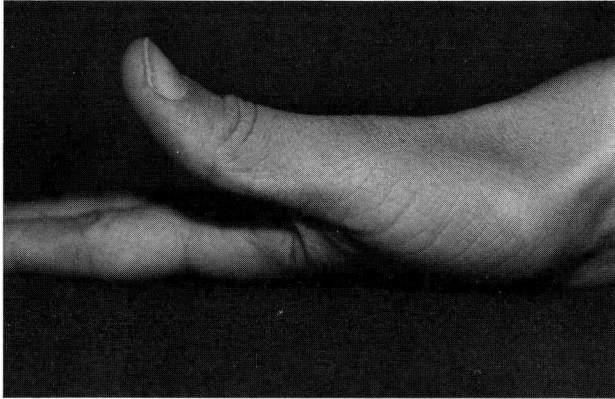

Fig. 4-12 The extensor pollicis longus tendon is tested by placing the patient's hand flat on the examining table and asking him to lift the thumb off the table. The extensor pollicis longus can then be visualized and palpated.

are tested by asking the patient to make a tight fist and to strongly dorsiflex the wrist. The two tendons are then palpated by the examiner (Fig. 4-11).

The extensor pollicis longus runs in the third dorsal compartment. This tendon extends the interphalangeal joint of the thumb as well as adducts the first ray. The tendon passes sharply around Lister's tubercle and may rupture spontaneously after a Colles fracture or in rheumatoid arthritis.[37] Its function is tested by placing the patient's hand flat on the examining table and having him lift only the thumb off the table. The extensor pollicis longus can be visualized and palpated (Fig. 4-12).

The area of the wrist just distal to the radial styloid and bounded by the extensor pollicis longus ulnarly and the abductor pollicis longus and extensor pollicis brevis radially is known as the anatomic snuffbox. In this area runs the deep branch of the radial artery. The carpal scaphoid can be palpated in the base of the snuffbox. Tenderness in this area is suggestive of an acute scaphoid fracture or a painful scaphoid nonunion.

The fourth dorsal compartment contains the extensor indicis proprius and the extensor digitorum communis. These tendons are responsible for extension of the MP joints of the fingers. The extensor indicis proprius allows independent extension of the index MP joint. The extensor indicis proprius is tested by having the patient extend the index finger while the other fingers are flexed into a fist. The mass action of the extensor digitorum communis tendons is tested by having the patient extend the MP joints (Fig. 4-13). This test is performed with the interphalangeal joints flexed, because the PIP joints are extended by the intrinsic muscles and not the long extensors of the hand. This may be a source of confusion to an uninitiated examiner, especially in a patient who has a high radial nerve palsy yet is still able to extend his interphalangeal joints.

The fifth dorsal compartment contains the extensor digiti quinti, which is responsible for independent extension of the MP joint of the little finger. It is tested by having the patient extend the fifth finger while the others are flexed. Because the extensor digiti quinti and the extensor indicis proprius work independently of the communis tendons, most examiners test them simultaneously by having the patient extend the index and fifth fingers while the middle and ring fingers are flexed (Fig. 4-14).

The sixth dorsal compartment contains the extensor carpi ulnaris, which inserts into the base of the fifth metacarpal and helps dorsiflex the wrist in an ulnar direction. This is tested by having the patient pull the hand dorsally and in an ulnar direction while the examiner palpates the tendon (Fig. 4-15).

Intrinsic muscle testing. The intrinsic musculature of the hand consists of the thenar and hypothenar muscles, as well as the lumbricals and the interossei. All of these muscles originate and insert within the hand. There is a delicate balance between the intrinsic and extrinsic muscles, which is necessary for normal functioning of the hand.

The thenar muscles consist of the abductor pollicis brevis, the flexor pollicis brevis, the opponens pollicis, and the adductor pollicis. These muscles position the thumb and help perform the complex motions of opposition and adduction of the thumb.[27] Opposition, according to Bunnell, takes place in the intercarpal, carpometacarpal, and MP

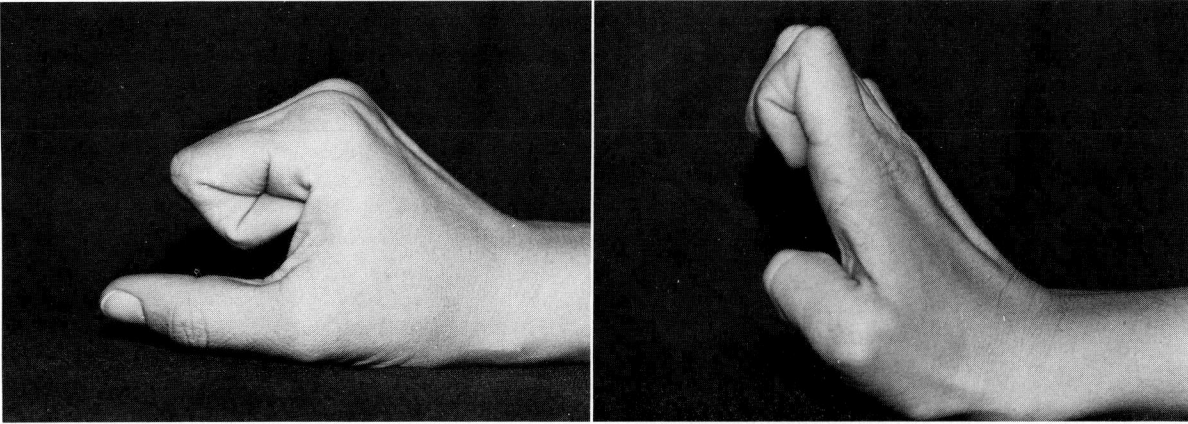

Fig. 4-13   The extensor digitorum communis tendons are tested by having the patient extend the metacarpophalangeal joints, with the proximal interphalangeal joints flexed.

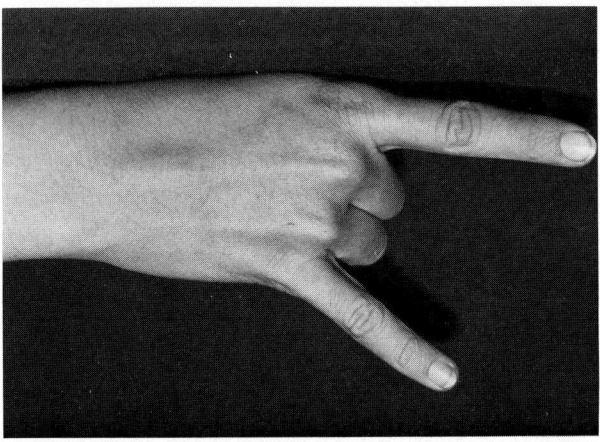

Fig. 4-14   The extensor digiti quinti and the extensor indicis proprius work independently of the communis tendons; they are tested by asking the patient to extend the index and fifth fingers while the middle and ring fingers are flexed.

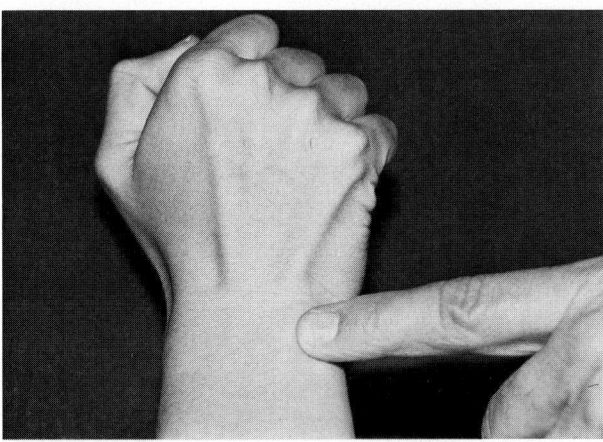

Fig. 4-15   The extensor carpi ulnaris can be visualized and palpated as it inserts on the base of the fifth metacarpal, while the patient dorsiflexes the wrist in an ulnar direction.

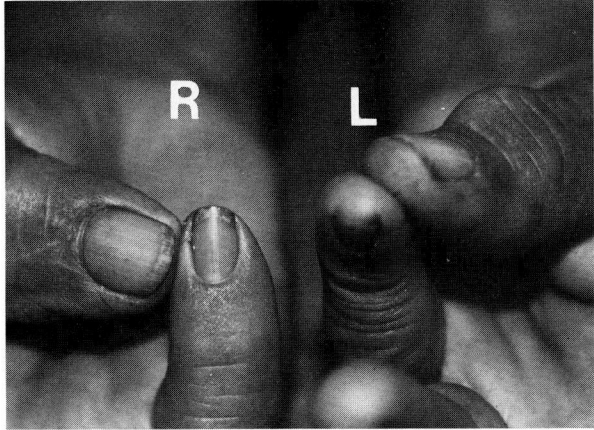

Fig. 4-16   Hands of a patient with a low median nerve palsy on the right side, resulting from a long-standing carpal tunnel syndrome. Notice that in attempted opposition, the nail plate is perpendicular to the plane of the metacarpals on the affected side *(R)*, while the nail plate is parallel to the plane of the metacarpals on the normal side *(L)*. Tip-to-tip pinch is impossible on the side with the loss of opposition.

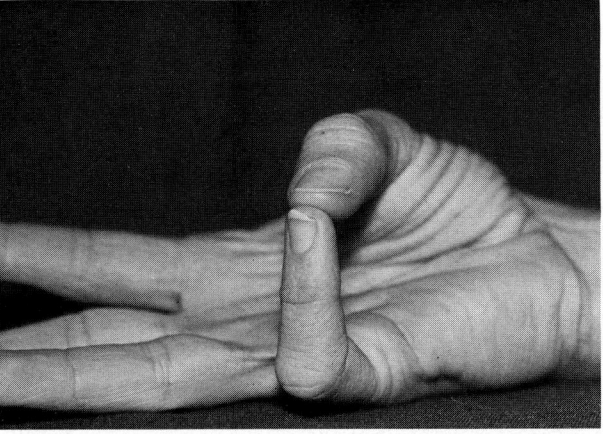

Fig. 4-17   Opposition of tip of thumb to tip of fifth digit. Notice tip-to-tip pinch and the relationship of the nail plate of the thumb to the plane of the metacarpals.

joints.[7] All three of these joints contribute to the angulatory and rotatory motions that produce true opposition. If one observes the thumb during opposition, it first abducts from the hand, and then it follows a semicircular path. The thumb pronates, and the proximal phalanx angulates radially on the first metacarpal. If the nail plate is observed, one can see that before beginning opposition, the thumbnail is perpendicular to the plane of the metacarpals. At the end of opposition, the thumbnail is parallel to the plane of the metacarpals. During adduction, the thumb sweeps across the palm without following the semicircular path. The nail plate remains at all times perpendicular to the plane of the metacarpals. Because opposition is median nerve innervated and adduction is usually ulnar nerve innervated, one can easily see the difference between these two motions by comparing the hands of a patient with a long-standing low median nerve palsy on one side (Fig. 4-16).

Opposition is tested by having the patient touch the tip of the thumb to the tip of the little finger (Fig. 4-17). At the end of opposition, the thumbnail should be perpendicular to the nail of the little finger and parallel to the plane of the metacarpals.

The abductor pollicis brevis, which is the most radial and superficial of the thenar muscles, is usually the first to atrophy with a low median nerve palsy, such as that resulting from a long-standing carpal tunnel syndrome. This muscle can be tested by having the patient abduct the thumb while the examiner palpates the muscle.

Thumb adduction is performed by the adductor pollicis, which is an ulnar nerve–innervated muscle. This muscle, in combination with the first dorsal interosseus, is necessary for strong pinch. The adductor stabilizes the thumb during pinch and also helps extend the interphalangeal joint of the thumb through its attachment into the dorsal apparatus. Thumb adduction can be tested by having the patient forcibly hold a piece of paper between his thumb and the radial side of the proximal phalanx of the index finger. When adduction is weak or nonfunctional, the interphalangeal joint of the thumb flexes during this maneuver; this is known as Froment's sign (1915).[25] Froment's sign is an indication of weak or absent adductor function. Jeanne's sign (1915) is hyper-

extension of the MP joint of the thumb during pinch.[25] (Fig. 4-18.)

The hypothenar muscles consist of the abductor digiti minimi, the flexor digiti minimi, and the opponens digiti minimi. The abductor and flexor aid in abduction of the fifth digit and in MP joint flexion of that digit. The deeper opponens digiti minimi aids in adduction and in rotating the fifth metacarpal during opposition of the thumb to the fifth finger. This helps cup the hand during grip and opposition. The hypothenar muscles are tested as one unit by having the patient abduct the little finger while the examiner palpates the muscle mass (Fig. 4-19).

The anatomy of the interossei is very complex, with much variation in their origins and insertions. There are seven interossei, four dorsal and three palmar. These muscles arise from the metacarpal shafts but have variable insertions. The palmar interossei almost always insert into the dorsal apparatus of the finger. The first dorsal interosseus almost always inserts into bone. The remaining dorsal interossei have varying insertions. (Refer to the work of Eyler and Markee for a more detailed description of the anatomy.[12]) The interossei are usually ulnar nerve–innervated, with a few exceptions.

There are four lumbricals, which originate on the radial side of the profundus tendons and usually insert on the dorsal apparatus. Occasionally a few fibers insert into the base of the proximal phalanges. Because these muscles are a link between the extrinsic flexor and extrinsic extensor mechanisms, they act as a modulator between flexion and extension of the interphalangeal joints.[28]

The interossei are much stronger than the lumbricals; however, both muscle groups work in conjunction. All of these muscle groups are of fundamental importance in extension of the interphalangeal joints and flexion of the MP joints. The interossei also abduct and adduct the fingers. It

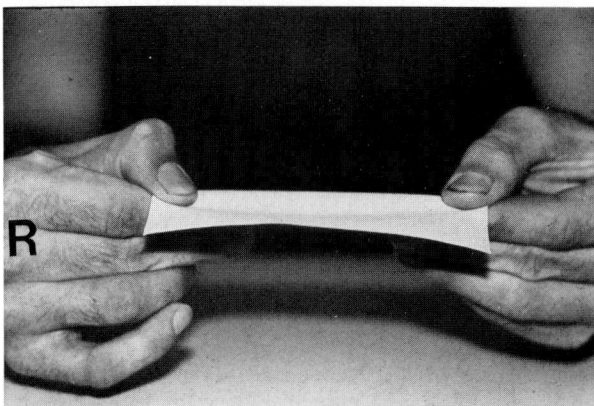
Fig. 4-18 Patient with low ulnar nerve palsy on the right. Weakness of pinch is demonstrated by Froment's and Jeanne's signs on the affected side *(R)*.

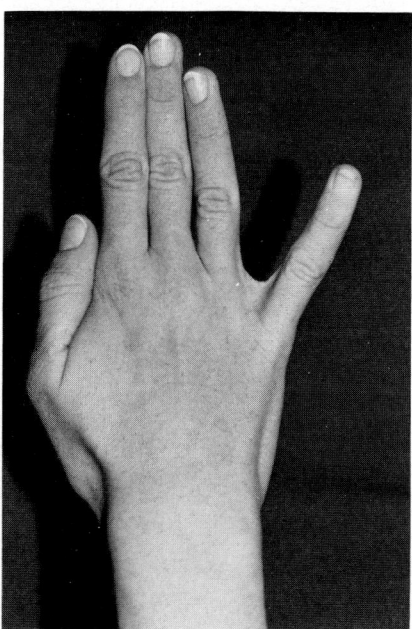
Fig. 4-19 Testing function of the hypothenar muscles by having patient abduct fifth digit.

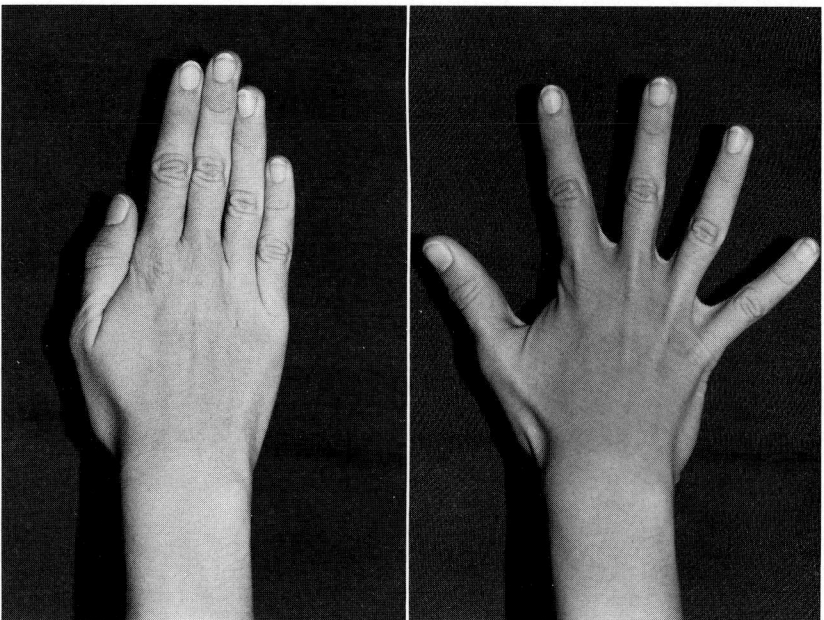

Fig. 4-20 Testing function of the interossei. With the hand flat on a table, the patient is asked to spread his fingers apart. Abduction and adduction are assessed from the relationship of the digits to the axis of the third metacarpal.

is believed that the dorsal interossei are the primary abductors and the volar interossei the primary adductors of the fingers.

The preceding statements are an oversimplification of the anatomy and functional significance of the interossei and the lumbricals. The clinical examination of these two groups of muscles is, however, rather easy.

To test interossei function, one should ask the patient to spread his fingers apart. This is best done with the hand flat on the examining table to eliminate the action of the long extensors, which can simulate the function of the dorsal interossei (Fig. 4-20). To supplement this test, one can have the patient radially and ulnarly deviate the middle finger while it is flexed. This cannot be performed if the interossei are paralyzed; this test is known as Egawa's sign (1959).[25]

The first dorsal interosseus is a very strong radial abductor of the index finger and plays an important role in stabilizing that digit during pinch. It can be tested separately by having

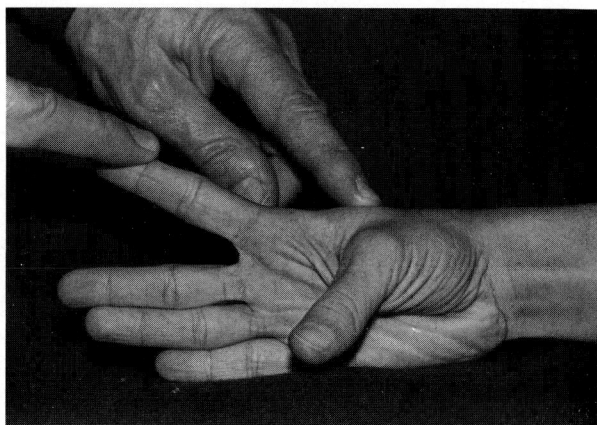

Fig. 4-21 On abduction of the patient's index finger, the examiner can palpate the first dorsal interosseus. This is the last muscle to receive innervation from the ulnar nerve.

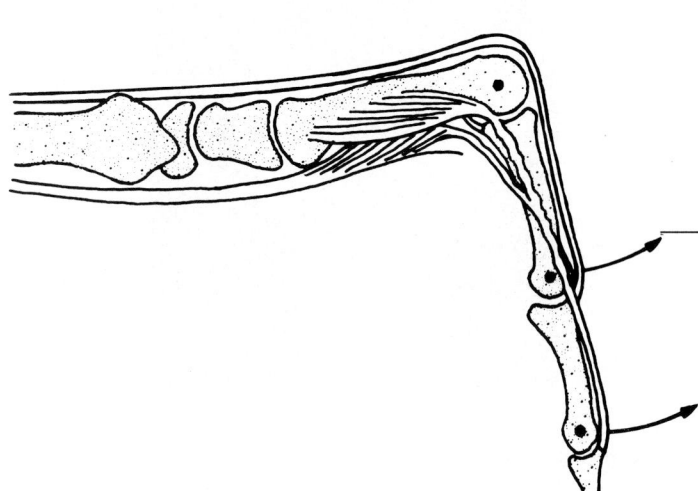

Fig. 4-22 The intrinsic muscles, by means of their attachment into the lateral bands and proximal phalanges, produce flexion of the metacarpophalangeal joints and extension of the proximal interphalangeal joints. The function of the lumbricals and interossei is tested by having the patient extend the proximal interphalangeal joints of the digits while the metacarpophalangeal joints are held in flexion by the examiner. (Redrawn from Tubiana R: The hand, Philadelphia, 1973, WB Saunders Co.)

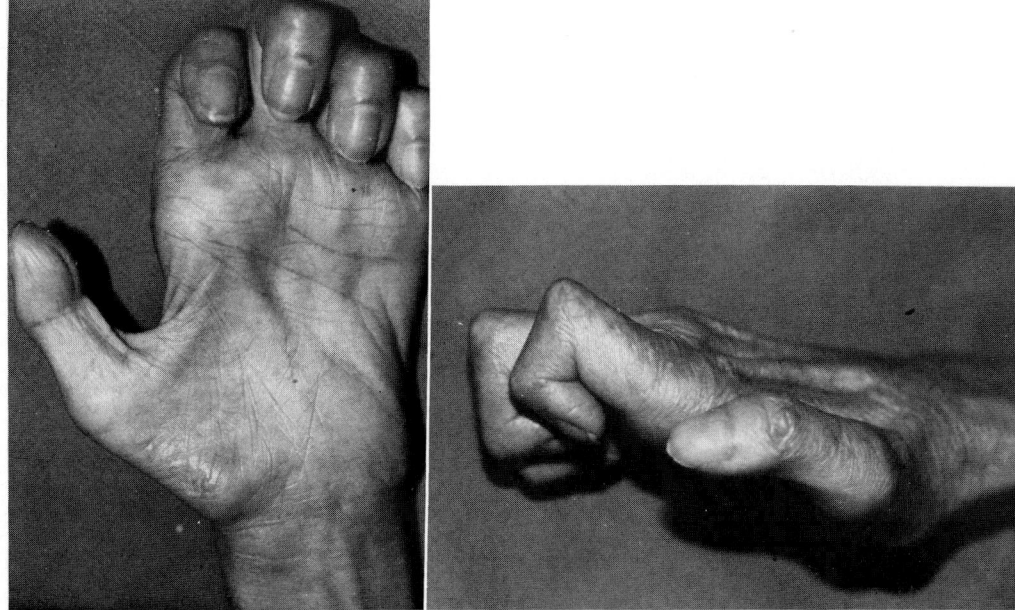

Fig. 4-23   Intrinsic-minus hand resulting from a long-standing low median and ulnar palsy. Notice loss of normal arches of the hand and wasting of all intrinsic musculature.

the patient strongly abduct the index finger in a radial direction while the examiner palpates the muscle belly (Fig. 4-21). The interphalangeal extension function of the lumbricals and interossei is tested by having the patient extend the PIP joints of the digits while the MP joints are held in flexion by the examiner (Fig. 4-22).

If all the interossei and lumbricals are functioning properly, the patient will be able to put his hand into the "intrinsic-plus position;" that is, the MP joints are flexed and the PIP joints are in full extension. J.I.P. James has recommended this as the position of immobilization for the injured hand.[17]

Injuries to the median or ulnar nerves, or both, or a crushing injury to the hand can result in paralysis or contractures of the intrinsic muscles. A hand without intrinsic function is known as the "intrinsic-minus hand."[8,14] This hand will have lost the normal cupping of the hand. The arches of the hand will disappear, and there will be wasting of all intrinsic musculature (Fig. 4-23). There will be clawing of the fingers, as described by Duchenne in 1867.[25] The claw deformity is defined as hyperextension of the MP joints and flexion of the PIP and DIP joints (Fig. 4-24). This is the result of an imbalance between the intrinsic and extrinsic muscles of the hand.[47] The extrinsic extensors hyperextend the MP joints, and the extrinsic flexors flex the PIP and DIP joints. The flexion vector, induced by the intrinsics, across the MP joint is lost.[29] In time, the volar capsular-ligamentous structures will stretch out, and the claw deformity will increase in severity.[32]

Injury to the intrinsics, which can be caused by ischemia, crushing injuries, or other pathologic states (such as rheumatoid arthritis), can result in tightness of the intrinsic muscles. A test for intrinsic tightness was first described by Finochetto in 1920.[53] Later, Bunnell and then Littler redescribed this test.[9] The intrinsic tightness test is performed

by having the examiner hold the patient's MP joint in extension (stretching the intrinsics) and then passively flexing the PIP joint. Then the MP joint is held in flexion (relaxing the intrinsics), and the examiner passively flexes the PIP joint again. If the PIP joint can be passively flexed more when the MP joint is in flexion than when it is in extension, there is tightness of the intrinsic muscles.[9,44,53] (Fig. 4-25.) In patients with rheumatoid arthritis, intrinsic tightness is common and may result in a swan-neck deformity.[34] The swan neck is a result of the strong pull of the contracted intrinsics on the lateral bands, which subsequently sublux

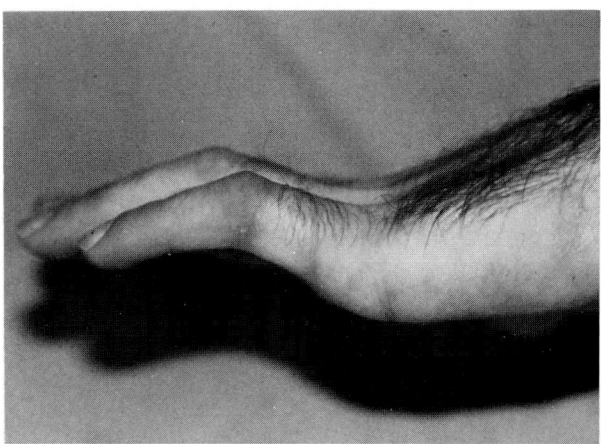

Fig. 4-24   Ulnar claw hand resulting from ulnar nerve laceration at the wrist. Notice hyperextension of the metacarpophalangeal joints and flexion of the proximal and distal interphalangeal joints because of an imbalance of the extrinsic flexor and extensor systems as a result of paralysis of the ulnar innervated intrinsic muscles.

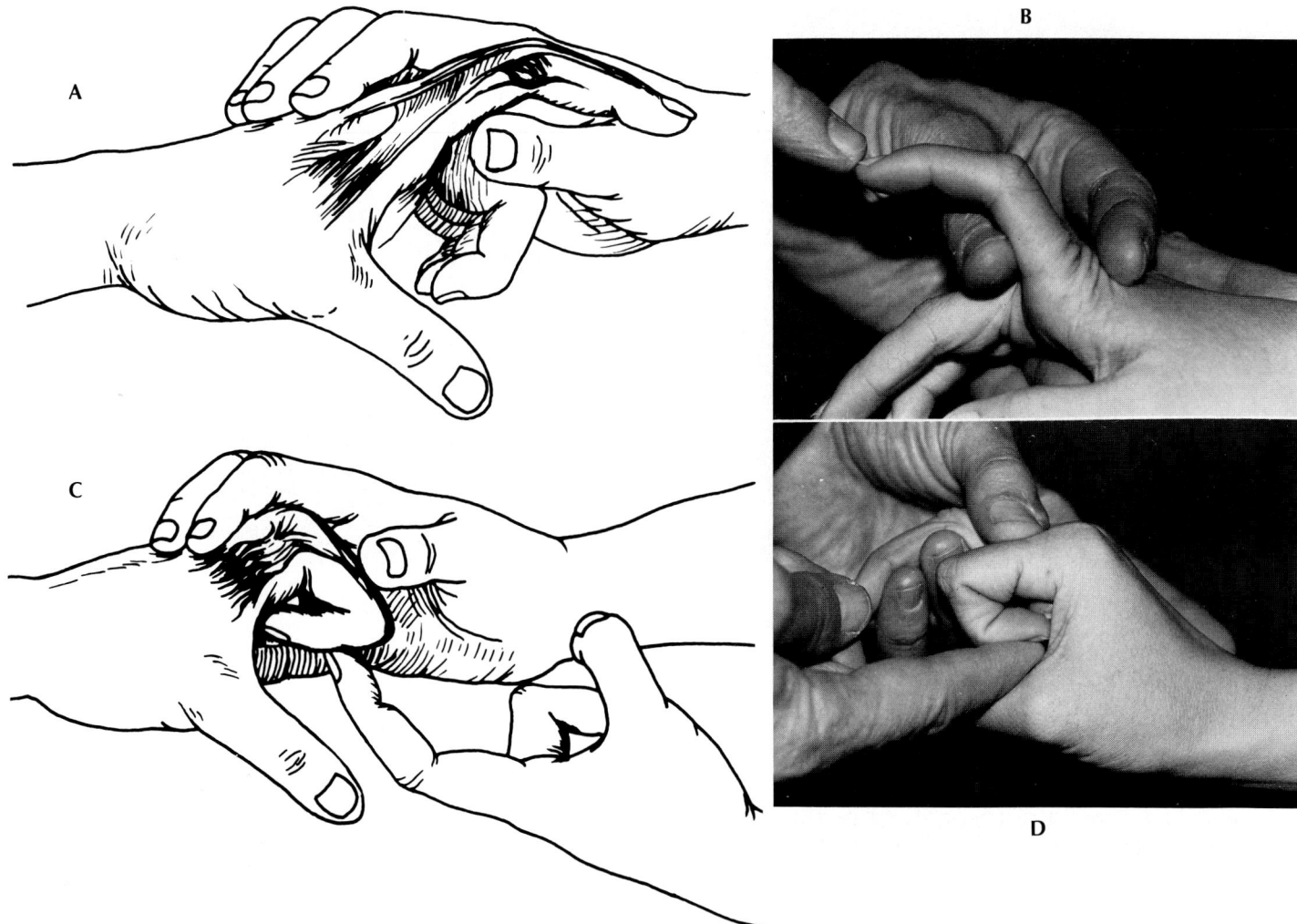

Fig. 4-25   Intrinsic tightness test. In **A** and **B,** the intrinsics are put on stretch by the examiner, who then passively flexes the proximal interphalangeal joint. The intrinsics are then relaxed by flexing the metacarpophalangeal joint, **C** and **D**. If the proximal interphalangeal joint can be passively flexed more with the metacarpophalangeal joint in flexion than when it is in extension, there is tightness of the intrinsic muscles. (Redrawn from Hoppenfeld S: Physical examination of the spine and extremities, New York, 1976, Appleton-Century-Crofts.)

dorsal to the axis of rotation of the PIP joint. The resultant deformity is one of hyperextension at the PIP joint and flexion at the DIP joint (Fig. 4-26). The boutonnière deformity may also occur in patients with rheumatoid arthritis.[33,52]

Occasionally there is confusion as to the cause of limited PIP joint motion. Is the condition a result of intrinsic tightness, of extrinsic tightness (for example, scarring of the long extensors proximal to the PIP joint), or of the joint itself (that is, collateral ligament tightness)? Three simple tests will clarify the situation. The intrinsic tightness tests will help one either rule out or identify intrinsic muscle problems. The extrinsic tightness test is just the opposite of the intrinsic test. Again the examiner holds the MP joint in extension and passively flexes the PIP joint and notes the amount of flexion. He or she then flexes the MP joint and passively flexes the PIP joint again. If there is extrinsic

tightness (because the long extensors are scarred), there will be more passive flexion of the PIP joint when the MP joint is held in extension than when it is held in flexion. Holding the MP joint in extension functionally lengthens the extrinsic extensor, whereas holding it in flexion relatively shortens it. If the motion of the PIP joint is unchanged regardless of the position of the MP joint, there is a joint contracture (Fig. 4-27).

OBLIQUE RETINACULAR LIGAMENT TEST

Occasionally a patient will exhibit a lack of flexion at the DIP joint. This loss of flexion may be caused by a joint contracture or a contracture of the oblique retinacular ligament.[21] The oblique retinacular ligament arises from the volar lateral ridge of the proximal phalanx and has a common origin with the distal A_2 and C_1 pulleys. It then traverses distally and dorsally to attach to the dorsal apparatus near

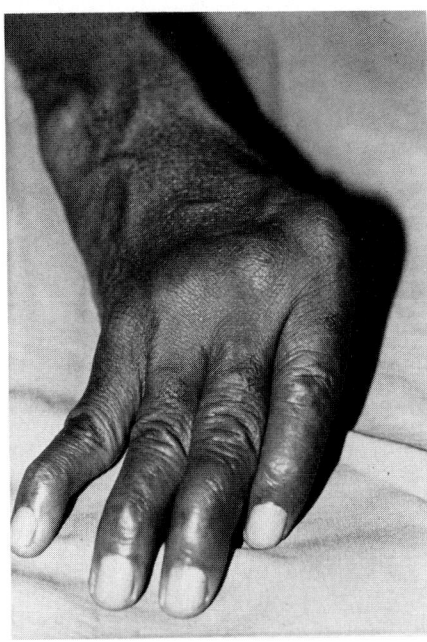

Fig. 4-26 Swan-neck deformity in a patient with rheumatoid arthritis. The swan-neck deformity is caused by intrinsic tightness, which causes the lateral bands to sublux dorsal to the axis of rotation of the proximal interphalangeal joint.

the DIP joint (Fig. 4-28). As pointed out by Shrewsbury and Johnson, the tendon varies in its development and occurrence.[43] It is, however, consistently made taut by flexion of the DIP joint. If this ligament is contracted, passive DIP motion will be limited. The oblique retinacular ligament tightness test is performed by passively flexing the DIP joint with the PIP joint in extension and then repeating this with the PIP joint in flexion. If there is greater motion when the PIP joint is flexed than when it is extended, there is a contracture of the ligament (Fig. 4-29). Equal loss of flexion indicates a joint contracture.

GRIP AND PINCH STRENGTH

The next step after evaluation of intrinsic and extrinsic musculature of the hand is determination of gross grip and pinch strength of the injured hand versus the noninjured hand. There are several commercially available devices for objective measurement of grip strength. The grip dynamometer (Fig. 4-30) with adjustable handle spacings provides an accurate evaluation of the force of grip.[4] This dynamometer has five adjustable spacings—at 1, 1½, 2, 2½, and 3 inches. The patient is shown how to grasp the dynamometer and is requested to grasp it with his maximum force. The grip is measured at each of the five handle spacings. The right and left hands are tested alternately, and the force of each is recorded. The test is paced at a rate to

Fig. 4-27 Proximal interphalangeal joint contracture. Collateral ligament tightness will limit proximal phalangeal joint motion, regardless of the position of the metacarpophalangeal joint.

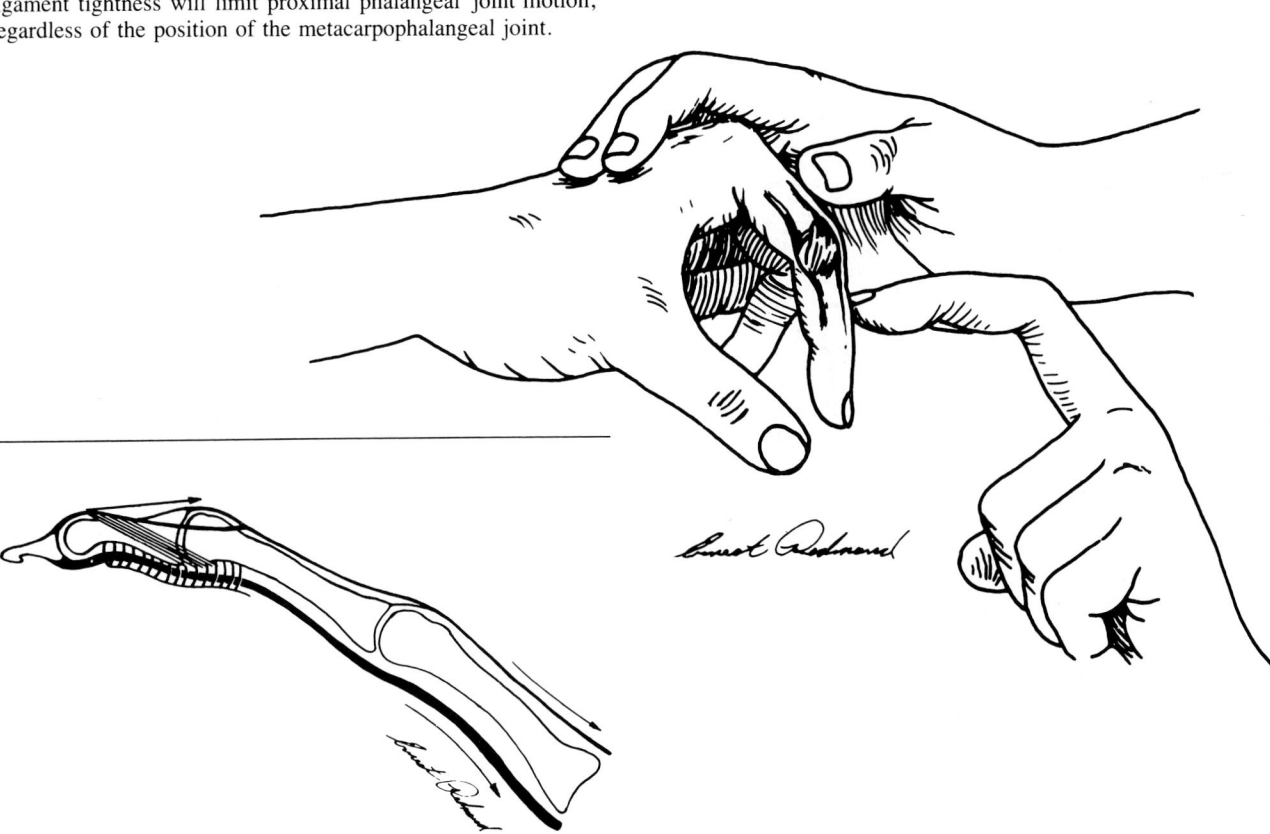

Fig. 4-28 Oblique retinacular ligament. (Redrawn from Tubiana R: The hand, Philadelphia, 1981, WB Saunders Co.)

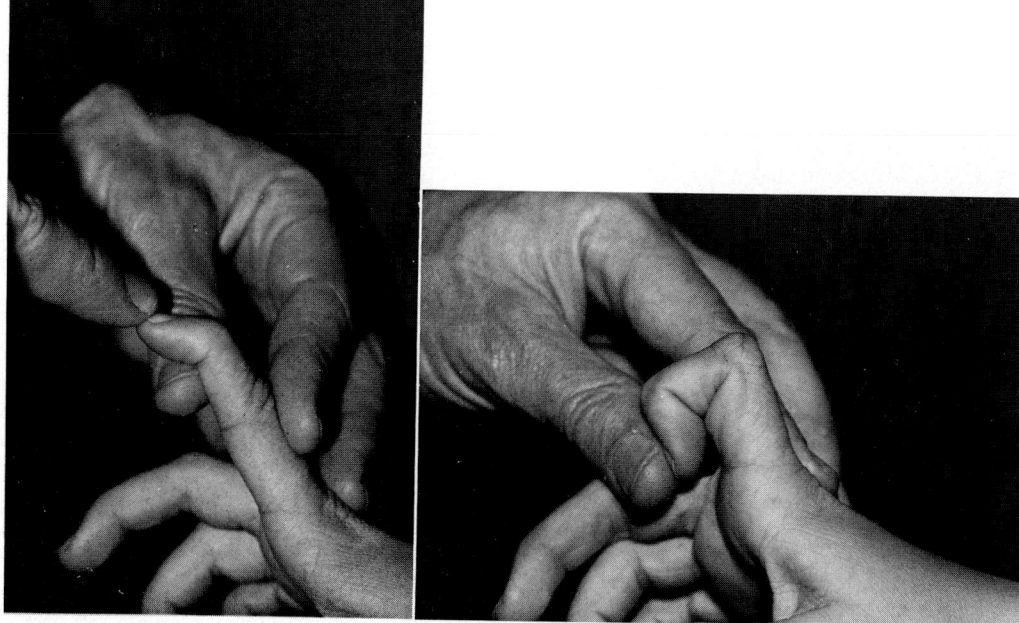

Fig. 4-29   The oblique retinacular ligament tightness test. The distal interphalangeal joint is passively flexed with the proximal interphalangeal joint held in extension. The distal interphalangeal joint is then passively flexed with the proximal interphalangeal joint flexed. If there is greater motion when the proximal interphalangeal joint is flexed than when it is extended, there is a contracture of the ligament. Equal loss of distal interphalangeal joint motion regardless of proximal interphalangeal joint position indicates a joint contracture.

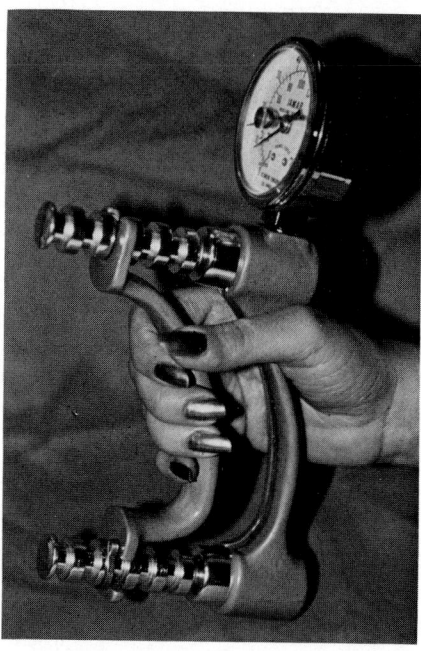

Fig. 4-30   Jamar grip dynamometer with five adjustable spacings. (Asimow Engineering Co, Los Angeles, Calif.)

eliminate fatigue. According to Bechtol, there is usually a 5% to 10% difference between the dominant hand and the nondominant hand.[4] Patients who use a less than maximal effort can be identified in two ways. First, if the test is repeated, a patient who applies less than maximal effort is usually not able to duplicate his previous performance. The discrepancy will be greater than 20% and sometimes as great as 100%.[4] Second, there is a normal bell curve of grip strength; the strength is greatest at the middle spacings and weakest at each end (for example, level I, 20 pounds; level II, 25 pounds; level III, 35 pounds; level IV, 25 pounds; and level V, 20 pounds). A patient who applies less than maximal effort will usually have a flat curve, with all values being approximately the same. If a patient has pain in the hand or forearm, of course the strength will be decreased. However, the bell curve pattern is usually still present. (Fig. 4-31.)

There are three basic types of pinch: chuck, or three-fingered pinch; lateral, or key pinch; and tip pinch (Fig. 4-32). These can be tested with a pinch meter (Fig. 4-33). Many disease processes can affect pinch power: basilar arthritis of the thumb, ulnar nerve palsy, and anterior interosseus nerve palsy, to mention a few.

NERVE SUPPLY OF THE HAND—MOTOR AND SENSORY MOTOR

Three nerves provide motor and sensory function to the hand: the median, radial, and ulnar nerves (Fig. 4-34). The motor and sensory innervation of the hand is also subject to much variation, as pointed out by Rowntree.[40] However, we will discuss the usual textbook innervation and ignore the variations.

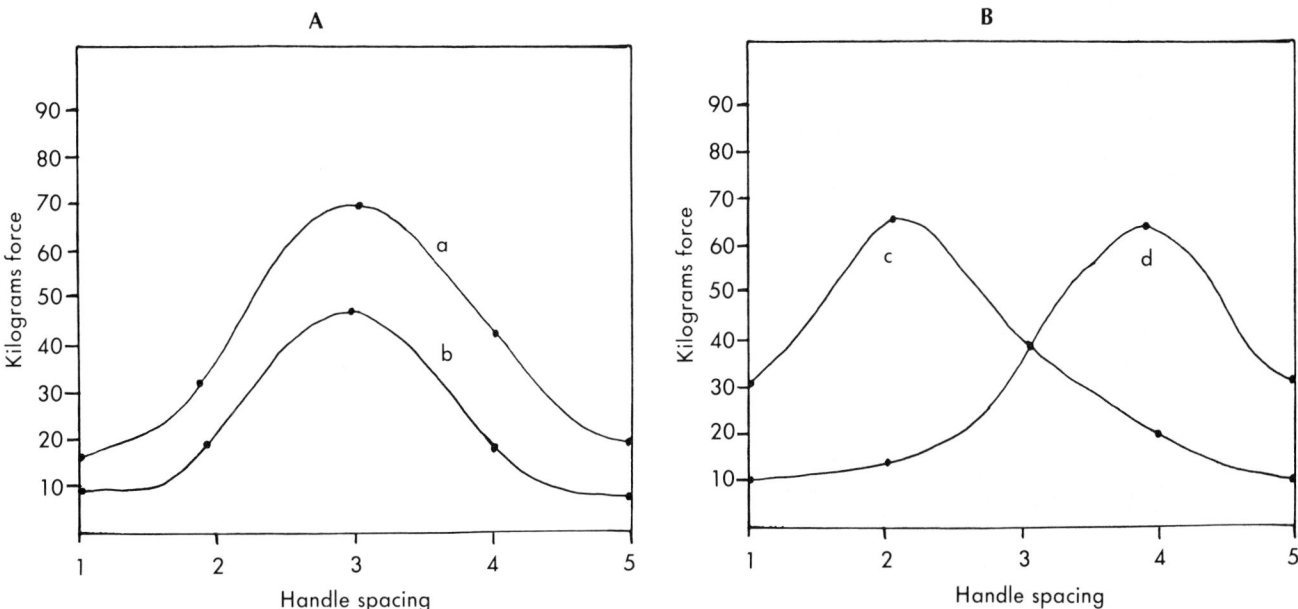

Fig. 4-31   A, The grip strengths of a patient's uninjured hand *(a)* and injured hand *(b)* are plotted. Despite the patient's decrease in grip strength because of injury, curve *b* maintains a bell-shaped pattern and parallels that of the normal hand. These curves are reproducible in repeated examinations, with minimal change in values. A great fluctuation in the size of the curve or absence of a bell-shaped pattern casts doubt on the patient's compliance with the examination and may indicate malingering. **B,** If the patient has an exceptionally large hand, the curve will shift to the right *(d);* with a very small hand, the curve will shift to the left *(c).* Notice, however, that the bell-shaped pattern is maintained despite the curve's shift in direction.

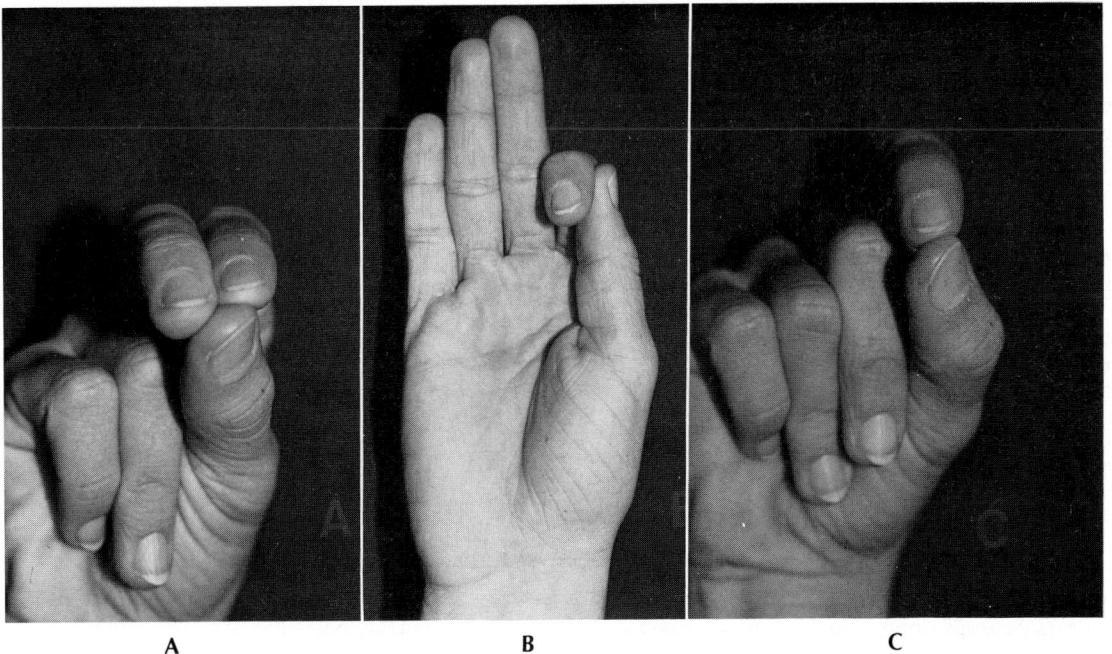

Fig. 4-32   A, Chuck, or three-fingered, pinch. **B,** lateral, or key, pinch. **C,** Tip pinch.

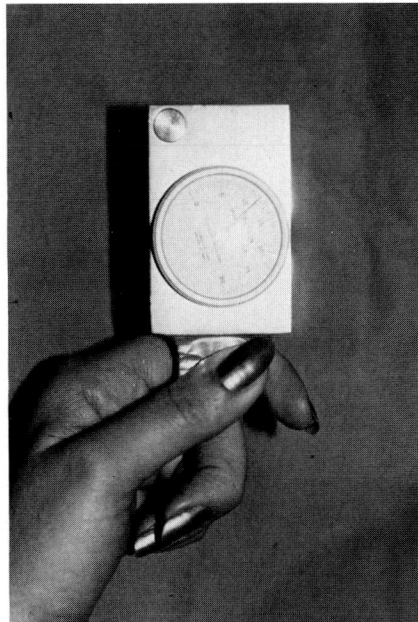

Fig. 4-33 Preston pinch gauge. (JA Preston Corp, New York, NY.)

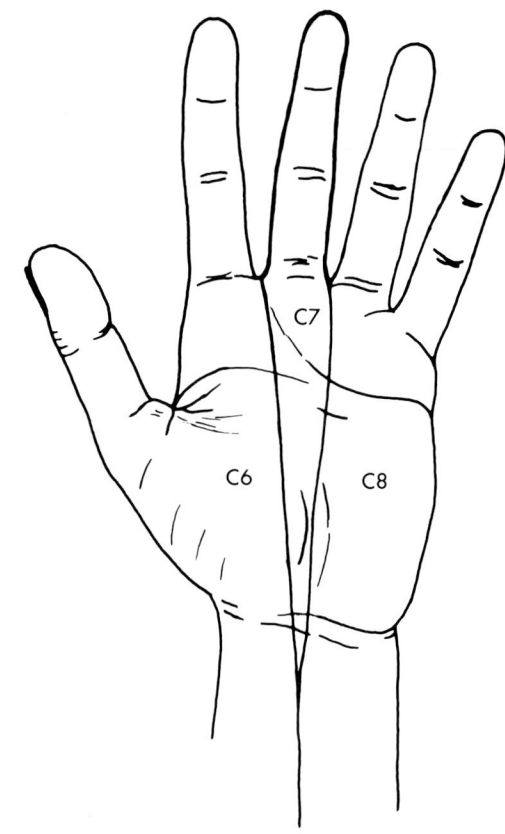

Fig. 4-34 Sensory dermatomes of the hand, by neurologic levels. (Redrawn from Hoppenfeld S: Physical examination of the spine and extremities, New York, 1976, Appleton-Century-Crofts.)

The median, radial, and ulnar nerves are peripheral branches of the brachial plexus. The radial nerve is formed from the C_6 and C_7 nerve roots. The median nerve is formed by branches of the C_7, C_8, and T_1 nerve roots. The ulnar nerve is formed from branches of the C_8 and T_1 nerve roots. The terminal branches of the median, radial, and ulnar nerves are shown in Fig. 4-35. It is necessary to have a fundamental knowledge of the branches and their sequence of innervation to appropriately place the level of an injury or to follow the path of a regenerating nerve.

These three nerves enter the forearm through various muscle and fascial planes and have multiple potential sources of entrapment. Entrapment of these nerves results in classic clinical presentations, with loss of motor function and paresthesias in the distribution of each nerve.

The median nerve may be entrapped as it enters the forearm at the level of the pronator teres muscle, the lacertus fibrosus, or the superficialis arch.[15,18,46] As it enters the hand, it may be entrapped at the level of the carpal tunnel.[38] This common neuropathy has been termed "carpal tunnel syndrome." Patients with carpal tunnel syndrome often complain of numbness in the thumb and the radial two and one-half fingers, as well as night pain, weakness of grip, and dropping of objects. With a long-standing compression, there will be marked thenar atrophy and loss of thumb opposition.[36,38,49]

Compression of the median nerve at the wrist was first described by Paget in 1854.[36] A number of authors since then have reported this entity and have recommended division of the transverse carpal ligament. Phalen has most clearly defined this entity as a syndrome; in 1966 he reported his experience with 654 cases of carpal tunnel syndrome.[36] Phalen found that in a high percentage of cases, the wrist flexion test, now commonly known as Phalen's test, had a positive result and that Tinel's sign was present.

When performing Phalen's test, the patient holds his forearms vertically and allows both hands to drop into complete flexion at the wrist for approximately 1 minute. In this position, the median nerve is compressed between the transverse carpal ligament and the adjacent flexor tendons. This maneuver causes almost immediate aggravation of numbness and paresthesias in the fingers.

Percussion of the median nerve at the wrist will produce paresthesias in the distribution of the nerve; this is known as Tinel's sign (Fig. 4-36). Tinel's sign will be present not only in compressive neuropathies of nerves but also in partial and complete lacerations of nerves and in areas where neuromas have formed.[19,31,50]

The presence of thenar atrophy, paresthesias in the median nerve distribution, a positive Phalen's test, and Tinel's sign, in association with a history of night pain, is pathognomonic for a compressive neuropathy of the median nerve in the carpal tunnel.

The ulnar and radial nerves are also subject to compression as they enter the arm and hand. The ulnar nerve can be compressed near the medial intermuscular septum, the cubital tunnel, or at the wrist (in Guyon's canal).[16,20,42,51] The radial nerve is subject to compression at the radial tunnel and as it passes between the two heads of the supinator muscle in an area known as the arcade of Frohse, or it can be compressed superficially at the wrist.* As with

---

*References 6, 23, 24, 39, 41, 45.

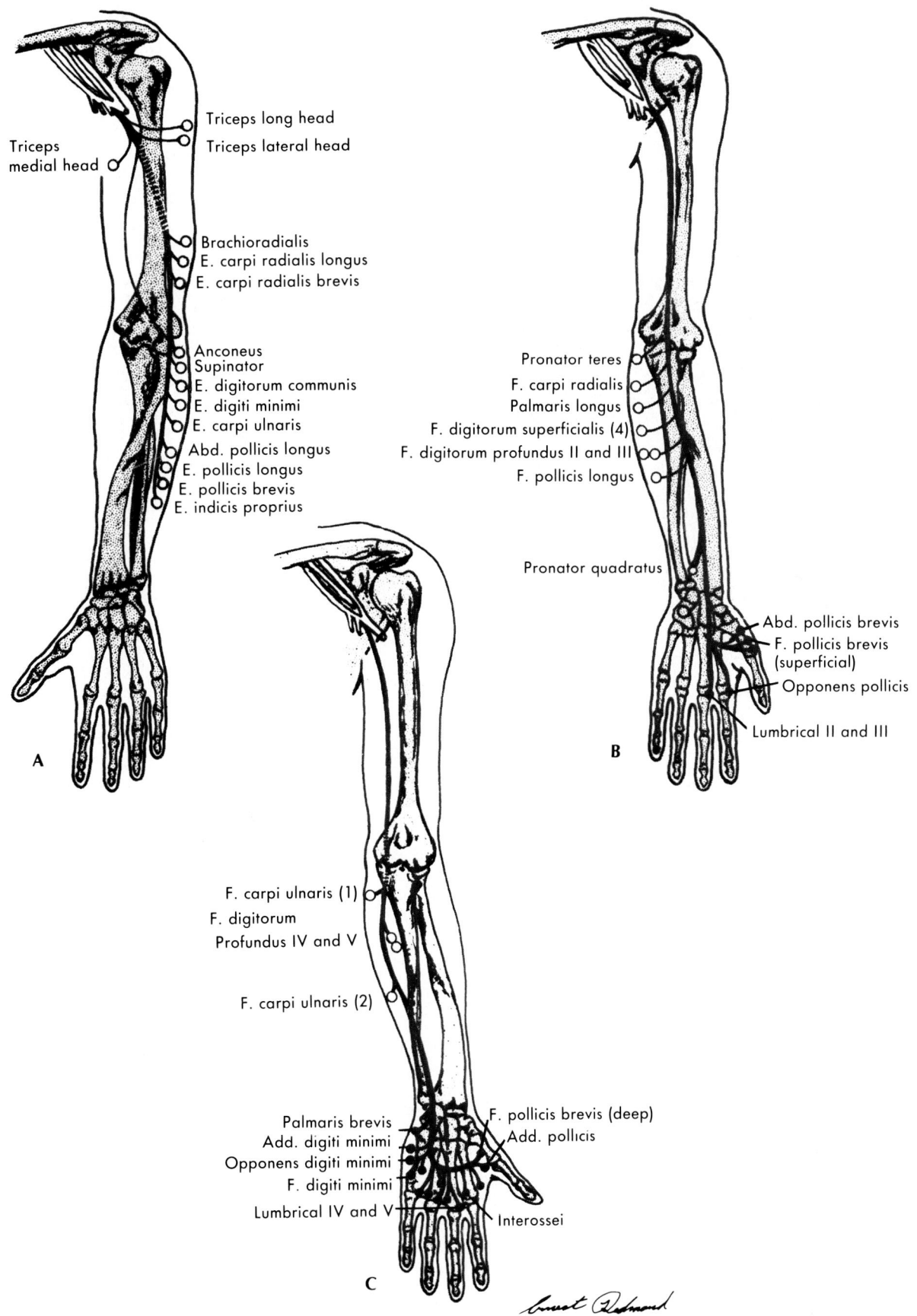

Fig. 4-35 Terminal branches of the radial, **A,** median, **B,** and ulnar, **C,** nerves. (Redrawn from American Society for Surgery of the Hand: The hand, examination and diagnosis, Aurora, Colo, 1978, The Society.)

compression of the median nerve, patients will complain of paresthesias in the sensory distribution of the irritated nerve and may have a positive Tinel's sign. In long-standing or severe acute compressive neuropathies, there will be atrophy or even paralysis of the muscles innervated distal to the area of compression. If one is aware of the sequence of innervation of each nerve and performs a good manual motor examination, it is usually not hard to make a diagnosis of a nerve entrapment.

Patients with carpal tunnel syndrome, especially post-menopausal women, may have pain at the base of the thumb, which may be thought to be caused by a compressive neuropathy. In this particular patient population, osteoarthritis of the metacarpal trapezial joint is frequent. The diagnosis can be made by performing the "grind test" and of course by radiographic examination. The grind test (Fig. 4-37) is performed by manipulating the patient's thumb with mild axial compression and gentle rotation. This maneuver will

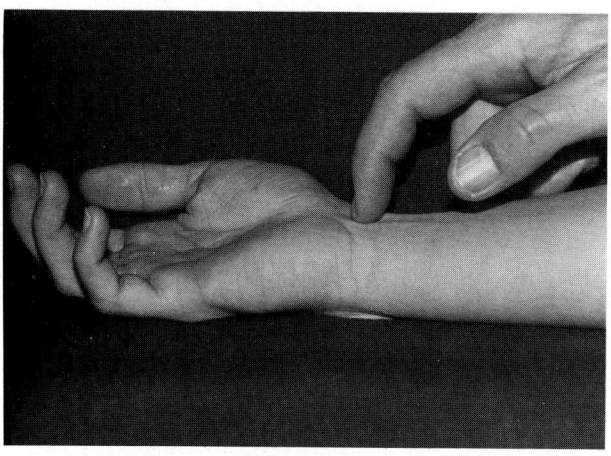

Fig. 4-36 Percussion of the median nerve at the wrist will elicit Tinel's sign in the presence of carpal tunnel syndrome.

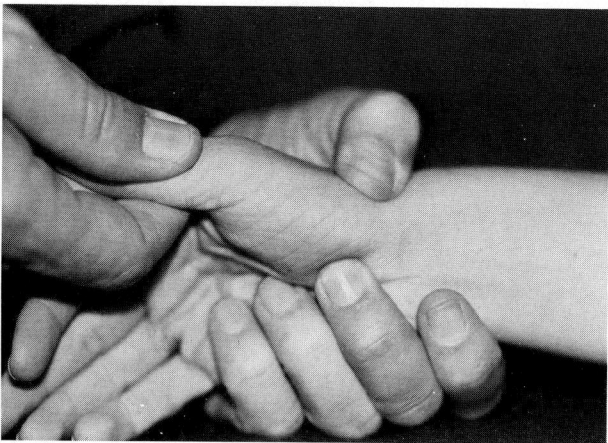

Fig. 4-37 The "grind test." Mild axial compression and gentle rotation of the thumb will elicit pain in the trapezial metacarpal joint if osteoarthritis is present.

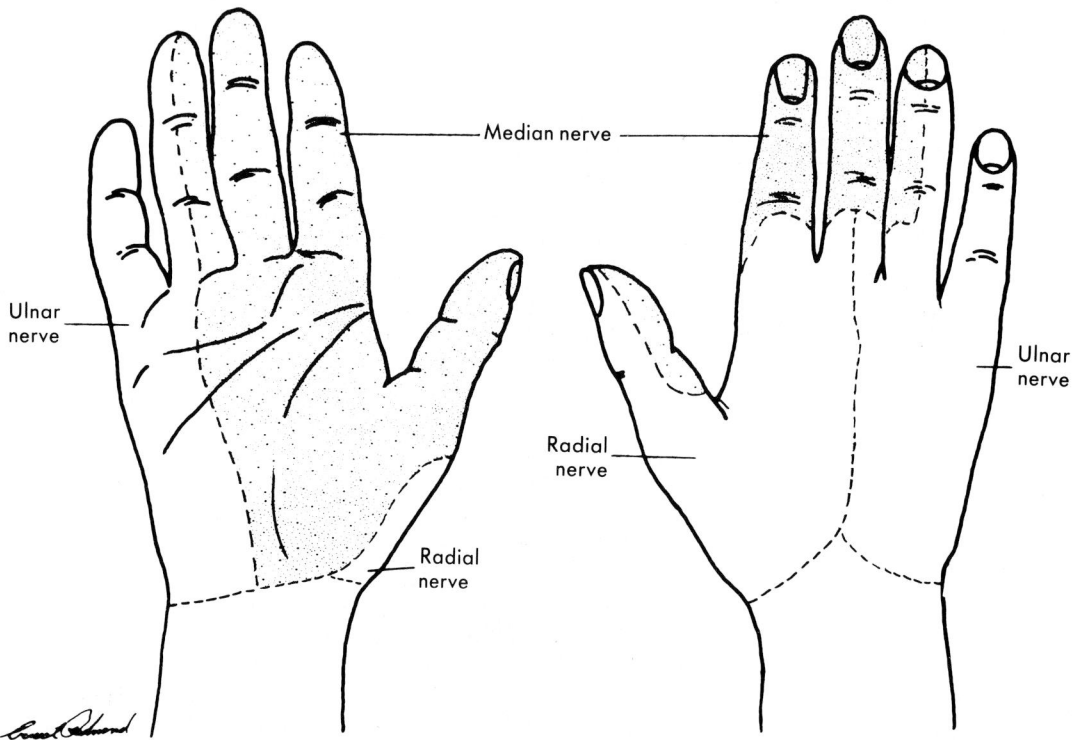

Fig. 4-38 Sensory distribution of the median, radial, and ulnar nerves in the hand. (Redrawn from Weeks PM, and Wray RC: Management of acute hand injuries: a biological approach, St Louis, 1973, The CV Mosby Co.)

induce pain in the metacarpal trapezial joint if degenerative joint disease is present. Often carpal tunnel syndrome and metacarpal trapezial arthritis will coexist, and it is sometimes difficult to identify the pain-causing lesion. The test performed for carpal tunnel syndrome and the grind test will help clarify the situation.[48]

CUTANEOUS SENSIBILITY

Normal sensibility is a prerequisite to normal hand function. A patient with a median nerve injury has essentially a "blind hand" and is greatly disabled, even if all motor function is present. The assessment of sensibility is therefore an integral and important part of the examination of the hand.

The distribution of sensory nerves is subject to as much variation as the distribution of the motor branches.[40] The classic distribution of the median, ulnar, and radial nerves is shown in Fig. 4-38.

There are many ways to assess sensibility: von Frey filaments, Moberg's Pickup Test, Seddon's coin test, the moving two-point discrimination test described by Dellon, and Weber's two-point discrimination test, to mention a few.[5,11,22,30] Each test has its supporters and detractors. Other chapters in this book will deal in detail with sensibility testing and sensory reeducation.

From a practical standpoint, an adequate sensibility examination can be performed by utilizing the two-point discrimination test and by careful examination of the patient's skin. Skin that has been deinnervated has lost its autonomic input and sudomotor function (that is, it does not sweat). The finger pulp becomes atrophic, smooth, and dry, with relative loss of dermal ridges. Deinnervated skin will not wrinkle when placed in warm water (the "wrinkle test").[30] Tinel's sign will be present at the site of a nerve injury. (Fig. 4-39.)

The two-point discrimination test is performed with a

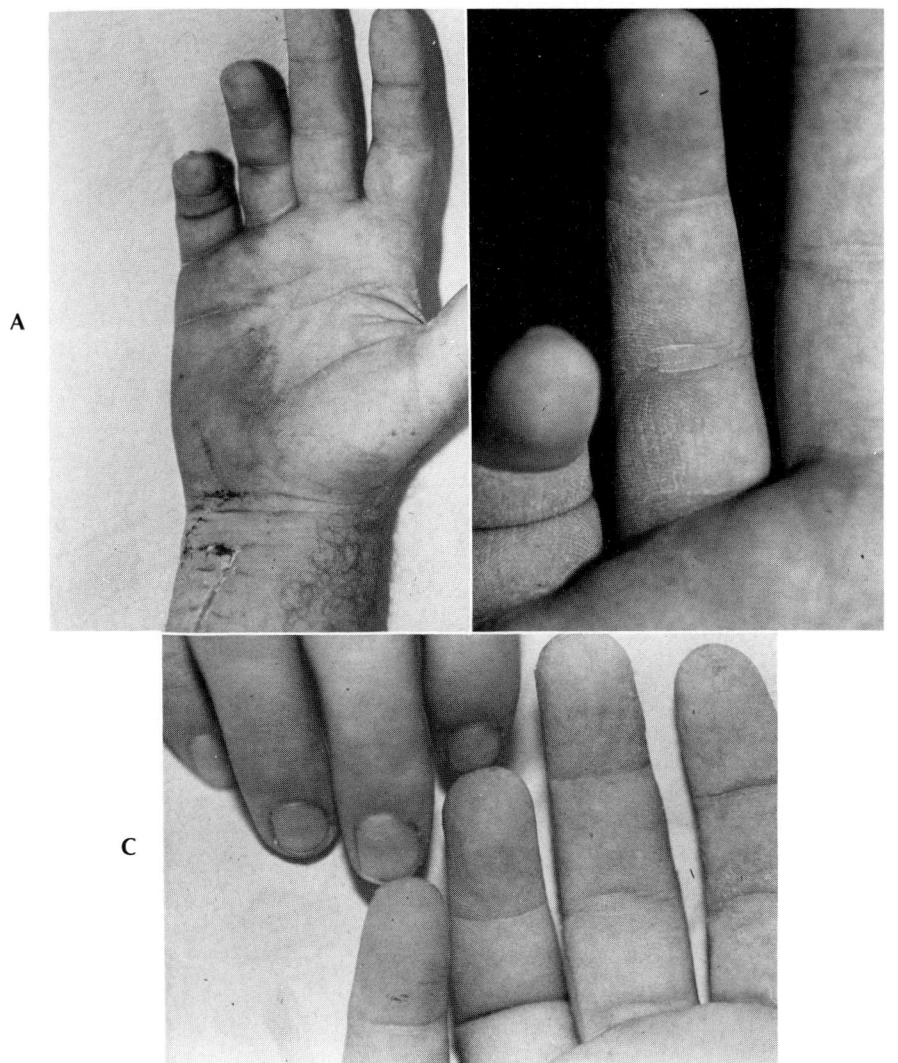

Fig. 4-39 Photographs illustrating loss of autonomic function after a peripheral nerve injury. **A,** The injury level to the ulnar nerve at the wrist is seen. The accumulated dry skin after the first postoperative dressing change can be seen in the classic ulnar nerve distribution. **B,** Closer view of the dry skin, which indicates a loss of sudomotor function. Notice how the fourth ray is split. **C,** Positive result of "wrinkle test" in same patient.

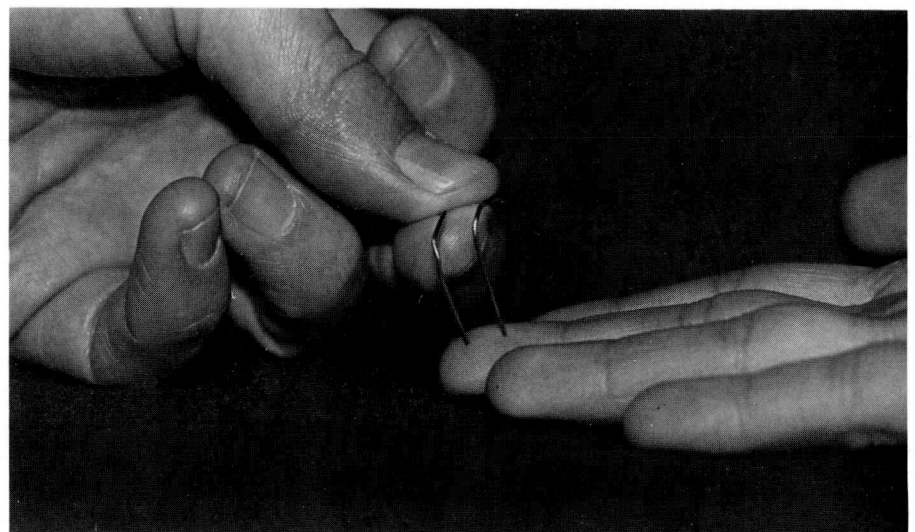

Fig. 4-40   Two-point discrimination test using a bent paper clip.

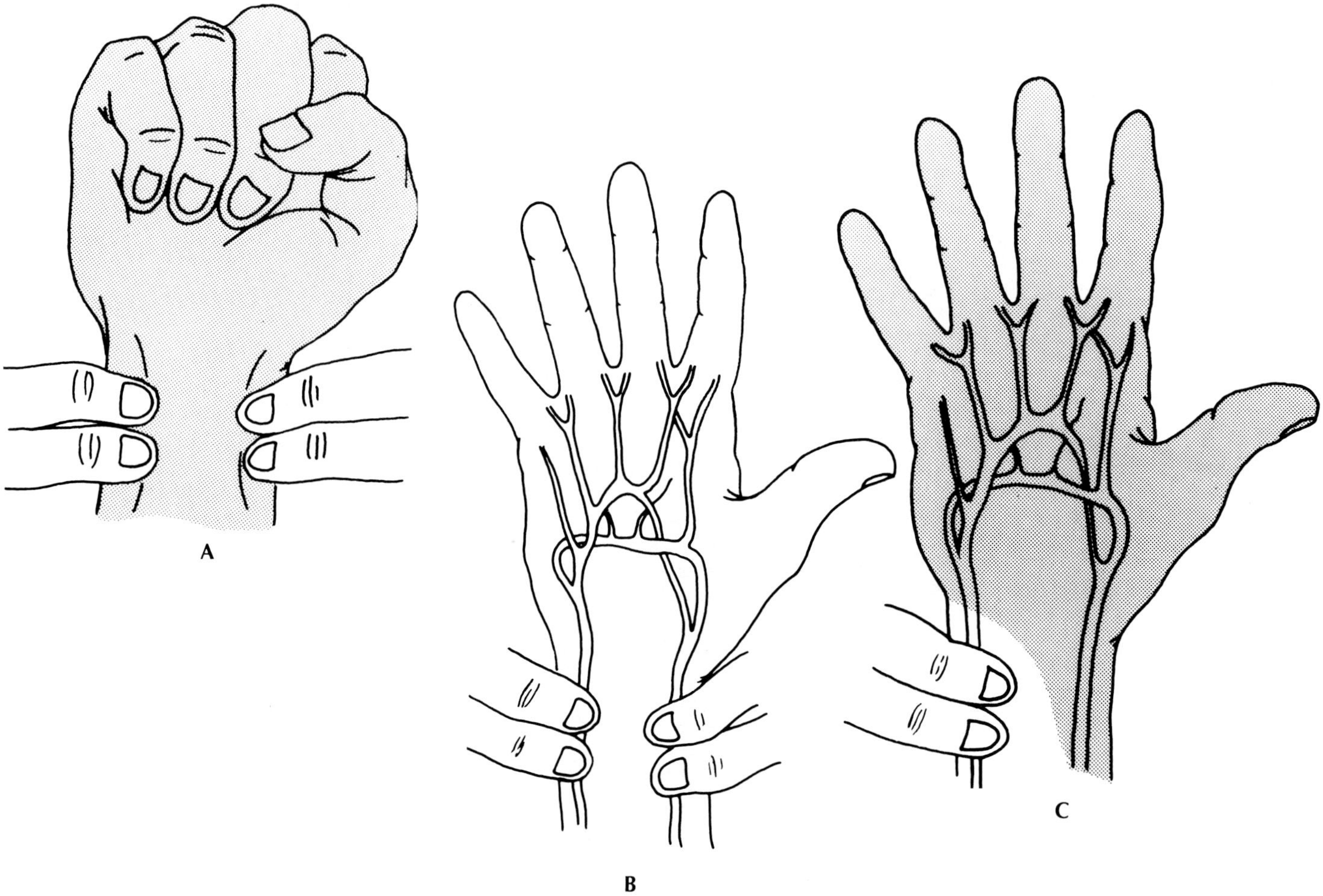

A

B

C

Fig. 4-41   Allen's test for arterial patency. **A,** The examiner places his fingers over the ulnar and radial arteries at the wrist. **B,** The patient then forcibly opens and closes his hand to exsanguinate it while the examiner occludes the radial and ulnar arteries. **C,** Next the patient opens his hand, and the examiner releases one artery and observes the flushing of the hand. The steps are then repeated, and the other artery is tested for patency. (Redrawn from American Society for Surgery of the Hand: The hand, examination and diagnosis, Aurora, Colo, 1978, The Society.)

paper clip that has been bent into a caliper. With the patient's eyes closed and his hand cradled in the examiner's, the examiner gently places the caliper on the skin in a longitudinal direction—that is, on either the ulnar or the radial side of the digit. The ends of the paper clip must touch the skin lightly, just to the point of blanching. The ends should be smooth and not barbed. The patient is then asked whether he feels one point or two. Gradually the points are brought closer together and reapplied until the patient feels only one point. Normal two-point discrimination at a fingertip is 6 mm or less (Fig. 4-40). Although this is not the most sensitive of tests and the result does not correlate with function of the hand, it is an adequate screening test and is much less time consuming than the more involved tests described.

VASCULARITY OF THE HAND

The vascular supply of the hand is usually extensive; however, it should be carefully evaluated before any surgery of the hand. The primary blood supply to the hand is through the radial and ulnar arteries. In some individuals, the dominant blood supply to the hand can be from one artery. The ulnar artery gives rise to the superficial palmar arch, and the radial artery gives rise to the deep arch. These arches usually have extensive anastomoses.[10,26] The superficial palmar arch gives rise to four common digital arteries, which then branch to form the proper digital arteries. The superficial arch may supply blood to the thumb, or the thumb may be completely vascularized by a branch of the radial artery known as the princeps pollicis artery. To assess blood supply to the hand, one should check the color of the hand (pale, red, or cyanotic), digital capillary reflux, and the radial and ulnar pulses at the wrist, and perform Allen's test. Allen in 1929 described a simple clinical test to determine the patency of the radial and ulnar arteries in thromboangiitis obliterans.[1] This test is performed by having the patient make a tight fist to exsanguinate the hand. The examiner occludes the radial and ulnar arteries at the wrist with digital pressure. The patient then opens his hand, which will be white and blanched. The examiner then releases either the ulnar or the radial artery and watches for revascularization of the hand. If the hand does not flush, the artery is occluded. This test is then repeated with the opposite artery (Fig. 4-41).

A modification of Allen's test can be performed on a single digit.[2] The steps are the same as just outlined except that the examiner occludes and releases the radial and ulnar digital arteries.

CONCLUSION

In this chapter, we have presented an organized approach to clinical examination of the hand. The books and articles listed at the end of this chapter will provide more detailed descriptions of the tests and clinical entities that have been presented here. Clinical examination is an art that will improve with practice and experience.

ACKNOWLEDGMENTS

We thank Cynthia DuPuy for her assistance in preparation of the illustrations and Mavis Stinus for her secretarial assistance in the preparation of this chapter.

REFERENCES

1. Allen E: Thromboangitis obliterans: methods of diagnosis of chronic occlusive arterial lesions distal to the wrist with illustrative cases, Am J Med Sci 178:237, 1929.
2. Ashbell T, Kutz J, and Kleinert H: The digital Allen test, Plast Reconstr Surg 39:311, 1967.
3. Baker D and others: The little finger superficialis—clinical investigation of its anatomical and functional shortcomings. J Hand Surg 6:374, 1981.
4. Bechtol C: Grip test: the use of a dynamometer with adjustable handle spacings, J Bone Joint Surg 36A:820, 832, 1954.
5. Bowden R and Napier J: The assessment of hand function after peripheral nerve injuries, J Bone Joint Surg 43B:481, 1961.
6. Braidwood A: Superficial radial neuropathy, J Bone Joint Surg 57B:380, 1975.
7. Bunnell S: Opposition of the thumb, J Bone Joint Surg 20:269, 1938.
8. Bunnell S: Surgery of the intrinsic muscles of the hand other than those producing opposition of the thumb, J Bone Joint Surg 24:1, 1942.
9. Bunnell S: Ischaemic contracture, local, in the hand, J Bone Joint Surg 35A:88, 1953.
10. Coleman S and Anson B: Arterial patterns in the hand based upon a study of 650 specimens, Surg Gynecol Obstet 113:408, 1961.
11. Dellon A: The moving two-point discrimination test: clinical evaluation of the quickly adapting fiber-receptor system, J Hand Surg 3:474, 1978.
12. Eyler D and Markee J: The anatomy and function of the intrinsic musculature of the fingers, J Bone Joint Surg 36A:1, 18, 1954.
13. Finkelstein H: Stenosing tenovaginitis at the radial styloid process, J Bone Joint Surg 12:509, 1930.
14. Harris C and Riordan D: Intrinsic contracture in the hand and its surgical treatment, J Bone Joint Surg 36A:10, 1954.
15. Hartz C and others: The pronator teres syndrome: compressive neuropathy of the median nerve, J Bone Joint Surg 63A:885, 1981.
16. Hunt JR: Occupation neuritis of the deep palmar branch of the ulnar nerve: a well-defined clinical type of professional palsy of the hand, J Nerv and Ment Dis 35:673, 1908.
17. James JIP: The assessment and management of the injured hand, Hand 2:97, 1970.
18. Johnson RK, Spinner M, and Shrewsbury MM: Median nerve entrapment syndrome in the proximal forearm, J Hand Surg 4:48, 1979.
19. Kaplan E: Translation of J. Tinel's "Four millement" paper. In Spinner M: Injuries to the major branches of peripheral nerves of the forearm, ed 2, Philadelphia, 1978, WB Saunders Co.
20. Kleinert H and Hayes J: The ulnar tunnel syndrome, Plast Reconstr Surg 47:21, 1971.
21. Landsmeer JMF: The anatomy of the dorsal aponeurosis of the human finger and its functional significance, Anat Rec 104:31, 1949.
22. Levin S, Pearsall G, and Ruderman R: Von Frey's method of measuring pressure sensibility in the hand: an engineering analysis of the Weinstein-Semmes pressure aesthesiometer, J Hand Surg 3:211, 1978.
23. Linscheid R: Injuries to radial nerve at the wrist, Arch Surg 91:942, 1965.
24. Lister GD, Belsole RB, and Kleinert HE: The radial tunnel syndrome, J Hand Surg 4:52, 1979.
25. Mannerfelt L: Studies on the hand in ulnar nerve paralysis: a clinical-experimental investigation in normal and anomalous innervation, Acta Orthop Scand [Suppl.] 87:1, 1966.
26. Markee J and Wray J: Circulation of the hand: injection-corrosion studies, J Bone Joint Surg 41A:673, 1959.
27. McFarlane R: Observations on the functional anatomy of the intrinsic muscles of the thumb, J Bone Joint Surg 44A:1073, 1962.
28. Mehta H and Gardner W: A study of lumbrical muscles in the human hand, Am J Anat 109:227, 1961.
29. Micks J, Reswick J, and Hager DL: The mechanism of the intrinsic-minus finger: a biomechanical study, J Hand Surg 3:333, 1978.
30. Moberg E: Objective methods for determining the functional value of sensibility in the hand, J Bone Joint Surg 40B:454, 1958.
31. Moldaver J: Tinel's sign: its characteristics and significance, J Bone Joint Surg 60A:412, 1978.
32. Mulder J and Landsmeer J: The mechanism of the claw finger, J Bone Joint Surg 50B:664, 1968.
33. Nalebuff E and Millender L: Surgical treatment of the boutonniere deformity in rheumatoid arthritis, Orthop Clin North Am 6:753, 1975.
34. Nalebuff E and Millender L: Surgical treatment of the swan-neck deformity in rheumatoid arthritis, Orthop Clin North Am 6:733, 1975.

35. Noer H and Pratt D: A goniometer designed for the hand, J Bone Joint Surg 40A:1154, 1958.
36. Phalen G: The carpal tunnel syndrome: seventeen years' experience in diagnosis and treatment of 654 hands, J Bone Joint Surg 48A:211, 1966.
37. Riddell D: Spontaneous rupture of the extensor pollicis longus: the results of tendon transfer, J Bone Joint Surg 45B:506, 1963.
38. Robbins H: Anatomical study of the median nerve in the carpal tunnel and etiologies of the carpal tunnel syndrome, J Bone Joint Surg 45A:953, 1963.
39. Roles N and Maudsley R: Radial tunnel syndrome: resistant tennis elbow as a nerve entrapment, J Bone Joint Surg 54B:499, 1972.
40. Rowntree T: Anomalous innervation of the hand muscles, J Bone Joint Surg 31B:505, 1949.
41. Shaw J and Sakellarides H: Radial nerve paralysis associated with fractures of the humerus: a review of forty-five cases, J Bone Joint Surg 49A:899, 1967.
42. Shea J and McClain E: Ulnar nerve compression syndromes at and below the wrist, J Bone Joint Surg 51A:1095, 1969.
43. Shrewsbury M and Johnson R: A systematic study of the oblique retinacular ligament of the human finger: its structure and function, J Hand Surg 2:194, 1977.
44. Smith R: Non-ischemic contractures of the intrinsic muscles of the hand, J Bone Joint Surg 53A:1313, 1971.
45. Spinner M: The arcade of Frohse and its relationship to posterior interosseous nerve paralysis, J Bone Joint Surg 50B:809, 1968.
46. Spinner M: The anterior interosseous nerve syndrome with special attention to its variations, J Bone Joint Surg 52A:84, 1970.
47. Srinivasan H: Clinical features of paralytic claw fingers, J Bone Joint Surg 61A:1060, 1063, 1979.
48. Swanson A: Disabling arthritis at the base of the thumb: treatment by resection of the trapezium and flexible (silicon) implant arthroplasty, J Bone Joint Surg 54A:456, 1972.
49. Tanzer R: The carpal tunnel syndrome: a clinical and anatomical study, J Bone Joint Surg 41A:626, 1959.
50. Tinel J: Le signe du "fourmillement" dans les lesions des nerfs peripheriques, Press Med 47:388, October 1915.
51. Uriburu I, Morchio F, and Marin J: Compression syndrome of the deep motor branch of the ulnar nerve (Piso-Hamate hiatus syndrome), J Bone Joint Surg 58A:145, 1976.
52. Vaughn-Jackson O: Rheumatoid hand deformities considered in the light of tendon imbalance, J Bone Joint Surg 44B:764, 1962.
53. Zancolli E: Structural and dynamic basis of hand surgery, Philadelphia, 1968, JB Lippincott Co, p 136.

5

Documentation: essential elements of an upper extremity assessment battery

Elaine Ewing Fess

"I often say that when you can measure what you are speaking about and express it in numbers, you know something about it; but, when you cannot measure it in numbers your knowledge is of a meagre and unsatisfactory kind; it may be the beginning of knowledge but have scarcely in your thought advanced to the stage of science whatever the matter may be."

LORD KELVIN

Objective measurements provide a foundation for hand rehabilitation efforts by delineating baseline pathology, from which patient progress and treatment methods may be evaluated. A thorough and unbiased assessment procedure furnishes information that helps predict the rehabilitation potential of the diseased or injured hand, provides data with which subsequent measurements may be compared, and allows the medical specialist to plan and evaluate treatment programs and techniques. Conclusions gained from evaluation procedures aid in ordering treatment priorities, provide both patient and staff incentive, and define functional capacity when rehabilitative efforts reach an end point. Assessment, through analysis and integration of data, also serves as the vehicle for professional communication, eventually influencing the comprehensive body of knowledge of the profession.

Because the quality of information depends on the level of sophistication, predictability, and accuracy of the instruments used in gathering data, it is of utmost importance to choose assessment tools with care and forethought. Dependable, precise tools allow the clinician to reach conclusions that are minimally skewed by extraneous factors or

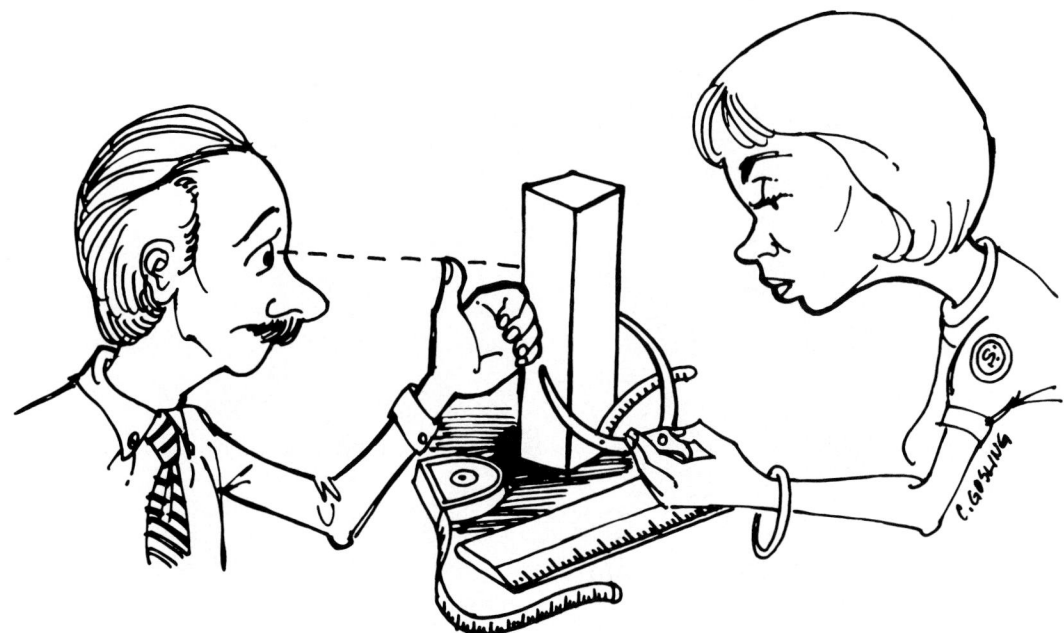

"ARE WE SPEAKING THE SAME LANGUAGE ?"

Fig. 5-1 Assessment with calibrated instruments provides accurate information and leads to a more thorough understanding of what is measured.

biases, thus diminishing the chances of subjective error and facilitating an objective and more accurate level of understanding. An instrument that measures diffusely produces undelineated and nonspecific data, while an instrument that has been proved to measure with precision yields more accurate and selective information (Fig. 5-1).

In addition to knowledge of the specific characteristics of assessment tools, it is important to identify how the manner in which they are used may affect resultant data. First and foremost, to maintain validity it is critical that assessment instruments never be used as practice tools for patients in therapy. Information obtained from a tool that has been used as part of the training process is radically skewed, rendering it invalid and meaningless. Other factors that may alter test results include patient fatigue, the patient's potential for physiologic adaptation, the degree of difficulty, and the length of time required to complete the test. To avoid possible tainting of test data through physiologic adaptation, sensory testing should be completed before the evaluation of gross grasp or pinch; and if appropriate rest periods are not provided, fatigue may diminish test scores. In addition, frustration thresholds may be inadvertently exceeded if difficult portions of the testing battery are scheduled early in the assessment session. The testing procedure must, therefore, reflect understanding of testing protocol as well as instrumentation requirements.

Although many variables influence the selection and use of assessment instruments, the underlying rationale for conducting evaluation procedures is communication. The acquisition and transmission of knowledge, which are fundamental to patient treatment and professional growth, can be enhanced through the development and use of a common professional language based on strict criteria for assessment instrument selection. In an age of consumer awareness and accountability it is no longer sufficient to rely on "home-brewed," nonvalidated evaluation tools, which almost universally produce meaningless splinter data (Fig. 5-2). Thus the purposes of this chapter are to (1) define testing terminology and criteria, (2) identify key factors that influence the development of an upper extremity assessment battery, (3) review currently utilized hand assessment instruments, and (4) provide samples of assessment forms. It is not within the scope of this chapter to recommend the use of one test or instrument over another; instead readers are encouraged to choose those instruments or protocols that will best meet the specific needs of their own practices.

ASSESSMENT TERMINOLOGY AND CRITERIA

Standardized tests, which represent the most sophisticated level of assessment tools, have been statistically proved to be both valid and reliable. This means that they appropriately measure what they purport to measure and that they measure consistently within their measurement unit, between examiners, and from trial to trial. "Reliability deals with whether a measurement consistently reflects something, whereas validity deals with how the measurement is used."[51] The few standardized tests currently available in the field of hand rehabilitation are limited to instruments that evaluate hand coordination, dexterity, and work tolerance; and unfortunately only a small number of these meet all the requirements of standardization. The remaining hand assessment instruments fall at varying levels along the validity and reliability continuums according to how closely their inherent properties coincide with those of standardized tools.

To qualify as a standardized test, an instrument must have all of the following elements: (1) a statement that defines the purpose or intent of the test; (2) correlation statistics or

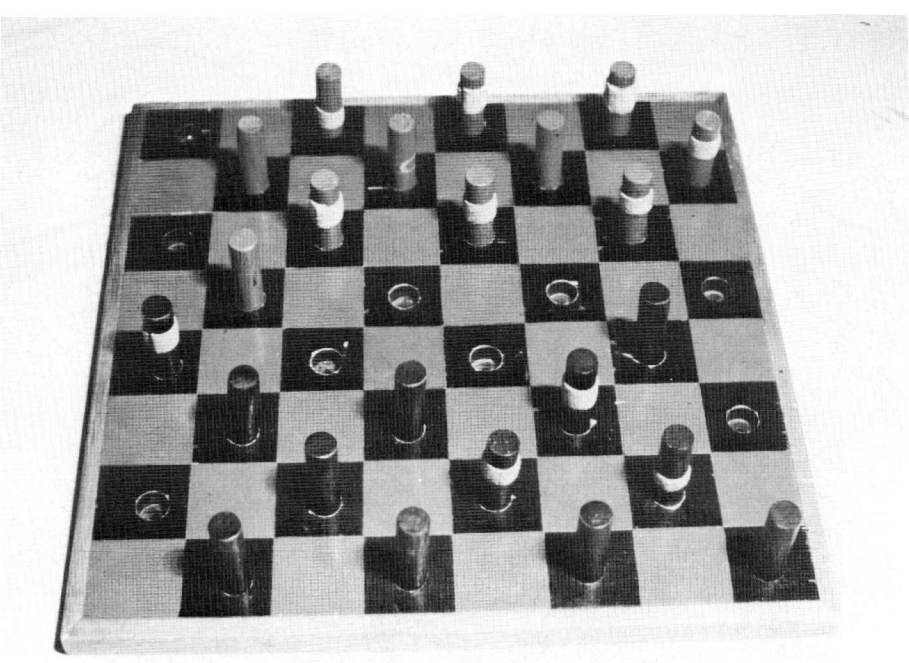

Fig. 5-2 Tests should be statistically proved to be reliable and valid before they are used for clinical assessment. "Home-brewed" tests should not be relied on to document patient progress.

another appropriate measure of instrument validity; (3) correlation statistics or another appropriate measure of instrument reliability; (4) detailed descriptions of the equipment utilized in the test; (5) normative data, drawn from a large population sample, which is divided into categories according to appropriate variables, such as hand dominance, age, sex, or occupation; and (6) specific instructions for administering, scoring and interpreting the test. A bibliography of related literature may also be included. It is important to note that although they claim to be standardized, many tests lack true validity and reliability coefficients, relying instead on mean or "average" values. Such tests are not standardized and actually have no foundation for justifying their consistency of measurement and their ability to assess that for which they were designed. Since relatively few hand evaluation tools fully meet standardization criteria,[24] instrument selection should be predicated on satisfying as many of the standardization requisites as possible, thus ensuring an identifiable level of quality control.

Through interpretation, standardized tests provide information that may be used to deduce or predict how a patient will perform in normal daily tasks. For example, if "patient no. 3" achieves "X" functional rating on a standardized test, it may be predicted that he should be able to perform at an equivalent of the "75th percentile" of "normal assembly line workers." Standardized hand function tests also allow the clinician to make statements about changes in patient status: "Yes, this patient's hand dexterity is improved as the result of this tendon transfer."

Other types of tests also provide significant information when they are used properly. Most important are the observational tests, producing responses on a yes-no performance continuum. An activities-of-daily-living (ADL) evaluation is an example of an observational test; it consists of various tasks, and the patient is graded on whether he can accomplish the tasks under specific conditions (for example, independent, independent with equipment, needs assistance). The ADL test tells the examiner "Yes, the patient can pick up a 12-ounce aluminum beer can with his right hand." This knowledge, however, cannot be used to predict the patient's performance in picking up potatoes or opening a ketchup bottle. An observational test is used to assess progress through comparisons of subsequent testing trials, and it is limited to longitudinal, item-to-item contrast: "The patient is now able to accomplish 'task Z,' which he was unable to do 3 weeks ago." Further assumptions or predictions are invalid and meaningless. Observational tests have a definite role in an upper extremity assessment battery, as long as they are used appropriately.

DEVELOPMENT OF AN ASSESSMENT BATTERY
General considerations

Development of an upper extremity assessment battery cannot be undertaken without a thorough understanding of the conditions that will influence its use. The types of patients to be evaluated, expectations about the acquired data, the way the data will be used, and physical setting must be carefully considered to ensure that an assessment battery meets the unique needs of a particular hand practice. Age, diagnosis, intelligence, socioeconomic background, language, and other patient population variables are important in the selection of assessment instruments. For example,

tests requiring high degrees of patient cooperation may not be appropriate for a practice that deals primarily with young children, mentally retarded individuals, or persons whose language skills are limited. The intent or reason for gathering information also plays a significant role in the creation of an assessment battery. Because the need for exacting precision and sophistication in the collection of research data is paramount, requirements are often more stringent for research evaluation instruments than for instruments used in daily clinical testing. An assessment battery should reflect the scope and demands of the practice, including staff qualifications, physical plan, and fiscal parameters. In addition, through licensure regulations, state or federal legislation is often influential in determining the selection of test instruments.

Specific considerations

To be complete, an assessment battery should address the total spectrum of upper extremity performance and condition, including physical status, motion, sensation, and function. A history is also an important part of the patient's permanent record. This information not only is essential to identifying and understanding a pathologic condition, but provides the medical specialist with pertinent occupational and vocational facts that allow subsequent intervention to be tailored to meet the specific needs of the patient. In addition, an assessment battery may contain relevant administrative information (Fig. 5-3) and specialized tests such as an upper extremity prosthetic checkout or a splint evaluation (Fig. 5-4).

Because there is no universal hand assessment instrument, the clinician must rely on a variety of tools to measure the various parameters of hand condition and performance. The four main divisions—physical status, motion, sensation, and function—should be represented through the selection of a minimum of one instrument per area. Although this minimum-requirement assessment battery is sufficient for a cursory evaluation, it is preferable, in those practices specializing in hand dysfunction, to include several instruments within each category, producing gradation and verification of information.

The American Society for Surgery of the Hand (ASSH)[3] and the American Society of Hand Therapists (ASHT)[2] have established guidelines for clinical assessment of the hand; these guidelines include recommendations for measurement of range of motion, strength, sensation (ASSH), volume (ASHT), dexterity and coordination (ASHT), and vascular status (ASSH). Representing the first major steps taken by recognized professional hand societies toward creating a common assessment language, these recommendations are milestones in the history of hand rehabilitation. To enhance the quality of professional communication and understanding of hand dysfunction, it is important that individuals responsible for developing evaluation protocols seriously consider these guidelines and generate assessment batteries that reflect the recommendations of these two societies.

TIMING AND USE OF ASSESSMENT TESTS

Not all patients who are evaluated need to be given all of the tests within an assessment battery. Most hand specialists use a few quick tests to check hand function initially and add the more sophisticated testing procedures as dictated by the patient's condition. For example, if on interrogation the patient reports no loss of sensation, and this is verified by a normal two-point discrimination test, in most instances it is not necessary to administer the remainder of the sensory tests. To conserve time and decrease frustration levels, tests within each area should be ordered according to type of information provided and degree of difficulty of administration, beginning with an easy, dependable test that will supply basic data and working toward the more esoteric instruments.

Initial and final evaluations are usually comprehensive in scope, whereas the intervening evaluations are less formal and concentrate on assessing progress in specific areas of dysfunction according to the problems exhibited by each patient. The frequency of reevaluation sessions depends entirely on the patient, the progress demonstrated, and the nature of the test itself. It is not unusual to measure range of motion in an early postoperative tenolysis patient three or four times a day. However, measurement of grip strength in the same patient may not be appropriate, because of wound healing and tensile strength limitations,[38] until 7 or 8 weeks postoperatively, and then strength, because of the time required to effect change, would not be measured as frequently as would motion.

The actual recording of assessment data also varies with the situation. For the tenolysis patient described previously, unless significant problems were encountered and frequent documentation was necessary to demonstrate lack of cooperation or other mitigating variables, only one set of range-of-motion measurements would usually be recorded per day even though multiple readings were taken. As change occurs less rapidly, motion values may be recorded two or three times a week, eventually decreasing to once every 2 weeks, once a month, and so on. The important concept is that change in status be documented with objective measurements at appropriate intervals.

Text continued on p. 62.

SPLINTING AND HAND THERAPY REFERRAL

Name: _____

Address: _____

Phone number: _____

Diagnosis:

Referral for extremity: ☐Right ☐Left

☐ Evaluation and report
☐ Evaluation and treatment
   ☐ Range of motion
   ☐ Strengthening
   ☐ Dexterity
   ☐ Sensory reeducation
   ☐ Desensitization
   ☐ Activities of daily living
   ☐ Work/home evaluation
   ☐ Joint protection (arthritic program)
   ☐ Upper extremity prosthetic training
   ☐ Upper extremity Jobst garment measurement and fitting
   ☐ Transcutaneous stimulation
   ☐ Upper extremity Jobst pump
   ☐ Other (specify): _____
☐ Splint fabrication:

A

Fig. 5-3 Administrative forms are essential to the organization of a hand rehabilitation center. Forms such as these may also be helpful in retrieval of data for research purposes. **A,** Referral form. **B,** Daily patient log. (**A** from Fess E and Philips C: Hand splinting: principles and methods, ed 2, St Louis, 1987, The CV Mosby Co.)

SPLINTING AND HAND THERAPY REFERRAL — cont'd

Check joints desired to be incorporated in splint*:

Immobilize (specify position of joint in degrees)							Mobilize				
						Elbow					
						Ext					
						Flex					
						Wrist					
						Ext					
						Flex					
						UD					
						RD					
					TH		TH				
						CMC					
						Ext					
						Flex					
						Abd					
Ind	**Long**	**Ring**	**Sm**	**Th**			**Th**	**Ind**	**Long**	**Ring**	**Sm**
						MP					
						Ext					
						Flex					
						RD					
						UD					
						PIP (IP)					
						Ext					
						Flex					
						DIP					
						Ext					
						Flex					

*Ext, Extension; *Flex*, flexion; *RD*, radial deviation; *UD*, ulnar deviation; *MP*, metacarpophalangeal; *PIP*, proximal interphalangeal; *DIP*, distal interphalangeal; *ABD*, abduction; *Th*, thumb; *Ind*, index; *Sm*, small.

A

Fig. 5-3, cont'd   For legend see opposite page.   *Continued.*

A

> ## SPLINTING AND HAND THERAPY REFERRAL—cont'd
> Describe the function you would like the splint or splints to provide:
>
> The correct fabrication of the splint is important. Therefore, please call for any specific instructions (phone number _____).

B

DATE: _____ am
pm

UPPER EXTREMITY ASSESSMENT BATTERY
DAILY PATIENT LOG

NAME:

EVALUATION
- VOLUME
- TEMPERATURE
- RANGE OF MOTION
- MUSCLE TEST
- SENSIBILITY
- COORDINATION
- ADL/HOMEMAKING
- EMPLOYMENT
- PROSTHETIC
- SPLINT
- JOBST MEASUREMENT
- EMG
- NCV
- OTHER
- INITIAL
- PROGRESS
- FINAL

TREATMENT
- PASSIVE EXERCISE
- ACTIVE EXERCISE
- RESISTIVE EXERCISE
- FUNCTIONAL ACTIVITY
- EARLY MOBILIZATION
- JOINT MOBILIZATION
- DESENSITIZATION
- SENSORY REEDUCATION
- DEBRIDEMENT
- JOINT PROTECTION
- HOME PROGRAM
- OTHER

MODALITIES
- BIOFEEDBACK
- ELEC STIMULATION
- TNS
- WHIRLPOOL
- HOT PACKS
- PARAFFIN
- FLUIDOTHERAPY
- INTERMIT PRESSURE
- OTHER

SPLINTS
- IMMOBILIZATION
- MOBILIZATION
- SIMPLE
- COMPOUND
- COMPLEX
- EQUIPMENT
- OTHER

THERAPIST: _____

Fig. 5-3, cont'd For legend see p. 56.

UPPER EXTREMITY FUNCTIONAL ASSESSMENT BATTERY

Upper extremity amputee prosthesis checkout

Amputee type: R _____ L _____ BE _____ AE _____ SD _____ WD _____ ED _____ Other _____

	Test	Performance	Standard
I	Conformance to prescription		Conform to written prescription
II	Workmanship and appearance		
III	Control system efficiency	Hook Hand	
	1. Force applied at terminal device	_____ lb _____ lb	B/E should be 70% or greater.
	2. Force applied at harness	_____ lb _____ lb	A/E should be 50% or greater.
	3. Efficiency = $\dfrac{\text{Force at T.D.}}{\text{Force at harness}}$	_____ % _____ %	
IV	Compression fit and comfort		Socket compression should cause no pain or discomfort.
V	Tension stability	_____ in displacement	50 lb (or ⅓ body weight) axial pull should not displace socket more than 1 in. Harness should not fail.
VI	Terminal device—opening and closing	Hook Hand	Full opening and closing should be obtained with forearm at 90°.
	1. Mechanical range	_____ in _____ in	
	2. Active range (forearm at 90°)	_____ in _____ in	B/E 70% (A/E 50%) opening at mouth and waist.
	3. Active range (waist)	_____ in _____ in	
	4. Active range (mouth)	_____ in _____ in	

Date: _____   Patient: _____

A

Upper extremity amputee prosthesis checkout

Additional below-elbow specifications

VII	Amount of forearm	Prosthesis off _____ Prosthesis on _____	Should be within 10° of range with prosthesis off, except for very short stumps
VIII	Amount of forearm rotation	Prosthesis off _____ Prosthesis on _____	Total rotation with prosthesis should be half that with prosthesis off (Practical only for long B/E and W/D)
IX	Placement of artificial elbow		Should be not more than below normal elbow on adult
X	Range of glenohumeral motion with prosthesis on	Abduction Flexion Extension Rotation	90° ⎫ 90° ⎬ Prosthesis on 30° ⎭ Variable
XI	Glenohumeral flexion required to flex forearm fully	_____ °	Should not exceed 45°
	Prosthetic elbow—mechanical range	_____ °	To 135°
	Prosthetic elbow—active range	_____ °	To 135°
XII	Force required to initiate forearm flexion from a position of 90° flexed	_____ lb	Should not exceed the force necessary to open terminal device or 10 lb
XIII	Socket rotation stability		Resist force of 3 lb 12 in from elbow center Applied laterally and medially

Prosthesis passed _____   Prosthesis rejected _____

Returned for following reasons: _____

_____

_____

Patient _____

Fig. 5-4 An assessment battery may contain specialized forms such as, **A,** upper extremity prosthetic checkout, designed by Prosthetic-Orthotic Department at Northwestern University, Chicago, or, **B,** splint check-out. (**B** from Fess E and Philips C: Hand splinting: principles and methods, ed 2, St Louis, 1987, The CV Mosby Co.)

Continued.

SPLINT CHECKOUT FORM

	Yes	No	Comments
DESIGN			
Does the splint meet general design concepts, including adaptation for:			
1. Individual patient factors			
2. Total utilization time			
3. Simplicity			
4. Optimum function			
5. Optimum sensation			
6. Efficient construction and fit			
7. Ease of application and removal			
8. Exercise regimen			
Does the splint meet specific design concepts, including adaptation for:			
9. Influencing key joints			
10. Attaining purpose			
a. Augment passive motion			
b. Substitute for active motion			
11. Types of forces used			
12. Surface of application			
13. Anatomic variables			
14. Material properties			
MECHANICS			
Does the splint meet specific mechanical concepts, including adaptation for:			
1. Reduction of pressure			
2. Increased mechanical advantage (Ratio of FA to RA)			
3. Optimum rotational force (90°)			
4. Torque			
5. Variance of passive mobility of successive joints			
6. Optimum utilization of parallel forces			
7. Material strength			
8. Elimination of friction			

B

Fig. 5-4, cont'd For legend see p. 59.

SPLINT CHECKOUT FORM—cont'd

	Yes	No	Comments
CONSTRUCTION			
Has the splint been fabricated appropriately to provide:			
1. Good cosmesis			
2. Rounded corners			
3. Smooth edges and surfaces			
4. Stable joints			
5. Finished rivets			
6. Ventilation			
7. Secure padding			
8. Secure straps			
FIT			
Has the splint been fitted appropriately to adapt to:			
1. Bony prominences			
2. Dual obliquity			
3. Ligamentous stress			
4. Arches			
5. Joint axis alignment			
6. Skin creases			
7. Kinematic changes			
8. Kinetic concepts			
DYNAMIC ASSIST(S)			
Does each dynamic assist meet appropriate requisites for:			
1. Magnitude of force application			
2. Physical properties correlated with patient needs			
3. Physical properties correlated with splint design			
4. Mechanical concepts			
a. 90° rotational force			
b. Torque			
c. Pressure			
5. Fit			
a. Ligamentous stress			
b. Kinematic changes			
c. Kinetic changes			
6. Maintenance of force magnitude			

B

Fig. 5-4, cont'd For legend see p. 59.

HISTORY AND PHYSICAL STATUS
History

In addition to noting the patient's current condition, the initial history should contain information regarding how and when the injury occurred, including specifics as to time and place. Questions about how the patient's vocational, avocational, and ADL skills have been changed by the disability are important, as is close observation of the patient's spontaneous use of the extremity during the evaluation session. The patient's subjective assessment of the pain may also provide insight into his attitude and ability to cope with his situation, and it is helpful to attempt to determine the cause of pain and its perceived intensity.

Obtaining a history is not only the amassing of facts; it is the time in which the first steps are taken toward building a firm foundation of trust and communication between the patient and the examiner. Each must feel that the other is being honest and open. Genuine concern and an unhurried manner on the part of the examiner will facilitate discussion, eventually netting returns in cooperation and understanding as the patient participates in the rehabilitation process.

Examination

The detail in which this portion of the assessment battery is pursued, and by whom, depends on the clinical setting in which patients are evaluated, and to a large extent on the division of duties between the surgeons and the therapists. Regardless of who is responsible for conducting the intake evaluation, each patient is assessed for general configuration of the extremity; condition of skin and soft tissue; skeletal stability; articular motion and integrity; tendon continuity and glide; neurovascular status, including isolated muscle function, sensation, and vessel patency; and finally for general function, coordination, and dexterity. (Refer to Chapter 4 for further details.)

It is the combination of careful clinical examination and precise measurement (Fig. 5-5) that allows the examiner to identify and make judgments about the patient's rehabilitative potential and the need for therapeutic intervention. Assessment instruments outline the problem in terms of data expressed as specific numerical values, quantifying and adding dimension to knowledge and understanding. Without measurement, perceptions are diffuse and unclear.

CURRENT HAND ASSESSMENT INSTRUMENTS

Hand evaluation instruments may be divided into four basic groups according to the entity measured: extremity condition, motion, sensibility, and function. Condition involves the neurovascular system as it pertains to tissue viability, nutrition, patency of vessels, and arterial, venous, and lymphatic flow. Through noninvasive monitoring of hand volume, skin temperature, and arterial pulses, impor-

```
TENDON
    FUNCTION
        Connect motor to support system
        Glide = Active motion
```

ETIOLOGY OF DYSFUNCTION	SYMPTOM	EVALUATION MEASUREMENT	OBSERVATION
Loss of continuity	Loss of AROM	A & P ROM	Posture/use
Early inflammation	Swelling/edema	Volume/circum	Dec. wrinkling
	Decreased motion	A & P ROM	Posture/use
Loss of motor	Loss of AROM	A & P ROM	Posture/use
	Weakness	EMG	"
		Manual Muscle	
		Dynamometer	
		Pinchometer	
Denervation	Atrophy (late)	Volume/circum	Trophic changes
Adhesion	Decreased AROM	A & P ROM	Posture/use
	Tenodesis effect	"	
Change of position,	Bowstringing	"	
angle of pull	Subluxation	"	
	Dislocation	"	
	Decreased motion	"	Posture/use
Inflammation	Swelling/edema	Volume/circum	Dec. wrinkling
	Decreased motion	A & P ROM	Posture/use
	Crepitation		Palpation
	Triggering		"
	Tenodesis effect		"
	Pain		"
Infection	Swelling/edema	Volume/circum	Dec. wrinkling
	Decreased motion	A & P ROM	Posture/use
	Pain		Palpation

Note: The above tendon problems influence composite hand function and may require dexterity/coordination, ADL or vocational assessment.

Fig. 5-5 Clinical examination and objective measurements are combined to provide better understanding of the underlying pathologic condition.

tant clues are provided about the status of the skin and subcutaneous tissues and about neurovascular function. The measurement of motion depends on muscle-tendon continuity, contractile and gliding capacity, neuromuscular communication, and volutional control. Techniques for evaluating hand motion include goniometric measurements and the determination of isolated muscle strength. Relying on neural continuity, impulse transmission, receptor acuity, and cortical perception, assessment of sensibility may be divided into sudomotor or sympathetic response and the abilities to detect, discriminate, quantify, and identify stimuli.[35] Hand function reflects the integration of all systems and is measured in terms of grip and pinch, coordination and dexterity, and ability to participate in ADLs and vocational and avocational tasks.

Condition assessment instruments

The volumeter, as designed by Brand and Wood,[15] is based on Archimedes' principle of water displacement; it measures composite hand mass (Fig. 5-6). Commercially available in several dimensions,[17] volumeters may be used to assess changes in hand size, including atrophy, local swelling, and generalized edema, provided that immersion of the extremity in water is not contraindicated. Waylett and Seibly[61] found a commercial hand volumeter to be accurate to within 10 ml when used according to the manufacturer's specifications. Variables that were implicated in reducing accuracy included use of an aerated hose or faucet to fill the tank, wrist or forearm motion once the hand is immersed in the tank, inconsistency of pressure applied to the horizontal stop rod, and inconsistent placement of the volumeter during successive measurements. Normal comparison values may be obtained by measuring the contralateral extremity. Measurements from both extremities should be recorded in the chart initially, and successive measurements of the symptomatic extremity should be noted at appropriate intervals (Fig. 5-7).

Circumferential measurements, by means of a flexible tape measure, are also employed to evaluate upper extremity size. Although the accuracy of this technique depends on consistency of placement[54] and tension of the tape, circumferential measurement provides a quick means of assessment; it is especially applicable in situations in which the use of a volumeter would be awkward or inappropriate. Serial measurements should be taken and recorded (Fig. 5-7) at appropriate intervals, as dictated by patient requirements and progress.

An external caliper, calibrated in millimeters, offers an additional method of assessing localized swelling—measuring the diameter of a segment. As with circumferential measurement, the accuracy of diameter readings is subject to error through inconsistent placement and tension. This technique provides greater measurement reliability on smaller-diameter segments; it is usually employed to evaluate change in digital size. (Refer to Chapter 13 for further details.)

Because skin temperature is directly related to digital vessel patency, it is a valuable indicator of tissue viability; temperature is used to monitor the status of revascularized hands or digits during the early postoperative period. Cutaneous temperature gauges are placed on the dressing, on a revascularized digit, and on a normal adjacent or corresponding digit to monitor room temperature, the temperature of the area in question, and the temperature of a matching, normal area. It is important to note any decrease in temperature in the revascularized segment, with critical temperature considered to be 30° C; lower readings indicate possible vascular compromise. Normal digital temperature ranges between 30° and 35° C.[16]

A Doppler scanner is used to map arterial flow through

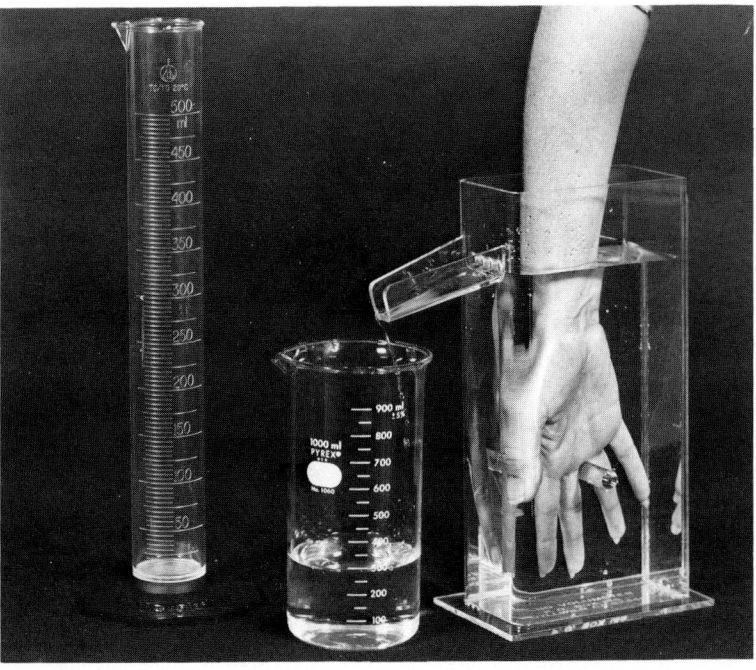

Fig. 5-6 Volumeter accuracy has been shown to be within 10 ml when used according to instructions.

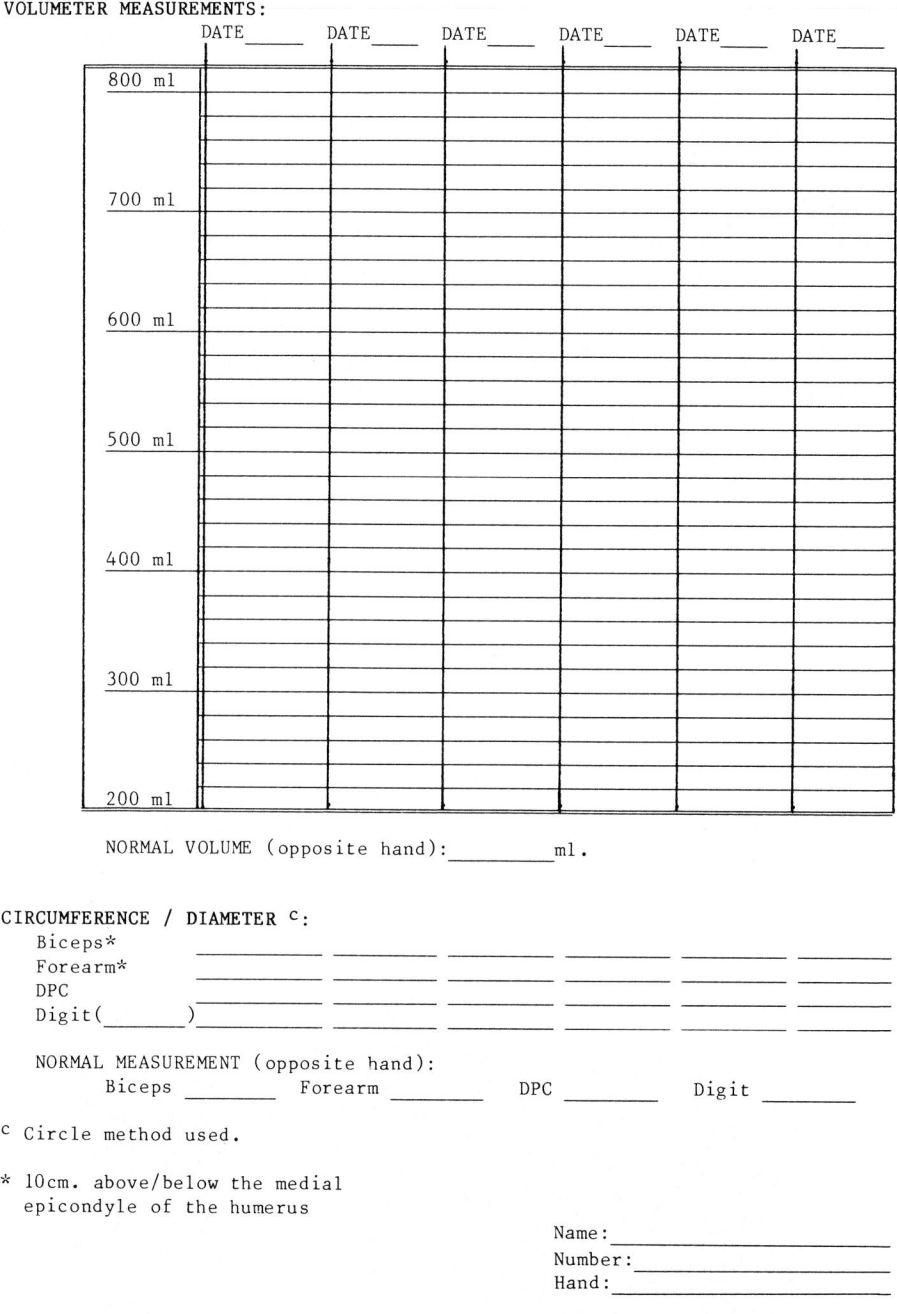

UPPER EXTREMITY ASSESSMENT BATTERY

VOLUME

VOLUMETER MEASUREMENTS:

DATE_____ DATE_____ DATE_____ DATE_____ DATE_____ DATE_____

800 ml

700 ml

600 ml

500 ml

400 ml

300 ml

200 ml

NORMAL VOLUME (opposite hand):_____ml.

CIRCUMFERENCE / DIAMETER c:
   Biceps*
   Forearm*
   DPC
   Digit(_____)

   NORMAL MEASUREMENT (opposite hand):
      Biceps _____ Forearm _____ DPC _____ Digit _____

c Circle method used.

* 10cm. above/below the medial
  epicondyle of the humerus

                        Name:_____
                        Number:_____
                        Hand:_____

Fig. 5-7 Recording of volumetric data on a graph facilitates explanations of progress for patients and students.

audible ultrasonic response to arterial pulsing. Although inconsistencies continue to plague attempts to quantify Doppler readings, to date the scanner is accepted as an important noninvasive tool in the evaluation of arterial patency.

Motion assessment instruments

Goniometric evaluation of the upper extremity is essential to monitoring articular motion and musculotendinous func-

tion (Fig. 5-8). Passive range-of-motion measurements reflect the ability of a joint to be moved through its normal arc of motion; limitations in passive motion are generally indicative of problems within the joint itself or involvement of capsular structures surrounding the joint. Active range-of-motion measurements reflect the muscle's ability to effect motion via its tendinous link to the osseous kinetic chain. Limitations in active motion may be caused by lack of tendon continuity; adhesions between the tendon and sur-

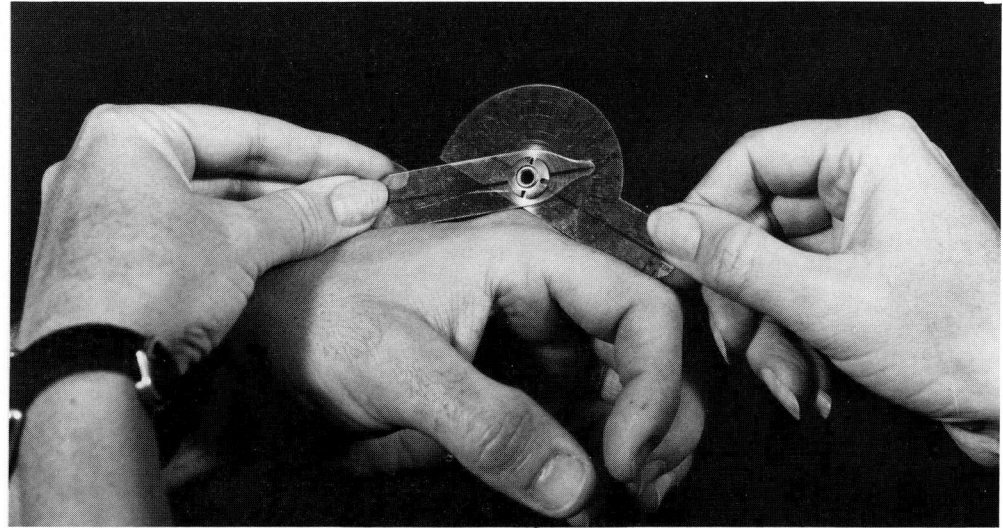

Fig. 5-8   A shortened goniometer facilitates range-of-motion measurements on the small joints of the hand.

rounding structures; constriction of the tendon sheath; inflammation of the tendon; subluxation, dislocation, or bowstringing of the tendon; or tendon attenuation. In the presence of diminished articular motion (passive), active range of motion may seem to be impaired even though tendon amplitude and muscular contraction are normal. Conversely, normal joint motion may seem to be limited when tendon gliding is reduced. Because active motion cannot exceed the passive capacity of joint motion, it is essential that both active and passive range of motion be assessed and recorded (Fig. 5-9) in a patient with upper extremity dysfunction. It is also important that the etiology of the limitation be analyzed and thoroughly understood, thus providing proper direction for therapeutic intervention.

Although influenced by a number of factors, the use of a goniometer has been shown to be more precise than visual estimates,[30,37] and reliability of goniometric measurements has been found to be accurate providing standard procedures are followed.[22,29,50,52] Accuracy of goniometric measurements has also been shown to differ according to the complexity of the joint being measured,[30,37] between active and passive measurements,[4,12,60] between the same examiner and multiple examiners,[13,29,38] and according to patient diagnosis.[5,29] Although further study is needed to address the validity of using a fixed axis device to assess joints with nonfixed axes of motion that are influenced by articular glide and rotation,[56] most clinicians accept the assumption of rotation around a central point axis when assessing joint motion.

Goniometric measurement is not technically a standardized assessment tool, but it does provide reliable and accurate information for which norms have been established.[1]

As an adjunct to the recording of individual joint motion, composite digital motion values may be computed as "total active motion" (TAM) and "total passive motion" (TPM).[3] TAM equals the sum of active flexion measurements of the metacarpophalangeal, proximal interphalangeal, and distal interphalangeal joints of a digit, minus the active extension deficits of the same three joints (Fig. 5-10). TPM is computed in a similar manner, except that passive flexion and

extension measurements are used. In addition TAM and TPM are expressed as a single numerical value, "total motion," which reflects both the extension and the flexion capacities of a single digit and thus provides a comprehensive assessment of function. (Refer to Chapter 6 for further details.)

Torque-angle range of motion, as described by Brand,[14] applies a series of increasing forces to a stiff joint to quantify measurement of passive range of motion. When translated into torque-angle curves, the composite mechanical qualities of the restraining tissues may be better understood (Fig. 5-11). Having an excellent level of repeatability, this technique provides a quantifiable method of predicting and monitoring joint response to therapeutic intervention.

The determination of isolated muscle strength through manual muscle testing[33] (Fig. 5-12) may be used to evaluate nerve lesions and the regeneration of nerves after injuries, and for preoperative evaluation for potential tendon transfers. Although criteria for grading muscle strength have been improved, eliminating much of the chance for subjective error, portions of the test continue to be subject to interpretation by the examiner. To increase interrater reliability, concentrated efforts should be made to establish a common method of conducting and interpreting manual muscle examinations. Various grading systems exist, but the two most commonly used are a numerical system (from 0 to 5) established by Seddon[54] and the ratings of "zero," "trace," "poor," "fair," "good," and "normal," recommended by the Committee on After-Effects, National Foundation for Infantile Paralysis.[33] The latter is further refined by a plus-minus system, involving the determination of half-ranges. It is important to note that because of fluctuation of muscle tone and altered reflex activity, testing of isolated muscle strength is of little value in upper motor neuron lesions such as cerebral palsy or cerebrovascular accidents.

Sensibility assessment instruments

Volitional participation is required for motor, sensibility, and dexterity testing, but the problem is compounded in the assessment of sensibility because the stimulus, when received, is also interpreted by the patient, resulting in test information that is vulnerable to bias. Although the majority of patients are cooperative, occasions arise when one is dealing with children, patients who have language problems or who exhibit mental confusion, or patients whose motives may be suspect, in which the use of a test that relies on sudomotor or sympathetic response may be helpful.[42,54,58]

The ninhydrin test identifies areas of disturbance of sweat secretion after peripheral nerve disruption. Because of the involvement of sympathetic fibers in a peripheral nerve injury, denervated skin does not produce a sweat reaction, resulting in dry skin in the distribution area of the involved nerve. Ninhydrin spray is a clear colorimetric agent that turns purple when it reacts with a small concentration of sweat. Unfortunately, sympathetic return after a peripheral nerve injury is variable, and on long-term follow-up sudomotor response does not correlate with sensibility return.[44]

Text continued on p. 74.

UPPER EXTREMITY ASSESSMENT BATTERY

RANGE OF MOTION

HAND

DATE: ———	THUMB	CHANGE +/−	INDEX	CHANGE +/−	LONG	CHANGE +/−	RING	CHANGE +/−	SMALL	CHANGE +/−
MP	( )	( )	( )	( )	( )	( )	( )	( )	( )	( )
PIP	IP ( )	( )	( )	( )	( )	( )	( )	( )	( )	( )
DIP	CMC ( )	( )	( )	( )	( )	( )	( )	( )	( )	( )
TAM (TPM)	( )	( )	( )	( )	( )	( )	( )	( )	( )	( )

DATE: ———	THUMB	CHANGE +/−	INDEX	CHANGE +/−	LONG	CHANGE +/−	RING	CHANGE +/−	SMALL	CHANGE +/−
MP	( )	( )	( )	( )	( )	( )	( )	( )	( )	( )
PIP	IP ( )	( )	( )	( )	( )	( )	( )	( )	( )	( )
DIP	CMC ( )	( )	( )	( )	( )	( )	( )	( )	( )	( )
TAM (TPM)	( )	( )	( )	( )	( )	( )	( )	( )	( )	( )

DATE: ———	THUMB	CHANGE +/−	INDEX	CHANGE +/−	LONG	CHANGE +/−	RING	CHANGE +/−	SMALL	CHANGE +/−
MP	( )	( )	( )	( )	( )	( )	( )	( )	( )	( )
PIP	IP ( )	( )	( )	( )	( )	( )	( )	( )	( )	( )
DIP	CMC ( )	( )	( )	( )	( )	( )	( )	( )	( )	( )
TAM (TPM)	( )	( )	( )	( )	( )	( )	( )	( )	( )	( )

KEY:

Active: extension/flexion

Passive: (extension/flexion)

Thumb CMC: adduction/abduction

Change: record in red

Name: _____

Number: _____

Hand: _____

Fig. 5-9 Active and passive range-of-motion and total-motion values should be recorded at appropriate intervals. Improvements or losses in motion may be expressed as plus or minus the amount of change, such as +15 or −5.

UPPER EXTREMITY ASSESSMENT BATTERY

RANGE OF MOTION

WRIST, FOREARM, ELBOW, SHOULDER

		DATE:_____	CHANGE +/−	DATE:_____	CHANGE +/−	DATE:_____	CHANGE +/−
W R I S T	EXTENSION	( )( )		( )( )		( )( )	
	FLEXION	( )( )		( )( )		( )( )	
	RADIAL DEVIATION	( )( )		( )( )		( )( )	
	ULNAR DEVIATION	( )( )		( )( )		( )( )	
F O R E A R M **E L B O W**	SUPINATION	( )( )		( )( )		( )( )	
	PRONATION	( )( )		( )( )		( )( )	
	EXTENSION	( )( )		( )( )		( )( )	
	FLEXION	( )( )		( )( )		( )( )	
S H O U L D E R	EXTENSION	( )( )		( )( )		( )( )	
	FLEXION	( )( )		( )( )		( )( )	
	ABDUCTION	( )( )		( )( )		( )( )	
	INTERNAL ROTATION	( )( )		( )( )		( )( )	
	EXTERNAL ROTATION	( )( )		( )( )		( )( )	

KEY:
Active: #°
Passive: (#°)
Change: Record in red

Name:_____
Number:_____
Extremity:_____

Fig. 5-9, cont'd   For legend see opposite page.

DATE: 6-1-82	THUMB	CHANGE +/−	INDEX	CHANGE +/−	LONG	CHANGE +/−	RING	CHANGE +/−	SMALL	CHANGE +/−
MP	( ) ( )		10/30 ( ) ( )		( ) ( )		( ) ( )		( ) ( )	
PIP	IP ( ) ( )		30/45 ( ) ( )		( ) ( )		( ) ( )		( ) ( )	
DIP	CMC ( ) ( )		0/75 ( ) ( )		( ) ( )		( ) ( )		( ) ( )	
TAM (TPM)	( ) ( )		110 ( ) ( )		( ) ( )		( ) ( )		( ) ( )	

Fig. 5-10   Total motion provides a single numerical value for composite digital motion: summation of digit flexion (30 + 45 + 75 = 150); summation of digit-extension deficits (10 + 30 + 0 = 40); flexion sum minus extension deficit sum (150 − 40 = 110); total active motion of digit = 110 degrees.

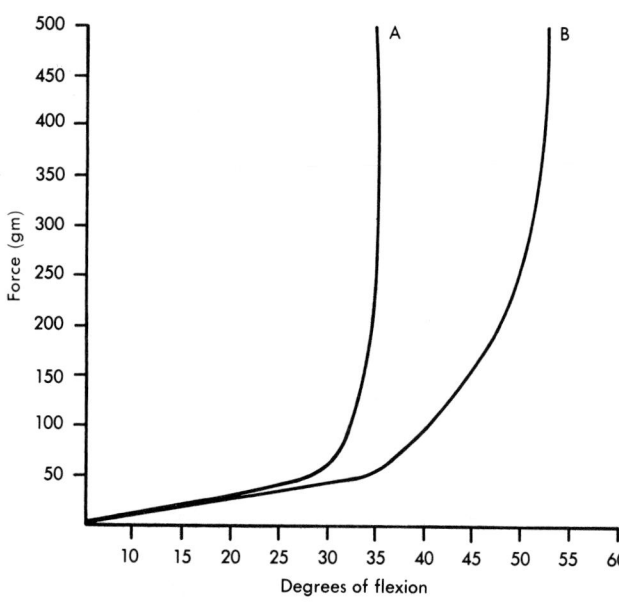

Fig. 5-11 This torque-angle, range-of-motion graph reveals that the long finger proximal interphalangeal joint, *B*, has more passive "give" than that of the index finger, *A*, indicating that the long finger may respond more readily to splinting and exercise programs. (From Fess EE and Philips CA: Hand splinting: principles and methods, ed 2, St Louis, 1987, The CV Mosby Co.)

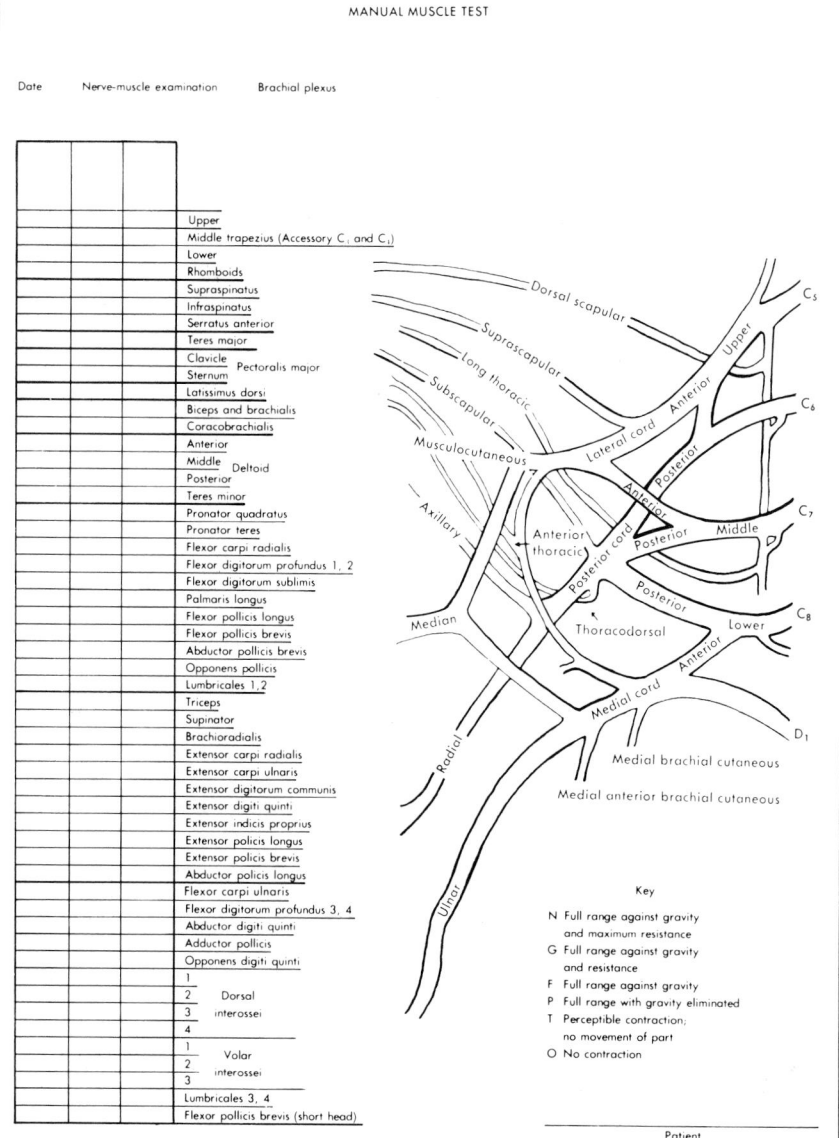

Fig. 5-12 Basic concept of this manual muscle test was inspired by a form designed by Dr. Lorraine F. Lake, Ph.D., Assistant Professor of Physical Therapy and Anatomy and Associate Director of Irene Walter Johnson Institute of Rehabilitation Medicine, Washington University School of Medicine, St Louis, Mo.

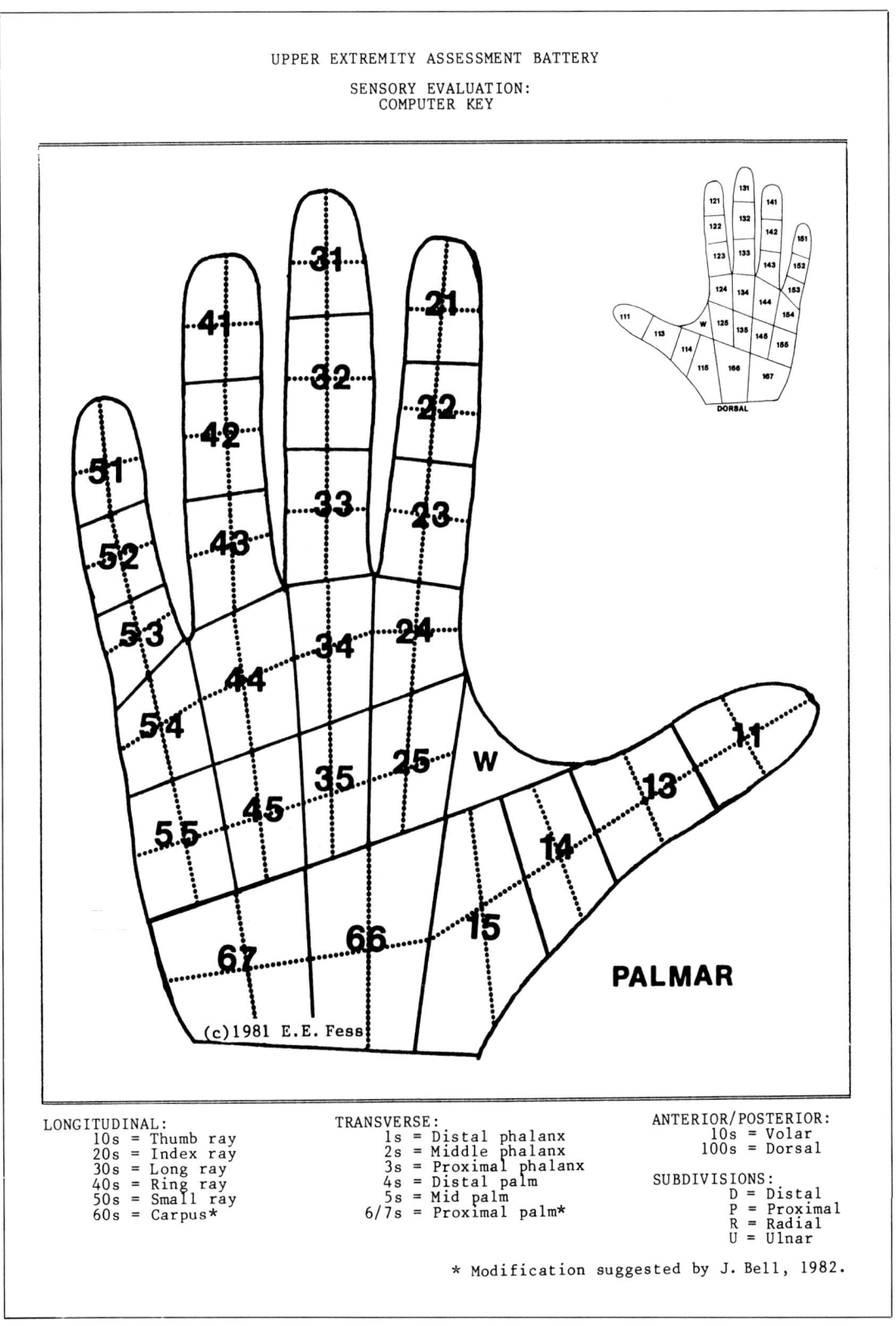

UPPER EXTREMITY ASSESSMENT BATTERY

SENSORY EVALUATION:
COMPUTER KEY

PALMAR

(c)1981 E.E. Fess

LONGITUDINAL:
    10s = Thumb ray
    20s = Index ray
    30s = Long ray
    40s = Ring ray
    50s = Small ray
    60s = Carpus*

TRANSVERSE:
    1s = Distal phalanx
    2s = Middle phalanx
    3s = Proximal phalanx
    4s = Distal palm
    5s = Mid palm
    6/7s = Proximal palm*

ANTERIOR/POSTERIOR:
    10s = Volar
    100s = Dorsal

SUBDIVISIONS:
    D = Distal
    P = Proximal
    R = Radial
    U = Ulnar

* Modification suggested by J. Bell, 1982.

Fig. 5-13   A range of sensibility tests provides a more thorough understanding of the level of dysfunction.

Continued.

UPPER EXTREMITY ASSESSMENT BATTERY

SENSORY EVALUATION:
TINEL'S SIGN & TROPHIC CHANGES

TINEL'S SIGN	NINHYDRIN/WRINKLE
DATE_____	
DATE_____	
DATE_____	

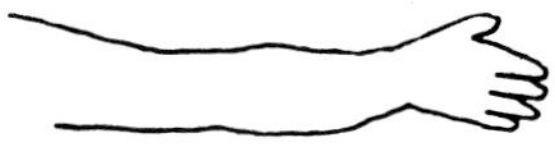

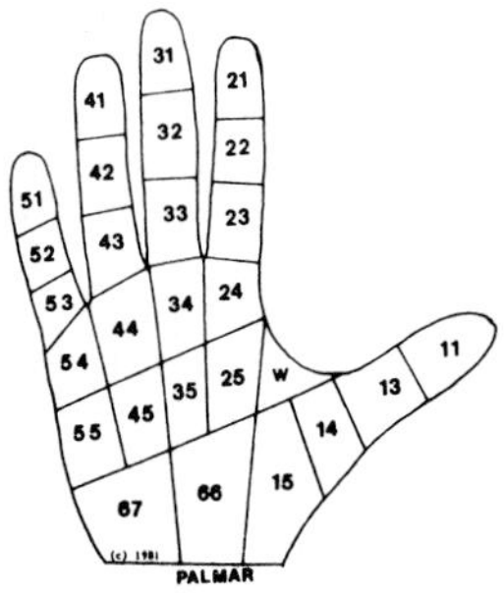

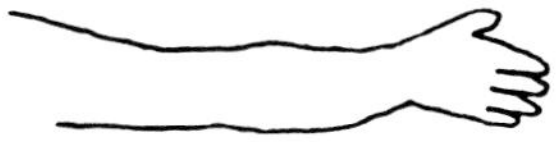

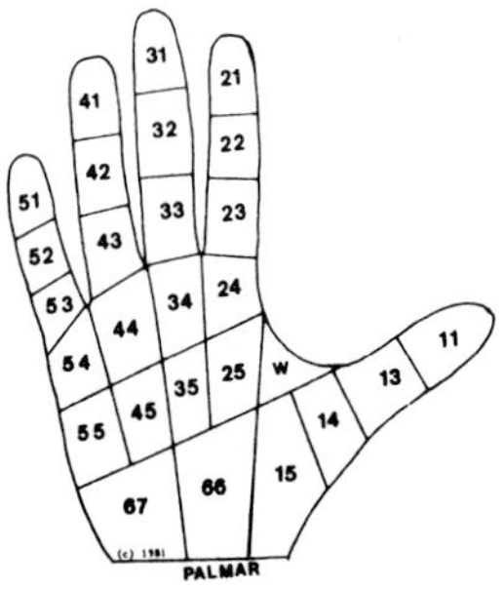

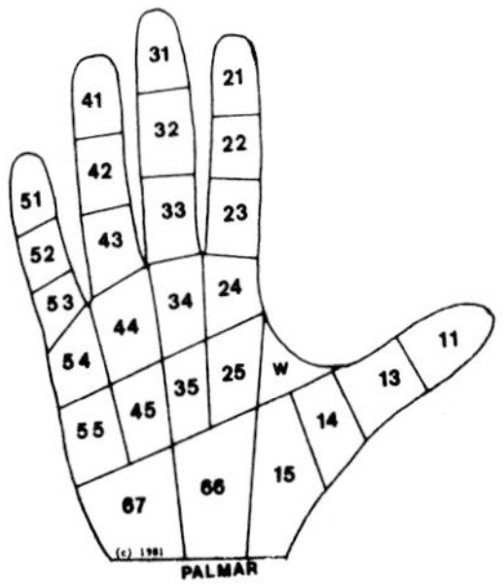

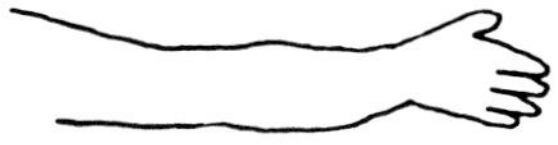

KEY:

[X] Tinel's

[:::] Ninhydrin

[///] Wrinkle

NAME_____

NUMBER_____

HAND_____

Fig. 5-13, cont'd For legend see p. 69.   *Continued.*

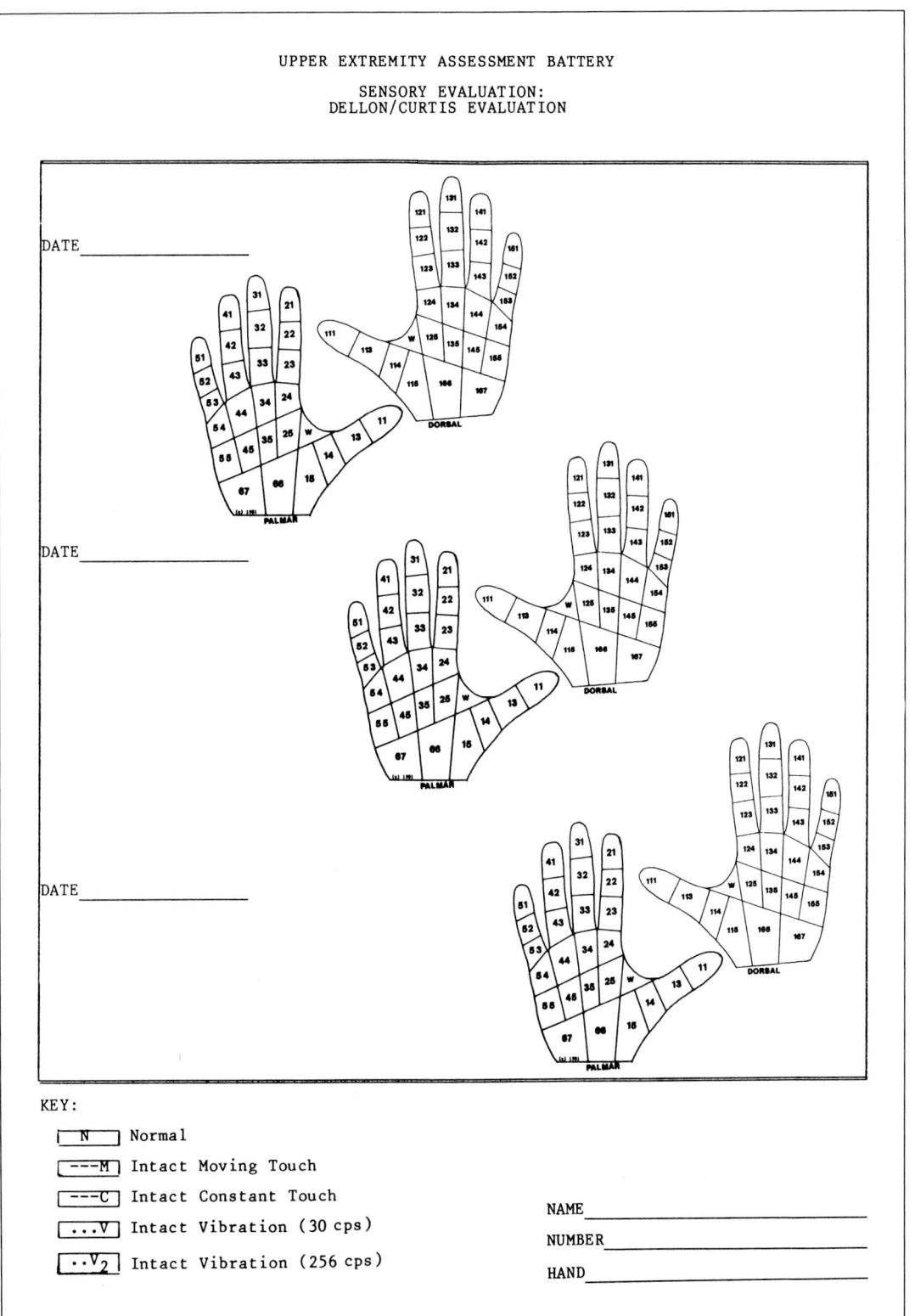

Fig. 5-13, cont'd   For legend see p. 69.   *Continued.*

UPPER EXTREMITY ASSESSMENT BATTERY

SENSORY EVALUATION:
SEMMES-WEINSTEIN CALIBRATED MONOFILAMENTS

PALMAR/DORSAL (circle):

DATE:	THUMB 1 U – R	INDEX 2 U – R	LONG 3 U – R	RING 4 U – R	SMALL 5 U – R
1					
2					
3					
4					
5					
6/7	///// 6_			6_	

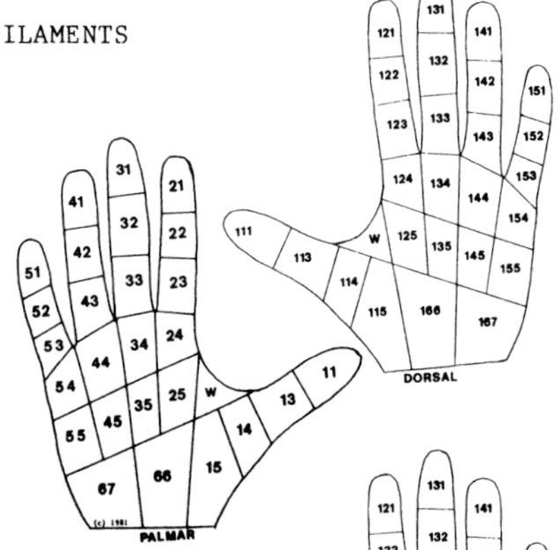

PALMAR/DORSAL (circle):

DATE:	THUMB 1 U – R	INDEX 2 U – R	LONG 3 U – R	RING 4 U – R	SMALL 5 U – R
1					
2					
3					
4					
5					
6/7	///// 6_			6_	

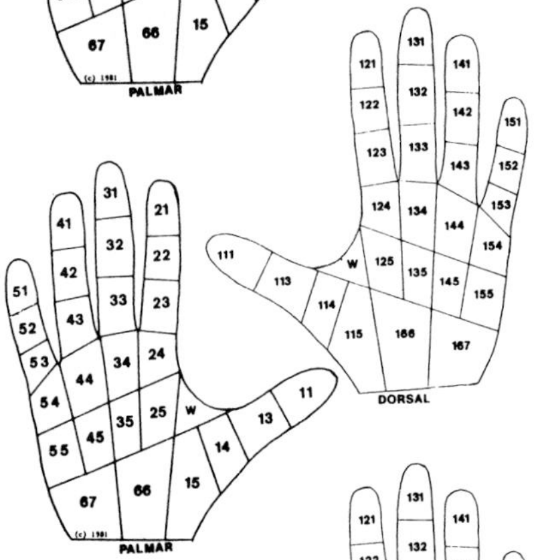

PALMAR/DORSAL (circle):

DATE:	THUMB 1 U – R	INDEX 2 U – R	LONG 3 U – R	RING 4 U – R	SMALL 5 U – R
1					
2					
3					
4					
5					
6/7	///// 6_			6_	

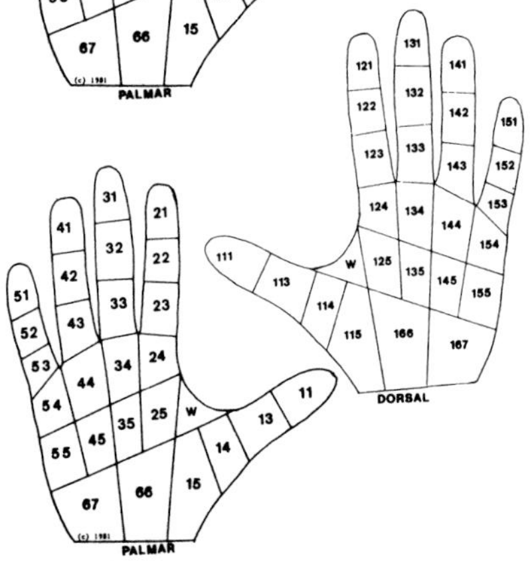

KEY:*

		Filament	Pressure (gm/mm^2)
	Normal	1.65-2.83	1.45- 4.86
Blue	Diminished light touch	3.22-3.61	11.1 - 17.7
Purple	Diminished protective sensation	3.84-4.31	19.3 - 33.1
Red	Loss of protective sensation	4.56-6.65	47.3 -439.0
Red-lined	Untestable	6.65	439.0

*Levine, S., Pearsall, G., & Ruderman, R.: J Hand Surg, 3:211, 1978.

NAME_____

NUMBER_____

HAND_____

Fig. 5-13, cont'd For legend see p. 69.

UPPER EXTREMITY ASSESSMENT BATTERY

SENSORY EVALUATION:
2 POINT DISCRIMINATION

PALMAR/DORSAL (circle):

DATE:	THUMB 1		INDEX 2		LONG 3		RING 4		SMALL 5	
	U	R	U	R	U	R	U	R	U	R
1										
2										
3										
4										
5										
6/7	/////		6				6			

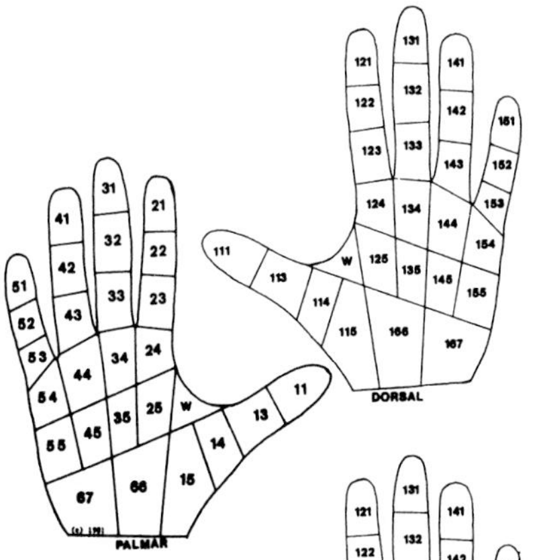

PALMAR/DORSAL (circle):

DATE:	THUMB 1		INDEX 2		LONG 3		RING 4		SMALL 5	
	U	R	U	R	U	R	U	R	U	R
1										
2										
3										
4										
5										
6/7	/////		6				6			

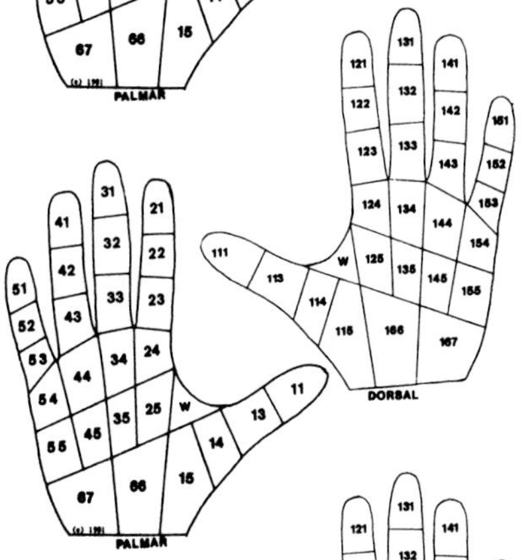

PALMAR/DORSAL (circle):

DATE:	THUMB 1		INDEX 2		LONG 3		RING 4		SMALL 5	
	U	R	U	R	U	R	U	R	U	R
1										
2										
3										
4										
5										
6/7	/////		6				6			

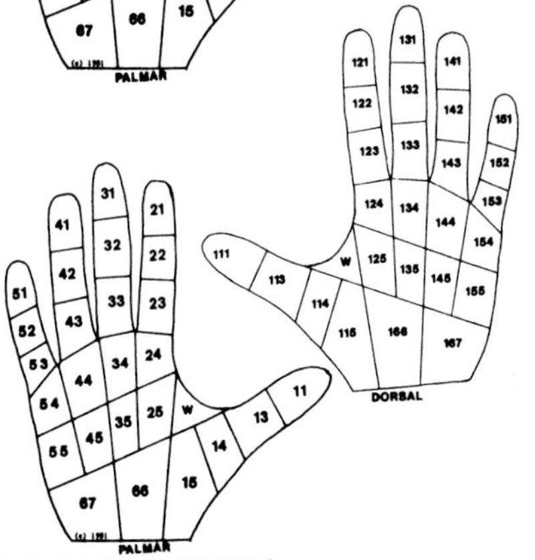

KEY:*

	Normal	Less than 6mm
Blue	Fair	6-10 mm
Purple	Poor	11-15 mm
Orange	Protective	One point perceived
Orange-lined	Anesthetic	No point perceived

*ASSH: The hand — examination and diagnosis, Aurora, Colorado, 1978.

NAME_____

NUMBER_____

HAND_____

Fig. 5-13, cont'd   For legend see p. 69.

Continued.

The wrinkle test[45] is based on a similar concept of sympathetic fiber involvement in peripheral nerve injuries, in that denervated palmar skin, as opposed to normal skin, does not wrinkle when soaked in warm water. As with sweating, palmar wrinkling has diminishing correlation to sensory function as the postinjury period increases, and has no correlation to sensory capacity in nerve compression injuries.[46] Inclusion of a sympathetic response test in an assessment battery (Fig. 5-13) for use with specific patients is helpful, but it should not be relied on as a primary sensibility assessment instrument.

The ability to detect a punctate stimulus is the initial and most simple level of function in the hierarchy of sensibility capacity of the hand. *Detection* requires that the patient be able to distinguish a single-point stimulus from normal-ly occurring atmospheric background stimuli. The normal touch force threshold (using Semmes-Weinstein monofilaments[55]) (Fig. 5-14) is considered to be approximately 4.86 g/mm^2 (note: this is pressure, not force); to be completely valid, a touch force assessment instrument should be able to produce stimuli that measure less than the normal threshold level. As testing instruments the monofilaments are unique in their abilities to actually control the amount of force applied, and as such are important to the hand specialist's assessment armamentarium[7] (Fig. 5-15). Bell and Tomancik[11] have shown that from set to set and from examiner to examiner the monofilaments produce consistently repeatable forces within a predictable range, providing their lengths and diameters are correct. They also noted that "the heaviest and lightest application forces of

UPPER EXTREMITY ASSESSMENT BATTERY

SENSORY EVALUATION:
MOVING 2 POINT DISCRIMINATION & RIDGE TEST

MOVING TWO POINT DISCRIMINATION

RIDGE TEST

PALMAR/DORSAL (circle):

DATE:	THUMB 1 U — R	INDEX 2 U — R	LONG 3 U — R	RING 4 U — R	SMALL 5 U — R
1					
2					
3					
4					
5					
6/7	//// 6 —		6 —		

PALMAR/DORSAL (circle):

DATE:	THUMB 1 U — R	INDEX 2 U — R	LONG 3 U — R	RING 4 U — R	SMALL 5 U — R
1					
2					
3					
4					
5					
6/7	//// 6 —		6 —		

PALMAR/DORSAL (circle):

DATE:	THUMB 1 U — R	INDEX 2 U — R	LONG 3 U — R	RING 4 U — R	SMALL 5 U — R
1					
2					
3					
4					
5					
6/7	//// 6 —		6 —		

(mm)

PALMAR/DORSAL (circle):

DATE:	THUMB 1 U — R	INDEX 2 U — R	LONG 3 U — R	RING 4 U — R	SMALL 5 U — R
1					
2					
3					
4					
5					
6/7	//// 6 —		6 —		

PALMAR/DORSAL (circle):

DATE:	THUMB 1 U — R	INDEX 2 U — R	LONG 3 U — R	RING 4 U — R	SMALL 5 U — R
1					
2					
3					
4					
5					
6/7	//// 6 —		6 —		

PALMAR/DORSAL (circle):

DATE:	THUMB 1 U — R	INDEX 2 U — R	LONG 3 U — R	RING 4 U — R	SMALL 5 U — R
1					
2					
3					
4					
5					
6/7	//// 6 —		6 —		

(cm)

NAME _____

NUMBER _____

HAND _____

Fig. 5-13, cont'd For legend see p. 69.

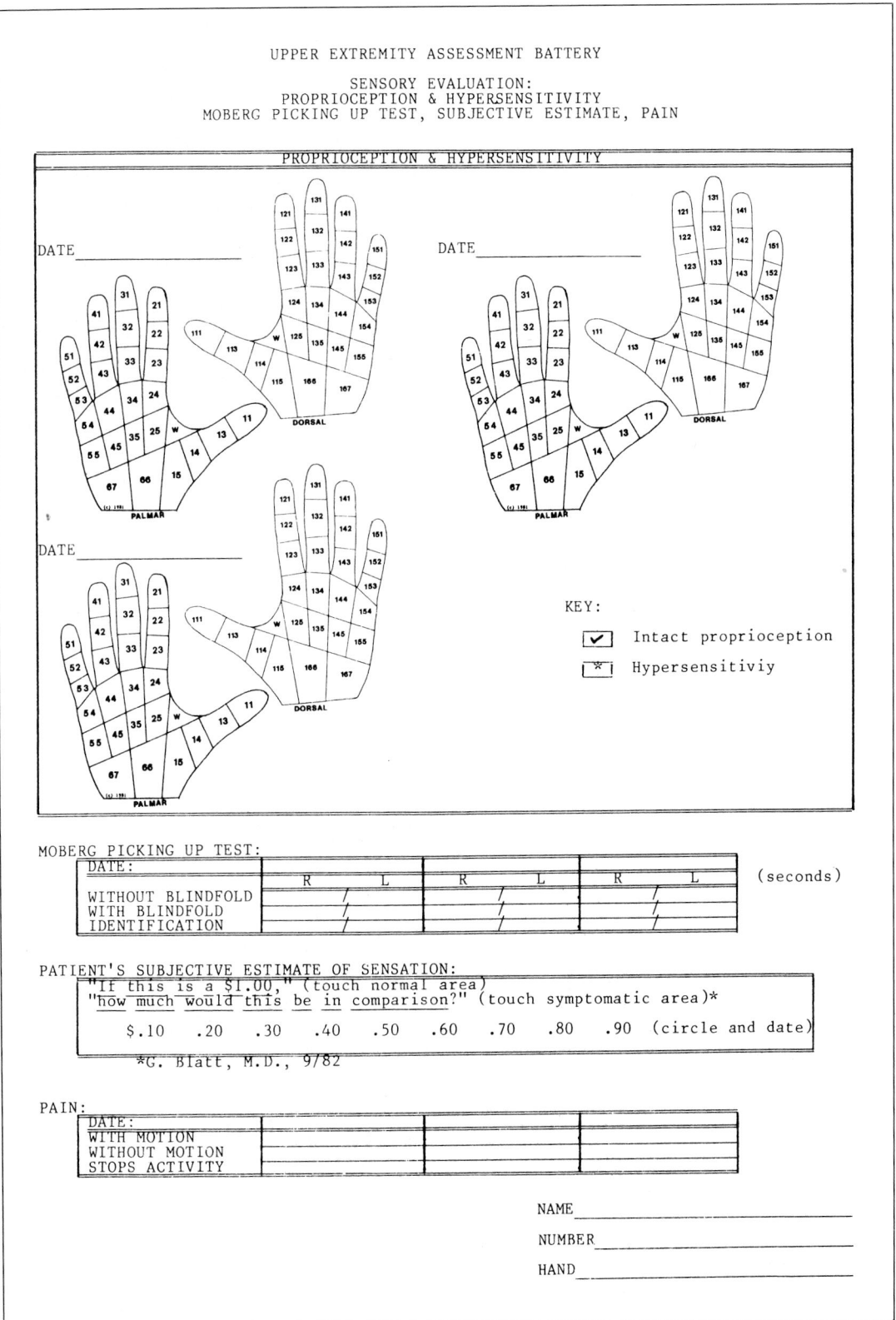

UPPER EXTREMITY ASSESSMENT BATTERY

SENSORY EVALUATION:
PROPRIOCEPTION & HYPERSENSITIVITY
MOBERG PICKING UP TEST, SUBJECTIVE ESTIMATE, PAIN

PROPRIOCEPTION & HYPERSENSITIVITY

DATE_____

DATE_____

DATE_____

KEY:

☑ Intact proprioception
[*] Hypersensitiviy

MOBERG PICKING UP TEST:

DATE:	R	L	R	L	R	L	(seconds)
WITHOUT BLINDFOLD							
WITH BLINDFOLD							
IDENTIFICATION							

PATIENT'S SUBJECTIVE ESTIMATE OF SENSATION:
"If this is a $1.00," (touch normal area)
"how much would this be in comparison?" (touch symptomatic area)*

$.10   .20   .30   .40   .50   .60   .70   .80   .90   (circle and date)

*G. Blatt, M.D., 9/82

PAIN:

DATE:			
WITH MOTION			
WITHOUT MOTION			
STOPS ACTIVITY			

NAME_____

NUMBER_____

HAND_____

Fig. 5-13, cont'd   For legend see p. 69.

Fig. 5-14 The monofilament collapses when a given force, dependent on filament diameter and length, is reached, controlling the magnitude of the applied touch pressure.

some filaments overlapped with those of their neighbors, lending support to the concept that the use of fewer filaments does not necessarily result in loss of test sensitivity, and, in fact, can make the test more reproducible." The monofilaments are now available in the original 20-filament set and also in a 5-filament mini set.*

Although the monofilaments produce the most sensitive and reliable data of all the clinical sensibility assessment instruments currently available, they are not without problems, including variance in tip geometry,[8] and force changes with atmospheric conditions.[36,41]

The Dellon-Curtis evaluation[19] consists of four categories, which assess moving touch, constant touch, flutter (30 cps vibration), and vibration (256 cps vibration). Controversy exists concerning this examination, with some neurophysiologists and neurologists questioning the use of vibration, because of a lack of stimulus specificity, to evaluate nerve status in a relatively small and confined space such as the

*North Coast Medical, Inc., Campbell, Calif.

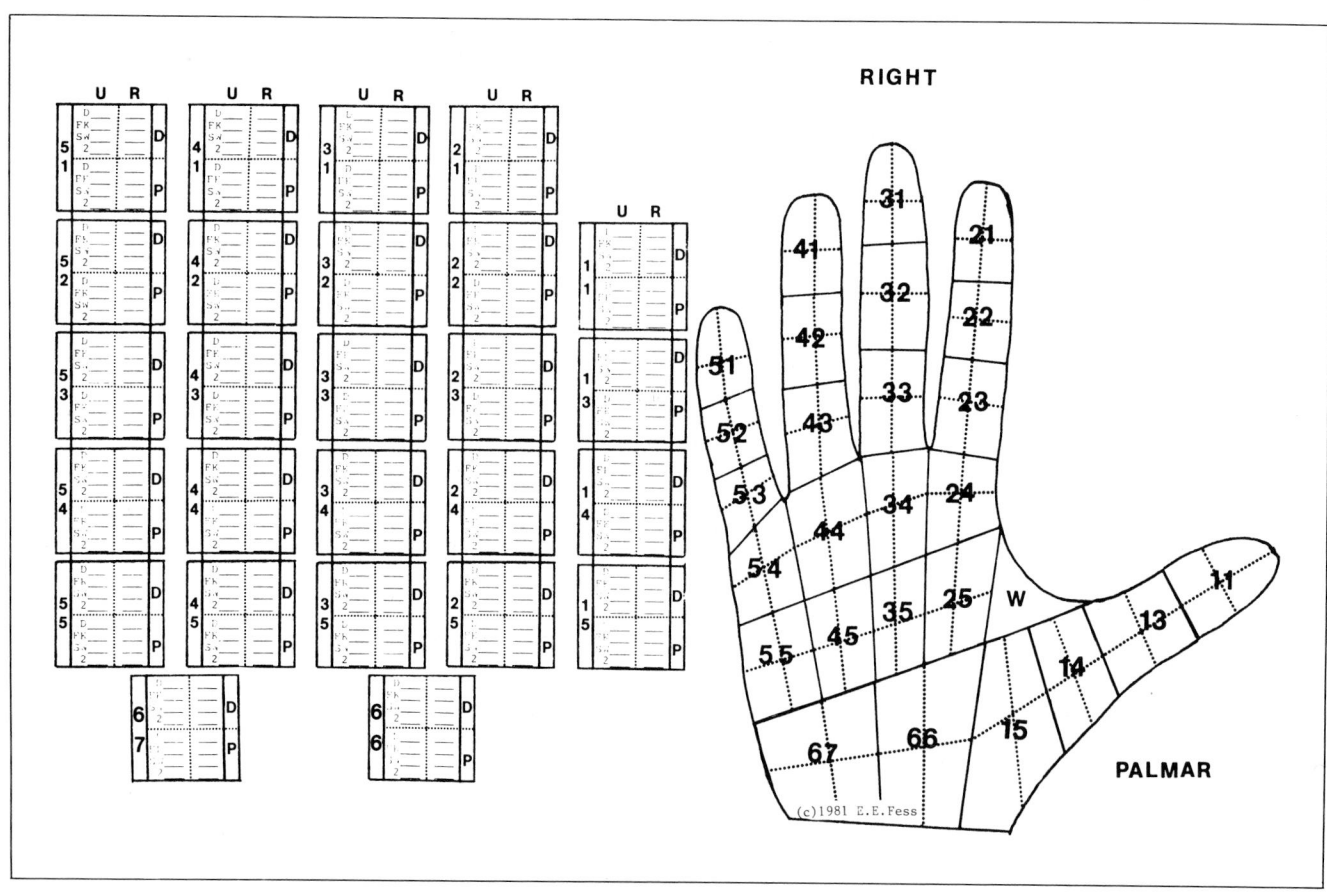

Fig. 5-15 Research forms may differ from those used for patient treatment. This form, used for a sensibility instrumentation study, requires explicit data on four instruments. Data from follow-up evaluations for research are often recorded on separate forms, whereas clinical follow-up data are included in an adjacent area on the form used for the initial evaluation.

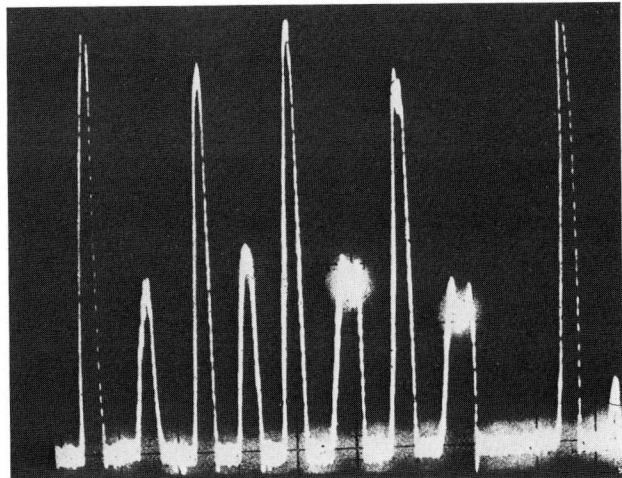

Fig. 5-16 Monitoring the applied force between one and two points, a transducer and oscilloscope graphically show the discrepancies in the amount of force applied between one and two points in a two-point discrimination test by an experienced hand specialist using skin deformation and lack of blanching as the clinical criteria. (Courtesy Judith A. Bell and W. Buford, Carville, La.)

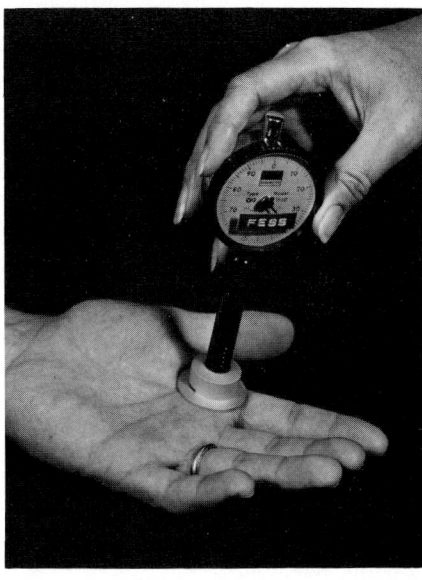

Fig. 5-17 A search for an instrument that will measure skin hardness involves instrumentation studies for reliability and validity.

hand.[21,35] Bell-Krotoski and Buford[10] found that the applied force produced by either size tuning fork is uncontrolled and oscillation is influenced by the random vibration of the hand of the person holding the instrument, by the strike force used to start oscillation, and by how long oscillation persists. Additionally, they noted that force amplitude of a tuning fork is more uncontrolled with side application than with tip application. Physicists also report that the use of a tuning fork in attitudes other than perpendicular to the surface of application changes the fine harmonic vibratory stimulus to a compression stimulus,[41] which may elicit a pain response.

Discrimination is the second level in the sensibility assessment continuum. The ability to perceive that stimulus A differs from stimulus B involves the capacity to detect each stimulus as a separate entity and to distinguish between them. Discrimination requires finer reception acuity and more judgment on the part of the patient than does detection, which is the first level in the continuum.

The two-point discrimination test[3,57,62] is the most commonly used method of assessing sensibility of the hand. In the performance of the test, there is some disagreement as to whether it is preferable to begin the test with a great distance or a small distance between the two points, and the number of correct responses required varies slightly among examiners. Moving two-point discrimination, described by Dellon,[18] adds the variable of motion to the test.

The two-point discrimination tests have some problems in regard to instrumentation criteria. Bell and Buford[9,10] found that even among experienced hand surgeons and therapists, the differences between the amount of force applied to the one point and that applied to two points easily exceeded the resolution or sensitivity threshold for normal sensation (Fig. 5-16). This lack of force consistency is amplified with the introduction of motion in the moving two-point test. Directly influenced by cutaneous topography,

applied forces were found to be 400 times the sensitivity of normal cutaneous receptors. They also discovered that because of the varying pressures applied, interrater reliability was poor, perhaps explaining the lack of agreement in reporting, and the multiplicity of current clinical sensibility assessment tools.

In contrast, Dellon and others[20] reported high interrater reliability using standard testing methods and a commercially available disk two-point discriminator instrument. However, their study involved only two examiners. More study is needed using multiple examiners in different conditions before conclusive statements may be made about interrater reliability. Even more important, before examiner reliability can be addressed, instrument reliability must first be documented in the laboratory. If this is not done, inherent flaws will be propagated and probably amplified because of less stringent controls throughout the process of investigating the clinical issues of examiner reliability, test validity, and the gathering of normative data.[27]

The Ridge device[47,49] introduces the important concept of control of the amount of tissue displacement instead of control of applied force. Sensibility instruments should control either the force variable or the displacement variable; and although most aesthesiometers are oriented toward regulation of force, the ridge device is unique among currently available assessment tools because of its displacement design. Consisting of a rectangular piece of plastic, from the center of which a narrow ridge gradually rises to a height of 1.5 mm, the ridge device is believed to be useful in identifying patients whose two-point discrimination is between 8 mm and 12 mm. Instrumentation problems with the ridge device include validity and reliability issues. Renfrew[49] reported that intelligence directly skewed test results, with more intelligent patients achieving better scores. Additionally, lack of specificity relating to measurement of the amount of tissue deformation is a detracting factor, in that the ridge rises from 0 to 1.5 mm without interruption, significantly decreasing the potential for accuracy and precision of readings and thus limiting interrater reliability.

Quantification is the third level of the sensory capacity; it involves the organizing of tactile stimuli according to degree. For example, a patient may be asked which of several alternatives is roughest, most irregular, or smoothest. *Recognition,* the final and most complicated sensibility level, is the ability to identify objects. Currently there are no sensibility instruments specific to these two areas, although some of the sensory reeducation methods that are used as treatment techniques[63] incorporate the basic concepts of quantification and recognition. For example, the Moberg picking-up test[42] requires the patient to pick up a series of 10 to 12 small objects of various sizes from a table surface and place them in a small container, using first the normal hand and then the symptomatic hand. The picking-up test, which may be adapted to include recognition variables, is an excellent example of a timed observational test in which the patient is his own normal.

The major problem in assessing sensibility is cortical modification of thresholds. With the exception of the sudomotor tests, all of the clinical sensibility evaluation instruments currently available have the potential for producing subjective, biased information. Another variable is callous formation (Fig. 5-17) or the hardness of the cutaneous surface. Influencing the amount of force transferred to sensory receptors, keratin layers decrease the applied force of a stimulus by increasing the area of force application. Therefore, the patient's occupation becomes a factor in the assessment of hand sensibility. Age and intelligence should also be considered. In addition, recent studies indicate that specific receptors cannot be isolated with the unrefined assessment instruments of today's technology.[9,21]

Sensibility assessment instrumentation is in an early developmental phase. Representing a final frontier that should be given a high priority, the generation of instruments that better evaluate sensibility of the hand will significantly influence the scope and direction of the profession in the next several decades. The inherent properties of instruments, current and future, must be analyzed and evaluated in terms of statistical reliability and validity. To progress, we must first be able to measure. To measure, we must look carefully at our tools. (Refer to Chapters 42, 43, and 44 for specific test protocols.)

Function assessment instruments

Grip strength may be measured with a commercially available hydraulic dynamometer (Fig. 5-18). Developed by Bechtol[6] and recommended in a study of grip assessment instruments by the California Medical Association,[34] the Jamar dynamometer has been shown to be a reliable test instrument, providing calibration is maintained[25] and standard positioning of test subjects is followed.[2,39,40] In a recent study of 51 Jamar dynamometers, 20 new and 31 used, 16 of the new dynamometers had laboratory intrainstrument reliability correlation coefficients ranging from $+0.9999$ to $+0.9994$, indicating a high degree of reliability. However, the same study found that of the 51 dynamometers evaluated, 54% of the used and 23% of the new dynamometers needed to be recalibrated.[26] Schmidt and Toews[53] reported proportional correlations between grip strength and height, weight, and age, and noted that the grip strength of the minor hand was equal to or stronger than that of the dominant hand in 28% of the normal population. Pryce[48] studied the effects of wrist position on grip strength and found that the strongest grips occurred with the wrist in 0 to 15 degrees extension. In 1978 the Clinical Assessment Committee of the American Society for Surgery of the Hand recommended that the second handle position be used in determining grip strength and that the average of three trials be recorded.[3]. Fatigue has been shown not to be an influencing factor in protocols if a 5-minute rest is provided after completion of each three-trial series.[23] Of significant importance is the concept that grip strength changes according to the size of the object being grasped. Normal adult grip values for the five consecutive handle positions consistently create a bell-shaped curve, with the first position being the least advantageous for strong grip, followed by the fifth and fourth positions; the strongest grip values occur at the third and second handle positions.[6,23,43] If inconsistent handle positions are used to assess patient progress, normal alterations in grip readings may be erroneously interpreted as advances or declines in progress. Knowledge of this normal grip curve may also be of assistance in identifying patients whose motivation is questionable. Strokes and Murray[43] describe a clinical correspondence between "flat" handle position curves and patients who were found to have "significant personality problems."

The Jamar's capacity as an evaluation instrument, the effects of protocol, and the ramifications of the instrument's use have been analyzed by many investigators over the years. Although not a standardized assessment tool, it does provide consistent and accurate information, when calibration is maintained. A major drawback is the lack of large population norms for the commercially available model. Unfortunately, the Schmidt-Toews study of 1200 subjects was based on Jamar dynamometers that were altered with an application of a sand-paint mixture to the handles. This invalidates the use of the resultant norms, except when

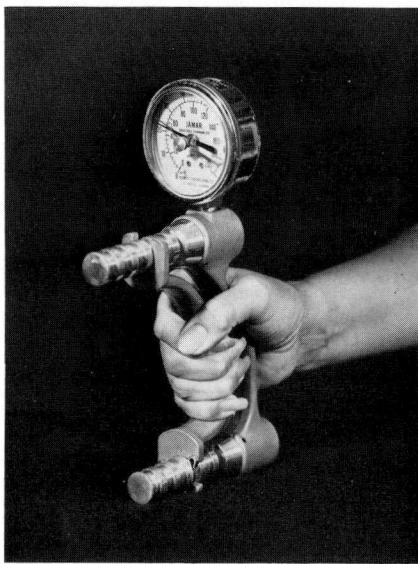

Fig. 5-18 The Jamar dynamometer provides reliable and accurate measurement of grip strength.

compared with values from a similarly altered dynamometer.

Pinch strength may be measured with a commercially available pinchometer. Three types of pinch are usually assessed: (1) prehension of the thumb pulp to the lateral aspect of the index middle phalanx (key, lateral, or pulp-to-side); (2) pulp of the thumb to pulps of the index and long fingers (three-jaw chuck, three-point chuck); and (3) thumb tip to the tip of index finger (tip-to-tip). Lateral is the strongest of the three types of pinch, followed by three-jaw chuck. Tip-to-tip is a positioning pinch used in activities requiring fine coordination rather than power. As with grip measurements, the mean value of three trials is recorded, and comparisons are made with the opposite hand.

Standardized tests for assessing manual dexterity and coordination are available in several levels of difficulty, allowing the examiner to screen and choose instruments that best suit the needs and abilities of individual patients. When a standardized instrument is being used, it is imperative not to deviate from the method, equipment, and sequencing delineated in the test instructions. The calibration, reliability, and validity of the test are determined using defined items and techniques, and any change in the stipulated pattern renders the resultant information invalid and meaningless. Utilizing a standardized test as a teaching or training device in therapy also excludes its use as an assessment instrument, because of skewing of data.

Of the tests available, the Jebson-Taylor[32] hand function test requires the least amount of extremity coordination, and it is inexpensive to assemble and easy to administer and score. The test consists of seven subtests: (1) writing, (2) card turning, (3) picking up small objects, (4) simulated feeding, (5) stacking, (6) picking up large light-weight objects, and (7) picking up large heavy objects. The Jebson norms are categorized according to maximum time, hand dominance, age, and gender. The capacity to measure gross coordination makes this test an excellent instrument to assess individuals whose severity of involvement precludes the use of many of the other coordination tests, which often require very fine prehension patterns.

Based on placing blocks into spaces on a board, the Minnesota Rate of Manipulation Tests (MRMT) include five activities: (1) placing, (2) turning, (3) displacing, (4) one-hand turning and placing, and (5) two-hand turning and placing. The MRMT, originally designed for assessment of personnel for jobs requiring arm-hand dexterity, is another excellent example of a test that measures gross coordination and dexterity, making it applicable to many of the needs encountered in hand rehabilitation. The norms of this instrument are based on more than 11,000 subjects.

Requiring prehension of small pins, washers, and collars, the Purdue Pegboard Test[59] evaluates finer coordination than the previously discussed instruments. This test's assessment categories are (1) right hand, (2) left hand, (3) both hands, (4) right, left, and both, and (5) assembly. The normative data are presented in categories based on gender and type of job: male and female applicants for assembly jobs, male and femal applicants for general factory work, female applicants for electronics production work, male utility service workers, and so on.

In terms of a psychomotor taxonomy, all of the previously described tests assess activities that are classified as skilled movements. Evaluating compound adaptive skills, the Crawford Small Parts Dexterity Test adds another dimension to hand function assessment by introducing tools into the test protocol. Increasing the level of difficulty, this test requires subjects to control implements in addition to their hands. The test involves the use of tweezers and screwdriver to assemble pins, collars, and small screws on the test board. This test is related to activities requiring very fine coordination, such as engraving and the assembly or adjustment of clocks, watches, office machines, and other intricate devices. The O'Connor[31] also requires the use of a tool to manipulate small pegs on a pegboard.

Other hand coordination and dexterity testing instruments are available. These should be carefully evaluated in terms of the criteria for standardization previously outlined in this chapter, to ensure that they have been proved to measure appropriately and accurately. Although many tests claim to be standardized, close scrutiny often indicates that they are not. (Refer to Chapter 7.)

The extent to which activities of daily living are assessed depends on the type of clientele treated by the particular rehabilitation center. In a situation oriented toward treatment of trauma injuries, the need for extensive ADL evaluation and training would not be as great as it would in a center whose case load consisted primarily of arthritic patients. To date, ADL tests have not been standardized, and they are limited to observational types of tests, the results of which may be quantified by timing specific tasks. A general ADL test may easily be refined to include only those activities that require the use of the upper extremities. If this is done, however, it is important to make provisions for assessment and treatment of lower extremity problems noted during the course of the test.

Assessment of a patient's potential to return to work is generally based on a combination of standardized and observational tests, knowledge of the specific work situation, insight into the patient's motivational and psychologic references, and understanding of the complexities of normal and disabled hands in general. Although its importance has been acknowledged in the past, vocational assessment of the upper extremity injury patient is being given a higher priority in many of the major hand centers in the country. Treatment no longer ends with the achievement of skeletal stability, wound healing, and a plateau of motion and sensibility. This shift in emphasis has been the result, in large part, of the contributions of the Hand Rehabilitation Center in Philadelphia, and of the hand therapist who is in charge of its physical capacity area, Patricia Baxter, O.T.R. Chapters 7 and 95 in this book describe the specific programs that she has been instrumental in developing.

CONCLUSION

Evaluation with instruments that measure accurately allows physicians and therapists to correctly identify hand pathology and dysfunction, assess the effects of treatment, and realistically apprise patients of their progress. Accurate assessment data also permit analysis of treatment modalities for effectiveness, provide a foundation for professional communication through research, and eventually influence the scope and direction of the profession as a whole. Because of their relationship to the kind of information obtained, assessment tools cannot be chosen irresponsibly. The choice of tools will directly influence the quality of individual treatment and the quality of understanding between hand specialists. Criteria exist for identifying instruments that can be depended on to measure accurately when used by different evaluators, and from session to session. Unless the results of a "home-brewed" test are statistically analyzed, the test is tried on large numbers of normal subjects, and the results are analyzed again, it is naive to assume that such a test provides meaningful information. Current tools may be better understood by checking their reliability and validity levels with bioengineering technology, and statisticians may be of assistance in devising protocols that will lead to more refined and accurate information. We as hand specialists have a responsibility to our patients and to our colleagues to continue to critique the instruments we use in terms of their capacities as measurement tools. Without assessment, we cannot treat, we cannot communicate, and we cannot progress.

REFERENCES

1. American Academy of Orthopedic Surgeons: Joint motion: method of measuring and recording, Chicago, 1965, The Academy.
2. American Society of Hand Therapists: Clinical assessment recommendations, Garner, NC, 1981, The Society.
3. American Society for Surgery of the Hand: The hand: examination and diagnosis, New York, 1983, Churchill Livingstone.
4. Amis AA and Miller JH: The elbow, Clin Rheum Dis 8:571, 1982.
5. Ashton BB, Pickles B, and Roll JW: Reliability of goniometric measurements of hip motion in spastic cerebral palsy, Dev Med Child Neurol 20:87, 1978.
6. Bechtol CD: Grip test: use of a dynamometer with adjustable handle spacing, J Bone Joint Surg 36A:820, 1954.
7. Bell J: Sensibility evaluation. In Hunter J, Schneider L, Mackin E, and Callahan A, editors: Rehabilitation of the hand, ed 2, St Louis, 1984, The CV Mosby Co.
8. Bell J: Symposium: assessment of levels of cutaneous sensibility, United States Public Health Service Hospital, Carville, La, 1980.
9. Bell J and Buford W: The force/time relationship of clinically used sensory testing instruments. Presented at the thirty-seventh annual meeting of the American Society for Surgery of the Hand, New Orleans, 1982.
10. Bell-Krotoski J and Buford WL: The force/time relationship of clinically used sensory testing instruments, J Hand Ther 1:76, 1988.
11. Bell J and Tomancik E: Repeatability of testing with Semmes-Weinstein monofilaments, J Hand Surg 12A:155, 1987.
12. Bird HA and Stowe J: The wrist, Clin Rheum Dis 8:559, 1982.
13. Boone DC: Reliability of goniometric measurements, Phys Ther 58:1355, 1978.
14. Brand P: Clinical mechanics of the hand, St Louis, 1985, The CV Mosby Co.
15. Brand P and Wood H: Hand volumeter instruction sheet, U.S. Public Health Service Hospital, Carville La.
16. Bright D and Wright S: Postoperative management in replantation. In American Academy of Orthopedic Surgeons: Symposium on microsurgery: practical use in orthopaedics, St Louis, 1979, The CV Mosby Co.
17. Creelnan G: Report on hand volumeter: accuracy and sensitivity of measurements, Idyllwild, Calif, 1979, Engraving Experts, Medical Supply Division.
18. Dellon A: The moving two-point discrimination test: clinical evaluation of the quickly-adapting fiber receptor system, J Hand Surg 3:474, 1978.
19. Dellon A, Curtis R, and Edgerton M: Reeducation of sensation in the hand after nerve injury and repair, Plast Reconstr Surg 53:297, 1974.
20. Dellon AL, Mackinnon SE, and Crosby PM: Reliability of two-point discrimination measurements, J Hand Surg 12A:693, 1987.
21. Dyck PJ and others: Clinical vs quantitative evaluation of cutaneous sensation, Arch Neurol 33:651, 1976.
22. Ekstrand J and others: Lower extremity goniometric measurements: a study to determine their reliability, Arch Phys Med Rehabil 63:171, 1982.
23. Fess EE: The effects of Jamar dynamometer handle position and test protocol on normal grip strength. Procedures of the American Society of Hand Therapists, J Hand Surg 7:308, 1982.
24. Fess EE: The need for reliability and validity in hand assessment instruments, J Hand Surg 11A:621, 1986.
25. Fess EE: A method for checking Jamar dynamometer calibration, J Hand Ther 1:28, 1987.
26. Fess EE: Intra-instrument reliability of the Jamar dynamometer, submitted for publication.
27. Fess EE: Reply to letter to the editor, J Hand Ther 2:219, 1988.
28. Hamilton GF: Reliability of goniometers in assessing finger joint angle, Phys Ther 49:465, 1969.
29. Harris SR, Smith LH, and Krukowski L: Goniometric reliability for a child with spastic quadriplegia, J Pediatr Orthop 5:348, 1985.
30. Hillenbrandt FA, Duvall EN, and Moore ML: The measurement of joint motion. III, Reliability of goniometry, Phys Ther Rev 29:302, 1949.
31. Hines M and O'Connor J: A measure of finger dexterity, Personnel J 4:379, 1926.
32. Jebson R and others: An objective and standardized test of hand function, Arch Phys Med Rehabil 50:311, 1969.
33. Kendall H, Kendall F, and Wadsworth G: Muscle testing and function, Baltimore, 1971, The Williams & Wilkins Co.
34. Kirkpatrick J: Evaluation of grip loss: a factor of permanent partial disability in California, Industr Med Surg 26:285, 1957.
35. LaMotte R: Symposium: assessment of levels of cutaneous sensibility, United States Public Health Service Hospital, Carville, La, 1980.
36. Levin S, Pearsall C, and Ruderman R: Von Frey's method of measuring pressure sensibility in the hand: an engineering analysis of the Weinstein-Semmes pressure aesthesiometer, J Hand Surg 3:211, 1978.
37. Low JL: The reliability of joint measurement, Physiotherapy 62:227, 1976.
38. Madden J, and Arem A: Wound healing: biologic and clinical features. In Sabiston J: Davis-Christopher textbook of surgery, ed 12, Philadelphia, 1981, WB Saunders Co.
39. Mathiowetz V, Rennells MS, and Donahoe L: Effect of elbow position on grip and key pinch strength, J Hand Surg 10A:694, 1985.
40. Mathiowetz V and others: Reliability and validity of grip and pinch strength evaluation, J Hand Surg 9A:222, 1984.
41. Mitchell E: Symposium: assessment of levels of cutaneous sensibility, United States Public Health Service Hospital, Carville, La, 1980.
42. Moberg E: Objective methods of determining the functional value of sensibility in the hand, J Bone Joint Surg 40B:454, 1958.
43. Murray J: The patient with the injured hand. Presidential address, American Society for Surgery of the Hand, J Hand Surg 7:543, 1982.
44. Onne L: Recovery of sensibility and sudomotor activity in the hand after severe injury, Acta Chir Scand [Suppl] 1:300, 1962.
45. O'Rain S: New and simple test for nerve function in the hand, Br Med J 3:615, 1973.
46. Phelps P, and Walker E: Comparison of the finger wrinkling test results to establish sensory tests in peripheral nerve injury, Am J Occup Ther 31:565, 1977.
47. Poppen N and others: Recovery of sensibility after suture of digital nerves, J Hand Surg 4:212, 1979.
48. Pryce J: The wrist position between neutral and ulnar deviation that facilitates maximum power grip strength, J Biomech 13:505, 1980.
49. Renfrew S: Fingertip sensation: a routine neurological test, Lancet 1:396, 1969.
50. Rothstein JM, Miller PJ, and Roetiger RF: Goniometric reliability in a clinical setting: elbow and knee measurements, Phys Ther 63:1611, 1983.
51. Rothstein JM: Measurement and clinical practice: theory and application. In Rothstein JM, editor: measurement in physical therapy: clinics in physical therapy, New York, 1985, Churchill Livingstone Inc.
52. Salter N: Methods of measurements of muscle and joint functions, J Bone Joint Surg 37B:474, 1955.
53. Schmidt R and Toews J: Grip strength as measured by the Jaymar dynamometer, Arch Phys Med Rehabil June 1970, p. 321.
54. Seddon H: Surgical disorders of the peripheral nerves, ed 2, New York, 1975, Churchill Livingstone.
55. Semmes J and others: Somatosensory changes after penetrating brain wounds in man, Cambridge, 1960, Harvard University Press.
56. Smidt, GL: Biomechanical analysis of knee flexion and extension, J Biomech 6:79, 1973.

57. Smith R: Clinical examination. In Lamb D and Kuezynski K, editors: The practice of hand surgery, Boston, 1981, Blackwell Scientific Publications, Inc.

58. Sunderland S: Nerves and nerve injuries, ed 2, New York, 1978, Churchill Livingstone.

59. Tiffin J and Asher E: The Purdue Pegboard: norms and studies of reliability and validity, J Appl Psychol 32:234, 1948.

60. Wagner C: Determination of the rotary flexibility of the elbow joint, Eur J Appl Physiol 37:47, 1977.

61. Waylett J and Seibly D: A study to determine the average deviation accuracy of a commercially available volumeter, J Hand Surg 6:300, 1981.

62. Weber E: Data cited by Sherrington CS in Shafer's textbook of physiology, Edinburgh, 1900, Young J. Pentland.

63. Yerxa EJ and others: Development of a hand sensitivity test for the hypersensitive hand, Am J Occup Ther 37:176, 1983.

6

Range-of-motion measurements of the hand

Catherine A. Cambridge

Rarely, if ever, is assessment of hand function discussed without some reference to the range of motion (ROM) of the involved extremity. In each edition of *Rehabilitation of the Hand*, chapters on evaluation have included range of motion as an essential component. Swanson and others relied significantly on limitation of motion in assessing impairment of the hand.[17] Fess and others gave range of motion prominence.[4] (See Chapters 4, 5, and 8.) In *The Hand—Examination and Diagnosis* by the American Society for Surgery of the Hand and in *Clinical Assessment Recommendations* published by the American Society of Hand Therapists, joint motion measurements are given much consideration.[5,7] Why? Because range of motion is considered by many clinicians to be a measurable, definable entity. Norms for motion of the various joints have been established in *Joint Motion: Method of Measuring and Recording*, allowing the examiner to compare readily the involved joint with the patient's own uninvolved contralateral joint or established values.[12]

But is the range of motion really reliable as an assessment tool? Does it really meet the criteria of being objective, measurable, and unbiased? Is the use of a goniometer necessary or are estimated motion measurements as reliable?[12] If a goniometer is used, does dorsal or lateral positioning change the measurement? Many such questions arise when health professionals involved in evaluation and treatment of patients with hand injuries discuss the role of range-of-motion measurements. One needs to answer these questions to determine the role of range of motion in the battery of assessment tools available to help evaluate the injured hand. The goal here is to address some of the questions about range of motion and to describe some of the more common methods to determine range of motion in the hand and wrist.

REVIEW OF THE LITERATURE
Range of motion—examiner estimation versus use of a goniometer

Opinions about the importance of the use of a goniometer in measuring joint range of motion vary.[13,14] In the literature little information was found comparing the accuracy of joint motion measured with and without a goniometer. In *Joint Motion: Method of Measuring and Recording*, the use of a goniometer is left up to the surgeon's discretion.[12] In *The Reliability of Joint Measurement*, 50 examiners estimated and then measured a fully flexed elbow and a completely extended wrist. The mean error in estimated elbow flexion was 9.3 degrees, compared with a 5-degree mean error in measured flexion. The mean estimated error for wrist extension was 12.8 degrees, with the measured mean error of 7.8 degrees.[13] No statistical analysis was completed to de-

research needs to be done before any firm conclusions can be reached, but the indication from this starting point is that reliability is improved by use of a goniometer, at least at the wrist and elbow.

The reliability of ROM measurements made with a goniometer has been assessed by more researchers than the previous topic. One of the earlier works was "Reliability of Goniometry," which found that a skilled observer varied 3 degrees or less in 70% of his or her measurements and 7 degrees or less in 95% of measurements when 780 paired observations were compared. The eight representative physical therapists were found to be within 7 degrees or less of their first measurements in duplicate trials in 62% to 72% of their observations. Statistical comparisons showed the average therapist to be reliable in duplicating measurements made by a highly skilled observer.[8] Hamilton and Lachenbruch also found a statistically significant level of reliability among investigators measuring the joint motion of the metacarpophalangeal (MP), proximal interphalangeal (PIP), and distal interphalangeal (DIP) joints of the hand.[6] "Reliability of Goniometric Measurements," by Boone and co-workers, compared four testers' measurements taken at the shoulder, elbow, and wrist and the hip, knee, and foot. They found reliability was greater for the three upper extremity movements than for the lower extremity movements. Their upper-extremity-motions intratester reliability compared favorably with the earlier work by Hellebrandt and others, "Reliability of Goniometry."[1,8]

Lateral goniometer placement compared with dorsal goniometer placement

Only one study that compared lateral and dorsal goniometric measurements of the hand was found. Hamilton and Lackenbruch investigated three types of goniometers: a 180-degree finger goniometer for dorsal placement, a 360-degree universal goniometer for lateral placement, and a pendulum type of goniometer that is also placed dorsally on the digit. Statistical analysis indicated equal reliability among all three goniometers. The authors then discussed factors, such as edema and deformity, that would influence the choice of instrument and may make one type more reliable than another given such complications. Choice of lateral or dorsal placement should be based on the experience of the tester and considerations of the injury, such as edema, dressing, and deformity.[6]

Intratester error compared with intertester error

The four studies mentioned were in agreement that the margin of error was greater when more than one tester was used to measure range of motion on the same patient.[1,6,8,13]

The intertester error averaged for measurement of the shoulder, elbow, and wrist by Boone and coworkers was comparable with the Hellebrandt findings.[1,8] Both intratester and intertester errors in the Boone and coworkers and the Hellebrandt studies were less than in the Low work.[1,8,13] The difference is not surprising, because both Boone's and Hellebrandt's testers had definite protocols to follow, whereas Low allowed each tester to use whatever technique the tester wished.

The conclusion drawn by the authors of the papers cited is that intratester reliability is greater than intertester reliability and that, when possible, serial measurements of a joint should be done by the same examiner. The greater degree of intertester error in Low's study appears to indicate that the more specific the protocol used by the various testers for measuring joint motion, the lesser the degree of intertester error.[1,6,8,13]

Total active motion, total passive motion, and fingertip to distal palmar crease measurements

Total motion values allow one number to represent the total motion capacity of a finger. The total extension deficits of a finger, including hyperextension, are added. This sum is subtracted from the total flexion capacity. The joint flexion measurements are taken with the fingers in the "fisted" position of maximum MP, PIP, and DIP flexion. The extension-motion measurements are taken with all three joints in extension.[5]

The difference between total active motion and total passive motion is in the force causing the movement. The term *active motion* indicates the motion achieved by the patient's own muscle power, whereas *passive motion* refers to the freedom of movement at a joint when an external force is applied.[10] Because the fisted position is used to measure both total active and total passive range of motion, the total passive range-of-motion readings may not correlate with the sum of passive motion measurements taken where each joint was evaluated individually. An example is a patient with a shortened extrinsic flexor tendon to the index finger. The passive range of motion in degrees could be MP, 0/90; PIP, 0/95; and DIP, 0/70, indicating that each joint has the capacity for full extension. The total passive extension deficit as measured in degrees in the completely extended position of the finger could be MP, 20; PIP, 30; and DIP, 20, equal to a total of 70 degrees. Then the sum of 70 degrees is subtracted from the sum of MP, 90; PIP, 95; and DIP, 70 (total passive flexion in degrees), giving a total passive motion of 185 degrees. Each type of measurement gives a specific type of information. The passive range-of-motion figures tell us that the joints are not inherently stiff, whereas the total passive motion figures indicate that as a functioning unit the finger lacks full motion. Total active and passive motion sums also facilitate statistical analysis of range-of-motion progression or regression for an entire finger, because only one numerical value per finger is involved. However, as the Clinical Assessment Committee of the American Society for Surgery of the Hand points out, total active motion values are not valid as part of a comparison of movement in determining a percentage of the norm (see Chapter 5).

Another measurement technique that illustrates the lack of overall finger flexion is measuring the distance from the

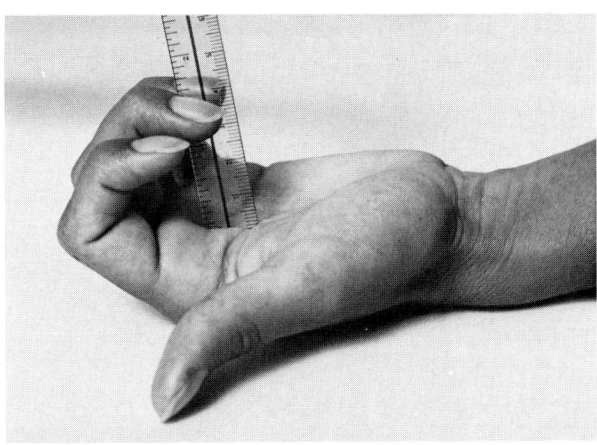

Fig. 6-1 Measuring from pulp of distal phalanx to distal palmar crease gives an easily understood value indicating the limitation of total finger flexion.

finger pulp to the distal palmar crease with the hand fisted.[5] This measurement gives an approximation of the total digital motion and is more comprehensible to many patients than motion measured in degrees (see Chapter 5). Centimeters or inches can be used to record the distance, with zero indicating full flexion to the distal palmar crease (Fig. 6-1).

TECHNIQUES FOR MEASURING RANGE OF MOTION OF WRIST AND HAND USING A GONIOMETER
General considerations for all joints

The patient should be as comfortable as possible without sacrificing joint positioning or musculotendinous dynamics. A clear understanding of the motion he is to perform during active range of motion is necessary if the patient is to cooperate. He should also know that the movement is to take place only in the assigned joints, to avoid substitution of motions.[10,15] During passive range of motion he should be as relaxed as possible, avoiding the problem of tensing muscles around the joint being measured.

The force exerted on a joint during passive motion should be minimal and consistent from one test to another. Swanson suggests that a pressure of 1 pound applied to the middle of the adjacent distal phalanx is adequate for evaluation of passive motion in the fingers.[18] Brand suggested that a therapist should check the amount of pressure that he or she is applying to the moving segment by using a pressure-gauging device. Such a check helps ensure consistent, gentle pressure.[2]

Range of motion—appropriateness of active and passive motion measurements. According to Hurt, "There are two primary purposes in measuring joint motion: to determine the degree of motion which can be accomplished in a joint by the active contraction of the governing muscle, and to determine the freedom existing at a joint by measuring the range through which it can be moved when all the muscles are relaxed."[10] Unless there are medical contraindications to active motion, the patient is first instructed in active motion to determine the available range of the joint when powered by its own musculature.[10] When the patient has full active excursion of a joint, passive motion values

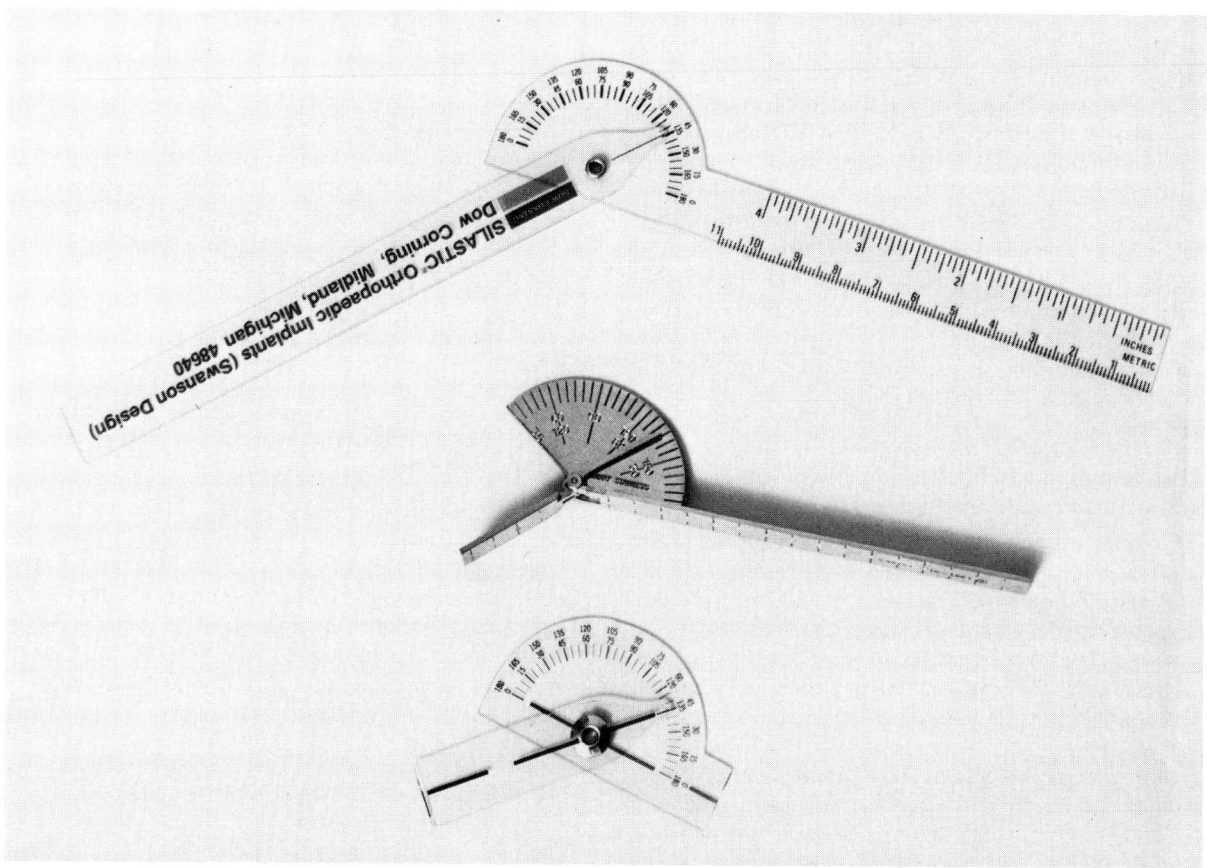

Fig. 6-2 Goniometer size and design should be appropriate for size of joint being measured and the technique being used.

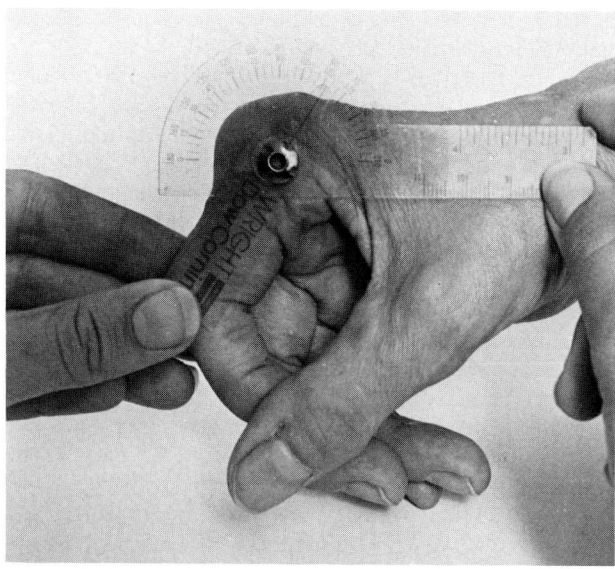

Fig. 6-3 Lateral placement of goniometer to measure active metacarpophalangeal flexion of a patient with rheumatoid arthritis.

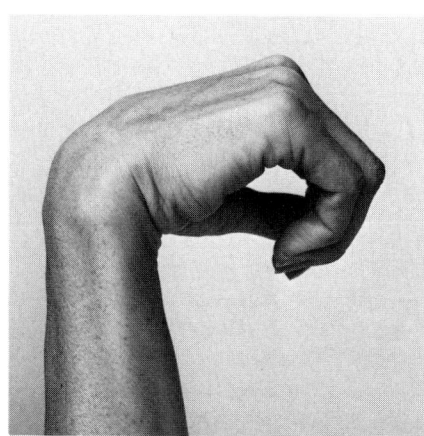

Fig. 6-4 Because of elongation of the extrinsic finger extensors over the fully flexed wrist, the remaining available excursion is inadequate to allow for full finger flexion.

need not be taken. A joint that has full active range will have full passive range as well. However, if the patient cannot actively move through the full range, the passive motion measurements become necessary to gain an accurate picture of a joint's movement.[10,15]

Goniometer size and placement. Goniometers are manufactured in a variety of forms and sizes. The size of the goniometer should be appropriate for the joint being measured. The wrist and forearm motions are adequately measured with a standard 14.5 cm–length arm.[3] (See also Chapter 5.) The finger joints are more easily measured by use of a commercially available finger goniometer made for dorsal alignment or by shortening of the arms on a small goniometer. Such an adapted goniometer is suitable for lateral or dorsal measurements of the finger joints (Fig. 6-2).

When a lateral measurement is being made, the goniometer should be placed so that the arms are parallel to the long axis of the adjacent bones forming the joint. The fulcrum should be as close to the axis of motion of the joint as possible[3,10] (Fig. 6-3). When a goniometer is placed dorsally on a digit, the fulcrum should be centered over the joint with the arm lying dorsally along the long axis of the adjacent bones.[10]

In the case of a multiarticular joint complex, such as the wrist, an anatomic landmark often is used for an approximate axis of motion. In the wrist, the styloid process of the radius laterally and the capitate dorsally and volarly are such landmarks.

Limiting the effects of positioning on ROM values. Hurt states further that "the resting length of a 2-joint muscle is insufficient to allow full motion in the direction away from itself simultaneously in both joints over which it passes"[9] (Fig. 6-4). However, full motion is available at either joint with relaxation of the other.[9] The extrinsic finger flexors and extensors cross one or more finger joints and the wrist. In the case of the flexor digitorum superficialis and the extensor digitorum communis, the elbow is crossed

as well just distal to their origins. To avoid having a resting-length insufficiency interfere with ROM readings, *Clinical Assessment Recommendations* suggests that the wrist should be neutral when digital motion measurements are taken. They also suggest that to limit the influence of forearm positioning on wrist measurements, the forearm should be pronated[4] (see Chapter 5 and Fig. 6-5).

Recording range-of-motion measurements. Lack of uniformity exists regarding how range-of-motion measurements should be recorded so that other professionals can accurately interpret the results. Several authors cited in this chapter comment on the importance of clearly defining a motion as being within the realm of normal flexion and extension or as an abnormal movement, such as hyperextension,[3,7,12,18] (see also Chapters 8 and 73) but exact guidelines for unequivocal interpretation are not given. The American Academy of Orthopaedic Surgeons[12] and the American Society for Surgery of the Hand[7] recommend a system of notation in which all motions are measured from a 0-degree (neutral) starting position. Flexion measurements are recorded as positive numbers; extension and hyperextension beyond the 0-degree starting position are recorded as negative numbers. Thus 15/110 passive motion of the PIP joint indicates a 15-degree flexion contracture and full passive flexion. Similarly, −15/110 indicates 15-degree hyperextension and full passive flexion. Written statements can be used to indicate rotation and alignment deformities[18,20] (see also Chapter 73).

Because of the lack of uniformity in recording motion measurements, it is important that a statement accompany ROM records explaining the notation system used. Otherwise, accurate data could be interpreted inaccurately.

Methods for measuring joint motion

Pronation and supination of the forearm. Measuring rotational movements at the radioulnar joints is difficult because of the long axis of movement and the lack of stable

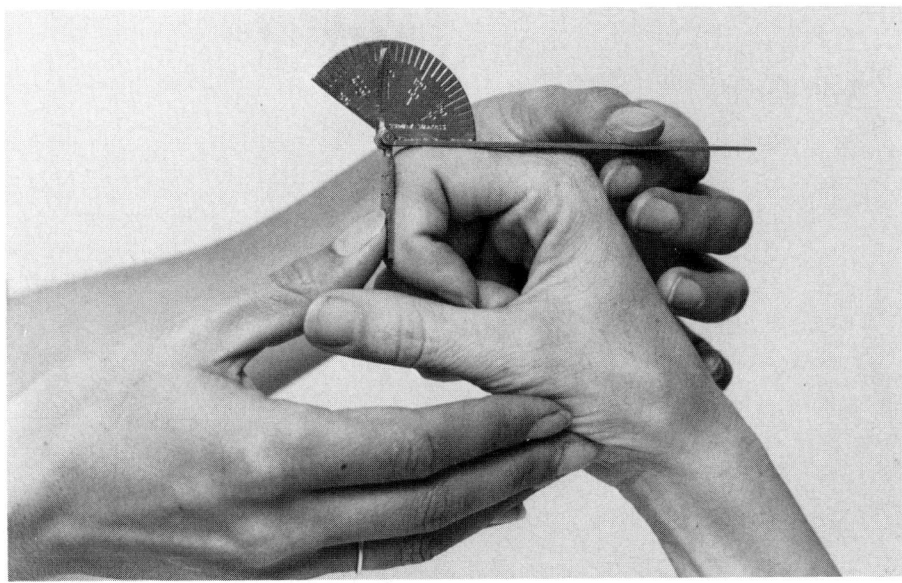

Fig. 6-5 Taking digital motion measurements with wrist in neutral and forearm in pronation eliminates possible effects of normal tendon-excursion limitation on range-of-motion measurements.

anatomic lever arms with which to align the goniometer. The method used by Downer of the Ohio State University incorporates the salient points of other techniques and does not require special equipment other than a standard goniometer.[3,10,15]

The patient may be sitting or standing, but the elbow must be flexed to 90 degrees with the arm close to the side of the body. The arm position is important to avoid substitution movements of the shoulder.[3,11] The forearm should be in midposition, with the palm vertical in relation to the floor. This position is defined as zero degrees.[12]

For measurement of supination, the patient rotates the hand and forearm to its maximum palm-up position without extending the elbow or abducting the upper arm. The stationary arm of the goniometer is aligned with the humerus or held perpendicular to the floor.[3] The movable arm is placed on edge across the volar aspect of the wrist at the level of the ulnar styloid. The axis of the goniometer is just medial to the ulnar styloid (Fig. 6-6). Normal range of motion in supination is 0 to 80 or 90 degrees.[12]

The starting position for pronation is the same as for supination. The patient rotates the hand and forearm into the maximum palm-down position. The stationary arm again is aligned with the humerus or perpendicular to the floor. The only change is the position of the movable arm, which is now on the dorsum of the wrist at the level of the styloid processes.[15] Normal motion is from 0 to 80 or 90 degrees.[12]

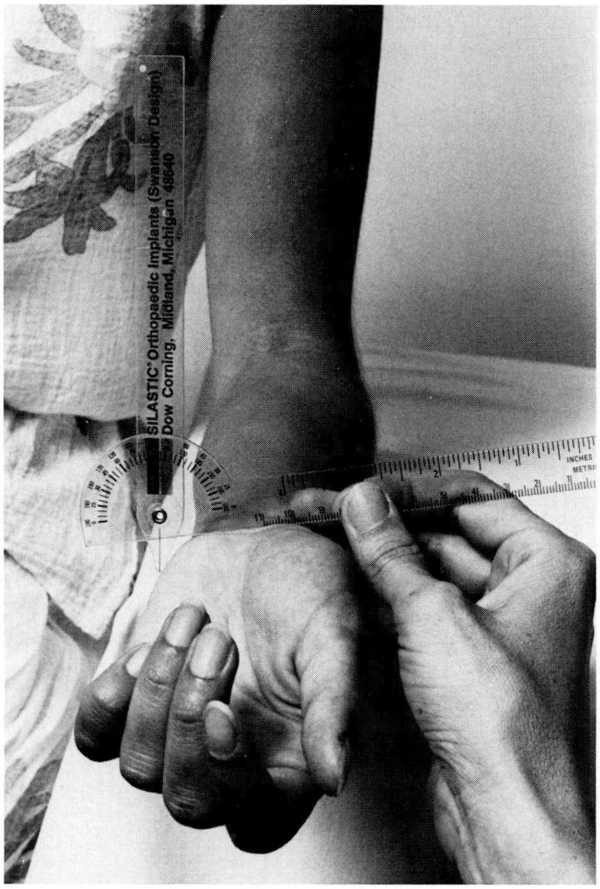

Motion at the wrist. The wrist motions usually measured are flexion, extension, and radial and ulnar deviation. Wrist circumduction cannot be measured accurately.[12]

Flexion. Wrist flexion can be measured with the goniometer placed dorsally on the wrist,[5,18] or laterally along the radial border of the forearm and second metacarpal.[11,15] Placement of the goniometer along the ulnar border of the wrist and the fifth metacarpal also has been suggested.[3,15] However, the mobility of the carpometacarpal joints of the fourth and fifth metacarpals could skew the measurements of wrist flexion when an ulnar placement is used.[5]

For measurement of wrist flexion (volar flexion) on the radial aspect of the forearm, the elbow is flexed and the forearm and wrist are placed in neutral for the starting position. The wrist is flexed, and the stationary arm of the goniometer is aligned with the radius while the movable arm is aligned with the second metacarpal.[11] The axis of motion of the goniometer is approximately at the level of the radial styloid (Fig. 6-7).

Wrist flexion (volar flexion), with the goniometer placed dorsally, requires the elbow to be flexed and the forearm in pronation with the wrist in neutral as the starting position. The wrist is flexed with the fingers relaxed. The stationary arm of the goniometer is aligned with the long axis of the forearm while the movable arm is aligned with the third metacarpal.[5] The fulcrum of the goniometer is approximately at the level of the capitate (Fig. 6-8). According to *Joint Motion: Method of Measuring and Recording,* the normal arc of motion for wrist flexion is 0 to 80 degrees.[12]

Extension. For measuring wrist extension (dorsiflexion) using the lateral placement, the wrist is extended with the

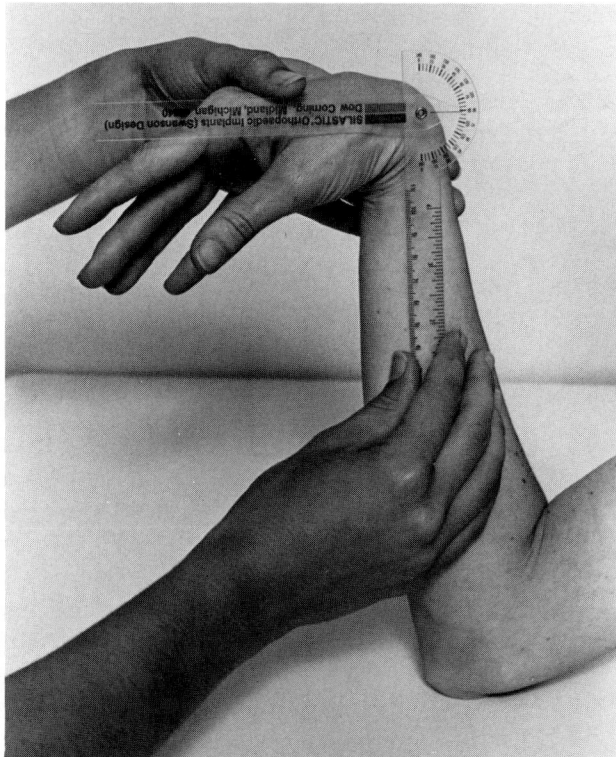

Fig. 6-6 Abduction of shoulder or extension of elbow will allow substitution of shoulder movement for true supination or pronation.

Fig. 6-7 Lateral measurement on radial aspect of wrist is preferred because of stability of second carpometacarpal joint.

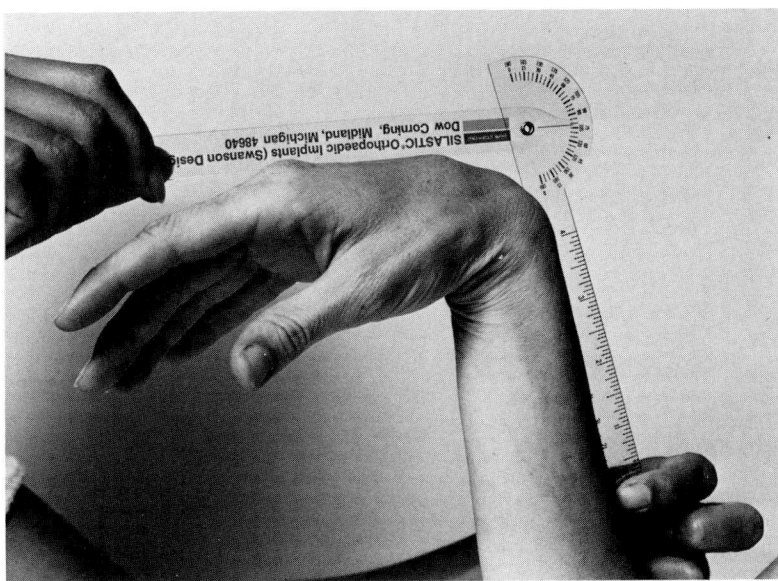

Fig. 6-8 The third carpometacarpal joint is stable and allows the metacarpal to be used for alignment of the dorsally placed goniometer.

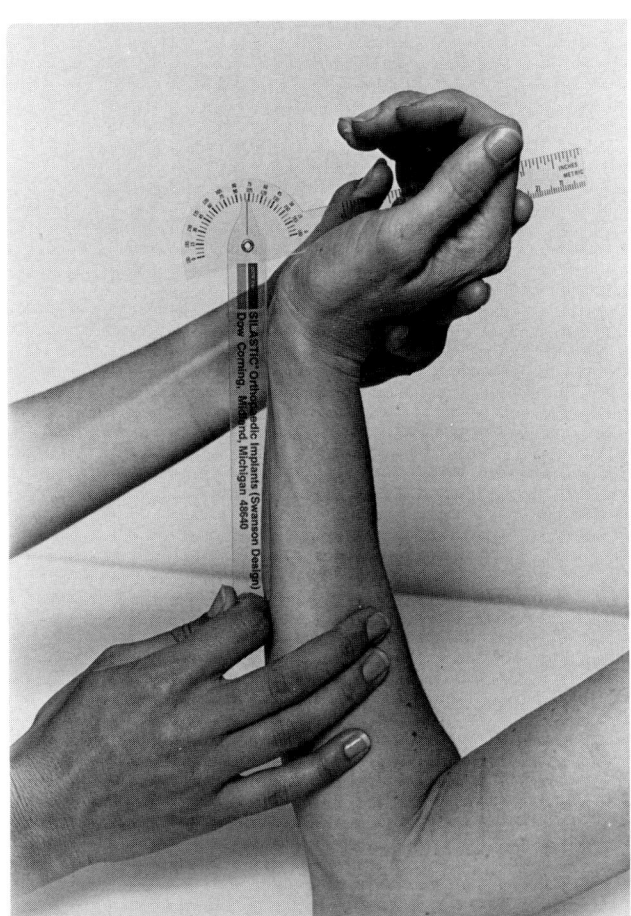

Fig. 6-9 The movable arm of the goniometer will be over the third metacarpal bridging the palmar arc.

fingers allowed to flex passively.[11] The normal arc of motion is 0 to 70 degrees.[12]

For measurement of wrist extension with the goniometer volarly placed, the starting position of the arm is the same as for wrist flexion. However, goniometer placement is different. Once the wrist is extended, the stationary arm is aligned with the long axis of the forearm on the volar surface and the movable arm is aligned with the volar surface of the third metacarpal.[5] The fingers should be relaxed (Fig. 6-9).

Radial and ulnar deviation. The starting positions for taking measurements of radial and ulnar deviation are the same. The forearm is in pronation, and the goniometer is placed dorsally.[5] The zero position is with the wrist in neutral.[12] The stationary arm is aligned in midposition along the forearm. The capitate and lateral epicondyle of the elbow can be used as reference points for the stationary arm, and the movable arm is placed along the third metacarpal[15] (Fig. 6-10). In both radial and ulnar deviation, wrist flexion and extension need to be avoided. The wrist is angled toward the thumb for radial deviation (Fig. 6-11) or angled toward the fifth finger for ulnar deviation.[3,11,15] The normal range of radial deviation is 0 to 20 degrees and of ulnar deviation 0 to 30 degrees.[12]

Motion of the fingers. The wrist should be in neutral to allow full tendon excursion of the long finger flexors and extensors when one is measuring the motion of the MP, PIP, and DIP joints.[5] This is true for both active and passive motion studies. At the Hand Rehabilitation Center in Philadelphia, active ROM values for flexion are taken with all three joints of each finger actively flexed to their maximum. For the measurement of extension, all three joints are actively extended to their maximum. Simultaneous flexion or extension of the finger joints during measurement gives the examiner a better picture of the musculotendinous limitations affecting active motion of the joints.

Passive motion is measured on a joint-by-joint basis with the adjacent joint or joints in neutral so that the musculo-

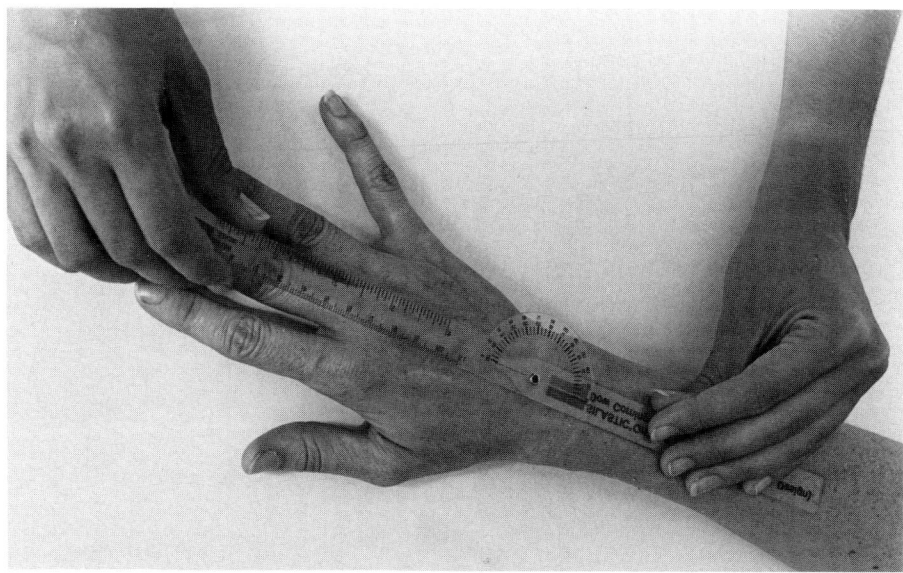

Fig. 6-10 The starting position for the measurement of radial and ulnar deviation requires the wrist to be in neutral in both planes of motion—flexion-extension and radial and ulnar deviation.

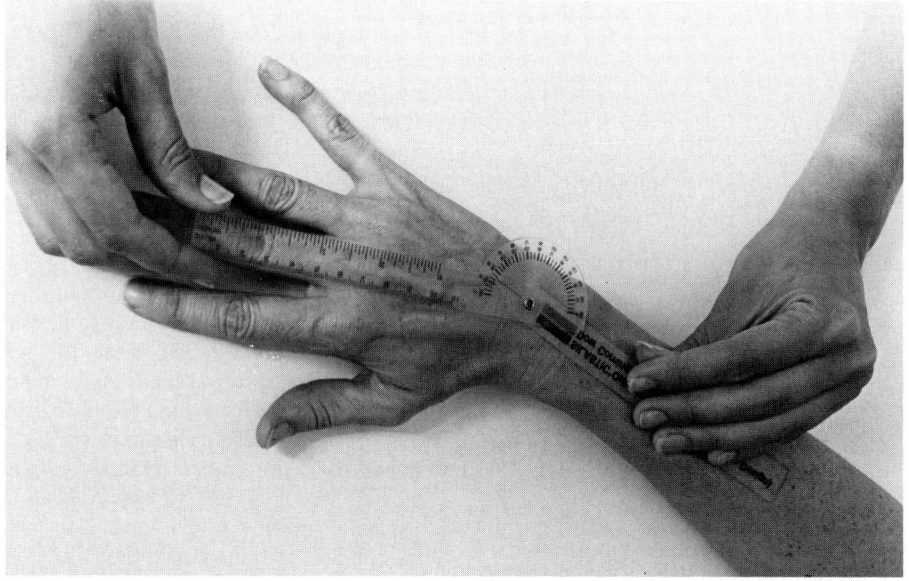

Fig. 6-11 It is important that the movable arm be aligned with the third metacarpal and not the third finger.

tendinous effects are minimized and only the excursion of the joint is being measured.[10]

Metacarpophalangeal joint. MP joint motion can be measured laterally or dorsally. The landmarks used for lateral measurement of joint flexion and extension are the same. For lateral placement of the goniometer on the index or middle fingers, the stationary arm is aligned with the lateral longitudinal axis of the second metacarpal. The moving arm is aligned with the lateral longitudinal axis of the first phalanx (Fig. 6-12). In the case of the middle finger, this requires the examiner to have the index MP joint slightly extended so that the middle finger can be clearly sighted

(Fig. 6-13). The ring and little fingers are measured from the ulnar border of the hand with the same techniques.

Dorsal placement of the goniometer to measure MP joint flexion and extension is the same for both. The stationary arm is placed over the dorsum of the metacarpal, the fulcrum is superior to the joint axis, and the movable arm is placed over the dorsum of the adjacent phalanx.[11] The arc of motion usually evaluated when one is measuring MP joint motion is 0 to 90 degrees, but hyperextension of as much as 45 degrees is also normal.[12]

Flexion and extension of the proximal and distal interphalangeal joints. The techniques used for measurement of

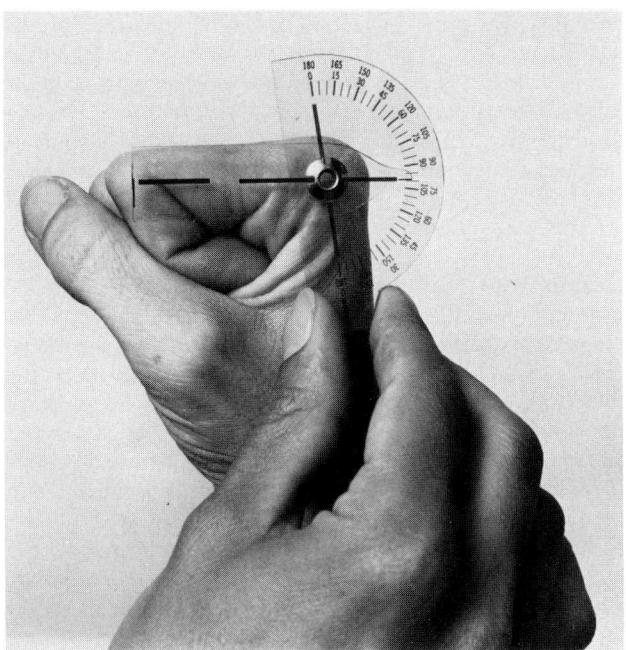

Fig. 6-12   The thumb should be held in abduction or adduction and slight extension when one is laterally measuring metacarpophalangeal motion of the index finger, so as not to block full metacarpophalangeal flexion of the index finger.

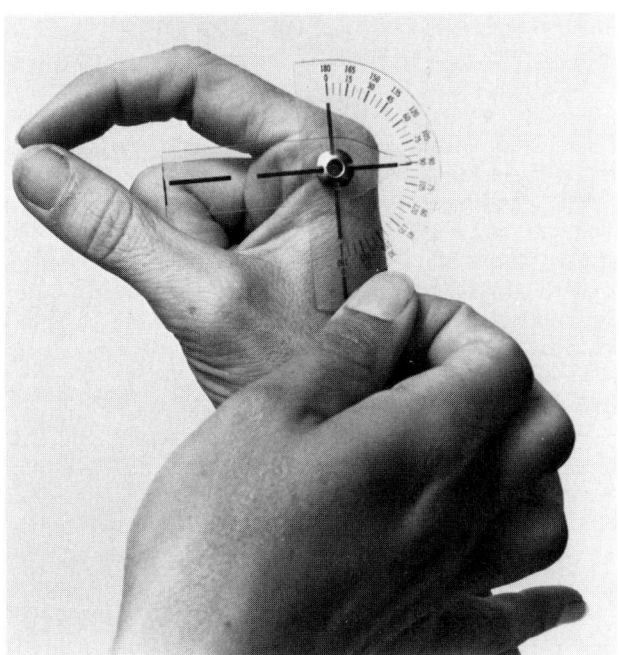

Fig. 6-13   Movable phalanx needs to be sighted as clearly as possible for an accurate measurement.

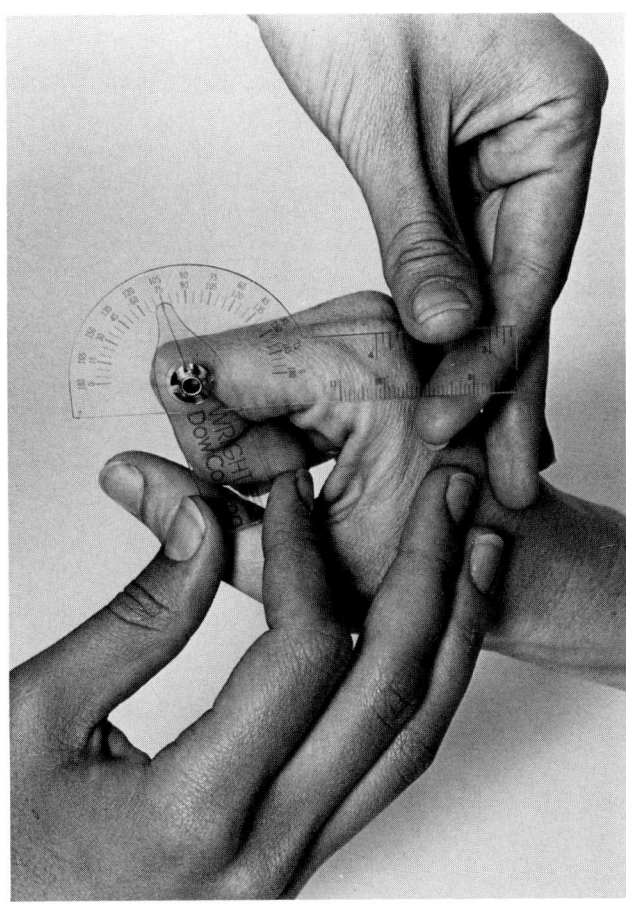

Fig. 6-14   Lateral placement of goniometer with shortened arms is suitable for finger joint measurements.

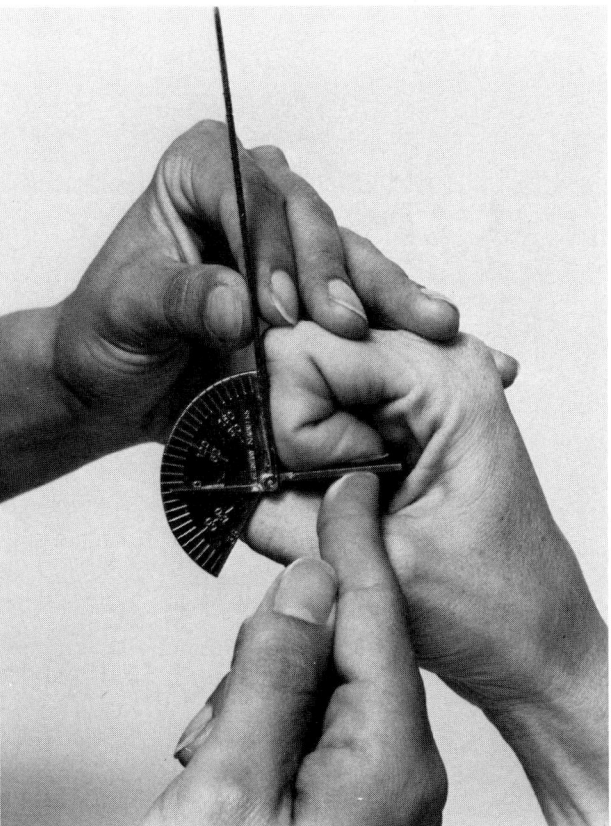

Fig. 6-15   Slight metacarpophalangeal extension allows full excursion of goniometer without interference by touching palm.

joint motion at the PIP and DIP joints are very similar; therefore they will be described together. The use of a commercially available finger goniometer for dorsal placement or a small goniometer in which the arms have been shortened for dorsal or lateral placement helps with the measurement of the finger joints (see also Chapter 5 and Fig. 6-2).

For lateral measurements, the stationary arm is placed along the long axis of the proximal phalanx, and the moving arm is placed along the long axis of the adjacent distal phalanx. The fulcrum approximates the axis of motion of the joint[16] (Fig. 6-14). The MP joints may have to be extended slightly when one is measuring the DIP flexion to allow the goniometer to clear the palm during full active flexion.

When one is measuring extension of the PIP and DIP joints, the same goniometer placement along the lateral long axis of the adjacent phalanges is used after the joints have been extended. Dorsal measurements of PIP and DIP flexion are made by placing the stationary arm on the dorsal long axis of the proximal phalanx and the movable arm on the dorsum of the adjacent distal phalanx.[3,11] The examiner should keep the goniometer in as complete contact with the dorsal finger surface as possible to avoid errors in measurement[16] (Fig. 6-5). As with lateral placement, slight MP extension may be necessary for measurement of the DIP flexion if total active flexion is complete or nearly so (Fig. 6-15).

The placement of the arms of the goniometer remains the same when one measures the extension of the PIP and DIP joints, except that the joints are in maximum extension

dorsally.[11] The range of motion of the PIP joints is 0 to 110 degrees and that of the DIP joints 0 to 60 or 70 degrees.[12]

Abduction and adduction of the metacarpophalangeal joints. Joint Motion: Method of Measuring and Recording does not give norms for finger abduction and adduction. It suggests measuring the distance from fingertip to fingertip in inches or centimeters. These measurements can be used for pretreatment and posttreatment comparisons only[12] (Fig. 6-16).

Thumb motions. The thumb's movement pattern is the most complex of all the digits because of its highly mobile carpometacarpal (CMC) joint. Flexion describes the movement across the palm that terminates with the tip of the thumb at the base of the fifth finger. It involves flexion of the CMC, metacarpal and interphalangeal joints for full excursion. Extension of the thumb involves the same joints in a movement away from the second metacarpal, again in the plane of the palm.[12]

Thumb flexion and extension can be measured with a goniometer placed laterally or dorsally along the appropriate adjacent bones. CMC flexion requires the stationary arm to be aligned with the lateral or dorsal long axis of the radius with the movable arm aligned with the first metacarpal. The approximate axis of motion is level with the anatomic snuffbox. Flexion of the CMC joint is 15 degrees.[12] CMC extension can be measured with the stationary arm aligned with the second metacarpal and the movable arm aligned over the first metacarpal (Fig. 6-17). MP and interphalangeal flexion and extension can be measured with the same lateral or dorsal technique appropriate for the index finger

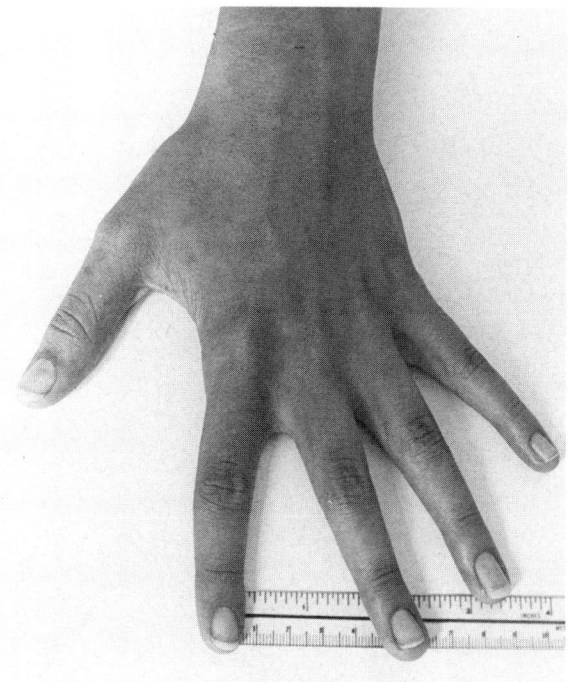

Fig. 6-16 Measuring distance between midpulps of adjacent maximally abducted fingers will allow for comparisons of abduction to help in evaluation of treatment effectiveness.

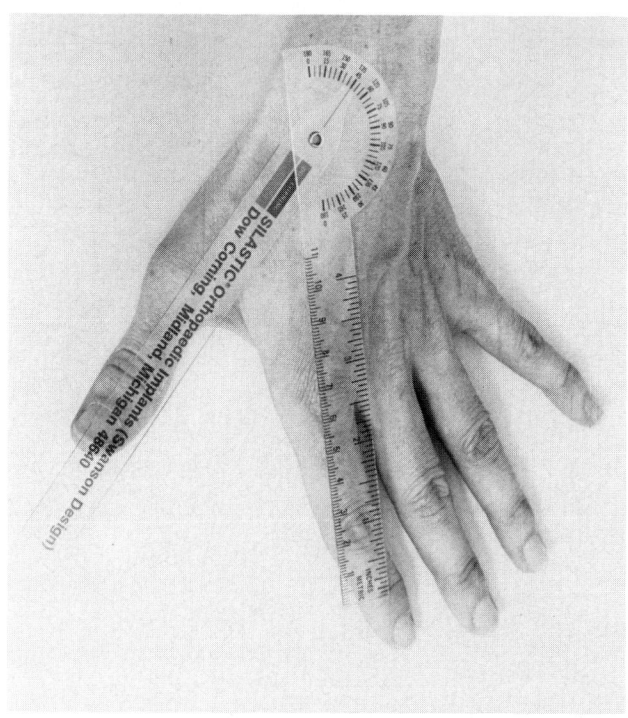

Fig. 6-17 Measurement of thumb extension is done with thumb in plane of palm. (From American Academy of Orthopaedic Surgeons: Joint motion: method of measuring and recording, Chicago, 1965, The Academy.)

MP and PIP joints. Thumb MP motion is 0 to 50 degrees and interphalangeal excursion is 0 to 80 degrees.[12] The interphalangeal joint of the thumb has varying degrees of hypertension and should be compared with the contralateral thumb if a pathologic condition is suspected.

Thumb abduction and adduction occur in a plane perpendicular to the palm and involve only movement of the CMC joint normally. Norms for abduction have not been established by the American Academy of Orthopaedic Surgeons, but the measurement can be compared with that of the contralateral hand. Adduction is defined as the thumb in line with the radius lying immediately beside the second metacarpal, whereas abduction is the angle that occurs as the thumb moves perpendicularly away from the plane of the palm.[12] This angle can be measured in degrees with a goniometer. The stationary arm is aligned with the lateral aspect of the second metacarpal, and the moving arm is placed dorsally along the long axis of the first metacarpal.[11] An alternative method is to measure in inches or centimeters the distance from the distal palmar crease of the index finger to the pulp or interphalangeal crease of the thumb[12] (Fig. 6-18). Other methods of measurement using special measuring devices, such as dental calipers, have been suggested

in the hand literature and may be helpful in specific circumstances (see Chapter 8).

Thumb opposition is a composite motion comprising abduction, rotation, and flexion. Measurement of opposition is usually done in inches or centimeters between the thumbtip and the tip or base of the fifth finger[12] (Fig. 6-19). For true opposition and not just thumb flexion, the thumb must move out and away from the plane of the palm with the thumbnail approximately parallel to the plane of the palm.

CONCLUSION

The limited research done on assessment of the reliability of measuring joint motion by use of a goniometer indicates that it can be an accurate, reproducible method for evaluation of motion. The use of the same tester for serial motion studies increases the reliability. When the same tester is not available, the use of the same goniometer technique may help improve reliability. The single study that evaluated lateral versus dorsal goniometer placement in the fingers did not find one method more accurate than the other.

The methods for measuring joint motion presented in this chapter are for the evaluation of hands without major deformities that cause excessive joint deviations, subluxations,

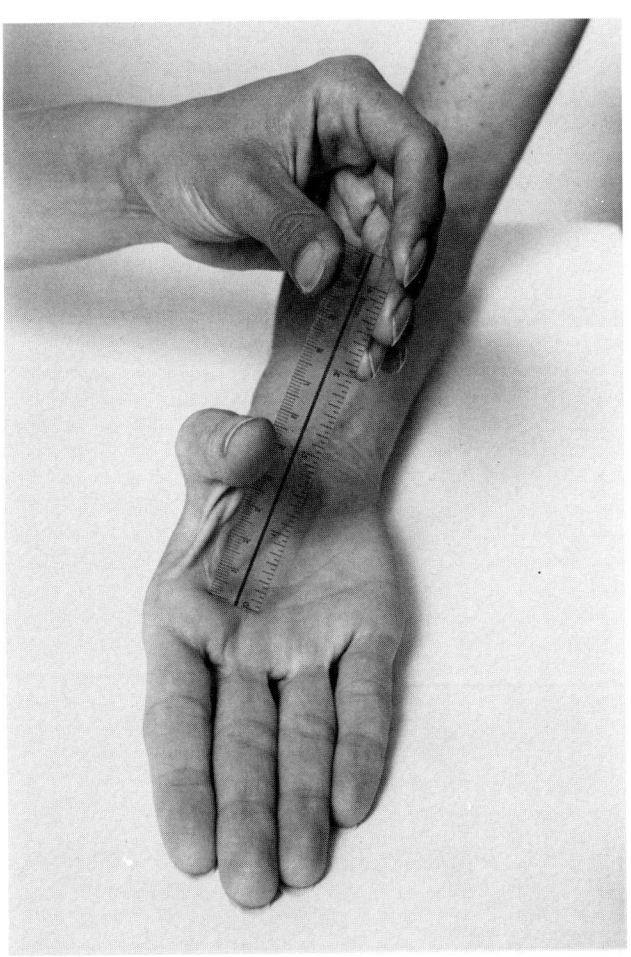

Fig. 6-18 Thumb abduction is measured in a plane perpendicular to palm. (From American Academy of Orthopaedic Surgeons: Joint motion: method of measuring and recording, Chicago, 1965, The Academy.)

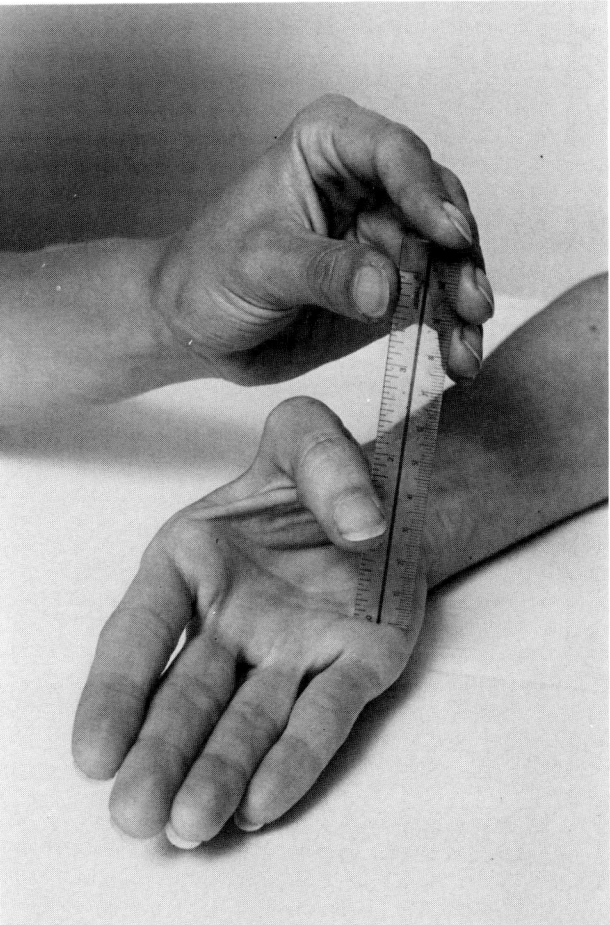

Fig. 6-19 During opposition, thumb must move out of plane of palm while approaching fifth finger.

and dislocations, such as advanced rheumatoid arthritis. Refer to the chapters on arthritis and specifically to those written by Swanson for the evaluation of the arthritic hand.

REFERENCES

1. Boone DC and others: Reliability of goniometric measurements, Phys Ther 58:1355, 1978.
2. Brand P and Costa P: Principles of dynamic splinting, Symposium and Workshop on Hand Rehabilitation Correlated with Hand Surgery, March 1981.
3. Downer A: Goniometry: measurement of joint range of motion, Columbus, 1982, Ohio State University Press (unpublished).
4. Fess EE and others: Evaluation of the hand by objective measurement. In Hunter JM and others, editors: Rehabilitation of the hand, St Louis, 1978, The CV Mosby Co.
5. Fess EE aned Moran CA: Clinical assessment recommendations, Aurora, Colo, 1981, American Society of Hand Therapists.
6. Hamilton GF and Lachenbruch PA: The reliability of goniometry in assessing finger joint angle, Phys Ther 49:465, 1969.
7. The hand—examination and diagnosis, Aurora, Colo, 1978, American Society for Surgery of the Hand.
8. Hellebrandt FA, Duvall EN, and Moore ML: The measurement of joint motion. Part III. Reliability of goniometry, Phys Ther Rev 29:302, 1949.
9. Hurt SP: Considerations in muscle function and their application to disability evaluation and treatment, Am J Occup Ther 1:69, 1947.
10. Hurt SP: Considerations in muscle function and their application to disability evaluation and treatment. Part I. Am J Occup Ther 1:209, 1947.
11. Hurt SP: Considerations in muscle function and their application to disability evaluation and treatment: joint measurement. Part II. Am J Occup Ther 1:281, 1947.
12. Joint motion: method of measuring and recording, Chicago, 1965, American Academy of Orthopaedic Surgeons.
13. Low JL: The reliability of joint measurement, Physiotherapy 62:227, 1976.
14. Moore ML: The measurement of joint motion. Part I. Introductory review of the literature, Phys Ther Rev 29:195, 1949.
15. Moore ML: The measurement of joint motion. Part II. The technic of goniometry, Phys Ther Rev 29:256, 1949.
16. Perry JF and Bevin AG: Evaluation procedures for patient with hand injuries, Phys Ther 54:593, 1974.
17. Swanson AB, Göran-Hagert C, and Swanson G: Evaluation of impairment of hand function. In Hunter JM and others, editors: Rehabilitation of the hand, St Louis, 1978, The CV Mosby Co.
18. Swanson AB: Flexible implant resection arthroplasty in the hand and extremities, St Louis, 1973, The CV Mosby Co.

7

Physical capacity evaluation

Patricia L. Baxter-Petralia, Laura A. Bruening, Susan M. Blackmore, and Pamela M. McEntee

Physicians and therapists who treat patients with hand injuries often are faced with the question of whether these patients will return to their previous occupations. The physical capacity evaluation has been developed to provide definitive information to assist in the determination of working capabilities. This chapter describes the tests used by therapists at the Hand Rehabilitation Center of Philadelphia to assess the hand-injured worker's ability to return to his or her previous occupation or to a modified job.

Before the evaluation, the patient is informed of its purpose and duration. The evaluation takes approximately 4 hours to administer, and 1 hour is needed to interpret the results and write a report. No two physical capacity evaluations are alike. The tests selected are based on the physical demands included in the patient's job description when return to former employment appears feasible. If the patient cannot return to his former job, capabilities and limitations are outlined.

The physical capacity evaluation has five parts: (1) medical history and identifying information, (2) a hand function evaluation, (3) observation of performance of physical demands of work, (4) administration of standardized tests, and (5) comparative sequential testing to assess the patient's consistency in performance among various tests. A variety of equipment is used for each subtest, and comparisons are made among the different subtests to evaluate the consistency of a patient's performance. The patient is instructed to work at his maximum ability during testing but is cautioned to work within his pain and fatigue tolerance. Subjective reports of pain and fatigue are documented with each task.

MEDICAL HISTORY AND IDENTIFYING INFORMATION

A full review of medical information is documented, including the mechanism of injury, surgical intervention, and therapeutic management. After the medical history is reviewed, the patient's job history is obtained. There are several resources to assist the therapist compile information regarding the patient's job requirements.

The therapist obtains the patient's job description from *The Dictionary of Occupational Titles*.[10] Within this publication there is a narrative description for jobs. The physical demands of each job can be found in the *Selected Characteristics of Occupations Defined in The Dictionary of Occupational Titles*.[11]

It is recommended that the therapist visit each patient's job site. If an on-site visit cannot be made, the therapist requests a complete job analysis from the patient's rehabilitation specialist or personnel manager. These sources and a thorough patient interview provide the therapist with the necessary information to select appropriate tests to complete the evaluation.

HAND FUNCTION EVALUATION

The physical capacity evaluation begins with a hand function assessment. Range of motion, pinch and grip strength, edema measurement, activities of daily living assessment, and sensibility testing constitute this part of the evaluation. One or all of these assessments may be used, depending on the patient's condition.

Active range of motion is measured with a goniometer according to the standard methods of measurement and recording as described in *Joint Motion* published by the American Academy of Orthopedic Surgeons.[1] Lateral, tip, and three-point pinch are measured on the Pinch Gauge.* Grip strength is tested on the Jamar Adjustable Dynamometer.† This dynamometer has five handle positions to allow the patient to perform a full-fisted grip on the first position and a successively wider grip on each of the remaining four positions.

Hand edema is recorded before the patient performs the remaining parts of the physical capacity evaluation and after he has completed the 4-hour test. The Volumeter‡ is used for measuring edema.[4] The patient is instructed to submerge his hand in the volumeter, and hand edema is measured by the amount of water displaced into a graduated cylinder.

When the sensibility function of the patient's injured hand is questioned, tests, such as two-point discrimination, light touch/deep pressure perception, and the Moberg Pickup Test are essential components of the hand function evaluation (see Chapter 44).

OBSERVATION OF PERFORMANCE OF THE PHYSICAL DEMANDS OF WORK

The third part of the physical capacity evaluation is the observation of the patient performing the physical demands of his or her job. The therapist must refer to the patient's job requirements to accurately simulate the physical demands of the patient's job. Physical demands are defined as those physical activities required of a worker in a job.[11] The patient must have physical capabilities at least equal to the physical demands required for the job to be released for work. Table 7-1 lists and defines the physical demands inherent in many jobs. Guidelines for the tools needed and

---

*Pinch Gauge, B&L Engineering, Santa Fe Springs, Calif.
†Jamar Dynamometer, Asimow Engineering Co., Los Angeles.
‡Volumeter Unlimited, Idyllwild, Calif.

Table 7-1 Guidelines for the work performance evaluation

Physical demands	Tools	Technique
Lifting: raising or lowering object from one level to another*	Box with weights: use maximum weight required on job: start with 10 pounds and progress to maximum weight	Observe patient performing repetitive weight lifting unilaterally and bilaterally for up to 1 hour depending on patient's job
Pushing: exerting force upon object so that object moves away from force*	Box with weights, dolly or pulley	Observe repetitive pushing and pulling on a table top, pulley, or dolly for up to 1 hour depending on patient's job
	Work Simulator	Observe patient on Work Simulator using handle nos. 801, 701, 901, and 111
Pulling: exerting force on object so that the object moves toward the force*	Same tools as used for physical demand of pushing	Same techniques as used for physical demands of pushing
Climbing: ascending or descending using feet, legs, hands, or arms*	Stairs	Observe patient ascend and descend stairs three times
	Ladder	Observe patient ascend and descend ladder three times
Stooping: bending body downward and forward by bending spine at waist*	1- and 3-pound cans	Observe patient transferring cans from table to floor while bending body downward at waist
	Valpar Whole Body Range of Motion Work Sample	Standardized technique of Valpar Whole Body Range of Motion Work Sample
Kneeling: bending legs at knees to come to rest on knees*	1- and 3-pound cans	Observe patient transferring cans from table to floor while he is kneeling for 3 minutes
	Valpar Whole Body Range of Motion Work Sample	Standardized technique of Valpar Whole Body Range of Motion Work Sample
Crouching	1- and 3-pound cans	Observe patient transferring cans from table to floor while crouching for 3 minutes
	Valpar Whole Body Range of Motion Work Sample	Standardized technique of Valpar Whole Body Range of Motion Work Sample
Crawling		Observe patient crawl 10 feet
Sitting		Observe patient sitting during test
Standing		Observe patient standing during test
Walking		Observe patient walking during test
Reaching	Box, 1-pound cans	Observe patient reaching overhead to place cans in box; repeat with box at waist level and on the floor
	Valpar Work Samples: Whole Body Range of Motion Upper Extremity Range of Motion Simulated Assembly Work Sample	Standardized technique of Valpar Work Samples
	Work Simulator	Observe patient on Work Simulator attachments 801, 701, 131, 901, and 141 in automatic mode

techniques used for this part of the evaluation are also included.

The therapist can perform this section of the evaluation through observation of the patient doing physical tasks (Fig. 7-1). However, we recommend that such observation be combined with standardized tests. The use of standardized tests provides quantitative information on the patient's ability to perform job tasks.

OBSERVATIONS FOR TESTING THE PHYSICAL DEMANDS OF WORK

Observations often made while testing the physical demands follow. These can serve to enhance and qualify the test results.

Lifting/carrying

For bilateral lifting and carrying, the patient is instructed to load weights into a box; for unilateral lifting and carrying, he is instructed to load weights into a bucket. He moves the box or bucket 10 feet with each trial and adds weight until he reaches his self-estimated maximal comfortable level for lifting and carrying weight.

Compensatory postures are noted, such as when the box is supported against the thighs or abdomen. When carrying is assessed, comments also include the patient's trunk compensation for the increasing load; for example, the patient may rest the box on his hip instead of bearing weight equally with both arms.

Table 7-1   Guidelines for the work performance evaluation—cont'd

Physical demands	Tools	Technique
Handling: seizing, holding, grasping, turning, primarily with hand or hands*	Tools and pipe structure	Observe patient handling tools while assembling and disassembling pipe structure
	Minnesota Rate of Manipulation Test	Standardized technique of Minnesota Rate of Manipulation Test
	Valpar Work Samples: Simulated Assembly Small Tools Mechanical Upper Extremity Range of Motion Whole Body Range of Motion	Standardized techniques of Valpar Work Samples
	Work Simulator	Observe patient on Work Simulator attachments 302, 501, 502, 503, 601, 701, 111, 901, and 161 in automatic mode
Manipulating: picking, pinching, or otherwise working with fingers primarily*	Small nuts and bolts: small tools	Observe patient manipulating small objects with and without tools
	Valpar Work Samples: Upper Extremity Range of Motion Small Tools Mechanical Whole Body Range of Motion Simulated Assembly	Standardized techniques of Valpar Work Samples
	Work Simulator	Use Work Simulator attachments 101, 102, 201, 400, and 151 in automatic mode
Feeling: perceiving such attributes of objects and materials as size, shape, temperature, and texture, by means of receptors in skin, particularly to fingertips*	Moberg Pickup Test	Observe patient's prehension pattern with vision occluded
	Valpar Work Samples: Upper Extremity Range of Motion Whole Body Range of Motion	Standardized technique of Valpar Work Samples
Talking, hearing, and seeing: Endurance: ability to work over a period of time		Observation of patient
	Valpar Work Samples: Whole Body Range of Motion Simulated Assembly Small Tools Mechanical	Standardized techniques of Valpar Work Samples
	Work Simulator	Use Work Simulator in automatic mode for 3 minutes with the tool attachments appropriate to patient's job

*US Department of Labor: Dictionary of occupational titles, ed 3, Washington, DC, 1968, US Government Printing Office.

Pushing/pulling

With this technique, the evaluator observes the following: full hand grasp on the item, trunk substitution for upper extremity motion, and asymmetry. More than one task is administered, and the results are compared to check for consistency. In addition, the patient can be observed for the ability to pull open doors, push off from a chair to stand, or push weighted bags aside to clear an area to work.

Climbing

Observations are recorded regarding reciprocal climbing motions with the upper extremities, the patient's ability to hold his weight with his injured arm, and the grasp patterns used for climbing a ladder.

When the patient is stair climbing, it should be noted if he or she displayed any difficulty with managing the hand rail, balancing while climbing, or climbing high steps.

Kneeling, crouching, crawling, and stooping

The patient is observed for the ability to assume the position and regain standing. Physical complaints are documented. Crawling is often difficult for the hand-injured patient. The technique used to support the body weight on the hand should be documented, that is, weightbearing on the proximal phalanges, fingertips, or palm.

This information can be compared with observations made during the setup on an activity or during standardized tests.

Standing, sitting, walking

The patient is observed throughout the evaluation and allowed to alternate positions. Any abnormal postures or difficulty is documented.

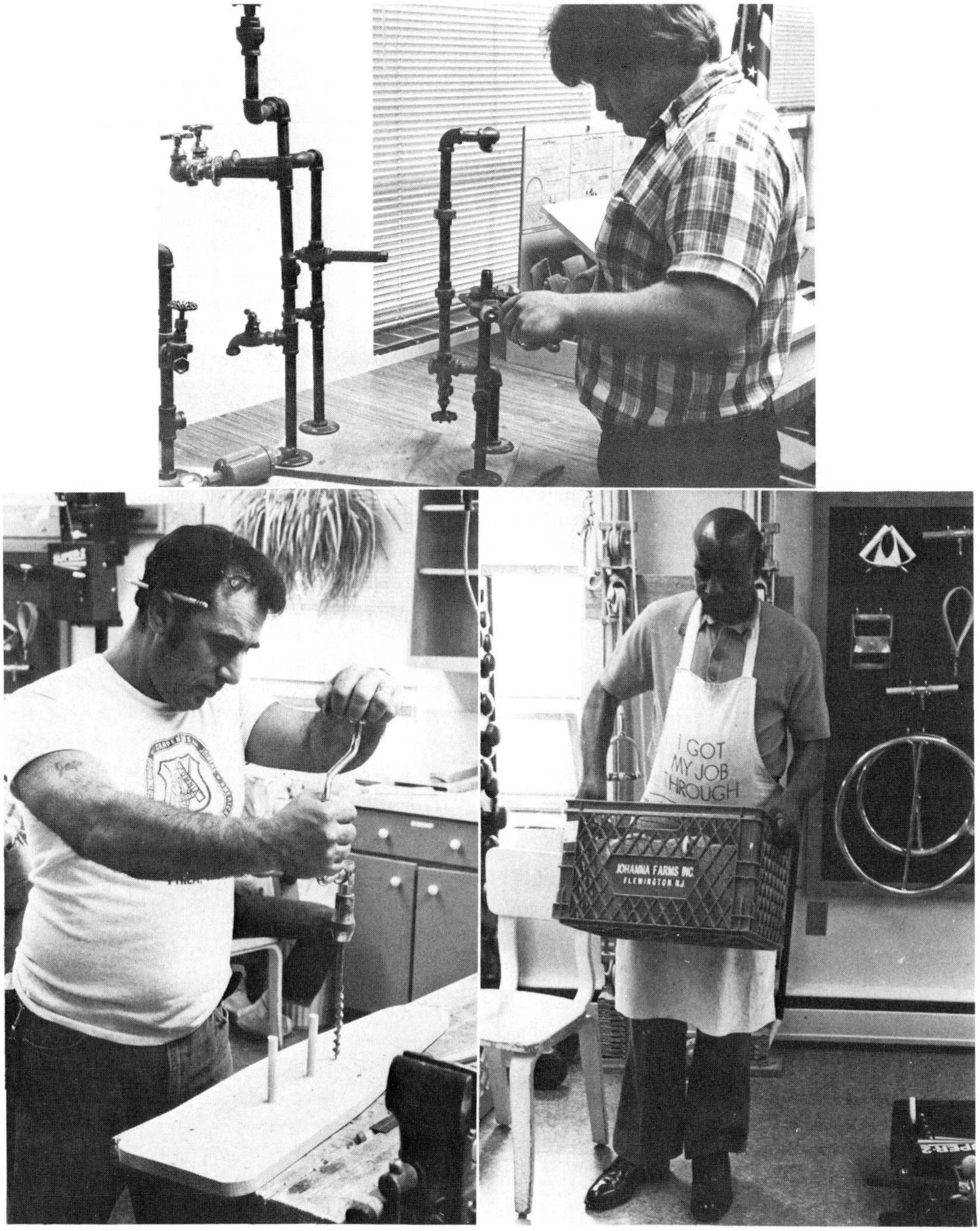

Fig. 7-1 Patients are observed as they perform the physical demands of their jobs.

Reaching

Observations are made regarding trunk and upper extremity substitution, body asymmetry, and pallor of the hand during prolonged overhead reaching. Discussion of reaching tasks should include the location and description of any discomfort during reaching within that specific range. Also, discussion can include the patient's ability to reach and manipulate, to reach to obtain heavy objects, or to sustain reaching.

Handling

For the observation of handling skills, the examiner notes the patient's method of grasping a tool, that is, lists deficits of full grasping abilities, coordination of movement, and frequency of dropped objects. Also documented is the patient's ability to cross midline; that is, during the Minnesota Rate of Manipulation Test, any postural substitution for distal deficits is noted, as is the patient's ability to display bilateral integration. If applicable, the examiner observes for equivalent grasp patterns bilaterally. Also noted is whether the patient can use the injured extremity similar to the uninjured one in bilateral tasks. Comments are made regarding his ability when his vision is occluded, such as during testing with the Valpar Whole Body Range of Motion Work Sample (Fig. 7-2).

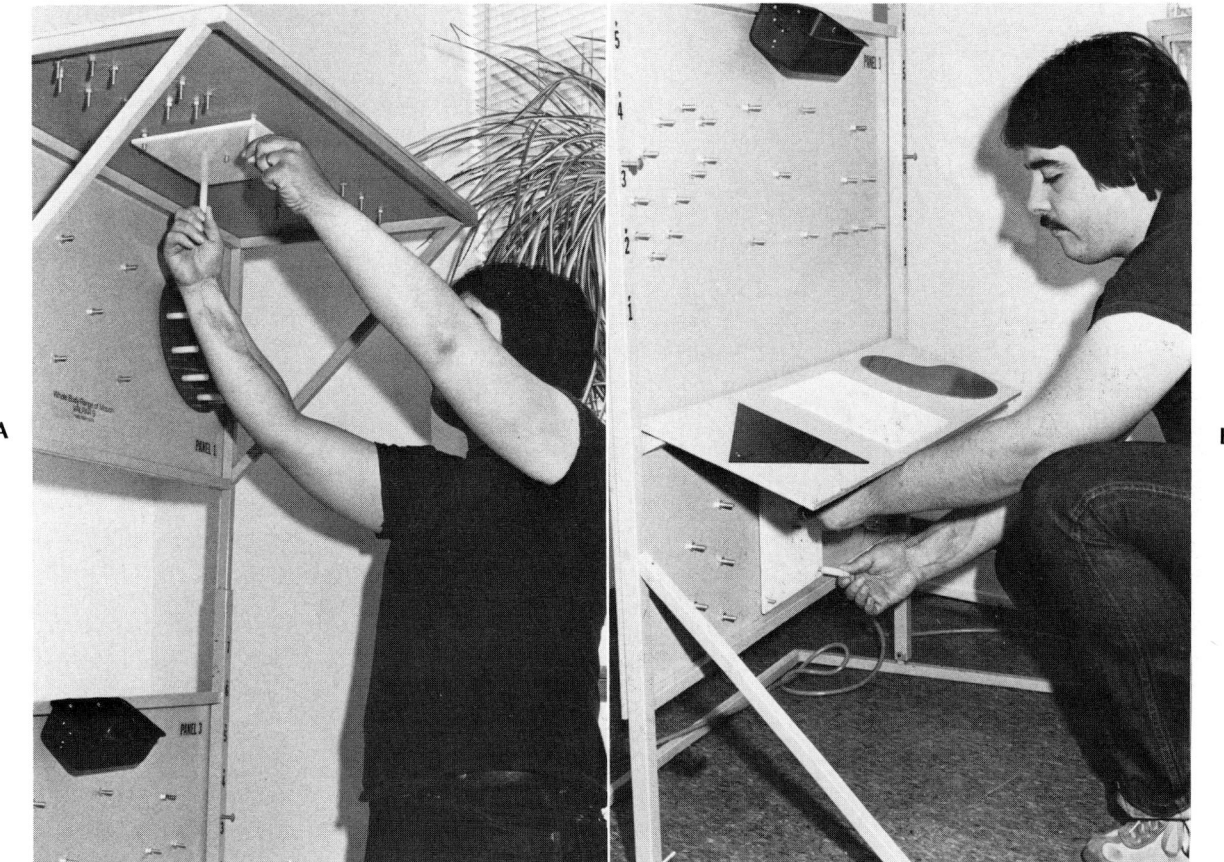

Fig. 7-2   A, Patient's endurance in overhead work is tested with this Valpar work sample. **B,** Patient stoops as he manipulates objects with his vision occluded.

Manipulation

The observations for manipulation are similar to those for handling skills. In addition, the patient's preferred prehension patterns are assessed.

Talking, hearing, seeing

During standardized evaluations, deficits in the ability to follow verbal and written instructions are noted. During the initial interview, the patient's ability to clearly communicate with the examiner is documented.

During all observations, the examiner documents any inconsistency between measurements of the same physical demand, such as the patient who displays an inability to achieve full shoulder flexion when measured with the goniometer but can complete the motion when reaching overhead on the Valpar Whole Body Range of Motion Work Sample.

ADMINISTRATION OF STANDARDIZED TESTS

This section of the physical capacity evaluation permits comparison of the patient's abilities with normative data.

Jebson-Taylor Hand Function Test

The Jebson-Taylor Hand Function Test[7] was developed to assess both prehension and manipulation skills with functional tasks. The test allows for the comparison of dominant and nondominant hands. Normative data are available with

divisions relative to age and sex. There are seven subtests that assess the patient's ability to write, turn cards, manipulate small common objects, use a spoon, manipulate small disks, and achieve a wide grasp around both empty and full 1-pound cans. Written instructions are read to the patient. A stopwatch is needed with test administration (Fig. 7-3).

An advantage of the test is that it can provide the examiner with measurable data regarding functional hand use within the short time it takes to administer. The test is easily constructed with readily available materials.

However, the Jebson-Taylor Hand Function Test does not test bilateral integration for functional tasks. The test does not emphasize a need to document altered prehension and manipulation patterns, because the scores are based on completion time in seconds. The documentation on altered prehension is extremely valuable and is included in the observation section within the physical capacity evaluation.

Minnesota Rate of Manipulation Test

The Minnesota Rate of Manipulation Test (MRMT)[6] was originally designed in 1933 to provide employers with a tool to improve personnel selection for jobs requiring manual dexterity. The source for normative data was an unemployed older-adult group before 1946 and young adults in 1957.

The test can be administered either individually or to a group. In a group, the motivation to complete the test

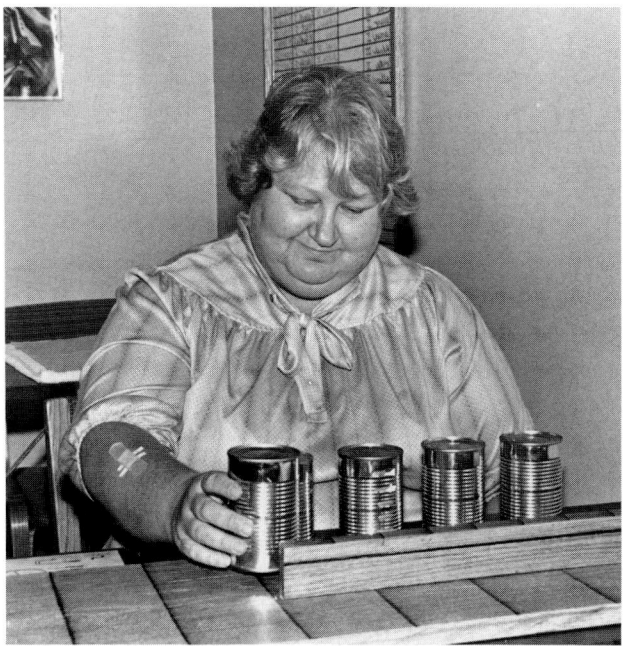

Fig. 7-3 Ability to perform prehension tasks is assessed with the Jebson Hand Function Test.

quickly is high. The examiner is responsible to motivate the patients during the test if administered individually. The materials needed to administer the test include the testing board, disks, stopwatch, and the instruction manual.

The test consists of five subtests that can assess both unilateral and bilateral manipulation. These include unilateral placing test, turning test, displacing test, turning and placing test, and the bilateral turning and placing test.

The advantages of the MRMT include: (1) the test allows for the evaluation of endurance with manipulation tasks if many of the subtests are assessed during one evaluation period; (2) only one of the subtests can be administered if desired; (3) sustained reaching at shoulder height can be observed during testing; and (4) the test can provide the astute examiner an opportunity to observe the patient's attitude, assurance, ability to follow instructions, and planning skills.[6]

There are also some disadvantages with this test. The test provides information about only one type of hand manipulation skill, such as managing 1-inch disks. If proximal range-of-motion limitations are present, the distal function may not be measured accurately.

Purdue Pegboard Test

The Purdue Pegboard Test[9] was designed in 1948 to test the dexterity needed for potential employees to perform jobs, such as assembly work, packing, or machine operation. Tip-pinch dexterity and the ability to reach when seated at table height are assessed. The equipment needed includes a stopwatch, the testing board with the pieces, and the standardized instruction manual. The pegboard has a row of four recessed cups that contain pegs, washers, and collars. The latest normative data available are based on a one-trial procedure. The normative sample was drawn from both men and women, primarily in the eastern half of the United States. The norms are categorized by sex,

specific jobs, such as assembly workers, and hand dominance. Additional norms are available for children, for those who are mentally disabled, and for candidates for vocational rehabilitation.[9]

There are four subtests in which both unilateral and bilateral prehension can be assessed. Both a comparison between hands and bilateral integration can be measured. The subtests include (1) prehension tests for the right hand, left hand, and both hands, and (2) an assembly task for both hands. Each of the subtests can be performed one to three times. The test takes approximately 15 minutes.

The benefits of the Purdue Pegboard Test include the following: (1) the test can be administered within a short time and can be given to a group of patients at one time if several testing boards are available, and (2) it allows the examiner to observe the patient for any limitations in sensory function in the median nerve–innervated area.

The limitations of the test include (1) a limited application to functional hand use, because the score depends on the speed of manipulation and not the quality of prehension, and (2) the normative data are based on specific occupations, so patients not employed in those types of industries cannot be expected to perform within norms.

Valpar Work Samples

The Valpar Work Samples* are a group of standardized tests used at the Hand Rehabilitation Center of Philadelphia to provide quantitative measurement of a patient's ability to perform job-related tasks. These standardized tests are designed to evaluate specific physical demands that are inherent in many industrial jobs, such as reaching, handling, and manipulating various objects.

The use of standardized norms facilitates comparison of the patient's work performance with that of the uninjured worker population. During performance of a work sample, a patient is given the opportunity to report physical discomfort or fatigue he experiences, and this information is recorded on a chart designed by the Valpar Corporation (Fig. 7-4). The work samples also provide the therapist the opportunity to document worker characteristics, such as ability to complete tasks according to instructions.

The Valpar Corporation has developed 19 work samples used by therapists and vocational evaluators. The following four work samples are used most frequently for physical capacity evaluations at the Hand Rehabilitation Center of Philadelphia. Careful analysis of the prevalent occupations of the patient population was used to determine the appropriate work samples chosen for the facility.

The Valpar Work Samples are used for evaluation of speed of coordination and evaluation of performance of physical demands, including reaching, handling, manipulating, and feeling. One or several of the work samples are chosen, depending on each patient's job requirements. Each Valpar Work Sample evaluates endurance and requires 20 minutes to 2 hours to administer. Therefore the evaluator must carefully select the work sample that will provide pertinent information, because time constraints do not allow administration of all four work samples.

The Valpar Upper Extremity Range of Motion Work Sam-

---

*Valpar Work Samples, Valpar Corporation, Tucson.

BODY POSITION CHART

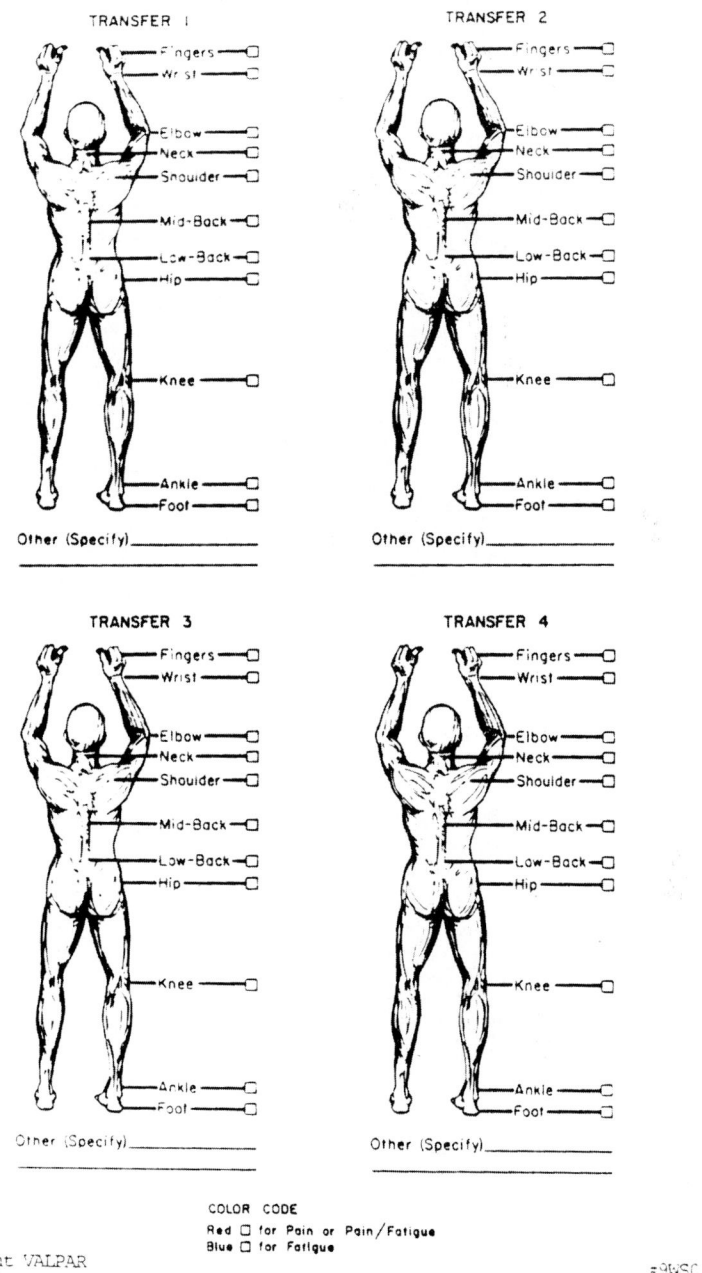

Fig. 7-4   Valpar Body Position Chart is used to record the patient's subjective complaints.

ple evaluates an individual's ability to reach into a 1-foot-square box and manipulate small and large nuts onto bolts. This work sample requires the individual to flex, extend, and radially and ulnarly deviate the wrist. Scores are calculated for the dominant and nondominant hands. Norms for employed workers are available to assess an individual's speed of coordination in comparison with a large random sample of employed workers. The test requires manipulation of the small objects with vision occluded. Therefore this test provides valuable information concerning the patient's ability to compensate for sensory deficits (Fig. 7-5).

The Valpar Whole Body Range of Motion Work Sample requires the individual to reach at shoulder level, overhead, at knee level, and at floor level to manipulate nuts onto bolts to move three plastic shapes from each of four panels of the work sample. Body postures required during the test include standing, stooping, and bending. Bilateral hand use is recommended; therefore scores for the dominant hand cannot be compared with scores for the nondominant hand. Because the work sample requires approximately 30 minutes to administer, endurance is evaluated. This work sample is chosen if the patient's job requires the physical demands of standing, stooping, crouching, reaching, handling, and manipulating. This work sample also requires manipulating objects with vision occluded (see Fig. 7-2).

The Valpar Small Tools Mechanical Work Sample is cho-

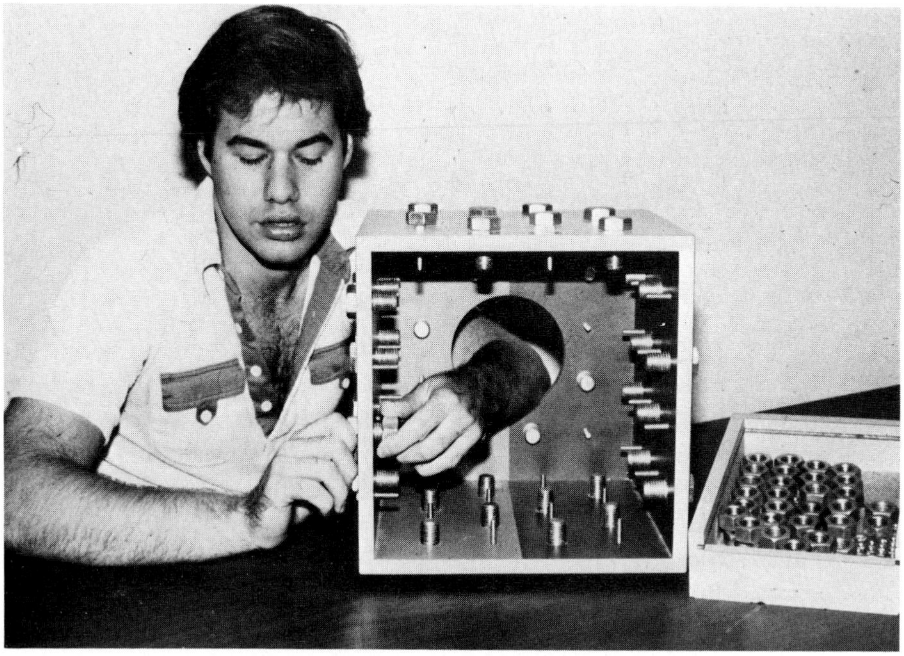

Fig. 7-5   Valpar Upper Extremity Range of Motion Work Sample assesses manipulative ability.

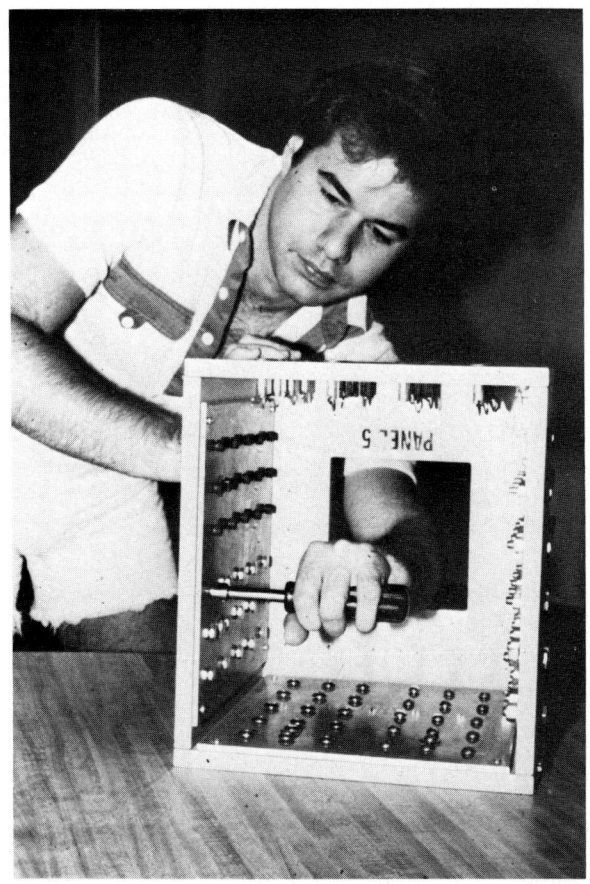

Fig. 7-6   Tool handling is assessed through this Valpar work sample.

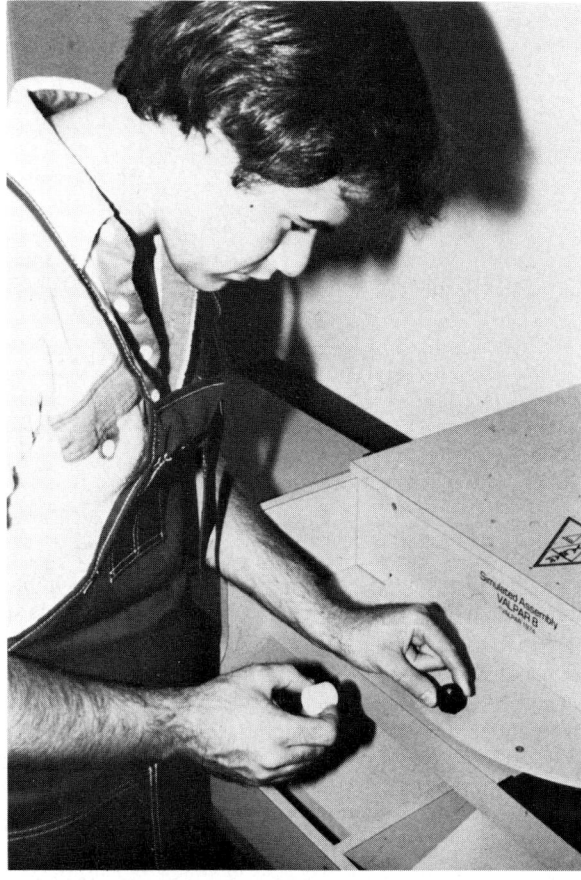

Fig. 7-7   Patient performs repetitive assembly tasks on this Valpar work sample.

sen to evaluate coordination, dexterity, and hand tool use. Appropriate candidates for this work sample include electrical workers, mechanics, and those who repair appliances and machines. The hand tools used in this work sample include pliers, screwdrivers, nut drivers, Allen wrenches, and other wrenches. The test can be administered for one or all five of the panels of the work sample. The patient must reach into a 1-foot box to manipulate the evaluation parts with the tools. The patient may work with either hand to perform the tasks; thus comparison of the dominant and nondominant hand speed cannot be made from this work sample (Fig. 7-6).

The Valpar Simulated Assembly Work Sample is designed to evaluate prolonged performance of a three-part assembly task on a simulated assembly line. The work sample includes a rotary wheel assembly line that is operated by a small motor. The individual performing the task must place a pin and two disks into a hole on the rotating wheel as it passes in front of him. This test is timed for 20 minutes and requires bilateral hand usage. Evaluation of the physical demands of standing, reaching, handling, and manipulating are observed during this test. This work sample is recommended for the patient who performs jobs such as assembly line work, inspecting work, or machine tending (Fig. 7-7).

THE WORK SIMULATOR

The BTE Work Simulator* is used to test the patient's ability to perform the physical demands of his job (Fig. 7-8). Designed to simulate upper-extremity motions required during performance of job tasks, the Work Simulator is a mechanical device with 18 tool attachments (see Chapter 100).

Tool attachments are selected to simulate the patient's job. These attachments are numbered to promote universal

---

*Work Simulator, Baltimore Therapeutic Equipment Co., Baltimore.

Table 7-2 Work Simulator tool attachments

Tool attachment numbers	Function of tool attachment
101	Small tip pinch
102	Medium tip pinch
201	Small lateral pinch
202	Medium lateral pinch
151	Three-point prehension
161	Power grip
111	Power grip, elbow flexion and extension
131	Combined upper-extremity motion with power grip (car steering wheel)
141	Combined upper-extremity motion with power grip (truck steering wheel)
302	Precision grip, wrist ulnar deviation (jar lid)
400	Lateral pinch and wrist circumduction (crank)
501	Small power grip with supination and pronation (small screwdriver)
502	Medium power grip with supination and pronation (medium screwdriver)
503	Large power grip with supination and pronation (large screwdriver)
601	Power grip with supintion and pronation
701	Elbow flexion and extension with power grip
801	Elbow flexion and extension and shoulder motion with power grip
901	Two-handed shoulder and elbow motion with T handle

use of the tools and to facilitate research that can be conducted in multiple clinical studies. Tool attachment numbers and the function of each of the tools are listed in Table 7-2 and will enable the therapist to follow the guidelines for evaluating the patient's performance of the physical demands for his job, which are listed in Table 7-1.

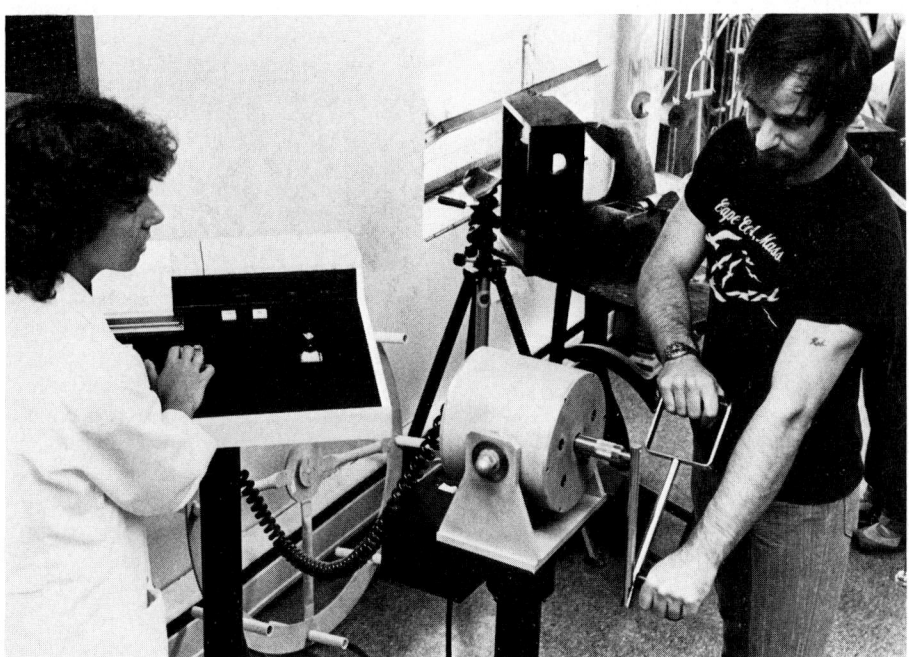

Fig. 7-8 Work Simulator assesses each patient's ability to perform his job tasks.

The Work Simulator has a calibrated electrical braking mechanism into which a tool is inserted so that the patient can work against resistance. The patient must exert force equal to the resistance set on the Work Simulator to move the tool attachment.

As the patient moves the tool attachment, the Work Simulator calculates the work output produced by the patient by multiplying the force he exerted by the distance he moved the tool attached to the shaft.[5] The Work Simulator also calculates the patient's endurance, or power output, by dividing the work produced by the amount of time worked.

The patient is instructed to exert his maximum effort as he moves the tool attachment for a 2-minute test period. The dominant hand and the nondominant hand are tested in the same manner. The numerical calculations for the work and endurance of each hand are compared. The results are interpreted by comparing the injured hand with the uninjured hand. Comparison between hands is calculated as a percent of difference for each hand for work and endurance capacity. The Work Simulator provides information that can be used to identify the patient's limitations relative to upper-extremity motions inherent in his job.

SEQUENTIAL TESTING

Comparative sequential testing is performed to determine the patient's consistent performance among various tests. The Work Simulator can be used to evaluate consistent performance of force output, according to the research by Vermette and Berlin.[3] The following procedure is used:
1. Place the Work Simulator on the manual static mode.
2. Use tool 161 for the test session.
3. Insert the tool in the brake mechanism of the Work Simulator and follow this procedure:
    a. Have the patient exert the maximum isometric force he is capable of on the 161 tool for 5 seconds. A stopwatch is used to time the patient's performance.
    b. Obtain a printout by ending the test.
    c. Perform the test three times with each hand.
    d. Add the forces for each hand. Using a calculator with statistical functions, find the mean and the standard deviation of the mean; divide standard deviation by the mean; then multiply by 100 to obtain the coefficient of variance. For men, according to Vermette and Berlin, the coefficient of variance should be no greater than 12%. For women tested in the same research project, the coefficient of variance should be no greater than 15% for tool 161.

The following format is used to report the results of the sequential testing on the Work Simulator:

Sequential testing was performed on the Work Simulator. According to the research by Vermette and Berlin in 1985 on sequential tests, the coefficient of variance should be less than 12% for men and less than 15% for women. (Patient's name) scored a _____ % coefficient of variance on the tool involving static gripping with the right hand. The patient scored a _____ % coefficient of variance with the left hand. This indicates that the patient demonstrated _____ (consistent or inconsistent) performance on sequential testing with his injured hand. The patient demonstrated _____ (consistent or inconsistent) performance with the noninjured hand.

Sequential testing using the Jamar Dynamometer was developed by Bechtol in 1954.[2] The method of sequential grip testing involved the patient in the following procedure:
1. The patient is instructed to apply his maximum force on the second or third level of the Jamar Dynamometer with each hand for three repetitions at three separate times.
2. The handle level is selected for each hand based on the patient's maximum grip strength, which is recorded before this test on all five levels of the handle of the Jamar Dynamometer. The second level of the handle is frequently the level women perform at their highest grip strength, whereas men perform higher on the third level of the Jamar Dynamometer handle.
3. A coefficient of variance is calculated for each hand based on the three grip strengths recorded during the sequential testing. The three numbers are added; then the mean and standard deviation are calculated. The mean is divided by the standard deviation and multiplied by 100 to obtain the coefficient of variance.

According to Bechtol, the coefficient of variance for sequential grip tests should be less than 10% for men or women.[2] To report on the sequential grip strength tests, the following format is used:

Grip strength was measured sequentially on the Jamar dynamometer on three occasions during the evaluation. According to the research of Bechtol in 1954, the coefficient of variance of sequential grip tests should be less than 10%. The patient scored _____ (less than or more than)10% with the right hand. He scored _____ (less than or more than)10% with the left hand. This indicates _____ (consistent or inconsistent) performance on sequential testing with the left hand.

Finally, grip strength measurements can be recorded on each of the five levels of the Jamar Dynamometer. Stokes in 1983[8] reported that if a patient is exerting maximum effort on each grip test on each position of the Jamar Dynamometer, the measurements will be lowest for the first and fifth levels and highest on the second to fourth levels. If all the measurements are similar, the patient may not be exerting his maximum effort.

SUMMARY

When all data have been analyzed, a summary of the physical capacity evaluation is formulated. This contains a brief review of the patient's demographic data, medical history, and former job status. Based on the patient's strength, speed, coordination, endurance, safety during performance, and the physical demands of work, the therapist and physician devise a summary with recommendations.

Recommendations can include return to work on a full-time basis if the patient performs all aspects of the physical capacity evaluation without difficulty. If the patient has low endurance, the therapist may arrange part-time work, which allows the patient to continue therapy.

Patients with permanent impairment, such as diminished sensibility or amputation of digits, often return to their previous jobs if modification of work tasks is permitted by their employers. If restrictions are necessary, these are outlined in the summary. For example, a carpenter may return to work but may need ergonomically designed tools.

If modifications are not available or if the patient cannot

perform the majority of the required job tasks, a referral to vocational assessment may be indicated. In this case, both the patient's abilities and limitations are listed to provide information for an alternative job search. Abilities and limitations are described in terms of the physical demands of work. For example, a patient may be able to lift 50 pounds to chest height, but repetitive lifting may not be recommended. In the instance where inconsistent test responses were obtained, this is noted; however, the physician, not the therapist, interprets the results. Recommendations for work restrictions are based on the U.S. Department of Labor Work Levels (see box above).

Sample reports follow. Names are deleted to ensure confidentiality.

SAMPLE REPORT I

The following illustrates test performance of a patient that resulted in the recommendation of return to work.

Physical capacity evaluation

Name	Mr. X
Date	March 1988
Evaluator	Therapist A

Medical history and identifying information

This 36-year-old, right-hand–dominant man was employed at a steel fabrication company. On October 6, 1986, Mr. X sustained lacerations to his left long and ring digits while at work. Surgery was performed by Dr. A and Dr. B. Mr. X was followed in therapy at the Hand Rehabilitation Center since October 1986. At present, Mr. X continues therapy. He has not worked since the injury. At the time of this evaluation, he was 3 months postoperative extensor tenolysis of the extensor tendon system from the wrist to the middle phalanx of the left long finger and dorsal capsulotomy of the metacarpophalangeal joint of the left long finger.

Mr. X indicated that he is married with three children. He indicated he is independent in self-care activities. He reported he has difficulty using his injured left hand to grasp objects, because his left third and fourth fingers do not extend completely and frequently knock objects over. He also reported he cannot grip heavy objects and cannot manipulate objects with the left hand. Additional medical history is significant for a back sprain approximately 10 years ago. The patient stated he is taking Inderal for migraine headaches.

Job history

Mr. X was employed as a blanking line operator for 6 years. An on-site visit was made on March 7, 1988, by his rehabilitation specialist. A job analysis and a video tape of an operator performing this job was presented to the therapist before evaluation of the patient. Job simulation was performed during this evaluation to simulate the patient's specific job tasks in his work as a blanking line operator.

As seen in the video and as described on the job analysis, left hand use during this work requires lifting and attaching chains to hoists, controlling the hoists, pushing a lever, using both hands to pick up various guides to set up the machine, turning knobs, holding and pushing wood pieces through a table saw, picking up the metal coil and pulling it to the second component of the machine, pushing roller coils, pulling stacked steel on the roller coils, pulling skids, lifting, bending, and cutting cardboard into shape, and applying wire to the steel bundles and cranking the metal bander with the left hand. The right hand performs fine manipulation and operates a hoist as well as performs bilateral lifting with the left hand.

According to the job analysis completed by the rehabilitation specialist, maximum lifting requirements include 20 pounds occasionally and 10 pounds frequently, using both hands. The work is done in various body postures, such as kneeling frequently, standing, and walking continuously, and continuous grasping and handling while reaching. The work environment includes indoor work with cold temperature indoors during the winter. Fumes, dust, and noise are minimal.

Mr. X reported an additional job history that included work as a stockman, sand blaster operator, crane operator, and loader.

Dr. A ordered the physical capacity evaluation to determine if Mr. X could return to his present job and to identify the level of work he could accomplish given his physical abilities and limitations. The physical capacity evaluation consists of three key components: hand function evaluation, administration of standardized tests, and observation of performance of physical demands and job simulation.

Hand function evaluation

Grip strength taken on the Jamar Dynamometer was as follows:

Jamar dynamometer	Right	Left
Level I (tight grip)	78 lbs.	20 lbs.
Level II	82 lbs.	27 lbs.
Level III	81 lbs.	28 lbs.
Level IV	64 lbs.	25 lbs.
Level V (wide grip)	75 lbs.	30 lbs.

The patient complained of pain in his left fourth proximal interphalangeal joint when he performed the wide-grip test. Pinch measurements were recorded with the pinch gauge and were as follows:

Pinch	Right	Left
Lateral pinch		
Thumb-index	30 lbs.	22 lbs.
Tip pinch		
Thumb-index	16 lbs.	11 lbs.
Thumb-long	22 lbs.	7 lbs.
Thumb-ring	13 lbs.	5 lbs.
Thumb-little	8 lbs.	7 lbs.

Active range-of-motion measurements were recorded by measuring the distance from the fingertips to the distal palmar crease. With the right digits, the patient could touch his palmar crease without difficulty. With the left digits, he lacked 3 cm touching the distal palmar crease with his long finger, 4 cm with his ring finger, and 0.5 cm with his little finger. The left index finger could touch the distal palmar crease.

Volumetric measurements taken before and after the physical capacity evaluation demonstrated that there was a mild increase in hand volume in the right and left hands after the patient worked for 3 hours. The right-hand volume increased from 550 ml to 570 ml. The left-hand volume increased from 560 ml to 565 ml.

Sensibility was evaluated by testing light touch/deep pressure sensation, two-point discrimination, and speed of prehension with vision occluded. The patient demonstrated normal sensibility in all areas of the right and left hands. Light touch/deep pressure and two-point discrimination was slightly diminished in the left hand compared with the right hand with vision occluded. The left hand required 15.9 seconds to pick up and place seven objects in a box, whereas the right hand completed this task in 11.6 seconds.

Administration of standardized tests

The Valpar Whole Body Range of Motion Work Sample was used to assess the patient's ability to handle and manipulate objects while working in various body positions, including bending, kneeling, and stooping with vision occluded. Mr. X scored in the 95th percentile using the Valpar San Diego Employed Worker Norms. This score is an above-average score, because the Employed Worker Norms range from 0% to 100%.

The Valpar Small Tools Mechanical Work Sample measures a patient's ability to work with small tools. On this test the patient was required to handle wrenches, because this is required in his work. Mr. X scored in the 95th percentile using San Diego Employed Worker Method Timed Motion Standards. This score is an entry level performance score, because Employed Worker Method Timed Motion Standards range from 0% to 150% with 100% indicative of entry level performance.

Observation of performance of physical demands of work

Physical task and observations

Lifting/carrying. Mr. X could lift and carry 28 pounds with the left arm and 57 pounds with the right arm a distance of 25 feet. He could lift and carry 30 pounds with both arms.

Pushing/pulling. Mr. X could push and pull a weighted box with 48 pounds with the left arm and 93 pounds with the right arm.

Reaching. Mr. X could reach overhead, forward, and to floor level without difficulty. However, he complained of fatigue in the right shoulder with prolonged overhead reaching.

Grasping/handling. Mr. X could use his right hand for grasping and handling of small, light, and heavy objects without difficulty. He could use his left hand for grasping and handling of light objects without difficulty. He experienced difficulty handling small and heavy objects with his left hand.

Manipulation. Fine manipulation was below normal limits with the right and left hand when tested on the Nine-Hole Peg Test by Mathiowetz. However, manipulation on the Valpar Work Samples indicated the patient had above-average speed of coordination when using both hands together. With the right hand, the patient was observed cutting with a razor knife without difficulty. With the left hand, he experienced some difficulty controlling the razor knife.

Standing/sitting/walking. Standing, sitting, and walking tolerance was estimated by the patient to be 8 hours with breaks. There was normal body posture observed.

Climbing stairs. Mr. X could climb stairs without difficulty.

Kneeling/crouching. Mr. X could kneel, crouch, and stoop frequently without difficulty.

Endurance. Endurance was tested using the Work Simulator—a computerized evaluation instrument that can measure the amount of power emitted by the hands and arms with a variety of tools. The test compared tool use between hands for 3 minutes. With the tool that simulates use of pliers, the patient's right hand measured 73% greater endurance than his left hand. On the tool that simulates pushing and pulling levers overhead, the right hand demonstrated 50% greater endurance than the left hand. On the tool that simulates turning knobs, the patient's right hand demonstrated 79% greater endurance than his left hand.

Comment

Sequential testing was performed on the Work Simulator to analyze the patient's consistent effort. According to Berlin and Vermette in 1985, the coefficient of variance on sequential tests should be no greater than 12% for men. The patient scored 5.4% with his right hand and 12% with his left hand, which indicated that he was performing with consistent effort with both hands.

Summary and recommendations

Based on Mr. X's test response, it is recommended that he can perform the job requirements of a blanking operator. He can lift and carry the work load required in this job. He can push and pull and handle objects as is required at work. The patient can perform the job duties of a blanking line operator, because the work does not require heavy lifting or repetitive tight grip of the left hand.

Mr. X demonstrated weak grasp of the left hand, weak pinch, limited range of motion of the left third and fourth digits, and mild swelling of both hands. However, because of his job requirements, he is physically able to perform light work of lifting less than 20 pounds occasionally and 10 pounds frequently.

He also can push and pull the heavy steel coils by grasping the handles on the pallets. He can use his left hand to move the hoist and place the chain on the hoist without difficulty. He may experience some mild difficulty pulling the steel to the second machine with his left hand. However, he could compensate and perform this task adequately with both hands.

It is recommended that Mr. X be released to return to his former job as a blanking line operator. With performance of work activities, it is believed that he will continue to increase his strength and endurance.

SAMPLE REPORT II

This report illustrates a recommendation for the patient to participate in a work tolerance program to recover strength and endurance in the right upper extremity.

Physical capacity evaluation

Name	Ms. Y
Claim no.	000-1
Date	July 7, 1988
Evaluator	Therapist A

Medical history and identifying information

This 19-year-old, right-hand–dominant woman was employed as a donut packer. On December 21, 1987, she sustained a crush injury to her right forearm while at work. The injury resulted in fractures in her right radius and ulna that required plating at Hospital A. Dr. A closed the wound secondarily a few days after the initial injury. Because of nonhealing of the fracture, replating and bone grafting of the fractures were performed by Dr. B a week after the initial injury. The patient has not returned to work since the date of injury.

Ms. Y indicated that she is single with one child. She indicated she is independent in self-care and home-care activities; however, she experiences difficulty using her right hand for any activities requiring strength and manipulation, such as buttoning, zipping, bathing her son, pulling her clothes on, and lifting trash bags. She stated her leisure activities included biking and working out at a spa. She reported she has been unable to participate in these activities since her injury.

Ms. Y indicated her major physical difficulties with her injured arm include limited motion, limited strength, discomfort with reaching, numbness around the scar, and fatigue of the arm. She described discomfort when reaching as a pulling sensation radiating from the forearm up her arm. She did not report any additional medical history or use of any medication at this time.

Job history

Ms. Y was employed as a donut packer for 6 weeks. *The Dictionary of Occupational Titles* defines this job as medium work requiring lifting, carrying, pushing, and pulling of 50 pounds, with frequent reaching, handling, and manipulating required. Ms. Y described the job requirements as rapid packing of donuts in cartons, opening cartons, pushing and pulling cartons, and working in a damp, cool environment.

Dr. B ordered a physical capacity evaluation to determine if Ms. Y can return to her present job and to identify her physical capabilities and limitations. The physical capacity evaluation consists of three key components: hand function evaluation, administration of standardized tests, and observation of performance of physical demands and job simulation.

Hand function evaluation

Grip strength taken on the Jamar Dynamometer was as follows:

Jamar Dynamometer	Right	Left
Level I (tight grip)	6 lbs.	20 lbs.
Level II	18 lbs.	37 lbs.
Level III	17 lbs.	47 lbs.
Level IV	20 lbs.	40 lbs.
Level V (wide grip)	18 lbs.	34 lbs.

Pinch measurements were recorded with the pinch gauge and were as follows:

Pinch	Right	Left
Lateral pinch	9½ lbs.	12 lbs.
3 point pinch	7 lbs.	12 lbs.
Tip pinch		
Thumb-index	7 lbs.	8 lbs.
Thumb-long	7½ lbs.	9 lbs.
Thumb-ring	6 lbs.	6 lbs.
Thumb-little	5½ lbs.	3½ lbs.

Active range-of-motion measurements were recorded with a goniometer as follows: right elbow lacked 20 degrees of flexion, right forearm lacked 20 degrees of supination, right wrist lacked 40 degrees of flexion and 40 degrees of extension. Radial deviation was restricted by 5 degrees, and ulnar deviation was restricted by 10 degrees.

Volumetric measurements taken before and after the physical capacity evaluation demonstrated that there was a significant increase in hand volume in the right hand. This indicated that the patient did not tolerate 3 hours of manual work without swelling in her right hand. Hand volume decreased in the left hand after this evaluation.

Administration of standardized tests

Coordination and dexterity were assessed using the Jebson-Taylor Hand Function Test. This test measures the patient's ability to write, turn cards over, manipulate small, lightweight objects, and pick up large, circumferential objects. Ms. Y scored within normal limits on four of the seven test components with her injured right hand. She scored below normal limits on picking up small objects, eating, and lifting 1-pound objects. She scored within normal limits on all seven of the test components with her left hand.

The Minnesota Rate of Manipulation Test was used to measure the patient's speed of manipulation. On the placing test, the patient scored in the 1st percentile with her right hand and 1st percentile with her left hand. This indicates her speed of coordination for reaching and handling is extremely slow.

The Valpar Upper Extremity Range of Motion Work Sample was used to assess the reaching, handling, and manipulating ability of each hand. Ms. Y scored in the 5th percentile with her right hand and the 10th percentile with her left hand. These scores are below average, because the San Diego Employed Worker Norms range from 0% to 100%.

Observation of performance of physical demands of work

Physical task and observation

Lifting/carrying. Ms. Y could lift and carry 7 pounds with her right hand and 17 pounds with her left hand a distance of 25 feet. She could lift 17 pounds using both hands. When lifting overhead, however, Ms. Y's maximum weight tolerated was 10 pounds. She complained of discomfort in her right wrist when she attempted to lift overhead.

Pushing/pulling. Ms. Y could push and pull ten pounds with her right arm using a wall pulley for 3 minutes. Using her left arm, she was able to push and pull 60 pounds.

Reaching. Ms. Y could reach forward, overhead, and to floor level with the right and left hands without difficulty. However, she reported a pulling sensation radiating from her hand to her right shoulder when she attempted to reach overhead.

Grasping/handling. Ms. Y could use her right hand for grasping and handling of small and lightweight objects without difficulty when speed was not required. She experienced difficulty lifting objects weighing more than 4 pounds with her right hand when reaching overhead or at waist level was required. She could use her left hand for grasping and handling of small, light, and heavy objects without difficulty.

Manipulation. Fine manipulation was below normal limits with the right and left hands. See results of standardized test.

Standing/sitting/walking. Ms. Y estimated her standing tolerance to be 8 hours daily. Her walking tolerance was estimated to be 8 hours with no restrictions. Abnormal posture was not observed during this evaluation. She estimated she could walk 5 miles without difficulty.

Climbing stairs. Ms. Y was observed climbing three flights of stairs without difficulty.

Kneeling/crouching/stooping. Ms. Y could kneel, crouch, and stoop frequently without difficulty.

Endurance. Endurance was tested using the Work Simulator—a computerized evaluation instrument that can measure the amount of power emitted by the hands and arms with a variety of tools. The test compared tool use between hands for 3 minutes. With a tool that simulates repetitive gripping of pliers, the left hand demonstrated 48% greater endurance than the right hand. On the tool that simulates pushing and pulling objects, the left hand demonstrated 24% greater endurance than the right hand. On the tool that requires gripping with repetitive supination and pronation of the forearm, the left hand demonstrated 32% greater endurance than the right hand. On the tool that requires pulling objects, the left hand demonstrated 11% greater endurance than the right hand.

Sequential testing. Sequential testing was performed to assess the patient's consistent effort on the Work Simulator and on the grip test with the Jamar Dynamometer. On the sequential test, Ms. Y performed within the coefficient of variance of less than 10% for grip strength and less than 15% for the work simulator. This indicates she exerted her consistent effort during testing.

Summary

This 19-year-old, right-hand–dominant woman sustained a fracture of her radius and ulna on December 22, 1987, while at work. Surgical procedures included plating, bone grafting, and replating. She has not worked since the date of injury. She complained of difficulty using her right arm for activities that require strength or repetitive use. She complained of swelling, limited motion, limited strength, numbness around the scar, and fatigue.

Based on the test results of this evaluation, Ms. Y cannot return to her former job as a donut maker. She is unable to perform the physical demands of this job, which include lifting of 50 pounds, pushing and pulling of 50 pounds, rapid manipulation for packing donuts into containers, opening containers, and opening boxes. The patient's right arm swelled after 3 hours of manual work.

Grip strength of the right hand measured 20 pounds maximum as compared with 47 pounds maximum in the left hand. Lateral pinch with the right thumb measured 7 pounds as compared with 12 pounds in the left thumb. Tip pinch of the right index measured 7 pounds as compared with 8 pounds in the left index finger. Range of motion was normal in the left arm, wrist, and hand. Range of motion was decreased in the right forearm, elbow, and wrist.

Manipulation was below normal limits in both the right and left hands. Maximum lifting ability was 7 pounds with the right hand compared with 17 pounds with the left hand. Pushing and pulling were restricted in the right arm to 10 pounds as compared with 60 pounds in the left arm.

The patient had difficulty with the right arm grasping and handling objects weighing more than 1 pound. With the left arm, she could grasp and handle small, heavy, and light objects without difficulty. Endurance was decreased in the right arm compared with the left arm. The patient demonstrated consistent effort on sequential testing on the Work Simulator and on the Jamar Dynamometer grip test.

It is recommended that this patient participate in 4 to 6 weeks of therapy to recover strength and endurance in her right arm. The patient can perform sedentary or light work that does not require rapid manipulation with the right arm. She has good ability to stand, sit, walk, stoop, kneel, or crouch. She can reach at waist level and to floor level with the right arm without difficulty. She complained of painful sensation in her right arm when she attempted to reach overhead. She can grasp and handle small or light objects with the right or left hand. It would be advisable for the patient to attend therapy even if she is returning to sedentary or light work.

SAMPLE REPORT III

This sample is an example of a report that recommends placement in modified work.

Physical capacity evaluation

Name	Mr. Z
Date	July 7, 1988
Evaluator	Therapist A

Medical history and identifying information

This 29-year-old, right-hand–dominant man was employed as a service technician for a medical supply company. On July 21, 1987, Mr. Z sustained an injury to his left wrist while lifting a dental chair with one other person. He stated that he felt a sharp pain in his wrist while performing this lifting activity at work.

On April 7, 1988, Dr. A performed an excision of a ganglion cyst of the left wrist. The patient was followed in therapy at another center for 2 months after surgery. At present, he is discharged from therapy. The patient reported that he returned to work for 1 week after his injury in July 1987 and has not worked for almost a year.

Mr. Z indicated that he is single with no children. He indicated that he is independent in self-care activities and home-care activities. His leisure activities include fishing, and he has been able to do this after surgery.

The patient indicated that his major difficulties now include swelling after strenuous activity, occasional wrist pain and soreness, and decreased wrist flexion. He reported that he had severe pain before surgery and now feels "much better." The patient reported no other medical history. He stated that he takes allergy medication and occasionally aspirin or Tylenol for wrist pain.

Job history

Mr. Z was employed as a service technician at Company X. *The Dictionary of Occupational Titles* defines this job as medium work involving reaching, handling, fingering, feeling, talking, hearing, and seeing. Medium work is described as occasional lifting of 50 pounds and frequent lifting of 25 pounds.

The patient also has attended school and is trained as an electronics technician. The job of an electronics technician is defined by *The Dictionary of Occupational Titles* as light work requiring occasional lifting of 20 pounds with frequent lifting of as much as 10 pounds. It also involves use of tools and test equipment involving reaching, handling, fingering, and feeling.

The patient described the requirements of his job as a service technician as installing dental equipment. He stated that his lifting requirements ranged from very light objects to very heavy objects. He occasionally was required to lift dental chairs with the assistance of another person. A dental chair may weigh up as much as 500 pounds. He was responsible for use of tools, including drills, hammers, pliers, screwdrivers, and wrenches. He occasionally was responsible for unloading trucks. The patient stated that he was fired from this job after his injury. The patient reported additional job history included work as a computer technician, manager of a car wash, and driver of a lumber truck.

Dr. B ordered the physical capacity evaluation to determine Mr. Z's physical capabilities and limitations. The physical capacity evaluation consists of three components: hand function evaluation, administration of standardized tests, and observation of performance of physical demands and job simulation.

Hand function evaluation

Measurements of grip strength taken with the Jamar Dynamometer were as follows:

Jamar Dynamometer	Right	Left
Level I (tight grip)	115 lbs.	85 lbs.
Level II	134 lbs.	118 lbs.
Level III	120 lbs.	99 lbs.
Level IV	105 lbs.	91 lbs.
Level V (wide grip)	89 lbs.	79 lbs.

Pinch measurements were taken on a pinch gauge as follows:

Pinch	Right	Left
Lateral pinch	26 lbs.	23 lbs.
Tip pinch		
Thumb to index	17 lbs.	16 lbs.
Thumb to long	19 lbs.	17 lbs.
Thumb to ring	10 lbs.	10 lbs.
Thumb to little	5½ lbs.	4 lbs.

Measurements of active range of motion were recorded with a goniometer as follows: right wrist extension, 65 degrees; right wrist flexion, 70 degrees; left wrist extension, 60 degrees; and left wrist flexion, 35 degrees. No limitations were noted in digital range of motion, and the patient could make a full fist.

Volumetric measurements were taken before and after the physical capacity evaluation. These measurements demonstrated that there was no significant increase in hand volume: the patient tolerated 3 hours of manual work without swelling in the hand.

Administration of standardized tests

The Valpar Upper Extremity Range of Motion Work Sample was used to assess the reaching, handling, and manipulating ability of each hand. The test was performed in a confined space with vision occluded. Mr. Z scored in the 95th percentile with the right hand and in the 70th percentile with the left hand. His score for the injured left hand is a below-average score compared with San Diego Employed Worker Norms ranging from 0% to 100%. The patient worked slowly and experienced pain while working on the panel of the assembly task that required extreme wrist flexion. He did not demonstrate difficulty with the other panels.

The Valpar Small Tools Mechanical Work Sample measures a patient's ability to work with small tools. The patient assembled the panel requiring use of the Allen wrench and nutdriver with the left hand. The patient scored 110% with the left hand, which is an average score compared with Method Timed Motion scores, which range from 0% to 150%. Mr. Z complained of no pain after this activity.

The Purdue Pegboard Test was used to measure fine fingertip dexterity. The patient could manipulate 17 pegs in 30 seconds with the right hand. This score fell in the 30th percentile compared with standardized norms. He also could manipulate 17 pegs in 30 seconds with the left hand. This score falls in the 50th percentile. Scores with both hands fell below average compared with standardized norms. However, it is believed that the patient has functional fine dexterity in the injured left hand, because he scored as high as the noninjured right hand.

Observation of performance of physical demands of work

Physical task and observation

Lifting/carrying. The patient could lift and carry (in a bucket over a distance of 25 feet) 51 pounds with the right arm and 32 pounds with the left arm. He could lift and carry 66 pounds holding a box at waist height with both arms. He could lift 25 pounds using both hands to an overhead height. He could lift 45 pounds to waist height and floor level.

Pushing/pulling. The patient could push and pull 60 pounds repetitively at waist height with the right hand and 45 pounds using the left hand for 3 minutes.

Reaching. The patient could reach forward, overhead, and to floor level with no difficulty with either hand.

Grasping/handling. The patient could use both hands to grasp and handle small, light, and heavy objects without difficulty.

Manipulation. Fine manipulation was observed to be within normal limits for both hands. The patient had difficulty manipulating objects with the wrist in a flexed position.

Standing/sitting/walking. During the 3-hour evaluation, the patient was observed to have no difficulty with standing, walking, or sitting. Normal gait and body posture were observed.

Climbing stairs/ladder. The patient reported no difficulty climbing stairs. He could climb a ladder without difficulty and could support his body weight on his injured left hand.

Kneeling/crouching/crawling/stooping. The patient could kneel, crouch, and stoop without difficulty. During crawling he reported pain in his wrist when asked to support his body weight on his wrist in a fully extended position.

Endurance. Endurance was tested using the Work Simulator—a computerized evaluation instrument that can measure the amount of power emitted by the hands and arms with a variety of tools. The test compared tool use between hands for 3 minutes. With a tool that simulates repetitive gripping of pliers, the right hand showed 22% more power than the left hand. The patient was also tested with a tool that simulates repetitive wrist motions as in using a screwdriver; however, the patient could not obtain a power reading with either hand using this tool.

Sequential testing. Sequential testing was performed on the Work Simulator. According to the research of Vermette and Berlin in 1985, on sequential tests, the coefficient of variance should be less than 12% for men. The patient scored 1% with the left hand and 1% with the right hand. This indicates that he demonstrated consistent performance on sequential testing with both hands.

Grip strength was measured sequentially on the Jamar Dynamometer on two occasions during the physical capacity evaluation. According to the research of Bechtol in 1954, the coefficient of variance on sequential grip tests should be less than 10%. Mr. Z scored 1% and 4% with the right hand. He scored 1% and 5% with the left hand. This indicates that he showed consistent performance with both hands.

Summary and recommendations

Mr. Z is a 29-year-old, right-hand–dominant man who injured his left wrist at work on 7/21/87. On April 7, 1988, the patient underwent excision of a ganglion cyst of the left wrist.

The patient reported no difficulties with activities of daily living. He complained of swelling after strenuous activity; however, no swelling was noted after the 3-hour physical capacity evaluation. The patient reported frequent soreness in his wrist and occasional pain.

The patient showed functional strength in both hands. The right hand measured 134 pounds of grip strength compared with 118 pounds in the left hand. Wrist flexion was limited in the left wrist to 35 degrees compared with 75 degrees in the right wrist.

Standardized testing was performed. The patient showed decreased ability to manipulate objects in a position of wrist flexion. Fine manipulation and tool use were within normal limits. The patient's lifting ability was tested to be 66 pounds bilaterally. The patient was able to lift 51 pounds with the right hand compared with 32 pounds with the left hand.

The patient stated that he will not be returning to his former job as a service technician. The patient's medical chart contained job descriptions from a vocational rehabilitation service. The first of these jobs is as a factory helper requiring 20 pounds lifting, simple grasping, and fine manipulation. The patient would have the physical abilities to perform this job. The second job involves installing car stereos. The patient would have difficulty using tools in enclosed spaces where he is required to use extremes of wrist flexion. The patient does have the fine motor ability to perform electronics work that does not require extremes of wrist flexion.

Based on the results of this evaluation, it is recommended that Mr. Z seek employment in the medium work category with maximum lifting of 50 pounds. He has been trained in electronics work, and it is believed that he could return to this work with limitations of working in extreme wrist flexion.

REFERENCES

1. American Academy of Orthopaedic Surgeons: Joint motion, method of measuring and recording, Chicago 1965.
2. Bechtol C: The use of a dynamometer with adjustable hand spacings, J Bone Joint Surg. 34A, 4, 1954.
3. Berlin S and Vermette J: An exploratory study of work simulator norms for grip and wrist flexion, Vocational evaluation and work adjustment bulletin, Summer 1985.
4. Brand P and Wood H: Hand volumeter instruction sheet, US Public Health Service Hospital, Carville, LA, 1978.
5. Curtis RM and Engalitcheff J Jr: A work simulator for rehabilitating the upper extremity—preliminary report, J Hand Surg 6:499, 1981.
6. Instruction for the 32023(4207) Minnesota Manual Dexterity Test: Lafayette Instrument Co., Sagamore and North Ninth Street, Lafayette, Ind.
7. Jebsen RH and others: An objective and standardized test of hand function, Arch Phys Med Rehab 50:311, 1969.
8. Stokes M: The seriously uninjured hand—weakness of grip, J Occup Med 25, 9, 1983.
9. Tiffin J: Purdue Pegboard examiner manual, Chicago, 1968, Science Research Assoc, Inc.
10. US Department of Labor: Dictionary of occupational titles, ed 4, Washington, DC, 1977, US Government Printing Office.
11. US Department of Labor: Selected characteristics of occupations defined in the dictionary of occupational titles, Washington, DC, 1981, US Government Printing Office.

BIBLIOGRAPHY

American Society for Surgery of the Hand: The hand—examination and diagnosis, Aurora, Colo, 1987.
Bly B and Michael R: On-the-job evaluations in a general hospital, Rehab Lit 34:364, 1973.
Bolton B, editor: Measurements and evaluation in rehabilitation, Baltimore, 1976, University Park Press.
Chaffin D: Ergonomic guide for the assessment of human static strength, Am Ind Hyg Assoc J Occup Ther 13:1, 1959.
Cromwell F: A procedure for pre-vocational evaluation, Am J Occup Ther 13:1, 1959.
DeVore G and Hamilton G: Volume measuring of the severely injured hand, Am J Occup Ther 22:16, 1968.
Institute for the Crippled and Disabled: TOWER: testing, orientation and work evaluation in rehabilitation, New York, 1967.
Kellor M and others: Hand strength and dexterity, Am J Occup Ther 25:77, 1971.
Kirkpatrick JE: Evaluation of grip loss: A factor of permanent partial disability in California, Industr Med Surg 26:285, 1957.
Tiffin J, and Asher EJ: The Purdue Pegboard: norms and studies of reliability and validity, J Appl Psychol 32:234, 1948.
Wegg LS: The essentials of work evaluation, Am J Occup Ther 14:65, 1960.

8

Evaluation of impairment of hand function

Alfred B. Swanson, Genevieve de Groot Swanson, and Carl Göran-Hagert

There are millions of persons in the world who are suffering the residual effects of injury or destructive diseases to the hand and upper extremity. Physicians interested in treating disabilities of the hand should accept the responsibility for accurate evaluation of the patient's physical condition, both local and general, and be able to compute the permanent anatomic and functional impairment resulting from these deficiencies. This evaluation is usually limited to the analysis of the anatomic, functional, and cosmetic effect loss after optimal surgical and physical rehabilitation have been achieved. The physician is responsible for a medical evaluation of impairment, not a rating of disability. The latter is an administrative function that relates to the patient's ability to engage in gainful activity as this affects his social and economic standard of living.

Determination of treatment programs and proper evaluation of the results depend on accurate and complete patient records. Records of examinations, operations, and treatment on these patients are increasingly under review. Insurance companies, law courts, and other judicial bodies are frequently required to evaluate the results of trauma and disease to the hand. Techniques for recording the history and for measuring anatomic, functional, and cosmetic deficits should be standard and routine and are facilitated by an orderly and convenient method of examination. Evaluations should be made after consistent and thorough histories are taken and careful observations, examinations, and tests are performed.

The proper evaluation of impairment of the injured limb presumes a knowledge of the normal functional anatomy of the part. It requires an appraisal of the resultant loss of function as it relates to activities of daily living and work and the more specialized hand activities. It is usually a determination of loss of structure, limitation, motion, strength, pain, and/or loss of sensibility as compared with the opposite normal limb; if both are impaired, comparison with an average limb is made.

In 1966 Dr. Swanson was chairman of a special committee of the International Federation of Societies for Surgery of the Hand, whose charge was to develop a system for evaluation of physical impairment in the hand and upper extremity that would be reliable and easy to use. The authors have brought together systems of medical societies and classic works, and with the participation of many hand surgeons, they have refined and extended the evaluation methods of physical impairment of the hand and upper extremity. The system developed has been tested and used by many hand surgeons around the world and was approved for international application by the International Federation of Societies for Surgery of the Hand at their first Congress, held in Rotterdam, Holland, in 1980. It recently has been approved by the American Medical Association for national usage and has been included in the *Guide to the Evaluation of Permanent Impairment of the Extremities and Back*.

EVALUATION METHODS

Methods of evaluation of the condition of the upper extremity can be arbitrarily divided into anatomic, cosmetic, and functional categories. We believe that a combination of these methods is necessary to show an accurate profile of the patient's condition. Their effect on the patient's psychologic, sociologic, environmental, and economic status must also be considered. The *physical evaluation* is necessary to determine the anatomic impairment for preoperative and postoperative surgical considerations. It is based on the history and a detailed examination of the upper extremity and patient. The *cosmetic evaluation* concerns the patient's and society's reaction to his impairment or the result of the surgical treatment. The *functional evaluation* is much more involved and of the greatest importance; it relates to the quality of function and the ability to perform activities of daily living. Functional evaluation studies are becoming increasingly sophisticated and may add greatly to the evaluation process.

A complete and detailed examination of the upper extremity is facilitated by the use of a printed chart that lists in an orderly fashion the various tests and measurements. A sketch of the hand with dorsal and palmar views simplifies the description of loss of parts and the location of scars or other defects. The printed charts used for hand evaluation for both the traumatized and rheumatoid hand are shown in Fig. 8-1. The evaluation record includes a checklist for the common information necessary to record the history, type of disease, onset, duration, distribution of disease process, laboratory tests, and treatment. Organized columns are provided to record the range of motion and strength of each joint, prehensile patterns, ability to perform activities of daily living, and ambulatory status. Specific clinical abnormalities, such as ulnar drift or lateral deviation, rotation, subluxation, and deformities secondary to tendon loss or imbalance, are recorded through the use of a coded number system. Arbitrary classifications—mild, moderate, and severe—were devised to help determine the degree of involvement or index of severity of each particular deformity (see boxed material on p. 112). For example, a moderate degree of ulnar drift is recorded as 7-b. A special section is provided in this record to describe the previous and current medical and surgical treatment.

RHEUMATOID ARTHRITIS EVALUATION RECORD
PREOPERATIVE SILASTIC^N IMPLANTS

Name _____ Sex: [ ] Male [ ] Female Date _____ Birth date _____

Address

Occupation _____ Dominant hand: [ ] R [ ] L [ ] Hospital _____ Examiner _____

Diagnosis: [ ] Juvenile rheumatoid [ ] Adult rheumatoid [ ] Erosive arthritis [ ] Osteoarthritis [ ] Psoriatic arthritis
[ ] Ankylosing spondylitis [ ] Sjögren's syndrome [ ] Systemic lupus erythematosus [ ] Trauma

Onset date _____ Sedimentation rate: [ ] Wintrobe [ ] Westergren [ ] Rourke _____ Rheumatoid test [ ] (+) [ ] (−)

Onset distribution [ ] Peripheral [ ] Central [ ] Both: Remission [ ] Yes [ ] No: Anemia [ ] Yes [ ] No Family Hx [ ] (+) [ ] (−)

Check if the following has been completed: [ ] X-rays [ ] Photographs [ ] Movies [ ] Cineradiography

Range of motion (ROM) use neutral   zero method of American Academy of Orthopedic Surgeons 1965.

Codes 1-25 represent observed and measured abnormalities. Use as indicated in appropriate sections.

Severity indices mild, moderate, and severe are represented by a, b, & c and further categorize codes 1-25.

The code 1-25 is below on this sheet. Severity indices are on separate detachable sheet.

This evaluation record has been designed for computer analysis. Responses must be complete.

Codes to use for thumb
1, 2, 3, 9-14, 19, & 22

Abd (degrees)
Add (cm)
Opp (cm)

Code   Joints   ROM
R   L   R   L

Thumb   MC Abd
              Add
              Opp
          MP
          IP

Finger codes 3-15, 19, 22-25   ROM

Index   MP
          PIP
          DIP
   Flex DIP crease to palmar crease (cm)

Middle   MP
          PIP
          DIP
   Flex DIP crease to palmar crease (cm)

Ring   MP
          PIP
          DIP
   Flex DIP crease to palmar crease (cm)

Little   MP
          PIP
          DIP
   Flex DIP crease to palmar crease (cm)
   Codes 3, 7-14, 19, 20, 22, 23

Wrist   Flex
          Ext
          U. Dev
          R. Dev

Prehensile patterns: Check if able to perform   R   L
Grasp:
Cylinders
   2.5 cm
   5 cm
   7.5 cm
   10 cm
Spheres
   5 cm
   7.5 cm
   10 cm
   12.5 cm

Strength: [ ] Lb [ ] Kg [ ] mm Hg   R   L
          Index
Pulp   Middle
pinch   Ring
          Little
Lateral or key pinch
Grip

ADL: I Independent A Assisted U Unable

Dressing   I A U   Hygiene   I A U
  Upper ext   Teeth
  Trunk   Hair
  Lower ext   Shave
Bath   Pickup coin
Shower   Turn key
Eating   Doorknob
Toilet   Car door
Telephone   Screw top jar
Typewrite   Aerosol can
Write   Fasteners

Ambulatory status:
[ ] Independent   [ ] Wheelchair with partial walking
[ ] Assisted walk [ ] Bedfast

Ambulatory status:
[ ] Independent   [ ] Wheelchair with partial walking
[ ] Assisted walk [ ] Bedfast

Code for clinical abnormality
1—Thumb swan neck
2—Thumb boutonniere
3—Subluxation—dislocation
4—Swan neck, finger
5—Boutonniere, finger
6—Intrinsic tightness
7—Ulnar drift
8—Radial drift
9—Ankylosis
10—Instability
11—Tendon rupture
12—Constrictive tenosynovitis
13—Synovial hypertrophy
14—Crepitation with motion
15—Extensor tendon subluxation
16—Varus angle
17—Valgus angle
18—Rotational deformity
19—Erosions
20—Joint narrowing
21—Subchondral sclerosis
22—Painful joint with motion
23—Nerve compression—M, U, R
24—Vasculitis
25—Nodules

Severity index
a—Mild
b—Moderate
c—Severe

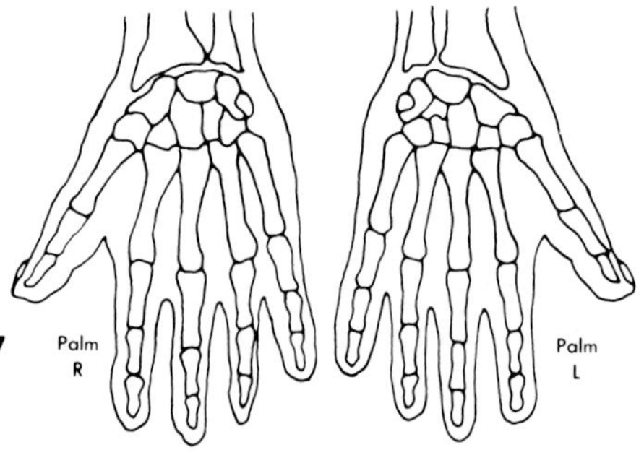

Sketch implant into appropriate site

Palm R   Palm L

Fig. 8-1 Preoperative evaluation record. **A,** This form is designed for evaluation of rheumatoid and arthritic hands. (From Swanson AB: Flexible implant resection arthroplasty in the hand and extremities, St Louis, 1973, The CV Mosby Co.)

HAND EVALUATION RECORD

Name _____ Age _____ Date _____ Major hand _____
Occupation _____ X-rays _____ Photographs _____
History:

Shoulder:	L	R		Wrist:				Circ:		
For	___	___		DF	___	___		Biceps	___	___
Back	___	___		PF	___	___		Forearm	___	___
Abd	___	___		RD	___	___		Grip: L	___	___
Add	___	___		UD	___	___		R	___	___
Rotation Int	___	___		Elbow: Ext	___	___		Forearm: Pro	___	___
Ext	___	___		Flex	___	___		Sup	___	___

		MP	IP			% Impairment
Thumb	Ext			Abd		
	Flex			Add		
	Ankylosis			Opp		

		MP	PIP	DIP	Flex pulp to midpalmar crease	
Index	Ext					
	Flex					
	Ankylosis					
Middle	Ext					
	Flex					
	Ankylosis					
Ring	Ext					
	Flex					
	Ankylosis					
Little	Ext					
	Flex					
	Ankylosis					

Total % _____

B

Chart:
1. Amputations
2. Scars
3. Skin—subcutaneous loss
4. Nail bed injury
5. Major nerve loss: R, M, U
6. Digital bundle loss
7. Neuroma
8. Pain and tenderness
9. Bone damage
10. Joint damage
11. Flexor tendon loss
12. Extensor tendon loss
13. Ligament injury
14. Sensibility—pickup
        two-point
        Ninhydrin
15. Prehension:
    Grasp—small
            large
    Pinch—pulp
            tip
            lateral
    Hook—distal
            proximal
    Scoop
16. Maximum improvement
17. Rehabilitation needed
18. Further treatment
19. Classification
NOTE: Degrees of motion recorded as left/right

Dorsum R hand or Palmar L hand   Dorsum L hand or Palmar R hand

Fig. 8-1, cont'd   B, This form is designed for posttraumatic conditions and other disorders of the hand.

SEVERITY INDEX ARBITRARILY CLASSIFIES COMMON DEFORMITIES AND DEGREE OF INVOLVEMENT AS MILD, MODERATE, OR SEVERE

Thumb swan neck—flexion limit of MCP joint
 a. Mild = MCP ROM +10° to 50°
 b. Moderate = MCP ROM +20° to 30°
 c. Severe = MCP ROM +30° to 10°
Thumb boutonniere—extension limit of MCP joint
 a. Mild = MCP −5° to −20°
 b. Moderate = MCP −20° to −40°
 c. Severe = MCP more than −40°
Swan-neck fingers—flexion limit of PIP joint
 a. Mild = PIP ROM +10° to 50°
 b. Moderate = PIP ROM +20° to 30°
 c. Severe = PIP ROM +30° to 10°
Boutonniere, fingers—extension limit of PIP joint
 a. Mild = PIP ext limit −5° to −10°
 b. Moderate = PIP ext limit −10° to −30°
 c. Severe = PIP ext limit more than −30°
Instability—measure excess of passive mediolateral motion compared with a normal joint
 a. Mild = less than 10°
 b. Moderate = 10° to 20°
 c. Severe = more than 20°
Subluxation to dislocation
 a. Mild = capable of reduction manually
 b. Moderate = incomplete reduction manually
 c. Severe = irreducible dislocation
Ulnar or radial joint deviation
 a. Mild = less than 10°
 b. Moderate = 10° to 30°
 c. Severe = more than 30°
Rotational deformity—fingers
 a. Mild = less than 15°
 b. Moderate = 15° to 30°
 c. Severe = more than 30°
Lateral deviation—wrist or elbow
 a. Mild = less than 20°
 b. Moderate = 20° to 30°
 c. Severe = more than 30°
Crepitation with motion
 a. Mild = inconstant during active ROM
 b. Moderate = constant during active ROM
 c. Severe = constant during passive ROM

Synovial hypertrophy
 a. Mild = visual increase in joint size
 b. Moderate = palpable increase in joint size
 c. Severe = more than 10% increase in joint size by measure
Constrictive tenosynovitis
 a. Mild = inconstant triggering during active ROM
 b. Moderate = constant triggering during active ROM
 c. Severe = prevents active ROM
Intrinsic tightness—with MCP joint extended
 a. Mild = PIP flexion more than 60°
 b. Moderate = PIP flexion 20° to 60°
 c. Severe = PIP flexion less than 20°
Extensor tendon subluxation
 a. Mild = subluxes on MCP flexion
 b. Moderate = reducible subluxation in intermetacarpal groove
 c. Severe = nonreducible subluxation in intermetacarpal groove
Painful joint with motion
 a. Mild = pain with active motion
 b. Moderate = pain with active motion that interferes with activity
 c. Severe = pain at rest and prevents activity
Subchondral sclerosis
 a. Mild, when present
Erosions—x-ray examination
 a. Mild = one erosion
 b. Moderate = two erosions
 c. Severe = three or more erosions
Joint narrowing—x-ray examination
 a. Mild = ⅓ narrowing
 b. Moderate = ⅔ narrowing
 c. Severe = obliteration of joint space
Vasculitis
 a. Mild = paronychial hemorrhages and/or subcutaneous nodules
 b. Moderate = peripheral neuropathy
 c. Severe = cutaneous gangrene
Nodules
 a. Mild = one nodule, mobile, and nontender
 b. Moderate = two nodules, fixed and tender
 c. Severe = more than three nodules, fixed, tender, and with skin breakdown

PRINCIPLES AND METHODS OF HISTORY TAKING

History taking should record the necessary information: identification, vital statistics, diagnosis, and history of the disease. Additionally, in the case of trauma, it should narrate the accident, how and where it happened, the mechanics of the injury, the degree of the injury, and the time sequence of treatment relative to emergency care, definitive care, and post-operative therapy. The present complaint of how the residual difficulty affects the patient's activities should be recorded in his own words. Any history of previous difficulty in the same extremity should be noted also. Any general condition that would influence the patient's recovery also is indicated. In disorders of the hand, such as arthritis,

neuromuscular diseases, and Dupuytren's contracture, an appropriate history should be recorded.

The patient's hand can be observed as the examiner is taking a history and measuring the upper portion of the limb. The general posture of the hand, the position of its various joints as active motion of the upper extremity is carried out, and the state of nutrition, color, moisture, swelling, or muscle weakness can be subtly checked without the patient's awareness.

Malingering or psychogenic overlay may make it difficult to obtain an accurate estimation of impairment. The patient whose complaints are not justified by objective findings or whose response to testing varies widely from time to time should put the examiner on guard. It may be impossible to identify the malingerer without the help of evidence gathered outside the examining room when the patient does not think he is being observed.

PHOTOGRAPHIC RECORD

Photographs are an important part of the record. A set of standard position photographs of the hand is essential for consistent and accurate interpretation of the hand disability. Suggested sequences should include views of the hand from various positions, carrying out flexion-extension of the fingers and the functions of grasp and pinch. Film sequences may also be used to evaluate the patient's adaptation to his needs of daily living. Manipulating buttons and safety pins, threading a needle, turning the screw-top lid of a jar, writing, picking up and releasing objects, and turning a nut on and off a bolt are but a few of the activities that are suitable for recording on film.

RADIOLOGIC EVALUATION

A standard series of roentgenograms including anterior, posterior, lateral, and oblique views of the hand and wrist should be part of the record. Films of the other joints of the upper extremity may also be included. The films should be taken without jewelry or other items about the extremity. The anatomic extended position is desired but must not be forced, so that the degree of deformity can also be evaluated on the roentgenogram. Roentgenographic views should be less than 3 months old. Evaluation of the range of motion of the skeleton may also be aided by cineradiography, which can show the degree of movement of the digits and wrist.

ANATOMIC EVALUATION

The hand is primarily a grasping or prehensile organ. The action of the shoulder, elbow, and wrist joints enables the hand to be placed at almost any area of the body. The hand can be pulled toward or pushed away from the body through considerably more than a hemisphere. It is obvious, therefore, that every examination should include an evaluation of the entire limb.

The condition of all the structures of the extremity including skin and neurovascular structures, muscles, tendons, bones, and joints should be considered. Joint instability and ligamentous injury, deformities secondary to tendon loss, or imbalance are noted. Circumferential measurement of the extremity as compared with the opposite member should be recorded.

The skin covering the hand should be evaluated as to the presence of scars, loss of subcutaneous tissue, fixation, and adherence to deeper structures and their effect on hand function. The temperature, color, swelling, texture, and tenderness should be noted. Nail bed deformities should be described.

For each joint the presence and degree of synovitis, instability, subluxation, ankylosis, contracture, lateral deviation, and rotation should be recorded. Circumferential measurement of individual joints should be measured in centimeters, and angulation and rotation should be measured in degrees. The presence and severity of collapse deformities are noted for each digit. The status of the tendinous system is recorded by stating the presence of tendon ruptures, constrictive tenosynovitis, and extensor tendon subluxations. Description of the thumb should include length, mobility,

stability, and capacity for placement to the rest of the hand. Flexibility and depth of the thumb web are noted.

Intrinsic tightness in the hand may be demonstrated by a test described by Bunnell.[3] Hyperextension of the metacarpophalangeal (MP) joint in a normal hand still allows passive flexion of the proximal interphalangeal (PIP) joint. If the intrinsic muscles are tight or contracted, the available stretch of these muscles is taken up by the hyperextended position of the MP joint, and passive flexion of the PIP joint will be difficult.

It is important to describe the posture of the hand as it relates to the normal arches. Any disturbance of the normal carpal and metacarpal transverse arches and the longitudinal arches of the digital rays should be noted. Collapse of these arches from joint instability, skeletal malalignment, or muscle imbalance contributes to the loss of function. The thumb ray on one side and the ring and little finger rays on the other side normally move widely around the firmly fixed, stable axis of the index and middle metacarpals. The normal longitudinal arch of the digit ray is especially necessary for small-object prehension.

A complete anatomic evaluation should also include measurement of the range of motion of individual joints, strength of pinch and grasp, muscle testing, sensory evaluation, and assessment of pain.

Some of the equipment necessary for evaluating the extremity is shown in Fig. 8-2. Important tools for a good examination include goniometer, dynamometer, pinch meter, ruler, sensory testing devices, a two-point compass, familiar objects for tactile identification and the pickup test, and cylinders of various sizes to measure the effective grasp.

Prehension and strength measurements

One can make measurements of strength of pinch and grasp by comparing the force with that of the examiner and measuring the size of the arms, forearms, and hands for estimating atrophy; dynamometers are also used. The mechanical dynamometer may be too gross to measure the grasp in the weak arthritic hand. A sphygmomanometer may be used to record grips of lesser power. The blood pressure cuff is rolled to a 5 cm diameter and inflated to 50 mm Hg; the cuff is then squeezed and the change of millimeters of mercury from 50 mm is recorded as the power of grip. An electronic pinch meter based on the strain-gauge principle has been used by us for measuring the strength of pinch in pounds or kilograms of pressure. Other devices used for pinch or grasp measurement include a variety of mechanical pinch meters and the force-pressure measuring device of Mannerfelt.[8]

Many factors, including fatigue, handedness, time of day, age, state of nutrition, pain, and cooperation of the patient, influence the strength of the grip. It has been shown that tests repeated at intervals during the examination are reliable if there is less than a 20% variation in the reading. If there is more than 20%, one can assume that the patient is not exerting his full effort. The test is usually repeated three times with each hand at different times during the examination and then recorded and later compared.

Although strength is one of the important characteristics of a normal hand, this factor is not given enough attention in reconstructive surgery as compared with other parameters of motion and sensibility. A baseline of normal grip and

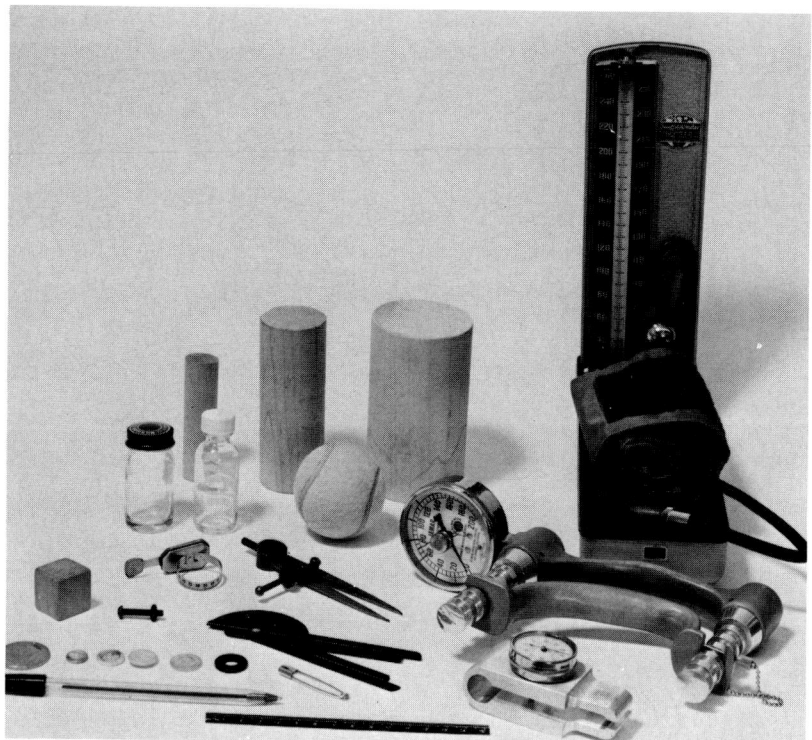

Fig. 8-2 Equipment suggested for evaluation of upper extremity. (From Swanson AB: Flexible implant resection arthroplasty in the hand and extremities, St Louis, 1973, The CV Mosby Co.)

pinch strength was studied in our clinic by testing a group of 100 healthy persons. Because it is necessary to know the normal to appreciate the abnormal, a parallel evaluation of the disabled hand could further define the degree of impairment present. The strength of the normal hand was recorded as applied in basic hand patterns: grasp, chuck, pinch (three-digit pinch), pulp pinch with separate fingers, and lateral pinch. Measurements were expressed in kilograms of force units. The force of grip was recorded with a hydraulic dynamometer. The strength of chuck, pulp, and lateral pinch was tested with an electronic pinch meter based on the strain-gauge principle. However, similar findings were obtained with the standard pinch meter.

The strength of the grip was measured with the adjustable handle of a Jamar dynamometer spaced at 6 cm. Most subjects were comfortable at this breadth of grip and could apply maximal force when tested. The minimal and maximal strength of the grip measurement ranged from 30.4 to 70.4 kg in the male group and 14 to 38.6 kg in the female group. Table 8-1 shows the average strength of grip listed by occupation, measured with the extremity unsupported. Table 8-2 shows the average strength of grip listed by age.

The majority of patients preferred chuck pinch to any other type of pinch for applying the most force. Table 8-3 shows the average strength of chuck pinch for the various groups examined. It is interesting to note that the interphalangeal joint of the thumb was hyperextended in most cases when maximal force of chuck pinch was applied.

The strength of pulp pinch with separate fingers was determined (Table 8-4). A tendency to hyperextend either the PIP or the distal interphalangeal (DIP) joints was evident

Table 8-1 Average strength of grip (unsupported) listed by occupation (100 subjects)

| | Unsupported grip (kg) | | | |
| | Male hand | | Female hand | |
Occupation	Major	Minor	Major	Minor
Skilled	47.0	45.4	26.8	24.4
Sedentary	47.2	44.1	23.1	21.1
Manual	48.5	44.6	24.2	22.0
AVERAGE	47.6	45.0	24.6	22.4

Table 8-2 Average strength of grip listed by age (100 subjects)

| | Grip (kg) | | | |
| | Male hand | | Female hand | |
Age	Major	Minor	Major	Minor
20	45.2	42.6	23.8	22.8
20-30	48.5	46.2	24.6	22.7
30-40	49.2	44.5	30.8	28.0
40-50	49.0	47.3	23.4	21.5
50-60	45.9	43.5	22.3	18.2

when maximal pinch force was applied. For the PIP joint, this tendency increased from the radial to the ulnar sides of the hand. Lateral pinch is a very strong type of pinch as noted in Table 8-5; it may be an important adaptation in the disabled hand and may provide a very useful function when pulp pinch is lost.

In the comparison of major and minor hands, the major hand was usually stronger in heavy manual workers; however, the minor hand may be stronger in a significant percentage of other individuals tested. On the average, grip strength of the minor hand was weaker in 5.4% of males and 8.9% of females. The strength of pinch in the minor hand was weaker by only 4% in males and 6% in females. The data obtained in our study indicated that there is less difference in strength of the major and minor hands than has generally been thought. It has been demonstrated that

Table 8-3   Average strength of chuck pinch by occupation (100 subjects)

| | Chuck pinch (kg) | | | |
| | Male hand | | Female hand | |
Occupation	Major	Minor	Major	Minor
Skilled	7.3	7.2	5.4	4.6
Sedentary	8.4	7.3	4.2	4.0
Manual	8.5	7.6	6.1	5.6
AVERAGE	7.9	7.5	5.2	4.9

Table 8-4   Average strength of pulp pinch with separate digits (100 subjects)

| | Pulp pinch (kg) | | | |
| | Male hand | | Female hand | |
Digit	Major	Minor	Major	Minor
II	5.3	4.8	3.6	3.3
III	5.6	5.7	3.8	3.4
IV	3.8	3.6	2.5	2.4
V	2.3	2.2	1.7	1.6

Table 8-5   Average strength of lateral pinch by occupation (100 subjects)

| | Lateral pinch (kg) | | | |
| | Male hand | | Female hand | |
Occupation	Major	Minor	Major	Minor
Skilled	6.6	6.4	4.4	4.3
Sedentary	6.3	6.1	4.1	3.9
Manual	8.5	7.7	6.0	5.5
AVERAGE	7.5	7.1	4.9	4.7

approximately 4 kg of force is needed for adequate grip to perform 90% of the activities of daily living. Patients can usually manipulate the objects of their environment, such as door handles, if they have this degree of strength. The majority of simple activities can be accomplished with approximately 1 kg of pinch strength. However, an adequate examination of a person, as far as the necessity for strength of the hand, should include an evaluation of his personal environment and how his hand strength can help him.

Muscle testing

Muscle testing may be an important part of evaluating impairment in the hand disabled by paralysis or paresis resulting from a proximal or peripheral nerve lesion. Manual muscle testing is based on the ability to raise the distal part through its range of motion against gravity and to hold the part against resistance. The determination of muscle strength impairment will be based on the therapist's or physician's interpretation as to whether the strength is (1) normal (no impairment of strength)—complete range of motion against gravity with full resistance; (2) good (1% to 25% impairment of strength)—complete range of motion against gravity with some resistance; (3) fair (26% to 50% impairment of strength)—range of motion against gravity; (4) poor (51% to 75% impairment of strength)—complete range of motion with gravity eliminated; (5) trace (76% to 99% impairment of strength)—evidence of slight contractility, no joint motion; and (6) zero (100% impairment of strength)—no evidence of contractility. When evaluating impairment for paralysis or paresis and associated sensory defects, it is not necessary to include impairment values for loss of motion or ankylosis of parts. This would result in a duplication of rating impairment.

Range of motion

The range of motion should be recorded on the principle that neutral position equals 0 degrees, as accepted by the American Academy of Orthopaedic Surgeons in 1975[1] (Fig. 8-3). In this method all motions of the joint are measured from defined zero as the starting position: The "extended anatomic position" of an extremity is therefore accepted as 0 rather than 180 degrees. Thus the degree of motion of a joint is added in the direction the joint moves from the zero starting position. Active motion is that motion obtained at the joints with full flexion or extension muscle force. Passive motion is the motion that is measured after normal soft tissue resistance to movement is overcome; in the finger joints this is approximately 0.5 kg of force.

A distinction should be made between the terms *extension* and *hyperextension*. Extension is used for motions opposite to that of flexion to the zero or neutral starting position. If motion opposite to flexion exceeds the zero or neutral starting position, such as that seen at the finger joint, elbow, or knee, it may be referred to as hyperextension. Motion of hyperextension is to be given a plus value. Incomplete motion of extension from a flexed position to zero starting position is reported as a negative or minus degree from zero. EXAMPLE: Finger joint flexion contracture of 15 degrees with flexion available to 45 degrees would be recorded as a range of motion of 30 degrees, in other words—15 to 45 degrees. This therefore refers to a lack of extension of 15 degrees to the zero position. A finger joint that has 15

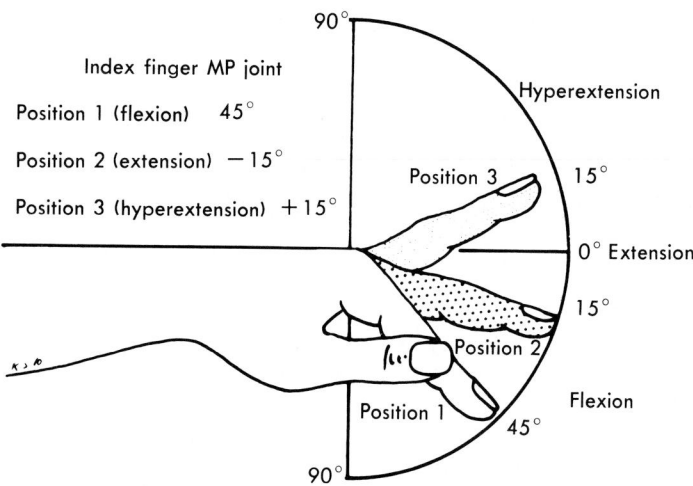

Index finger MP joint

Position 1 (flexion)   45°

Position 2 (extension)   −15°

Position 3 (hyperextension) +15°

Fig. 8-3   Range of motion of index finger. Measure hyperextension as (+) value, extension lag as (−) value, and neutral position as O degrees, as suggested by the American Academy of Orthopaedic Surgeons.

degrees of hyperextension available to 45 degrees of flexion would be recorded as a joint motion of +15 to 45 degrees.

The method of assigning the value of the angle within the sector of hyperextension as a "plus" or "minus" is a somewhat controversial subject. However, the method that we present employs the traditional terminology and is easily

understood by most clinicians and therefore has the greatest validity.

Measurement of individual joints should be recorded in table form and expressed in degrees. Proximal joints should be in neutral or straight-line position when one is measuring the distal joints (Fig. 8-4, *A* to *C*). Ankylosis contractures and active motion should be noted. Digits are named rather than numbered, according to the terms *thumb, index, middle (long), ring,* and *little* fingers. Deformity of the fingers as to rotation and alignment should be noted. The spread of the fingers and the strength of the spreading can be measured.

The method described by Boyes[2] of measuring maximal finger flexion by noting the distance that the pulp of the finger lacks in touching the distal palmar crease should be included in evaluating finger flexion (Fig. 8-4, *D*). This is the most simple and informative basis for impairment evaluation. The range of motion of the individual joints of the digit should also be included for completeness of reporting and as an alternative method of evaluating impairment. Further description of the thumb should include a measurement of radial abduction, adduction, flexion, extension, opposition, anteposition (palmar abduction), and retroposition (Fig. 8-5).

The motion of the wrist in dorsal and palmar flexions and radial and ulnar deviations should be measured. Range of motion at the elbow in flexion, extension, pronation, and supination should be checked. Shoulder motion in flexion, extension, abduction, adduction, and internal and external rotation should be measured also.

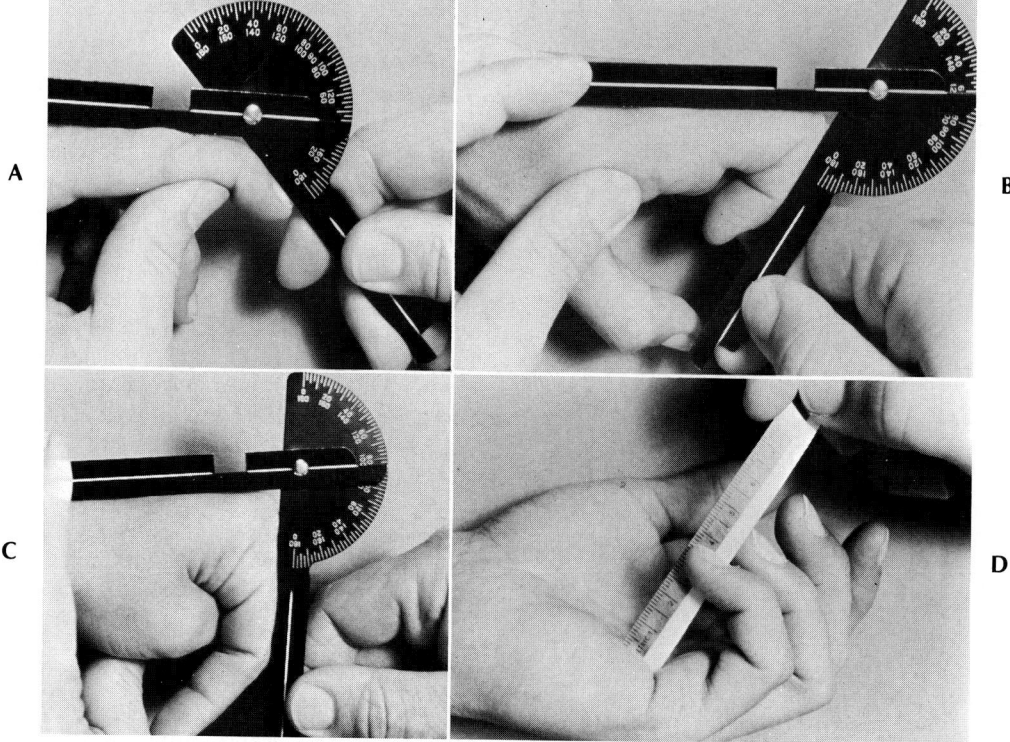

Fig. 8-4   Techniques of measurement of digital joints. **A,** Distal interphalangeal joint. **B,** Proximal interphalangeal joint. **C,** Metacarpophalangeal joint. **D,** Maximal flexion distance measured by Boyes' method as distance pulp of finger lack of touching distal palmer crease. (From Swanson AB: Flexible implant resection arthroplasty in the hand and extremities, St Louis, 1973, The CV Mosby Co.)

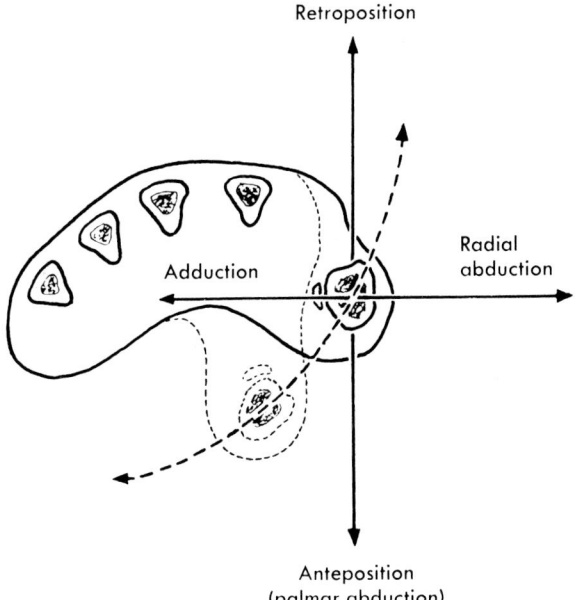

Fig. 8-5 Movements of thumb are adduction and radial abduction, anteposition or palmar abduction, and retroposition. Opposition *(dotted line)* is accomplished by movements of axial rotation, abduction, and flexion of all three joints of thumb, which result in rotation of thumb in position to present its palmar pad to pad of any finger. (Redrawn after Tubiana R: Surg Clin North Am 48:967-977, 1968.)

Neurologic examination

The presence of neurologic disorders, and brachial, radial, ulnar, and median nerve palsies, as they are evidenced by motor and sensory disturbances in the hand, is noted. Digital nerve loss and the presence and localization of neuromas should be evaluated. Tenderness, sensitivity, and painful states, such as the causalgias and other sympathetic dystrophies, should be appraised. A complete sensory examination should be done.

The Ninhydrin test for sudomotor function can be a useful method for documenting the interruption of the digital nerves. However, it has limitations in evaluating the "recovering" nerve, because there is not a direct relationship between return of sudomotor function and return of tactile gnosis. A two-point discrimination test can help determine functional loss of tactile gnosis. More than 18 to 20 mm in two-point discrimination testing is considered a total loss of this function. Functional isolation of the finger, as noted in the blindfolded pickup test, will aid the examiner in determining the presence or absence of any useful sensation in the digit.

Pain evaluation

Pain is difficult for the examiner to evaluate, because it is a subjective symptom. Pain can be defined as a disagreeable sensation that has as its basis a highly variable complex made up of afferent nerve stimuli interacting with the emotional state of the individual and modified by his experience, motivation, and state of mind. Pain may be verified and the intensity of pain may be evaluated in a thorough physical examination. Pretended pain may be detected by tests that

confuse the patient into responding with signs that are contradictory to the usual clinical examination. Examination can further demonstrate whether the pain has an anatomic background or if it is associated with other signs of nerve dysfunction. Permanence of the loss of function because of pain or discomfort is described as a condition that exists after optimum physiologic adjustment and maximum medical rehabilitation have been administered. Subjective complaints of pain that cannot be substantiated along these lines should not be considered for impairment.

It is important to have an impairment classification for pain and discomfort in order to clarify subjective symptoms that interfere with the patient's activities. Such a classification must be set on arbitrary baselines. Pain associated with peripheral spinal nerve disorders can be classified according to how the pain interferes with the individual's performance of his activities: (1) Minimal—is it annoying (0% to 25%)? (2) Slight—does it interfere with activity (26% to 50%)? (3) Moderate—does it prevent activity (51% to 75%)? (4) Severe—does it prevent activity and also cause distress (76% to 100%)? The percentage of impairment of the part caused by pain or discomfort can be calculated the same as when one is evaluating for loss of sensation or amputation of the part (for example, in a severe causalgia there may be 100% loss of usefulness of the extremity). Partial impairment can be taken as a percentage of the whole part, by using the amputation tables to obtain the relative value of each part to the larger part.

COSMETIC EFFECT OF THE HAND

It should be remembered that the cosmetic effect of a hand implies both a passive and an active element: The *passive* cosmetic effect of the normal hand at rest may be simulated by certain artificial hands that are now available. They are made of plastic materials that closely resemble skin; however, the moment the patient moves the hand in space, the normal postures and slight movements that a hand normally assumes are absent and the hand loses some of its cosmetic effect. The *active* cosmetic effect concerns movements that are characteristic of the normal hand during performance. The movements provide a certain grace and elegance that give a pleasing effect to the hand. These movements may compensate for other losses in the hand.

Our method of evaluating the cosmetic effect is described as follows: (1) evaluate the cosmetic result according to the general appearance of the hand at rest and on activity, (2) consider the aspect of the scar, the stiffness, residual joint imbalance, rotational deformities, and coordination, and (3) using the cosmetic improvement "point system," rate the number of points for the degree of cosmetic improvement at rest and on activity from both the patient's and the examiner's point of view; the maximum possible points are 12 (Table 8-6).

FUNCTIONAL EVALUATION AND MEASUREMENTS

Evaluation of an accurate profile of a patient's condition requires an appraisal of the resultant loss of function as it relates to activities of daily living and the more specialized hand activities common to all persons. In the evaluation of the functional capacity of a patient, it is important to determine his ambulatory status and his ability to perform

Table 8-6 Cosmetic result—example rating of a hand adding to a total of 11 of a possible 12 points

Examiner		Cosmetic improvement		Patient	
Rest	Activity			Rest	Activity
	2	Minimum	(1 point)		
		Moderate	(2 points)		
3		Marked	(3 points)	3	3

certain basic activities in either an independent or an assisted fashion, or not at all. A special questionnaire is provided to rate his performance in dressing, personal hygiene, eating, communicating, opening doors and jars, and using aerosol cans as shown in Fig. 8-1, *A*.

The functional evaluation of the hand includes mainly the functional tests for activities of daily living and the motion-time-measurement method that is discussed later in this chapter.

The use of graduated sizes of cylinders and spheres to determine the ability to open the hand and to grasp and hold these objects can be a useful method of measuring grasp functions. Recording the size of the sphere or cylinder grasped can give a picture of the patient's functional ability. The end of the cylinder can be used to simulate the shape of the sphere. If the patient is cooperative, the use of these devices can be worthwhile in examining the disabled hand for strength and stability of the hand and wrist.

The examination should describe the ability of the patient to perform small and large grasp; pulp, tip, and lateral pinch; distal and proximal hook; and scoop functions. One should note whether further treatment is needed or further improvement will occur.

Functional evaluation systems

Most systems for evaluation of physical impairment attempt to establish a numerical deficit from normality by weighing factors such as missing or nonfunctional portions of the body. The resultant figure provides an index of anatomic impairment. However, this does not provide sophisticated insight into the effect the impairment will have or has had on the individual patient.

Most commonly, the physician is asked to judge physical impairment to permit a nonphysician or third-party judicial body to rate the patient's disability. Physical impairment, along with many other factors, such as motivation, fatigue, and pain, is a most important factor in disability. In a way, the anatomic impairment evaluation is what the patient is able to put into a functional situation. The evaluation of disability should hinge to a degree on a measure of the patient's motor performance of functional activities.

Industrial engineers have been evaluating the motor performance of normal man in the industrial setting for many years. A person can be analyzed according to his ability to perform a given task composed of any given motion element and by matching his performance at a selected performance level. Therefore from a synthetic test of performance ability, performance in an industrial setting can be predicted. A performance index can be described for specific tasks. An example of how a disabled person might perform certain

activities is a man who has lost his left upper extremity and is totally disabled as a pianist; however, he is very capable and essentially nondisabled as a radio announcer. Most injuries and vocational situations are less clear, however. It would be useful to be able to indicate that an injured worker could perform 10% of normal on job A and 90% of normal on job B. It should also be possible to analyze job A to determine how that task could be altered to take advantage of the worker's abilities while minimizing his disabilities and thereby improving his work performance.

The disability index should also be a measure of performance that could change from motivation, fatigue, pain, coordination, and strength. Because only the output is measured, it could have an important place in the evaluation of the improvement of the patient's ability.

The system of analysis of motor performance, motion-time measurements, is concerned with the physical aspect of disability. It basically allows evaluation of general manual dexterity and helps predict specific skills. In the ideal evaluation there should be (1) a representation of all skills required by specific, available jobs and (2) a determination of all the significant manual skills possessed by the patient being tested. This method is contained in a predetermined motion-time system (PMTS) and is used widely in industry in the improvement, analysis, and timing of industrial work.

Sophisticated derivatives of motion-time study have been developed that can (1) define the subunits of the elements of motion that compose virtually any test performance, (2) time the performance of these motion elements, and (3) relate the timed individual performance of these motion elements to the established "norms" of performance.

One of these systems is *methods-time-measurement (MTM)* system. MTM is a procedure that analyzes any manual operation or method into the basic motion elements required to perform it and assigns to each motion element a predetermined time standard that is determined by the nature of the motion and the conditions under which it is made. The system implies that the time involved in task performance is meaningless unless a manner of task performance is defined.

The principal elements employed in MTM are various degrees and purposes of reaching, grasping, moving, turning, applying pressure, and positioning. For complex analyses, there are guides, for example, for motion that can or cannot be performed simultaneously by two hands, for eye-travel time, for eye-focus time, for principal gross body movements, for walking, and for side-stepping.

An index of disability that will allow a numerical figure to compare the disabled person with a normal person can be obtained. The use of MTM elements should make it possible to evaluate the impaired hand from trauma or disease and to give it some index of impairment of function, which, combined with the physical impairment, can more fairly attest to the patient's true condition of disability. Further work and research are required in this area to develop the methods and personnel requirements to use the well-established MTM system in disability evaluation. We are now attempting to do this in our department.

PRINCIPLES AND METHODS OF IMPAIRMENT EVALUATION

The most practical and useful approach to the evaluation of digit impairment is through comparison of the loss of function found to be present with that resulting from amputation. Most schedules of evaluation consider the upper limb as a unit of the whole person and divide it into hand, wrist, elbow, and shoulder. The hand is further separated into digits and their parts.

Total loss of motion of a digit or total loss of sensation, or ankylosis and severe malposition that would render the digit essentially useless, are considered about the same as amputation of the part.

Ankylosis in the optimum functional position of joints is given the least disability on the charts. The majority of

functional activities of the hand require a 5 cm opening in the fingers and thumb, and therefore this degree of opening should be considered favorably in the impairment charts. The ability to flex the fingers to within 1 or 2 cm of the distal palmar crease is indicative of a useful range of motion and should also be considered favorably in the charts for impairment.

We will describe the methods for evaluation of amputation impairment, sensory impairment, finger range of motion, and ankylosis impairment. The principles for evaluating combined impairments of the entire extremity or a part will be defined. We will also present impairment charts for the fingers, thumb, wrist, elbow, and shoulder and describe the methods for their use.

AMPUTATION IMPAIRMENT EVALUATION

Amputation of the entire extremity or 100% loss of the limb is considered 60% impairment of the whole man. Amputations at levels below the elbow, distal to the biceps insertion and proximal to the MP level are considered a 95% loss of the total limb (Fig. 8-6).

Prehension and sensation are, in essence, the sum of roles played by the separate digits. Sensation and prehension of the palmar aspect of the palm and wrist are so gross that

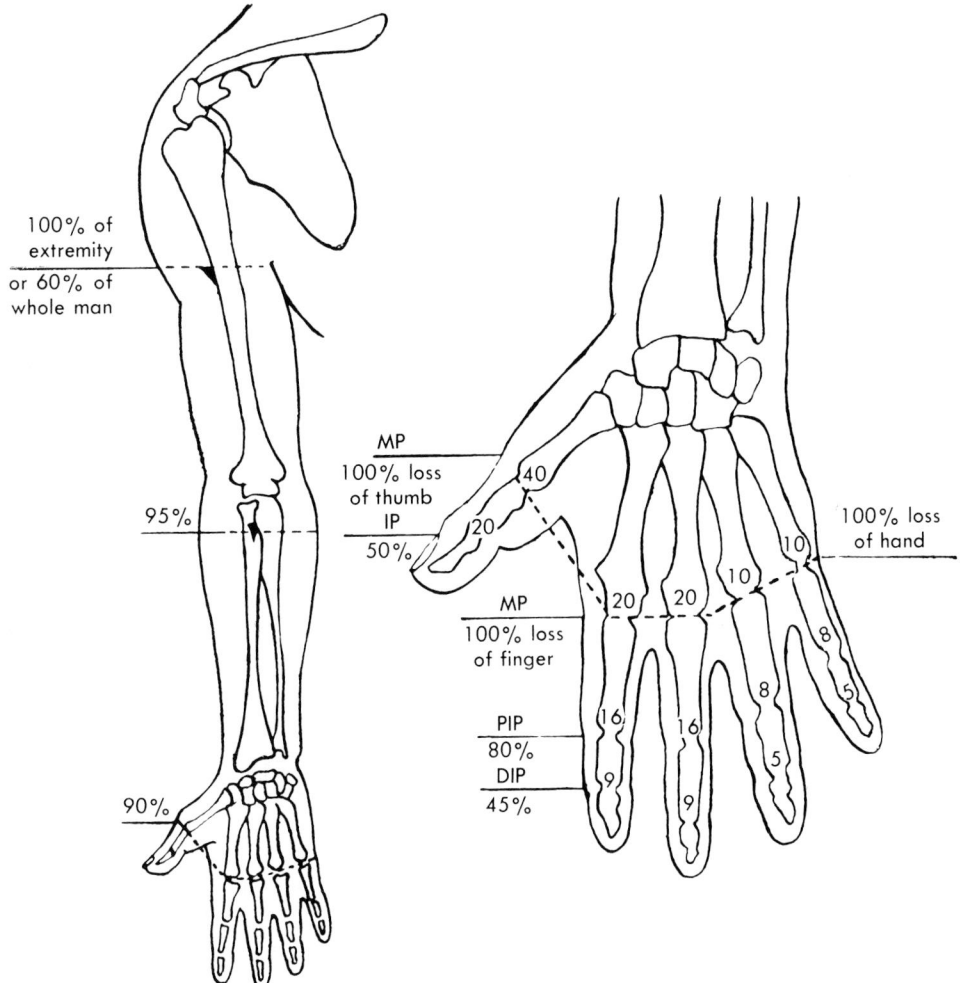

Fig. 8-6 Amputation impairment. Percentage of impairments related to whole body, extremity, hand, or digit. *MP*, Metacarpophalangeal; *IP*, interphalangeal; *PIP*, proximal interphalangeal; *DIP*, distal interphalangeal.

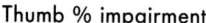

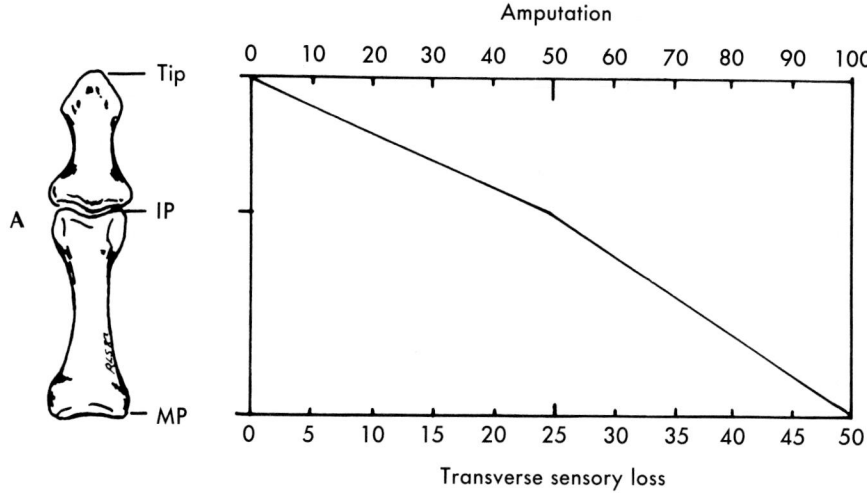

Fig. 8-7 Percentages of impairment to digit in **A,** thumb or **B,** finger. The scale at the top of each graph shows the amputation impairment scale (up to 100%). The scale at the bottom of each graph represents the transverse sensory loss impairment (up to 50%).

they are of no particular industrial use. Amputation of the fingers and thumb removes the most essential parts and is considered 100% impairment to the hand or 90% impairment to the total limb; because loss of the entire limb would equal 60% impairment to the whole person, 90% impairment of the limb would equal 54% impairment to the person. Using this principle of progressive multiplication of percentage values, the impairment of each digit or portion thereof can be related to the hand, the upper limb, and eventually to the whole man.

The digits represent five coordinated units into which all hand function is unequally divided. When evaluating the impaired function of the whole hand, one first has to evaluate each finger and the thumb separately according to the 100% scale in relation to the entire digit. Each of the digits is then weighed according to its respective value to the total hand as follows: thumb, 40%; index and middle finger 20% each; and ring and little finger 10% each as shown in Fig. 8-6. Any portion of the digit is taken as a percentage of the whole digit (Fig. 8-7). Amputation through the MP joint equals 100% loss of the finger; amputation through the PIP joint equals 80% loss to the finger; amputation through the DIP joint equals 45% loss to the finger, and amputation through the interphalangeal joint of the thumb equals 50% loss to the thumb. The value of each portion of a digit can be related to the whole hand by multiplying it by its respective value to the hand. For example, amputation of the index finger equals 20% loss to the hand and amputation through the PIP joint represents 80% loss of the index finger, resulting in an 80% × 20% loss to the hand or 16%. The values relating the loss of each part of each digit to the whole hand have been calculated as above and are shown in Fig. 8-6. Multiple digit losses are calculated as a sum of

parts and are related to the whole hand. Because the hand represents 90% to the upper extremity, hand impairment values are multiplied by 90% to obtain upper extremity impairment and then by 60% to obtain the impairment to the whole person. For example, amputation of the entire thumb (40% loss to the hand) with amputation through the DIP joint of the index finger (9% loss to the hand) equals 49% total impairment to the whole hand or 49% × 90% = 44% to the upper extremity, and 44% × 60% = 26% to the whole person.

SENSORY IMPAIRMENT EVALUATION

Any loss resulting from sensory deficit, pain, or discomfort that contributes to permanent impairment must be unequivocal and permanent. Loss of sensation on the dorsal surface of the digits is not considered disabling. Sensation on the palmar surface of the distal segment contributes to the function of the digit. Sensory loss on the least often opposed surfaces of the fingers and thumb should be given less value than the more important surfaces used in the usual pinch and grasp activities.

Complete loss of palmar sensation of the part is considered a 50% deficit of functional capacity. It is calculated therefore as 50% that of an amputation; for example, loss of both digital nerves of the thumb is considered one half of an amputation loss, which equals half of 40%, or 20%, loss to the hand. Complete loss of sensation of the index or middle fingers equals 10% loss to the hand each, and complete loss of sensation of the ring and little fingers equals 5% loss to the hand each (Fig. 8-8).

Partial transverse sensory loss can be calculated as a percentage value of a portion of the digit; for example, sensory loss of the distal phalanx of the thumb equals one

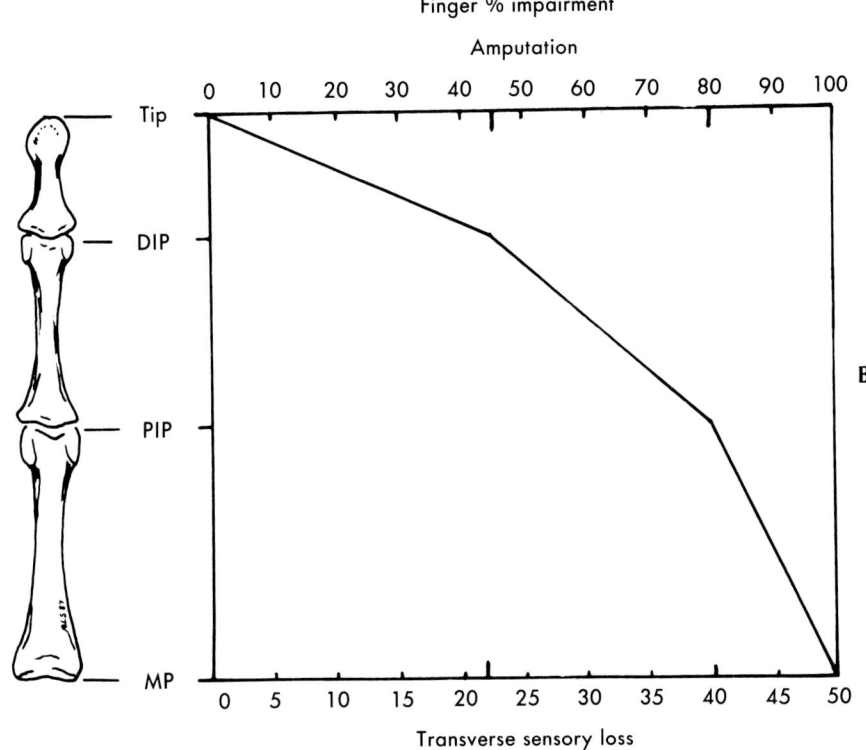

Finger % impairment

Amputation

half of the value assigned for amputation through the interphalangeal joint, or 25% impairment to the thumb, or 10% impairment to the hand. The values for each transverse level of sensory loss can be easily calculated from the amputation values reported on Fig. 8-6 and Fig. 8-7.

Partial longitudinal loss is figured on the relative importance of the side of the digit for sensory function. Loss of sensibility of the radial half of the thumb is given 40% deficiency to the thumb, and loss of the ulnar half of the thumb is given 60% loss to the thumb. Sensory loss on the ulnar half of the fingers is given 40% finger sensory impairment and on the radial half, 60%, except for the little finger where sensation on the ulnar border is more important. The impairment value for longitudinal sensory deficit of each digit is converted to hand impairment by multiplying it by the digit's sensory relative value to the hand (half of its amputation relative value to the hand). For example, 100% loss of thumb sensation corresponds to a 20% hand impairment; longitudinal sensory loss on the ulnar side of the thumb represents a 60% thumb sensory impairment or 12% hand impairment (40% × 50% = 20% × 60% = 12%). The values for radial and ulnar longitudinal sensory impairment to the hand for each digit are shown in Fig. 8-8.

FINGER MOTION IMPAIRMENT EVALUATION

There has been a variety of methods proposed for evaluation of flexor tendon repair. The method suggested by Boyes[2] of a *linear measurement* from the fingertip to the distal palmar crease has been used by many. Litchman and Paslay[7] have attempted to give values of impairment of the finger function as related to a linear distance from fingertip to distal palmar crease. Van't Hof and Heiple[11] proposed a

method for evaluation of lack of extension as a linear measurement from the rim of the nail to the point to which the nail is expected to reach in case of full extension. White[12] used a numerical sum of the angles in maximum flexion of the three finger joints. Swanson[9] in 1964 proposed a method for evaluating impairment caused by loss of flexion motion

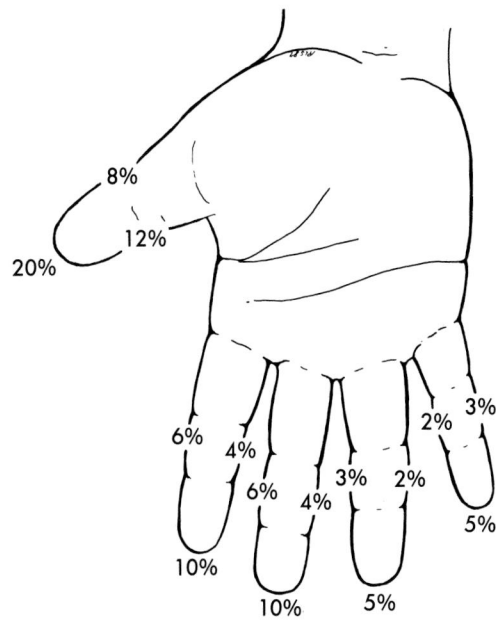

Fig. 8-8   Sensory impairment: relative value to whole hand for total sensory loss of digit and comparative loss of radial and ulnar sides. Sensory loss is calculated as 50% that of amputation.

based on a *combined angular measurement principle*. The individual values for impairment of finger function caused by ankylosis and lack of flexion were obtained from the American Medical Association's *Guide for Evaluation of Permanent Impairment of the Extremities and Back*.[6] A system based on the formula:

$$A\% + B\%(100\% - A\%) = \text{the combined values of } A\% + B\%$$

was developed and used to add the combined values of impairment as is explained later in the text. Swanson also correlated the *combined angular measurement with the linear measurement of Boyes* and presented charts that could be used for everyday clinical practice[9] (Fig. 8-9). The Committee on Impairment Evaluation of the American Medical Association proposed the use of combining joint angles. Tubiana, Michon, and Thomine[10] have also proposed methods of evaluation of results after operations for Dupuytren's contracture.

Most impairment evaluations arbitrarily classify results as excellent, good, fair, and poor. We will not attempt to compare result evaluation according to the different methods, but we believe that arbitrary classifications that fail to

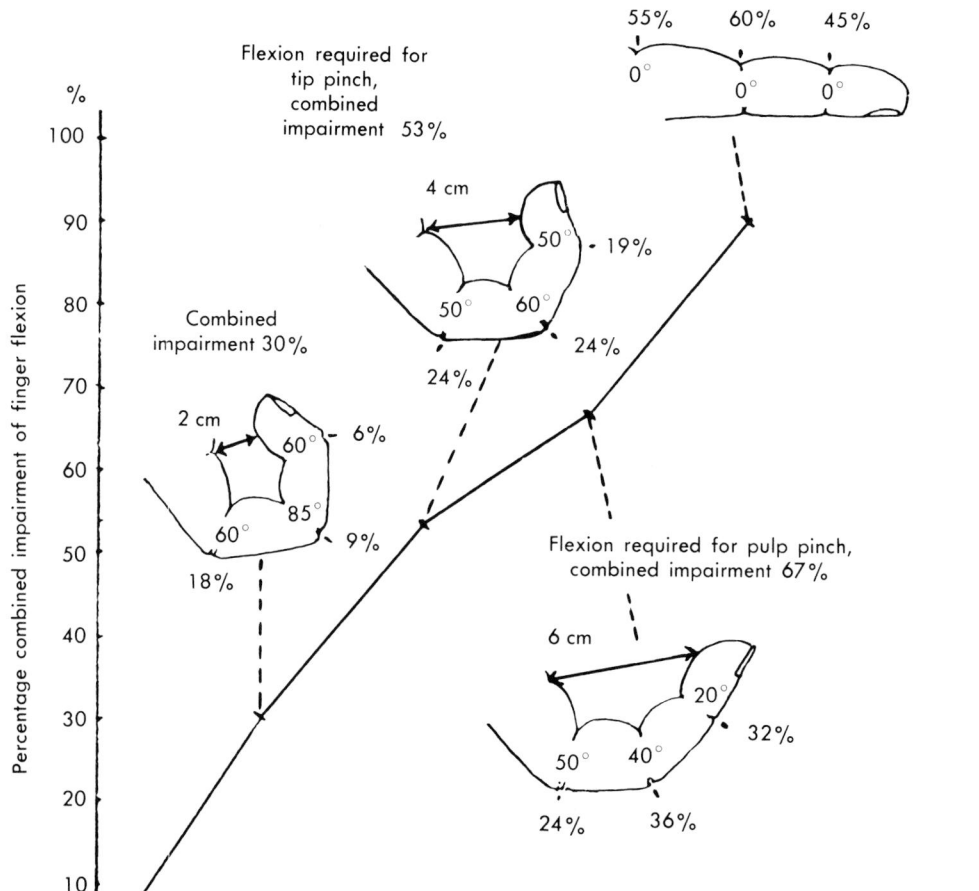

Fig. 8-9 Boyes' linear measurement of distance between finger pulp and middle palmar crease is the simplest method for rating finger flexion capacity. Several common functional postures of fingers are noted. The impairment values to digit for loss of flexion of each joint in these positions are shown. Combined impairment values for each posture are also represented and were calculated from formula "A% + B% (100% − A%) = combined impairment value for finger." This figure correlates Boyes' linear measurements with combined angular measurement of finger flexion. For example, linear measurement of 6 cm lack of flexion from fingertip to palmar crease corresponds to 67% impairment according to Boyes' linear chart. For same position, ankylosis impairment can be obtained for each joint (MP at 50 degrees = 24%, PIP at 40 degrees = 36%, DIP at 20 degrees = 32%) and added according to above formula: 24% + 36% (100% − 24%) = 51%; 51% + 32% (100% − 51%) = 67%. Note good correlation between linear and angular measurements of impairment. (From Swanson AB: Surg Clin North AM 44:925-940, 1964.)

consider joint motion in flexion and extension are incomplete and that the only reasonable approach to evaluation of finger function is to determine impaired motion in terms of percentage of impairment as this relates to the normal hand. Of course, hand function is very complex and depends not only on motion but on sensibility, strength, and coordination. The anatomic evaluation presented is a more important area of disability. However, the functional capacity must be considered also.

"A = E + F" METHOD FOR FINGER IMPAIRMENT EVALUATION

The evaluation of impaired joint motion that is presented here is based on the American Medical Association's *Guide to the Evaluation of Permanent Impairment of the Extremities and Back*[6] and the work of Swanson,[9] which has been widely used. In these studies values for ankylosis and impaired flexion are calculated on the assumption that the normal extension for the MP and interphalangeal joints is 0 degrees. Previously, impairment values for lack of extension have not been adequately considered and for that reason a method for evaluating the lack of extension impairment values has been formulated and is presented here.

The range of motion of a joint is the number of degrees of movement traced by an arc from maximum extension to maximum flexion. To determine the range of motion, one must measure the two angles of extreme motion; they are represented by a small *v*. Flexion is the motion toward achieving the largest possible angle, and extension is the motion toward achieving the smallest possible angle. These values can be represented as follows:

Flexion v (v_{flex}) = largest possible angle to achieve by flexion
Extension v (v_{ext}) = smallest possible angle to achieve by extension

Assuming an MP joint has a normal range of motion (ROM) from 0 degrees to 90 degrees, the largest possible angle to achieve by flexion is 90 degrees and the smallest

possible angle to achieve by extension is 0 degrees. When v_{flex} = 90 degrees and v_{ext} = 0 degrees, there is no impairment of joint motion. Considerations for normal hyperextension of the MP joints are discussed later.

Assuming a decrease of joint flexion from 90 degrees to 60 degrees while extension remains unchanged at 0 degrees, v_{flex} now equals 60 degrees and v_{ext} equals 0 degrees, as illustrated in Fig. 8-10. The lost flexion is represented by *F* and is equal to the theoretically largest v_{flex} minus the measured value of v_{flex}. For an MP joint extending from 0 degrees to 60 degrees flexion, the lack of flexion can be expressed as follows:

$$F = 90°(v_{flex} \text{ largest}) - 60°(v_{flex} \text{ measured}) = 30°$$

Assuming there is a lack of extension of 20 degrees, v_{ext} equals 20 degrees, as illustrated in Fig. 8-11. The lost motion of extension is represented by *E* and is equal to the measured value of v_{ext} minus the theoretically smallest value of v_{ext}. For an MP joint lacking 20 degrees of extension, the lost extension can be expressed as follows:

$$E = 20°(v_{ext} \text{ measured}) - 0°(v_{ext} \text{ smallest}) = 20°$$

With decreased flexion there is a decrease in v_{flex}, and with impaired extension there is an increase of v_{ext}; these two values will finally meet each other. In other words, v_{ext} and v_{flex} will be located at the same point of the arc or $v_{flex} = v_{ext}$. This situation is illustrated in Fig. 8-12. As can be seen, there is ankylosis. The total loss of joint motion is represented by *A*. This does *not refer to the angle of the arc of motion* at which a joint is ankylosed but to the *sum of the lack of extension (E) and the lack of flexion (F)* resulting from this ankylosis. The total loss of joint motion can be expressed as: A = E + F. If the joint is ankylosed at 40 degrees as shown in Fig. 8-12:

$$v_{ext} = v_{flex} = 40°$$
$$E \text{ (extension loss)} = 40°$$
$$F \text{ (flexion loss)} = 90° - 40° = 50°$$
$$A \text{ (total motion loss)} = 40° + 50° = 90°$$

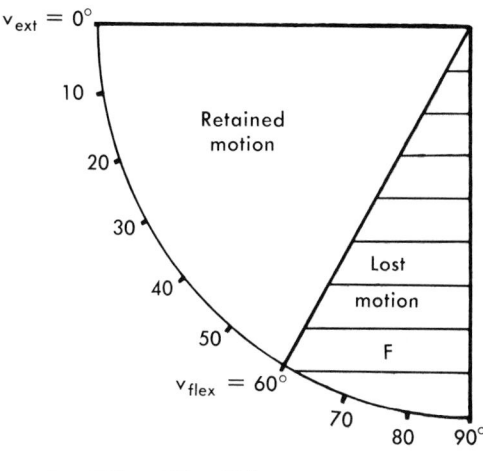

$$F = 90° - 60° = 30°$$

Fig. 8-10   Example of metacarpophalangeal joint presenting motion from 0 degrees extension to 60 degrees flexion; lost flexion, *F*, is equal to theoretically largest possible angle of flexion (90 degrees) minus measured flexion angle (v_{flex} = 60 degrees), or F = 90 degrees − 60 degrees = 30 degrees.

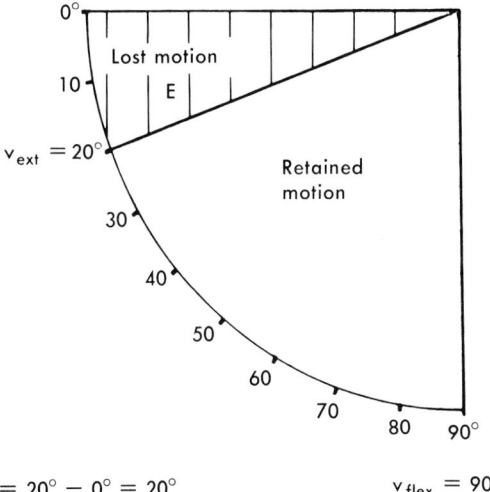

$$E = 20° - 0° = 20°$$

Fig. 8-11   Example of metacarpophalangeal joint presenting motion from 20 degrees extension lag to 90 degrees flexion; lost extension, *E*, is equal to measured extension angle (v_{ext} = 20 degrees) minus theoretically smallest possible extension angle (0 degrees), or E = 20 degrees.

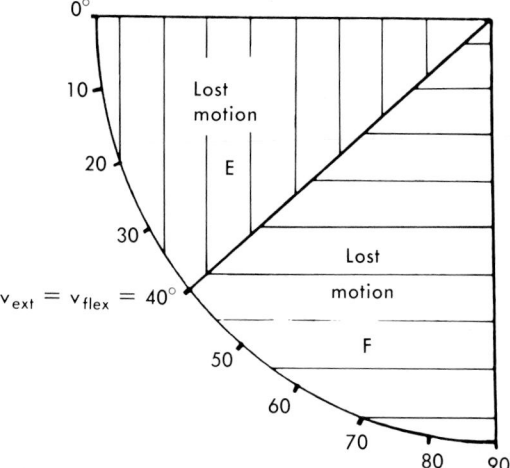

Fig. 8-12 When no motion is retained, ankylosis is present—in this example at 40 degrees. As can be seen, *total motion lost to ankylosis (A)* is equal to 40 degrees lack of extension, *E*, plus 50 degrees lack of flexion, *F*; sum of E (40 degrees) and F (50 degrees) equals A (90 degrees).

One should observe that the value A represents a total loss of joint motion and is always equal to the same number of degrees as the normal full range of motion of that joint. For an MP joint, A always equals 90 degrees, no matter where in the arc of motion the ankylosis has occurred as long as v_{flex} equals v_{ext}.

Ankylosis at 30°: A = 30°(E) + 60°(F) = 90°
Ankylosis at 80°: A = 80°(E) + 10°(F) = 90°

The above formula is of basic importance in the following discussion. Restricted joint motion will, of course, result in a certain degree of impaired function. Note that when we are referring to *lack of motion*, we are discussing *lack of function* and its evaluation. Impairment of finger function may be caused by lack of extension (E) with or without lack of flexion (F) or ankylosis (A). The restricted motion in terms of percentage impairment of finger function may then be called I_E, I_F, and I_A, respectively. These are functions of v, the angle measured at examination. More specifically, the percentage of impairment can be expressed in the following way:

I_E is a function of v_{ext} (smallest angle measured for extension) and goes to 0% when v_{ext} reaches its theoretically smallest value (for example, 0 degrees for the MP joint).

I_F is a function of v_{flex} (largest angle measured for flexion) and goes to 0% when v_{flex} reaches its theoretically largest value (for example, 90 degrees for the MP joint).

I_A is a function of v when v_{ext} = v_{flex} and similarly I_A = I_E + I_F

The function impairment is expressed in a percentage and relates the loss of function (for example, flexion) to the part affected (for example, the finger) on the 100% scale. From the AMA's *Guide to the Evaluation of Permanent Impairment of the Extremities and Back,*[6] we now have percentage values for impairment of finger function at the MP joint from 0 degrees to 90 degrees because of lack of flexion, F, and ankylosis, A, called I_F and I_A respectively. These values are shown on Tables 8-7 and 8-8 and can also be expressed

Table 8-7 Impairment percentage* attributable to loss of flexion of the MP joint from a neutral position (0°)

Flexion from 0° to	Degrees lost motion (F)	Percent impairment
0°	90	55
10°	80	49
20°	70	43
30°	60	37
40°	50	31
50°	40	24
60°	30	18
70°	20	12
80°	10	6
90°	0	0

*These figures are from the American Medical Association "Guide to the Evaluation of Permanent Impairment of the Extremities and Back."

Table 8-8 Impairment* attributable to MP joint ankylosis

Degrees joint ankylosed	Percent impaired finger function
0	55
10	52
20	48
30	45
40	54
50	63
60	72
70	82
80	91
90	100

*These figures are from the American Medical Association "Guide to the Evaluation of Permanent Impairment of the Extremities and Back."

as illustrated in Fig. 8-13 and 8-14. According to the formula previously described, A = E + F, which can also be written, E = A − F, we can derive the value for extension impairment, I_E, at each given angle according to the following formula: I_E = I_A − I_F. For example, at an angle of 30 degrees, I_A equals 45% according to the presented AMA chart (Table 8-8), and I_F equals 37% (Table 8-7); the value of I_E can be derived according to the above formula and is found to be: 45% (I_A) − 37% (I_F) = 8% (I_E). This same process can be applied to each angle of the arc of motion from 0 degrees to 90 degrees to derive the values of I_E from the AMA percentage impairment values (Fig. 8-15). However, notice that the AMA guide has made no considerations for values of hyperextension; therefore we have slightly modified the values for I_F from the AMA guide (Table 8-7) to account for values of hyperextension of the MP joint up to 20 degrees, which can be considered normal. The modified values are represented for the MP joint in Fig. 8-16. For an angle of ankylosis of 30 degrees, the I_E is calculated according to the usual formula, giving I_F a value of 33%

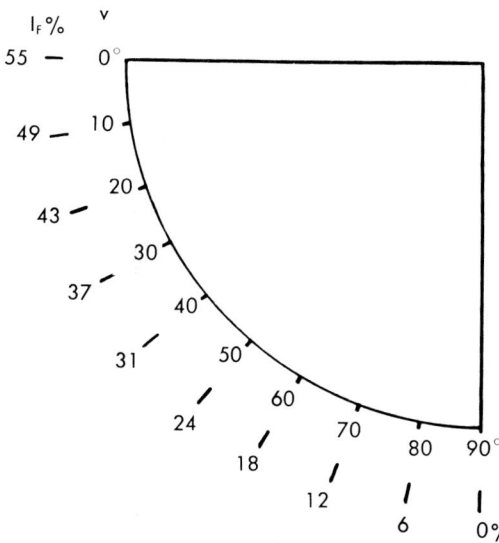

Fig. 8-13 Percentage impairment of finger function caused by lack of flexion (F) is expressed as I_F; here AMA values of I_F shown in Table 8-7 have been transposed to arc of motion. If $v_{flex} = 40$ degrees, F is 50 degrees and corresponds to $I_F = 31\%$. Note that I_F is function of v_{flex} and reaches 0% when v_{flex} equals 90 degrees or F goes to 0 degrees.

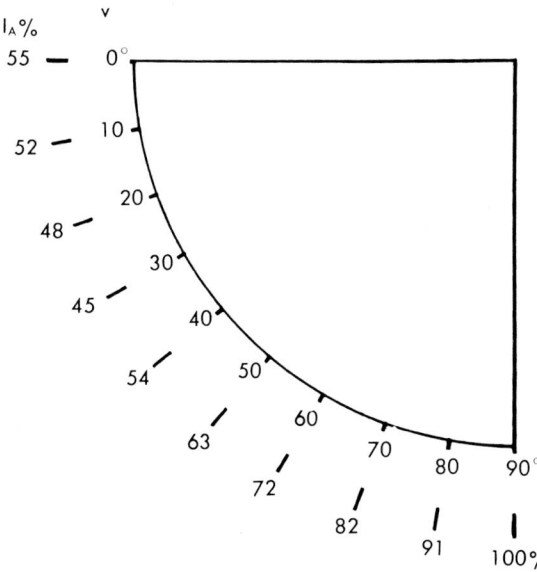

Fig. 8-14 Percentage impairment of finger function because of ankylosis (A) is expressed as I_A. Here AMA values of I_A shown in Table 8-8 have been transposed to arc of motion. If joint is ankylosed at 40 degrees, A = E (40 degrees) + F (50 degrees) = 90 degrees and $I_A = 54\%$.

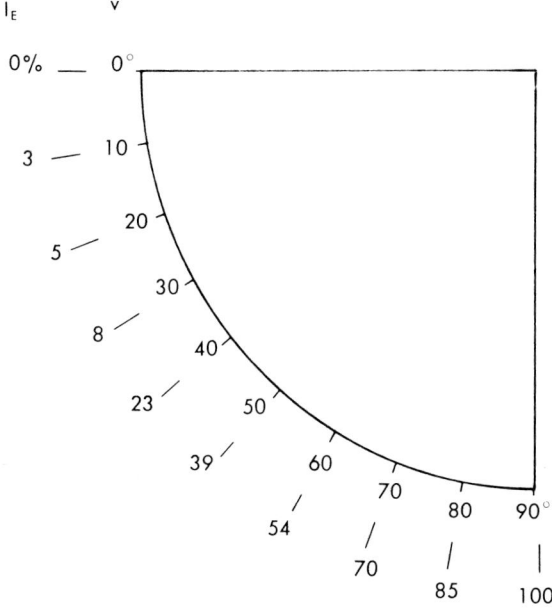

Fig. 8-15 Value of I_E can be derived for each angle from formula $I_A = I_E + I_F$, or $I_E = I_A - I_F$. When a metacarpophalangeal joint presents an extension lag of 40 degrees, $I_E = 54\%$ $(I_A) - 31\%$ $(I_F) = 23\%$. I_E is a function of v_{ext} and reaches 0% when $v_{ext} = 0$ degrees or E goes to 0 degrees.

instead of 37% as in the American Medical Association guide (Table 8-7):

$$I_E = I_A - I_F \text{ or } I_E = 45\% - 33\% = 12\%$$

The derivation of I_E is of fundamental importance for adequate evaluation of function impairment resulting from limitation of joint motion. This allows us to have values for both I_E and I_F to estimate the correct percentage of functional impairment relating not only to the degrees of lost movement but, most important, to the location of the impairment in the arc of finger motion.

Because the relative value of the MP joint to the finger is 100%, the maximum motion impairment value at this level reaches 100%.

By referring to Fig. 8-16, one can easily understand the following examples. Assuming a situation where the MP joint has 30 degrees of retained motion, one can see that this motion takes place between 10 degrees extension lag to 40 degrees flexion. The percentage of functional impairment is not as severe as it would be if the preserved motion occurred from 50 degrees extension lag to 80 degrees flexion. For an MP joint extending from -10 degrees and flexing to 40 degrees $I_E = 7\%$, and $I_F = 27\%$, for a total impairment of $7\% + 27\% = 34\%$. For an MP joint extending from -50 degrees to 80 degrees flexion $I_E = 41\%$, and $I_F = 6\%$, for a total impairment of $41\% + 6\% = 47\%$. From Fig. 8-16 one can see also that ankylosis of the MP joint at 30 degrees or the position of function would equal 12% (I_E) $+ 33\%$ (I_F) $= 45\%$ or the lowest value for I_A; it is obvious also that ankylosis at 80 degrees would represent a more severe degree of impairment 85% (I_E) $+ 6\%$ (I_F) $= 91\%$ (I_A).

The principles for evaluating impairment from ankylosis, loss of flexion, and/or loss of extension should now be clearly understood. Impairment tables for loss of function of the fingers, thumb, wrist, elbow, and shoulder have been derived from the basic formula discussed above and are presented.

Table 8-9 Combined values for impairment increments of 1%*

	1	2	3	4	5	6	7	8	9	10	11	12	13	14	15	16	17	18	19	20	21	22	23	24	25	26	27	28	29	30
1	2	3	4	5	6	7	8	9	10	11	12	13	14	15	16	17	18	19	20	21	22	23	24	25	26	27	28	29	30	31
2	3	4	5	6	7	8	9	10	11	12	13	14	15	16	17	18	19	20	21	22	23	24	25	26	27	27	28	29	30	31
3	4	5	6	7	8	9	10	11	12	13	14	15	16	17	18	19	19	29	21	22	23	24	25	26	27	28	29	30	31	32
4	5	6	7	8	9	10	11	12	13	14	15	16	16	17	18	19	20	21	22	23	24	25	26	27	28	29	30	31	32	33
5	6	7	8	9	10	11	12	13	14	15	15	16	17	18	19	20	21	22	23	24	25	26	27	28	29	30	31	32	33	34
6	7	8	9	10	11	12	13	14	14	15	16	17	18	19	20	21	22	23	24	25	26	27	28	29	30	30	31	32	33	34
7	8	9	10	11	12	13	14	14	15	16	17	18	29	20	21	22	23	24	25	26	27	27	28	29	30	31	32	33	34	35
8	9	10	11	12	13	14	14	15	16	17	18	19	20	21	22	23	24	25	25	26	27	28	29	30	31	32	33	34	35	36
9	10	11	12	13	14	14	15	16	17	18	19	29	21	22	23	24	24	25	26	27	28	29	30	31	32	33	34	34	35	36
10	11	12	13	14	15	15	16	17	18	19	20	21	22	23	24	24	25	26	27	28	29	30	31	32	33	33	34	35	36	37
11	12	13	14	15	15	16	17	18	19	20	21	22	23	23	24	25	26	27	28	29	30	31	31	32	33	34	35	36	37	38
12	13	14	15	16	16	17	18	19	20	21	22	23	23	24	25	26	27	28	29	30	30	31	32	33	34	35	36	37	38	38
13	14	15	16	16	17	18	19	20	21	22	23	23	24	25	26	27	28	29	30	30	31	32	33	34	35	36	36	37	38	39
14	15	16	17	17	18	19	20	21	22	23	23	24	25	26	27	28	29	29	30	31	32	33	34	35	36	36	37	38	39	40
15	16	17	18	18	19	20	21	22	23	24	24	25	26	27	28	29	29	30	31	32	33	34	35	35	36	37	38	39	40	41
16	17	18	19	19	20	21	22	23	24	24	25	26	27	28	29	29	30	31	32	33	34	34	35	36	37	38	39	40	40	41
17	18	19	19	20	21	22	23	24	24	25	26	27	28	29	29	30	31	32	33	34	34	35	36	37	38	39	39	40	41	42
18	19	20	20	21	22	23	24	25	25	26	27	28	29	29	30	31	32	33	34	34	35	36	37	38	39	39	40	41	42	43
19	20	21	21	22	23	24	25	25	26	27	28	29	30	30	31	32	33	34	34	35	36	37	38	38	39	40	41	42	42	43
20	21	22	22	23	24	25	26	26	27	28	29	30	30	31	32	33	34	34	35	36	37	38	38	39	40	41	42	42	43	44
21	22	23	23	24	25	26	27	27	28	29	30	30	31	32	33	34	34	35	36	37	38	38	39	40	41	42	42	43	44	45
22	23	24	24	25	26	27	27	28	29	30	31	31	32	33	34	34	35	36	37	38	38	39	40	41	42	42	43	44	45	45
23	24	25	25	26	27	28	28	29	30	31	31	32	33	34	35	35	36	37	38	38	39	40	41	41	42	43	44	45	45	46
24	25	26	26	27	28	29	29	30	31	32	32	33	34	35	35	36	37	38	38	39	40	41	41	42	43	44	45	45	46	47
25	26	27	27	28	29	30	30	31	32	33	33	34	35	36	36	37	38	39	39	40	41	42	42	43	44	45	45	46	47	48
26	27	27	28	29	30	30	31	32	33	33	34	35	36	36	37	38	39	39	40	41	42	42	43	44	45	45	46	47	47	48
27	28	28	29	30	31	31	32	33	34	34	35	36	36	37	38	39	39	40	41	42	42	43	44	45	45	46	47	47	48	49
28	29	29	30	31	32	32	33	34	34	35	36	37	37	38	39	40	40	41	42	42	43	44	45	45	46	47	47	48	49	50
29	30	30	31	32	33	33	34	35	35	36	37	38	38	39	40	40	41	42	42	43	44	45	45	46	47	47	48	49	50	50
30	31	31	32	33	34	34	35	36	36	37	38	38	39	40	41	41	42	43	43	44	45	45	46	47	48	48	49	50	50	51

*Based on the formula: $A\% + B\% (100\% - A\%)$ = the combined values of $A\% + B\%$. If three or more values are to be combined, two may be selected and their combined value found. This combined value and the third value are combined to give the total figure. This process can be repeated indefinitely, with the value obtained in each case being a combination of all the previous values. After having the two values, one enters the table at one value horizontally and at the other value vertically, and the combined value will be read at intersections. This combined value must then be combined with the third value to give a final combined value, for example, 30% impairment to DIP, 20% impairment to PIP, and 25% impairment to MP; this would add as follows on this chart: 30% DIP + 20% PIP = 44% to the digit. The following step is calculated on Table 8-8: 44% digit + 25% MP = 59% combined impairment to digit.

IMPAIRMENT ESTIMATION FOR COMBINED VALUES

When multiple impairments may involve the whole finger, the principle of relating the smaller part of the next larger part to obtain a combined value is useful. The method to combine various impairments is based on the principle that each impairment acts not on the whole part (for example, the whole finger) but on the portion that remains (for example, the PIP joint and proximally) after the preceding impairment has acted (for example, on the DIP joint). When there is more than one impairment to a given part, these impairments must be combined before the conversion to a larger part is made. The combined values determination is based on the formula:

$$A\% + B\% (100\% - A\%) = \text{the combined values of } A\% + B\%$$

When this formula is used, all percentages combined must be expressed on a common denominator. For example, multiple impairments of a finger are combined as expressed on the 100% relative value of the finger. The combined value is rounded to the nearest 5% and converted to the next larger part, for example, the hand. If three or more values are to be combined, two may be selected and their combined value found. This combined value and the third value are combined to give the total value. This procedure can be repeated indefinitely, with the value obtained in each case being a combination of all the previous values. Combined value tables for ease of determination are provided in Tables 8-9 and 8-10. Increments of 1% of impairment value are shown in Table 8-9 for values to 30%; values greater than 30% are figured by increments of 5%, such as shown in Table 8-10; combined values obtained represent the impairment to the total finger. This can then be related to the hand, the extremity, and the whole person.

For example, an index finger presents an amputation at the DIP joint and ankylosis of the PIP joint at 90 degrees; the combined impairment to the index finger can be computed according to the formula as follows: amputation of the DIP joint represents a 45% impairment to the index finger (see Fig. 8-6), and ankylosis of the PIP joint at 90 degrees represents a 75% impairment to the index finger. These can be added:

$$45\% + 75\%(100\% - 45\%) =$$
$$45\% + 75\%(55\%) = 45\% + 41\% =$$
$$86\% \text{ impairment to the index finger}$$

The index finger represents 20% to the hand, and the above impairment would represent a 20% × 86% impairment to the hand, or 17%. The combined impairment value of the above example can also be found quickly in Table 8-10 at the intersection of the vertical and horizontal coordinates represented by 45% and 75% finger impairment.

IMPAIRMENT EVALUATION TABLES AND HOW TO USE THEM
Finger impairment

Based on the previous discussion, the material for the evaluation of any finger joint is presented in Figs. 8-16 to 8-18 and shows the three different impaired functions (I_A, I_F, and I_E) for each of the three finger joints (MP, PIP, DIP). Note that the maximum impairment value for each joint is the same as the amputation value through that joint. This value reaches 100% for the MP joint (Fig. 8-16), 80% for the PIP joint (Fig. 8-17), and 45% for the DIP joint (Fig. 8-18). I_A gives the impairment of finger function attributable to ankylosis at any angle; I_E and I_F give the impairment of finger function attributable to lack of extension and lack of flexion, respectively. The positions of function in each joint are taken from the AMA guide, and hyperextension has been added to this material. This explains the slight differences in impairment values found when the values shown in Fig. 8-16 are compared with the AMA values shown in Table 8-7 (for example, $I_F = 55\%$ at 0° in Table 8-7, whereas $I_F = 49\%$ at 0° in Fig. 8-16). In a normal hand the MP joint can usefully hyperextend to 20 degrees. A very small percentage of impairment has been assigned to loss

Table 8-10 Combined impairment values representing increments of 5%

	5	10	15	20	25	30	35	40	45	50	55	60	65	70	75	80	85	90	95
5	10	15	19	24	29	34	48	43	48	52	57	62	67	72	76	81	86	91	95
10	15	19	24	28	33	37	42	46	51	55	60	64	69	73	78	82	87	91	96
15	19	24	28	32	36	41	45	49	53	58	62	66	70	75	79	83	87	92	96
20	24	28	32	36	40	44	48	52	56	60	64	68	72	76	80	84	88	92	96
25	29	33	36	40	44	48	51	55	59	63	66	70	73	78	81	85	89	93	96
30	34	37	41	44	48	51	55	58	62	65	69	72	76	79	83	86	90	93	97
35	38	42	45	48	51	55	58	61	64	68	71	74	77	81	84	87	90	94	97
40	43	46	49	52	55	58	61	64	67	70	73	76	79	82	85	88	91	94	97
45	48	51	53	56	59	62	64	67	70	73	75	78	81	84	86	89	92	95	97
50	52	55	58	60	63	65	68	70	73	75	78	80	83	85	88	90	93	95	98
55	57	60	62	64	66	69	71	73	75	78	80	82	84	87	89	91	93	96	98
60	62	64	66	68	70	72	74	76	78	80	82	84	86	88	90	92	94	96	98
65	67	69	70	72	73	76	77	79	81	83	84	86	88	90	91	93	95	97	98
70	72	73	75	76	78	79	81	82	84	85	87	88	90	91	93	94	96	97	99
75	76	78	79	80	81	83	84	85	86	88	89	90	91	93	94	95	96	98	99
80	81	82	83	84	85	86	87	88	89	90	91	92	93	94	95	96	97	98	99
85	86	87	87	88	89	90	90	91	92	93	93	94	95	96	96	97	98	99	99
90	91	91	92	92	93	93	94	94	95	95	96	96	97	97	98	98	99	99	100
95	95	96	96	96	96	97	97	97	97	98	98	98	98	99	99	99	99	100	100

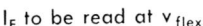

I_E to be read at v_{ext}

I_F to be read at v_{flex}

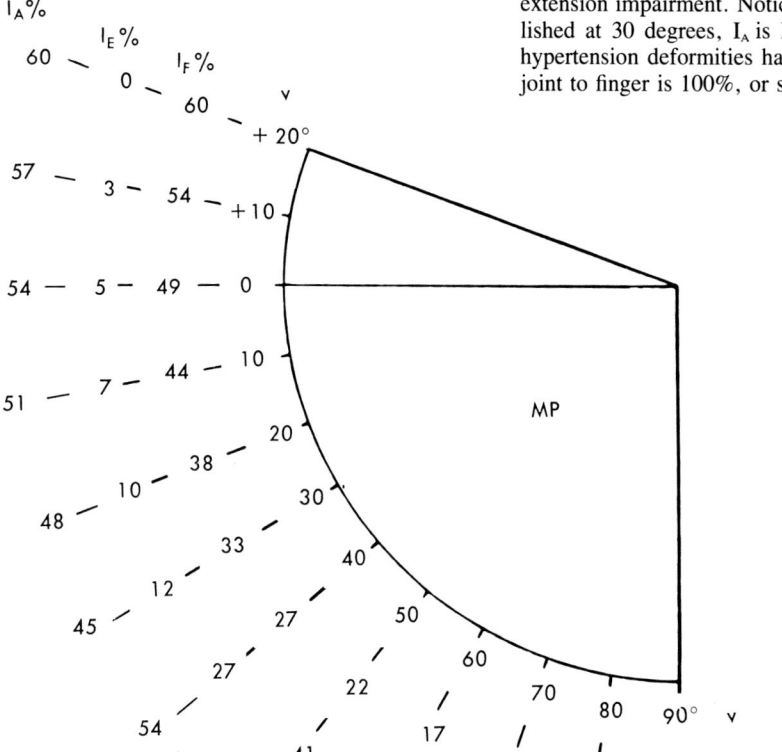

Fig. 8-16 Impairment of function for metacarpophalangeal joint (MP). I_A represents ankylosis impairment. I_F represents flexion impairment, and I_E represents extension impairment. Notice that when position of function of MP joint is established at 30 degrees, I_A is lowest, or 45% at this angle. Impairment values for hypertension deformities have been included in this chart. Relative value of MP joint to finger is 100%, or same as amputation through joint.

of this normal hyperextension as seen on this chart: at 0 degrees extension of the MP joint $I_E = 5\%$. Note that for the PIP and the DIP joints, the normal functional extension is to 0°; consequently, $I_E = 0\%$ at 0° extension for these joints; between 0° and +30°, the impairment values for the PIP and the DIP joints are given for lack of flexion and not for hyperextension. However, consideration for hyperextension angles now allows us to rate impairment of flexion when ankylosis in a hyperextended position occurs; for example, PIP joint ankylosis at +30° rated 80% impairment.

Note that for each joint the percentage of impairment ankylosis, or I_A, is at the lowest at the angle of position of function; I_A at 30° = 45% for the MP joint, I_A at 40° = 50% for the PIP joint, and I_A at 20° = 30% for the DIP joint.

These diagrams are used in the following way: measure the range of motion, for example, 20 degrees of extension lag to 60 degrees of flexion for the MP joint. The impairment corresponding to this angle is found in the row headed I_E or 10% extension impairment for 20 degrees extension lag, and the impairment corresponding to 60 degrees of flexion

is found under the row headed I_F or 17%. The impairment resulting from the above range of motion totals 10% + 17% = 27%.

Thumb impairment

The thumb represents 40% of the whole hand; it is considered to have four different functional units, each contributing to its total motion function: (1) flexion-extension of the MP and interphalangeal joints, (2) adduction, (3) radial abduction, and (4) opposition. Adduction is measured as the smallest possible distance in centimeters from the flexor crease of the interphalangeal joint of the thumb to the distal palmar crease at the level of the fifth MP joint. Radial abduction is measured as the largest possible angle in degrees formed by the first and second metacarpals during maximum active radial abduction. Opposition is measured in centimeters as the largest distance possible to achieve between the flexor crease at the interphalangeal joint of the thumb to the distal palmar crease over the third MP joint.

Combined flexion/extension of the MP and interphalangeal joints contribute 20% to thumb function. On the 100%

Fig. 8-17 Impairment of function for PIP joint. Note that when position of function of PIP joint is established at 40 degrees, I_A is lowest, or 50%, at this angle. Values for hypertension deformities have been included in this chart. Relative value of PIP joint to finger is 80%, or same as amputation through joint.

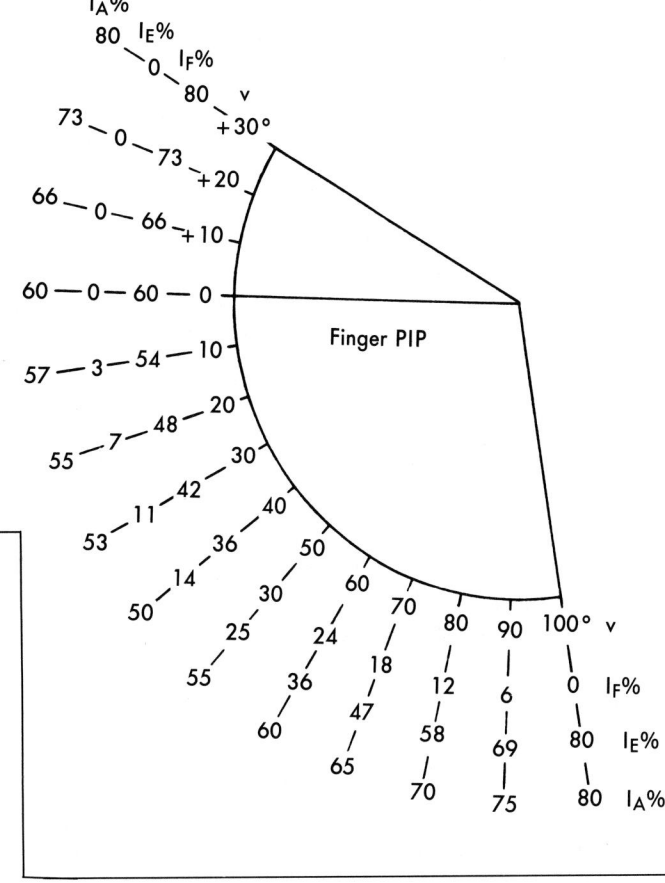

I_E to be read at v_{ext}

I_F to be read at v_{flex}

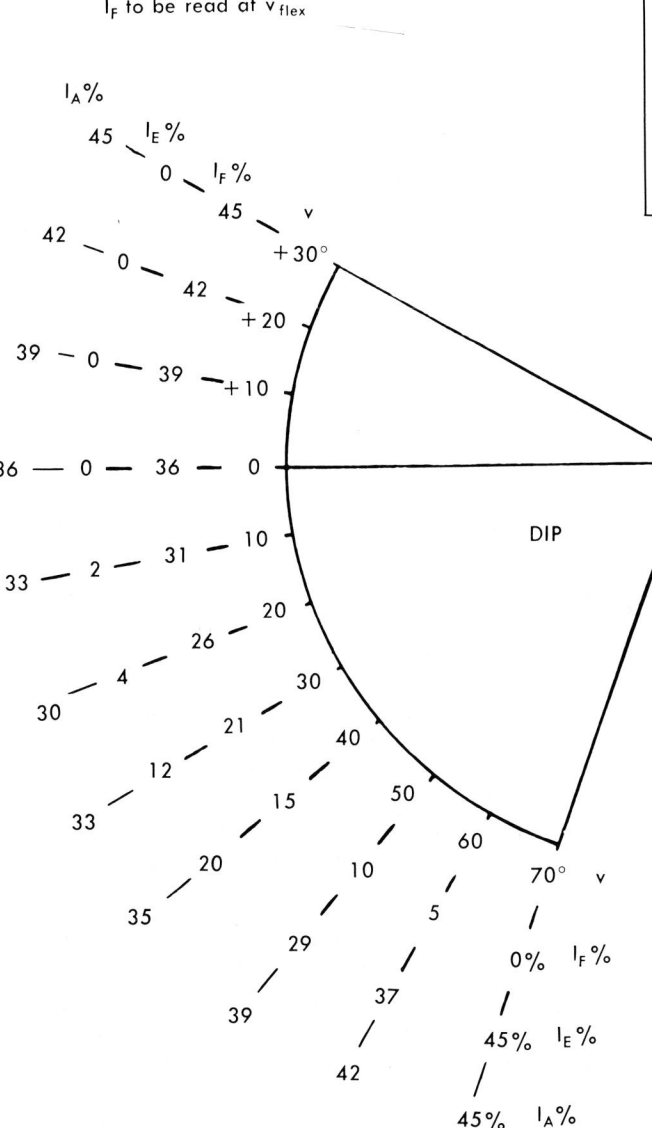

Fig. 8-18 Functional impairment of distal interphalangeal (DIP) joint. Notice that when position of function of DIP joint is established at 20 degrees, I_A is 30%, or is lowest at this angle. Relative value of DIP joint to finger is 45%, or same as amputation through joint.

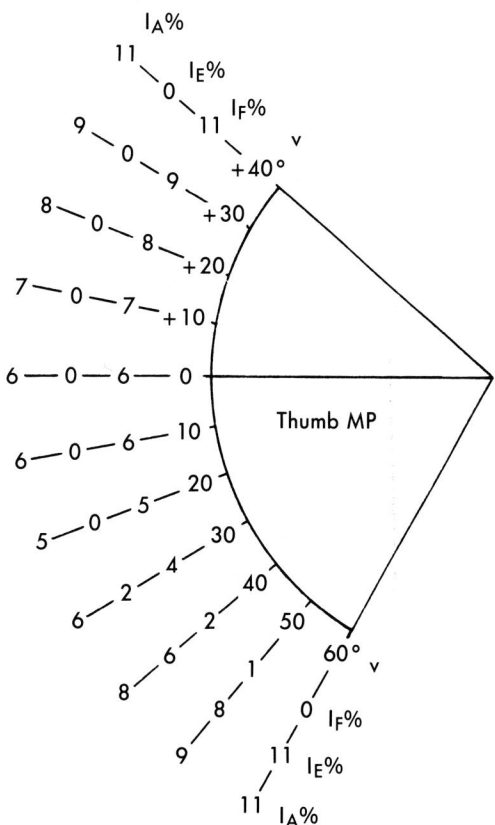

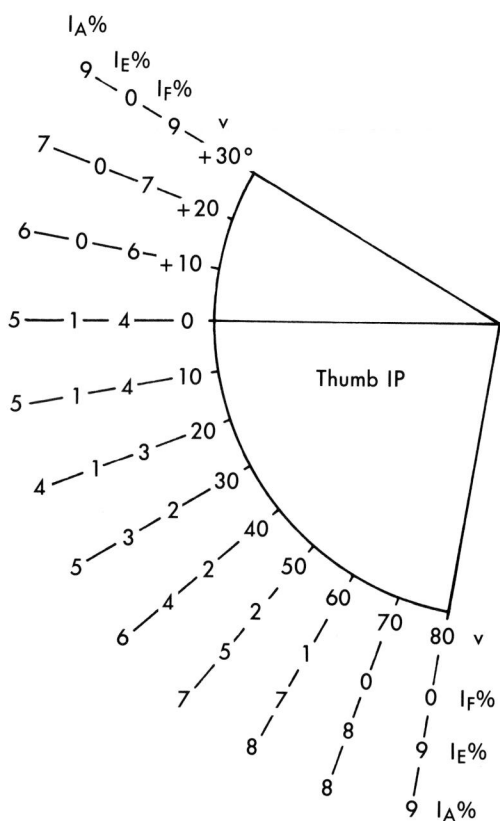

Fig. 8-19 Thumb MP joint: impairment percentages to thumb for loss of flexion, extension, and for ankylosis of MP. Functional position has been established at 20 degrees. Thumb flexion/extension represents 20% of motion units. Of this, a value of 11% is given to the MP joint, and of 9% to the IP joint.

Fig. 8-20 Thumb IP joint: impairment percentages to thumb for loss of flexion, extension, and for ankylosis of IP. Functional position has been established at 20 degrees. Thumb flexion/extension represents 20% of motion units. Of this, a value of 11% is given to the MP joint, and of 9% to the IP joint.

scale, the relative functional value of the MP joint is 55% and of the interphalangeal joint, 45%. This is equivalent to 55% × 20% = 11% relative value for MP joint motion, and 45% × 20% = 9% relative value for interphalangeal joint motion. These values have been considered in the Thumb Motion Impairment Charts (Figs. 8-19 and 8-20). Note that the functional position of the MP and interphalangeal joints is 20°, hence the I_A values are the lowest at this angle. For example, thumb MP ankylosis at 20° flexion equals 5% impairment ankylosis (I_A), and interphalangeal ankylosis at 20° flexion equals 4% impairment ankylosis (I_A).

Adduction contributes 20% to the thumb function, and impairment values have been calculated, considering this factor. The adduction impairment curve is shown in Fig. 8-21. For example, adduction to 4 cm represents a 20% impairment of adduction (Fig. 8-21), or 20% × 20% (4% impairment to the entire thumb) (Table 8-11).

Radial abduction contributes 10% to the thumb motion value, and impairment values have been calculated, considering this factor (Table 8-12). Note that ankylosis in any position of radial abduction corresponds to a complete impairment of this function, because prehension is not possible without some opposition component.

Opposition contributes 50% to the thumb function. Its

impairment curve and calculated values for loss of motion or ankylosis are shown in Fig. 8-22 and Table 8-13.

The values derived for each thumb motion impairment are added numerically to obtain the total motion impairment of the thumb. The combined table is not used. Hand impairment values are obtained by multiplying the thumb values by the thumb's relative value to the hand (40%).

Wrist, elbow, and shoulder impairment

The usefulness of the joints of the upper extremity in placing the hand in space for functional adaptations has great importance. The segments of the extremity have a value that may be calculated in terms of impairment to the total extremity and, from that, to the body. A definite percentage factor for impairment may be given to defects such as awkwardness, incapacity, disturbance of function, and necessary overactivity of the remaining joints resulting from total loss of function of one of the extremity segments. The shoulder segment is given 60% of the total extremity; the elbow, 70%; and the wrist, 60%.

Wrist joint. Evaluation of impairment of the wrist joint is reflected in loss of motion or ankylosis. Dorsal and palmar flexion are given a 70% value to the total range of joint motion, and radial and ulnar deviation are given a 30% value. The usual range of motion of the wrist is from 60

Table 8-11 Thumb adduction impairment (values in % thumb motion impairment*)

Lack of adduction (CM)	Thumb impairment %	
	Lost motion	Ankylosis
0	0	20
1	0	19
2	1	17
3	3	15
4	4	10
5	6	15
6	8	17
7	13	19
8	20	20

*Considering that adduction contributes 20% to thumb function

Table 8-12 Thumb radial abduction impairment (values in % thumb motion impairment*)

Measured radial abduction (degrees)	Thumb impairment %	
	Lost motion	Ankylosis
50	0	10
40	1	10
30	3	10
20	7	10
10	9	10
0	10	10

*Considering that radial abduction contributes 10% to thumb function

Table 8-13 Thumb opposition impairment (values in % thumb motion impairment*)

Measured opposition (CM)	Thumb impairment %	
	Lost motion	Ankylosis
0	50	50
1	35	45
2	25	40
3	15	35
4	10	30
5	6	25
6	3	27
7	1	30
8	0	32

*Considering that opposition contributes 50% to thumb function

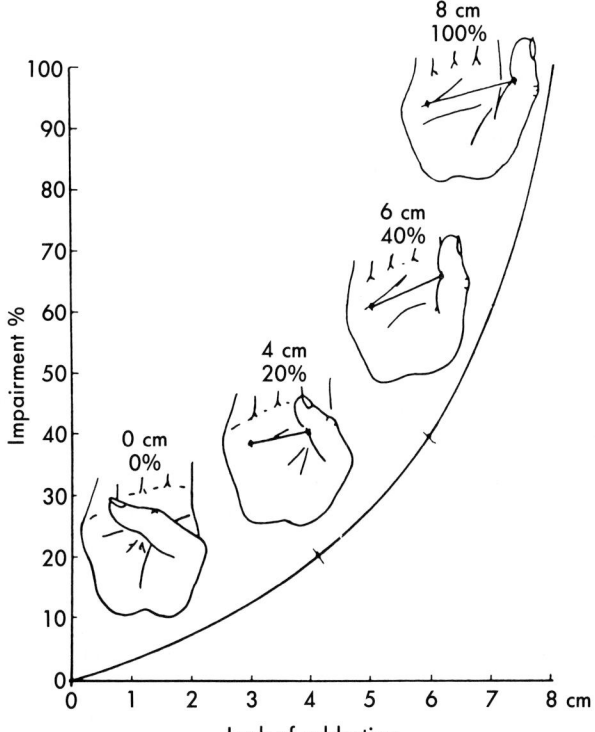

Fig. 8-21 Adduction is measured as distance from flexor crease of interphalangeal joint of thumb to distal palmar crease over metacarpophalangeal joint of fifth finger. Graph represents percentage value for lack of adduction relative to this function and not to whole thumb function. Adduction contributes to 20% of thumb function, and impairments shown must be multiplied by 20% to obtain impairment percentage to entire thumb function, such as shown in Table 8-11.

Fig. 8-22 Opposition is measured as largest possible distance from flexor crease of interphalangeal joint to distal palmar crease over third metacarpophalangeal joint. Impairment value curve for lack of opposition is shown relative to this function. Opposition contributes to 50% of entire thumb function, and values of impairment shown must be multiplied by 50% to obtain impairment percentage to entire thumb function such as shown in Table 8-13.

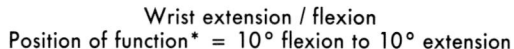

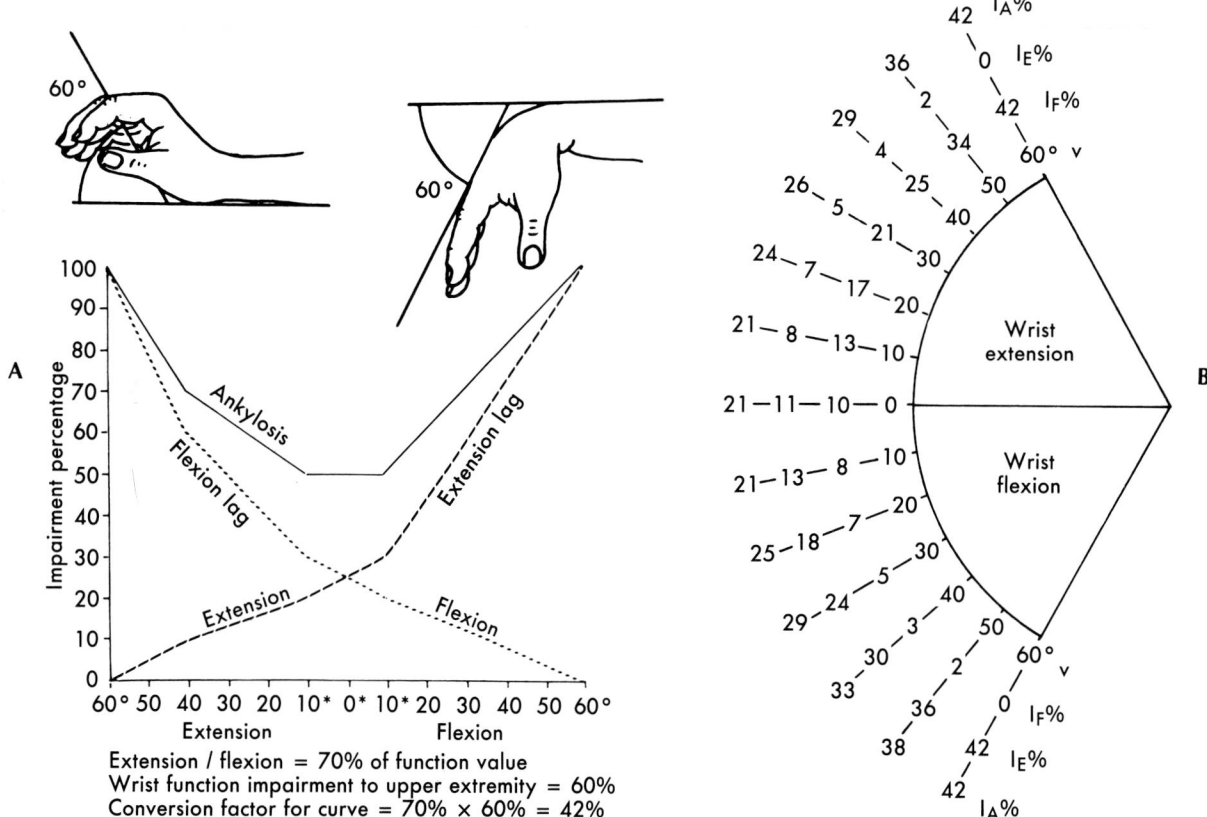

Fig. 8-23 **A,** Wrist flexion and extension impairment curves shown relative to this function. Note that usual ROM is from 60% dorsiflexion to 60% palmar flexion; position of function is from 10 degrees palmar flexion to 10 degrees dorsiflexion, and values for impairment ankylosis reach their lowest between these two angles, or I_A is 50%. **B,** Wrist flexion/extension impairments in upper extremity values. Flexion/extension is given 70% of the wrist functional value. The wrist represents 60% to the upper extremity function; therefore conversion factor for curve shown in Fig. 8-23, **A** is: 70% × 60% = 42% upper extremity impairment.

degrees dorsiflexion to 60 degrees palmar flexion; the position of function is from 10 degrees palmar flexion to 10 degrees dorsiflexion. The usual range of deviation of motion of the wrist is from 20 degrees of radial deviation to 30 degrees of ulnar deviation; the position of function in lateral deviation is from 0 to 10 degrees of ulnar deviation.

The dorsiflexion/palmar flexion impairment curve is shown in Fig. 8-23, *A*. These values were converted to upper extremity impairment values, taking into consideration that this motion contributes 70% to the wrist function and that wrist function contributes 60% to the upper extremity impairment. The conversion factor for this curve is 70% × 60% = 42% upper extremity impairment (Fig. 8-23, *B*).

The lateral deviation motion impairment curve is shown in Fig. 8-24, *A*. These values were converted to upper extremity values, considering that this motion contributes 30% to wrist function. The conversion factor for this curve is 30% × 60% = 18% upper extremity impairment (Fig. 8-24, *B*).

Upper extremity impairment caused by loss of wrist mo-

tion is calculated by adding the flexion/extension and lateral deviation percentages.

Example: Wrist motion 20° extension, 30° flexion, 5° radial deviation, 15° ulnar deviation:

$$I_E\ (7\%)\ +\ I_F\ (5\%)\ +\ I_{RD}\ (3\%)\ +\ I_{UD}\ (3\%)\ =$$
18% upper extremity impairment

Elbow impairment

The elbow functional unit represents 70% to the upper extremity. On a scale of 100%, elbow flexion/extension is given 60% of this value, and pronation/supination is given 40%. The conversion factor for flexion/extension curve is 60% × 70% = 42% upper extremity impairment (Fig. 8-25, *A*). The conversion factor for pronation/supination curve is 40% × 70% = 28% upper extremity impairment (Fig. 8-25, *B*).

The average normal range of motion in the elbow is assumed to be from 0 degrees to 140 degrees of flexion/extension. The position of function is 80 degrees of flexion. The most useful range of motion from the functional view-

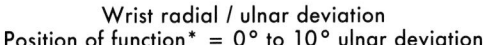

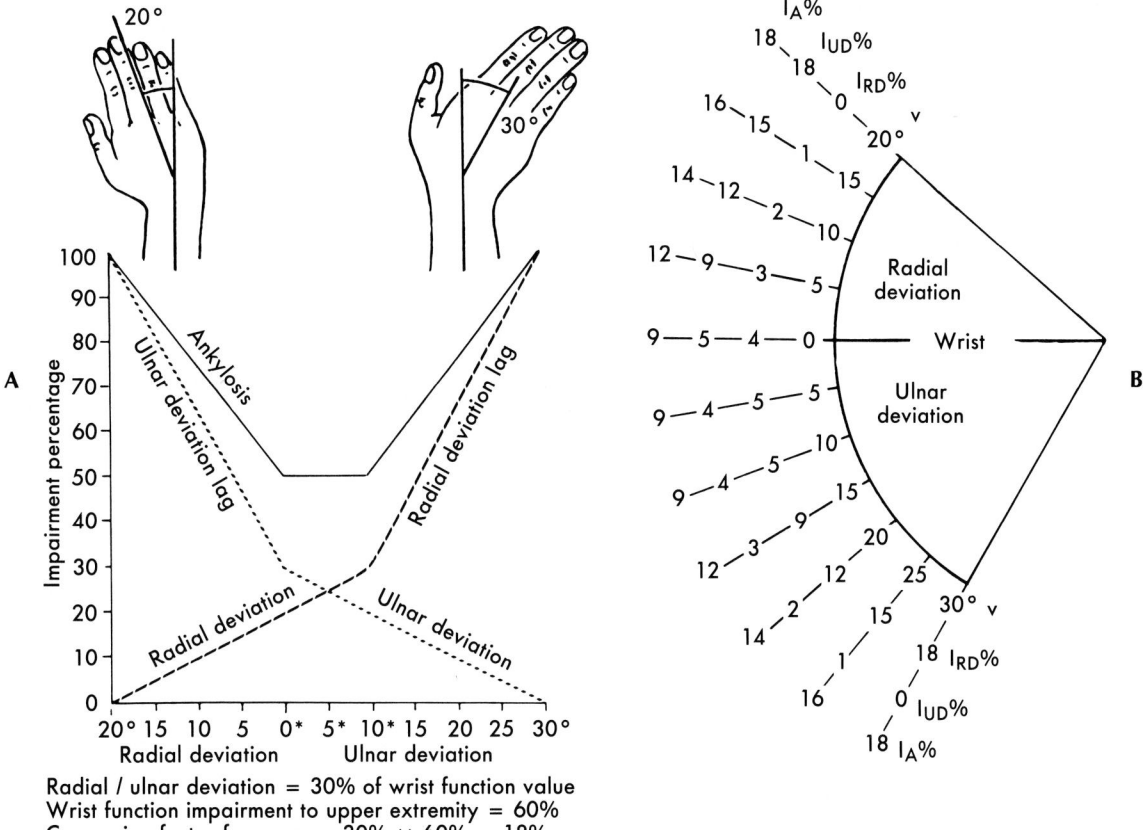

Wrist radial / ulnar deviation
Position of function* = 0° to 10° ulnar deviation

Radial / ulnar deviation = 30% of wrist function value
Wrist function impairment to upper extremity = 60%
Conversion factor for curve = 30% × 60% = 18%

Fig. 8-24 **A,** Wrist radial and ulnar deviation impairment curves shown relative to this function. Note that usual ROM is from 20 degrees radial deviation to 30 degrees ulnar deviation and that position of function is from 0 to 10 degrees ulnar deviation. Ankylosis impairment values reach their lowest point between these angles, or 50%. **B,** Wrist radial/ulnar deviation impairments in upper extremity values. Radial/ulnar deviation is given 30% of the wrist functional value. The wrist represents 60% to the upper extremity function. Therefore the conversion factor for curve shown in Fig. 8-24, **A** is: 30% × 60% = 18% upper extremity impairment.

point is considered to be from 45 degrees to 110 degrees of flexion. Lack of extension less than 45 degrees, and lack of flexion from 110 to 140 degrees are therefore considered to give a relatively small impairment of function. The usual range of rotation is from 80 degrees supination to 80 degrees pronation. The position of function is considered to be in 20 degrees of pronation (Fig. 8-26).

Upper extremity impairment caused by loss of elbow motion is calculated by adding the flexion/extension and pronation/supination percentages.

Example: Elbow motion −30° extension, 110° flexion, 60° pronation, 40° supination:

$$I_E \ (3\%) + I_F \ (4\%) + I_p \ (1\%) + I_s \ (2\%) =$$
$$10\% \text{ upper extremity impairment}$$

Shoulder impairment

The shoulder functional unit represents 60% to the upper extremity. The motion units and their relative value to the shoulder function on a 100% scale are as follows: flexion

(40%), extension (10%), abduction (20%), adduction, (10%), and internal/external rotation (20%). The conversion factor for the flexion/extension curve is 50% × 60% = 30% upper extremity impairment (Fig. 8-27). The conversion factor for the abduction/adduction curve is 30% × 60% = 18% upper extremity impairment (Fig. 8-28). The conversion factor for the rotation curve is 20% × 60% = 12% upper extremity impairment (Fig. 8-29).

In each of these three functions, the position of function has been chosen according to the recommendations in the literature concerning arthrodesis of the glenohumeral joint, even though motions of different joints are involved in each function (glenohumeral joint, acromioclavicular joint, sternoclavicular joint, and the movement between the scapula and the chest wall).[4,5]

The average normal range of shoulder motion is assumed to be from 50 degrees extension to 180 degrees flexion, the position of function being 25 degrees flexion. Ankylosis in the position of function gives 50% impairment of function,

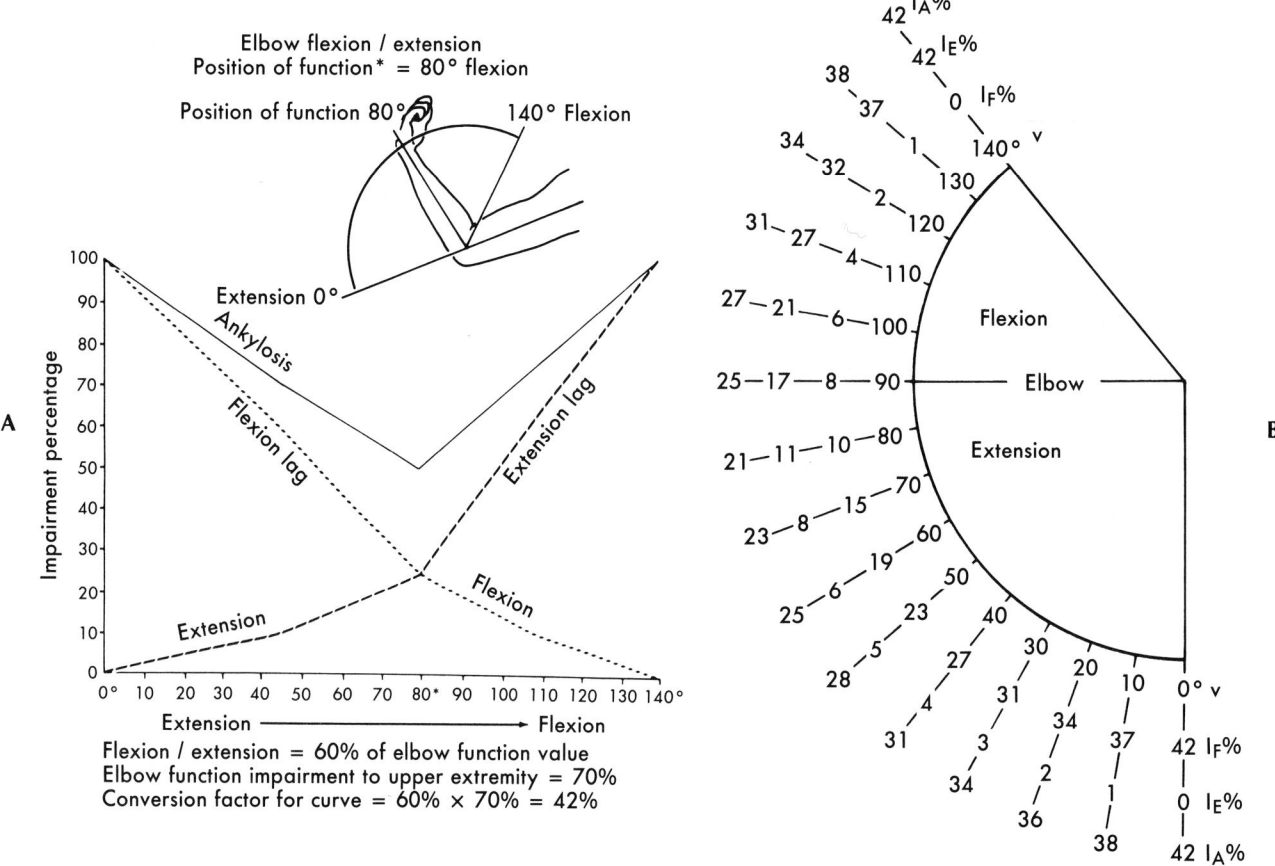

Fig. 8-25 **A,** Elbow flexion/extension impairment: curves shown relative to this function. Range of motion of elbow is usually from 0 degrees extension to 140 degrees flexion, and position of function is 80 degrees flexion. Note that impairment ankylosis percentage is lowest for position of function, or 50%. **B,** Elbow flexion/extension impairments in upper extremity values. Flexion/extension is given 60% of the elbow functional value. The elbow represents 70% to the upper extremity function. Therefore the conversion factor for curve shown in Fig. 8-25, **A** is: 60% × 70% = 42% upper extremity impairment.

ankylosis in 0 degrees gives 80% impairment, and ankylosis in 90 degrees flexion gives 90% impairment (Fig. 8-27, A). The most important range of flexion is from 0 degrees to the position of function with a decrease of impairment from 70% at 0 degrees, to 40% at 25 degrees. From there, the flexion curve relatively flattens to end at 0% of impairment at 180 degrees flexion. The most important range of extension is to bring the arm from 90 degrees flexion to the position of function; the impairment consequently decreases from 70% at 90 degrees, to 10% at 25 degrees. Extension from the position of function to 50 degrees is of less importance, and the extension curve goes relatively flat within this range.

The average normal range of shoulder motion is considered to be from 50 degrees adduction to 180 degrees abduction; the position of function being 50 degrees abduction. Ankylosis in the position of function gives 50% of impairment; ankylosis in 0 degrees abduction gives 80% impairment, and ankylosis in 90 degrees abduction gives 90% impairment (Fig. 8-28, A). Abduction from 0 degrees to the position of function (50 degrees abduction) is considered to be the most important part of abduction with a decrease of impairment from 70% at a position of 0 degrees to 35%

at the position of function (Fig. 8-28, A). From there, the abduction curve goes relatively more flat to 0% impairment at 180 degrees abduction. The most import function of adduction is to bring the arm from 90 degrees abduction down to the position of function with a decrease of the impairment from 65% at 90 degrees, to 15% at 50 degrees. Adduction from the position of function to 50 degrees adduction is considered to be of less importance, and the adduction curve goes relatively flat within this range.

The average normal range of shoulder motion is assumed to be 90 degrees internal rotation and 90 degrees external rotation, the position of function being 20 degrees external rotation. Ankylosis in the position of function gives 50% impairment; ankylosis in 50 degrees external rotation and 40 degrees internal rotation gives the same impairment, or 90% (Fig. 8-29, A). The most important range of external rotation is from 40 degrees internal rotation to the position of function (20 degrees external rotation), with a decrease of impairment from 80% to 20%. The most important range of internal rotation is from 50 degrees external rotation to the position of function, with a decrease of the impairment from 80% to 25%.

Upper extremity impairment because of loss of shoulder

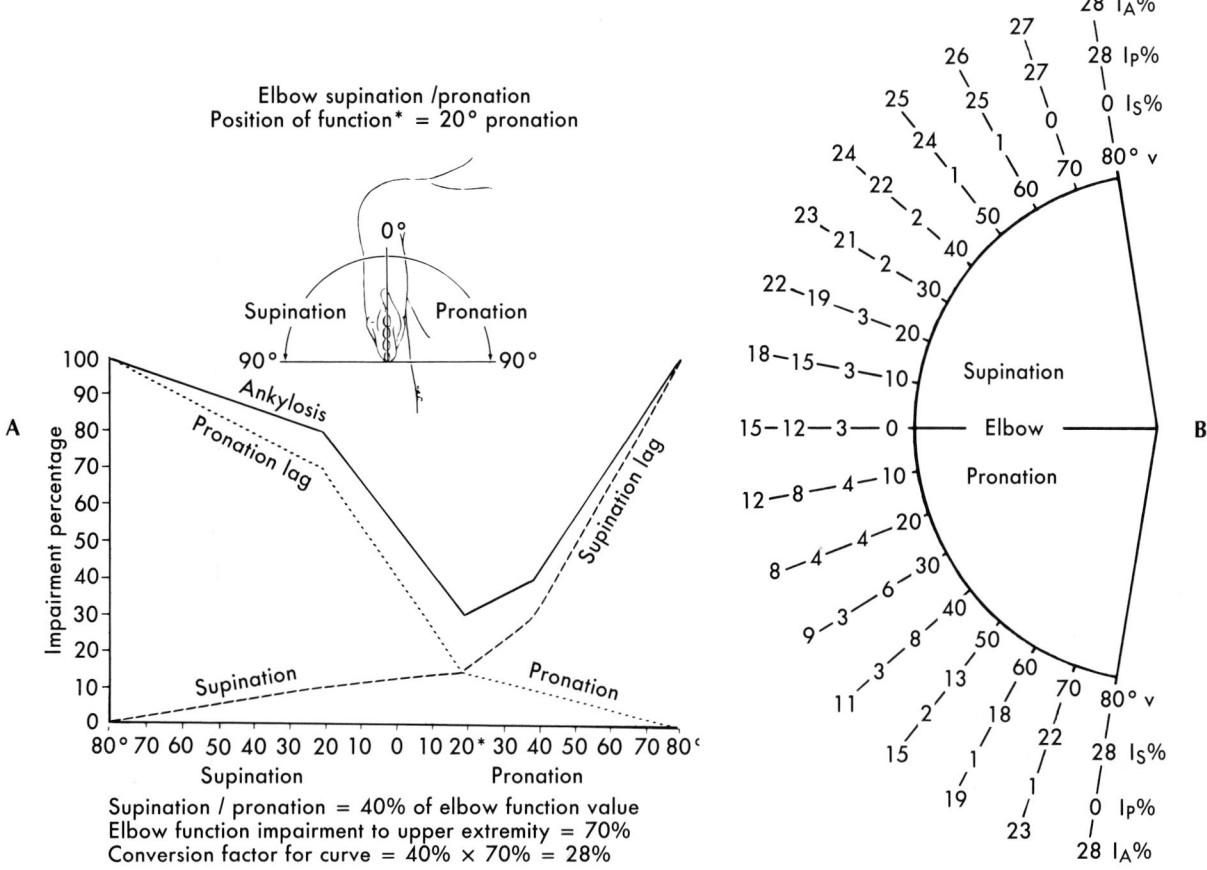

Fig. 8-26 **A,** Rotation of forearm impairment: curves shown relative to this function. Usual range of rotation is from 80-degree supination to 80-degree pronation, and position of function is considered to be 20-degree pronation. Note that impairment ankylosis percentage is lowest for position of function, or 30%. **B,** Elbow pronation/supination impairments in upper extremity values. Pronation/supination is given 40% of the elbow functional value. The elbow represents 70% to the upper extremity function. Therefore the conversion factor for curve shown in Fig. 8-26, **A** is: 40% × 70% = 28% upper extremity impairment.

motion is calculated by adding flexion/extension, abduction/adduction, and rotation percentages.

Example: Shoulder motion: flexion 110°, extension 20°, abduction 70°, adduction 40°, internal rotation 20°, external rotation 10°:

$$I_F (5\%) + I_E (2\%) + I_{ABD} (5\%) + I_{ADD} (0\%) + I_{IR}$$
$$(2\%) + I_{ER} (4\%) = 18\% \text{ upper extremity impairment}$$

HOW TO COMBINE UPPER EXTREMITY IMPAIRMENT

For each level of involvement, impairments from amputation, motion loss, sensory loss, pain, strength, and other derangements must be expressed in the same denominator before combining their value with the combined values principle (Tables 8-11 and 8-12).

When multiple joints or multiple impairments are present in a finger, they are combined with the combined values principles.

Thumb functional impairments at the level of the CMC, MP, and IP joints are added directly together, because the relative value of each thumb level has been figured on a 100% scale to the thumb (CMC, 80%; MP, 11%; IP, 9%).

Note that these values differ from the thumb amputation values (MP, 100% and IP, 50%) (Fig. 8-5).

When multiple digits are involved, each digit impairment is expressed in terms of hand impairment by multiplying it by the relative value of the digit to the hand. The relative value of each digit has been figured on a 100% scale to the hand (thumb, 40%; index, 20%; middle, 20%; ring, 10%; and little, 10%) (Fig. 8-5). Therefore hand impairment values derived for each digit are added directly together.

When there is involvement at multiple levels of the extremity, for example, hand, wrist, elbow, or shoulder, the impairment percentage for each level is converted in upper extremity impairment values. These are then combined using the combined values principle.

DISCUSSION OF IMPAIRMENT EVALUATION METHODS

It is noted in the diagrams that the impairment has been given a linear configuration that is of practical benefit. It might have been of greater accuracy to note greater changes of impairment immediately around the positions of function for the various joints discussed. It should be observed that the angle of ankylosis has its lowest impairment at the po-

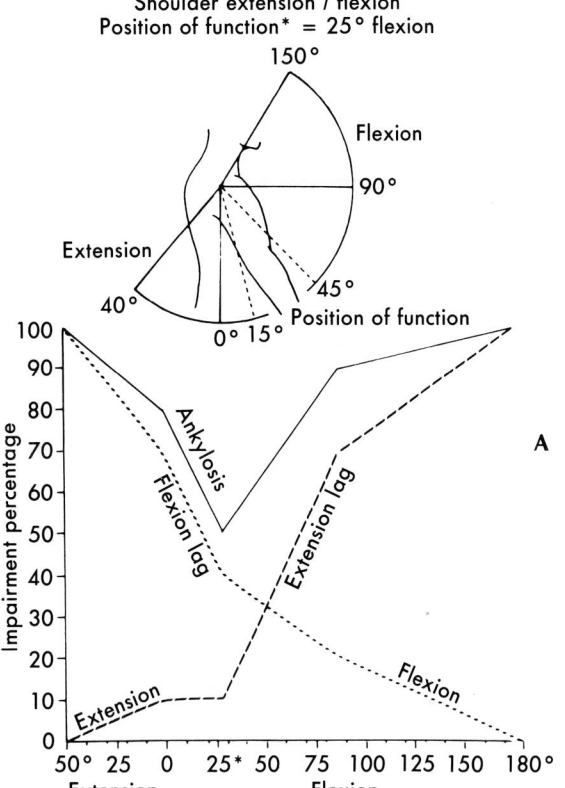

Shoulder extension / flexion
Position of function* = 25° flexion

Extension = 10% / flexion = 40% of shoulder function value
Extension / flexion = 50% of shoulder function
Shoulder function impairment to upper extremity = 60%
Conversion factor for curve = 50% × 60% = 30%

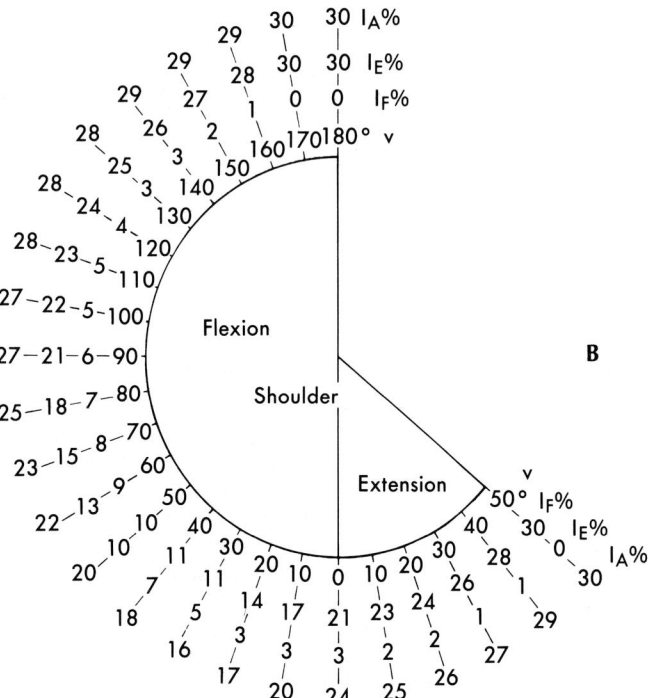

Fig. 8-27 **A,** Shoulder flexion/extension impairment curves shown relative to this function. Position of function has been established at 25 degrees flexion. **B,** Shoulder flexion/extension impairments in upper extremity values. Extension is given 10% and flexion 40% of shoulder functional value, or 50% for the combined motion. The shoulder represents 60% to the upper extremity function. Therefore the conversion factor for the curve shown in Fig. 8-27, **A** is: 50% × 60% = 30% upper extremity impairment.

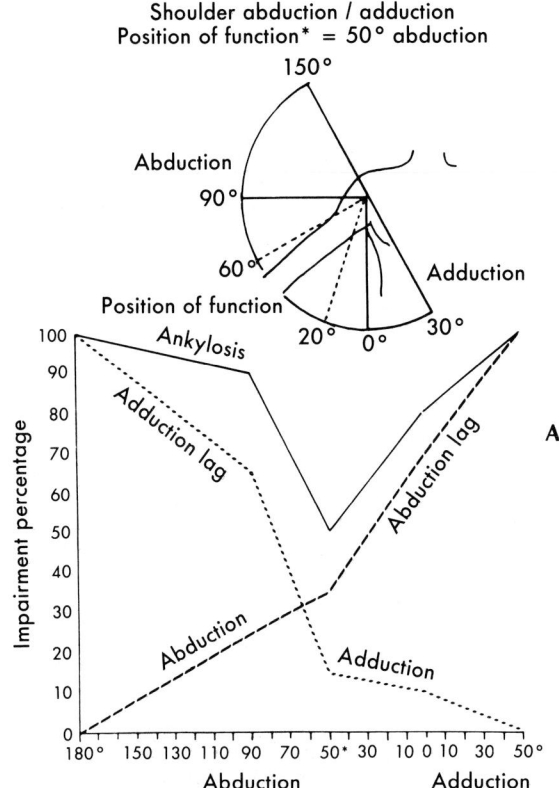

Shoulder abduction / adduction
Position of function* = 50° abduction

Abduction = 20% / adduction = 10% of shoulder function value
Abduction / adduction = 30% of shoulder function value
Shoulder function impairment to upper extremity = 60%
Conversion factor for curve = 30% × 60% = 18%

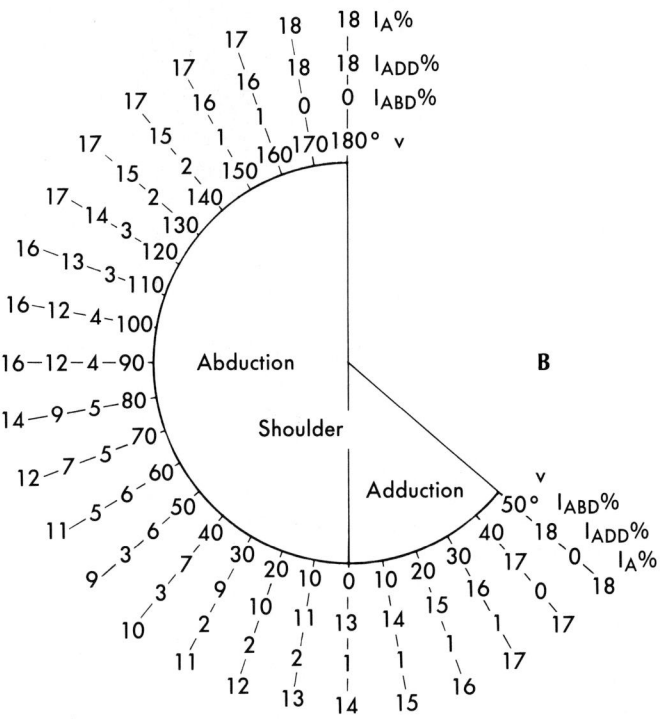

Fig. 8-28 **A,** Shoulder abduction/adduction impairment curves shown relative to this function. Position of function is 50 degrees abduction. **B,** Shoulder abduction/adduction impairments in upper extremity values. Abduction is given 20% and adduction 10% of shoulder functional value, or 30% for the combined motion. The shoulder represents 60% to the upper extremity function. Therefore the conversion factor for the curve shown in Fig. 8-28, **A** is: 30% × 60% = 18% upper extremity impairment.

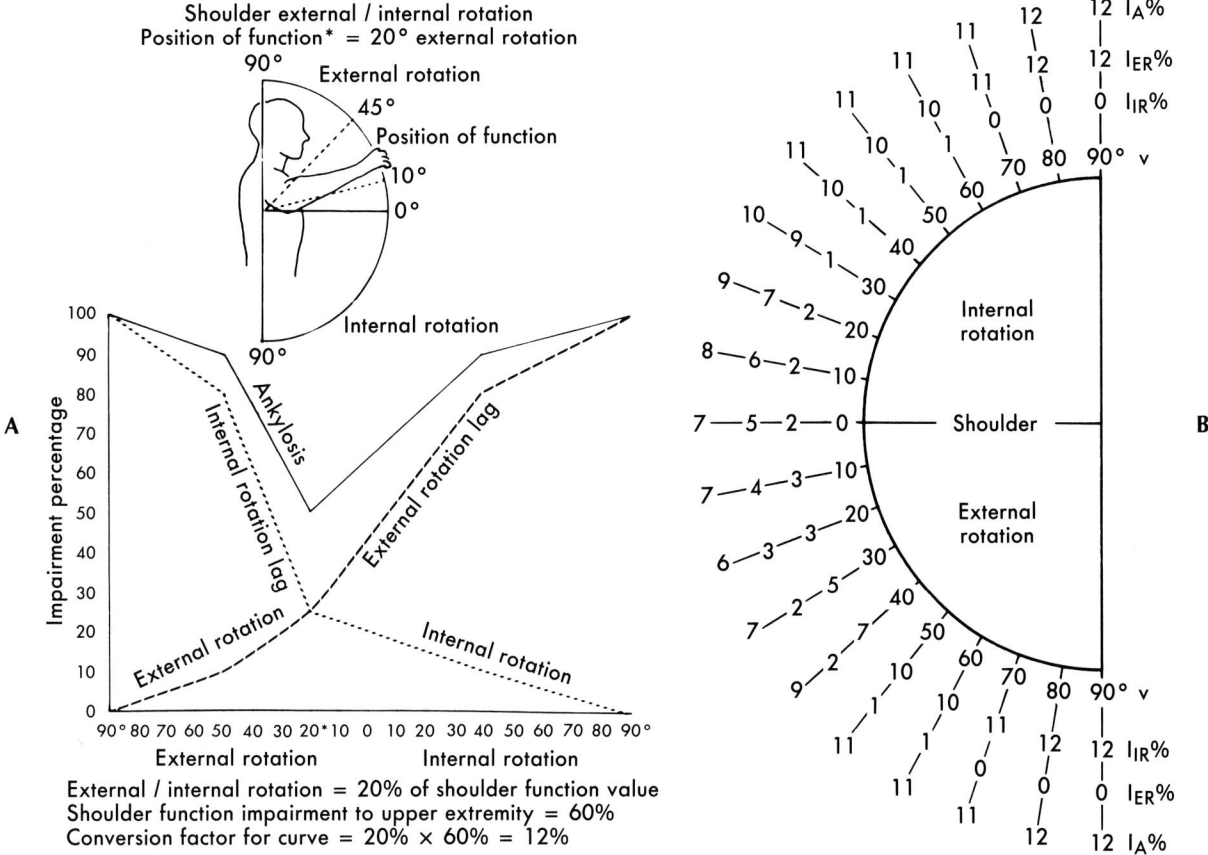

Fig. 8-29 **A,** Shoulder internal/external rotation impairment curves shown relative to this function. Position of function is 20 degrees external rotation. **B,** Shoulder internal/external rotation impairments in upper extremity values. Rotation motion is given 20% of shoulder function value. The shoulder represents 60% to the upper extremity function. Therefore the conversion factor for the curve shown in Fig. 8-29, **A** is: 20% × 60% = 12% upper extremity impairment.

sition of function; we have used the recommendation of the American Medical Association of 30 degrees for the MP joint, 40 degrees for the PIP joint, and 20 degrees for the DIP joint in reference to their respective positions of function.

Values for hyperextension of the finger joints have been included in the charts presented here; these were not included in the American Medical Association guide or in our previous work. We consider about 20 degrees of hyperextension in the MP joint to be normal and of some functional importance to open the hand completely. Lack of this hyperextension in the MP joint is therefore considered to give some impairment. The linear function representing ankylosis, I_A, has simply been extended to include 20 degrees of hyperextension. Hyperextension in the PIP and DIP joint is, however, considered unnatural, at least without importance functionally. Lack of hyperextension in these joints will therefore of course not give any impairment. Consequently, in the formula presented, $I_A = I_E + I_F$, I_A and I_F therefore are equal when I_E is 0, and so their functions coincide within the sector of hyperextension. We consider ankylosis or severely limited flexion within this sector, as in severe swan-neck deformity, to give a more pronounced impairment and have therefore drawn the functions more steeply within this sector.

For the evaluation of impairment of the basal joint of the thumb, two motions are measured, namely, thumb opposition and adduction. The difficulty in measuring the angles of the complex thumb movements make this simplified method logical.

SUMMARY

The responsibility of recording, evaluating, and assessing impairment of the upper extremity resulting from trauma and disease is a true medical entity. The method of measuring these defects, the mechanism of estimating impairment, and relating this physical loss of each anatomic segment to the body are presented. The mathematical principles of estimating incapacity are shown.

The common impairments are placed in table form for easier use. A new method of evaluating lack of extension and relating it to ankylosis and lack of flexion is described. A plea is made for the consideration of research into better functional evaluations, including the use of the motion-time-measurement method.

The principles presented and the methods outlined should aid the physician examiner as he attempts to assess impairment in the upper extremity and hand.

REFERENCES

1. American Academy of Orthopaedic Surgeons: Joint motion, method of measuring and recording, Chicago, 1965.
2. Boyes JH: Bunnell's surgery of the hand, ed 5, Philadelphia, 1970, JB Lippincott Co.
3. Bunnell S: The management of the non-functional hand—reconstruction vs. prosthesis, Artif Limbs 4:76, 1957.
4. Crenshaw AH, editor: Campbell's operative orthopaedics, ed 5, St. Louis, 1971, The CV Mosby Co.
5. de Palma A: Surgery of the shoulder, ed 2, Philadelphia, 1973, JB Lippincott Co.
6. Guide to the evaluation of permanent impairment of the extremities and back, JAMA 166:February 16, 1958 (Special edition).
7. Litchman HM and Paslay PR: Determination of finger-motion impairment by linear measurement, J Bone Joint Surg 56A:85, 1974.
8. Mannerfelt L: Studies on the hand in ulnar nerve paralysis, Acta Orthop Scand (Suppl.) 87:63, 1966.
9. Swanson AB: Evaluation of impairment of function in the hand, Surg Clin North Am 44:925, 1964.
10. Tubiana R, Michon J, and Thomine J: Scheme for assessment of deformities of Dupuytren's disease, Surg Clin North Am 48:979, 1968.
11. Van't Hof A, and Heiple KG: Flexor tendon injuries of the fingers and thumb: a comparative study, J Bone Joint Surg 40A:256, 1958.
12. White W: Personal communication, 1965, Pittsburgh.

BIBLIOGRAPHY

American Rheumatism Association: Primer on the rheumatic diseases, JAMA 171:1205, 1345, 1680, 1959.

American Society for Surgery of the Hand, Committee on Hand Evaluation, Richard Eaton, Chairman.

Bateman JE: Disability evaluation about the shoulder, Surg Clin North Am 43:1721, 1963.

Beasley WC: Quantitative muscle testing: principles and applications to research and clinical services, Arch Physiol Med 42:398, 1961.

Bechtol CO: Grip test, the use of a dynamometer with adjustable handle spacings, J Bone Joint Surg 36A:820, 1954.

Bertelsen A and Capener N: Fingers, compensation and King Canute, J Bone Joint Surg 42B:390, 1960.

Boyes JH: Flexor tendon grafts in the fingers and thumb, J Bone Joint Surg 32A:489, 1950.

Carroll D: A quantitative test of upper extremity function, J Chron Dis 18:479, 1965.

Flatt AE: Rheumatoid Hand Research Project (Booklets), Department of Orthopaedics, University of Iowa, 1963.

Flatt AE: The care of the rheumatoid hand, ed 3, St. Louis, 1974, The CV Mosby Co.

Garrett JW: The adult human hand; some anthropometric and biomechanic considerations, Hum Factors 13:117, 1971.

Guides to the evaluation of permanent impairment of the peripheral spinal nerves, American Medical Association Committee on Medical Rating of Physical Impairment, 1962.

Guides to the evaluation of permanent impairment, American Medical Association, ed 3, Engelberg, A. editor, 1988, pp 13-40.

Hamasaki K: The study of the hand, lost digit, Acta Med Kyushu University, 31:53, 1961.

Hollander JL: Arthritis and allied conditions, a textbook of rheumatology, ed 8, Philadelphia, 1972, Lea & Febiger.

Hunter JM and Salisbury RF: Flexor tendon reconstruction in severely damaged hands, J Bone Joint Surg 53A:829, 1971.

Karger DW and Bayha FH: Engineered work measurement, ed 2, New York, 1965, Industrial Press Inc.

Kirkpatrick EJ: Evaluation of grip loss, Calif Med 85:314, 1956.

Kroemer KHE and Howard JM: Towards standardization of muscle strength testing, Med Sci Sports 2:224, 1970.

Lewey FH, Kuhn WG, and Juditski JT: A standardized method for assessing the strength of hand and foot muscles, Surg Gynecol Obstet 85:785, 1947.

Littler JW: The physiology and dynamic function of the hand, Surg Clin North Am 40:259, 1960.

McBride ED: Disability evaluation, ed 6, Philadelphia, 1963, JB Lippincott Co.

McCormack RM: Reconstructive surgery and immediate care of the badly injured hand, Clin Orthop 13:78, 1959.

Moberg E: Objective methods for determining the functional value of sensibility in the hand, J Bone Joint Surg 40B:454, 1958.

Moberg E: Dressings, splints and postoperative care in hand surgery, Surg Clin North Am 44:35, 941, 1964.

Parry CBW: Rehabilitation of the hand, ed 2, London, 1966, Butterworth & Co (Publishers) Ltd.

Patterson HMcL: Grip measurements as a part of the pre-placement evaluation, Ind Med Surg 34:555, 1965.

Rattner IN: Injury ratings, New York, 1970, Crescent Publishing Co.

Slocum DB: Amputations of the fingers and the hand, Clin Orthop 15:35, 1959.

Slocum DB and Pratt DR: The principles of amputation of the fingers and hand, J Bone Joint Surg 26:535, 1944.

Slocum DB and Pratt DR: Disability evaluation for the hand, J Bone Joint Surg 28:491, 1946.

Smith HB: Smith hand function evaluation, Am J Occup Ther 27:244, 1973.

Smith WC: Principles of disability evaluation, Philadelphia, 1959, JB Lippincott Co.

Stack G, editor: Internal publication. International Federation of Societies for Surgery of the Hand, 1970.

Swanson AB: Multiple finger amputations: concepts of treatment, J Mich Med Soc 61:316, 1962.

Swanson AB: Restoration of hand function by the use of partial or total prosthetic replacement, J Bone Joint Surg 45A:276, 1963.

Swanson AB: The Krukenberg procedure in the juvenile amputee, J Bone Joint Surg 46A(7):1540, 1964.

Swanson AB: Surgery of the hand in cerebral palsy and the swan-neck deformity, J Bone Joint Surg 42A:951, 1960.

Swanson AB: Levels of amputation of fingers and hand: considerations for treatment, Surg Clin North Am 44:1115, 1964.

Swanson AB, Mays JD, and Yamauchi Y: A rheumatoid arthritis evaluation record for the upper extremity, Surg Clin North Am 48:1003, 1968.

Swanson AB, Matev IB, and deGroot G: The strength of the hand, Bull Prosthet Res, p. 145, Fall, 1970. Swanson AB: Flexible implant resection arthroplasty in the hand and extremities, St. Louis, 1973, The CV Mosby Co.

Taylor CL: Biomechanics of the normal and the amputated upper extremity. In Klopsteg PE and Wilson PD, editors: Human limbs and their substitutes, New York, 1954, McGraw-Hill Book Co.

Taylor CL and Schwartz RJ: The anatomy and mechanics of the human hand, Artif Limbs 2:22, 1955.

Wechesser EC: Reconstruction of a grasping mechanism following loss of digits, Clin Orthop 15:69, 1959.

9

Application of biomechanics for evaluation of the hand

Judith A. Bell-Krotoski, Donna E. Breger, and Robert B. Beach

Surgeons and therapists historically have had to deal with surgical tendon transfers, soft tissue problems, splinting, and measurement techniques largely based on educated experience and intuitive judgment. Only recently has there been a growing interest in use and application of biomechanical terms and principles in treatment and in measurement techniques that are truly objective.* One advantage in the recent climate of litigation and reimbursement problems is that more individuals are referring to hand surgery and hand therapy in quantifiable, objective terms.

A new member of the rehabilitation team is adding insight into hand function and principles of measurement: the biomedical engineer. This person adds depth to our understanding of hand function and principles of objective measurement that can be directly applied in clinical hand practice.

Dr. Paul Brand has long believed the biomedical engineer to be a needed member of the surgical/therapy team, and has spent much of his professional life fostering this concept. He demonstrated the value of the engineer in the rehabilitation research laboratory he established in Carville, La.† The information in this chapter is a result in large part of knowledge gained through interaction with Brand, his colleagues, engineers, and other therapists on a rehabilitation team.[5]

This material has been selected specifically to heighten the clinician's awareness and appreciation of basic principles of soft tissue mechanics, hand mechanics, and materials mechanics and to show how such understanding can improve the accuracy and repeatability of clinical measurements. Understanding alone is not enough. The application of newly understood mechanical principles in clinical practice is needed also.

Elements of soft tissue and materials mechanics are discussed first, followed by examples of how this knowledge can be used in practice in routine clinical measurements. Such application in clinical practice rewards the clinician by clinical records that are more objective, repeatable, and comparable with subsequent examinations and other tests and measures; by elimination of some of the guesswork in clinical measurements and treatment; and by clinical treatment that is both safe and efficient.

MECHANICS OF FORCE/PRESSURE ON SKIN

When discussing the biomechanics of soft tissue, we are first concerned with the force, or pressure (force per unit area), applied to the skin and other soft tissue. The skin and other soft tissues were designed to cushion the skeleton, to absorb certain amounts of impact, and to be flexible enough to allow free movement of joints and tendons. Some stress of skin (stress occurs in the skin when a force is applied) is normal and, in fact, is needed to help maintain normal healthy tissue. Skin that does not receive stress becomes thin and shiny and tears easily. Skin that receives repetitive stress can react by forming callus and becoming tougher. But as with all things, there are limits to how much stress the skin can tolerate before its integrity is compromised. The therapist's understanding of these limits is important in measurement. It is important also in providing safe and efficient treatment, such as rubber-band traction for improved range of motion.

Before one considers actual measurement of force that acts on the skin, it is important to understand exactly how skin reacts to force by the internal stress created in the skin and under what mechanical stress skin and other soft tissue is damaged. Brand points out that every pressure sore results from excessive mechanical force. With this understanding, we can modify and control the mechanical environment so that pressure problems from too much stress can be prevented.

There are at least four ways in which living skin and soft tissue can be injured or destroyed by mechanical force. These four ways are associated with (1) varying degrees, (2) duration, (3) repetition, and (4) direction of force. In addition, the effect that force has on skin and soft tissue will vary according to the condition of the tissue. Tissue that has changed in quality by disuse or injury has lost some of its ability to sustain stress. The condition of skin must then be considered when judgments are made as to "safe" amounts of force the skin can sustain.

DEGREE OF STRESS

The *degree* (amount) of stress that occurs in the tissue is important in determining whether tissue will be damaged. High stress may be acceptable for a short period and low stress acceptable for a long period. But how much stress is too much, and when is an applied force sufficiently low so that the resulting stress is acceptable for splint traction?

Low stress

Normally the skin has a protective mechanism against sustained low-pressure ischemia (pressure that is not immediately uncomfortable but enough to cause some decrease in capillary flow and to eventually cause ischemia). At some point before actual tissue damage, an ischemic area begins to become uncomfortable. The normal reaction of the in-

---

*References 1, 2, 33, 48, 57, 69.

†Paul W. Brand Research Laboratory, US Public Health Service, Gillis W. Long Hansen's Disease Ctr., Carville, La.

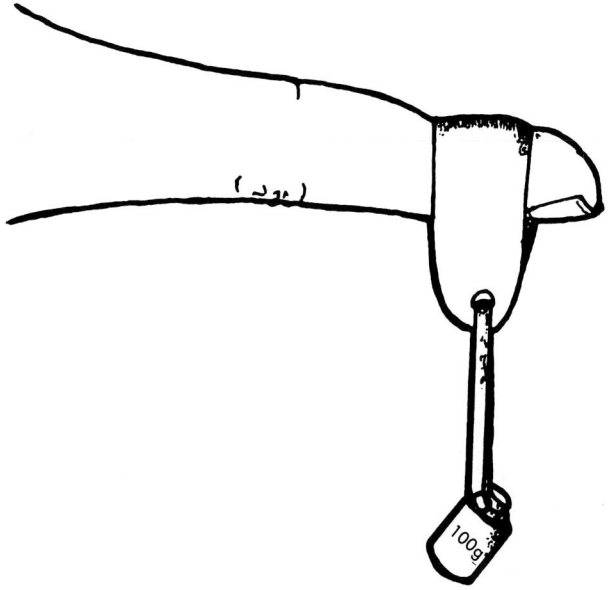

Fig. 9-1 Low force × time. Low force over time can cause ischemia, hyperemia on release of force, swelling, and cellular damage.

dividual is to move and redistribute the pressure. This is why most people do not get bed sores from sleeping. They must first have some other factor that overrides the normal protective response, such as generalized or specific muscle weakness, sensory impairment, or sedation.[21]

Low stress can be damaging to tissue if it is continuous for a long *duration* and can eventually result in ischemic necrosis (Fig. 9-1). We can see the effect of continuous, low force under constricting circumferential bandages, splint straps, and areas of splint contact. Capillary flow in the skin will be obstructed with very little pressure—30 to 50 mm Hg.[79] To prevent ischemic necrosis, it is necessary to control either the degree of pressure or the duration of pressure or both.[17,29,38]

When attempting to mobilize a stiff joint by dynamic splinting, the forces acting on the skin are the limiting factors in most cases; the tendon and bone can usually withstand additional torque (force multiplied by distance from which the force is applied). More force for traction could be used then if the skin under the traction could safely sustain higher force.

Other factors affecting the onset of ischemic necrosis of the skin include degree of stiffness/pliability, of tissue, and temperature. Tissue that is tense and more rigid from edema will more quickly develop ischemic necrosis, as will inflamed tissue. Skin overlying stiff joints will more quickly develop ischemic necrosis because of the absence of joint movement, which would help redistribute the pressure on the skin.

An easy experiment to demonstrate ischemic pressure on the skin can be done by pressing a glass slide against a fingertip. Blanching of the skin will occur at a very low force. This blanching begins with the weight of the slide against the fingertip and increases as the force against the skin is increased by the examiner's finger until capillary action ceases. The skin was not meant to sustain constant low pressure causing such ischemia. The skin's capillary

action is vital to its adequate nutrition and survival and is even more critical to healing tissue.

Another experiment to demonstrate the effects of ischemic pressure is to wrap clear plastic tape around each of three fingers. Apply the first just short of blanching; the second to mottled blanching; and the third to full blanching. Note the time it takes for each to become uncomfortable. One would not think of wearing either of the tapes that cause blanching for any extended period. But this is often what is asked of patients undergoing traction splinting. Care must be taken to distribute pressure throughout as broad an area as possible and to splint to tissue tolerance, where sustained low stress, or force/area, will not cause sustained skin blanching. When a patient experiences discomfort from a splint, there may be areas of ischemic pressure, which he cannot explain.

Moderate stress

As discussed, low stress of relatively short duration can easily be tolerated by normal healthy tissue and is a part of everyday use of the skin that contributes to its health. Moderate stress (generally, enough stress to occlude capillary action in a relatively short period compared with low stress) is also not harmful and can be considered beneficial unless it is too repetitive.

Moderate stress can be damaging to tissue if it is *repetitive* (stress of multiple repetitions), causing inflammation of tissue and resultant breakdown. (Of course, moderate stress can also cause ischemic damage from prolonged duration of stress.) At first the stress may be acceptable and harmless for a number of repetitions. If this is followed by continued repetitive moderate stress, it will eventually result in tissue necrosis and there will be an inflammatory response.[17] The inflammation will come first unless the tissue gets mechanically torn apart (pulverized, where vascular tissue and skin cells are torn apart before an inflammation response can occur).

The signs of inflammation are redness, swelling, and heat. An important finding by Brand and others from soft tissue studies in our lab showed that once swelling and heat from repetitive stress occurred on one day, it took far less time and amount of stress for the swelling and heat to recur on the second day. This effect was long-lasting into the next couple of weeks.[21] The tissue had in essence become sensitized by the previous stress (force per unit area that develops within a structure in response to stress) (Fig. 9-2). In these cases histologic changes were seen microscopically, even when no obvious signs of tissue inflammation or swelling were seen before the tissue was further stressed.

The effect of repetitive stress can be seen on the fingertip of a patient undergoing rubber-band traction if the patient continually flexes the finger against the cuff and rubber band. A seemingly moderate force at some point can eventually become inflammatory. We adjust rubber-band traction "to tissue tolerance" for this reason, relaxing or discontinuing the force of traction if evidence of inflammatory response is seen, then continuing traction with a reduced force once obvious redness has subsided. (Because once an inflammatory response has occurred and it takes much less force to produce the same amount of inflammatory response in the next few days, it is better to start traction with a low force and gradually increase the force if the tissue tolerates

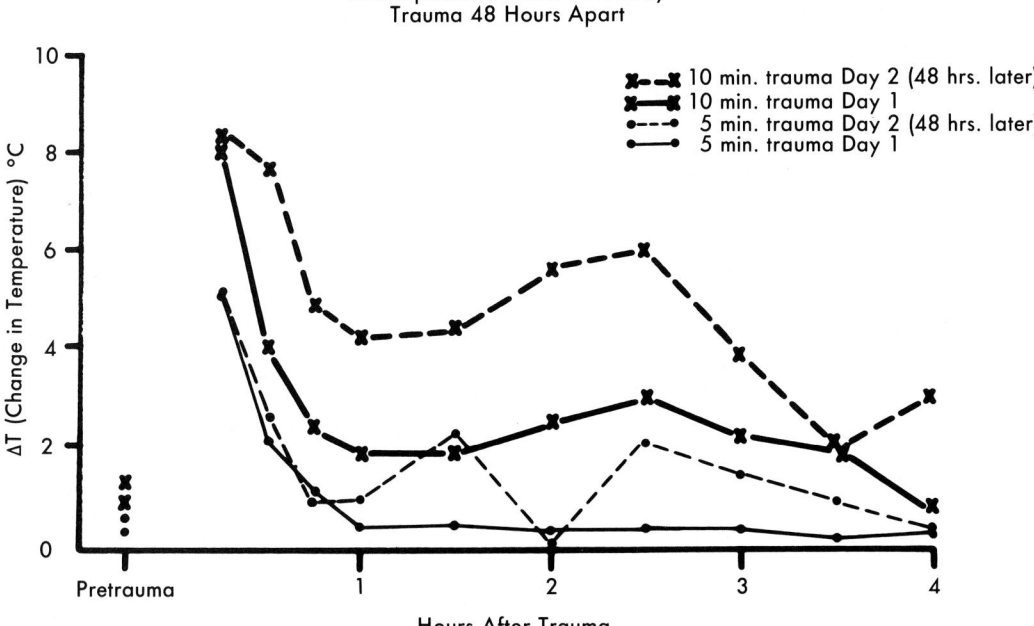

Fig. 9-2 Repetitive force. Moderate force of short duration can be damaging if it is repetitive. Note the temperature elevation that occurred because of the repetitive force of two different durations. The effect of repetitive stress on tissue can be long lasting and may continue several weeks. (From Brand PW, Sabin TD, and Burke JF: Sensory denervation: a study of its cause and its prevention in leprosy and of management of insensitive limbs. Final Report, Carville, La USPHS Hospital, SRS Project No. RC-40-M, Aug. 1, 1966 through June 30, 1970.)

the traction for a day or a few days, than to begin traction with too great a force and have to reduce it.) Often it is necessary to reduce traction force from that otherwise used if repetitive use of the finger is required, particularly if the skin has become sensitized for any reason.

It is emphasized again that not all stress is bad and some stress on skin tissue is needed to maintain normal healthy tissue and build callus in areas of high stress. But excessive stress, and in this case too much repetitive stress, can be harmful. Patients with nerve injuries can develop fingertip changes of scar tissue, tissue absorption, and decreased vascularity even without breaking the skin or developing infection. This happens by repetitive stress on already sensitized tissue. The sensitivity of obviously inflamed tissue is striking. A measured amount of stress on inflamed tissue can be shown to yield skin breakdown at low stress levels that would have little effect on noninflammed skin.[17] If the early stages of traumatic inflammation are recognized, further injury may be prevented.

There are objective monitors of heat and swelling to measure inflammation from moderate stress. Thermography (measurement of heat) and volumetry (measurement of swelling by water displacement) were described by Brand[69] and are reviewed later in this chapter. The examiner must remember to look at the tissue. Hyperemia and the length of time hyperemia persists after pressure removal (longer than 15 minutes) are evidence of inflammation from pressure (unless an infective process is present).[17]

High stress

High stress (stress sufficiently high to tear and destroy tissue) can destroy tissue by direct excessive stress in a short

period. This degree of stress results in what is often referred to clinically as traumatic injury. Human skin can resist stresses of 100 Kg/cm² according to Yamada.[79] High stress may be as high as 1000 times the amount of pressure that causes ischemia. High stress can result from an impact against the skin from any object, but the smaller the object or edge of the object, the greater the stress produced. A pin prick is an injury of great stress, because the force is concentrated on the small area at its tip, producing very high stresses sufficient to penetrate the skin.[12]

DIRECTION OF STRESS

The degree of stress, the duration of stress, and the repetition of stress have been mentioned as important in the mechanical damage of skin and soft tissue. A fourth way mechanical force can damage skin and soft tissue is by the direction of stress.

Normal, or direct stress

The most commonly recognized stress of the skin is what is referred to as normal, or direct, stress (perpendicular to the surface). Normal stress approaches the skin surface at right angles and has degrees of magnitude from low to high. Many examiners think primarily of this type of stress when considering force that could result in damage to the skin and soft tissue. This type of stress is often clinically called pressure. Pressure to the skin is the result of the force directly applied.

Shear stress

Studies have shown that the most damaging type of stress to the skin is not normal stress (perpendicular to the surface),

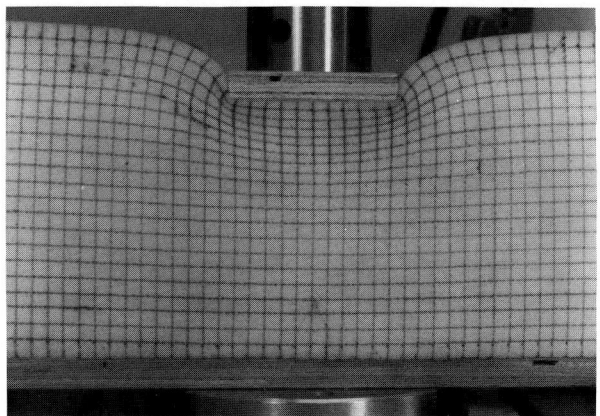

Fig. 9-3 Direction of force. Shear force that is tangential is more damaging than normal force that is direct. As a piston and block compress a foam model, compare the twisting and angulation of squares created at the edge of the block with compressed rectangular "cells" underneath the block. (Photograph by David E. Thompson, Ph.D., Louisiana State University, Baton Rouge.)

but *shear* stress (produced by lateral forces).[17,24,70] This is the stress that occurs where edges of objects, such as splints, come into contact with the skin and have a force component parallel to or tangent to the surface (Fig. 9-3). Shear has a rotational effect on the skin cells and can tear and deform skin cells. Shear stress can cause damage before injury in a normal hand is perceived. An example is the blister that

often occurs in the palm when a screwdriver or other hand tool is used. The twisting of the handle grabs the skin and twists and tears it from other soft tissue. The shearing force separates the outer skin layers, making the blister. Seemingly low shear can be damaging. The skin can absorb relatively high, direct impact but does not so readily accommodate shear stress.

Shear stress is produced near concentrations of high force, such as splint holes or edges, because the force is concentrated in a small area. If a "doughnut" is made to pad a skin area, the skin in the middle of the hole will herniate into the hole, and the skin is injured by the shear stress caused at the inner edge of the hole where the skin angulates around it. The shear effect can be reduced by rounding the edges of the doughnut, thereby increasing the contact area and spreading force over a larger area.

Shear stress occurs as a normal part of everyday use of hands but should be kept to a minimum in splinting by avoiding doughnuts, by rounding splint edges, and, in general, by spreading out contact force over as broad an area as possible. In the treatment of insensitive hands, shear stress from objects can be minimized by padding and enlarging handles and contact areas, such as edges of keys. Sharp objects should be avoided or the skin protected against them; edges of objects should be rounded, particularly splint edges.

Localized pressure and shear from splinting occur when contact force on the skin is concentrated at any small area, such as over a bony prominence or over any area with a small radius. If an elastic bandage is wrapped around the hand, the areas of greatest pressure are at the lateral sides

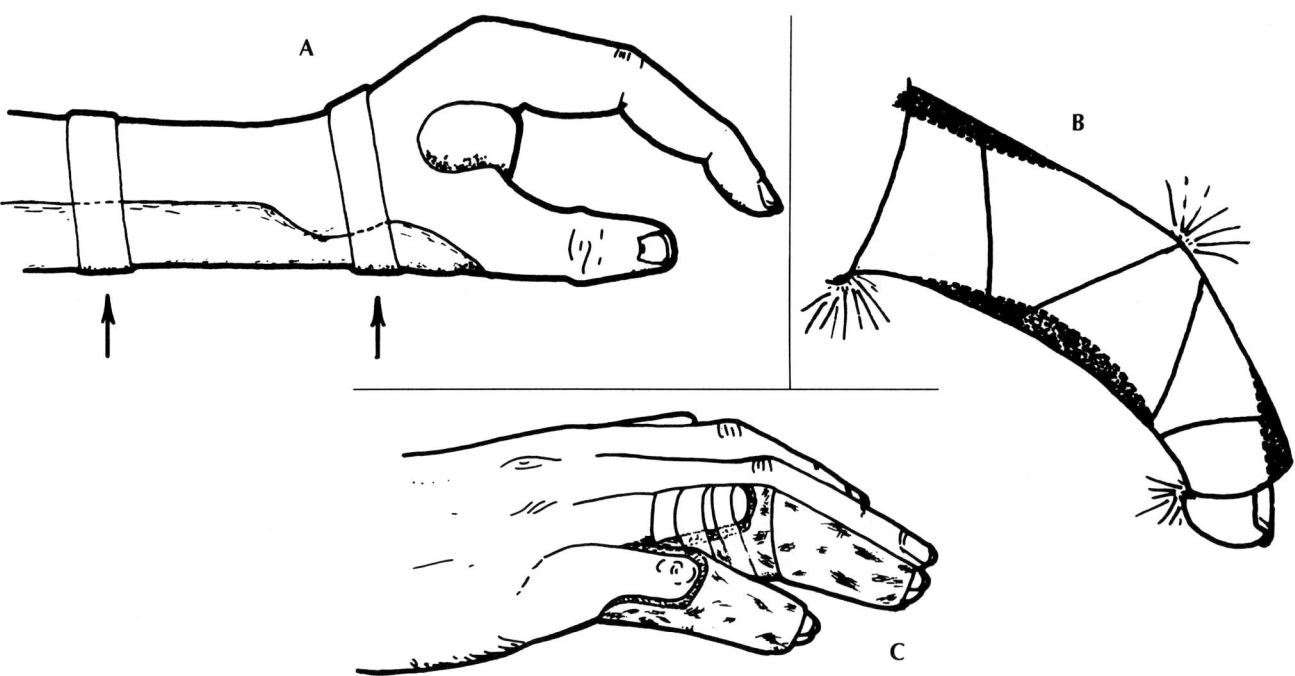

Fig. 9-4 Reduction of shear. Shear stress on hands can be minimized by rounding edges and increasing surface contact areas of objects, and avoiding areas of concentrated force at edges and pressure around small radii such as the sides of fingers, hands, and bony prominences. **A,** Splints should lift straps away from sides of hand and fingers. **B,** Casts should have minimal padding and be changed when loose, so the hand does not move under the cast and receive shear stress. **C,** Windows in casts should be filled in to equalize pressure on skin, or be avoided entirely to eliminate shear at edges.

of the index and little fingers and over the dorsum of joints such as the metacarpophalangeal (MP) joints where the tendons are prominent. These areas are curved and have a small radius, and pressure is concentrated at their most prominent point (Fig. 9-4). Damage from direct pressure is likely, but is even more likely if movement occurs under the straps, casts, or splints and increases shear.

Every therapist knows the problems that arise when he or she tries to position a splint strap over a bony prominence. Splint straps also can cause localized pressure as they course around fingers and the hand. This makes it necessary to design a splint that lifts the straps away from the sides of the hand and fingers (Fig. 9-4, *A*). The hand then is anchored by more direct and anterior/posterior pressure over a broader area of the hand than that of the side of the fingers and hand.

A frequent mistake in splinting is padding over an area of localized concentrated pressure, such as an area of abrasion from a cast. This often results in increased concentration of the pressure rather than the intended relief of pressure. Usually the splint needs to be relieved (readjusted to fit) rather than padded.

MECHANICS OF SKIN AND SOFT TISSUE

The skin and associated soft tissue have inherent physical properties that make them ideal coverings for the intricate mechanics of the skeletal system. The skin absorbs impact, cushions and molds around objects, and expands to meet the limits of joint range of motion, returning to its normal resting position. Engineers call these characteristics plastic (degree of moldability) and viscoelastic properties (degree

of viscosity and elasticity).[8,71,75] The skin's plastic characteristic allows it to mold and reshape to various surfaces. Both the plastic and viscoelastic properties of the skin enable it to resist breaking down under stress in normal situations.

Engineers have measured the viscoelastic properties of skin in experimental studies. Strength-testing of skin reveals much about its characteristics. When a tensile elongation or compression load is applied to the skin, there is at first a gradual increase of stress in the skin. Within a range, the skin has a capacity for elastic deformation (can be elongated or compressed and then return to normal resting length without injury or deformity when the elongation or compression load is discontinued). With increasing load, stress in the skin increases. At a certain point, stress in the skin begins to occur rapidly (as it begins to approach the limits of its accommodation), and if the load is continued, the skin becomes tense and begins to break down. Beyond a certain point, the skin will fatigue (break down) and may undergo plastic deformation, or creep (is permanently deformed and loses its ability to return to normal resting length). If load is further increased, the skin will eventually rupture.

The stress versus strain (change in length) that occurs as the skin is subjected to increasing load is plotted on a curve called a stress/strain curve (Fig. 9-5). (Stress in this case refers to the amount of load force/unit area applied to the skin.) The slope of the curve is important to engineers in analysis of the viscoelastic properties of the tissue and is referred to as the "elastic modulus." Analysis of the elastic modulus of various tissues tells how different tissues respond to elongation or compression. The elastic modulus of bone or tendon is very high (steeper) when compared

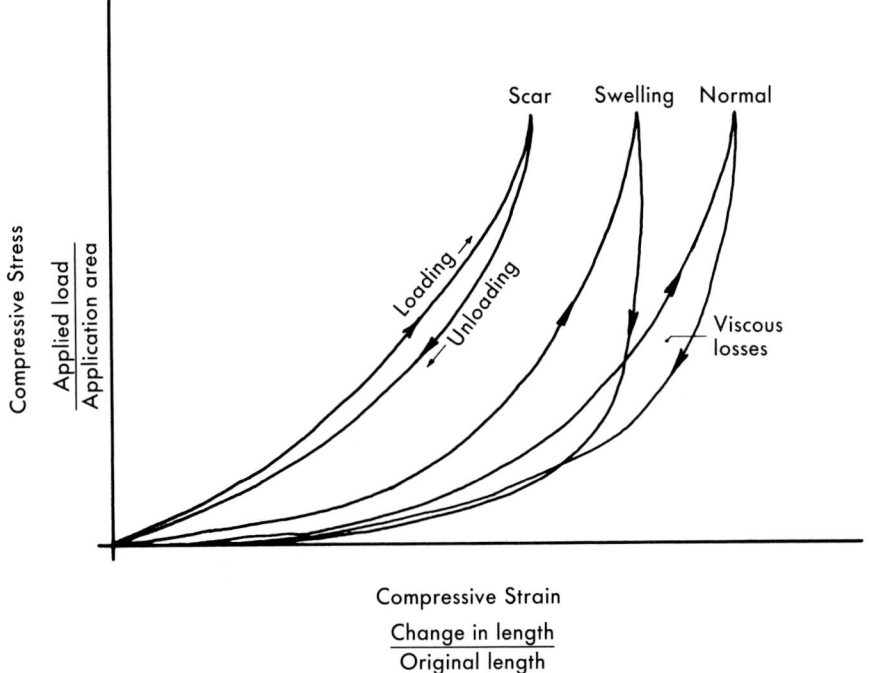

Fig. 9-5   Normal tissue is pliable and has viscous and elastic components. Minimal force results in significant strain until the skin's elastic limit is reached. Scar tissue, in comparison, builds stress rapidly, producing increasing strain and a steeper curve. Swelling increases the viscous content of tissue, producing a steeper stress/strain curve and a greater distance between loading and unloading curves than does normal tissue. (Researched by William Buford, BME, Ph.D., Chief, Rehabilitation Research Dept. Gillis W. Long Hansen's Disease Center; and David E. Thompson, Ph.D., Professor of Mechanical Engineering, Louisiana State University, Baton Rouge.)

with that of skin, which is much more elastic and the testing of which results in a curve that is lower and more relaxed. All tissues have their own elastic modulus relative to the degree of their viscoelasticity (as do orthotic and other materials—even steel). Yamada published excellent information regarding the relative elasticity of various tissues from measurement of every tissue in the body of a lion.[79]

MECHANICAL CHANGES IN SOFT TISSUE WITH SCAR

The ability of the skin to serve as a cushion for deeper structures and to elongate and contract for joint range of motion is changed dramatically with the introduction of scar tissue. Scar tissue does not react like normal tissue, and the more it develops in tissue, the more the tissue changes in its normal inherent plastic and viscoelastic properties. Scar tissue is more rigid and less elastic in comparison with normal healthy tissue and results in areas of high stress concentration in the skin.[70] Scarred tissue is more vulnerable to injury from areas of stress concentration and reduced compliance.

The relative inelasticity of scar tissue can be understood on a stress/strain curve as compared with normal tissue (Fig. 9-5). The resulting curve is a steeper slope (higher modulus of elasticity) compared with normal, healthy tissue, which has a lower elastic modulus. Scar limits joint range of motion by reduced capacity for excursion of skin with load from force of muscles and excursion of tendons.

MECHANICAL CHANGES IN SOFT TISSUE WITH EDEMA

Normal soft tissue that is plastic (flexible and compliant) and elastic undergoes mechanical changes with the increased viscous fluid volume that accompanies swollen tissue. These changes are directly related to the amount of fluid volume in the tissues and can be reduced or eliminated in direct relationship to a corresponding reduction in the fluid volume. Permanent deformity of the tissue or tissue remodeling does not occur unless swelling is prolonged or excessive.

Swollen skin, joints, and tendons have an increase in friction relative to their amount of increased fluid. More resistance to movement is present in tissue that is swollen. The faster fluid is moved, the more resistance there is to movement. (Healthy joints and tendons have minimal friction.)

Intercellular swelling (intercellular increase in fluid volume) can change the apparent elastic modulus of the skin and soft tissue by the increased tension in the tissue; thus it has the effect of making tissue more impacted and rigid. Edema serves as a cushion (as if cells were balloons) of passive material (collection of water and electrolytes) that requires energy to move. Edema limits longitudinal movement of collagen fibers by their reorientation in a transverse direction.[17] Swollen tissue, then, in addition to increased viscosity is limited in its ability to be elongated, compressed, or compliant. This is why a hand will never have a normal range of motion as long as there is edema in the tissue in and under the skin.

INTERFACE OF SOFT TISSUE WITH MATERIALS

Just as an understanding of the mechanical properties of skin is important for safe and efficient treatment, knowledge of the mechanical properties of materials that are used on the skin is also important. Materials used for splinting also have degrees of plasticity and viscoelastic properties.[74]

Mechanical properties of materials

Although at first seemingly unimportant to the surgeon or therapist, knowledge of materials' properties can be an advantage in patient treatment. Certain materials are rigid and nonconforming in comparison with other materials. If we understand the stresses that can injure skin and other soft tissue, our splints and casts can be made to minimize tissue stress. For instance, in engineering tests of commonly used splinting materials in our laboratory, it was found that Spenco elastic (cloth-covered microcellular rubber) most nearly simulated the elastic quality of normal human skin but lacked the moldability of skin.* This material has been used with success for shoe insoles and may be adaptable to the interface between skin and hard, rigid materials used in hand splinting, to reduce shear stress on the skin.

Soft splints, which have semirigidity but some pliability, may be more common in the future as we fully understand the desirable properties of such materials. Splints must be supportive along certain planes of movement but flexible in others. Soft splints have become imperative in sports medicine because of the physical contact nature of games and potential injury to others from rigid splints. Other applications include the treatment of children and patients with insensitivity who are much more vulnerable to injury. Materials for soft splints include Aliplast, Plastazote, and Spenco elastic.* These materials can be combined and laminated to each other to provide more intimate tissue contact and cushioning.

Mechanics of pressure under bandages

Bandages create varying amounts of pressure on the skin and underlying tissue, depending on how they are applied. It is easy to appreciate that bandages are wrapped in a figure-of-eight fashion if possible, rather than in a circular manner, to avoid areas of tissue constriction. If a circular wrap is used, pressure can be uneven, because one point of the wrap may be two layers thick and another point one or three.

The amount of pressure from bandaging is not easily appreciated. A nonexpandable bandage material (material not cut on a bias or with little if any elasticity) will apply more pressure than a bias-cut material or elastic material. Usually a bias-cut or elastic material is preferred for use on the hand to permit some expansion if swelling occurs. Some hand treatment centers order large rolls of bias-cut stockinette and trim it to desired strips for bandages.

Elastic bandages can cause excessive amounts of pressure, both at specific sites as described and over large areas, thereby causing vascular and lymphatic constriction. They should be used with careful consideration of the amount of pressure intended. With the second wrap of an elastic bandage, the pressure under the bandage is doubled. With the third wrap, the pressure is tripled, and so on (every layer carries with it the pressure from the elastic).[7] This is true even when the bandage is wrapped in a figure-of-eight fashion, although the crossed wrapping helps distribute the pressure evenly and it is less likely to be constrictive and allows

---

*Alimed, Inc., Dedham, Mass.

some room for tissue expansion with swelling as individual layers slide over each other.

Movement of the hand in the bandage can further concentrate pressure, particularly over prominent areas. The circumference of a wrist, for instance, is greater when the wrist is in extension rather than in neutral, and pressure around the wrist will be greater when the wrist is in extension if the bandage has been wrapped with the wrist in neutral. Pressure can be enough to damage the dorsum of the wrist if bending creates folds of material, which further concentrate the stresses.

Coban* self-adhesive, disposable elastic bandages have the potential to create more internal tissue pressure with swelling and on bending at joints than regular elastic bandage and should be used with caution. The individual layers of the Coban material stick together, resulting in higher surface skin pressure if the underlying tissue expands while the material layers do not expand because they are adhering.

Mechanics of pressure under cuffs

When a patient who has sensibility complains about a splint or will not wear a splint, it is often related to low-level ischemia that is ocurring. Actual pressure necrosis from splinting is likely only in patients with insensitive hands. Patients with sensitivity will remove cuffs (slings) if they become too uncomfortable.

The force that is necessary to gradually reduce a joint contracture is a slow, steady tension. This often results in too much pressure on the skin from the traction cuff. Because the skin is the limiting factor in most cases (tendon and bone can withstand more torque), larger amounts of traction torque may be tolerated by the patient if ways are found to reduce the pressure on the skin. Cuff materials and mechanics then, are very important.[18]

A traction cuff made of very flexible material will bend so much that it causes high shear at the sides of the finger and will conform so closely that it causes vascular compromise throughout its contact arc. A firm cuff may tilt through other than perpendicular angles (90 degrees) of traction and cause high shear stress at its edge. If the line of rubber-band traction is angulated and the cuff is thereby tilted, the edge pressure of the cuff can more than triple.

Most therapists choose materials between the extremes

---

*Minnesota Mining and Manufacturing Company (3M), North Coast Medical Inc., Campbell, Calif.

of too much flexibility and too much rigidity but do not alwas know why. Leather makes a good material for a traction cuff, because it simulates normal skin somewhat and can be flexble while being firm enough to reduce shear at the sides and edges of the contact arc. The loop of the cuff should not be too shallow, because this increases the contact area of shear stress at the sides of the finger. A loop length extending at least 2 to 2.5 cm beyond the finger is desirable.

The width of the cuff is also important, because thin cuffs will increase skin pressure by their limited contact area, thereby causing shear at edges. Generally the cuff should be as wide as is possible to distribute pressure over as wide an area as possible without causing shear as the fingers move. Cuffs should be no less than 1 cm wide and preferably larger.

Brand suggests a way for safe use of rigid cuffs that will spread pressure over larger areas without causing edge shear.[17] He suggests using a small plaster shell (two to three layers) molded around the finger. Once this cuff is firm, a loop of thread can be added to the center back of the cuff. The thread loop is used for rubber-band or spring traction (Fig. 9-6). If the angle of traction pull on the thread is changed, there is no tilting of the total contact cuff, because the force is stabilized by applying it at the back of the cuff. There is limited shear at the finger edges, because the firm cuff does not tilt. The cuff serves to lift the thread away from the lateral sides of the finger where it otherwise could cause high shear.

The approximate pressure of cuffs can be measured in terms of the pressure they produce on the skin. The force of a spring or rubber band can be measured and also the area of cuff contact. Pressure is simply force divided by unit area of contact.

It has been suggested that as a rule, traction force on the skin by typical traction cuffs should not exceed 300 g.[46] (For more description on measurement of pressure under cuffs, see discussion of rubber-band traction measurement.) A 300 g traction force for a semirigid leather cuff, that is 2 cm wide and contacts the skin for 2 cm length, thus provides a 4 cm² contact area, which would not exceed 75 g/cm² (or 0.025 psi, 13 mm Hg.).

$$300 \text{ divided by } 4 \text{ cm}^2 = 75 \text{ g/cm}^2$$

This is a guideline for an estimate of traction. Were the same cuff only 1.5 cm wide, pressure on the skin would be higher, so the traction force might need to be reduced to accommodate the thinner cuff.

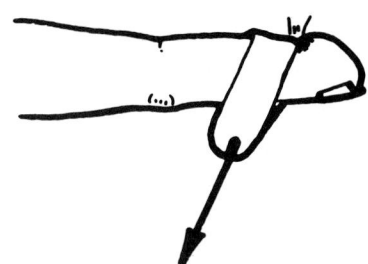 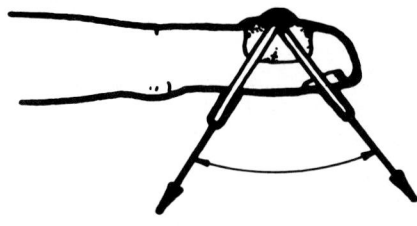

Fig. 9-6 Traditional cuff versus Brand cuff. Traditional cuffs can tilt and angulate as the hand moves in the splint, causing shear at the edge of the cuff. Brand has suggested a plaster molded cuff fitted directly on the finger, the back of which has an attachment in midposition for a traction thread of string or elastic. This cuff tilts with the finger when it moves. Pressure is disbursed throughout the cuff area rather than being concentrated at any one point or edge.

$$300 \text{ divided by } 3 \text{ cm}^2 = 100 \text{ g/cm}^2$$

The condition of the skin must be considered and checked for areas of sustained redness after periods of traction. A period of hyperemia follows ischemia when capillary flow returns. This is why it is important to visually check the tissue's response to traction to adjust the splint to skin tolerance. It is safer to underestimate beginning traction force and to increase it slowly over a few days than to overestimate and to need to reduce the force because of the skin sensitivity induced by inflammation (see discussion that follows).

MEASUREMENT OF FORCE/PRESSURE ON SKIN
Pressure transducers

Measurement of pressure under materials can be assessed by small pressure transducers attached to a recording device (Fig. 9-7). These transducers are not without their problems. Used with their limitations in mind, they can be helpful in determining relative amounts of pressure. Basically, the commercially available transducers were designed to function in fluid mediums where pressure on them is evenly distributed. Taken out of a fluid medium, they are subject to variability depending on where the pressure is on their surface. The transducer force readings also can differ as the rigidity of the material differs. For repeat measurements, they should be used under the same conditions and in the same position.[41]

Another measurement problem with pressure transducers is their thickness. To measure pressures on skin, transducers need to be as thin as possible to avoid creating pressure problems on their own. To measure pressure under materials, they also need to be as thin as possible or incorporated as a part of the material tested.

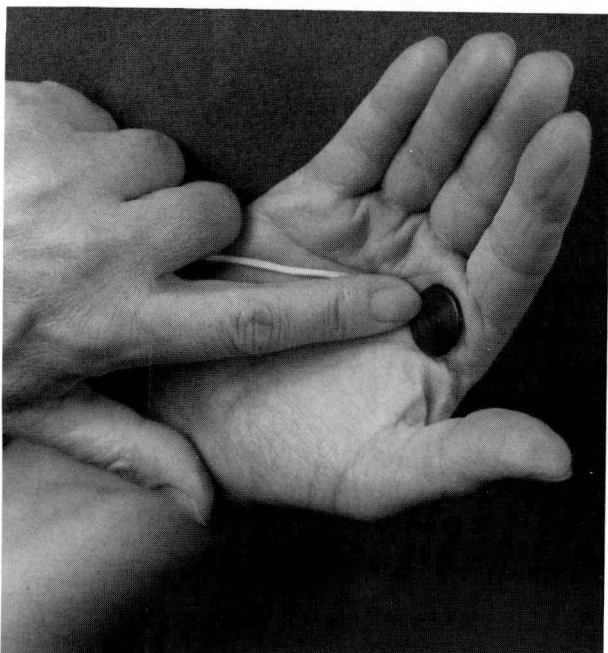

Fig. 9-7 Hercules pressure transducer. Pressure transducers, within some limitations, can be used experimentally to measure pressure distribution on the hand during use, that is, pressure on the hand from splints.

In our laboratory, such transducers have been used experimentally to study a number of contact pressure problems related to the hand and foot. Transducers have been attached to the fingertips of gloves or other hand areas to determine pressure at the fingertips while gripping before and after surgery, to measure pressure under a splint, or to measure the relative pressure of various contact areas. They would be useful in routine clinical measurements for determining the amount of pressure a patient uses on tools, if currently available transducers were not so fragile and expensive. If used more often where mass-production would be economically feasible, durable but sensitive transducers might be made available at acceptable lower costs.

The FILPIP (Franklin Institute Laboratory Pressure Indicating Patch) was used for our early studies. Unfortunately, this is no longer produced. Another that has similarly been useful in skin pressure studies is the Hercules model.* Smaller models would be helpful if as accurate.

Pressure-sensitive microcapsule gloves

Gloves impregnated with pressure-sensitive capsules have been used in our laboratory to demonstrate relative differences in pressure when a hand is used.[19] This technique was first used for determining localized pressures on insensitive feet in shoes. The technique of pressure determination has also been helpful in demonstrating high localized pressure on the hand, such as from an instrument or tool a patient uses. The small dye capsules burst at high compressive or shear pressures and are used to line the inner surface of gloves. Stress between the hand and glove results in a release of dye of different amounts. It takes time to prepare gloves and other materials, but the technique lends well to photographic record (Fig. 9-8).

Gloves are made of open-cell polyurethane foam with a cotton liase outer cover impregnated with dye-filled microcapsules. Staining of the glove occurs as the weakly acidic bromophenol solution contacts the alkaline powder (used as an activator) that is dusted over the inner surface of the glove. Unbroken capsules remain yellow. A few broken capsules stains light blue, and complete breakage stains dark blue. This differential staining provides an "objective index of the location and distribution of stress."[20,21] A quantitative assessment of magnitude of stress is not possible. "The microcapsules are broken by a single application of a large force—60 pounds per square inch (psi)—or by repetition of smaller forces—20 to 30 psi."[66]

The microcapsules and powder must be stored in separate sealed-lid glass containers (prolonged humidity can ruin the material). Thin, uncut polyurethane material† can be obtained in rolls to make the gloves. Gloves can be prepared in advance and sprinkled with microcapsules at the time of study.

Harris mat grid

A rubber-mat grid first used to measure pressure distribution on the feet has been adapted to determine pressure distribution of the hand.[56] The mat contains a grid with

---

*Hercules model F4-4R Orthoflex Pressure Transducers, Hercules, Inc, Aerospace Products Group, Allegany Ballistics, Cumberland, Md.

†Polyester Foam—white, Curon 508D, Reeves Brothers, Curon division, Cornelius, NC.

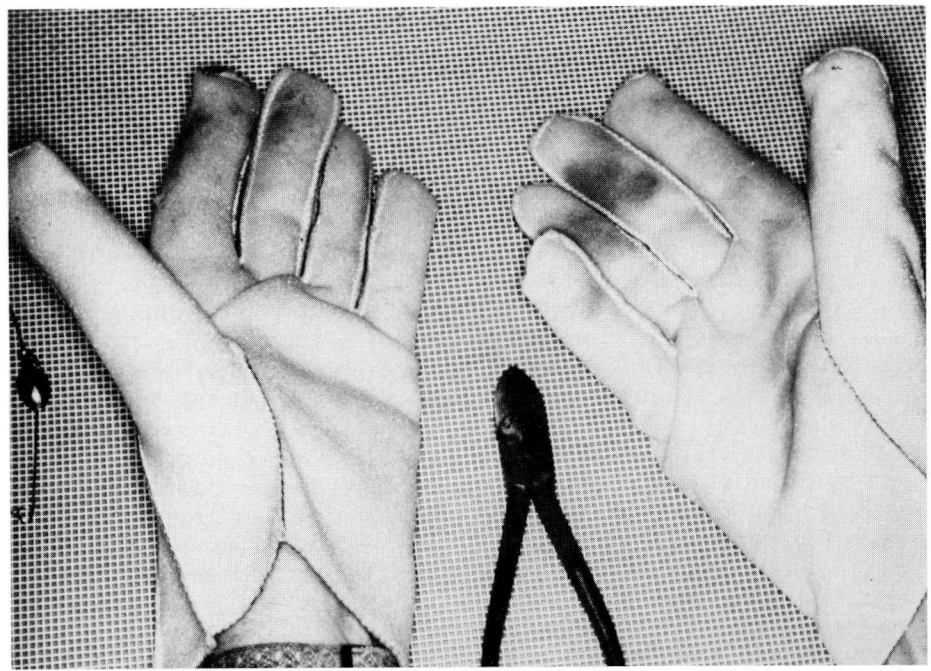

Fig. 9-8 Pressure-sensitive microcapsule gloves. Note staining in the area of high pressure where the tool was used in the hand.

squares of various sizes and heights. The more direct pressure exerted against the pad, the more the details of the grid will show in the final paper print record. The use of the mat has been beneficial in demonstrating contact areas of cylinder grip.[59] It is not considered helpful in defining regions of high shear force.

The mat is trimmed and glued with contact cement to a 1-, 2-, or 3-inch cylinder (wood or other material). The pad is inked with black printer's ink. The surface of the mat cylinder is rubbed lightly with cotton to distribute the ink evenly. A piece of paper cut to the size of the cylinder is carefully wrapped around the cylinder. The patient then grasps the clinder firmly. With a felt pen, the examiner outlines the patient's fingers. The paper is carefully removed from the cylinder and laid flat (Fig. 9-9).

In treatment of patients with insensitive hands, the mat is helpful in identifying and demonstrating contact areas. Forces on the fingertips are increased by patient compensation for disturbed sensory feedback. Patients with intrinsic muscle weakness will demonstrate increased force concentration on the fingertips rather than the more normal even pressure distribution over the contact area. These concentrations of force can result in direct and indirect tissue damage. Repeat mat stains after tendon rebalancing procedures will demonstrate increased finger and palm contact areas and a more uniform pressure distribution.

Cylinder contact

An alternate way to assess contact areas on a cylinder is simply to number the phalanges that come into contact with a 1-, 2-, or 3-inch cylinder. This is done before and after surgery or other treatment to show changes in contact areas after tendon rebalancing or casting for contractures. The cylinders can be weighted if desired to assess grip contact

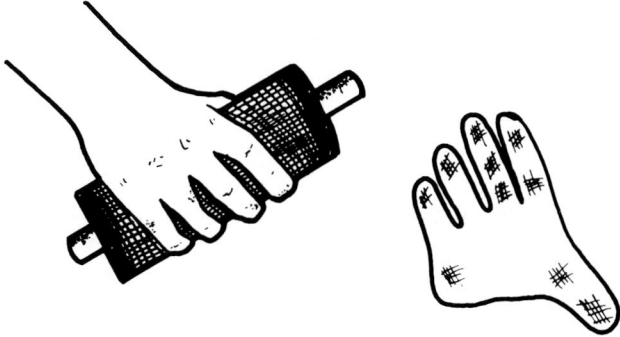

Fig. 9-9 Harris mat grid. A cylinder grid with squares of various sizes and heights can be used to determine areas of pressure distribution of the hand on the grip. The more direct pressure is exerted against the pad, the more details of the grid will show.

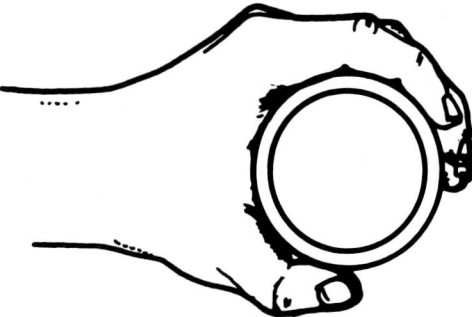

Fig. 9-10 Cylinder contact. Counting the number of phalanges that come into contact on cylinders of different sizes can help quantify pressure concentration on fingers and, therefore, quantify changes in contact grip area when surgical tendon transfer rebalancing has been performed.

at progressive weights by attaching lead weights to the bottom of the cylinders. Weighted cylinders are particularly helpful in loading finger grasp and pinch in hands with muscle imbalances where a light pinch or grasp may appear normal, yet when the fingers are loaded with a weight, the fingers collapse (Fig. 9-10).

REMODELING AND REGROWTH OF SOFT TISSUE

One must have an understanding of the remodeling and regrowth capacity of soft tissue to fully understand what is happening in the skin in response to traction and methods that attempt to increase joint range of motion. The skin and other soft tissue is alive and reacts biologically to demands placed on it.

Brand described the mechanics of the remodeling of soft tissue.[11] He explained that the body seeks a homeostatic balance of tension in the skin and muscles. The skin will change to adjust to the tension that is required of it. Just as the skin can lose length, as in a contracture, and be remodeled, it can increase in length by growing new cells. This is a gradual change and is not one that occurs by stretching. (Stretching can result in creep and permanent deformity of tissue.) Remodeling occurs from a low, gentle, constant tension (not enough tension to cause deformation or to rupture skin cells). The slightly increased tension over normal resting tension serves as a cue to the cells that more length is required. The physiologic response is to grow new cells, thereby restoring normal resting tension.

It is the skin's viscoelastic properties that give it the ability to elongate and retract. When "stretch" results in the rupture of cellular material, this cellular rupture causes the release of protein material, which will create scar. Scar tissue creates major changes in the viscoelastic properties of the skin. Therapists' attempts to treat contractures, then, should include minimal stretching of skin and soft tissue—only a gentle elongation within the skin's elastic limit. Therapists learn to work within the skin's elastic limit when doing massage and mobilization techniques.

What is necessary to make skin remodel and grow is not often understood. Many therapists are taught that they must do stretching exercises or hold tissue under moderate or high stress to remodel. What is not realized is that actual stretching of the skin is often harmful and results in more scar in the tissue.

Massage and range of motion used together are often enough to restore skin mobility if minimal changes have occurred, but these alone are usually not enough to make the skin remodel. When skin is elongated to its elastic limit, it will have a low tension increase. It will return to its original position unless it has been stretched beyond its elastic limit and has become deformed. This is always true. Skin can be elongated only so far. But if the skin is held at the end of its elastic limit for 1 or 2 days, the initial tension created by the elongation will diminish. What is critical to understand is that as the skin grows, new cells grow to accommodate the increased load and the tension slowly drops to its original resting tension. A new elastic limit has been created! The skin may then be elongated again. Gradual remodeling of the skin occurs as this process is repeated again and again through such techniques as serial cylinder casting for improved joint range of motion or application of pressure garments for scar remodeling.

Important to realize is that remodeling cannot occur in an hour's treatment session or even in several hours. It takes time for skin to grow, just as it takes time for the skin to become contracted and lose tissue cells initially. Thus a therapist cannot cause a contracture to regrow by stretch in one treatment session.

For optimal regrowth to occur, the applied tension must be continuous or almost continuous. Any interruption of tension will slow the process. If dynamic traction is used, care must be taken to assure the tension is uniform and continuous for a 24-hour period. Exercise between treatment or cast changes is recommended to keep the skin pliable and to maintain gliding surfaces, but time of reduced tension should be kept minimal. Skin that has contracted tends to return toward contracture very quickly. (When interphalangeal (IP) flexion contractures are casted, removal of a cast for longer than 30 minutes will sometimes prevent a finger from slipping back into the same cast.) This tendency for the contracture to recur continues while the remodeling process continues and even beyond for a period. Retainer splints (for the same reason they are necessary in dentistry) are sometimes necessary until the tendency for recurrence of the contracture is lost.

Use of a normal hand through a full range of motion is enough to keep the skin and other soft tissue structures healthy and pliable.[50,51,60,66] Joint contractures particularly are likely in the small joints of the fingers when the joints are no longer functioning in their full range of motion. Forces acting on the skin and other soft tissue structures are changed. Skin and other soft tissue contract (remodel and lose tissue cells) when they are not required to assume their normal range of motion; even ligaments and blood vessels contract.

In joints with flexion contractures, the skin over the dorsum of the joints will grow and become redundant because of the sustained increased elongation tension on the skin. On the volar surface, skin is reabsorbed because of the sustained decreased tension for elongation. This change in the skin occurs regardless of the initial cause of the contracture. Even a contracture develops because of joint remodeling. The result of changes in the forces acting on the skin and soft tissue is remodeling (either contracture or regrowth) (Fig. 9-11).

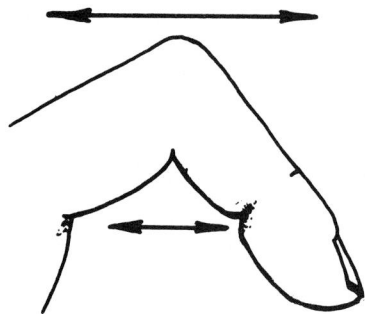

Fig. 9-11 Remodeling of skin tissue with contracture. Whatever the initiating cause of joint contracture, without specific treatment the result will be an increase of skin tissue on the surface where skin stress is increased and a loss of skin tissue where skin stress is lessened. Cylinder casting and other splinting attempt to reverse this process and remold the skin and other soft tissue away from the contracture.

With the technique of serial casting for contracted joints, changes in forces acting on the skin are reversed by casting.[10,58] The unwanted change in force is reversed in the opposite direction. Thus in a casted flexion contracture, increased skin elongation tension is created on the volar surface, and elongation tension is relaxed on the dorsal surface. The cast is usually changed every other day or twice a week if time for return visits is a problem. For quickest results, every other day is recommended. The cast must be changed at least once a week. (See Chapter 91.)

MOVEMENT, STRESS, AND WOUNDS
Effect of movement on wounds

Much has been written about the way wounds heal, but relatively little has been written about the effect of mechanical stress on wound healing. The effect of movement can be detrimental to wound healing because of the stress placed on fragile new tissue. Progressive mobilization of injured tissue and careful assessment of tissue response are indicated whether the wound has been traumatic or controlled, such as in elective surgery. In many cases, a cast or splint should not just be removed and the hand returned to function, but instead, immobilization restraints should be "weaned away" as the hand becomes more mobilized. The tissue response to mobilization can be evaluated by volume and temperature measurements described in this chapter.

Infections need immobilization

Mechanical stress can be even more damaging to healing tissue if infection is present. When tendons and joints move through their normal range of motion, blood and other tissue fluids are forced into motion. It is generally recognized that with movement, some infections will migrate to other sites in the hand through communicating pathways. But in general, the effect of movement on infected tissue, particularly impacted tissue, is to drive the infection deeper into other tissue 'areas, thereby increasing the area of infection and delaying healing.

The adverse effect of movement on wound healing is seen most dramatically in patients with insensitive limbs. In these patients, the normal mechanism by which the injured hand is functionally splinted and protected by pain is lost. Because of the unrestrained mechanical stress placed on the healing tissue, patients with insensitive hands have wounds that, even when routinely treated with antibiotics, do not easily improve. It is not uncommon to see infections extending into the axillae in many untreated patients. When the same hands are immobilized in functional positions, erythema quickly subsides, and the wounds become localized in small areas of primary infection.

Movement of infected tissue in any hand can cause further tissue damage. Often it is better to completely immobilize the infected part (one joint higher than the infection) for a few days and then allow gentle range of motion to maintain tendon and joint planes of movement than it is to daily move an infected hand enough to maintain normal or partial range of motion. The result of moving the infected hand in the initial stages of infection may be to extend the course of treatment of the hand, which could have been casted a few days and then moved without danger of further tissue damage.

Measurement of wound circumference

The circumference of a wound decreases as the wound scar contracts. The edges of the wound can be recorded relative to the amount and range of contraction by tracing the wound on plastic sheets, such as expired x-ray film. Serial tracings can be used for photographs and records.

TRACTION, DYNAMIC ASSISTS, AND RELATED MEASUREMENTS

"Dynamic assists are the fuel or power for mobilization splints," but tissue damage and ineffective treatment may occur with incorrect traction.[46] Too much force, torque, or pressure may cause additional inflammation, scarring, and deformity of skin. Too little force may prevent the patient from reaching full rehabilitative potential from treatment.

Rubber bands

Mechanical properties of rubber bands. Rubber bands, like soft tissue and other splinting materials, have viscoelastic properties. The elastic restraint component is the

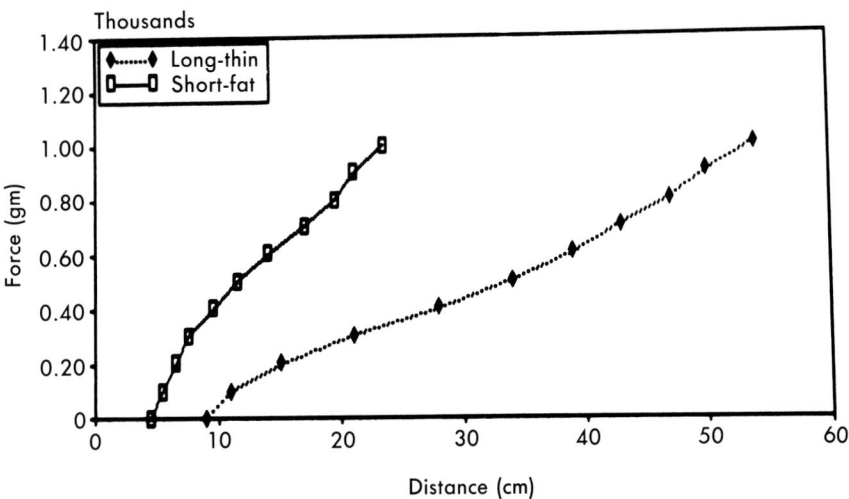

Fig. 9-12   Stress/strain curve of rubber bands. Each rubber band of a different length and width will have its own stress/strain curve, which can be measured. Short, fat bands produce high force with limited elongation, compared with the long, thin bands.

tension we see in the rubber band. The tension of rubber bands is determined by their length and thickness. Short, thick bands produce high forces, and long, thin bands produce relatively low forces.

There is a relationship between the elongation and tension of a given rubber band. When there is a change in length of the rubber band, there is a relative change in the tension it produces. A graph of this tension versus elongation is called a length/tension curve, and each band of a different length and width will have its own tension-producing capacity (Fig. 9-12). Excursion of the bands is important, because limited excursion will limit joint range of motion. Short bands in general produce a large amount of tension with a limited excursion. For this reason, long bands are usually desirable for traction. Our length/tension measurements indicate longer bands that are not too thick (1 to 3 mm) and have a more desirable length/tension ratio for traction splinting.[32]

Another physical property of rubber bands is their hysteresis. Hysteresis is the change that occurs in the bands with loading and unloading. The tension (elastic restraint component) during loading (stretching) is more than the tension that occurs during unloading. This adds to the indeterminant force production of the stretched rubber band at any given length of the band. The hysteresis is variable, depending on the size, material, and age of the band. There is less control over actual applied force. New bands are less affected by hysteresis. Bands should be replaced often and old ones discarded, because they fatigue easily.

While Fess found that a given size and quality of rubber band can have a fairly predictable force spectrum, rubber bands tested by Buford in our laboratory were found to demonstrate as much as 200 g of tension difference between bands of the same batch.[32,43] Variations in the size of bands in the same batch accounted for much of the variation in force. Rubber bands tested were size 33, which is a commonly used rubber-band size for splinting. For consistent

traction then, it is important to pick bands of the same relative size and tension even within a given batch. Mildenberger and others published a valuable systematic approach to selection of rubber-band traction.[62]

Fess tested selection of rubber-band tension chosen by experienced and inexperienced therapists.[46] Therapists with experience in dynamic splinting were much more likely to select bands of appropriate length and tension than inexperienced therapists and students. Most often, if there was a mistake made in choice, it was toward selecting bands of too much tension rather than too little. Inexperienced therapists may be well advised to use bands of less tension at first and to check band tension and skin tolerance frequently.

Force measurement of rubber bands. Rubber-band force should be measured directly on the splint. This can be done as the splint is fitted. For finger traction, Brand recommends starting with a force from 100 to 300 g. There is no way to guess the force: it must be measured. If the cuff is wider, more force might be possible. If thinner, less is necessary. It is emphasized that there is no such thing as a "safe" amount of force against the skin. The tissue needs to be examined for areas of sustained redness an hour after traction has been applied and again the next day. As with any force on the skin, the mechanical properties of the skin and the quality of the skin will make the end determination of the amount of rubber-band force that can be used.

The static force exerted by rubber bands while on a splint can be determined by measuring the length of the band while on the splint, then removing the cuff and recreating the same length by pulling the cuff with the measurement arm of the Haldex gauge* and reading the resultant force.[34] The distance of the rubber band is measured with a ruler from its attachment point on the splint to its attacment point on the traction cuff. The cuff is removed from the finger. The

---

*Be OK Sammons, Inc, Bessell Healthcare Co, Brookfield, Ill.

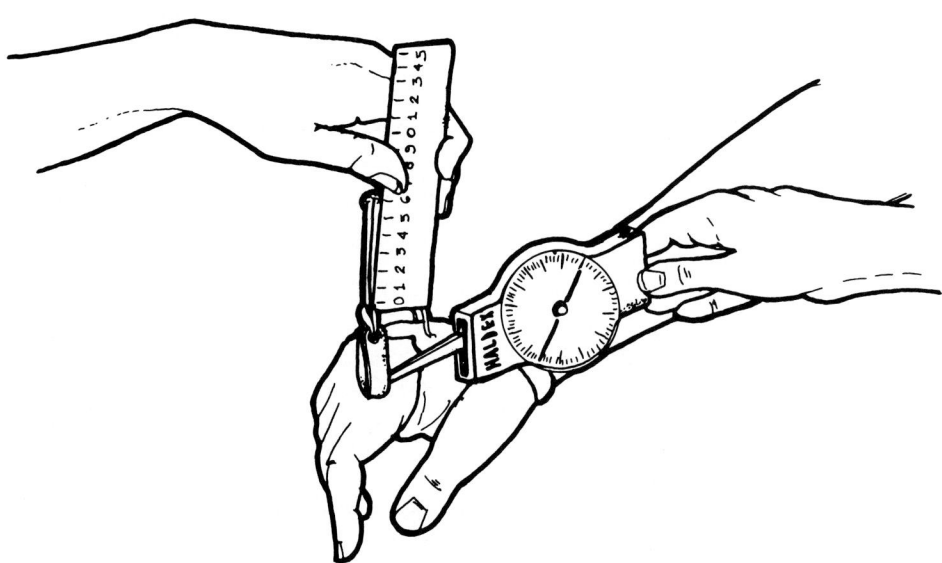

Fig. 9-13 Measurement of rubber-band traction force. Rubber band traction force must be measured on the splint in the same position that will be used for traction. (From Buford WL: Clinical evaluation of orthotic devices. Proc. 13th Ann Meeting US Public Health Service, Commissioned Officer's Association, Atlanta, March 1978.)

tip of the Haldex orthotic gauge arm is inserted into a mid-position on the cuff, and the rubber band/cuff unit is then extended in the same direction it was on the finger. The band is pulled by the gauge arm to the same length it was when the cuff was on the finger, reproducing in this way the same band tension to be measured. The resultant measurement force is read on the gauge while the band continues to be extended. Other measurements of rubber-band force can be made, but in determining tension of the rubber bands for static traction in an individualized splint, this is the most useful measurement of force (Fig. 9-13).

Similarly, the maximum force that will be exerted on the fingers at extremes of range of motion can be calculated. This measurement will provide the maximum force exerted when the patient fully extends or flexes the splinted joint or finger. The amount of safe force will vary according to amount of wearing time and other variables described. The bands should be measured at the longest length at which they will exert pressure against the skin. Higher forces may be acceptable at extremes of joint motion (full flexion or full extension) if intermittent and do not cause damage from repetitive stress.

For force comparison among bands, weights can be hung from ends of bands hung from a post. One might use a 300 g weight and measure the resultant elongation (length) of the bands. Once bands used on a splint are selected and measured, replacement bands of the same tension can be identified by the length they hang with the weight as compared with the selected band. This process can be used in the clinic to have replacement bands of the same tension ready (Fig. 9-14).

Springs

Mechanical properties of springs. Quantification of traction force in dynamic splinting has been advocated by

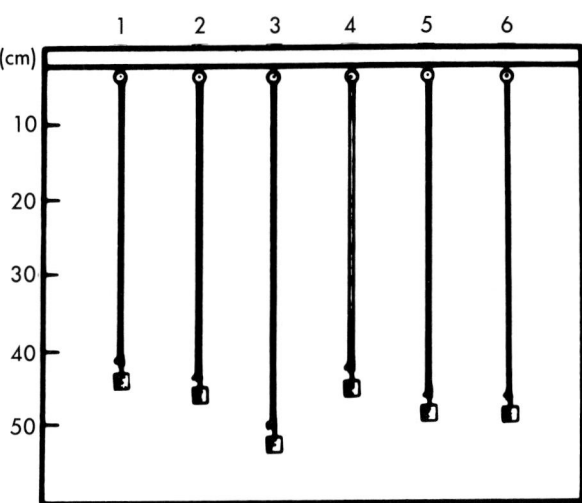

Fig. 9-14 Measurement of rubber-band batches for desired tension producing capacity. Weights (e.g., 100 g) can be attached to rubber bands, and the bands then hung on a measuring board to determine their relative tension-producing capacity. Once a particular band has been selected, similar bands can be identified quickly (a similar band will produce the same length on the board when attached to an equal weight).

Brand, Fess, and Malick.[63] There is a new and growing interest in the use of springs for traction and dynamic assists.[30] Springs are more durable, their shelf life is excellent, and they provide a consistent and controlled force. In contrast, the elastic properties of rubber bands can change rapidly. They exhibit variability, lack of durability, and are fatigue- and technique-dependent. The use of graded springs may be an improvement over rubber bands.

Force measurement of springs. A wide range of spring forces suitable for splinting is available commercially as a kit. Springs in the SCOMAC Low Profile Outrigger Kit developed by Rouzaud and Allieu[64] are color-coded for specific force, and range from 50 to 2000 g* (Fig. 9-15). Length/tension measurements of the springs were made by the manufacturer and are published in a table for reference. Using the table, springs of specific force can be selected for traction and changed to increase or decrease the force during the course of splinting. Other sources of springs providing graduated forces are becoming available.

Roberson and others in an independent study tested the SCOMAC springs for their length/tension relationships, creep, hysteresis, and fatigue.[63] One kit was tested with three springs for each increment of force up to 800 g. The sample springs were found to be linear and consistent within each force set. The increment in force from one spring to the next was nearly consistent throughout the range tested. Variability of length/tension measurements of the sample springs was low. The springs were consistent in length/tension measurements among those studied and the forces specified by the manufacturer. There was no creep (deformity causing changes in force) found in the tested springs, indicating reliability of the force exerted at a given length after a given amount of time. There was little hysteresis found; the springs provided a controlled, repeatable force at each length, whether the spring was stretching or contracting. There was no detectable fatigue when subjected to durability testing. With repeated elongation they maintained their original length/tension measurements and did not break or bend.

Mechanical properties of outriggers

Drag is a biomechanical term encompassing both frictional and tissue restraint, such as seen in adhesions. It is any factor within the limb that tends to prevent or hinder the free motion of a joint. In the case of dynamic assists, we can see the effect of external drag when the rubber band or nylon thread is moving around an outrigger, with friction caused by the actual materials used.

Friction can cause a band or nylon thread around the bar to move like a ratchet in slips and starts. The result is additional and unwanted force that directly can affect the skin and cause ischemic pressure.[23] Ratchetlike movement from friction is seen when rubber bands or nylon thread passes over an outrigger that is made from thermoplastic materials or when hook Velcro is used to provide retainers to hold thread in place.

It is desirable to use a free and frictionless bar. It is even better to use a wheel pulley or smooth steel bar, both of which are available as prefabricated splint accessories.

---

*Available through WFR/Aquaplast Corporation, Ramsey, NJ.

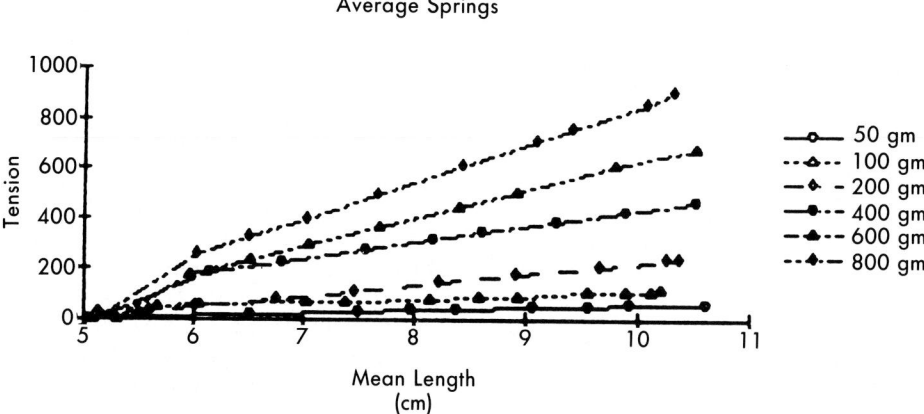

Fig. 9-15 Spring measurement. Springs for splint traction are now becoming available in calibrated kits. Springs of specific lengths and forces can be selected and progressively increased in specific increments of tension.

Mechanics of reaction bars

Reaction bars used to stabilize parts of fingers and joints to supply traction to other joints are common components of splinting. The "lumbrical bar" is one of the most common reaction bar stabilizers and is also one of the most frequent areas for splint pressure problems (Fig. 9-16, *A*). In a system where there is tension, such as in dynamic splinting, any movement is toward the tension. If a joint is stiff, the rubber band will pull or tilt the whole finger toward the outrigger. For example, in a dorsal splint with a proximal phalanx block built into the body of the splint, the MP joints will move away from the inside surface of the splint. To secure the MP joints in the splint, a strap with moldable insert pad is recommended (Fig. 9-16, *B*). A flexible strap will still allow the hand at the MP joints to move away from the inside surface of the splint. The semirigid mold can fit into the hollow of the palm and secure the hand.

Direct pressure, which can be ischemic, and shear forces from the edge of the splint occur on the dorsum of the fingers in contact with the lumbrical bar. Pressure problems occur because for every gram of force exerted by the rubber-band traction, there is at least twice as much force pushing down on the reaction bar. (The application of rubber-band force occurs at some distance from the reaction bar, creating a long lever arm to increase force at the reaction bar.) The surface of the bar should be curved to fit the shape of the fingers to prevent concentration of pressure on the small area on the dorsum of the fingers. The bar can be made as wide as possible and padded. If the hand fits into the splint well, the skin can take the even pressure over a larger area from both directions.

SPLINT MECHANICS

The new insight into the biomechanics of soft tisse and biomechanics of hand functions makes it necessary to redefine the concept of static and dynamic splints. This is important to measurement and evaluation of treatment, because a splint may not be doing as much or, in some cases,

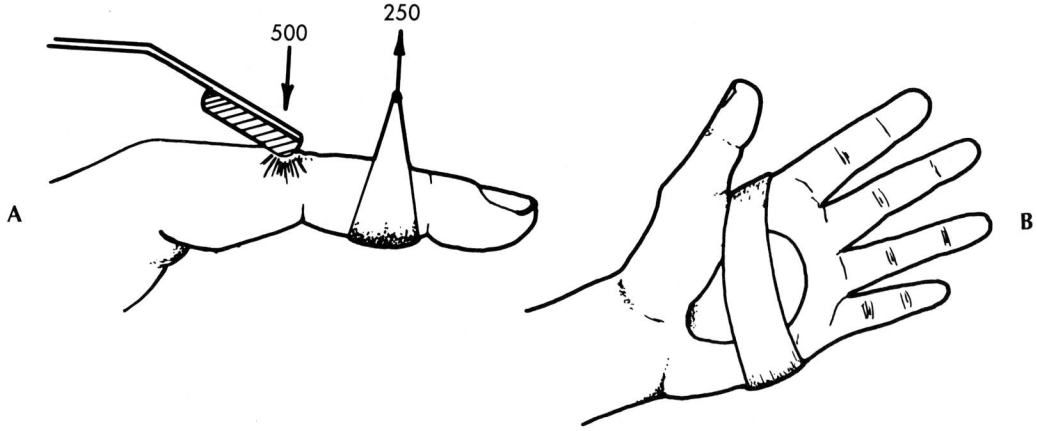

Fig. 9-16 Reaction bars. To counterbalance the traction force of splint traction and have the traction applied efficiently to the desired joint(s), reaction bars are sometimes necessary. The most typical is the so-called lumbrical bar. **A,** Unless secured sufficiently, the hand or fingers will rotate in the direction of traction, causing shear pressure at distal edges or reaction bars and structures that function as reaction bars (distal edge of the splint). Reaction bars should disburse pressure throughout as large an area as possible and, therefore, should be curved around the finger or part and should be padded. **B,** A semirigid palmar arch pad molded to the palm of the hand is usually necessary to sufficiently secure the hand in a splint.

may be doing more than intended. A static splint may not be static in its function. A splint that immobilizes one joint can dynamically affect the action at another joint. For instance, casting of the distal interphalangeal (DIP) joint of a finger transfers the flexion force of the flexor digitorum profundus more proximally to the proximal interphalangeal (PIP) joint, thus increasing the flexion force acting at the PIP joint.[11]

The realization of the dynamic transfer of force is important, because it can be a distinct help, particularly in the treatment of stiff joints. Because after an injury to a joint, such as the PIP joint, the joints with the least resistance to glide will be the first to move, the injured PIP joint would likely be the last to move and thus increase its stiffness over time. Were the DIP joint casted, the increased force of flexion at the PIP joint would likely overcome resistance and restore full flexion range of motion until the stiffness subsided.

When tendon repairs are functioning primarily at the distal joints, casting or splinting the distal joints periodically (with removable casts) will encourage normal range of motion at the more proximal joints. In the reverse, casting of the more proximal joints will transfer power of motion force to the more distal joints. This is what happens when a therapist blocks the more proximal joints to concentrate movement at the distal joints. For instance, after a boutonnière repair, the IP joint that most easily moves in flexion is the PIP joint. This is, in fact, dangerous to the repair at the level of the dorsum of the PIP joint, because the repair can be given too much tension too early. By casting the PIP joint, the therapist dynamically decreases flexion there and shifts the flexion power of the flexor digitorum profundus, which normally flexes two joints, to the DIP joint.

Without realizing the dynamic transfer of force that occurs with splinting, the surgeon or therapist can be causing undesirable results. Often the results of joint fusions are not satisfactory, but it is not always understood why. The normally balanced biomechanics of the flexors and extensors is disrupted by a fused joint, and the force that was acting on that joint is often transferred to other joints. Fusion of a joint affects biomechanics of the thumb even more than of the fingers, because the thumb has (in addition) more rotational forces. The effect of this transfer in force needs to be evaluated over time, because it may not be as apparent for the first few months or a year and the examiner can be lulled into thinking that there is no problem. Fusions of the IP joints of the fingers often result over time in progressive flexion contractures at the DIP joints. The flexion force then works only at the DIP joint and is unopposed by the extensors that were disrupted during surgery. Thus a mechanical imbalance can be created at surgery.

As we learn more about the biomechanics of the hand, we will understand more how to rebalance externally that which has become internally mechanically imbalanced through disease and injury. Splinting is most efficient and effective with the internal dynamics of the hand in mind.

"TORQUE" RANGE-OF-MOTION MEASUREMENTS
Rationale for use

Joint torque range-of-motion measurements are "windows into the mechanics of the joint."[25] This method can be used to differentiate joint stiffness caused by adhesions around tendons from that caused by stiffness around joints and to differentiate elastic from viscous restraints.[28] Torque range-of-motion measurements can be used to determine (1) the type of therapy to recommend, (2) whether conservative treatment may be a waste of time, or (3) when surgery is indicated.

Careful clinical measurements of range of motion may provide significant insights into etiology and treatment of joint problems. They may be used to monitor changes as a result of pathologic conditions, or to evaluate effectiveness of treatment modalities as well as the rebalancing of muscle power on joints introduced by tendon transfers.

Almost all stiffness is caused by ligaments, capsules, skin, or scar.[76,77] Salter, in studies on constant passive motion in joints, demonstrated that both lubrication and structural integrity of joint cartilage are improved by motion.[66] It is important to identify and quantifiably demonstrate the improvement that range-of-motion treatment (exercise or splinting) has on abnormal tissue restraints.

Passive range-of-motion measurement is a fundamental tool for evaluation of joint mobility and is clinically used as a gross measurement of the degree of joint stiffness. The need for more objective monitoring of range of motion led Brand to suggest torque range-of-motion measurements. This method controls two large variables affecting measurement accuracy: the twisting moment, or torque, applied to the joint and the posture of adjacent joints during measurement.

Range-of-motion measurements should be repeatable whether done by the experienced or inexperienced therapist. Traditional goniometric measurements performed by therapists are subject to error, because they are technique dependent. They vary according to amount of force used at a joint during the measurement. Because small range-of-motion changes may dictate changes in treatment, repeatable measurements are necessary for prompt intervention.

Torque is what occurs at the joint as the force is applied at a given distance from the joint axis. Fortunately, because torque is force multiplied by distance if the distance is kept constant, examiners have to worry only about measuring the force that is applied when doing torque range-of-motion measurements. The same amount of force when applied to different distances from the joint will result in variable torque, and the torque will be higher the farther the measurement is made from the joint (as the moment for torque or lever arm is increased). To keep the distance constant in measurements, a non-water-soluble ink can be marked at the level of the inside edge of the traction loop (cuff), and the loop can be placed at the level of joint creases.

The position of other joints during measurement also can cause a tremendous difference in the position of the joint being measured. For instance, measurements of the IP joint will often be different if the wrist is placed in flexion, neutral, or extension. For truly objective measurement then, it becomes important to describe the position of the other joints or to keep their position constant from one measurement to another.

Although torque range-of-motion measurement may seem excessively tedious at first, it is much easier than it seems. Range-of-motion measurements would be immediately more objective if only one force were selected for posi-

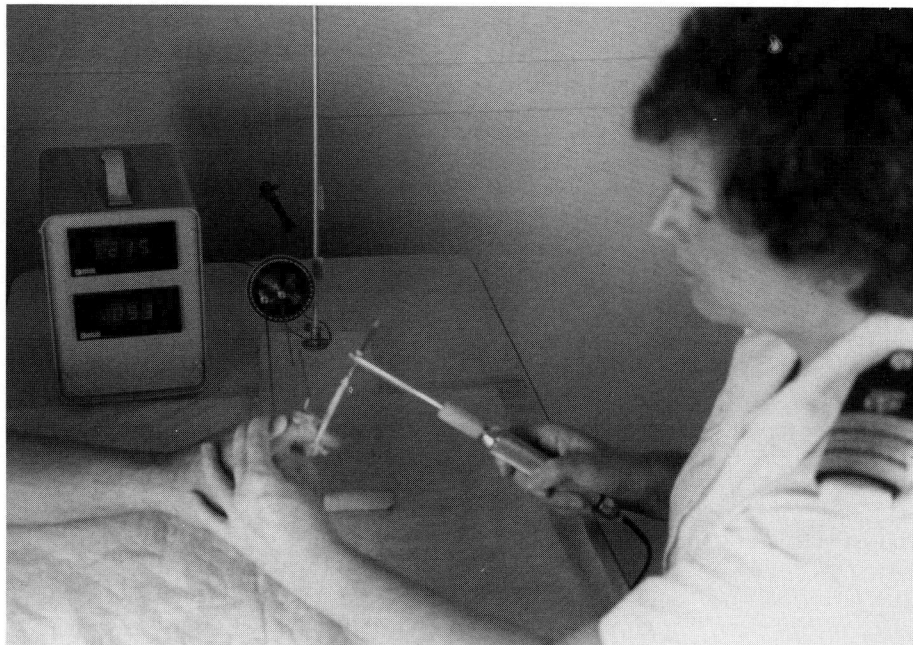

Fig. 9-17 "Rabbit ear" electrogoniometer. An experimental electrogoniometer for measuring torque range of motion.

tioning the measured joint with the other joints held consistently in only one position.

Experimental instrumentation

Instrumentation for measuring torque range of motion can be complicated or simple, but the measurement principles remain the same.[53] In our laboratory, engineers have been developing instrumentation. The objective is a simple instrument that can be used both for research and in the clinic. Sensitive experimental instruments have been tested by Buford. He developed a cantilever, beamtype force transducer with instrumentation and digital readout that is essentially an analogue device for use in the clinic. This device is currently one-of-a-kind. It is used with an electric goniometer, known as "rabbit ears," and a strain gauge. This device was developed to objectively measure angular excursion and to increase the amount of objective information on descriptive mechanics of the joint[27] (Fig. 9-17).

Clinical instrumentation

Torque range-of-motion measurements can be done in the clinic using a standard goniometer, a strain gauge (Haldex orthotic gauge), and a finger loop (cuff) (Fig. 9-18, A). To stabilize the wrist in flexion, neutral, or extension for finger joint measurements, it has also been found helpful to fabricate a universal type of cock-up splint (Fig. 9-18, B). This splint has been made with minimal support for wrist extension and with thumb extension tongues on both sides so the splint can fit either the right or left hand. A tape recorder is also helpful to record the resultant joint angle measurements of the different forces applied. (Hands need to be free to do the measurements.)

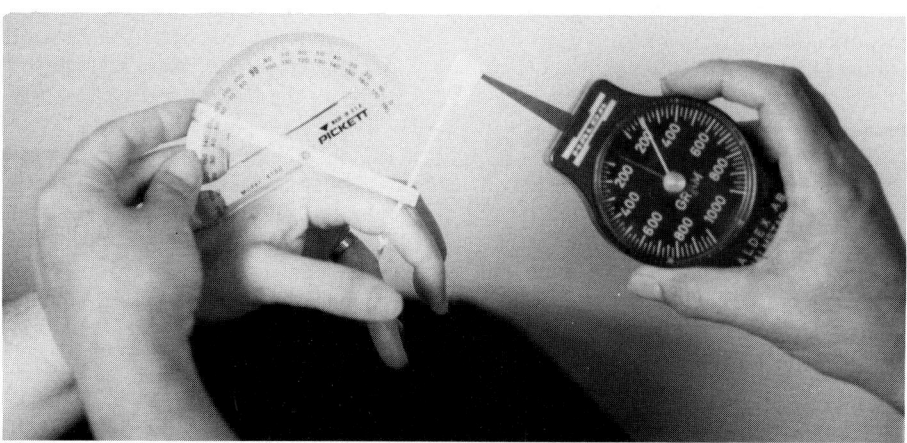

Fig. 9-18 Measurement of torque range of motion. Clinical instrumentation for measuring torque range of motion.

Procedure

It is important to use the same technique for every measurement. It is not necessary to measure the distance (lever arm or moment arm) every time a force is applied. Repeatability is assured if the same anatomic markers are used for every measurement, such as the same flexion crease.

> EXAMPLE: For measurement of the PIP joint in extension, the crease of the DIP joint can be used for the loop moving the PIP joint into extension. The Haldex orthotic gauge is used with a loop of thick string attached to the most distal part of the device. The gauge measures the grams of force applied. A finger goniometer is placed over the dorsum of the finger in the usual method to read the range of motion. The traction must be maintained at right angles to the segment distal to the joint measured (Fig. 9-18).
>
> To measure PIP flexion, the arm of the Haldex orthotic gauge is applied to the finger using a pencil eraser tip (eraser has been attached to the gauge for this purpose). The dorsum of the middle phalanx opposite the finger distal flexion crease is used to determine a repeatable distance through which the force is applied. The direction of application of force must be at right angles to the segment of the digit that is to move. The position of the MP joints and the wrist should be noted and maintained constant for each measurement.

Description of measurements

Torque "angle." It is not necessary to do measurements at several force levels on every patient. Range-of-motion measurements are immediately more objective if a standard force (torque at joint) is used to measure every joint. One torque angle refers to the resultant angle measurement at a specific force. This method of testing is clinically expedient when there is not time for more detailed testing or when more detailed testing is not needed.

Torque angle measurements. More useful information about the mechanical quality (elasticity or inelasticity) of the joint tissues may be obtained by making a succession of torque angle measurements at different levels of force (at the same distance from the axis).[28,31,78] Torque angle measurements refer to a sequence of torques applied in increments to the joint, noting the angular changes that result. The forces may be applied at from 100 to 800 g. The maximum amount of safe force varies according to the size of the hand and the pathologic condition. With small, fragile hands the force should not exceed 300 to 600 g. The greatest changes in angle should be produced with the lower levels of force (100 to 400 g), with higher forces producing little change, so it is not always necessary to use the higher forces. Arthritic joints or joints with instability should not be measured with more than enough force to gently straighten the joint if possible (100 to 200 g).

Brand recommends use of four forces in equal increments in obtaining a torque angle curve. For the sake of time, another variation of the measurement is for only two measures to be used, for example, 200 and 600 g of force.

Torque angle curve. A torque angle curve is a line plot of the torque angle measurements of a joint. A graph can be made by recording measurement for force on the vertical axis and angle on the horizontal axis (Fig. 9-19). The viscoelasticity of the joint's restraining tissue is revealed in the

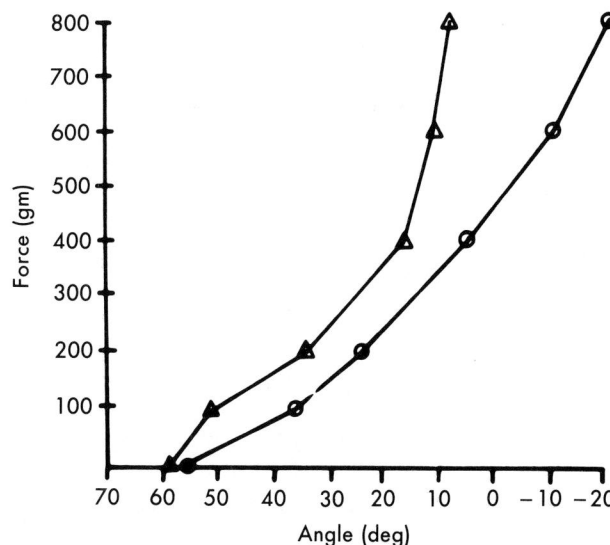

Fig. 9-19 Typical "normal" torque angle curves for the proximal interphalangeal joint and the metacarpophalangeal-joint extension. (Note the similarities in slope with the earlier stress/strain curve of normal tissue in Fig. 9-5, and rubber bands in Fig. 9-12).

curve. Curves can be serially compared for changes during the course of therapy or surgical treatment.

Interpretation of measurements

Normal versus abnormal torque angle curve. A torque angle curve of a normal individual joint shows it has a soft end-feel (springiness), which varies according to the joint. A curve that is made by plotting the force versus angle begins in a soft slope that changes quickly with increased gram load (Fig. 9-19). In contrast, a fixed, contracted joint comes to a rather abrupt halt in slope and has a steep curve with increasing load (Fig. 9-20).

Pretreatment and posttreatment. The viscosity of normal joints changes with elevation or dependent positioning and time of day. This change is even more dramatic after hand injury and disease, and the amount of fluid can change the torque angle curve. Arthritic patients who have morning stiffness have an increase in viscosity. For this reason, repeat measurements should be taken at the same time of day and with the hand in the same relative position.

Torque range-of-motion measurements before and after whirlpool, elevation, massage, exercise, and other modalities make an objective, permanent record and help determine the efficacy of the treatment.[7,31,63]

An example is shown of a patient treated with paraffin for joint stiffness (Fig. 9-20):

	Before	After
At 200 force	39 degrees	55 degrees
400 g force	47 degrees	64 degrees
600 g force	54 degrees	71 degrees

Presplinting and postsplinting. We see patients presurgically who may require a certain amount of serial casting to remodel and elongate the tissues of contracted joints. Changes in joint angle with casting or other splinting can be demonstrated with torque angle curves.[6,47,49,58] If the joint shows little change during the course of treatment, we may be dealing with a bony block, a tenodesis, or excessive scar

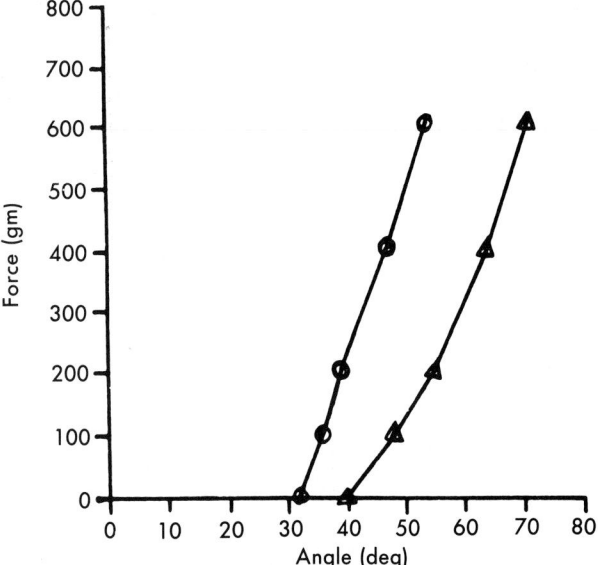

Fig. 9-20 Abnormal torque angle curves for proximal interphalangeal joint flexion before and after paraffin treatment. An abnormal curve will be steeper when increased force produces less change in the joint angle. Note the angle improvement and softening of the curve following paraffin treatment of an index proximal interphalangeal joint. Measurements such as these can help document efficacy of treatment.

around the tendon. Torque angle measurements will continue to show little change in joint angle measurements with increased load. In those patients who do have a change, the change will be reflected in the torque angle curve by improvement in angle measurements for the same gram loads in previous measurements. Minimal change in the curves and steepening of the curves will predict when joints have reached their maximum potential from casting or other splinting.

Muscle tendon unit tightness. Tightness of the flexor superficialis and/or profundus, which can occur after median or ulnar nerve injury, inhibits a good surgical result after a tendon transfer. This can be treated before surgery by splinting with the wrist and fingers progressively in extension (starting from a neutral position or less). Torque angle curves can objectively determine the amount of flexor tightness. This is done by comparing the torque angle measurements of each finger taken first with the wrist flexed, then wrist extended.

HAND VOLUME MEASUREMENT
Rationale for use

Any edema in a hand signals trouble and can be difficult to assess accurately without objective measures. Swelling can be one of the greatest treatment complications after surgery. The hand can be swollen from too much use, and the hand can be swollen from too little use; the therapist and surgeon must be attuned to the differences. If the edema is of the water type from inactivity or dependent positioning, there will be a hand volume change in a short period after elevation of the extremity. This is the type of edema that responds to string wrapping, elastic bandage wrapping, or

some other type of compressive treatment to the hand. Exercise, if possible, is indicated to help pump the fluids out of the hand.

If the edema is from too much movement too soon, there are often other signs of irritation, such as heat or redness. The hand volume in the case of this type of inflammatory edema will not show a change in a short period but may after a few hours as the tissue slowly increases in fluid volume. Treatment indicated in this case is rest or at least a slow-down in activity.

Infection is an ever-present possibility after surgery and is usually signaled by swelling, redness, and temperature elevation. The hand volume will slowly increase or decrease. Early serial measurements of hand volume may signal whether the infection is subsiding or exacerbating. Treatment, in addition to appropriate medications, is rest and protection until signs of inflammation have subsided. Exercise limited to only that which is necessary to maintain joint and tendon gliding may be allowed but complete immobilization should be considered to avoid spreading the infection by gliding tendons squeezing infected tissue (as discussed under Movement, Stress, and Wounds in this chapter).

Brand introduced a way to measure changes in hand volume objectively.[4,17,24,26] The hand volumeter he designed* (see Chapter 13) was developed over several years through clinical studies in India and with therapists and engineers in our laboratory. The volumeter measures hand volume by water displacement and is commercially available. Specifications are available from the Paul W. Brand Research Laboratory in Carville, La. Brand recommends establishing a baseline measurement for patients before instituting treatment, particularly before surgery. In this way, postoperative measurements can be compared.

The volumeter helps examiners recognize signs and direction of treatment early. There is often a 10 ml difference between right and left hands. There is a 10 ml difference between the dominant and nondominant hands, but fluid volume changes are often 30 to 50 ml or more between one measurement and the next if swelling is a problem. Waylett and Seibly studied the average deviation accuracy of the Brand-designed volumeter and reported 10 ml or less of measurement variation with one examiner and 10 to 15 ml variation between examiners.[76] The size, shape, and spout of the volumeter are extremely important to its efficiency. The design for the commercially available volumeter was carefully developed from many variations to optimize the change in volume for various hand sizes. Other volumeters have been used, and each design will have its own deviations in milliliters from one measurement to another. Barclay,[3] Devore and Hamilton,[37] Eccles,[39] and Greenhill[55] reported on the use and reliablity of similar volumeters.

Equipment
- Plastic hand volumeter*
- 500 ml graduated cylinder
- Small bucket or container
- Elevated support for hand volumeter
- Chair

---

*Volumeters Unlimited, Idyllwild, Calif.

Procedure

The patient's hand is measured while he or she is seated with back against chair and feet flat on floor. The hand is positioned with palm in anatomic position, and the patient is instructed to slowly lower the hand into the volumeter, which has been filled with water until it has slightly overflowed and the spout has stopped dripping. (Silicone spray on the dry spout will facilitate overflow water to stop when the hand is fully lowered and, if applied to the inside of the dry tank, will eliminate the surface water meniscus, which can be an error factor.) The hand is lowered until the dowel of the volumeter rests between the web of the middle and ring fingers. The hand remains until water no longer flows from the spout. The patient then lifts his hand and is given a towel. The measurement is read in milliliters at eye level on the graduated cylinder. The chair is reversed and the procedure repeated for the opposite hand.

If the hand cannot be positioned in the standard way on the dowel because of, for example, contractures, location of the dowel between any finger is acceptable. Subsequent measurements of the same patient must be made with the hand in the same position for repeatability.

Graphs and serial volume measurements

Serial measurements can be plotted on a graph. Because volume changes can occur with, for example, exercise, positioning, or time of day, a graph will help identify trends in measurements. A graph will resemble an electrocardiogram somewhat, with peaks and valleys. The peaks can be associated with reasons for increased swelling, such as lack of exercise or lack of elevation, and the valleys associated with improvement, such as a change in treatment program or compression wrapping.

Circumferential measurements

One problem in repeat measurements of volume is that a hand could have a fluid change in distinct areas, such as from palm to fingers, and still maintain the same volume. For this reason it is sometimes important also to do circumferential measurements of the hand and fingers at joints or areas of swelling. Tapes for measuring the circumference of the hand or fingers are available commercially.* The exact location measured should be noted and subsequent measurements made at the same sites. Non-water-soluble ink can be used to mark the site, for example, the location of the distal edge of the measurement tape. Solder wire, which is flexible, can be used to measure around a swollen joint or area. The wire can be cut to fit, then opened and laid flat to measure. The "ring" can then be refashioned and kept as a visual record or given to the patient to check his swelling at home.

TEMPERATURE ASSESSMENT
Rationale for measurement

The difference between swelling from disuse and swelling from too much use of a hand, particularly a postoperative hand, can be determined by temperature. An elevation in skin temperature that is prolonged is the soft tissue's response to too much stress.[14,17,54] Any exercise of the hand will result in some temperature elevation, but this elevation

*North Coast Medical, Inc., Campbell, Calif.

should be of short duration. A hand that has swelling from disuse or too little use will be cool by comparison.

Thermistors are not always needed to recognize an area of apparent inflammation, only to quantify the amount of inflammation. Temperature can be felt easily by the back of the examiner's fingers. The examiner can learn to discern changes in temperature by regularly checking the skin temperature of patients.

It is important to identify relative changes in temperature (hot spots). If one area has a temperature elevation when the same area of the other hand or other areas on the same hand are cooler, an area of localized inflammation is indicated. Temperature differentials (called Δ-T) are the important consideration and are much more important than the absolute temperature. Normally, there is a Δ-T within 1°C between one skin area and the same area on the other hand. If the difference in temperature is greater than this, an elevated temperature is indicated. It is important that a skin area of elevated temperature is referenced with similar skin areas, because the skin temperature can vary, particularly from the dorsal to volar surfaces of the hand.

When the whole hand is warm, no temperature differential may be indicated, because the patient will not under normal circumstances rise above his core body temperature.[17] This is particularly true when a hand has been warmed in a glove or bandage or has been exercising a lot. It is sometimes necessary, then, to cool the extremity before measurement. A cold pack can be wrapped in a towel and placed on the hand, or the hand can be wrapped in a damp, cool towel. The skin temperature changes rapidly, and it is therefore not necessary to cool the extremity for more than 5 minutes. Too much exposure to cold can result in hyperemia after warming and should be avoided.

A healing wound or injury will have an elevated temperature when compared with other tissue.[15] It is important to establish a baseline measurement in these cases so that increases in temperature differential can be recognized. For instance, if an injured joint that is exercised in therapy has a several-degree Δ-T in the hours or day after being exercised in therapy, the indication is that it was exercised too much. In contrast, so long as repeated measurements show only a degree or two Δ-T in the hours or day after being exercised in therapy, the exercise level is within tolerance of the tissue and could possibly be increased.

Infections result in the greatest Δ-T in skin areas, sometimes as high as 7°C difference. An area with a large Δ-T is suspect for infection, and the hand should be examined closely for other clinical signs indicating infection. These include hyperemia, puncture wounds, drainage, foul odor, pus, discoloration, and necrosis.

Chronic ulcers are a different problem. In chronic ulcers the initial inflammatory stage of healing has subsided and the wound may actually be cool in comparison with other skin areas. Not all temperature elevation is bad. The temperature elevation of the infected wound indicates that activity is going on to heal the wound. Absence of temperature elevation in the wound signals that the infection is chronic or that the tissue has little blood supply with not very much healing activity. Sometimes it is even necessary to abrade the chronic wound slightly with a piece of sterile gauze to create a slightly inflammatory process to promote healing. (Abrading a wound should be done only with the concurrence of a physician and when the wound looks clean and the granulation bed looks good, but epithelialization is not progressing.)

Experimental instruments

Thermography, or infrared heat photography, has been available for research for several years.*[14] A thermogram easily demonstrates differences in warmer and cooler skin areas by an isotherm mapping generated in colors from cool through hot (Fig. 9-21). Hot spots can easily be identified by the warm colors of red, orange, and white, as opposed to cooler colors of green, blue, and purple.

Unfortunately, the high cost and bulky equipment of the thermography instruments makes it impractical for most programs other than research institutions. Thermography has been available to our clinic for the past 15 years and has given much insight into the relationship of temperature with wounds and healing. Unfortunately, the cost of the instrumentation makes its use prohibitive for the routine clinic in most cases, and other forms of temperature instruments must be used.

Clinical instruments

One conclusion of our clinical research with thermography is that once the relationship of temperature with wound healing was learned, thermography, while still helpful, was

---

*AGA 680 Thermovision Unit, AGA Corporation, Secaucus, NJ.

not as necessary to understand the significance of temperature differentials. Much clinical information can be obtained from small skin thermistors commercially available at much less cost.

Surface skin thermometers are available for measuring surface skin temperature. They are inexpensive but unfortunately not very practical. Skin thermometers take several minutes to measure each area. This makes relative readings difficult, because to have repeatable measurements, they must be taken for the same length of time.

Thermistors measure absolute skin temperature in degrees within seconds, and they are easy to use and to read (Fig. 9-22). A color mapping with separate colors for separate degrees could be made for demonstrating relative temperature differences by using standard colors for each temperature degree. The best currently available instrument is a hand-held radiometer,* but more standard temperature probe instruments work very well.† These are battery-operated.

STRENGTH
Quantification of strength

Most strength measurements in the clinic are of available external strength or performance against something outside the body. Manual muscle tests were developed in attempts to make muscle grading objective. These are greatly subject to examiner experience and subjective interpretation. They

---

*Mikron Infrared Thermometer, Mikron Instrument Co, Inc., Midland Park, NJ.

†Model KM 900, Probe KS, Measurements, Inc., New Orleans.

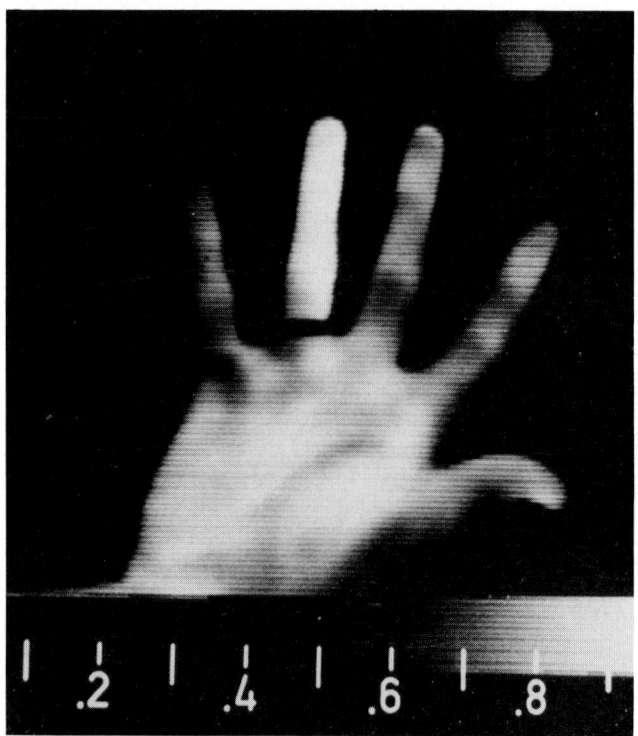

Fig. 9-21 Thermogram. Experimental infrared heat photography demonstrates differences in warmer and cooler skin areas which can be used for monitoring the status of infections, trauma, tendinitis, postsurgical exercise, and circulation.

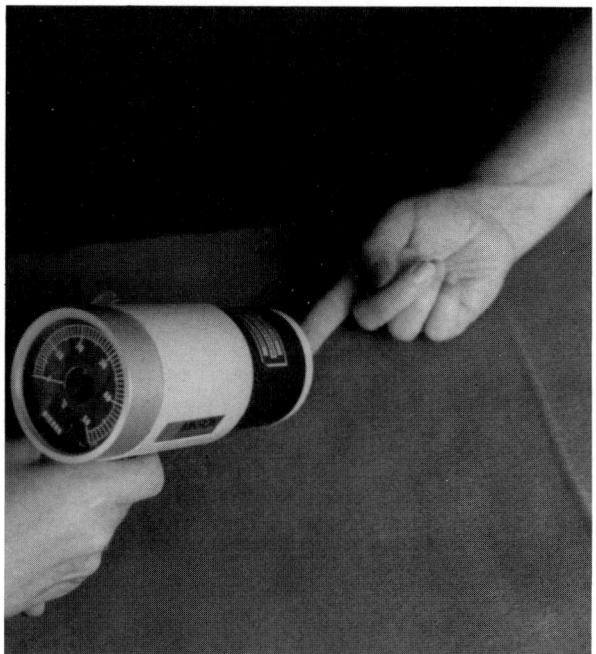

Fig. 9-22 Hand held radiometer. Clinical instrumentation for measuring surface skin temperature and monitoring such things as clinical status of infections.

are most repeatable if the same examiner does subsequent examinations. Other examiners may have different interpretations of patient muscle performance. Ways of further quantifying strength would be helpful.

Strength of a muscle is the tension a muscle can develop and is related to the cross-sectional area of its fibers and its excursion.[22,68] Excursion is the distance through which the strength can be used and is related to work capacity of the muscle itself.[16,40] Strength of a muscle provided at a given joint depends, in addition, on how far it is from the joint axis and on the number of joints it is crossing. The distance the muscle or tendon is from the axis in part determines the usable "external strength" of the individual, which is not the same as the strength or tension produced by the muscle.

Grip-strength measurements are used as a collective measure of patient overall strength or weakness. Innumerable studies have been made on grip strength in different populations. Although populations vary in mean grip strength, grip strength can be measured in absolute values on an instrument such as the Jamar dynamometer.[9,61] The Jamar dynamometer has been shown to be a sensitive and repeatable test instrument when calibrated correctly and used in a procedure that is in itself repeatable.[44] It is most useful when the patient can be used as his own control, such as in comparing right and left hands, and when comparing baseline measurements with subsequent measurements.

One disadvantage of grip-strength measurement with current instruments is that it cannot be individualized to different muscles or fingers. Experimental instruments have been explored for this purpose and could become available for clinical use were a market established. A gyroscopic grip-strength dynamometer with force transducers for each finger was designed experimentally at the National Institutes of Health by a therapist formerly associated with our laboratory during its early years.[67] Engineers at the National Rehabilitation Institute were involved in this and similar projects.

The Instron Materials Testing Instrument* used for studies of viscoelastic properties of materials has been adapted experimentally to test strength of individual muscles or fingers (Fig. 9-23). This instrument is essentially a large-scale stress/strain gauge that can be connected to an instrument with a calibrated graph readout. The flexion strength of a ring finger before and after a sublimis transfer has been tested in this fashion, as have the radial wrist extensors before and after use for an intrinsic replacement procedure. This testing is position dependent, therefore it requires identical positioning for repeat testing.

Similar testing can be devised in the clinic with strain gauges, such as the Haldex orthotic gauge. The gauge can be mounted, and positioning devices can be made that would ensure repeatable positioning. For instance, weak radial wrist extension can be measured as to the exact load it can resist before it can no longer extend beyond neutral. Then on subsequent measurements, a numerical reference would be available to judge progressive improvement or weakness.

Electromyography is another traditional way of numerically grading muscle strength and viability. This testing, too, depends on the experience and interpretation of the examiner. An integrating monitor can remove some subjectivity. The amplitude of the signal is considered more important than the wave form for strength (because the abnormal wave forms are the basis for noting pathologic conditions with electromyography). A weak strength of signal (amplitude) indicates weak muscle fiber contraction ac-

---

*Instron Materials Testing Instrument Model 1122, Instron Instruments and Systems, Houston.

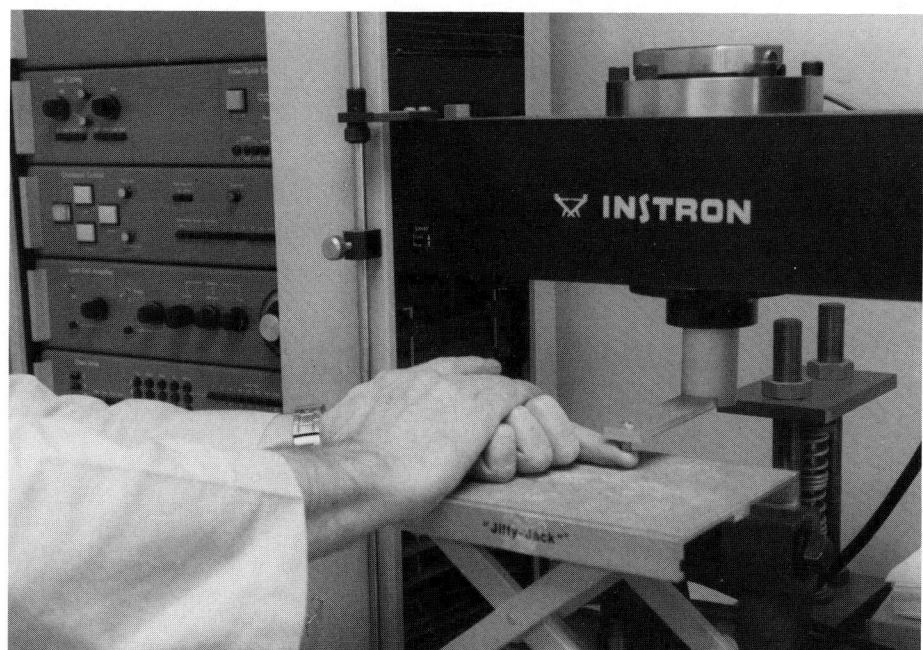

Fig. 9-23   Instron materials testing instrument. Experimental instrument for testing viscoelastic properties of materials and soft tissue, adapted experimentally to measure individual finger strength and wrist strength.

tivity. The duration or continued muscle activity over time is also important, because some muscles will at first show a good amount of contraction activity but drop off quickly.

As a measure of strength and duration of strength of a muscle, Brand suggested the use of selected gram weights moved by the patient to the timing of a musical metronome while the examiner counts the number of possible contractions through full range of motion. For example, the number of wrist extensions possible with a 2-pound weight (at a given speed timed to the metronome) can be counted and recorded to measure the strength and endurance of returning wrist extensors after a radial nerve injury.

Relative strength of muscles

Brand and others believe actual strength is so variable in different populations that a list of average muscle performance values are meaningful only for limited groups of similar individuals. Consider the multitude of grip-strength studies and the confusion as to what study norms should be used for different patients. Whose measurements are used as norms? Brand, like Bunnell in describing muscle balance and imbalance, considers the relative strength to be more important than absolute strength. He has found the relative muscle strength in most normal individual forearms and hands to be fairly constant and published this with Beach and Thompson in a review of 15 cadaver specimens.[22] The study did not measure "muscle strength" in cadavers but implied strength or relative tension based on a cross-sectional area.

Brand and colleagues found that the fiber length of the muscles are about equal when the muscles are displayed with the fibers aligned, based on geometric descriptions of muscle fibers by Steno,[68] and that all fibers reach from tendon of origin to tendon of insertion. This is important, because it means the fiber mass and lengths can be measured to determine the relative strengths of the muscles.

Elftman,[40] after the work of Blix,[16] previously demonstrated the relationship between fiber length, tension, and excursion. Weber and Fick[47] found muscle mass or volume proportional to total work capacity. Brand and others confirmed and added to these earlier studies.

The fiber length of a muscle is proportional to its potential excursion. Muscles with short fibers do not move far, whereas muscles with long fibers have long excursions. Muscles with short fibers and with large mass will be powerful muscles, but for short distances. Muscles with long fibers but with small mass will move relatively long distances, but with relatively little strength. The relative mean fiber resting lengths were determined for each muscle in the hand and forearm and published in a table.[22]

The relative muscle mass for each muscle could be determined by weighing the muscles individually. Some muscles would have many short fibers but potentially have the same relative volume, thus have the total work capacity as muscles with long fibers with less volume. A relative muscle-mass table was developed for all of the muscles of the hand and forearm. Each muscle has its own "mass fraction," that is, the individual muscle mass percentage of total muscle mass of all muscles of hand and forearm (% total mass).

The cross-sectional area of all fibers is proportional to the maximum tension, or tension-producing capacity of the muscles. Mass was converted to volume (mass = 1.02 vol for muscle) and divided by mean fiber length to determine the physiologic cross-sectional area of a muscle). A relative muscle-tension table was developed for all of the muscles of the forearm and hand. Each muscle has its own "tension fraction," or individual muscle percentage of total cross-sectional areas for muscles of hand and forearm (% total cross-sectional area).

These tables can be used in considerations of tendon transfers for rebalancing hands with more weakness or loss. They give a truer indication of potential versus available

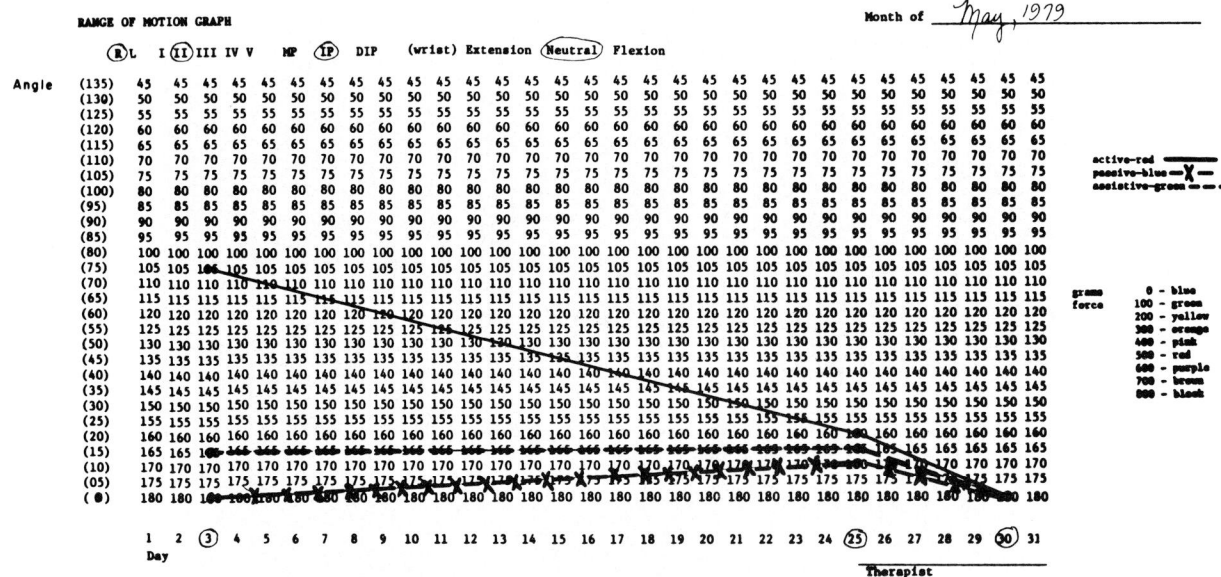

Fig. 9-24 Simplified measurement graphs. Example of premade measurement graph listing full range of data expected for serial monitoring of patient status. Exact numerical measurement can be recorded to reduce error sometimes made when recording data points. Data are reduced to the specific item monitored. Changes in status over time can be reviewed and compared with treatment versus treatment interruption. Graphs could be used as recording forms.

tension and excursion of the muscles than manual muscle tests. They also add insight into the biomechanics of the muscle-tendon units and relative relationships of muscle groups.

MEASUREMENT GRAPHS

Graphs of patient performance are helpful and understandable to the patient as well as to the therapist, surgeon, and employer. Patients can even be involved in keeping their own graphs of performance as their measurements change from one treatment session to another. Graphs need not be complicated, but can be line plots. The resultant peaks can be associated with improvement and the valleys with regression, or vice versa.

One disadvantage of graphs is the time required to make them. If the graph forms can be premade for the range of particular measurements, considerable time is saved. Almost everyone is familiar with the premade temperature graphs found on medical charts. New measurements can be made quickly and simply by noting specific degrees of temperature and the date recorded. This type of recording can be done with almost any type of routine measurement, such as joint range of motion.

Simplified graphs can be made by listing in columns the pertinent numerical data range on prepared forms[10] (Fig. 9-24). These graphs are sometimes easier to record and read quickly.

INTERACTIVE SURGICAL WORK STATIONS

Computer models of the hand are being developed to advance both knowledge of hand biomechanics and the teaching of biomechanics (Fig. 9-25). These models should potentially aid understanding and measurement of abnor-

mality by providing normal hand models that can be adjusted with abnormal clinical data, such as an intrinsic muscle loss with retention of remaining extrinsic musculature. Research in this area seems promising and is now several years underway.[35,52,72,73] Once an interactive workstation is available for clinical use, the clinician can develop accelerated knowledge of biomechanics. By changing the normal balance of muscles in and around joints of a computer model, the resultant imbalance is recreated on the screen. The surgeon's understanding will be enhanced by his ability to propose and plan surgical transfers using preprogrammed data of patient relative muscle strength and excursion. The therapist can then design splints to correct biomechanical imbalances efficiently and test new ideas. A most important realization is that even the interactive workstation must be developed and programmed to include data from objective clinical measurements.

NEED FOR IMPROVED MEASUREMENT INSTRUMENTS

Information presented in this chapter underlines the need for objective instruments. To describe and analyze clinical problems accurately, data must be recorded in terms other than subjective.[18] There is no substitute for experience and educated intuition. The value of an experienced clinician should not be belittled, because it is by experience and intuition that surgeons and therapists skillfully employ their knowledge. But the assessment of patient performance and degree of patient problems requires sensitive and repeatable measures. How else can patient performance be compared with normal subjects, with prior performance, or with patients in other treatment programs?

Many of our clinical tests and treatments are unstand-

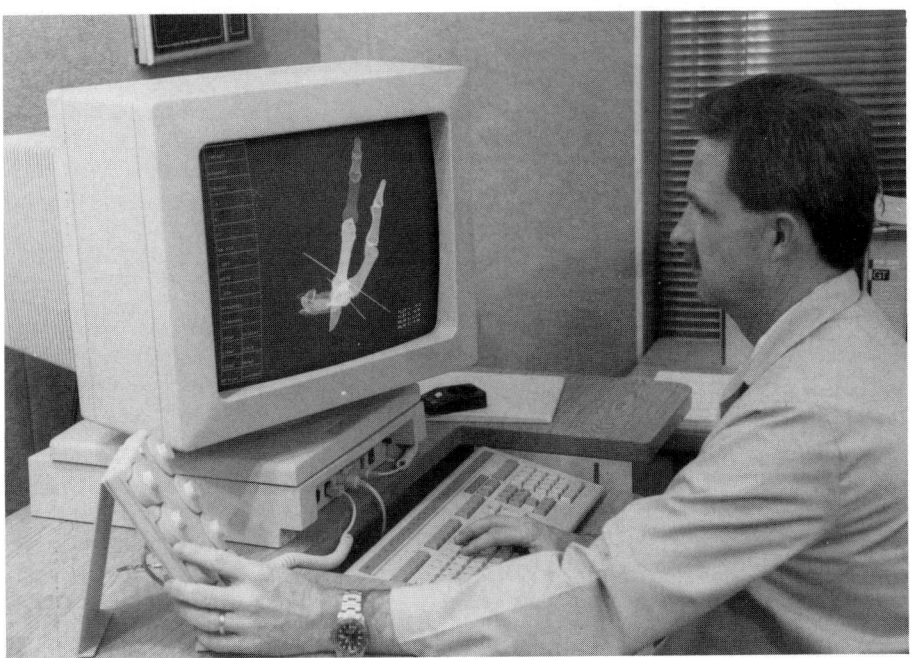

Fig. 9-25   Computer workstation. Computer modeling of the hand on the computer for an interactive workstation in hand biomechanics (in progress). The model simulates normal hand function and abnormal hand function, based on patient clinical data. It will be used for teaching biomechanics of the hand, for biomechanical analysis of clinical problems such as surgical tendon transfers, and to design biomechanically sound equipment and prostheses.

ardized but have been accepted into common clinical practice by their popularity and frequent use.[12,13,42,45] The first step in changing this is for examiners to be more critical of available instruments by asking several questions:

1. How sensitive is an instrument or technique?
2. Is it as sensitive as it needs to be?
3. Is it calibrated or quantified?
4. How repeatable is it?
5. Is it repeatable for serial measurements, and is it repeatable among examiners?
6. Is it technique-dependent?
7. Has the instrument or technique been studied, or has it just been used and reported in studies? (There is a great difference between an instrument that has become "standard," and one that has been standardized through accepted clinical trials.)
8. What are the variables in terms of being hand-held,[12] changes from one instrument to another, changes in the time the patient is tested, and how much is or could be subjective?[36]

These questions should at least be asked and variables in tests and measurements controlled as much as possible.

When clinicians demand more objective instruments, more will become available. When clinicians check the calibration of instruments and return those out of calibration, manufacturers will be more exacting and more concerned about design specifications.

NEED FOR CLINICAL RESEARCH BY CLINICIANS

As objective measures are becoming more available in the clinic, clinical problems and specific treatment techniques can be followed more objectively and compared with other patients and programs. Data from objective measures can be reviewed retroactively at any time. Protocols that eliminate variables can be developed and improved for clinical studies.

It is often thought that there is not time in the clinic to do clinical studies. The opposite is true if objective measures are available and some of the guesswork is removed from practice. Every patient is his or her own clinical study. It is from patients and their clinical abnormalities that we learn clinical treatment. The clinician is continually reapplying and altering treatment techniques to fit particular patient problems. What seems to work is probably used again, and what does not work is soon omitted.

SUMMARY

An understanding of biomechanics and objective measurement is on the forefront of new knowledge in hand therapy and surgery. Biomedical engineers are adding depth to our understanding of hand function and principles of measurement that can be directly applied in clinical hand practice. The clinician is ever challenged to think, develop, discover, and rediscover, but with new tools that will aid in solving clinical problems. Advances in treatment depend on objective measurements and subsequent clinical research integrated with clinical treatment.

This chapter is incomplete—and will always be incomplete. As new knowledge of the hand and biomechanics is developing, clinical measures will change and improve. Measurement techniques need further analysis and devel-

opment by clinicians who are sensitive and attentive to biomechanical principles and who are experienced in clinical treatment.

DEFINITION OF TERMS AS USED IN THIS CHAPTER[65]

compression   Force loading acting in opposite directions to push the material together

creep   Continued and progressive deformation of soft tissue from constant loading over extended time (as opposed to remodeling of tissue, which involves growth of tissue)

elasticity   That property by which a material returns to its original form after deformation

elastic deformation   A deformation that is reversible when loading is released

fatigue   Failure of material under loading

force   The direct or indirect action of one body on another

friction   Tangential force acting between two structures in contact that opposes motion or impending motion (static friction if the structures are at rest, kinetic friction if the structures are in relative motion)

length/tension relationship   Variation in length with variation in tension (force loading in opposite directions)

load   Force or stress applied to a structure

modulus of elasticity   Slope of the curve in the elastic region produced by graphing a ratio of stress versus strain; stiff materials have higher elastic moduli than soft materials

normal stress   Direct or perpendicular stress that occurs in soft tissue

plasticity   That property by which a material retains its form after deformation; a plastic material is moldable

plastic deformation   A strain in a material that is not recoverable when loading is released

pressure   Force/unit area acting on a structure from a load

shear stress   Angular stress that occurs tangentially in soft tissue

strain   Change in length of a structure under loading

stress   Tensile or compressive force/unit area that develops within a structure in response to externally applied load

stress/strain relationship   Variation in strain output (length or angle) with variation in stress (force/unit area) input

tangential force   Force that occurs at angles to the surface of tissue and has lateral and rotational components that produce shear

tension   Force loading acting in opposite directions, which tends to pull an object apart

tissue remodeling   Growth and relaxation of tissue held under low constant tension, thereby returning to its homeostatic resting state

transducer   A device that converts one form of energy to another, such as pressure to electrical energy, where it can be measured and quantified

torque   Force times distance from center of joint axis

torque angle curve   A graph of torque versus angle for passive joint measurement; the steeper and higher the curve, the stiffer the joint measured

torque range of motion   Objective measure of range of motion where a constant force (at a constant distance from the joint axis) is applied to the joints being measured

viscoelastic properties   The viscous and elastic properties of soft tissue and materials that give them relative degrees of stiffness and elasticity

ACKNOWLEDGMENTS

The authors acknowledge with appreciation the review and critique of this chapter by the entire staff of the Paul W. Brand Research Laboratory, U.S. Public Health Service, Gillis W. Long Hansen's Disease Center, Carville, La. Acknowledged in particular is the assistance of William Buford, M.E., Ph.D., Chief, Paul W. Brand Research Laboratory, and David E. Thompson, Ph.D., Professor of Electrical Engineering, Louisiana State University.

REFERENCES

1. Agee M, Brand W, and Thompson E: The moment arms of the carpometacarpal joint of the thumb: their laboratory determinations and clinical application, Proc. of the 37th Annual Meeting, American Society for Surgery of the Hand, New Orleans, Jan 1982.
2. An KN, Chao EY, and Cooney WP: Normative model of human hand for biomechanical analysis, J Biomech 12:775, 1979.
3. Barclay TL: Edema following operation for Dupuytrens's contracture. Plast Reconstr Surg 23(4):348, 1959.
4. Beach RB: Measurement of extremity volume by water displacement, Phys Ther 57(3):286, 1977.
5. Beach RB: The rehabilitation research department, The Star 38:7, 1979; 38(8):8, 1979.
6. Beach RB and Bell JA: Torque range-of-motion curve: an objective method for passive joint range of motion measurement. Proceedings of the American Society of Hand Therapists, Fifth Annual Meeting, J Hand Surg 7(3):308, 1982.
7. Beach RB and Bell JA: Ace, Coban, and bias stockinette: pressures resulting from their use, Proceedings of the American Society of Hand Therapists' Sixth Annual Meeting, J Hand Surg 8(5):627, 1983.
8. Beach RB and Thompson DE: Selected soft-tissue research: an overview from Carville, Phys Ther 59(1):30, 1979.
9. Bechtol CD: Grip test: use of a dynamometer with adjustable handle spacing, J Bone Joint Surg 36A:820, 1954.
10. Bell JA: Simplified measurement graphs: a new approach. Proceedings American Society of Hand Surg 8(5):626, 1983.
11. Bell JA: Plaster casting for the remodeling of soft tissue. In Fess EF and Philips CA, editors: Hand splinting: principles and methods, ed 2, St. Louis, 1987, The CV Mosby Co.
12. Bell-Krotoski JA and Tomancik E: Repeatability of testing with the Semmes-Weinstein monofilaments, J Hand Surg 12A:155, 1987.
13. Bell Krotoski JA and Buford WL: The force/time relationship of clinically used sensory testing instruments, J Hand Ther 1(2):76, 1988.
14. Bergtholdt HT and Brand PW: Thermography: an aid in the management of insensitive feet and stumps, Arch Phys Med Rehabil 56:205, 1975.
15. Blakeney AB, Bergtholdt HT, and Wood HL: Injury splinting and temperature assessment of the insensitive hand, Proc 12th Ann Meeting US Public Health Service, Commissioned Officers Professional Association, San Francisco, April 1977.
16. Blix M: Die Lange und die spannung des Muskels, skand. Arch Physiol 3:295, 1891.
17. Brand PW: Clinical mechanics of the hand, St. Louis, 1985, The CV Mosby Co.
18. Brand PW: Mechanics of dynamic splinting. In Boswich JA, editor: Current concepts in hand surgery, Philadelphia, 1983, Lea & Febiger.
19. Brand PW and Ebner JD: Pressure sensitive devices for denervated hands and feet: a preliminary communication, J Bone Joint Surg 51A:109, 1969.
20. Brand PW: The slipper sock footprint test. Monograph, published by GW Long Hansen's Disease Center, Rehabilitation Branch, Carville, Louisiana, USA, 1970.
21. Brand PW: Pathomechanics of pressure ulceration. In Symposium on the neurological aspects of plastic surgery, vol 17, St. Louis, 1978, The CV Mosby Co.
22. Brand PW, Beach RB, and Thompson DE: Relative tension and potential excursion of muscles in the forearm and hand, J Hand Surg 6(3):209, 1981.
23. Brand PW: The forces of dynamic splinting: ten questions before applying a dynamic splint to the hand. In Hunter JM and others, editors: Rehabilitation of the hand, ed 2, St. Louis, 1984, The CV Mosby Co.
24. Brand PW, Sabin TD, and Burke JF: Sensory denervation: a study of its cause and its prevention in leprosy and of management of insensitive limbs, Final Report, Carville, LA USPHS Hospital, SRS Project No. RC-40-M, Aug. 1, 1966 through June 30, 1970.
25. Brand PW, Thompson DE, and Micks JE: The biomechanics of the interphalangeal joint: the proximal interphalangeal joint, London, 1987, Churchill & Livingstone.
26. Brand PW and Wood H: Hand volumeter instruction sheet, US Public Health Service Hospital, Carville, La.
27. Brandsma JW: Preoperative and postoperative evaluation of the hand with intrinsic paralysis, Proceedings of the International Conf on Biomechanics and Clinical Kinesiology of Hand and Foot, IIT Madras, India, Dec 1985.
28. Brandsma JW and Brand PW: Quantification and analysis of joint stiffness: Proceedings of the International Conference on Biomechanics and Clinical Kinesiology of Hand and Foot, IIT Madras, India, Dec 1986.
29. Branemark PI: Microvascular function at reduced flow rates. In Kenedi RM, Cowden JM, and Scales JT, editors: Bed sore biomechanics, Strathclyde Bioengineering Seminars, New York, 1976, Macmillan Press, Ltd.
30. Breger DE: Biomechanics of splinting, Am Soc Hand Therapists' 11th Annual Meeting, San Antonio, Sept, 1987.
31. Breger DE: Torque range of motion: quantification of joint stiffness, Proceedings of 22nd Annual US Public Health Service, Commissioned Officer's Assoc Professional Meeting, Nov. 1987.
32. Buford WL: Clinical evaluation of orthotic devices. Proc 13th Ann Meeting US Public Health Service, Commissioned Officer's Association, Atlanta, March 1978.
33. Buford WL: An interactive three-dimensional simulation of the kinematics of the human thumb, doctoral dissertation, Science, 1984, Louisiana State Univ; also University Microfilms, Ann Arbor, 1985.
34. Buford WL and Bell JA: Working analysis of dynamic splinting. Proc 14th Ann Meeting US Public Health Service, Commissioned Officer's Association, Phoenix, April 1979.
35. Buford WL, Myers L, and Thompson DE: A computer graphics system for musculoskeletal modeling, Proc 8th Annual EMBS Conference, 1, Fort Worth, 1986.
36. Cromwell L, Weibell J, and Pfeiffer, EA, editors: Biomedical instrumentation and measurements, ed 2, Englewood Cliffs, NJ, 1980, Prentice Hall.
37. DeVore GL and Hamilton GF: Volume measuring of the severely injured hand, Am J Occup Ther 22(1):16, 1968.
38. Daly CH and others: The effect of pressure loading on the blood flow rate in human skin. In Kenedi RM, Cowden JM, and Scales JT, editors: Bed sore biomechanics, New York, 1976, Macmillan Press, Ltd.
39. Eccles MV: Hand volumetrics, Br J Phys Med 19:5, 1956.
40. Elftman H: Biomechanics of muscle, J Bone Joint Surg 48A:363, 1966.
41. Fernie G: Instrumentation in studies of the effects of pressure on soft tissue, Proc Workshop on Effects of Pressure on Human Tissue, Brand PW and Mooney V, editors, Carville, LA, March 1977.
42. Fess EE: The need for reliability and validity in hand assessment instruments, J Hand Surg 11A:621, 1986.
43. Fess EE: Rubber-band traction: physical properties, splint design, and identification of force magnitude, Proceedings of the American Society of Hand Therapists' Seventh Annual Meeting, J Hand Surg 9A:610, 1984.
44. Fess EE: A method for checking Jamar dynamometer calibration, J Hand Ther 1(1):28, 1987.
45. Fess EE and others: Evaluation of the hand by objective measurement. In Hunter JM and others, editors: Rehabilitation of the hand, St. Louis, 1978, The CV Mosby Co.
46. Fess EE and Philips C: Principles of using dynamic assists for mobilization. In Hand splinting: principles and methods, ed 2, St. Louis, 1987, The CV Mosby Co.
47. Fick A: Statische Betrachtung der Muskulatur des Oberschenkels, Z rationelle Med 9:94, 1850.
48. Flatt AE and Fischer GW: Biomechanical factors in the replacement of rheumatoid joints, Ann Rheum Dist 28:36, 1969.
49. Flowers KR and Pheasant SD: The use of torque angle curves in the assessment of digital joint stiffness, J Hand Ther 1(2):69, 1988.
50. Frank C and others: Physiology and therapeutic value of passive joint motion, Clin Orthop 185:113, 1984.
51. Fung YCB: Biomechanics: mechanical properties of living tissues, New York, 1981, Springer-Verlag.
52. Giurintano DJ and Thompson DE: A kinematic model for the flexor tendons of the hand, Proc IEEE/EMBS, Paper 40.330.4, Nov 1987.
53. Goddard R and others: The measurement of stiffness in human joints, Rheological Acta Band S Heft 229, 1969.
54. Goller H, Lewis DW, and McLaughlin RE: Thermographic studies of human skin subjected to localized pressure, Am J Roentgenol Radium Ther Nucl Med 113:749, 1971.
55. Greenhill A: Clinical note: the hand volumeter, Physio Ther Canada 31(1):34, 1979.
56. Harris JR, and Brand PW: Patterns of disintegration of tarsus in anaesthetic foot, J Bone Joint Surg 48B:4, 1966.
57. Hazelton FT and others: The influence of wrist position on the force produced by the finger flexors, J Biomech 8:301, 1975.
58. Kolumban SL: The role of static and dynamic splints: physiotherapy techniques and time in straightening contracted interphalangeal joints, Lepr India 41:323, 1969.

59. Kumar RP and Brandsma JW: A method to determine pressure distribution of the hand, Lep Rev 57:39, 1986.
60. Malcom LL: Frictional and deformational responses of articular cartilage interfaces to static and dynamic loading, doctoral dissertation, La Jolla, CA, 1976, University of California.
61. Mathiowetz V and others: Reliability and validity of grip and pinch strength evaluations, J Hand Surg 9A:222, 1984.
62. Mildenberger LA, Amadio PC, and An KN: Dynamic splinting: systematic approach to the selection of elastic traction, Arch Phys Med Rehab 67:241, 1986.
63. Roberson L and others: Analysis of the physical properties of scomac springs and their potential for use in dynamic splinting, J Hand Ther 1(3):110, 1988.
64. Rouzaud JC and Allieu Y: L'assistant dynamique chiffre par ressort spirale etalonne dans l'orthese de la main, Orthese De La Main 6(3):256, 1987.
65. Rodgers MM and Cavanagh PR: Glossary of biomechanical terms, concepts, and units, J Phys Ther 64(12):1886, 1984.
66. Salter RB and others: The biological effect of continuous passive motion on the healing of full-thickness defects in articular cartilage: an experimental investigation in the rabbit, J Bone Joint Surg 62A(8):1232, 1980.
67. Schneiderwind W: A new method for simultaneously evaluating individual finger function during power grip, master's thesis, Boston, 1972, Boston University.
68. Steno N: Elementorum nyologiae specimen s. musculi descriptio geometrica, 1667. In Maar V, editor: Opera philosophico, Copenhagen, 1910, vol 2 p 108. Quoted in Bastholm, E: The history of muscle physiology, Copenhagen, 1950, Ejnar Munksgaard.
69. Swanson AB: Pathomechanics of deformities in hand and wrist. In Flexible implant resection arthroplasty in the hand and extremities, St. Louis, 1973, The CV Mosby Co.
70. Thompson DE: Mechanical principles. In Fee EE and Philips CA, editors: Hand splinting: principles and methods, ed 2, St. Louis, 1987, The CV Mosby Co.
71. Thompson DE: The effects of mechanical stress on soft tissue. In Levin ME and O'Neal LW, editors: The diabetic food, ed 3, St. Louis, 1988, The CV Mosby Co.
72. Thompson DE and others: Simulating hand surgery: a work in progress, SOMA 2(2):6, 1987.
73. Thompson DE and others: A hand biomechanics workstation, Proc ACM/SIGGRAPH Conference, Atlanta, GA Aug 1988, and ACM Computer Graphics, 1988 (in press).
74. Thompson DE and Hussin HMB: Characteristics of orthotic materials by mechanical impedance method, Proceedings of the 30th ACEMB, Los Angeles, 1977.
75. Thompson DE, Hussein HMB, and Perritt R: Point impedance characterization of soft tissue in vivo, Proceedings of Second International Symposium for Bioengineering of the Skin, Cardiff, Wales, 1979.
76. Waylett J and Seibly D: A study to determine the average deviation accuracy of a commercially available volumeter, J Hand Surg 6:3, 1981.
77. Wright V, Dowson D, and Longfield M: Joint stiffness: its characterization and significance, Biomed Engineering 4:8, 1969.
78. Wright V and Johns R: Quantitative and qualitative analysis of joint stiffness in normal subjects and in patients with connective tissue diseases, Ann Rheum Dis 20:36, 1961.
79. Yamada H: Strength of biological materials. Baltimore, 1970, Williams & Wilkins (Edited by FG Evans).

III
TRAUMA

10

Wound classification and management

William E. Burkhalter

All extremity wounds regardless of the wounding agent have three similarities and differ only in matter of degree. Host tissue injury, contamination by living organisms, and the presence of foreign bodies exist in all wounds. A cleanly incised wound secondary to a knife laceration in a relatively clean hand with a relatively clean knife has limited host injury and minimal contamination with foreign bodies and bacteria. A crush injury in a farmyard environment has widespread severe host injury with considerable foreign bodies and dangerous bacterial contamination. The term *tidy wound* has been applied to the first example, whereas the term *untidy* is definitely applicable to the second. These terms have definite therapeutic implications to the surgeon called on to treat the wounds. The role of the surgeon in wound management is to obtain primary intention wound healing with minimal host tissue reaction.[1] In the tidy wound this should be relatively easy, whereas in the more severe untidy wounds this could be quite complicated.

HISTORY OF INJURY

What tools are available to the surgeon to use in his desire to obtain wound healing with minimal reaction? First, there is the history of injury. A split in the skin of the finger without flexor tendon function may be secondary to a sharp laceration with a knife or secondary to a crush injury. In the first instance, the area of injury is in proximity to the wound tract, and the host injury is highly localized. In the crush injury, the finger has been split open from maximal compression of bone and soft tissue, and the host injury is widespread throughout the entire digit. Was the wound inflicted by a relatively clean knife in a kitchen or in an operating room or was it inflicted by the blade of a knife contaminated by a foreign body or many living organisms? The kitchen knife, though relatively free of pathogenic bacteria, may be contaminated by foreign protein from cutting raw pork or chicken. The blade of a rotary lawn mower is traveling at an extremely high velocity when the wound is inflicted and the wound has the same characteristics as a high-velocity bullet wound. In addition to the velocity of the injury, there is considerable contamination of the wound by living soil organisms and foreign bodies from the ground. So, although the wound is a laceration, it is definitely an untidy wound and one that is prone to develop wound infection without proper management.

By history, then, the treating surgeon can determine to a large extent what he will find when he begins his initial wound management.

WOUND MANAGEMENT

Adequate light, instruments, assistants, and anesthesia are required for all wound management. Tetanus prophylaxis is mandatory, and the use of antibiotics varies with the wound and the surgeon.

Wound management begins with the careful and meticulous preparation of the skin to reduce the foreign bodies and bacterial concentration in the area of the wound. Next, wound exploration under tourniquet ischemia determines the extent of the injury. "Débridement" is a word that means different things to different people, and its definitions vary. Nevertheless, the removal of anything in the wound that is detrimental to wound healing is functional débridement. This may include actual excision of necrotic muscle from a crush injury or a bullet wound; it may include the removal of a visible foreign body and wound irrigation to reduce both the foreign body and bacterial contamination. These are all part of wound débridement. Vital structures such as blood vessels, nerves, and tendons are obviously not excised no matter how badly contaminated but are superficially debrided surgically and copiously irrigated.

Débridement is usually felt to be complete when no visible foreign body or necrotic tissue is present within a wound. At this point, if the wound was secondary to a clean knife laceration with minimal foreign body and necrotic tissue and if only minimal débridement was necessary, the wound cound be simply closed by sutures. Before this, however, repair of deep tissue may be carried out if there was damage. In this type of wound, tendon repairs, nerve repairs, and internal fixation of fractures can be carried out before actual closure of the wound; that is, wound débridement has been followed by repair of deep structures and primary closure of the wound. If, on the other hand, there has been widespread injury as occurs with a bullet wound, crush injury, or rotary lawn mower blade, the amount of host injury is great and located away from the actual wound tract. Widespread host injury plus high concentrations of foreign body and bacteria make the wound prone to infection. The surgery of débridement in this must be extensive, generally requiring additional incisions for exploration and the removal of necrotic tissue and foreign body. In this type of wound, the surgeon is frequently not able to say that his débridement is complete. He may be unable to state exactly what tissue is necrotic. In this situation, primary wound closures should not be carried out. The expectations of wound infection in primary closure of this type of wound is high. Even if frank suppuration does not occur, a highly reactive wound with

A B C

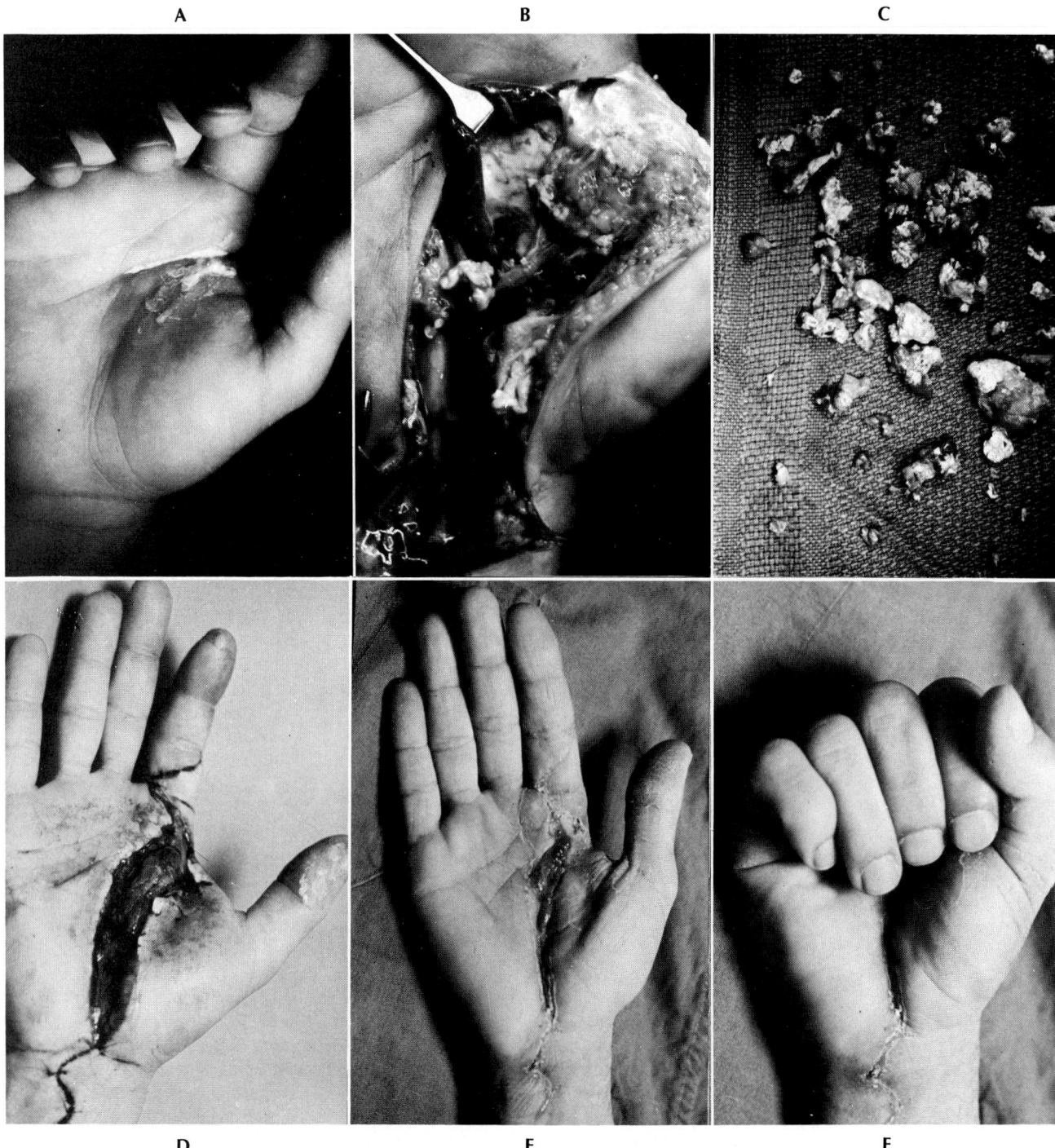

D E F

Fig. 10-1 Patient incurred paint-injection injury to radial aspect of index finger 3 hours before this initial photograph. **A,** Again note diffuse injury with foreign body exuding from injection site. **B,** At exploration and debridement additional incisions were required volarly and dorsally. **C,** Considerable foreign material was removed from palm and digit. **D,** It was believed that wound closure was not indicated because of diffuse injury, residual foreign body, and bacterial contamination. **E** and **F,** Wound gradually closed by secondary intention during which time active use of hand in a light dressing was allowed. Range of motion seen at 3 weeks.

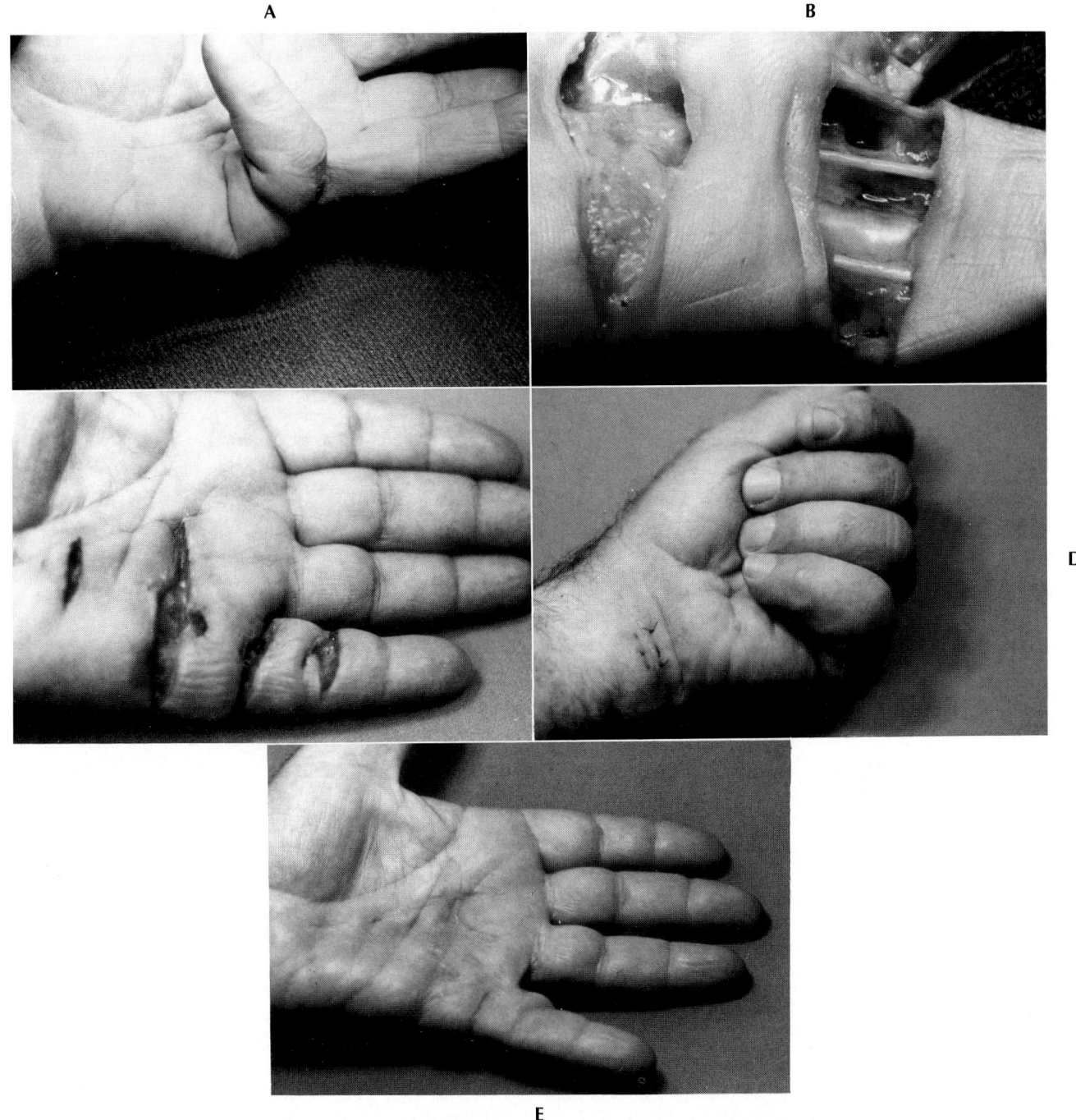

Fig. 10-2   A, A 65-year-old dentist with Dupuytren's contracture of many years involving both MP and PIP joints. **B,** Surgery consisted of releases through multiple transverse incisions in the palm and finger. Note exposure of the digital vessels and nerves even though these structures were open in the base of the wound. There was no real loss of sensibility. **C,** At 10 days the wounds are healing, and the patient has full flexion of his fingers. **D,** Sutures at the wrist were used for exposure of the ulnar nerve for direct injection of xylocaine as an adjunct to the brachial block anesthesia. **E,** At 1 year wounds were well healed, scars are acceptable, and function is full.

considerable edema and redness will persist for many weeks. The wound closure should be delayed.

DELAYED WOUND CLOSURE

Immediately after débridement a dressing should be applied to the open wound and an occlusive hand dressing added to this. Clinically and experimentally it has been shown that delayed primary wound closure of contaminated wounds is more successful than primary closure. The optimum time of wound closure appears to be 4 or 5 days after initial wound surgery.[3,4] Thus 4 to 5 days after the initial wound surgery, the patient is returned to the operating room for wound exploration. At this time, removal of initially questionable tissue can be carried out, and if definite necrosis is seen, further wound irrigation and search for the foreign body are carried out. At this point, wound closure may be accomplished. However, remember that wound closure is an elective surgical operation that should be carried out only when all possible chances for success exist. This second look before wound closure allows the surgeon to evaluate the adequacy of the initial surgery and to redébride if necessary before wound closure. In addition, delayed primary repair of deep structures may also be carried out. Tendons and nerves may be repaired. Fractures may be internally fixed in an environment that has already demonstrated its freedom from necrotic tissue and foreign bodies. In this situation wound healing should occur with minimal tissue reaction.[2]

SECONDARY INTENTION HEALING

In certain wounds, generally the untidy type, wound closure may not be indicated for many days or perhaps it is believed that wound closure is not indicated at all. In this case wound closure occurs by secondary intention healing. Wounds in this category may include burns of the hand and wounds that occur after drainage and débridement of infections. In the latter cases healing by secondary intention is the usual method of management. Sometimes in elective surgery, wound closure by secondary intention healing is chosen by the surgeon. In Dupuytren's contracture, Mc-Cash[5] and many others have written extensively about the excision of the contracting band through transverse incisions in the palm. We have also used the same technique in the fingers with good success. In both cases wound healing by secondary intention is accepted. This is done so that the complications of skin slough, hematoma, and loss of motion are reduced. In all these situations—the hand burn, the postoperative hand infection, and the postoperative Dupuytren's contracture—wound healing occurs by secondary intention. The key to success in all these situations is active motion during wound healing. It has been said many times that allowing a wound of the hand to heal by secondary

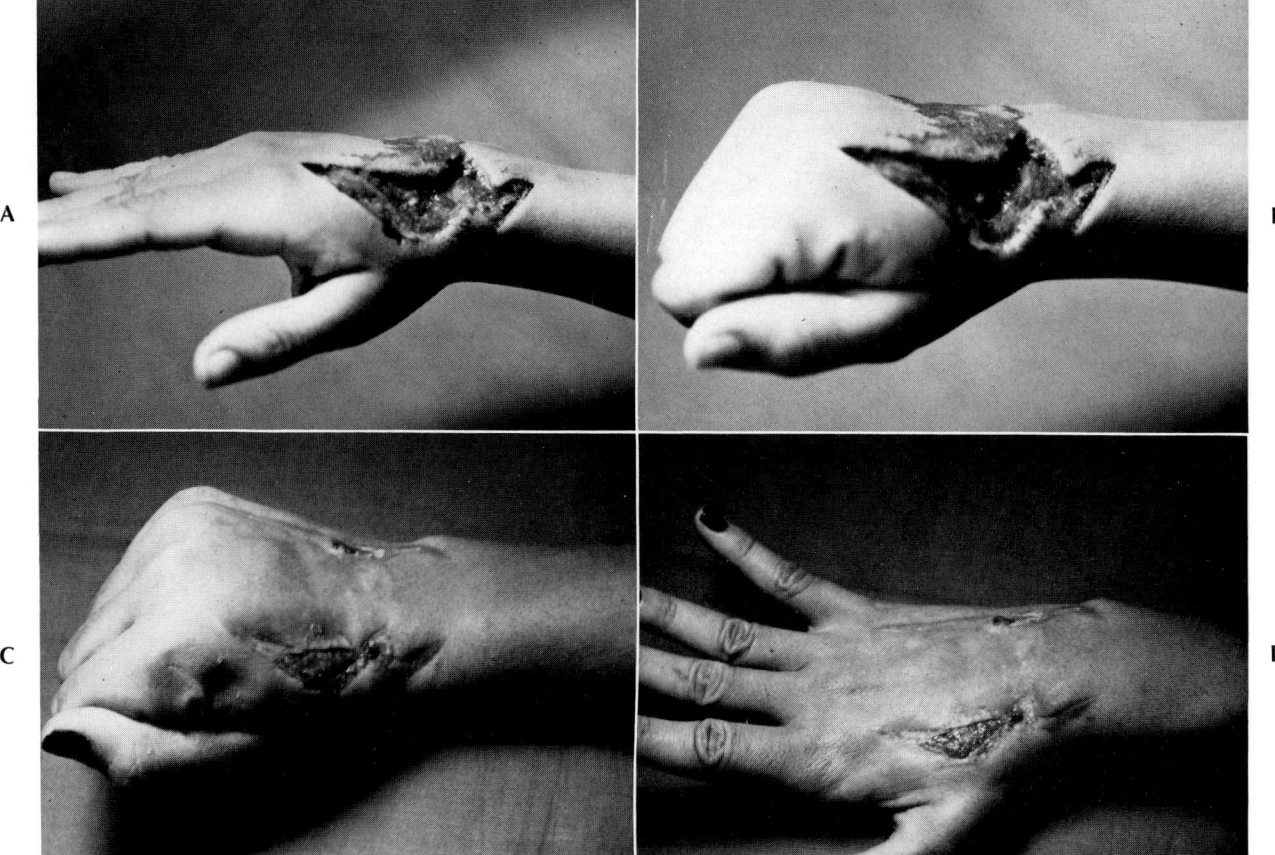

Fig. 10-3   **A** and **B,** Subcutaneous dorsal infection treated by débridement plus early motion. **C** and **D,** Healing progressed while the patient actively exercised the hand.

intention will give extreme stiffness and deformity. Certainly this may be true if there has been actual loss of skin and active motion cannot be instituted because of skeletal instability. However, with active motion, proper splinting, and proper explanation to the patient extremely functional hands can be regained from infections, burns, or Dupuytren's contracture with secondary intention wound healing (Figs. 10-1 and 10-2). Once again, wound closure is an elective procedure that should be carried out when the surgeon believes that the wound will accept closure. It should not be carried out on any rigid time schedule.

If secondary intention wound healing is deemed to be the safest for the patient as a method of obtaining a closed wound, we believe that function must be added as well. As stated before, to allow healing to occur without function is to invite disaster in the form of stiffness. Many times we have heard that immobilization must be maintained until solid wound healing is achieved. This is absolute nonsense and again courts stiffness. Here a question of timing arises. When is function instituted? How early is early function? In the case of the burn patient or the infection or the Dupuytren's patient that we have used before as examples of secondary intention wound healing, we believe that motion should be instituted within 24 to 48 hours of injury or operation. The undamaged structures in the hand will only deteriorate with immobilization and will be caught in the glue that accompanies injury without function. So then, early function is function within 1 to 2 days of accident or surgical insult and this function must take precedence over wound closure. If wound closure and function can be instituted simultaneously, fine, but if the two are the least bit prejudicial, motion and function must be achieved before wound closure whether this be carried out by suture, skin graft, pedicle flap, or secondary intention healing.

Fig. 10-3 shows a dorsal infection of the hand treated by incision and drainage and active motion of the flexors and extensors within 24 hours. Notice that the patient initially had an extensor lag but then gradually regained full motion. To wait for secondary intention wound healing before instituting function would have been to prejudice the ultimate functional recovery of this hand. As is seen, wound healing progressed as function continued to improve. Once again, wound closure is an elective procedure that should be carried out when the surgeon believes that the wound will accept closure. It should not be carried out on any rigid time schedule.

REFERENCES

1. Boyes JH: A philosophy of care of the injured hand, Bull Am Coll Surg 50:341, 1965.
2. Burkhalter W and others: Experiences with delayed primary closure of war wounds of the hand in Viet Nam, J Bone Joint Surg 50A:945, 1968.
3. DeMuth WE Jr and Smith JM: High velocity bullet wounds of muscle and bone: the basis of rational early treatment, J Trauma 6:744, 1966.
4. Lowry KF and Curtis GM: Delayed suture in the management of wounds, analysis of 721 traumatic wounds illustrating the influence of time interval in wound repair, Am J Surg 80:280, 1950.
5. McCash CR: The open palm technique in Dupuytren's contracture, Br J Plast Surg 17:271, 1964.

11

Wound care for the hand patient

Kevin L. Smith

Since the dawn of man, wound care has figured prominently in daily life, religion, and ritual. Man has treated wounds with potions and poisons, nostrums and hokums, and with substances as far ranging as ashes, animal excrement, boiling oil, and salves of earthworms in turpentine added to puppies boiled in oil of lilies.[9] In view of the myriad products on today's market, there is probably no best wound dressing or technique.

Wound management is often an emotional issue, guided more by experience than scientific basis. As long as the dressing material or technique does not harm the wound, healing will occur (given conditions such as sufficient time, adequate state of nutrition, and lack of disease). The purpose of this chapter is to provide an overview of wound management and dressing techniques based on sound biologic principles. With this background, effective dressings can be chosen to facilitate wound healing and, it is hoped, hasten rehabilitation.

The patient with a posttraumatic or postoperative hand wound has problems that are unique to hand surgery. For most wounds, an optimum environment for healing usually requires immobilization, but total immobility can run counter to the successful maintenance of gliding surfaces. The goals of conservative débridement and aggressive therapy are often difficult to balance in the presence of an unstable wound. Although the decision to institute therapy is made with the surgeon, it is necessary for the therapist to be able to diagnose and appropriately treat wounds ranging from clean to dirty.

WOUND HEALING

Whether a wound is incised or excised and regardless of the amount of tissue lost, the four phases of wound healing are the same. During all phases of wound healing, the process can be facilitated by the appropriate choice and application of dressings.

Phase I: inflammatory

The inflammatory phase is the immediate response to injury caused by the release of intracellular materials from damaged cells. These substances cause vasodilation, and they increase the vascular permeability leading to localized tissue edema. Normal blood vessels are not thrombogenic, but damage causes exposure of subendothelial collagen, which stimulates platelet adherence. Platelet agglutination initiates the coagulation sequence, and a clot is formed within injured vessels. Diapedesis then becomes the primary route by which leukocytes and macrophages enter the extravascular space.

Phase II: cellular

Polymorphonuclear leukocytes and macrophages are attracted to the area of injury during the inflammatory phase, and their action begins the cellular or destructive phase. The inflammatory phase lasts 2 to 3 days, at which time the phagocytic cells begin to defend against bacteria and begin the process of repair by clearing necrotic debris, damaged cells, and blood clot. The enzymatic breakdown of cellular debris and increased osmolarity of the local tissue fluid attract more water by osmosis, and further swelling occurs. If the inflammatory phase is reduced by such means as steroid administration or chronic debilitation, this cellular phase is reduced and wound healing is prolonged. In an untidy wound with a large amount of cellular debris or one in which an aggressive infection is ongoing, a prolonged inflammatory phase occurs and the next phase is delayed until the debris is eliminated. This phase can also be lengthened by iatrogenic tissue trauma caused by heavyhanded tissue handling, traumatic therapy, excess suture material, foreign body, or inadequate débridement.[21,29]

Phase III: proliferative

The proliferative or fibroplastic phase of repair lasts from 2 to 6 weeks, depending on the extent of the wound. This phase begins 3 to 5 days after wounding and consists of fibroblastic proliferation, which is accompanied by endothelial budding of new capillary growth. On a framework of fibrin and fibronectin, the fibroblasts begin to lay down collagen on which the fragile capillary buds grow, and together they form granulation tissue. During this period, immobilization helps prevent collagen fiber disruption and consequent delay in the increase in tensile strength of the wound.[21,29]

It is the granulation tissue bed on which epithelial cells migrate in a centripetal fashion, thereby resurfacing the wound with immature "scar" epithelium. This newly formed epithelium is characterized by its lack of dense attachment to an underlying dermis, causing it to be thin and fragile.[21] Traumatic handling during therapy or pressure points from dressings should be avoided. This will lead to blistering and deepithelialization. Epithelialization occurs independent of but usually in concert with contraction. Peacock defines contraction as "an active process which attempts to close a wound in which a loss of tissue has occurred."[21] Contracture on the other hand refers to a result that may or may not be caused by contraction. Contraction proceeds even after epithelial coverage is achieved, but to a lesser degree. The only way to effectively reduce wound contraction is to close the wound (for instance,

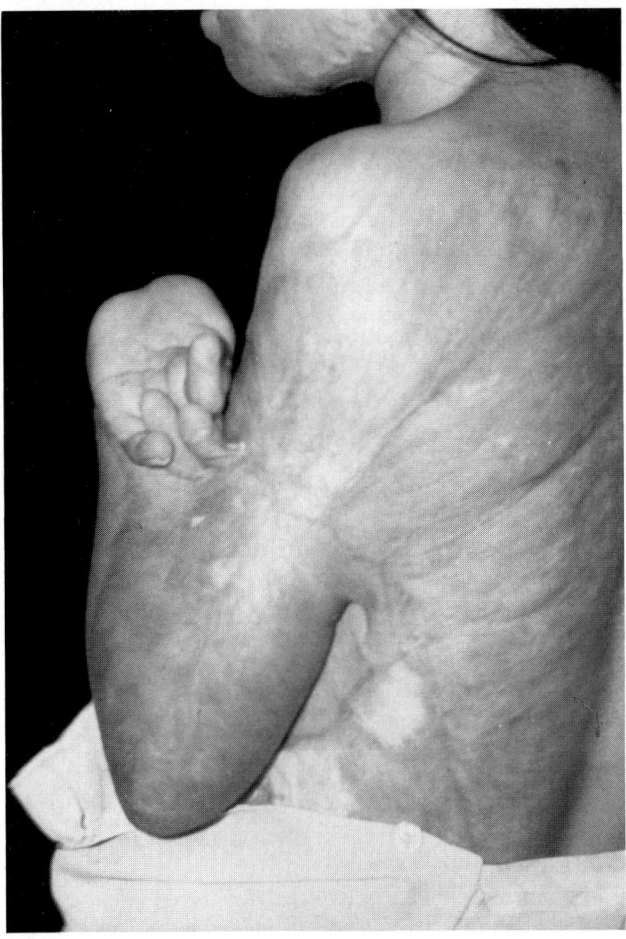

Fig. 11-1 An example of end-stage wound contracture caused by allowing a burn wound to heal without treatment by wound contraction and secondary epithelialization.

by skin graft) and maintain appropriate splinting regimens.[3,14] If coverage is inadequate and splinting is ignored, contracture can reach unreconstructable degrees (Fig. 11-1). The thickness of the skin graft is important. Split-grafted wounds contract 25% more than full-thickness skin-grafted wounds.[24] Therefore the dermis plays the key role in reduction of wound contraction. However, recent studies have shown that Biobrane—a synthetic, temporary, polypeptide-coated, nylon-silicone fabric—when applied to an open wound inhibits contraction as well. The mechanism for this is not elucidated.[7] Skin wounds contract by the stretching of surrounding skin to close the defect and not by the production of new skin.

Phase IV: maturation

The maturation phase continues for as long as 1 year after injury. Tensile strength progressively increases, with approximately 50% of normal tensile strength regained by 6 weeks.[29] Early, the new scar is red, raised, thick, and rigid. Given time, scar maturation proceeds and the scar softens and becomes more pliable and thin.

SURGICALLY CLOSED WOUNDS

In a surgically closed wound, there is minimal debris, and reepithelialization seals the wound by 48 hours.[14] The

basal layer of the epithelial cells at each margin of the wound multiplies and migrates over the defect over a "bridge" provided by accurate dermal approximation.

These wounds are not usually problems for the patient, therapist, or surgeon. Barring the formation of an abscess or marginal tissue necrosis necessitating débridement in a surgically closed wound, minimal dressings are required. For the first 24 hours after surgery, a light gauze dressing moistened with saline serves to absorb wound exudate by capillarity. This leads to a clean wound that is free of crust.[2] On the morning of the first postoperative day, this light dressing can be removed and the wound can safely be washed with mild soap and water without increased wound complications.[20] A light dressing of bland antibiotic ointment, such as Neosporin or Polysporin, can be applied to the wound with or without a light gauze dressing, which will allow better fit of a splint and full potential for range of motion to facilitate hand therapy if it is to be started this early.

THE OPEN WOUND

When the patient with a hand wound is left with an open wound or unstable wound after a surgical procedure or trauma, it is necessary to accurately assess the wound to determine its stage of healing and to prescribe an appropriate dressing.

The evaluation of surface tissue viability is all-important. The wound should be completely undressed, and the presence of necrotic debris, drainage, odor, eschar, or protein coagulum should be noted. The color of the surrounding skin and the presence or absence of granulation tissue in the wound should be appreciated. The warmth of the tissue should be assessed. The sensibility of the tissues should be determined (providing nerve damage has not occurred), because its presence implies viable tissue. An assessment of vascularity should be made by the observation of direct dermal or wound bed bleeding and the "blanch and blush" of capillary refill. The latter can be a deceptive sign, and a comparison should be made with a normal control tissue. Too rapid capillary refill implies venous congestion and that the viability of the tissues may be in jeopardy. Dangerous venous congestion is further indicated by an increased tissue turgor and even a peau d'ange appearance. A sound foundation in the anatomic structures involved is necessary to know what adjacent tissues risk exposure and further injury. This knowledge will guide the aggressiveness with which the wound will be treated.

Débridement

Wound healing will not progress in the presence of active infection or excessive necrotic debris. Any open wound needs to be kept meticulously free of dead material and exudate to facilitate healing. This can be accomplished by any one of several means.

A "natural dressing," such as a scab, which is made of dried blood and protein coagulum, or an eschar, which is a thick covering of denatured collagen, is protective and can be left in place and the wounds treated by this "exposure" method. As the epithelium migrating from the wound margins separates the scab or eschar aided by elaboration of collagenases, the scab or eschar can be trimmed. As long as there is no drainage or purulent liquefaction below the

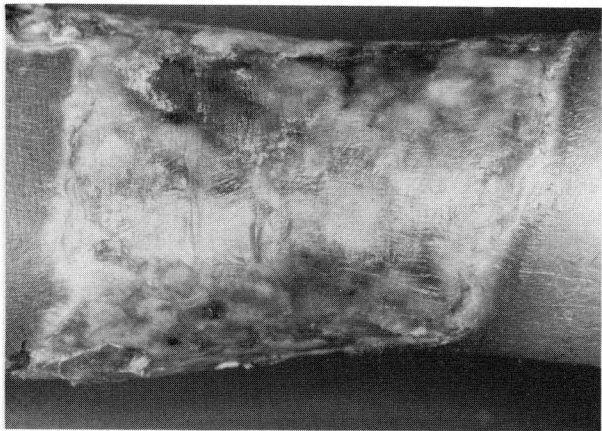

Fig. 11-2 This full-thickness burn shows an overlying eschar, which is made up of denatured collagen and protein coagulum. Providing this remains clean and devoid of infection and subeschar liquefaction, this eschar can be maintained as a dressing using the "open treatment" technique. At first sign of eschar separation or infection, this eschar should be debrided and the wound treated with wet dressings until the wound is sufficiently clean to progress to a three-layered, nonadherent, clean wound dressing.

eschar, this method is suitable. If this occurs, débridement is mandatory (Fig. 11-2).

Adherent eschar or large patches of necrotic material must be mechanically debrided, using fine forceps and sharp scissors or a knife blade. Hydrotherapy or wet dressings can soften this debris and ease its removal. It must be remembered that the débridement is generally not painful to the patient, because only the nonviable tissue is excised. When the wound is filled with numerous small patches of necrotic debris, mechanical débridement with forceps and scissors can be tedious. In this case, frequent wet dressings, by their adherence to the debris and wick action, can effectively remove these smaller fragments (Fig. 11-3).

In the hand wound, it is not uncommon to see tendons exposed. A single exception to the rule of aggressive débridement of nonviable tissue exists when tendons are considered. Even though a tendon may be devitalized by the loss of its peritenon, if it is protected and not allowed to dessicate, the stability of the collagen matrix remains and this devitalized tendon can serve in much the same manner as a tendon graft. If the wound is treated and closed with the devitalized tendon placed beneath adequate skin and soft tissue, ultimately the tendon will be cellularized and have the potential for good function[21] (Fig. 11-4).

Separation of eschars, scabs, or fibrinous coagulum can also be hastened by commercially available proteolytic enzyme ointments, such as Travase (Flint Pharmaceuticals—bacillus subtilis protease) and Elase (Parke-Davis Pharmaceuticals—fibrinolysin and desoxyribonuclease). These are useful for short-term use to hydrolyze the protein-rich fibrinous coagulum found on many draining wounds. Although these enzymes may interfere with leukocyte phagocytosis, they do not appear to interfere with wound healing.[23] Some have even suggested that these enzymes spare viable tissue.[8,32] I suggest that these enzyme preparations should be used sparingly and only after the evaluation of the char-

acter of the wound debris before each use. These preparations are sometimes painful to the patient on application and can cause a burning sensation. Their action seems to be facilitated by their application under an occlusive dressing.

Bacteria and wound infection

The presence of bacteria can be demonstrated in any open wound, and sterilization of the wound can be achieved only by closure—not drugs or dressings. The factors that determine clinical infection are the number of bacteria, their virulence, and host resistance. Resistance relates to systemic factors as well as local factors, such as amounts of wound debris, foreign body, and compromised tissue. Quantitative tissue cultures, the bacterial count per gram of sampled tissue, are necessary to determine infection. It is considered a clinical infection if the concentration of bacteria is greater than 10^5 per gram. If closure is attempted with bacteria counts greater than 10^5, it is likely to fail, especially if the organism is *Staphylococcus* or *Pseudomonas*. Most organisms can be reduced in number by adequate débridement and an effective dressing regimen. Occasionally the topical application of antimicrobial or antiseptic agents is useful. The exception to this is for β-hemolytic streptococcus, which produces wound lysins: streptokinase and streptodornase. This organism must be eliminated before wound closure, and fortunately *Streptococcus* is very sensitive to systemic penicillin.[17,30]

WOUND DRESSING
Functions of a dressing

When a dressing is prescribed for a patient, there are many factors that are considered, including the patient, the wound, and the goals of treatment. In all cases, the dressing should adhere to basic criterion and can then be adjusted to meet the specific needs of each patient (see Box below). The ideal dressing should be designed to *protect* the wound from the external environment, isolating it from trauma, exogenous bacteria, and temperature changes in the environment. By being *supportive*, the dressing immobilizes the wound, which facilitates wound healing. Motion, by disruption of immature fibrin scaffolding and capillary budding, increases inflammation and ultimately increases scarring and extends the wound-healing process.[2] In the treat-

---

A dressing should:

Be protective
Be supportive but not restrictive
Control the microenvironment
Be nontoxic
Provide comfort
Serve aesthetic and symbolic function

A dressing may:

Absorb
Debride
Apply topical medicaments
Be adherent or nonadherent
Be wet or dry
Be compressive

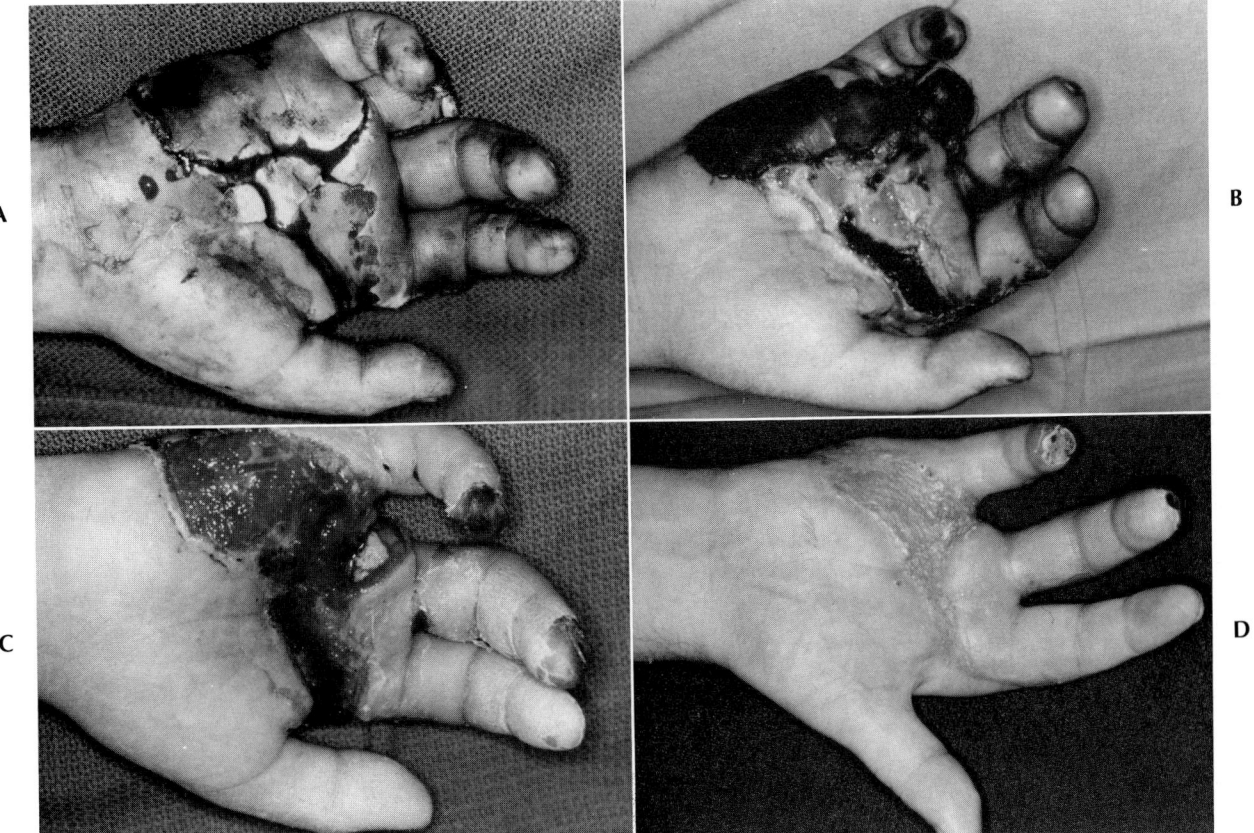

Fig. 11-3   **A,** Printing press crush with extensive soft tissue injury before the first débridement. **B,** Five days later, "second look" débridement necessitates a fourth ray amputation. **C,** After 10 days of wet dressings allowing aggressive hand therapy, the granulating bed of the wound and marginal epithelial migration denotes readiness for closure with skin graft. **D,** Six weeks after injury the wounds are healed with skin graft. Hand therapy was suspended only during the initial five days after skin grafting.

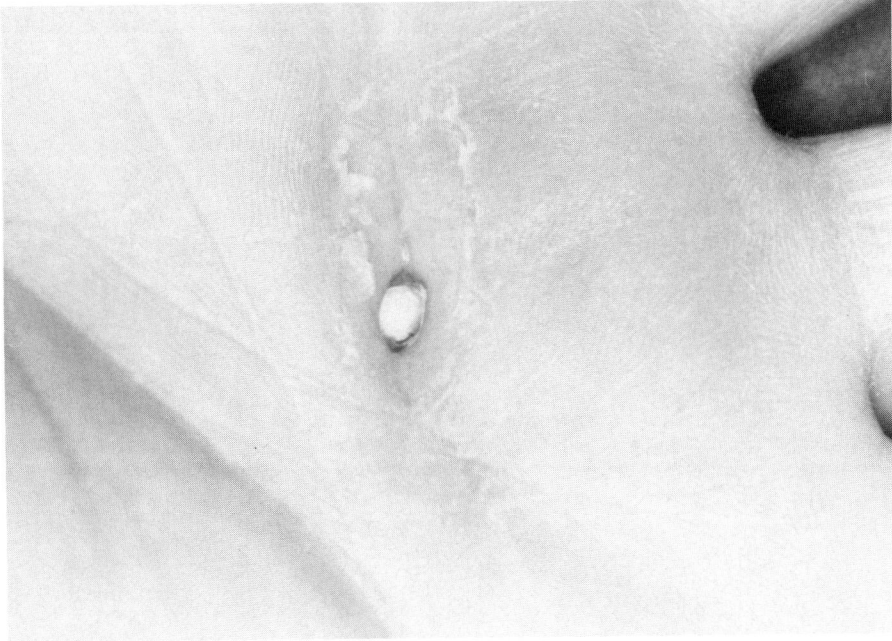

Fig. 11-4   Some wounds such as this, an exposed superficialis tendon following trigger finger release, will heal spontaneously, providing the wound is not allowed to dessicate. This exposed tendon is best managed by continuous wet dressings until closure is obtained. In this case the wound closed in 14 days.

ment of the hand, splinting becomes an integral part of wound immobilization and support. The dressing for the hand should be designed to immobilize the wound and provide protective positioning in whatever position is dictated by the injury. This dressing should also be nonrestrictive to allow motion in the noninjured portions of the hand.

The ideal dressing can *control the microenvironment* of the wound. Healing proceeds best in a moist environment.[4] A drying wound will extend tissue damage, and the resultant denatured collagen and dessicated protein coagulum will create an impermeable scab, which will retard epithelialization. The epithelialization will be forced to proceed at a deeper level at the junction of the live tissue with the dead. A moist environment also allows gaseous exchange, which is necessary to maintain Po_2 and a pH at optimum levels.[27] By the hydrostatic characteristics of the dressings, the level of moisture can be controlled. Too wet an environment will cause maceration and possibly enhance bacterial proliferation.[19] Too dry an environment will encourage further tissue loss caused by dessication.

The ideal dressing provides *comfort* during its application and removal and when it is in place. It also provides the *psychologic purpose* of reminding the patient he has a wound and reporting the same to the people he contacts. A dressing also serves to cover, aesthetically, a highly visible wound to decrease associated anxiety. An expertly applied dressing also can increase the confidence a patient has in those who are caring for him. Most important, the dressing *should do no harm* to the wound and should not impede the healing process.

Special wounds and dressing requirements

After the nature of a wound is assessed, the dressing is prescribed accordingly. A dressing may need to be *absorptive* for use on the secreting or draining wound. It may be designed to *debride* the wound or apply topical medicaments, or both. It may be *adherent or nonadherent* or *wet or dry*. The dressing may be designed to be *compressive* to help minimize scar volume.[6,19]

As a wound progresses through the healing process, the

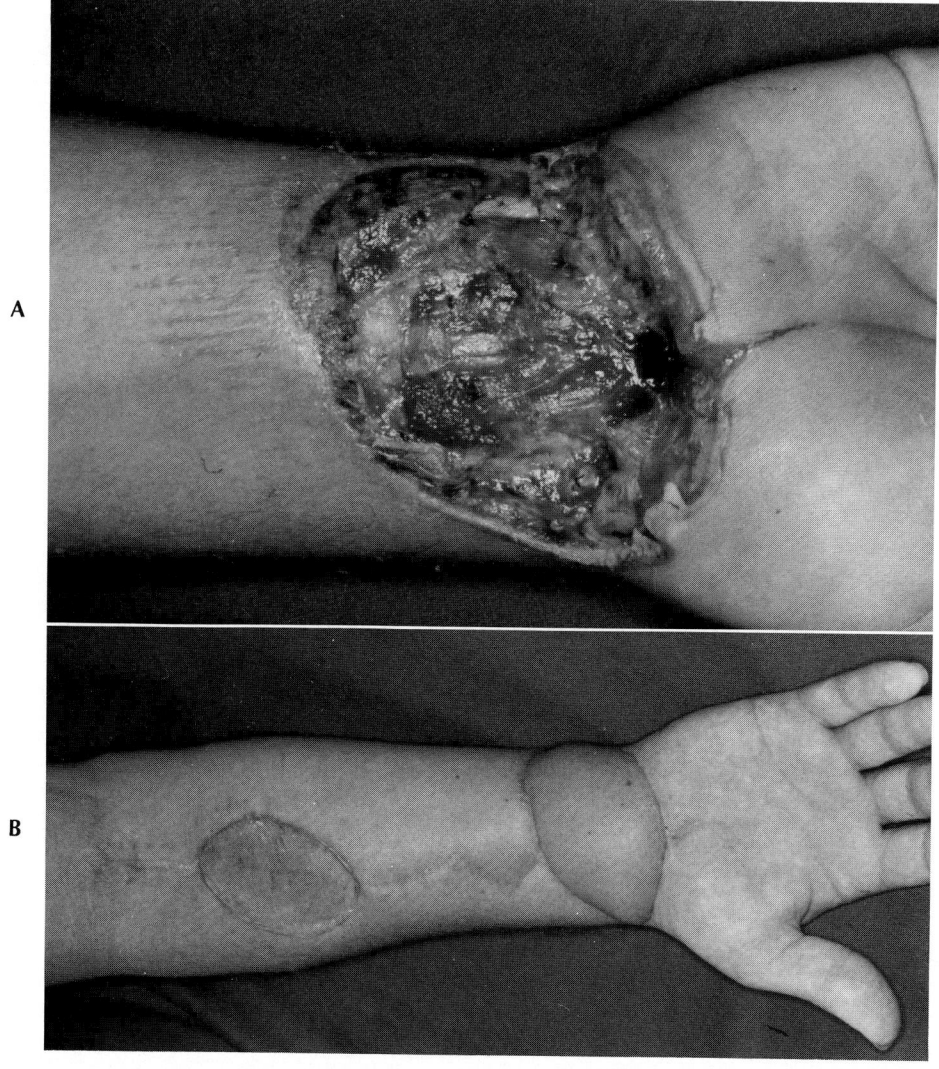

Fig. 11-5   A, This 55-year-old man sustained a hot roller crush/burn to his right wrist. Three weeks following injury there are exposed tendons and nerves and a dirty, infected wound bed. **B,** Two days following débridement and wet dressings every 4 hours, a distally based radial forearm flap is applied to allow healing by first intention.

method of dressing should change according to the requirements of the wound. One dressing style will not be sufficient for the entire healing phase.

The dirty or infected wound

The dirty or infected wound (Fig. 11-5) is first treated by adequate surgical débridement. Then dressings are applied with the intention of hastening further removal of necrotic debris or drainage. In this instance, personal preference and tradition have frequently dictated which dressing is used. A *dry dressing* of wide mesh gauze (standard 4 × 4s) is absorptive and serves to remove the transudate or exudate from the wound. Also this dressing will adhere to loose necrotic debris, which is then removed with the dressing. Frequency of dressing changes is determined by the amount of drainage and debris and should be performed before the dressing is saturated. The usual interval of dressing change is about every 4 to 6 hours. Disadvantages of the dry (dry to dry) dressings are the pain they create with removal, the possibility that they may cause dessication and worsen the wound, and, last, that viable cells may be removed and fragile healing epithelium damaged with the dressing changes.[19]

Wet dressings can be used and are an effective means of softening adherent crusts and debris. The wet wide mesh gauze has greater capillarity than dry dressings[18] and can enhance the removal of wound drainage. There is less adherence of the dressing to the wound, and consequently less pain is caused with its removal, but this affords relatively less debriding action than dry dressings. A moist physiologic environment provided by a wet dressing encourages reepithelialization,[31] and the topical application of gentle heat or cold over the dressing is better transmitted to the wound. These dressings should be changed frequently (every 2 to 4 hours) and can be kept wet with a variety of solutions—the best being lactated Ringer's solution warmed to body temperature. The wet dressing can also be saturated with topical medicaments to provide bacteriostatic or bactericidal action.[19]

Although wet dressings provide a moist physiologic environment for healing, bacteria can flourish in this situation, complicating healing. Also, the constantly wet dressing may macerate intact skin and thus effect an unwanted keratolytic action.

Topical medicaments in the wet dressing

A decided advantage of the wet dressing technique is the ability to apply topical antibiotics or nonspecific antimicrobial solutions directly to the wound surface. Most solutions in use today are efficacious bacteriocidal agents, but recent studies have shown that many have significant cytotoxic properties in commonly used concentrations.[10–12,28]

These solutions should be applied at frequent intervals (at least every 4 hours) to keep the dressing wet. If the wound has little exudate and the dressing remains clean, the dressing need not be changed each time it is moistened. Care must be taken to avoid the drying of these dressings, because evaporation can yield medicament concentrations that are toxic. Occlusive overwraps, such as Saran, can be helpful to prevent evaporation.

The choice of topical antibiotics should be governed by specific wound cultures, and antibiotics, which are rarely given systemically, should be used to avoid the risk of compromising further parenteral therapy. Preference should be given to those drugs that have been shown to be effective, such as neomycin, kanamycin, cephaloridine, and bacitracin (penicillin, ampicillin, and cephalothin are possibly effective). These drugs should be used in concentrations 2 to 4 times the minimum inhibitory concentration (MIC).[22,26]

Nonspecific antimicrobials such as 1% povidone-iodine (Betadine), 0.5% sodium hypochlorite (Dakin's solution), 0.25% acetic acid, and 3% hydrogen peroxide, can all be toxic to some degree at full strength. Of these, there was *no* bactericidal concentration of acetic acid, hydrogen peroxide, or sodium hypochlorite that was not cytotoxic.[10,12] Therefore it is recommended that these solutions be abandoned for dressing care. Though 1% povidone-iodine did not appear to disturb the normal wound healing process,[28] fibroblast toxicity was apparent until dilutions of .001% (1:1000)—a level at which bactericidal activity was maintained.[12]

The wet to dry dressing

A combination of these two dressing techniques is the commonly used "wet to dry" dressing. The same wide mesh gauze is placed on the dirty wound and is applied wet. The dressing is then allowed to dry. The wick action pulls necrotic material, exudate, or transudate into the gauze, which is removed with the gauze during dressing changes every 4 to 6 hours. Unfortunately, the débridement is indiscriminate, and healthy granulation and immature epithelium is removed with the dressing, causing pain, bleeding, and damage to the wound.[19] This technique is perhaps the most widely used dressing technique, and though it is effective in debriding a dirty wound, it is not surpassed by careful surgical débridement and a wet dressing regimen.

Wound packing

Packing of a wound is indicated when the wound has significant dead space and the superficial portions of the wound need to be kept open while the deeper recesses are allowed to contract. The packing must be in contact with all wound edges, and the wound cavity should not be packed too tightly. A tight packing will retard drainage, create tissue ischemia, and cause the wound to behave in a similar fashion as the abscess that created it.

Many materials can be used in wound packing, the most common being wide mesh gauze, such as 4 × 4s or Kling, or fine mesh strip gauze commercially available as Nugauze. Rarely, however, does a hand wound require packing, and generally the aforementioned dressings will suffice.

Use of topical creams and ointments

Aside from simple suture line care, there are a few special instances where topical creams—primarily silver sulfadiazine—have been useful. Generally, the cream is placed on the wound directly and then covered with gauze wraps to hold it in place. For burns of the hand, the wounds are coated with silver sulfadiazine and then the hand is placed within an appropriately sized plastic bag (10 × 18 inches) (Fig. 11-6). Motion is then encouraged, and hand therapy is instituted immediately. The patient is encouraged to manage his own activities of daily living and is kept out of any protective splinting during times of exercise, meals, and

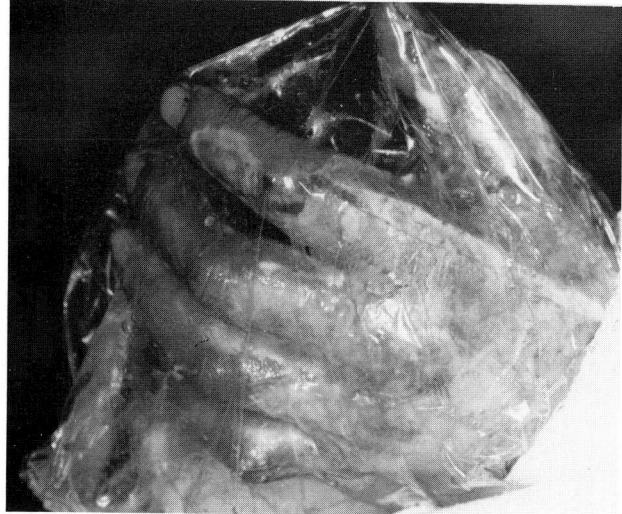

Fig. 11-6   This acutely burned hand has been placed in a plastic bag dressing with silver sulfadiazine following initial débridement and escharotomy. This allows close application of the protective positional splint and also allows the hand to be used for activities of daily living. The dressing is comfortable and does not interfere with hand therapy.

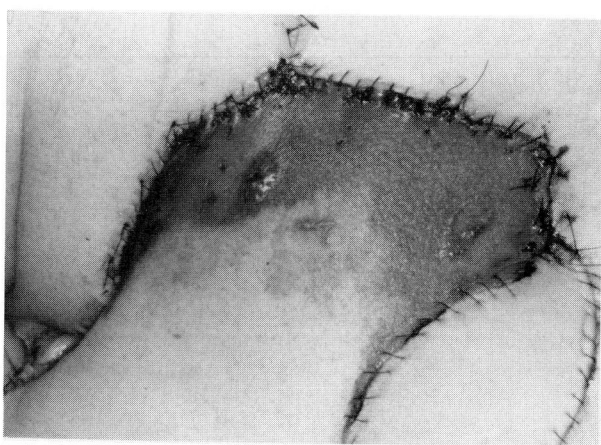

Fig. 11-7   Pedicle flap clearly showing ischemic changes in its distal margin with a clear line of demarcation marked by deep blue coloration and early epidermolysis. Just proximal to the line of demarcation, venous congestion with too brisk capillary refill and slow bleeding can be seen. Experience has shown that a flap such as this can be partially salvaged by the application of topical dressings (silver sulfadiazine). Experiments have shown that this is likely to be because of the dressing being occlusive.[33]

hygiene. The hand is fitted for proper splints while in the plastic bag "dressing," thereby allowing closer fit without the interference of bulky dressings.[1,25] Of interest, commercially available plastic bags are sterile as a result of the manufacturing process and require no further preparation off the shelf.[15,25]

Topical silver sulfadiazine has also been used in attempts to salvage some or all portions of "questionable" flaps (Fig. 11-7). Treatment of the compromised margin of the flaps with topical antibacterial creams applied under dry gauze twice daily reduced the depth of tissue loss and consequently increased the surviving length of experimental flaps. This dressing regimen seemed to improve survival by the prevention of dessication and not by the inherent augmentation of vascularity. Although bacterial counts were three logarithms higher in flaps treated with only inactive vehicles, there was no appreciable difference in survival between flaps treated with topical antibiotic and not.[16] I continue to use Silvadene dressings as a last resort for compromised flaps, under the assumption that a three-logarithm decrease in bacterial load may decrease potential wound complications associated with flap failure.

The clean open wound

The distinguishing feature of a clean open wound is that it demonstrates a uniform presence of flat, healthy granulation tissue with evidence of epithelial proliferation and migration at the wound margin (Fig. 11-8). A wound such as this requires a different dressing than does the dirty or infected wound. This dressing should most of all be *nonadherent* and designed to maintain a moist environment for healing (Fig. 11-9).

The dressing for the clean wound starts with a contact layer. This layer determines how the dressing will interact with the wound. The contact layer must be sterile, it must

contact all surfaces of the wound by conforming to its contours, and there must be no gaps to allow collections of serum, blood, or pus to form. The nonadherent contact layer should be of gauze mesh sufficiently fine to prevent the growth of granulations within the interstices but open enough to allow drainage to pass through into the overlying absorbent layer of the dressing. This layer must also be occlusive. Though occlusion—partial or complete—has decreased wound pain and promoted reepithelialization, there is the theoretic potential of increased maceration and infection.[5] In general, occlusive dressings are used only in those clean superficial wounds with little or no drainage in which healing by reepithelialization is expected. Examples of these wounds are the superficial burn and the skin graft

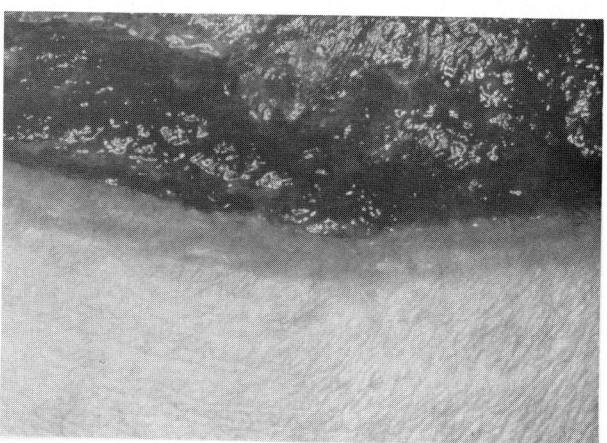

Fig. 11-8   Clean, open wound revealing a uniform bed of granulation tissue with an advancing epithelial margin at the skin/wound junction.

donor site. Even in these wounds, a malodorous exudate (pus) can collect beneath the occlusive dressing, but this is not clinical infection and does not slow the healing process.[5] The comparative increased healing rates shown by wounds under occlusive dressings may be a result of their more efficient prevention of secondary wound dessication.[13]

The choice of a nonadherent contact layer is dictated by the character of the wound drainage. If the wound has little or no drainage, this layer need only be *nonadherent.* If moderate drainage exists, the contact layer must allow the passage of some of the fluid into the overlying absorptive

dressing. Most medicated dressings are made by impregnating fine mesh rayon or cotton gauze, and common examples are Vaseline gauze, Xeroform, scarlet red, and Adaptic. Other nonadherent dressings combine a permeable or perforated polymeric film, which allows immediate strike through and an absorptive intermediate layer. Examples of these products are Telfa, Exudry, and Dermasel. Of the above, Xeroform, Vaseline gauze, and scarlet red tend to allow less drainage, and wound maceration is more likely in a heavily draining wound.

The central or intermediate layer in the dressing for a

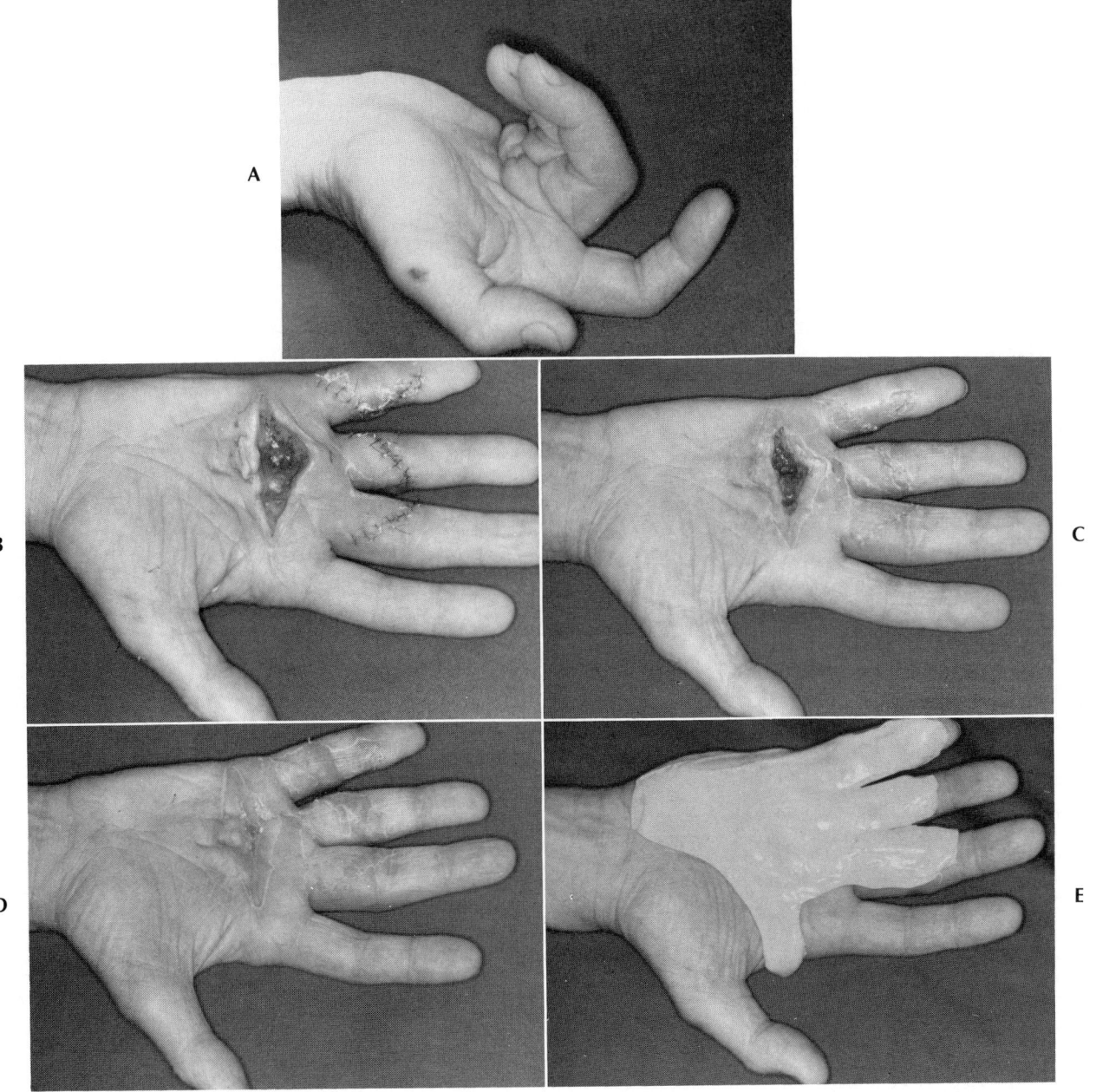

Fig. 11-9 **A,** Sixty-seven-year-old patient with Dupuytren's contracture. **B,** Three days after release using open technique. **C,** This clean open wound is managed with Xeroform, fluff gauze, and Kling wraps with range-of-motion therapy four times daily and continuous splinting in extension. **D,** Twenty-two days after surgery the wound is closed and splinting is reduced to nighttime only in extension. **E,** Compression is applied to the wound and is directed by using silastic 382 medical grade Elastomer (Dow Corning Corp., Midland, Mich.) with continued extension splinting at night.

clean wound is *absorptive* to the degree necessary for the wound. This layer is also *protective and supportive*. It is commonly "fluffed" gauze, mechanics waste, or cotton or dacron batting. This is changed as often as is necessary before saturation. Improved wicking is achieved if the material (most frequently, wide mesh gauze 4 × 4s) is applied moist. Antibiotics or antimicrobials can be effectively used in this layer.

The final layer of a dressing for the clean wound binds the dressing and holds it in place. This layer may incorporate a rigid splint or may be elastic. In either case it stabilizes the dressing and the underlying wound.

SUMMARY

This chapter has summarized basic dressing principles and has described dressings useful in many types of wounds. The injured hand presents unique problems to the surgeon and therapist that are different from wound problems in other areas of the body. Optimum care requires a coordinated effort among the surgeon, therapist, and patient to yield a maximally functioning hand with a healed wound.

After initial assessment of the patient with an open hand wound, the surgeon will either close the wound or apply the first dressing. For a severely injured hand, the patient frequently must be returned to the operating room for a "second look" to assess the viability of compromised tissues left during the initial conservative débridement. The patient is then referred to the hand therapist where the decision regarding appropriate dressing is made by the surgeon and therapist. If the wound is open and in need of débridement, wet dressings are prescribed. When the wound is sufficiently debrided by surgery or these dressings, the dressing is advanced to the three-layer nonadherent clean wound dressing. This is maintained until healing is completed by secondary intention or until the wound is closed by skin graft, flap, or delayed primary techniques. As long as the wound is maintained stable during the entire period that the hand is dressed, therapy can proceed and will not delay wound healing.

The open wound should not therefore cause a delay in therapy, and wound dressing is an important part of the care of the patient from injury to complete rehabilitation.

REFERENCES

1. Beasley RW: Hand injuries, Philadelphia, 1981, WB Saunders Co.
2. Brody GS: Dressings, splints and casts. In Goldwyn RM, editor: The unfavorable result in plastic surgery: avoidance and treatment, ed 2, vol 1, Boston, 1984, Little, Brown & Co, Inc.
3. Donoff RB and Grillo HC: The effects of skin grafting on healing open wounds in rabbits, J Surg Res 19:163, 1975.
4. Eaglestein WH: The effect of occlusive dressings on collagen synthesis and re-epithelialization in superficial wounds. In Ryan TJ, editor: An environment for healing: the role of occlusion, London, 1984, Royal Society of Medicine.
5. Eaglestein WH, Mertz PM, and Falanga V: Occlusive dressings, Am Fam Physician 35(3):211, 1987.
6. Finley JM: Practical wound management: a manual of dressings, Chicago, 1981, Yearbook Medical Publishers, Inc.
7. Frank DH and Bonaldi LC: Inhibition of wound contraction: comparison of full-thickness skin grafts, Biobraine, and aspartate membranes, Ann Plast Surg 14(2):103, 1985.
8. Harmel RP, Vane DP, and King DR: Burn care in children: special considerations, Clin Plast Surg 13(1):95, 1986.
9. Knight B: The history of wound treatment. In Westaby S, editor: Wound care, London, 1985, William Heinemann Medical Books, Ltd.
10. Kozol RA, Gillies C, and Elgebaly SA: Effects of sodium hypochlorite (Dakin's solution) on cells of the wound module, Arch Surg 123:420, 1988.
11. Lineweaver W and others: Antimicrobial toxicity, Arch Surg 120:267, 1985.
12. Lineweaver W and others: Cellular and bacterial toxicities of topical antimicrobials, Plast Reconstr Surg 75(3):394, 1985.
13. Linsky CB, Rovee DT, and Dow T: Effects of dressings on wound inflammation and scar tissue. In Hildick-Smith G, editor: The surgical wound, Philadelphia, 1981, Lea & Febiger.
14. Madden JW: Wound healing: biological and clinical features. In Sabiston DC Jr, editor: Davis-Christopher textbook of surgery: the biological basis of modern surgical practice, Philadelphia, 1977, WB Saunders Co.
15. Matthews DC: Unpublished observations, 1982.
16. McGrath MH: How topical dressings salvage "questionable" flaps: experimental study, Plast Reconstr Surg 67(5):653, 1981.
17. McKinney P and Cunningham BL: Handbook of plastic surgery, Baltimore, 1981, Williams & Wilkins.
18. Noe JM & Kalish S: The mechanisms of capillarity in surgical dressings, Surg Gynecol Obstet 143:454, 1976.
19. Noe JM and Kalish S: Dressing materials and their selection. In Rudolph R and Noe JM, editors: Chronic problem wounds, Boston, 1983, Little, Brown, & Co.
20. Noe JM and Keller M: Can stitches get wet? Plast Reconstr Surg 81(1):82, 1988.
21. Peacock EE Jr: Wound repair, ed 3, Philadelphia, 1984, WB Saunders Co.
22. Polk HC and Finn MP: Chemoprophylaxis and immunoprophylaxis in surgical wound infection. In Simmons RL and Howard RJ, editors: Surgical infectious disease, New York, 1982, Appleton-Century-Crofts.
23. Rodeheaver G and others: Side-effects of topical proteolytic enzyme treatment, Surg Gynecol Obstet 148:562, 1979.
24. Sawhney CP and Monga HL: Wound contraction in rabbits and the effectiveness of skin grafts in preventing it, Br J Plast Surg 23(4):318, 1970.
25. Slater RM and Hughes NC: A simplified method of treating burns of the hands, Br J Plast Surg 24(3):396, 1971.
26. Tobin GR: The compromised bed technique: an improved method for skin grafting problem wounds, Surg Clin North Am 64(4):653, 1984.
27. Turner TD: Which dressing and why? In Westaby S, editor: Wound care, London, 1985, William Heinemann Medical Books, Ltd.
28. Viljanto J: Disinfection of surgical wounds without inhibition of normal wound healing, Arch Surg 115:253, 1980.
29. Westaby S: Fundamentals of wound healing. In Westaby S, editor: Wound care, London, 1985, William Heinemann Medical Books, Ltd.
30. Westaby S and White S: Wound infection. In Westaby S, editor: Wound care, London, 1985, William Heinemann Medical Books, Ltd.
31. Wheeland RG: The newer surgical dressings and wound healing, Dermatol Clin 5(2):393, 1987.
32. Zawacki BE: The effect of Travase on heat injured skin, Surgery 77:132, 1975.

12

Wound healing: the biological basis of hand surgery

John W. Madden

In order to manipulate our environment effectively, the hand performs feats which, on superficial analysis, seem incompatible. The hand changes shape in thousands of subtle ways, adapting physical configuration to the requirements of the moment. Equally important, however, the hand becomes a stable transmitter of powerful forces on demand. This unique combination of strength, movement, and stability is inherent in the anatomic configurations of epidermal and mesenchymal tissues that comprise the hand. Almost all hand structures are dense connective tissues, the strongest of animal products. Movement is achieved by allowing architectural components to move relative to one another. Stability is obtained by arranging periarticular structures to allow movement in one plane and to resist movement in another, or by adding forces to create stability through active muscle contraction. Thus the key to normal hand function is the ability of strong, dense connective tissue structures to glide relative to one another.

Gliding depends on precise placement of blood vessels, fascial septa, areolar tissue, tendons, ligaments, and fascial sheaths. The physical properties of all normal hand structures are adapted to gliding. Any alteration in macroscopic anatomy that changes the physical characteristics or anatomic arrangement of tissues prevents relative gliding and reduces hand functions significantly. Because the basic reaction of tissue to injury alters physical properties by replacing normal structures with scar, a thorough understanding of wound healing reactions and scar formation forms the biologic foundation on which hand surgery rests.

SCAR FORMATION

The normal anatomic events occurring during the early phases of wound healing are familiar to most surgeons and will be reviewed only briefly. Within minutes after planned or accidental tissue disruption, the wound space fills with clotted blood. Within hours, a typical acute inflammatory response is well established: marked vasodilation occurs with accompanying local edema, white blood cells migrate through the walls of blood vessels, and fixed tissue macrophages become actively mobile. The initial cell population is predominantly polymorphonuclear leukocytes. Within a few days, however, monocytic macrophages become the most frequently encountered cell type. The removal of dead tissue fragments and foreign bodies, including bacteria, by

Reprinted with permission from *Clinics in Plastic Surgery*, vol. 3, no. 1, Jan. 1976. The author's work reported in this article supported by National Institute of Arthritis, Metabolism, and Digestive Diseases, Grant No. AM14047, National Institutes of Health, Bethesda, Maryland.

phagocytic cells seems an obligatory part of the wound-healing process. Recent data suggest that late stages of wound healing can be influenced significantly by the effectiveness of cellular phagocytosis.[28] If tissues are incised sharply and reapproximated quickly with minimal tissue damage, the inflammatory phase of wound healing is completed within a few days. If tissues are damaged significantly or if the wound becomes contaminated with bacteria, the inflammatory phase can last indefinitely.

As the inflammatory response evolves in the deeper portions of the wound, significant events occur at the wound surface. Epithelial cells along the margins of skin wounds begin to undergo dramatic changes within hours of injury. Fixed basal cells at the wound edge begin migrating down and across the surface, using fibrin strands as walkways.[50] Within 48 hours, cleanly incised, sutured wounds are completely epithelialized. Over several weeks, the epithelial surface becomes multilayered, thickens, and the restoration of the epithelial surface is obvious to the naked eye.

Within the first 72 hours, spindle-shaped cells associated with small blood vessels in the periphery of the wound begin to divide, and daughter cells invade the wound space.[49] By the end of the first week, this new cell type, the fibroblast, begins replacing the macrophage as the most frequent cell type. By the second week, the wound space is completely filled by these actively metabolizing cells. As fibroblasts migrate into the wound space, small blood vessels proximal to the area of injury begin to bud and growing capillaries follow the migration. Although collagen fibers comprise the majority of the mature scar, fibers cannot be visualized by the light microscope until the fourth or fifth day following injury. Once fibers appear, however, collagen accumulates in the wound rapidly. Thus, by the end of the second week, the wound is filled with a rich capillary network, large numbers of fibroblasts, and a moderate number of newly synthesized collagen fibers.

Morphologic changes occurring during the early phases of healing are dramatic and rapid. From a physiologic point of view, changes occurring after the second or third week are equally dramatic, but morphology changes at a more leisurely pace. From the third to the sixth week after injury, the number of fibroblasts and blood vessels within the wound space diminishes slowly. As the cell population decreases, scar collagen fibers increase. Gradually, the wound changes from predominantly cellular structure to a predominantly extracellular tissue. Because morphology changes so slowly during later stages, many biologists have been lulled into feeling that wound healing begins abruptly and ends within 1 month of injury. Nothing could be farther from the truth.

Scars remain metabolically active for years, slowly changing in size, shape, color, texture, and strength.

Although wounds become stronger with time, gain in strength follows a sequence of time, gain in strenght follows a sequence of physical changes not reflected precisely in macroscopic appearance. Because hand function ultimately depends on the physical properties of scar tissue, the kinetics of physical change is as important to the surgeon as morphology.

Within the first few days, cohesive forces between epithelial cells, fibroblasts, and endothelial cells add some strength to healing wounds.[51] Intercellular forces, however, are weak, and wounds may be disrupted with ease at this stage. When collagen fibers appear, wounds begin to gain strength rapidly. Although scars are composed of many chemical constituents, collagen fibers are responsible for the characteristic physical properties of scars.[1] Indeed, collagen is the basic structural protein of all animals, and the physical properties of mesenchymal tissues, from strong tendons to loose areolar tissues, depend on the physical characteristics and weave of collagen fibers. By 3 weeks, the normal incised and sutured wound has less than 15% of its ultimate tensile strength.[29] Strength of an incised wound increases linearly for at least 3 months in animals and probably much longer in man. Lacerated and repaired tendons gain strength at an even slower rate.[41] Factors responsible for this prolonged increase in strength will be discussed in a later section.

During the early phases of wound healing, the wound space is filled completely with cells and randomly oriented collagen fibers. Although surgeons attempt to compartmentalize wounds by carefully reapproximating fascial layers, histologic study reveals that during the early phases of healing the scar is a single unit invading all areas of the wound space regardless of careful stitchwork.[43] Thus all injured tissues are bound together in a single unit by the newly synthesized scar tissue.

Rapidly uniting all injured tissues into a single strong mass has homeostatis advantages, reestablishing integrity and strength quickly and effectively. In some instances, a single massive scar produces an excellent functional outcome. As an example, the abdomen functions normally in the presence of a scar, welding peritoneum, muscle, fascia, subcutaneous tissue, and skin into a single unit. In the hand, however, scars of this nature are never satisfactory. The characteristic feature of hand architecture is strong collagenous structures moving freely relative to fixed units. Binding mobile and immobile units together limits function. For example, a wound binding skin, palmar fascia, lumbrical muscle, tendon, and bone into a single unit prevents active motion completely. In order to reestablish satisfactory function, cut tendon ends must be linked together by strong scar tissue, but the character of scar joining tendon with surrounding immobile structures must be altered to permit tendon gliding. During the later phases of wound healing, scars can and do change anatomic arrangement. This phenomenon, the remodeling of scar tissue, determines success or failure of reconstructive surgical procedures on the hand.

The "one wound" concept is useful in planning elective hand incisions or in routine tendon transfers and grafts. When a choice is possible, gliding structures must be placed next to tissues that also move. Tendon transfers and grafts should be placed in subcutaneous tissue away from skin incisions, old scars, or other fixed structures. If all injured tissues are free to move, less reliance need be placed on the remodeling process to restore normal function.

SCAR CHEMISTRY

Because collagen fibers determine the physical characteristics of scar tissue, an understanding of wound healing requires some familiarity with this unique protein. The collagen molecule is a long, straight, rigid, rodlike structure, measuring 3000 Å in length and 14 Å in width.[6] Individual molecules are composed of three polypeptide chains wound around each other in a helical fashion. The molecule is synthesized initially in precursor form. Individual chains, synthesized within fibroblasts on large polyribosomes, are composed of several sections. Chains come together within the cell to form the precursor molecule, procollagen. Procollagen has a large, nonhelical portion at the aminoterminal end; a long, rigid central section; and a small, nonhelical portion at the carboxy-terminal end.[7] After excretion into the extracellular space, the large, nonhelical portion of procollagen is deleted under enzymatic control, producing the typical helical molecules that comprise normal fibers.

Collagen is one of the few proteins synthesized by animal cells that is designed to become insoluble. When collagen molecules are brought together under physiologic conditions, even in the absence of cells, they aggregate quickly, forming a random mat of fibrils. Under normal physiologic conditions, collagen molecules aggregate in a three-dimensional array, overlapping each adjoining molecule by one quarter. Quarter staggering is responsible for the typical 640 Å band periodicity of collagen fibers seen in electron micrographs.

Initially, aggregated collagen molecules are held together by hydrogen bonds and other weak physical forces. New fibrils rupture easily when stressed. Within a matter of hours, however, fibrils demonstrate a marked increase in tensile strength. As fibrils mature, weak intermolecular forces are supplemented by the formation of strong covalent bonds.[25] Covalent bonding occurs between individual peptide chains within the molecule (intramolecular bonds) and between adjacent molecules (intermolecular bonds). Again, this process occurs even in the absence of living cells. Ultimately, collagen fibers become giant polymers, each molecule linked to neighbors by strong covalent bonds. Aggregation and covalent bonding produce a strong, flexible fiber that can be woven into many different tissue patterns.

The nature of covalent bonding between collagen molecules is still under intense investigation.[56] Although several types of bonding may be involved, the principal bond between adjacent molecules seems to be a reaction between aldehyde groups.[8] If crossbonding is prevented, collagen molecules aggregate, form fibrils, but fail to develop the characteristic strength of native collagen.[55] Thus collagen synthesis, aggregation, and crossbonding are the chemical events that alter the physical properties of injured tissues. The quantity of scar collagen, the anatomic configuration of the fibers, and the density of covalent bonding determine the physical characteristics of the injured hand.

The collagen content of incised and sutured wounds increases rapidly during the first 3 weeks.[36] Following this initial rapid accumulation, however, total collagen content stabilizes and remains constant for long intervals. Histologically, the wound appears as a dynamic structure during the first 3 to 4 weeks, but undergoes few morphologic changes thereafter. How do wounds gain strength for prolonged intervals while maintaining a stable chemical and histologic appearance? Recent experiments on the kinetic chemistry of scar collagen have helped to resolve this paradox. Direct measurements of rate of new collagen deposition in primary and secondary wounds have demonstrated that scar collagen remains metabolically active for prolonged periods in spite of stable collagen content and histologic picture.[35,38] Fibroblasts within the wound area begin synthesizing collagen on the third day. The rate of new collagen deposition increased rapidly to a maximum between the second and fourth weeks but remains elevated for prolonged intervals. Even 4 months after wounding, new collagen is being deposited at a significantly higher rate in the scar than in normal skin. Rapid collagen synthesis and deposition in the presence of stable amounts of scar collagen indicate simultaneous and rapid collagen destruction.[36] Thus scar collagen content represents an equilibrium, the product of the destruction and removal of old collagen molecules, and the synthesis and deposition of new molecules. The prolonged and rapid metabolic turnover of scar collagen provides the chemical mechanism responsible for scar remodeling and seems to account for a variety of abnormal wound-healing reactions.[48]

In addition to collagen, scar tissue contains large amounts of glycosaminoglycans.[44] These large, sulphated mucopolysaccharides are synthesized locally within the wound space, presumably by fibroblasts. The precise role of the glycosaminoglycans in wound healing remains unknown. Under laboratory conditions, the size, weave, and physical characteristics of collagen fibers can be controlled, in part, by the character of the glycosaminoglycans in the environment. In all probability, glycosaminoglycans play a significant role in the organization of collagen molecules within normal and scarred tissues. Defining how the glycosaminoglycans influence wound healing and scar remodeling remains a significant challenge to interested investigators.

SCAR REMODELING

All wounds undergo remarkable changes in color, texture, firmness, and bulk with time. A well-healed wound, 2 months following injury, bears little resemblance to the same wound 1 year later. As we have discussed, measurable physical properties of sutured wounds (tensile strength, burst strength, tear strength, etc.) change slowly for many months. Physical changes seem to be caused by alterations in the architecture of scar collagen fibers and by alterations in the density of covalent bonding between collagen molecules. Studies using the scanning electron microscope, in addition to the light microscopic observations, indicate that the organization of collagen fibers within the wound changes with time.[18,19]

Striking alterations in scar architecture occur in situations where gliding function is reestablished following injury. The randomly matted collagen fibrils uniting all injured structures during the early phases of healing become oriented in more specific ways with time.[43] Scar collagen between tendon ends becomes oriented in parallel bundles resembling normal tendon. Parallel organization establishes a strong

union between tendon ends capable of transmitting powerful longitudinal forces. As a part of the same process, collagen fibers lying adjacent to gliding surfaces enlarge but retain their random orientation, creating a loose areolar configuration. Blood vessels present in the peritendinous scar become coiled and tortuous, permitting movement without loss of vessel integrity. Over many months, scar tissue initially deposited in a random configuration becomes rewoven into structures that resemble the preinjury condition (parallel collagen bundles between tendon ends, peritenon-like structures surrounding gliding surfaces). In contrast, examining injured tendons that fail to regain gliding demonstrates an entirely different scar architecture. Instead of remodeling to resemble peritenon, scar tissue organizes into firm collagenous adhesions with parallel collagen fibers uniting the gliding surfaces firmly to fixed surrounding structures. The physical characteristics of these adhesions prevent tendon gliding completely.

Demonstrating prolonged and rapid metabolic turnover of scar collagen establishes the chemical mechanism responsible for the remodeling of scars but provides no clues as to why scar collagen in one wound remodels to permit gliding while scar in another becomes an ever stronger unit uniting mobile and immobile structures into an unyielding mass. Controlling the factors responsible for morphologic change in scar tissue seems to be the key to perfect restoration of the injured hand. If morphologic changes could be controlled precisely, all tendon repairs and grafts would be successful, all joint replacements would move freely, and all wounds would heal with minimal functional abnormalities.

Although factors controlling the morphogenic aspects of scar remodeling are poorly understood, certain biologic observations seem pertinent. Experimental and clinical evidence indicates that longitudinal and shearing stresses are responsible for the remodeling of bone.[3] The clinical behavior of scars supports the concept that physical forces play an equally important role in the remodeling of scar tissue. As an example, skin wounds placed across lines of changing dimension slowly but irrevocably hypertrophy. In contrast, scars placed along the midaxial line of a finger or parallel to lines of changing dimension, become insignificant with time. Recently, the influence of tension on remodeling scar tissue has been demonstrated experimentally.[2] As yet, however, how the magnitude, rate of application, frequency, duration, and direction of stress application influence and ultimate size and physical properties of scar tissue remain unknown. Although every clinician uses the controlled application of stress to regain motion following tendon injury, treatment programs are empirical. If we knew precisely how to apply stresses, postoperative therapy could become more efficient and productive.

A variety of factors other than stress influence the remodeling of scars. The surfaces against which scar tissue is deposited influence the nature of remodeling. Scar deposited in the presence of cut tendon ends remodels to mimic the organization of tendon bundles; scar collagen adjacent to an uninjured tendon surface tends to remodel to resemble peritenon. How adjacent structures induce architectural changes is unknown.

Age seems to influence scar remodeling. Younger animals tend to remodel scar tissue more effectively than older animals. Although young children seem to produce more reactive scars than adults, remodeling is rapid and effective. An increase in the rate of metabolic turnover may be responsible for the excellent restoration of gliding seen in young patients undergoing tendon repair.

The total quantity of scar deposited seems to influence the remodeling process. The larger the scar, the less likelihood of effective restoration of physiologic function. Because the quantity of scar deposited is related directly to the quantity of tissue injured, atraumatic surgical technique and careful débridement yield better restoration of function. Rough surgical technique and retained foreign bodies, including injured tissue, prolong the initial phases of healing and produce large amounts of scar tissue. In this case, remodeling reactions are insufficient to reestablish proper scar architecture.

These observations may provide a rationale for the excellent results reported in two-stage flexor tendon grafts. Some authors claim that preliminary implantation of Silastic rod provides a smooth surface against which grafts may glide. Actually, the rod may serve only as a method of establishing tendon continuity with minimal tissue damage. At the first stage, extensive tissue dissection and injury initiate a normal wound healing response. After several months, the rate of new collagen deposition has slowed appreciably. At the second stage, only the tissues at either end of the tendon graft are disturbed. Restoration of the blood supply to the grafted tendon occurs in an environment in which fibrous protein synthesis is minimized. Without the extensive operative trauma and tissue damage, less new collagenous tissue is formed and remodeling occurs more effectively.

The presence of excessive quantities of old scar within a new wound has detrimental effects on remodeling. Although scar tissue remains metabolically active for years, the ability to change morphology is lost with time. Old scar, firmly bound to immobile structures, provides an unsatisfactory bed for subsequent gliding. To maximize remodeling potential, all old scar tissue should be excised prior to repairing gliding structures. In tendon transfers, old scars should be avoided and tendons placed in beds containing a minimal amount of scar tissue.

Finally, the biologic condition of tissues at the time of injury influences scar remodeling. Because wounds remain dynamic structures for prolonged periods, a second injury during this active metabolic period increases scar collagen synthesis.[38] Performing restorative procedures while the injured hand remains reactive produces unsatisfactory results. Although initial reconstructive procedures are often performed 6 to 8 weeks following injury, clinical and experimental evidence suggests that a much longer interval is advisable. The physical characteristics of injured tissues provide clues to their metabolic state. As long as wounds feel hard and immobile, attempts at secondary reconstruction should be avoided.

WOUND CONTRACTION

The biologic events described in the preceding sections are characteristic of sharply incised and primarily closed wounds. Open wounds, with or without tissue loss, present different clinical problems. Although the basic morphologic and the chemical processes operating in closed wounds par-

ticipate, wound contraction becomes an important feature and epithelialization assumes a more prominent role.

Full-thickness defects in any mobile area of mammalian skin undergo dramatic changes in size and shape. After a 2- or 3-day latent period, wounds begin to contract actively and by 2 or 3 weeks are less than 20 percent of their original area.[4] In areas where skin is relatively loose and mobile structures are not nearby, wound contraction produces minimal deformity. In the hand, however, where no "extra skin" exists, wound contraction produces disastrous results. The forces of contraction act to close the wound until balanced by equal tension in the surrounding skin. Although tension in surrounding tissue may lessen with time, for all practical purposes a wound contracts until fixed tissues prevent further contraction. In the hand the mobility of the small joints permits open wounds to contract until joints become fixed in abnormal positions. For example, a 4 × 4 cm defect on the dorsum contracting to a 2 × 2 cm scar fixes the metacarpophalangeal joints in extension. If joints are allowed to remain in abnormal positions for any length of time, secondary changes in the periarticular tissues produce permanent joint stiffness. Because of these potential disasters, minimizing wound contraction is critical to the proper management of open hand wounds.

Experimental data support the concept that living cells, rather than alterations in extracellular mesenchymal material, supply the force moving wound edges together.[57] Recently, Gabbiani and co-workers have identified a specific cell type in granulation tissue which may represent the contractile element.[22] This unique cell combines the ultrastructural features of the fibroblast and smooth muscle cell. Modified fibroblasts (myofibroblasts) have been identified in contracting tissues from several animal species and in a variety of human fibrocontractive diseases.[30,31] Although it is impossible to prove that atypical cells, identifiable by ultrastructural criteria alone, supply the motive force for wound contraction, a variety of data supports this interpretation. Biochemical measurements demonstrate that granulation tissue from contracting wounds contains as much actomyosin as uterus.[21] Human antismooth muscle sera label the cytoplasm of myofibroblasts.[23] Granulation tissue containing significant numbers of myofibroblasts contracts actively in vitro, behaving as vascular smooth muscle tissue.[40] Finally, topically applied antismooth muscle agents inhibit wound contraction completely.[34]

Although the use of smooth muscle antagonists or other methods of controlling the contraction process offer promise for the future, the only practical method of influencing contraction at the moment is the immediate replacement of missing skin with thick skin grafts or pedicle flaps. Contrary to popular opinion, epithelialization per se does not inhibit contraction.[53] Replacing missing tissue immediately does not prevent contraction, but the ultimate area of the defect is much larger following immediate coverage.[52] Once contraction has begun, however, replacing missing skin is less effective in inhibiting the process.[54] A combination of immediate coverage plus mechanical splinting, by skeletal structures in the area or by external devices, is the most effective method of minimizing wound contraction.[39] All open wounds of the hand must be covered as quickly as possible to prevent permanent residual deformities.

CONTROLLING THE WOUND-HEALING PROCESS

Several novel solutions to the problems created by scar formation in the injured hand are being evaluated experimentally. Although all tissue injury produces scarring and potentially limits gliding, the location of newly deposited scar tissue can be controlled. As an example, the entire digital theca can be removed from cadavers and transplanted to animals as a single unit. Although the cellular components of the graft die and the extracellular components seem to be replaced by host protein, the architectural arrangement of the transplant is retained.[42] The blood supply to the tendinous structures is reestablished by connections between the local tissue and outer fibrous sheath. An intense wound-healing reaction occurs but at the outer surface of the transplant protecting the gliding structures. The specialized mesenteric structures within the fibrous envelope and the gliding surfaces remain uninvolved in the scarring process. Several centers have reported encouraging long-term results using allografts in human fingers.[20,24,46] Unfortunately, grafts are inconvenient to obtain. Attempts are being made to lyophilize human flexor mechanisms and produce a product that can be stored indefinitely and used conveniently.[9]

Another approach to the problem of healing and gliding involves fundamental manipulations of collagen chemistry. As we have discussed, the physical properties of collagen fibers, not the presence of scar tissue per se, prevent gliding in poorly remodeled wounds. The physical properties of individual collagen fibers are determined by their covalent bonding patterns. Inhibiting covalent bonding produces a fibril without significant tensile strength. A class of chemical compounds called osteolathyrogens specifically inhibit the enzyme responsible for intermolecular crosslinking.[55] Betaaminoproprionitrile (BAPN), the most powerful known osteolathyrogen, reduces the tensile strength of experimental wounds, improves gliding following experimental tendon injury, prevents esophageal stenosis following lye burns, and restores esophageal diameter in fixed esophageal stenosis.[15,17,33,45] BAPN has been administered to human beings in clinical trials.[26,37,47] The agent causes significant biochemical and physical effects on newly synthesized scar collagen. Whether or not lathyrogenic effects produce significant improvement in gliding, however, awaits further clinical investigation.

Inhibiting the synthesis and deposition of scar collagen specifically and selectively could control the healing process. The hydroxylation of proline is a unique and requisite step in collagen synthesis. The enzyme responsible for hydroxylation, peptidylproline hydroxylase, requires ferrous iron as a cofactor.[11] Chelating ferrous iron produces specific inhibition of collagen synthesis without effecting noncollagenous protein synthesis.[10,13] Although this technique has been used effectively in vitro, available chelators seem too toxic to be applied clinically.[14] Analogues of proline can also inhibit collagen synthesis specifically.[6] Several authors have claimed that administering proline analogues to animals inhibits collagen synthesis and improves tendon gliding.[5,16,27] The effects of proline analogues in vivo, however, are controversial and the effects in human beings remain unknown.[12,32]

Effective control of the healing process in man has not been achieved. However, experimental data suggest that clinical control of the healing process is feasible. Over the next decade, the development of clinically useful methods of controlling scar formation and wound contraction will be developed. Until these tools are in our possession, the skillful surgeon must utilize the biologic information covered in this article to regain maximum function in the injured hand. At the moment, we have no pharmacologic crutch to support poor wound management.

REFERENCES

1. Adamsons R, Musco F, and Enquist I: The relationship of collagen content to wound strength in normal and scorbutic animals, Surg Gynec Obstet 119:323, 1964.
2. Arem AJ and Madden JW: Effects of stress on healing wounds. I. Intermittent noncyclical tension, J Surg Res 20(2):93, 1976.
3. Bassett CA: The effect of force on skeletal tissues. In Downey JA and Darling RC, editors: Physiological basis of rehabilitation medicine, Philadelphia, 1971, WB Saunders Co.
4. Billingham RE and Russell PS: Studies on wound healing, with special reference to contracture in experimental wounds in rabbits' skin, Ann Surg 144:961, 1956.
5. Bora RF Jr, Lane MM, and Prockop DJ: Inhibitors of collagen biosynthesis as a means of controlling scar formation in tendon injury, J Bone Joint Surg 54A:1501, 1972.
6. Bornstein P: The biosynthesis of collagen, Ann Rev Biochem 43:567, 1974.
7. Bornstein P and others: Structure, synthesis and secretion of procollagen. In Slavkin HC and Gruelich RC, editors: Extracellular matrix influences on gene expression, New York, 1975, Academic Press.
8. Bornstein P and Piez KA: The nature of the intramolecular crosslinks in collagen. The separation and characterization of peptides from the crosslink region of rat skin collagen, Biochemistry 5:3460, 1966.
9. Cameron RR, Contrad RN, and Latham WD: Preserved composite tendon allografts. Acceptance and survival in the injured finger. Presented at the forty-ninth annual meeting of the American Association of Plastic Surgeons, Colorado Springs, 1970.
10. Chvapil M, Hurych J, and Ehrlichova E: Effects of long term in vivo application of phenanthroline, penicillamine and further chelating agents on the synthesis of collagenous and noncollagenous proteins in fibrotic liver and wound granulation tissue, Hoppe Seyler Z Physiol Chem 349:218, 1968.
11. Chvapil M and others: Mechanism of the action of chelating agents on proline hydroxylation and its incorporation into collagenous and noncollagenous proteins, Eur J Biochem 2:229, 1967.
12. Chvapil M and others: Effect of cis-hydroxyproline on collagen and other proteins in skin wounds, granuloma tissue, and liver of mice and rats, Exp Mol Pathol 20:363, 1974.
13. Chvapil M and others: In vivo effect of 1,10-phenanthroline and desferrioxamine on peptidyl proline hydroxylase and hydroxylation of collagen in rats, Biochem Pharmacol 23:2165, 1974.
14. Chvapil M and others: Effect of chelating agents, proline analogs, and oxygen tension in in vivo and in vitro experiments on hydroxylation, transport, degradation, and accumulation of collagen. In Vogel HG, ed: Connective tissue and aging, vol I. International Congress Series, No 264, Amsterdam, 1973, Excerpta Medica.
15. Craver JM, Madden JW, and Peacock EE Jr: Biological control of physical properties of tendon adhesions. Effect of beta-aminoproprionitrile in chickens, Ann Surg 167:697, 1968.
16. Daly JM and others: Inhibition of collagen synthesis by the proline analogue cis-4-hydroxyproline, J Surg Res 14:551, 1973.
17. Davis JM, Madden JW, and Peacock EE Jr: A new approach to the esophageal stenosis, Ann Surg 176:469, 1972.
18. Forrester JC and others: Tape closed and sutured wounds: a comparison by tensiometry and scanning electron microscopy, Br J Surg 57:729, 1970.
19. Forrester JC and others: Wolff's law in relation to the healing skin wound, J Trauma 10:770, 1970.
20. Furlow LT Jr: Homologous flexor mechanism replacement in four fingers of one hand, Plast Reconstr Surg 43:531, 1969.
21. Gabbiani G and others: Granulation tissue as a contractile organ: a study of structure and function, J Exp Med 135:719, 1972.
22. Gabbiani G, Ryan GB, and Majno G: Presence of modified fibroblasts in granulation tissue and their possible role in wound contraction, Experimentia 27:549, 1971.

23. Hirschel BJ and others: Fibroblasts of granulation tissue: immunofluorescent staining with anti-smooth muscle serum, Proc Soc Exp Biol Med 138:466, 1971.
24. Heuston JT, Hubble B, and Rigg BR: Homografts of the digital flexor tendon system, Aust N Z J Surg 36:269, 1967.
25. Jackson DS and Bentley JP: On the significance of the extractable collagens, J Biophys Biochem Cytol 7:37, 1960.
26. Keiser HR and Sjoerdsma A: Studies on beta-aminoproprionitrile in patients with scleroderma, Clin Pharmacol Ther 8:593, 1967.
27. Lane JM and others: Inhibition of scar formation by the proline analog cis-hydroxyproline, J Surg Res 13:135, 1972.
28. Leibovich SJ and Ross R: The role of the macrophage in wound repair, Am J Pathol 78:71, 1975.
29. Levenson SM and others: The healing of rat skin wounds, Ann Surg 161:293, 1965.
30. Madden JW: On "the contractile fibroblast," Plast Reconstr Surg 52:291, 1973.
31. Madden JW, Carlson EC, and Hines J: Presence of modified fibroblasts in ischemic contracture of intrinsic musculature of the hand, Surg Gynecol Obstet 140:509, 1975.
32. Madden JW and others: Toxicity and metabolic effects of 3,4-dehydroproline in mice, J Tox Appl Pharmacol 26:426, 1973.
33. Madden JW and others: Experimental esophageal lye burns. 2. Correcting establishing strictures with beta-aminoproprionitrile and bougienage, Ann Surg 178:277, 1973.
34. Madden JW, Morton D Jr, and Peacock EE Jr: Contraction of experimental wounds. I. Inhibiting wound contraction by using a topical smooth muscle antagonist, Surgery 76:8, 1974.
35. Madden JW and Peacock EE Jr: Studies on the biology of collagen during wound healing. I. Rate of collagen synthesis and deposition in cutaneous wounds of the rat, Surgery 64:288, 1968.
36. Madden JW and Peacock EE Jr: Studies on the biology of collagen during wound healing. III. Dynamic metabolism of scar collagen and remodeling of dermal wounds, Ann Surg 174:511, 1971.
37. Madden JW and others: Unpublished results, 1974.
38. Madden JW and Smith HC: Studies on the biology of collagen during wound healing. II. The rate of collagen synthesis and deposition in dehisced and resutured wounds, Surg Gynecol Obstet 130:487, 1970.
39. Madden JW and Stone PA: Biological factors affecting wound contraction, Surg Fourm 26:547, 1975.
40. Majno G and others: Contraction of granulation tissue in vitro: similarity to smooth muscle, Science 173:548, 1971.
41. Mason ML and Allen HS: The rate of healing of tendons, Ann Surg 113:424, 1941.
42. Peacock EE Jr: Restoration of finger flexion with homologous composite tissue tendon grafts, Am Surg 26:564, 1960.
43. Peacock EE Jr: Fundamental aspects of wound healing relating to the restoration of gliding function after tendon repair, Surg Gynecol Obstet 119:241, 1961.
44. Peacock EE Jr: Dynamic aspects of collagen biology, J Surg Res 7:433, 1967.
45. Peacock EE Jr and Madden JW: Some studies on the effect of beta-aminoproprionitrile on collagen in healing wounds, Surgery 60:7, 1966.
46. Peacock EE Jr and Madden JW: Human composite flexor tendon allografts, Ann Surg 166:624, 1967.
47. Peacock EE Jr and Madden JW: Some studies on the effects of beta-aminoproprionitrile in patients with injured flexor tendons, Surgery 66:215, 1969.
48. Peacock EE Jr, Madden JW, and Trier WC: Biologic basis for the treatment of keloids and hypertrophic scars, South Med J 63:755, 1970.
49. Ross R: The fibroblast and wound repair, Biol Rev 43:51, 1968.
50. Ross R and Odland G: Fine structure observations in human skin wounds and fibrogenesis. In Dynphy JE and Van Winkle W, eds: Repair and regeneration, New York, 1969, McGraw-Hill Book Co.
51. Rovee DT and Miller CA: Epidermal role in the breaking strength of wounds, Arch Surg 96:43, 1968.
52. Sawhney CP and Monga HL: Wound contraction in rabbits and the effectiveness of skin grafts in preventing it, Br J Plast Surg 23:318, 1970.
53. Stone PA and Madden JW: Contraction of experimental wounds. II. The role of epithelialization (in press).
54. Stone PA and Madden JW: Effect of primary and delayed splint skin grafting in wound contraction, Surg Forum 25:41, 1974.
55. Tanzer ML: Experimental lathyrism, Int Rev Connect Tissue Res 3:91, 1965.
56. Tanzer ML: Cross-linking of collagen, Science 180:561, 1973.
57. Van Winkle W Jr: Wound contraction, Surg Gynecol Obstet 125:131, 1967.

13

Management of edema

James M. Hunter and Evelyn J. Mackin

Because it delays healing and causes pain and stiffness, thereby compromising functional results, the problem of edema should represent a constant challenge to concerned hand surgeons and hand therapists.

In the *normal* extremity mild edema of the hand may be produced in a few hours by immobilizing the upper extremity with the hand in a dependent position (sling). The addition of a dropped, unsplinted wrist and tight elastic bandage on the forearm can produced marked (balloonlike) swelling of the hand and fingers (Fig. 13-1). Edema produces bloating of the skin on the back of the hand, which results in flattening of the hand and loss of the longitudinal and transverse arches (Fig. 13-2).[5]

In the hand, afferent blood flow occurs on the volar surface controlled by arterial blood pressure. The major portion of the return blood flow takes place on the dorsal surface through the lymphatic and venous systems. The return systems require active movement of the hand to compress and produce retrograde venous and lymphatic flow by joint movement and compression of the fascial compartments. The dynamics of return flow are further augmented by motion of the elbow and shoulder.[11]

The picture of reduced dynamics becomes more alarming in chronic edema as soft tissues become fibrosed from foreign body tissue reaction. The greater the edema fluid and the longer it persists, the more extensive the scarring will be. All tissues—vessels, nerves, joints, and intrinsic muscles—become involved in a state of reduced nutrition and inelasticity. Although a certain amount of edema is reversible, fibrosis of moving tissue planes is not, and if edema is associated with injury and poor position, a "stiff" hand will result. *The prevention and treatment of edema are of paramount importance during all phases of management of the injured hand.*[5]

PREVENTION OF EDEMA

After severe injury the hand should be immobilized immediately in "the position of function" and maintained in this position except for a few special exceptions. Postinjury dressings should be bulky and firm and evenly placed from fingertip to the upper forearm (Fig. 13-3). According to Boyes,[2] firm optimal pressure implies that the pressure has been applied with judgment and discrimination. The fingers should be separated. A splint should support the hand and wrist in the functional position, offering comfortable immobilization. Volar or dorsal splints should be carefully padded to avoid pressure at bony prominences or over the dorsal venous system. The dressed, splinted hand should be elevated comfortably on pillows or in a canvas hand support. Cooling with ice bags will be helpful early if properly applied and arranged so that the weight of the bag is not carried on the hand. The initial dressing should remain undisturbed for the first 3 to 5 days, followed by débridement, daily open wound care, and skin grafting.[5]

The use of proteolytic enzymes given orally to reduce postoperative edema has not been effective in the controlled clinical situation. Hunter and Salisbury[6] studied 62 patients undergoing hand surgery who were given Orenzyme or a placebo in a double-blind study. No significant difference was noted in the postoperative course of edema or wound healing in the two groups.

Once established, edema should be approached with an active hand therapy program of supported elevation and supervised exercises, depending on the condition of the wound. The practice of making stab wounds or incisions over the dorsum of the hand to "drain the edema" is mentioned only to be condemned. Such techniques merely insult and open more tissue, provoking further inflammation and swelling.[5]

PATIENT EDUCATION

Edema is the first and most obvious reaction of the hand to injury. Most wounds have an excess of fluid content early in the healing process. The therapist should not be alarmed at this type of edema as long as the principles of elevation and active motion are observed.[10]

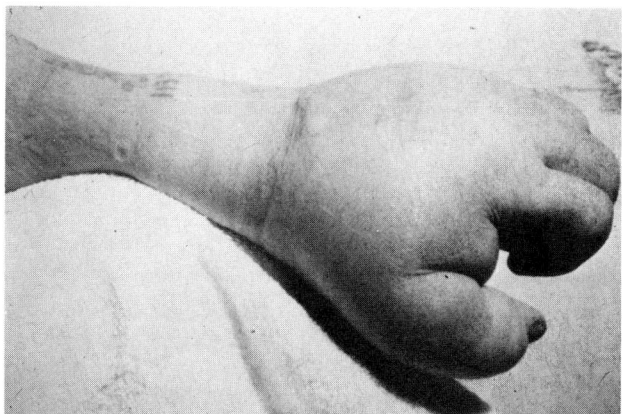

Fig. 13-1 "Balloon edema" of hand in 32-year-old man from chronic lymphatic and venous obstruction. This patient apparently, for purposes of secondary gain, methodically applied tight elastic bandage to midforearm over 3 to 4 months. Notice that healed incisions over dorsum of hand represent attempts to "drain edema."

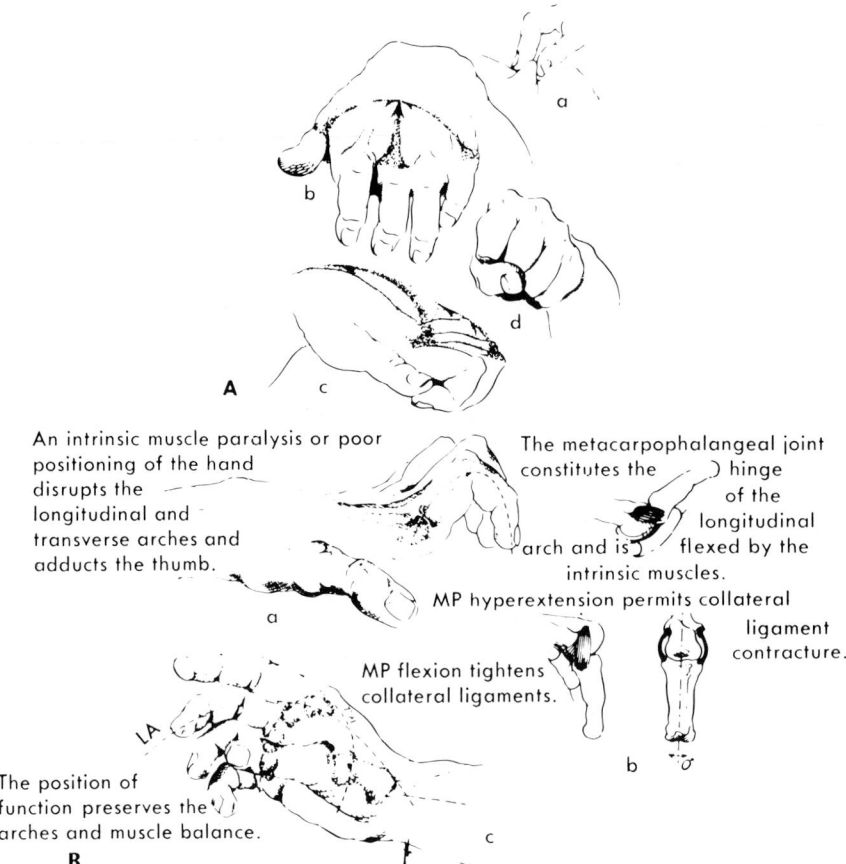

An intrinsic muscle paralysis or poor positioning of the hand disrupts the longitudinal and transverse arches and adducts the thumb.

The metacarpophalangeal joint constitutes the hinge of the longitudinal arch and is flexed by the intrinsic muscles.

MP hyperextension permits collateral ligament contracture.

MP flexion tightens collateral ligaments.

The position of function preserves the arches and muscle balance.

Fig. 13-2   **A,** *Edema* producing poor functional position, *b* and *c*, by obliterating soft tissue stretch on dorsum of hand. Functional use of hand, *d*, is in jeopardy. **B,** Loss of function of arches of hand by intrinsic paralysis, *a*. Contracture of relaxed collateral ligaments of joints produces fixed deformity. Objective of hand rehabilitation: a functioning hand, *c*. **A** from Littler JGW: In Converse JM: Reconstructive plastic surgery, Philadelphia, 1977, WB Saunders Co; **B** from Hunter JM: Am J Surg 92:1427, 1956.

The edema that must concern the therapist generally occurs 1 to 2 weeks after surgery and presents itself as an ongoing problem unless early intervention is applied. It will engulf the joint capsules, collateral ligaments, and other fibroelastic components of the injured hand. If the edema is allowed to persist in conjunction with immobilization, the patient will ultimately develop a stiff hand. Structures will continue to swell, thicken, shorten, and eventually be replaced by dense fibrous tissue.[10,16]

Edema is reversible. If edema can be controlled early, subsequent scar formation is minimized in comparison with the scar that forms if edema is prolonged and brawny. Postoperative efforts are directed toward minimizing edema and promoting uncomplicated wound healing. Patient education is vital. Beginning with the initial treatment in the hospital or clinic, the patient must be made aware of the factors that can exacerbate or alleviate edema.

Elevation

Elevation of the hand above the heart until the tendency for swelling ceases means immediate postoperative elevation of the splinted hand in a supportive sling. For elevation to be effective, the distal part of the extremity must be above the proximal part and the proximal part must be above the heart. Elevation with the hand above the elbow and the elbow above the shoulder can also be accomplished by resting the hand comfortably on pillows during the day or at night in bed.[8]

If elevation causes ischemia of the extremity, then the level of elevation will need to be altered. The point of reference for elevation of the replanted hand is the right atrium of the heart; the part should be 10 to 20 cm above this level. However, the extremity may be raised or lowered depending on the color changes that may occur. Healthy replanted digits are warm and pinker than normal digits. Arterial occlusion should be suspected if the digit becomes cool and pale. Venous obstruction is usually present if the finger takes on a bluish purple hue and has a drop in temperature. Adjustment of the position of the arm will improve its circulation. When arterial occlusion is diagnosed, the arm should be lowered below the heart. When venous occlusion is diagnosed, the extremity should be elevated.[13] Care must be taken to ensure that the elbow is not overflexed, creating an obstruction to venous drainage. A sudden increase in edema or an alteration in color or temperature should be reported immediately to the surgeon.[10]

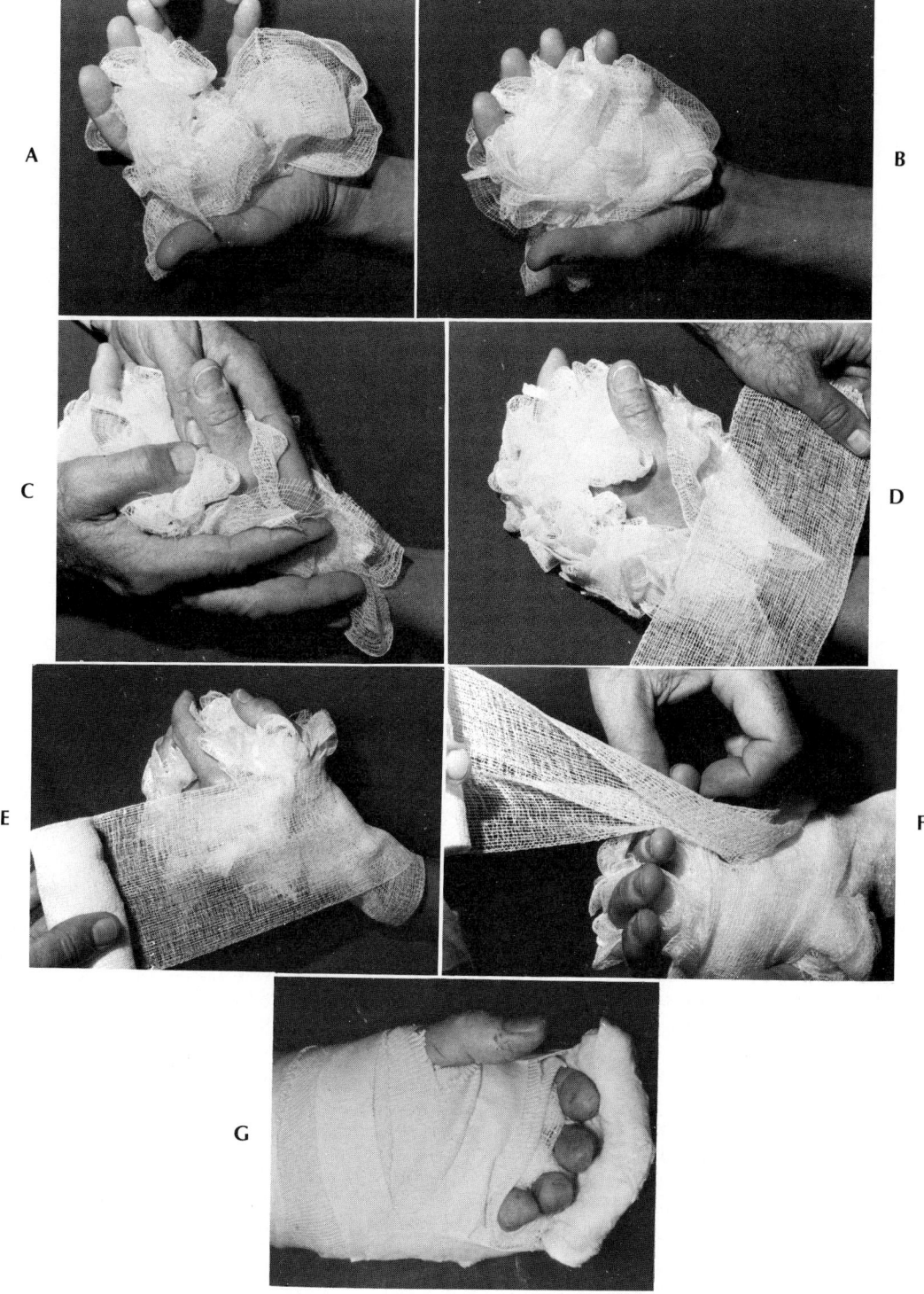

Fig. 13-3   Postinjury dressings. **A,** Light gauze fluffs pressed gently between fingers. **B,** Additional gauze fluffs placed in palm and thumb web. **C,** Fluffy gauze molded in palm and around thumb. **D,** Kling elastic gauze bandage (Johnson & Johnson, New Brunswick, N.J.) gently held in open position by ungloved hand. **E,** Bandage gently anchored at wrist and moved in oblique figure-of-eight manner throughout entire dressing. **F,** Bandage tension maintained by left hand as roll is flipped 180 degrees to compress bandage between each finger. **G,** Completed dressing should be comfortable, permitting tight finger motion and unrestricted by splint or cast. Splint support for wrist is usually placed on dorsum.

Active motion

Active motion must be forceful as illustrated by the blanching of skin over our knuckles with grasp. Wiggling of the fingers is totally ineffectual in combatting edema, as can be observed in the dorsal veins. Wiggling not only fails to blanch the skin but also does not even empty the dorsal veins. The interphalangeal joints must move through a full range of motion and the fingers must make a firm fist in order to propel fluids effectively assisting return flow circulation. An effective exercise that incorporates elevation and active motion is to have the patient elevate both arms over his head and make firm fists at least 25 repetitions each hour. Moberg states that by having his patients perform this exercise hourly he has never had a patient develop a reflex sympathetic dystrophy.[12]

Although immobilization of a fracture is necessary to ensure union, the uninvolved fingers must be actively moved. Joints should never be immobilized needlessly, for if they become stiffened in a poor position, months of effort are necessary to regain motion. Early active digital motion prevents the adherence of tendons at the fracture site, diminishes edema by pumping the fluid from the fingers, and decreases ligament contracture. If the cast unnecessarily prevents full range of motion at any joint, it should be trimmed by the surgeon at the first postoperative visit. Attention to cast application and the initiation of early active motion of the uninvolved fingers in elevation must be a primary goal of the therapist in the postoperative management of wrist and hand fractures.[10]

Active exercises should also include full range of motion to both shoulders. The shoulder of the involved extremity should be put through a full range of motion several times a day to prevent shoulder-hand syndrome or "frozen shoulder." "Overhead fisting" exercises effectively incorporate the important shoulder range of motion with the active digital motion.[1,10]

ASSESSMENT OF EDEMA

Observing changes in the amount of fluid in the patient's hand is of utmost importance in the management of edema.

Volumeter

The volumeter* provides the hand therapist with a method to measure edema by submerging the patient's hand in a specifically designed water-filled container and measuring the water displacement (Fig. 13-4). Patients are assessed when wounds permit on their initial visit and thereafter checked routinely for changes in hand size from edema.

The concept of the volumeter to measure swelling by water displacement was designed by Dr. Paul Brand and Helen Wood, O.T.R., at the United States Public Health Service Hospital at Carville, Louisiana. The technique is as follows:

Purpose: To measure edema in the hand
Equipment needed
1. Plastic hand volumeter (Fig. 13-4, *A*)
2. Graduated cylinder, 500 ml
3. Small bucket or container
4. Elevated wooden support for hand volumeter
5. Chair

Measurement procedure
1. The hand volumeter and graduated cylinder are properly positioned on the elevated wooden support, and water is poured into the hand volumeter from a small bucket or container until the water overflows and discontinues dripping into the graduated cylinder. Thoroughly empty the cylinder.
2. A chair is placed in a preset position at a height that easily allows the lowering of one third of the forearm into the plastic hand volumeter.
3. The patient is instructed to sit with the back well against the chair and the feet flat on the floor.
4. The hand is positioned with the palm in the anatomic position,* and the patient is instructed to lower the hand slowly so as not to spill water over the rim of the graduated cylinder (Fig. 13-4, *B*).
5. The hand should go down until the stop dowel rests between the web of the middle and ring fingers† (Fig. 13-4, *C*).
6. The hand is kept in this position until the water no longer flows from the spout.‡ The graduated cylinder is then removed and the patient is told to remove the hand from the water.§
7. Reading the water level in the graduated cylinder is accomplished on a flat surface that should be marked so that subsequent readings will always be taken at the same spot. Because of the water tension, it will appear that two lines are visible. Determine which line you will read and thereafter be consistent.
8. The chair is reversed and the same procedure is repeated for the opposite hand.

Circumferential measurements

Another technique for measurement of edema is circumferential measurements of the hand and forearm. Measurements are taken with a tape measure before and after treatment. To allow more valid comparison of sequential measurements, anatomic landmarks are used as reference points for placement of the tape.

TECHNIQUES FOR REDUCTION OF EDEMA

The therapist may use one or more of the following techniques in attempting to reduce edema and facilitate venous flow: (1) retrograde massage, (2) intermittent compression pump, (3) string wrapping, (4) Coban wrapping, (5) elastic bandage wraps, and (6) Isotoner glove.

---

*If the patient is unable to lower the hand into the hand volumeter in the anatomic position, he may reverse the position of the palm.
†If the patient has gross contractures or digits missing and cannot position the stop dowel on the web between the ring and middle fingers, a location between any finger will be acceptable if the test is done the same way at every reading.
‡If water continues to drip from the spout of the hand volumeter when the hand has reached the stop dowel, dry the spout thoroughly and spray a light coat of silicone on it.
§If it appears that a hand will measure more than 500 ml of water, have the patient stop lowering the hand in the hand volumeter before 500 ml is reached on the graduated cylinder. Raise the hand slightly and hold this position until the cylinder has been removed and the reading taken. Empty the water thoroughly and return the cylinder to its position. Instruct the patient to continue lowering the hand until the stop dowel is reached. Remove the cylinder and record the sum of the two readings. Each department should statistically analyze its own apparatus for error.

---

*Volumeters Unlimited, Idyllwild Calif.

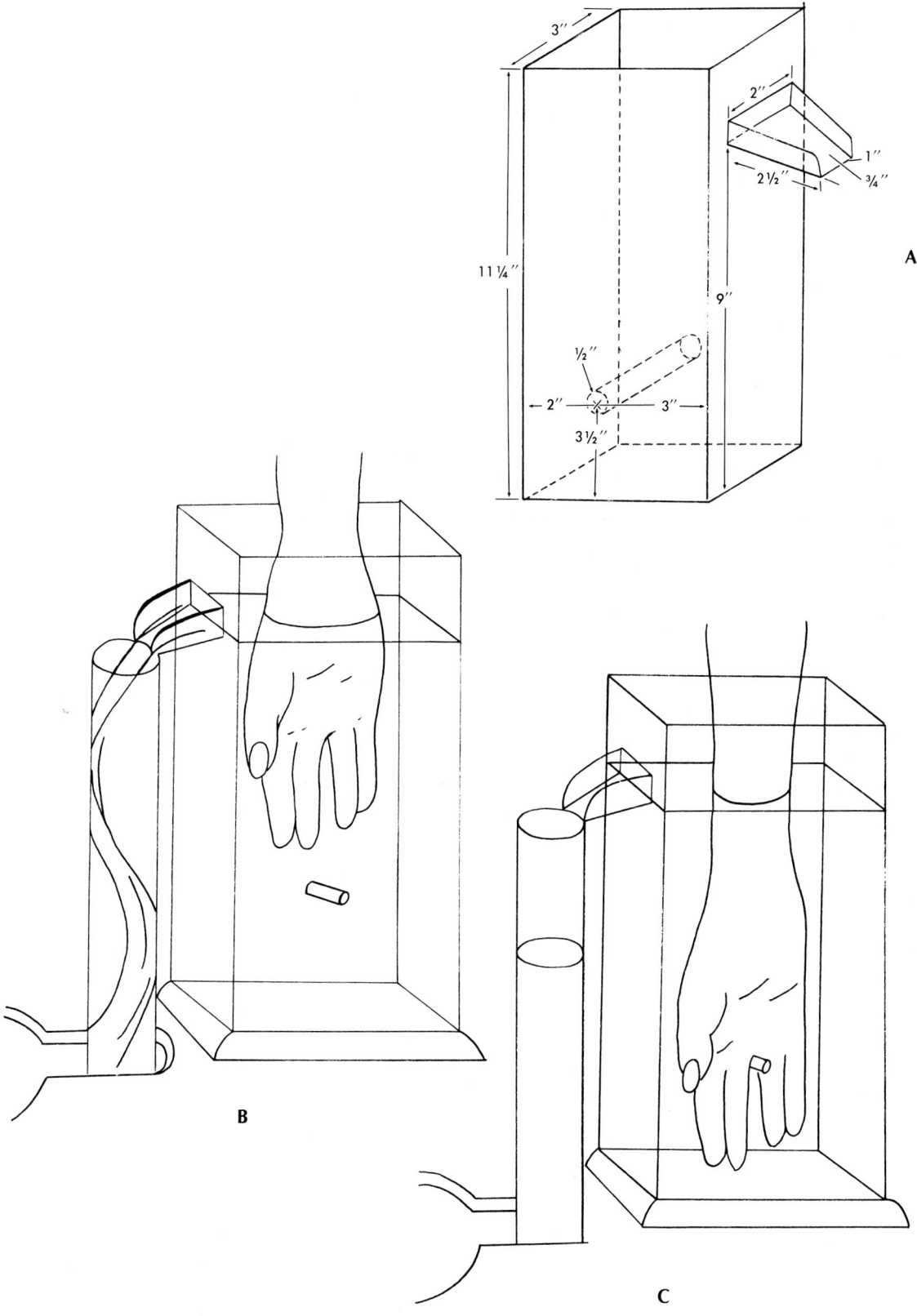

Fig. 13-4   **A,** Plastic hand volumeter. All measurements are inside measurements. **B,** Patient is instructed to lower hand slowly so as not to spill water over rim of graduated cylinder. **C,** Hand should go down until stop dowel rests between web of middle and ring fingers.

Retrograde massage

Probably the greatest single indication for massage is to overcome the swelling and induration that frequently occur after trauma. To assist the return flow circulation of blood and lymph the stroke should always be in a centripetal direction.[9]

Intermittent compression pump

An intermittent compression pump may be used to reduce edema. Intermittent mechanical compression is applied by a pneumatic sleeve that is inflated under pressure and then deflated. The treatment is applied for periods of 15 minutes to 2 hours. The intermittent pressure increases interstitial pressure, thereby driving lymphatic fluid back into the venous system.

Intermittent compression can be very beneficial in acute edema after surgery or severe trauma. An edematous crushed hand may be placed in the arm pneumatic appliance as early as the first day after the trauma or surgery. The extremity is elevated on a table or pillows to an angle of 30 to 45 degrees to take advantage of the flow of gravity while the intermittent pressure is being applied.

The amount of pressure must be adjusted according to each patient's diagnosis and condition. Acute conditions, such as fractures, begin with a low amount of pressure and are supervised carefully by the therapist. The pressure of open wounds does not prohibit intermittent pressure as long as sterile dressings are used. Felt pads can be positioned around pins to prevent pressure on them.

The pressure at the initial treatment might be as low as 30 mm Hg for 30 minutes. To be effective, the pressure must be greater than capillary pressure, that is, 25 mm Hg. However, for safety, it must be kept lower than diastolic pressure at all times. Time and pressure can be gradually increased when sufficient healing has occurred to allow the tissues to tolerate increased pressure.

After the mechanical massage by the intermittent compression unit, retrograde manual massage is applied by the therapist in a further attempt to push the extracellular fluid out of the hand.

String wrapping

An easy, inexpensive, and effective means to remove edema fluid is by string wrapping (Fig. 13-5, *A*). Soft cord should be used. Starting at the distal end of the index finger, the cord is wrapped closely and firmly around the finger (Fig. 13-5, *B*) to give good edema reduction. The string wrapping should progress distally to proximally until all the fingers and hand are wrapped proximally to the area of edema. The hand is then placed in elevation. The cord remains on the hand for 5 minutes (Fig. 13-5, *C*). When the cord is removed, the patient is instructed to make a fist 10 times. Most of the time string wrapping produces the following results.

1. Circumferential measurements taken before (Fig. 13-5, *D*) and after (Fig. 13-5, *E*) the string wrapping indicate a decrease in edema.
2. The patient will find fist making easier.
3. Measurements taken of the patient's active range of motion will show an increase in active flexion of the finger pulp to the distal palmar crease.

The beneficial effects induced by the string wrapping may last only a short time at first. The treatment should be repeated three times a day until return flow circulation is restored adequately.

Flowers reported that massage and string wrapping are equally effective in the reduction of edema, but a combination of the two, that is, retrograde massage to the hand while the string is in place, is more effective than either technique used alone.[4]

Coban* wrapping

For constant, light compression the digit or hand can be gently wrapped in Coban elasticized paper tape to reduce edema. A 1 inch wide tape is used to wrap the digit from distal to proximal in a spiral fashion. The direction of the wrapping pushes the lymphatic fluid proximally into the venous system. Care must be taken not to apply tension to the tape while wrapping, because this can result in too much restriction of circulation.

The patient must be instructed to observe for any signs of the Coban wrapped too tightly, for example, change in color, coldness, or numbness in the fingertip. If this occurs, the Coban should be removed. This becomes particularly important when the patient is performing his own wrapping at home. The Coban will not prevent the patient from carrying out his exercise program, and in most instances it will make exercising easier.

Elastic bandage wraps

A 3 or 4 inch wide elastic (Ace) bandage may be used to form a tube around the digit. The bandage is cut to fit the digit and the two ends are sewn together. These are easy to apply and very effective in postoperative swelling after implant arthroplasty surgery in the rheumatoid fingers when it may be necessary to wrap all the digits.

Isotoner glove

The Aris Isotoner glove† is effective in applying external pressure to an edematous hand. It is made of a washable blend of Antron-nylon-Lycra-Spandex. Inexpensive and readily available at department stores, the glove should be worn continuously day and night except for personal hygiene. As with compressive bandages, the patient must be instructed to observe for signs of restriction of capillary flow.

HEAT MODALITIES
Paraffin dips

It is generally agreed that heat is contraindicated in edema; however, if the physiologic effects of heat and conforming pressure are desired and there are no open wounds, paraffin dips may be used if the edema is mild. Heat is transferred from the paraffin to the skin by conduction. G. Keith Stillwell[14] reported that by the addition of one part of light mineral oil to seven parts of paraffin, the melting point of the wax is lowered to about 52° C (125.6° F). Because its specific heat is only 0.5, the paraffin may be applied directly

---

*Coban, Medical Products Division, Minnesota Mining & Manufacturing Co., St. Paul, Minn.
†Aris Isotoner Glove, New York, NY.

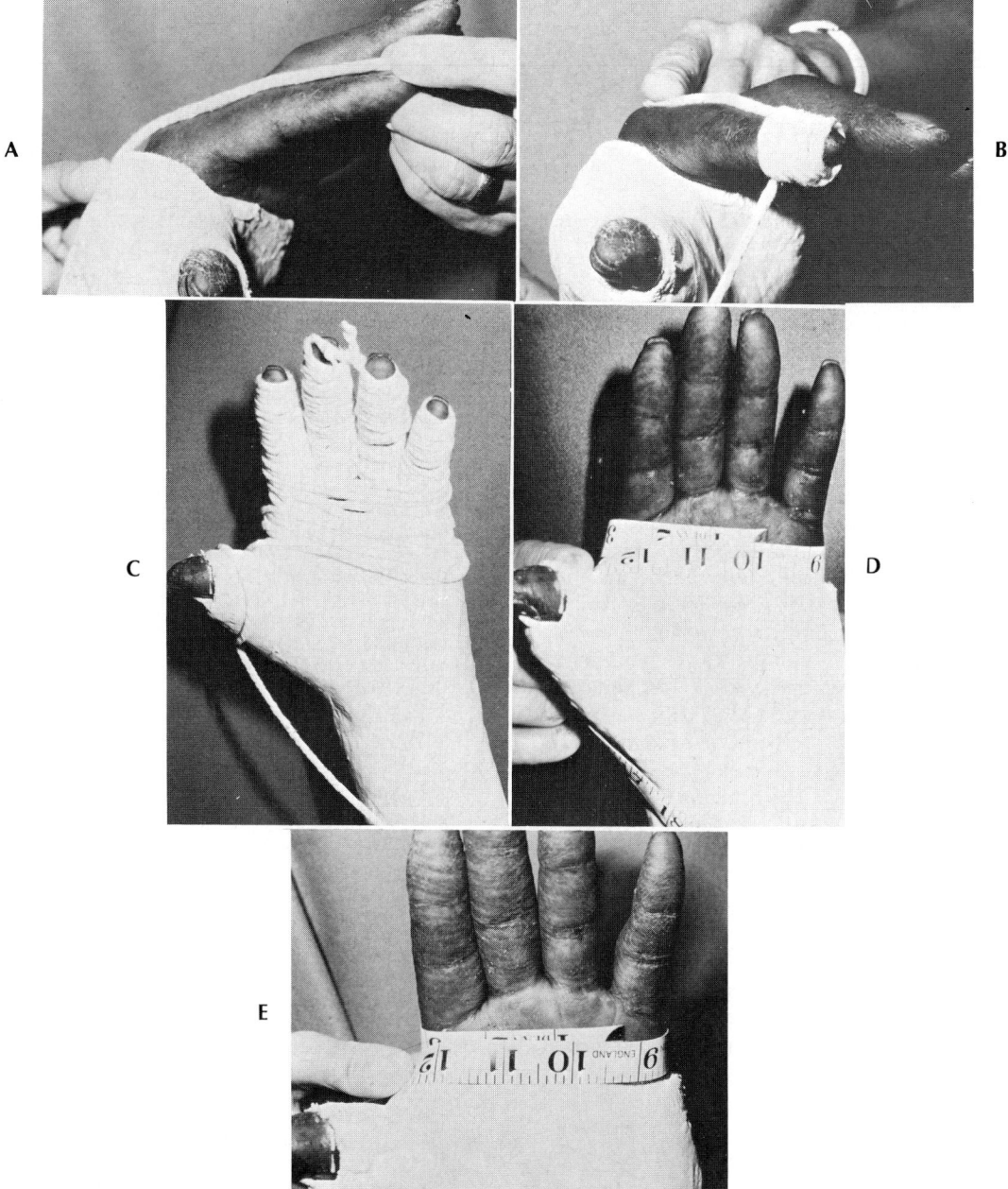

Fig. 13-5 **A,** String wrapping may be started while patient is in cast to begin early reduction of edema. **B,** Starting at distal end of index finger, cord is wrapped closely and firmly around finger. **C,** Patient's hand is placed in elevation. Cord remains on hand for 5 minutes. String wrapping is followed by active fist-making. **D** and **E,** Circumferential measurements taken before and after string wrapping with retrograde massage indicate decrease in edema.

to the skin at this temperature if the circulation is normal. Patients with open wounds should never be given paraffin as a treatment. The advantage of paraffin is that it may be applied and then the extremity can be placed in elevation. The heat should be followed by massage with emphasis on distal to proximal stroking. Heat and massage should always be followed by active exercise.

Small paraffin baths are commercially available for home use. They are effective, safe, easy to use, and thermostatically controlled to hold the wax at a safe 126° to 130° F.

Patients unable to purchase a commercial unit may, with care, improvise a paraffin bath at home.

Materials required

Four pounds of paraffin

One cup of light mineral oil

Procedure

1. Place paraffin and light mineral oil in the top of a double boiler.
2. Heat slowly until the paraffin is completely melted.
3. Remove from heat and let the paraffin cool. *When a*

thin film forms on the top of the paraffin, it is a safe temperature for use (126° to 130° F). The temperature may be measured with a candy thermometer.

4. Dip the hand quickly into the paraffin with the hand relaxed.
5. When the coat of paraffin hardens slightly, dip the hand again. Dip the hand about 12 times, until a layer of paraffin is built up.
6. Wrap the paraffin-covered hand with waxed paper and a towel.
7. Elevate the arm.
8. Exercise the fingers with the parrafin on.
9. When the paraffin has cooled (about 20 minutes), it may be removed and returned to the pan for reuse.
10. Treatment may be repeated twice a day.

Whirlpool

Surgery is based on the assumption of obtaining uncomplicated healing in the postoperative wound. Thus meticulous postoperative management of wounds is essential.

The whirlpool bath offers water temperature control in combination with the mechanical effects of the agitating water, providing heat and gentle massage. It can be the best method of cleansing and debriding open wounds. As a heat modality it is of benefit if it contributes to more active motion and if it is used properly. The adage "the hotter the better" does not apply to the injured hand. Hot water promotes swelling and serves only to perpetuate the disability. Water temperature should be between 92° and 96° F depending on the vascular status. The patient's elbow should be flexed to avoid as much as possible the dependent position of the forearm. Actively, gently exercising the hand while it is in the whirlpool helps to minimize increase in swelling.[1,10]

If whirlpool for débridement is desired, it should be of short duration to minimize the time the hand is in a dependent position. Byron and Muntzer[3] recommend that the patient remove his hand from the whirlpool every 3 minutes, raise it overhead, and make as strong a fist as possible, if permitted, for 1 minute to counteract the effects of the dependent position.

Walsh[15] reported that elevation during the whirlpool treatment had no significant effect on edema occurring after the treatment. If, however, the physiologic effects of heat are desired, for example, whirlpool for débridement, clinical experience indicates that attention to the position of the hand in the whirlpool, "overhead fisting" during the treatment, and the recommended water temperature may help to minimize an increase in edema.

COLD

Cooling with cold packs is helpful in the reduction of edema and the alleviation of pain in some patients. Although many patients seem to prefer the warmth of heat before an exercise session, there are those who benefit more from cold when properly applied. Careful attention is given to the vascular status when cold packs are used. (For full discussion of cold as a treatment modality, refer to Chapter 14.)

SUMMARY

The prevention of edema is of vital importance in the care of the injured or surgical hand. Good early care should emphasize the principles of functional support dressing splints and elevation before surgery, atraumatic surgical techniques and skillfully applied postoperative dressings during surgery, and comfortable elevation and cooling with supervised early movement of uninjured parts after surgery. Once established, the assessment and application of techniques to reduce edema must be the prime concern of the surgeon and therapist in order to restore good hand function.

ACKNOWLEDGMENTS

Photographs by Earl Spangenberg, Audiovisual Department, Jefferson Medical College of Thomas Jefferson University, and Larry Kradle, Department of Orthopaedic Surgery, Jefferson Medical College of Thomas Jefferson University, Philadelphia, Pa.

REFERENCES

1. Beasley RW: Vascular injuries. In Hand injuries, Philadelphia, 1981, WB Saunders Co.
2. Boyes JH: A philosophy of care of the injured hand, Bull Am Coll Surgeons 50:341, 1965.
3. Byron TM and Muntzer EM: Therapist's management of the mutilated hand. In Mackin EJ, editor: Hand rehabilitation, hand clinics, vol. 2, no. 1, Philadelphia, 1986, WB Saunders Co.
4. Flowers K: String wrapping versus massage for reducing digital volume, J Hand Surg 10A:583, 1985.
5. Hunter JM: Salvage of the burned hand, Surg Clin North Am 47(5):1060, 1967.
6. Hunter JM and Salisbury RE: Evaluation of oral trypsin-chymotrypsin for prevention of swelling after hand surgery, Plast Reconstr Surg 49(2):171, 1972.
7. Kanavel AB: Infections of the hand, ed 7, Philadelphia, 1943, Lea & Febiger.
8. Knapp ME: Aftercare of fractures. In Krusen FH, editor: Handbook of physical medicine and rehabilitation, ed 2, Philadelphia, 1971, WB Saunders Co, p 579.
9. Knapp ME: Massage. In Krusen FH, editor: Handbook of physical medicine and rehabilitation, ed 2, Philadelphia, 1971, WB Saunders Co, p 382.
10. Mackin EJ: Prevention of complications in hand therapy. In Complications of hand surgery, hand clinics, vol. 2, no. 2, May 1986.
11. Moberg E: Shoulder-hand finger syndrome, Surg Clin North Am 40:365, 1960.
12. Moberg E: Personal communication, 1977.
13. Steichen JB and Idler RS: Surgical aspects of replantation and revascularization. In Hunter JM, Schneider LH, Mackin EJ, and Callahan AD, eds: Rehabilitation of the hand, ed 2, St Louis, 1984, The CV Mosby Co, p 547.
14. Stillwell GK: Therapeutic heat and cold. In Krusen FH, editor: Handbook of physical medicine and rehabilitation, ed 2, Philadelphia, 1971, WB Saunders Co, p 264.
15. Walsh M: Relationship of hand edema to upper extremity position and water temperature during whirlpool, J Hand Surg 9A:609, 1984.
16. Weeks P and Wray RC: Management of the stiff hand. In Management of acute hand injuries, St Louis, 1978, The CV Mosby Co.

14

Use of therapeutic modalities in upper extremity rehabilitation

Patricia A. Taylor Mullins

This chapter is a brief review of the vast information on various therapeutic modalities. It is advisable to investigate state licensure laws to determine individual professional limitations before applying these concepts in the clinic.

THERAPEUTIC HEAT

Heat has long been used as a therapeutic agent. Of the many therapeutic agents in ancient times, few have been used as continuously and in as many forms as heat.

Many primitive people exposed themselves to fire to drive out the demons of disease. For some this meant applying smoldering plant materials to skin, whereas others walked on glowing coals. It was a relatively easy step from these acts to the use of cautery with heated metal. The use of this procedure by physicians was reported by the Egyptians as early as 3000 BC.[40] The use of therapeutic heat has a long and wonderful history with the Egyptians, who used burial of patients in hot sand for treatment of obesity and joint pain.[9] Hippocrates applied flat earthenware dishes filled with boiling water to the chest for treatment of congestion.

The first clinical study documenting the use of therapeutic heat was performed by Guyot in France about 1840. He constructed a hot-air cabinet in which he could maintain an environmental temperature between 30° and 70° C. He found that when the temperature was maintained at 30° C, he witnessed increased wound healing.[25,40]

Some of the more recent studies that relate to the use of therapeutic heat in the clinic are those performed by Justus Lehmann. With his intense studies, he discusses heat not as a cure for disease entities but rather as a valuable adjunct in the management of specific symptoms.[42]

It is generally accepted by contemporary therapists that heat has the following effects:
1. It increases extensibility of collagen tissue and decreases joint stiffness.
2. It produces pain relief.
3. It reduces muscle spasm.
4. It assists in the resolution of inflammatory infiltrates.
5. It increases blood flow.

Connective tissue effects

In hand therapy, the most recognized effects of therapeutic heat are increased collagen tissue extensibility and decreased joint stiffness. Effective use of heat for these goals depends on a number of factors, including the amount of time the tissue is heated, the depth of the tissue heated, the degree of heat achieved, and the degree of stretch applied after heat.

Studies have shown that temperatures greater than 50° C are destructive to collagen and actually cause the fibers to shrink and melt. At lower temperatures (41° to 45° C), tissue reacts differently, and these effects can be therapeutic. Tendon normally has an elastic behavior, and at normal tissue temperature, if the tendon is stretched or elongated, the tension of the tendon is increased. This increased tension is held for the duration of the stretch. When released, the tendon will return to the original length.[67] In contrast, if the tendon is heated to therapeutic temperatures of 45° C before stretch, tension increases initially, but this initial increase is quickly followed by a decrease in tension[45] (Fig. 14-1).

Further studies show that at 45° C, different loads of tension produce varying degrees of elongation and with increasing stress cause residual elongation after stress is removed. These same stress levels do not produce residual elongation if tissue is maintained at normal tissue temperature. If elevation of temperature is produced with no stress applied, there occurs no residual elongation[45,47] (Fig. 14-2). It is from these studies that the decisions for treatment in the clinic evolve. Such studies imply that it is necessary to perform range of motion to tight structures immediately after or during heat application. Less force is needed to achieve increased motion when heat is applied before stretch or range of motion. If heat is applied but no follow-up exercise is performed, no increase in range of motion is seen.

Vascular effects

If the desired result from therapeutic heat is to increase blood flow, consideration should be given to the depth of tissue to which increased blood flow is desired. The control of blood flow to different structures, such as skin and skeletal muscle, is quite different in response to varying types and degrees of temperature. Blood flow changes involve vasodilation of skin after heat application and can occur both through the direct effect of elevated temperature on cellular and tissue function and partly through axon and spinal cord reflexes. Cutaneous thermoreceptors carry afferent impulses to the spinal cord; some of these impulses are carried through branches toward the skin blood vessels, causing a vasodilation response through axon reflex.

The spinal cord reflex is seen when afferent fibers stimulated by heat travel to the spinal cord, resulting in a decreased postganglionic sympathetic response to cause a vasodilation. This response also causes a contralateral reflex response in areas not heated, such as in the opposite extremities.[23]

The cellular response occurs when applied heat causes a release of histamine and bradykinen, producing vasodila-

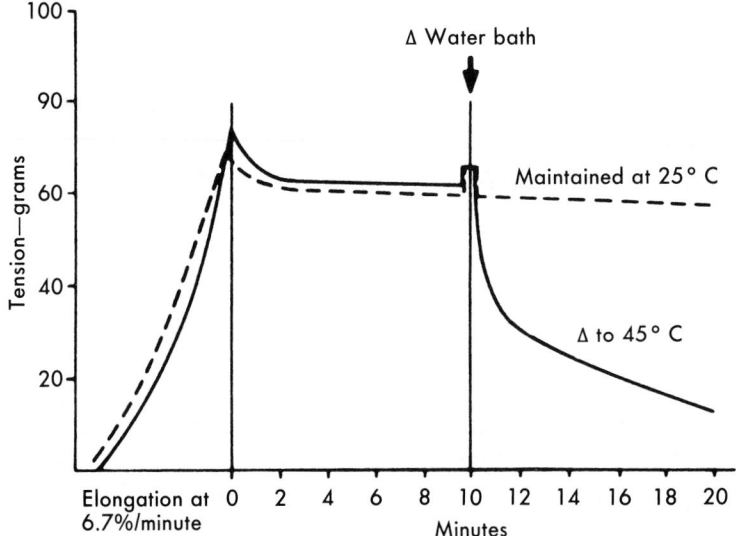

Fig. 14-1 Relaxation of tension in tendon after application of heat compared with nonheated tissue. (From Lehmann JF: Therapeutic heat and cold, ed 3, Baltimore, 1982, Williams & Wilkins.)

tion. The increasing capillary hydrostatic pressure caused by this response allows the flow of fluid from vascular to extravascular space, thus increasing interstitial fluid and producing edema. Increased edema caused by application of heat is a concern. Elevation during heat application may aid in venous return.

Superficial forms of heat have little effect on muscular blood flow. The vasodilation response at the skin dissipates most heat forms before there is increased blood flow in the muscle.[120]

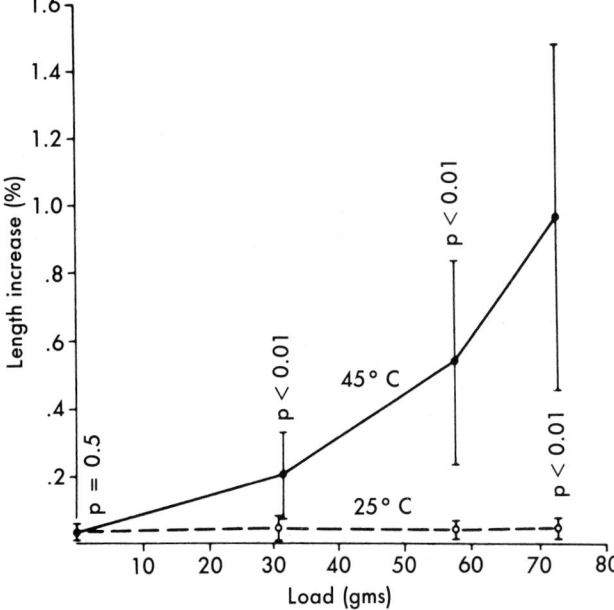

Fig. 14-2 Increase in tendon lengths is shown after application of heat and varying load of stress. (From Lehmann JF: Therapeutic heat and cold, ed 3, Baltimore, 1982, Williams & Wilkins.)

Pain and muscle spasm

Although the precise mechanisms are not totally understood, it is reported that heat is helpful in decreasing pain and muscle spasm. This appears to be related to the ability of heat to alter nerve conduction velocity, elevate the pain threshold, and also change the firing rates of muscle spindles.[42]

In many musculoskeletal problems, pain may be the result of protective or guarding spasms. With these spasms, pain is thought to be caused by ischemia, which can be relieved by heat application. Heat can also be applied as a counterirritant; in effect, the pain cessation is, as explained by Melzack and Wall, the gate-control theory.[53] Heat can also have an effect on muscle spasm by changing the firing rates of the muscle spindle. When pain triggers a tonic muscle contraction, increased firing is seen in the muscle spindle II afferents. Elevation of muscle temperature to therapeutic range decreases firing rate of II afferents and increases firing of Ib fibers of the Golgi tendon organs. This reversal of activity causes a decreased firing of alpha motoneurons and reduces the tonic contraction.[54]

Heat modalities that produce only superficial increases in temperature (rather than increases in muscle temperature) produce the same effects by indirect means. Studies have shown that heating of the skin decreases gamma fiber activity, producing less stretch on the muscle spindle and reduced afferent firing from the muscle spindles.[23] This again decreases firing in the alpha motoneuron.

Another consideration is that muscle strength and endurance can be affected by application of heat. Edwards has shown that by using immersion in warm water at 44° C for 45 minutes, quadricep strength and endurance are reduced.[20] The muscle temperature after this heat application was elevated to 38.6° C from a normal value of 35.1° C. A later study by Chastain using a deep-heating modality of shortwave diathermy over the quadriceps showed isometric strength to be decreased during the first 30 minutes after discontinuing the heat. An actual increase in strength occurred in the subsequent 2 hours.[12] A study performed by Grose showed that after an 8-minute immersion of the arm in water at 48° C, initial strength was unchanged but total work output of the forearm was significantly reduced.[27]

These effects should always be considered when performing strength and endurance evaluations in the clinic.

Modes of transfer

There are three ways in which heat is transferred to tissue.
1. Conduction: Transfer of heat between two objects, such as hot packs and paraffin baths.
2. Convection: Transfer of heat between a surface and a moving medium. It is actually a form of conduction with added variables of velocity of movement, viscosity, and thermal conductivity. Examples of this type of heating include whirlpool and Fluidotherapy.
3. Conversion: Penetration of various types of nonthermal energy to deeper tissue and conversion into heat. The most commonly used form of conversion heat is ultrasound (Fig. 14-3).

In determining which heat modality to use, one must decide whether a vigorous or mild effect from the heat is desired. One must determine also the depth of the pathologic condition that is being treated and what results one wants from treatment. In general, vigorous heating is used in chronic conditions, such as joint contractures, or in chronic inflammatory processes. Vigorous heating actually would be contraindicated in acute inflammatory processes, because the mild inflammatory heat response mentioned earlier may superimpose already existing inflammatory response, causing damage. Mild heating would be appropriate in acute inflammatory processes to aid in pain reduction.[47]

Mild heating usually raises temperature at the site of the pathology to less than 40° C and is believed to have more of a soothing effect.[78] Vigorous heating raises the temperature to between 40° and 45° C. The depth of the pathology

is important; a superficial heat, such as hot packs, may be a form of vigorous heat in the PIP joint but only a mild form of heat over the radial head. A comparison of mild and vigorous heat is as shown in Fig. 14-4.

In clinical decision making, consider the case of rheumatoid patients. In an acute phase, vigorous deep heating is likely to penetrate too deeply and aggravate the inflammatory reaction, whereas a mild form of superficial heat may decrease pain, muscle spasm, and joint stiffness. In contrast, consider a patient with rheumatoid disease who has a burnt out, contracted joint. Vigorous heat is needed to produce increased extensibility of the collagen tissue.[40]

Superficial heat

Decisions regarding heat modalities revolve around the desired effects of heat and the level of penetration. If the area to be treated is a deep-seated joint or muscle belly, many heat modalities are not effective. When superficial structures, such as adherent incisions, are involved, the more superficial heat modalities are indicated (see Fig. 14-3).

Changes in tissue temperature from superficial heat depend on the intensity of the heat applied, the duration, and the type of heat modality applied. Superficial heating elevates tissue temperature within 0.5 cm from the surface to the greatest degree; the maximum temperature will be reached within 6 to 8 minutes.[46] Muscle temperature at a depth of 1 to 2 cm will require approximately 15 to 30 minutes to reach the maximum temperature and will be heated to a lesser degree.[1]

Hot packs. Probably the most widely used form of superficial heat is the use of hot packs, which is a type of heat by conduction.

The most important consideration regarding hot packs is that the temperature of the water in the hydrocollator ranges from 61.1° to 79.4° C, which is well above the level of

Modes of heat transfer	Conduction	Convection	Conversion
Modality	Hot packs Paraffin bath	Fluidotherapy Whirlpool	Ultrasound
	Superficial heat		Deep heat

Fig. 14-3 Models of heat transfer.

Mild and vigorous heating

	Temperature elevation at site of pathology	Degree of temperature increase	Rate of rise of temperature	Duration of peak temperature elevation
Mild	Low	Up to 40° c	Slow	Relatively short period
Vigorous	High	40° c to 45° c	Rapid	Relatively long period

Fig. 14-4 Comparison of mild and vigorous heating. (Adapted from Micholivitz SL, ed: Thermal agents in rehabilitation, Philadelphia, 1986, FA Davis Co.)

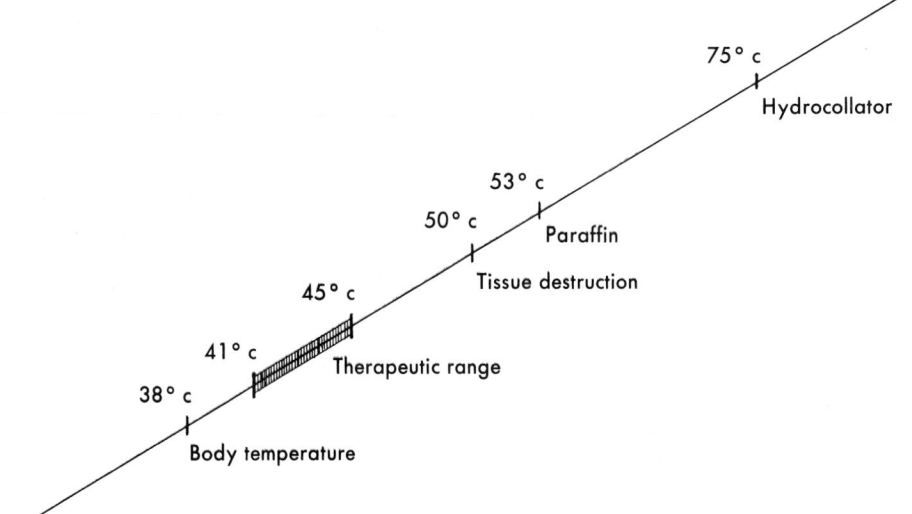

Fig. 14-5   Temperature levels of common modalities are compared with therapeutic temperature range.

tissue destruction (Fig. 14-5). The packs are *never* applied directly to the skin; it is necessary to apply 8 to 10 layers of toweling to bring heat down to a therapeutic range and provide insulation to maintain the heat of the pack. It is best to check the temperature inside the hot pack setup to measure the heat that is being transferred. Though the treatment lasts for 20 to 30 minutes, the highest skin temperature is reached after 8 to 10 minutes.[46] Temperature elevations at a depth of 1 cm remain elevated for approximately 45 to 60 minutes before the associated increased blood flow causes a decreased temperature. This allows adequate time for stretch from passive and active range of motion after heat application to achieve tissue elongation before cool down.

Lehmann's report of increased tissue elongation with heat and stretch applied together allows great variations of application in the clinic to achieve this result (Fig. 14-6). In zones IV and V extensor tendon lacerations, when the healing time is adequate to allow passive stretch into flexion, a patient can be positioned to achieve stretching during heat. The hand is draped over a roll, placing the wrist in flexion, and heat is applied dorsally. The weight of the hot pack actually applies stress during application.

Contraindications. The major contraindication of applying hot packs is the presence of decreased circulation and decreased sensation. The appropriate timing of application in the healing process is also quite important.

Hot packs can be used safely in the presence of peripheral nerve involvement, but great caution must be used. Not only is sensation inadequate to report when heat is too great, but the associated sympathetic involvement slows the circulatory response to dissipate the heat. For these patients, do not rely on the uninjured fingers to serve as a guideline; check the temperature of the hot pack. Appropriate timing of application relates to adequate healing time, in which the heat with stretch can be applied to healing structures. As mentioned earlier, with the extensor tendon lacerations, the hot packs should be applied at a time in which passive stretch is appropriate. Care should be taken in the proper positioning

of postsurgical problems, as well as in the avoidance of unwanted stresses.

Paraffin. Another form of conductive heat is the use of paraffin. With treatment of joint contractures, paraffin often can provide a greater temperature rise in the joints of the fingers than with hot packs because of the circumferential coating of the paraffin. Although the temperature of a paraffin bath is not as high above the level of tissue destruction (Fig. 14-5) as is the hydrocollator, caution should nonetheless be taken to monitor the paraffin bath temperature. The melting point of paraffin is 54.5° C. When mixed with mineral oil, the oil lowers the melting point to 47.8° C, and this combination has a low specific heat.[55] The result is that application of paraffin can be tolerated at temperature levels of 51.7° to 54.4° C.[71] These temperatures can be tolerated better than water at the same temperature. If heat were applied with water at this same level, tissue destruction could occur. Paraffin has a low heat-carrying capacity and thermal conductivity when compared with water.

There are two methods of paraffin application, the dip method and the immersion method. In the dip method, the hand and wrist are dipped quickly in and out of the tank, with six to eight repetitions, until a "glove" is formed. The hand is then placed inside a plastic bag and covered with a towel to maintain the heat. This is maintained for 20 to 30 minutes. The immersion method is performed by repeated dipping to form the "glove" and then reimmersion into the tank for 20 to 30 minutes. Of the two methods, the dip method is considered to be a mild heat method, and the immersion method is a more vigorous method. Skin temperatures of 46° C have been recorded with the immersion technique.[2]

Again, the heat and stretch method can be used in gaining IP flexion, either individually or in mass flexion. The finger is held in mass flexion using an elastic wrapping material, such as Coban, and then dipped into the paraffin and wrapped to maintain the heat (Fig. 14-7). As the heat stretches the joints, the elasticity of the Coban pulls the digit further into flexion.

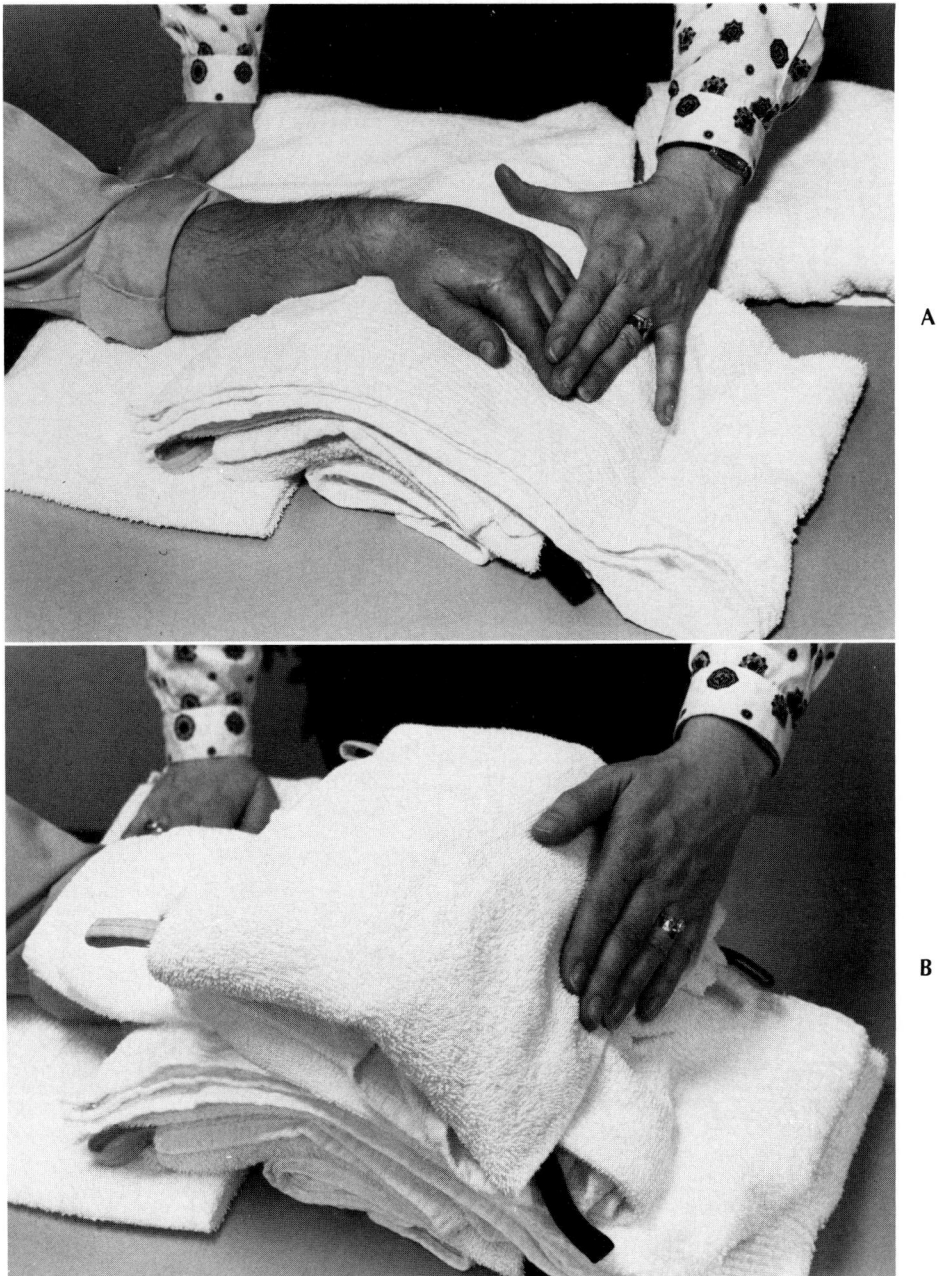

Fig. 14-6   **A,** Hand is positioned to cause stretch of the injured structures. **B,** Dorsal hot pack is applied to the hand to maintain light pressure on the position.

Precautions. Paraffin should not be applied to open wounds because of the risk of infection or burns. Caution also needs to be used with insensate hands and recently healed burns, because the ability to dissipate the heat through sympathetic response is greatly reduced.

Whirlpool. A type of convection heat is whirlpool. Though an excellent aid in debridement and as stimulation in the healing of open wounds, whirlpool is not a highly recommended form of heat for the upper extremity.

Studies performed by Magness[51] with a group of normal volunteers and patients using whirlpool showed a significant increase in volume in the upper extremity, which was di-

rectly related to increased water temperature. This increase was seen in both normal volunteers and patients, with a significantly higher increase in volume seen in patients. What is more interesting is that the water temperature used for the patient group was in the standard accepted range for whirlpool treatment (37.8° to 40° C), which is below Lehmann's reported therapeutic temperature range.

Many have advocated use of active exercise or elevation during whirlpool to prevent edema. In a study by Schultz,[69] a group of normal subjects and upper extremity patients were evaluated after whirlpool at temperatures of 37° C administered while performing active exercise. No signifi-

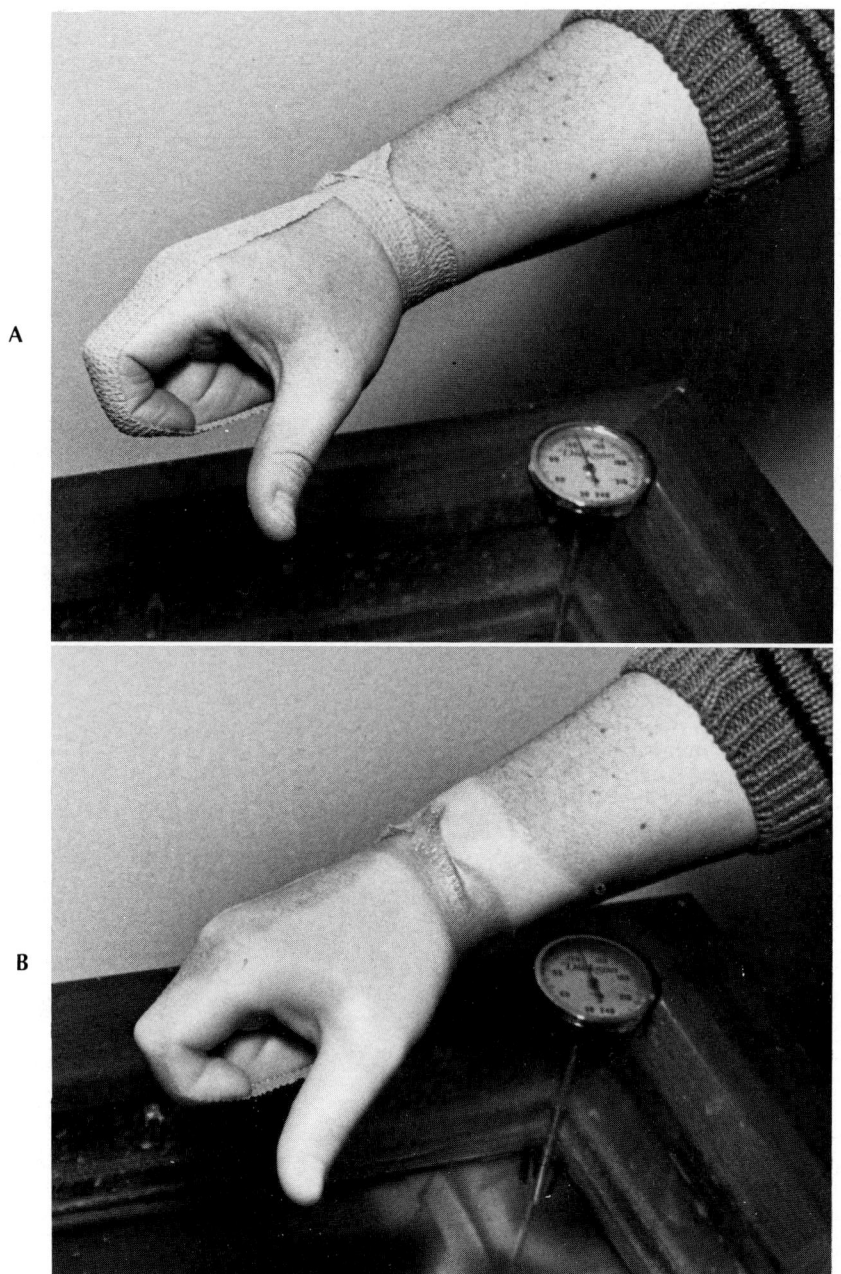

Fig. 14-7 **A,** Hand is wrapped into a stretched position with Coban. **B,** Hand is dipped in paraffin to apply heat in conjunction with stretch.

cant difference in edema formation was found when comparing active exercises with no active exercise during whirlpool with both the normal subjects and the patients. Walsh[77] performed an evaluation of 30 normal volunteers receiving whirlpool at 37.6° and 40° C, compiling the effect of elevation of the arm during immersion and nonelevation. An increase in edema was found at 40° C. Though not statistically significant, the data supported the theory of need for elevation during whirlpool for prevention of edema. These studies would suggest precaution in application of whirlpool to patients with edema.

If whirlpool is used to aid in cleansing and debridement of open wounds, provide padding between the axilla and the edge of the whirlpool to prevent constriction of circulation (Fig. 14-8).

Fluidotherapy. Fluidotherapy is another convection heating agent. In this therapy, dry particles of corn husk are used much in the same way whirlpool uses water. Treatment involves inserting the hand into the circulating medium at temperature ranges of 110° to 120° F for 20 to 30 minutes. Circulation of dry particles allows higher temperature than water, because the thermal conductance of these particles is not as great as that of water (Fig. 14-9).

Borrell[8] performed a study in which Fluidotherapy was applied at a temperature of 47.8° C and found temperature rises in the joints of the hands of 9° C. He compared the Fluidotherapy treatment with dip paraffin and whirlpool, which showed a rise of 7.5° C and 6° C, respectively. No comparison was made with hot packs.

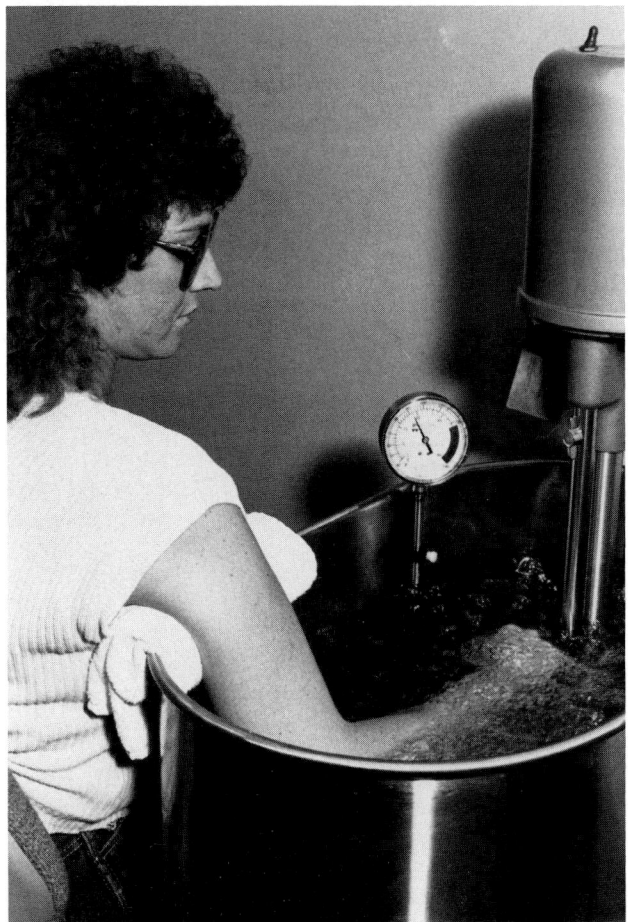

Fig. 14-8 Towel is placed in axilla to aid in comfort during whirlpool.

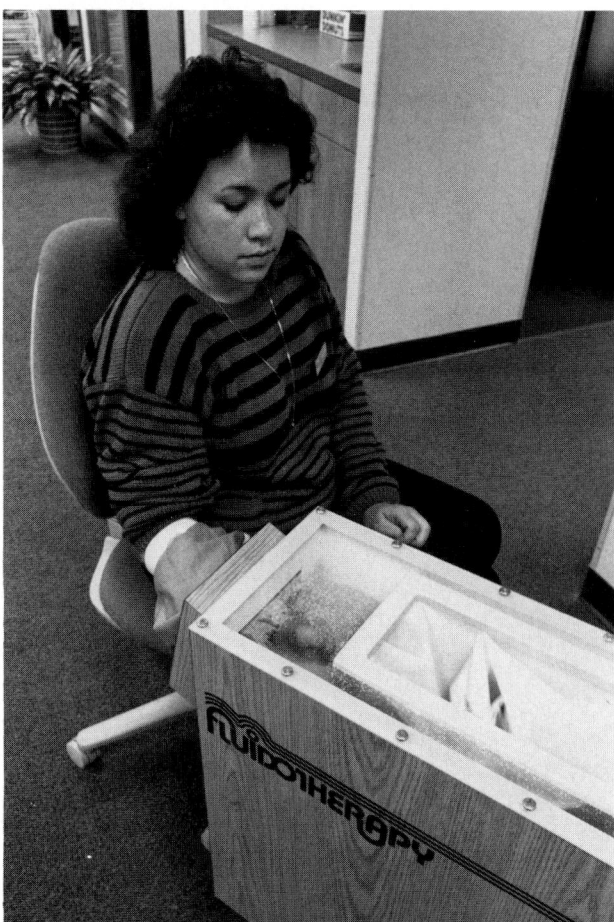

Fig. 14-9 Heated particles circulate around the hand during Fluidotherapy treatment.

Another subjective report is a decrease in pain and hypersensitivity in hands. This could be because heat raises the pain threshold. If desensitization is desired but edema is a problem, the heat can be left at low levels during circulation of the particles.

Deep heat

In treatment of deep levels of pathology, it is necessary to find a modality to heat tissue at depths of 3 cm or more without causing excessive heating of the overlying superficial tissue.

Ultrasound. The most commonly used form of deep heat is ultrasound. A form of conversion heat, ultrasound uses high-frequency soundwaves, which convert into heat when applied to tissue. This conversion takes place as the soundwaves are absorbed and cause molecules to vibrate, setting neighboring molecules into motion. This particle movement produces heat.

The number of vibrations a molecule undergoes in 1 second is expressed in hertz (Hz). The human ear is capable of hearing sound frequency between 16 Hz and 20,000 Hz. Sound with higher frequency than this is ultrasound.

For therapy consideration, 1.0 megahertz is the frequency of sound most often used. Ultrasound at higher frequency than this can result in so much internal friction in the tissue

that the sound cannot penetrate beyond the superficial tissues. The soundwave for ultrasound is produced by applying electrical current to a piezoelectric crystal within the soundhead, which converts the electrical current to sound energy at such high frequency that it becomes ultrasound. The frequency is generated by an oscillator circuit, which can have the capabilities to be an interrupted circuit to produce a pulsed ultrasound. This frequency is set by the manufacturer. The intensity is determined by the electrical voltage applied to the crystal. This is controlled by the therapist.

Ultrasound is a dimension of the acoustic spectrum in contrast to the earlier described heat modalities, which are dimensions of the electromagnetic spectrum. This point is important, because acoustic energy travels better through liquids than does electromagnetic energy (Fig. 14-10). Because soft tissue in the body is 70% to 80% water, it is an excellent transmitter for ultrasound, with depths of penetration at 5 to 6 cm. Though these depths are reported, at 5 cm the intensity value is one half the intensity at the point of application. Past this point, the intensity continues to decrease.[96]

An advantage of ultrasound in clinical use is that the more homogenous the tissue, the less the absorption. Subcutaneous fat is a highly homogenous tissue and often presents problems with electromagnetic energies, because it acts as

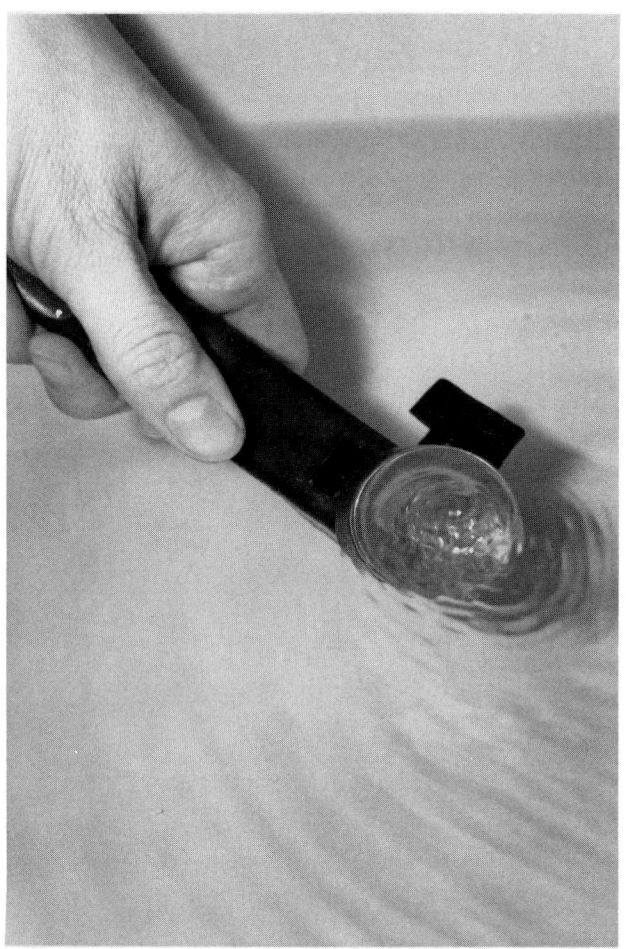

Fig. 14-10 Passage of soundwaves underwater is shown with soundhead immersed.

The effects of ultrasound have been divided into those felt to be thermal effects and those felt to be nonthermal effects.

The thermal effects are those produced also by the other heating modalities. Some of these include increased blood flow, increased metabolic rate, alteration of nerve conduction, increased tendon extensibility, assistance in resolution of inflammation and edema, and decreased pain. Though these same effects can be seen with other modalities, the effects from ultrasound have been shown to occur more rapidly and be more long-lasting than with the electromagnetic spectrum. The nonthermal effects are less established but should be mentioned. These include membrane permeability changes accelerating the rate of diffusion and gaseous cavitation.

The ability to increase membrane permeability is believed to be the result of the stringing of the soundwaves through tissue, which increases the grading of concentration of ions and other materials across the cell membrane, thus accelerating the rate of diffusion. This makes possible "phonophoresis," that is, using the soundwaves to diffuse an analgesic or antiinflammatory agent into tissue when applied topically.

Gaseous cavitation is a phenomenon that occurs when soundwaves cause gas bubbles to be produced in tissue fluid during the rarefaction phase of the soundwave, which collapses in the subsequent phase of compression. This collapse may expand to the extent that it causes a tear in tissue. Cavitation can be prevented by firm application of external pressure during the treatment. The external pressure is applied with the soundhead.

Application. The most common techniques of application of ultrasound are direct contact with either a moving or stationary soundhead and the immersion method. In applying ultrasound with direct contact, a coupling agent is mandatory to minimize the trapping of air bubbles at the skin surface during treatment. It is important to remember that ultrasound is an acoustic energy and does not pass through gases, and the coupling agent also decreases friction of the soundhead over the skin. There are many commercially available gels on the market for use with ultrasound; other effective coupling agents include mineral oil, lotion, or glycerin.

Direct contact ultrasound is most commonly applied with the soundhead kept in continuous motion. This allows a higher intensity to be used without periosteal overheating and will also allow a greater area of coverage during treatment (Fig. 14-11). A slow, circular motion at approximately 4 cm per second is the most effective uniform heating pattern.[36]

If the problem being treated is very localized, a stationary contact technique can be used. However, this is not commonly recommended because of the greatly increased risk of periosteal overheating. Intensity must be kept very low, and a coupling agent with high viscosity must be used. Close observation of a patient is necessary: if pain should occur, the intensity should be lowered.

The immersion technique involves use of the soundhead under water and is used when areas to be treated involve bony prominences, such as the dorsum of the hand and fingers (Fig. 14-12). This provides better contact for the soundhead, because it is not "bouncing" off the promi-

an insulator and prevents deep tissue temperature rise. With ultrasound, the depth of penetration, plus the ease of use with the subcutaneous fat layers, makes it the most effective heat modality for deeply seated joints. It is also capable of heating deep structures more quickly, because it penetrates directly and does not first heat more superficial structures.[26]

As sound is propagated through tissue, it is absorbed and converted to heat. Absorption is higher in tissue with a higher amount of protein or collagen. Temperature rises are greatest in cortical bone, with a rise of approximately 5° to 6° C. Subcutaneous fat has the lowest temperature rise at approximately half that of muscle temperature rise, which is approximately 1° to 2° C.[41]

When discussing deep temperature rises, it is important to remember that there is a considerable amount of reflection at any tissue interface, such as a tendon-bone interface.[43] This reflection causes greater intensity of temperature in a more superficial layer of tissue, particularly from the higher-density tissue. Reflection from bone to tendon or to the periosteum can raise temperatures to damaging levels very quickly. If the patient has decreased sensation, he may not be able to report the burning sensation. Therefore minimal levels of intensity should be maintained. In a patient with normal sensation, the pain should be an immediate indicator to decrease the intensity before damage occurs.

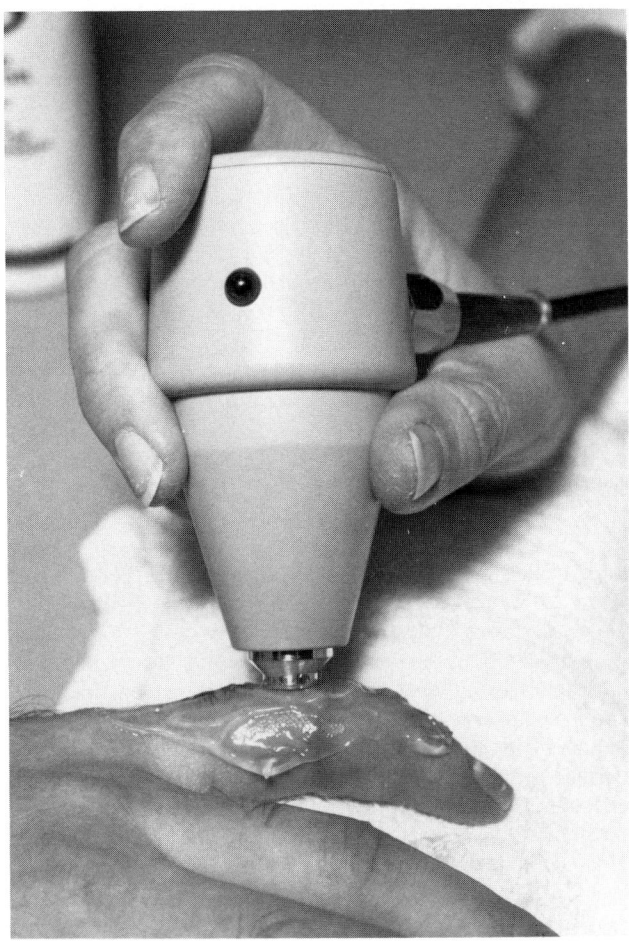

Fig. 14-11 Direct contact application of ultrasound is shown using a small soundhead directly over the PIP joint.

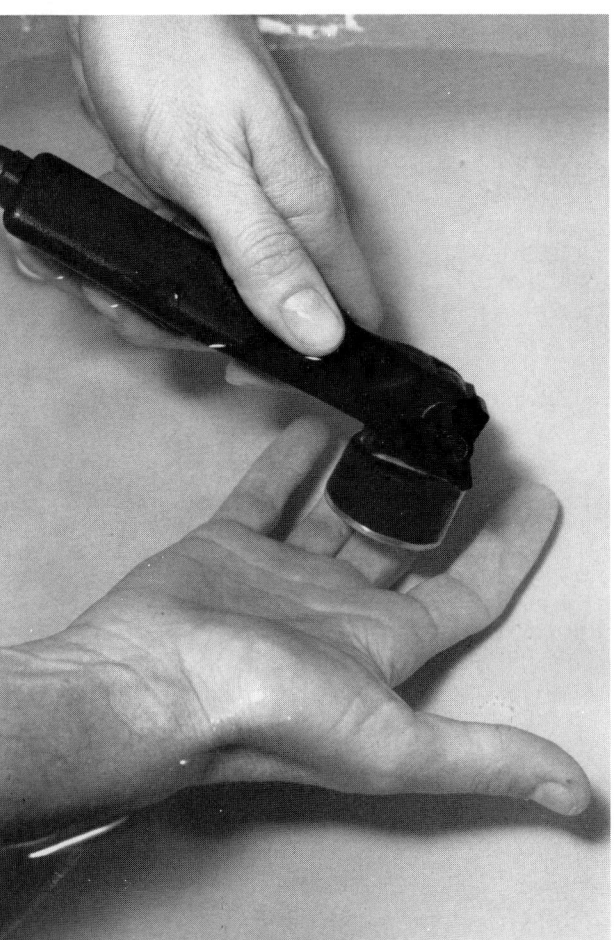

Fig. 14-12 For easy application of ultrasound over uneven surfaces, the soundhead can be immersed in water for replacement of coupling agent.

nences, which would allow air between the soundhead and the skin. With this method, the soundhead is held approximately ½ inch from the skin over the area to be treated. Air bubbles should be brushed from the skin and the soundhead with the hand in immersion, because these gases will impede the sound.

Intensity. Intensity selection is based on the depth of the pathology and the amount of area treated. Patient comfort is an important indicator of overheating deep tissue, such as the periosteum. When areas that have thick soft tissue covering the bone, such as in the extensor mass of the forearm, are treated, intensities of 1.5 to 2.0 W/cm² are used comfortably. In areas of less tissue coverage, such as over bone in the dorsum of the hand, a lower intensity of 0.5 to 1.0 W/cm² is indicated. These intensities will need to be adjusted as a function of varying sizes and of area treated, or of varying sizes of tranducer heads. For instance, if a 5 cm² head is covering 10 cm² of tissue, the exposure of sound energy is one half of that produced by a 10 cm² tranducer head to the same area. A smaller head necessitates more movement over the tissue with less efficient heating.

The most important factor of the intensity selection is patient comfort. Instruction should be given that a gentle warmth will be felt. Any report of a delayed onset of pain

after ultrasound should be an indication to decrease the intensity during the next session, and of course any complaint of pain during treatment should be an immediate indication for decrease in intensity. Higher intensity of 1.5 W/cm² to 2.5 W/cm² is tolerated with moving direct contact or immersion technique. When using stationary technique, intensity is not often tolerated more than 0.5 W/cm².

Ultrasound can also be given in continuous wave form or pulsed wave form. The pulsed wave form gives sound a designated percentage of on-time with pulsed off-time (Fig. 14-13). This allows concentration in a smaller area with higher intensity. Pulsed soundwave can be expressed by the percentage of on time compared with off time. This is called the duty cycle. The most common range of a duty cycle is 0.2 (20%) to 0.5 (50%).

Ultrasound is an excellent choice of heat when deep scar tissue is believed to be preventing tendon gliding, such as in zone IV flexor tendon injuries or zone V extensor tendon injuries. Placing tissue on a stretch during application of ultrasound and leaving the tissue in the position for 5 to 10 minutes after treatment once again ties into Lehmann's heat and stretch report (Fig. 14-14).

Contraindications. Recent studies by Roberts, Rutherford, and Harris[64] have shown ultrasound to have an adverse

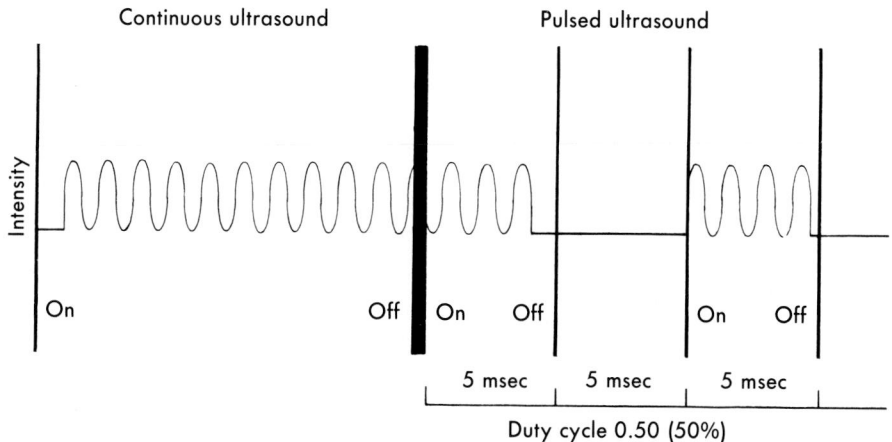

Continuous ultrasound   Pulsed ultrasound

Fig. 14-13 A comparison of continuous and pulsed ultrasound.

effect on healing rabbit tendons. In their studies, tendons receiving ultrasound before 6 weeks after repair, compared with controlled groups, are shown to have lower tensile strength. Though this was not a human study, most advocates of the use of ultrasound with tendon repair suggest a delay of use until after 8 weeks, when the tendon is thought

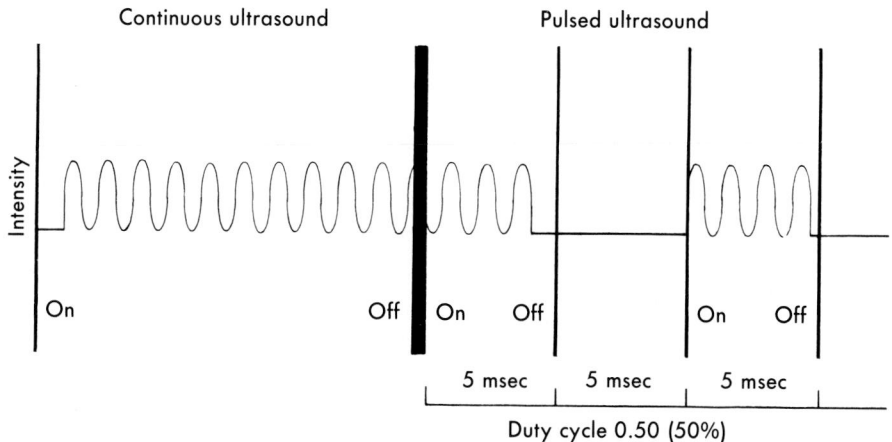

Fig. 14-14 Hand is placed in stretch position before applying ultrasound to combine heat application with stretch.

to be healed. With tendon grafts, there is a further delay to 10 to 12 weeks after surgery, because the avascularity of the graft causes a slower healing time.

Another contraindication of ultrasound is that of using ultrasound in patients with open growth centers in bone. Until recently, it was believed that absorption of this type of energy in the cells of the growth center tended to disrupt normal growth.[17] Other studies have shown that minimal exposure to ultrasound in the epiphyseal areas is safe. Until further studies are performed, when increased extensibility of tissue is desired in children, another form of heat should be used.[75]

It has also been suggested to avoid use of ultrasound in areas of malignancy, because the sound waves may cause cellular detachment and metastasis.[7]

Other contraindications include those of typical heat precautions, such as lack of sensation and the presence of impaired circulation.

Phonophoresis. Phonophoresis is the application of ultrasound to a topical agent on the skin to drive medication into the tissue. As mentioned earlier, this phenomenon is believed to be the result of increased membrane permeability after treatment of ultrasound. Cortisol has been driven to depths of 5 to 6 cm subcutaneously into skeletal tissue, skeletal muscle, and peripheral nerve after phonophoresis.[61] Another study revealed that more lidocaine was extracted from rabbit tissue after ultrasound than when lidocaine was applied topically and not followed by ultrasound.[63]

When hydrocortisone ointment is used, a 10% solution, which is prepared pharmaceutically, is appropriate. The ointment is applied directly to the skin and then covered with a coupling agent for transmission. If bony prominences are prohibitive of direct application to the skin, the ointment can be applied to the skin, and the ultrasound transmitted under water. Higher intensities of application may be necessary, because the use of the hydrocortisone ointment decreases transmission of the ultrasound.[79]

Other medications have been administered with phonophoresis, such as aspirin, and the ointment used in this instance is Myoflex. The reported use is common, but no formal reports have been made.

Another use of phonophoresis is the application of ultrasound after intramuscular or intraarticular injection of hydrocortisone. Relief of symptoms was reportedly increased when ultrasound was applied after injection; this is believed to be a result of increased membrane permeability and increased diffusion.[3]

Indications

As with other heat modalities, ultrasound is used when thermal effects of heat are desired in the tissue. There have been some reports of increased transmission with greater deep tissue temperature rise when ultrasound is used after hot packs.[57] This would be particularly beneficial when hot packs are applied before phonophoresis, thus increasing blood flow both superficially and deep to aid in diffusion of medication.

Ultrasound has shown specific improvement in Dupuytren's contractures, with relaxation of the tight palmar fascia after administration.[26] Ultrasound can also be applied to the hypertrophic scar tissue often seen after Dupuytren's release and subsequent healing.[58] Exposure to ultrasound is an effective means of gaining range of motion when limitation is caused by hypertrophic scar tissue, also seen in newly healed burn patients.[7] Distinction should be made between hypertrophic scarring and keloid formation, because ultrasound does not seem effective in releasing tissues bound by keloid.[83]

Relief of pain has been reported with administration of ultrasound in those patients with neuromas. The relief is believed to be from nonthermal effects, because the patient group studied reported no relief from other heat modalities.[66]

Application of ultrasound can speed resorption of organized hematoma by increased deep tissue blood flow and cell permeability.[60] Ultrasound should not, however, be applied in the area of suspected venous thrombus, because the clot may be dislodged into the blood stream.

The indication or contraindication of ultrasound over fracture sites has been discussed. Recent studies have shown that pulsed ultrasound may accelerate fracture healing.[19] Further studies are warranted. Ultrasound can be used in the presence of surgical metal implants, with no report of selective heating of the implants;[44] no effects are seen with use in the presence of silastic implants.[11a]

CASE STUDY

A 43-year-old man is referred to rehabilitation after laceration from broken glass, which resulted in multiple flexor tendon lacerations in zone IV. He was treated initially with cast immobilization in a protected position for 3½ weeks. The major problem is lack of full tendon excursion caused by scar formation.

On referral at 3½ weeks after surgery, decision was made to begin moist heat to aid in tendon extensibility. Because the injury also involved a median nerve laceration, extreme caution was taken with the degree of heat applied to the injured hand. Hot packs was the heat of choice, and the hand was positioned with the wrist in flexion so that no passive extension was applied across the repair site.

This use of heat followed by active range of motion (AROM) was continued until 7 to 8 weeks after surgery. At this time, it was safe to add ultrasound to the treatment program to heat deeper scar tissue to aid in softening adhesion formation.

Because passive extension is allowed at 7 to 8 weeks after surgery, both the hot packs and the ultrasound were applied in a stretched position of extension.

Appropriate electrical modalities were applied also, as indicated.

CRYOTHERAPY

As with the application of heat, the application of cold or cryotherapy involves the alteration of tissue temperature to achieve desired therapeutic effects.

Hippocrates, according to the writings of medical historians, recommended cold drinks to reduce fever. The eighteenth-century reports of the Curries[15] told of positive results using cold baths to reduce fever, which subsequently sparked an interest in cold therapy.

Evaporative cooling methods, now popular in techniques of treating myofascial pain, were introduced in 1850 by Vollemier. He cooled patients' foreheads by evaporating ether from the skin.[82] In 1832 the effects of cooling on the contralateral extremity were reported in observations of Edwards when he noted that if one hand was plunged into cold water, the temperature of the opposite hand would fall.[21]

Vascular effects

The initial response after application of cold is that of vasoconstriction. Associated decrease in blood flow is brought about not only by the decrease in vessel diameter, but also by the resistance of the flow of the cooled blood because of its increased viscosity.

When the temperature of tissue is reduced for an extended period, there occurs a period of vasodilation. The sudden reddening and warming of the cooled areas is known as the Hunting reaction and was first described in 1930 by Lewis.[49] He discovered that when fingers were immersed in water at 10° to 12° C, skin temperature decreased during the initial 15 minutes but then began cycling with periods of warming and cooling. Though skin temperature would rise with vasodilation, it would not reach the preimmersion temperature.

Skin and joint temperature changes

The application of cold will obviously reduce skin temperature. Reported studies reveal a wide range of temperature changes as a result of the application of cold. This variation may be explained by the fact that these studies used different application methods, application times, and temperatures of the cold application.

Such studies include that by Bugaj,[10] who noted that an application of ice massage of the gastrocnemius area for 10 minutes would result in a fall of skin temperature of 26.6° C. Waylonis[77] reported a decrease of skin temperature of 18.2° C for the same period. A decrease in skin temperature of 29.5° C after an immersion for 193 minutes in water of 4° C was reported by Abramson,[22] whereas Migliattea[56] reported a decrease of 19.5° C in water emersion of 7° C for 30 minutes.

As with cold application to the skin, application of cold to a joint causes vasoconstriction and decreased intraarticular temperature.[14] Cryokinetics, or the alternation of cold and exercise, is gaining popularity because of the belief that there occurs a cold-induced vasodilation, which brings more blood flow to the joint. Knight and Londeree[36] performed a study in which blood flow was measured in the ankle under several different conditions, such as hot packs, cold packs, heat and exercise, and cold and exercise. Results showed that blood flow was greater with heat application than with cold application. Relative to cold and exercise, there was greater blood flow seen with this method of application than with heat alone. This would suggest that the increased blood flow comes from the exercise and not from a cold-induced vasodilation.

Inflammation and edema

It has long been stated that cold is the treatment of choice for acute injuries, 24 to 48 hours after onset. Cold is advocated for reduction in both edema and inflammation.

As with heat, it has been shown that the degree of cold temperature applied has much effect on the outcome. In a study by Farry,[22] cold was applied to an experimental group of pigs with clinically induced ligament injuries. The results of the treatment revealed a decrease in the histologic evidence of inflammation.

In this same study, the effects of cold on edema were not as positive. The amount of edema in the cold-treated limbs was actually greater, not only with the injured limbs but also with the uninjured controls.

Farry further studied the effects of cold application by combining the cold with compression, as is the procedure with most first aid. After this method, residual edema was decreased. The question raised from these results is the degree to which compression, rather than cold, caused the reduction.

McMaster and Liddle[52] examined not only cold application, but also the degree of cold as it affected edema. Using a group of crush injuries with rabbits, cold immersion at 20° C was applied for 1 hour after trauma. The degree of edema measured at 4, 6, and 24 hours after immersion showed an increased volume compared with the control group measures at 20° C. A group measured with the same technique at 30° C showed consistently less edema throughout the observation.

In the clinic, consideration must be given in the application of cold so not to cause undesired effects. Temperature changes should not be severe, because this may actually increase edema. Such an increase in edema is thought to be the result of increased permeability of lymph vessels, which is seen at about 15° C.[49] The increased performance and decreased pain reported from cryotherapy after sports injuries, such as tendinitis and sprains, are seen when cold is applied in combination with compression, exercise, or massage.[33,74]

Connective tissue extensibility

Cold application decreases the extensibility of collagen by increasing the stiffness through a decrease in plastic deformation and increased viscosity of tissue.[47] A decrease in range of motion of the MP joint after cold immersion was reported by Wright.[84] A similar finding was also described by Hunter[34] and was thought to be a result of increased viscosity within the joint. LeBlanc[38] showed a direct relationship between decreased finger flexion and decreased dexterity with increased synovial fluid viscosity when the temperature was lowered.

Neuromuscular effects

Cooling has been reported to affect almost every component of the neuromuscular complex, including the muscle spindle, the extrafusal fibers of the muscle, and nerve conduction velocity.

Motor and sensory nerve conduction velocity has been shown to progressively decrease proportionately with the degree of application of cold until tissue temperature reaches 10° to 15° C.[24] The rate of firing of muscle spindle afferents also decreases when spindles or the entire muscle are cooled.[62]

Spasticity has also been shown to decrease after application of cold. In contrast to findings in treatment of edema, it has not been shown that exercise or stretch increases the effectiveness more than ice alone.

Pain

When sensory nerve conduction is decreased, the application of cold has been shown to be effective in providing analgesia and relief of pain. Evidence reveals that to achieve this analgesic affect, the skin temperature needs to be approximately 10° to 15° C. Bugaj[11] applied needle pricking to patients during cooling stages and found that when skin temperature fell below 10° C, all subjects had analgesia.

Travell[74] has long used the combination of Fluori-Methane spray and stretch technique in relieving musculoskeletal or myofascial pain. Reports of increased range of motion from stretching or mobilization during this cold-induced anesthesia have accompanied these techniques.

Modes of transfer

There are two primary modes of transfer for cold: conduction and evaporation. As with heat, conduction is the transfer of temperature from direct contact between two objects. Conductive agents of cooling include ice massage,

Modes of transfer	Conduction	Evaporation
Modality	Ice massage	Flouri-methane spray
	Cold packs	Ethyl chloride
	Ice towels	
	Cold bath	

Fig. 14-15 Modes of transfer for cryotherapy.

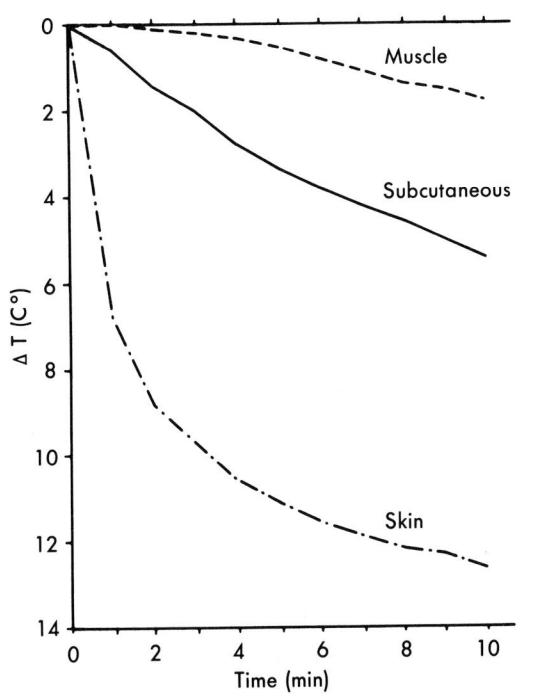

Change of skin, subcutaneous, and muscle temperatures during topical (thigh) ice application in a person with greater than 1 cm of subcutaneous fat.

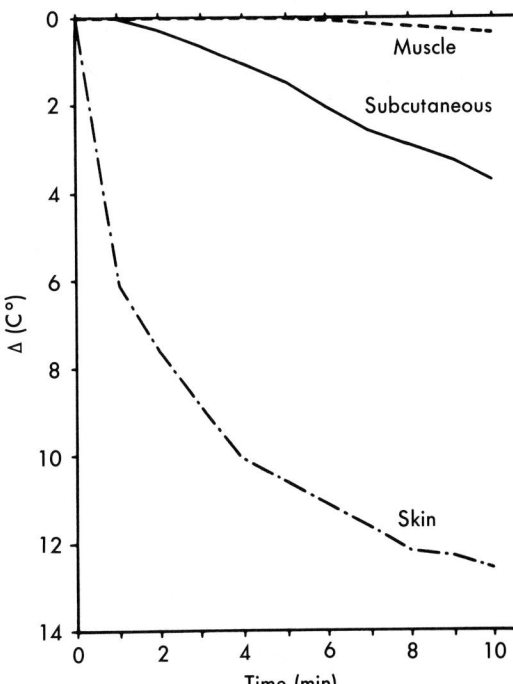

Change of skin, subcutaneous, and muscle temperatures during topical (thigh) ice application in a person with greater than 2 cm of subcutaneous fat.

Fig. 14-16   Change of tissue temperature with application of cold. (From Lehmann JF: Therapeutic heat and cold, ed 3, Baltimore, 1982, Williams & Wilkins.)

cold packs, ice towels, or cold-bath immersion. In the case of cryotherapy, cold-bath immersion is considered conduction rather than convection, because the fluid is not moving across the skin as with whirlpool or fluidotherapy (Fig. 14-15).

Evaporative cooling occurs when a vapocoolant spray, such as Fluori-Methane or ethyl chloride, is applied to the skin; the spray rapidly evaporates and causes a cooling of the skin. Like alcohol, these sprays evaporate much more quickly than water.

Application of cold

The choice of which agent to use for cryotherapy is determined by consideration of the patient's medical condition, the treatment area, and the body part under treatment. Cooling by conduction is applied for 10 to 30 minutes, depending on the depth of tissue to be treated. Subcutaneous tissue is an insulator, preventing deep tissue cooling; as subcutaneous tissue depth increases, the time of exposure must also increase to achieve deep tissue cooling[47] (Fig. 14-16).

After initial application of cold, the patient will feel intense cold; the skin will redden. This is caused by secondary hyperemia—a greater amount of blood to the area. The next sensations will be burning and then a deep aching. Analgesia, the final sensation, begins 10 to 15 minutes after application. Activities after this analgesia should be performed with caution, because the patient may be prone to reinjury or overuse as a result of pain-free status.

Ice massage. Easy and inexpensive to make in the clinical setting, ice massage is effective in the treatment of small areas, such as muscle belly or tendon, as in the case of lateral epicondylitis or first dorsal compartment tendinitis. Small paper cups are filled with water and frozen. For application, the upper edge of the cup is torn away leaving a cover over the ice for the therapist to hold (Fig. 14-17). The ice is slowly rubbed in small circles over the affected area for approximately 10 minutes. When a level of analgesia is reached, the massage is ceased.

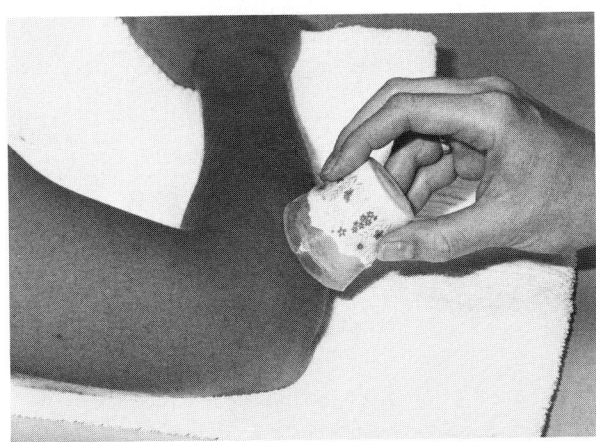

Fig. 14-17   Ice massage is applied directly to the skin in a circular manner for effective cooling.

A certain amount of discomfort is expected on initial application, with the aforementioned burning and aching occurring before total analgesia is reached. If these stages do not pass within the initial 3 to 4 minutes of treatment, the problem may be that too large an area is being covered. Waylonis[80] reports that an area as large as 10 cm × 15 cm can be treated effectively. With this mode of cryotherapy, risk of tissue damage is minimal, because skin temperature is usually no lower than 15° C.

Cold packs. Cold packs are effective in coverage of larger areas and can be obtained commercially or made in the clinic. The commercial packs are a plastic shell filled with silica gel, much like hydrocollator packs. They are stored before use in either a standard freezer or a special unit produced by the manufacturer.

Packs are easily made in the clinic by filling a tight self-sealing plastic bag with a mixture of isopropyl alcohol and water in a 1:3 ratio and freezing it. The alcohol prevents the water from solidifying, and the packs remain pliable for ease and comfort of application. When applying the packs to skin, it is best first to cover the skin with a lukewarm moist towel (Fig. 14-18). This prevents air from being trapped between the skin and the pack and is also more comfortable for the initial placement. Application of cryotherapy with this method should last for 15 to 20 minutes.

Ice towels. Though not commonly used, application of

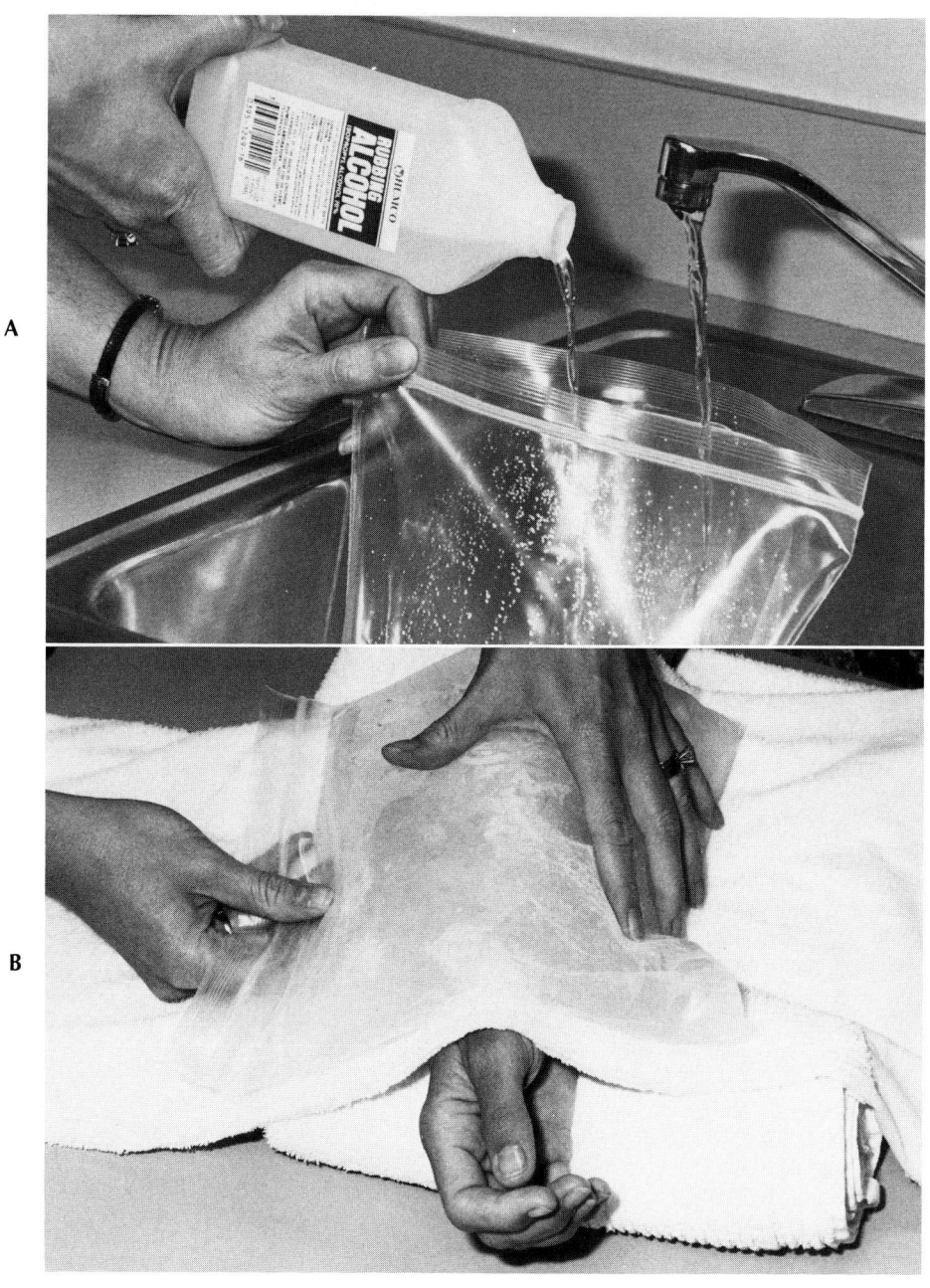

Fig. 14-18   A, Self-sealing bag is filled with mixture of isopropyl alcohol and water. **B,** Following freezing, the mixture remains pliable for conforming to body parts.

iced towels allows a large circumferential application of cold. Towels are dipped in a mixture of ice and water, wrung out, and wrapped around an extremity.

This application is quite effective in the reduction of spasticity, in which case the towels can be applied before stretching. The disadvantage to this method is that the towels do not maintain cold temperature levels for long and need to be changed every 5 to 6 minutes.

Vapocoolant sprays. As mentioned, vapocoolant sprays lower tissue temperature by evaporation. The most commonly used spray is Fluori-Methane. As the spray is directed across the skin, evaporation rapidly occurs, which extracts heat from the tissue.

Vapocoolant sprays are most often used with spray followed by stretch techniques. These techniques are used in the treatment of myofascial pain, which is discussed in detail in Chapter 57 of this book.

Contraindications. The major precaution with use of cryotherapy is the possibility of development of cold hypersensitivity or urticaria. After application of cold, certain patients will develop local areas of wheals, with reddened borders and blanched centers. This is accompanied by histamine release into the area and may include systemic reactions of increased heart rate, decreased blood pressure, and syncope. Patients should be monitored during initial application of cold for development of symptoms related to cold hypersensitivity.

Cryotherapy should be avoided also in those patients suffering from Raynaud's phenomenon. Application of cold with these individuals may precipitate Raynaud's symptoms, with blanching, cyanosis, or numbness.

Because of the effects of vasoconstriction, cold should not be applied to healing wounds. Studies have shown impaired healing with decreased wound tensile strength with cold application. Lundgren[50] demonstrated a 20% decrease in wound tensile strength in wounds of rabbits existing in temperatures of 12° C compared with a group existing in temperatures of 20° C. Because of this and similar studies, cold should not be applied to areas of wound healing before 3 weeks.

One major precaution to hand therapists is to avoid cold application in patients after revascularization or replantation. With the patient already in a vasocompromised state, the resultant vasoconstriction may cause tissue damage. This precaution should also apply to all patients with peripheral vascular diseases, such as is present in individuals who have diabetes.

Application of heat versus cold

As demonstrated in this reading, there are indications in which either heat or cold may be used successfully. In addition, there are indications in which use of one modality may be appropriate, whereas the other may not.

Both heat and cold decrease muscle spasm caused by injury. In upper motor neuron lesions, both modalities are effective, but heat does not have as long an effect as does cold.

In contrast, blood flow is increased with heat and decreased with cold. Heat increases tissue extensibility, allowing decreased resistance to stretching tissue, whereas cold decreases tissue extensibility and increases joint stiffness, causing an increased resistance to stretching tissue. A difference is also noted in muscle strength after applications of thermal modalities, with cold decreasing strength and heat increasing strength (Fig. 14-19).

Individual variations of clinical problems should be considered in addition to the diagnosis in the decision-making process of therapeutic thermal intervention. Outcome of rehabilitation can be further enhanced by appropriate application of thermal modalities.

CASE STUDY

A 23-year-old woman, employed as a data entry technician at a local banking institution, is referred for rehabilitation after a chronic de Quervain's condition. She has been treated initially in a conservative manner with immobilization and anti-inflammatory medication.

Upon referral, the primary goal for treatment is to begin a strengthening and endurance program to prepare the patient for return to work. The major precaution is to monitor the patient's activities for return of symptoms.

Before exercise, moist heat is applied to increase tissue extensibility. After heat, exercise is begun, consisting of active range of motion, progressing to functional activities,

Heat vs. Cold

	Heat	Cold
Blood flow	↑	↓
Tissue temperature	↑	↓
Tissue extensibility	↑	↓
Joint stiffness	↓	↑
Muscle strength	↑	↓
Muscle spasm	↓	↓

Fig. 14-19 Tissue changes seen with application of heat or cold.

such as pegboard and small assembly tasks. As these activities are tolerated, typing is added. After the increasing periods of work hardening, ice massage is applied over the area of the first dorsal compartment to relieve any recurrent inflammation.

ELECTROTHERAPEUTIC CURRENTS

Though the use of electricity as a therapeutic agent was not reported as early as the use of heat, the history of electrical treatment is just as fascinating. Many of the devices we think of as new were used more than a century ago.

In 1744, after being inspired by the lectures of a professor suggesting the possible usefulness of electricity in paralyzed limbs, Kratzenstein reported use of electrification in patients and stated, "I enabled a learned man, after a single electrification, to play the piano again with his two paralyzed fingers."[72] Seiler in 1860 reported improvement in cases of scoliosis after electrical stimulation, whereas the concept of ion transfer, or iontophoresis, was first claimed by DeLuc in 1908.[72]

Before discussing individual electrical modalities, it is important to review the most basic concepts of electrotherapeutic currents.

Physiology

To understand which types of currents are appropriate to apply to individual cases in the clinic, it is important to understand the excitability of nerve and muscle tissue and the effects of electrical stimulation on tissues in the path of its current.

In the normal state, muscle and nerve cells are encased in a membrane that separates a charge from the inside of the cell to the outside of the cell. This charge is found in its resting state to be approximately −60 mV, with the inside of the cell negative in respect to the outside (Fig. 14-20). This charge is a result of the unequal concentration of sodium (Na^+) and potassium (K^+) ions on either side of the membrane. In normal muscle and nerve tissue, K^+ is higher on the inside of the cell and Na^+ is higher on the outside of the cell. This negative charge is because of differences in concentration and permeability of these ions across the membrane. The concentration differences are maintained by an active pump across the membrane that eliminates Na^+ ions from the cell and receives K^+ ions. There is also passive diffusion of ions across the membrane that occurs in an attempt to equalize ion concentration. The excitable cell membrane has greater permeability to K^+, and the diffusion process is greater with the K^+ ions. As K^+ ions flow out of the cell, a negative charge develops. When this charge increases, there is a force on the outside of the cell to return K^+ ions to create an equal exchange of the K^+ ions. If equal diffusion or exchange of K^+ is achieved, the cell membrane charge would be approximately −100 mV. In the typical resting membrane state, at about −60 mV, there is not equal flow of K+ ions, and more K^+ ions leave the cell than enter the cell.

At the same time K^+ ions diffuse in and out of the cell, Na^+ ions will also be diffusing across the membrane into the cell in an attempt to equalize those Na^+ ions being actively pumped out of the cell. The diffusion of the Na^+ is not as great as K^+ diffusion because of lower membrane

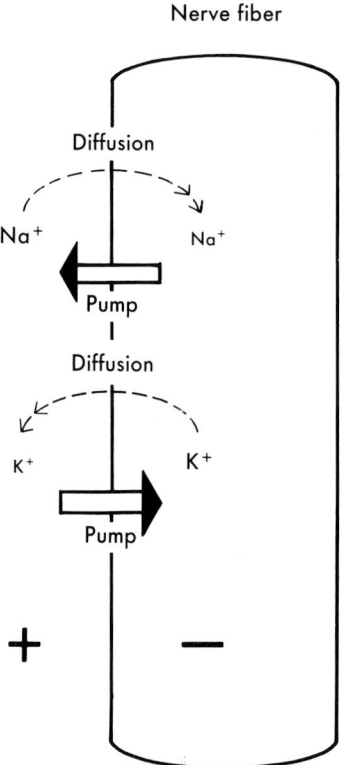

Fig. 14-20 Depiction of active movement and passive diffusion of Na^+ and K^+.

permeability to Na^+. If the Na^+ flow was equal, the membrane charge would be about +50 mV inside the cell compared with outside the cell. The limited flow of sodium ions does reduce the negative charge caused by outward diffusion of K^+ ion and prevents K^+ equality or equilibrium from occurring. This steady flow of both ions across the membrane creates the resting membrane potential of −60 mV.

If excitable cells are stimulated, there is an increased permeability to Na^+ ions. As this inward flow of Na^+ ions continues, there will be a reduction in the negative charge of the cell, or depolarization. As the charge decreases, the permeability increases and Na^+ ions flow rapidly into the cell, causing the membrane potential to change to +25 mV. This state of increased permeability lasts only a brief time.

As the permeability to Na^+ increases, so does permeability to K^+, but at a slower rate. Although this increase in permeability to K^+ occurs at a slower rate, it lasts longer than the Na^+ permeability. This sustained K^+ flow allows equilibrium to be achieved, and the membrane potential becomes −100mV, or reaches the state of hyperpolarization. This state of flow does not last long either, and the active ion pump will return the membrane to its resting potential. This brief change in the membrane's potential is known as the action potential.

If a stimulus is not applied at a level sufficient to cause a rapid depolarization, thus maintaining a slow flow of Na^+ for a long period of time, an action potential may never occur. After such a sustained subthreshold stimulus, a greater amount of depolarization is needed for the action potential, and the stimulus will have to be increased beyond

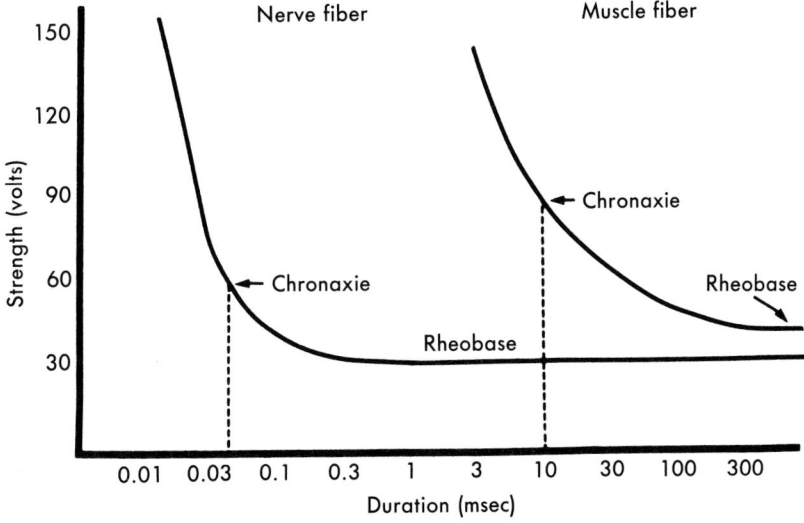

Fig. 14-21 Strength duration curve of nerve and muscle fiber.

the normal threshold necessary for firing. This adjustment to the stimulus is called accommodation.

The stimulus causing the action potential may come from various sources, such as electrical, thermal, chemical, or mechanical. To be effective, this stimulus needs to be of sufficient intensity and of sufficient duration to surpass the excitation threshold for the tissue. With regard to electrical stimulation, different types of tissue have different thresholds of excitation. The combination of the required minimum intensity and duration is represented as a strength-duration curve (Fig. 14-21). For excitation, current of short duration requires a higher intensity of application, whereas lower intensity current requires a longer duration of application. Rheobase is the minimal intensity of current sufficient to cause excitation with prolonged duration of current. When this intensity is doubled, the amount of duration required before excitation is called chronaxie. An extreme can be reached in which a short duration of current will require an intensity that cannot be used in the clinic or, if an intensity is too low, the duration could be infinite and no response would occur.

With each action potential, the cell membrane needs time to recover its normal resting potential before another action potential can be elicited. This time is referred to as the absolute refractory time. As well, there is a period before full recovery when application of a higher stimulus will elicit an action potential. This period is called the relative refractory time. The recovery time for the cell membrane limits the effective frequency of pulses in electrical stimulation. Even if duration and intensity are sufficient, the cell may not react to every pulse given if adequate time is not allowed for recovery.

Stimulation of nerve and muscle

In normal muscle, contraction occurs with electrical stimulation via excitation of the nerve rather than by excitation of muscle fiber. As shown in Fig. 14-21, the nerve and muscle tissue do not respond in an equal manner to electrical stimulation. Nerve fibers need only a low intensity, short duration of current before response, whereas muscle fibers

need a longer duration and higher intensity of current before response.

Stimulation of denervated muscle. After peripheral nerve injury, it has been shown that the usual response of muscle is atrophy of individual muscle fibers with eventual infiltration of fibrous connective tissue. This process does not occur until 30 to 36 months after denervation.[12] Once deterioration has occurred to this extent, no contractile response will result from any type of current.

Many have advocated the use of direct current to denervated muscle to prevent or delay this occurrence. Much controversy surrounds this belief, with questions raised as to the actual cause of muscle fiber degeneration. Sunderland speculated that degeneration of muscle fibers is a result not only directly of denervation, but indirectly by intramusculature vascular stasis.[73] Denervation leads to both vasoconstrictor paralysis and loss of muscle-pump action. This stasis, if prolonged, impairs the nutrition of the muscle fibers, which then degenerate. Another theory is that, as a result of the impaired nutritional status, the muscle fibers are more prone to trauma and cumulative minor trauma during the denervated state, leading to increased degeneration.[4] These clinicians advocated limiting edema and stasis, maintaining flexibility, and avoiding further injury to prevent degeneration of muscle fibers.

More direct studies on the effects of electrical stimulation have had varying results, with poorly defined recordings of the type of current used, duration of pulse, number of treatment sessions per day, and number of muscle contractions per session. One study by Wakim and Krusen[76] examined the effects of electrical stimulation on strength and endurance in denervated muscle groups of rats. They found that 30 minutes of stimulation given once daily to be of some benefit, with increased frequency of times of stimulation, that is, as long as 5 minutes every 30 minutes of an 8 hour day, more beneficial. In another study by Gutmann and Guttmann,[70] the effect of 20-minute treatments of galvanic current to denervated muscle groups in rabbits was studied. They reported finding diminished or delayed atrophy, as well as larger muscle fibers with less connective tissue invasion histologically. In addition, they reported that rate of reinnervation was neither retarded or hastened by the treatment.

In a study of rats as long as 7 weeks after denervation, Schmrigk, McLaughlin, and Gruninger reported histologic changes suggesting delayed reinnervation of treated muscle,[68a] raising more concerns about deleterious effects.

In summary, for nearly every report advocating use of electrical stimulation in denervated muscle,[13,25] a contradictory report has also appeared.[29,32]

Where does that leave clinicians who are treating these patients? The evidence of deleterious effects of electrical stimulation to denervated muscles should not be ignored. If the level of lesion is such that reinnervation would be expected in 15 to 18 months, the application of electrical stimulation based on the theory that degeneration will be retarded is not necessary, because degeneration will not occur by that time. Reports involving two human studies have shown that recovery of non-stimulated muscle can equal that of stimulated muscle during this period.[18,60] The patient in whom regeneration is not expected for 2 to 3 years is at issue. This is the patient for whom degeneration and fibrosis are a major concern. As mentioned earlier in the studies of Wakin and Krusen, the stimulation needed requires frequent application during each day for a long period; patient compliance is of question in these instances. Until further human studies reveal more conclusive evidence of positive gains with use of electrical stimulation in long-standing denervation, the efficacy of this treatment is questioned. It is better to utilize the benefits of known improvement in using electrical stimulation on normally innervated muscles.

Stimulation of innervated muscle. Most of the recent research in the use of electrical stimulation on healthy muscle involves the effect of electrical stimulation on increased strength. This is largely a result of the work of the Russian scientist Yadov M. Kots.[16] He instituted the addition of a program of electrical stimulation with the traditional training programs of the Russian olympic team at the 1976 Olympic Games in Montreal. His claim of 30% to 40% strength increases in trained athletes using electrical stimulation sparked new research in the use of electrical stimulation. Although most of these claims remained unverified to the extent reported by Kots, researchers in the United States were left with much information on the effects of electrical stimulation on healthy muscle.

Laughman[37] studied the effect of electrical stimulation on increased quadriceps strength with three groups of subjects. These groups consisted of a control group, an isometric exercise group, and a group receiving electrical stimulation. After 5 weeks, the control group showed a 2% increase in strength, the isometric exercise only group showed an 18% increase, and the electrical stimulation group increased strength by 22%.

Using a method similar to the above-mentioned study, Currier and Mann produced similar findings in the quadriceps muscle.[59] Their comparison groups consisted of an isometric exercise group, an electrical stimulation group, and a group performing isometric exercises and receiving electrical stimulation at the same time. The isometric group showed a 30% increase in strength, the electrical stimulation group increased 17%, and the combination group gained

25%. Clinical application of these studies will be described with later discussion of the various clinical stimulators.

Therapeutic currents

With the constant flow of "new" electrical stimulators, it has become increasingly confusing to discriminate among the different stimulators available to the clinician. Each stimulator is recognized by commercial names such as interferential, Russian, transcutaneous electrical nerve stimulator (TENS), functional electrical stimulation (FES), high voltage, low voltage, galvanic, or faradic. These names do little to describe the type of current received or the physiologic response elicited. To make these classifications even more confusing, these stimulators are all essentially TENS stimulators. They all electrically stimulate the nerves transcutaneously, whether the gain is decreased pain, muscle facilitation, or induction of ions. What discriminates one stimulator from another is the characteristics of the current received.

Direct current. In direct current (DC), polarity does not change once it is established. This current is applied in a continuous manner (Fig. 14-22). Variables can be applied to DC by changing the rate of rise of the current, which causes the maximum current to be reached gradually and then sustained, followed by either a sudden release or a gradual release. This is called a surge, or more recently a ramp, hence the terms *ramp-up* and *ramp-down*.

Pulsating currents. In comparison with the unidirectional DC, all other currents are considered pulsating currents. These are defined as pulses of current lasting only a few milliseconds, rather than the 1-second duration of DC. The distinctions of these currents then lie in the shape of the pulse or wave form. Wave forms can be classified under

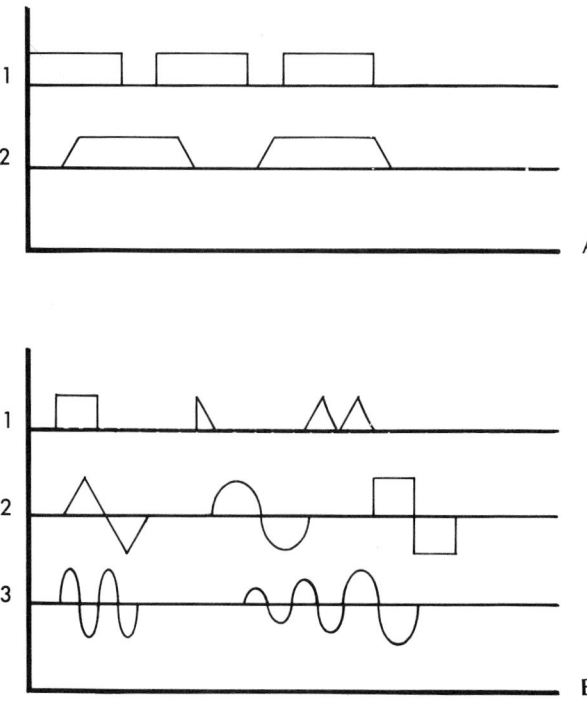

Fig. 14-22 **A,** Direct current. *1,* Interrupted DC; *2,* Ramped DC. **B,** Wave forms. *1,* Monophasic; *2,* Biphasic; *3,* Polyphasic.

three categories: monophasic, biphasic, or polyphasic (Fig. 14-22).

Monophasic wave forms are essentially rapidly pulsed DC. Polarity does not change; current flow is unidirectional. In biphasic wave forms, each pulse has two phases that cross the zero line of polarity; these can be either symmetric or asymmetric in shape. Sinusoidal wave form, or classical alternating current (AC), is a biphasic wave form. Pulses containing three or more phases are called polyphasic. A common example of a stimulator using this wave form is the interferential current. Actually, these currents are likely to be clumpings of symmetrical biphasic pulses.

Duration. Duration can be described as the duration of the phase, which is the time the current leaves the zero line until it returns to the zero line. It is also described as the pulse duration, which is the time elapsed in both phases of a biphasic pulse. The sum of the duration of all the pulses in the group provides duration of a polyphasic pulse.

Intensity. When the intensity of a monophasic pulse is measured, the highest point of the phase is referred to as peak current or peak phase. When intensity measurements are taken for biphasic pulses, the distance from the zero line of one phase and the distance between the zero line of the other phase are combined for a peak-to-peak intensity.

Frequency. Frequency or pulse rate of a pulsatile current is determined by the addition of time of all phases of a pulse; this occurs regardless of whether the current is monophasic or polyphasic in determining the number of pulses per second or cycles per second.

Duty cycle. In many applications of therapeutic current, it is desirable to alternate periods of electrical stimulation with periods of nonstimulation. The ratio of stimulation to nonstimulation is called the duty cycle. An example of an expressed ratio would be 1:5; in such a situation, 1 second of stimulation is followed by 5 seconds of nonstimulation, or rest.

Modulation. Modulation is another term that has gained recent use and has caused much confusion. Modulation simply means that certain parameters within the current applied or characteristics of the pulse are set to be automatically varied, either increased or decreased. This modulation, when applied to the pulse, can be seen as a modulation of phase or pulse duration, pulse intensity, or pulse frequency (Fig. 14-23).

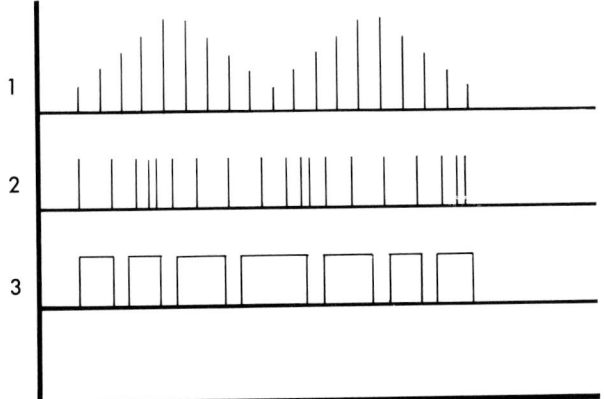

Fig. 14-23 Modulations of pulse characteristics. *1,* Intensity; *2,* frequency; *3,* duration.

When modulation is applied to the current, it is seen as either interruption in the current or ramping of the current. The term *burst* comes from a modulation of the current; bursts of pulses flow for a few milliseconds and then are interrupted for a few milliseconds. A true interrupted current occurs when pulses flow for 1 second or more and then are interrupted for 1 second or more. This point is very confusing; the reader should remember that bursts do not allow true interruption of muscle contraction. This is very important in the clinic, because most clinic stimulators provide adjustable interrupted cycles of 1 to 60 seconds. Techniques of application for increased strength, tendon excursion, or edema control require true interruption of muscle contraction. It would not be appropriate to use a stimulator with a bursting current for a contract-relax technique of muscle facilitation.

The characteristics of current involving pulse width, intensity, and duration are often what distinguish one clinic stimulator from another. A stimulator classically referred to as TENS, often used for pain relief, applies a modulated current of bursts. FES applies a modulated current of true interruptions, allowing release of muscle contraction. Other characteristics of TENS involve phase durations or pulse widths that are short (40 to 400 µsec), and peak intensities that are low (50 to 100 mA). The FES has wider pulse widths (200 to 300 µsec) and higher peak intensity (100 to 150 mA).

Although the concepts presented can be confusing, the way electrical stimulation is applied has ramifications on the effects achieved in the clinic. Understanding the combinations of parameters aids in clinical decision making.

Stimulator components

All stimulators have basic components in common, whether they are high-voltage, low-voltage, AC, or DC. The flow of current to the patient must come from a power source. The two common sources for power that are seen in electrical stimulators are the battery pack or the alternating 115v house current. These sources are not appropriate for direct clinical application and must be converted within the stimulator to the appropriate current.

With the formation of the appropriate current to the clinical application, there must be a complete circuit from the stimulator through leads to the electrodes, which connect to the patient. To have a complete circuit for conduction of electric current, there must be at least two separate leads with electrodes.

In DC, one lead will be positive with respect to the other electrode. The recognition of lead polarity is important where a treatment method requires a specific polarity. The negative electrode, or cathode, attracts positive ions from the tissue, and the anode, or positive electrode, attracts negative ions from the tissue. In eliciting a depolarized state in the tissue, the cathode is referred to as the active electrode and the anode is referred to as the inactive electrode.

With AC wave form, each electrode is alternatively the anode and the cathode. This alternation of polarity occurs so rapidly that there is essentially no polarity to consider with the individual electrode. To attain an "active" electrode with AC, it may be necessary to apply electrodes of different sizes to the area stimulated, thus increasing current density under the smaller electrode and thereby obtaining a stronger tissue response. Much clinical consideration is needed in electrode size and placement, and further reading is recommended for full understanding.[84]

Clinical electrotherapeutic stimulators

Further discussion of electrical modalities will describe various stimulators used in the clinic, explaining differences in their characteristics and the indications for which they would be valuable.

Functional electrical stimulation. Functional Electrical Stimulation (FES) is a general term describing a group of stimulators that use pulsating AC for stimulation of innervated musculature. Use of this type of stimulation has been reported in maintaining or gaining range of motion, facilitating muscle contraction, and substituting for orthoses.

With regard to use in muscle education or facilitation, LeDoux and Quinones[39] evaluated muscle facilitation for adduction of the great toe. They compared a group using a program of FES with a group receiving only verbal instruction and feedback and reported greater adduction in the group receiving FES.

In a project by Rancho Los Amigos,[6] application of FES was used to alleviate the need of orthotic assistance in the prevention of shoulder subluxation of hemiparetic patients. It was believed in those patients expectant of reinnervation of the shoulder capsule that stimulation of the posterior deltoid and supraspinatus muscles helped prevent stretching of the shoulder capsule until adequate strength of the involved muscles could restore proper alignment.

In hand rehabilitation, use of FES for muscle facilitation can be very beneficial. In postsurgical tendon repairs or tenolysis, FES can be applied to the affected muscle group to aid in strong muscle contraction, thus assisting in tendon gliding. In these cases, proper timing with application is extremely important. After tendon repair, application of FES at high intensity is the equivalent of performing resistive activities. It would be necessary to wait 5 1/2 to 6 weeks after operative repair before applying FES at a level to elicit strong muscle contraction. After tenolysis, FES may be applied earlier, at 7 to 10 days after surgery, but care should be taken not to overexercise the involved tendon, thereby causing an inflammatory response.

Application of FES to muscle groups in state of disuse may facilitate a more functional use of the muscle. Those patients unable to actively extend the wrist without assistance from the finger extensors may benefit from an isolated stimulation program to the wrist extensors.

When FES is used to maintain or increase range of motion, the area is treated by stimulating the prime mover of a limited joint. In the case of stimulating previously immobilized muscle, the stimulation will facilitate increased muscle strength, allowing the patient to eventually use voluntary contraction for the same response.

Various manufacturers produce FES units. The units are usually battery-supplied with two electrodes, one active and one dispersive. Some stimulators have the capacity for two channels of electrodes, allowing application in a reciprocating mode to two different muscle groups. Most stimulators allow the clinician various levels of parameter control, such as duty cycle, rise time, and pulse rate (Fig. 14-24).

Clinical application. The application of the FES requires proper placement of the active electrode over the motor point

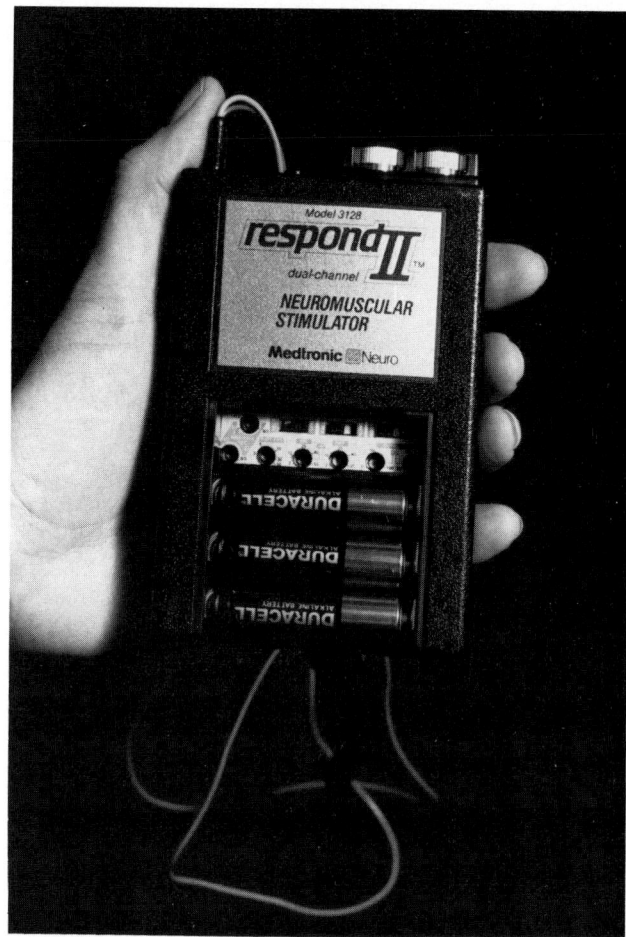

Fig. 14-24 Neuromuscular stimulator shown with available adjustments to current parameters.

of the target muscle with application of the dispersive electrode in an adjacent area. Some common electrode placement sites are demonstrated in Fig. 14-25. To prevent stimulation of muscle under the dispersive electrode, it is best to have the dispersive or inactive electrode be a larger electrode, which thereby increases current density under the active electrode and decreases current density under the inactive electrode. Thus a stimulus adequate to elicit muscle contraction with the active electrode is not sufficient for contraction under the inactive electrode.

The duty cycle of the stimulus is an important factor in the prevention of muscle fatigue. It has been suggested that the duty off should be 2 to 3 times that of the duty on, such as 7 seconds of stimulus followed by 15 to 20 seconds of rest.[6]

High-voltage galvanic stimulation. High-voltage galvanic stimulation (HVGS) is a form of stimulation that has gained popularity since the 1970s. Some of the symptoms treated successfully with HVGS are pain, edema, and wound healing.

This stimulator is an interrupted monophasic wave form and should more correctly be called high-voltage pulsed galvanic stimulation. The voltage of the stimulator is greater than 100 volts, classifying it in the high-voltage range. The duration of pulses are fixed (approximately 200 μsec), but

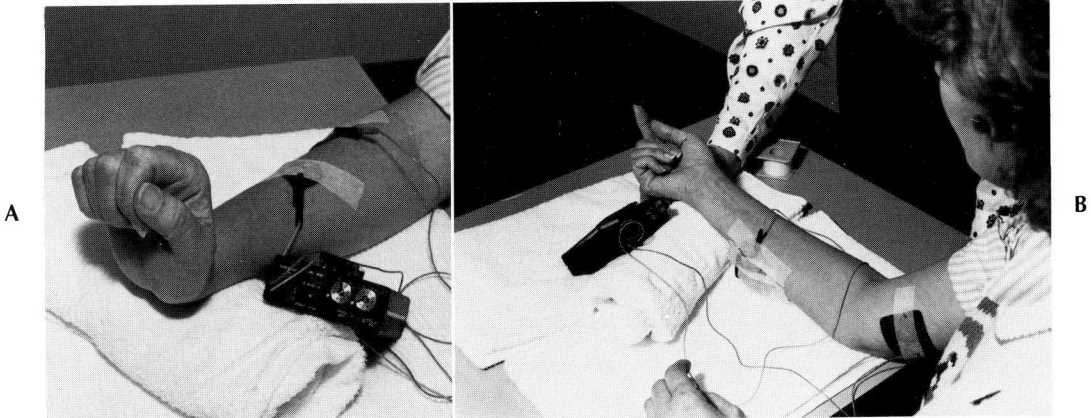

Fig. 14-25   **A,** Common placement of the wrist extensors. **B,** Placement of the ulnar flexor digitorum profundus.

pulse frequency, intensity, and polarity are controlled by the clinician. The mode of application can be established as continuous, whereby a constant pulsing current is applied without variation, or as a reciprocate, where two active electrodes are used and the current alternates between the two electrodes (Fig. 14-26).

Indications. HVGS is an excellent choice of modality for treatment of chronic edema, such as in forearm fractures after cast removal. Another clinical indication appropriate for HVGS is soft-tissue injury with organized hematoma or fibrous edema of a long-standing nature. Also effective in the treatment of pain, HVGS has some of the same current characteristics as those TENS units with monophasic pulsating currents.

Contraindications. It is not advised to use HVGS in patients with reported dysrythmias of the heart. Also to be noted is that HGVS is not effective in stimulation of denervated muscle because of the interrupted current or in iontophoresis because of the high voltage parameters. Other contraindications will be mentioned under individual clinical applications.

Edema control. If edema is present as a result of long-standing vascular stasis from inactivity or physical disruption of vessels, this may be alleviated with HVGS by cre-

ating a muscle-pump action. Polarity of the current applied may also assist in removal, because blood and plasma cells are negatively charged and proper application of electrical current can repel these cells from the treated area.[81] The protocol for edema control is as follows:

*   Frequency: Low-frequency rates of 2 to 8 pulses per second (pps)
*   Polarity: Negative
*   Mode: Continuous unless it is desirable to stimulate opposing muscle groups, in which case a reciprocating mode of treatment can be used
*   Intensity: Minimal muscle contraction
*   Duty cycle: 1:4 or 1:5 to prevent fatigue of muscles
*   Duration of treatment: 20-30 minutes

Applications with this mode of treatment can be used in early management of patients with forearm fractures after cast removal. It facilitates blood flow in disuse conditions of the hand.

In the presence of crush injuries, the use of HVGS can facilitate muscle activity and aid in resolution of established hematomas.[81]

A precaution for the use of HVGS for edema control would be to not apply intensity to the level of the muscle contraction if postsurgical protocols in tissue would not be appropriate for active muscle contraction, such as in early tendon repairs.

Pain relief. There are two methods of applying HVGS for relief of pain, one for the treatment of acute pain and the other for the treatment of chronic pain. It has been found that a high-frequency stimulus of HVGS produces relief for acute pain, whereas a lower-frequency stimulus brings relief for more chronic pain. A trial period of treatment with each protocol should be used to assess the better method of pain relief. The protocol for treatment of acute pain is as follows:

*   Frequency: High-frequency rates of 50-120 pps
*   Polarity: Positive or negative
*   Mode: Continuous
*   Intensity: Sensory stimulation, below muscle contraction
*   Duration of treatment: 20-30 minutes

The protocol for treatment of chronic pain is as follows:

*   Frequency: Low-frequency rates of 5-15 pps
*   Polarity: Positive or negative

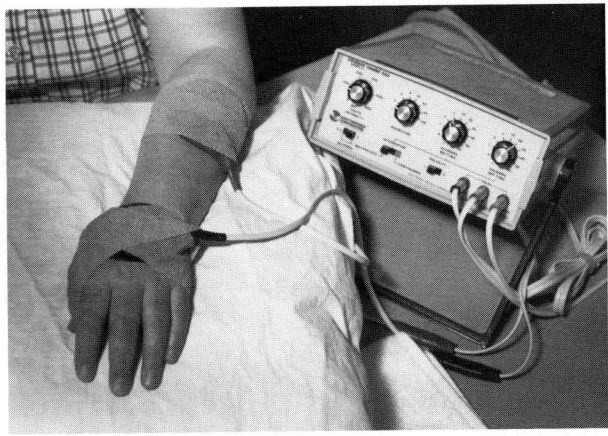

Fig. 14-26   High-voltage galvanic stimulation is applied for muscle-pump action.

Ion (source)	Polarity	Clinical indications
Dexamethasone (Decadron)	Positive	Inflammatory conditions (tendonitis, bursitis, arthritis)
Iodine (iodine)	Negative	Sclerolytic (adhesions, scar formation)
Salicylate (sodium salicylate)	Negative	Arthritis
Xylocaine (Xylocaine)	Positive	Analgesic needs

Fig. 14-27 Common ions used in iontophoresis.

- Mode: Continuous
- Intensity: Intense sensory stimulation
- Duration of treatment: 5-10 minutes

Wound healing. Though not used regularly in hand rehabilitation, HVGS has been shown to have effects on wound healing, both in decreased growth of organisms[5,65] and in increased migration of epithelial cells.[30] These two desired effects require differences in protocol with regard to polarity, because the negative polarity retards the growth of microorganisms and positive polarity causes increase in epithelial cells. Please see references for more explicit information in this area. The protocol for wound healing is as follows:

- Frequency: Rates of 8-20 pps
- Polarity
  a. Negative polarity if microorganisms are present
  b. Positive polarity if the wound is culture free
- Mode: Continuous
- Intensity: Sensory stimulation, below muscle contraction.

Contraindications. Caution should be taken with application of HVGS for this purpose without detailed study in safe application

Iontophoresis. Iontophoresis is the induction of topically applied ions into the tissue by application of a low-voltage direct galvanic current. This transfer of ions can be effective in the treatment of inflammatory conditions or scar formation when the proper ion is introduced for the condition. The occurrence of iontophoresis is based on the principle that an electrically charged electrode will repel a similarly charged ion, much as magnets of like polarity repel.

Continuous low-voltage direct current is the current of choice for iontophoresis. Other forms of current, such as HVGS or FES, are not effective in ion transfer. One disadvantage of the application of galvanic current is the risk of an electrochemical burn under the electrode. This is the result of the sustained application of unidirectional current. Normal skin can tolerate current densities to 1.0 mA/cm^2 when applying continuous DC. If electrodes are of the same size, the current density under each electrode will be the same. When the size is not equal, current density will be greater under the smaller electrode. With galvanic current, alkaline reactions under the cathode, or active, electrode is much more irritating than the inactive, or anode, electrode. If the size of the cathode electrode is larger, current density and chemical irritation will be less. When applying ionto-

phoresis, keep the cathode twice the size of the anode to further reduce likelihood of skin burns.

Selection of ion and proper transfer is based on knowledge of effective ions and their polarity. Several ions have been identified as effective in treatment of medical conditions (Fig. 14-27). After the proper ion is selected, it is applied superficially to the affected area. An electrode is then constructed that consists of several layers of moistened gauze cut to the size of the area; the medication must be present under the entire area of gauze. This is followed by application of a metal electrode of tin or aluminum foil. This metal electrode is cut slightly smaller than the gauze to prevent direct metal contact with the skin (Fig. 14-28). If the ion is in liquid form and cannot be applied topically, the gauze may be soaked in the solution. A similar electrode without the topical solution is applied as a dispersive pad. Both electrodes are secured with straps or adhesive tape: good uniform contact must be made.

After application of the electrodes, the lead wires are clipped to the electrodes and current is begun with proper polarity based on type of medication (Fig. 14-28). As mentioned, the desired current is approximately 0.5 mA/cm^2 to 1 mA/cm^2 of the surface of the electrode. The patient may report a tingling in the area of the electrode, but any discomfort would warrant discontinuing the current and investigating for lack of uniform contact. Duration of treatment is usually 20 minutes.

A simpler method of application is through the use of a stimulator specifically designed for iontophoresis. This stimulator comes with electrode bubbles for injection of the ion solution. This bubble is then applied to the skin as an electrode (Fig. 14-29). It can also be used for application of topical creams by removing the electrode bubble and clipping the lead wire to an aluminum foil electrode. This machine allows for ease of application, but any low-voltage galvanic stimulator in the clinic may be used.

Clinical indications. Several clinical conditions can be treated effectively with iontophoresis. In hand rehabilitation, the two most common conditions are acute inflammatory conditions and scar formation.

Inflammatory conditions. Studies have shown that it is possible to induce dexamethasone with iontophoresis into tendon and cartilage[25] and thus offer an effective treatment for inflammatory conditions. For use with dexamethasone, xylocaine is mixed with the steroid on a 1 ml dexamethasone to 2 ml xylocaine ratio. In a study by Harris, 50 patients

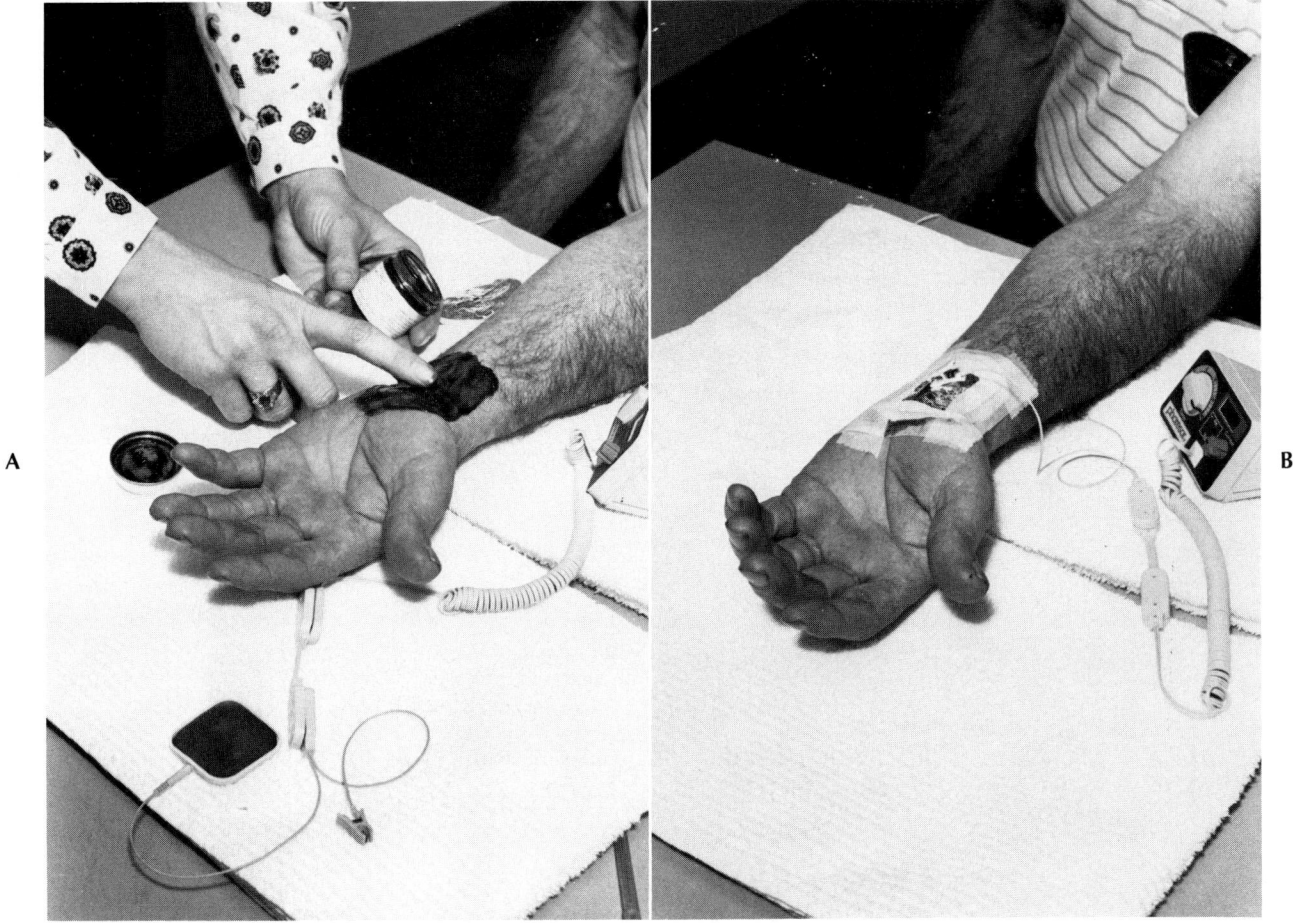

Fig. 14-28   A, Iodex ointment is applied to the skin in preparation for iontophoresis. **B,** Electrode is attached to the unit with proper polarity.

with various musculoskeletel problems were treated with iontophoresis-induced dexamethasone. Of the group, 38 patients reported excellent relief, 7 reported moderate relief, and 5 reported little or no relief.[31]

In hand rehabilitation, use of iontophoresis with steroids is effective with acute conditions of De Quervain's syndrome, lateral epicondylitis, and carpal tunnel syndrome.

Ease of application of this iontophoretic treatment is possible by using the commercial Phoresor and the bubble electrodes. On placement of an empty electrode on the skin, the air is aspirated with the syringe and the medication injected. The protocol for treatment of inflammatory conditions is as follows:
- Polarity: Positive
- Medication: 1 ml of dexamethasone, 2 ml of xylocaine hydrochloride
- Intensity: The current is gradually increased in 1 mA increments until level of 4 mA current is reached
- Duration of treatment: After level of 5 mA current is reached, treatment continues for 20 minutes; treatments are given three times weekly for five to seven sessions as necessary for relief
- Caution: Because of publicized side effects of corticosteroids, caution should be used in clinical use of

these agents. The application of the steroid through the skin can lighten pigmented skin areas, much like steroid injections

Scar formation. The use of iontophoresis in treatment of scar formation is gaining popularity. Iodine ion has been suggested as a sclerolytic agent when delivered with iontophoretic current. Conditions treated in the clinic are postsurgical Dupuytren's releases, and over-adherent incision and laceration sites that cause decreased tendon gliding. Scar formation seldom matches the size of the prefabricated iontophoretic bubbles. For treatment of these areas, it is better to apply iodine in a topical form, such as Iodex. This area is then covered in the previously described method of gauze and electrode. The protocol is as follows:
- Polarity: Negative
- Medication: Iodex with methyl salicylate applied topically
- Intensity: 0.5 mA to 1 mA, depending on size of electrode and area covered
- Duration of treatment: 20 minutes

Contraindications. Iontophoresis cannot be used over metal implants. Other contraindications include use over skin abrasions or open lacerations. Because medication is being introduced into the body, it is advised to question

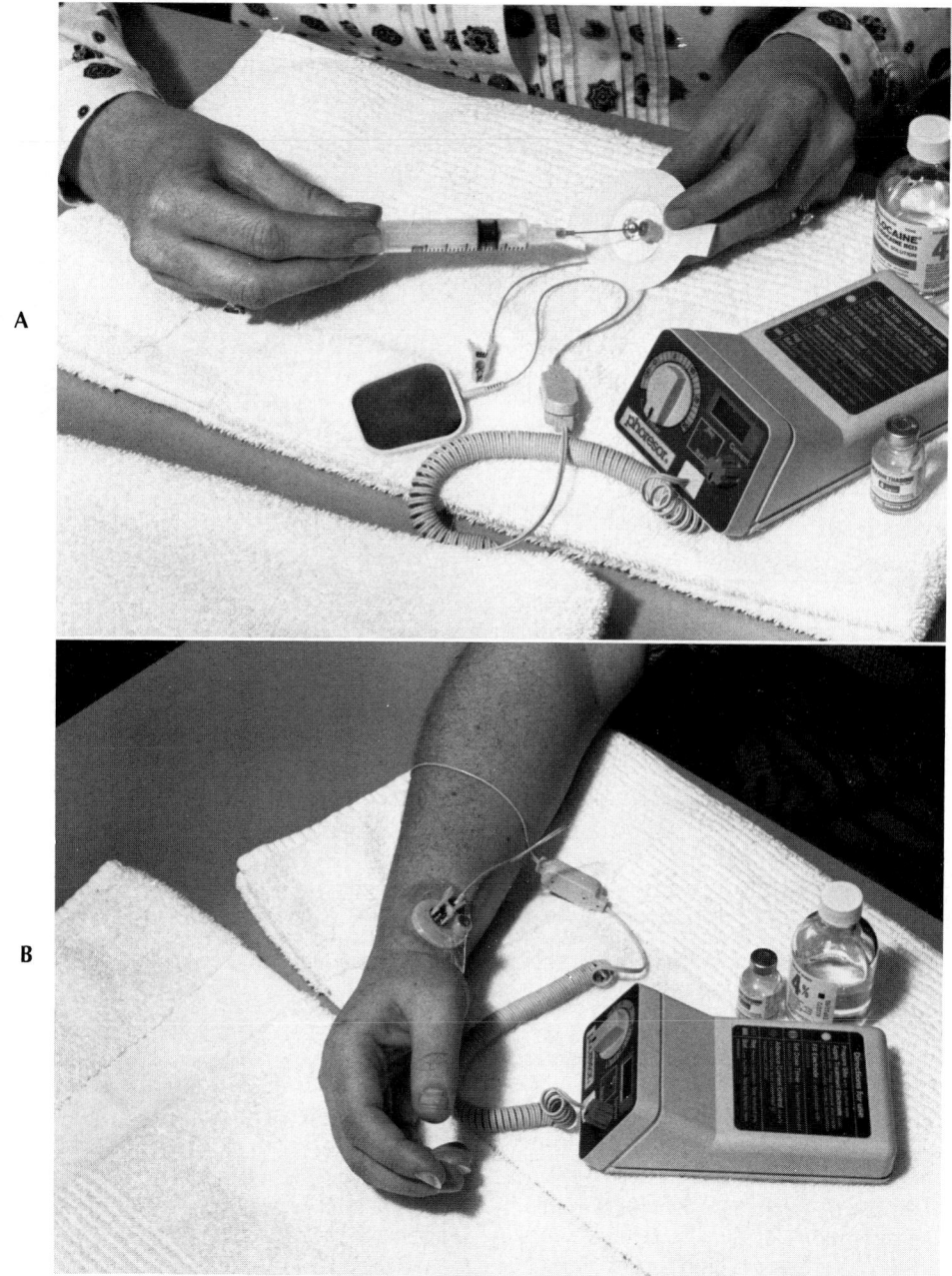

Fig. 14-29 **A,** Solution is injected into bubble electrode. **B,** Electrode is applied to the skin and current is begun.

patients regarding allergies and to discontinue treatment if any skin wheals or whelps develop after treatment.

In the application of Iodex with iontophoresis in treatment of adherent tendons after repair, no clinical studies have been performed to determine the effects of iodine on healing structures. Caution should be taken in these situations, and it is suggested to apply iontophoresis with iodine no sooner than 6 weeks after tendon repair.

CASE STUDY

A 62-year-old woman was referred to rehabilitation after cast removal for treatment of Colles' fracture. The major problems were chronic edema, lack of wrist and forearm motion, and loss of strength.

On referral, decision was made to use high-voltage galvanic stimulation to aid in edema by muscle-pump action. The treatment mode of choice was continuous stimulation with low-frequency rate to allow true interruption of muscle contraction.

During examination it was noted that patient had inability to extend the wrist without assistance of the finger extensors. When finger extension is prevented, the wrist extensors do not have adequate strength to extend the wrist. Decision was made to apply FES to the individual wrist extensors to facilitate a stronger contraction and to strengthen the individual muscles. Appropriate heat modalities were also applied as indicated.

SUMMARY

When applied appropriately, thermal modalities can enhance therapeutic intervention. Heat modalities can be effective in increasing tissue extensibility and decreasing joint stiffness. Inflammation and edema can be reduced with proper use of cryotherapy. Both thermal modalities can be useful in temporary relief of muscle spasm and pain.

Electrical current has been in therapeutic use for more than a century. Basic understanding of the differences in characteristics of current is essential for appropriate use of electric current in the clinic. The characteristics of the current used in commercial TENS units elicit relief of pain, while the low-voltage galvanic current producing iontophoresis causes ion transfer through tissue.

Innervated and denervated muscle can be facilitated through stimulation by either AC or DC, respectively.

To aid in proper decision making regarding use of modalities, the clinician must have an understanding of tissue healing and disease process. Inappropriate application of thermal or electrical modalities may impair healing. This should not discourage the use of these various modalities, because the benefits from their use can improve outcome of rehabilitation.

REFERENCES

1. Abramson DI and others: Changes in blood flow, oxygen uptake and tissue temperatures produced by the topical application of wet heat, Arch Phys Med Rehabil 42:305, 1961.
2. Abramson DI and others: Effect of paraffin bath and hot fomentations on local tissue temperatures, Arch Phys Med Rehabil 45:87, 1964.
3. Aldes JH and Jadeson WJ: Ultrasonic therapy in treatment of hypertrophic arthritis in elderly patients, Ann West Med Surg 6:545, 1952.
4. Axelsson J and Thesleff S: A study of supersensitivity in denervated mammalian skeletal muscle, J Physiol 147:178, 1959.
5. Barranco SD, Spadero JA, and Berger TJ: In vitro effect of weak direct current on staphylococcus aureus, Clin Orthop 100:250, 1974.
6. Benton LA and others: Functional electrical stimulation, Rancho Los Amigos, 1980, Downey.
7. Bierman W: Therapeutic use of cold, JAMA 157:1189, 1955.
8. Borrell RM and others: Fluidotherapy: evaluation of a new heat modality, Arch Phys Med Rehabil 58:69, 1977.
9. Breasted JH: The Edwin Smith Surgical Papyrus, Chicago, 1930.
10. Brunner GD and others: Can ultrasound be used in the presence of surgical metal implants: an experimental approach, Phys Ther Rev 38:823, 1958.
11. Bugaj R: The cooling, analgesic, and rewarding effects of ice massage on localized skin, Phys Ther 55:11, 1975.
11a. Caputo L, Krulewitz D, and Gerbert J: Effects of ultrasonic energy on the physical properties of Silastic, J Am Podiatr Assoc 72:145, 1982.
12. Chastain PB: The effect of deep heat on isometric strength, Phys Ther 58:543, 1978.
13. Cobbold AF and Lewis OJ: Blood flow to the knee joint of the dog: effect of heating, cooling, and adrenaline, J Physiol 132:379, 1956.
14. Chor H, Cleveland D, and Davenport HA: Atrophy and regeneration of the gastrocnemius-soleus muscles, JAMA 113:1029, 1939.
15. Currie WA: Observations on the causes and cure of remitting or bilious fevers, Philadelphia, 1798.
16. Currier DP and Mann R: Muscular strength development by electrical stimulation in healthy individuals, Phys Ther 59:1508, 1979.
17. DeForest RE, Herrick JF, and Jones JM: Effect of ultrasound on growing bone: an experimental study, Arch Phys Med Rehabil 34:21, 1953.
18. Doupe J, Barnes R, and Kerr AS: Studies in denervation: the effect of electrical stimulation on the circulation and recovery of denervated muscle, J Neurol Psych 6:136, 1943.
19. Dyson M and Brookes M: Stimulation of bone repair by ultrasound, Ultrasound Med Biol 8:50, 1982.
20. Edwards HT and others: Effect of temperature on muscle energy metabolism and endurance during successive isometric contractions sustained to fatigue of the quadriceps muscle in man, J Physiol 220:335, 1972.
21. Edwards WF: On the influence of physical agents on life, London, 1832.
22. Farry PJ and others: Ice treatment of injured ligaments: an experimental model, NZ Med J 91:12, 1980.
23. Fischer E and Solomon S: Physiological responses to heat and cold. In Licht S, editor: Therapeutic heat and cold, Baltimore, 1965, Waverly Press.
24. Fox RH and Wyatt HT: Cold-induced vasodilatation in various areas of the body surface of man, J Physiol 162:289, 1962.
25. Girlanda R, Dattola R, and Vita G: Effect of electrotherapy on denervated muscles in rabbits: an electrophysiological and morphological study, Exp Neurol 77:483, 1982.
26. Griffin JE, Karselis TC, and Currier DP: Physical agents for physical therapists, ed 2, Springfield, 1982, Charles C. Thomas, Publisher.
27. Grose J: Depression of muscle fatigue curves by heat and cold, Res Q Am Assoc Health Phys Educ 29:19, 1958.
28. Guyot J: Traite' de l'Incubation et son, Influence Therapeutique, Paris 1840.
29. Halle JS, Scoville CR, and Greathouse DG: Ultrasound's effect on the conduction latency of the superficial radial nerve in man, Phys Ther 61:345, 1981.
30. Harrington DB, Meyer R, and Klein RM: Effects of small amounts of electric current at the cellular level, Ann NY Acad Sci 238:300, 1974.
31. Harris PR: Iontophoresis: clinical research in musculoskeletal inflammatory conditions, J Ortho Sports Phy Ther 4:109, 1982.
32. Herbison GJ, Teng C-S, and Gordon EE: Electrical stimulation of reinnervating rat muscle, Arch Phys Med Rehabil 54:156, 1973.
33. Hocutt JE and others: Cryotherapy in ankle sprains, Am J Sports Med 10:316, 1982.
34. Hunter J, Kerr EH, and Whillans MG: The relation between joint stiffness upon exposure to cold and the characteristics of synovial fluid, Can J Med Sci 30:367, 1952.
35. Knight KL and Londeree BR: Comparison of blood flow in the ankle of uninjured subjects during therapeutic applications of heat, cold, and exercise, Med Sci Sports Exerc 12:76, 1980.
36. Kramer JF: Ultrasound: evaluation of its mechanical and thermal effects, Arch Phys Med Rehabil 65:223, 1984.
37. Laughman RK, Yondas JW, and Garrett TF: Strength changes in the normal quadriceps femoris muscle as a result of electrical stimulation, Phys Ther 63:494, 1983.
38. LeBlanc JSJ: Impairment of manual dexterity by cold, J Appl Physiol 9:62, 1956.
39. LeDoux J and Quinones MA: An investigation of the use of percutaneous electrical stimulation in muscle reeducation, Phys Ther 61:678, 1981.
40. Lehmann JF: Therapeutic heat and cold, ed 3, Baltimore, 1982, Williams & Wilkins.
41. Lehmann JF: Temperature distributions upon exposure to ultrasonic energy, Arch Phys Med Rehabil 48:662, 1967.
42. Lehmann JF, Brunner GD, and Stow RW: Pain threshold measurements after therapeutic application of ultrasound, microwaves, and infrared, Arch Phys Med Rehabil 39:560, 1958.
43. Lehmann JF and others: Heating produced by ultrasound in bone and soft tissue, Arch Phys Med Rehabil 48:397, 1967.
44. Lehmann JF and others: Influence of surgical metal implants on the distribution of the intensity in the ultrasonic field, Arch Phys Med Rehabil 39:756, 1958.
45. Lehmann JF and others: Effect of therapeutic temperatures on tendon extensibility, Arch Phys Med Rehab 51:481, 1970.
46. Lehmann JF and others: Temperature distributions in the human thigh, produced by infrared, hot pack and microwave applications, Arch Phys Med Rehabil 47:291, 1966.
47. Lehmann JF, Warren CG, and Scham SM: Therapeutic heat and cold, Clin Orthop 99:207, 1974.
48. Lewis T: Observations upon the reactions of the vessels of the human skin to cold, Heart 15:177, 1930.
49. Lievens P and Leduc A: Cryotherapy and sports, Int J Sports Med 5:37, 1984.
50. Lundergren C, Muren A, and Zederfeldt B: Effect of cold vasoconstriction on wound healing in the rabbit, Acta Chir Scand 118:1, 1959.
51. Magness J, Garrett T, and Erickson D: Swelling of the upper extremity during whirlpool baths, Arch Phys Med Rehabil 51:297, 1970.

52. McMaster WC, Liddle S, and Waugh TR: Laboratory evalution of various cold therapy modalities, Am J Sports Med 6:291, 1978.

53. Melzack R and Wall PD: Pain mechanisms: a new theory, Science 150:971, 1965.

54. Mense S: Effects of temperature on the discharges of muscle spindles and tendon organs, Pflugers Arch 374:159, 1978.

55. Micholivitz SL, editor: Thermal agents in rehabilitation, Philadelphia, 1986, FA Davis Co.

56. Miglietta O: Action of cold on spasticity, Am J Phys Med 52:198, 1973.

57. Miller LE and others: Sequential use of hot packs and ultrasound, Phys Ther 59:559, 1979.

58. Miller LE, Markham DE, and Wood MR: Ultrasound for Dupuytren's contracture, Physiotherapy, 66(2):55, 1980.

59. Nelson RM and Currier DP: Clinical electrotherapy, Norwalk, 1987, Appleton & Lange.

60. Newman WK, Berris JM, and Bohn SS: Management of facial paralysis by physical methods, Arch Phys Ther 21:270, 1940.

61. Newman MK, Kill M, and Frampton G: Effects of ultrasound alone and combined with hydrocortisone injections by needle or hydrospray, Am J Phys Med 37:206, 1958.

62. Newton MJ and Lehmkuhl D: Muscle spindle response to body heating and localized muscle cooling: implications for relief of spasticity, J Am Phys Ther Assoc 45:91, 1965.

63. Novak EJ: Experimental transmission of lidocaine through intact skin by ultrasound, Arch Phys Med Rehabil 45:231, 1964.

64. Roberts M, Rutherford JH, and Harris D: The effect of ultrasound on flexor tendon repairs in the rabbit, Hand 14:17, 1982.

65. Rowley BA: Electrical current effects on E coli growth rates, Proc Soc Exp Biol Med 139:929, 1972.

66. Rubin D, Magovern G, and Kallenberger R: Application of ultrasound to experimentally induced neuromas in dogs, Arch Phys Med Rehabil 38:377, 1957.

67. Sapega AA: Biophysical factors in range of motion exercises, Phys Sports Med 9:57, 1981.

68. Sawyer M and Zbieranek C: The treatment of soft tissue after spinal injury, Clin Sports Med 5:387, 1986.

68a. Schimrigk K, McLaughlin J, and Gruninger W: The effect of electrical stimulation on the experimentally denervated rat muscle, Scand J Rehabil Med 9:55, 1977.

69. Schultz KS: The effect of active exercise on edema, J Hand Surg 8(5):625, 1983.

70. Sprilholtz N: Electrical stimulation of denervated muscle. In Clinical electrotherapy, Norwalk, 1987, Appleton & Lange.

71. Stillwell GK: General principles of thermotherapy. In Licht S, editor: Therapeutic heat and cold, ed 2, Baltimore, 1965, Waverly Press.

72. Stillwell GK: History of electrotherapy. In Therapeutic electricity and ultraviolet radiation, Baltimore, 1983, Williams & Wilkins.

73. Sunderland S: Nerves and nerve injuries, ed 2, Edinburgh, 1978, Churchill Livingstone, Inc.

74. Travell J: Ethyl chloride spray for painful muscle spasm, Arch Phys Med Rehabil 32:291, 1952.

75. Vaugheu JL and Bender LF: Effects of ultrasound on growing bone, Arch Phys Med Rehabil 40:158, 1959.

76. Wakim KG and Krusen FH: The influence of electrical stimulation on the work output and endurance of denervated muscle, Arch Phys Med Rehabil 32:523, 1951.

77. Walsh M: Hydrotherapy: the use of water as a therapeutic agent. In Michlovitz SL, editor: Thermal agents in rehabilitation, Philadelphia, 1986, FA Davis Co.

78. Warren CG: The use of heat and cold in the treatment of common musculoskeletal disorders. In Kessler RM and Hertling D, editors: Management of common musculoskeletal disorders, Philadelphia, 1983, Harper & Row Publishers, Inc.

79. Warren CG, Koblanski JN, and Sigelmann PA: Ultrasound coupling media: their relative transmissivity, Arch Phys Med Rehabil 57:218, 1976.

80. Waylonis GW: The physiologic effect of ice massage, Arch Phys Med Rehabil 48:37, 1967.

81. Williams R and Carey L: Studies in the production of standard venous thrombosis, Ann Surg 149:381, 1959.

82. Wise TA: Review of the history of medicine, London, 1867.

83. Wright ET and Haase KH: Treatment of keloids with ultrasound, Arch Phys Med Rehabil 52:280, 1971.

84. Wright V and Johns RJ: Physical factors concerned with the stiffness of normal and diseased joints, Johns Hopkins Hosp Bull 106:215, 1960.

ADDITIONAL READINGS

Abramson DI and others: Effect of tissue temperatures and blood flow on motor nerve conduction velocity, JAMA 198(10):156, 1966.

Bierman W: Ultrasound in the treatment of scars, Arch Phys Med Rehabil 35:209, 1954.

Borrell RM and others: Comparison of in vivo temperatures produced by hydrotherapy, paraffin wax treatment, and Fluidotherapy, Phys Ther 60:1273, 1980.

Bowden RE and Gutmann E: Denervation and reinnervation of human voluntary muscle, Brain 67:273, 1944.

Bundt FB: Ultrasound therapy in supraspinatus bursitis, Phys Ther Rev 38:826, 1958.

Conger AD, Zizkin MC, and Wittels H: Ultrasonic effects on mammalian multicellular tumor spheroids, J Clin Ultrasound 9:167, 1981.

Coakley WT: Biophysical effects of ultrasound at therapeutic intensities, Physiotherapy 64:166, 1978.

Elhtag M and others: The anti-inflammatory effects of dexamethasone and therapeutic ultrasound in oral surgery, Br J Oral Maxillofac Surg 23:17, 1985.

Fisk GH: Ultrasonic energy in physical medicine, Can Med Assoc J 69:533, 1953.

Gersten JW: Muscle shortening produced by ultrasound, Arch Phys Med Rehabil 38:83, 1957.

Glass JM, Stephen RL, and Jacobsen SC: The quantity and distribution of radiolabeled dexamethasone delivered to tissues by iontophoresis, Int J Dermatol, 19:519, 1980.

Griffin JE: Transmissiveness of ultrasound through tap water, glycerin, and mineral oil, Phys Ther 60:1010, 1980.

Griffin JE: Physiologic effects of ultrasonic energy as it is used clinically, Phys Ther 46:18, 1966.

Harada Y, Nakano K, and Fujiwara M: Effects of electrical stimulation on the denervated rat muscle, Acta Med Hyogensia 4:129, 1979.

Hashish W and others: Anti-inflammatory effects of ultrasound therapy: evidence for a major placebo effect, Br J Rheum 25:77, 1986.

Hillman SK and Delforge G: The use of physical agents in rehabilitation of athletic injuries, Clin Sports Med 4:431, 1985.

Kahn J: Iontophoresis and ultrasound for postsurgical temporomandibular trismus and paresthesia, Phys Ther 60:307, 1980.

Lane C: Therapy for the occupationally injured hand, Hand Clin 2:593, 1986.

Lee JM and Warren MP: Ice, relaxation and exercise in reduction of muscle spasticity, Physiotherapy, 60:296, 1974.

Lehamnn JF and Biegler R: Changes of potentials and temperature gradients in membranes caused by ultrasound, Arch Phys Med Rehabil 35:287, 1954.

Lehmann JP, DeLateur BJ, and Silvermann DR: Selective heating effects of ultrasound in human beings, Arch Phys Med Rehabil 47:331, 1966.

Lehmann JF and others: Therapeutic temperature distribution produced by ultrasound as modified by dosage and volume of tissue exposed, Arch Phys Med Rehabil 48:662, 1967.

Lehmann JF and others: Heating of joint structures by ultrasound, Arch Phys Med Rehabil 49:28, 1968.

Lehmann JF and Krusen FH: Effect of pulsed and continuous application of ultrasound on transport of ions through biologic membranes, Arch Phys Med Rehabil 35:20, 1954.

Oakley EM: Application of continuous beam ultrasound at therapeutic levels, Physiotherapy 64:169, 1978.

Oakley EM: Dangers and contraindications of therapeutic ultrasound, Physiotherapy 64:173, 1978.

Rudd E: Physiatric management of osteoarthritis, Clin Rheum Dis 11:433, 1985.

Schoenbach SF and Song IC: Ultrasonic debridement: a new approach in the treatment of burn wounds, Plast Reconstr Surg 66:34, 1980.

Schwartz FF: Ultrasonics in medicine, J Med Assoc Alabama 26:200, 1957.

Sela M and others: Maxillofacial prosthetics and iontophoresis in management of burned ears, J Prosthet Dent 53:226, 1985.

Stanitski CL: Rehabilitation following knee injury, Clin Sports Med 4:495, 1985.

Stewart HF, Abzug JL, and Harris GR: Considerations in ultrasound therapy and equipment performance, Phys Ther 60:424, 1980.

Valenza J and others: A clinical study of a new heat modality, J Am Podiatr Med Assoc 69:440, 1979.

Wyper DJ and McNiven DR: Effects of some physiotherapeutic agents on skeletal muscle blood flow, Physiotherapy 62:83, 1976.

Yung P, Unsworth A, and Haslock I: Measurement of stiffness in the metacarpophalangeal joint: the effects of physiotherapy, Clin Phys Physiol Meas 7:147, 1986.

15

Mutilating injuries of the hand

William E. Burkhalter

Mutilating injuries of the hand are untidy, widely variable injuries that result in varying degrees of tissue loss as well as loss of parts of the hand. The etiology of these injuries may be burn, crush, explosion, or severe infection. Reid[42] classified mutilating injuries of the hand into five categories based on what is injured: grade I, dorsal injury; grade II, volar injury; grade III, radial hemiamputation; grade IV, ulnar hemiamputation; and grade V, transverse tissue loss in the hand—not just in the fingers. It is obvious from this classification that the dorsal injury with completely intact volar structures has the best prognosis, whereas the volar injury with loss of digital nerves, flexor tendons, and skin may have the worst functional recovery. Radial hemiamputation with loss of thumb or thumb and index suggests a poor result, but if a reconstructive procedure can be performed to give a radial digit, excellent function may result. Loss of the ulnar two fingers may give a very useful hand—one with good prehension but obviously not one with gross grasp. A transverse amputation in these untidy injuries usually precludes vascular reconstruction, but if the wound is such, a revascularization or replantation is possible.

By definition, these are complex injuries with varying tissue loss in various locations within the hand. The circumstances of the injury should influence decisions about débridement and wound closure. Barnyard injuries all carry the threat of clostridial infection, and much care should be taken when these wounds are repaired. Likewise, many injuries result from boating accidents and, again, infection from waterborne organisms must constantly be considered. An initial wound exploration cannot be done in the emergency room; after the patient is seen and evaluated, the wound must be splinted and protected from further contamination. A detailed physical examination to determine, for example, what nerve or vessel is intact is not indicated in the emergency room and merely causes unnecessary discomfort to the patient. Wound cultures, if they can be taken in the emergency room, may be useful, but perhaps even this can be postponed until the patient is in the operating room. After the patient has been scheduled for surgery, antibiotics may be started. Tetanus prophylaxis is always appropriate in these patients, even though the patient has had active immunization in the past. It is in the tetanus-prone wound, which many of these are, that passive immunization should be added. It is usually not worthwhile in the emergency room to obtain x-ray films. The best quality films can usually be obtained in the operating room with the patient anesthetized, immediately before starting the surgical preparation. Only with good quality x-ray films can the osseous structures be evaluated relative to dislocations and bone loss injuries.

Débridement is an operative procedure in which anything detrimental to wound healing is removed. Bacterial contamination must be reduced. Necrotic tissue and foreign bodies must be removed. Initial surgery should consist mainly of decompression of fascial compartments and excision of the enveloping fascia of these muscle compartments. This is an important portion of the initial operative procedure in that fascia tolerates sepsis poorly because of its poor blood supply, and its enveloping characteristics reduce the ability of swollen muscle to perfuse itself. In the hand there is very little muscle that can be removed without significantly compromising its overall usefulness; so the débridement of musculature structure in the hand must be conservative initially.

Wound exploration requires incisions along physiologic lines rather than through perforating injuries. After removal of as much visible necrotic tissue and foreign body as possible, low-pressure jet lavage may be used to further reduce bacterial contamination.* After the wound has been surgically debrided, jet lavaged, and recultured, revascularization should be considered. If there is significant lack of vascularity of certain areas of the hand, this should be improved if possible. There is reluctance to revascularize in the presence of an unstable skeleton; if revascularization is indicated in the hand or distal forearm injury, some type of internal stability to the fractures is required before revascularization. Only if arterial repair is going to be performed, do we feel that internal fixation should be done at this time.

In general, we perform internal fixation at the second-look procedure, usually in 2 or 3 days, which allows us to better determine viable from nonviable tissue.[10,20] We believe that the application of plates and screws, internal fixation devices, and even bone grafts at the second-look procedure is preferred (Fig. 15-1).

Because of the extent of soft tissue injury in these wounds, the simple Kirschner wire (K-wire) is inadequate. Excellent stability is needed, not as much to obtain osseous union, but to obtain a stable base from which the functioning muscles and tendon systems can move. Only with a stable fixation can function be instituted. Intact soft tissue and external means cannot be used to achieve a stable skeleton in these wounds. We feel that with a second-look procedure in 3 or 4 days, internal fixation with plates, screws, and bone grafts should be considered if the wound is reasonably clean. Spacer wires have been used, but I think more sophisticated internal fixation of bone grafts is worthwhile.[39] Our results with delayed primary bone grafts in more than 150 cases have suggested that infection is not a problem.[14] Additional surgery may be required because of adhesions,

---

*References 1, 4, 7, 8, 13, 15, 17, 22, 25, 37, 45, 49.

but our only failures have been those cases in which we could not achieve a satisfactory stability of the fracture because of the fracture geography. When we obtained satisfactory rigidity of the fracture at the time of the delayed primary bone grafting, our results were good. Therefore no primary closures are performed at first operation. At the second procedure we can reevaluate the adequacy of the débridement, and debride additionally if required, and internally fix the fracture.

At the second-look procedure, if satisfactory stability can be obtained, wound closure should be considered. It is obvious that function is not contingent upon wound closure,

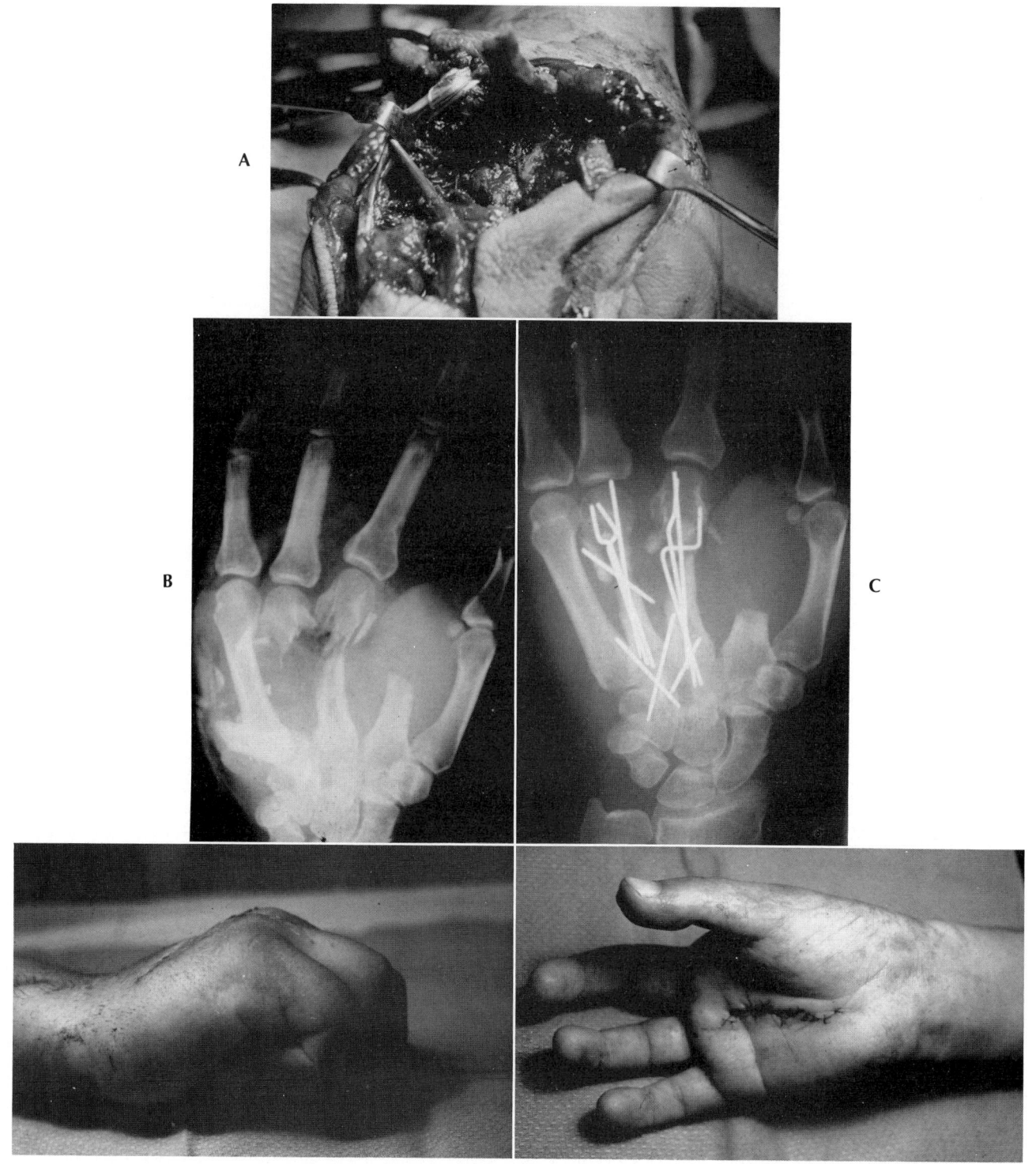

Fig. 15-1, A-E   A gunshot wound of the palm in a patient with a previous index ray deletion treated by débridement, skeletal stabilization with Kirschner wires, delayed primary closure of the wound and early motion. At 10 days the function is improving, and a healing wound is present. (From Burkhalter W: Hand Clin 2:47, 1986, by permission of WB Saunders Co.)

but if the wound is ready for closure, this should be done—not in any particular time frame but based on the quality of the wounded tissue itself. Four or five days after the initial wound cultures, antibiotic therapy should be evaluated relative to initial cultures. If this assessment as well as the appearance of the wound seem satisfactory, the wound should be closed.* If there is a probability that wound closure will not be successful, it should be avoided.[54]

---

*References 18, 23, 24, 35, 44, 51.

The reason for stabilizing the skeleton is to enable motion, and motion in the presence of open wound is not unknown to the hand surgeon. The treatment of the burned hand and the use of the open palm and digit technique in Dupuytren's contracture are examples of motion in the presence of an open wound. The same can be said here, and it is certainly preferable to have a stable skeleton in the moving hand than a stable skeleton in the infected one[2,9] (Fig. 15-2).

As the severity and complexity of the injury increase, one needs to be concerned about salvaging a basic hand—not

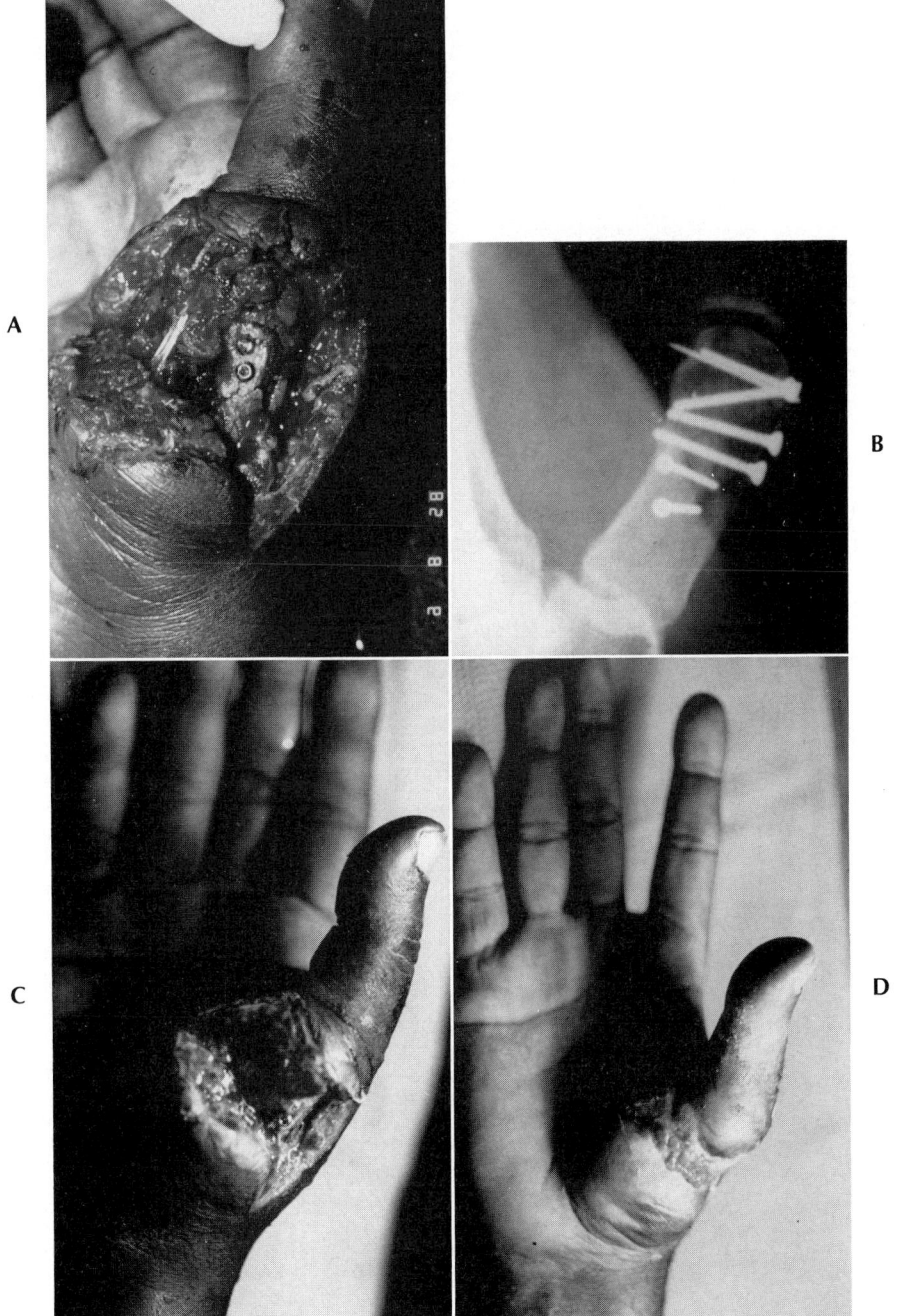

Fig. 15-2, A-D Using delayed primary bone grafting of this thumb bone-loss injury and internal fixation without wound closure, a functional thumb resulted. The dynamics of the healing wound actually drew the abductor pollicis brevis muscle belly distally allowing far better function of the muscle. Final photograph was taken 6 weeks after injury.

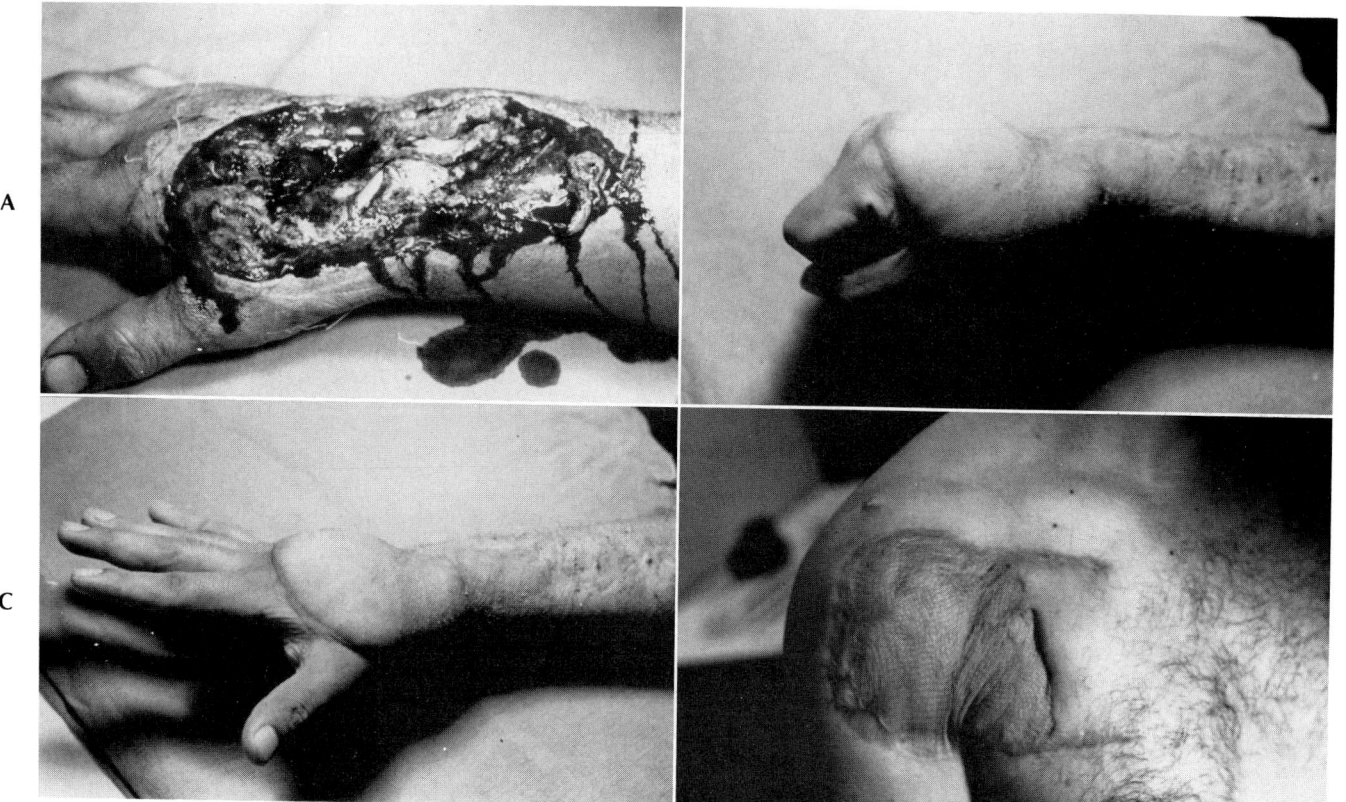

Fig. 15-3, A-D Deltopectoral flap coverage of this dorsal injury resulted in extremely good functional result, but the skin-grafted anterior chest wall was a cosmetic problem for the patient.

so much restoration of normal hand function, but salvaging a basic hand. A basic hand is composed of at least two nonpainful digits with adequate cover, durability, and sensibility. The two digits should be able to touch each other with some power, and at least one of the digits should be capable of motion to open for grasp.

Wound closure in these groups of patients is difficult. The usual techniques of simply suturing the intact skin are rarely applicable in this type of injury. At the least, various split-thickness skin grafts, finger fillets, and rotation flaps are required to cover important structures. Regardless of the method of closure, one must not put the hand in a non-functional position; that is, the usual abdominal pedicle flap that allows the wrist to drop into flexion and the MP joints to be in full extension should not be used in this group of patients. This type of coverage will result in loss of motion and poor position. Some alternative method should be used to ensure that the hand is in a functional position. Attempts to correct a nonfunctional position have been extensive. The deltopectoral flap was used early in the Vietnam War because it could be rotated 180 degrees. The flap could be elevated without delay, it was thin, and the hand could be elevated at application. The advantages of this flap coverage were almost outweighed by the cosmetic defect that it created on the anterior chest wall (Fig. 15-3). The quality of coverage of the hand, although excellent, created an anterior chest wall defect covered with split graft. This deltopectoral flap fell into disfavor and has been replaced by other axial pattern

flaps, such as the groin flap. With a few days' delay, the groin flap can be extended from its axial pattern into a random portion more posteriorly, giving more skin. In this way the forearm may be placed into supination so that increased mobility is possible. The patient is able to move the wrist and fingers much more easily.

The retrograde radial artery flap, which has been used extensively, also gives excellent coverage but creates a considerable defect in the forearm. An alternative to this flap is the use of the retrograde radial artery fascial flap, which was described to me by Partega.[38] Since that time, we have done a number of these retrograde radial artery fascial flaps. The radial artery and vein are ligated proximally, freed in a distal direction with attached forearm and muscle fascia, and placed over the dorsal or volar defect. This coverage can then be covered with a split-thickness skin graft (Fig. 15-4). This avoids removal of skin from the forearm with the subsequent split-graft–covered defect. An advantage to the use of this flap is that the coverage is very thin and not bulky on the hand, with excellent qualities of gliding beneath. Although this flap does not require microsurgical technique, the retrograde radial artery flap may have compromised venous return. There are many questions about how the blood exits from this flap. At inset time, one of the larger veins taken with the flap may be sutured to one of the larger veins on the dorsum of the hand or wrist. This has improved enormously the venous return of this flap.

In addition to these axial pattern skin flaps or fascial flaps,

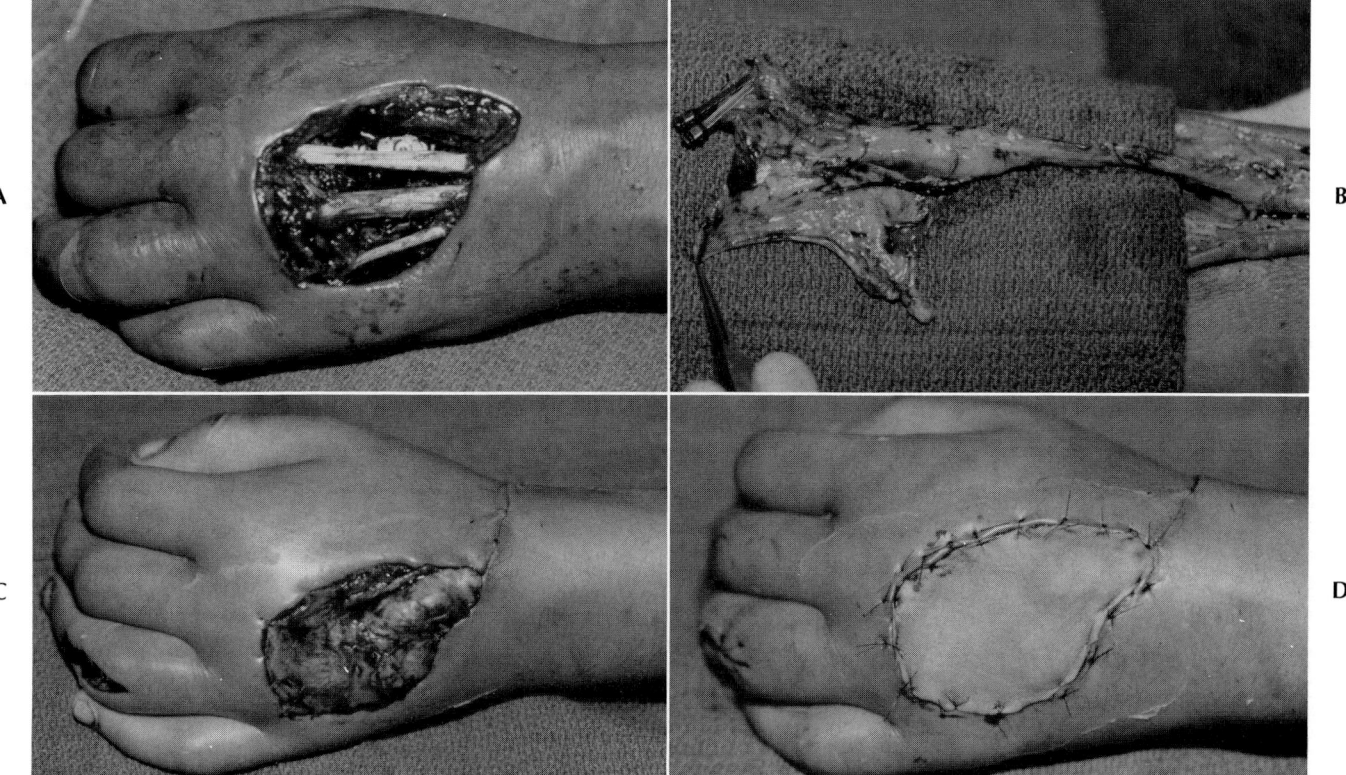

Fig. 15-4, A-D The radial artery fascial flap gives excellent coverage with good gliding beneath the fascia. Split grafting of the fascia allows only a linear defect in the forearm. This flap can be used both volarly and dorsally and even distally in the fingers to improve the overall functional result of flap coverage in the hand. (From Burkhalter W: Hand Clin 2:47, 1986, by permission of WB Saunders Co.)

free flaps may be used for cover. These have the advantages of (1) requiring no particular positioning of the hand and forearm, (2) allowing the patient to begin motion relatively early, and (3) avoiding many of the problems associated with usual coverage. In certain cases, extensor tendons from the dorsum of the foot have been moved with a dorsalis pedis flap to compensate for losses of tissue and skin. All of these innovative techniques for coverage, in addition to incorporating bone or tendon, allow for early reconstruction and rehabilitation, before development of extreme stiffness in a mangled hand.

Because of the advantages of free-flap transfer in certain mutilating injuries, we have used the lateral arm flap carried on the branches of the profunda brachii artery. The donor site can usually be closed primarily, and there is adequate skin for most hand defects. Multiple other free flaps are available, but none really seem to have the quality of skin and the ease of obtaining that the skin of the lateral arm flap has.

If the operative procedures of débridement, skeletal stabilization, and wound closure have been successful within a week or less of injury, active motion of the damaged parts can begin. At this point we have closed unreactive wounds, stabilized the skeleton, and provided at least a potential for motion. Only by starting early to move extensor and flexor tendons and other gliding structures within the hand, can we hope to avoid terrible problems of stiffness, which is usually associated with these diffuse injuries.

DORSAL INJURIES

Dorsal injuries, perhaps in many respects the least destructive of hand function, can be quite spectacular. They are usually associated with grinding-type wounds or roller injuries of the hand in which the skin, tendons, and osseous structures are frequently exposed. In most of these, the palmar surface is completely normal. The flexor tendons are normal, usually the MP joints are normal, and certainly all of the vessels and nerve structures volarly are normal. The problem is to stabilize the wrist early and get the intrinsics and active digital flexors working the fingers into flexion. In spite of much dorsal injury with, for example, loss of tendon, the real problem is stiff MP joints—that is, loss of flexion. The stumps of the remaining tendons get entrapped in this dorsal scar and limit flexion. In addition, flap coverage is usually believed to be necessary immediately. The flaps, unless carefully designed, usually result in limitation of flexion of the MP joints and a flexion deformity of the wrist. This combination is a bad dynamic balance for the hand. Because of the grinding nature of some of these injuries, the carpus itself is so badly damaged that the patient cannot use the wrist extensors even when they are present. In many of these, the proper management might be immediate arthrodesis of the wrist. This could be followed by coverage and tendon replacement, using care early to avoid stiffness of MP joints. If the wrist extensors are intact, arthrodesis should not be done, but with significant osseous injury to the carpal bones, primary fusion in this case is often warranted and ultimately is the best way to manage these rather complex injuries. The timing of reconstructive procedures is critical in the management of these injuries. Once wound control has been obtained and if an arthrodesis is required based on the destruction of the carpal joints, the fusion should be done within a few days of the initial operative procedure. This will allow a stable base from which to maintain simultaneous three-joint digital flexion of the fingers and thumb (Fig. 15-5).

Now the problem of tendon reconstruction and coverage becomes paramount. Placing tendons into a situation that requires immobilization invites stiffness. Although Hentz reported transposition of extensor tendons with a dorsalis pedis flap as a single entity done acutely, we do not have experience with this procedure.[19] It seems that stabilization of the wrist, coverage, and maintenance of MP joint flexion until the hand is unreactive is probably preferable. There is no set time to do tendon grafts for digital extension. In general, function is the best guideline, not time or tissue equilibrium. If the patient can maintain simultaneous three-joint flexion without external splintage for 3 or 4 weeks, he is ready for the relative immobilization required of the tendon graft. For a tendon graft to be successful in these patients, a good motor that has normal excursion is required, especially with a fused wrist. The only motor really available is the flexor digitorum superficialis. After wrist fusion, the present flexor carpi radialis (FCR) and flexor carpi ulnaris (FCU) volarly may not have adequate excursion to be used

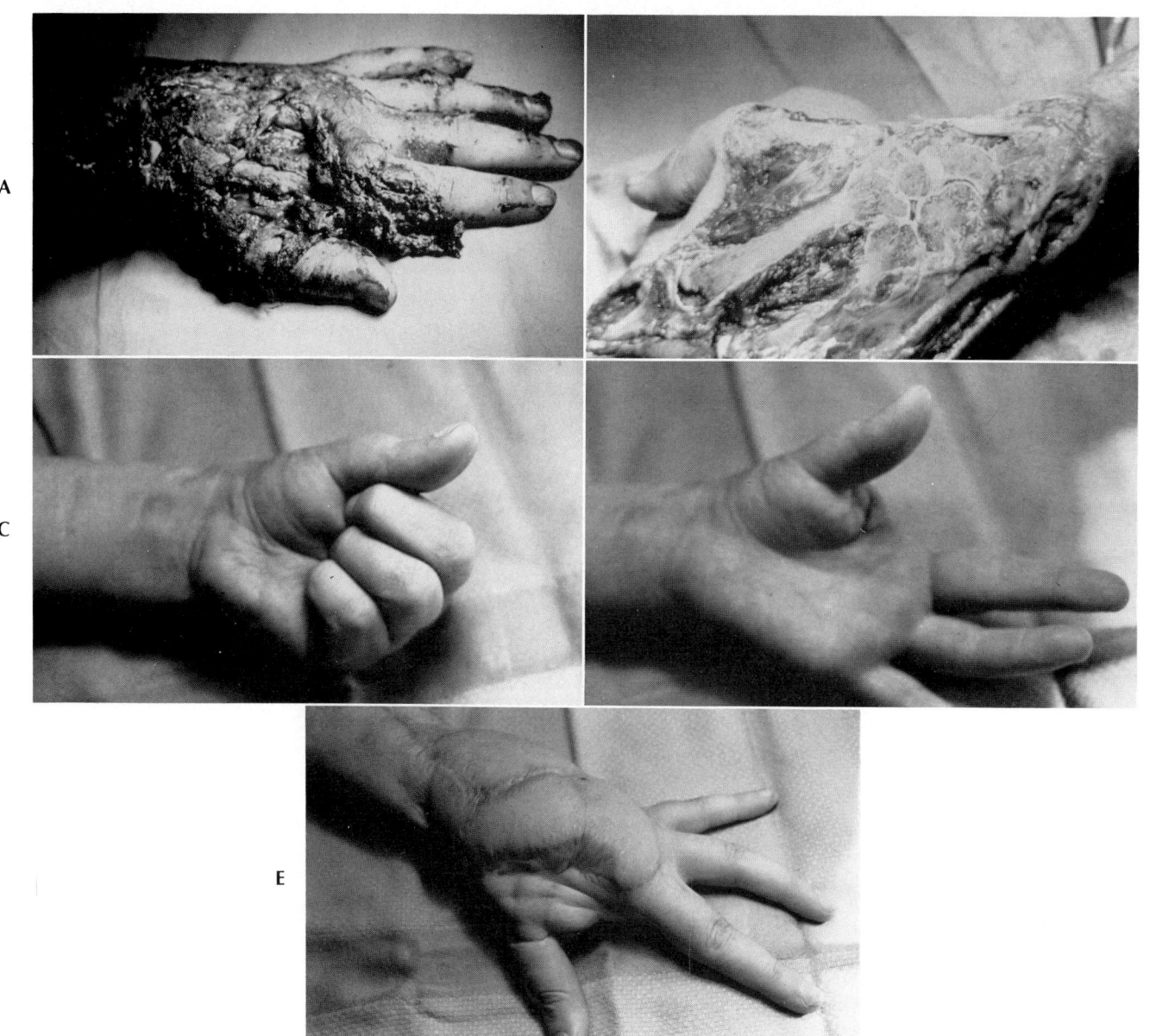

A   B   C   D   E

Fig. 15-5, A-E   A severe dorsal grinding injury resulting in loss of skin, tendon, and bone treated by wrist arthrodesis, tendon grafts, and flap coverage as well as deletion of the index finger. Dorsal skin coverage can be improved by alternate coverage methods.

for digital extension. With the tendon loss, very little useful tendon on the dorsum of the hand will be available. Probably the only muscle tendon unit that will be of adequate length and excursion is the flexor digitorum superficialis. This is a difficult transfer to relearn, especially as the patient gets older, but it does avoid the tendon graft and perhaps avoids using a motor with limited excursion. Certainly the selection of motor is much easier if arthrodesis of the wrist is not necessary; that is, if the injury was more superficial and did not involve the carpal joints, maintenance of a useful wrist allows wrist flexors to motor tendon grafts brought from the volar surface, much as one would in a radial nerve paralysis. Here the FCU or FCR can be transferred after extension with grafts to motor the individual fingers. A mobile wrist

makes rehabilitation of the fingers far easier. However, again it must be remembered that even though the wrist is normal and has good control, MP joint stiffness remains a major problem both early and late in these patients.

Total immobilization of the fingers in the postoperative tendon graft transfer period, however, is not necessary. Evans[12] showed that managing complex dorsal injuries early and late with protected passive and active motion can reduce adhesions and the necessity for subsequent tendolysis. Just as protected motion in the immediate postoperative period has improved our results with flexor tendon injuries, so has protected motion improved our results dorsally. The technique allows limited MP joint flexion with the interphalangeal joint in extension. This MP joint flexion is calculated

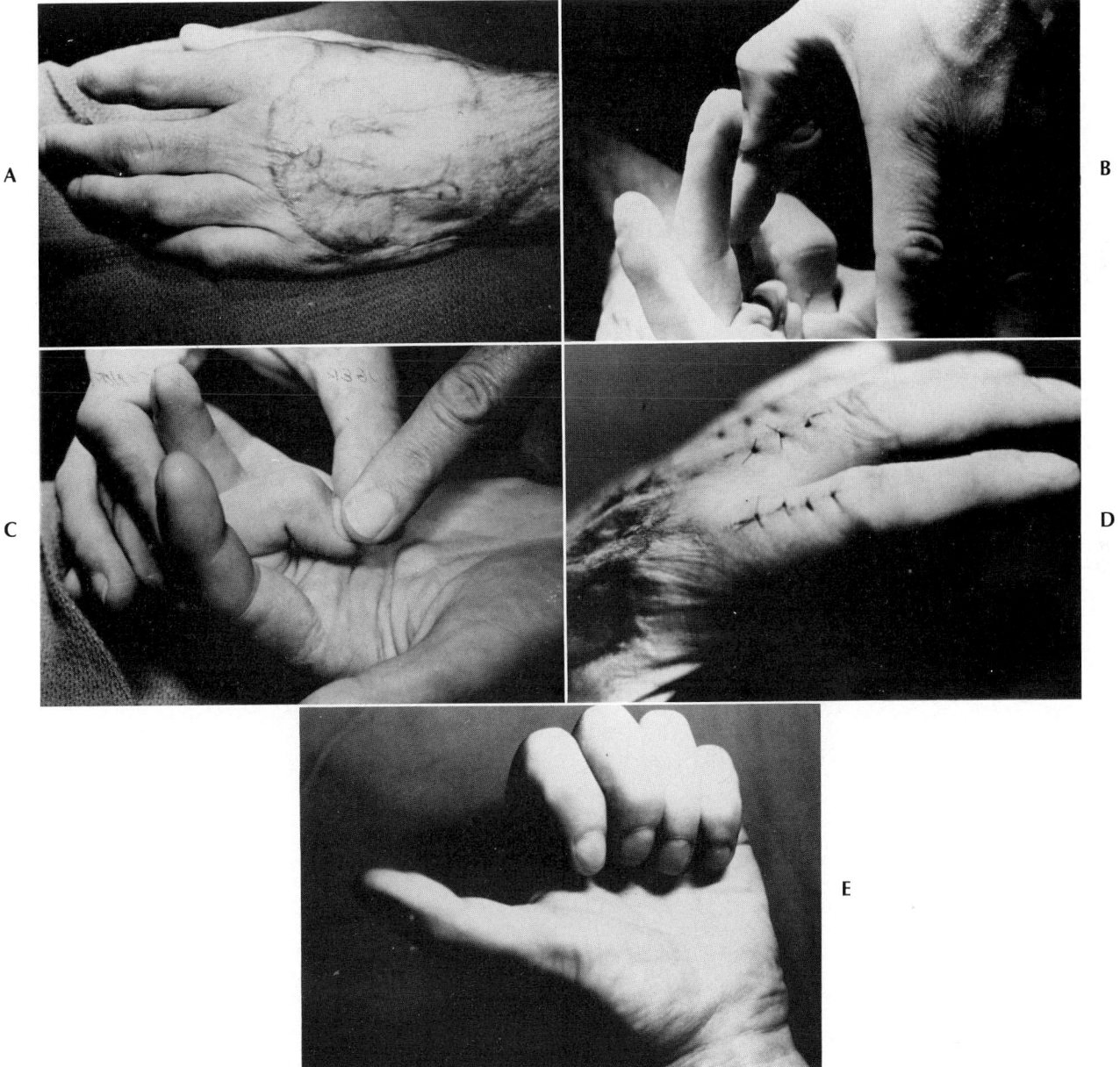

A B C D E

Fig. 15-6, A-E Poor skin over the dorsum of the hand, without joint stiffness but with tendons adherence, may be treated by tenotomy of the extensor mechanism over the proximal phalanx. This separates intrinsic from extrinsic extensors. This patient with a burn and infection on the dorsum of the hand had limited tendon excursion but good joint motion. Tenotomy over the proximal phalanx resulted in maintenance of full MP motion and improvement in interphalangeal joint flexion without loss of extension.

based on achieving 3 to 5 mm of tendon motion. The amount of motion is slightly variable but is 30 to 40 degrees more than the MP joint. Elastic traction returns the digits to full extension. The interphalangeal joints are actually flexed fully with the MP joints held passively in full extension. Using this technique, the entire extensor mechanism can be kept mobile during the healing period, and stress can be added in a controlled fashion to the healing juncture of tendon repair or graft.

In addition, if the flexor digitorum superficialis transfer is utilized with a fused wrist, the route to the dorsum should be subcutaneous around the forearm either radially or ulnarly. This has the advantage of placing the muscle belly of the transfer immediately beneath the skin. Because relearning the transfer is difficult, various biofeedback techniques can be used to help the patient relearn the action of the flexor digitorum superficialis with this subcutaneous location of the muscle.

If the functional result after transfer is less than optimal, tenolysis of the grafts or transfers should be considered. We do not hesitate to do tenolysis of flexor or extensor tendon repairs to equalize active and passive joint motion. Why then not do the same with transfers? Not only can range be improved, but strength can be improved. The old adage of a transferred muscle losing one grade of strength postoperatively is not related to something inherent in the muscle but to adhesions, which can be freed, thereby improving strength (Fig. 15-6).

Similarly, separating the intrinsic and extrinsic tendon system as initially described by Littler can improve digital flexion.[8] If the extensor tendon adherence is over the dorsum of the hand or more proximally if the wrist is fused, a tenotomy over the proximal phalanx separates the two systems. The tenotomy should not involve the lateral bands but only the extensor digitorum tendon over the proximal phalanx distal to the MP joint, usually in its midportion. This procedure has merit if full flexion of the MP joint brings the distal joints into full extension, which can be overcome only by allowing the MP joint to extend. This dorsal rein can also be treated by tenolysis, obviously, if adequate skin is present dorsally.

RADIAL HEMIAMPUTATION

Radial tissue loss in the hand implies loss of the thumb or portions of the thumb, but in these types of injuries, other digits or portions of index or index and long may also be lost. There is no question that in these cases revascularization or replantations should be the primary treatment options. The results of thumb replantation almost routinely are good functionally, especially with remaining intrinsic muscle and a good basilar joint. Wound exploration and débridement should always be the first concern. Vascular failure almost always will occur if infection occurs in the operative area. In this type of wound with widespread injury, a vein graft probably will be needed. Internal fixation of fractures and coverage also will be required, which places great demands on the ability to obtain wound control ini-

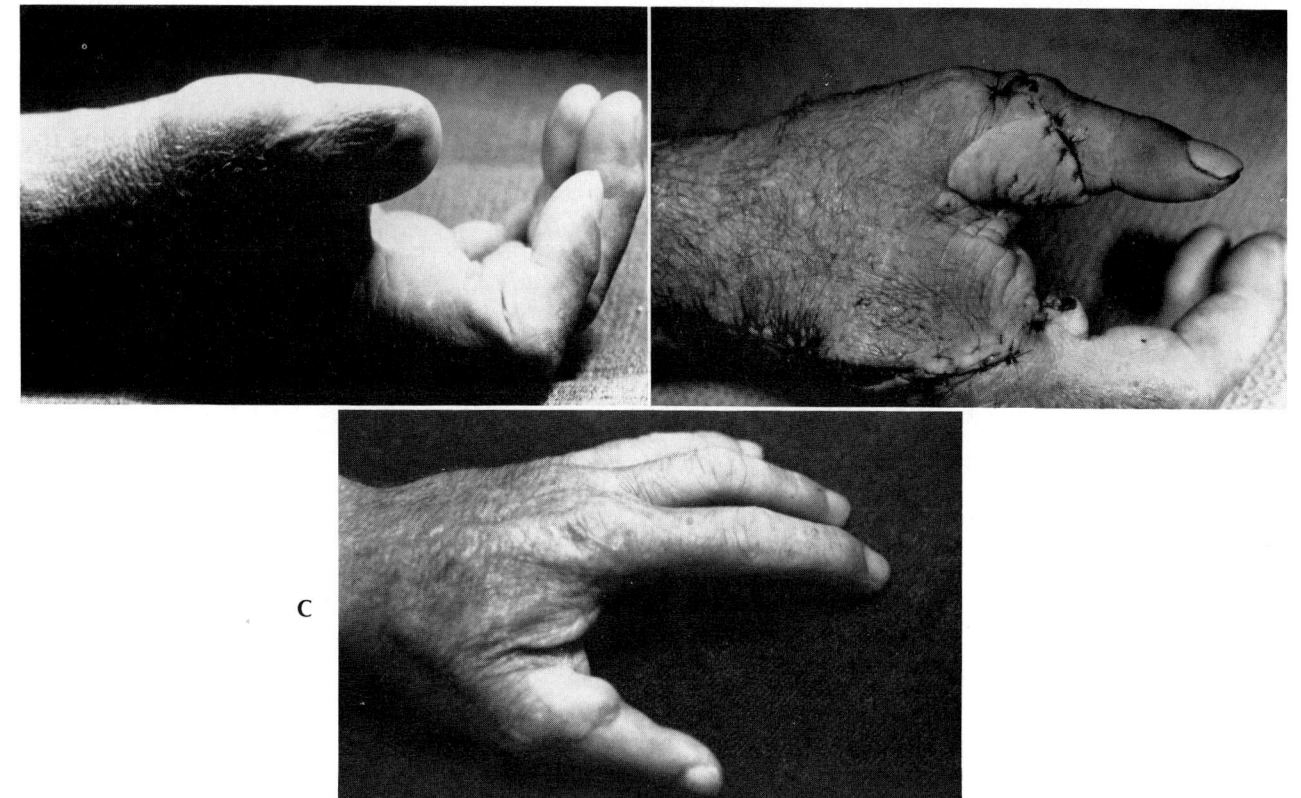

Fig. 15-7, A-C   A stiff index finger with loss of a single nerve and vessel and a short thumb can both be used to improve the overall function of the hand. Deletion of the stiff index ray and thumb lengthening resulted in marked improvement in function.

tially. If the replantations or revascularization is successful, there is no longer a mutilated hand, but if the vascular surgery is unsuccessful because of sepsis or diffuse crush, there is tissue loss that may need replacement. Certainly isolated thumb loss, partially or completely, does not always mean a thumb reconstructive procedure.

There are many techniques for thumb reconstruction, and care should be taken to avoid having a favorite operation looking for a patient. Thumb reconstruction is an elective procedure that should be undertaken only when the remaining hand is completely rehabilitated from the injury. In addition, the patient must volunteer a need or at least ask for information regarding a new thumb.

Available are techniques of metacarpal lengthening, partial or complete pollicization,[16,43] island pedicle tissue transfer with bone graft, and pedicle tissue.[30] Various microsurgical procedures, such as wraparound plasty and great or small toe transfer, also bring tissue from a distance[31] (Fig. 15-7). All have their advantages and disadvantages.[47] The patient should be as completely informed as possible before making the decision. The information must include functional and cosmetic expectations and the probabilities of the reconstruction looking thumblike . The latter concern is an individual consideration. Meyer, when considering a second toe transfer on a group of patients, constructed a photomontage of the toe and placed it photographically in the thumb position. In this way the patient could see the appearance of the transposed toe. The majority of this preselected group of patients rejected the proposed operative procedure on the basis of cosmesis.[28]

Cosmesis in the hand is obviously important, at least from the patient's standpoint. Loss of tissue is, however, not always difficult to hide. Others see what they expect to see.

They expect to see symmetry. Lack of symmetric blending of one structure into another calls attention to the defect. Loss of a single digit in a hand is rarely appreciated by a viewer if the symmetry is preserved by ray resection, whereas loss of the ring finger at the PIP joint creates asymmetry and is immediately obvious. Must symmetry be created surgically by ray resection of the ring finger in the example above? Certainly not. Symmetry may be created by aesthetic protheses that are capable of some passive function. Jean Pillet in 1974 at the Annual Meeting of the American Society for Surgery of the Hand in Dallas, Texas, opened all eyes to truly beautiful, aesthetic prostheses for tissue loss in the hand. These devices have excellent color match, texture, and enough stiffness to impart a lifelike quality to the part. With elastic memory, some of these devices are capable of passive function. In addition to substituting for loss, they may be fabricated to cover existing functional structures to improve the contour and symmetry. These prostheses have been added even to second toe transfers for thumb reconstruction to improve the overall symmetry[41] (Fig. 15-8). Michon pointed out that with isolated thumb loss, pollicization is preferable to free tissue for thumb reconstruction.[29] However, as the index is added to the loss, the advantage shifts toward toe transfer as a method of improving hand function. Add thumb, index, and long to the list of tissues lost, and there is little question that improved function will result with tissue added from a distance. This becomes more basic than simple thumb reconstruction and becomes salvage of the basic hand. The transposed toe will have some motor function, but motion will be incomplete, and sensibility in the adult will be far from perfect. Motion, strength, and sensation will come from the remaining ulnar border digits, ring and small. It

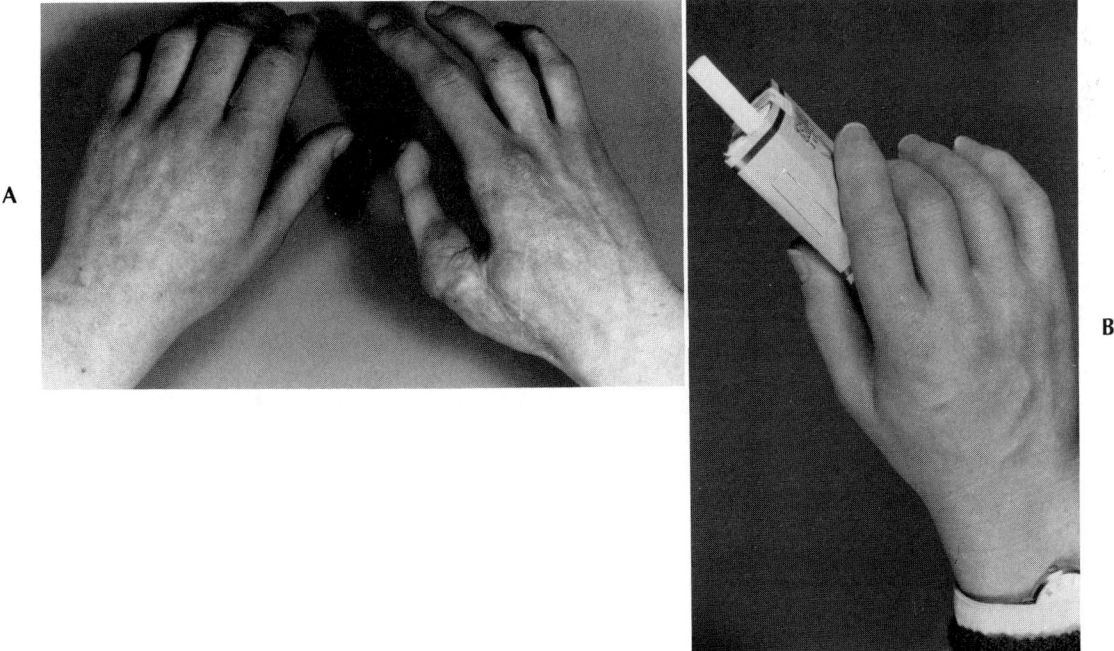

Fig. 15-8, A-B In spite of improved function, following second toe microvascular transfer, this patient was hesitant to use the thumb. With improved cosmesis from a prosthetic cover, the patient was more at ease with functional activities.

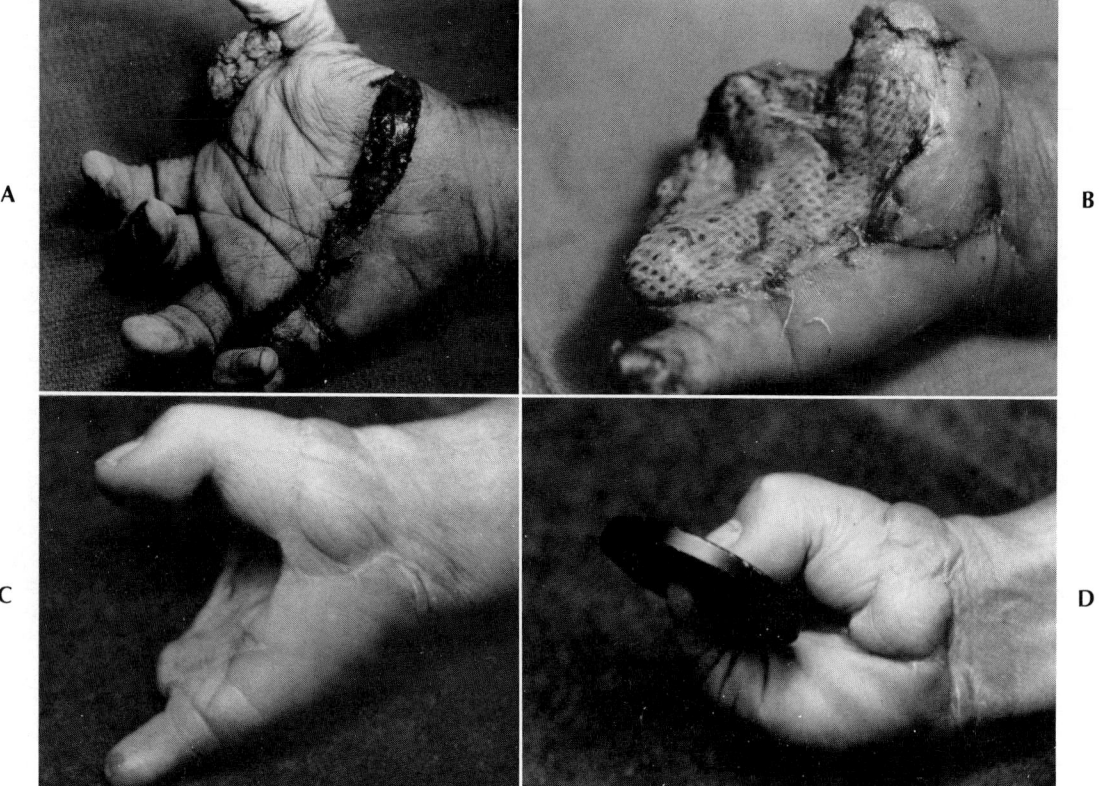

Fig. 15-9, A-D   A 25-year-old man whose hand was crushed in a cement mixer. A failed revascularization resulted in loss of thumb, index, long, and ring finger with only a portion of the small remaining. Great toe transfer and maintenance of full mobility in the remaining portion of the small finger resulted in a functional hand.

is obvious from this that once tissue has been lost from the hand, the most important consideration is to avoid compromising the intact portions. Full motion must be maintained in the remaining digits by active motion. Splintage, plaster-of-paris casts, and joint positioning by K-wires may be necessary to avoid the function-robbing contractures in the remaining parts (Fig. 15-9).

In addition to free transfer and pollicization, there are several other techniques for thumb reconstruction that should be considered. None of these require microsurgical technique and have been used for congenital as well as acquired tissue loss. Osteoplastic reconstruction must be considered. This procedure has a poor reputation because of graft absorption and perhaps fracture, and because multiple stages may be required to achieve a functional thumb. However, Morgan and Stein[30] have used osteoplastic reconstruction as a single operative procedure. They applied directly a neurovascular island flap from one of the adjacent fingers to a corticocancellous graft, which was placed to lengthen the thumb. Dorsal coverage of this bone graft was achieved by a pedicle flap of a random type: the vascularity and neurologic function were supplied by the transposed neurovascular island flap. Initially Morgan and Stein used a deltopectoral flap, but any random flap or axial pattern flap can be used to surface the dorsum of the thumb. In many of these cases, the bone graft seems to be actively bleeding at the time of detachment of the dorsal flap coverage (Fig. 15-10). In general, our experience with this method has been good. No fractures or absorption of the

graft have resulted from this one-stage technique in our experience, although it has been reported by other authors. Graft fractures, however, should be expected. It seems that this bone, actually unsupported by muscle tissue to act as an absorber of energy, undergoes excessive stress. Normal bone will easily fracture if overloaded, and the reason for absence of frequent fracture is normal muscle, which protects the skeleton. Without muscle support in the transposed graft to the thumb position, fracture is almost inevitable, certainly within the first year or so.

If one is concerned only about additional length of the thumb with normally functioning intrinsic muscles and good basilar joint, the remaining metacarpal or metacarpal and proximal phalanx can be lengthened using an external fixator. Although this technique was initially used in congenital short thumb deformities, it is now used on traumatic amputations with excellent results.[21,26] In the adult, however, bone graft is usually required to achieve solid union once length has been regained. In addition, this lengthening technique brings distal migration of the thumb-index web space; therefore some type of deepening of the web space is required after obtaining desired length of the thumb. It was initially believed that in trauma cases, the distal scar would melt away with pressure from the bone beneath and the external fixator, but this has not occurred. With a reasonably mature and nonadherence scar, exposure of the distal bone has not been seen. Considerable length can be obtained by this technique. Because the thumb is lengthened in a strictly linear fashion, flexion can be added to the thumb at the time

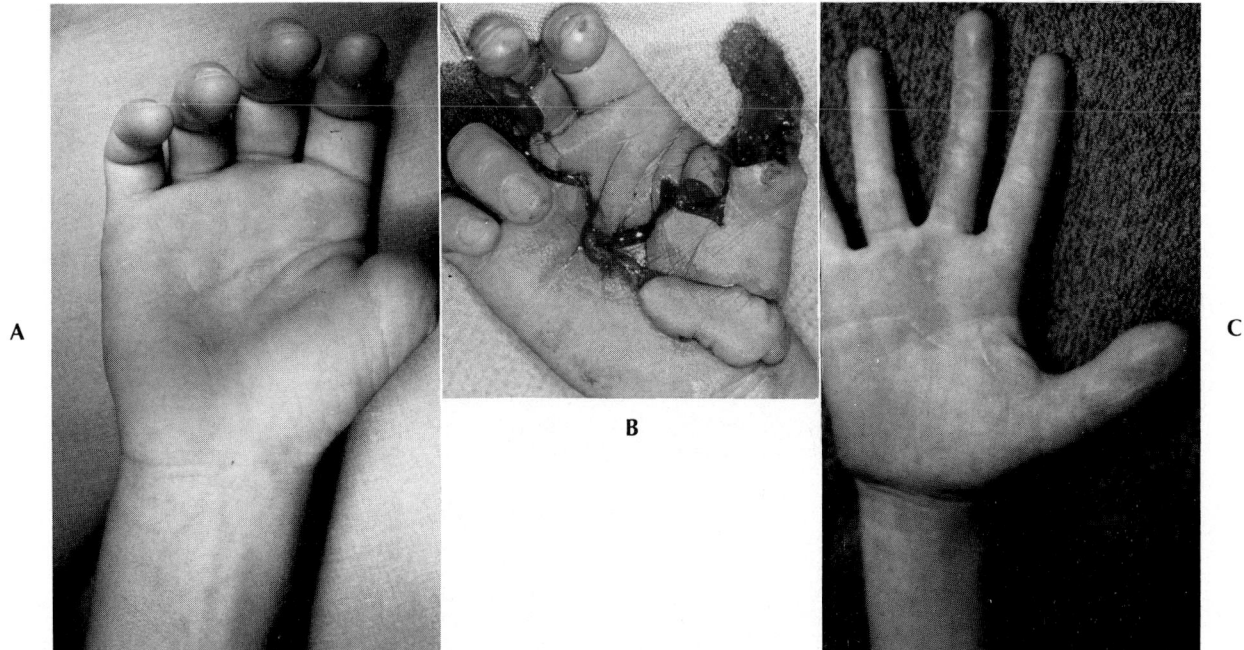

Fig. 15-10, A-C   Increased thumb length may be obtained by a one-stage procedure. This uses dorsal flap coverage, volar island pedicle flap coverage to an iliac bone graft. Good vascularity and nerve function in this thumb reconstruction make it especially applicable to the younger patient.

of inset of the bone graft. Without this flexion, the thumb, although of adequate length, may not have adequate flexion to reach the fingers, which likewise may have some compromised mobility.

One of the most cosmetically appealing microsurgical thumb reconstructions, however, is Morrison's wraparound plasty. This utilizes a portion of the nail, bone, and skin from the great toe. The procedure consists of elongating the remaining thumb with an iliac bone graft and surrounding this graft with a portion of the great toe skin and portion of the nail, and this is all supported by a microsurgical anastomosis of arteries, veins, and nerves. Not all of the great toe skin is required, nor is all of the nail. Although no motion is present in the thumb, the function is improved by extra length, by restored sensibility, which can be achieved by nerve suture, and by extraordinary cosmesis: the thumb has almost a normal appearance from the dorsum. Cosmetically this is probably superior to either a pollicization or a second toe transfer.

ULNAR HEMIAMPUTATION

Loss of digits on the ulnar border of the hand may require little reconstruction (Fig. 15-11). In this case the basic hand with the thumb, index, and long finger remain with good sensibility. The major functional loss is one of loss of power grip. Prehension is still available, and the hand is certainly much more than a helper. With these injuries, the major problem might be coverage that has some degree of sensibility. The application of a flap to the ulnar border of the hand, with its position of relative dependency and exposure to external damage, may create a problem early, until some sensibility returns to the ulnar border. Using fillet skin in

these cases is far preferable to flap coverage from a distance, with its instability and inadequate sensibility. Injuries here are generally a problem only if the wound goes far enough proximally to involve the motor branch of the ulnar nerve. Then the loss of interosseous function and adductor function to the thumb may severely compromise a relatively good-looking radial border; that is, the pinch mechanism, which is really the remaining function in this type of tissue loss, will be severely weakened because of the nerve injury to the deep branch of the ulnar nerve (Fig. 15-12). With this injury, grafting or certainly repairing the motor branch and the ulnar nerve to restore power to the pinch mechanism should be considered. Failing this, tendon transfers, if there are available motors with satisfactory excursion and length, should be done to improve pinch.

VOLAR SURFACE INJURY

Other than actual loss of parts, probably the most devastating injuries are to the volar surface of the hand. These are usually avulsions from rollers or explosion in character. In addition to skin loss, there is usually loss of tendon with nerve and vessel. The dorsum is normal, and the circulation to the dorsum of the hand is usually adequate to supply the dorsal skin plus bones and joints (Fig. 15-13). However, the volar side is completely denuded of all soft tissue. If the thumb and all fingers are involved, the ability to regain useful function is limited. However, in certain patients, some type of useful hand function might be achieved. The initial feeling is, after wound débridement, to obtain coverage volarly. Groin flap coverage preserving all fingers at full length gives unstable skin volarly without sensibility and without any real improvement in the vascularity. Al-

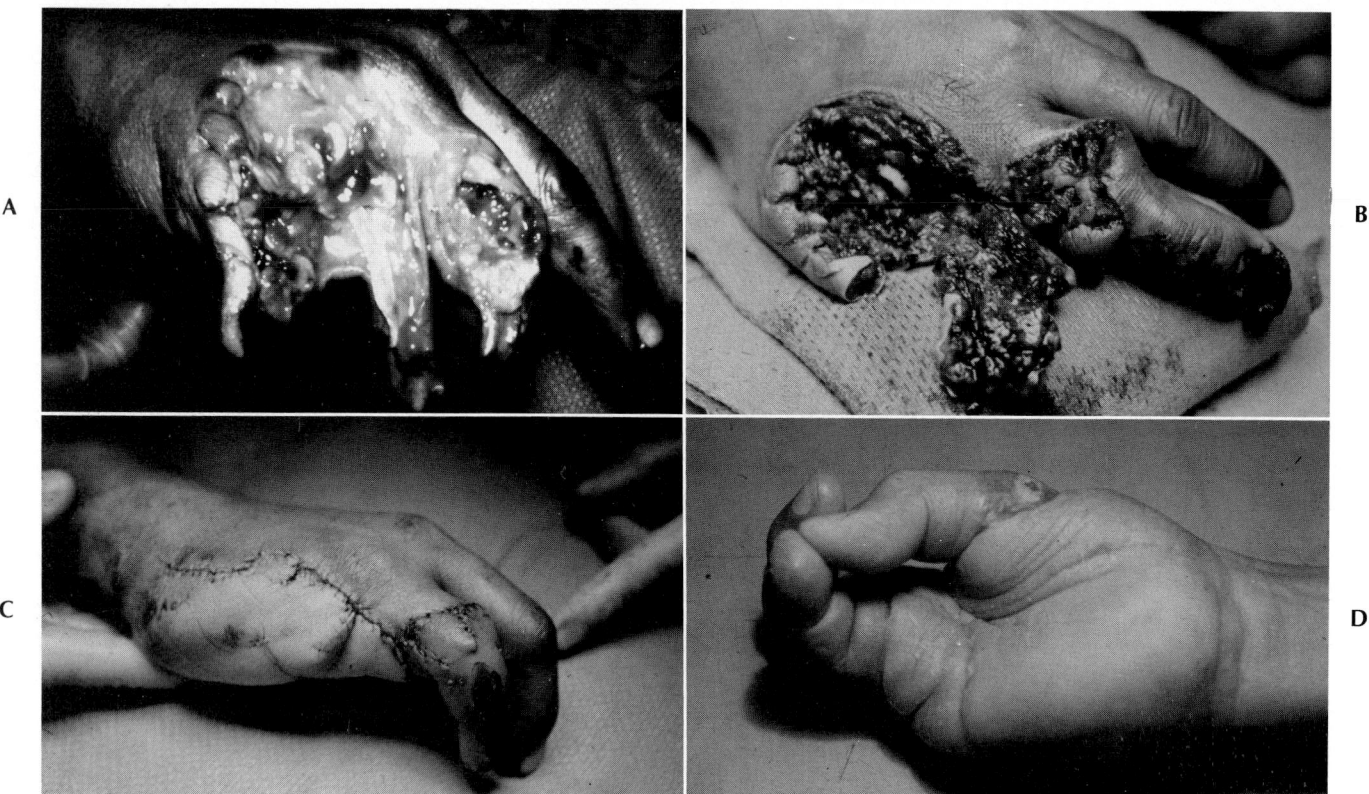

Fig. 15-11, A-D Ulnar border amputations with three good remaining digits and without damage to the ulnar nerve result in a hand capable of prehension, but no power grip. (From Burkhalter W: Hand Clin 2:57, 1986, by permission of WB Saunders Publishing Co.)

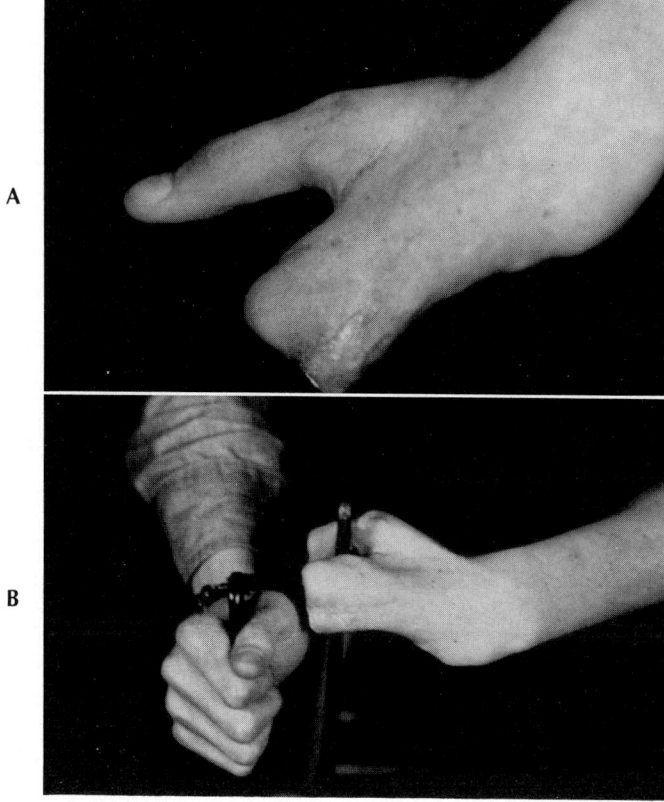

Fig. 15-12, A-B A basic hand with metacarpals remaining on the ulnar side and a mobile thumb radially. Even with function loss of the thumb adductor as a result of ulnar nerve injury, overuse of the flexor pollicis and good sensibility in the thumb make this a basic functional hand.

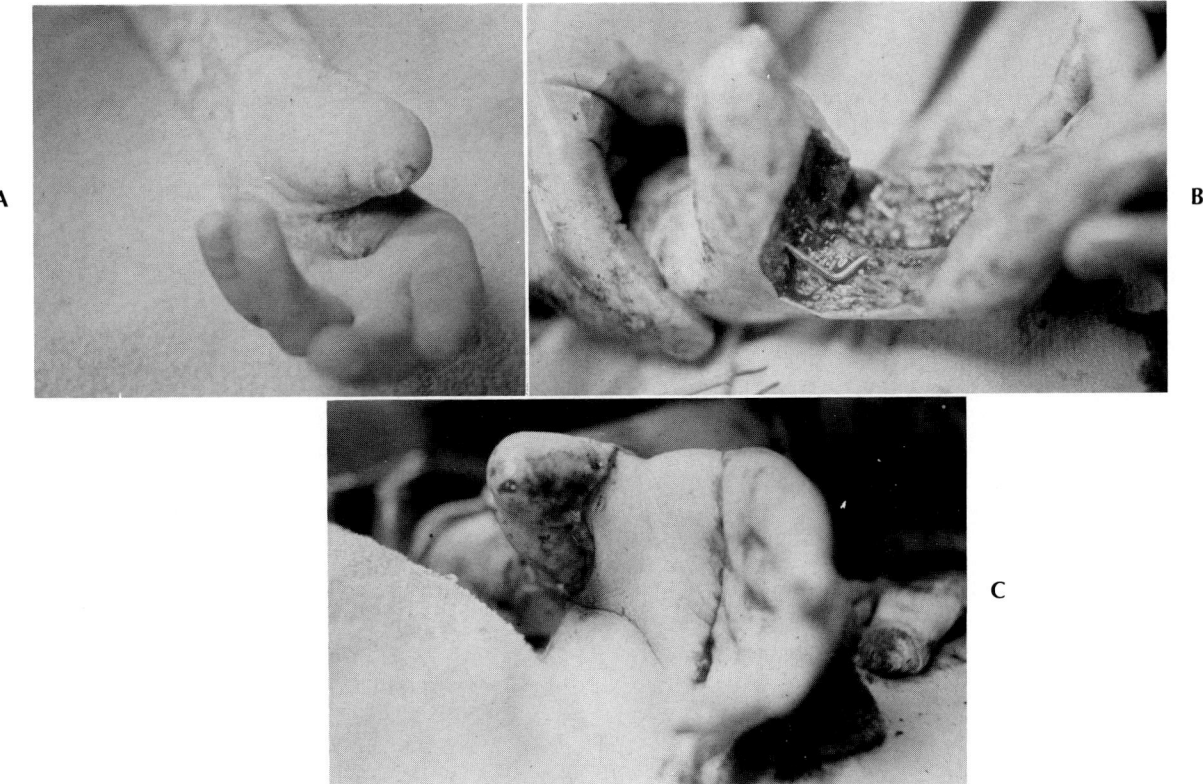

Fig. 15-13, A-C   With volar tissue loss, although coverage can be achieved, only metacarpophalangeal joint motion is possible. Here the unstable skin from the distant site may compromise function. Interphalangeal joint flexion is not possible for this patient, even with attempted use of tendon prostheses and tendon grafts. (From Burkhalter W: Hand Clin 2:65, 1986, with permission from WB Saunders Publishing Co.)

though the fingers may be later divided so that there are individual digits remaining, this is not very useful. They will have only limited MP joint function, unstable volar skin, and poor sensibility. I think there is an alternative when there has been loss of palmar skin but a maintenance of some thumb function.

Because interphalangeal joint motion is not likely, there will be little power grip or power grasp in this hand. Precision will be used, so the MP joint movement should be started early. Arthrodesis of the PIP joint can be done through the volar wound for stability. This surgical approach maintains normal dorsal circulation. With this stability and probably some intrinsic muscles, MP joint motion can be started. In the severely involved hand, loss of MP joint motion will seriously compromise the ultimate result. Rather than using skin that has no sensibility and no vascularity of its own, volar skin coverage can be accomplished by finger fillet. Fillet of two peripheral fingers allows the normal dorsal skin, which has some sensibility and certainly better vascularity, to cover the volar side of the ring and long finger; that is, with a good thumb, the skin of the dorsal surface of the index could be used to resurface the volar side of the long, and the dorsal side of the small could be used to resurface the volar side of the ring finger as required. In addition, if there were a requirement for some palmar skin, ray deletions of the index and small fingers (although narrowing the palm considerably) would reduce the size of the defect, and this could be covered more easily by these lateral flaps. In this way, the amount of tissue that needs

coverage is reduced, and the quality of the coverage is improved.[51] The stability from the arthrodesis allows the patients to begin early MP joint motion, and the tendency for stiffness is reduced in this group. An alternative to finger fillet and using the dorsal skin to achieve volar coverage is the use of very thin, free tissue transfers that can bring some innervated skin to the palm of the hand. Such tissue transfers as the dorsalis pedis flap can be carried with neural tissue, which can be sutured to the median and/or ulnar nerves proximally to give some sensibility to the palm of the hand. However, there is usually inadequate tissue to resurface all four fingers using such a flap, and the stability of the skin, I think, is still open to some question regarding the quality of sensibility that might be recovered in such a situation. Therefore, although it is certainly possible to cover such a defect with dorsalis pedis skin, the functional improvement is only problematic.

An interesting phenomenon can occur in these volar injuries in which there has been loss of tendons and proximal migration of the flexor tendon system and/or lumbricals into the carpal tunnel. A patient may complain of severe pain with no way of evaluating the sensibility in the hand. In multiple digit amputations, either transverse or with loss of substance and proximal migration of the flexor system, the development of carpal tunnel should be considered if pain is a problem with rehabilitation. With a normal functioning thumb, sensory conduction velocity to the digital nerves of the thumb can be carried out as can motor conduction velocity. However, the problem is that the usual symptoms, such as night pain and tingling, that are associated with carpal tunnel are usually absent, and a carpal tunnel diagnosis may be overlooked. As with many diagnoses, thinking about it is the major problem. When one thinks about the possibility of the development of a carpal tunnel in these patients, the diagnosis can usually be made without much difficulty.

SINGLE DIGIT INJURIES

Partial or complete single digital amputations perhaps are not a true mutilation of the hand but certainly may affect the cosmesis as well as the overall function. One may actually have a combination of distal loss plus proximal joint stiffness. The classic example of this is the older patient with a fingertip injury who loses proximal joint function both at the PIP joint and MP joint. Therefore, after the initial surgery, the primary concern of the distal amputation should be maintenance of proximal joint motion. In addition to this distal injury or distal amputation, more proximal joint injury may occur. What is then left is a combination of a distal amputation with proximal joint stiffness. In this situation, two potential complications should be considered. One has already been mentioned: the development of a carpal tunnel syndrome. Although this usually develops in multiple finger amputations, it certainly may occur with single digit loss. The other complication in single digits with limited motion may be limited motion of undamaged fingers. This is the so-called quadregia effect (Fig. 15-14). In its

full-blown status, it is easy to diagnose, but in its more subtle form, the diagnosis may be difficult to make. The reason is that it may not be as much loss of digital motion as it is loss of digital strength at the extremes of tendon excursion. With widespread injury and the lack of full flexion in relatively undamaged fingers, this problem should definitely be considered.[34] The offending stiff finger is usually the long or the ring. The index or small finger, even though stiff, does not compromise motion in the remaining digits.

When confronted with loss of strength or motion, look to the contralateral undamaged hand to help in the diagnosis. When one stabilizes an interphalangeal joint of a ring finger or a long finger in varying degrees of extension, with or without full MP joint flexion, and notices loss of digital motion, this is true quadregia. However, if there is just limited excursion but almost full motion, the quadregia may be more subtle and simply give limited strength. This quadregia effect is one of the reasons for the dissatisfaction with PIP joint fusion, especially in the long and ring finger. Many patients with these stiff interior fingers have suggested to surgeons that the stiff digit be removed. An alternative to this, if there is a reason for keeping the digit, is tenotomy of the profundus tendon to free the single muscle belly from its limited excursion proximally. To maintain some distal joint motion in those patients who have just a stiff PIP joint, transfer of the proximal superficialis to the distal profundus in the palm or perhaps the forearm will give increased

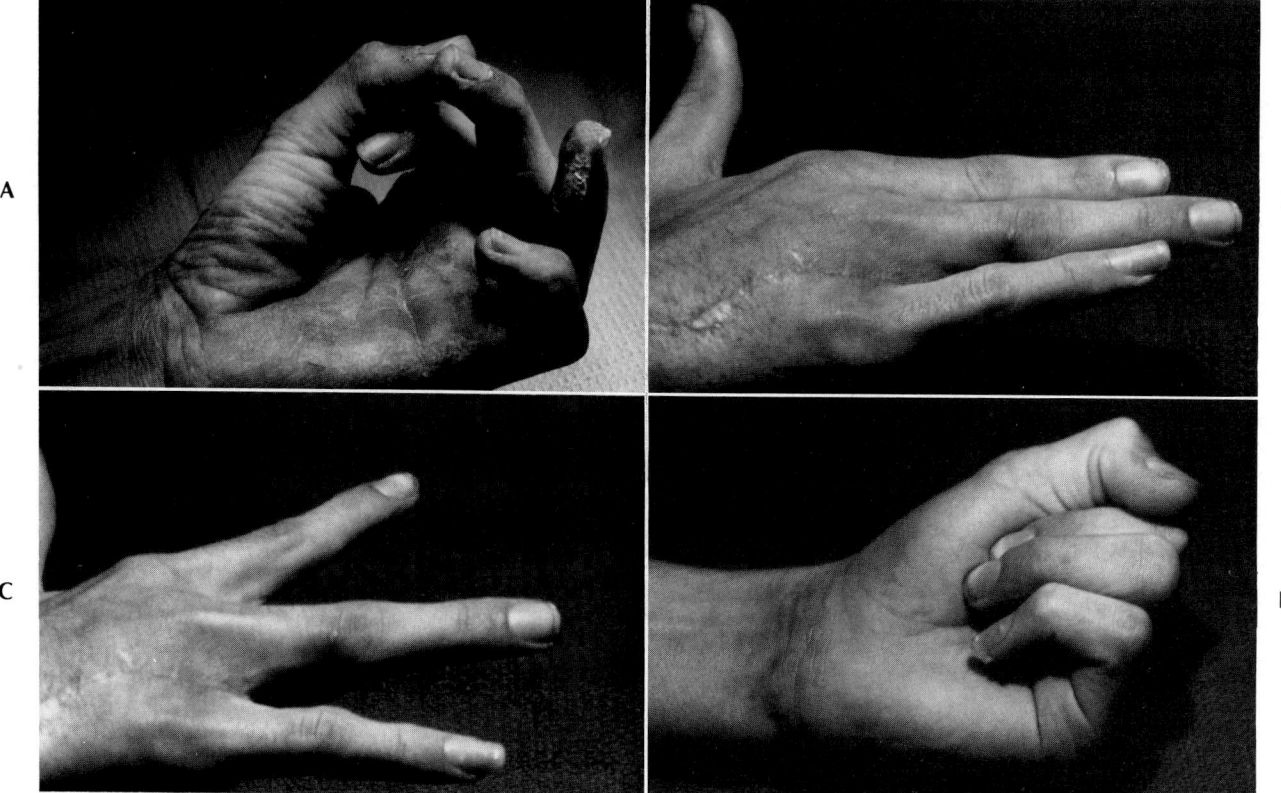

Fig. 15-14, A-D   This patient incurred a gun shot wound that fractured the metacarpophalangeal joint and proximal phalanx of the ring finger. Early on severe quadregia was noted as the patient attempted to close the hand. The ring finger was removed and a simple ray resection without osteotomy was performed. After 4 weeks the hand shows excellent function and cosmesis.

strength to this finger and will still relieve the quadregia effect.

When elective amputation of the long or ring finger in the management of a quadregia is discussed, thoughts of money, for example, falling through the fingers immediately come to mind. This hole, however, or defect in the palm exists only if there is loss of length at the level of the MP joint. Amputations at the midportion of the proximal phalanx do not create a gap within the palm. Whether to perform a ray resection or amputate through the proximal phalanx is definitely an elective operative decision, and before the patient decides, he should recover from his initial injury, gain maximum function, and live with the problem. Ray resection reduces the flexor strength in the hand but also narrows the surface over which that strength operates, and so there is a significant loss of power grip with a combination of flexor tendon loss and a narrow palm. The cosmesis and the general symmetry of the hand are markedly improved by ray resection and digital transposition. With the restoration of this symmetry, the amputation of a stiff finger becomes far less obvious. With damage to a ring finger and a desire for ray deletion, two surgical options are available. The ring metacarpal has no wrist extensor or flexor attached to its surface, and therefore a basilar disarticulation is possible. With removal of this ring finger metacarpal, the fifth metacarpal actually moves into the defect, and with removal of the intrinsic muscles and suture of the deep intermetacarpal ligament or deep intervolar plate ligament, the hand achieves an appropriate shape and configuration. Instability of the base of the fifth metacarpal is not a problem, and there is no requirement for the union of fracture, and no postoperative immobilization is necessary.

An alternative to the disarticulation just discussed is digital transfer by osteotomies of the base of the fourth and fifth metacarpal with removal of the ring finger ray distal to the osteotomy. The small ray with the entire small finger then is transferred to the base of the ring finger metacarpal. This osteotomy is then internally fixed. The advantages of this seem to be that the length of the small finger is increased so there is not a great disparity between small finger and long finger length cosmetically when the fingers are held in full extension.[40] Attempting to lengthen this small finger through the metacarpal, however, increases tension on the intrinsic muscles and impedes fracture union, which must occur. There is also the possibility of tendon adherence and nonunion.

With deletion of the long finger ray, there are also two surgical options. Simple basilar dislocation is not done because of the extensive insertion of the powerful extensor carpi radialis brevis muscle and also because this metacarpal is a central block for stability for the hand. An osteotomy can be created at the base of the long metacarpal and the long metacarpal with its remaning intrinsics and extrinsics is removed. The base remains stable with the wrist extensor attached. At this time, the index metacarpal may be osteotomized to its base and transferred with its intrinsic muscles to the base of the third metacarpal. The osteotomy may then be internally fixed with plate or K-wires. Here again, the same problem occurs with union of the fracture and adherence of the extensor mechanism. An alternative to this suggested by Steichen[46] is to determine whether the metacarpal heads of the index and ring, as they approach one another,

scissor, or cross over. If the gap is gone and scissoring is not present, strong repair of the deep intervolar plate ligament with heavy sutures can be performed. In addition, dermodesis by excision of tissue from the dorsum will reduce the problem with scissoring, or crossing over, of the fingers with MP joint flexion. The latter procedure, if it can be done, is far easier to rehabilitate and is cosmetically as appealing. The transfer of the index metacarpal to the long metacarpal is a classic method of managing this long finger metacarpal deletion, but at the time of the transfer, this index and long segment must be shortened because of the increasing tension on the dorsal interosseous muscle and because this muscle will become tight as the insertion is actually transferred ulnarward. Previous attempts with this osteotomy and inadequate fixation with K-wires have convinced me that rigid internal fixation with plates and screws is the method of choice. Certainly motion should be started early to avoid joint stiffness, and motion should be through full three-joint digital flexion.

Amputation of the index ray does not require transposition of the metacarpal or sophisticated bone surgery but does require patient evaluation and attention to detail. Neuroma is a problem here. This broad thumb index web space is prone to develop symptomatic neuroma, either from the radial sensory nerve or from the median nerve sensory branches in the palm. If one of the reasons for the amputation is a symptomatic neuroma, one must look at the problem differently. A stiff finger with painful neuromas can be kept out of harm's way, and remaining fingers can perform their function. If, however, these neuromas remain symptomatic after index ray deletion, they are now in the web space between thumb and long finger, and overall hand function will be compromised. Although the cosmesis of the hand may be much improved by deletion of the index ray, neuromas that are symptomatic in this web space may severely compromise the overall usefulness of the hand. These neuromas should be transferred into the adductor muscle substance or into the first dorsal interosseous muscle, but in some patients even this is unsatisfactory, and long-term problems without satisfactory long-term solutions may become obvious.[32]

In the small finger, proximal amputations to improve the cosmesis are probably not indicated. If a small portion of the proximal phalanx remains and has a voluntary control, it should not be amputated. Intrinsic muscles attach to the fifth metacarpal shaft throughout its entire length. These intrinsic muscles of the hypothenar area flex the CMC joint, which in many patients has 40 to 45 degrees of flexion. This cupping action of the hand is important; to voluntarily remove this for cosmesis is not indicated.

With multiple digital amputations, one again must think of basic hand function—not of restoring normal hand function. If the central fingers have been lost but portions or all of the peripheral digits remain, little surgery is required to restore basic hand function. A normal thumb will reach metacarpals for pinch activities, assuming that these metacarpals are covered with durable skin. If peripheral digits cannot reach one another, two possibilities exist. Either shorten the central metacarpals so that the peripherals can approach one another and then bring about some sort of prehension activities, lengthen or reposition the peripheral metacarpals. Lengthening techniques, as mentioned with

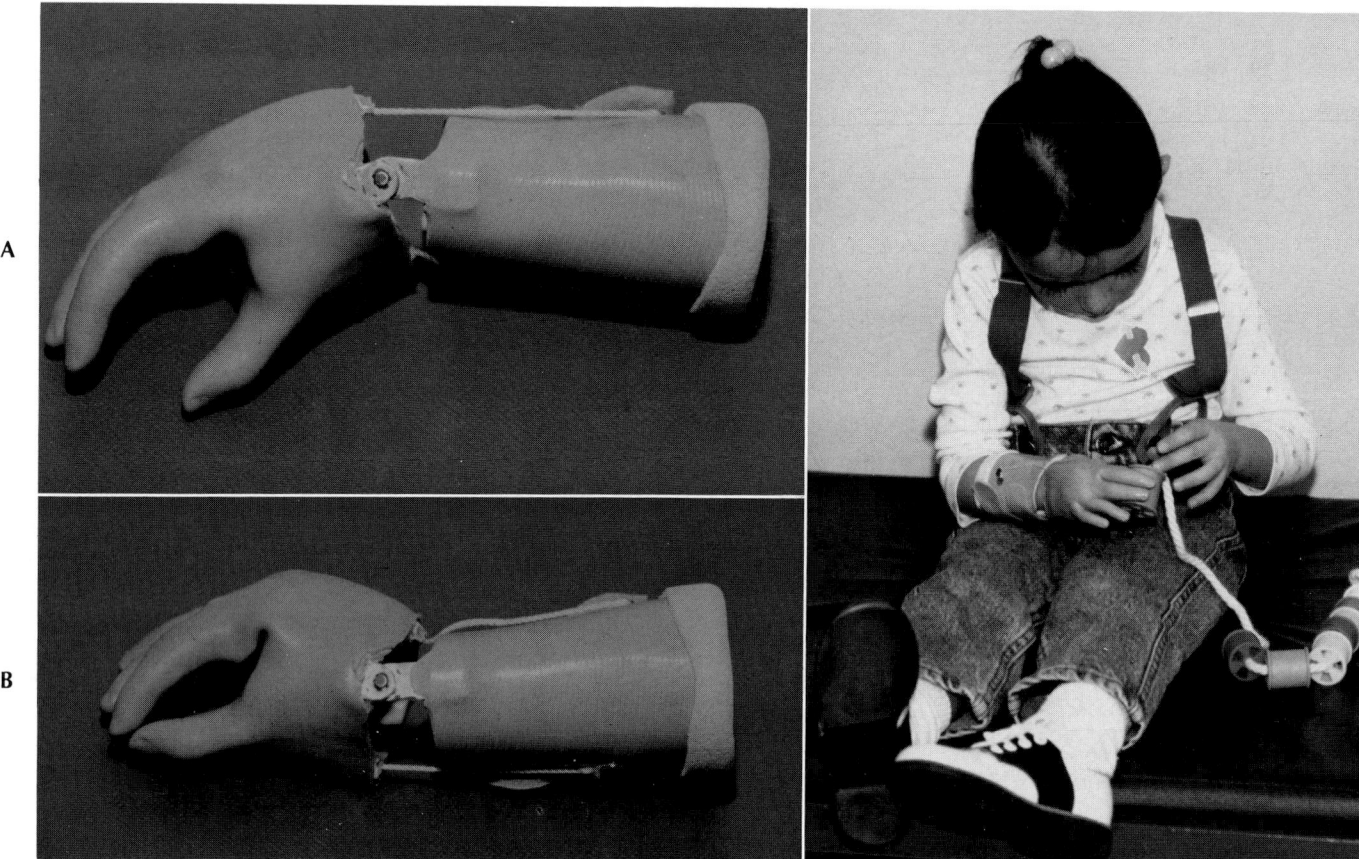

Fig. 15-15, A-C A wrist-driven flexor hinge hand. A functional wrist joint without satisfactory metacarpal length to allow any type of digital function may be a real frustration to a patient. However, adding a terminal device that is opened and closed by active flexion and extension of the wrist allows markedly improved hand function.

thumb reconstruction, are available as well as the transfer of portions of the central metacarpal. In the thumb, lengthening may occur by index ray deletion. However, in addition to merely excising the metacarpal, a portion of the index metacarpal bone may be transferred with a strip of volar skin containing metacarpal artery and palmar digital nerve. In this way the index can be used to lengthen the thumb and at the same time give greater space between the thumb and the remaining metacarpals.[28] In addition, the more peripheral part of the hand in the hypothenar area can be altered by rotation or flexion osteotomy of the fifth metacarpal.[36,53] This will allow the peripheral metacarpals to come together for some type of gross hand function.

With only metacarpals remaining in the hand, what can be done by microsurgery to increase function?[5] A toe transfer to each metacarpal can give length and improve strength and prehension. If the basilar joints are normal and there is remaining intrinsic function, function will be improved but probably not cosmesis. However, if cosmesis is a problem, a cosmetic prosthesis as mentioned before may be fitted. This prosthesis will allow the patient to better use the remaining metacarpal motion for active function. A third alternative is to disregard metacarpal motion and simply to fit the patient with a wrist-driven flexor hinge prosthesis. That is a terminal device driven by wrist motion[11] (Fig. 15-15). The cosmesis may be good and function would probably

be much better, but the decision is difficult both for patient and doctor.[3] There is no rush; it must be remembered that all surgery and prosthetic devices in this situation are elective. It might be best to try a prosthetic device and see what the patient thinks of its functional characteristics and cosmesis.

What is the role of prosthetics in mutilating injuries of the hand? The functional prosthesis or hook has been available since the 1940s. This has been a voluntary opening device with rubber bands of varying thickness used for closing. These are body powered, using a shoulder harness and flexion of the shoulder to open the prosthesis. In the below-elbow amputee of the younger patient, the acceptance rate was good; with the addition of immediate or early post-surgical fitting, the results seem actually to improve.[7] The myoelectric prosthesis has achieved enthusiasm in recent years, and the myoelectric mechanism has become free from mechanical and electric failures and is capable of function in a wider variety of areas than the body-powered prosthesis. For instance, opening a body-powered below-elbow prosthesis overhead is difficult. This is not a problem with a myoelectric prosthesis, which has both voluntary opening and closing. Within certain limits, more closing pressure can be exerted by the prosthetic wearer as he sends more myoelectric signals to the electric motor. To some extent there is an element of feedback in patients using the myo-

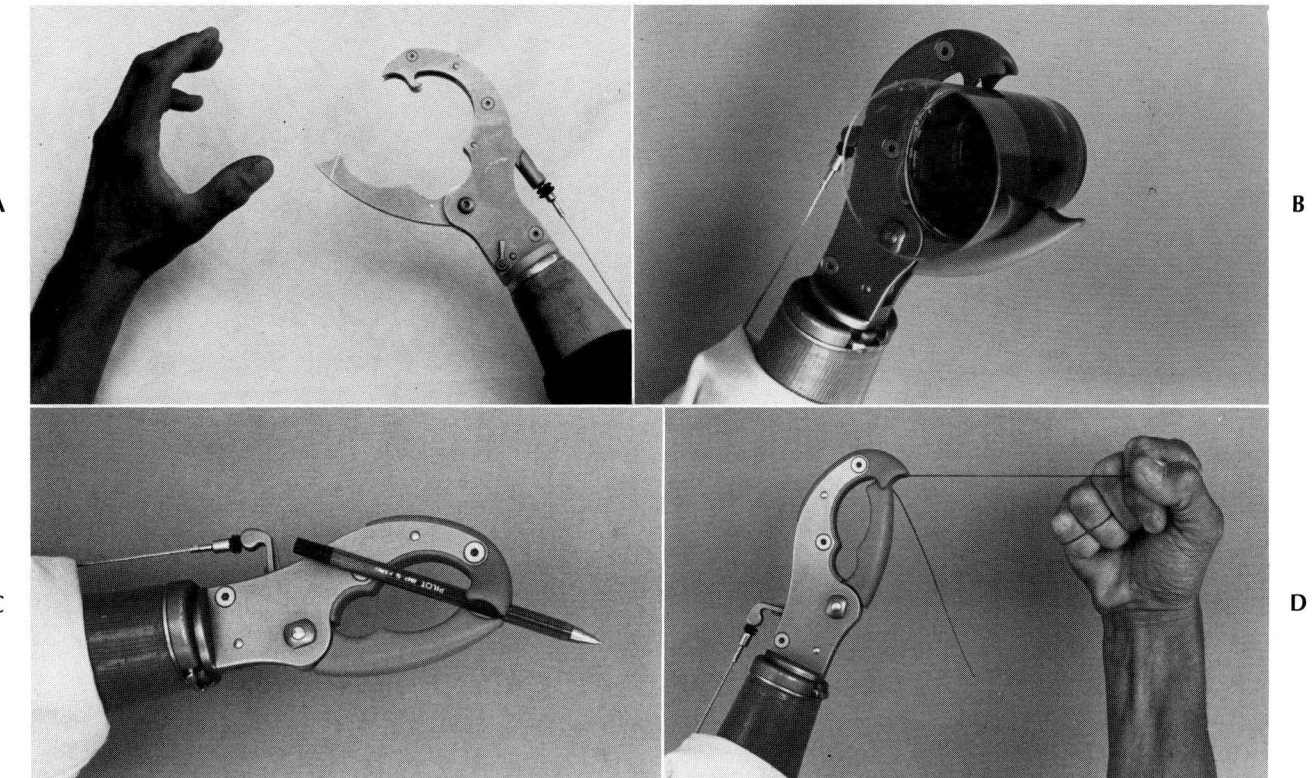

Fig. 15-16, A-D   A voluntary-closing prosthesis. The feedback the patient receives as a result of the voluntary-closing principle makes this the best body-powered prosthesis. Such feedback is not achieved with the conventional voluntary-opening hook.

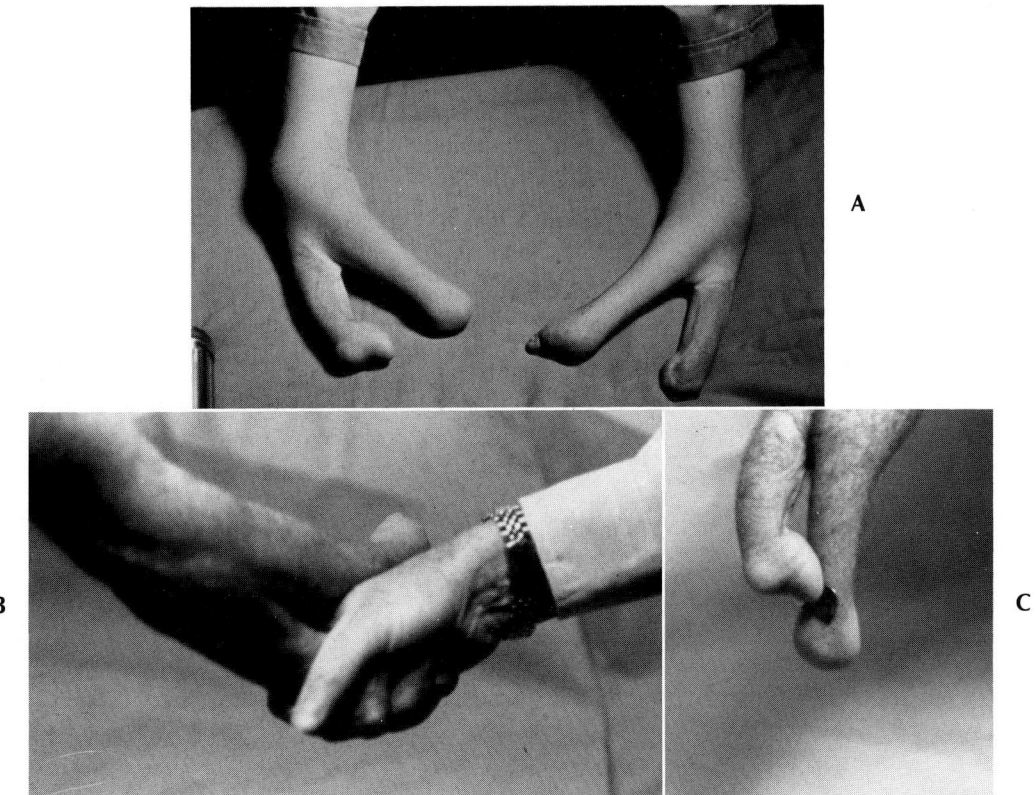

Fig. 15-17, A-C   A 7-year-old boy with a Krukenberg amputation done bilaterally 3 years before. A follow-up photo taken 18 years later shows continued power grip and excellent prehension in spite of the discrepancy in length between the radius and ulna. Maintenance of the small tissue tag adds immeasureably to the prehension of this Krukenberg stump.

electric prosthesis that is absent in the classic body-powered terminal device. More recently, Therapeutic Recreation Systems of Boulder, Colorado has developed a voluntary closing device similar to the World War II American Prosthetic Research Laboratory (APRL) hand, but one that can be used harder without failure (Fig. 15-16). Although the experience with fitting patients with this device is somewhat limited, the closing pressure can easily be adjusted by the patient so that he can use it in various prehension endeavors. In spite of the usefulness of the voluntary closing hook device, most amputees now seem to prefer the myoelectric hand, both functionally and cosmetically.

Discussion of upper extremity mutilations should include the Krukenberg procedure. Initially the Krukenberg procedure was indicated for blind, bilateral below-elbow amputees (Fig. 15-17). The procedure has been used, however, in children with absence of hands and has been widely used in certain countries for unilateral amputees with normal sight.[33,48,52] Although there has been much concern about the cosmesis of the stump, the amount of function that is possible in these patients is amazing. The Krukenberg stump functions by forearm rotation rather than by actual abduction and adduction of the radius and ulna. Therefore forearm rotation must be normal or close to normal for there to be adequate mobility of the phalangized radius and ulna. This stump can be fitted with a standard hook or hand prosthesis, either functional or cosmetic if required. I think there is little enthusiasm for the Krukenberg amputation in this country and that this is because of our lack of experience and understanding of the procedure and what really can be done functionally with the Krukenberg amputation in a well-trained individual.

CONCLUSIONS

Mutilating injuries of the upper extremity are highly individualized wounds that result in loss of various portions of the hand and affect the patient, both because of loss of function and because of altered cosmetic appreciation by the patient and those who see him. The usual modalities of wound care need to be addressed, but almost always, further surgery is needed to improve function or cosmesis or both. In this situation the patient's needs, desires, and expectations take precedence over the surgeon's enthusiasm for any particular operative procedure. Surgeons are usually devotees of a particular surgical technique and are constantly looking for patients who need this procedure. They must constantly think in terms of the needs of the patients rather than their needs as surgeons to manage a severely injured patient-hand relationship.

REFERENCES

1. Brown PW: The prevention of infection in open wounds, Clin Orthop 96:42, 1973.
2. Brown PW: The fate of exposed bone, Am J Surg 137:464, 1979.
3. Brown PW: Sacrifice of the unsatisfactory hand, J Hand Surg 4:417, 1979.
4. Brunner JM: Cornpicker injuries of the hand, Plast Reconstr Surg 21:306, 1958.
5. Burkhalter WE: Increasing finger flexion by tenotomy—the extensor digitorum communis over the proximal phalanx. Presented at the American Society for Surgery of the Hand, Atlanta, Feb 1984.
6. Burkhalter WE and others: Experience with delayed primary closure of war wounds of the hand in Vietnam, J Bone Joint Surg 50A:945, 1968.
7. Burkhalter WE, Mayfield G, and Carmona L: The upper extremity amputee early and immediate post-surgical fitting, J Bone Joint Surg 58A:46, 1976.
8. Butler B Jr: Initial management of hand wounds, Milit Med 134:1, 1969.
9. Caulkins M, Burkhalter WE, and Reyes F: Exposed bone grafts in the upper extremity. Presented at the AAOS, Las Vegas, Jan 1985.
10. DeMuth WE Jr and Smith JM: High velocity bullet wounds of muscle and bone: the basis of rational early treatment, J Trauma 6:744, 1966.
11. Dick T, Lamb D, and Douglas W: A wrist powered hand prosthesis, J Bone Joint Surg 66B:742, 1984.
12. Evans R and Burkhalter WE: A study of the dynamic anatomy of extensor tendons and implications for treatment, J Hand Surg 11A:774, 1986.
13. Fitzgerald R: Bacterial colonization of mutilating hand injuries and its treatment, J Hand Surg 2:85, 1977.
14. Freeland JM, Burkhalter WE, and Chavez A: Delayed primary bone grafting in the hand and wrist, J Hand Surg 9:22, 1984.
15. Gross A, Cutright DE, and Bhaskar SM: Effectiveness of pulsating water jet lavage in treatment of contaminated crushed wounds, Am J Surg 124:373, 1972.
16. Harkins PD and Rafferty JE: Digital transposition in the injured hand, J Bone Joint Surg 54A:1064, 1972.
17. Haury B and others: Débridement: an essential component of traumatic wound care, Am J Surg 135:238, 1978.
18. Heggers JP, Robson MC, and Ristroph JD: A rapid method of performing quantitative wound cultures, Milit Med 134:666, 1969.
19. Hentz V: Free dorsalis pedis flap with extensor tendons in hand reconstruction. Presented 2nd International Federation of Societies for Surgery of the Hand, Boston, 1984.
20. Jabaley ME and Peterson HD: Early treatment of war wounds of the hand and forearm in Vietnam, Ann Surg 177:163, 1973.
21. Kessler I, Hecht O, and Baruch A: Distraction lengthening of digitated rays in the management of the injured hand, J Bone Joint Surg 61A:83, 1979.
22. Kleinert HE and Williams DJ: Blast injuries of the hand, J Trauma 2:10, 1962.
23. Krizek TJ and Robson MC: Evolution of quantitative bacteriology in wound management, Am J Surg 130:579, 1975.
24. Lowry KF and Curtis GM: Delayed suture in the management of wounds: analysis of 721 traumatic wounds illustrating the influences of time interval in wound repair, Am J Surg 80:280, 1950.
25. Marshall KA and others: Quantitative microbiology: its application to hand injuries, Am J Surg 131:730, 1976.
26. Matev I: Thumb reconstruction through metacarpal bone lengthening, J Hand Surg 5:482, 1980.
27. May J and others: Thumb reconstruction in the burned hand by advancement pollicization of the second ray remnant. Presented at American Society for Surgery of Hand Annual Meeting, Anaheim, CA, March 1983.
28. Meyer V: Personal commmunications.
29. Michon J and others: Functional comparison between pollicization and toe transfer for thumb reconstruction. Presented at American Society for Surgery of the Hand Annual Meeting, Las Vegas, NV, Feb 1981.
30. Morgan LR and Stein F: Method for a rapid and good thumb reconstruction, Plast Reconstr Surg 5:131, 1972.
31. Morrison WA, O'Brien BM, and MacLeod AM: Thumb reconstruction with a free neurovascular wrap around flap from the big toe, J Hand Surg 5:575, 1980.
32. Murray J, Carman W, and MacKenzie J: Transmetacarpal amputation of the index finger: actual assessment of hand strength and complications, J Hand Surg 2:471, 1977.
33. Nathan PA and BuTrung N: The Krukenberg operation of modified technique avoiding skin grafts, J Hand Surg 2:127, 1977.
34. Neu B, Murray J, and MacKenzie J: Profundus tendon blockage in finger amputations. Presented at the Annual Meeting of the American Society for Surgery of the Hand, Atlanta, Feb 1984.
35. Omer GE Jr: The early management of gunshot wounds of the extremities, South Dakota J Med 9:340, 1956.
36. Onne L: Rotary angulatory osteology of the metacarpal bones of mutilated hands, Acta Chir Scand 108:268, 1954.
37. Paradies LH and Gregory CF: The early treatment of close range gunshot wounds to the extremities, J Bone Joint Surg 48A:425, 1966.
38. Partega B: Personal communication (Ersteoberartze Hand Chirugila Unit) 1984.
39. Peimer C, Smith R, and Leffert R: Distraction-fixation in the primary treatment of metacarpal bone loss, J Hand Surg 6:111, 1981.

40. Posner MA: Ray transposition for central digital loss, J Hand Surg 4:242, 1979.
41. Pillet J: Personal communications.
42. Reid DAC: The severely mutilated hand. In Reid DA and Gosset J, editors: Mutilating injuries of the hand, New York, 1979, Churchill Livingstone, Inc.
43. Reid DAC: Thumb reconstruction in the mutilated hand with special reference to pollicization. In Reid, DA and Gosset J, editors: Mutilating injuries of the hand, New York, 1979, Churchill Livingstone, Inc.
44. Robson MC and Heggers JP: Bacterial quantification, Milit Med 134:19, 1969.
45. Rodeheaver GT, Pettry D, and Thacker, JG: Wound cleansing by high pressure irrigation, Surg Gynecol Obstet 141:357, 1975.
46. Steichen J and Idler R: Results of central ray resection without bony transposition, J Hand Surg 11A:466, 1986.
47. Strickland JW: Thumb reconstruction. In Green DS, editor: Operative hand surgery, New York, 1982, Livingstone, Inc.
48. Swanson AB: The Krukenberg procedure in the juvenile amputee, J Bone Joint Surg 46A:1540, 1964.
49. Swanson AB: The treatment of war wounds of the hand, Clin Plast Surg 2:615, 1975.
50. Tajima T: Treatment of open crushing type of industrial injuries of the hand and forearm: degloving open circumferential, heat press and nail bed injuries, J Trauma 14:995, 1974.
51. Thoresby FP and Darlow HM: The mechanism of primary infection of bullet wounds, Br J Surg 54:359, 1967.
52. Tubiana R, Stack HG, and Hakistan RW: Restoration of prehension after severe mutilation of the hand, J Bone Joint Surg 48B:455, 1966.
53. Weckesser EC: Reconstruction of the grasping mechanism following extensive loss of digits, Clin Orthop 15:60, 1959.
54. Whelan TJ Jr, Burkhalter WE, and Gomez A: Management of war wounds. In Welch CE, editor: Advances in surgery, vol 3, Chicago, 1968, Year Book Medical Publishers, Inc.

16

Therapist's management of the mutilated hand

Karen M. Stewart

A mutilating injury encompasses multiple system trauma: skeletal, neurovascular, and many soft tissue structures may all be involved. The injury may include amputation, crush, laceration, and avulsion in a single extremity and so presents a problem in management. It is essential that patient, surgeon, and therapist work together closely to coordinate their efforts in this demanding course of treatment.

The goal of all hand rehabilitation is satisfaction of the patient's need for a hand that is functional and aesthetically acceptable. All our efforts are in vain if the patient does not use his hand. From a psychologic standpoint, we must recognize and address the patient's difficulties with con-

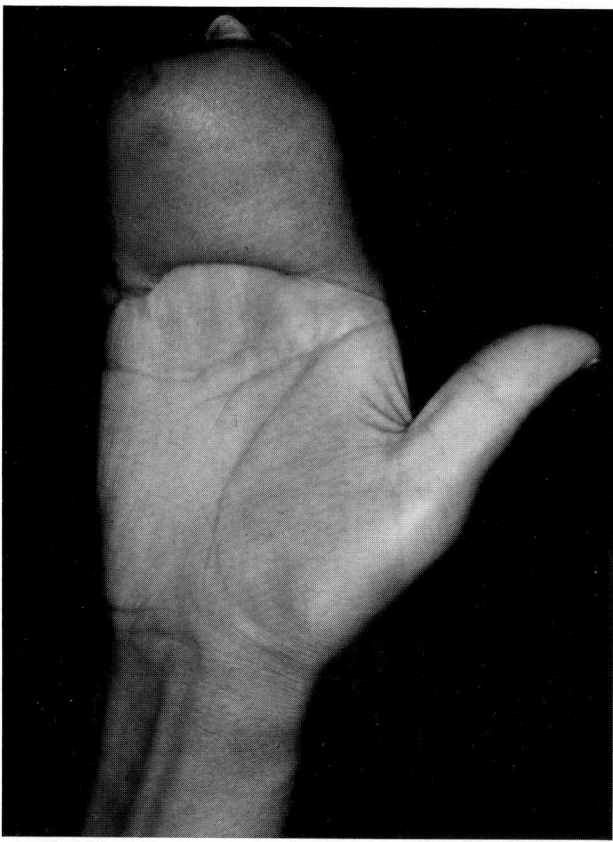

Fig. 16-1 Although skin coverage was accomplished in this degloved hand, the result was unattractive and nonfunctional because of excessive tissue bulk and syndactyly. The surgical plan was for delayed separation and defatting of each finger (three separate procedures), which ultimately produced a functional and cosmetically acceptable hand. Intensive therapy preceded and followed each surgical procedure.

fronting the injury and reintegrating the hand into normal use. From a physical standpoint, we must restore functional motion, strength, and sensibility to the hand. In both cases, we must control the formation and remodeling of scar tissue, which can render a hand both ugly and useless (Fig. 16-1).

Normal hand function requires strong tissue repairs with free gliding between neighboring structures. Uncontrolled scar will adhere tissues to one another, rendering them immobile, but insufficient scar formation at the repair site will not withstand the demands of normal hand use. Therefore management of the complex hand injury necessitates selective control of healing, ensuring stable, durable scar where strength is needed and long, mobile, elastic scar where motion is crucial between adjacent tissues.

The most difficult aspect of scar management in mutilating injuries is the coordination of treatment of the various systems and tissues injured. In addition to basic knowledge of hand anatomy, physiology, and kinesiology and a wide repertoire of therapeutic skills, the therapist must possess a thorough comprehension of the phases of normal and pathologic healing of each type of tissue injured and an understanding of the relationships among the various systems. The key to treating the mutilated hand is careful evaluation of the individual systems and a treatment plan based on logical analysis of the problems identified.

Toward that end, this chapter will first present an overview of wound healing and the appropriate focus of treatment in each of its phases. We will then consider the various tissues and special considerations for their treatment as dictated by such factors as anatomy, surgical-medical management, and mechanism of healing. This will be followed by a review of treatment modalities, giving more emphasis to those techniques not covered in other chapters of this book. We will then explore the early, intermediate, and late stages of rehabilitation, with guidelines for evaluation and treatment at each stage.

WOUND HEALING

Wound healing has been described in detail elsewhere in this volume, and the reader is advised to study the process carefully before proceeding further. In brief, however, all wounds, in whatever type of tissue, heal in the same manner. The time frame given here applies to uncomplicated soft tissue healing. Times vary from one tissue to another, and are never absolutely exact, because healing is a continuum, with the phases overlapping. In addition, mutilating injuries are characterized by untidy and extensive wounds, often contaminated or subject to other influences that considerably alter the timing of wound healing.

The *inflammatory phase* of healing begins within hours of trauma and continues for at least 3 days, though it may persist for days or weeks, especially in mutilating injuries. Local vasodilation permits the leakage of blood and plasma into the injured area, creating increased edema, heat, redness, and pain, the classic signs of inflammation. The edematous exudate contains leukocytes and macrophages, which remove bacteria and dead cells from the area. The superficial wound begins epithelialization from the margins inward, usually completely covering small, clean wounds within 3 days.

The phase of *fibroplasia*, or *collagen deposition*, begins at 3 to 4 days. New capillaries are laid down to supply nutrition to the area. By now wound contraction has begun to decrease significantly the size of the superficial wound, also exerting traction on surrounding tissue. Fibroblasts begin to outnumber other types of cell within the wound. They synthesize collagen at a rapid rate, filling in the wound. The tensile strength of the wound is very low at this stage, and excessive tension can rupture the fragile bonds.

Collagen fibers soon begin to outnumber fibroblasts. By the end of the third week or so, the collagen content of the wound stabilizes, as old collagen fibers are destroyed to make way for new. Collagen production continues to be very active for many months.

This brings us into the *scar maturation* or *remodeling phase*, when the dynamic turnover of collagen provides for differentiation of scar to accommodate to the tissue type and the stresses under which it is placed. This lasts from about 3 weeks until 6 months at its most active, with further remodeling continuing for at least a year at a reduced rate.

Initially, all tissues involved in a wound develop a single massive scar, with randomly oriented collagen fibers. In the remodeling phase, fibers reorient and scars assume some of the characteristics of the tissues being healed.

Stresses placed on healing tissues have been shown to increase scar strength.[1] It has also been noted that controlled stress and motion appear to encourage remodeling of scar tissue to selectively increase strength in some scars and decrease adherence between others.[3,6,7,8] However, it is not yet known how much stress is necessary and at exactly what time and manner it must be applied to any given type of scar tissue to produce a desired change.

During the *inflammatory phase*, our efforts are directed toward minimizing pain and edema and promoting uncomplicated wound healing. Any complications could exacerbate or prolong the inflammatory reaction and lead to increased scar formation. During the *fibroplasia phase*, we continue to minimize edema and avoid undue stress to the injured area, again preventing provocation of an inflammatory response. Depending on the nature of the injury and the tissues injured, we may begin some form of controlled stress to further decrease edema and increase or maintain joint and soft tissue mobility. During the *remodeling phase*, we gradually increase our focus on mobility, and as healing allows, begin strengthening, dexterity training, and other intervention aimed toward return to former activity.

It should be emphasized that although the phases are described as discrete entities, they overlap considerably and treatment should always take this into account. For example, although as fibroplasia begins we may initiate gentle controlled stress, we know that the inflammatory response may still be quite active. Careful evaluation of wound status helps us modify treatment accordingly.

INDIVIDUAL TISSUES
Skin and superficial soft tissue

Skin wounds heal relatively quickly, with a simple sutured wound tolerating mobilization within a few days. Sutures can be removed in 7 to 21 days, depending on the wound and the stresses to which it is subject. Flaps and grafts need more protection, the timing of which depends on the type of coverage. Areas left open and allowed to heal by secondary intention may take several weeks, depending on the size of the wound.

In most cases, it is better to leave dressings undisturbed for the first week to avoid trauma to healing tissues. Some surgeons prefer to change dressings themselves during this critical early phase.

Superficial scar management begins with early wound care, avoiding trauma that could prolong or exacerbate the inflammatory response and stimulate overproduction of scar. Scar adhesions between superficial and deep soft tissues can limit motion severely. This is particularly true of the dorsum of the hand, where the normal skin redundancy allows more mobility.

Blood vessels

Blood vessels require 2 weeks of protection. Generally this is provided by the immobilization necessary for protection of other tissues. Close attention should be paid to signs of arterial or venous insufficiency during this phase, and bandages should be nonconstrictive. Venous return can be assisted by elevation of the hand above heart level, which also assists lymphatic drainage and thus minimizes the compression placed on vessels by excessive edema. However, if arteries have been repaired, they should not be required to work too hard against gravity, and so elevation should be modified accordingly.

Nerves

Although the soft tissue healing at the wound site is similar to the healing of other tissues, peripheral nerve healing involves the very different process of axonal regeneration, which is described in Chapter 37. We judge our protection of nerve repairs according to the status of the suture site, where the usual phases of soft tissue healing apply, but we expect return of sensory or motor innervation to vary depending on the location of the injury.

A completely transected and repaired nerve requires 3 to 4 weeks of protection from stress. This stress includes anything that might increase scar formation. In any nerve repair exact end-to-end repair of the correct axons is impossible to ascertain, and a certain percentage of nerve function is therefore destined to be lost. Any scar formation could impede axonal regeneration and diminish the success of the repair. Causes of scar formation include direct compression on the nerve, positioning in excessive stretch, or intermittent stretch and compression through too early mobilization of the affected part. In addition, if the hand is immobilized so that the nerve heals in an excessively shortened position, later mobilization will stretch the nerve.

If the nerve is incompletely transected or is only contused, then little or no immobilization may be needed. If a nerve was avulsed, or a portion of the nerve was destroyed, leaving a gap, the nerve may be left unrepaired or may be grafted primarily or secondarily. In the first case, any insensate areas must be carefully protected. In the second case, the two suture sites must be protected appropriately.

In the case of motor nerve injury, treatment must take into account the functional imbalance produced by loss of specific muscle function. Such imbalance can lead to development of secondary deformity during the lag time required for nerve regeneration. In the case of sensory nerve injury, patients must be taught to protect insensate areas from injury.

Even if a nerve were perfectly repaired, with the two halves of each axon approximated precisely, axonal regeneration would take a long time (1 mm per day, following a 3 to 4 week latent period, according to Seddon[17]). The management of the peripheral nerve injury requires regular reevaluation of affected sensory and motor function, with adaptation of the treatment plan as needed. Because nerve regeneration is slow, this aspect of recovery can be neglected, to the great detriment of the patient.

Following an amputation or other injury in which a nerve is transected and left unrepaired, neuroma formation is the inevitable result. Neuromas can be asymptomatic, but in many cases they are quite painful. They should be addressed promptly to avoid functional limitations. In cases when neuroma formation is likely, hypersensitivity may be minimized or prevented by prompt initiation of desensitization and use of the affected hand.

An aspect often ignored in treatment of nerve injuries is preservation or restoration of nerve gliding through scar control. Gliding is just as important for nerves as for tendons and other soft tissues. An adherent nerve is subject to both compression and stretch, both of which may produce internal scar and impede transmission of nerve impulses.

Muscles and tendons

Much has been written and much is still unknown about the mechanism of tendon healing. There is controversy over the extent to which intrinsic and extrinsic mechanisms contribute to healing. Most authorities now say that both intrinsic and extrinsic mechanisms play a part, to a different extent in different cases.

In the inflammatory phase the repair site is very weak, relying on the sutures to maintain continuity. In the fibroplasia phase tensile strength increases steadily as collagen is laid down (although in the second week, the suture site grows weaker and must be treated with greater caution). As noted above, the quantity of collagen stabilizes by about 3 weeks. During the remodeling phase, destruction and replacement of collagen allows for differential reorientation of fibers. The parallel orientation of fibers within the tendon provides increased tensile strength, and the random orientation of peritendinous fibers produces long, gliding adhesions.

In general, repaired tendons have sufficient tensile strength to withstand gentle active motion at 3 to 4 weeks, and they can tolerate light resistance after another 2 to 3 weeks. However, these are *very general* guidelines; the specifics of each case should be carefully considered in timing the progression of treatment. A tendon with poor vascularity might be protected longer, as would a tendon that demonstrated excellent gliding, evidence of few tendon adhesions. A badly adherent tendon or a tendon at risk for heavy scarring should be mobilized earlier and more aggressively if early motion is not contraindicated by other factors.

An injury to the richly vascularized muscle belly or musculotendinous junction heals more quickly and easily. Adhesions at this level can be strong but are much less of a problem than are tendon adhesions, since less gliding is demanded between muscle belly and surrounding tissues than between tendon and peritendinous tissues.

Bone and articular structures

As with other tissues, there are three phases of bone healing. During the inflammatory phase a fracture hematoma is formed and cellular debris is cleared away. The next phase is the formation of a bulky bony callus, which bridges the gap between the ends of intact bone. Through osteogenesis the endosteum produces an internal callus and the periosteum an external callus. This callus, although joining fracture fragments, is not strong, forming what is known as a "clinical union," not sufficiently solid to be visible by x-ray films. Often motion of a healing bone is begun during this stage, because a clinically healed bone shows no motion at the site of fracture and *controlled* stress is therefore safe. In many cases, though, we must wait until radiographic healing can be seen, to assure stability in difficult fractures. This occurs during the remodeling phase, when true cortical and cancellous bone is formed and gradually increases in strength in response to longitudinal and shearing stresses.

Remodeling may begin within a month and continue for several years. The healing rate of fractures varies tremendously throughout the body. In the hand, a fracture may be considered clinically healed at as early as 2 to 5 weeks, or it may need several months of immobilization. The type of fracture and fracture fixation naturally also affect the course of treatment. For these reasons it is extremely important to discuss each case with the attending surgeon and consult the literature for specific information regarding any unusual fractures or fractures one has not encountered before.

Articular cartilage does not regenerate as bone does, but rather forms a fibrocartilage that tends to be less elastic than the original tissue. Ligaments present a different set of problems. In injured ligaments scar tissue contraction can limit considerably the available motion of a joint. In addition, in an edematous joint, collagen is deposited around ligaments and the scar thus formed can diminish the elasticity of uninjured ligaments and produce joint contractures. Therefore, whenever possible, the injured hand should not be immobilized for long periods with ligaments in a shortened position.

OVERVIEW OF TREATMENT TECHNIQUES
Patient education

After sustaining a mutilating injury, many patients are overwhelmed by the gravity of the situation. The recovery of function depends on psychological, as well as physical, recuperation, and patient education is crucial. From the very first visit patient education must be oriented toward both current status and future return to a normal way of life.

The complexity of the injury usually demands complex and time-consuming therapy. It is important to keep the home program as clear and simple as possible, so that the patient can and will follow through on his own. This means tailoring the program not only to the patient's physical needs but also to his psychosocial status. How complex a program can he understand? How much time does he have during the day? What are the other demands on his time? It is important to adapt the program as needed, beginning with a very simple program, adding items as the patient becomes ready, subtracting portions that are no longer necessary. The program must include frequent enough exercise but must not dominate the patient's life.

The home program must be written out, demonstrated to the patient, and discussed thoroughly. The patient should then read his program and demonstrate to the therapist a full understanding of all instruction. This should be repeated at each successive visit and with each addition or change to the program, until the therapist is satisfied that the patient is following through well at home.

The patient may be coming to therapy for months or years, with a series of surgical reconstructions and postoperative rehabilitation. Over time, some patients become dependent on coming to the hand center as a way of life. This dependence can be minimized or eliminated by careful patient education and early enlistment of family support. Referral to a psychologist or social worker may also be indicated.

Wound care

Careful wound care can minimize scar formation and thus result in a more cosmetically acceptable hand with greater mobility and function. Early wound care includes *very careful* conservative débridement, removing only dead tissues that come away easily. This can be accomplished either manually, using sterile forceps, scissors, and gauze, or with gentle whirlpools.

Whirlpools should be short (no more than 15 or 20 minutes) to minimize the time spent with the hand in a dependent position, because this could increase edema. Every 3 minutes the patient should raise the hand overhead and, if healing structures permit, make several strong fists to aid venous and lymphatic return and counteract the effects of dependent

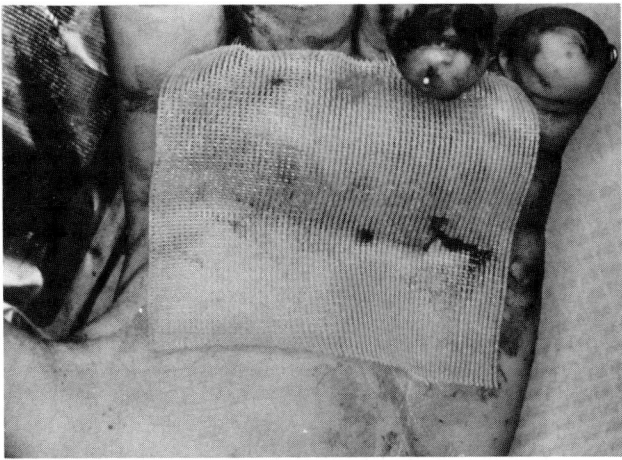

Fig. 16-2 Nonstick dressings prevent disturbance of healing open wounds. This piece of dressing, placed over a fragile skin flap, was then trimmed to size to avoid maceration of surrounding healthy skin.

positioning. While in the whirlpool, the hand should be kept moving gently. Walsh[20] found that elevation during whirlpool treatment had no significant effect on edema occurring after whirlpool treatment, and Schultz[16] found no significant difference produced by active motion. However, there is insufficient literature regarding the effect of combined elevation and active motion, which clinical experience validates as efficacious (see also Edema Reduction Techniques, p. 245). Studies have found that whirlpool temperatures significantly affect edema.[9,21] A temperature of 32° to 35° C is recommended.

Since research results so far have been equivocal concerning the effectiveness of bactericidal additives, whirlpools should be used with great caution in the care of open wounds to minimize the chances of infection.[15,18] Walsh recommends sodium hypochlorite 5.25% (household bleach) or a povidone-iodine solution prepared for whirlpool use, with a dilution of 1:120 to reduce the chances of tissue irritation or harmful vapors.[21] A useful precaution is rinsing the open area under running water after whirlpool, to remove any surface contaminants. The presence of sutures, exposed K-wires, or other hardware may be considered a contraindication, since these provide a route for infection to travel into the extremity.

Whirlpools may also be contraindicated in the early care of grafts and flaps, when it is, in fact, often better to leave dressings undisturbed if possible, to ensure graft or flap take. When whirlpools are used, they should be of short duration (5 minutes), agitation should be kept low, and the water should not be too cold, because this could produce vasoconstriction and ischemia.

Patients can perform saline soaks at home as an adjunct to whirlpool treatments, with the same precautions to keep the hand moving to control edema.

Dressings are a controversial topic. Although the simple sutured wound is best kept clean and dry, many open wounds may be best treated with moist, occlusive dressings. The practice varies from center to center. It is best to follow the practice of the referring surgeon.

Whether the wound is kept moist or dry, the basic principle is to keep it as clean as possible without undue stress to healing or newly healed areas. Forceful removal of an adherent dressing, for example, can inflict trauma to the tissues and prolong the inflammatory response. This is especially important with grafts and flaps. Graft "take" involves the establishment of new vascular supply to the graft, and this tenuous developing circulation is very easily disrupted. In addition, even after vascularity is established, the scar interface between graft and bed is weak in early stages. Therefore shearing force and pressure must be avoided until at least 2 weeks following grafting. There are several types of nonstick dressings on the market that can prevent adherence to grafts or open areas and also provide antibiotic protection (Fig. 16-2).

All gauze bandages should be nonconstrictive, wrapped in a figure eight from distal to proximal to minimize the chances of creating a tourniquet with a circular wrap. Revascularizations, flaps awaiting division, free flaps and composite tissue transfers, and replanted parts present a more difficult problem in dressing application, but in these cases it is doubly important to avoid all constriction during the early stages when vascularity is being established. Skin color and temperature must be carefully monitored for signs of ischemia or venous congestion after all microsurgical vascular procedures and any problems immediately reported to the attending surgeon.

Many patients with more simple wound care needs can perform dressing changes at home. If any external hardware is present, this provides a direct route for entrance of infection, and therefore all fixators should be cleaned one or two times a day by the patient, using clean cotton swabs. Each pin or wire should be cleaned first with hydrogen peroxide and the swab discarded. A second swab should be used to finish the cleaning with alcohol. Some surgeons prefer to follow cleaning with application of antibiotic ointment and/or a light dressing.

Patients should be instructed to monitor pin sites and all wounds for signs of infection: increased local redness or warmth, pain, or exudate. A fever may also be present. If the patient has any doubts, he should contact the therapist or doctor at once, and if the therapist identifies a possible infection, it should be reported immediately to the attending physician. A culture may be necessary to determine the appropriate antibiotic treatment.

Scar management

Deep transverse friction massage, crossing the grain of tightening connective tissue, helps to mobilize superficial scar by stretching its adhesions to underlying tissues. Heat applied before massage increases the elasticity of the tissues and thus increases the effectiveness of the massage (see also Heat and Cold, p. 247).

Continuous pressure over a bulky superficial scar flattens it and may make it softer, more elastic, and more cosmetically acceptable to the patient. This has been dramatically demonstrated in the clinic in the case of hypertrophic scar in burn patients.[10] While such clinical experience seems to support the use of pressure for scar control,[19] Peacock[14] questions its use. He considers it only temporarily effective and resulting as much from short-lived scar dehydration as from the mechanical effects of compression. Although research is hindered by the difficulty of reliably measuring scar bulk, adherence, and rigidity, further investigation is obviously needed.[4]

In the hand continuous pressure can be provided with elasticized gloves such as Jobst gloves,* by Coban elasticized paper bandage,† or, for firmer and more localized pressure, by the use of Elastomer,‡ prosthetic foam,§ or Spenco gel sheets or dermal pads.‖

Elastomer or prosthetic foam is mixed with a catalyst and spread onto the scar (Fig. 16-3). The mixture is then allowed to set, forming an exact mold of the scar and all the skin creases. Prosthetic foam is more rubbery and elastic in texture; Elastomer does not have air bubbles and is consequently less elastic. A combination of the two can be used to good effect for filling in larger spaces such as the palm, where the bulk of prosthetic foam combines with the better conforming properties of Elastomer. The pad is worn con-

*Jobst Co., Toledo.
†Coban, Medical Products Div., 3M, St. Paul.
‡Silicon Elastomer, Smith & Nephew Rolyan, Inc., Menomonee Falls, Wis.
§Q74290 Prosthetic Foam, Dow Corning Corp., Midland, Mich.
‖Spenco Medical Corp., Waco, Tex.

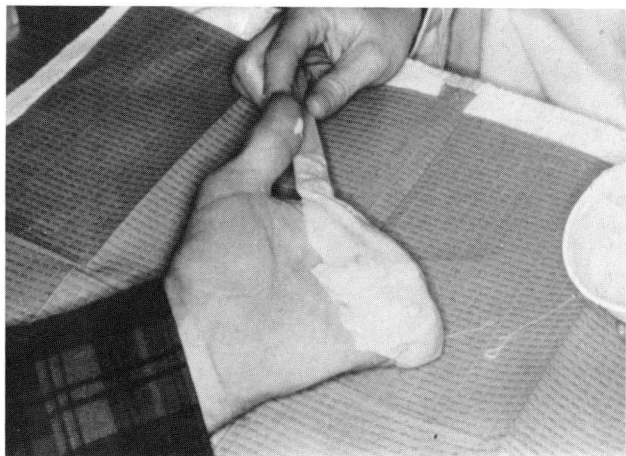

Fig. 16-3 After thoroughly mixing in the catalyst, Elastomer is spread over the scar, and all edges smoothed down for comfort. Once set, the pad can be trimmed with scissors if needed.

stantly if possible, for best results, and is held in place by a closely fitting splint or Coban wrapping. As the scar compresses over time, new molds must be made to accommodate to changes.

A scar in a normally mobile area such as the palm or crossing the wrist is not a good candidate for elastomer or prosthetic foam pressure, unless the pressure is applied under a splint that holds the part immobile. When the wrist flexes and extends or the hand is opened and closed, the scar moves and stretches and the mold is no longer exact. In this case, Spenco gel sheets or dermal pads (⅛ inch thick) are preferable. Although these do not conform as exactly to the shape of the scar, they do provide very close pressure that is flexible and adapts to motion of the scar.

All three materials or firm foam rubber can also be used to form a doughnut-shaped pad to protect a hypersensitive area by transferring pressure to the surrounding area. Many patients find relief also through constant gentle pressure to the hypersensitive area. Dermal pads or gel sheets are particularly helpful for this.

In the case of amputations, stump care is an important part of scar management. The stump must be massaged frequently to soften scars and prevent hypersensitivity caused by avoidance of contact (see also Desensitization and Sensory Reeducation, p. 245). "Dogears," or corners, must be softened and rounded, because they may be either hypersensitive or bulky enough to impede sensibility. Pressure can be provided, using Coban for stump wrapping, with some form of pressure pad if necessary for unusually bulky or malformed stumps. To wrap a stump, the Coban is first wrapped across the tip, then back across to completely cover the tip, and then in a figure eight fashion, wrapped from distal to proximal only as far as necessary to anchor the wrapping (Figs. 16-4 and 16-5).

In all wrapping and pressure pads for scar control and protection, a balance must be struck between scar management and overprotection. The patient must grow accustomed to using an amputated digit unprotected to fully desensitize it and use available sensibility. At some point, the constant

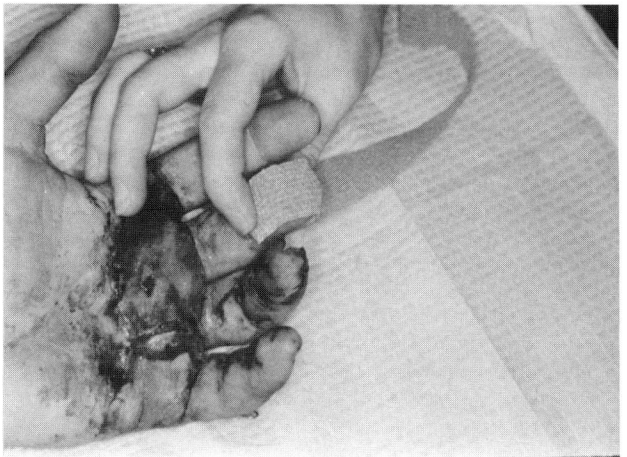

Fig. 16-4 Stump wrapping, step 1. Coban 1-inch bandage is placed across the tip of the stump to apply conforming pressure.

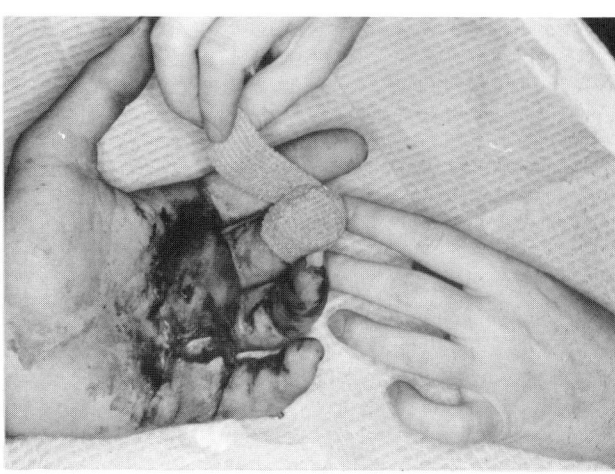

Fig. 16-5 Stump wrapping, step 2. Once the tip is completely covered, the stump is wrapped from distal to proximal only as far as necessary to secure the wrapping.

pressure necessary for effective scar remodeling must be abandoned to allow greater function.

Ultrasound is known to affect collagen cross-linking, when applied at sufficiently high levels, *above* therapeutic dosage levels. It is as yet unclear what nonthermal effects are produced by ultrasound applied to scar at therapeutic levels. This is discussed more thoroughly in Chapter 14.

Desensitization and sensory reeducation

Although commonly viewed separately, desensitization and sensory reeducation programs often blend together in practice. The topics are covered in Chapters 45 and 56. It is important to stress here, however, that most patients with mutilating injuries need some form of both programs.

Neuromas and hypersensitive scars are a common outcome of complex soft tissue injuries. Often a prophylactic desensitization program appears to forestall severe hypersensitivity.

Because sensory nerve return is extremely slow, it is easy to neglect sensory reeducation in a hand with many other needs. Yet all our efforts at gaining mobility will be wasted in a hand that is nonfunctional because of poor sensory return.

Edema reduction techniques

Edema reduction is crucial to minimizing scar formation and maximizing mobility. The edema produced during the inflammatory phase contains the fibroblasts that produce the collagen making up scar tissue. Wherever edema is present, scar tissue will be laid down, and the longer the edema is present, the harder it is to remove, as it becomes thicker with the continued formation of collagen. During the inflammatory and fibroplasia phases, edema can be described as "pitting." A fingertip pressed into the edematous area leaves a dent or pit that remains for at least several seconds. At this stage, edema is still easy to mobilize. Chronic edema, however, becomes "brawny," or fibrous, and is very difficult to mobilize.

In the traumatized hand, edema typically collects on the dorsum, where the skin is loose. Dorsal edema pulls the metacarpophalangeal (MP) joints into extension, which produces compensatory flexion at the proximal interphalangeal (PIP) joints and the wrist. Likewise, edema over the dorsum of the first web space pulls the thumb into adduction. This is the classic wounded hand position and can lead to severe joint contractures and functional limitations as edema becomes fibrotic.

Specific edema reduction techniques are discussed in greater depth in Chapter 13. The most important means of edema control is elevation of the hand above heart level, preferably with the whole extremity raised, hand above elbow and elbow above heart. The patient should avoid using a sling, because this rarely achieves acceptable elevation, and positions the shoulder in adduction, internal rotation, and flexion and the elbow in flexion, putting them at unnecessary risk for stiffness and pain. Elevation is particularly important at night, when the patient is not using or exercising the hand, and edema has a greater opportunity to pool in the hand.

Elevation may be *contraindicated* in certain cases. Following microsurgical procedures such as replantations, free flaps, or revascularizations, elevation above heart level may place too great a burden on the arterial anastomoses, resulting in ischemia. However, venous congestion may result from insufficient elevation. Therefore the position of the extremity should be carefully monitored. Elevation may also be contraindicated in the presence of infection not yet controlled by antibiotics. When in doubt, the therapist should always consult the attending surgeon.

In the inflammatory phase and early fibroplasia phase, cold may be useful for reduction of edema (see Heat and Cold, p. 247).

When healing structures develop sufficient strength, active and resistive exercise can be initiated for edema control. The intermittent compression produced by muscle contraction acts as a pump to assist the overburdened venous and lymphatic drainage systems. Elevation and active exercise can be combined in "pumping" exercises. Every waking hour the patient makes 5 or 10 strong fists with his hand raised as high overhead as possible.

Prehension activities can be performed with the hand in elevation, and many patients find this a pleasant and motivating means of combining lightly resistive exercise with elevation. Even lightly resistive tasks should be performed with caution, however, because the patient may very easily overdo such activities in the early stages, provoking a renewed inflammatory reaction and thereby increasing, rather than decreasing, edema.

External mechanical compression also aids edema reduction. This can include compressive wrapping or gloves, retrograde massage, or intermittent compression devices such as the Jobst or Flowtron* pumps. To use intermittent compression devices, the patient inserts his hand and arm in a sleeve attached to a pneumatic pump, which alternately inflates and deflates the sleeve, applying intermittent pressure to the entire extremity to expel excess interstitial fluid. Caution should be exercised when using these devices, which have the potential for overstressing healing structures. Pressure levels and inflation/deflation ratios should be carefully monitored and kept within the manufacturer's guidelines and the bounds of good clinical judgment. Generally, 55 mmHg is the pressure limit for the upper extremity, and the ratio of inflation to deflation time is 3:1.

For constant light compression the hand can be gently wrapped in Coban elasticized paper tape to reduce edema. The 1-inch wide bandage is wrapped from distal to proximal in a spiral or figure eight fashion, taking care not to stretch the tape, but rather to lay it on. This avoids a tourniquet effect, and when the wrap is initially applied, interstitial fluid is gently pushed proximally by the direction of wrapping. Such wrapping can be done only by a reliable patient, who will check carefully for any signs of wrapping too tightly (cyanosis, cold or numb fingertips). An alternative means of applying Coban is to use the 3 or 4 inch wide size to form a tube around the finger. A seam is formed on the back of the finger, trimmed to 1/2 inch wide, and laid flat. This is less bulky and easier to apply when all the fingers must be wrapped, but it does not have the advantages of the distal-to-proximal wrapping. Prefabricated finger sleeves are now available commercially, and these are a convenient alternative.

Because it is difficult to wrap an entire hand with even pressure, sometimes gloves may be a better alternative. There are several different types of prefabricated gloves available; if prefabricated gloves do not fit the patient because of edema or deformity, gloves can be custom-made by the Jobst Company. All gloves should leave fingertips exposed to allow the patient to monitor fingertip color, sensibility, and temperature.

Ideally, gloves or compressive bandages should be worn continuously day and night. They should be removed once a day for careful hygiene, and the patient should have spare gloves or bandages so that they can be changed periodically. If gloves or bandages interfere with hand mobility, they should be removed for exercise or perhaps worn only at night.

As with all parts of the home program, the patient should demonstrate to the therapist that he understands precautions and can apply and remove gloves or dressings correctly. The patient *should not wear* compressive gloves or wrappings if he does not appear able to follow these instructions. It has been shown that even with careful application by an experienced therapist, pressure gradation is greatly affected by the amount of overlapping, the number of layers, and any joint motion occurring while pressure bandages are worn. Injudicious use can result in obstruction of capillary flow.[2]

A temporary form of compressive wrapping is string wrapping, described in Chapter 13, which should always be followed by retrograde massage and fistmaking. Flowers[5] found that massage and string wrapping were equally effective in reducing edema, but a combination of the two was more effective than either technique used alone.

Retrograde massage should be performed at least once a day for 5 minutes, preferably before exercises. It is more effective for mobile or "pitting" edema than for chronic, fibrous edema. Deep, firm, long strokes milk the excess interstitial fluid from distal to proximal.

Active range of motion

Active exercise not only decreases overall stiffness and edema but also preserves or increases gliding between tendons, nerves, and other soft tissue structures that would otherwise become entrapped in scar. The patient should exercise not only the injured hand but also the entire upper extremity, to prevent stiffness and weakness caused by disuse and protective positioning. Whole body conditioning completes the program: following an injury that disrupts the normal pattern of life, patients invariably become less active and less physically fit, and this has profound effects on their emotional outlooks, as well as on their general health.

Exercises should be simple and comprehensive, moving all necessary structures. As far as possible, different motions should be combined into one exercise.

Blocking exercises involve stabilizing of the finger proximal to the joint being exercised, thus isolating motion to that joint. This promotes gliding of specific tendons and increases the range of motion (ROM) available at the isolated joint by exerting active force on tight soft tissue structures. For example, isolated distal interphalangeal (DIP) joint flexion requires differential gliding of the flexor digitorum profundus tendon, while stretching tight oblique retinacular ligaments and extensor tendons.

Among the digits, the thumb accounts for the greatest percentage of function in the normal hand. If the fingers are severely injured, the thumb carries an even greater burden, so maximum thumb motion is critical. The functional value of the thumb is a result of its mobility in several planes; this mobility must therefore be maintained or attained through exercises in all planes of motion.

Functional electrical muscle stimulation may be used as an adjunct to active exercise. It can serve to reinforce a weak muscle contraction or provide a "rhythm" to exercise. Biofeedback can also aid in active and resistive exercise by encouraging a patient to use a stronger muscle contraction or to relax the antagonist muscles when cocontraction is a problem.

When initiating active motion, the healing of *all* affected tissues should be considered. Just because the tendon is ready for active motion does not mean the coexisting fracture

---

*Flowtron, Huntleigh Technology, Aberdeen, NJ.

is sufficiently stable; we may want to get those adherent flexor tendons gliding but need to protect a fragile extensor tendon repair.

Passive range of motion

Joints are passively ranged very gently at first, and later with greater firmness, to stretch tightening soft tissues and thus increase available motion. Gentle traction should be applied to distract joint surfaces before moving the joint passively. This prevents compressive or shearing forces to the joint surfaces. More aggressive joint mobilization should not be performed without specific training in this skill.

The status of all healing tissues must be considered when performing passive range of motion (PROM): for example, passive finger flexion stretches the dorsal apparatus and joint structures, so extensor tendon healing must be sufficiently advanced to allow any such stretch. As a precautionary measure, adjacent joints can be held in extension during passive flexion (for example, MP and DIP extension during PIP flexion).

Heat and cold

Heat modalities can be effectively used as adjuncts to passive and active range of motion, either in combination with or preceding mobilization. Superficial heat agents used in the hand may actually increase temperatures of deeper structures, including joints, if applied at sufficiently high temperatures and for sufficiently long periods (20 minutes or more). This is because of the relatively thin layers of insulating adipose tissue in the hand. Superficial heat agents include paraffin, heat packs, hydrotherapy, and fluidotherapy. Deeper heat is provided by ultrasound, which is discussed in Chapter 14. All heat and cold should be applied with caution in the hand with sensory nerve or vascular injury.

Local superficial heat application produces vasodilation and increased blood flow, which improves nutrition and may aid healing after the acute inflammatory phase of healing is completed. However, heat may increase acute inflammation and so must be used with great caution. At any phase it may increase edema and so must be applied with the hand in elevation if edema is a current concern. Cold, on the other hand, may aid in control of edema and acute inflammation.

Although the actual mechanism is not known, heat and cold both relieve pain, with some patients being more amenable to one than to the other. Therefore it is often helpful to apply heat or cold before potentially painful treatments such as motion of stiff joints.

In addition to minimizing pain associated with passive stretch, heat augments the effectiveness of stretch in attaining plastic deformation of connective tissues. It is unclear how heat assists stretch, but the phenomenon has been well demonstrated both clinically and through in vivo and in vitro study. Zarro,[22] Newton,[13] and Michlovitz[11,12] have provided excellent surveys of the current literature regarding the effects of heat and cold on pain, edema, and other responses to injury.

Splinting

Static splints are used for rest and support, for protection, and to position for prevention of deformity. If possible, a resting splint in the early stages should position the wrist in 10 to 20 degrees of extension, with 70 to 80 degrees of MP flexion, from 0 to 15 degrees of IP flexion, and thumb palmar abduction. This position counteracts the typical joint contractures of the mutilated hand, which produce a deformity of PIP flexion, MP extension, thumb adduction, and wrist flexion. All injured structures must be taken into account and the splint design modified accordingly. For example, an extensor digitorum communis injury would demand greater extension of both wrist and MP joints, whereas a coexisting MP collateral ligament injury would need extra protection against lateral stress and carefully determined MP flexion to prevent ligament healing in a shortened position.

Early postoperative splints should be wrapped with elastic wrap or bias-cut bandage, wrapping distally to proximally in a figure eight fashion, to avoid the tourniquet effect of constrictive circular straps or bandages. Splints and straps should also be cut and modified to protect external hardware.

Passive stretch is most effective when applied with low intensity over a long period. Connective tissue is viscoelastic. This means that not only does it include elastic elements, which will stretch and then return to the original length, but it also includes viscous elements, which respond to stretch with plastic (permanent) deformation. Prolonged low intensity stretch produces plastic change in the form of increased length.

Serial-static and dynamic splints are the best means available for providing prolonged low intensity stretch. Serial-

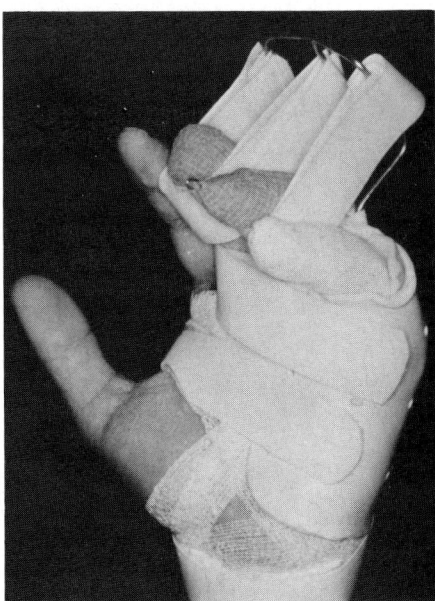

Fig. 16-6   This splint allows active motion of the fifth digit interphalangeal joints, while protecting a newly healed fifth metacarpal head fracture by immobilizing the metacarpophalangeal joint. At the same time, serially adjusted, low-intensity static pull is exerted on the middle phalanges of the third and fourth digits, to increase extension at the proximal interphalangeal joints. Note that a Kirschner wire immobilizes the fourth digit distal interphalangeal (DIP) joint. The strap is therefore carefully positioned at the DIP joint level, rather than distal or proximal to the joint, to protect joint immobilization. The third digit is amputated at the DIP joint.

static splints are static splints that are periodically adjusted or refabricated to accommodate for increases in available motion. Examples are periodically remade web stretchers and cylinder casts and serially adjusted flexion gloves. Fig. 16-6 illustrates a splint that combines protective static splinting with serially adjusted static positioning to increase joint motion.

No dynamic or serially adjusted splint should be used unless healing structures are clearly strong enough to withstand such stress, however gentle. It is vital that patients understand precisely how to apply and remove splints, how long to wear them, and how to check for signs of incorrect fit or pressure problems. This is particularly important in the insensate hand.

Prosthetics

Although it is beyond the scope of this chapter to discuss prosthetics, it should be noted here that prosthetic planning and training begin very early. In the mutilated hand there is often a need for a partial hand prosthesis, replacing the thumb in a partial radial hand amputation, or replacing the fingers in an ulnar amputation. Using splinting materials, the therapist can fabricate prototypes for prostheses to be fabricated later after the design has been refined and functional limitations delineated. If there is a need for a functional aesthetic prosthesis (see Chapter 82), planning may begin early, since the condition of the stump is vital to prosthesis fit.

Muscle strengthening

Effective strengthening exercise must involve resistance that elicits the strongest muscle contraction that can safely be demanded. As strength increases over time, resistance likewise must be increased as tolerated. Pain, edema, and strength must be carefully monitored to help determine the appropriate amount of resistance in a given session. If edema increases notably following exercise, for example, resistance should not be increased in the next session, and the exercise or activity must be modified to incorporate elevation.

Purposeful activity

In the use of activities for dexterity training, job simulation, and other purposes, care must be taken to avoid overwork. Endurance must be increased slowly to meet the demands of daily life.

With job simulation we can observe the patient performing work activities and design any necessary tool or task adaptations. The patient spends increasing amounts of time in therapy to improve his endurance and prepare him for return to the rigors of a full work day. Not only will he be physically prepared for his usual work, but he will also have demonstrated to himself that he is able to do so.

PHASES OF TREATMENT
Early

This stage of treatment includes the early inflammatory phase of wound healing. It is also applicable to a short period of preparation of a wound for soft tissue coverage or other early reconstructive procedures. The emphasis of treatment is on minimizing edema and either promoting uncomplicated wound healing or cleansing the wound in preparation for further procedures. At the same time, as far as possible, range of motion is maintained.

In the first treatment session the focus is on helping the patient understand the injury, fabricating any necessary splints, and introducing a simple home program. This session is usually very tiring and confusing for the patient and so should be kept short. Evaluation may be brief and subjective, with more detailed measurement in successive sessions.

Before seeing the patient the therapist should gather as much information as possible from the surgeon, including operative reports, precautions, and a look at the x-ray films. Specific advice should be sought about any unusual aspects such as special dressings or unfamiliar surgical procedures. The therapist should know exactly what structures should be immobilized or protected and in what positions, and the purpose of any splints or specific treatments requested by the surgeon.

Evaluation. In a mutilated hand there are many injuries, necessitating a comprehensive evaluation. A thorough medical, occupational, and psychosocial history should be taken so that all factors are considered in planning treatment. It may be helpful to take photographs or draw diagrams of the hand, including wounds, incisions, hardware, and amputations, and indicating insensate areas or other special problems.

The wound is evaluated for width, length, depth, and characteristics such as granulation tissue, bleeding, contaminants, or exposed vital tissues. The therapist notes the presence of sutures or external fixators and signs of infection such as foul odor, thick exudate, or erythematous, warm skin surrounding the wound.

Edema is evaluated by circumferential measurement rather than volumeter, since in the presence of open wounds the hand should not be immersed in water except for any sterile whirlpools or soaks necessary for débridement. Edema should be monitored at the same point in each treatment session, preferably before treatment. Later it will be helpful to measure hand volume both before and after any intervention that may increase edema.

Range of motion is evaluated within any limits imposed by immobilization. Uninvolved joints should not be neglected, especially the shoulder and elbow if a sling has been worn. Passive range of motion should always be evaluated with great care at this early stage, especially in an insensate hand.

Sensory status should be ascertained as far as possible. It is better to delay a full objective sensory assessment until wounds are better healed and edema has subsided, because both pain and edema can interfere with evaluation and it is unlikely that there will be a great change in sensory status in the first week or so. Nonetheless, a good subjective evaluation is essential, along with brief objective evaluation to alert the therapist to any insensate areas needing protection or any paresthesias or other signs of nerve compression. Such signs may indicate either the need for surgical decompression of a nerve or problems with bandaging, casting, or splinting.

Pain should be evaluated: Is there constant pain, or pain only with motion? Is it sharp or dull? Is it relieved by elevation of the hand?

An evaluation of activities of daily living should begin

now, as the patient first encounters problems with using only one hand.

Treatment. Patient education is the most pervasive element of early treatment. During the entire session, the therapist should explain and demonstrate, listen to the patient's questions and anxieties, and use every opportunity to set an example for home therapy.

The patient must learn the difference between normal posttraumatic pain and discomfort and the sharp pain with motion that indicates excessive force. He must learn not to be afraid of dull pain and the feeling of mild stretch that accompanies early motion, but he must also realize that sharp or persistent pain is a danger sign.

He must key in to the signs of fatigue and overwork and also be aware that he cannot always rely on his body to tell him when he is overworking. Often too many repetitions of an apparently innocuous and easy exercise produce great discomfort 1 or 2 days later. On the other hand, too few repetitions or sessions and halfhearted muscle contractions prolong stiffness. If the patient learns now to follow his home program exactly, without adding or subtracting, he will lay the foundations for a smooth recovery.

Because the patient has a lot of new information to take in and is under the stress of pain and fatigue, his home program should be simple to begin with. It is a good idea to add a new element to the program every session or so, giving the patient time to integrate each part in turn.

If the patient has a severe pain problem, the physician should be consulted to ascertain the cause of the pain and any possible intervention. Pain medication makes many patients drowsy and poses the risks of dependence and masking of pain that is useful as a danger sign. A transcutaneal electrical nerve stimulation (TENS) unit may be a more appropriate means of pain control, but even here there is a risk of psychological dependence. Pain is always a difficult issue, because we must strike a balance between acceptable pain and pain that interferes with a patient's physical performance and emotional well-being.

If the hand is insensate, there may be no pain even with excessive pressure or motion. The patient must be taught to avoid overzealous pursuit of the home program and thus prevent inadvertent damage to the hand.

Wound care includes whirlpools *if necessary* for débridement or cleansing of the wound, conservative manual débridement, and dressings, as well as pin care and monitoring of the wounds for signs of infection or unusual inflammatory response.

Edema control at this stage concentrates on elevation and active motion. If vessels were reconstructed, consult the referring surgeon about limiting elevation to heart level to avoid overburdening fragile structures. Retrograde massage is restricted to areas where there are no open wounds and where massage will not disturb adjacent healing. Compressive wrapping may be contraindicated because of grafts, flaps, or unusually unstable structures. In the presence of active infection, elevation above heart level, compressive wrapping, and retrograde massage are all contraindicated to avoid spreading the infection proximally.

At this stage we stress active over passive motion, although both are done. Active motion tends to be gentler to healing structures, so passive exercise is restricted to those motions that are actively weak and that must be performed to avoid stiffness and eventual deformity. Both active and passive exercises are performed only as allowed by all applicable precautions, to protect injured structures.

To reduce edema, strong fisting is always a part of the program *when not contraindicated,* and exercise should be performed with the hand in elevation. Exercises concentrate on preserving gliding of soft tissues and motion of all joints, especially in those areas where the nature of injury indicates there will be the greatest problems. This generally includes MP flexion, PIP extension, wrist extension, and thumb palmar abduction, all of which are commonly limited following mutilating injuries with notable edema.

Uninvolved joints should also be ranged to prevent problems caused by disuse. Exercise sessions should be short and frequent, maintaining mobility, but avoiding fatigue: three to five repetitions, every 1 or 2 hours.

Splinting will vary according to the individual injury, but generally it will be limited to static splinting to immobilize, rest, and support affected joints. Dynamic splinting for protected early passive mobilization of tendons may also be initiated. If splints are fabricated during the patient's first visit, other treatment and evaluation should be kept to a minimum to keep the session short. It is helpful to perform any range-of-motion exercises before splint fabrication, to decrease stiffness before positioning the hand for splinting.

All patients benefit from discussion of problems they encounter in activities of daily living (ADL). Some will need adaptive equipment; others use adaptive techniques. The discussion itself is helpful because it focuses the patient's attention on how he can and will get on with his normal life.

Intermediate

This phase begins at the start of fibroplasia (3 to 4 days after injury) and continues through the end of the third week, by which time collagen content is at its peak. As the inflammatory response ends, we are able to treat somewhat more aggressively, focusing not only on continued wound healing, but also on scar management and increasing motion. It must be borne in mind, however, that tensile strength of healing wounds is still very low, and there is always the danger of provoking a renewed inflammatory response through excessive stress and resultant microscopic trauma.

Evaluation. We continue to monitor pain, wounds, and edema, particularly noting changes in response to changes in treatment. Range of motion is monitored with special attention to any developing joint contractures.

A full sensory evaluation can be performed for the first time in this period, if indicated. Splints are checked closely for pressure problems and for changes in fit as edema decreases and dressings are debulked. Each splint should also be reevaluated regularly to determine whether it still serves the patient well. Are the splint's goals still valid for this patient?

The therapist should frequently reevaluate the patient's comprehension and performance of the home program, along with any progress or problems with ADL.

Treatment. Sutures will be removed in this period, and as wounds heal, transverse friction massage should be instituted for all scars, along with more extensive retrograde massage. Massage is gentle at first, to avoid inflicting microscopic trauma, but over time deeper pressure should be

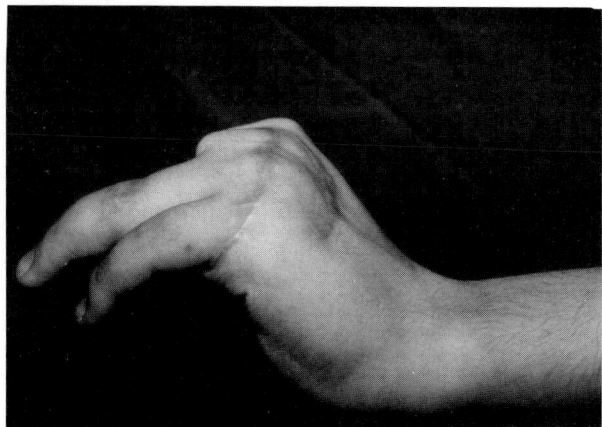

Fig. 16-7 In this child with revascularized ring and small fingers, active flexion could be limited by any of a number of factors. Joint stiffness or ankylosis and flexor or extensor tendon adhesions are the most likely causes.

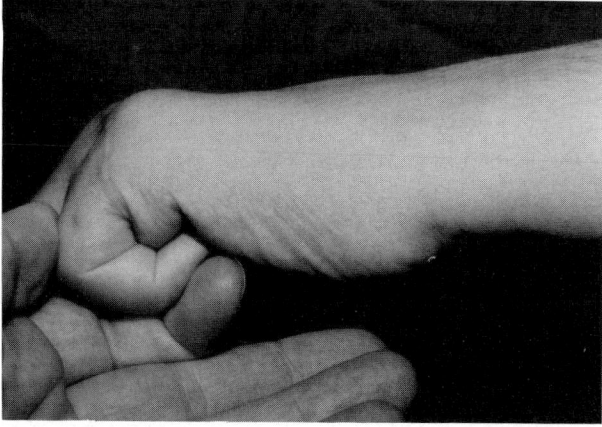

Fig. 16-8 Passive flexion of the small finger is complete, indicating that flexor tendon adhesions are the major culprit limiting active flexion of this finger.

applied. Massage serves also for relaxation before exercise, for desensitization, and as a time for building patient-therapist rapport. A formal desensitization program may also begin.

If not contraindicated (for example, in grafts, before 2 weeks), compressive wrapping may be initiated now, along with use of compression pumps. Elastomer or other pressure pads should be fabricated as early as possible, to influence collagen formation in its early stages.

If there are no contraindications and there is sufficient active motion, the patient may now begin light prehension tasks such as macrame, performed in elevation, to control edema and begin functional hand use. Passive range of motion is added to the program as passive limitations become apparent. These are also addressed through splinting.

The hand is still elevated when not active, but the need to elevate the hand or to wear splints or compressive wrappings should not interfere unduly with opportunities for active hand use. Problems will arise as the patient attempts to resume activities for the first time, and the therapist must promptly address these problems through adaptive techniques and equipment.

Late

This stage corresponds roughly with the scar maturation or remodeling phase of wound healing. From 3 weeks until discharge, therapy focuses on scar remodeling at all levels: to strengthen repairs, to facilitate gliding of soft tissues, and to improve function and cosmesis. For some patients this may be an intermediate stage of preparation for further reconstructive surgery, but our ultimate goal is always the same: return to former vocational or avocational activities.

Evaluation. Until all wounds are healed we are alert to any signs of infection. We continue to monitor changes in edema in response to treatment.

Regular evaluation of superficial scar and deep adhesions will reveal the relative success of scar management techniques and dictate changes in approach. In the mutilated hand it is especially important to understand the etiology of any problems. For example, a deficit in digit extension could

be caused by any of the following: adherence or shortening of long flexor tendons; secondary joint contractures; adherence, stretch, denervation, weakness, or rupture of long extensor tendons; denervation of the intrinsics; or pain. There could also be a combination of several problems. If we do not identify precisely the source of the limitation, we cannot effectively plan our treatment (Figs. 16-7 and 16-8).

Beginning about 1½ to 2 months after injury, sensory evaluation may reveal nerve regeneration. Monthly re-evaluation reveals not only regeneration, but also the results of sensory reeducation. Progress of desensitization and sensory reeducation programs must be closely monitored, because they require great dedication on the part of the patient.

As we begin to address muscle strength, endurance, and dexterity, periodic evaluation helps quantify progress and pinpoint problems. Towards the end of therapy, a physical capacity evaluation, possibly coupled with an on-site job evaluation, helps determine the patient's readiness to return to work and dictate changes in discharge planning (see Chapter 7).

Treatment. Scar management becomes more aggressive in this phase. It is particularly important to use evaluation results to identify problems and adapt treatment accordingly. Especially bulky or adherent scars should receive longer and firmer massages, as well as continued application of pressure pads. As edema becomes less of a problem, heat modalities come into their own, as an adjunct to active and passive exercise and soft tissue mobilization.

Active and passive range-of-motion limitations become harder and harder to deal with in this phase, if not treated promptly. This may be the first time we can move some structures, and since this initial motion is occurring when collagen content is high, more stiffness can be expected the later we begin motion and more joint contractures secondary to immobilization.

Sensory reeducation begins and desensitization continues, facilitated also by functional activities. Muscle strengthening and endurance and dexterity training all start gradually, stepping up in intensity according to tissue healing and

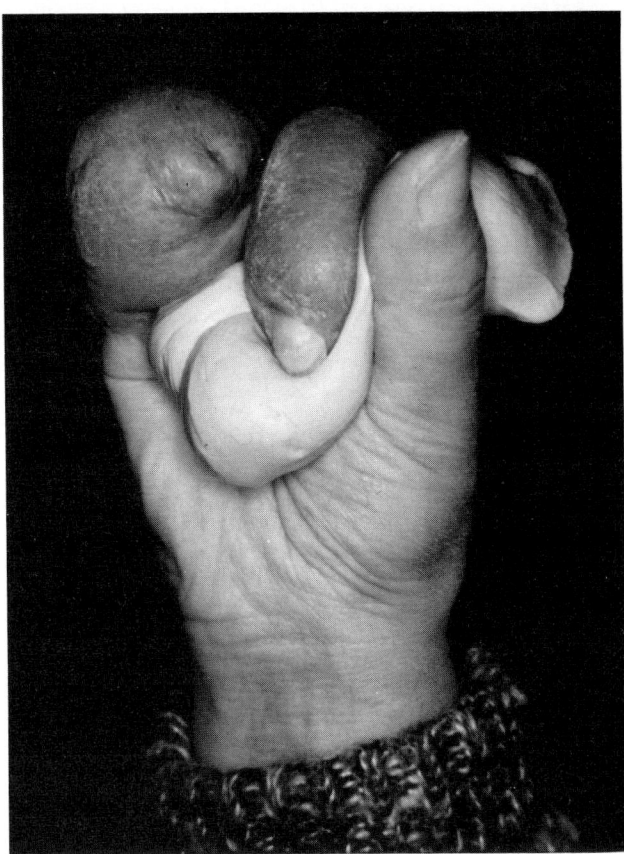

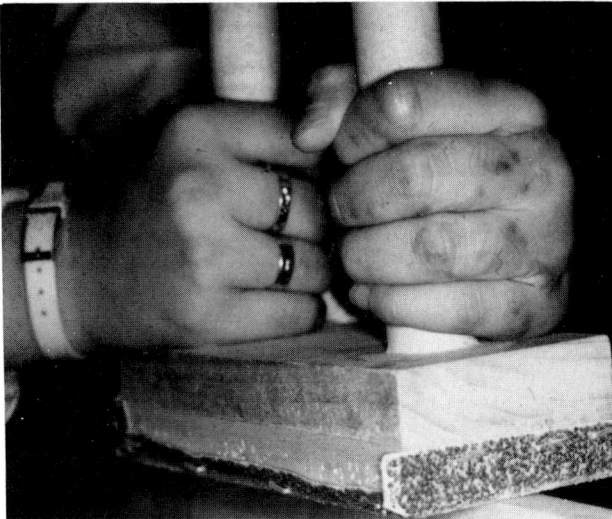

Fig. 16-10 Sustained grip activities such as use of a modified sander are an effective way of initiating resisted finger flexion while exercising the entire upper extremity.

Fig. 16-9 Therapy putty was used for resisted prehension, fisting, and isolated finger flexion in this patient (see Fig. 16-1), shown here at approximately 4 weeks after separation and defatting of the index finger.

evaluation results (Figs. 16-9 and 16-10). In the later stages, job simulation begins. Training in ADL focuses on specific problems as they emerge (Fig. 16-11).

A common problem is overwork, which provokes an inflammatory response. Many patients, encouraged by their returning abilities, will overdo some apparently easy activity such as writing a letter; even 15 minutes of this light but repetitive prehension may not hurt today but could leave the hand edematous and sore tomorrow. This is especially true of resistive exercise, such as in use of grip exercisers while watching television. The patient loses count of repetitions and doesn't even realize he has overdone the exercise. It cannot be overemphasized to the patient that not only is this uncomfortable, but it also represents a step backward, because the inflammatory response leads to further scarring. Cold, elevation, and a temporary return to short, frequent exercise sessions can alleviate the pain and edema, but prevention is infinitely preferable.

Splinting in this phase focuses on increasing motion and function. Serial-static and dynamic splinting provide prolonged low intensity stretch, and dynamic splints assist weak motions while resisting antagonistic motions. Dynamic and static splints augment function.

Because the mutilated hand has such complex needs, it is all too easy to make splints of matching complexity. The patient is unlikely to wear large, complicated splints or

follow confusing schedules involving many splint changes (Figs. 16-12 and 16-13). We assign priority to splint needs in response to frequent evaluation.

Throughout the late stage of therapy, the focus must be on present and future simultaneously. If the patient can see not only his current status, but also his future possibilities, he will make a smoother transition back into his normal life.

SUMMARY

There are no easy formulas or protocols for rehabilitation of the mutilated hand. Each component of injury is evaluated and each intervention designed both individually and in the

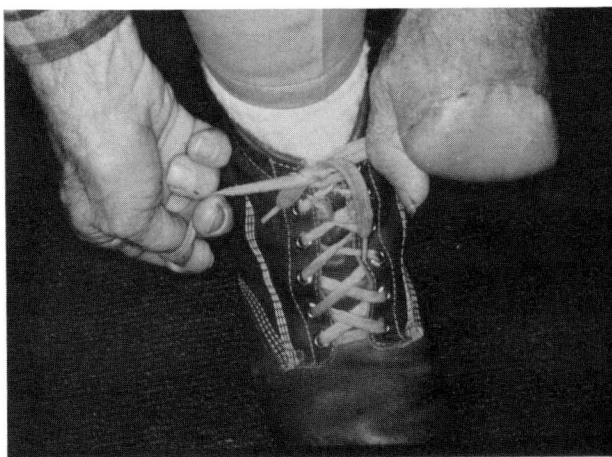

Fig. 16-11 In the absence of the second through fifth digits distal to the metacarpophalangeal joints, this patient regained functional prehension sufficient for independence in activities of daily living. His functional potential was particularly good because the injury was to his nondominant hand and spared the thumb.

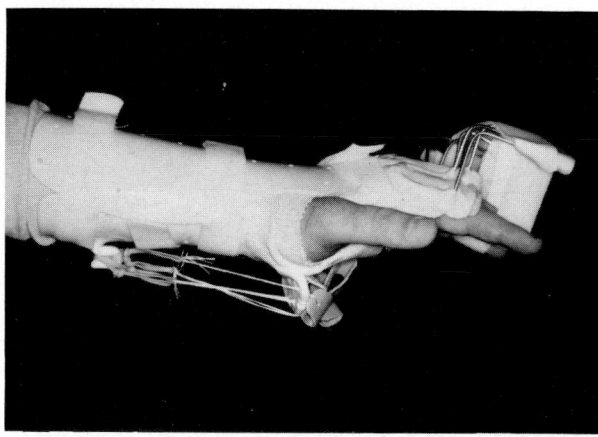

Fig. 16-12 Patient's hand shown after replant of long, ring, and small fingers, followed by extensor and flexor tenolysis and metacarpophalangeal capsulotomies. Because he had complex splinting needs, one splint was designed to meet his two most pressing needs. Here can be seen serial-static extension to the proximal interphalangeal joints, which exhibited a hard endfeel.

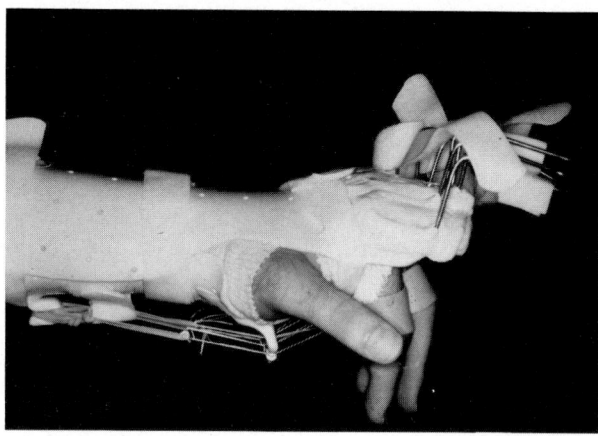

Fig. 16-13 This part of the splint provided dynamic flexion to the metacarpophalangeal joints, which had a more elastic endfeel.

context of the entire complex injury. The psychosocial needs of the patient can be profound and must not be overshadowed by the physical injury. Key elements in therapy are the therapist's understanding of normal and pathological healing of each injured tissue, logical application of this knowledge to evaluation and treatment planning, and constant, close communication between the three members of the rehabilitation team: patient, surgeon, and therapist.

REFERENCES

1. Arem AJ and Madden JW: Effects of stress on healing wounds. I. Intermittent noncyclical tension, J Surg Res 20:93, 1976.
2. Beach RB and Bell J: Ace, Coban and bias stockinette: pressures resulting from their use, J Hand Surg 8:627, 1983.
3. Byron PM and Muntzer EM: Therapist's management of the mutilated hand. In Mackin EJ, editor: Hand clinics, vol 2, no 1, Philadelphia, 1986, WB Saunders Co.
4. English CB and others: Reliability of the durometer for testing scar softening, J Hand Surg 8:625, 1983.
5. Flowers K: String wrapping versus massage for reducing digital volume, J Hand Surg 10A:583, 1985.
6. Heppenstall RB: Fracture and cartilage repair. In Hunt TK and Dunphy JE, editors: Fundamentals of wound management, New York, 1979, Appleton-Century-Crofts.
7. Hunt TK and Van Winkle W Jr: Normal repair. In Hunt TK and Dunphy JE, editors: Fundamentals of wound management, New York, 1979, Appleton-Century-Crofts.
8. Madden JW: Wound healing: the biological basis of hand surgery, Clin Plast Surg 3(1):3, 1976.
9. Magness J, Garrett T, and Erickson D: Swelling of the upper extremity during whirlpool baths, Arch Phys Med Rehabil 51:297, 1970.
10. Malick MH and Carr JA: Manual on management of the burn patient. Pittsburgh, 1982, Harmarville Rehabilitation Center Educational Resource Division.
11. Michlovitz SL: Biophysical principles of heating and superficial heat agents. In Michlovitz SL, editor: Thermal agents in rehabilitation, Philadelphia, 1986, FA Davis Co.
12. Michlovitz SL: Cryotherapy: the use of cold as a therapeutic agent. In Michlovitz SL, editor: Thermal agents in rehabilitation, Philadelphia, 1986, FA Davis Co.
13. Newton RA: Contemporary views on pain and the role played by thermal agents in managing pain symptoms. In Michlovitz SL, editor: Thermal agents in rehabilitation, Philadelphia, 1986, FA Davis Co.
14. Peacock EE Jr: Wound repair, ed 3, Philadelphia, 1984, WB Saunders Co.
15. Rodeheaver G and others: Bactericidal activity and toxicity of iodine-containing solutions in wounds, Arch Surg 117:181, 1982.
16. Schultz K: The effect of active exercise on edema, J Hand Surg 8:625, 1983.
17. Seddon HJ: Surgical disorders of the peripheral nerves, ed 2, Edinburgh, 1975, Churchill Livingstone.
18. Simonetti A, Miller R, and Gristina J: Efficacy of povidone-iodine in the disinfection of whirlpool baths and hubbard tanks, Phys Ther 52:450, 1972.
19. Sullivan J: Scar management techniques with the use of pressure contact dressings postreconstructive surgery, J Hand Surg 9A:610, 1984.
20. Walsh M: Relationship of hand edema to upper extremity position and water temperature during whirlpool, J Hand Surg 9A:609, 1984.
21. Walsh M: Hydrotherapy: the use of water as a therapeutic agent. In Michlovitz SL, editor: Thermal agents in rehabilitation, Philadelphia, 1986, FA Davis Co.
22. Zarro VJ: Mechanisms of inflammation and repair. In Michlovitz SL, editor: Thermal agents in rehabilitation, Philadelphia, 1986, FA Davis Co.

ADDITIONAL READINGS

Brand PW: Clinical mechanics of the hand, St Louis, 1985, The CV Mosby Co.

Fess EE and Philips CA: Hand splinting: principles and methods, St Louis, 1987, The CV Mosby Co.

Hardy M: Preserving function in the inflamed and acutely injured hand. In Moran C, editor: Hand rehabilitation, Clinics in physical therapy, vol 9, New York, 1986, Churchill Livingstone, Inc.

Miles W: Soft tissue trauma. In Mackin EJ, editor: Hand clinics, vol 2, no 1, Philadelphia, 1986, WB Saunders Co.

Rosenblum NI and Robinson SJ: Advances in flexor and extensor tendon management. In Moran C, editor: Hand rehabilitation, Clinics in physical therapy, vol 9, New York, 1986, Churchill Livingstone, Inc.

Sorenson MK: Fractures of the wrist and hand. In Moran C, editor: Hand rehabilitation, Clinics in physical therapy, vol 9, New York, 1986, Churchill Livingstone, Inc.

Ziskin MC and Michlovitz SL: Therapeutic ultrasound. In Michlovitz SL, editor: Thermal agents in rehabilitation, Philadelphia, 1986, FA Davis Co.

17

Management of skin grafts and flaps

Daniel I. Singer, John H. Moore, Jr., and Patricia M. Byron

Soft tissue coverage of the upper extremity may present a problem to the reconstructive surgeon. Aside from aesthetic aspects, vital structures that include arteries, veins, nerves, tendon, and bone may need to be protected. In various situations, reconstructive options may be as simple as allowing the wound to close by secondary intention or as complex as free tissue transfer. Each method has its proper place, but the key elements are conscientious decision making, intraoperative technique, and careful postoperative care to ensure optimal results.

Small open wounds (usually less than 1.5 cm in diameter) may be allowed to close by secondary intention. This technique is most commonly used on fingertips where closure can be accomplished in 3 to 4 weeks without sacrifice of function. This is perhaps the oldest technique for wound closure and is still applicable in situations where function will not be compromised by scar contracture.

The history of attempted wound closure dates to 1817 when Sir Ashley Cooper successfully grafted skin from an amputated thumb to cover the stump. Many successful reports of skin grafting followed, but it was Ollier in 1872 who first realized the importance of the dermis.[20] In 1886 Thiersch described a thin, split-thickness skin graft to cover large wounds. In contrast to contracture noted in split-thickness skin grafts, in 1876 Wolfe noted that full-thickness skin grafts retained their shape and size better.[41] During this time, new horizons were being seen in soft tissue reconstruction with the advent of the flap. In 1889 Manchot described and defined anatomically the cutaneous vascular pattern[26] that Halsted subsequently used in his "waltzing" flaps.[16] The first myocutaneous flap was used by Tansini in 1906 for breast reconstruction.[47] In 1919, Davis wrote about pedicle flap principles,[10] and 2 years later, Blair described the delay phenomenon in flaps.[4]

The next major advance came in 1972 when McGregor and Jackson described the first axial flap, the groin flap, and noted its clinical usefulness in upper extremity reconstruction.[31] In the following year, a new era of reconstructive surgery was defined with microvascular free tissue transfer.[8,18,38] Multiple free and pedicled flaps have since been described. These new flaps fulfill the requirements of the recipient defect and have acceptable donor morbidity.

DEFINING FLAPS

The physician and therapist supervising the postoperative recovery of a patient who has undergone reconstruction should understand the anatomy and physiology of the donor flap or graft if the functional and cosmetic potential of the hand is to be realized.

Classification systems are useful to organize and simplify information. Unfortunately, there is not one classification method that is both simple and complete for flaps. Flaps can be classified according to donor site, either local or distant. They can also be classified according to the tissue that is transferred, with combinations of skin, subcutaneous tissue, fascia, muscle, and bone. Finally, they can be classified according to the nature of their blood supply. We have chosen to use vascularity as the method of classifying in this chapter because vascularity directly determines much of the postoperative management of flaps.

The following classification system is used throughout this chapter:

I. Nonvascular skin transfers
   A. Split-thickness skin graft
   B. Full-thickness skin graft
II. Pedicled flaps
   A. Random
   B. Axial
   C. Island
   D. Fasciocutaneous
   E. Myocutaneous
III. Free vascularized tissue transfer

NONVASCULAR SKIN TRANSFERS
Skin grafts

Nonvascular skin transfers may be divided into two groups: split-thickness skin grafts and full-thickness skin grafts. In general, a split-thickness skin graft is one that includes the epidermis and any portion of the dermis. These grafts vary between 0.01 and 0.022 inches in thickness. A full-thickness graft is one that includes the epidermis and entire dermis.

A split-thickness skin graft is generally obtained from the thigh, buttock, or abdomen. Advantages of these grafts include a large supply of donor areas, ease of harvesting, reusable donor sites, decreased primary (or early) contracture, and the ability to cover large surface areas. Disadvantages include cosmetic inferiority to full-thickness grafts, hyperpigmentation, decreased durability, and increased secondary (or late) contracture. Primary contracture refers to the shrinkage of the graft immediately as it is removed from its bed. The split-thickness graft undergoes secondary contracture when it contracts as it heals, pulling the wound margins in.

For upper extremity reconstruction, full-thickness skin grafts are generally obtained from the hypothenar eminence, medial aspect of the arm, or groin. Advantages include improved cosmesis and color match, increased durability,

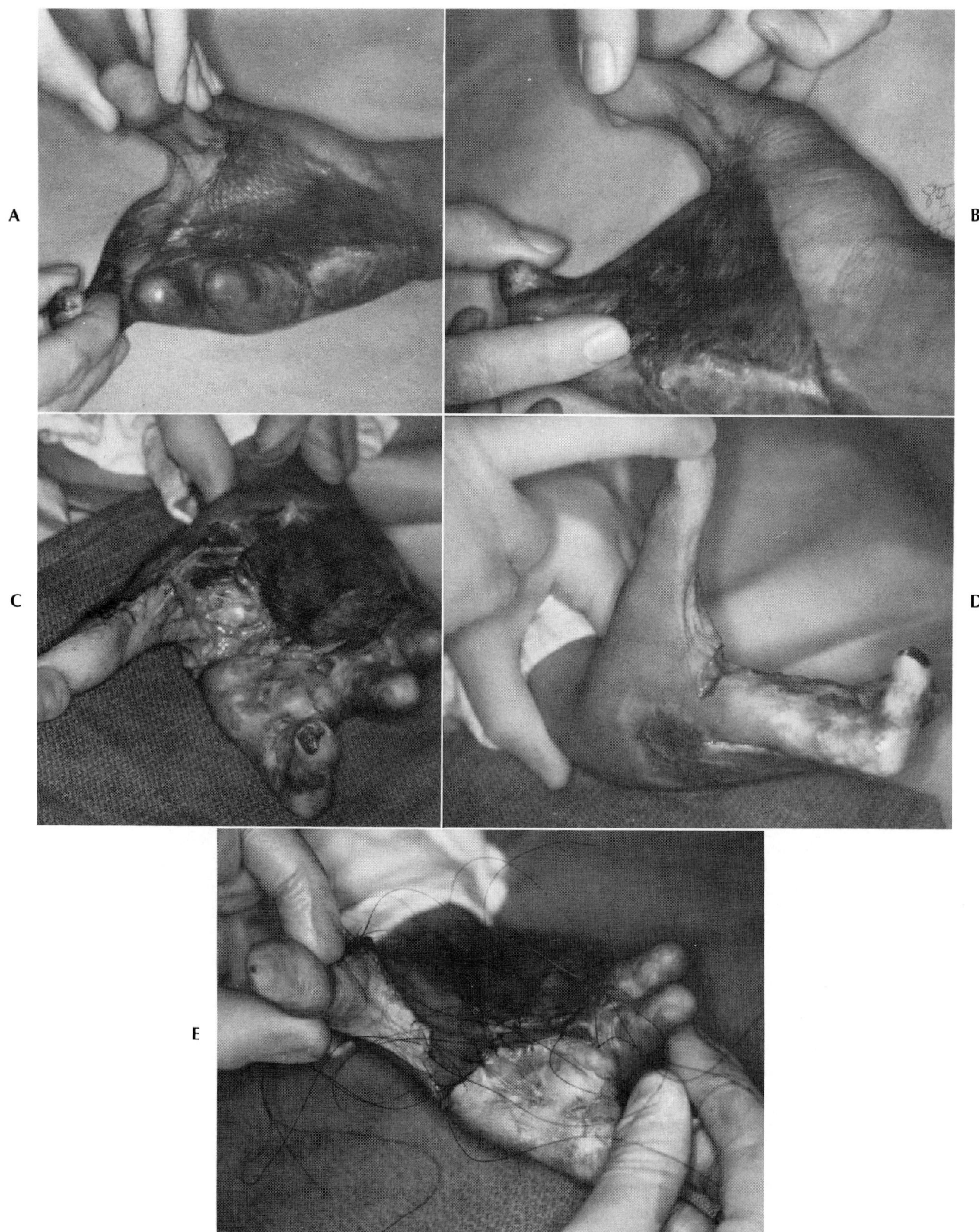

Fig. 17-1   A and **B,** This patient with a roller-crush injury was initially treated with split-thickness skin grafts to the palm and thumb web space. His use of splints, pressure garment, and inserts was sporadic in the postoperative period. **C** and **D,** Three months after the initial surgery the patient underwent scar revision and contracture release. **E,** The split-thickness grafts were replaced with full-thickness grafts.

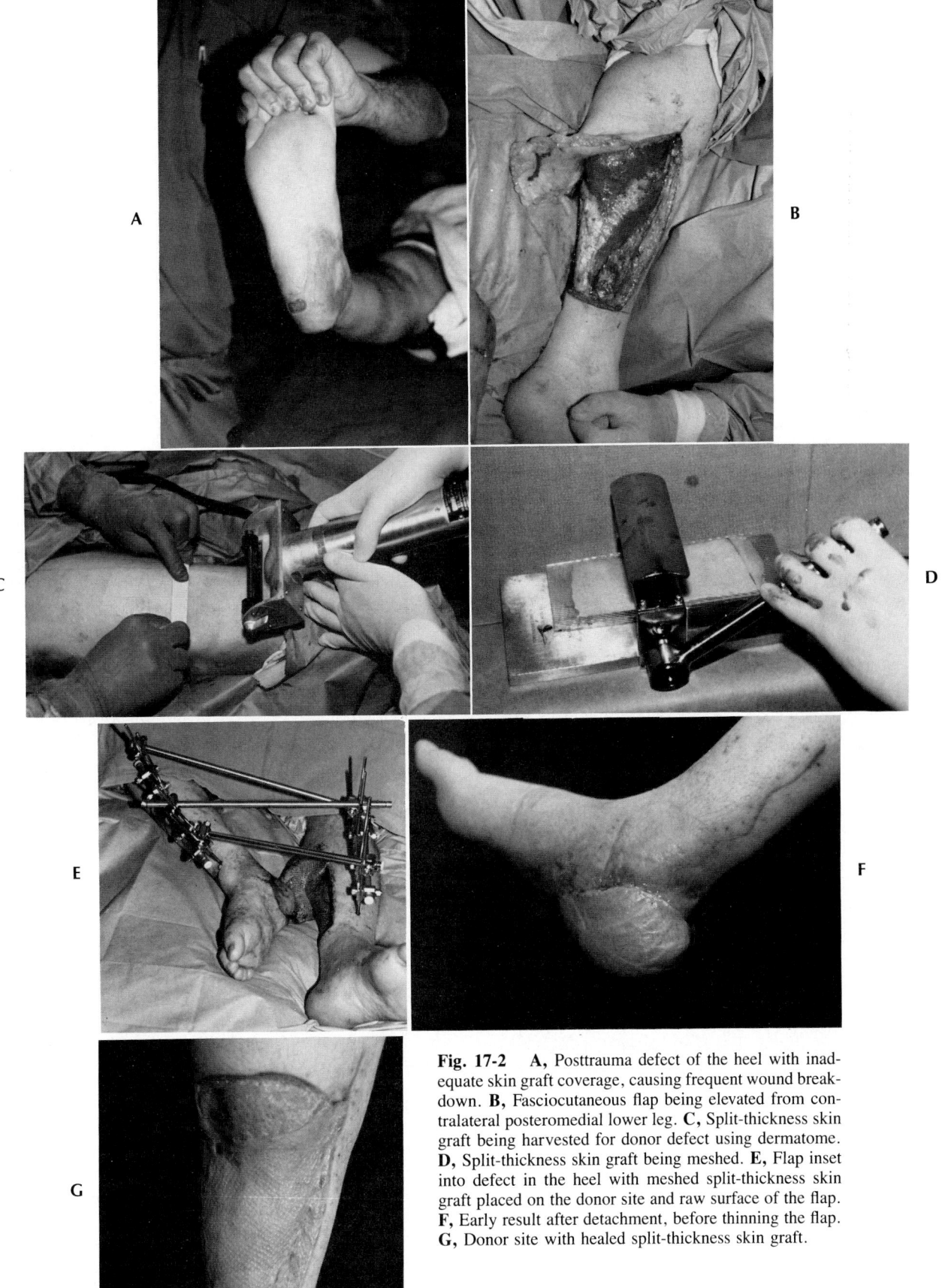

Fig. 17-2   A, Posttrauma defect of the heel with inadequate skin graft coverage, causing frequent wound breakdown. **B,** Fasciocutaneous flap being elevated from contralateral posteromedial lower leg. **C,** Split-thickness skin graft being harvested for donor defect using dermatome. **D,** Split-thickness skin graft being meshed. **E,** Flap inset into defect in the heel with meshed split-thickness skin graft placed on the donor site and raw surface of the flap. **F,** Early result after detachment, before thinning the flap. **G,** Donor site with healed split-thickness skin graft.

and decreased secondary contracture. Disadvantages include limited donor sites, increased primary contracture, and the need for an optimal bed for survival ("take") of the graft (Fig. 17-1).

Split-thickness skin grafts are generally taken with instruments designed to cut tissue to a specified depth (Fig. 17-2. Once harvested, they can be meshed to expand the graft surface area and improve the chances of survival of the graft in a suboptimal bed. "Take" of the graft is usually noted by the fourth or fifth postoperative day. The donor site is dressed either with nonadherent gauze that permits a scab or with a semipermeable membrane that improves epithelialization in a moist environment. For most patients, the semipermeable membrane is more comfortable.

Full-thickness skin grafts are usually taken free-hand. All subcutaneous fat is removed from the dermis to improve the survival of the graft. The donor site is closed primarily, which limits the size of the graft. Common donor sites include the groin and the medial aspect of the arm because the residual scar is hidden.

Split-thickness and full-thickness skin grafts are tissues that have been detached from their native blood supply. They depend totally on the recipient bed for their revascularization. Recipient beds with good blood supply improve the survival of the grafts. In contrast, recipient beds with poor blood supply are generally less successful. Inappropriate beds that will not support graft survival include exposed cortical bone, cartilage, and tendon. Suboptimal graft beds that are likely to restrict function or be prone to breakdown include cancellous bone, mesotendon, nerves, and vessels. Optimal beds include muscle and fascia.

With both types of grafts, the recipient bed needs to be adequately prepared to ensure optimum survival of the graft. This includes débridement of the necrotic and infected material and hemostasis. Both types of grafts can be held in

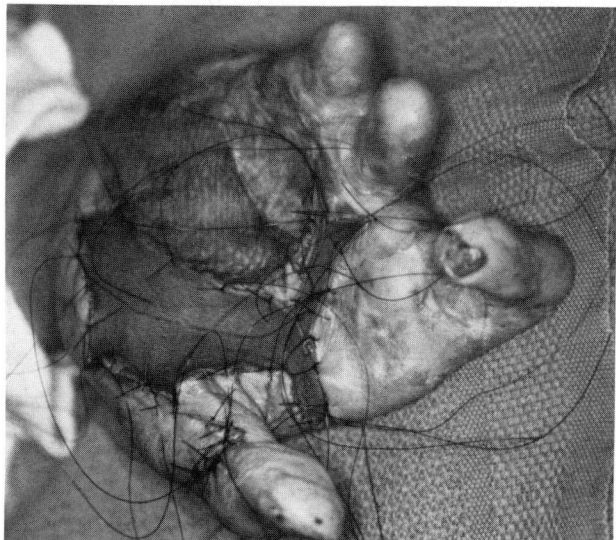

Fig. 17-3 Graft prepared for application of a tie-over bolus dressing. Nonadherent gauze is placed next to the graft. A bolus of saline-soaked cotton is placed over the gauze, and the sutures are tied to hold it in place.

place with sutures, staples, or tape. Meshing the graft is helpful in improving survival where moderate serous drainage is expected. Where grafts may be exposed to shear forces, "tie-over" dressings are useful (Fig. 17-3).

Postoperative management

The grafts are usually left undisturbed for 4 or 5 days postoperatively, unless there is concern about purulence or fluid collection beneath the graft. During the first 48 hours post-operatively, grafts survive on the imbibition of plasma. During this time, a delicate fibrin network is laid down to improve contact. The next phase of inosculation and neovascularization occurs, and at this time, the graft turns pink. Lymphatic connections usually occur about the fifth postoperative day.[52] Loss of the graft is usually the result of shear forces, fluid accumulation under the graft, tension, or purulence.

When the graft is noted to be surviving by the fifth postoperative day, daily dressing changes with nonadherent gauze are instituted.[13] Gentle range-of-motion exercises may begin by the seventh postoperative day under the supervision of a trained therapist. If small open areas are noted, Mercurochrome is helpful in promoting wound contracture and hastening the reepithelialization process.

Although the healing graft is generally well-vascularized by the seventh to tenth postoperative day, there is little tensile strength in the wound, making it prone to injury by shearing forces for another 10 days. This must be kept in mind in dressing application and in initiating guarded range of motion. A dressing that slips or rubs may harm rather than protect the healing wound. For this reason it may even be advisable to exercise without dressings during this phase of healing. Elevation is used initially to control edema. Compression wraps are not applied until the graft appears to have taken well; usually by about 2 weeks postoperatively the graft will be pink and adherent over its area. Pressure should not be applied without consulting the treating physician. In cases where graft take is poor or where spotty loss has occurred by about 1 week, whirlpool and saline soaks may be used to clean the wound and to stimulate local circulation. Saline soaks are prepared by adding 1 tablespoon of table salt to every quart of boiling water, and allowing the water to cool to lukewarm before use.

Grafted areas are often dry and tight as they heal because of lack of natural lubrication. This condition may be improved by regular application of a topical lubricant once the wound is closed. This helps prevent skin breakdown that can occur when range of motion is begun. In the later stages of healing (generally 3 to 4 weeks postoperatively), gentle massage is used on a regular basis to keep the skin pliable, to mobilize the skin and underlying scar, and to assist with early desensitization in the presence of any hypersensitivity.

Late contracture may be a significant complication in the management of grafts, especially split-thickness grafts. It can be minimized by the early use of pressure garments initiated by 10 to 14 days after the graft. Care must be taken in application to prevent shearing forces. If commercial pressure garments are used, zippers are helpful. Pressure garments should not be prescribed until edema is decreased, because a decrease in edema will decrease the garment's ability to apply firm pressure over the grafted area. Inserts such as Elastomer or Otoform are molded directly over the graft area and improve distribution of force to the entire scar. Splints may be applied over the pressure garment or insert to maintain the grafted part in its maximally lengthened position. The importance of regular wear of the appliance cannot be overemphasized if success is to be achieved.[21]

The patient should be cautioned against exposure of either graft donor or recipient sites to the sun for at least 6 months. Permanent discoloration can occur because the graft is more susceptible to sunburn. Pressure garments are helpful in protecting the graft from exposure. Sunscreens are also recommended.

Some return of sensation can be expected in grafted areas. This will be quicker in areas covered by thinner grafts.[11] Some recovery of sensation may be noted as early as 5 weeks after grafting, and it continues to improve for up to 2 years. This recovery may be facilitated by sensory reeducation techniques.

Management of donor sites

Split-thickness skin graft donor sites are usually managed by the application of a fine-mesh gauze impregnated with a compound such as glycerin. Dry dressings are placed over this gauze intraoperatively. These absorb the initial bleeding from the donor site and are removed after the first day. This permits the use of a heat lamp intermittently that dries the coagulum that has oozed through the gauze. The lamp may be used for about 10 minutes three times daily. This "seals" the donor site and minimizes the risk of infection. After 2 to 3 days, migration of epithelial cells from sweat glands

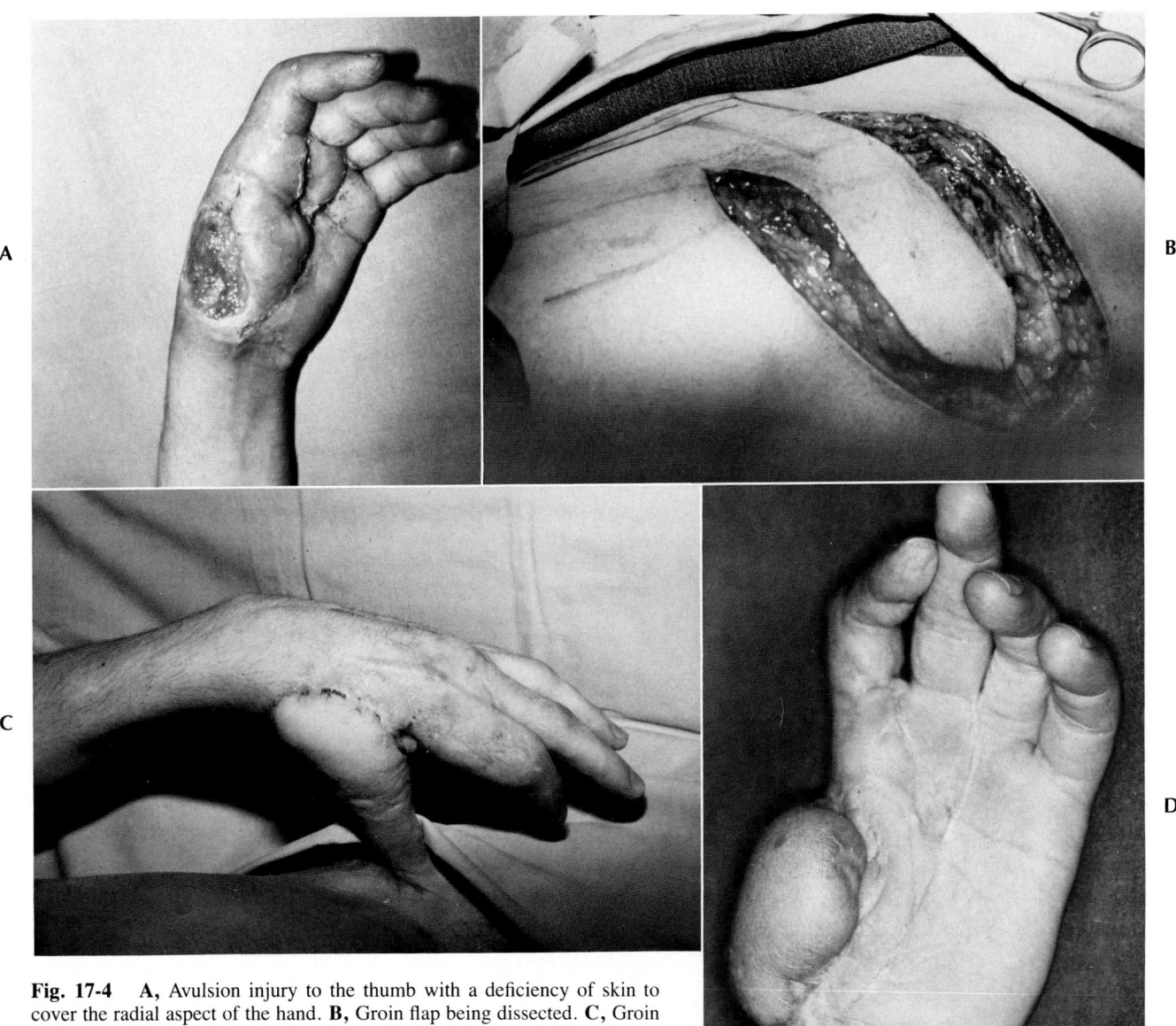

Fig. 17-4 **A,** Avulsion injury to the thumb with a deficiency of skin to cover the radial aspect of the hand. **B,** Groin flap being dissected. **C,** Groin flap attached to radial aspect of the hand. **D,** Healed flap providing closure and extra skin for secondary reconstruction of a thumb.

and hair shafts begins beneath the gauze. Usually within 5 to 10 days, epithelialization is completed and the gauze will gradually fall away from the donor site. Donor sites should be monitored for the appearance of hypertrophic scarring. Application of pressure, as outlined above, is useful if this develops. Also, massage with a topical lubricant will improve patient comfort after initial reepithelialization has occurred.

Full-thickness skin graft donor sites are treated as any sutured wound. The suture line is kept dry and clean and monitored for signs of infection. Sutures are removed at 7 to 10 days. Massage may be initiated 2 to 3 days after suture removal to help soften the scar area.

PEDICLED FLAPS
Indications

In situations where there is bone devoid of periosteum, tendon devoid of paratenon, cartilage devoid of perichon-drium, or exposed vital structures, skin grafts will not provide suitable coverage. In these instances, a flap will be necessary for wound coverage. A flap is a portion of skin and/or subcutaneous tissue and muscle that contains its own vascular supply. Thus, survival of the tissue does not initially depend on the status of the vascularity of the recipient bed. Blood to the flap is supplied through the segmental vessels to the perforating vessels. From there, branches of the cutaneouos vessels supply the dermal-subdermal plexus.[9]

A random flap is a pedicled flap that receives its blood supply from the dermal-subdermal plexus.[32] There is no anatomically recognized arterial or venous system. Examples include Z-plasty, W-plasty, V-Y advancement, rotation, and transposition flaps. In general, flaps are always viable in a length-to-width ratio of 1:1. They may be extended further on various cutaneous territories. Survival is based on blood flow through the dermal-subdermal plexus.

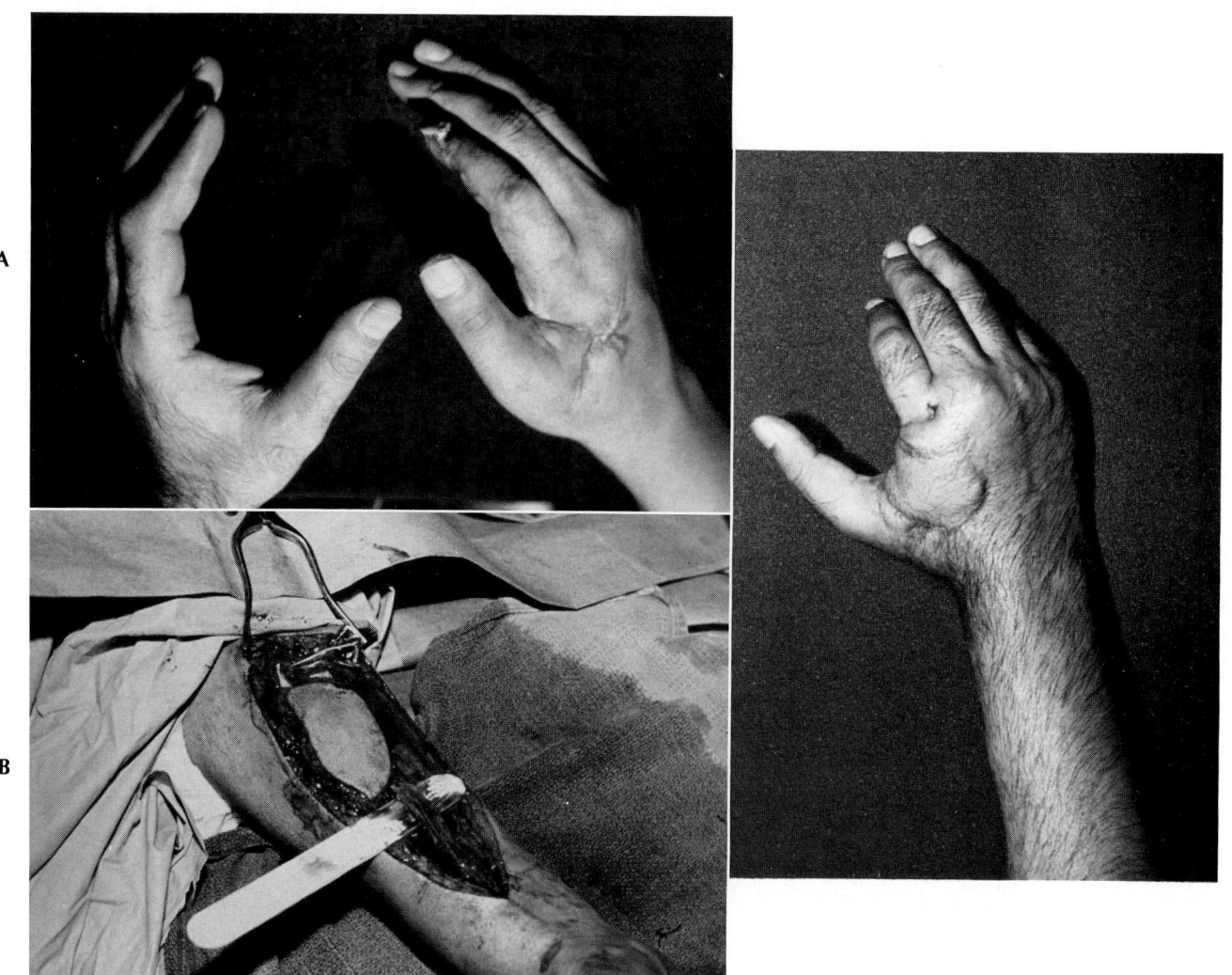

A

B

C

Fig. 17-5   **A,** Secondary healing of a gunshot wound in the first web space caused a severe thumb-index web space adduction contracture. **B,** A radial forearm fasciocutaneous flap is dissected as an island flap, based on its retrograde blood supply from the radial artery and veins. **C,** Result of inset flap showing improved thumb abduction.

Axial, island, and myocutaneous flaps differ from random flaps in that there is an anatomically recognized arterial and venous system. In axial and island flaps a direct cutaneous vascular bundle is noted, whereas in a muscle or myocutaneous flap there is a direct vascular pedicle to the underlying muscle.[32] In myocutaneous flaps, the cutaneous portion is supplied by direct cutaneous perforators from the muscle to the dermal-subdermal plexus. These flaps have the advantage of greatly increasing the length-to-width ratio of the flap because of their intrinsic blood supply.[29,30]

Axial flaps may be converted to island flaps by skeletonizing the vascular pedicle. This decreases the base of the flap to a single vascular bundle at the time of transposition. Examples of an axial flap include the groin flap and deltopectoral flap (Fig. 17-4). An example of an island flap is a neurovascular digital island flap.

Fasciocutaneous flaps are based on the vascular plexus of the deep fascia.[7,39] Average length-to-width ratio is 2.5:1 (see Fig. 17-2). Advantages of these flaps are ease of elevation, decreased soft tissue bulk, and lack of any functional impairment. The donor site is often unaesthetic because it requires a skin graft for closure. Examples of a fasciocutaneous flap are the radial artery flap (Fig. 17-5) and the lateral arm flaps. In many instances, these flaps are also useful as free vascularized flaps.

Muscle and myocutaneous flaps are superb sources of vascularized tissue. In general, muscle flaps have less bulk than myocutaneous flaps. Their blood supply is predictable, as are the cutaneous territories over the muscle that are supplied by the muscle perforators. These are most often used to cover vital exposed tissue in contaminated or previously infected wounds, because muscle is the most effective tissue in fighting off infection in contaminated wounds.

In all situations where the flap is used, initially there is moderate swelling of the flap because of some disruption of the venous and lymphatic collaterals. This increases soft tissue bulk, which occurs early in the postoperative period and gradually subsides over the next few months. Once skin

is deemed stable, by 1 to 2 weeks, gentle compression, such as elastic wrap, may help with the final results.

When a groin flap is planned, the patient should be prepared as much as possible before surgery. This includes instruction in one-handed techniques and information regarding the type of clothing that will best accommodate the arm while it is attached. Sweat pants with a draw-string, not elastic waist, or overalls, are recommended.

Postoperative management

The axial flap is generally left attached for 2 to 4 weeks. During this time the involved area must be kept well supported to prevent stress on the flap. In the case of the groin flap, an adapted shoulder immobilizer, or a sling–elastic wrap combination may be used (Fig. 17-6). The shoulder immobilizer consists of an elastic chest band with cotton web humeral and wrist cuffs. The cuff position on the immobilizer may need to be changed to accommodate the flap. The flap should be inspected following securing of the support to be sure that no kinking of vessels or tension in the flap has occurred through positioning.

Maceration may be a problem in areas where the extremity rests against the body. (Fig. 17-7) Gauze pads should be placed between these areas. These pads are changed regularly.

Edema is most significant when positioning for the flap requires dependence of the extremity. String wrapping using soft cotton string may be applied to free digits if this does not stress the attachment.[33] Retrograde massage is used also to mobilize the edema (Fig. 17-8).

Every effort must be made to maintain motion in uninvolved joints. This includes available active and passive motion that does not stress the flap (Fig. 17-9).

Therapy goals following flap detachment include: wound healing, edema control, regaining active and passive motion in uninvolved joints, and reestablishing active and passive motion in the involved joint. The donor site is monitored for healing and development of hypertropic scar.

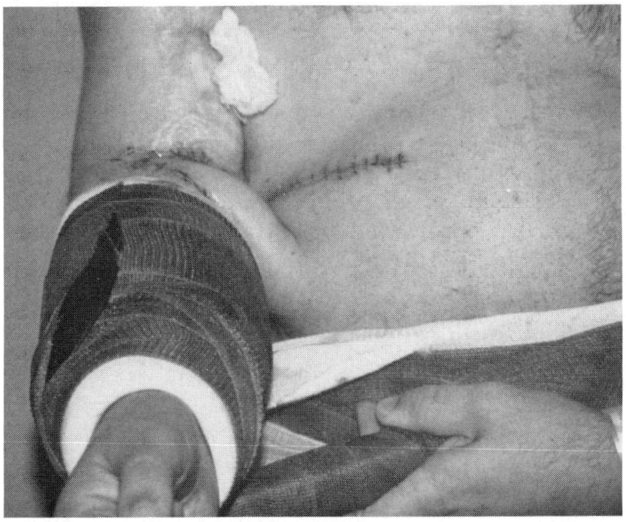

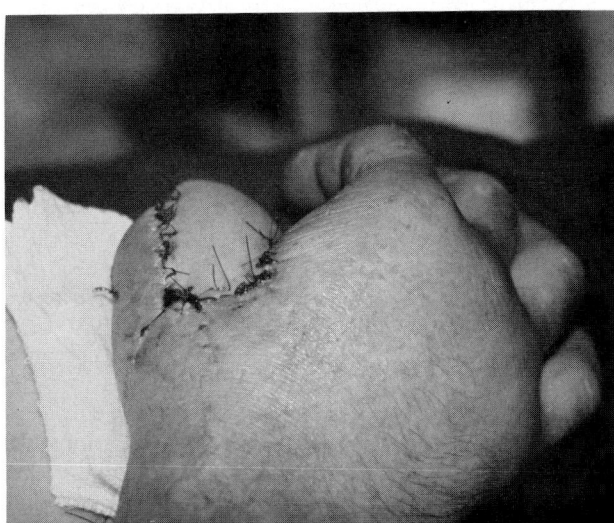

Fig. 17-6 A fiberglass support with waist and forearm segments was used to protect the flap for this patient. This stable positioning permitted motion of the digits.

Fig. 17-7 Sterile gauze pads are used to prevent maceration caused by the attached hand resting on the abdomen.

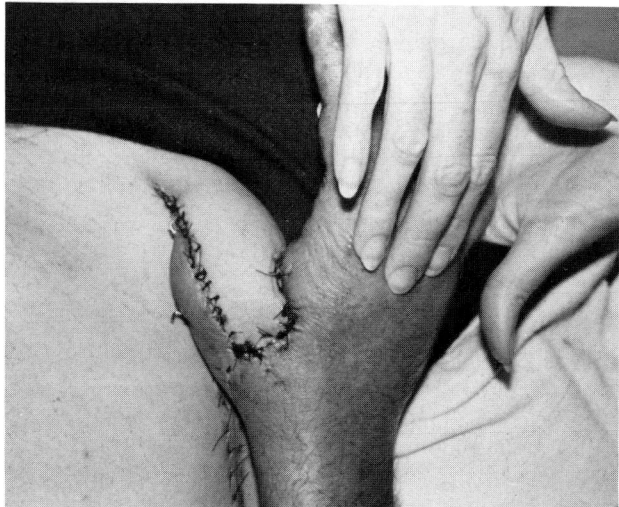

Fig. 17-8 Retrograde massage is performed with the patient in a supine position.

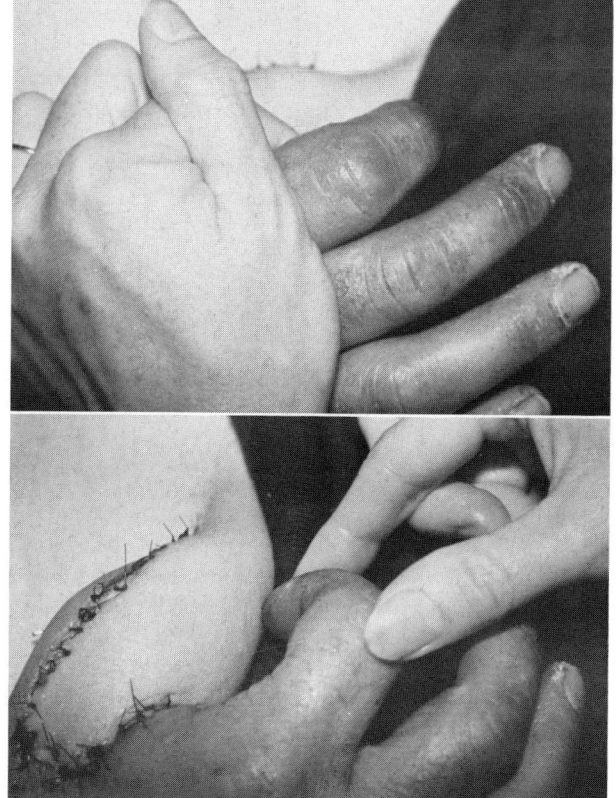

Fig. 17-9 **A** and **B,** Gentle, protected active and passive range-of-motion exercises that do not stress the flap are performed in therapy.

FREE TISSUE TRANSFER

Free vascularized tissue transfer was first described by Daniels and Taylor in 1973.[8] This new method of reconstruction was an outgrowth of two advances in the field of surgery that preceded it. The first was the identification of an axial pattern flap that could be skeletonized into an island flap.[31,32] The second was the advances in microsurgical techniques over the proceeding 15 years that made the technique of a 1 mm vascular anastomosis reliable. This technique had been refined for replantation surgery. The term *free flap* has become acceptable terminology to describe an island flap that is transferred on its vascular pedicle to another area by vascular anastomosis.

A free flap is really three surgical procedures done at one operative setting. The first is to debride the site where the tissue is to be transferred (the recipient site) and identify appropriate vessels at this site for subsequent microvascular anastomosis. Next (or concurrently if two surgical teams are working simultaneously) the flap is dissected as an island flap based on its vascular pedicle. Finally the vascular pedicle is cut, the microvascular anastomoses are performed at the recipient site, and the flap is inset.

There are multiple advantages of free flaps. They bring a new blood supply to the injured recipient area, thereby improving the potential for healing, especially in a poorly vascularized, scarred bed. Conversely, both pedicled flaps and grafts must ultimately obtain their vascularity from the recipient bed. In pedicled flaps, the donor and recipient sites must be brought together anywhere from 10 to 28 days before division of the flap. This is necessary to allow new vascular ingrowth to the flap from the recipient bed. Often this positioning interferes with early therapy. Finally, with the increasing number of free flaps identified as being appropriate for free tissue transfer, often the match between tissue available and recipient requirements is better after free than pedicle flaps.

The disadvantages of free flap transfer are that the surgical procedures are long and technically demanding. Failures after free flap transfers often result in a dramatic loss of the entire tissue transfer. This contrasts with pedicled transfers, which rarely become completely necrotic, although partial tip necrosis can occur. Free flaps must be closely observed in the postoperative period for vascular thrombosis, and the surgeon must be available to return the patient to the operating room on an emergency basis if there is circulatory embarrassment.

When evaluating a tissue defect, the surgeon tries to reconstruct the defect using the simplest available method that will still reliably close the defect and provide a satisfactory functional and cosmetic result. If a skin graft will accomplish the desired result, then there is no need to do anything more complicated. Next, local flaps are evaluated for their appropriateness. Then distant flaps are evaluated if there is no local flap that fills the surgeon's criteria. Finally, free flaps should be evaluated if simpler methods are deemed inappropriate or less than satisfactory. The patient should be an active participant in the decision-making process because the patient has to help determine his functional and cosmetic goals and what he is willing to sacrifice in regard to time, risk, and donor defect to obtain these goals.

Free tissue transfers in the hand fall into two general categories. The first involves composite transfers that reconstruct lost thumbs or digits. These are most often harvested from the toes, although rarely they can be harvested from the opposite hand.[50] The entire great toe, including

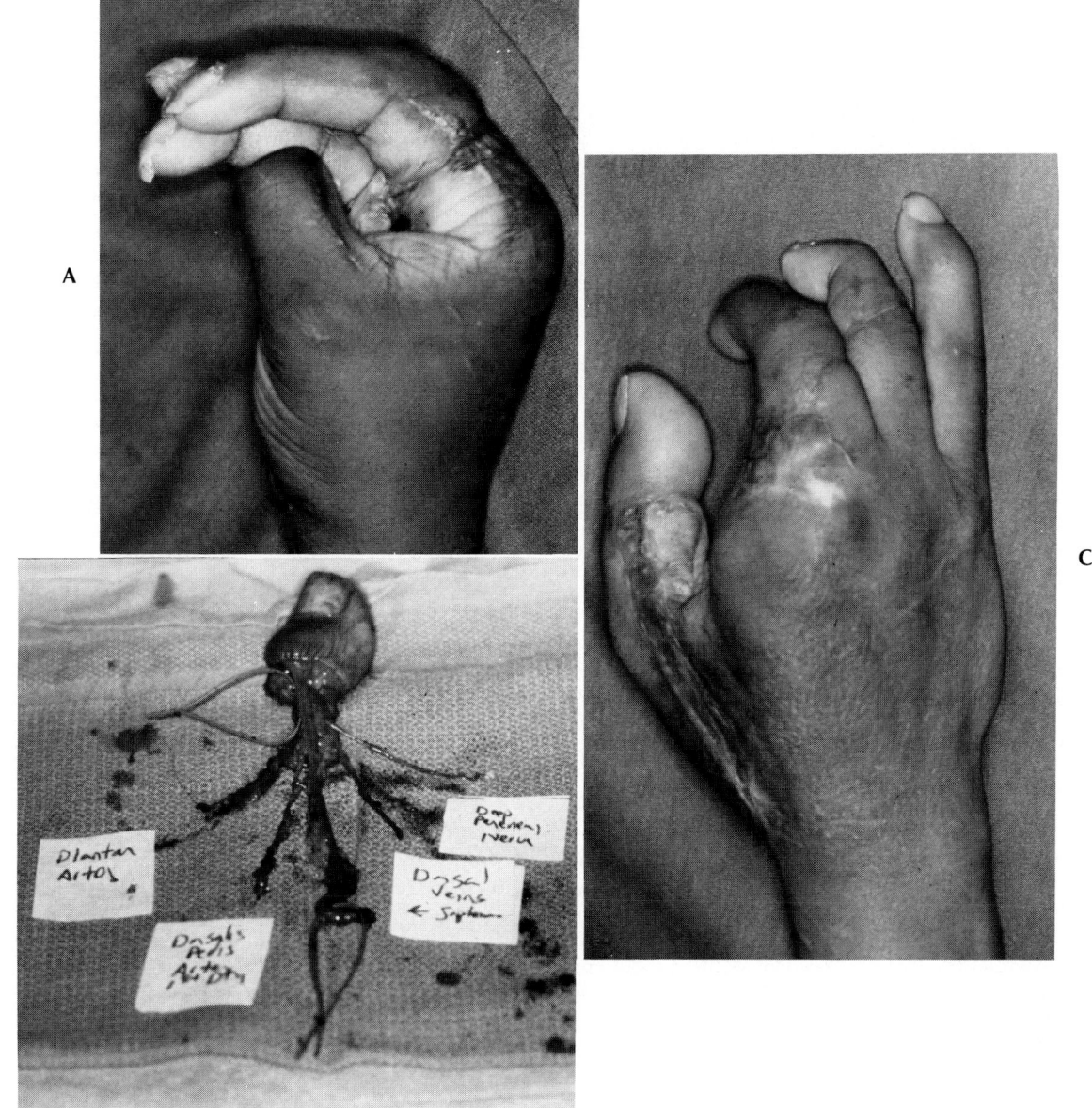

Fig. 17-10 **A,** Posttrauma loss of thumb tip with stiffness of the replanted digits preventing the thumb from opposing the digits. Thumb tip and finger were unreplantable. **B,** Dissected great toe with labeled neurovascular structures. **C,** Result of toe transfer with restoration of strong pinch (16-pound key pinch).

bone, vessels, tendons, nerve, and skin, may be used to reconstruct the thumb[6] (Fig. 17-10). Conversely, the skin of the great toe with its nail bed and neurovascular bundle can be used to reconstruct the thumb, using the thumb's own skeleton or replacing that skeleton with bone graft (commonly known as the wraparound flap).[12,25,34] Even just the pulp of the thumb can be replaced by part of the pulp of the great toe.[28,46] The second and third toes are most often used to reconstruct a digit or digits when a functioning thumb has no digits to pinch against. An opposite ring finger can also be used, especially if it is already injured, but the donor defect must be carefully evaluated and discussed with the patient.[35]

The other major type of free tissue transfer used in the upper extremity is most commonly a soft tissue and/or bony

flap used to reconstruct large defects after trauma or tumor resection. This chapter concentrates on soft tissue transfers. In the hand, thin flaps are usually preferable to prevent a pancakelike appearance. This contrasts with the forearm, where sometimes bulky muscle and myocutaneous flaps better restore contour after deep tissue loss.

There are many available donor flaps for the hand; however, none match the specialized skin on the volar aspect of the hand, nor do they match the extraordinarily thin skin and subcutaneous tissue on the dorsum of the hand and still leave an acceptable donor defect. Certainly, the plantar skin of the foot is an excellent match for palmar skin and dorsal foot skin matches dorsal hand skin. However, in spite of the technical feasibility of transferring this skin as a free flap, they are rarely if ever indicated because of the rather severe donor defect they leave behind that may ultimately interfere with painless gait. Presently, commonly used, relatively thin, free flaps include the radial forearm flap,[45,53] the ulnar forearm flap,[24] the lateral arm flap,[22,43,44] the scapular flap,[3,14,17,42,51] the parascapular flap,[37] and the peroneal artery flap[54]; perhaps the groin flap could be included in this group. Each flap has its relative advantages and disadvantages, including such things as ease of dissection; size, length, and predictability of vascular pedicle; potential for innervation; thinness and hairiness of flap; and donor defect. Choosing the most appropriate flap is a joint decision between surgeon and patient.

The importance of preoperative patient preparation cannot be overemphasized, because the same procedure performed in both a prepared and an unprepared patient may have drastically different outcomes.

Postoperatively, the vascular status of the flap is critical. This is closely monitored for the first several days. During this time the flap patient and room are kept warm. The patient abstains from caffeine and nicotine. Some edema is expected. Elevation is to heart level only, because extensive elevation may impair arterial inflow.

If the early healing period is uneventful, the flap should be stable by 8 to 10 days. The patient may be referred to therapy at this time. Early therapy goals include: (1) wound care for both donor and recipient sites, (2) monitoring of vascularity, (3) edema control, and (4) AROM. If the wounds are dry and healing well, minimal dressing is required. If wound healing is not progressing well, whirlpool may be initiated once the flap is thought to be stable by the treating physician. Care must be taken during the whirlpool to position the arm in a way that does not increase edema. Edema control is limited to elevation until the third postoperative week to prevent vascular compromise. More aggressive edema control such as elastic wraps or Coban wrap may be started after this time. Vascular status is monitored by observing the color, temperature, and capillary refill time. AROM should be started for uninvolved joints as early as possible. Motion at involved joints is initiated as soon as vascular status permits (usually by 14 days).

An alternative to a thin skin and subcutaneous flap is a free fascial flap that is skin grafted. The advantage of this flap is that it is thin. It forms a vascular bed wherein a split-thickness or full-thickness skin graft can successfully survive and still allow gliding of tendons beneath the fascial flap. Of course, this flap is used in situations where a skin graft would not take (such as directly on a tendon or cortical bone) or where a skin graft would prevent required motion even if it did take. Examples of free fascial flaps include the superficial temporal fascial flap[1,5] and the dorsal thoracic fascia[23] and the radial forearm flap.

Initially the postoperative treatment for fascial flaps is dictated by the need to monitor its vascularity and optimize conditions for take of the overlying skin graft. Usually the area is rested for the first 5 to 7 days. Thereafter, early motion can begin under the guidance of physician and therapist to make sure the skin graft is not sheared off the flap during movement. Although edema of the flap is usually not a problem, pressure dressings can be started after 3 weeks to prevent hypertrophic scarring and contracture of the skin graft.

Muscle flaps and muscle flaps with overlying skin (myo-cutaneous flaps) are most commonly used to fill in contour defects in the forearm and arm. Free muscle can also be transferred as a functional muscle transfer when local tendon transfers are not available to restore active motion. Requirements for functional muscle transfer also include an available motor donor nerve. Furthermore, great care must be taken to set the muscle at its appropriate tension at its new origin and insertion. Commonly used muscle and myo-cutaneous transfers include the latissimus dorsi,[2,15] the rectus abdominis,[48,49] and the gracilis.[19,27] Other available donor muscles that can be harvested include the internal oblique abdominis[40] and the tensor fascia lata.[36]

Where a functional muscle flap is to be performed on a nonemergency basis, the patient should be referred to therapy preoperatively to maximize passive range of motion of the involved joints and to strengthen the muscle selected for the transfer.

Following a period of immobilization (usually about 3 weeks) in a position that places the transplanted muscle in a relaxed position, gentle passive stretching exercises are initiated. During the immobilization phase for the transplanted muscle, care is taken to maintain good passive range of motion in uninvolved joints. This can be initiated once vascular stability is achieved, usually by 1 or 2 weeks. This should be cleared with the surgeon before initiation. Preoperative passive range of motion should be achieved by about 6 to 8 weeks after surgery. Passive range must be regained slowly through gentle prolonged stretching. This may be accomplished through either serial static or dynamic splinting. This stretching is begun as soon as possible to reduce adhesions and overcome myotonic contracture.[27] The clinical signs of reinnervation should be present in 2 to 4 months. As reinnervation is noted, active range-of-motion exercises are initiated. This is accomplished in the gravity-eliminated position through the use of a powder board or through active assisted range of motion initially. As strength improves, the patient is progressed to working against gravity. Full range of excursion can be expected to develop between 6 and 12 months after surgery. Muscle stimulation may be used to facilitate strengthening. Resistive exercises are initiated and progressed as tolerated. The patient can be expected to show improvements in strength for up to 2 years with final strength measures of about 50% of normal.

SUMMARY

In summary, the role of pedicled flaps and nonvascular skin grafts has been not diminished but augmented by the increased incidence of free tissue transfers. Each has a particular place in a given situation. Advances in the last 15 years have enabled the reconstructive surgeon to salvage devastating upper extremity injuries. The success rate of the tissue transfers continues to improve with increased experience on the part of the surgeon and development of improved techniques. Repeated communication between the therapist and surgeon is essential to obtain the best possible outcome with maintenance of function and cosmesis.

REFERENCES

1. Abul-Hassan HS, Ascher GD, and Acland RD: Surgical anatomy and blood supply of the fascial layers of the temporal region, Plast Reconstr Surg 77:17, 1986.
2. Bartlett SP, May JW, and Yaremchuk MJ: The latissimus dorsi muscle: a fresh cadaver study of the primary neurovascular pedicle, Plast Reconstr Surg 67:631, 1981.

3. Barwick WJ, Goodkind DJ, and Serafin DS: The free scapular flap, Plast Reconstr Surg 69:779, 1982.
4. Blair VP: Delayed transfer of long pedicle flaps in plastic surgery (face), Surg Gynecol Obstet 33:261, 1921.
5. Brent B and others: Experience with the temporoparietal fascial free flap, Plast Reconstr Surg 76:177, 1985.
6. Buncke HJ and others: Thumb replacement: great toe transportation by microvascular anastomosis, Br J Plast Surg 26:195, 1973.
7. Cormack GC and Lamberty BGH: A classification of fascio-cutaneous flaps according to their patterns of vascularization, Br J Plast Surg 37:80, 1984.
8. Daniel RK and Taylor GI: Distant transfer of an island flap by microvascular anastomosis, Plast Reconstr Surg 52:111, 1973.
9. Daniel RK and Williams HB: The free transfer of skin flaps by microvascular anastomosis: an experimental study and a reappraisal. I. The vascular supply of the skin, Plast Reconstr Surg 52:16, 1973.
10. Davis JS: Plastic surgery: principles and practice, Philadelphia, 1919, Blakiston & Co.
11. Dellon AL: Evaluation of sensibility and re-education of sensation in the hand, Baltimore, 1981, Williams & Wilkins.
12. Doi K and others: New procedure on making a thumb: one-stage reconstruction with free neurovascular flap and iliac bone graft, J Hand Surg 6A:346, 1981.
13. Epstein E and Epstein E Jr: Skin surgery, Philadelphia, 1987, WB Saunders Co.
14. Gilbert A and Tect L: The free scapula flap, Plast Reconstr Surg 69:601, 1982.
15. Gordon L, Buncke HJ, and Alpert BS: Free latissimus dorsi muscle flap with split-thickness skin graft cover: a report of 16 cases, Plast Reconstr Surg 70:173, 1982.
16. Halsted WS: Three cases of plastic surgery, Bull Johns Hopkins Hosp 7:25, 1896.
17. Hamilton SGL and Morrison WA: The scapular free flap, Br J Plast Surg 35:2, 1982.
18. Hani K and Ohmori S: Use of the gastroepiploic velles as recipient or donor vessels in the free transfer of composite flaps by microvascular anastomosis, Plast Reconstr Surg 52:541, 1973.
19. Harii K, Ohmori K, and Toril S: Free gracilis muscle transplantation with microvascular anastomosis for the treatment of facial paralysis, Plast Reconstr Surg 57:133, 1976.
20. Hauben DJ, Baruchin A, and Mahler D: On the history of the free skin graft, Ann Plast Surg 9:242, 1982.
21. Johnson CL: Physical therapists as scar modifiers, Phys Ther 64:1381, 1984.
22. Katsaros J and others: The lateral upper arm flap: anatomy and clinical applications, Ann Plast Surg 12:489, 1984.
23. Kim PS and others: The dorsal thoracic fascia: anatomic significance with clinical applications in reconstructive microsurgery, Plast Reconstr Surg 79:72, 1987.
24. Lovie MJ, Duncan GM, and Glasson DW: The ulnar artery forearm free flap, Br J Plast Surg 37:486, 1984.
25. Lowdon IMR and others: The wrap-around procedure for thumb and finger reconstruction, Microsurgery 8:154, 1987.
26. Manchot C: Die Hautarterien des Medschlichen Koerpers, Leipzig, 1889, Bogel.
27. Manktelow RT: Free muscle transplantation to provide active finger flexion, J Hand Surg 3:416, 1978.
28. May JW and others: Free neurovascular flap from the first web of the foot in hand reconstruction, J Hand Surg 2:387, 1977.
29. McCraw JB and Dibbell DG: Experimental definition of independent myocutaneous vascular territories, Plast Reconstr Surg 60:212, 1977.
30. McCraw JB, Dibbell DG, and Carraway JH: Clinical definition of independent myocutaneous vascular territories, Plast Reconstr Surg 60:341, 1977.
31. McGregor IA and Jackson IT: The groin flap, Br J Plast Surg 25:3, 1972.
32. McGregor IA and Morgan G: Axial and random pattern flaps, Br J Plast Surg 26:202, 1963.
33. Miles W: Soft tissue trauma. In Mackin EJ, editor: Hand clinics, hand rehabilitation, Philadelphia, 1986, WB Saunders.
34. Morrison WA, O'Brien BMcC, and Macleod AM: Thumb reconstruction with a free neurovascular wrap-around flap from the big toe, J Hand Surg 5:575, 1980.
35. Morrison WA, O'Brien BMcC, and Macleod AM: Ring finger transfer in reconstruction of transmetacarpal amputation, J Hand Surg 9A:4, 1984.
36. Nahai F and others: The tensor fascia lata musculocutaneous flap, Ann Plast Surg 1:372, 1978.
37. Nassif TM and others: The parascapular flap: a new cutaneous microsurgical free flap, Plast Reconstr Surg 69:591, 1982.
38. O'Brien B and others: Successful transfer of a large island flap from the groin to the foot by microvascular anastomosis, Plast Reconstr Surg 52:271, 1973.
39. Ponten B: The fasciocutaneous flap: its use in soft tissue defects of the lower leg, Br J Plast Surg 34:215, 1981.
40. Ramasastry SS, Tucker JB, and Swartz WM: The internal oblique muscle flap: an anatomic and clinical study, Plast Reconstr Surg 73:721, 1984.
41. Rudolf F and Klein L: Healing processes in skin grafts, Surg Gynecol Obstet 136:41, 1973.
42. Santos LF: Dos retallro escapular: um novo retallro livre microcirurgico, Rev Bras Cir 70:133, 1980.
43. Scheker LR, Kleinart HE, and Hanel DP: Lateral arm composite tissue transfer to ipsilateral hand defects, J Hand Surg 12A:665, 1987.
44. Song R and others: The upper arm free flap, Clin Plast Surg 9:27, 1982.
45. Soutar DS and Tanner SB: The radial forearm flap in the management of soft tissue injuries to the hand, Br J Plast Surg 37:18, 1984.
46. Stern PJ: Free neurovascular cutaneous toe pulp transfer for thumb reconstruction, Microsurgery 8:158, 1987.
47. Tansini I: Sopra il mio nuovo processo di amputazione della mammella, Gazzetta Medica Italiana 57:141, 1906.
48. Taylor GI, Corlett RJ, and Boyd JB: The extended deep inferior epigastric flap: a clinical technique, Plast Reconstr Surg 72:751, 1983.
49. Taylor GI, Corlett RJ, and Boyd JB: The versatile deep inferior epigastric (inferior rectus abdominis) flap, Br J Plast Surg 37:330, 1984.
50. Urbaniak JR: Thumb reconstruction by microsurgery. In Murray JA, editor: Instructional Course Lectures, St. Louis, 1984, The CV Mosby Co.
51. Urbaniak JR and others: The vascularized cutaneous scapular flap, Plast Reconstr Surg 69:772, 1982.
52. Vistnes LM: Grafting of skin, Surg Clin North Am 57:939, 1977.
53. Yang G and others: Forearm free skin flap transplantation, Nat Med J China 61:139, 1981.
54. Yoshimura M and others: Peroneal island flap for skin defects in the lower extremity, J Bone Joint Surg 67A:935, 1985.

IV
FRACTURES

18

Fractures and traumatic conditions of the wrist

Gary K. Frykman and Elvert F. Nelson

The wrist is a complex joint with 21 separate articulations and a network of ligaments. This unique joint complex produces flexion and extension, radial and ulnar deviation, and axial rotation. Powerful proximal forearm muscles are transmitted across this joint to move finger joints delicately and place the hand in an almost infinite number of spatial orientations. Nowhere else in the body are so many tendons, nerves, and vessels confined to such a concentrated area. A fall on the outstretched hand is so common that a large variety of wrist injuries can occur. A great deal of force must be absorbed by a very limited area, making the wrist vulnerable to injury. The frequency of wrist injuries, the variety of injury mechanisms, and confusing multiple roentgenographic patterns make exact diagnosis of traumatic wrist injuries sometimes difficult even for the experienced clinician.

Unlike many other conditions, a careful history and physical examination on a patient with a wrist injury is not always helpful to the clinician attempting to make a diagnosis. Frequently the history is vague and incomplete and the physical examination may show diffuse swelling, generalized tenderness, and variable limitations in wrist motion. Deformity, shortening of the wrist, and point tenderness make the diagnosis easier. Usually one must rely primarily upon roentgenograms to make the exact diagnosis. Familiarity with normal bony anatomy and carpal alignment is essential if one expects to identify subtle malalignment and fractures with superimposed images (Figs. 18-1 and 18-2). The diagnosis of a wrist sprain must be made with extreme caution. When the wrist has sustained a significant injury, it must be treated in spite of normal roentgenograms. When serial clinical and roentgenographic follow-ups have failed to demonstrate any serious condition, the wrist can be treated symptomatically.

It is helpful to be acquainted with the possible traumatic wrist conditions and the frequency of their occurrence. Large series of carpal injuries show the following breakdown: 60% to 70% scaphoid fractures, 10% carpal dislocations and fracture dislocations (traumatic carpal instability), 10% dorsal chip fractures, 3% lunate fractures, and 7% all other carpal fractures.[22]

PREVENTION OF COMPLICATIONS

A great deal can be done to prevent or minimize complications after wrist injuries. An accurate early diagnosis with adequate reduction and immobolization not only minimizes discomfort but also decreases swelling. Edema can be decreased by early cooling and elevation of the injured extremity. A well-molded cast avoiding extreme palmar flexion and ulnar deviation will help diminish compression of the median nerve in the carpal tunnel. Early active finger motion must be started. It is essential that the form of immobilization used allows full metacarpophalangeal flexion of all the fingers (Figs. 18-3 and 18-4). The problem of neural or vascular compromise early in the course of injury can be avoided by use of a sugar-tong cast. When reduction is lost in comminuted or unstable distal radius fractures, prompt application of a self-contained traction apparatus will not only frequently anatomically reduce the fracture but also allow unrestricted finger and thumb motion. Frequent follow-up and serial roentgenograms with remanipulation or operative intervention when indicated will minimize malunion and possible carpal instability.

Stiffness of the shoulder, elbow, and hand can usually be averted by proper education and avoidance of a sling. Although a sling has traditionally been used for patients with traumatic wrist conditions, it discourages movement of the entire extremity. The shoulder-hand-finger syndrome may occur because of inadequate muscular activity with subsequent venous stasis.[65] It is the responsibility of the physician to educate the injured patient in frequent, regular active range-of-motion exercises to all the nonimmobilized joints in the upper extremity from the shoulder to the fingers. From the beginning the patient is taught to place the injured hand over the head at least 50 times a day and perform active range of motion of the fingers a thousand times a day. When watching television, he is told to move his fingers at least 10 times with each commercial. This kind of exaggeration will get the point across that we are serious about keeping the free joints moving actively and keeping the injured upper extremity elevated.

DISTAL RADIUS FRACTURES
Colles' fracture

The distal radius fracture is one of the most common fractures of the human skeleton. It was originally accurately described by an Irish surgeon, Abraham Colles, as a nonarticular fracture occurring 1½ inches proximally to the radiocarpal joint.[16] The eponym "Colles' fracture" is generally used to describe any fracture involving the distal radius with dorsal displacement. It is caused by a fall on the outstretched hand, producing a variety of fracture patterns. A practical classification of these fractures is by Frykman,[26] who distinguished between extra-articular and intra-articular fractures and stressed the importance of the ulnar side of the wrist. The diagnosis is easily made when one finds a painful swollen wrist where the dorsally displaced distal radius gives the appearance of an upside-down dinner

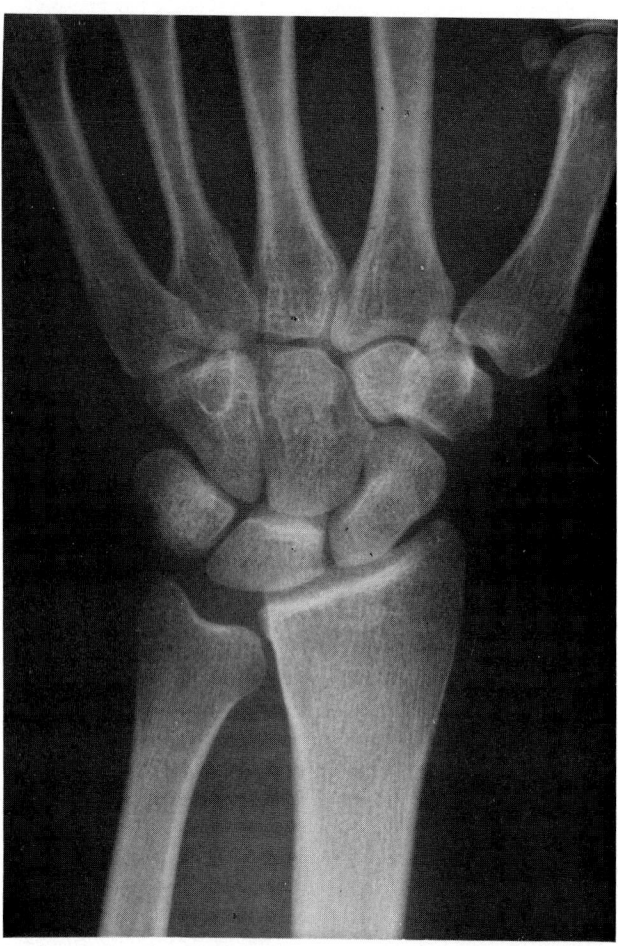

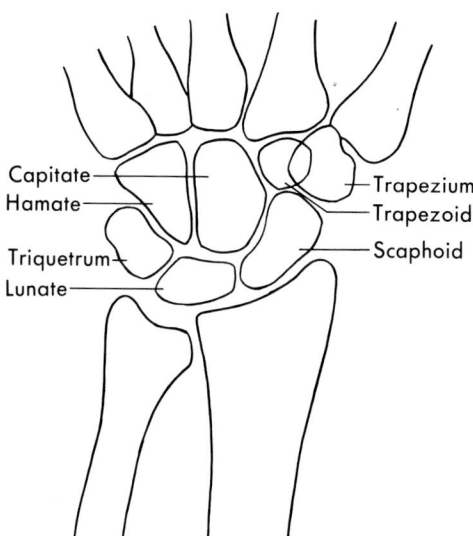

Fig. 18-1 Anteroposterior roentgenogram of a normal wrist. Radial styloid is distal to ulnar styloid with an ulnar-slope articular surface of distal radius. There is normally a wide space on roentgenogram between the distal ulna and the lunate and triquetrum. Scaphoid spans proximal and distal carpal row. There is an equal space between each carpal bone with overlapping of trapezium and trapezoid. Lunate is quadrilateral, and scaphoid is peanut or canoe shaped.

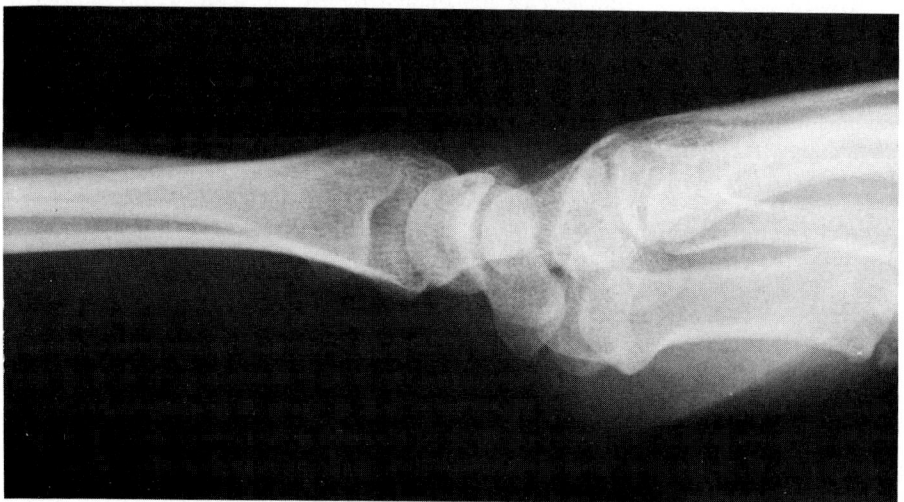

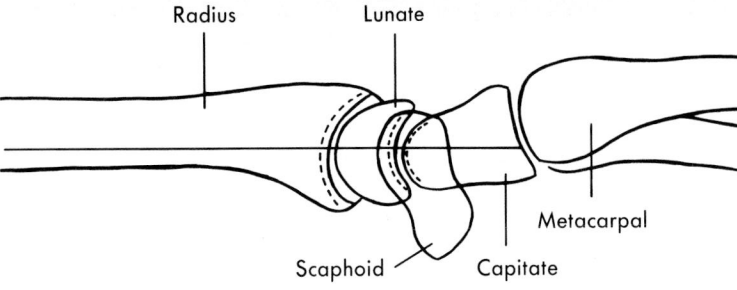

Fig. 18-2 Lateral roentgenogram of normal wrist. There is a slight volar tilt to distal radius articular surface. Because radial styloid extends distally, it is superimposed on lunate. Long axis of distal radius, lunate, capitate, and metacarpal bones are colinear. Articular surfaces of distal radius, lunate, and capitate fit together like multiple C's facing same direction.

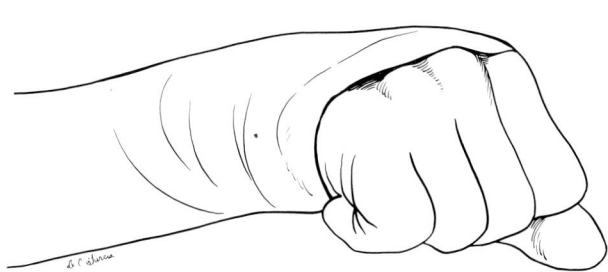

Fig. 18-3 Wrist immobilization. Volarly, cast or splint should extend only to distal palmar crease allowing full metacarpophalangeal flexion. This fitting not only keeps the joints from getting stiff but decreases finger edema by allowing active finger motion during wrist immobilization.

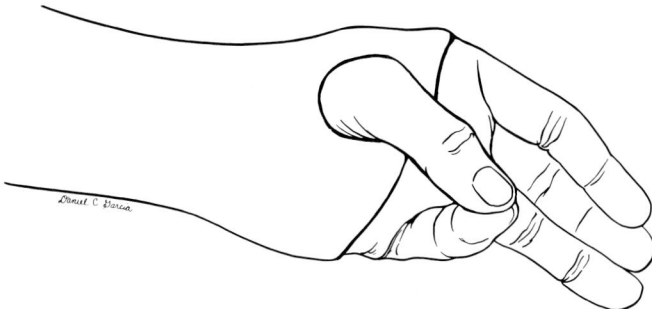

Fig. 18-4 Wrist immobilization. Except for injuries involving thumb axis or scaphoid, thumb should be free during wrist immobilization. Plaster and padding should not cover thumb metacarpal to allow full opposition.

fork. Palpation reveals a tense, tender wrist with a prominent ulnar styloid and frequently with the radial styloid at the same level as the distal ulna. Roentgenograms in two planes confirm the diagnosis (Fig. 18-5). Care must be exercised to avoid missing an associated carpal fracture, carpal dislocation, or subluxation of the distal radioulnar joint.

Treatment of Colles' fractures is considerably more controversial than its diagnosis. Over 85% of these fractures require some form of reduction.[41,59] General anesthesia, regional block anesthesia, or local anesthesia injected into the fracture hematoma are required before manipulation. Once radial length is restored by traction or manipulation, the dorsal angulation may be corrected by a palmar-directed manipulation of the distal radius. The reduction is then maintained by dorsal and palmar padded plaster splints molded so that three-point pressure is applied dorsally over the distal fragment and the midforearm and palmarly over the distal aspect of the proximal fragment.[14] The wrist is placed in a slight palmar flexion and ulnar deviation. There is controversy about whether the forearm should be immobilized in pronation[52] or supination.[74] We prefer the more pronated position because if forearm rotation is lost permanently, it is more functional for the forearm to be in pronation. Successful noninvasive immobilization techniques include sugar-tong splints, short-arm casts, long-arm casts, and functional bracing. One method has not been shown to be statistically superior. Regardless of which form of immobilization is used, full finger motion must be permitted, significant edema or neurologic symptoms must be avoided, and frequent clinical follow-up is mandatory. Settling and displacement of the distal radius may occur during the first 3 weeks.[71] Remanipulation during this time is sometimes necessary.

The exact clinical and roentgenographic criteria for an acceptable fracture reduction are not established. There is good correlation between anatomic and functional results. Radial shortening is the most disabling deformity and must be corrected if possible.[26,29] It contributes to distal radioulnar problems and compromises hand mobility and power. Dorsal tilting is the most difficult deformity to correct but the least disabling, with up to 25 degrees of residual angulation associated with a good functional result.[52] If there has been no loss of reduction during the first 3 weeks, the elbow is usually freed by application of a short-arm cast for another

2 to 4 weeks. Immobilization is discontinued when point tenderness at the fracture site no longer exists and roentgenographic evidence of fracture consolidation is present.

The reductions of severely comminuted, unstable, or intraarticular distal radius fractures are extremely difficult to hold with simple plaster immobilization. Various self-contained skeletal traction systems have been developed to hold the unstable fracture out to length (Fig. 18-6). Percutaneous pins are placed proximal and distal to the fracture site through the metacarpal and proximal forearm bones.[71] Fracture reduction can be maintained by incorporation of pins into the plaster of a short-arm cast.[92] We have found that external fixation devices have been as effective as pins in plaster in maintaining reduction but also have the advantage of being lighter in weight, are less restrictive in allowing finger mobilization, and seem to decrease edema formation more than pins in plaster.[94] During the 8 weeks of immobilization that these fractures require, the elbow and fingers can be free to maintain their mobility. Since Bohler[5] first used external fixation to treat unstable Colles' fractures, numerous modifications have improved overall results.[18,35] At least 11 different external fixators are available for treating wrist injuries with rigidity varying as much as tenfold from the least to the most rigid.[28] However, similar functional results are reported independent of the type of fixator used.[17,25,67,102] Improved pin design,[34] the use of open pin insertion, precise pin placement using image intensification, and avoidance of excessive ligamentotaxis have all contributed to reducing complications. Wrist stiffness, however, tends to occur with the 8 weeks of external fixation required.

Dynamic external fixators are now available to allow early wrist flexion and extension while maintaining radial length. Applying the external fixator to allow wrist motion requires considerable care. Patient cooperation and the absence of osteoporosis are required for success. One study shows improved wrist motion with a dynamic external fixator.[15]

To unload the wrist, the external fixator can be used to treat conditions independent of unstable Colles' fractures. Preliminary studies report favorable results using wrist frames in stage I Kienbock's disease[85] and as an adjunct to open reduction and internal fixation of complex carpal dislocations.[24]

Complications. Complications of Colles' fractures are common; they include the following:

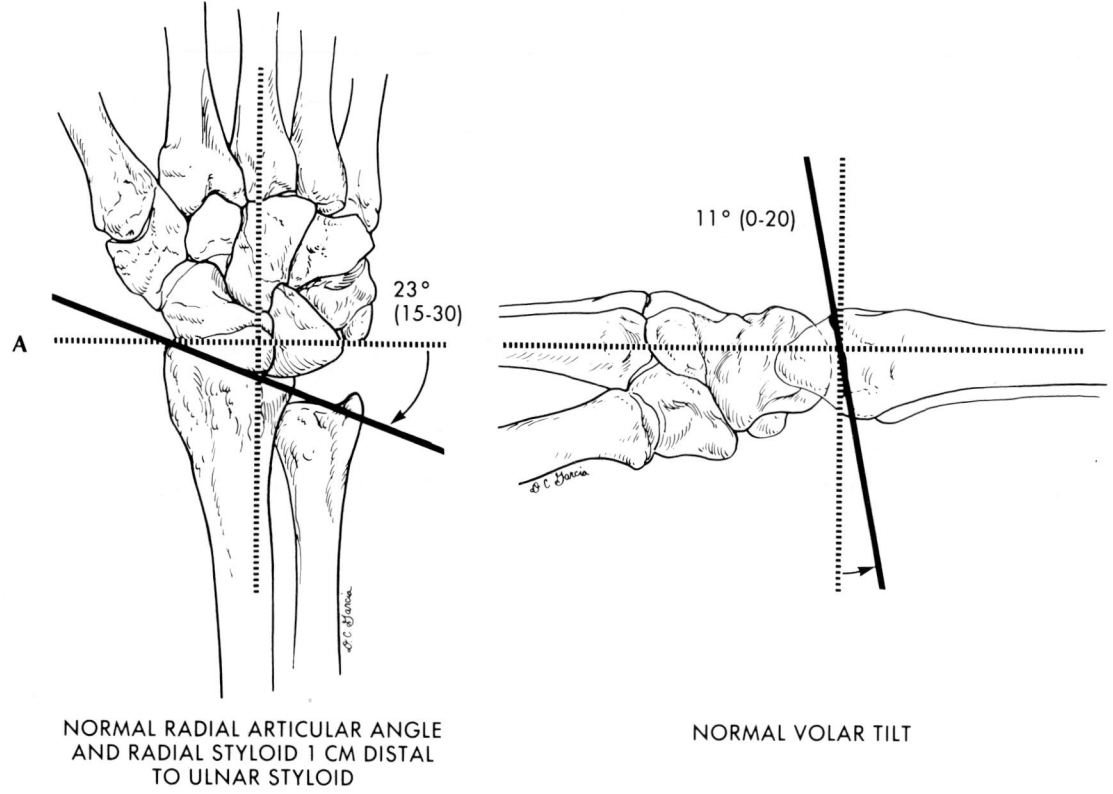

NORMAL RADIAL ARTICULAR ANGLE
AND RADIAL STYLOID 1 CM DISTAL
TO ULNAR STYLOID

NORMAL VOLAR TILT

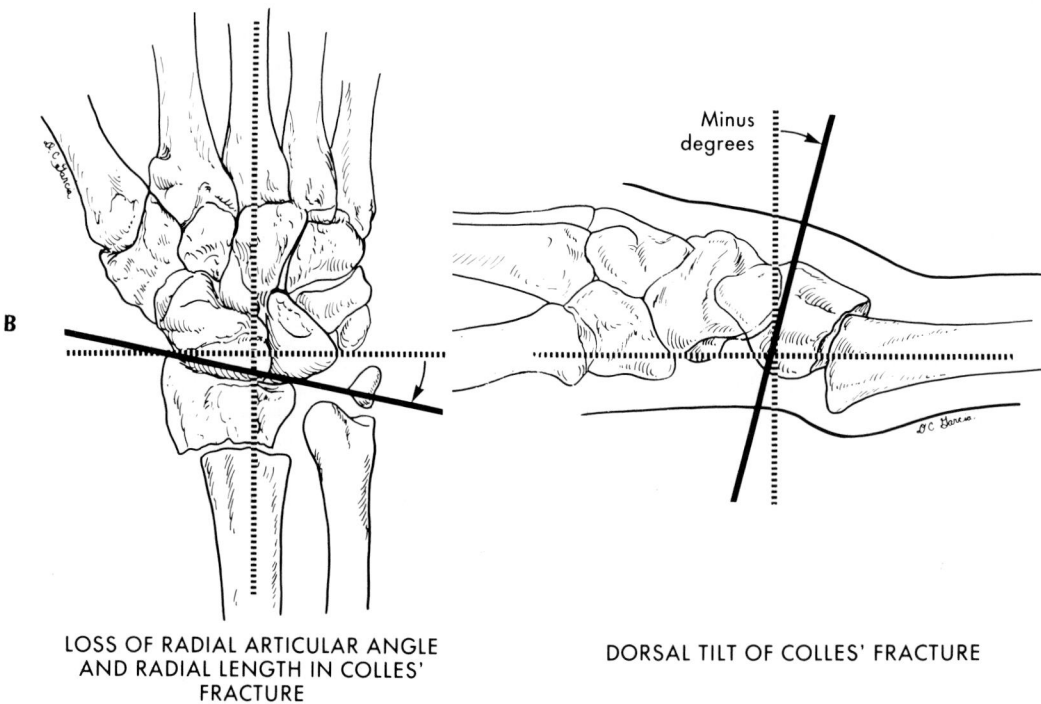

LOSS OF RADIAL ARTICULAR ANGLE
AND RADIAL LENGTH IN COLLES'
FRACTURE

DORSAL TILT OF COLLES' FRACTURE

Fig. 18-5 **A,** Normal wrist. Normal ulnar tilt of distal radius is 23 degrees to a line perpendicular to long axis of radius. Normal volar tilt is 11 degrees to a line perpendicular to long axis of radius. **B,** Colles' fracture.

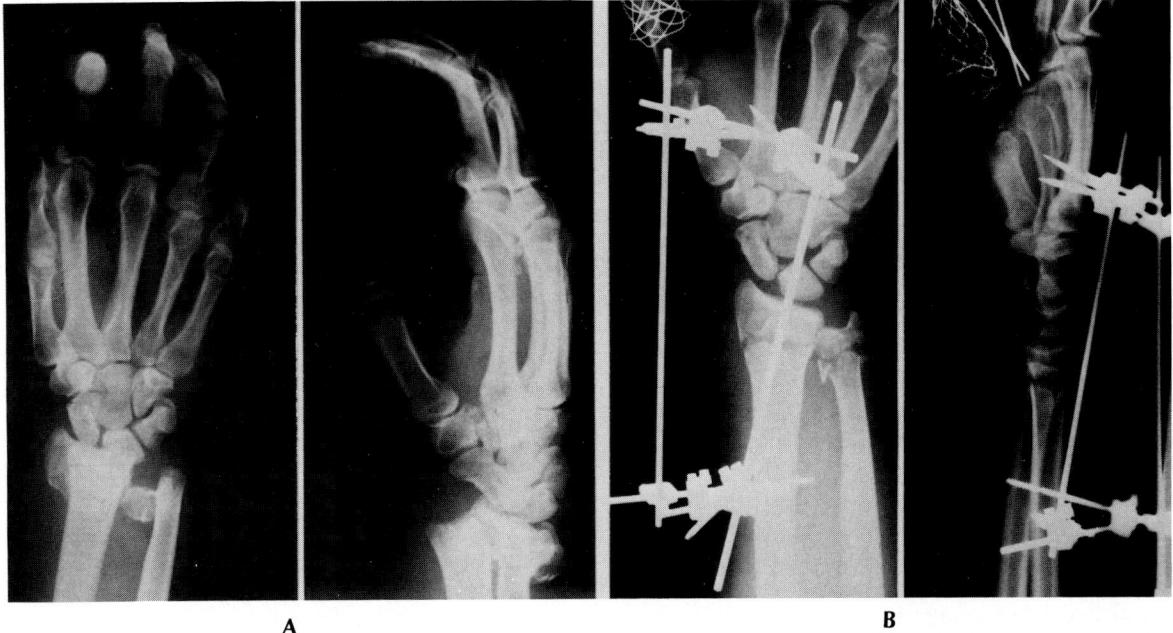

Fig. 18-6   Comminuted distal radius fracture. **A,** This severely comminuted distal radius and ulna fracture was not amenable to a closed reduction and plaster immobilization. **B,** Hoffman external fixator. Fracture was reduced and length reestablished with finger trap traction. External system was applied to maintain the reduction, and distraction was released.

Stiffness of finger, wrist, forearm, elbow, and shoulder
Carpal tunnel syndrome
Malunion
Weakness of grip
Radiocarpal arthritis
Distal radioulnar dysfunction
Extensor pollicis longus rupture
Posttraumatic reflex sympathetic dystrophy
Intrinsic contracture

Twenty percent of patients have residual symptoms and 10% have significant functional impairment.[52] The last complication listed, intrinsic contracture, deserves additional comment. Although rarely mentioned in the literature as a complication of wrist fractures, we have found intrinsic tightness in most cases where there has been considerable swelling after wrist trauma. We hypothesize that this is a limited intrinsic ischemic contracture caused by excessive swelling and pressure in the interosseous compartments of the hand. It may be resistant to hand therapy and splinting and may require surgical release of the interossei.[12]

The poorest results can be expected in cases of intra-articular involvement, pronounced initial displacement, severe comminution, and evidence of damage to the ulnar side of the wrist.[26] The young adult with vigorous functional demands who sustains a severe distal radius fracture has a guarded prognosis.

Smith's fracture

Smith's fracture of the distal radius is frequently called a "reverse Colles' fracture."[77] It occurs in a younger age group and is less frequent than the Colles' fracture. The mechanism of injury was classically believed to be a fall on the back of the hand. Other proposed mechanisms include a fall on the supinated wrist followed by pronation of the upper limb, and motorcycle injuries where the knuckles of the hand gripping the handlebar sustain a dorsal blow.

Three clinical types of Smith's fractures have been noted by Thomas based on the obliquity of the fracture line.[88] The patient presents with the hand and wrist palmarly displaced in reference to the forearm giving the appearance of a "garden spade." Compared with Colles' fractures, these injuries have dorsal displacement of the ulnar head and less noticeable subcutaneous crepitance. Lateral roentgenograms confirm the palmarly displaced distal radius (Fig. 18-7).

Treatment of Smith's fractures consists of longitudinal traction, manual manipulation with a dorsally direct force applied to the distal radius, and immobilization in supination and neutral wrist position.[104] For many years the wrist was immobilized in dorsiflexion,[6] but recently it has been shown that this position placed the radiocarpal joint contact area volarly so that the deformity is increased,[88] and thus slight palmar flexion is recommended. Similar to Colles' fractures, loss of reduction or severe comminution requires remanipulation and possible self-contained traction. Uncomplicated Smith's fractures require long-arm plaster immobilization for 3 weeks followed by a short-arm cast for another 2 to 3 weeks. Complications of these palmarly displaced fractures are essentially similar to Colles' fractures. Median nerve injury is more common in Smith's fracture. Making up only 5% to 10% of distal radius fractures, these injuries are not regularly seen, and misinterpretation of the initial roentgenogram along with incomplete reduction is a problem leading to a worse prognosis compared to the Colles' fracture.[41,100]

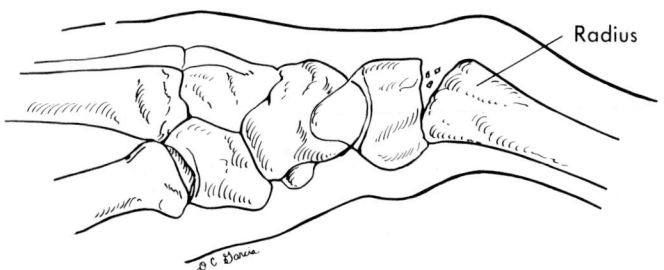

Fig. 18-7 Smith's fracture.

Barton's fracture

John Barton described this injury as "a subluxation of the wrist consequent to a fracture through the articular surface of the carpal extremity of the radius."[3] This original description refers to dorsal and volar marginal articular fractures, but Barton believed the former was more common. Later, confusion arose about whether a Barton's fracture involved the dorsal or volar articular margin, perhaps because the dorsal injury occurs less frequently.[5] The volar marginal fracture is actually a type III Smith's fracture described by Thomas.[88] Nevertheless, these injuries are called "dorsal Barton's" and "volar Barton's fractures" in current literature (Fig. 18-8).[89]

The mechanism of injury and the clinical presentation are similar to those of either the Colles' or Smith's fractures. The diagnosis can usually be confirmed with a lateral roentgenogram, but occasionally oblique films may be necessary to clarify the extent of articular involvement and displacement.

A common mistake is to treat the dorsal Barton's like a Colles' fracture. Immobilization of the wrist in *palmar flexion* allows the lunate to press against the unstable dorsal fragment and push it proximally and dorsally. The tendency for redislocation after manipulative reduction is actually increased because the longitudinal axis of the carpus is directed into the fracture site, creating instability.[89] This concept has been referred to as "Barton's enigma."

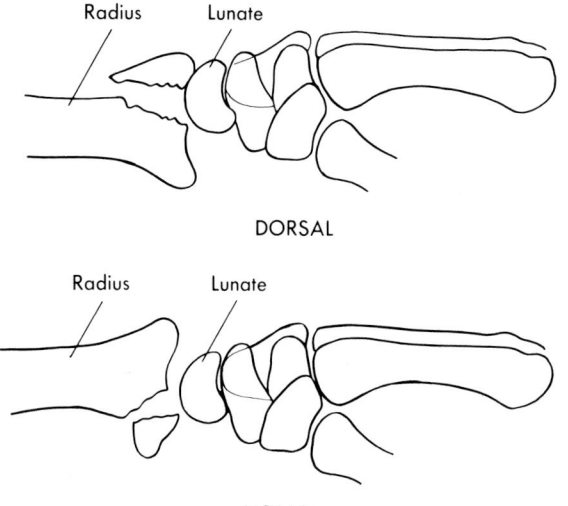

Fig. 18-8 Barton's fracture.

To achieve a stable reduction the wrist is immobilized toward the fracture. This places the lunate and the longitudinal axis of the carpus against the intact articular surface of the distal radius. The dorsal Barton's fracture is immobilized in slight dorsiflexion, and the volar Barton's fracture is immobilized in slight palmar flexion. Open reduction and internal fixation are indicated in both fracture types if there is involvement of a large portion of the articular surface or inability to obtain and maintain satisfactory joint congruity after manipulative reduction.[20,22,89] Operative modalities include T-plate, percutaneous pin fixation, or bone screws. The joint can be explored, loose cartilaginous fragments removed, and anatomic reduction obtained. If good stability is achieved surgically, early active wrist motion can be started.

CARPAL FRACTURES
Scaphoid fractures

Carpal fractures are about one tenth as frequent as distal radius fractures. Scaphoid fractures account for over 60% of all carpal injuries.[5] The scaphoid is the preferred term for the carpal navicular bone; it is canoe shaped with four of its six surfaces covered with articular cartilage. It spans the proximal and distal carpal row. It is the principle bone block to extreme wrist dorsiflexion, making it particularly vulnerable to injury. The blood supply to the scaphoid enters largely distally through dorsal and lateral volar vessels.[86] This diminished blood supply to the proximal scaphoid makes fractures in this area susceptible to avascular necrosis.

The mechanism of injury is similar to the mechanism of distal radius fractures. A fall on the outstretched hand forces the scaphoid between the dorsal lip of the distal radius and the palmar radiocapitate ligament. Point tenderness in the anatomic snuffbox is a constant and dependable physical finding in patients with scaphoid fractures. Negative roentgenographic findings do not exclude a scaphoid fracture. All patients with injury to the wrist and point tenderness in the scaphoid region should be treated as if they had a fracture until it has been disproved by negative roentgenograms and clinical findings at 2 and 4 weeks.[22]

Classification of scaphoid fractures is based on anatomic location. The four usual sites of fractures are distally through the tuberosity, the distal third, the waist (Fig. 18-9), and through the proximal pole. The waist fractures in the middle third are most common, making up about 70% of all scaphoid fractures. Prognosis for healing is related to the site, obliquity of the fracture, promptness of diagnosis, and treatment.

The more horizontal the fracture line in relation to the long axis of the scaphoid, the more rapidly healing will occur. There is a great variation in healing times between the anatomic location and the fracture types. The richly nourished distal tuberosity fractures heal in 5 to 6 weeks, while the relatively avascular proximal third fractures may require 20 weeks or longer to heal. The acute scaphoid fracture must be immobilized. The most frequent type of support is the short-arm guantlet type of cast from the thumb proximal phalanx to the proximal forearm with the wrist in slight dorsiflexion and radial deviation.[72] There is no agreement about whether the elbow or the entire thumb should be immobilized during fracture healing. The duration of

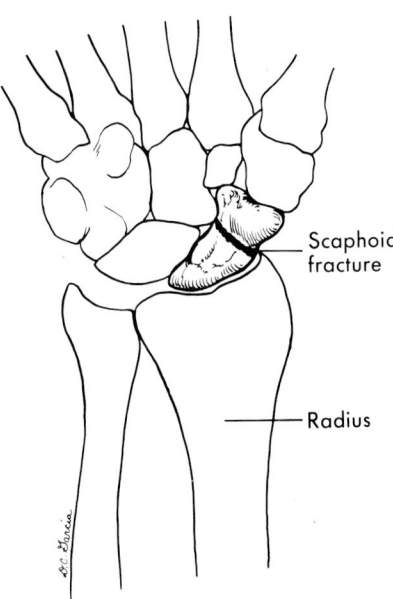

Fig. 18-9   Scaphoid fracture. This fracture is in waist, the most common site.

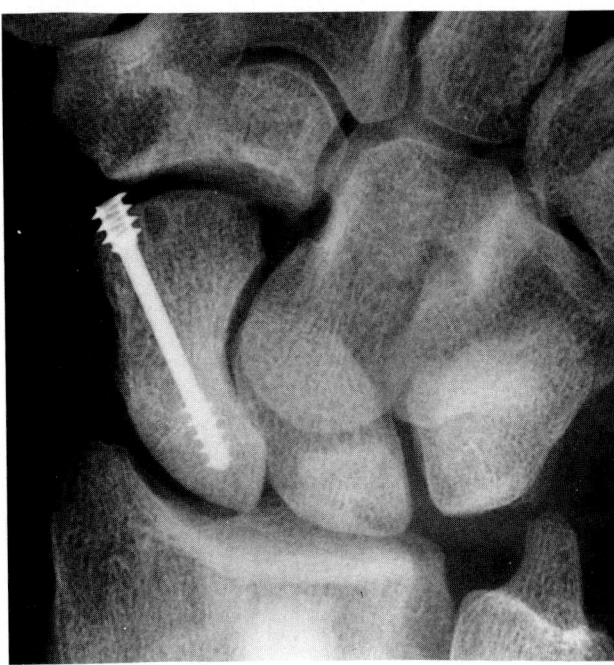

Fig. 18-10   Healed scaphoid fracture after Herbert screw.

immobilization is dependent on roentgenographic evidence of trabeculae across the fracture site and the absence of point tenderness in the scaphoid region. In spite of the well-recognized problems of scaphoid nonunions, 90% of these fractures heal without complications if treated early and casted properly.[56,60]

Nonunion is the most frequent and disabling complication associated with scaphoid fractures. Differentiating between a delayed union and an established nonunion taxes even the most astute clinician. Roentgenographic evidence of delayed union includes absorption at the fracture line, cystic changes, and sclerosis[60] adjacent to the fracture. Many delayed unions will eventually heal if properly immobilized for a long enough interval. The scaphoid nonunion is a fracture that fails to show roentgenographic evidence of healing on three separate monthly examinations. Not all scaphoid nonunions are symptomatic or disabling. It is not uncommon to see an untreated ununited scaphoid fracture on an individual unaware of the problem.

The real value of treating asymptomatic scaphoid nonunions has been questioned. However, recent long-term studies on untreated scaphoid fractures reveal a progressive deterioration of the wrist from carpal instability to periscaphoid arthritis.[57,93]

In the absence of periscaphoid arthritis, nonunions require operative intervention with bone grafting through either a dorsal or volar approach.[36,72] Until recently, internal fixation of scaphoid nonunions had not gained popularity. Consistent, reliable results are difficult to obtain, because the internal fixation is technically rigorous and firm fixation is not always possible.[39,58] Herbert has developed a new bone screw that seems to offer several advantages over conventional compression screws.[42] The Herbert screw is smaller in diameter, with different pitched threads on each end. It

provides firm fixation by causing compression when tightened (Fig. 18-10). Implant removal is not necessary.

Electrical stimulation of scaphoid nonunions is a viable nonsurgical treatment alternative.[10] The treatment of nonunion scaphoid fractures by pulsed electromagnetic field (PEMF) and thumb spica cast immobilization is a simple, low-risk, reliable method associated with an 80% union.[27] The PEMF method is considered for undisplaced, nonunited fractures in the absence of carpal instability that are less than 5 years after injury.

When local degenerative changes are present, different salvage procedures may be necessary. Radiocarpal or intercarpal fusion is usually reserved for the young patient with extreme functional demands. Scaphoid replacement arthroplasty is better suited to the older patient with limited wrist stress.[81] Other operative modalities include radial styloidectomy,[76] excision of one or both fragments,[22] proximal row carpectomy,[41,45] and wrist arthrodesis.

Triquetrum fractures

Fractures of the triquetrum are the second most common carpal fractures. Located on the ulnar side of the proximal carpal row, the triquetrum forms one of the anchors of the wrist with strong volar and dorsal attachments. Excessive wrist dorsiflexion and ulnar deviation produce the common dorsal avulsion fracture when the hamate shears the posteroradial projection.[11] Pain and swelling on the dorsal ulnar aspect of the wrist help make the diagnosis, and a lateral roentgenogram of the wrist in flexion usually shows the avulsion fracture. It may be easily overlooked on the anteroposterior roentgenogram. The isolated ligamentous avulsions respond well to 4 to 6 weeks of immobilization with a short-arm cast in wrist dorsiflexion. If there is considerable displacement, some of these chip fractures do not heal and require excision and ligamentous repair. Rarer triquetral body fractures are caused by impingement or direct blows and are easily identifiable and heal with 6 weeks of immobilization.[4]

Lunate injuries

Accounting for about 7% of all carpal injuries, lunate fractures are the third most common carpal fractures. A fall on the outstretched hand produces a translational compression force when the lunate is caught between the capitate and the dorsal aspect of the distal radius articular surface. If a dislocation does not occur, the lunate will fracture. Initial roentgenograms may be misinterpreted as normal unless one carefully searches for a thin lucent line across the proximal pole of the lunate on the anteroposterior film. Roentgenographic diagnosis may be difficult. If the diagnosis of lunate fracture can be made initially, immobilization in a short-arm cast until healing is well established in 6 to 8 weeks decreases the long-term morbidity.

Kienbock's disease. Lunate sclerosis, fragmentation, collapse, or shortening, commonly termed lunatomalacia, was originally recognized by Kienbock in 1910.[46] This interesting condition has achieved considerable attention in medical literature during the past 75 years. The cause remains obscure[48] and a reliable method of treatment has not been clearly established. There is a significant association between Kienbock's disease and negative ulnar variance.[30,44] In most normal wrists, the distal articular surface of the radius and ulna are at the same level with even loading across the proximal surface of the lunate (Fig. 18-11). In the negative ulnar variant wrist, the ulna is proximal to the radius. The ulnar half of the lunate lacks protective support and is subject to uneven compression. With the wrist in dorsiflexion, the lunate is subject to a nutcracker effect between the ulnar border of the radius and the capitate. In extreme dorsiflexion, the lunate is subject to opposite tensile forces of the volar radiolunate and lunotriquetral ligaments.[2] The relative significance of these observations to the cause of Kienbock's disease is not known. Lunatomalacia is probably the result of a combination of factors, including repetitive compression leading to a stress fracture. The uneven stress across the lunate and the nutcracker effect interrupt normal fracture healing and lead to eventual collapse and fragmentation.

Patient's with Kienbock's disease may initially have varying degrees of disability. The usual clinical pattern consists of wrist pain, limitation of dorsiflexion, point tenderness over the dorsal aspect of the lunate, and weakness of grip. Roentgenograms confirm the diagnosis of Kienbock's disease, which is classified into four stages[51] based on roentgenographic changes in the lunate. In stage I the roentgenograms are normal or show a transverse linear fracture. In stage II the density of a normally shaped lunate is increased. Stage III (Fig. 18-12) shows lunate collapse and fragmentation with proximal migration of the capitate. In stage IV perilunate osteoarthritis exists.

Several treatment alternatives have been proposed since the condition was recognized. These include hot compresses,[46] prolonged immobilization,[78] lunate excision,[46,82] insertion of a lunate implant,[50] ulnar[80] lengthening,[2] radial shortening,[1] proximal row carpectomy,[45] limited wrist arthrodesis,[101] and total wrist arthrodesis.[33] The treatment alternatives depend on the roentgenographic stage of the disease.[51] In stage I the lunate can be unloaded with an external fixator and stimulated electrically or unloaded with a joint-leveling operation consisting of radial shortening or ulnar lengthening.[85] In stage II the lunate is fragmented but not collapsed, and a joint-leveling operation is indicated. With stage III, combined lunate fragmentation and collapse with

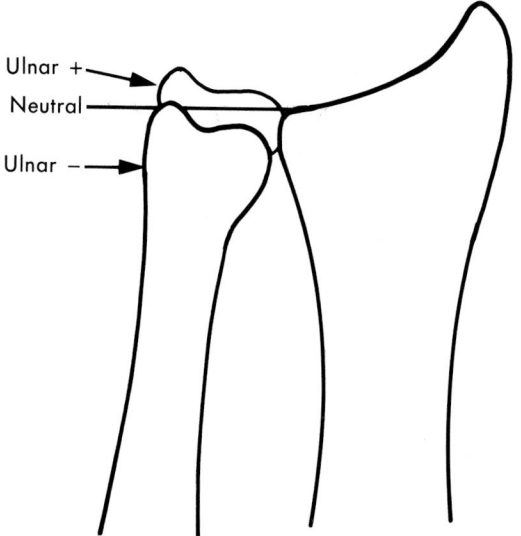

Fig. 18-11 Ulnar variance. Most people have the distal ulnar articular surface even with the distal radius. The ulnar minus individuals have a higher incidence of Kienböck's disease. Those individuals with ulnar plus variance may have ulnocarpal impingement.

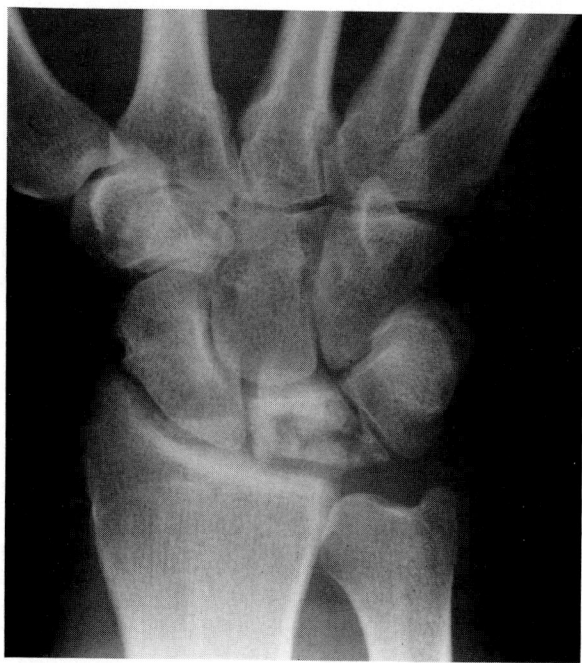

Fig. 18-12 Kienböck's disease stage III. In this stage there is fragmentation, change in shape of the lunate, and in later stages, proximal migration of the capitate.

carpal instability occur. Silastic or tendon replacement of the lunate must be combined with a midcarpal limited arthrodesis to correct both problems.[101] In stage IV, the aggressiveness of the salvage procedure depends on the severity of the perilunate osteoarthritis. In milder cases, a formal wrist arthrodesis can be avoided by combining a lunate implant with an appropriate scaphotrapezium-trapezoid arthrodesis. The treatment options are clearly greater, and the results are better when the diagnosis is made early. None of the treatment options in use gives uniformly excellent results.

Other carpal fractures

The remainder of carpal fractures are rare with the clinical and roentgenographic diagnosis difficult. Fractures of the trapezium are usually associated with fracture-dislocation of the thumb metacarpal base (Bennett's fracture). Capitate fractures are rare. The central position of this bone in the carpus protects it between the proximal carpal row and stable central metacarpal bones. Pisiform and hamate fractures may occur from a direct fall on the outstretched hand or a direct blow from the handle of rackets, golf clubs, or baseball bats.[8,91] Ulnar nerve symptoms may be present. The diagnosis may be missed, since routine roentgenograms are normal. Point tenderness over the pisiform or hook of the

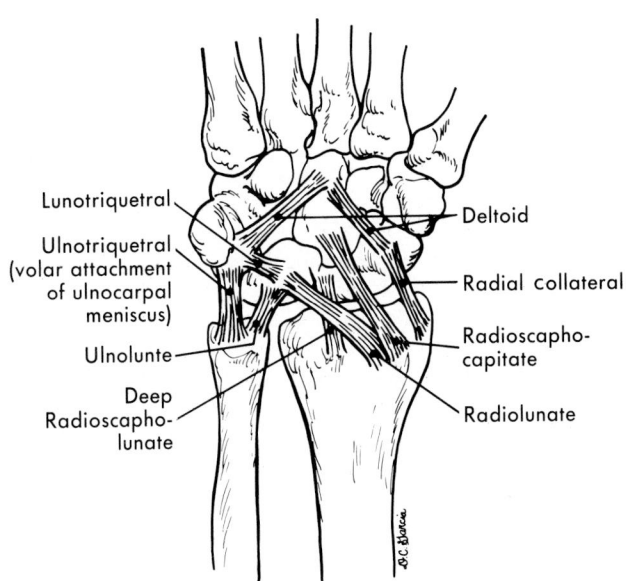

Fig. 18-13 Palmar carpal ligaments. This schematic representation of volar wrist ligaments shows a proximal and distal V-shaped system. Majority of these intracapsular ligaments originate on radius laterally and triquetrum medially and insert on their adjacent carpal bones.

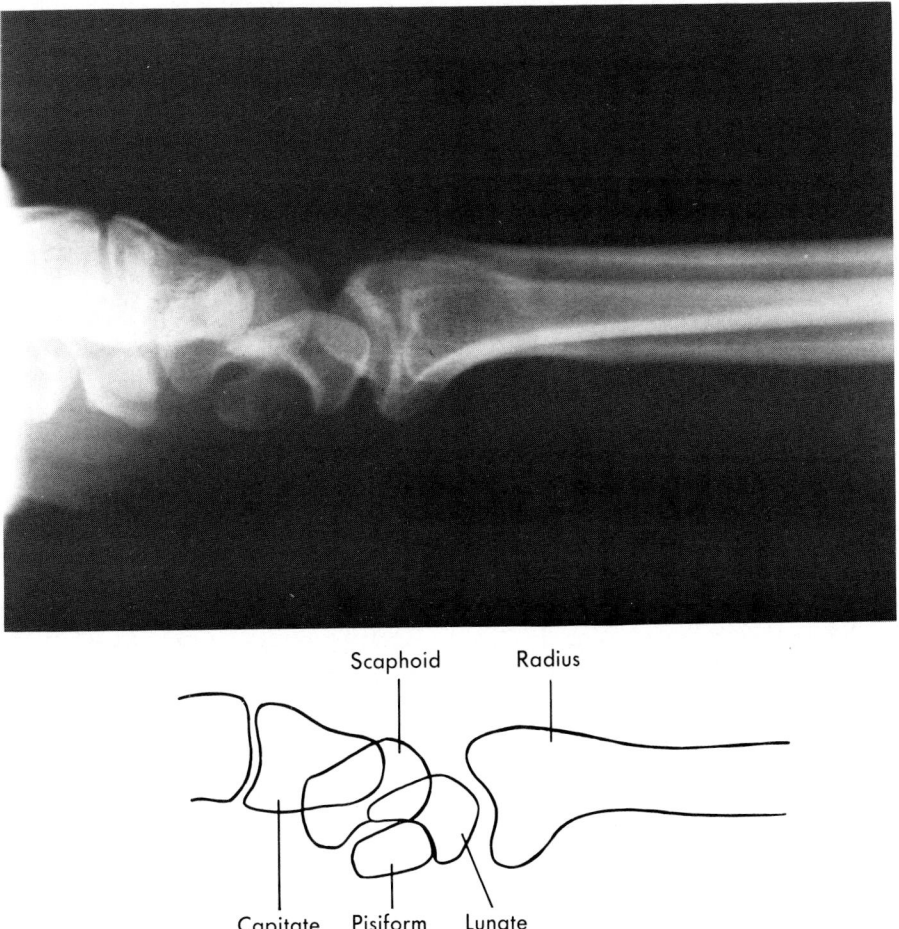

Fig. 18-14 Dorsal perilunate dislocation. Lateral roentgenogram of this injury shows scaphoid and capitate displaced dorsally to lunate.

hamate and a carpal tunnel view will help make the diagnosis. Excision of the painful fragment may be necessary if casting does not help.[79]

CARPAL DISLOCATIONS

Before any discussion of carpal dislocation, a description of the normal complex intercarpal relationships is essential (Figs. 18-1 and 18-2). The most important film when examining suspected carpal dislocations is the lateral wrist roentgenogram.

Carpal instability depends on the maintenance of bony architecture interlaced with ligaments. The volar wrist ligaments (Fig. 18-13) are intracapsular and more substantial than the dorsal ligaments. The scaphoid is supported proximally by the volar radioscaphoid and scaphoid lunate ligaments and distally by the radial collateral, radiocapitate, and deltoid ligaments. The triquetrum is important in volar ulnar stability, with all ligaments converging on this bone like the spokes of a wheel from their origins in the lunate (lunotriquetral), the ulna (ulnotriquetral), and the capitate (deltoid ligament).[83] The general configuration of the volar ligaments is a double V-shaped structure with an area of potential weakness between them lying directly over the capitate-lunate articulation.[37] The dorsal wrist ligaments are weaker and less clearly defined.

Perilunate dislocations

Most carpal dislocations are of the dorsal perilunate type (Fig. 18-14). The lunate is the usual bone around which the remainder of the carpus dislocates. It, like most wrist injuries, occurs from violent hyperextension. Rarely do any physical findings point to the diagnosis. Median nerve paresthesias may increase the index of suspicion.[13] Since dislocation occurs at the midcarpal joint, the scaphoid that bridges both must either sustain ligamentous disruption proximally and follow the capitate or fracture through its waist, producing the transscaphoid perilunate dislocation.[96]

If these injuries are seen within the first 3 weeks, closed reduction after adequate muscle relaxation can usually be accomplished by distraction of the carpus and manipulation. Dorsally directed pressure on the palmarly dislocated lunate plus pressure directed palmarward on the dorsally dislocated capitate is the maneuver needed to achieve reduction. If *anatomic reduction* is confirmed by good quality roentgenograms, the wrist is immobilized in a short-arm cast with slight palmar flexion from 6 to 8 weeks. If the reduction is not maintained by casting alone, percutaneous pinning is necessary. If reduction cannot be obtained, open reduction, internal fixation, and ligament repair are necessary.

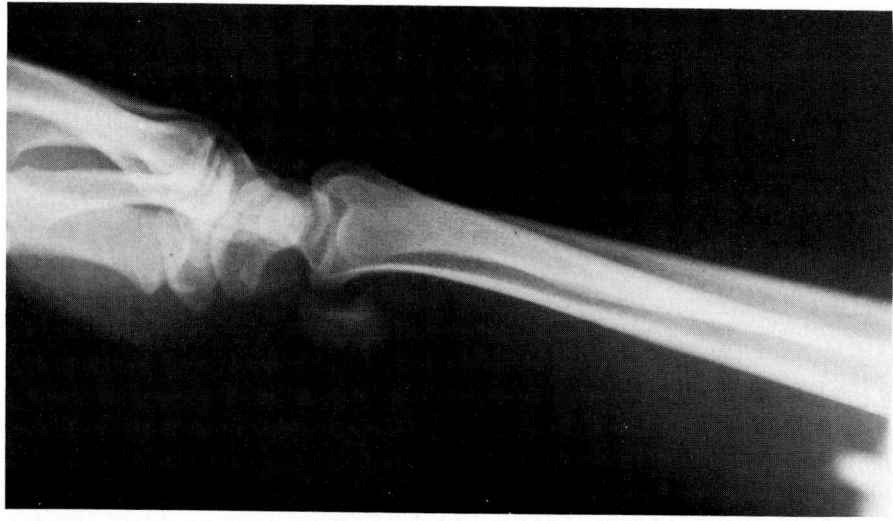

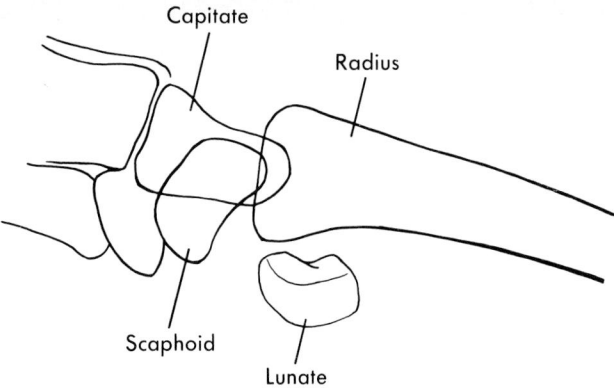

Fig. 18-15 Lunate dislocation. Lunate is displaced volarly to other carpal bones or distal radius. Wrist is shortened with capitate articulating with radius.

Lunate dislocations

The volar lunate dislocations occur from the same mechanism as the perilunate dislocation. Many consider the lunate dislocation to be the end stage of a perilunate dislocation. Many variations are frequently seen between the two common dislocations, making it easy to believe the injuries are different roentgenographic manifestations of the same injury.

Lunate dislocation frequently causes median nerve compression. On the anteroposterior roentgenogram the lunate appears triangular and there is a peculiar space between the scaphoid and the triquetrum. The appearance of this dislocation on the lateral roentgenogram is fairly typical (Fig. 18-15). Closed reduction can be achieved if the injury is seen early. Atraumatic closed reduction with muscle relaxation is attempted after a period of sustained traction. With the wrist in extension, digital pressure is exerted over the volarly dislocated lunate. Once reduced, the wrist is brought into flexion and immobilized for 6 to 8 weeks.[102] Since there is a tendency for the reduction to be lost with time, percutaneous pinning of the lunate in its reduced position or open reduction is recommended.

CARPAL INSTABILITY

Since Linscheid and coauthors[54] published their classic work on traumatic instability of the wrist in 1972, knowledge[84] and treatment methods have flourished in attempting to identify practical and predictable procedures for treating these challenging problems.

In the normal lateral wrist roentgenogram there is a colinear alignment of the long axis of the radius, lunate, and capitate (see Fig. 18-2). The carpal bones are spring-loaded like a jack-in-the-box and kept under control by ligament restraints[97] (see Fig. 18-13). When these ligaments are torn, the lunate, balanced between the forearm and hand, collapses. The lunate or intercalated segment subsequently forms an unstable radiolunate-capitate zigzag alignment. When the lunate rotates dorsally, the term *dorsal intercalated segment instability* (DISI) is used (Fig. 18-16). With volar or palmar flexion of the lunate, the condition is called *volar intercalated segment instability* (VISI). Dynamic forms of carpal instability require a high index of suspicion, because routine wrist roentgenograms are normal. The diagnosis is confirmed with cineradiographs, ulnar deviation, radial deviation, and clenched fist anteroposterior roentgenographs. The loose or "lax" ligamentous restraints may be evident only when the wrist is stressed.

Taleisnik[84] has classified wrist instability patterns into the lateral, medial, and proximal columns. The lunate, capitate, trapezium and trapezoid make up the central column and separate the scaphoid (lateral column) from the triquetrum (medial column). Proximal carpal instability occurs between the articular surfaces of the distal radioulnar joint and the carpus.

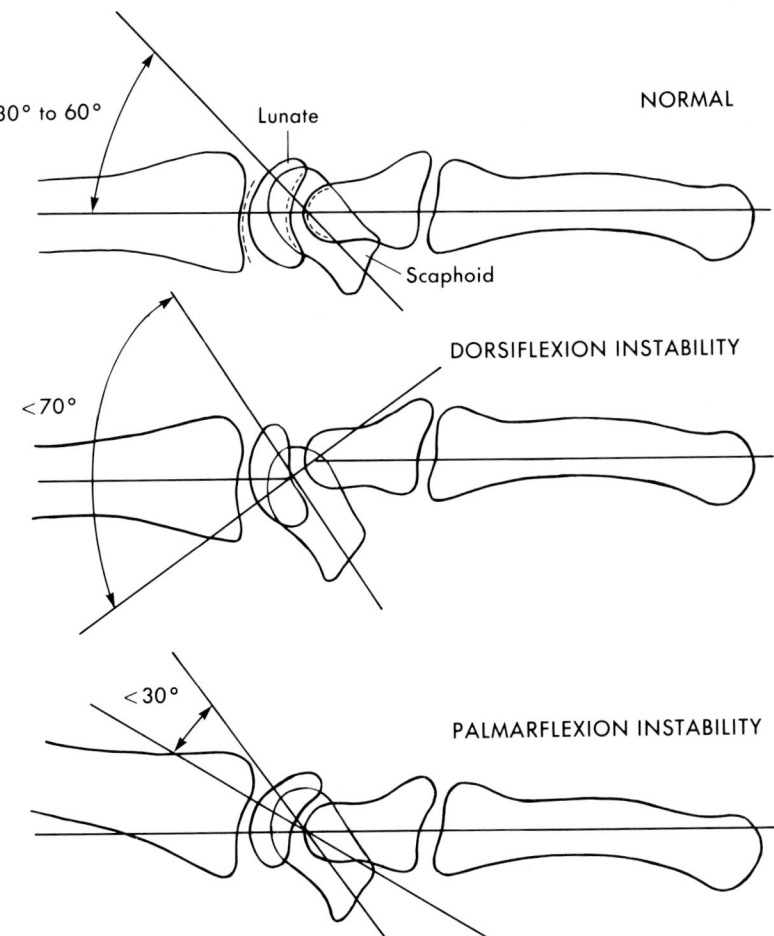

Fig. 18-16 Posttraumatic wrist instability patterns. When wrist is in neutral position on lateral roentgenogram, normal scapholunate angle is from 30 to 60 degrees. When lunate faces dorsally, scapholunate angle is greater than 60 degrees (usually about 100 degrees). This angle indicates a dorsiflexion instability pattern (DISI). When lunate faces palmarly and scapholunate angle is less than 30 degrees, palmar flexion instability pattern (VISI) is demonstrated.

Scapholunate dissociation is the most common form of carpal instability. The ligaments supporting the proximal pole of the scaphoid are torn. The scaphoid palmar flexes, and the lunate dorsiflexes simultaneously, producing a DISI pattern. A fall on the dorsiflexed, ulnarly deviated wrist typically produces this injury. It may occur secondary to a perilunate dislocation or to rheumatoid arthritis. Early diagnosis of this condition offers the greatest opportunity for a successful result. The condition is frequently incorrectly diagnosed as a "wrist sprain." If roentgenographs fail to show the characteristically increased scapholunate gap (Fig. 18-17) and DISI pattern cineradiographs may be necessary. When the diagnosis is made early, closed reduction and percutaneous pinning or an open reduction through a dorsal and/or volar approach is indicated. The volar capsular tear is repaired and the reduced scaphoid pinned to the capitate and lunate with Kirschner wires.[55] Chronic scapholunate dissociation without osteoarthritis is disabling. Surgical reconstruction of the scapholunate ligament with a tendon graft has been disappointing[31,68] except in the patient with skeletal immaturity, rheumatoid arthritis, or ligamentous laxity.[85] Recently most chronic scapholunate instability pat-

terns have been treated with a fusion of the scaphoid and the trapezium-trapezoid (STT) joints[98] (Fig. 18-18). Excellent grip strength is regained after this triscaphoid fusion, with 20% loss of dorsiflexion-palmar flexion range and 30% loss of radial-ulnar deviation noted.[47] The altered biomechanics of the wrist with scapholunate dissociation may rapidly lead to articular damage of the radioscaphoid joint. Recognition of early degenerative changes in the radioscaphoid joint is possible with wrist arthroscopy. An STT fusion in the presence of radioscaphoid joint degeneration will not relieve the wrist pain.

Watson described a pattern of combined carpal instability and degenerative arthritis called scapholunate advanced collapse, or SLAC wrist.[99] He recommended treating the SLAC wrist with a scaphoid implant arthroplasty and lunocapitate fusion. This procedure is theoretically attractive, because it eliminates the pathologic joints and provides a stable central column to bear the wrist loading and reduce the load bearing on the prosthesis. Alternative procedures include radial styloidectomy, proximal row carpectomy, and wrist arthrodesis.

There are two types of medial carpal instability[51]: triquetrolunate and triquetrohamate dissociation. These less frequent instability patterns develop when ligamentous disruption occurs between the triquetrum and the lunate, or hamate. Both patterns are difficult to recognize and must be considered in the differential diagnosis of ulnar wrist pain. Triquetrolunate dissociation is a static type of VISI pattern where the unrestrained lunate follows the volar flexed posture of the scaphoid and the triquetrum is distal in relationship to the hamate. This pattern, occasionally seen in the rheumatoid wrist, can be treated with tenodesis using the distally attached flexor carpi ulnaris or a radiounate fusion.[53] Triquetrohamate dissociation is a dynamic form of midcar-

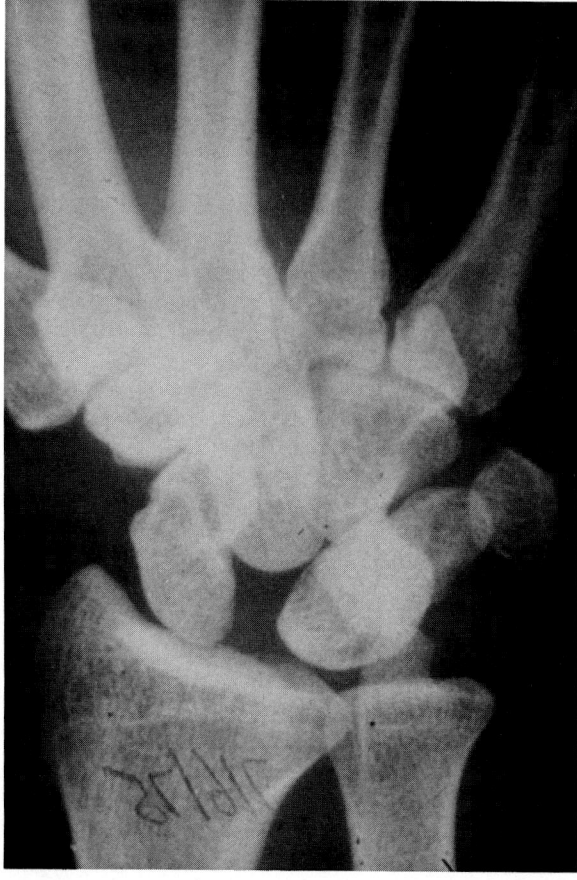

Fig. 18-17 Scapholunate dissociation. Scaphoid is tilted dorsally. It is oval in contour rather than having normal canoe shape. Because one is looking down long axis of scaphoid, there is a double density or cortical "ring" shadow of tuberosity. Scapholunate gap (normally 2 mm or less) is increased. This gap is popularly called "Terry Thomas sign" and refers to the British actor with a wide gap between his front teeth.

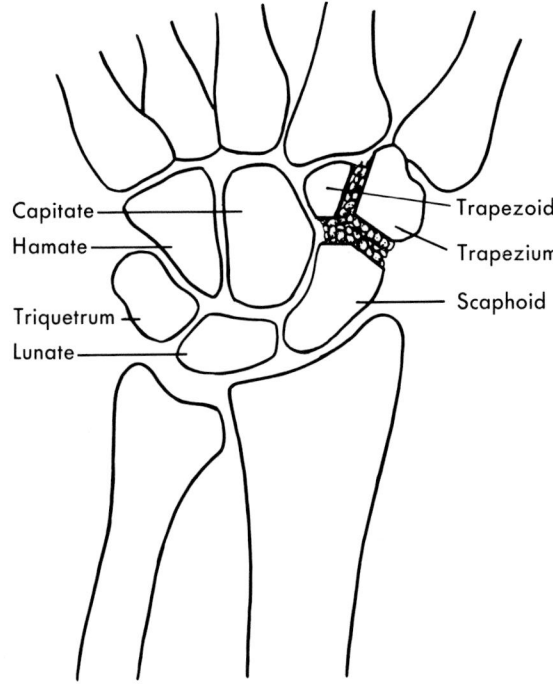

Fig. 18-18 STT Fusion. This procedure arthrodeses the scaphoid to the trapezium and trapezoid with bone graft and pinning.

pal instability in which the palmar intercarpal or V ligament medially has lost its integrity.[51] This ligament supports the ulnar half of the midcarpal joint. It is responsible for a concurrent palmar shift and dorsiflexion of the lunate during wrist ulnar deviation. It maintains the colinear relationship between the radius and capitate. With loss of the V ligament, the lunate pivots on its own axis of rotation and a zigzag collapse pattern is observed. The capitate is displaced dorsal to the radius on ulnar deviation in the dynamic DISI variety or displaced volar to the radius on radial deviation in the dynamic VISI pattern. The presenting complaint may be a painful, snapping wrist and midcarpal tenderness. Lateral roentgenographs of the wrist in pronation and ulnar deviation demonstrate the dynamic instability pattern. The colinear relationship between the radius and the capitate is lost. When nonsurgical management is no longer successful, surgical treatment is needed. In the low-demand wrist, a tenodesis is preferred. In the wrist requiring heavy activity, a radiolunate fusion is a viable alternative.

Proximal carpal instability is a result of radiocarpal ligamentous disruption or abnormal changes in the alignment of the distal radiocarpal articulation.[84] In this category two main types of instability occur: radiocarpal and midcarpal. In the radiocarpal type of instability an abnormal relationship exists between the distal radiocarpal joint and the carpus. The carpus can be translocated ulnarly, dorsally, or volarly. Ulnar translocation is usually associated with rheumatoid arthritis but can be associated with other conditions including aggressive distal ulnar resection. In the absence of radiocarpal osteoarthritis, the lunate is relocated and fused to the distal radius. Dorsal carpal translocation may follow malunited fractures of the distal radius. The dorsally directed radial articular slope results in a true carpal dorsal subluxation. Excellent success can be achieved with a dorsal openwedge osteotomy of the distal radius, bone grafting, and internal fixation.[23,87] Conversely, volar carpal translocation is possible with malunited Barton's or Smith's fractures. Treatment should focus on correcting the original deformity when feasible. If radiocarpal degeneration is present, a fusion limited to the radius, scaphoid, and lunate may leave limited motion to the midcarpal joints. Infrequently, a midcarpal instability pattern develops with a malunited fracture of the distal radius. When the normal palmar tilt of the distal radius is lost, the carpus shifts dorsally, the weak dorsal ligaments are unable to compensate, and a dynamic DISI pattern may develop. Occasionally scapholunate dissociation follows malunited fractures of the distal radius. Surgical treatment consists of realigning the palmar slope of the distal radius.[23]

DISTAL RADIOULNAR INJURIES

Our understanding of ulnar wrist disorders have increased dramatically in the past 10 years. This can be attributed to a better understanding of the functional anatomy of the ulnar carpal area.[70] Improved diagnostic studies include wrist arthrography,[49] stress roentgenographs, fluoroscopy, computerized tomography,[64] and arthroscopy.[7]

The distal radioulnar joint is stabilized by two complex ligamentous structures: the triangular fibrocartilage (TFC)[103] (Fig. 18-19) and the ulnocarpal ligament complex (UCLC).[69] The semicylindrical head of the ulna articulates radially 270 degrees with the ulnar concave face of the distal radius, or sigmoid notch. The TFC and UCLC are two perpendicular ligamentous triangles that suspend the radius and carpus above the distal ulna. Additional local stability is provided by the extensor carpi ulnaris unit dorsally and the pronator quadratus volarly.

Recognition of distal radioulnar disorders is difficult and frequently overlooked when treating common fractures of the distal radius.[95] Frykman recognized the importance of the distal radioulnar joint in his wrist fracture classification.[26] It should not be assumed that the distal radioulnar joint derangement will "do well" if attention is devoted only to the length and volar articular tilt of the radius.[9]

In acute intraarticular fractures of the sigmoid notch of the radius an anatomic reduction must be obtained, either indirectly with external pin fixation,[18] or directly if the fracture is amenable to internal fixation. Ulnar styloid fractures are ligamentous avulsion injuries, usually part of the spectrum of distal radius fractures. When they occur independently and displacement is present, the TFC-UCLC styloid may be opened, repaired, and internally fixed.

Traumatic disruption of the distal radioulnar joint ligaments (TFC-UCLC) is frequently associated with other fractures or dislocations.[43,61] When the primary proximal radius or ulna fracture is internally fixed, the distal radioulnar disruption can usually be managed with immobilization of the forearm in midrotation and the wrist in slight ulnar deviation and volar flexion.

Isolated distal radioulnar joint dislocation occasionally occurs. Careful attention to the true lateral wrist roentgenogram should help identify the isolated volar or dorsal dislocation of the ulna. However, if one is still not certain of the distal radioulnar joint relationship on roentgenogram, computerized tomography of both wrists is most helpful. Dislocation of the volar ulna is reduced by pronation and dorsal ulnar dislocation by supination.[40] Six weeks of long-

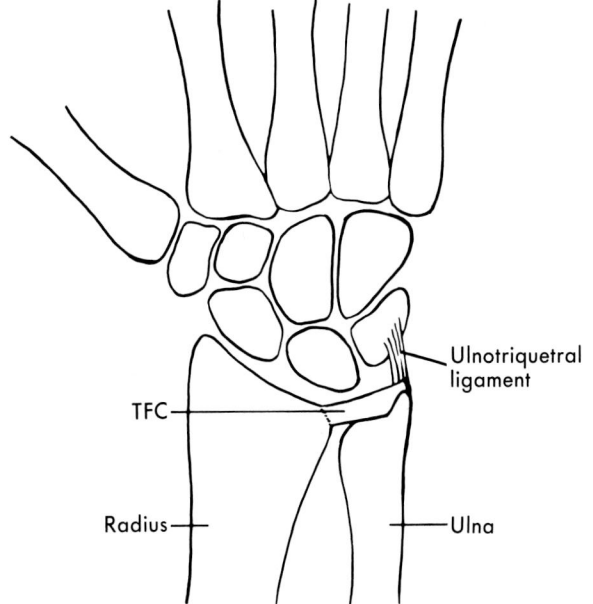

Fig. 18-19 TFC is the triangular fibrocartilage. It fills the space between the ulna and the carpal bones and attaches to the ulnotriquetral ligament, the strongest attachment of the ulna to the carpus.

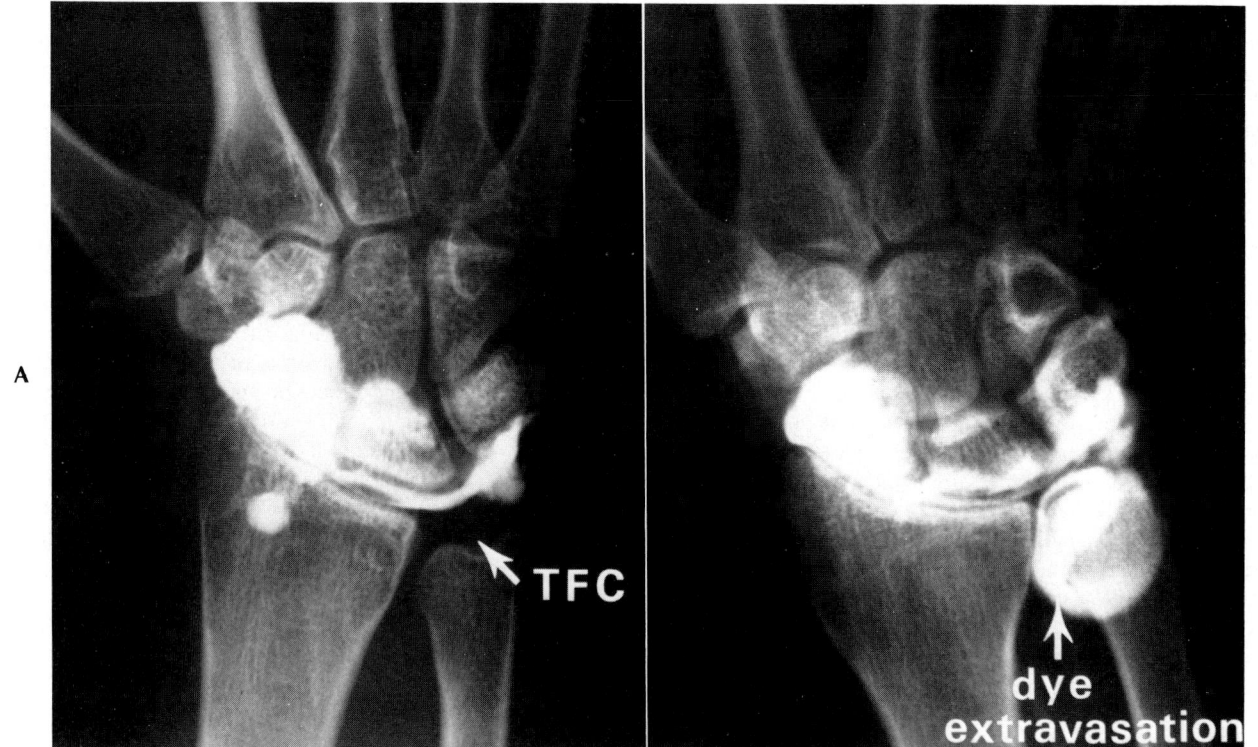

Fig. 18-20 Wrist arthrogram. **A,** In normal persons dye is confined to radiocarpal joint. Triangular fibrocartilage (TFC) is clearly seen. **B,** A torn TFC with contrast material leaking into distal radioulnar joint.

arm cast immobilization is required. A locked or irreducible periulnar dislocation requires an open reduction and repair of the TFC-UCLC.

Before our better understanding of the TFC-UCLC, ulnar wrist pain and clicking were attributed to tears of the so-called wrist disk. Arthrography and wrist arthroscopy have brought to light an interesting differential diagnosis. Local ulnar wrist pathology includes isolated TFC disruptions, dislocating ECU tendon, pisotriquetral arthritis, and lunate-triquetral ligament disruptions. Isolated TFC disruptions do occur (Fig. 18-20). Unless a tear can be unequivocally identified, TFC excision is discouraged.[66]

Mikic[62] clearly describes an age-related attritional degeneration of the TFC. This occurs commonly on the ulnar side of the TFC, then follows on the carpal side of the complex with lunate-triquetral ligament disruption. Chondromalacia of the ulna head convex surface is a frequent cause of distal radioulnar joint pain. When conservative treatment has been exhausted, the surgical options include resection of the distal ulna,[21,63] hemiresection-interposition arthroplasty,[26] distal ulnar recession,[19] hemireplacement arthroplasty,[81] and ulnar pseudoarthrosis procedures.[32] The properly executed distal ulna resection as described by Darrach remains a viable option. Arthroscopic debridement of the TFC is gaining in popularity but long-term results have not been reported.

WRIST SPRAIN

The diagnosis of wrist sprain is incorrectly made all too frequently by those inexperienced with traumatic wrist conditions. There definitely are wrist sprains consisting of minor radiocarpal or intercarpal ligamentous tears. Basically the diagnosis of wrist sprain is one of exclusion. It can be accurately made only after careful exclusion of scaphoid or lunate fractures, dorsal chip carpal fractures, traumatic wrist instability patterns, and other carpal fractures. Frequently, repeat roentgenograms are required at weekly intervals after wrist immobilization to identify fractures suspected but only confirmed on initial roentgenographic evaluation. A history of minor trauma with mild generalized diffuse pain or swelling lasting 2 to 3 weeks with all other more serious conditions ruled out is the pattern required for an accurate diagnosis of a wrist sprain.

SECRETAN'S DISEASE

Secretan described a curious condition where minor trauma to the dorsum of the hand is followed by brawny non-pitting edema.[75,90] The extensor tendons become embedded in a mass of organizing fibrous tissue containing macrophages and hemosiderin. There is no bony injury or ecchymosis present. This chronic condition with an obscure cause is believed to be a self-inflicted entity producing prolonged disability in patients who have a possible claim for occupational injury. Since the condition is believed to be a form of reflex sympathetic dystrophy, treatment consists of benign neglect. Surgical intervention, heat, massage, and passive manipulations are not helpful.[73,90]

GENERAL PRINCIPLES FOR REHABILITATION OF WRIST INJURIES

All wrist injuries require some form of rehabilitation. Although a great variation exists in the type and severity of wrist injuries, the general principles of rehabilitation are the same. There are specific limitations for each injury. Good communication between the physician and the therapist can help incorporate these limitations into the rehabilitation plan. Pain is one limiting factor. It dictates the duration of immobilization yet limits exercises designed to mobilize and strengthen the wrist.

Edema of the injured wrist is always present to some degree. It involves the hand but may extend proximally to involve the entire upper extremity. Functional disuse of the hand in itself may result in edema. The required immobilization inhibits the pumping action of the muscles with subsequent venous stasis and edema. The most important preventive measures are elevation and active motion of the uninjured joints. When in bed, the patient must elevate the injured wrist on pillows. The patient is taught to rest his elbow on the arm of a chair with the hand elevated above the elbow in the upright position; dependency must be avoided. A comfortable sling or arm immobilizer is fitted to assist the patient in keeping the area of injury elevated. Active motion of uninjured joints must be done regularly and frequently. Exaggerated instructions are a good way to get the point across.

Chronic edema associated with traumatic wrist injuries is a difficult problem to treat. The Jobst Intermittent Compression Unit "pumps" the lymphedema out of the hand and arm. Alternating rest intervals allow for the lymph flow and venous return. The standard treatment consists of wearing the Jobst sleeve for 45 minutes with a pressure of 66 mm Hg in 60 second–30 second compression-rest intervals. Depending on the patient's tolerance, adjustments can be made in the duration of treatment, position of the hand during compression, pressure during compression, and the compression-rest interval.

Massage of the hand, another useful modality to treat chronic edema, assists venous and lymphatic circulation by its mechanical effects on the tissues. Massage should be performed with the patient comfortably seated and the arm resting in a softer surface with the hand elevated and the elbow extended. A skin lubricant is used to aid the long flowing strokes from a distal to proximal direction. The forearm is rotated frequently during massage.

The wrist is always stiff after immobilization for more than a few weeks. Mobilizing the stiff wrist cannot be started until the injured tissue has healed enough to provide some degree of stability. The longer the required immobilization, the greater the degree of wrist stiffness. The problem of wrist stiffness increases with age and the severity of the injury. If the type of immobilization used is properly applied and active exercises performed during the healing phase, joint stiffness proximal and distal to the wrist should not be a problem. Active wrist range of motion exercises should be started as soon as the cast is removed. Patients do not usually recognize that the wrist normally moves through both the dorsal palmar and the radial ulnar planes. They must be instructed to include these motions in their exercise program. Pronation and supination should not be overlooked. Active assisted range-of-motion exercises should be started when the wrist motion is not increasing with active exercises. Pain is a guide when one is deciding how soon and how aggressive active assisted exercises should be started. The hand can be rested flat on a table and the wrist slowly moved forward and backward. Wrist dorsiflexion can

be improved by putting both palms together in the praying position and moving the forearm to the horizontal position. Similarly palmar flexion can be assisted by putting the dorsum of each hand together. Turning a door handle against resistance or turning the hand over repeatedly in gloves with the fingers and palms sewn together are exercises to regain lost pronation and supination.

In most traumatic wrist injuries it is desirable to start mobilizing the joint before the bone and soft tissues are completely healed. This requires the use of various splints to protect and support the wrist in its final stage of healing. A static wrist splint in the neutral or slightly dorsiflexed position is worn at night during the first few days or weeks after the cast is removed. During the day it is more desirable to fit the patient with a dynamic wrist splint. This increases the functional use of the wrist while stabilizing and strengthening it. The patient has the security of wrist support while attempting to regain motion.

Once the wrist is healed, edema controlled, and motion improved, the muscles crossing the wrist must be strengthened. Even vigorous athletic youths lose muscle mass quickly when immobilized for any length of time. One can best achieve strengthening by returning the patient to some type of functional activity. This may initially be the activities of daily living such as dressing, personal hygiene, or light housework. Before the patient is returned to his preinjury level of activity, progressive resistive exercises are necessary. The wrist flexors and extensors are actively contracted against maximum resistance through a full arc of motion. The hand is held over the edge of a table with a slight incline. Weights are attached to the hand. The supinated wrist is flexed to strengthen the wrist palmar flexors, and the pronated wrist is extended to strengthen the wrist dorsiflexors. Functional activities have the advantage of easy accessibility and usefulness and are less boring to the patient.

REFERENCES

1. Almquist EE and Burn JF: Radial shortening for the treatment of Kienbock's disease: a 5 to 10 year follow-up, J Hand Surg 7:348, 1982.
2. Armistead RB and others: Ulnar lengthening in the treatment of Kienbock's disease, J Bone Joint Surg 64:170, 1982.
3. Barton JR: Views and treatment of an important injury to the wrist, Philadelphia Med Exam 1:365, 1838.
4. Bartone NF and Grieco RV: Fractures of the triquetrum, J Bone Joint Surg 38A:353, 1956.
5. Bohler L: The treatment of fractures, ed 4, Baltimore, 1942, William Wood & Co.
6. Bohler L: Treatment of fractures, Bristol, England, 1956, A John Wright & Sons, Ltd.
7. Bora FW: Wrist arthroscope, J Hand Surg 10A:308, 1985.
8. Bowen TL: Injuries to the hamate bone, Hand 5:235, 1973.
9. Bowers WH: Distal radioulnar joint. In Green DP, editor: Operative hand surgery, vol 1, New York, 1982, Churchill Livingstone.
10. Brighton CT: Treatment of nonunion with constant direct current, Clin Orthop 124:106, 1977.
11. Bryan R and Dobyns JH: Fractures of the carpal bones other than the lunate and navicular, Clin Orthop 149:107, 1980.
12. Bunnell S: Ischemic contracture, local in the hand, J Bone Joint Surg 35A:88, 1953.
13. Campbell RD, Lance EM, and Yeoh CB: Lunate and perilunate dislocations, J Bone Joint Surg 46B:55, 1964.
14. Charnley J: The closed treatment of common fractures, ed 3, Baltimore, 1961, Williams & Wilkins.
15. Clyburn TA: Dynamic external fixation for comminuted intra-articular fractures of the distal end of the radius, J Bone Joint Surg 69A:248, 1987.

16. Colles A: On the fractures of the carpal extremity of the radius, Edinb Med Surg J 10:182, 1814.
17. Cooney WP: External fixation of distal radial fractures, Clin Orthop 180:44, 1983.
18. Cooney WP III, Linscheid RL, and Dobyns JH: External pin fixation for unstable Colles' fractures, J Bone Joint Surg 61A:840, 1979.
19. Darrow JC and others: Distal ulnar recession for disorders of the radioulnar joint, J Hand Surg 10:482, 1985.
20. DeOliveira JC: Barton's fracture, J Bone Joint Surg 55A:586, 1973.
21. Dingman PVC: Resection of the distal end of the ulna (Darrach procedure), J Bone Joint Surg 39A:893, 1952.
22. Dobyns JH and Linscheid RL: Fractures and dislocations in the wrist. In Rockwood CA and Green DP, editors: Fractures in adults, ed 2, Philadelphia, 1984, JB Lippincott Co.
23. Fernandez DL: Correction of post-traumatic wrist deformity in adults by osteotomy, bone-grafting, and internal fixation, J Bone Joint Surg 64:1164, 1982.
24. Fernandez DL and Ghillani R: External fixation of complex carpal dislocations: a preliminary report, J Hand Surg 12A:335, 1987.
25. Foster DE and Kopta JA: Update on external fixators in the treatment of wrist fractures, Clin Orthop 204:177, 1986.
26. Frykman G: Fracture of the distal radius including sequelae-shoulder-hand-finger syndrome, disturbance in the distal radioulnar joint, and impairment of nerve function: a clinical and experimental study, Acta Orthop Scand Suppl 108:1, 1967.
27. Frykman G and others: Treatment of nonunited scaphoid fractures by pulsed electromagnetic fields and cast, J Hand Surg 11:344, 1986.
28. Frykman GK and others: Compression of 11 external fixators for unstable wrist fractures, J Hand Surg (in press).
29. Gartland JJ Jr and Werley CW: Evaluation of healed Colles' fractures, J Bone Joint Surg 43B:245, 1961.
30. Gelberman RH and others: The vascularity of the lunate bone and Kienbock's disease, J Hand Surg 5:272, 1980.
31. Glickel SZ and Lillender L: Results of ligamentous reconstruction for chronic intercarpal instability, Orthop Trans 6:167, 1982.
32. Goncalves D: Correction of disorders of the distal radio-ulnar joint by artificial pseudoarthrosis of the ulna, J Bone and Joint Surg 56B:462, 1974.
33. Graner O and others: Arthrodesis of the carpal bones, J Bone Joint Surg 48A:767, 1966.
34. Green CA and Matthews LS: The thermal effects of skeletal pin placement on human bone, Orthop Trans 5:261, 1981.
35. Green DP: Pins and plaster treatment of comminuted fractures of the distal end of the radius, J Bone Joint Surg 57A:304, 1975.
36. Green DP: The effect of avascular necrosis on Russe bone grafting for scaphoid nonunion, J Hand Surg 10A:597, 1985.
37. Green DP and O'Brien ET: Classification and management of carpal dislocations, Clin Orthop 149:55, 1980.
38. Hartz CR and Beckenbaugh RD: Long-term results of resection of the distal ulna for post-traumatic conditions, J Trauma 19:4, 1979.
39. Heim V and Pfeiffer KM: Small fragment set anual. technique recommended by the ASIF group, New York, 1974, Springer Verlag.
40. Heiple KG, Freehafer AA, and Van't Hoff A: Isolated traumatic dislocation of the distal end of the ulna or distal radio-ulnar joint, J Bone Surg 44A:1387, 1962.
41. Heppenstall RB: Fracture treatment and healing, Philadelphia, 1980, WB Saunders Co.
42. Herbert TJ and Fisher WE: Management of the fractured scaphoid using a new bone screw, J Bone Joint Surg 66B:114, 1984.
43. Hughston JC: Fractures of the distal radial shaft: mistakes in management, J Bone Joint Surg 39A:240, 1957.
44. Hulten O: Uber anatomische Variationen den Hand. Gelenkknochen, Acta Radiol Scand 9:155, 1928.
45. Inglis AE and Jones EC: Proximal row carpectomy for disease of the proximal row, J Bone Joint Surg 59A:460, 1977.
46. Kienbock R: Uber traumatishe Malazie des Mondbeins, und ihre Folgezustande Entartungsformen und kompressions Frakturen, Fortschr Roengenstr 16:77, 1910.
47. Kleinman WB, Steichen JB, and Strickland JW: Management of chronic rotatory subluxation of the scaphoid by scapho-trapezio-trapezoid arthrodesis, J Hand Surg 7:125, 1982.
48. Lee MLH: Interosseous arterial pattern of the carpal lunate bone and its relationship to avascular necrosis, Acta Orthop Scand 33:43, 1962.
49. Levinsohn EM and Palmar AK: Arthrography of the traumatized wrist, Radiology 146:647, 1983.
50. Lichtman DM and others: Kienbock's disease: the role of silicone replacement arthroplasty, J Bone Joint Surg 59A:899, 1977.
51. Lichtman DM and others: Ulnar midcarpal instability—clinical and laboratory analysis, J Hand Surg 6:515, 1981.
52. Lidstrom A: Fractures of the distal end of the radius: a clinical and statistical study of end results, Acta Orthop Scand Suppl 41:1, 1959.
53. Linscheid RL and Dobyns JH: Radiolunate arthrodesis, J Hand Surg 10A:821-828, 1985.
54. Linscheid RL and others: Traumatic instability of the wrist: diagnosis, classification and pathomechanics, J Bone Joint Surg 54A:1612, 1972.
55. Loeb TM, Urbaniak JR, and Goldner JL: Traumatic carpal instability: putting the pieces together, Orthop Trans 1:163, 1977.
56. London PS: The broken scaphoid bones: the case against pessimism, J Bone Joint Surg 42B:237, 1961.
57. Mack GR and others: The natural history of scaphoid nonunions, J Bone Joint Surg 66A:504, 1984.
58. Maudsley RH and Chen SC: Screw fixation in the management of the fractured carpal scaphoid, J Bone Joint Surg 54B:432, 1972.
59. Mayer JH: Colles' fractures, Br J Surg 27:629, 1940.
60. Mazet R and Hohl M: Fractures of the carpal navicular: analysis of 91 cases and review of the literature, J Bone Joint Surg 45A:82, 1967.
61. McDougall A and While J: Subluxation of the interior radio-ulnar joint complicating fractures of the radial head, J Bone Joint Surg 39B:287, 1957.
62. Mikic ZD: Age changes in the triangular fibrocartilage of the wrist joint, J Anatomy 126:367, 1978.
63. Milch H: Cuff resection of the ulna for *malunated* Colles fracture, J Bone Joint Surg 23:311, 1941.
64. Mino DE, Palmar A, and Levinsohn EM: Radiography and computerized tomography in the diagnosis of incongruity of the distal radio-ulnar joint, J Bone Joint Surg 67A:247, 1985.
65. Moberg E: The shoulder-hand-finger syndrome, Surg Clin North Am 40:367, 1960.
66. Mossing N: Isolated lesions of the radio-ulnar disc treated with excision, Scand J Plast Reconstr Surg 9:233, 1975.
67. Nakata RY and others: External fixators for wrist fractures: a biomechanical and clinical study, J Hand Surg 10A:845, 1985.
68. Palmar AK, Dobyns JH, and Linscheid RL: Management of post-traumatic instability of the wrist secondary to ligament rupture, J Hand Surg 3:507, 1978.
69. Palmer AK and Werner FW: The triangular fibrocartilage complex of the wrist—anatomy and function, J Hand Surg 6:153, 1981.
70. Palmer AK and Werner FW: Biomechanics of the distal radioulnar joint, Clin Orthop 187:26, 1984.
71. Parisen S: Settling in Colles' fracture: a review of the literature, Bull Hosp Joint Dis 34:117, 1973.
72. Russe O: Fracture of the carpal navicular, J Bone Joint Surg 42A:759, 1960.
73. Saferin EH: Secretan's disease, Plast Reconstr Surg 58:703, 1976.
74. Sarmiento A: The brachioradialis as a deforming force in Colles' fractures, Clin Orthop 38:86, 1965.
75. Secretan H: Hard edema and traumatic hyperplasia of the dorsum of metacarpus, Rev Med Suisse Romande 21:409, 1901.
76. Smith L and Friedman B: Treatment of ununited fractures of the scaphoid by styloidectomy of the radius, J Bone Joint Surg 38A:368, 1956.
77. Smith RW: A treatise on fractures in the vicinity of joints, and on certain forms of accidental and congenital dislocations, Dublin, 1854, Hodges & Smith.
78. Stahl F: On lunatomalacia (Kienbock's disease): a clinical and radiographic study especially on its pathogenesis and the late results of immobilization treatment, Acta Chir Scand 95 (suppl 126):1, 1947.
79. Stark HH and others: Fractures of the hamate in athletics, J Bone Joint Surg 59A:575, 1977.
80. Swanson AB: Silicone rubber implants for replacement of the carpal scaphoid and lunate bone, Orthop Clin North Am 1:299, 1970.
81. Swanson AB: Implant arthroplasty for disabilities of the distal radioulnar joint, Orthop Clin North Am 4:373, 1973.
82. Taine GJ: Excision of the lunate in Kienbock's disease, J Bone Joint Surg 47:599, 1965.
83. Taleisnik J: The ligaments of the wrist, J Hand Surg 1:110, 1976.
84. Taleisnik J: Post traumatic carpal instability, Clin Orthop 149:73, 1980.

85. Taleisnik J: The wrist, New York, 1982, Churchill Livingstone.
86. Taleisnik J and Kelly PJ: The extraosseous and intraosseous blood supply to the scaphoid bone, J Bone Joint Surg 48A:1126, 1966.
87. Taleisnik J and Watson HK: Midcarpal instability caused by malunited fractures of the distal radius, J Hand Surg 9A:350, 1984.
88. Thomas FB: Reduction of Smith's fractures, J Bone Joint Surg 39B:463, 1959.
89. Thompson GH: Barton's fractures—reverse Barton's fractures, Clin Orthop 122:210, 1977.
90. Van Demark RE: Peritendinous fibrosis of the dorsum of the hand, J Bone Joint Surg 30A:284, 1948.
91. Vasilas A, Gireco RV, and Baritone NF: Roentgen aspects of injuries of the pisiform bone and pisotriquetral joint, J Bone Joint Surg 42A:1317, 1960.
92. Vaughn PA and others: Treatment of unstable fractures of the distal radius by external fixation, J Bone Joint Surg 67B:385, 1985.
93. Vender MI and others: Degenerative changes in symptomatic scaphoid nonunion, J Hand Surg 12A:514, 1987.
94. Vidal J, Buscayret C, and Connes H: Treatment of articular fractures by "ligamentotaxis" with external fixation. In Brooker AF and Edwards CC, editors: External fixation: the current state of the art, Baltimore, 1979, Williams & Wilkins.
95. Vesely DG: The distal radioulnar joint, Clin Orthop 51:75, 1967.
96. Wagner CJ: Fracture-dislocation of the wrist, Clin Orthop 15:181, 1959.
97. Watson HK: Carpal instability, Cont Orthop 4:107, 1982.
98. Watson HK, Ryu J, and Akelman E: Limited triscaphoid intercarpal arthrodesis for rotatory subluxation of the scaphoid, J Bone Joint Surg 68A:345, 1986.
99. Watson HK and Ballet FL: The SLAC wrist: scapholunate advanced collapse pattern of degenerative arthritis, J Hand Surg 7:125, 1982.
100. Watson HK, Ryu J, and DiBella A: An approach to Kienbock's disease, triscaphe arthrodesis, J Hand Surg 10A:2179, 1985.
101. Watson JK: Limited wrist arthrodesis, Clin Orthop 149:126, 1980.
102. Watson-Jones R: Fractures and joint injuries, ed 5, Edinburgh, 1976, E & S Livingstone.
103. Weigl K and Spira E: The triangular fibrocartilage of the wrist joint, Reconstr Surg Traumatol 11:139, 1969.
104. Woodyard JE: Review of Smith's fractures, J Bone Joint Surg 51B:324, 1969.

19

Management of hand fractures

Robert Lee Wilson and Margaret S. Carter

Although fractures in the hand occur more frequently than in any other location, their significance is often underestimated. When hand fractures are incorrectly managed or associated with injuries to other tissues, stiffness, pain, or contracture may result and produce a loss of normal hand function. The two factors that most influence the end result after a digital fracture are the severity of the initial injury and the method of primary treatment. Although the seriousness of some injuries precludes a perfect result, our goal should be to recover maximal function in every injured hand.

More than one half of all hand fractures are sustained at work. Fractures occur with less frequency from motor vehicle accidents, recreational activities, and household mishaps. The location of fractures within the hand has been reviewed by several authors. Distal phalanx fractures are the most common (45% to 50%), followed by metacarpal (30% to 35%), proximal phalanx (15% to 20%), and last, middle phalanx fractures (8% to 12%).

In evaluating digital fractures, one must first consider the force that produced the injury and the extent of soft tissue involvement. The hand is examined for rotational deformities of the fingers, as well as angulation and fracture displacement. X-ray evaluation should include three views (anteroposterior, oblique, and a true lateral) of the digit. Lastly, the stability of the fracture must be assessed to determine the exact immobilization needed to obtain bony union.

The first principle in the treatment of hand fractures is *accurate fracture reduction*. As little as 5 degrees lateral angulation may create overlapping of the fingers. Although immobilization of the injured finger may be necessary to ensure union, the *uninvolved fingers must be actively moved* to prevent stiffness. *Elevation of the extremity* at all times is the best method to limit edema.

The fingers that are *immobilized should be placed in the "clam-digger," or intrinsic-positive position:* the wrist in 30 to 60 degrees extension, the metacarpophalangeal (MP) joints in 60 to 70 degrees flexion, and the interphalangeal joints in neutral to 10 degrees flexion. This position maintains the ligaments of the digital joints under maximal tension, and, it is hoped, prevents the most serious joint contractures. Immobilization of the wrist in extension produces synergistic flexion of the MP joints and overcomes the pain reflex position (wrist flexion and MP joint extension with clawed fingers). However, the clam-digger position invites intrinsic contracture, and intrinsic tendon stretching exercises should be initiated early (Fig. 19-1).

Early mobilization of the injured finger is necessary to prevent stiffness and should be started as soon as local pain and fracture healing permit. Motion prevents adherence of the tendons at the fracture site, diminishes edema by pumping fluid from the finger, and decreases ligament contracture (Fig. 19-2).

An *exercise program must be directed toward the particular problems* that are characteristic of each individual fracture. The *most important joint in the hand is the proximal interphalangeal (PIP) joint,* and many of the exercises will be aimed at preventing stiffness and preserving function in this most important articulation.

The treatment of specific hand fractures is adequately described in several texts.[1,3] In the remainder of this chapter, fracture treatment will be discussed for only the more common injuries, with an emphasis on the cause of the fracture deformities and the treatment of specific fracture problems that may occur following reduction or internal fixation.

DISTAL PHALANX FRACTURES

Fractures of the distal phalanx occur more frequently than any others in the hand and present themselves most commonly in the middle finger and thumb. A crushing force such as a punch press usually causes these fractures, and associated skin loss and nail injuries are frequent. The extreme pain following distal phalanx trauma results from swelling and hematoma formation within the septated compartments of the fingertip. Chronic pain after such an injury is produced by a secondary fibrosis. Several types of fracture can occur (Fig. 19-3). Comminuted tuft fractures do not become displaced, however, as no tendon pull is exerted beyond the distal phalanx base.

Treatment of distal phalanx fractures should be directed toward the soft tissues, much as in a fingertip injury. Fracture immobilization is rarely necessary; a short splint, however, will prevent the digit from reinjury and more discomfort. Two fractures deserve special attention. Open displaced distal phalanx fractures that lose soft tissue control of the fragments and displaced transverse basilar fractures may require reduction and pin stabilization for 3 to 4 weeks to achieve rapid union.

Articular fractures of the distal phalanx usually involve the dorsal surface and can be classified with the mallet or drop-finger deformity (Fig. 19-4). The most common injury producing this deformity is stretching of the terminal extensor tendon. The patient is first seen with a 20- to 35-degree extension lag at the distal joint, but some weak active extension remains. With complete tendon rupture, the tip is dropped 45 degrees. Occasionally, a fragment of bone from the site of extensor insertion is avulsed. On x-ray film the distance the tendon has retracted is indicated by the displacement of the bone chip. Fragments that are minimally displaced (3 mm or less) or extremely small should be

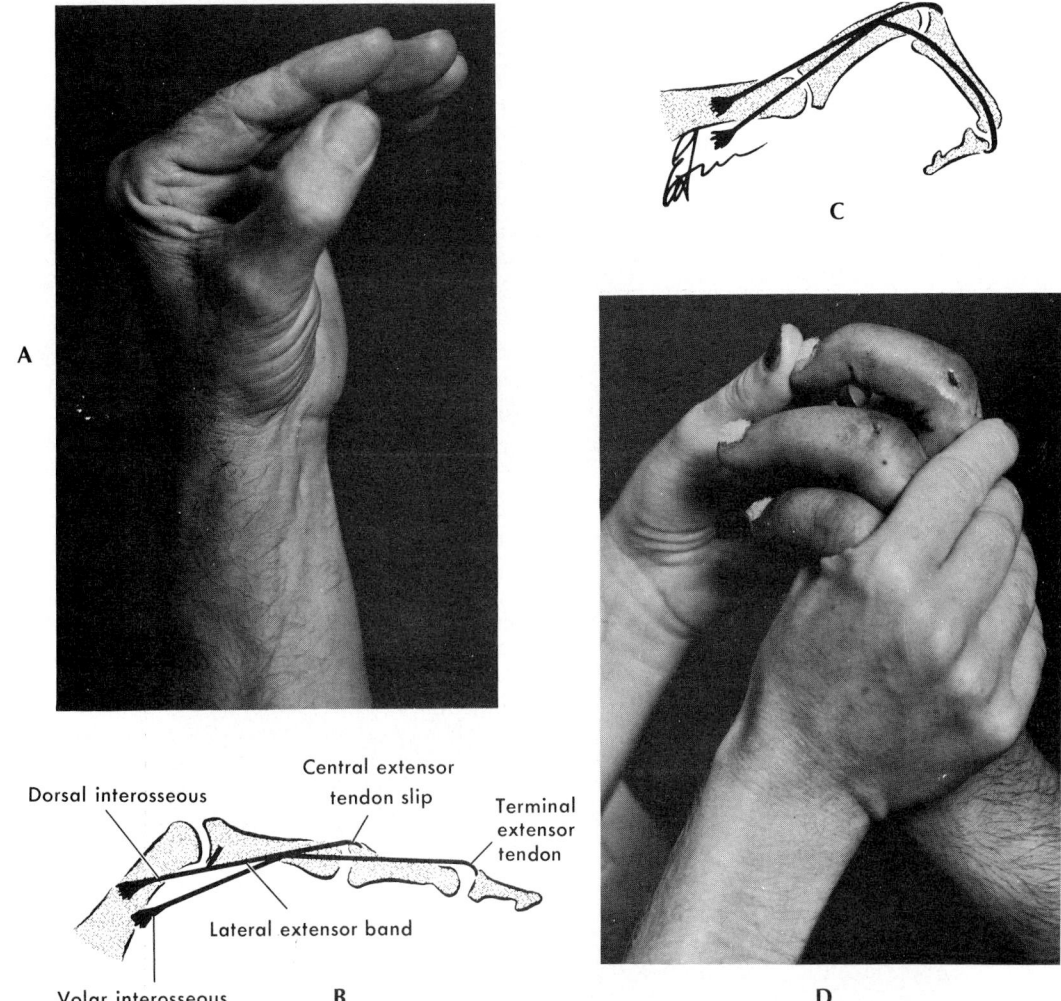

Dorsal interosseous
Central extensor tendon slip
Terminal extensor tendon
Lateral extensor band
Volar interosseous

Fig. 19-1   While "clam-digger" position, **A,** prevents joint contractures, intrinsic tendons are being maintained at their shortest length. **B.** To prevent intrinsic contracture, these tendons must be stretched, **C** and **D.**

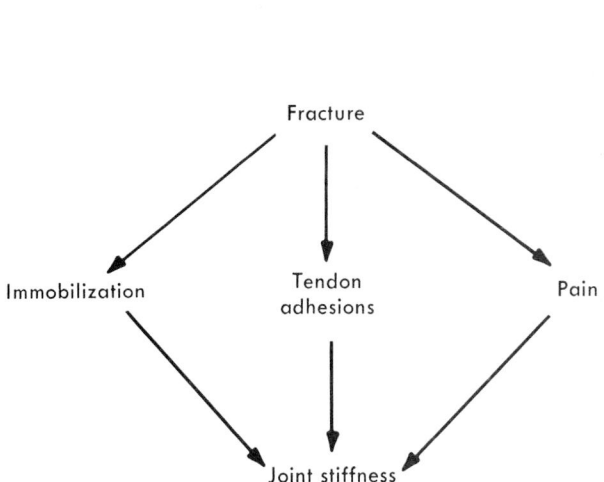

Fracture

Immobilization   Tendon adhesions   Pain

Joint stiffness

Fig. 19-2   Causes of joint stiffness.

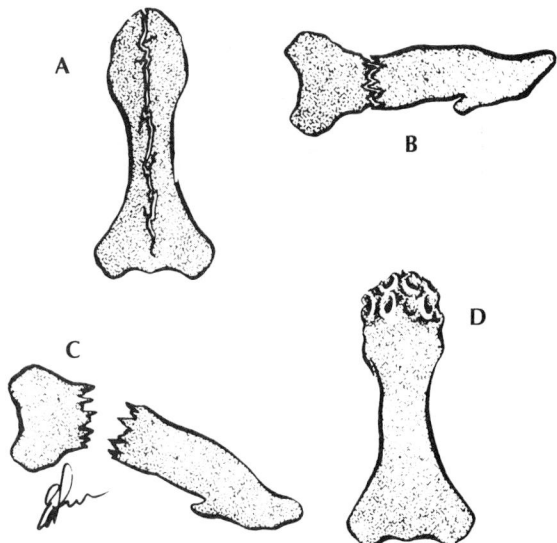

Fig. 19-3   Distal phalanx fractures may be, **A,** longitudinal, **B,** impacted, **C,** displaced transverse basilar, or **D,** tuft. The last is most common.

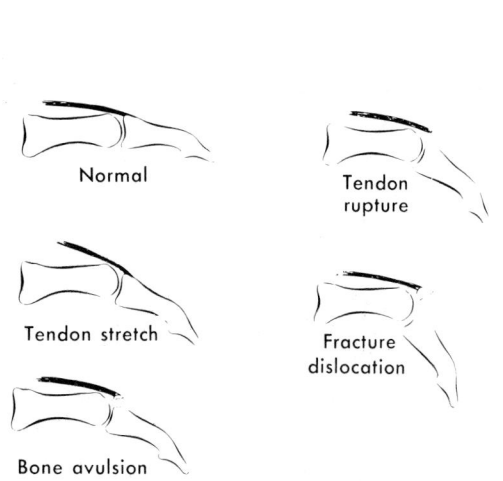

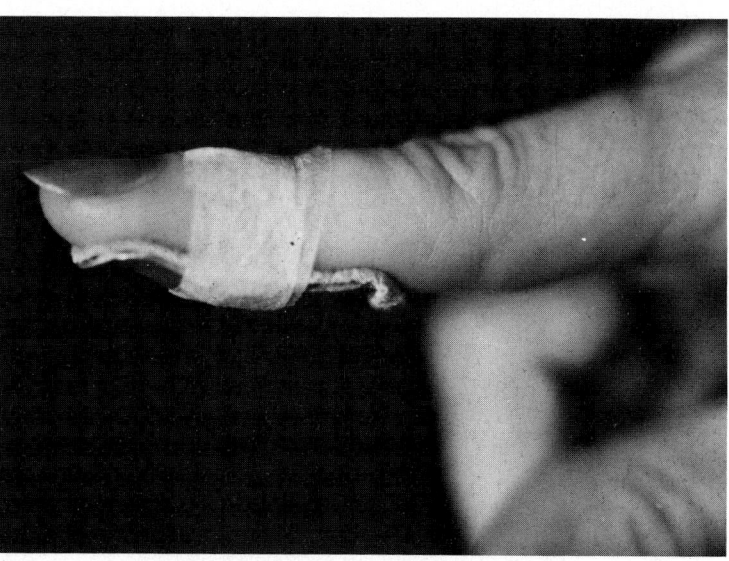

Fig. 19-4 Drop-finger deformity (mallet or baseball finger).

Normal

Tendon rupture

Tendon stretch

Fracture dislocation

Bone avulsion

Fig. 19-5 Volar padded metal splint bent to maintain slight distal joint extension can be simply applied and maintained.

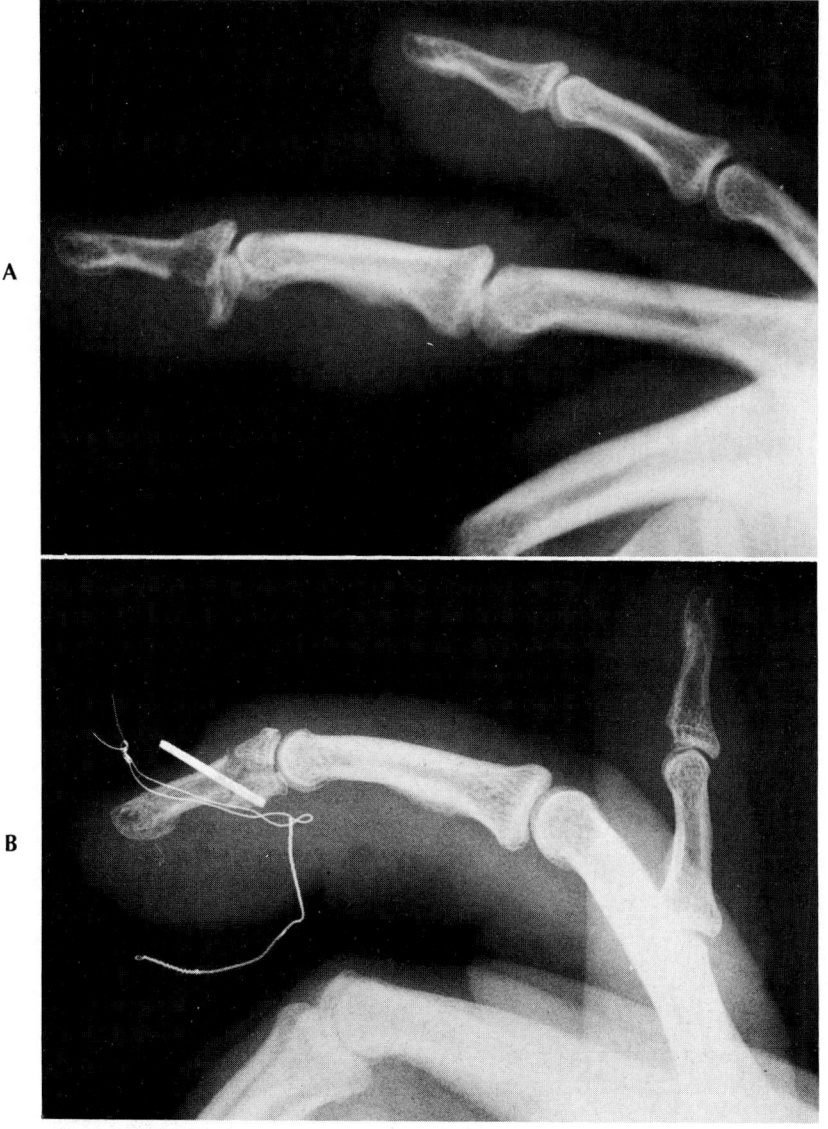

A

B

Fig. 19-6 Fractures of distal phalanx volar base can be associated with profundus avulsion, **A.** Sometimes bone fragment becomes displaced with tendon marking distance of retraction. Treatment includes fracture reduction with tendon advancement, **B.**

treated nonoperatively. A fracture involving one third or more of the articular surface can lead to dislocation of the distal joint, particularly with vigorous splinting into the hyperextended position.

Nonoperative treatment of mallet injuries consists of continuous distal joint immobilization in 10 degrees hyperextension for 6 weeks. Splints may be applied dorsally or volarly (Fig. 19-5). The PIP joint is not immobilized but should be exercised to prevent stiffness. Splinting at night is needed for an additional 2 or 3 weeks should an extensor lag occur.

One final distal phalanx injury to keep in mind is the "football jersey injury." This injury occurs when a football player accidentally grabs his opponent's jersey while missing a tackle, and his finger is forced into the extended position as the runner breaks away. The contracted profundus tendon becomes avulsed from the distal phalanx, often with a piece of bone. Profundus avulsion occurs most commonly in the ring finger and produces tremendous reaction within the tendon sheath. A lateral x-ray film of the digit may reveal a distal phalanx volar avulsion fracture that has retracted with the tendon (Fig. 19-6). Tendon reattachment within the first 2 weeks should restore nearly normal motion.

Therapy program

As soon as the distal phalanx can be mobilized, exercises should be directed toward regaining distal interphalangeal (DIP) motion and desensitizing the tip area. The more proximal joints of the finger are blocked to isolate flexor profundus and terminal extensor tendon activity. Desensitization of the tip is achieved through progressive activities that begin with rubbing and tapping and proceed to resistive pinching and grasping activities. A painful fingertip will not be incorporated in normal prehension patterns.

PROXIMAL AND MIDDLE PHALANX FRACTURES

Fractures of the proximal and middle phalanges are more difficult to treat than metacarpal or distal phalanx fractures, because of the frequent association of serious tendon and skin injuries, as well as instability resulting from lack of soft tissue support. Fracture displacement and angulation are determined by the mechanism of injury and the deforming forces of various tendons attached to each bone fragment. For instance, a direct blow to a digit may produce a transverse or comminuted fracture, whereas a twisting force results in an oblique or spiral fracture.

Proximal phalanx fractures occur most commonly on the radial side of the hand (thumb and index finger) and are usually located in a proximal or midshaft area. Such fractures are produced either by a fall or by a direct blunt injury. The characteristic deformity is volar angulation, the interossei flexing the proximal fragment and the central extensor tendon slip extending the distal portion (Fig. 19-7).

The major problem in the management of proximal phalanx fractures is the preservation of PIP joint motion. Stiffness of this joint occurs rapidly as the adjacent tendons become adherent to the fracture callus. A volar collapsed deformity will compound any potential flexion contracture as the extensor and intrinsic tendons are functionally lengthened, preventing full active PIP joint extension. Splint immobilization of the digit eliminates early motion and adds to the stiffness.

Middle phalanx fractures occur with the least frequency of all hand fractures. A crushing injury is the most common cause and the fracture is usually located in the distal portion of the shaft. Fractures of the middle phalanx are displaced by the central slip attachment to the proximal fragment and the broad volar superficialis insertion. Thus a distal fracture will angulate volarly, whereas a fracture near the phalanx base will have dorsal angulation. The major problem is to obtain union in a fracture that is frequently comminuted and open while maintaining PIP joint motion.

Before the appropriate treatment is selected, fracture stability must be assessed. The angle of the fracture is an important factor in determining this stability. Transverse fractures are frequently stable, whereas oblique fractures are inherently unstable. It is also important to know whether the fracture has been impacted or displaced and what deforming forces are acting on it. If there is any question of the fracture's stability, the digit is anesthetized and stress is applied. More than one half of all digital fractures are stable—that is, longitudinal fracture lines in the proximal phalanx (Fig. 19-8). *Such fractures should be started on early protected motion* as soon as pain subsides (within the first 3 to 5 days). Protection is provided by taping the injured finger to the adjacent digit (Fig. 19-9)—a form of dynamic splinting. It may be necessary to rest the finger intermittently in a metal or plaster splint to prevent reinjury while the patient is working or performing heavy activities.

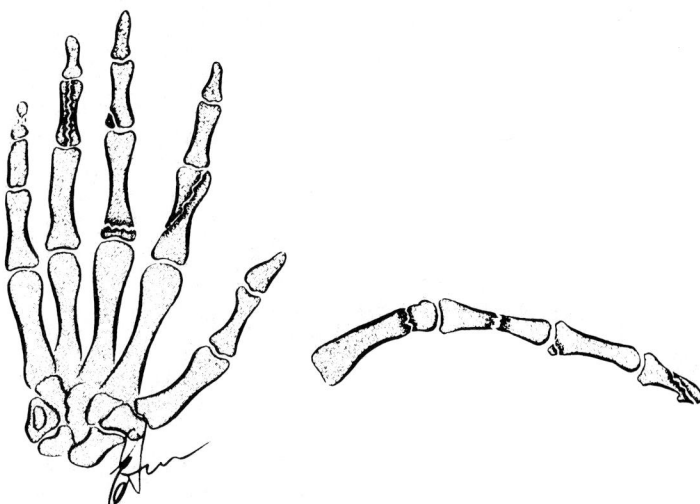

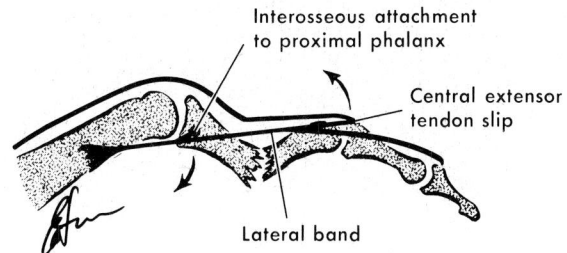

Fig. 19-7 Proximal phalanx fractures angulate volarly, interossei attached to proximal fragment flexing this portion. Central slip extends distal portion.

Fig. 19-8 Stable fractures should be mobilized as soon as pain subsides.

Interosseous attachment to proximal phalanx

Central extensor tendon slip

Lateral band

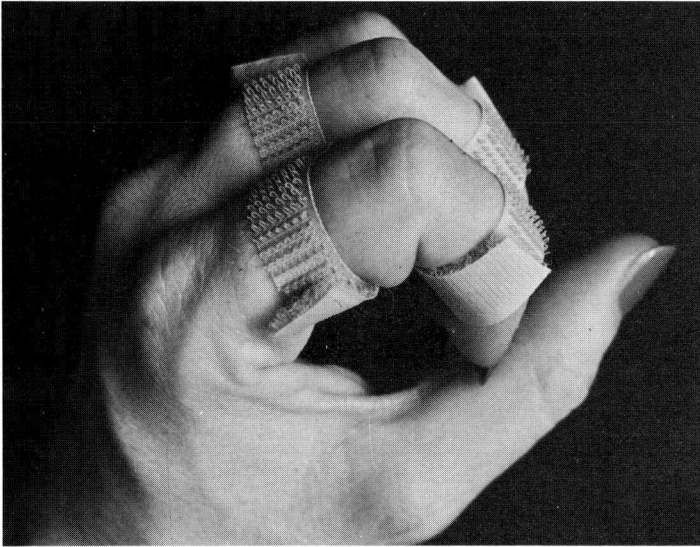

Fig. 19-9 Adjacent digit taping encourages motion while providing protection.

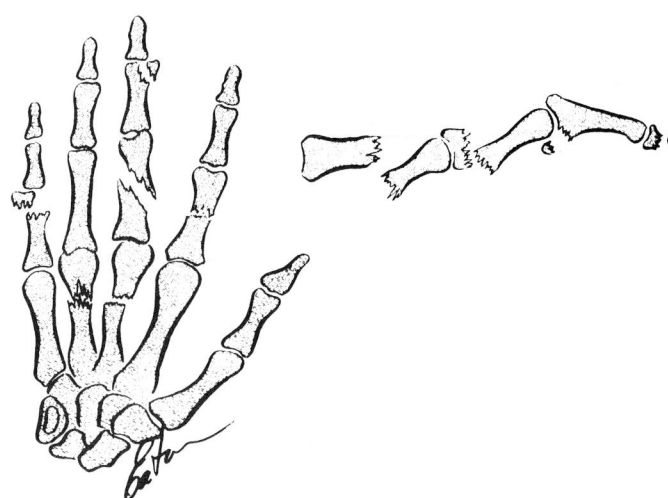

Fig. 19-10 Unstable fractures require reduction and immobilization. Pin fixation may be needed.

A type of fracture that is potentially unstable is an oblique but nondisplaced proximal phalanx fracture (Fig. 19-10). Early movement may well displace such a fracture, and the finger is best immobilized for 10 to 14 days. Then the digit should be reexamined and radiographed again, and a motion program should be started.

Many displaced fractures become converted to stable fractures after reduction. With sufficient anesthesia, the fracture is manipulated and the controllable distal fragment aligned with the proximal fragment. A splint is applied after reduction to stabilize and maintain this position. One form of immobilization is a plaster gutter that includes the adjacent noninjured finger for support and alignment and to judge rotation. The fingers are placed in the clam-digger position with the least amount of PIP flexion necessary to maintain reduction. A second technique is to incorporate a metal splint or padded bent wire into plaster and tape the finger to this splint. The advantage of this latter method is that the finger can be easily observed and radiographed for any shift of the fracture, since no plaster intervenes (Fig. 19-11).

Several other treatment techniques previously recommended have been discarded owing to the complications encountered. Traction is now indicated only when bone loss or severe comminution is being treated. Skin traction has been known to produce circulatory compromise and pulp traction necrosis, and nail traction often results in loss of the nail. Banjo splints, gauze rolls placed in the palm, and various commercial splints have been discredited.

Unstable fractures will require supplemental fixation, usually with a Kirschner wire or pin, to maintain the correct position. Closed reduction of some fractures is possible with pins inserted percutaneously to provide stabilization. Such a technique allows early motion and prevents the adhesions inherent with open reduction, when the extensor mechanism must be split and the periosteum reflected. Percutaneous pinning is best applied to proximal phalanx fractures. Pins may be started proximally at the wide metaphyseal flares and advanced distally across the fracture site. Transverse

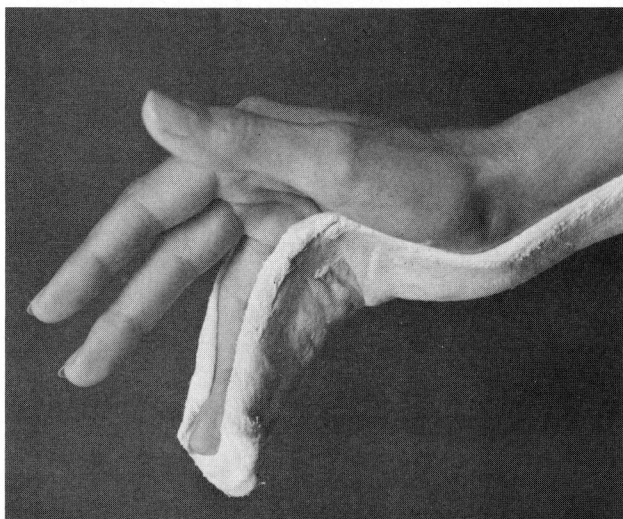

A

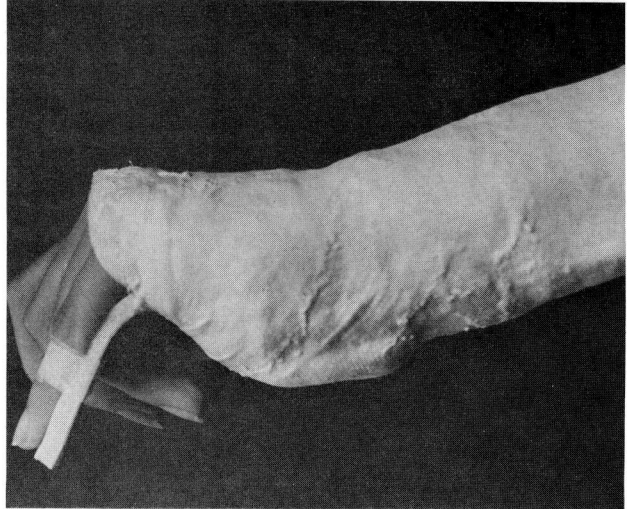

B

Fig. 19-11 Plaster gutter splint, **A,** can maintain reduction with adjacent finger for support and to control alignment. Metal splint, **B,** incorporated into plaster requires tape to maintain fracture position. X-ray reevaluation is more easily achieved.

A

B

C

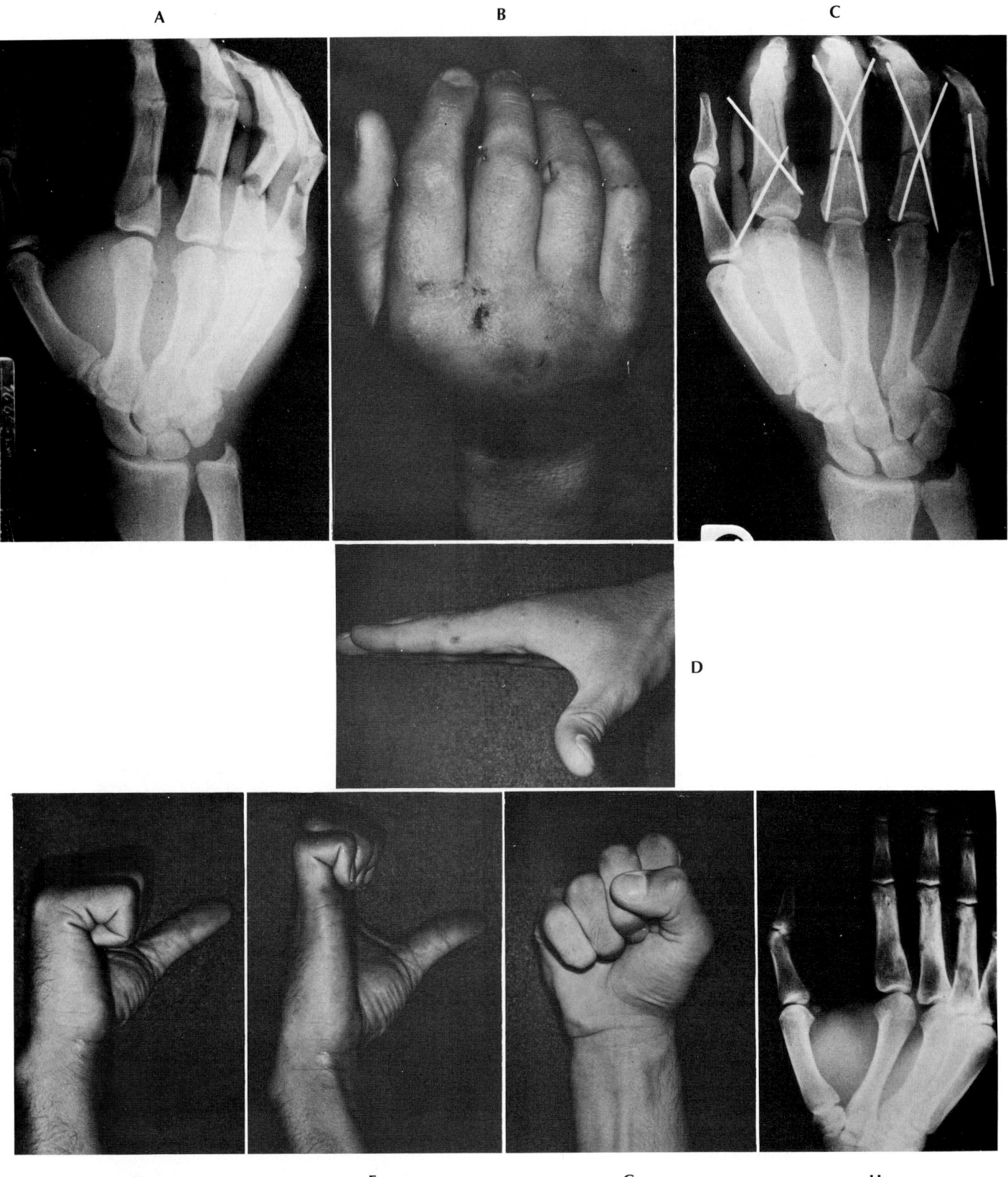

D

E

F

G

H

Fig. 19-12   M.H., 19-year-old male, sustained crush injury to right hand in hamburger machine, with displaced unstable transverse proximal phalanx fractures in all fingers, **A.** Closed reduction and percutaneous pin fixation, **B** and **C,** was followed by early (1-week) exercise program and split protection. At 9 weeks patient had regained near normal motion and returned to work, **D** to **H.**

fractures are difficult to treat using a percutaneous technique, and such treatment is contraindicated for comminuted or displaced intraarticular fractures (Fig. 19-12).

Open reduction is indicated in certain problem fractures, the most common being unstable fractures not amenable to closed reduction and splinting or percutaneous pinning (see list). In the proximal phalanx, this frequently includes basilar fractures with volar angulation greater than 25 degrees, displaced transverse shaft fractures, oblique fractures, and neck fractures. Displaced articular fractures (greater than 2 mm) and those that involve a single condyle with rotation will require internal fixation. Fractures incompletely reduced or with fragments poorly positioned such that malunion is likely need to undergo open reduction.

> *Hand fractures for which open reduction and fixation are indicated*
> Unstable fractures
> Inadequately reduced fractures
> Open fractures
> Associated soft tissue problems
> Multiple fractures
> Articular fractures
> Bone loss

Open fractures occur frequently (25% to 35%). If they are unstable or if tendon injuries or serious soft tissue management problems coexist, internal fixation is indicated. The presence of an open fracture in the hand is not a contraindication to pin or wire fixation as it might be with large-bone fractures. The fracture stabilization that can be provided by internal fixation will make treatment of a tendon injury easier. Attention may be directed toward the restoration of tendon gliding without fear of displacing the fracture. The management of soft tissue injuries such as a potential skin slough following a crush injury is only compounded by trying to maintain the fracture position with a plaster cast rather than utilizing pin fixation. Delayed closure is indicated in wounds with contamination or questionable tissue viability.

Multiple fractures in the hand occur more frequently (9%) than one might expect. Unless aggressively treated, stiffness of many digits will result. Pin or wire stabilization of fractures that are amenable to such treatment will greatly facilitate an early motion program.

Bone loss in the hand, such as is caused by gunshot wounds, is a subject that has received insufficient attention.

When a portion of a metacarpal is lost, temporary pin stabilization and delayed bone grafting are indicated. In the finger such reconstruction should be undertaken only when reasonably good eventual function can be anticipated. The goal of internal fixation is to achieve sufficient stabilization of fracture fragments to allow early protective motion.

The questions most frequently asked regarding fractures are: how long does it take to heal, when can motion be started, and how much splinting is necessary (and for how long)? The average time for a phalangeal fracture to show complete bone union on radiographs is 5 months, with a range of 1 to 14 months. The question is better phrased: when is a fracture solid enough to allow unprotected motion? For most closed nondisplaced fractures, motion should commence in the first 21 days, depending on stability. Immobilization for longer than 3 weeks will lead to stiffness and loss of hand function. Fractures of the tapered midshaft region of the phalanges, however, require a longer time to become consolidated (Fig. 19-13). In this area the cortical bone is thick, with minimal cancellous bone. Protection in the form of intermittent splinting for midshaft proximal phalanx fractures is needed for 5 to 7 weeks and in the middle phalanx for 10 to 14 weeks. Gentle motion protecting the fracture site is initiated at 3 weeks. The presence of pins stabilizing a fracture should not prevent an exercise program. Comminuted fractures and those requiring open reduction will take longer to become solid, and prolonged protection is necessary.

Therapy program

If internal fixation has provided satisfactory fracture stabilization, the patient is mobilized as soon as pain permits

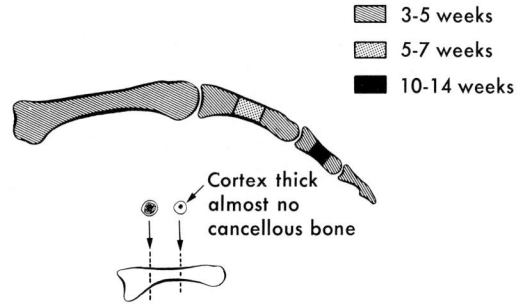

Fig. 19-13 Fracture consolidation varies within each segment of hand and is slowest where ratio of cortical to cancellous bone is highest (after Moberg).

Legend:
- 3-5 weeks
- 5-7 weeks
- 10-14 weeks

Cortex thick almost no cancellous bone

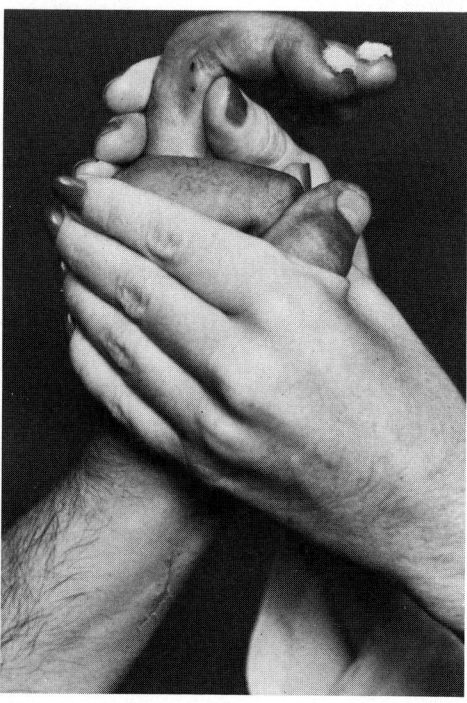

Fig. 19-14 Manual support of proximal phalanx fracture is provided by therapist while encouraging active proximal interphalangeal flexion by patient.

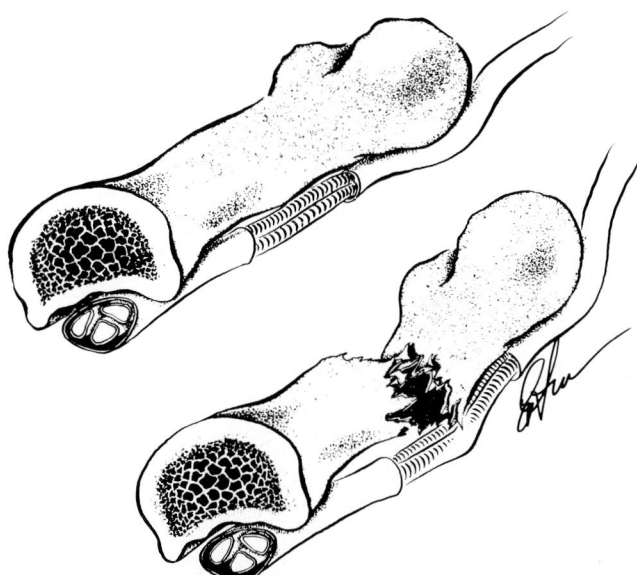

Fig. 19-15   Fracture disruption of fibro-osseous flexor tendon sheath will encourage tendon adherence at fracture site.

(5 to 15 days). Stable fractures or ones that have been splinted 3 weeks may be treated in a similar manner.

The goal in the treatment of proximal phalanx fractures is to attain maximal PIP joint motion while preventing a flexion contracture. Tendon adhesions at the fracture site are the main cause of joint stiffness. The therapist provides additional manual support at the level of the fracture while encouraging active PIP flexion and extension (Fig. 19-14). The injured digit is immobilized in the clam-digger position when not undergoing exercise, until the fracture is consolidated. Intrinsic stretching is mandatory to prevent contracture (Fig. 19-1). Although the dorsal and lateral tendons frequently adhere, the fibroosseous flexor sheath must be violated by the bone for flexor tendon adhesions to occur (Fig. 19-15). Thus the therapist, exercising a nondisplaced fracture, will encounter little difficulty in having the tendons glide by the fracture, while the converse is true of a markedly displaced fracture.

The most serious complication following a proximal phalanx fracture is a PIP joint flexion contracture. At rest, the hand assumes a position of PIP joint flexion, and this position can become fixed. The PIP joint must be splinted at neutral or as close to neutral as possible until the likelihood of a contracture ceases (usually by 5 weeks). When the fracture is considered solid (Fig. 19-13), a dynamic splinting program can commence, alternating dynamic flexion (flexion cuff) with extension (reverse finger knuckle bender or Capener splint).

The primary objective with middle phalanx fractures is to achieve full motion in the two more proximal joints, the MP and PIP joints. The goal is to achieve a "superficialis hand." If prolonged splinting includes the proximal phalanx, the PIP joint will become stiff. Thus fractures of the middle phalanx that will require longer than 3 weeks to consolidate should have pin stabilization to allow early motion. Later the distal joint will be exercised and the oblique retinacular ligament stretched to overcome contracture (Fig. 19-16).

METACARPAL FRACTURES

Fractures of the metacarpals can be classified for treatment by their location (head, neck, shaft, base). The event leading to a fracture in this area is usually a fight or a fall. Metacarpal fractures generally are more stable than phalangeal fractures because of the support provided the bones by the intrinsic musculature. Flexor and extensor tendons are not in close contact with the bone and become adherent less frequently. However, an intrinsic contracture can occur easily from swelling and direct trauma to the intrinsic muscles. The MP joint, unless carefully splinted, can develop an extension contracture.

The most common metacarpal fractures involve the neck, where the bone is weakest. Comminution of the volar cortex allows collapse into the flexed position. Reduction should be attempted by flexing the MP and PIP joints 90 degrees and pushing the metacarpal head into position. The PIP joint should never be left in this fixed position, because a flexion contracture may develop. It should be held with a plaster gutter or cast in the clam-digger position. Motion is begun at 2 to 3 weeks after removal of the splint, with further protection for 2 more weeks. With severe angulation of the fracture, clawing may result from collapse of the tendon system and will require fixation of the reduced fracture. Hunter has shown, however, that as much as 70 degrees volar angulation is acceptable as long as no malrotation is present.[2]

Transverse metacarpal shaft fractures develop dorsal angulation and are usually caused by a direct blow (Fig. 19-17). Fractures in the midshaft of the third and fourth metacarpals frequently occur simultaneously and will disrupt the transverse arch unless correctly reduced. Reduction of the fracture can be maintained with pin fixation. Stabilization should be attempted percutaneously with a longitudinal wire to control angulation and possibly a transverse pin to prevent malrotation.

Oblique metacarpal fractures are caused by a torque force with the finger acting as a lever arm. The result will be shortening and rotation but no angulation. The third and fourth metacarpals shorten least, owing to the tethering effect of the interossei and the transverse metacarpal ligament. Two to three millimeters of shortening is acceptable, but anything further requires internal fixation.

Comminuted metacarpal fractures are produced by crush injuries, such as those that occur in punch-press accidents. Sometimes such fractures are minimally displaced and can be treated with a gutter splint for 3 weeks, followed by gentle motion and 3 more weeks protection. Displaced or unstable fractures can be easily controlled with transverse pins.

Metacarpal bone loss, such as in a gunshot wound, will usually have an associated soft tissue problem that will command primary attention. Transverse and possibly longitudinal pins will control the fracture, and secondary bone grafting will make up for the bone loss.

Therapy program

The objectives of treatment in metacarpal fractures are elimination of edema, maintenance of architectural integrity, and prevention of contractures.

Excessive dorsal edema characterizes metacarpal fractures. Initially, constant elevation can lessen the swelling.

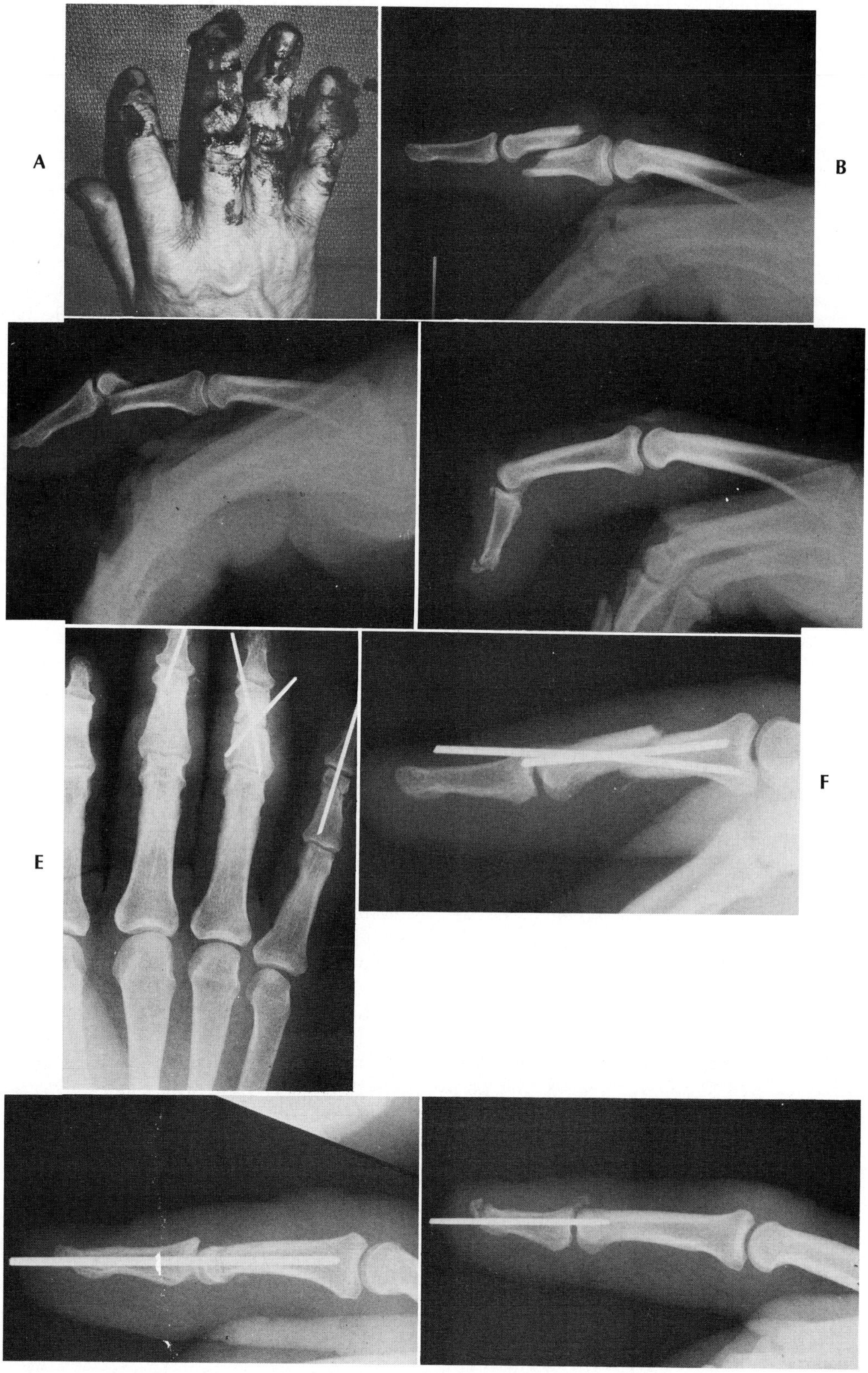

Fig. 19-16 C.F., 35-year-old machinist, sustained open middle phalanx fracture in ring, **B,** and little fingers, **C,** and extensor tendon disruption in middle finger, **A** and **D.** Fracture reduction (ring and little), **F** and **G,** and distal joint stabilization with extensor repair (middle), **H,** was followed with early (10 days) mobilization, **E.** At 3 weeks good proximal interphalangeal flexion was attained, **I** and **J,** and by 12 weeks patient had regained sufficient motion and strength to return to work, **K** to **M.**

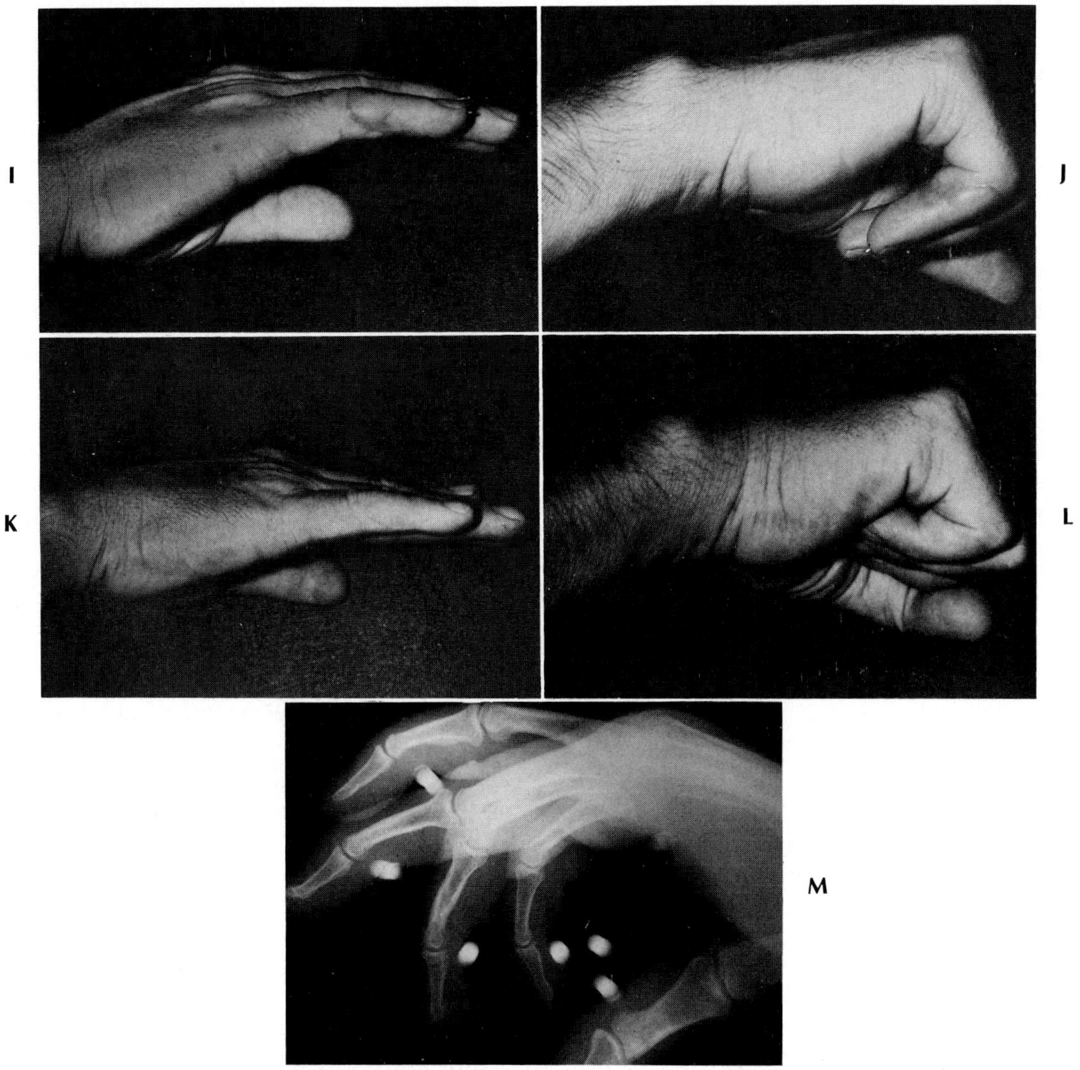

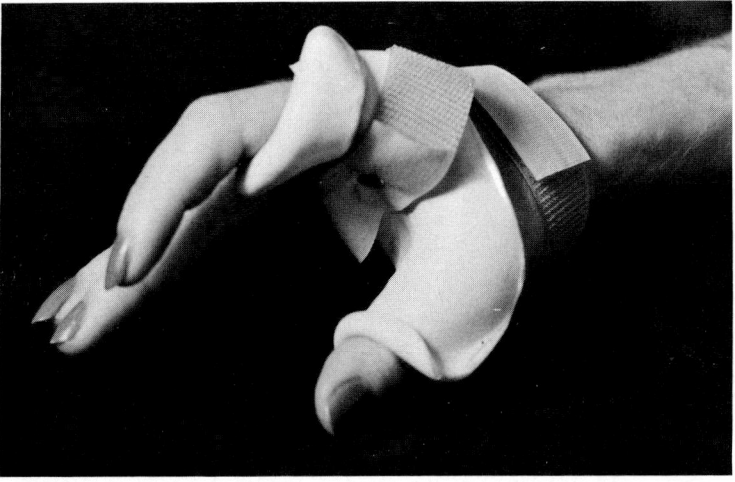

I

J

K

L

M

Fig. 19-16, cont'd   For legend see opposite page.

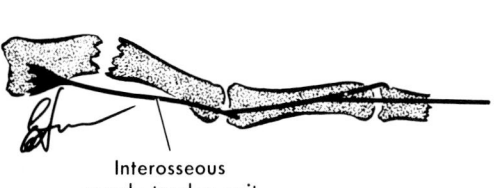

Interosseous
muscle-tendon unit

Fig. 19-17   Metacarpal fractures angulate dorsally as intrinsic muscles lie palmarward and tendons pass volar to axis of MP joint.

Fig. 19-18   Thumb web-space contracture can occur after any injury producing significant dorsal edema (that is, burn, crush, fracture). Resting splint can protect against such an occurrence.

Motion, massage, and intermittent compression will also reduce edema later in the therapy program.

With second- and third-metacarpal fractures, the transverse arch of the hand must be supported by the therapist during exercising and with a splint when the hand is at rest. After a fracture of the first metacarpal, the thumb web space must be protected with a splint to prevent contracture (Fig. 19-18).

Extension contractures of the MP joints can easily occur unless these joints are immobilized in 60 to 70 degrees flexion. This may require frequent fabrication of a new clam-digger splint as edema diminishes.

SUMMARY

Many of the serious complications that can occur after hand fractures (see list) may be prevented by observing a few basic principles. The safe position for immobilizing a fractured hand is the clam-digger, or intrinsic-positive, position. Early protective motion is the best means of preventing joint stiffness or contracture.

Complications following hand fractures
Joint stiffness
Joint contractures, especially flexion contractures
Pain
Weakness
Intrinsic contractures
Chronic edema
Tendon adherence
Malrotation
Associated injuries (for example, soft tissue loss, nerve, vascular)
Reflex sympathetic dystrophy
Infection
Nonunion

REFERENCES

1. Flynn JE: Hand surgery, ed 2, Philadelpha, 1975, Williams & Wilkins.
2. Hunter JM and Cowen NJ: Fifth metacarpal fractures in a compensation clinic population, J Bone Joint Surg 52A:1159, 1970.
3. Rockwood CA and Green DP: Fractures, Philadelphia, 1975, JB Lippincott Co.

BIBLIOGRAPHY

Barton N: Fractures of the phalanges of the hand, Hand 9:1, 1977.
Bloem JJAM: The treatment and prognosis of uncomplicated dislocated fractures of the metacarpals and phalanges, Arch Chir Neerl 23:55, 1971.
Borgeskov S: Conservative therapy for fractures of the phalanges and metacarpals, Acta Chir Scand 133:123, 1967.
Burton RI and Eaton RG: Common hand injuries in the athlete, Orthop Clin North Am 4:809, 1973.
Butt WD: Fractures of the hand. I. Description, Can Med Assoc J 86:731, 1962.
Butt WD: Fractures of the hand. II. Statistical review, Can Med Assoc J 86:775, 1962.
Butt WD: Fractures of the hand. III. Treatment and results, Can Med Assoc J 86:815, 1962.
Carroll RE and Match RM: Avulsion of the flexor profundus tendon insertion, J Trauma 10:1109, 1970.
Clinkscales GS Jr: Complications in the management of fractures in hand injuries, South Med J 63:704, 1970.
Coonrad RW and Pohlman MH: Impacted fractures in the proximal portion of the proximal phalanx of the finger, J Bone Joint Surg 51A:1291, 1969.
Crawford GP: Screw fixation for certain fractures of the phalanges and metacarpals, J Bone Joint Surg 58A:487, 1976.
Dobyns JH: Articular fractures of the hand, J Bone Joint Surg 48A:610, 1966.
Flatt AE: The care of minor hand injuries, ed 4, St. Louis, 1979, The CV Mosby Co.
Green DP and Anderson JR: Closed reduction and percutaneous pin fixation of the fractured phalanges, J Bone Joint Surg 55A:1651, 1973.
Howard LD Jr: Fractures of the small hand bones, Plast Reconstr Surg 29:334, 1962.
James JIP: Fractures of the proximal and middle phalanges of the fingers, Acta Orthop Scand 32:401, 1962.
James JIP: Common, simple errors in the management of hand injuries, Proc R Soc Med 63:69, 1970.
Kilbourne BC: Management of complicated hand fractures, Surg Clin North Am 48:201, 1968.
Lipscomb PR: Management of fractures of the hand, Am Surg 29:277, 1963.
Milford L: The hand. In Edmonson AS and Crenshaw AH, editors: Campbell's operative orthopedics, ed 6, St. Louis, 1980, The CV Mosby Co.
Moberg E: Emergency surgery of the hand, Edinburgh, 1968, E & S Livingstone.
Peacock EE: Management of conditions of the hand requiring immobilization, Surg Clin North Am 33:1297, 1953.
Riordan DC: Fractures about the hand, South Med J 50:637, 1957.
Ruedi TP, Burri C, and Pfeiffer KM: Stable internal fixation of fractures of the hand, J Trauma 11:381, 1971.
Smith FL and Rider DL: A study of the healing of one hundred consecutive phalangeal fractures, J Bone Joint Surg 17:9, 1935.
Stark HH: Troublesome fractures and dislocations of the hand. In AAOS: Instructional course lectures, vol 19, St. Louis, 1970, The CV Mosby Co, pp 130.
Sutro CJ: Fracture of metacarpal bones and proximal manual phalanges: treatment with emphasis on the prevention of rotational deformities, Am J Surg 81:327, 1951.
Swanson AB: Fractures involving the digits of the hand, Orthop Clin North Am 1:261, 1970.
Watson-Jones R: Fractures and joint injuries, ed 3, Edinburgh, 1943, E & S Livingstone.
Weeks PM and Wray RC: Management of acute hand injuries: a biological approach, ed 2, St. Louis, 1978, The CV Mosby Co.
Wright TA: Early mobilization in fractures of the metacarpals and phalanges, Can J Surg 11:491, 1968.

20

Joint injuries in the hand: preservation of proximal interphalangeal joint function

Robert Lee Wilson and Margaret S. Carter

Trauma to the small joints in the hand is frequently treated as a trivial injury. However, the stiffness, pain, and occasional instability that may occur in these joints after injury or prolonged immobilization may seriously restrict hand function. The most important small hand joints are the proximal interphalangeal (PIP) joints. This chapter will deal with trauma to this most critical articulation. Other sources provide a comprehensive view of injuries to the remaining joints in the hand.[2,3,5] First, to better understand the pathomechanics of PIP joint injuries, we review the anatomic features of this joint.

ANATOMY

The PIP joint is hinged in the sagittal plane and has considerable stability as contrasted to the metacarpophalangeal (MP) joint.[6,7] Lateral stability is provided by the bicondylar head of the proximal phalanx with its convex condyles and intercondylar groove, which articulate with the concave condyles and intercondylar ridge of the middle phalanx base. These articular surfaces are only slightly incongruous allowing minimal lateral and torsional movements.[8] The width of this joint is twice the vertical height. The collateral ligaments enclose both sides of the joint arising from the proximal phalanx condyles and attach to the volar base of the middle phalanx and volar plate. The PIP collateral ligaments are under constant tension throughout the entire arc of motion in contrast to those of the MP joint, which are relaxed in extension and tightened in flexion. The accessory collateral ligament, a more anterior continuation, attaches to and suspends the volar plate and flexor tendon

sheath. The accessory ligament is more flexible and folds during maximal joint flexion. The fibrocartilaginous volar plate surrounds the anterior aspect of the PIP joint, acting as a gliding surface for the proximal phalanx condyles on one side and the flexor tendons on the other. The proximal lateral portion of the volar plate is thickened and attached to the proximal phalanx to check or prevent joint hyperextension. Synovial recesses are present both dorsally and volarly. Prolonged joint immobilization, particularly in the flexed position, will obliterate these spaces with volar plate and collateral ligament adherence. Although the dorsal capsule may also become adherent, contracture in this more pliable dorsal tissue takes longer to develop. Therefore the recommended position for immobilization of the PIP joint is 0 to 15 degrees of flexion (Fig. 20-1).

The stability provided by this capsular-ligamentous structure is supplemented by several tendons passing around the joint. The central slip of the long extensor tendon inserts into the dorsal tubercle of the middle phalanx and extends the PIP joint. The lateral bands, receiving contributions from the intrinsic and the extrinsic extensor tendons, pass laterally about both sides of the joint and lie dorsal to the PIP joint axis. The transverse retinacular ligament runs from the anterior border of the lateral band to the flexor sheath at the level of the joint and prevents dorsal displacement of the lateral bands. Landsmeer's oblique retinacular ligament begins at the flexor sheath over the proximal phalanx, lies volar to the axis of motion of the PIP joint, and attaches to the terminal extensor tendon. With PIP joint extension the oblique retinacular ligament tightens, pulling the terminal

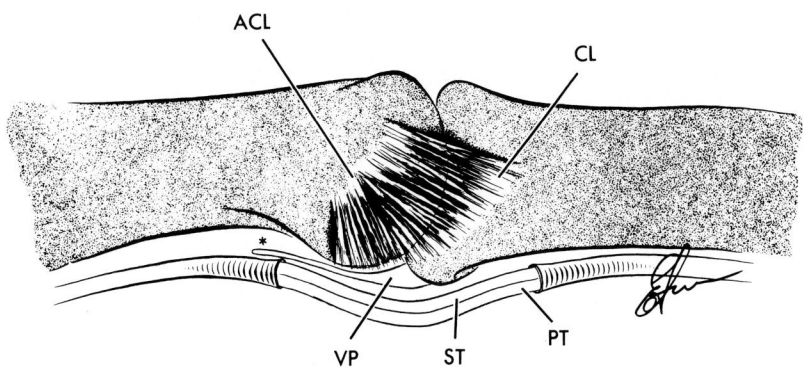

Fig. 20-1 Proximal interphalangeal joint in lateral view showing collateral, *CL,* and accessory collateral ligaments, *ACL,* attaching to middle phalanx and volar plate, *VP.* Flexor tendon sheath containing superficialis, *ST,* and profundus tendons, *PT,* is closely attached to periosteum of phalanges and volar plate. Recess (*) is present between volar plate and phalanx.

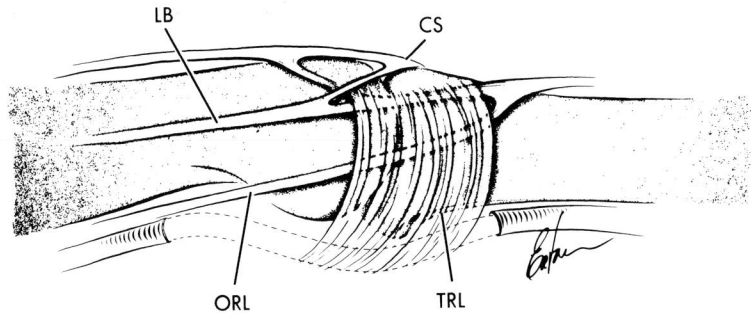

Fig. 20-2 Diagram of proximal interphalangeal joint, emphasizing digital extensor mechanism. Central extensor tendon slip, *CS*, extends PIP joint. Lateral bands, *LB*, are supported by transverse retinacular ligament, *TRL*, and along with oblique retinacular ligament, *ORL*, provide coordinated distal joint extension.

extensor tendon proximally and preventing passive distal joint flexion. This ligament also prevents PIP joint hyperextension (Fig. 20-2).

Thus a number of factors contribute to PIP joint stability, the most important being the base of the middle phalanx, the volar plate, and the collateral ligaments. The key point is where these three structures intersect. To dislocate the PIP joint, at least one and sometimes all three of these structures must be damaged.

However, it is the stability of the PIP joint that makes it susceptible to injury. The MP joint is anatomically dissimilar, having lateral movement and flexion and extension. Thus when the finger is struck at the tip, such as with a baseball, the force is dissipated at the MP joint because of the mobility but concentrated at the PIP joint.

EVALUATION

The first step in examining the patient who has sustained an injury about the PIP joint is to determine the mechanism of injury (hyperextension, lateral dislocation, and so on). The area about the PIP joint should be carefully palpated, especially over each collateral ligament and the volar plate, to localize any area of tenderness and tissue damage. Note that the radial collateral ligament is injured more frequently than the ulnar. A digital nerve block should be performed before one stresses the joint if the injured finger is painful. Each collateral ligament should be stressed, and confirmatory roentgenograms should be taken if there is any question of joint stability. Next, active flexion and extension of the injured digit by the patient will determine if joint stability is present throughout the full flexion arc. Frequently after hyperextension injuries, the joint will redislocate in the last 20 degrees of extension. If dislocation occurs with active motion, the joint is considered functionally unstable.

In the following discussion, injuries about the PIP joint have been arranged arbitrarily into six categories (see list). Although they are discussed individually, one must remember that these joint injuries can occur in combination.

Proximal interphalangeal joint injuries
1. Collateral ligaments
2. Dorsal dislocations
   a. Acute
   b. Chronic
3. Volar dislocations
4. Articular fractures
5. Boutonnière deformities
6. Pseudoboutonnière deformities

COLLATERAL LIGAMENT INJURIES

Unilateral stress to the extended finger can produce a collateral ligament injury. The injuries are of varying degrees of severity, from complete disruption to sprains (functionally intact ligament but with diffuse individual fiber disruption). Although stress testing will reveal the relatively infrequent complete ligament rupture, no clinical test can differentiate between minimal ligament injury and almost complete ligament disruption. Ligaments are notoriously slow to heal, and symptoms vary with the extent of ligament damage, persisting for many months.

Ligament sprains that are stable to stress and active motion testing are immobilized until the acute discomfort subsides—usually from 3 to 10 days. The joint and ligament are further protected when the injured finger is taped to the adjacent digit (Fig. 20-3). Easily adjustable Velcro loops may be substituted for adhesive tape. This protection may need to be continued for months to prevent minor reinjuries that can prolong the healing period and disability.

Partial or almost complete ligament tears may require immobilization up to 3 weeks. With any collateral ligament injury, the adjacent lateral band may adhere to the ligament (Fig. 20-4). To prevent this adherence from becoming a contracture, intrinsic stretching must be incorporated into the exercise program.

Lateral dislocations are produced by shear stress. The collateral ligament is ruptured at the PIP attachment and often is displaced into the joint. Incomplete transverse tears into the volar plate are associated with this injury. Treatment of complete ligament rupture remains controversial, with some authors recommending splinting of the reduced joint for 3 weeks and others advising immediate surgical repair.[12-14] Joints that are grossly unstable (that is, an additional 25 degrees or more of lateral deviation on stress testing) should be explored, and the extent of damage assessed. Volar plate repair and collateral ligament reattachment may be necessary. After surgery, the joint is immobilized for 3 weeks in the extended position and then gradually mobilized. Further splinting is usually necessary.

Therapy considerations

Successful management of collateral ligament injuries is largely the result of patient education. The principle objectives in a therapy program are mobilization of the joint to overcome stiffness, prevention of PIP flexion contractures, and protection from recurrent injuries. Patients are placed

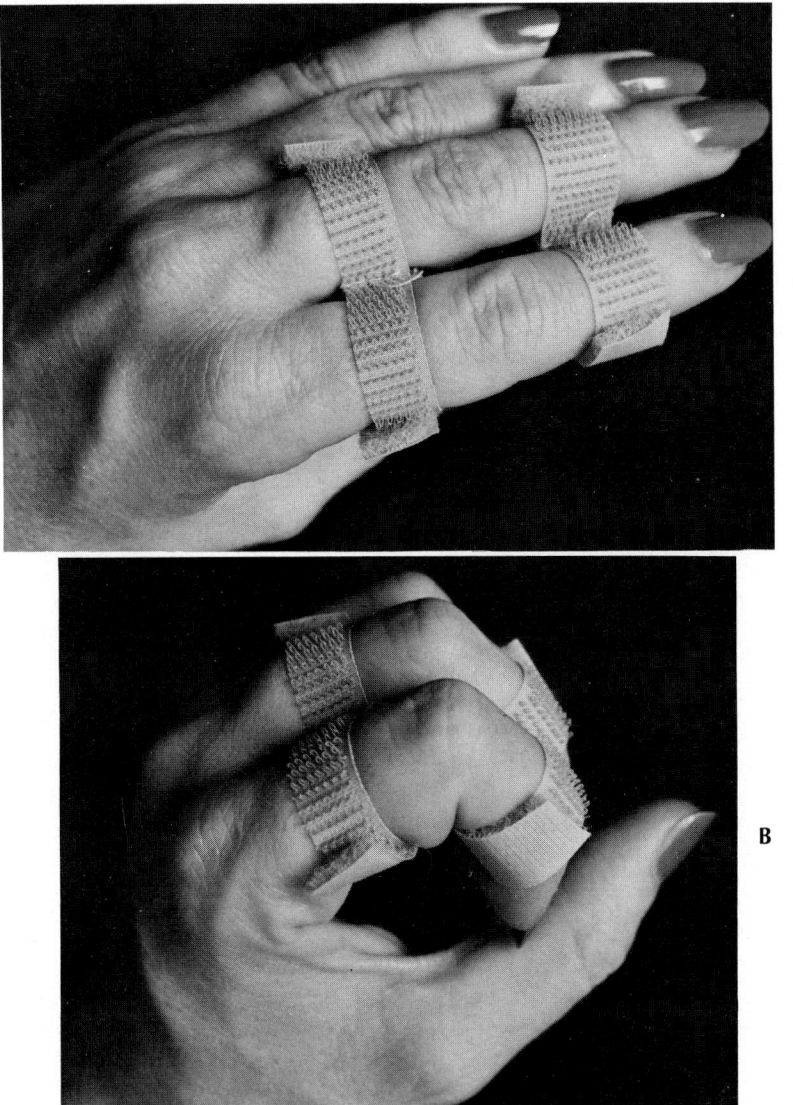

Fig. 20-3   Adjacent digit taping (seen here with Velcro loops) provides protection by keeping fingers together in extension, **A,** as well as flexion, **B.**

Fig. 20-4   Inflammatory response associated with partial or complete collateral ligament, *CL*, disruption can produce adhesions to lateral bands, *LB*, or oblique retinacular ligaments. To prevent any limitation of excursion of these structures, one must start stretching exercises early.

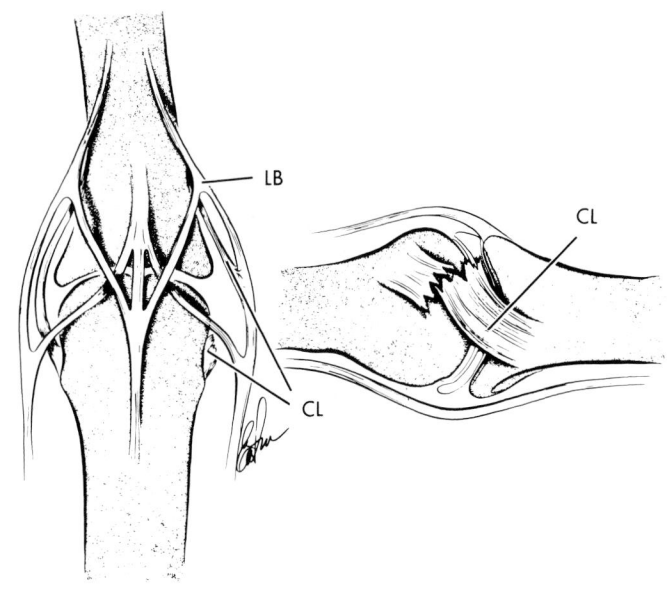

on a treatment program of specific exercises and splinting. Counseling regarding the potential seriousness of the injury and the length of time required for ligament healing must be provided early and reinforced frequently during the many months of healing. Reevaluation of joint motion and circumference measurements are made frequently, and the exercise program is altered accordingly. A directed exercise program includes stretching of the intrinsic tendons and retinacular ligaments, isolated intrinsic exercises, and a graduated progressive resistive exercise program to increase grip and pinch strength. Significant weakness of grip frequently accompanies ligament injuries.

All exercises are performed for 3 to 5 minutes and repeated every hour over the course of the day to prevent further joint swelling. Antiinflammatory agents (phenylbutazone, oxyphenbutazone) may decrease joint swelling but should only be used for a short course. When persistent pain or swelling becomes localized to one area, an injection of a cortisone type of drug is frequently beneficial. Edema of the digit and hand can be controlled through the use of the Jobst Intermittent Compression Unit, elevation, heat, and retrograde massage. A splinting regimen must provide protection, prevent flexion contractures, and increase active flexion and extension.

Dynamic daytime splinting besides the digital taping or Velcro loops might include a Capener splint (Fig. 20-5) because it provides ideal protection with the lateral wires adjacent to the collateral ligaments. The digital taping must be altered with a dynamic extension splint such as a reverse knuckle bender if a flexion contracture is noted.

Static night splinting with either a metal splint or serial finger cast (Fig. 20-6) cut out proximally and dorsally to accommodate joint swelling will rest the finger in an optimal position. Night splinting should be instituted with the appearance of any flexion contractures. To establish maximal PIP motion, one has the constant dilemma with either ex-

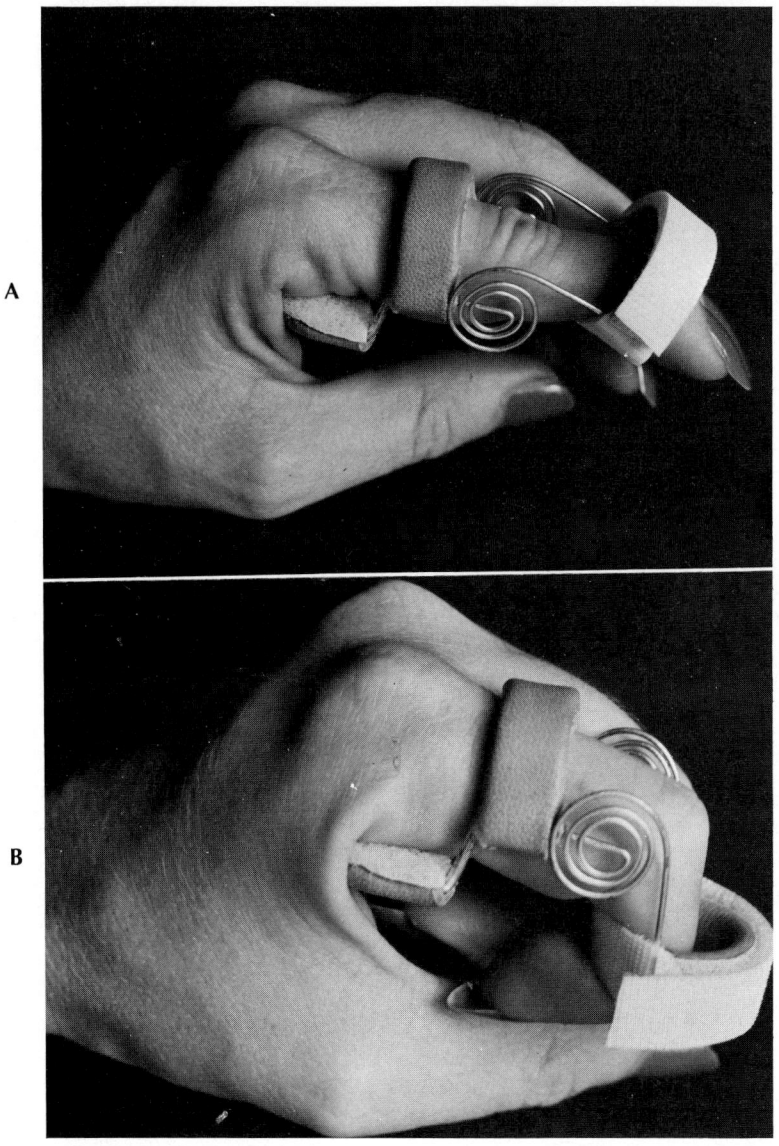

Fig. 20-5 Capener splint provides dynamic extension assist, with wires closely paralleling collateral ligaments in extension, **A,** and in flexion, **B.**

TREATMENT: ACUTE DORSAL DISLOCATIONS	
1. Stable: no fractures	Splint 25 degrees flexion—3 weeks
2. Stable: fracture nondisplaced	Splint 25 degrees flexion—3 weeks
3. Unstable: no fracture	Dorsal block—5 weeks
4. Unstable: fracture displaced	Open reduction or dorsal block
5. Comminuted fracture	Volar plate advancement

ercising or splinting of attaining full joint flexion while preventing a flexion deformity.

DORSAL DISLOCATIONS

Dorsal displacement of the PIP joint is the most common acute dislocation. This injury may occur in association with

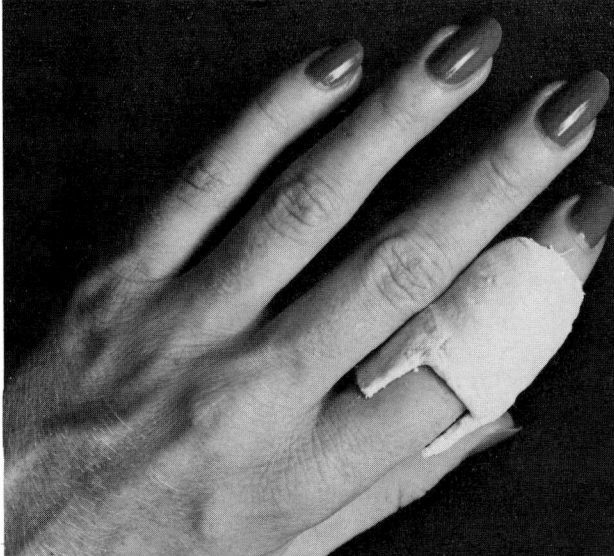

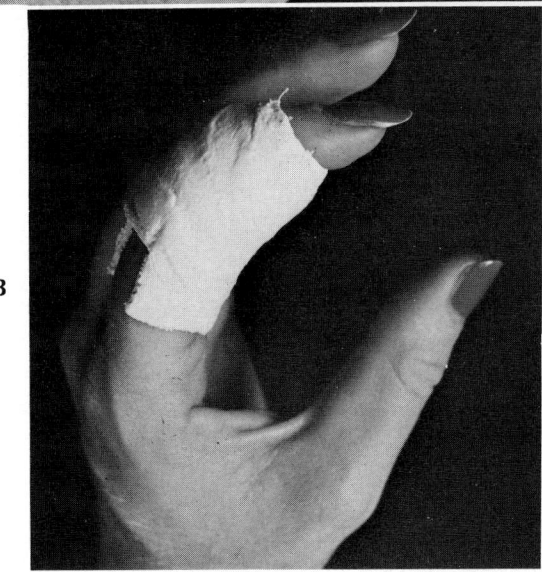

Fig. 20-6 Plaster finger casts are cut out dorsally, **A,** in order to slip past an enlarged joint. PIP joint is thus statically maintained in maximal extension, **B,** to combat any tendency for increasing flexion contracture.

a mallet finger injury. PIP joint dislocations can be produced by a longitudinal force on the extended finger, as when a baseball strikes the digit's tip with the interphalangeal joints in extension. The proximal phalangeal head divides the volar plate insertion at the middle phalangeal base. This injury may include an avulsion of the volar plate, a collateral ligament tear, or a middle phalangeal fracture. After roentgenographic evaluation and digital nerve block, the dislocation is reduced by traction and flexion. After postreduction roentgenograms, lateral stress testing determines collateral ligament integrity. Then joint stability through a full arc of flexion is assessed (see boxed material).

If the dislocation after reduction is stable and has no fracture, the PIP joint is splinted in 25 degrees flexion for 3 weeks to allow soft tissue healing. If the middle phalangeal base is fractured, but on postreduction roentgenograms the fracture fragment is not displaced and the joint is stable through an active range of motion, immobilization for 3 weeks should be sufficient. Fractures involving less than one quarter of the middle phalangeal base are usually stable.

The PIP joint that is unstable, redislocating with active extension but demonstrating no fracture, has disruption of both the volar plate and collateral ligaments. In the nonsurgical approach to this problem, a dorsal metal splint is incorporated in a plaster cast immobilizing the hand and wrist. The dorsal metal splint is bent so as to limit the last 25 degrees of PIP extension, thus blocking dorsal dislocation (Fig. 20-7). This splint should be continued for 5 weeks with the joint exercised by active flexion. This same program is also applicable to the stable injuries previously mentioned.

Unstable dorsal dislocations with displaced fractures require open reduction. The joint is best approached through a volar zigzag incision. Large fracture fragments are reattached to the middle of the phalanx with Kirschner wires. If multiple small fragments are present, these are excised and the volar plate is advanced into the middle phalangeal defect with a pullout wire. If the injury is old or the treatment is delayed, first the adherent dorsal capsule and extensor tendon must be released and then the contracted collateral ligaments divided to allow reduction (Fig. 20-8).

Volar plate advancement will prevent redislocation; the transarticular wire holds the joint surfaces in the reduced position. Three weeks after surgery this pin is removed, and the patient is started on active and active assisted proximal interphalangeal flexion exercises. By 5 weeks a dynamic flexion splint can usually be added, and at 7 weeks extension splinting is begun (Fig. 20-9).

A chronic dorsal subluxation or dislocation may occur if a middle phalangeal base fracture is unrecognized or untreated. If, at exploration, collapse of the middle phalanx is encountered and the amount of joint damage minimal, an

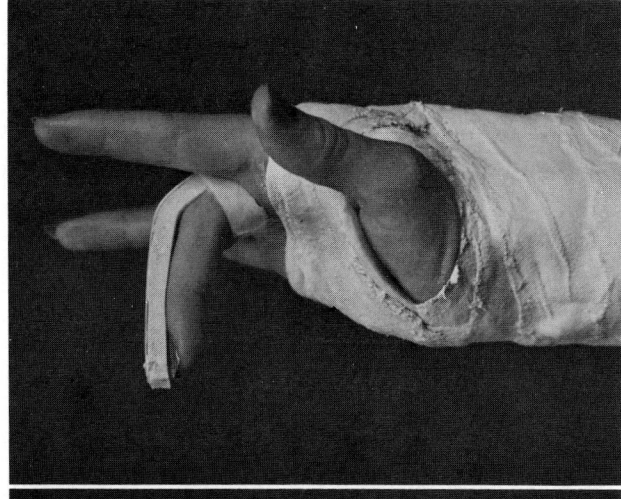

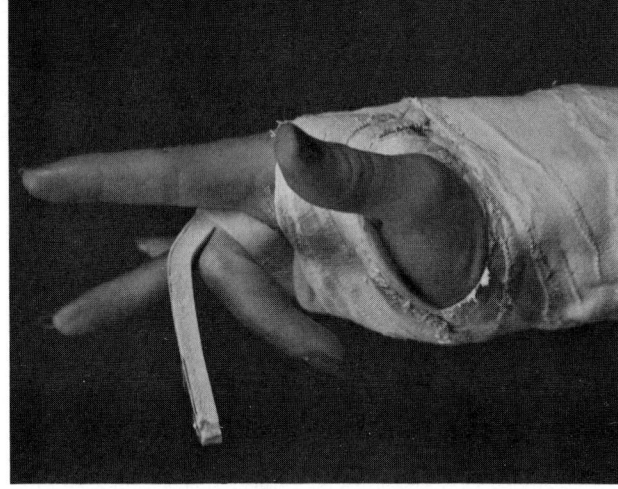

Fig. 20-7 With dorsal block splint, proximal phalanx is taped to splint, limiting extension, **A,** while allowing flexion, **B.**

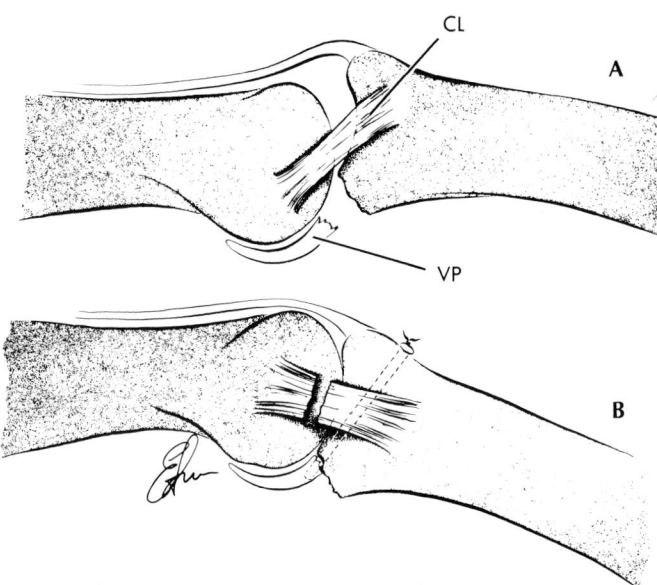

Fig. 20-8 To reduce dorsal dislocation, **A,** any dorsal capsule adhesions or collateral ligament, *CL,* contractures must be released. Small fracture fragments are removed and volar plate, *VP,* is advanced into defect with wire suture, **B.**

opening wedge osteotomy can reestablish the volar buttress. Frequently, the amount of articular damage is so severe that fragment excision and volar plate advancement arthroplasty are necessary.[1]

A common sequela of untreated PIP hyperextension injuries is the swan-neck deformity, which occurs from damage to the volar plate and collateral and retinacular ligaments. Surgery to correct this established deformity is indicated if the joint becomes locked in the hyperextended position. Pain produced by damage to the articular surface is a surgical contraindication to soft-tissue reconstruction alone. Numerous surgical procedures have been advocated. Curtis[2] recommends dividing one slip of the superficialis and attaching it to the proximal phalanx, producing a tenodesis effect. Littler[9] reconstructs the oblique retinacular ligament using a portion of the lateral band, which has been detached proximally, tunneled volarly to Cleland's ligament, and attached to the flexor tendon sheath over the proximal phalanx to prevent PIP hyperextension.

If painful partial ankylosis of the dislocated PIP joint is present, arthrodesis or implant arthroplasty may be indicated.

VOLAR DISLOCATIONS

Volar or anterior PIP joint dislocations are infrequent injuries. Experiments in which stress was applied to cadaver joints revealed that two forces are necessary to produce volar displacement. An angular or lateral force produced collateral ligament avulsion and a tear that extended through the transverse retinacular ligament and volar plate. A volarly or anteriorly directed force ruptured the central extensor tendon attachment to the middle phalanx and produced a boutonnière deformity.

Anterior or lateral dislocations may be irreducible with either the lateral band interposed or the proximal phalanx forced through the extensor mechanism and trapped. If this dislocation is capable of being reduced and the joint is congruent on follow-up examination with an extensor lag of 30 degrees or less, splinting the PIP joint in the extended position is the recommended treatment. More frequently, open reduction with repair of all injured structures will be necessary. Treatment for chronic anterior dislocation requires reconstruction of the collateral ligament and central tendon plus release of the tight retinacular ligaments. Thus what appears to be a straightforward boutonnière deformity may be a more complex injury with multiple structures damaged. Testing the collateral ligament and volar plate integrity may confirm this severe injury.

FRACTURES

Articular fractures can involve the PIP joint, the head of the proximal phalanx being the most common location (Fig. 20-10). To evaluate fully any injury to a small joint in the hand, one should take three roentgenograms (anteroposterior, lateral, and oblique) to rule out an obscure but potentially dangerous fracture. Joint fractures are classified by their stability, displacement, and amount of joint involve-

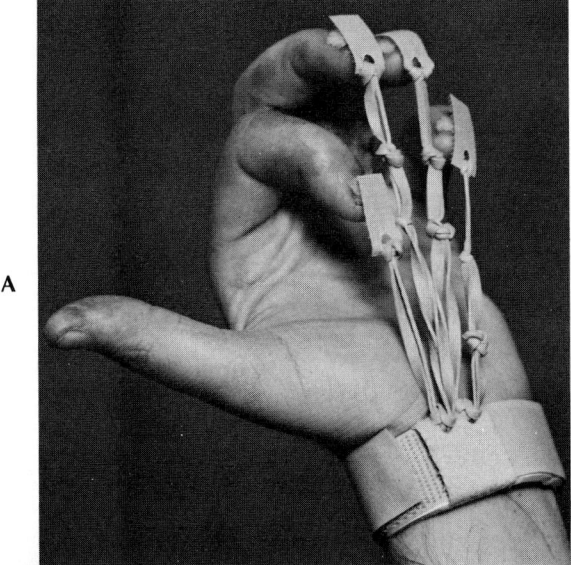

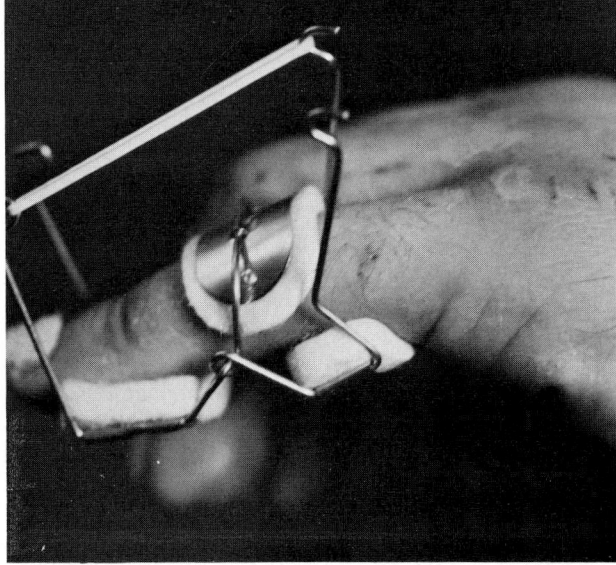

Fig. 20-9 **A,** Direction of pull of each finger should be toward scaphoid. **B,** Reverse finger knuckle bender can give dynamic extension.

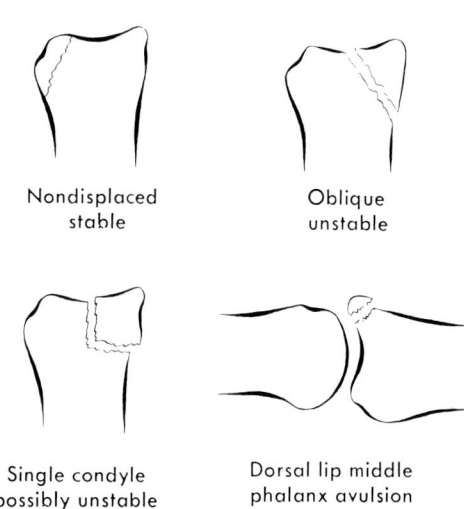

Fig. 20-10 Articular fractures of PIP joint can be nondisplaced, unstable, involve single condyle with rotation, or avulse central slip at middle phalanx base dorsally.

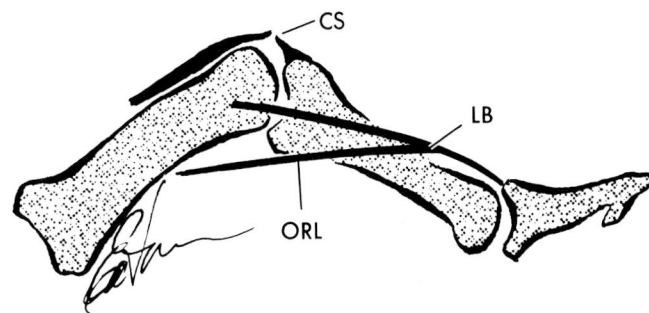

Fig. 20-11 In boutonnière deformity, lateral bands, *LB*, are displaced below axis of PIP joint. Any repair must recenter these bands and release any retinacular ligament, *ORL*, contracture. *CS*, Central extensor tendon slip.

ment. Stable, minimally displaced fractures should be immobilized for 3 weeks and then begun on gentle motion with further protection by splinting for 3 additional weeks. Unstable or displaced fractures are usually oblique; angulation and rotation can occur. Such a fracture will require open reduction through a dorsal approach, which divides the dorsal apparatus between the central tendon and the lateral band on the side of the fracture. After reduction the fracture is transfixed with small wires or a screw and protected for 10 to 14 days in the extended position before motion is begun. The extensor tendon must be protected by splinting for an additional 2 to 4 weeks.

Fractures involving a single condyle must be carefully evaluated because rotation can occur. A dorsal midphalangeal fracture requires open reduction and stabilization

with a wire or suture, with the PIP joint maintained in extension for 4 weeks before flexion is begun.

BOUTONNIÈRE DEFORMITY

The boutonnière deformity results from rupture or attenuation of the central extensor tendon over the PIP joint; the digit assumes a position of PIP flexion and distal joint extension (Fig. 20-11). The lateral bands slide volarly to the PIP joint axis, concentrating their extensor forces at the distal interphalangeal (DIP) joint. This inability to flex the distal joint is the most disabling aspect of the boutonnière deformity and will become fixed with time.

Closed boutonnière injuries are the most common and frequently occur when the digit's tip is struck with a ball. Treatment includes splinting of the PIP joint in the extended

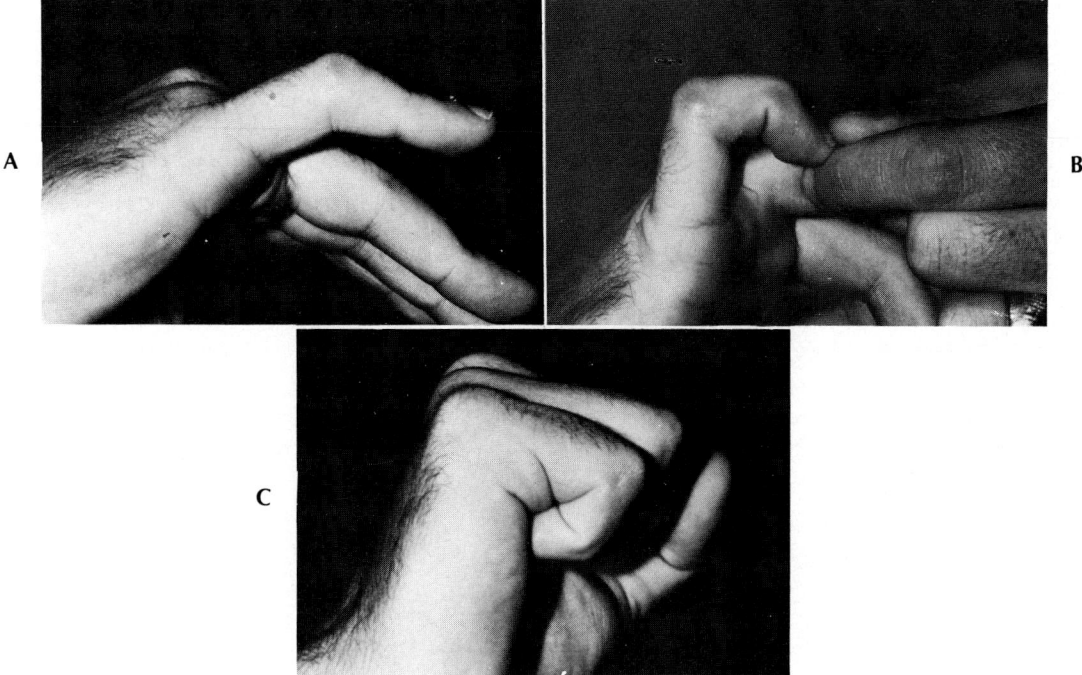

Fig. 20-12   Pseudoboutonnière deformity is seen as PIP flexion contracture, **A,** but with good passive, **B,** and active, **C,** flexion of distal joint.

position; the distal joint is left free for flexion exercises for prevention of lateral band adherence and retinacular ligament contracture. Open injuries (tendon lacerations) require suture of the extensor tendon with immobilization of the PIP joint in extension for 4 weeks.

Many different reconstructive procedures have been suggested to repair the established boutonnière deformity.[4,10,15] The purpose of any of these operations is to rebalance the extensor mechanisms either by directly repairing the central tendon or by reinforcing it with at least one lateral band. Before any surgery, full passive extension of the PIP joint should be obtained. This can be accomplished by splinting if necessary. The extensor tendon at the level of the PIP joint, whether repaired or reconstructed, must be immobilized for at least 4 weeks and then gradually moved with protection against an extensor lag for the total of 8 weeks.

PSEUDOBOUTONNIÈRE DEFORMITY

The term "pseudoboutonnière" has been suggested for a group of PIP hyperextension injuries, which present a boutonnière-like appearance (Fig. 20-12).[11] On examination a PIP flexion contracture is found, but the distal joint while positioned in extension is flexible. The extensor mechanism has not been damaged, but the volar plate's proximal attachment has been avulsed with subsequent scarring in the flexed position. It can be differentiated from the true boutonnière deformity by complete active and passive distal joint flexion. Flexion deformities of the PIP joint greater than 45 degrees may require surgical release.

In summary, proper management of injuries of the PIP joint can significantly reduce the stiffness and impairment all too often seen when a patient is uninformed and unsupervised in his treatment. A thorough knowledge of the

anatomy and understanding of all the injuries to this most important joint are required before one begins such treatment. In mobilizing the PIP joint, a gentle progressive exercise program should be closely monitored to prevent possible complications (that is, flexion contractures and increasing stiffness).

REFERENCES

 1. Adams JP: Correction of chronic dorsal subluxation of the proximal interphalangeal joint by means of a cross-cross volar graft, J Bone Joint Surg 41A:111, 1959.
 2. Curtis RM: Injuries to joints. In Flynn JE, editor: Hand surgery, ed 2, Baltimore, 1975, Williams & Wilkins.
 3. Eaton RG: Joint injuries of the hand, Springfield, Ill, 1971, Charles C Thomas, Publisher.
 4. Elliott RA: Boutonnière deformity. In Cramer IM and Chase RA, editors: Symposium on the hand, vol 3, St. Louis, 1971, The CV Mosby Co.
 5. Green DP and Rowland SA: Fractures and dislocations in the hand. In Rockwood CA Jr and Green DP, editors: Fractures, Philadelphia, 1975, JB Lippincott Co.
 6. Kuczynski K: The PIP joint: anatomy and causes of stiffness in the fingers, J Bone Joint Surg 50B:656, 1968.
 7. Kuczynski K: Less-known aspects of the proximal interphalangeal joint of the human hand, Hand 7:31, 1975.
 8. Landsmeer JMF: The proximal interphalangeal joint, Hand 7:30, 1975.
 9. Littler JW and Cooley SG: Restoration of the retinacular system in hyperextension deformity of the proximal interphalangeal joint, J Bone Joint Surg 47A:637, 1965.
10. Littler JW and Eaton RG: Redistribution of forces in the correction of boutonnière deformity, J Bone Joint Surg 49A:1267, 1967.
11. McCue FC, Honner R, Gleck JH and others: A pseudoboutonnière deformity, Hand 7:166, 1975.
12. Moberg E: Fracture and ligamentous injuries of the thumb and fingers, Surg Clin North Am 40:297, 1960.
13. Moberg E and Stener B: Injuries to the ligaments of the thumb and fingers, diagnosis, treatment and prognosis, Acta Chir Scand 106:166, 1953.

14. Redler L and Williams JT: Rupture of a collateral ligament of the proximal interphalangeal joint of the fingers, analysis of eighteen cases, J Bone Joint Surg 49A:322, 1967.
15. Souter WA: The problem of boutonnière deformity, Clin Orthop 104:116, 1974.

BIBLIOGRAPHY

Aufranco OE, Jones WN, and Bierbaum BE: Fracture dislocation of the proximal interphalangeal joint of the finger, JAMA 204:815, 1968.

Bate JT: An operation for the correction of locking of the proximal interphalangeal joint of finger in hyperextension, J Bone Joint Surg 27:142, 1945.

Brunelli G, Morelli E, and Salvi V: Traumatic lesions of tendons and ligaments of the proximal interphalangeal joint, Hand 7:43, 1975.

Howard LD: Treatment of posttraumatic recurvation deformity of the proximal interphalangeal joint with occasional locking but with other free joint mobility. In Cramer LM and Chase RA, editors: Symposium on the hand, vol 3, St. Louis, 1971, The CV Mosby Co.

Johnson FG and Greene MH: Another cause of irreducible dislocation of the proximal interphalangeal joint of a finger, J Bone Joint Surg 48A:542, 1966.

Kleinert HE and Kasdan ML: Reconstruction of chronically subluxed PIP finger joint, J Bone Joint Surg 47A:958, 1965.

Lee MLH: Intra-articular and peri-articular fractures of the phalanges, J Bone Joint Surg 45B:103, 1963.

London PS: Sprain and fractures involving the interphalangeal joints, Hand 3:155, 1971.

McCue FC, Honner R, Johnson M and others: Athletic injuries of the proximal interphalangeal joint requiring surgical treatment, J Bone Joint Surg 52A:937, 1970.

McElfresh EC, Dobyns J, and O'Brien ET: Management of fracture-dislocation of the proximal interphalangeal joints by extension-block splinting, J Bone Joint Surg 54A:1705, 1972.

Neviaser RJ and Wilson JN: Interposition of the extensor tendon resulting in persistent subluxation of the proximal interphalangeal joint of the finger, Clin Orthop 83:118, 1972.

Portis RB: Hyperextensibility of the proximal interphalangeal joint of the finger following trauma, J Bone Joint Surg 36A:1141, 1954.

Robertson RC, Cawley JJ, and Faris AM: Treatment of fracture-dislocation of the interphalangeal joints of the hand, J Bone Joint Surg 28:68, 1946.

Shrewsbury MM and Johnson RK: A systematic study of the oblique retinacular ligament of the human finger: its structure and function, J Hand Surg 2:194, 1977.

Spinner M and Choi BY: Anterior dislocation of the proximal interphalangeal joint, J Bone Joint Surg 52A:1329, 1970.

Stark HH: Troublesome fractures and dislocations of the hand. In AAOS: Instructional course lectures, vol 19, St. Louis, 1970. The CV Mosby Co.

Thompson JS and Eaton RG: Volar dislocations of the proximal interphalangeal joint, Orthop Trans 1:5, 1977.

Trojan E: Fracture dislocation of the bases of the proximal and middle phalanges of the fingers, Hand 4:60, 1972.

van der Meulen JCH: The treatment of prolapse and collapse of the proximal interphalangeal joint, Hand 4:154, 1972.

Wiley AM: Instability of the proximal interphalangeal joint following dislocation and fracture-dislocation: surgical repair, Hand 2:185, 1970.

Wilson JN and Rowland SA: Fracture-dislocation of the proximal interphalangeal joint of the finger, J Bone Joint Surg 48A:493, 1966.

21

De Quervain's disease

William H. Kirkpatrick

Since the first description of "washerwoman's sprain,"[5] tenosynovitis of the first dorsal compartment has become a commonly recognized inflammatory disorder. This most radial of the extensor compartments on the dorsum of the wrist is occupied by the tendons of the extensor pollicis brevis and abductor pollicis longus. The tendons are enveloped in an osseofibrous canal lined by synovium, which, when subjected to excessive or repetitive mechanical stresses, responds in a characteristic fashion distinguished by pain, swelling, and limitation of motion of the thumb. In 1895 de Quervain[6] was first credited with the recognition of this "disease" and hence it has borne his name. More accurately, though, Tillaux[31] and Gray[5] referred to the disorder before the work of de Quervain.

The most frequently cited cause is overuse of the hand and wrist. Finkelstein identified "chronic trauma and overexertion"[8] in his patients, and Muckart implicated activities involving "radial deviation movement with the thumb stabilized in the gripping position."[26] The resulting "acute angulations" of the tendons as they course from their restraining sheaths over the radial styloid to their insertions may be translated into greater stresses through the first dorsal compartment,[3,16] thus initiating an inflammatory response. As the inflammation persists, the overlying fibrous sheath thickens and stenosis develops.

Less frequent causes include direct trauma to the radial styloid, such as a sudden blow or acute strain as in lifting. Some cases may be related to a ganglion within the first dorsal compartment,[19,40] whereas other cases appear to be idiopathic. Metabolic abnormalities, though not demonstrated to be causative, may be associated with de Quervain's disease; they include diabetes, hyperuricemia, hypothyroidism, pregnancy, and rheumatoid arthritis. An anatomic predisposition has been suggested, especially in women whose "wrists normally angulate further than those of men."[18] Women appear to be three to ten times more frequently affected than men.[11,18,30]

Symptoms of de Quervain's disease generally include pain and swelling localized in the area of the radial styloid. Pain is especially aggravated by ulnar deviation of the wrist, by flexion and adduction of the thumb, or by simple adduction of the thumb. Supination has been reported to be more frequently painful than pronation.[8] The pain may occasionally radiate into the forearm or may be described as a constant ache over the dorsum of the thumb. Pain may also cause a sense of weakness with diminished grip and pinch strengths. Swelling in the area of discomfort is frequently present, especially in chronic cases.

On examination, tenderness is elicited with palpation over the first dorsal compartment. This tenderness may be worsened in the presence of contiguous inflammation involving the superficial radial nerve. In these infrequent cases, a positive Tinel test result with percussion over the radial styloid is present, suggesting a superficial nerve neuritis.[29]

A useful maneuver was proposed by Finkelstein[8] in 1930 and is found to be present in nearly all patients with de Quervain's disease. The thumb is held in full flexion-adduction, and the wrist is abruptly deviated in an ulnar direction. Excruciating pain in the region of the radial styloid is helpful in making the diagnosis but not pathognomonic. Other causes of pain with the maneuver must be excluded, keeping in mind that the test is often uncomfortable in normal wrists.

Discomfort may also be found with resisted thumb extension at the metacarpophalangeal (MP) joint—a positive "hitchhiker's" test result. Inflammation of the extensor pollicis brevis tendon in the first dorsal compartment can be suggested with this test though it does not exclude other diagnoses. Similarly, inflammation and thickening of the extensor pollicis brevis tendon distal to its sheath may cause limited thumb extension[26] compared with the uninvolved side. Triggering of the thumb as a result of the extensor pollicis brevis thickening has also been reported.[32]

Radiographic examination is usually unremarkable. Localized osteopenia in the radial styloid may be noted.[28] Calcifications in the area of the first dorsal compartment may also be identified, especially in chronic cases.

Radiographs may concomitantly demonstrate basal joint arthritis of the thumb, scaphoid nonunion, radioscaphoid or intercarpal arthrosis. Basil joint arthritis may be painful with thumb motion and may demonstrate a positive Finkelstein test result; however, it can usually be distinguished from de Quervain's disease by a positive axial compression test[4] and the absence of first dorsal compartment tenderness to palpation. However, the two may coexist.

Inflammation of the radial wrist flexor or extensor tendons must be differentially considered and excluded. The *intersection syndrome*[10] represents a tenosynovitis of the second dorsal compartment tendons in the area over which they are crossed by the muscle bellies of the abductor pollicis longus and the extensor pollicis brevis. This area is proximal to the usual site of de Quervain's disease and may demonstrate pain, swelling, and crepitation with wrist motion. Previously, other authors have referred to this syndrome as *peritendonitis crepitans*[12] and *abductor pollicis longus bursitis*.[34]

ANATOMY

The most radial tendon on the dorsum of the wrist is the abductor pollicis longus. Most commonly, it inserts into the radial side of the base of the first metacarpal although this may be variable. Other insertions include the transverse carpal ligament, the proximal phalanx of the thumb, the scaphoid or trapezium, and the abductor pollicis brevis or opponens pollicis.[3,13,15,20,30] Unlike standard anatomy depictions, the abductor pollicis longus is often present as multiple tendons, i.e., as two tendons or, less frequently, as three to five separate tendons. Reported incidences of more than one tendon range from 68% to 98% in cadaver studies.[3,14,30] When a second tendon is present, it usually inserts into the trapezium.[18]

The extensor pollicis brevis has less variability in its insertions or duplications. It is consistently narrower than the abductor pollicis longus and usually inserts into the base of the proximal phalanx. Les frequent insertions include the distal phalanx with the extensor pollicis longus tendon or to both the proximal and distal phalanges. It is more commonly present as a single tendon although duplication as an accessory tendon is reported in 8% to 11% of cases studied.[9,26,30]

Despite potential variability, the most common pattern in cadaver studies appears to be two abductor pollicis longus tendons and one extensor pollicis brevis tendon[13] (Fig. 21-1). Absence of the long abductor or short extensor tendon may be encountered and may represent a regressive tendency in the evolution of the human thumb.[16] Phylogenetically, both muscles are differentiations of a common muscle and are present as separate muscles in only humans and gorillas.[9,14,30]

Each of the tendons in the first dorsal compartment may be separated by one or more septations. Septations are any fibrous or osseofibrous divisions—not simply synovial divisions—between tendons, which create separate compartments and represent potential sites of stenosis. Most commonly found is a discreet fibrous septation extending obliquely from the extensor retinaculum of the first dorsal compartment to the radius, separating the dorsal extensor pollicis brevis from the volar abductor pollicis longus.[13,26]

An often unrecognized form of septation is the intramural presence of a tendon, such as the extensor pollicis brevis, dorsal to the abductor pollicis longus.

Septations may be incomplete, involving only the distal portion of the compartment.[13] They may even be entirely absent,[20] permitting the short extensor and long abductor tendons to occupy the same canal. Rarely is a septum found between the individual long abductor tendons. Occasionally an accessory abductor pollicis longus tendon may lie completely outside of the first dorsal compartment.[13,20]

As observed by Loomis,[20] septation is more common in patients with de Quervain's disease than in the general population. Likewise, in approximately 70% of patients with the disease, septation will be found.[26,32] The number of extensor pollicis brevis or abductor pollicis longus tendons present in the first dorsal compartment, however, does not seem to be significantly different.[13,20]

TREATMENT

The initial treatment of a symptomatic patient is premised on decreasing the inflammation in the first dorsal compartment. If cessation of provoking activities is not successful, simple immobilization of the wrist and thumb with the interphalangeal (IP) joint free in a thumb spica splint may be effective. Nonsteroidal anti-inflammatory medication may also be effective.

If symptoms persist after several weeks, a local injection of a steroid may be administered. Various water soluble steroid preparations with different potencies and durations of response are available. Comparison of products to determine the most efficacious, however, remains difficult.[23] Potential complications include subcutaneous fat atrophy, tendon deterioration, and skin depigmentation (Fig. 21-2). The latter may be lessened in incidence with betamethasone (Celestone), though this is unproven. The preferred preparation is 6 mg of betamethasone in 1 cc of 1% lidocaine.

Whether diagnostic or therapeutic, the injection should be administered into the synovial sheath of the first dorsal compartment. The sheath is located by gently inserting the needle to the bony surface of the radial styloid distal to the first dorsal compartment and alongside one of the palpable

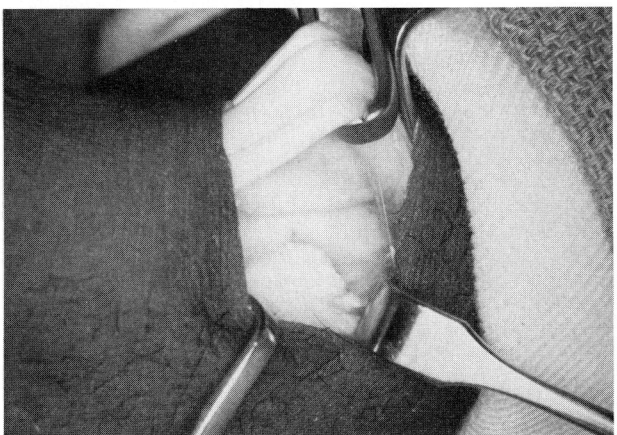

Fig. 21-1 Tendons within the first dorsal compartment. Through a transverse dorsoradial skin incision, the first dorsal compartment is exposed. Two abductor pollicis longus tendons and a single extensor pollicis brevis tendon are retracted from the released sheath.

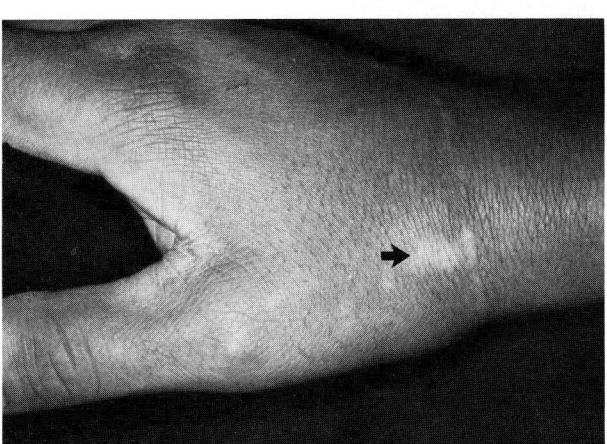

Fig. 21-2 Skin depigmentation *(arrow)* from a steroid injection for de Quervain's tenosynovitis. The type of steroid solution used was not known, and the injection site appears to be more distal than recommended.

tendons. The needle is then slowly retracted as pressure is simultaneously exerted on the plunger. Free flow of the solution indicates that the sheath has usually been entered.[24] Subcutaneous placement of the injectant may be revealed by diffuse filling in the immediate area, whereas injection into the sheath can often be palpated along the course of the sheath. Especially in chronic cases, peritendonous adhesions and constrictions may interfere with adequate placement of the steroid.

After injection, thumb spica splint immobilization is continued for approximately 1 week, or longer if symptoms persist. One or more repeated injections may be considered every 4 weeks; however, surgical decompression should be given consideration with recurrence after the second or third injection. For less severe cases though, approximately 90% of patients may expect relief with conservative management.[24,25]

Surgical decompression is indicated for symptoms that persist despite adequate conservative treatment. Some authors, however, prefer even earlier surgical treatment.[14,35] Under tourniquet control, a transverse incision is made 1 to 2 cm proximal to the tip of the radial styloid. A transverse incision is preferred to minimize scar formation in the area contacting the tendons of the first dorsal compartment. Some authors favor a longitudinal incision,[14,26] but problems may include scar hypertrophy and inadequate surgical exposure.[2,27] A longitudinally curved incision with the convexity volar has also been used successfully.[22] Care must be used to avoid damage by direct injury or vigorous retraction to the branches of the superficial radial nerve, which may be located immediately within the surgical field. Under direct visualization, the retinaculum overlying the first compartment is sharply incised along its dorsoradial length, which may be 1 to 4 cm. This leaves a volarly based flap that may assist in prevention of volar subluxation of the tendons postoperatively. Serous fluid, hemosiderin-pigmented synovium, and a thickened fibrous sheath may be encountered, although the pathologic changes vary in degree and with the chronicity of the disease.[19] With this retinacular incision, the extensor pollicis brevis tendon is generally first to be recognized because of its dorsal relationship to the abductor pollicis longus. The septation, which includes the abductor pollicis longus tendon or tendons, is then incised. Careful exploration and testing of tendon function may reveal an overlooked accessory tendon, especially if intramurally located. Though some recommend excision of the sheath, particularly if thickened, it does not appear to be necessary.[14,16,25] After careful hemostasis is obtained, the wound is closed with a subcuticular suture, and a thumb spica splint is applied with the wrist in slight extension for 3 to 5 days. At that time the splint is discontinued and early active motion is begun. (Some surgeons prefer not to immobilize the thumb in a splint and to initiate immediate early active motion.)

Variations in anatomy must be remembered, and each tendon must be identified and tested to determine its function and to ensure complete decompression. Simply noting the presence of two tendons in the first dorsal compartment after incision of its retinaculum does not ensure adequate treatment. An important cause of unsatisfactory results may be failure to identify accessory tendons in separate compartments.[3,7,9,21,30]

Complete relief of symptoms within several weeks has been reported in 92% to 100% of all patients.[19,25,30,35] Recurrence is unusual; however, in addition to incomplete surgical decompression with persistent symptoms, other less than satisfactory results have been reported.[2,9,17,21,30] These may be caused by an incorrect initial diagnosis, an unsightly scar, or a superficial radial nerve injury and neuroma. Tendon adherence and volar or dorsal tendon subluxation have also been encounterd.[1,33]

REFERENCES

1. Alegado RB and Meals RA: An unusual complication following surgical treatment of de Quervain's disease, J Hand Surg 4A(1):185, 1979.
2. Arons MS: de Quervain's release in working women, J Hand Surg 12A(4):540, 1987.
3. Baba MA: The accessory tendon of the abductor pollicis longus muscle, Anat Rec 119:541, 1954.
4. Burton RI: Basal joint arthrosis of the thumb, Orthop Clin North Am 4(2):331, 1973.
5. Gray's anatomy, ed 13, 1899.
6. de Quervain F: Correspondez—Blatt F. Schweizer Aerzte, uber eine form von chronicher tendovaginitis, 25:389, 1895.
7. Fenton R: Stenosing tendovaginitis at the radial styloid involving an accessory tendon sheath, Bull Hosp Joint Dis 11:90, 1950.
8. Finkelstein H: Stenosing tendovaginitis at the radial styloid process, J Bone Joint Surg 12:509, 1930.
9. Giles KW: Anatomical variations affecting the surgery of de Quervain's disease, J Bone Joint Surg 42B(2):352, 1960.
10. Grundberg AB and Reagan DS: Pathologic anatomy of the forearm: intersection syndrome, J Hand Surg 10A(2):299, 1985.
11. Hall CL: Chronic stenosing tenovaginitis of the wrist, J Int College Surg 14(1):48, 1950.
12. Howard NJ: Peritendinitis crepitans, J Bone Joint Surg 19(A):447, 1976.
13. Jackson WT and others: Anatomical variations in the first extensor compartment of the wrist, J Bone Joint Surg 68A(6):923, 1986.
14. Keon-Cohen B: de Quervain's disease, J Bone Joint Surg 33B(1):96, 1951.
15. Lacey T, Goldstein LA, and Tobin CE: Anatomical and clinical study of the variations in the insertions of the abductor pollicis longus tendon, associated with stenosing tendovaginitis, J Bone Joint Surg 33A(2):347, 1951.
16. Leao L: de Quervain's disease, J Bone Joint Surg 40A(5):1063, 1958.
17. Linscheid RL: Injuries to radial nerve at wrist, Arch Surg 91:942, 1965.
18. Lipscomb PR: Stenosing tenosynovitis at the radial styloid process, Ann Surg 134:110, 1951.
19. Lipscomb PR: Tenosynovitis of the hand and the wrist, carpal tunnel syndrome, de Quervain's disease, trigger digit, Clin Orthop 13:164, 1959.
20. Loomis LK: Variations of stenosing tenosynovitis at the radial styloid process, J Bone Joint Surg 33A(2):340, 1951.
21. Louis DS: Incomplete release of the first dorsal compartment—a diagnostic test, J Hand Surg 12A(1):87, 1987.
22. McFarland GB: Entrapment syndromes. In Evarts CM, editor: Surgery of the musculoskeletal system, New York, 1983, Churchill Livingstone, Inc.
23. McGrath MH: Local steroid therapy in the hand, J Hand Surg 9A(6):915, 1984.
24. McKenzie JMM: Conservative treatment of de Quervain's disease, Brit Med J 4:659, 1972.
25. Medl WT: Tendonitis, tenosynovitis, "trigger finger," and de Quervain's disease, Orthop Clin North Am 1(2):375, 1970.
26. Muckart RD: Stenosing tendovaginitis of abductor pollicis longus and extensor pollicis brevis at the radial styloid (de Quervain's disease), Clin Orthop 33:201, 1964.
27. Murphy ID: An unusual form of de Quervain's syndrome, J Bone Joint Surg 31A(4):858, 1949.
28. Nyska M, Floman Y, and Fast A: Osseous involvement in de Quervain's disease, Clin Orthop 186:159, 1984.
29. Rask MR: Superficial radial neuritis and de Quervain's disease, Clin Orthop 131:176, 1978.

30. Strandell G: Variations of the anatomy in stenosing tenosynovitis at the radial styloid process, Acta Chir Scan 113:234, 1957.
31. Tillaux P: Traite d'anatomie topographique. Avec applications a la Chirurgie, ed 7, Paris, 1892, Asselin et Houzeau.
32. Viegas SF: Trigger thumb of de Quervain's disease, J Hand Surg 11A(2):235, 1986.
33. White GM and Weiland AJ: Symptomatic palmar tendon subluxations after surgical release for de Quervain's disease: a case report, J Hand Surg 9A(5):705, 1984.
34. Wood M and Linscheid R: Abductor pollicis longus bursitis, Clin Orthop 93:293, 1973.
35. Woods THE: De Quervain's disease: a plea for early operation, Brit J Surg 51(5):358, 1964.

ADDITIONAL READINGS

Armstrong TJ and others: Ergonomics consideration in hand and wrist tendinitis, J Hand Surg 12A(5):830, 1987.
Brooker AF: Extensor carpi radialis tenosynovitis, an occupational affliction, Orthop Rev 6(5):99, 1977.
Conklin JE and White WL: Stenosing tenosynovitis, Surg Clinics North Am 40:531, 1960.
Froimson AI: Tenosynovitis and tennis elbow. In Green DP, editor: Operative hand surgery, ed 2, 1988.
Howard NJ: Peritendinitis crepitans, J Bone Joint Surg 14(2):447, 1937.
Lapidus PW and Fenton R: Stenosing tenovaginitis at the wrist and fingers, Arch Surg 64:475, 1952.
Muffly-Elsey D and Flinn-Wagner S: Proposed screening tool for the detection of cumulative trauma disorders of the upper extremity, J Hand Surg 12A(5):931, 1987.
Pick RY: De Quervain's disease: a clinical triad, Clin Orthop 143:165, 1979.

22

Therapist's management of de Quervain's disease

Patricia A. Totten

The versatile thumb provides the hand with flexibility, stabilization, and strength when performing activities that require manipulation, pinch, and grasp. The thumb's flexibility results from the nature of the carpometacarpal (CMC) and the metacarpophalangeal (MP) joints. These joints basically have two degrees of freedom in the direction of adduction-abduction, and flexion-extension. Axial rotation is accomplished by the elasticity of ligaments, which offers a third degree of freedom to both joints.[27] The aspects of strength and stability are accomplished by the coordinated efforts of tendon forces, constraining forces of the joint capsule and ligaments, and the articular compressive forces across the joint surfaces. In mechanical and anatomic studies by Cooney,[10] it was determined that during normal pinch and grasp activities, the thumb intrinsic muscle tendon forces are one and a half to three times the applied external force, whereas the thumb extrinsic muscle tendon forces are four to five times the applied external force.

Because the thumb plays a main role in hand function, it is subject to an "over-use" phenomenon, which was first identified in the 1893 edition of Gray's *Anatomy* as "washer-woman's sprain."[9] In 1895 this condition was further described by the Swiss surgeon Fritz de Quervain as a stenosing tenosynovitis in the first dorsal compartment, which contains the abductor pollicis longus and extensor pollicis brevis tendons.[40] The symptoms include tenderness over the radial styloid, aching over the dorsal aspect of the thumb, and pain over the radial aspect of the wrist, which are aggravated by wrist ulnar deviation, thumb flexion and adduction,[2] or thumb MP joint extension.

ANATOMY

A review of the anatomy relevant to de Quervain's disease must include an understanding of the first two extensor compartments on the dorsoradial aspect of the wrist (Fig. 22-1). The compartments are formed by an oblique fibrous band of tissue, the extensor retinaculum, which is attached medially to the distal ulna and the medial ligament and carpal bones of the wrist. Laterally, the extensor retinaculum attaches to the anterior border of the radius. Six tunnels or compartments are formed beneath the extensor retinaculum to allow for the excursion of extensor tendons of the wrist and hand as they pass from the forearm to the hand.[18] Associated with de Quervain's tenosynovitis, the first compartment houses the two tendons that form the lateral boundary of the anatomic snuff box: the abductor pollicis longus and the extensor pollicis brevis tendons (Fig. 22-2).[18] Sharing a common synovial sheath extending approximately 1 cm distal to the extensor retinaculum,[18] these tendons pass through a shallow groove over the prominence of the radial styloid.[7] During wrist motion, the tendons undergo as much as 105 degrees of angulation as they pass from the radius to the first metacarpal. Anatomically it has been pointed out that the greater angulations at the radial joint appear in women.[5] According to Brand, tendons transmit tension along a straight line and lie in synovial sheaths whenever they round a concave surface. As tendons angulate because of their route over a bony surface or their inclination caused by postural changes, tendons become subject to increased tension or friction. Synovial tendon sheaths secrete a lubricating fluid, which is "probably not improved by contin-

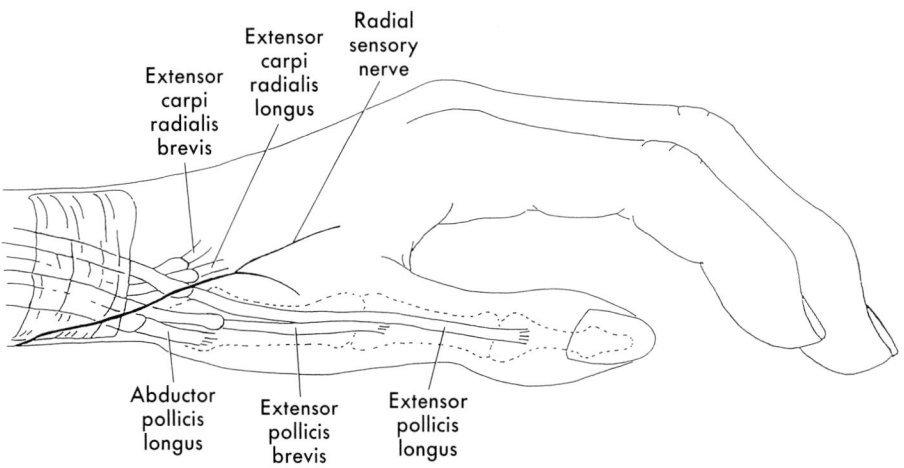

Fig. 22-1 The first two extensor compartments on the dorsoradial aspect of the wrist.

uous motion as it is in a joint. This is why fast, strong, continuous reciprocal motion results sometimes in tenosynovitis but rarely in joint synovitis."[6] De Quervain's tenosynovitis results from friction between the tendon, the tendon sheath, and the shearing of the tendons against the bony groove of the radius.[5]

Positioned most radially in the first dorsal compartment, the abductor pollicis longus inserts on the radial aspect of the base of the first metacarpal. Acting to abduct and extend the CMC joint of the thumb, as well as assist in wrist flexion and radial deviation of the hand, the abductor pollicis longus maintains the arch of pinch despite the strong influence of the thumb adductors and flexor pollicis longus.[6] Smaller and weaker than the abductor pollicis longus, the extensor pollicis brevis inserts in the dorsal aspect of the proximal phalanx of the thumb. This tendon extends to the CMC joint and the MP joint and acts to assist in radial deviation of the wrist and abduction of thumb.

The second extensor compartment contains the powerful extensor carpi radialis brevis tendon, which inserts on the carpus at the base of the third metacarpal. Referred to as the prime wrist extensor,[3] it can be noted beneath the skin during power grasp when the wrist is extended. The extensor carpi radialis longus tendon, inserting at the base of the second metacarpal, is also housed in the second compartment and assists in wrist extension and abduction.

Passing through the third dorsal compartment is the tendon of the extensor pollicis longus, which travels around Lister's tubercle to insert on the distal phalanx of the thumb. This tendon acts primarily to extend the interphalangeal (IP) joint of the thumb. However, it also assists in MP and CMC joint extension and wrist abduction and extension.[28] The compartment and its accompanying tendon is not included in the de Quervain's malady; however, it is worth mention for the purpose of understanding the reasons behind splinting treatment that will be addressed later in this chapter.

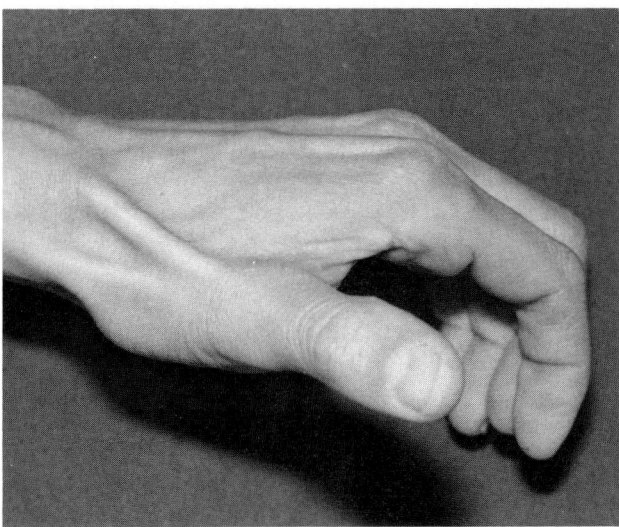

Fig. 22-2   The anatomical snuffbox becomes apparent with active extension-abduction of the thumb. The radial border is formed by the superficial extensor pollicis brevis and the deep-lying abductor pollicis longus. The ulnar boundary of the snuff box is formed by the extensor pollicus longus.

To complete the description of the de Quervain's scenario, the course of the radial sensory nerve must be acknowledged. Dividing approximately 8 cm proximal to the radial styloid, the terminal branch is separated into the medial branch and the superficial lateral branch. The medial branch innervates the dorsal radial aspect of the hand, the dorsal ulnar border of the thumb, the dorsal proximal phalanx of the index finger, and the dorsal radial aspect of the long finger. The superficial lateral branch travels in the area of the anatomic snuff box and supplies the dorsal aspect of the thumb with the exception of the distal tip.[24,50]

CAUSATION

The most frequently documented occurrences of de Quervain's disease are in manual laborers who combine pinch with wrist motion and forearm rotation.[5,23] The persistence of strain as these motions are performed rapidly and repetitively over the course of time is instrumental in the development of tenosynovitis. According to Hammer, "Human tendons will not tolerate more than 1500 to 2000 manipulations per hour."[19] Often classified as a cumulative trauma disorder (CTD), tenosynovitis may also be categorized under the term "nonimpact wrist disorder,"[26] which is attributable to "repetitive pressure; voluntary motions; overexertions; lifting objects; pulling objects; throwing objects; or nonspecific overextension."[26] Work involving grasp and repetitive manipulation of an instrument or tool may also contribute to hand injury, and, as documented by Hymovich, the dominant extremity is usually involved.[23] A surveillance of occupational injuries and illnesses in the United States reports that cumulative trauma disorders are the second most frequently reported category after skin disease.[48]

Although excessive use of the thumb is linked to the cause of de Quervain's disease, aberrant abductor pollicis longus tendons sharing a common sheath are also an important consideration in the development of de Quervain's symptoms.[5,31] In this instance the muscle of the abductor pollicis longus produces various amplitudes of tendon action.[5]

PATHOLOGY

Pathologically, as the tendons of the first dorsal compartments move, the synovial sheaths secrete a lubricating fluid, which may not increase in proportion to the amount of tendon use, thus resulting in tenosynovitis or inflammation of the tendon sheath.[6] Characterized first by congestion of serum and fibrin within the walls of the sheath, tenosynovitis occurs when serum is reabsorbed, thus contributing to adherence between the synovium and the tendons.[9,19] According to Conklin, the tendons may become flattened and thinned and covered with granulation tissue, which may cause the formation of connecting fibrous bands.[9] Usually about 0.75 mm in thickness, the ligamentous sheath may become two to four times its normal size.[5] As the fibrous sheath becomes further inflamed and edematous, the tendons are constricted in this area, but beyond this region they appear approximately normal.[9] As a sequela to these changes, a loss in blood flow may result affecting the nutritional status of the area.[43]

A roentgenographic view of soft tissue shows a lateral bulge of the skin near the radial styloid. The tendon sheath appears enlarged, and although views of the subcutaneous tissue planes are obliterated, no immediate bone changes

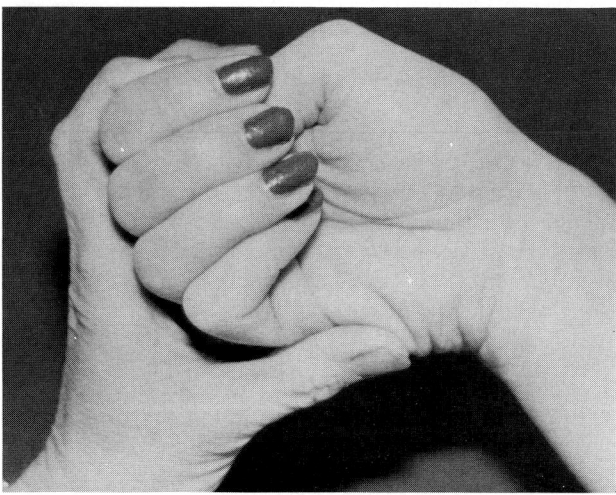

Fig. 22-3 Finkelstein test. The forearm is stabilized, and the patient is instructed to clasp the fingers over the flexed thumb. The examiner then passively deviates the wrist toward the ulnar. With this test the patient may complain of pain over the abductor pollicis longus tendon.

are demonstrated.[44] Later, Usoltseva points out that osteoporosis of the radial styloid process may become apparent.[52]

SYMPTOMS

A patient with de Quervain's disease complains of discomfort over the radial aspect of the wrist, which may radiate proximally up the forearm and distally into the thumb.[29] This pain is typically aggravated by thumb and wrist motions,[46] especially active or resistive extension and abduction of the thumb.[33] On palpation, the examiner may elicit localized tenderness approximately 1 cm proximal to the radial styloid,[33] and the area of the extensor sheath may appear and feel thickened.[2,42]

Usually used to test the presence of de Quervain's disease, the Finkelstein test (Fig. 22-3) first described by Eichoff in 1927, is performed by grasping the thumb with the fingers. The wrist is then passively deviated toward the ulna, which stretches the tendons further.[7] This test produces localized pain over the abductor pollicis longus tendon in the first dorsal compartment.[29] Hymovich recommends that the patient perform simultaneous Finkelstein maneuvers with both hands so that the resultant pain can be qualified.[23]

To rule out extensor pollicis longus involvement, the tester positions the wrist in neutral and stabilizes the CMC and MP joints of the thumb while testing resisted IP joint extension. Any discomfort reported by the patient should be noted, because this involvement of the third compartment will affect the treatment plan.

THERAPIST'S EVALUATION

On receiving a physician's referral of a patient with de Quervain's disease to the clinic, the therapist must proceed with a thorough interview. Notations are made about the patient's gender, age, hand dominance, date of onset of symptoms, as well as previous upper extremity problems. One must inquire about the patient's relevant job history and present occupation and the duration of time spent in

this capacity. Importantly, the therapist must inquire about positions, tools, and equipment that the patient may use to perform the job. Frequency of hand use must also be addressed. During the interview, the therapist must learn if the patient is required to wear cumbersome gloves at work. Gloves may pose external limitations on wrist and digital motion causing the worker to exert greater strains on his or her tendons to accomplish job tasks.

The ultimate goal of treatment is to return the patient to former capacity. If it is necessary to further understand job requirements, it is important to check with the *Dictionary of Occupational Titles** and the patient's employer. A job site visit is often beneficial in determining required tasks and possibly the implementation of modifications needed to optimally perform specific job duties.

No interview is complete unless an understanding of the patient's activity of daily living status is obtained. Postures that may exacerbate symptoms must be assessed. Former leisure activities that are now avoided are also documented.

The subject of pain must be dealt with rather than dwelt on. As therapists, we must try to qualify pain so that we establish a baseline gauge. A helpful guide is the 10 cm pain analog scale whereby the patient points out the present level of pain (equating the number 0 with no pain and 10 with maximal pain that would require immediate medical intervention). Other considerations in documenting pain include the area of pain, the time of day pain is felt, the corresponding activity that may elicit pain, the duration of pain, the posture of the extremity that reproduces pain symptoms,[54] and importantly, the patient's report of how he or she can effect a diminution of the pain response. Pain level is addressed only on a weekly basis as the therapist attempts to teach the patient to deemphasize pain.[11] The understanding of the theory that chronic pain may be associated with overprotection and thus the continuation of symptoms[12] assists the therapist in the treatment approach.

Visual inspection of the affected area and comparison with the nonaffected side is essential. The therapist should note the attitude of the thumb at rest and check for signs of edema on the radial aspect of the wrist, in the area of the first dorsal compartment, and throughout the thumb.

Objective measurements, again comparing the involved with the noninvolved side, must include documentation of edema. Volumetric readings comparing the measurements of both hands may elucidate edema. Comparative measurements with the circumferential gauge, Jobst tape measure,† or jeweler's rings may be taken at the usual thumb landmarks of the proximal phalanx and IP joint. A tape measure may be used to measure edema that may occur at the level of the wrist or distal palmar crease.

Motion of the affected thumb and wrist may be normal or slightly limited[2,5] and thus must be carefully measured with a goniometer. The ability of the thumb to oppose the fingertips and the volar head of the fifth metacarpal or ulnar aspect of the distal palmar crease is also documented. The first web space must also be assessed for a possible contracture.

An evaluation of range of motion must not be limited to

---

*Superintendent of Documents, US Government Printing Office, Washington, DC 20402.
†Jobst, Toledo.

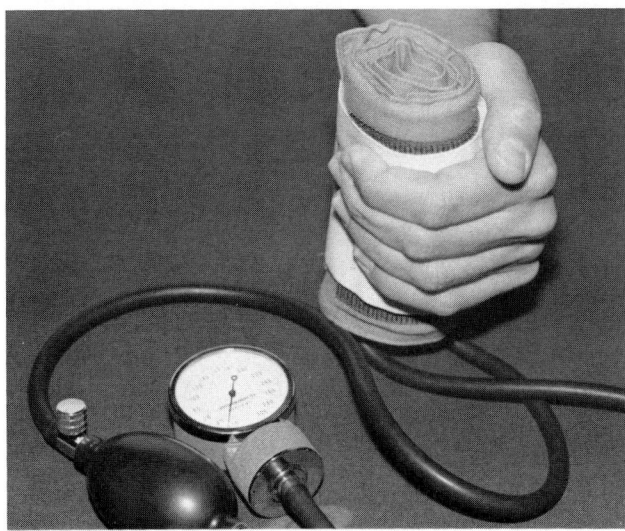

Fig. 22-4 The sphygmomanometer may be used to obtain an early baseline grip measurement. The thumb is stabilized next to the index finger, and the fingers exert pressure on the rolled blood pressure cuff.

the affected wrist and thumb, because proximal problems ranging from tennis elbow to shoulder capsulitis to neck pain frequently coexist with de Quervain's disease.[2,45]

Secondary to the patient's complaint of discomfort, strength testing is usually deferred or taken in an adaptive manner using the sphygmomanometer.[37] The thumb is positioned in a relatively quiet position, stabilized next to the index finger, while grasping the blood pressure cuff (Fig. 22-4).

TREATMENT
Conservative approach

Initial phase (1 to 4 weeks). When the patient is referred to therapy, communication must define the disease process as acute or chronic, outline the type of medical intervention, and make recommendations for therapeutic treatment. If the patient has had symptoms less than 6 months, a conservative treatment approach may be initiated.[9] Generally, in conjunction with the therapy program, the patient may receive from two to four steroid injections into the first dorsal compartment.[29,41] The therapist must advise the patient of the initial anesthetic perception, which may persist for 2 hours secondary to the accompanying anesthetic injected. The patient should also be informed of the heightened perception of pain, which may occur as the anesthesia wears off.[29]

Of paramount importance during this conservative phase is the focus on reduction of pain symptoms and inflammation. Rest for the tendons of the first dorsal compartment is indicated. The tendons of the adjacent second compartment must also be considered when designing a program for the patient having de Quervain's disease. Only if the physician specifies a diagnosis of an accompanying synovitis of the third compartment's extensor pollicis longus should the therapist include a rest program for this tendon, which powers IP joint extension of the thumb.

Rest to the proximal thumb and radial wrist extensors is provided by a forearm-based splint, which may be referred to as a long opponens or a long thumb spica splint. Although sometimes applied dorsally,[49] it is usually fabricated from a volar or radial approach. Its design immobilizes the wrist and the CMC and MP joints of the thumb (Fig. 22-5).[8,34,49,55] When fitting the splint, the superficial branch of the radial nerve and the ulnar digital nerve of the thumb[45] must be respected and be free of compression. Hand positioning is recommended as follows: the wrist should be placed in 15 degrees of extension, the CMC joint in 40 to 50 degrees of palmar abduction[49] and the MP joint in 5 to 10 degrees of flexion. This allows for the thumb to be in opposition for limited performance of light prehension activities. The IP joint is left free to perform active motion unless the extensor pollicis longus is involved. Various manufacturers have made available prefabricated thumb splints; however, care should be taken to ensure a precise fit. The therapist should

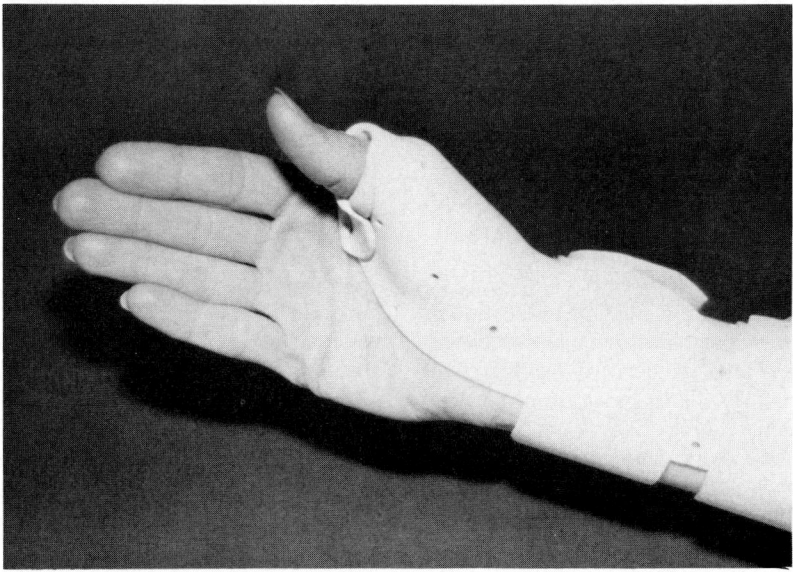

Fig. 22-5 The splint design for the patient with de Quervain's disease immobilizes the entire or radial aspect of the wrist and includes the carpometacarpal and metacarpal phalangeal joints of the thumb.

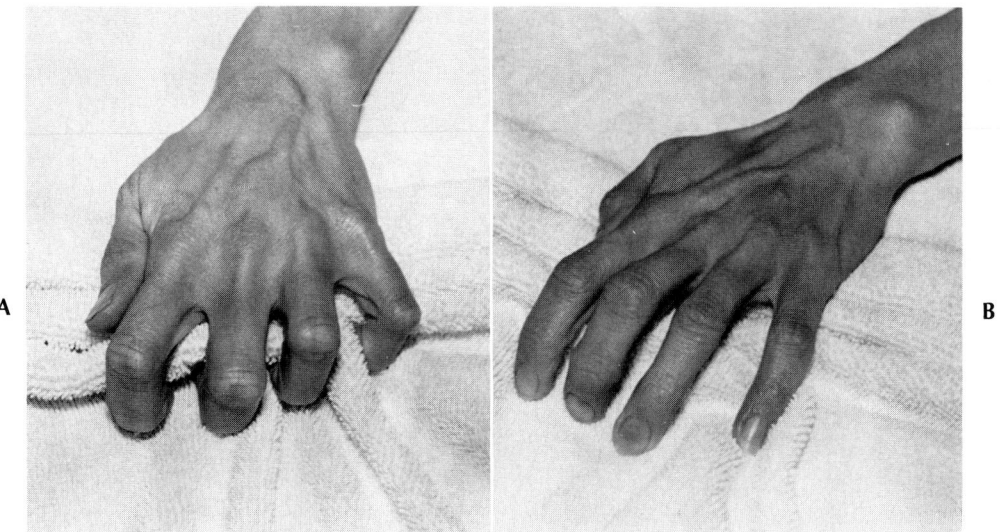

Fig. 22-6 **A,** Towel gathering may be performed by repetitively flexing and extending the fingers while gathering the material under the hand. The task may be initiated with the thumb resting next to the index, but as the patient progresses, the thumb may be actively involved. **B,** Towel unfolding may be performed by using the fingers to extend and stretch out the folds of a towel. Again, the task is initially performed with the thumb at rest. Then the patient is instructed in gradual extension-abduction of the thumb.

make recommendations that the splint be worn at all times with the exception of removal for hygiene and exercise purposes. On removal, the patient should be advised to gently stabilize the thumb against the lateral aspect of the index finger while bathing and performing other activities with the long, ring, and small fingers. The patient should be warned not to exacerbate symptoms by "testing out his/her hand" or performing maneuvers that include components of the Finkelstein test. The splint may be removed three times daily for short exercise periods.

Active range of motion (ROM) exercises are performed to prevent joint stiffness and the possible formation of adhesions between the tendons and the synovial sheath. Gentle passive and active wrist and thumb motions in all planes are encouraged, but the patient is advised not to forcibly push to maximal motion and to heed signs of discomfort. During the first week, only a light program of exercise is indicated. If the patient demonstrates the ability to withstand an increased number of repetitions in the days that follow, light prehension activities may be initiated. Again, forceful tendon excursion is discouraged as the patient begins grasp and release of small lightweight objects (foam pieces, cotton balls, spools, checkers) using various patterns of prehension. Other activities such as macramé may be initiated, but it is important to instruct the patient in varying the prehensile pattern to avoid overuse of the tendons of the first two compartments. A patient may also benefit from a towel gathering and unfolding activity (Fig. 22-6, *A* and *B*), which may later be advanced to a more resistive paper crumpling activity. During the first 4 weeks of treatment, short exercise periods ranging from 10 to 20 minutes should be stressed. Only as the patient demonstrates increased tolerance for activity should the program be expanded.

For the periods when the patient's splint is on, a proximal joint ROM program is provided to enhance circulation, min-

imize joint stiffness and protective posturing, and maintain functional motion of the affected extremity. Methods to monitor edema must be incorporated in the first day of treatment. While wearing the splint, the patient should be encouraged to maintain the affected hand above the heart level as much as possible, to perform overhead intermittent pumping of the fingers every hour, and to wear a compressive stockinette encompassing all MP joints, the wrist, and the forearm. Coban* wrapping applied in a distal-to-proximal fashion from the thumb to distal forearm level may also be considered. Although an Isotoner† glove may seem like a good method for edema reduction, de Quervain's patients have difficulty donning the glove over their affected thumb, thus incurring increased discomfort. A glove may be considered later in the treatment phase.

Other techniques used to assist with control of the inflammatory stage include retrograde lotion massage and cryotherapy. These methods can be employed at home four times per day. An ice pack application lasting from 10 to 15 minutes must be insulated with a thin moist towel. Ice massage, avoiding bony prominences, for a maximum duration of 5 minutes may assist in producing an initial vasoconstriction response immediately followed by a vasodilation response, which assists in removing inflammatory by-products.[39] Contrast baths performed in elevation have been a recommended treatment choice[53] because of their effect on increased metabolic and phagocytic activity. In the beginning stages of treatment the therapist may choose to modify the contrast bath treatment. Squeezing a sponge may be too resistive initially, and the patient is taught instead to gently move the thumb to the lateral aspect of the index

---

*3M Medical-Surgical Division, St. Paul.
†Aris Gloves, Inc., New York, NY.

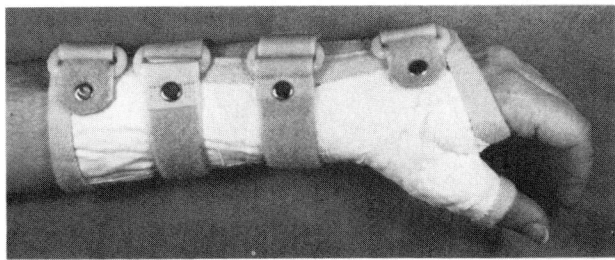

Fig. 22-7   A semiflexible support may be fabricated to limit extremes of motion. (From Henshaw J, Satren J, and Wrightsman JA: The semiflexible support: an alternative for the hand-injured worker, J Hand Ther 2(1), Jan-March, 1989).

finger while pumping the fingers in one bath. In the other bath, gentle wrist motion may be performed.

Phonophoresis is often used in acute and chronic inflammatory conditions.[14] It employs ultrasonic energy to drive an anti-inflammatory agent to a depth of approximately 5 cm to 6 cm subcutaneously.[17] Before the use of phonophoresis over the affected area, heat, which is thought to improve conduction through the skin, may be applied.[43] The choice of 10% hydrocortisone has been documented as being effective in the treatment of upper extremity disorders because it assists with decreasing edema and pain.[30] Generally, 10 to 12 daily treatment sessions of 5 minutes' duration[4] are given[20] to allow adequate permeation of the medication to assist in pain relief.[15,17]

Second phase (4 to 12 weeks). If documented progress occurs in edema reduction and pain-free motion, the patient advances to the second phase of treatment, which may span 4 to 12 weeks. As this phase is initiated, the patient is gradually weaned from his protective splint. The patient continues to wear the splint throughout the night and decreases wearing time during the day. Oftentimes, during the day, it is best to incorporate a semiflexible external support to limit extremes of motion. Some supports that include the thumb and wrist are commercially available. Others, such as one designed by the Petzoldt Clinic,[21] are custom made from adhesive tape and Coban wrapping (Fig. 22-7).

When this phase of treatment is begun, the patient is instructed in thumb protection techniques such as avoidance of prolonged pinch, forceful thumb flexion, repetitive thumb motions, and combined pinch or grip with repetitive wrist motion in any plane.[53] Activities of daily living are reviewed, and the patient is taught alternative methods to approach a task and to incorporate adaptive equipment such as built-up handles for writing. The patient is instructed to acknowledge symptoms of discomfort and be prepared to intervene with a treatment technique to prevent recurrence of the acute stage. The analysis of pinch and grip strength may be employed using conventional instruments if the patient is mindful not to exacerbate symptoms during the testing procedure. Quick assessments of coordination may be assessed using the Jebsen-Taylor hand function test,[25] the Block and Box Test,[35] the Nine Hole Peg Test,[36] the Purdue Pegboard Test,* or the Minnesota Rate of Manipulation Test.*

The patient may now elongate the light activity exercise session. Gentle isometric strengthening may be initiated for

---

*Lafayette Instrument Co., Lafayette, Ind.

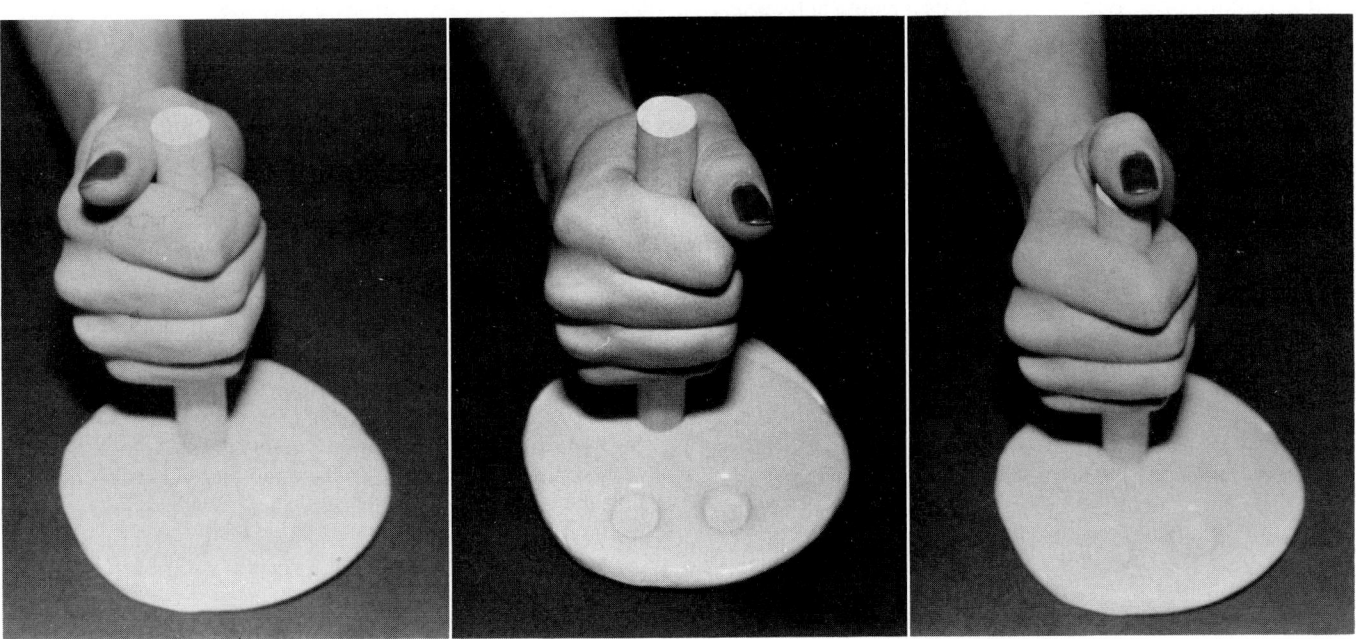

A   B   C

Fig. 22-8   Isometric strengthening may be initiated by pushing a dowel through putty. **A,** The thumb is first stabilized on the proximal phalanx of the index finger. **B,** Next, it is positioned around the dowel, this time stabilizing on the middle to distal portion of the index finger. **C,** Then the thumb is progressed to a position atop the dowel. These exercises are issued separately, beginning with position **A.** When the patient can perform multiple repetitions without pain, the patient advances to the next position.

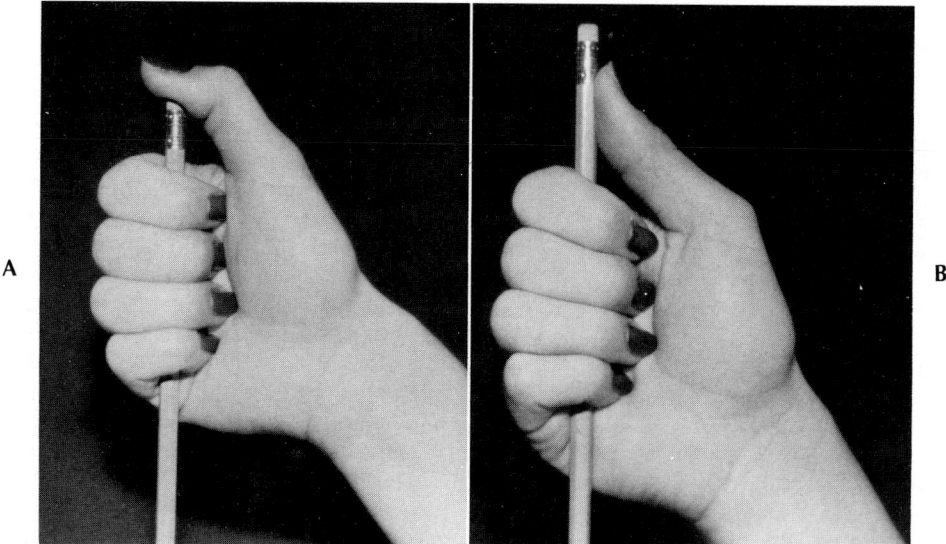

Fig. 22-9 Isotonic strengthening may be initiated by, **A,** pushing the thumb down on a pencil while the fingers provide graded resistance; then, **B,** actively using the thumb extensors to help push the pencil back up to its original position.

5 minutes three times a day. Various sized dowels may be pushed through putty while (a) first stabilizing the thumb on the proximal phalanx of the index finger, (b) progressing to a position where the thumb encompasses the dowel, and (c) pushing the dowel with the thumb (Fig. 22-8, *A*, *B*, and *C*). Isotonic strengthening for the thumb may be initiated by positioning the forearm and wrist in a neutral position and holding a dowel or pencil in the hand. The thumb then pushes down on the pencil as the fingers provide a graded resistance to the activity. The thumb then assists in returning the pencil back to the original position (Fig. 22-9, *A* and *B*). The use of syringes and commercially designed equipment such as the Thumbciser* assist in upgrading this exercise. Putty pinching, ceramics moulding, and link belt fabrication may be added to the program. It is advised that the patient accomplish lateral pinch asymptomatically before progressing to the more challenging positions of opposition pinch. An isometric wrist-strengthening program employing the grasp of 1 ounce to a 3-pound weight assists the patient in regaining muscle strength. An isometric program is initially performed because this method does not employ joint motion. Thus isometrics for the wrist produce only slight muscle fiber shortening and avoid repetitive tendon excursion over the radial styloid. When the patient demonstrates the ability to tolerate isometric exercises pain free, the program may be advanced to include an isotonic wrist-strengthening program, which produces changes in muscle length and joint motion. The program may include weights, a weight well, tools, or a BTE Work Simulator.†

Rather than add a full complement of exercises to the patient's program, it is imperative to issue exercises one at a time and assess the patient's reaction to them. Edema and pain-free ROM measurements may be taken before and after activity to gauge whether or not the patient may proceed

with further exercises. Symptom control by means of the aforementioned techniques must be continually maintained.

Interestingly, a dated report links de Quervain's symptomatology with a predisposition to rheumatoid arthritis or other collagen diseases.[35] Although current literature does not seem to support or refute this finding, the therapist may consider joint protection programs for patients on an individual basis.

Based on a review of the patient's job demands, exercises are provided for each portion of a job task before initiation of the task as a whole. Exercises requiring lifting, carrying, reaching, grasping, tool handling, and pinching are initiated[26] for short periods of time while using the affected wrist and thumb in midrange. As the patient becomes successful, actual distances are moved and graded weights are incorporated in the simulated job tasks. Frequently alternative methods of job completion are then added to the program. If the dominant hand was affected, the therapist should also consider assessment of the nondominant hand's ability to perform skills efficiently and safely.[47]

To successfully return a patient to work, the therapist must provide opportunities for the patient to upgrade his endurance.[22] Analyses of endurance for activity or tool use may be provided by the use of the Valpar battery of tests*; the BTE Work Simulator or the Bennett Hand Tool test.† As the date of discharge from therapy is anticipated, contact with the patient's employer is advised. It is helpful to understand the employer's expectations of the employee and whether or not adaptions may be allowed. Adaptions might include (1) returning to a shortened work day, (2) rotating work stations to ensure changes in hand positioning, (3) employing techniques to reduce ergonomic stresses,[1] (4) allowing the patient to use a flexible support during work, and (5) permitting the patient to attend therapy once a week

---

*Available through North Coast Medical Inc., Campbell, Calif.
†Baltimore Therapeutic Equipment Co., Baltimore.

*Pleasantville Educational Supply Corp., Pleasantville, NY.
†The Psychological Corp., Dallas, Tex.

for consultation and home program modification. It should be conveyed to the employer that returning to work midweek may be helpful in easing the patient's successful transition back to the work place.

During all stages of treatment the therapist must keep the physician informed of the patient's reaction to treatment because this will determine the physician's course of action, whether it be to return the patient to some phase of work or to proceed with surgery.

Postsurgical approach

If the patient does not report relief of symptoms after a trial treatment period of 3 to 6 weeks,[51] surgery may be considered. Surgical intervention involves a first dorsal compartment approach and careful guarding of the radial nerve. The gliding ability of the compartmental tendons is then appraised as the thumb is positioned in extension, adduction, and abduction.[52] The tendons are decompressed, analyzed, and surgically treated for abnormalities,[40] or, in the case of longstanding inflammation, adhesions are dissected.

After surgery, the wound is aseptically dressed. A splint is applied, which maintains the wrist in neutral to slight extension and the thumb in a neutral position, while allowing the fingers freedom of movement. The dressing is replaced on the second to third postoperative day,[13] and the patient is referred to therapy for a light exercise program as tolerated.

During the first postoperative visit, the therapist examines the surgical site for signs of infection, which may include warmth, redness, abnormal swelling, tenderness, and presence of an opaque exudate. Should these cardinal signs exist, the treating physician should be notified immediately. While the dressings are removed, general notations should be made regarding edema and nonstressful range of motion. If the assessing tools have been carefully cleansed, circumferential measurements and goniometric measurements may be taken

over the lightly dressed surgical area. Pain is also qualified during the initial visit.

A thermoplastic splint as previously described (see Fig. 22-4) may replace the surgical cast. The patient is instructed in nonresistive proximal upper extremity exercises and edema control techniques such as cold pack application four times per day and hourly overhead intermittent fisting of the uninvolved digits of the affected hand. The patient is advised to elevate his arm during activities of daily living and sleep. A moderately compressive stockinette may be worn at all times over the hand and forearm to assist with venous return, and the patient may be taught a home program of distal-to-proximal retrograde massage, avoiding the wound area. If the edema does not respond to this treatment, the clinical use of an intermittent compression pump may be indicated.

The patient is encouraged to perform tendon-gliding exercises of the uninvolved digits five times a day. Early, gentle, active motion exercises are recommended for the wrist and the thumb CMC, MP, and IP joints three times a day. Gentle, passive range-of-motion exercises may be initiated only if joint stiffness is noted. During the early stages of treatment, biofeedback may also be considered for some patients. A case study by Budic reports that biofeedback with auditory signals is sometimes useful after surgery in the patient with de Quervain's disease, because thumb extensors appear "more active than necessary, even at rest."[54]

After surgery, the patient may have paresthesias in the area supplied by the radial sensory nerve. This may occur secondary to anesthesia or traumatization of the nerve by retractors, and, according to Usoltseva[52] if no complications are present, resolution of symptoms may be seen within 3 weeks. However, if the patient has prolonged hypersensitivity in the area of the surgical site, a desensitization program is incorporated into the home program on an hourly basis. The program use tactile stimulation; the patient is taught to rub the area with a gradation of textures (refer to

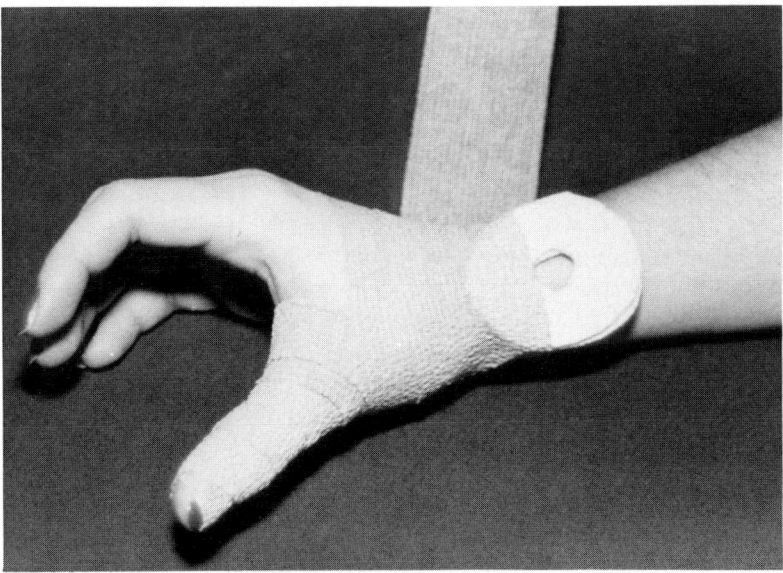

Fig. 22-10   If the patient experiences hypersensitivity in the scarred area, a foam doughnut may be applied before the applications of sturdier pressure stents.

Chapter 56). Rather than apply a pressure stent, the therapist may fabricate a soft foam doughnut for the patient who has discomfort with constant tactile input (Fig. 22-10). In this instance, a light bolus of cotton may be the first type of constant pressure stent applied. If treatment progresses and the patient does not report a diminution of pain, the therapist should consider the gate control theory proposed by Melzack and Wall.[38] The concept is that a neutral mechanism in the spinal cord may increase or decrease pain impulses from the periphery to the brain. It further proposes that when the sensory input is greater than or equal to the pain, the perception of pain is diminished. Methods of counter-irritation such as the use of heat, cold, and transcutaneous electric nerve stimulator (TENS) may be tried. The TENS unit has been recommended for cases involving the superficial radial nerve because irritation to this nerve may lead to reflex sympathetic dystrophy (RSD).[32]

After the sutures are removed between the eighth and tenth postoperative days,[52] tissue massage is recommended on the perimeter and later over the surgical site. Firm pressure massage applied for approximately 5 seconds per area is necessary to blanch out the underlying scar. A lanolin-rich lotion may be massaged into the skin when the wound is closed. Scar massage becomes an important component of the home program, and the patient is advised to perform this three times daily. As therapy progresses, various densities of pressure stents may be applied to compress scar. Lightweight foam may be upgraded to a denser foam or to a molded Otofoam* or silastic Elastomer† stent. These pressure pads may be held in place with Coban wrap or a compression stockinette. The patient should be advised to wear the pliable foam stents when performing activities and exercises and to incorporate the denser pads into the resting phase when the hand is relatively less mobile. As an adjunct to massage and pressure stents, ultrasound may be applied over the scar to assist in the disruption of the connective tissues polypeptide bonds.[16]

The remainder of the patient's postsurgical treatment is the same as that discussed previously for conservative management. As the patient progresses through various stages, his response to treatment is constantly assessed and treatment is modified or advanced.

SUMMARY

Throughout treatment the injured patient advances from the dependent role to one who becomes knowledgeable in the treatment of his hand. The patient appraises postures that may provoke symptoms, learns to implement adaptive approaches during job performance, and efficiently uses techniques to alleviate recurrence of symptoms.

---

*Dreze, Inc., Unna, West Germany
†Dow Corning Corp., Midland, Mich.

REFERENCES

1. Armstrong TJ and others: Ergonomics considerations in hand and wrist tendonitis, Am J Hand Surg 12A:830, 1987.
2. Arons MS: De Quervain's release in working women: a report of failure complications and associated diagnoses, J Hand Surg 12A(4):540, 1987.
3. Beasley RW: Hand injuries, Philadelphia, 1981, WB Saunders Co.
4. Bierman W: Ultrasound in the treatment of scars, Arch Phys Med 34:209, 1954.
5. Boyes JH: Bunnell's surgery of the hand, Philadelphia, 1970, JB Lippincott Co.
6. Brand PW: Clinical mechanics of the hand, St Louis, 1985, The CV Mosby Co.
7. Cailliet R: Hand pain and impairment, Philadelphia, 1982, FA Davis Co.
8. Cannon NM and others: Manual of hand splinting, New York, 1985, Churchill Livingstone.
9. Conklin JE and White WL: Stenosing tenosynovitis, Surg Clin North Am 40(2):531, 1960.
10. Cooney WP and Chao E: Biomechanical analysis of static forces in the thumb during hand function, J Bone Joint Surg 59A(1):27, 1977.
11. Curry RT: Patients with chronic pain syndromes. Conference on upper extremity inflammatory disorders, San Diego, Calif, Oct 21, 1988.
12. Fletcher C: Pain slowly surrenders its secrets as research seeks safer opiates, new class of analgesics, JAMA 252(23):3236, 1984.
13. Froimson AI: Tenosynovitis and tennis elbow. In Green DP, editor: Operative hand surgery, vol 2, New York, 1982, Churchill Livingstone.
14. Gould JA and Davies GJ: Orthopedic and sports physical therapy, vol 2, St Louis, 1985, The CV Mosby Co.
15. Griffin JE and others: Patients treated with ultrasonic driven hydrocortisone and with ultrasound alone, Phys Ther 47(7):595, 1967.
16. Griffin JE and Karselis T: Physical agents for physical therapists, Springfield, Ill, 1980, Charles C Thomas, Publisher.
17. Griffin JE and Touchstone JC: Effects of ultrasonic frequency on phonophoresis of cortisol into swine tissue, Am J Phys Med 51(2):62, 1972.
18. Hamilton WJ: Textbook of human anatomy, St Louis, 1976, The CV Mosby Co.
19. Hammer AW: Tenosynovitis, Med Record 140:353, 1934.
20. Hayes KW: Manual for physical agents, Chicago, Ill, 1979, Northwestern University Medical School, Program in Physical Therapy.
21. Henshaw J, Satren J, and Wrightsman JA: The semi-flexible support: an alternative for the hand injured worker, J Hand Ther 2(1):35, 1989.
22. Herbin M: Work capacity evaluation for occupational hand injuries, J Hand Surg 12A:958, 1987.
23. Hymovich L and Lindholm M: Hand, wrist, and forearm injuries, J Occup Med 8(11):573, 1966.
24. Jabaley ME and Heckler FR: Extensor tendon injuries. In Wolfort FG, editor: Acute hand injuries: a multidisciplinary approach, Boston, 1980, Little, Brown & Co.
25. Jebson RH and others: An objective and standardized test of hand function, Arch Phys Med Rehabil 50:311, 1969.
26. Jensen RC, Klein BP, and Sanderson LM: Motion-related wrist disorders traced to industries, occupational groups, Monthly Labor Re, p 13, Sept 1983.
27. Kapandji IA: The physiology of the joints, vol 1, Upper limb, New York, 1978, Churchill Livingstone.
28. Kendall FP and McCreary EK: Muscles, testing, and function, Baltimore, 1983, Williams & Wilkins.
29. Kilgore E and Graham W: The hand-surgical and non-surgical management, Philadelphia, 1977, Lea & Febiger.
30. Kleinkort JA and Wood F: Phonophoresis with one percent versus ten percent hydrocortisone, Phys Ther 55:1320, 1975.
31. Leao L: De Quervain's disease, J Bone Joint Surg 40-A(5):1063-1070, 1958.
32. Lee VH: The painful hand. In Moran C, editor: Hand rehabilitation, New York, 1986, Churchill Livingstone.
33. Lucas G: Examination of the hand, Springfield, Ill, 1972, Charles C Thomas, Publisher.
34. Malick MH: Manual on dynamic hand splinting with thermoplastic materials, Harmarville, Penn, 1978, Harmarville Rehabilitation Center.
35. Mathiowetz V and others: Adult norms for the box and block test, Am J Occup Ther 39:6, 1985.
36. Mathiowetz V and others: Adult norms for the nine hole peg test of finger dexterity, Occup Ther J Res 5:1, 1985.
37. Melvin JL: Rheumatic disease: occupational therapy and rehabiliation, Philadelphia, 1978, FA Davis Co.
38. Melzack R and Wall PD: Pain mechanics: a new theory, Science 150:971, 1965.
39. Michlovitz SL: Thermal agents in rehabilitation, Philadelphia, 1986, FA Davis Co.
40. Mosely LH: De Quervain's disease (stenosing tenosynovitis at the

radial styloid) and "trigger finger" stenosing tenosynovitis, Alexandria, Va.

41. Phalen G: Stenosing tenosynovitis. In Flynn JE, editor: Hand surgery, Baltimore, 1982, Williams & Wilkins.

42. Pick RY: De Quervain's disease: a clinical triad, Clin Orthop 143:165, 1979.

43. Poole B: Cumulative trauma disorder of the upper extremity from occupational stress, J Hand Ther 1(4):172, 1988.

44. Poznanski A: The hand in radiologic diagnosis, Philadelphia, 1984, WB Saunders Co.

45. Rayan GM and O'Donoghue DH: Ulnar digital compression neuropathy of the thumb caused by splinting, Clin Orthop 175:170, 1983.

46. Reid DAC and McGrouther DA: Surgery of the thumb, Boston, 1986, Butterworths.

47. Schultz-Johnson K: Assessment of upper extremity–injured persons return to work potential, J Hand Surg 12A(5)(part 2):950, 1987.

48. Tanaka S and others: Use of workers compensation claims data for surveillance of cumulative trauma disorders, J Occup Med 30(6):488, 1988.

49. Tenney CG and Lisak JM: Atlas of splinting, Boston, 1986, Little, Brown & Co.

50. Tubiana R: The hand, vol 2, Philadelphia, 1985, WB Saunders Co.

51. Urbaniak JR: Regional review course in hand surgery, rev ed, San Francisco, 1983, American Society of Surgery of the Hand.

52. Usoltseva EV and Mashkara KI: Surgery of diseases and injuries of the hand, St Louis, 1979, The CV Mosby Co.

53. Walker S: Treatment of inflammatory problems, from the office of RL Petzoldt. Presentation in San Jose Calif, April 15, 1982.

54. Walker SE and Rehm R: Hand therapy management for cumulative trauma disorders: acute phase through work capacity testing. Presentation for the National Safety Council, Nov 16, 1983.

55. Ziegler EM: Current concepts in orthotics, 1984, Rolyan Medical Products.

ADDITIONAL READINGS

Fine LJ and others: Detection of cumulative trauma disorders in the work place, J Occup Med, 28(8):674-680, 1986.

V
THE STIFF HAND

23

Management of the stiff hand

Raymond M. Curtis

The joints of the hand are the means by which the power of the muscles moving the bones of the hand bring about useful function. When these joints are stiffened by fibrosis, destroyed by disease, or deformed by dislocation or fracture, the function of the hand is impaired or even destroyed. This alteration in function may occur despite all our efforts; however, it more frequently occurs because of improper methods of treatment.

CAUSES OF JOINT STIFFENING IN THE HAND

The primary factors behind stiffening of the hand are (1) edema, (2) fibrosis, (3) collagen alteration,[17] (4) anatomic factors, and (5) disease. The patient with rheumatoid arthritis or dermatomyositis has a primary disease that leads to stiffness.

To prevent stiffness of the hand, the following principles should be followed: (1) elevation of the injured extremity, (2) mild compression dressing, (3) elimination of pain, (4) prevention of hematomas, (5) prevention of infection, and (6) understanding of the underlying emotional factors that occur with hand injuries.

Bunnell[2] has stated that all uninjured parts should be kept unrestrained and free to move. This is the functional treatment of fractures as described by Bohler[1] and Watson-Jones.[22] Moberg and Stener[15] have emphasized that contraction of the muscles pumps the tissue fluids through the limb, preventing edema and stasis and keeping the tissues nourished. Bunnell[2] has stated that "one should be alert to recognize early those cases that will go on to the edematous, immobile osteoporotic hand, by recognizing the signs of tropic disturbance and the disposition on the part of the patient to hold his hand completely immobile."

A pressure point produced by the dressing or cast will lead to edema and swelling of the injured or postoperative hand. For this reason, the dressing should be checked 12 to 24 hours after surgery and released at least along one border, much as one would do in splitting a cast. Any point where the patient complains abnormally about pressure and pain should also be checked.

Peacock[17] has stated on the basis of his clinical and experimental studies that the stiffness that follows simple immobilization is attributable to fixation of the joint ligaments to bone in areas normally meant to be free from such fixation and shortening of the ligaments by new collagen synthesis.

It is possible that with injury we may have an imbalance between fibrin formation and lysis of fibrin.

CONSERVATIVE METHODS OF TREATING STIFFENED JOINTS

Elevation. Elevation of the injured part is important in that it minimizes the degree of swelling. This should be used immediately after all surgery on the hand, and one should be sure that the patient, when ambulatory, keeps the hand elevated as well.

Elastic splints and elastic traction. Elastic splints and traction should be used early and continuously; the amount of tension used should not produce swelling.[18]

Molded plaster splints or casts. Molded plaster splints or casts can be applied and changed at regular intervals (daily is possible) to gradually stretch the finger joints or wrist joint into flexion or extension.

Intermittent compression unit. Intermittent compression therapy (with the Jobst Intermittent Compression Unit) has been very helpful in reducing swelling in the posttraumatic and postoperative hand and in mobilizing the stiff interphalangeal joints. The hand is placed in the sleeve with the fingers in extension for 10 minutes, under pressure, and then in flexion for 10 minutes. The amount of pressure that can be easily tolerated by the patient is used, with the time in the pneumatic sleeve being gradually increased from 30 minutes to 1 hour, one or more times a day, and with the pressure (in mm Hg) in the sleeve also being gradually increased.

The fact that the extracellular fluid is pressed out of the hand by the intermittent pressure and that the tight capsular ligaments are stretched first into extension and then into flexion makes it possible to mobilize some joints where splinting and other methods of treatment have failed.

Local heat therapy. Physiotherapy in the form of warm water soaks or whirlpool bath is helpful, as is hot wax therapy.

Stellate ganglion blocks and local nerve blocks. The local nerve blocks, or blocks with local anesthesia of the painful trigger areas, are very helpful. When indicated in sympathetic dystrophy, the stellate ganglion block or sympathectomy can be an aid in relieving pain and decreasing edema.

Active exercise. The need for active use of the hand in mobilizing stiff joints cannot be overemphasized.

Passive exercise. Passive exercises can be used to improve the range of motion in the stiff joints of the hand. The force applied must not increase the swelling or pain in the joints that are stiff.

Medical treatment. There are various drugs available for systemic use that may be helpful. Two of the most effective are phenylbutazone (Butazolidin) and prednisone. Triamcinolone may also be used in an amount of 2 mg injected intraarticularly into the small finger joints. Some tranquilizers seem to aid in the patient's recovery.

METACARPOPHALANGEAL JOINTS
Anatomy

The metacarpophalangeal (MP) joints of the four fingers can be flexed and extended. When the hand is open in extension, the fingers can also be abducted and adducted; thus they perform the four movements that make up circumduction and are called "condyloid joints." Grant[8] indicates that if it were not for the presence of ligaments, these joints would be ball-and-socket joints. When the joints are completely flexed, neither abduction nor adduction is possible. The reason is that the heads of the metacarpals, though rounded at their ends, are flattened in the front. Another reason is that the collateral ligaments, though slack on extension, are taut on flexion because of their eccentric attachments to the sides of the heads of the metacarpals and because the metacarpal head is broader volarly.

The collateral ligament is attached to a pit in front of the eccentrically placed tubercle on the head of the metacarpal; it is composed of two parts: a dorsally placed portion or "cord" ligament and a fan-shaped volar portion, the accessory collateral ligament, which extends from the metacarpal to the sides of the palmar or volar plate.

For allowance of flexion and extension, the anterior and posterior parts of the capsule must be lax. Dorsally there are no ligaments to these joints. Here the extensor or dorsal expansion of the extensor tendons effectively serves the part. The synovium of the joint closes the joint dorsally.

Anteriorly the capsule is replaced by a fibrocartilaginous plate, the palmar ligament or "volar accessory ligament." This plate is firmly united to the front edge of the phalanx and loosely attached to the metacarpal by areolar tissue.

Consequently, if a finger is wrenched off the hand, the platelike palmar ligament will part from the metacarpal and remain attached to the phalanx. Fibers of the collateral ligaments radiate to the sides of this plate and keep it firmly applied to the front of the head of its metacarpal, visor fashion.

The palmar or volar ligaments of the fingers are united to each other by three ligamentous bands, the deep transverse ligaments of the palm, which help to prevent the metacarpals from spreading.

Ankylosis

Anatomic structures that limit MP joint flexion are (1) adhesions of the extensor tendons over the dorsum of the hand or adhesions of the extensor hood mechanism over the MP joints, (2) thickening of the dorsal capsule of the MP joints, (3) contracture of the collateral ligament (cordlike portion), (4) insufficient skin coverage of scar of the skin over the dorsum of the hand, as in a burn, and (5) bony block within the joint.

Immobility of the MP joints for whatever reason, particularly if there is swelling with the deposition of edema fluid in the ligamentous tissue, leads to adhesions of the extensor mechanism, contracture and adhesions of the collateral lig-

aments, thickening of the entire capsular ligamentous structure, and the ankylosis so commonly seen in the MP joints.

This immobility is seen in hands in which there has been infection, trauma of all types, burns of the hand with burn-scar contracture over the dorsum of the hand, congenital aplasia of the MP joints, and certain systemic diseases such as rheumatoid arthritis and dermatomyositis.

The prevention of this very disabling abnormality is of primary importance. It can best be prevented by (1) early motion of the MP joints, (2) elevation of the injured extremity with prevention of edema, (3) elimination of plaster casts or splints, which immobilize the MP joint, and (4) early elastic band traction in patients who are developing this clinical entity.

Treatment by splinting and physiotherapy

In patients seen early after injury, attempts should be made to carry out rubber-band traction along with the use of a small volar plaster splint, worn 12 to 24 hours a day, or the practical Bunnell knuckle-bender splint, to determine what can be achieved with such conservative treatment.

This type of therapy can be coupled with various forms of physiotherapy. Alternating positive pressure with a compression unit can be of great help in reducing edema of the hand and mobilizing the joints. In addition, active exercise should be carried out.

If one is making progress with this form of treatment, the operative release should be delayed. If after several months of this type of conservative treatment there is no progress in the range of active or passive motion in the metacarpophalangeal joints, then there is an indication for surgical release of the MP joints.

It is important to point out that in most normal hands the MP joints passively flex 90 degrees. However, when one flexes the fingers for grasp, as in a closed fist, the index

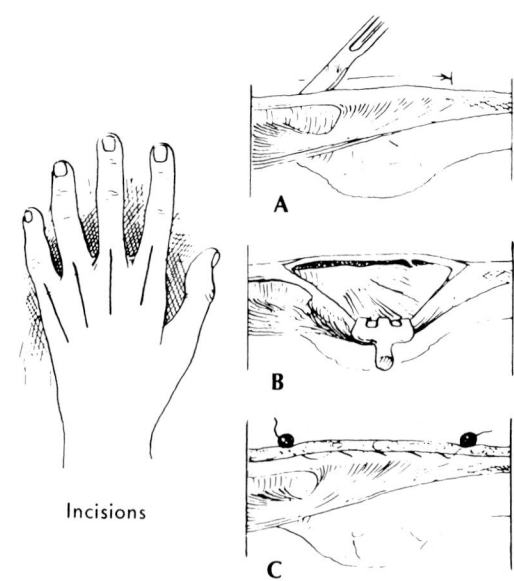

Fig. 23-1 Incisions for exposure of capsular ligaments of MP joints of fingers for capsulectomy. **A,** Splitting extensor tendon. **B,** Retraction of extensor hood to expose capsular ligament. **C,** Closure of extensor tendon with running 4-0 stainless-steel wire (redrawn from Bunnell). (From Curtis RM, as reported in Flynn JE: Hand surgery, Baltimore, 1966, Williams & Wilkins.)

finger actively flexes 75 degrees, the middle finger flexes 75 degrees, the ring finger flexes 80 degrees, and the little finger flexes 80 to 85 degrees. It is not necessary to achieve 90 degrees of active flexion in the MP joints to have a useful hand.

These ranges of motion should be remembered, for in a given hand it must be decided whether to proceed with surgical release in the patient who can flex somewhat at the MP joint. If the patient has no flexion at the MP joint but does have an intrinsically good joint, one can expect to achieve a good result from the release of the tight capsular ligaments and extensor tendon mechanism. If 75 degrees of active motion are approached in the MP joint, there is less indication for surgical intervention.

I do not perform capsulectomies on the MP joints if the patient flexes as much as 65 degrees in these joints. This patient should continue physiotherapy and special splinting. In patients whose hands are fixed in full extension or have a range of motion less than 65 degrees of flexion, sufficient improvement in the range of motion can be expected to warrant operative intervention.

Bunnell[2] has stated that the essentials for the success of capsulectomy are the presence of good surrounding tissue, good nerve supply and nutrition, redundant dorsal skin, good working muscles about the joints, and free extensor and intrinsic muscles or some correction for them to furnish strong flexion.

The choice between arthroplasty or capsulectomy in a given situation where there is an ankylosis in the MP joint will depend on the appearance of the metacarpal head and the base of the phalanx in the roentgenogram. Frequently, it is possible to salvage a good range of motion in the MP joint even in instances where by roentgenogram there has been considerable joint destruction.

Capsulectomy

Operative technique (Figs. 23-1 to 23-3). The extensor tendons are exposed by four straight longitudinal incisions over the metacarpals. The extensor tendon is then split longitudinally for a distance of approximately 2.5 cm on either side of the MP joint.[11] The aponeurotic hood, or extensor hood, is then retracted to either side, and the attachments of the extensor tendon to the base of the proximal phalanx are severed when they are present. The synovium, which forms the dorsal part of the capsule of the joint between the base of the phalanx and the head of the metacarpal, is excised, for this may be greatly thickened in severe cases. This dorsal capsule is excised from one collateral ligament across to the opposite collateral ligament over the dorsum of the joint.

Because the cordlike portion of the collateral ligament limits flexion, this can be released from its attachment just beneath the tubercle on either side of the head of the metacarpal, leaving it attached to the accessory collateral ligament, but freeing any adhesions that may have formed between the cord portion of the collateral ligament and the head of the metacarpal.[6] Pressure against the base of the proximal phalanx will then carry the proximal phalanx into flexion beneath the head of the metacarpal.

In those patients with much thickening in the collateral ligament, a section of the cordlike portion of the ligament should be removed near the tubercle on either side of the head of the metacarpal. The remainder of the cordlike portion of the collateral ligament should be left attached to the accessory collateral ligament. This will prevent ulnar deviation of the finger, which is seen when too much of the

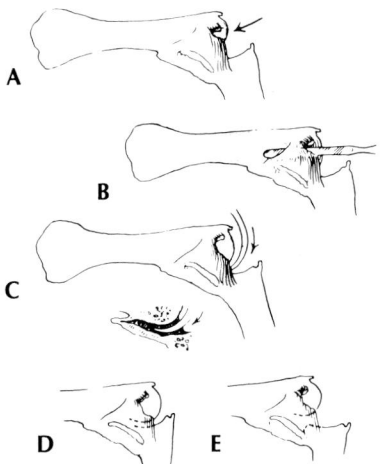

Fig. 23-3 Technique for capsulectomy with release of "cord" portion of ligament. Continuity is maintained between distal portion of "cord" ligament and accessory collateral ligament to prevent ulnar deviation even when small wedge of "cord" portion of ligament is excised. **A,** Dorsal capsule excised and "cord" portion released at point of attachment to metacarpal; accessory collateral ligament still intact. **B,** Elevator frees adhesions between ligament and head of metacarpal. **C,** Elevator releases adherent volar capsule and recreates normal pouch beneath metacarpal head. **D,** Proper relation of phalanx to metacarpal. **E,** With inadequate release of volar capsule, phalanx does not rest beneath head of metacarpal. (From Curtis RM, as reported in Flynn JE: Hand surgery, Baltimore, 1966, Williams & Wilkins.)

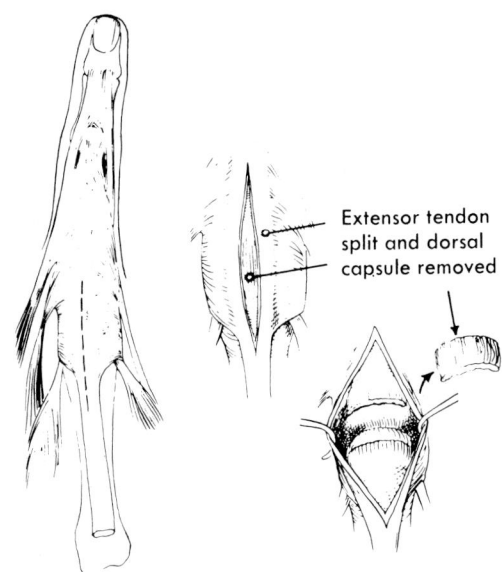

Extensor tendon split and dorsal capsule removed

Fig. 23-2 Exposure of joint by dorsal approach through extensor tendon, with excision of thickened synovium that forms dorsal part of capsule. (From Curtis RM, as reported in Flynn JE: Hand surgery, Baltimore, 1966, Williams & Wilkins.)

cord portion of the collateral ligament and its accessory ligament are removed.

This deviation is likely to occur in the patient with ulnar nerve palsy. One must also take care not to sever the attachment of the interosseous tendon into the base of the phalanx just distal to the attachment of the collateral ligament to the phalanx, because this may also lead to ulnar deviation of the fingers.

If the phalanx does not drop into flexion beneath the head of the metacarpal, a curved periosteal elevator should be inserted around the head of the metacarpal to recreate the volar pouch beneath the head of the metacarpal, because in long-standing cases this pouch becomes obliterated when the volar plate becomes adherent to the metacarpal head.

The excursion of the extensor tendons over the dorsum of the hand should be checked. If these are not gliding freely, they should be tendolyzed over the dorsum of the hand and, if necessary, over the dorsum of the wrist and into the forearm. In addition, it may be necessary to free the extensor hood well onto either side of the MP joint.

I prefer to place 2 mg of triamcinolone acetonide (Kenalog) into each joint before closing the extensor tendon and distribute another 10 mg beneath the extensor tendons on the dorsum of the hand if they have been tendolyzed.

The extensor tendon is closed with a running suture of 4-0 stainless steel wire. The hand is dressed in a pressure dressing with the MP joints in moderate flexion—however, not in such a severe degree of flexion as to cause the extensor tendons to open over the MP joint. This pressure dressing is left in place for 72 hours, at which time it is removed and a volar plaster splint applied so that one may begin rubber-band traction by leather loops about the proximal phalanges for flexion.

The elastic splinting must be continued as long as necessary, both day and night. After 4 to 6 weeks, a Bunnell knuckle-bender splint may be used. During the period of elastic splinting some active extension is allowed as well. If the patient has a problem with finger extension, a dynamic splint for extension is alternated with one for flexion.

Complications

Certain complications may occur after the operative procedure of capsulectomy.
1. Ulnar deviation of the fingers as a result of a too radical resection of the collateral ligament on the radial side, particularly in the presence of ulnar nerve palsy, may occur. Also, if one inadequately releases the collateral ligament on the ulnar side of the joint, ulnar deviation may result.
2. Disruption of the extensor tendons over the metacarpophalangeal joint may occur in those patients in whom one has not adequately tendolyzed the extensor tendons. It may also occur in those patients in whom there has been considerable shortening of the extensor muscles themselves. This latter complication can usually be prevented if the MP joints are not forced into full flexion immediately postoperatively instead of flexing with rubber-band traction as the tight extensor tendons gradually loosen.
3. Recurrence of the ankylosis may occur where the abnormality was inadequately corrected at surgery or where adequate rubber-band traction was not maintained after surgery. If a good result is not obtained, the procedure can be repeated after 4 to 6 months.

Arthroplasty

Arthroplasty with the use of a joint prosthesis may be the procedure of choice for patients who have such severe destruction of the metacarpal head or the base of the proximal phalanx that release of the capsular ligament may not provide a satisfactory range of motion.[7] It is indicated in the rheumatoid arthritic patient, where there has been such severe destruction of the metacarpal head that satisfactory stabilization cannot be accomplished in the MP joint by the usual imbrication of the extensor hood and reconstruction of the collateral ligaments.[21] In addition, it is used in osteoarthritic patients, in whom there is pronounced deformity in this joint, and in destruction of the joint after trauma.

The best arthroplasty result is obtained by the use of a joint prosthesis interposed between the metacarpal and the proximal phalanx.

PROXIMAL INTERPHALANGEAL JOINTS

When the surgeon treats a crippled hand, he is confronted frequently with a hand that fails to function properly because of limitation of flexion or extension in the interphalangeal joints. Bunnell[2] noted that it is the narrow joint space present in the interphalangeal joints that produces limitation of motion when there is even the slightest shortening of the capsular ligaments as might be produced by nonuse or edema of the ligaments and subsequent fibrosis.

This shortening, with limitation in motion, may occur despite the most rigid attention to proper splinting and physical and occupational therapy, with proper reduction of fractures or dislocations. However, it more often follows the improper use of these methods of treatment.[17]

Anatomy

The proximal interphalangeal (PIP) joint is constructed on essentially the same plan as the MP joint. It possesses collateral ligaments, a palmar fibrocartilage, and a loose dorsal capsule or synovial tissue guarded by an extensor expansion. This is considered a hinge joint, since movements are restricted to flexion and extension by the anteroposterior flattening of the ends of the bones.

An important fascial structure covers the collateral ligaments on either side of the joint. This has been described in detail by Landsmeer[13] as being composed of a transverse portion extending from the extensor tendon dorsally to the lateral border of the volar plate. The oblique portion of the ligament passes from the proximal phalanx to the extensor tendon over the middle phalanx. Stack[20] believes that this ligament is really a portion of the extensor tendon mechanism. Kaplan[12] has described this as a deep fascial cuff.

Sprains

Sprains may occur with varying amounts of injury to the capsular ligaments about the joint, from minute tears of the ligament to more extensive damage. The usual history is that of a patient having twisted or jammed the finger. There may be a hemarthrosis associated with the ligament injury. After the injury, there may be months of painful swelling of the joint, with stiffness on both flexion and extension.[16]

These injuries should receive careful attention in the acute stage; they should be splinted in slight flexion for 2 to 3 weeks. If possible, the splint should be removed periodically with careful flexion and extension, guarding against forced flexion and extension.

Local injection of the joint with triamcinolone acetonide (Kenalog) may be helpful in relieving pain in chronic cases and aid in mobilizing the joint.

In those cases seen late, with thickened capsular ligaments and stiffness on flexion and extension, the most careful splinting will be required to stretch the joint into full flexion and extension. For a severely ankylosed joint in extension or flexion a capsulectomy may be needed to restore function.

Ankylosis in extension

The surgeon about to correct a limitation of flexion of the PIP joint must have in mind the various anatomic structures in the finger that may limit this motion. These structures are (1) scar contracture of the skin over the dorsum of the finger, (2) contracted long extensor muscle or adherent extensor tendon, (3) contracted interosseous muscle or adherent interosseous tendon, (4) contracted capsular ligament, particularly the collateral ligament, (5) retinacular ligament adherent to capsular ligament, (6) bone block or exostosis, and (7) adherence of the flexor tendons within the finger.

Before surgically correcting the lack of flexion of the interphalangeal joint, it is important to determine first by clinical examination and roentgenogram just which anatomic structures are limiting flexion and to be certain that a true ankylosis or bony fusion is not present. Bunnell, Doherty, and Curtis[3] have described various test positions of the hand and fingers to determine which structures are to blame.

Operative technique. (Fig. 23-4). The PIP joint is approached by a dorsal curvilinear incision.[4] The incision is deepened through the skin and subcutaneous tissue to expose the transverse retinacular ligament.[13]

In some long-standing cases, the volar synovial pouch will have become obliterated and must be reformed with a small, curved elevator or by forcing of the base of the middle phalanx into flexion. When there is an associated contracture of the interosseous muscle, the interosseous tendon is lengthened by tenotomy at the point where the longitudinal fibers join the middle slip of the extensor tendon, allowed to slide proximally, and then resutured to the extensor aponeurosis. One can also overcome this interosseous contracture by excision of a triangle including the longitudinal fibers from the interosseous and lumbrical muscles, as recommended by Littler[14] in the Littler release procedure (see Harris and Riordan[9]).

If there is severe contracture of the interosseous muscle with flexion deformity at the MP joint as well, it may be necessary to tenotomize this tendon proximally to the MP joint and divide the volar capsular ligament of the MP joint. If necessary, the extensor tendon mechanism should be freed over the dorsum of the finger. The dissection and the freeing of all contracted tissues must continue until there is a free range of motion of the middle phalanx about the distal end of the proximal phalanx. This may necessitate freeing of the extensor tendon from the phalanx, opening of the dorsal synovium of the joint, resection of the collateral ligaments,

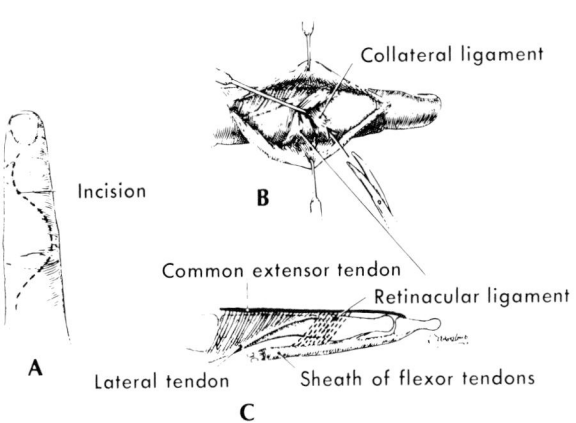

Fig. 23-4   Capsulectomy of PIP joint. **A,** Dorsal excision; dorsal skin is elevated and retracted. **B,** Retracted skin, with elevation of retinacular ligament exposes the collateral ligament, which is totally excised. **C,** Relationship of retinacular ligament to joint capsule and flexor and extensor tendons. (**A** from Curtis RM, first published in Adams JP, editor: Current practice in orthopaedic surgery, St. Louis, 1965, The CV Mosby Co.)

and a release of the contracted interosseous tendon mechanism.

One may elect to place 2 mg of triamcinolone acetonide (Kenalog) into the interphalangeal joint after this procedure.

The hand is placed in a dorsal plaster splint, using mechanics' waste and mild compression, with the fingers in moderate flexion at the PIP joints. Within 48 to 72 hours rubber-band traction is begun either by leather loops over the finger tips or by traction through the nail, pulling the fingers gradually into the flexed position. It may be necessary to alternate between rubber-band traction for flexion at the interphalangeal joints and rubber-band traction for extension of the fingers together with active exercise. Elastic splinting is continued until the patient is able to maintain by active and passive exercise the range of motion obtained at surgery. In some cases this necessitates part-time splinting for 3 or 4 months.

When the PIP joint may be actively flexed to 75 degrees or more, it is better judgment to rely on conservative measures such as physiotherapy and special splinting to achieve further flexion. In that group of patients who have a lesser degree of flexion, even in those whose fingers are held in rigid extension but without bony ankylosis, one can expect to improve flexion by this operative procedure. This was true in a series of patients even though capsulectomy had to be combined with other operative procedures when other anatomic structures were limiting flexion.

The results seem to indicate that the more anatomic structures there are involved in the limitation of motion, the poorer is the result.[4]

If the only limiting factor for flexion in the interphalangeal joint was a capsular ligament, capsulectomy of the collateral ligaments would produce a good result for both flexion and extension. However, if it was necessary to free the extensor tendon over the proximal phalanx to perform a tenotomy of the interosseous tendons and a capsulectomy of the collateral ligaments to obtain flexion of the PIP joint, the result achieved by surgery was not so successful. This was particularly true of the finger bound by cicatrix. In some of these patients the increase in motion was only 20 to 30 degrees, whereas in others the increase in motion was as much as 80 degrees beyond what existed before the operation. In many of these patients this increase meant the difference between a hand that could be used for work and one that could not. It cannot be expected that function will be restored completely by this procedure, but it can be expected to improve.

This approach is applicable to a joint stiff in extension, whether secondary to trauma or rheumatoid arthritis or whatever cause, if the joint surfaces are not too badly destroyed. In cases where there is extensive joint surface damage, an arthroplasty with a joint prosthesis is the procedure of choice.

Sprague[19] and Harrison[10] reported their results of the surgical treatment of the stiff PIP joint. Harrison recommends division only of the main collateral ligament and the dorsal capsule for the joint stiff in extension.

Ankylosis in flexion

The anatomic structure that limits extension of a finger at the PIP joint may be caused by these structures: (1) scar of the skin over the volar surface of the finger, (2) contraction of the superficial fascia in the finger, as in Dupuytren's contracture, (3) contracture of the flexor tendon sheath within the finger, (4) contracted flexor muscle or adherent flexor tendon, (5) contraction of the volar plate of the capsular ligament, (6) adherence of the retinacular ligaments of Landsmeer to the collateral ligaments, (7) adherence of the collateral ligaments with the finger in the flexed position, and (8) bony block or exostosis. Frequently, more than one structure is involved in this flexion contracture.

In congenital flexion contracture of the finger, all tissues from the skin to the joint capsule, and even the joint itself, may be involved. Interosseous function may be absent. Abnormal insertions of the lumbrical muscles have been reported.

Similarly, in the patient with Dupuytren's contracture that has existed for a long period of time and in whom there is pronounced flexion contracture of the PIP joints, the skin is contracted, there is a thick strand of contracted superficial fascia, the flexor superficialis tendon may be contracted, and the volar capsule and accessory collateral ligaments shorten in such a way as to prevent extension.

Operative technique. (Fig. 23-5). Operative release of the finger in an acutely flexed position is usually through a midlateral incision that is deepened to expose the flexor tendon sheath and the joint itself. (A Z-plasty on the flexor surface of the finger may be preferable in Dupuytren's contracture and congenital flexion contracture.) My initial approach is to excise a portion of the flexor tendon sheath distal to the A_2 pulley and see whether this simple excision will allow any extension. In some instances, it may be the only structure that is contracted.

This excision is then followed by checking of the flexor tendons to see whether they are adherent over the proximal phalanx or whether they are contracted. If they are severely contracted, it may be necessary to tenotomize and lengthen the flexor tendons in the forearm.

The retinacular ligament is freed from the lateral capsular ligament, and the volar capsule is then excised from the PIP joint. When necessary, the accessory collateral ligament is incised on either side of the proximal interphalangeal joint. Subluxation of the middle phalanx may occur if the cord portion of the lateral ligament is completely severed. In some instances, it will be necessary to divide the retinacular ligament of Landsmeer as well. The surgical release of the contracted structures will then allow extension of the PIP joint. The joint is fixed in moderate extension by a Kirschner wire across the PIP joint. The Kirschner wire is removed in 1 week, and active motion for flexion and extension is begun with rubber-band traction to improve the degree of extension and maintain the gain that was achieved operatively.

If a Dupuytren's contracture is present, a partial volar capsulectomy is performed with excision of the accessory collateral ligaments when excision of the thickened fascial band does not achieve complete extension of the joint.[5]

REFERENCES

1. Bohler L: The treatment of fractures, Baltimore, 1932, William Wood & Co.
2. Bunnell S: Surgery of the hand, ed 3, Philadelphia, 1948, JB Lippincott Co.
3. Bunnell S, Doherty EW, and Curtis RM: Ischemic contracture, local, in the hand, Plast Reconstruct Surg 3:424, 1948.
4. Curtis RM: Capsulectomy of the interphalangeal joints of the fingers, J Bone Joint Surg 36A:1219, 1954.
5. Curtis RM: Volar capsulectomy in Dupuytren's contracture. In Tubiana R and Hueston JT, editors: Les Monographies Du Groupe D'Etude de la Main, Paris, 1972, Expansion Scientifique Française.
6. Curtis RM: Joints of the hand. In Flynn JE, editor: Hand surgery, ed 2, Baltimore, 1975, Williams & Wilkins.
7. Fowler SB: Mobilization of metacarpophalangeal joint, arthroplasty and capsulotomy, J Bone Joint Surg 29:193, 1947.
8. Grant JCB: A method of anatomy, ed 4, Baltimore, 1948, Williams & Wilkins Co.
9. Harris C Jr and Riordan DC: Intrinsic contracture in the hand and its surgical treatment, J Bone Joint Surg 36A:10, 1954.
10. Harrison DH: The stiff interphalangeal joint, The Hand 9:102, 1977.
11. Howard LD: Cited by S. Bunnell in Surgery of the hand, ed 2, Philadelphia, 1948, JB Lippincott Co, p 301.
12. Kaplan EB: Functional and surgical anatomy of the hand, Philadelphia, 1953, JB Lippincott Co.
13. Landsmeer JMF: The anatomy of the dorsal aponeurosis of the human finger and its functional significance, Anat Rec 104:31, 1949.
14. Littler JW and Howorth MB: A textbook of orthopedics, Philadelphia, 1952, WB Saunders Co, p 251.

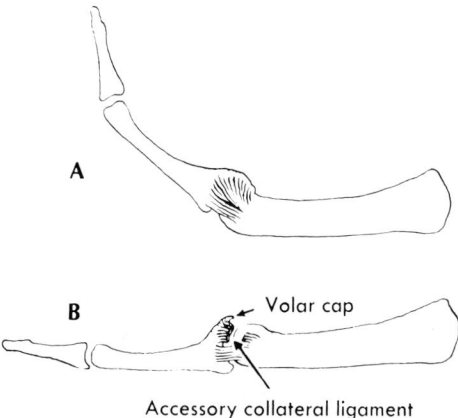

Fig. 23-5 Capsulectomy for release of flexion contracture of finger. **A,** Fixed flexion contracture. **B,** Excision of portion of volar capsule and release of accessory collateral ligament, with cord portion being left to maintain stability of joint. (From Curtis RM, as reported in Flynn JE: Hand surgery, Baltimore, 1966, Williams & Wilkins.)

15. Moberg E and Stener B: Injuries to the ligaments of the thumb and fingers: diagnosis, treatment, and prognosis, Acta Chir Scand 106:166, 1953.
16. Peacock EE Jr: Preservation of interphalangeal joint function: a basis for the early care of injured hands, South Med J 56:56, 1962.
17. Peacock EE Jr: Some biochemical and biophysical aspects of joint stiffness: role of collagen synthesis as opposed to altered molecular their treatment, Trauma 16:259, 1976.
18. Pratt DR: Joints of the hand and fingers—their stiffness, splinting and surgery, Calif Med 66:22, 1947.
19. Sprague BL: The proximal interphalangeal joint contractures and their treatment, Trauma 16:259, 1976.
20. Stack HG: Muscle function in the fingers, J Bone Joint Surg 44B:899, 1962.
21. Vainio K and Pulkki T: Surgical treatment of arthritis mutilans, Ann Chir et Gynaecol Fenniae 48:361, 1959.
22. Watson-Jones R: Fractures and other bone and joint injuries, Baltimore, 1940, Williams & Wilkins Co.

24

Therapist's management of the stiff hand

Pamela M. McEntee

Prevention of the stiff hand presents a challenge to the therapist, the surgeon, and the patient. An acutely stiff hand, characterized by pitting edema, pain, and decreased range of motion, can follow trauma to the hand whether minor or severe (Fig. 24-1). If left untreated, it can progress to a chronically stiff hand, characterized by brawny edema, soft-tissue fibrosis, and serious loss of hand function (Fig. 24-2). Early intervention by trained hand therapists is essential in remediation of the acutely stiff hand and prevention of the chronically stiff hand. The primary goal of treatment of the stiff hand is restoration of hand function. Evaluation, patient education, edema control, therapeutic exercise, therapeutic activities, and splinting are all avenues that lead to this goal (Fig. 24-3). The purpose of this chapter is to discuss the management of the stiff hand in both the acute and the chronic stages.

THE ACUTELY STIFF HAND

An acutely stiff hand is often seen after injuries such as a blow to the dorsum of the hand or a crush injury. The importance of early treatment for the acutely stiff hand cannot be overemphasized. A patient is often anxious about the condition of such a hand, because he fears it may restrict his ability to work or carry out activities of daily living. He has a natural inclination to protect the injured hand by complete immobilization. It is the responsibility of the therapist to assure the patient that early motion is essential for a quick recovery.

Evaluation

A thorough evaluation is essential before the initiation of treatment. It enables the therapist to formulate an innovative treatment plan to fit the individual patient's needs. Follow-up evaluations determine progress and the need for changes in the treatment program.

History. The evaluation begins with a detailed history, including the patient's age, occupation, hand dominance, description of injury, diagnosis, and previous surgeries. Pertinent psychosocial information, such as the patient's transportation and financial status, aids the therapist in determining the length and frequency of therapy visits.

Inspection. The patient's hand is closely examined for color, infection, and the presence of pain and edema. If edema is present, its area and extent are recorded before and after treatment. One method to measure edema objectively is to use a tape measure to compare the circumferences of the involved and uninvolved hands or fingers (Fig. 24-4). For tape measurements to be accurate, the same anatomic reference point is used for each sequential measurement. The volumeter[4] provides another method to evaluate edema. The patient's hand is submerged in a specifically designed water-filled container, and the amount of water displaced

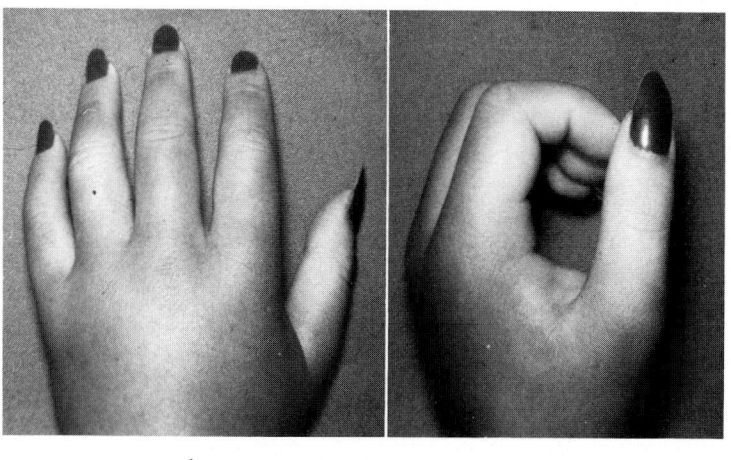

Fig. 24-1   **A,** "Pitting" edema in an acutely stiff hand. **B,** Pain and edema restrict active range of motion.

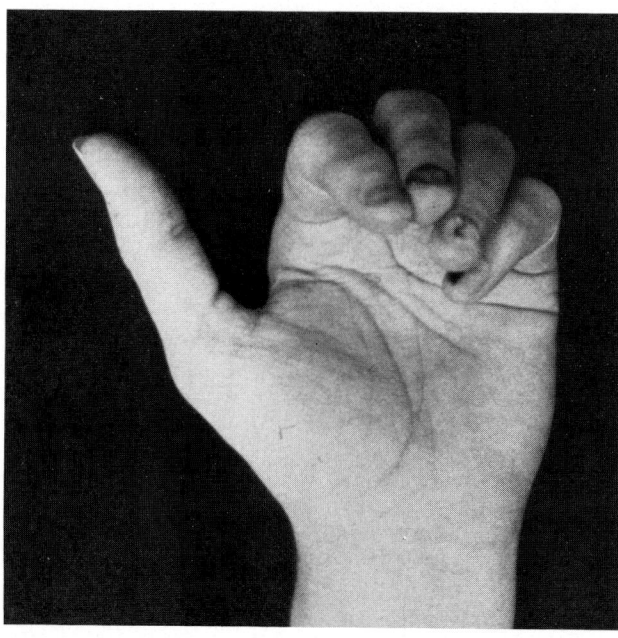

Fig. 24-2   In this chronically stiff hand, active flexion is restricted by malrotation of the fingers, joint contractures, and tendon adhesions.

328

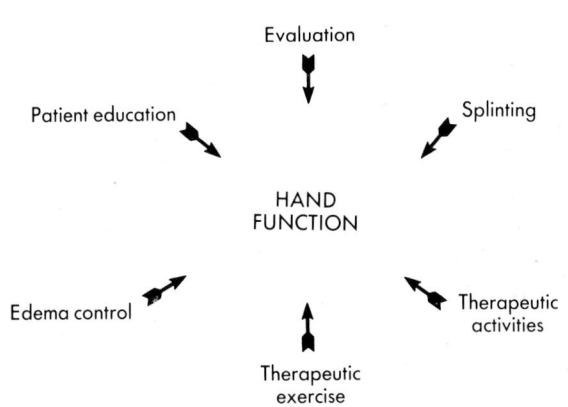

Fig. 24-3 Restoration of hand function is the primary goal in management of the stiff hand.

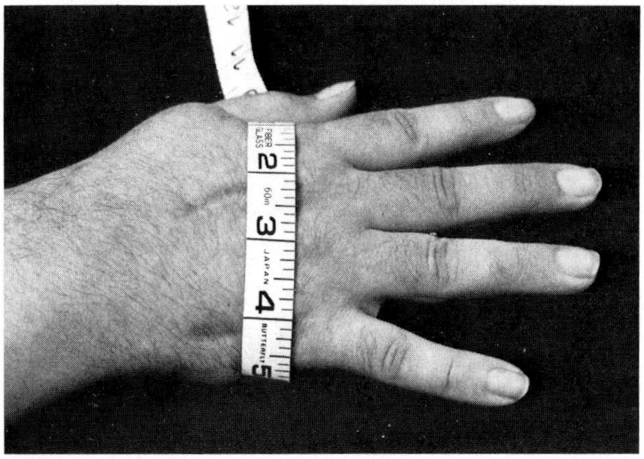

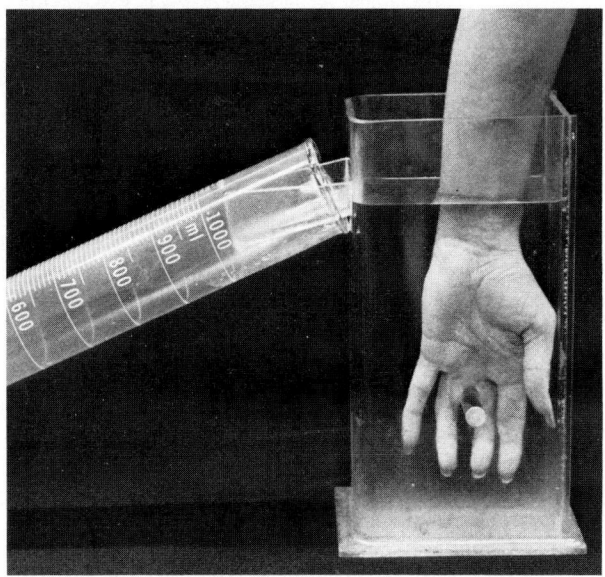

Fig. 24-4 Circumferential measurements are used as an indicator of edema.

by the submerged hand is measured (Fig. 24-5). Measurements before and after a therapy visit are often useful to teach the patient the beneficial effect of the elevation, massage, and active range of motion carried out in therapy.

Range of motion. The emphasis of the range-of-motion assessment in the acutely stiff hand is on active motion, because improvement in active motion will be the best indicator of progress in treatment. Active motion is measured by use of a finger goniometer, with the wrist positioned in neutral (Fig. 24-6).

Treatment guidelines

Edema control. A primary goal of treating the acutely stiff hand is the reduction of edema, because its presence can result in stiff and painful joints that lead to further loss of active motion. Elevation of the hand above the level of the heart allows gravity to assist in the reduction of the edema. This, along with active range of motion, is the most effective way to manage edema in the early stages. String wrapping of the hand distally to proximally for a period of 5 minutes (Fig. 24-7), followed by a retrograde massage and active fist making, is also an effective technique for managing edema. Other techniques that can be used include an intermittent pressure pump, Aris Isotoner Glove,* and elastic tape for wrapping of individual fingers or the entire hand. Wrapping should be in a figure-of-eight manner and pressure should be graded distal to proximal. (Refer to the discussion of edema and bandaging, Chapter 13.)

Therapeutic exercise. Active exercises within the patient's pain tolerance should always follow whatever edema control technique is used. Active exercises, such as fist making, produce a milking action in the deep veins of the hand. Active exercise of the hand is accompanied by gentle active range of motion of the shoulder, elbow, and wrist when severe swelling is present. Guarded passive range-of-motion exercises and graded resistive exercises are begun at the therapist's discretion, but they must not cause an increase in pain or edema. They include activities such as using a foam squeeze, squeezing putty, or using the Hand Helper.† In some cases, active exercise and edema control

---
* Aris Isotoner Glove, New York, NY.
† Hand Helper, Medex Corporation, Los Altos, Calif.

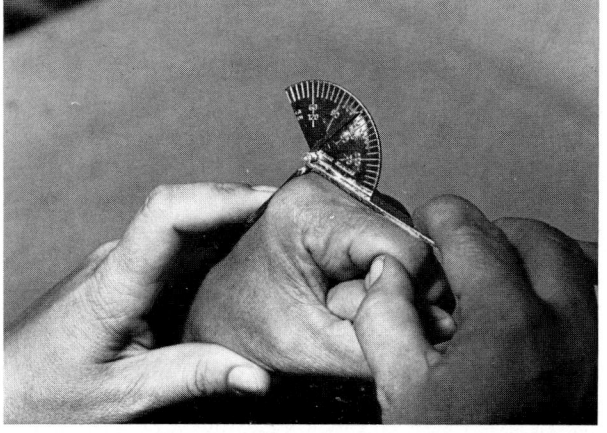

Fig. 24-5 The volumeter is used to measure edema in the stiff hand.

Fig. 24-6 Active range-of-motion measurements are taken using a finger goniometer.

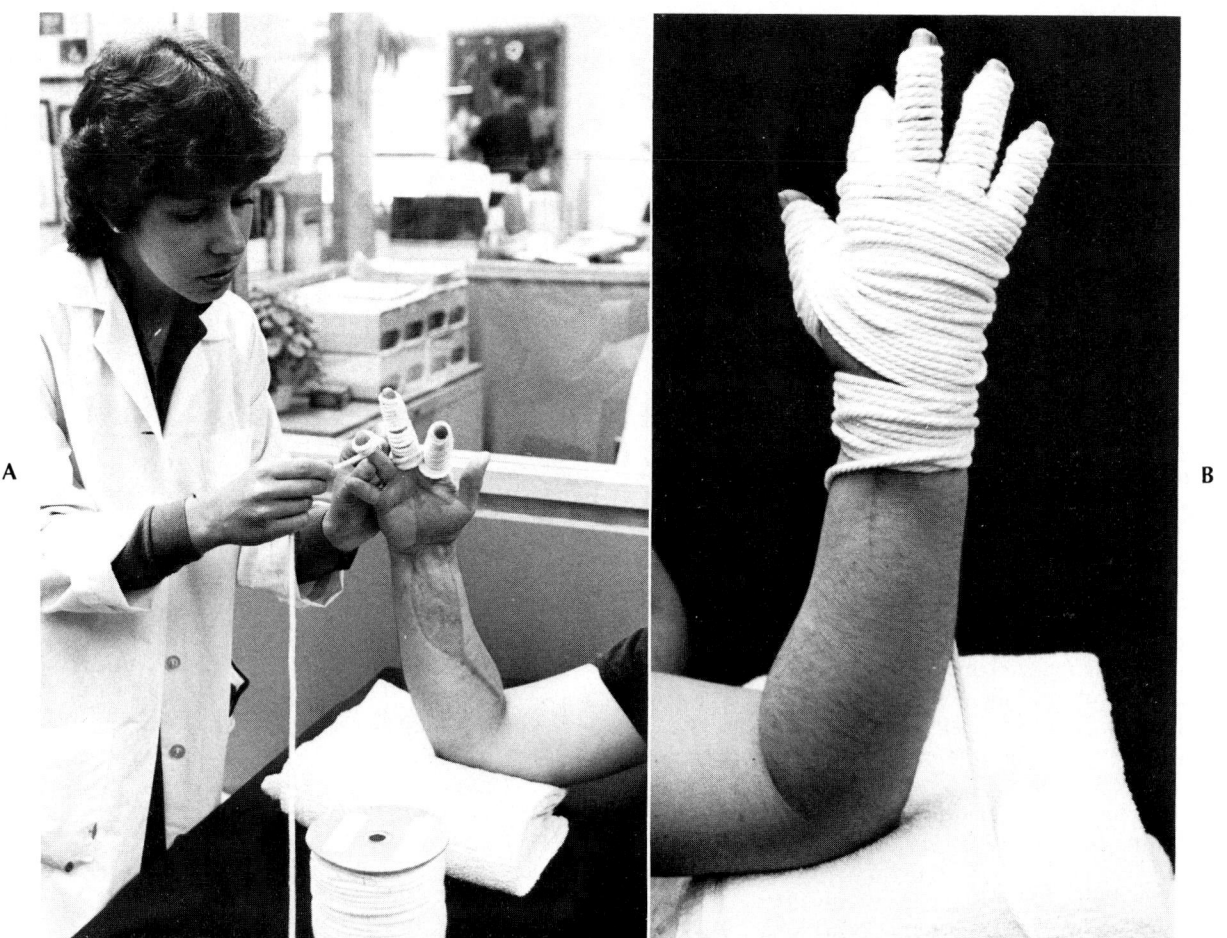

Fig. 24-7 **A,** Patient's hand is wrapped with string distal to proximal. **B,** Hand is then elevated for 5 minutes.

will reverse the cycle of immobilization and no further treatment will be needed.

Therapeutic activities. It is essential in the early stage of treatment that the patient begin using his hand even for the simplest activities. Prehension tasks (Fig. 24-8) such as light pick-ups, macramé, and light sanding are examples of activities that can be done in elevation and encourage range-of-motion exercise of all joints of the involved extremity.

Splinting. Supportive static splinting may be indicated to prevent strain of a severely swollen and painful hand. A functional resting splint worn at night or a wrist cockup splint worn during functional activities are two examples of splints that are used during the early stages of recovery. These splints are secured with a figure-of-eight elastic wrap when severe edema is present, so that pressure is distributed over a large area (Fig. 24-9). Static splinting can lead to greater stiffness, and therefore splints must be removed frequently to allow for range-of-motion exercises. Uncontrolled pitting edema is a contraindication for dynamic splinting.

Patient education. Each patient must be instructed on a home program that carries out the treatment techniques used during the therapy session. Exercises should be performed at least four times daily, with each exercise being slowly repeated five to ten times. Therapeutic activities such as macramé are carried out for three to five sessions daily

according to the patient's tolerance. The patient must be cautioned to follow the home program exactly as prescribed. Overzealous patients, who believe it is best to exercise constantly, may suffer an increase in pain and edema of their hand. Contrary to this, patients who are fearful that active exercise will be harmful to the hand will not perform their exercise program with the amount of frequency that is necessary to restore function. Home programs are written and reviewed at each therapy session. Illustrations of exercises are given to help clarify written instructions (Fig. 24-10).

Ongoing evaluation. In the treatment of an acutely stiff hand, a significant decrease in edema and an increase in active range of motion should be seen during the first week of treatment. If improvement is not noted, check to see if the patient is performing his home therapy program correctly. If he is, the initial treatment plan must be reevaluated and the patient's surgeon notified. After a discussion with the patient's surgeon, appropriate changes in the treatment program are made.

THE CHRONICALLY STIFF HAND

The patient with the chronically stiff hand requires a comprehensive therapy program in which there is ongoing communication between the patient, the therapist, and the surgeon. Examples of problems that commonly lead to a chronically stiff hand are fractures of the wrist or fingers,

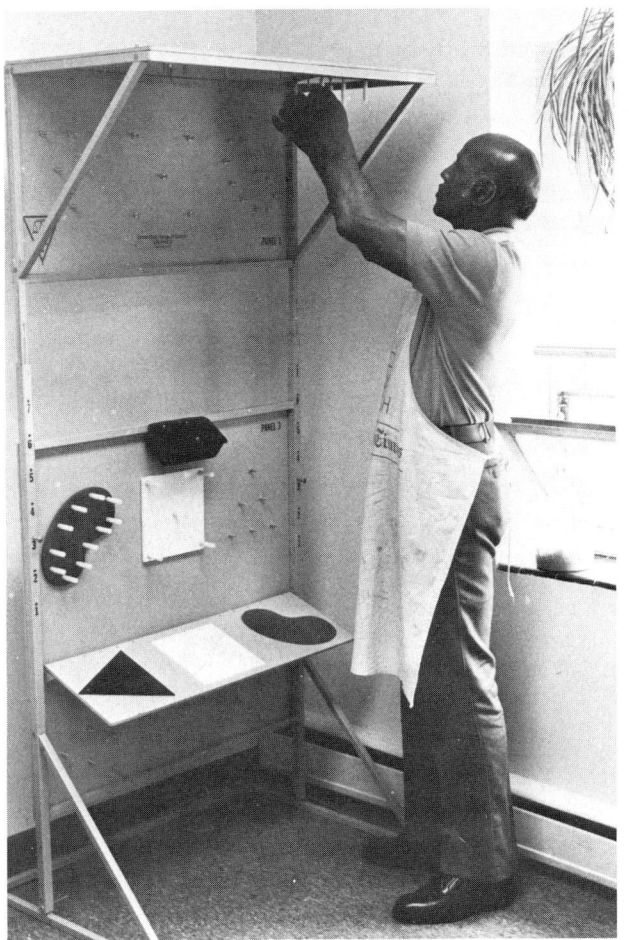

Fig. 24-8 Prehension activities performed with the extremity in elevation help reduce edema.

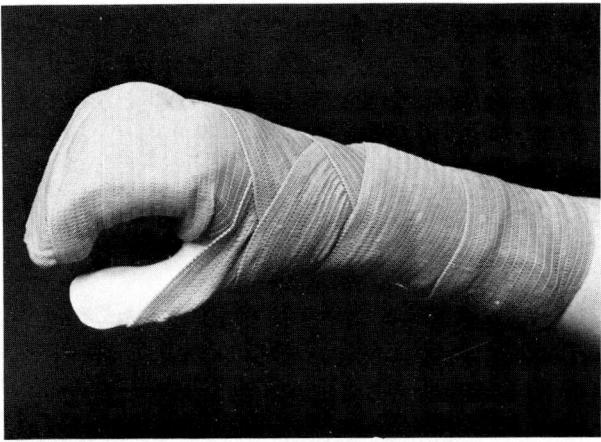

Fig. 24-9 A functional resting splint is secured with a figure-of-eight elastic wrap when severe edema is present, to help distribute pressure over a wide area.

to these structures should be incorporated in the treatment program. If the skin puckers when a stretch is applied, it indicates adherence to the underlying structures.

Active range of motion is measured by means of standard methods for measuring and recording, as described by the American Academy of Orthopaedic Surgeons.[1] If joint stiffness is present, closely examine the "end feel" of each joint before measuring passive range of motion with a goniometer. To do this, move the finger gently in the direction in which the joint motion is limited. If the joint comes to a slow stop and has a springy feel, the prognosis for improvement is good. However, if the joint moves freely to a certain

serious crush injuries, and acutely injured hands that were left untreated. The initial treatment session begins with an explanation about what has caused the patient's stiff hand and what must be done to restore function to it. The patient must understand that progress will be slow and strongly dependent on how motivated he is in consistently carrying out his therapy program.

Evaluation

Evaluation of the chronically stiff hand is more in-depth than that of the acutely stiff hand. As with the acutely stiff hand, a thorough history and hand inspection are done. Assessment of range of motion, strength, sensibility, and the patient's ability to perform activities of daily living completes the evaluation.

Range of motion. Knowledge of the causes of joint stiffness is essential before evaluation of the range of motion of the chronically stiff hand. Tests for skin tightness, joint range of motion, and intrinsic and extrinsic muscle tightness are routinely done.

Joint motion may be limited by tight skin around a joint or by a scar that crosses a joint. To evaluate this condition, one puts the joints adjacent to the joint being evaluated on slack before a passive stretch is applied. If blanching of the skin or scar occurs during passive motion of the joint, stretch

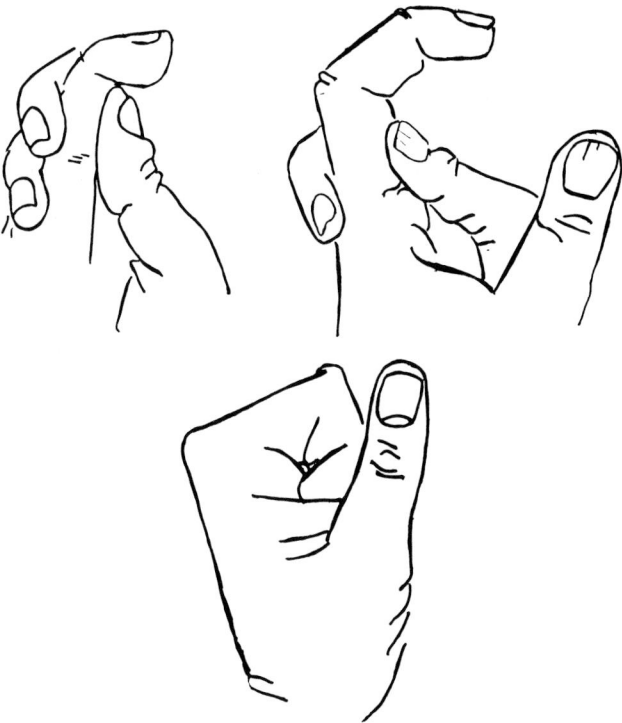

Fig. 24-10 Illustrations reinforce the written exercises given for patient's home program.

point and then stops abruptly, the prognosis for conservative treatment is poor. To measure passive joint motion with a finger goniometer, place the adjacent joints in whatever position is necessary to allow for maximum motion of the joint being measured, to eliminate influence from adherent tendons.

To complete the evaluation for range of motion, tests for intrinsic and extrinsic muscle tightness must be done. In-

trinsic tightness exists if the PIP and DIP joints can be passively flexed with the MP joint in flexion (Fig. 24-11, A) but cannot be fully flexed when the MP joint is extended[2] (Fig. 24-11, B). Extrinsic extensor tightness is present if the PIP and DIP joints will passively flex when the MP joint is extended (Fig. 24-12, A) but cannot be fully flexed when the MP joint is flexed[2] (Fig. 24-12, B). Extrinsic flexor tightness is present if the PIP and DIP joints will passively

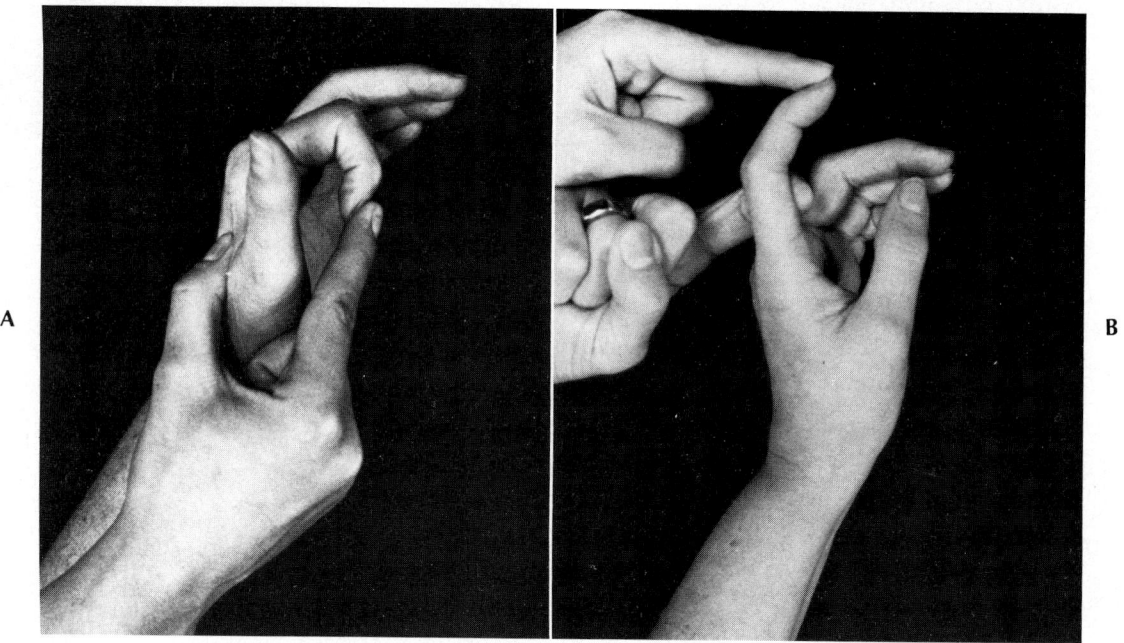

Fig. 24-11 Intrinsic tightness exists if the PIP and DIP joints can be passively flexed with the MP joint in flexion (**A**) but cannot be fully flexed when the MP joint is extended (**B**).

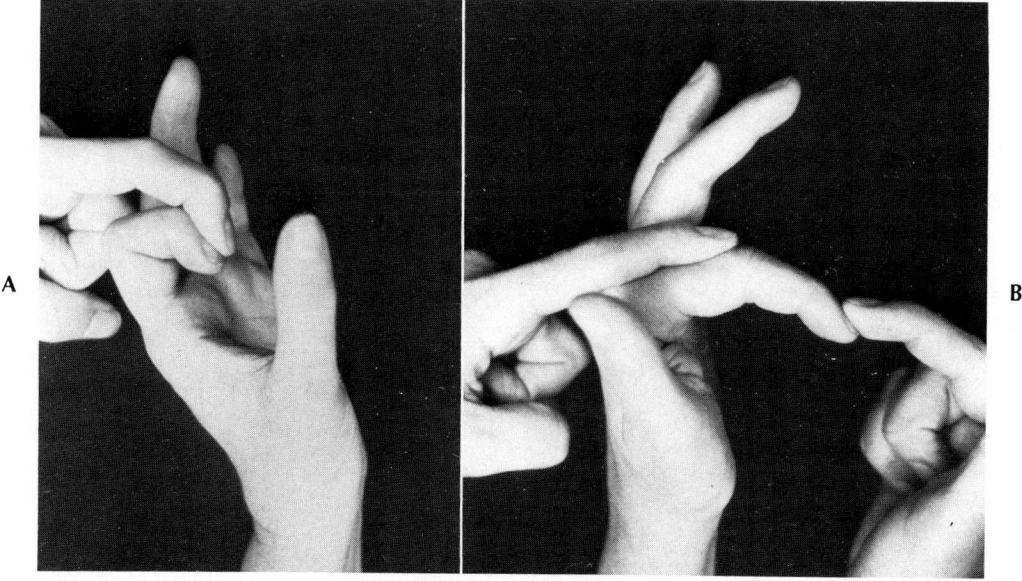

Fig. 24-12 Extrinsic extensor tightness is present if the PIP and DIP joints can be flexed when the MP joint is extended (**A**) but cannot be fully flexed when the MP joint is flexed (**B**).

extend with the MP joint flexed (Fig. 24-13, *A*) but cannot be fully extended when the MP joint is extended (Fig. 24-13, *B*). Tests for extrinsic muscle tightness will be affected by wrist position. Therefore the wrist must be positioned in neutral during testing.

Strength. Pinch and grip strength are measured on both extremities and compared. Grip strength is measured on all five handle positions of the adjustable Jamar* dynamometer (Fig. 24-14). Lateral, tip, and pulp pinch are measured on a pinch meter (Fig. 24-15). Individual muscle testing is done on selected patients to determine the motor function of a particular nerve and the relative strengths of the involved muscles.

*Jamar dynamometer, Asimow Engineering Co., Los Angeles.

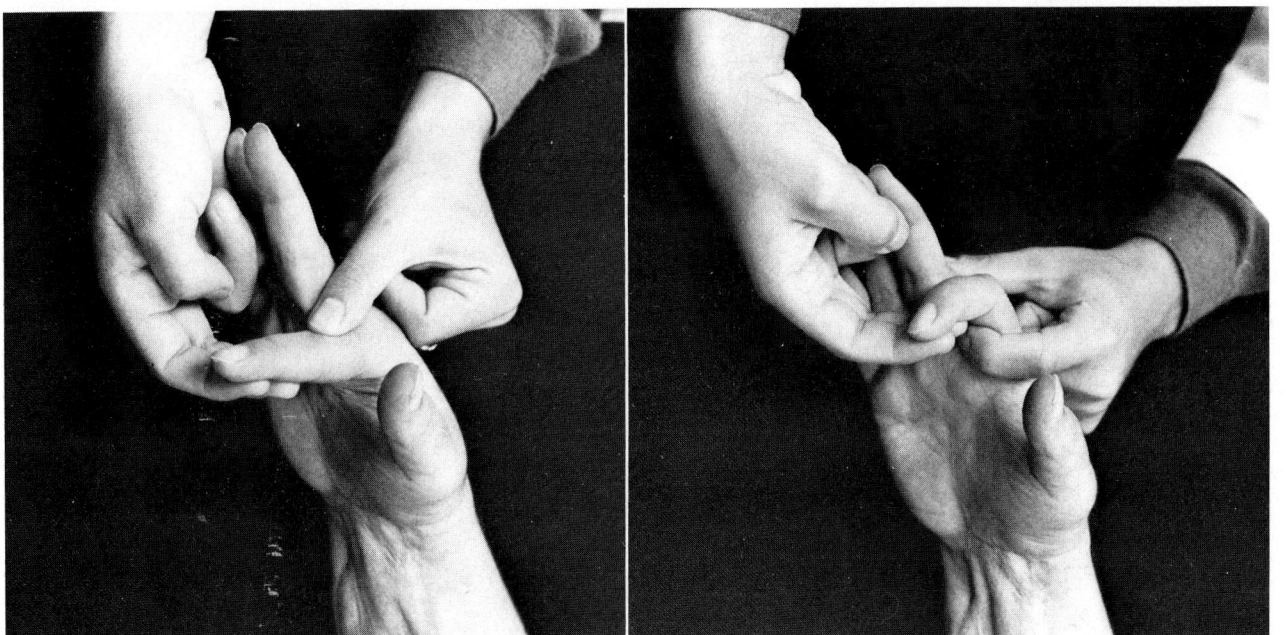

Fig. 24-13 Extrinsic flexor tightness is present if the PIP and DIP joints can be passively extended with the MP joint flexed (**A**) but cannot be extended as fully when the MP joint is extended (**B**).

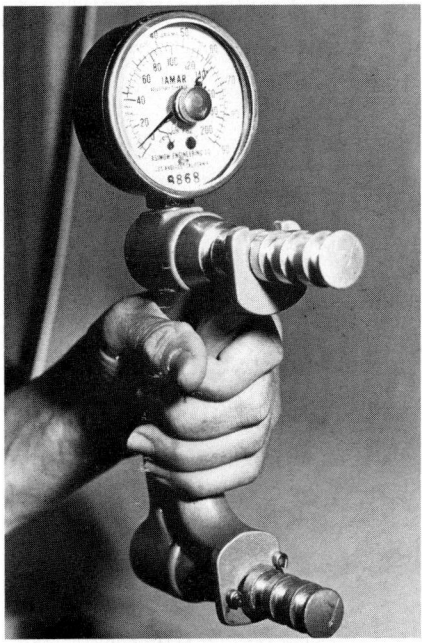

Fig. 24-14 The adjustable Jamar dynamometer is used to evaluate grip strength on five handle positions.

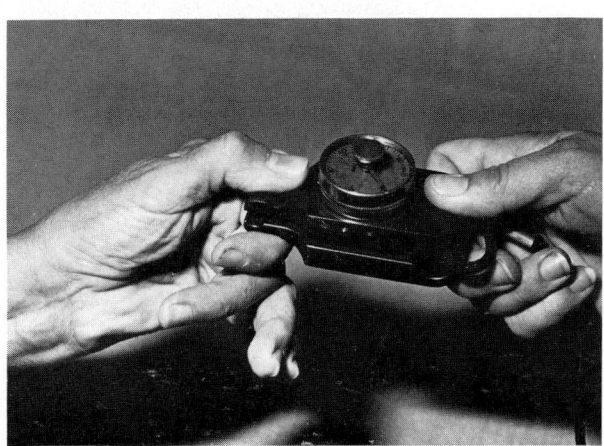

Fig. 24-15 Lateral, tip, and pulp pinch are measured on a pinch meter.

Sensibility. When indicated, tests for light touch and two-point discrimination are administered to determine the sensory function of a particular nerve.

Activities of daily living. An interview and the Jebson Hand Function Test[8] are used to determine the patient's ability to perform activities of daily living independently. The Jebson Hand Function Test assesses a person's ability to write, manage eating utensils, manipulate small objects, and manipulate both light and heavy objects.

Treatment guidelines

Edema control. In the chronically stiff hand, pitting edema has usually disappeared, but it leaves behind a brawny type of edema that is much more difficult to treat. Treatment for this brawny edema includes retrograde mas-

sage, active exercise, elasticized gloves, elasticized tape, and functional activities.

Massage done firmly in a retrograde manner is used in an attempt to mobilize edema and adherent tissues. Massage of the patient's hand by the therapist is an ideal way to begin the therapist-patient relationship. It gives the therapist an opportunity to transmit feelings of caring and understanding to the patient and at the same time allows the patient to become more relaxed and able to discuss any problems related to his hand injury. After massage tendon gliding exercises,[10] which encourage full tendon excursion, are performed in the hook, fist, and straight fist positions.

An Aris Isotoner glove may be used to provide external compression to a chronically swollen hand and can be effective in reducing dorsal edema. The patient wears the

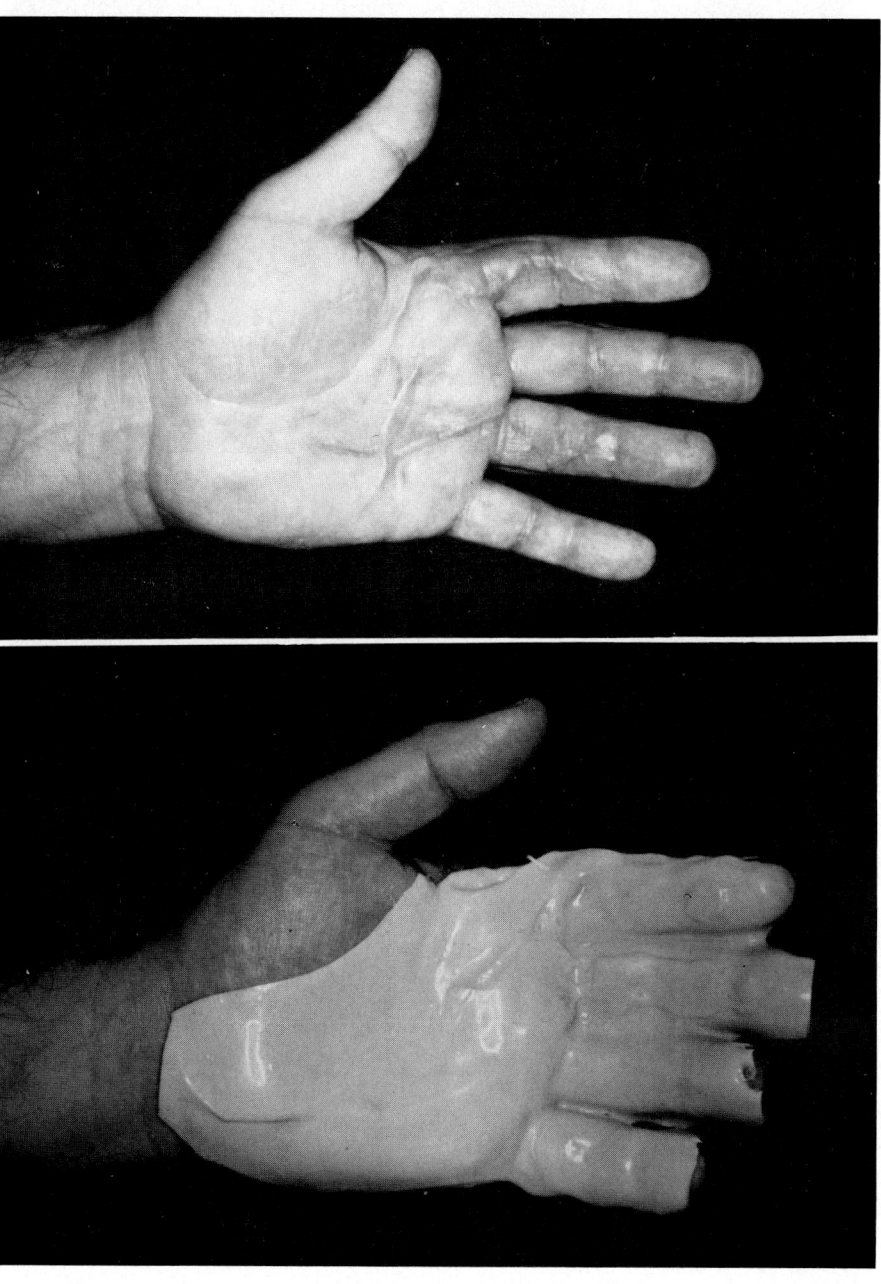

Fig. 24-16 Elastomer secured with an elasticized tape is used for scar management.

glove while performing activities of daily living and prehension tasks such as macramé and leather work.

Scar management

Scar formation often results in limitations in joint range of motion and tendon gliding (Fig. 24-16, *A*). Deep friction massage will help mobilize adherent scars from surrounding tissues. Elastomer* secured with an elasticized tape such as Coban† will apply pressure over scars, helping to flatten and improve their appearance (Fig. 24-16, *B*). Elastomer can be used in conjunction with splinting as is often done for scar management following Dupuytren's release.

---

*Elastomer, WFR/Aquaplast Corporation, Wyckoffi, NJ.
†Coban, Medical Products Division, Minnesota Mining & Manufacturing Co., St. Paul.

Therapeutic exercise

Passive range-of-motion exercises. Passive range-of-motion exercises are helpful before one begins active motion. In order for the effects of passive range-of-motion exercises to be of lasting benefit, they should be done for a prolonged period of time with a low to moderate amount of tension.[3,5,6,8] Sapega and coworkers have proposed that stretching be combined with a rise in tissue temperature. In vitro studies suggest that a prolonged stretch, accompanied by an elevated tissue temperature, assists lengthening of connective tissue.[9] The therapist can incorporate the principle of combining heat and stretch to a stiff hand in the following way. Using an elasticized tape, such as Coban, apply a stretch to the involved finger or fingers in the direction in which you wish to increase motion. Once the

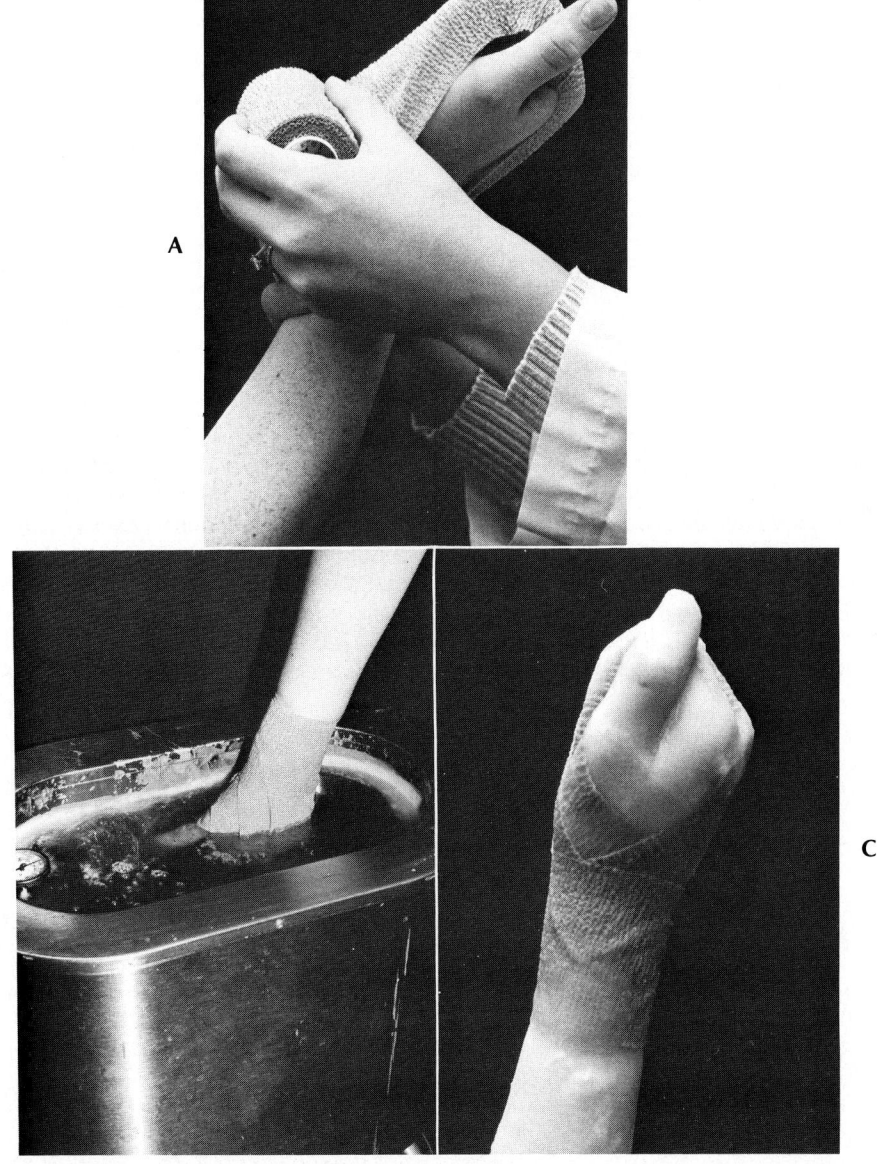

Fig. 24-17   **A,** Elasticized tape is used to gently stretch the fingers into flexion. **B** and **C,** Hand is then dipped in paraffin and placed in elevation under a hot pack for 30 minutes.

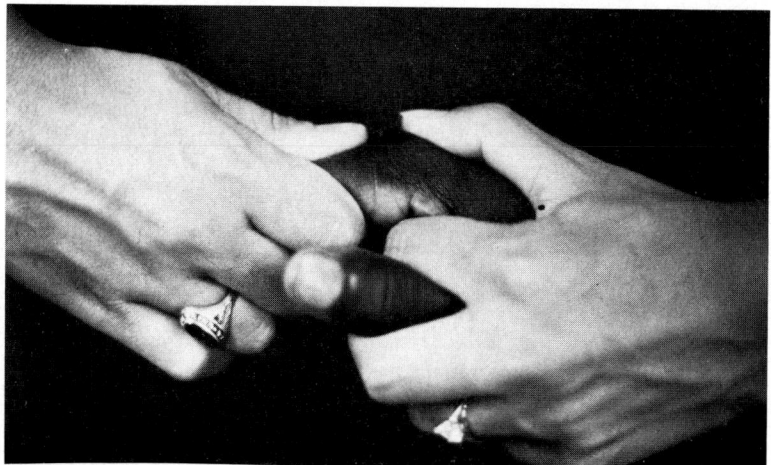

Fig. 24-18 To perform passive range-of-motion exercises, gently distract the joint being mobilized before flexing or extending it.

hand is stretched with the tape, dip it in paraffin, and place it under a hot pack for approximately 30 minutes (Fig. 24-17). Caution must be taken when applying heat to areas with decreased sensibility or poor skin quality. Active exercise should be done immediately after this procedure.

As an adjunct to prolonged stretch, manual passive range-of-motion exercises can be performed. To administer passive range-of-motion exercises, ask the patient to relax his hand, and place both of your hands close to the axis of the joint being mobilized. Gently distract the joints to avoid compression of the segments being mobilized, and move the joint in the direction desired (Fig. 24-18) until a slight resistance is felt; hold the joint in that position of stretch for several seconds, and then relax the joint and repeat. During the performance of passive range-of-motion exercises, it is important to teach the patient to distinguish between the sensation of pain and the sensation of stretch. Forceful manipulations are always contraindicated because they result in pain and swelling around the involved joints.

Active range-of-motion exercises. The patient's active exercise program includes motion of all joints of the involved extremity, because uninvolved joints quickly become stiff after trauma to the hand. The following exercises can be included:

1. Tendon gliding[10]
2. Blocking of the DIP and PIP joints of each finger to encourage isolated motion of the flexor digitorum profundus (Fig. 24-19).
3. Isolated motion of flexor digitorum superficialis
4. Extension, abduction, and adduction of the fingers
5. Opposition, abduction, flexion, and extension of the thumb
6. Wrist flexion and extension and ulnar and radial deviation
7. Pronation and supination of the forearm

When one is instructing patients in active range-of-motion exercises, they must be taught to perform the correct pattern of motion. For example, excessive attempts at finger flexion often result in simultaneous wrist flexion. To correct this problem, the patient is instructed to hold his wrist in slight extension when performing finger flexion. If the patient is unable to support voluntarily his wrist with finger flexion, an external wrist support is used for exercise until finger flexion is strengthened. Also, if the goal of exercise is to

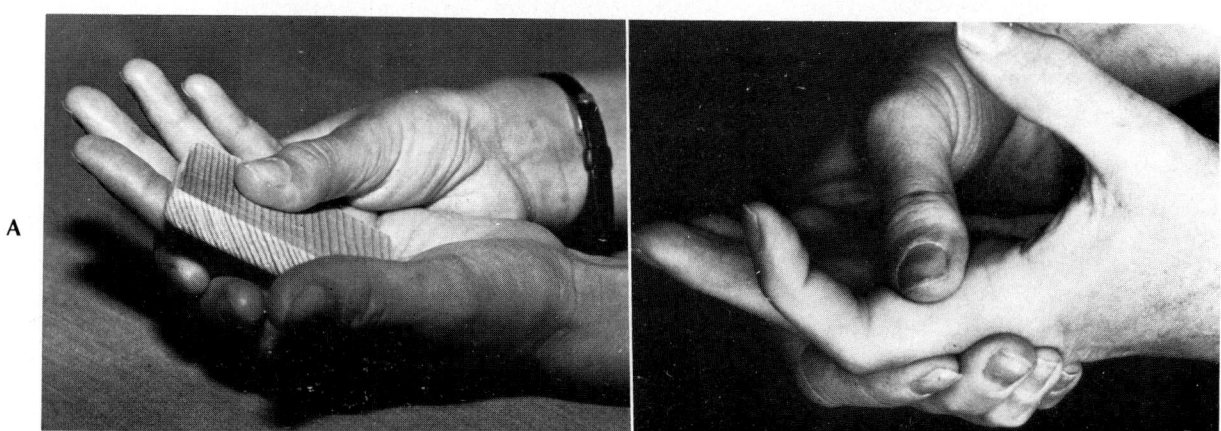

A

B

Fig. 24-19 A wood block (**A**) or finger block (**B**) is used to facilitate isolated pull-through of the long flexor tendons.

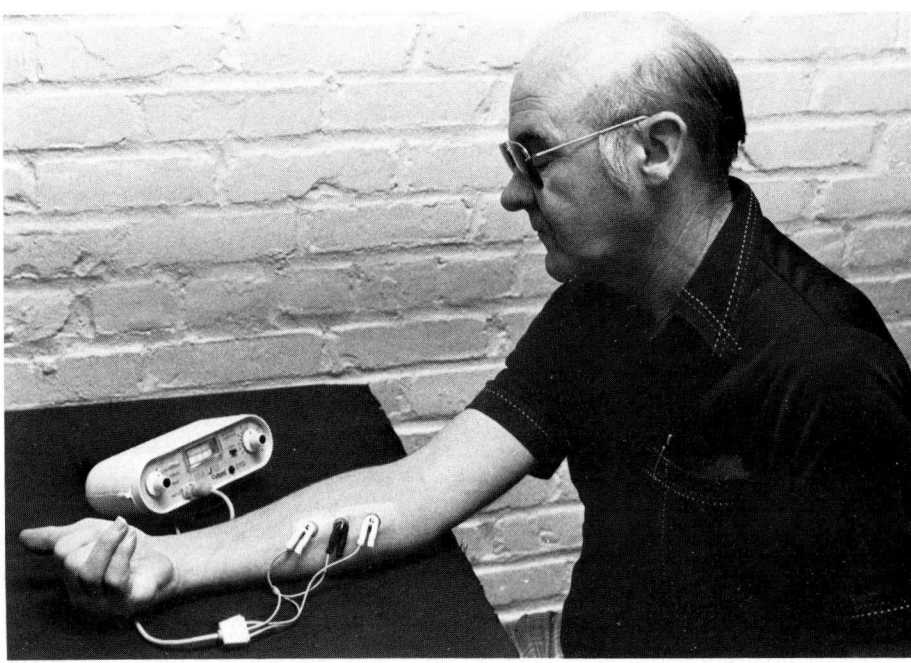

Fig. 24-20 Biofeedback is used to help prevent co-contraction during exercise sessions.

improve active motion of the long flexors, the patient must be taught to support the metacarpophalangeal joint in extension while flexing the distal joints, thereby eliminating the action of the intrinsic muscles.

It should be stressed to the patient that the correct motion is more important than the strength of motion. Often a patient will try so hard to perform a motion that he will co-contract the agonist and antagonistic muscles. The patient is taught to prevent co-contraction by relaxing the opposing muscles. Biofeedback can be used for this purpose by placing three surface electrodes on the opposing muscles and setting the machine to pick up the unwanted muscle activity. If the patient co-contracts his muscles, the machine will give off an auditory signal telling the patient he has performed the motion incorrectly (Fig. 24-20). Patients using biofeedback can work independently on their exercise programs.

Resistive exercises. For patients who have little or no pull-through of the flexor or extensor tendons because of adhesions or weakness, resistive exercises must be initiated immediately. Graded resistive activities progressing from a foam squeeze, putty, or the Hand Helper to progressive resistive weights, ceramics, woodworking, and the BTE Work Simulator* are some of the many activities selected to help increase strength of the hand.

Therapeutic activities. Therapeutic activities are used to help increase active motion, strength, and endurance of a chronically stiff hand. They are an integral part of the therapy program, since they encourage patients to again consider their hands as functional and working parts of their bodies. When a patient's dominant hand is injured, he is encouraged to write, dress, and eat with it, even if it requires the use

of a piece of adaptive equipment such as a built-up handle. Activities such as macramé and light pickups are used for patients who are not ready for heavy resistance. These activities can be done in elevation in the case of a swollen hand. Leatherwork and ceramics provide active motion and moderate resistance to a stiff hand, whereas woodworking and woodcarving are used to provide heavy resistance. It is important when the patient is performing his activities that the handle on the working tools be built up to the point where the fingers are able to maintain a sustained grip around them (Fig. 24-21). The patient's endurance for whatever activity he is performing is increased daily if the therapist has him perform the activity for longer periods of time each day.

Splinting. Dynamic splinting is the most effective modality that can be used to apply a low-to-moderate amount of tension to a stiff joint over a prolonged period of time. If evaluation reveals that limitation in the range of motion is strictly related to soft-tissue contracture around a particular joint, a splint must be designed to apply traction to that specific joint. Fig. 24-22 shows an example of a splint that is being used to apply passive flexion to a proximal interphalangeal joint stiff in extension. When evaluation reveals that restrictions in active range of motion are attributable to a combination of joint contracture and muscle tightness, a two-stage splinting program is required. Initially a splint is designed to increase the passive range of motion of the involved joint. Once this has been achieved, the splinting program is directed at providing a stretch to the involved intrinsic or extrinsic musculature. In the following chapter, Colditz provides a full review of the principles and methods of splinting the stiff hand.

"Quick splints" are named for the fact that they can be quickly and inexpensively fabricated. Situations may arise in which one or both of these factors necessitates the use

---

*Work Simulator, available from Baltimore Therapeutic Equipment, Baltimore.

of a quick splint. It is important to remember that they are not the answer to every splinting problem. The following are descriptions of the more commonly used quick splints.

1. Web strap. The web strap (Fig. 24-23) provides a passive stretch necessary to improve the range of motion from the finger pulp to the palmar crease. It is most effective in gaining the final degrees of proximal interphalangeal flexion. This strap is worn over the proximal interphalangeal joint and behind the metacarpophalangeal joint. The strap is fabricated from a 1-inch-wide lamb wick and a 1-inch-wide buckle.

2. Combination web strap. The combination web strap (Fig. 24-24) is effective when all joints of one or two fingers are stiff in extension. It is comfortable and

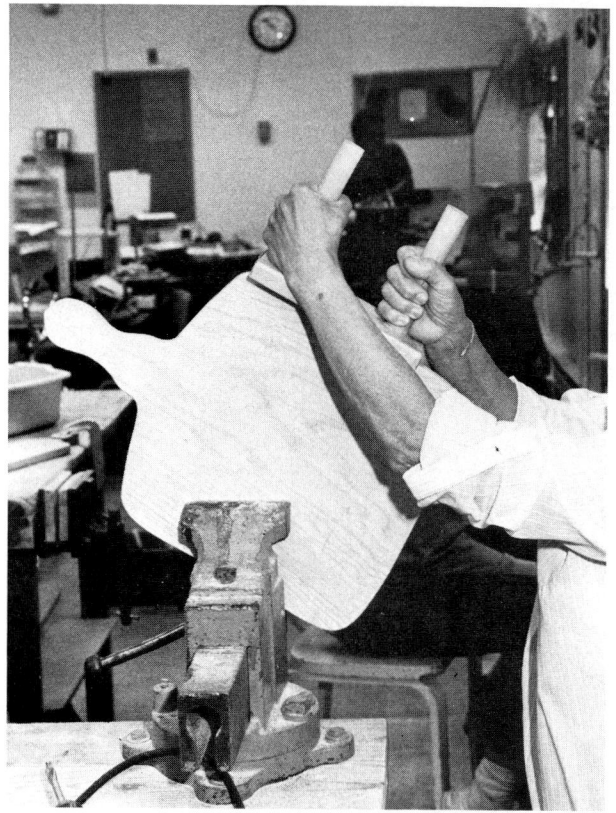

Fig. 24-21 Sustained-grip activities, such as wood sanding, are used to strengthen weakened muscles in the stiff hand.

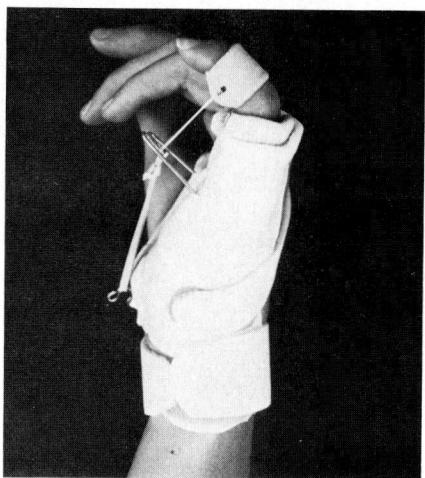

Fig. 24-22 A dynamic, hand-based splint is used to improve flexion of the PIP joint.

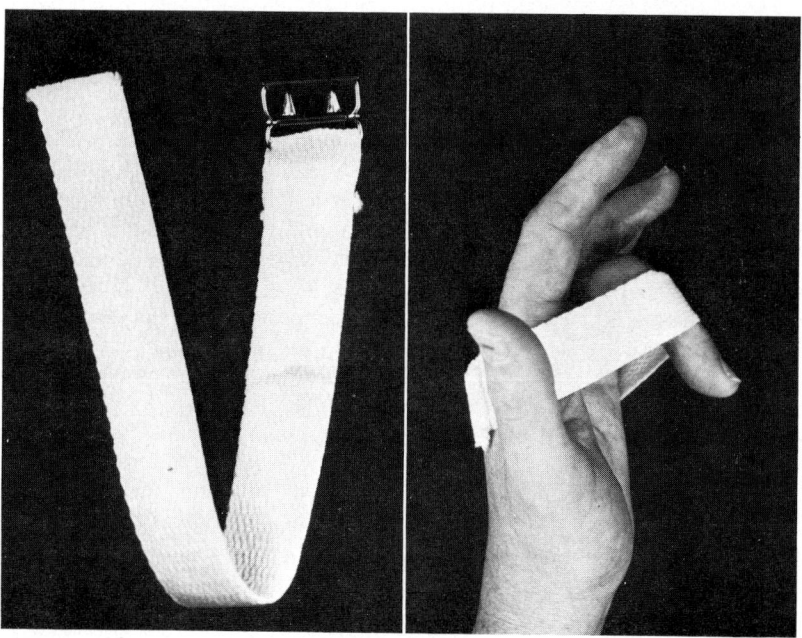

Fig. 24-23 The web strap is used to improve passive range-of-motion of the PIP joint.

easily adjusted and can be worn as a night splint. One should keep in mind that the combination web strap will be most effective on the joints that are least restricted. The combination web strap is not effective in gaining the final degrees of PIP or DIP joint motion. The materials necessary to construct the combination web strap are a Velcro* hook and loop and a 1-inch-wide D ring.

---

*Velcro USA, Inc., New York, NY.

3. Elastic flexion strap. The elastic flexion strap (Fig. 24-25) is used to obtain primarily DIP motion and, to a lesser extent, PIP motion of a stiff finger. The elastic flexion strap is worn over the DIP and PIP joints. To construct the strap, a piece of elastic with a width of three fourths of an inch and a length of 4 inches is fitted around the patient's interphalangeal joints while they are held in maximum flexion. A mark is made on the elastic at the point where the two ends of the elastic meet on the proximal phalanx, and the elastic

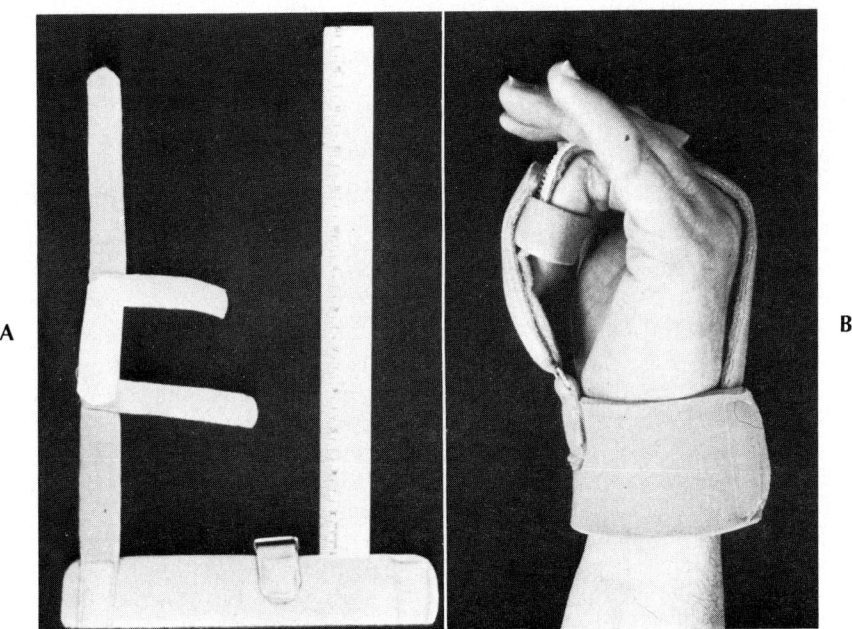

Fig. 24-24   **A,** Combination web strap. **B,** This strap is used when all joints of one or two fingers are stiff in extension, but it exerts its force most effectively at the least stiff joint.

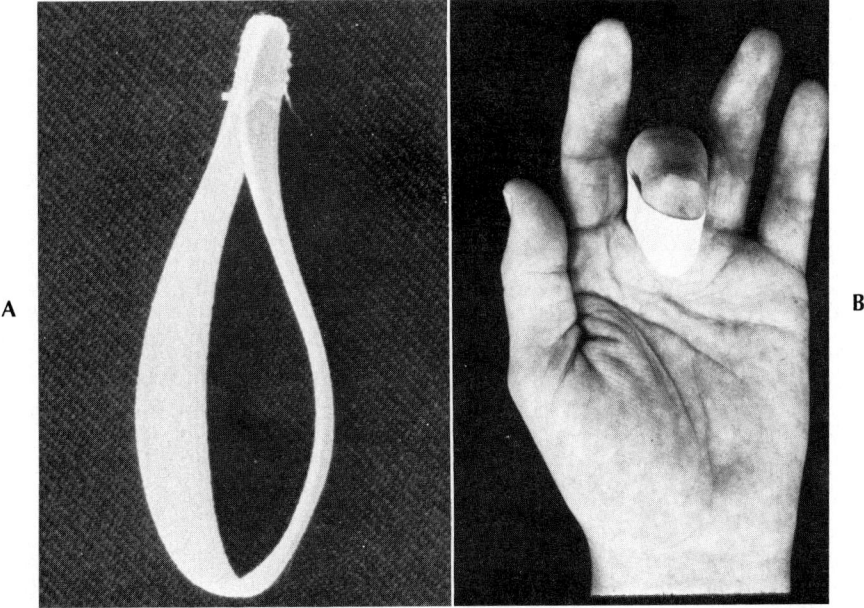

Fig. 24-25   To improve passive range of motion of the DIP joint, an elastic strap is worn periodically during the day over the interphalangeal joints.

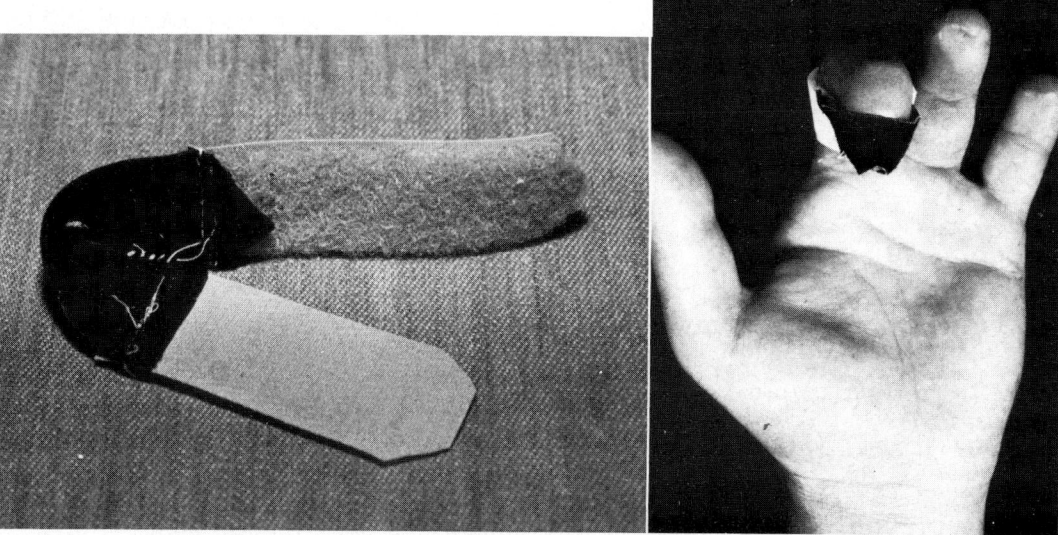

Fig. 24-26 The elastic strap is replaced at night with an adjustable DIP flexion strap, fabricated from leather and Velcro, to maintain gains made during the day.

is sewn together on that mark. At night, the elastic strap is replaced by a retaining splint that is similar in design to the elastic strap but, because its tension can be adjusted, is more comfortable to wear during sleep (Fig. 24-26).

Patient education. Restoration of hand function to a chronically stiff hand is strongly dependent on the patient's level of motivation. Therapeutic exercises and activities must be performed consistently at home. The patient must understand that any splint that has been prescribed will only be effective if it is worn for a long period of time with a low-to-moderate amount of tension. The home program should be written and reviewed at each therapy session.

Ongoing evaluation. Evaluation is an integral part of the treatment program. Ongoing evaluations assist the therapist in determining when changes in the treatment program are necessary and provide information regarding when the patient has plateaued in his therapy program. When the patient's progress has plateaued for a significant period of time, the surgeon must then determine if the patient has achieved maximum function or if surgical intervention is indicated. Surgical procedures that might be performed on a stiff hand include tenolysis, joint capsulectomies, and joint arthroplasties.

CASE STUDY: THE CHRONICALLY STIFF HAND

The following case study demonstrates the principles of treating the chronically stiff hand. The patient is a 46-year-old, right-handed housewife who injured her left shoulder in a fall 1 year before referral to the Hand Rehabilitation Center in Philadelphia. The patient initially sustained a tear to her rotator cuff muscles and underwent surgical repair 3 months after injury. The patient's shoulder was immobilized for 6 weeks, and she reported that during that time she developed severe swelling and limitation in the range of motion of her hand. The patient attended therapy at a local hospital for 6 months and stated that she received painful therapy to her shoulder and hand. The patient was referred

to the Hand Therapy Department at the Hand Rehabilitation Center 1 year after injury for rehabilitation of her left upper extremity. Evaluation revealed a painful, sensitive extremity with severe limitations in hand and shoulder range of motion and strength. Intrinsic muscle tightness and mild extrinsic extensor tightness were noted. The patient reported that she was only able to use her hand to assist in light activities of daily living.

Most of the first treatment session was used to help establish a trusting relationship. Once the patient realized that the philosophy of treatment stressed nonpainful therapy, she became more willing to participate actively in the program.

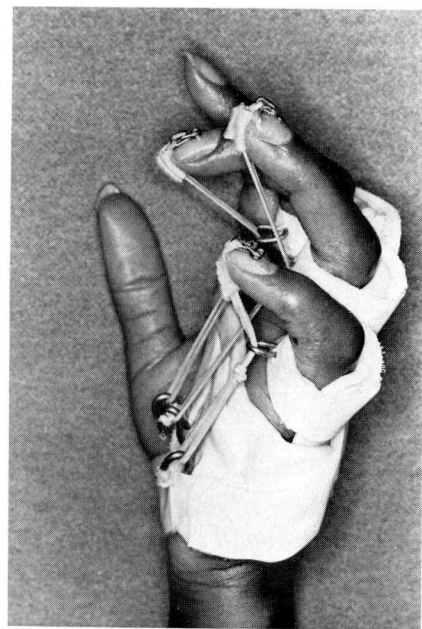

Fig. 24-27 An intrinsic stretching splint positions the MP joints in extension while flexing the interphalangeal joints.

The patient was given an Isotoner glove to help alleviate the internal pressure from brawny edema that she felt in her hand. She was instructed in desensitization techniques and contrast baths to help decrease the pain and sensitivity of her arm. Before exercise, the patient's hand was wrapped in an elasticized tape, pulling her fingers into flexion. The patient's hand was then dipped in paraffin and placed under a hot pack to retain the heat for a period of 30 minutes. Active and guarded passive range-of-motion exercises of all joints of the extremity were encouraged through the use of specific exercises and therapeutic activities. The patient was begun on macramé and light pick-ups to help increase shoulder and hand range of motion. In 1 month she progressed to a resistive weight program, woodworking, and the potter's wheel for strength and endurance.

A splinting program was initiated at the patient's second visit. Because the patient had severe intrinsic tightness, a splint was fabricated to stretch the intrinsics by holding the metacarpophalangeal joints in extension and applying moderate tension that pulled the PIP and DIP joints into flexion (Fig. 24-27). A timetable for a home program of exercise, functional use, and splinting was discussed with the patient and designed to fit her individual needs.

This patient attended therapy three times weekly for half-day sessions for a total of 6 months. At that time, the patient had regained the full range of motion of her hand. Shoulder range of motion, though occasionally painful, had improved significantly and was within functional limits. Grip strength of the involved hand, measured by the Jamar dynamometer, was 80% of that of the uninvolved hand.

SUMMARY

A patient with an acutely swollen, stiff hand who receives the proper treatment immediately after injury will not require long-term care. Once edema and pain have stabilized and active range of motion has been restored, the patient should be able to resume his normal activities. An acutely stiff hand, left untreated, will progress to a chronically stiff hand, with serious loss of hand function. Treatment of the chronically stiff hand may be long-term and will require innovative problem solving by the therapist. Evaluation techniques and treatment guidelines described in this chapter are intended to aid the therapist in designing a treatment program that fits the individual needs of each patient.

REFERENCES

1. American Academy of Orthopedic Surgeons: Joint motion, Chicago, 1965, The Academy.
2. American Society for Surgery of the Hand: The hand: examination and diagnosis, Aurora, Colo, 1978, The Society.
3. Becker AH: Traction for knee-flexion contractures, Phys Ther 59:1114, 1979.
4. Brand PW and Wood H: Hand volumeter instruction sheet, United States Public Health Service Hospital, Carville, La.
5. Glazer RM: Rehabilitation. In Happenstal RB, editor: Fracture treatment in healing, Philadelphia, 1980, WB Saunders Co.
6. Jackman RV: Device to stretch the achilles tendon, J Am Phys Ther Assoc 43:729, 1963.
7. Jebson RH and others: An objective and standardized test of hand function, Arch Phys Med Rehabil 50:311, 1969.
8. Kottke FJ, Pauley DL, and Ptak KA: The rationale for prolonged stretching for correction of shortening of connective tissue, Arch Phys Med Rehabil 47:345, 1966.
9. Sapega AA and others: Physiological factors in range-of-motion exercise, Phys Sports Med G:57, 1981.
10. Wehbé MA: Tendon gliding exercises, Occup Ther 41(3):164, 1987.

BIBLIOGRAPHY

Beasley RW: Hand injuries, Philadelphia, 1981, WB Saunders Co.
Curtis RM: Joints of the hand. In Flynn JE, editor: Hand surgery, ed 2, Baltimore, 1975, Williams Wilkins.
Harrison DH: The stiff proximal interphalangeal joint, Hand 9(2):102, 1977.
Peacock EE Jr: Preservation of interphalangeal joint function: a basis for the early care of injured hands, South Med J 56:56, 1962.
Peacock EE Jr: Some biochemical and biophysical aspects of joint stiffness: role of collagen synthesis as opposed to ultra-molecular binding, Ann Surg 164:1, 1966.
Pratt DR: Joints of the hand and fingers—their stiffness, splinting and surgery, Calif Med 66:22, 1947.

25

Dynamic splinting of the stiff hand

Judy C. Colditz

SPLINTING RATIONALE
Physiology of stiffness

Dynamic splinting of the injured hand is well accepted as a treatment modality in hand rehabilitation.* The unavoidable response to injury of edema production within the finely balanced tissues of the hand often demands a modality beyond pure active motion to regain the balance of motion. To understand the rationale of dynamic splinting, one must understand the physiology of stiffness. No one has stated it better than Sterling Bunnell in 1946:

> Hands are particular in that they are prone to become stiffened—evidently because the joint surfaces are so accurately approximated, and there are more close fitting, gliding parts than elsewhere in the body. Joint ligaments are just long enough, but not too long. If, from any cause, a hand remains swollen and immobile, the serum-soaked ligaments become short and thick, binding the joints. From the fluid of oedema, fibrin settles between the movable tissues and within them—muscles, tendons, and joints alike. Fibroblasts invade; the whole becomes organized and shrinks; and the hand becomes congealed.[9]

This process may be seen most vividly in the crushed hand with multiple tissue injuries, but stiffness secondary to immobility and edema production may also be demonstrated in a hand with minor trauma that has been immobilized excessively. In either case the combination of edema and immobilization has altered the balance of motion. Thus

*References 3, 9-11, 14, 18, 21.

splinting to stretch the tightness and reestablish the balance is frequently an appropriate tool of the therapist.

Splinting frequently may be a replacement for surgery.[18,20] For what can be quickly altered by the scalpel can often be slowly altered by the stress applied by a splint. Surgery to regain motion reestablishes the vicious cycle of edema and pain and requires again a period of initial immobilization to promote wound healing. Gaining motion by dynamic splinting allows increasing strength and tissue glide while gaining motion and thus avoids the stimulation of edema production. One must emphasize that dynamic splinting is only part of a comprehensive rehabilitation of the hand.[19,23] The splint helps gain passive motion by the stress applied, but only active and active resistive motion can reestablish a balance of power and glide. Dynamic splinting imposes immobility on the hand, since only one direction of motion can be gained at a time. Periods out of the splint must allow for other motions.

Static versus dynamic splinting

Static splints are those supporting a joint or joints in one position. Dynamic splints move a joint through application of the prolonged force of elastic traction. Serial static splints, although providing only one position for a joint or joints, is changed frequently and always applied at the maximum range of the joint motion. Serial static splinting, changed frequently, can effect change in joint motion just as does the sustained force applied by elastic traction in dynamic splinting.

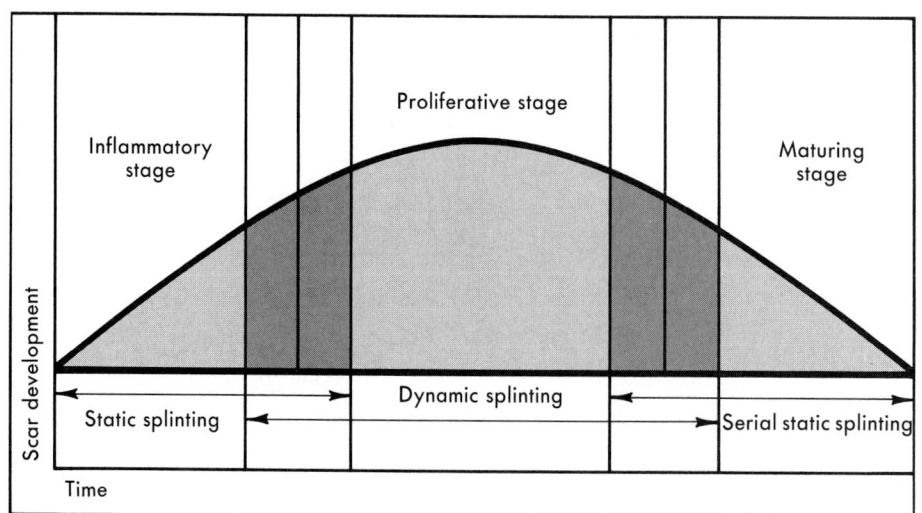

Fig. 25-1   Stages of scar maturation determine appropriate type of splinting.

342

The use of static, dynamic, or serial static splints is determined by the stage of tissue healing (Fig. 25-1).

Inflammatory stage. Healing tissue needs support and immobilization, and static splints are most useful in this stage. If early motion is desired, it is accomplished either during short periods of controlled exercise out of the splint or with a dynamic component that controls a specific motion while in the splint.

Static splinting is also preferred in the nerve-injured hand, because static splinting is the best biomechanical constraint for the hand imbalanced by loss of muscle power. (See Chapter 49.)

Proliferative stage. Dynamic splinting to gain motion is most appropriate to use during the proliferative stage of wound healing; as increased cellular activity occurs at the healing site, the gentle prolonged force of dynamic splinting influences the direction and alignment of collagen fibers. To be effective, dynamic splinting must not be applied until the inflammatory stage is subsiding so that the dynamic forces do not prolong the inflammatory response. If edema is still fluctuant, if joints continue to be red, or if joint motion creates edema and pain, static splinting should be continued with alternating periods of active motion, or one may be able to proceed with serial static splinting. The process of tissue healing and maturation proceeds at variable rates in individuals, and many persons demonstrate a prolonged inflammatory response.[5]

Dynamic splinting is clearly the technique of choice over serial static splinting when passive motion in the clinic is responsive to manual stretch and inflammation has subsided.[1,6-8,22] The great advantage of dynamic splinting is the ability to provide a specific force to specific tightness, be it joint tightness, tendon adhesions, skin tightness, muscle-tendon unit tightness, or any combination. Forces applied by a dynamic splint are translated easily to the loose joints of a paralyzed hand, but in the stiff hand they are directed specifically to the limiting structure.

Maturing scar. As scar tissue matures and the cells become more organized, the tissue resistance to the force applied by the dynamic splint increases. At times dynamic splinting can be effective in this stage, but the force must be such that the patient can wear the splint comfortably for the majority of the time. The best means to apply force to tight structures at this stage is through serial static splinting, which maintains a stretched position for prolonged periods of time, allowing the tissue to accommodate and "grow" to this new length.

Tissue response to splinting

The effectiveness of dynamic splinting is based on a sound physiologic theory: a long period of applied tension alters cell proliferation.[3,17,24,25] The tension must be of such low magnitude so as not to tear or force the tissues and thus stimulate the inflammatory response, causing more edema and then more fibrosis. It must be applied for a long enough period to alter the way in which new tissue is synthesized. This can be achieved by serial casting, in which a new tension is applied daily and the tissues accommodate to it, or by a dynamic splint, which accomplishes the same goal and can provide a constant tension over a longer period of time. It must be clear to the patient that the goal is not to tolerate increasing amounts of tension on the rubber band,

but rather to tolerate it for increasing periods of time. The hand may need an initial period of adjustment to the tension applied, but the time should slowly increase so that the patient is comfortable with the splint for hours at a time. The patient should be aware of a sensation of stretching, but it should not be painful.

Human tissue is viscoelastic; that is, it responds to the stress applied. The immediate response of the tissues is one of elasticity; tissue stretched will return to its original shape and length. Only with a period of prolonged stretch will one achieve a viscous or plastic response, in that the tissues now take on the shape to which they have been deformed by the force applied.[6] Thus it is the prolonged quality of the stretch that mobilizes stiffness. The analogy of a stretched rubber band is helpful when this phenomenon is described to patients: quickly stretch a rubber band and when you let it go it will return to its original length, but hold the rubber band stretched for a day and it will not contract to its original resting length and will then go the stretched distance with greater ease. This phenomenon is the principle of prolonged stretch, which mobilizes stiffness. Patients should report that the dynamic splint relieves a sense of tightness in the hand, which they are otherwise unable to affect, and they should demonstrate a certain eagerness about the splint in that wearing it relieves the internal tension. If this is not the case, the splint is ill fitting or the tension too great.

Like rubber, scar when inactive (cool) is tight and non-elastic. Heat (created by stretch or friction) allows it to become more elastic, and tension within the scar is decreased. This explains the phenomenon of morning stiffness, since the tissues have been immobile during sleep. For this reason, gentle prolonged stretch at night to produce motion in the direction with the greatest deficit is encouraged. After there has been a prolonged stretch at night, the plastic response (that is, changing shape) allows easier elastic response (that is, stretching the distance) during the day, and the potential for active motion is maximized. Extension splinting is generally more easily tolerated at night because flexion splinting may be somewhat constrictive. Therefore any flexion splinting at night needs to be of a lesser force than that applied during the day. This decreased force is true of all-night splinting, since distracting events during the day allow tension to be easily tolerated, but the lack of stimuli at night causes one to become much more aware of the stress. Additionally, during periods of rest and inactivity, the natural pumping assistance of active muscles is removed from the extremity, again clearly pointing up the need for a lesser tension so as not to constrict blood flow.

Because of the constant activity of cell multiplication and proliferation within a healing area, the use of a dynamic splint must be not only for long periods at a time but also over a long span of time. Many patients are encouraged by the rapid gains of motion from the fitting of a dynamic splint only to become discouraged when they remove the splint and the deformity recurs. When fitting a splint, one would be wise to instruct the patient that when he removes the splint for any long period he will be unable to retain what the splint has gained. It is only when he has worn the splint long enough to encourage cell proliferation in the direction and of the length needed that he can retain the motion without the splint. Explaining this at the time of splint fitting prevents the patient from being unnecessarily discouraged and increases compliance with the long-term need for splinting.

SPLINTMAKING
History

The art and science of splintmaking as we know it today is relatively new, but the word "splint" has its origin in the Middle Ages. Splints were the triangular parts of armor that allowed motion at the joints but offered protection from arrows and other missiles. Although the modern use of the word frequently refers to static immobilization, it is useful to remember that the original device allowed motion.

Many early devices for splintage of the upper extremity were reminiscent of armor design, undoubtedly fashioned by the village blacksmith. Although there are numerous isolated original splint designs published both before and after World War II, there is little written about the rationale for splinting except for the original work of Bunnell.[1,7,9,10] He was instrumental in organizing hand treatment centers within the United States military medical system and did much to document and standardize surgical treatment, immobilization, and rehabilitation techniques. Although the army had issued a manual on hand splints in 1917, it was Bunnell's chapter on splints in the *Orthopaedic Appliance Atlas* in 1952 that began the standardization of splint design.[1] In his first edition of *Surgery of the Hand* there is a chapter devoted to splints, splintmaking, and current materials.[10]

Many early splints had a somewhat homemade appearance, since there were no special materials available. Plaster of paris was often the material chosen for the splint base, since one could achieve a close-fitting mold with the hand. Ingenuity often replaced the sophisticated materials, and during World War II aluminum salvaged from wrecked airplanes was used, as were corset spring steel strips. Bunnell illustrates a splint with clock springs,[9] and Capener in England used window curtain springs.[13] The army hand centers frequently used brass wire as an outrigger incorporated into a plaster base, as described by Peacock.[21]

In many settings the orthotist made splints for hand patients, but the orthotist had no training in the therapy process. Construction time required for these permanent devices did not allow immediate fit. Fitting of the splint was a process removed from therapy. Adjustments of these permanent devices were then hardly encouraged. The metal and high-temperature plastics did not lend themselves to the intricate plasticity of the hand shape, and often these splints forced the hand into position rather than the hand dictating the splint needed. Capener described this problem well: "Surgical appliance making has been in the past and still is in the hands of the commercial craftsmen who have done a splendid work, yet who are often divorced from adequate medical guidance."[13]

In an attempt to standardize hand surgery and treatment many of Bunnell's original designs were made commercially available and still are widely used today. Unfortunately, the metal and felt used for commercial production did not offer a custom device. The era of polio influenced the thinking about upper extremity orthotics, and to standardize the language, splints were defined by the components in the splint system: lumbrical bar, C-bar, palmar bar, and so on. Un-

fortunately, the component system that effectively harnesses a hand with muscular imbalance has often become confused with the outrigger systems needed to stretch tight internal structures.

Advent of splinting materials

As hand surgery continued to establish itself as a specialty, it became clear that the fitting of the splint should be incorporated into the therapy treatment. A number of high-temperature plastics became available (Lucite, Nyloplex, Plexiglas, and Royalite), but these materials required such high temperatures to become workable that it required making a positive plaster mold from which to work. Thus construction time and easy adjustability remained a problem. These materials and the traditional plaster and metal did not encourage a timely response to a changing hand.

The advent of low-temperature materials designed specifically for splinting needs (such as Orthoplast, Polyform, K-splint, and Aquaplast) allowed dynamic splinting to become a more active part of hand therapy. Therapists now could quickly cut, mold, and finish even a complicated splint that was appropriate for use early in treatment and even with open wounds. With these new materials, alteration to accommodate increased motion, relieve a pressure area, or adjust tension could be immediate. The thermoplastic materials were responsive to the hand, instead of the hand being forced to respond to the material.

With the strong influence of commercial splints, the process of custom splinting of the hand has been poorly documented for indications, timing of applying splints, and design choices. It is now often the dilemma of the hand therapist to evaluate critically whether the time-saving fitting of a commercial splint or the application of a custom-made splint is the better treatment for the hand in question. Only as the hand therapist develops better skills at design and application of splints within the total framework of hand rehabilitation will this decision become clear.

READINESS FOR SPLINTING
Use of splint

The trained hand therapist must be thoroughly knowledgable about many treatment modalities to effect improvement in the injured hand. Dynamic splinting is only one of these. The use of the splint should complement the gains made during therapy visits. It not only prevents loss of motion because of contraction of the constantly tightening tissues, but it also can make passive gains beyond what is achieved during therapy. Therapy visits should concentrate on active pull-through and strengthening, thus reinforcing the passive gains made by the splint. Only very mild deformities, such as the slight proximal interphalangeal (PIP) joint flexion contracture resulting from a sprain of the collateral ligaments, respond to splinting without a strong complementary exercise program.

Edema control

The natural phenomenon of edema production is often the key to understanding the appropriate timing for splinting application.[19] The amount of edema produced varies depending on both the severity of the injury and the individual response the body makes to the injury. Because of these variations, there is no clear rule about the time to begin dynamic splinting after injury. Edema of the hand can be compared to the sausage skin stuffed full of sausage. Just as the sausage is difficult to bend, so are the joints of the hand until some of the "stuffing" is removed. Although the goal of early dynamic splinting is to prevent chronic stiffness, which requires more long-term treatment, the decision for application of the splint must be based on a state of good control of post injury edema and on the absence of gross fluctuations of the edema. Otherwise the constricting forces of the splint stimulate even more accumulation of edema in the hand. The dilemma of splinting for increased motion at the expense of aggravating edema is always the early problem. The acutely injured hand, with pitting edema, red swollen joints, and pain with motion, is a hand to be treated gently, elevated, and moved primarily with active motion between periods of rest in a static splint. At this stage the goal of edema and pain reduction far exceed any splinting goals. Any dynamic splint, no matter how well constructed, will by virtue of the force it is applying be a constrictive force to the already borderline circulatory and drainage status of the injured hand.

Tolerance to stretch

In addition to the hand demonstrating a reduction of edema, it is ready for dynamic splinting when there is a tolerance to both active motion and gentle prolonged passive stretch. Rarely is it appropriate to dynamically splint a stiff injured hand immediately out of the surgical dressing. A few days in therapy of gaining active pull-through, monitoring edema levels, and allowing the tissues to gain a tolerance to the stress of active and very gentle passive motion readies the hand to be very tolerant of a splinting program. Unfortunately, the few days of therapy may stretch into a longer period for those patients who demonstrate a hyperactive inflammatory response to injury.

In the evaluation of a hand for dynamic splinting it is helpful to gain a feel for the springiness of the tight tissues. Manual evaluation of the resistance within the tissues will indicate to the therapist whether splint gains will be rapid or long-term. A hand that responds well to a gentle passive stretch may not need the help of a splint, and a short period of active therapy may be appropriate before there is a final decision about splinting. On the contrary, a joint that has almost full range of motion but demonstrates significant resistance to stretch in the end ranges is an excellent candidate for splinting. It is the prolonged stretch at the end of the range that gives the patient full, easy joint motion. The more acutely one is able to apply the splint, the less the tension and the shorter the period of time the patient will need the splint. Patients seen late who have fibrotic stiffness often need months of splinting, and because the tissues are more organized, one must apply greater tension to effect reorganization of collagen. The longer the time between the injury and the splinting, generally the longer the patient will need to wear the splint.

Goniometric measurements

Accurate goniometric measurements are helpful in determining both the readiness for splinting and the indications for altering the splinting routine. Whenever full passive range of motion is not present, it is appropriate to consider splinting. However, if there is a large discrepancy between the active and passive range of motion, the emphasis should lie on active pull-through, with splinting being the secondary goal. If the active and passive range of motion is equal, concentration on the splinting program will allow passive gains to be made so that the potential for active motion is greater. The final result can only be as good as the passive potential.

One may also see early rapid improvements of joint motion with other clinical modalities, but one joint may plateau in its improvement, thus an indication of the appropriateness for splinting. Careful and frequent monitoring of goniometric measurements give precise direction for the splinting program.

PRINCIPLES OF SPLINTING
Positioning

Basic principles of splinting often refer to the "position of function"[9] which is slight wrist extension (usually 30 degrees) accompanied by metacarpophalangeal (MP) flexion and slight interphalangeal flexion and thumb abduction. It was not Bunnell's intent that this "position of function" be a rule for all splinting, but he advocated this as a position to be used during the period of initial immobilization and healing. The balance of motion could be maintained more easily than when the wrist was allowed to fall into a position of flexion creating the typical clawhand. Although it is good

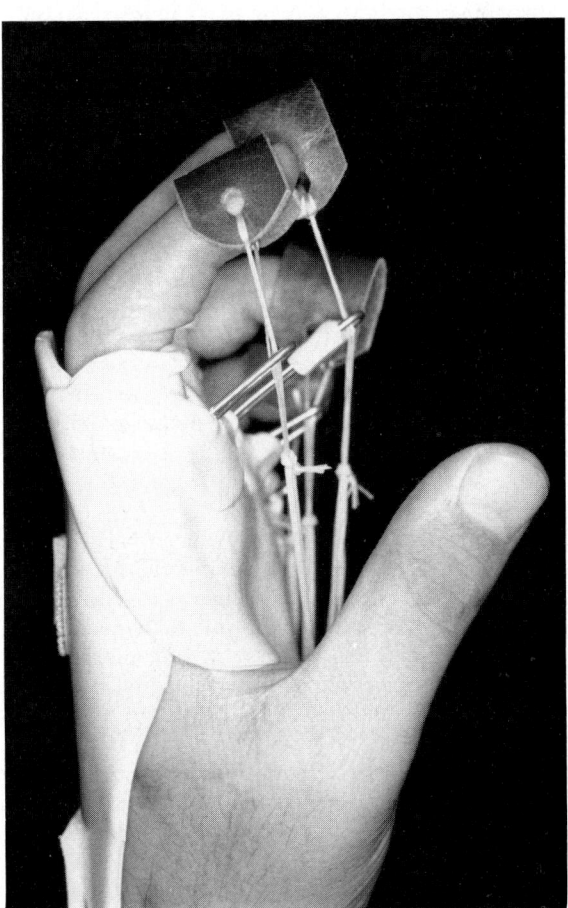

Fig. 25-2 Palmar bar is extended to stabilize metacarpophalangeal joint during dynamic flexion of the interphalangeal joints to stretch the intrinsic muscles.

to maintain this basic position whenever possible, the goal of dynamic splinting is to stretch the tight motions. This may mean that appropriately the wrist may need to be in flexion as when one flexes the fingers to stretch extrinsic extensor adherence proximal to the wrist or when one protects a newly repaired flexor tendon. Dynamic splints are not permanent devices but are intermittent, applying a specific force, and thus must position the hand as demanded by the specific tightness.[21]

Palmar bars are routinely designed to end proximally to the proximal palmar crease to allow full MP flexion. But if the goal of the splint is to gain PIP joint flexion with the MP joints stabilized, it may be appropriate to end the splint distally to the crease for better stability of the MP joint (Fig. 25-2). When blocking a proximal joint to stretch a more distal joint into flexion, one must stop the block well proximally to the skin creases, thus allowing for folding of the volar tissues.

This is only one example of the way in which dynamic splint designs may differ from basic principles of static splinting. Dynamic splints are supplying a specific force, and the splint must thus provide a specific good that outweighs the general constriction and immobility it demands.[4] Dynamic splints should be applied to effect the tightest structures, and this often demands an awkward position in the splint. The intermittent nature of the splinting allows these awkward positions to be tolerated, and the active therapy combines with the splinting program to regain the balance of motion.

Goal of dynamic splinting

A dynamic splint can only effectively achieve one motion at a time, although it may be able to achieve different motions on different fingers concurrently. For example, if one attempts concurrent flexion of the MP joints and extension of the interphalangeal joints, the effectiveness of the force will cancel itself. A splint may indeed be multipurpose in that one splint base can provide multiple outriggers so that joints can be stretched alternately in opposite directions or concurrently in the same direction. For example, one may continue to achieve a dynamic flexion force for MP tightness while stretching the interphalangeal joints into flexion, reducing extrinsic tightness (Fig. 25-3). The splint must be constructed with sound mechanical principles[3] to be effective.

Frequently one sees badly traumatized hands that have stiffness in multiple planes, and it is difficult to see priorities for the splinting needs. After a clinical assessment of the motion present it is reasonable to splint the motion that has the most resistance to passive stretch for this is the least likely motion to gain with only active and intermittent passive stretching. Additionally, it is helpful to remember the naturally weaker kinesiologic patterns of wrist extension, MP flexion, and interphalangeal extension, favoring these weaker motions. An example is the PIP joint, which lacks full flexion and extension. Because of the great mechanical advantage of the flexors arising from the ability to transmit power through the efficient pulley system, one expects the potential for gaining flexion to be greater than that for gaining extension through the inefficient and weaker extensor hood mechanism. One may begin a splinting program with this as a baseline approach, but the constantly changing

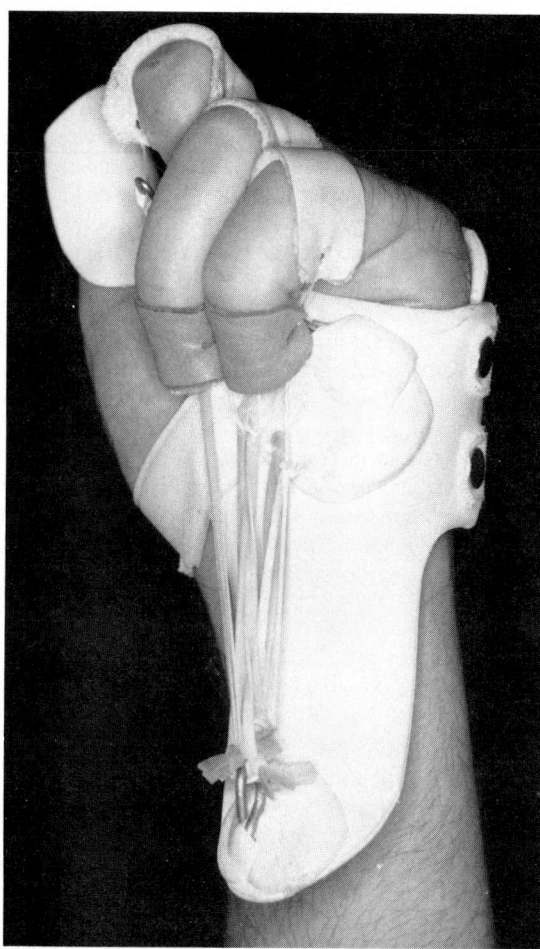

Fig. 25-3 Use of concurrent forces stretches both metacarpophalangeal joints and interphalangeal joints, thus effectively reducing metacarpophalangeal joint tightness and extrinsic extensor tightness.

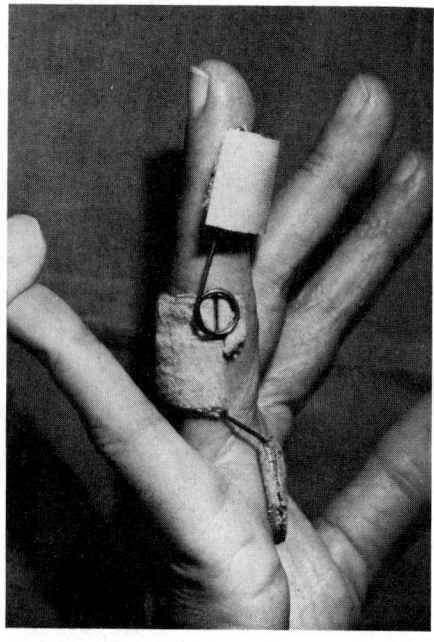

Fig. 25-4 Spring-wire splint (Capener design) for isolated tightness of proximal interphalangeal joint.

balance of motion may indicate a change of splinting priorities.

Evaluation for splinting

Proper splinting demands that the splint objective be based on the specific evaluation of impaired function.[12] Being able to determine whether there is a need for changing (1) skin tightness, (2) joint tightness, (3) tendon adherence, or (4) muscle-tendon unit tightness is of basic importance. Frequently the splint must be adapted for a combination of these problems.

One may determine skin tightness by applying a stretch to the area and observing blanching or palpable tightness of the scar line or skin graft and local immobility of the tissue bed. When the skin is placed in its shortest length, it should allow increased joint motion proximally or distally. This range of joint motion is diminished as the proximal joint is positioned so as to place a stretch on the skin. Any splinting program to stretch a tight scar or shortened skin must also position the joints at the proximal and distal ends of the tightness to allow elongation of the tissue. It is not the scar that is stretched so much as it is the normal skin at the end of the scar that accommodates to the stress of the stretched position. Unlike the other areas discussed below where tightness can frequently be best stretched by dynamic forces, pure skin tightness is best altered by a static splint that holds the skin at maximum length as it simultaneously provides direct positive pressure to the scar.

One best evaluates joint tightness by determining the easy passive range of the joint and then evaluating if this passive range changes as proximal and distal joint positions are changed. If the range of the joint motion does not change, there is isolated joint tightness, indicating the appropriateness of a splint that goes only proximally and distally to that specific joint (Fig. 25-4). In dynamic splinting one wishes to immobilize only the minimum number of joints possible.

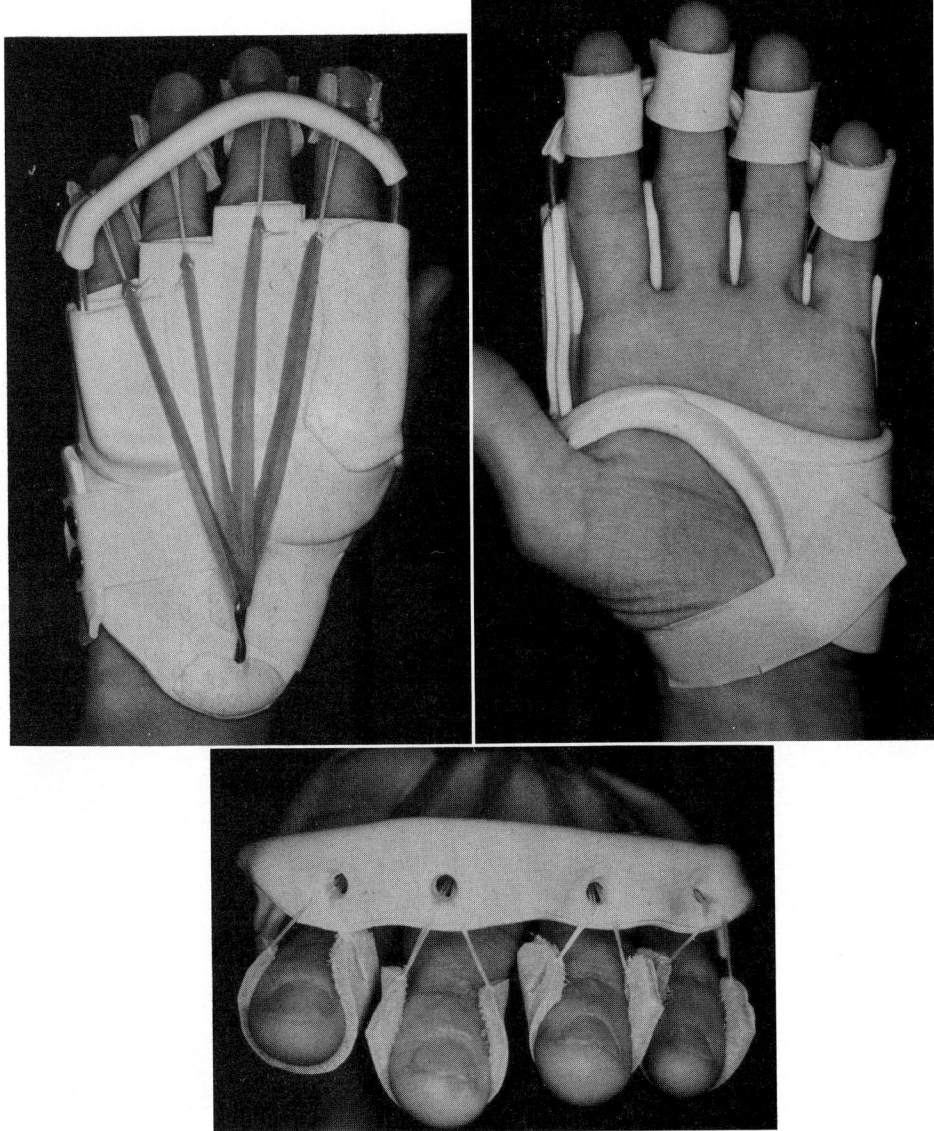

Fig. 25-5   Splint to stretch interphalangeal joints into extension without immobilization of wrist.

Tendon adherence and muscle-tendon unit tightness are both demonstrated by a distinct difference in the ease of distal joint motion when the proximal joints are positioned in either flexion or extension. Adherence may be present anywhere along the course of the muscle-tendon unit where there has been direct trauma, and therefore a difference in tightness is seen only distally to this point, requiring a splint only from this point distally. A good example is a flexor tendon lacerated within the middle portion of the flexor tendon sheath. If it is adherent within this sheath, limiting extension, the splint needs to come only proximally to the MP joint and not proximally to the wrist (Fig. 25-5). This can be proved by positioning the wrist in flexion and extension and demonstrating that there is no difference of the tightness within the finger.

When evaluating muscle-tendon unit tightness (which may or may not have an element of tendon adherence), one must evaluate the tightness of the unit from origin to insertion. The most proximal joint crossed by the unit is the key in determining tightness. With tightness of the extrinsic extensors the fingers will be unable to flex as far with the wrist in flexion as with the wrist in extension. Therefore a splint to stretch this tightness must include the wrist and position it in flexion. The opposite is true of extrinsic flexors in that with wrist extension finger extension is limited by the shortness of the unit, but when the wrist is dropped, the fingers can extend. To achieve an effective stretch to the extrinsic flexors, the wrist must be held in extension by the splint while the fingers are being dynamically extended (Fig. 25-6). The same principle holds true for the intrinsics of the hand, with the position of the MP joint being the key for determining tightness. Since the intrinsic tendons run volarly to the axis of the MP joint and dorsally to the axis of the PIP joint, the maximum stretch of this muscle-tendon unit occurs when the MP joints are held in maximum extension and the interphalangeal joints are flexed. If the range of interphalangeal joint flexion is less and demonstrably tighter when the MP joint is held in extension, the intrinsic muscles are tight. A splint to stretch this tightness thus need not include the wrist (see Fig. 25-2).

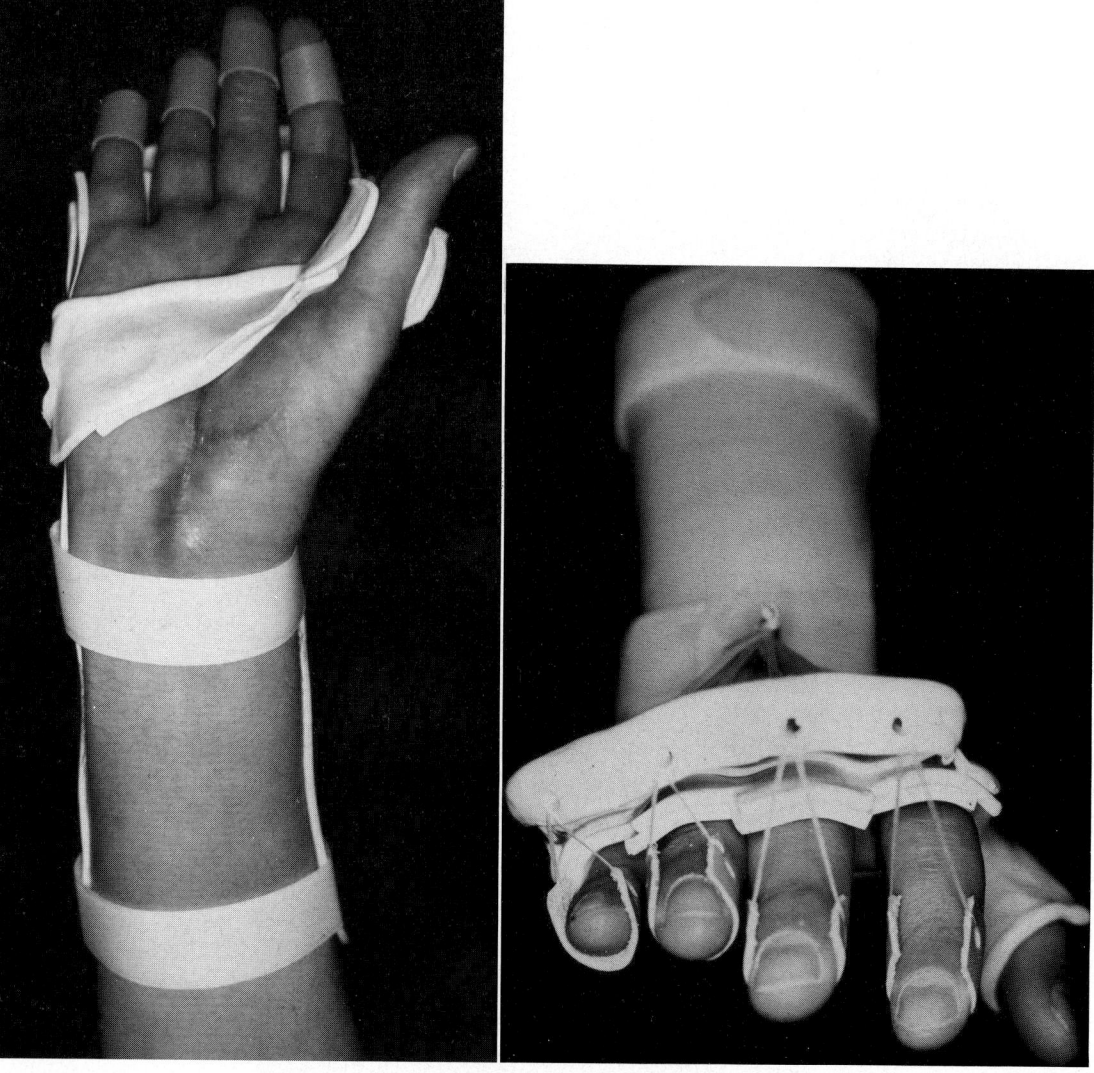

Fig. 25-6 Dynamic splint that positions wrist in extension while extending fingers to stretch adherence of flexor tendons proximal to wrist.

PRINCIPLES OF DESIGN
Analysis of forces

Analyzing the deficit in an injured hand and translating that need into a splint design is a critical skill for any hand therapist. Each and every splint should be approached as a unique device, and even though the splints will often fall into standard groups, it is a pitfall of the insecure therapist to try to fit the hand into a type of splint rather than design the splint totally based on the clinical evaluation of the hand. One of the easiest ways to determine a splint design is to simply hold the patient's hand and apply a passive stretch to the tight area. Analyze the specific joint positions and the points where the therapist's hands are applying stabilizing pressure and where they are applying stretching pressure. Translation of these forces into the splint design is the goal.

The hand is a three-dimensional structure, and frequently it is difficult for the therapist to position the hand on paper, mark the landmarks, and then draw a shape that will translate into a three-dimensional shape. Taking care and time to achieve a good basic splint pattern provides a specific, well-fitted device and saves material usage. Since one is applying a force with a dynamic splint, it is a basic requirement that the splint base be well designed so that it provides a stable base for attachment of outriggers. Force applied to a stiff joint will easily be transmitted to a poorly stabilized proximal joint with normal flexibility. Heating the splinting material so that it drapes to the true shape of the hand and paying attention that the splint achieves total contact are also basic requirements. No other aspect of hand therapy so well combines the elements of art and science as does splintmaking. Just as one can learn to be a skilled dressmaker by studying sewing principles, one can become an effective splintmaker by studying mechanical principles.

Effectiveness of splinting

Making a splint a comfortable device is of paramount importance if the splint is to be effective.[15] All details must be attended to, and pressure must be distributed over as large an area as possible. Listen to the patient; some minor detail may be the limiting factor for comfort, and the patient can easily point out what changes are needed. Making a device as streamlined as possible so as to interfere minimally with daily function and devising the splint so that it is easy to apply and remove aid in the patient's integration of the splint into a home therapy routine.[1,21]

As previously described, the usefulness of splinting is based on a prolonged stretch of the tissues. Rubber bands have long been the accepted means of applying this force.[11,21] The use of springs are now advocated by many because of their consistency of force. Although therapists have begun to measure the amount of force applied by dynamic splints, there is still no proved rationale for any specific amount of tension. Weeks and Wray describe the present problem well: ". . . we do not know the optimal amount of stress, the optimal length of time of application of stress, or the optimal method of application to bring about the most rapid favorable modification of scar tissue."[23] Brand agrees that we do not know how much force is needed to lengthen specific tissues and clarifies for us that the critical question is not the amount of force we are applying but rather the pressure exerted on the skin where we are applying

the force and this often becomes the limiting factor.[3] Although one can measure how much pressure can be tolerated before skin necrosis occurs, this is only indirectly of value, since dynamic splints allow motion and the force can be applied on an intermittent basis. Brand states that the pressure becomes relatively unimportant in the presence of intermittent application.[3,4]

Therapists should measure the amount of force applied to standardize their approach, but at the present time clinical observation is the only guideline to determine appropriate tension. Effort should be directed toward providing as consistent force as possible, either with rubber bands stretched for a long distance or spring coils.

A well-made splint that effectively stretches a tight area should not be painful. The patient may be aware of a pulling sensation, but he can clearly distinguish between the pull and a painful sensation. Tearing of fibrotic adhesions is not the goal. Patients often exhibit an eagerness about their dynamic splint in that it relieves a sensation of tightness they cannot otherwise effect. Rather than prescribing a specific hourly routine for splinting, instruct the patient to remove the splint when it reaches maximum tolerance. This period may be realistically short as one starts the splinting program, but if the patient cannot quickly increase splinting tolerance to 1 or 2 hours, the tension should be decreased.

Make it clear to the patient that the goal is to be able to tolerate the splint for longer periods of time and not at increasing tensions. If a patient cannot increase the splinting time, it is the result of a splint being ill fitted, applied too early or exerting too great a force.

To achieve increased motion, one must execute a good design and be keenly aware of the need for constant monitoring of the splint. The patient must understand the specific goals of the splint and should see splint changes as a reflection of improvement. Since the goal is to provide a 90-degree angle pull, the line of pull must be adjusted frequently to maintain the correct directional pull as the joint motion increases. Reminding patients to bring their splint to each therapy session encourages ease of adjustment. A good approach is to begin the therapy session frequently with a trying on of the splint, asking the patient if any area is uncomfortable, how long it can be worn continuously, and if he feels any adjustments would be helpful to increase tolerance.

CLINICAL APPLICATION
Design choice

The variety of splint designs is as limitless as human imagination. Simplicity of design and effective material utilization is of vital importance. In observing the normal hand one is able to use the normal kinesiologic and anatomic parameters as guidelines for splinting designs to approach specific tightness. Barr states: "It must be emphasized that the design of any sort of splint stems from the patient's own problems and has no other valid identity."[2]

In effecting joint motion it is the goal of the splint to provide a line of pull at a 90-degree angle to the axis of the long bone of the joint in question (Fig. 25-7).[14] It is of utmost importance that the splint be designed so that this 90-degree line of pull is achieved and easily maintained. Application of the force at the end of the bone (that is, maximum length of lever arm) allows efficiency for the

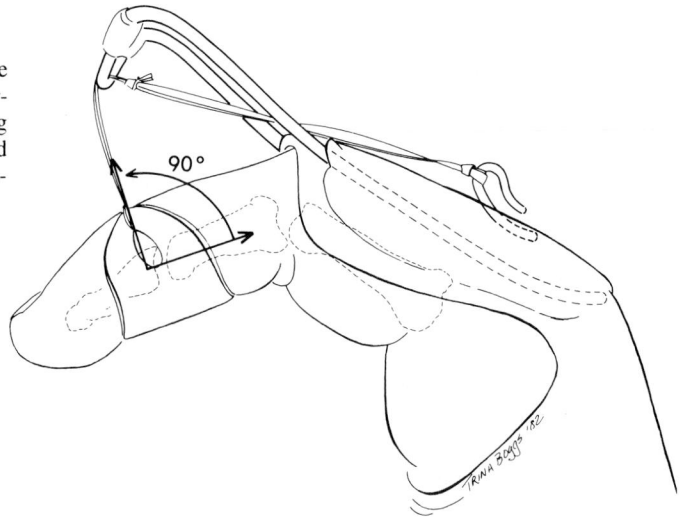

Fig. 25-7 Low-profile dynamic splint provides a 90-degree line of pull to distal end of middle phalanx to extend proximal interphalangeal joint. (From Colditz JC: Low profile dynamic splinting to the injured hand. Am J Occup Ther 37:182, 1983. Reprinted with the permission of the American Occupational Therapy Association, Inc. Copyright 1983.)

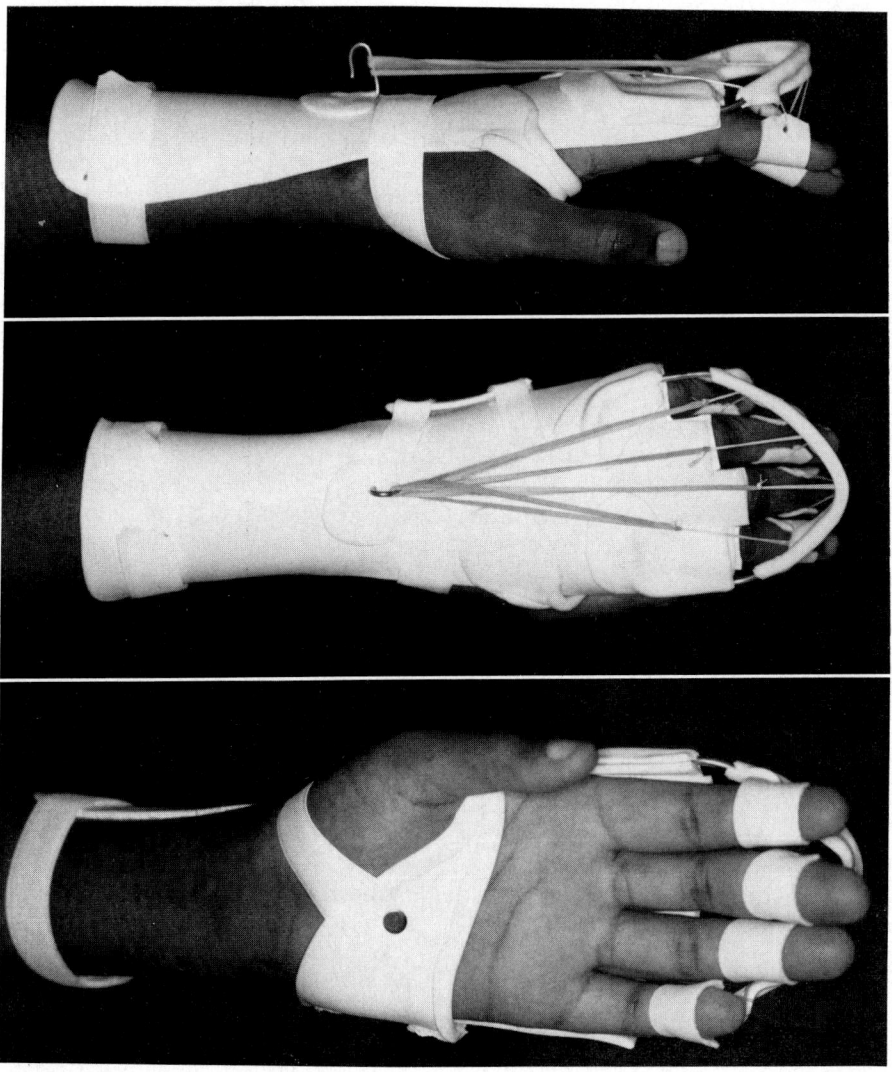

Fig. 25-8 Low-profile design splint for interphalangeal joint extension, with wrist and metacarpophalangeal joints stabilized.

force. Although it can be argued that application of the finger loop at maximum distance from the joint can supply a compressive force to the joint, this appears insignificant because of the intermittent nature of dynamic splinting. Normally dynamic splints are not used as exercise splints, since pulling against the force strengthens the opposite motion. A carefully supervised program of active and active resistive motion is mandatory to compliment the splinting program, which only increases the passive potential.

Low-profile designs

Use of a low-profile splint design where the line of pull is redirected by means of a pulley system and then carried parallel to the splint base is an effective means of applying the 90-degree line of pull without large bulky outrigger arms (Figs. 25-7 and 25-8). The device is kept as small as possible and patient compliance is particularly encouraged in climates where outer layers of clothing are frequently applied and removed.

Equally efficient is the use of the low-profile pulley system for the last ranges of PIP joint flexion (Fig. 25-9). The small pulley on the proximal phalanx "ring" allows specific direction of the line of pull on the middle phalanx and allows use of a long rubber band when the band is attached to the splint base at the wrist. Use of the pulley system is the only way to provide a force for the last ranges of PIP joint flexion, since there is no room in the palm for a traditional outrigger for rubber band attachment.

Use of wire (brass welding rod) as the outrigger base is perhaps the greatest advantage to a low-profile splinting system, since the correct line of pull may be maintained by a simple bend of the wire (Fig. 25-10). In the case of an increased extension range the wire is easily bent dorsally and proximally, maintaining the correct angle of pull. Conversely, a gain in the range of flexion may also be adjusted when the wire is bent more volarly and proximally.

The ease with which one can stabilize a proximal bone and apply force to the distal bone allows for minimum immobilization of the uninvolved joints. As with isolated MP joint flexion it is not necessary to immobilize the wrist, thumb, or other metacarpophalangeal joints in the splint; thus there is increasing patient compliance as the cumbersomeness of the splint is decreased (Fig. 25-11).

The system of pulleys is additionally useful for providing to the patient a specific feedback of gains of motion. A small mark on the string as it slides over the outrigger pulley provides a visual indication as the joint gains motion. If one desires, one may also harness active motion and provide visual feedback as the mark moves away from the pulley. In this case one must provide enough length of the string beyond the outrigger to allow sliding of the string without the knot where the rubber band is attached hanging on the pulley.

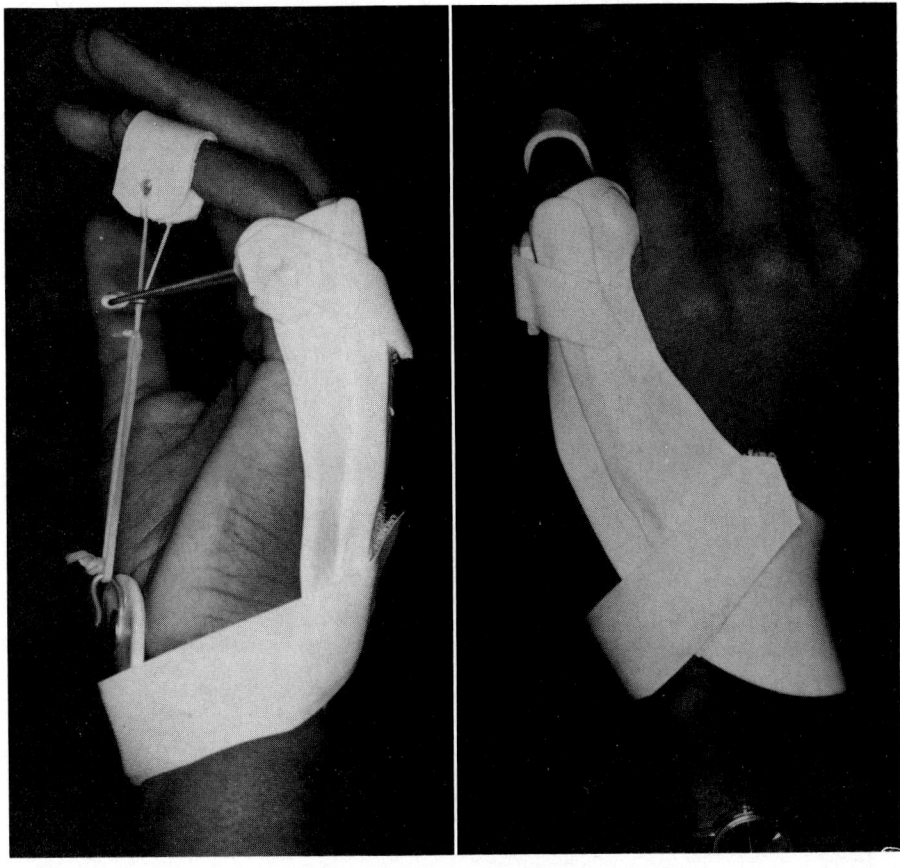

Fig. 25-9 Splint designed to gain last ranges of proximal interphalangeal joint flexion by blocking metacarpophalangeal joint flexion and directing line of pull by use of wire-loop pulley.

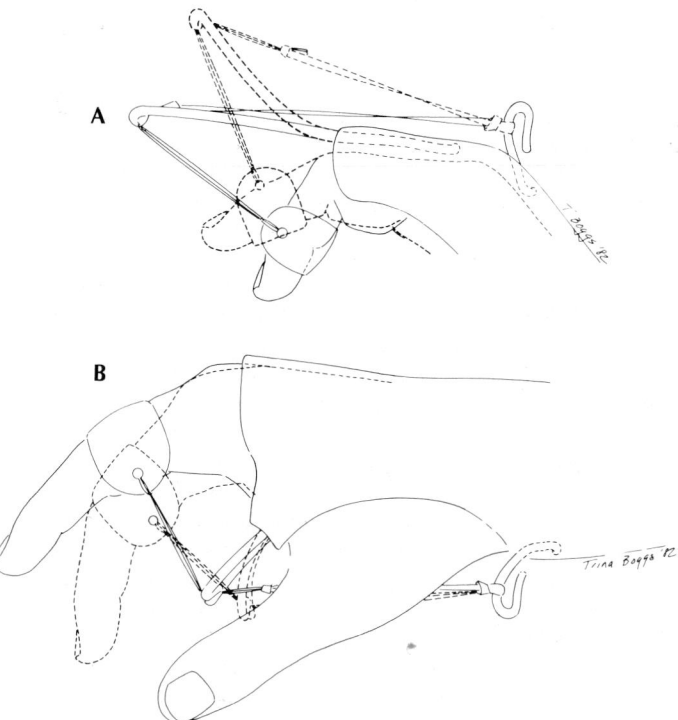

Fig. 25-10 Ease of adjustment of low-profile wire outrigger system is accomplished by simple bend of wire outrigger. This allows maintenance of 90-degree line of pull when either extension, **A,** or flexion, **B,** is accomplished. (From Colditz JC: Low profile dynamic splinting to the injured hand, Am J Occup Ther 37:182, 1983. Reprinted with the permission of the American Occupational Therapy Association, Inc. Copyright 1983.)

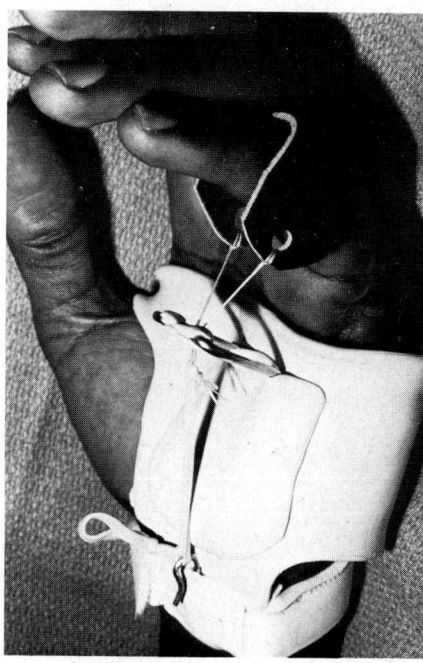

Fig. 25-11 Splint to stretch isolated metacarpophalangeal joint tightness. No other joints are immobilized with the low-profile technique.

CONCLUSION

Splintmaking is truly the ultimate combination of art and science. Effective dynamic splinting requires both the scientific knowledge of wound physiology and mechanical design and the creative ability to construct a splint based on these principles. It is a skilled hand therapist who can effectively assess to the injured hand, establish priorities for treatment, and then create a splint that is an effective tool in reestablishing motion. As hand surgery and hand therapy continue to develop as a well-recognized medical specialty, every hand therapist should continue to face the challenge of being accountable for effective splinting of the stiff hand.

REFERENCES

1. American Academy of Orthopaedic Surgeons (Office of the Surgeon General of the Army and Veteran's Administration): Orthopaedic appliance atlas, Ann Arbor, Mich, 1952, JW Edwards Co.
2. Barr N: The hand: principles and techniques of simple splintmaking in rehabilitation, Sevenoaks, Kent, 1975, Buttersworth & Co (Pubs), Ltd.
3. Brand P: Clinical mechanics of the hand, St Louis, 1985, The CV Mosby Co.
4. Brand P: The forces of dynamic splinting: ten questions before applying a dynamic splint to the hand. In Hunter JM and others, editors: Rehabilitation of the hand, St. Louis, 1984, The CV Mosby Co.
5. Bryant WH: Wound healing, Clin Symp 29(3):9, 1977.
6. Bunch WH and Keagy RD: Principles of orthotic treatment, St. Louis, 1976, The CV Mosby Co.
7. Bunnell S, editor: Hand surgery in World War II, Washington, DC, 1955, US Surgeon General's Office.
8. Bunnell S: Spring splint to supinate or pronate the hand, J Bone Joint Surg 31A:664, 1949.
9. Bunnell S: Active splinting of the hand, J Bone Joint Surg 28:732, 1946.
10. Bunnell S: Surgery of the hand, Philadelphia, 1944, JB Lippincott Co.
11. Bunnell S and Howard LD: Additional elastic hand splints, J Bone Joint Surg 32A:226, 1950.
12. Cailliet R: Hand pain and impairment, Philadelphia, 1971, FA Davis Co.
13. Capener N: Physiological rest, Br Med J 2:761, 1946.
14. Colditz JC: Low profile dynamic splinting of the injured hand, Am J Occup Ther 37(3):183, 1983.
15. Fess EE, Gettle K and Strickland J: Hand splinting: principles and methods, St. Louis, 1981, The CV Mosby Co.
16. Fess EE and Phillips C: Hand splinting: principles and methods, ed 2, St Louis, 1987, The CV Mosby Co.
17. Kottke FJ and Ptak RA: The rationale for prolonged stretching for correction of shortening of connective tissue, Arch Phys Med Rehabil 47:345, 1966.
18. Littler JW: Dynamic splinting and immobilization. In Littler JW, editor: Reconstructive plastic surgery, vol 4, Philadelphia, 1964, WB Saunders.
19. Littler JW: Tendon transfers and arthodesis in combined median and ulnar nerve paralysis, J Bone Joint Surg 31A:225, 1949.
20. Nachlas JW: A splint for the correction of extension contractures of the metacarpophalangeal joints, J Bone Joint Surg 27:507, 1945.
21. Peacock EE Jr: Dynamic splinting for the prevention and correction of hand deformities, J Bone Joint Surg 34A:789, 1952.
22. Pearson SO: Dynamic splinting. In Hunter JM and others, editors: Rehabilitation of the hand, St Louis 1978, The CV Mosby Co.
23. Weeks P and Wray RC: Management of acute hand injuries, St. Louis, 1973, The CV Mosby Co.
24. Wynn Parry CB: Stretching. In Rogoff JB, editor: Manipulation, traction and massage, ed 2, Baltimore, 1980, The Williams & Wilkins Co.
25. Wynn Parry CB: Rehabilitation of the hand, ed 3, Sevenoaks, Kent, 1978, Butterworth & Co (Pubs), Ltd.

26

Anatomic considerations for splinting the thumb

Judy C. Colditz

"On the length, strength, free lateral motion, and perfect mobility of the thumb, depends the power of the human hand."[1] So wrote Sir Charles Bell in 1833. The thumb encompasses an enormous range of motion when its three joint motions are combined. Most frequently it is considered a minimum of 50% of hand function when disability ratings of the hand are done.

Much has been written about splinting to facilitate the primary flexion and extension motion of the fingers, but the literature offers minimal specific references for splinting approaches to harness or reestablish the many complex motions of the thumb. Most often the thumb is left to progress on its own. When specific pathology or injury is localized to the thumb, one must have an in-depth understanding of the complex biomechanics of the thumb to splint it correctly.

MOTIONS OF THE THUMB

The thumb has many planes of motion, and the terminology is often confusing. Terms may describe specific isolated joint motions of flexion or extension or complex composite motions where flexion or extension is combined with rotary or abduction/adduction movements.

Motion of the interphalangeal joint

Flexion and extension are terms reserved for the biplane motion of the interphalangeal joint of the thumb, a stabile hinge joint. Flexion of the interphalangeal joint is in a plane perpendicular to the fingernail (Fig. 26-1). Extension of the thumb interphalangeal joint is in the opposite direction but identical plane.

Motion of the metacarpophalangeal joint

Although thought of as a hinge joint especially when compared with the multiplaned carpometacarpal (CMC) joint, the metacarpophalangeal (MP) joint demonstrates increased laxity as compared with the interphalangeal joint, thus allowing radial and ulnar deviation and some rotation as accessory motions to flexion and extension. The accessory motions of the MP joint are a reflection of the related motion at the CMC joint. When combined, they allow a greater functional range of motion for the thumb.

It is important to note that one cannot fully flex the MP and interphalangeal joints of the thumb while holding the CMC joint in an abducted or extended position, a relevant point when splinting.

Motion of the carpometacarpal joint

Zancolli describes retropulsion, antepulsion, adduction, and abduction as the four directions of movement possible at the saddle CMC joint.[3] When interphalangeal, MP, and

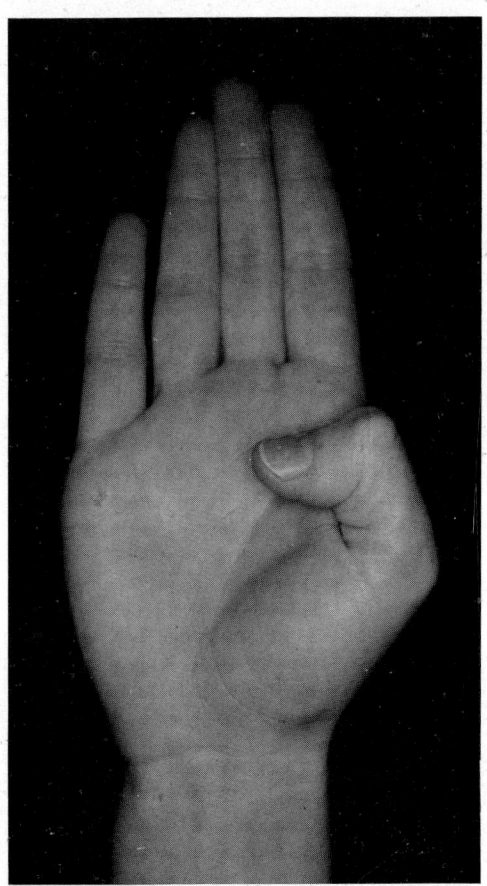

Fig. 26-1 Flexion of the thumb metacarpophalangeal and interphalangeal joints.

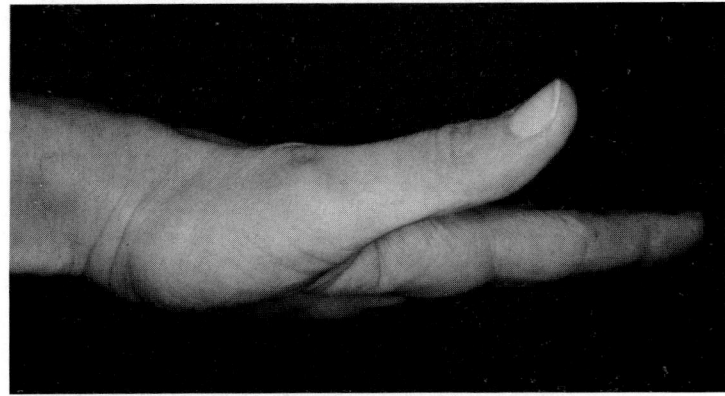

Fig. 26-2 Retropulsion (full extension and abduction) of the thumb.

353

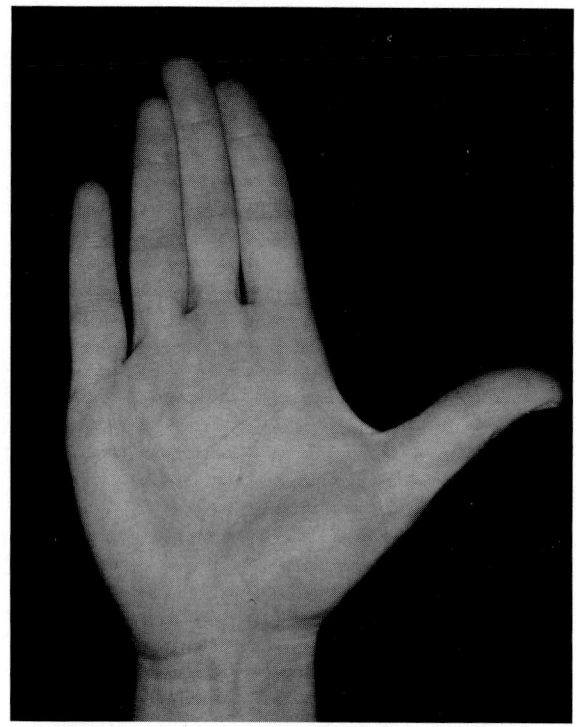

Fig. 26-3 Radial abduction of the thumb.

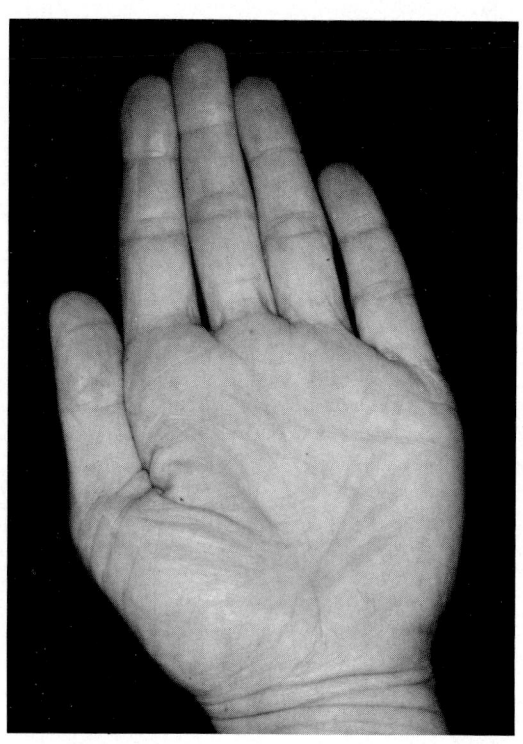

Fig. 26-4 Adduction of the thumb.

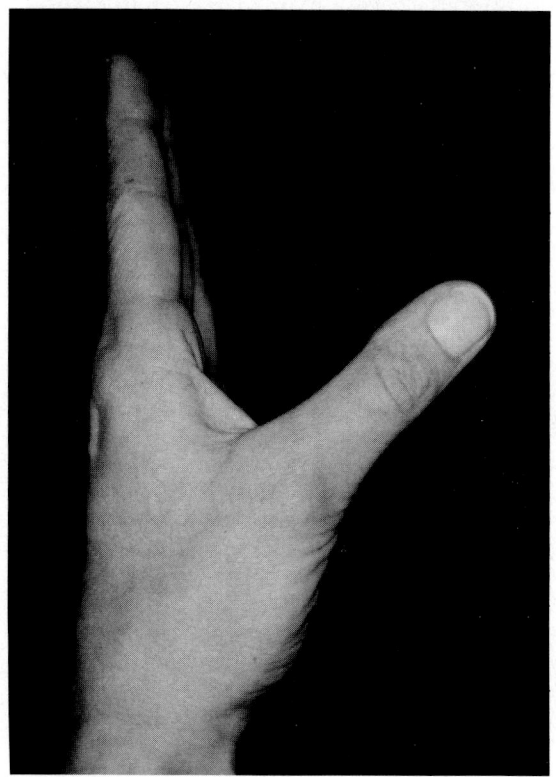

Fig. 26-5 Palmar abduction of the thumb.

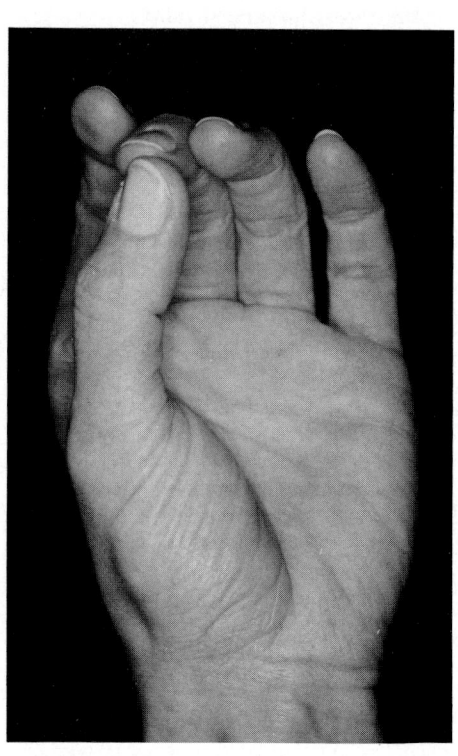

Fig. 26-6 Opposition of the thumb. Note the plane of the thumb-nail.

CMC motions are combined, the terms "opposition" and "circumduction" become relevant.

Retropulsion describes the position of the first metacarpal rising above the plane of the other metacarpals (Fig. 26-2). Clinically this motion is seen with full abduction and extension of the first metacarpal away from the second metacarpal with associated full extension of the MP and interphalangeal joints. This is commonly referred to as *extension/abduction*. When less than full retropulsion (extension/abduction) of the thumb is achieved but full abduction of the first metacarpal is achieved in the same plane as the other metacarpals, this may be referred to as "radial abduction" (Fig. 26-3).

When the thumb begins to move toward the fingertips, the terminology becomes more confusing and changes as the thumb moves toward the ulnar fingers. When the thumb rests against the index finger, it is described as zero position or "adduction" (Fig. 26-4). Note that this describes only the motion of the CMC joint. Some clinicians refer to palmar adduction when the thumb is held against the hand on the palmar surface of the index finger. These two positions reflect a change in the position of the interphalangeal joints, but the position of the CMC joint remains relatively unchanged. If the plane of the fingernail stays at a 90-degree angle to the plane of the palm of the hand and the thumb is pulled directly away from the index finger, this is termed "palmar abduction" (Fig. 26-5). As the thumb proceeds toward the tips of the ulnar fingers, rotation begins at the CMC joint. The angle of the thumbnail becomes almost parallel to the plane of the palm, creating a position of opposition (Fig. 26-6). When the thumb is touching the base of the ulnar digits and the fingernail is parallel to the plane of the palm (i.e., opposed) the CMC joint is maximally rotated and flexed, describing the position of antepulsion (Fig. 26-7).

The collective motion from the position of maximum radial abduction and extension (retropulsion) to the ulnar border (antepulsion) of the hand is called "circumduction."

SPECIFIC JOINT PROBLEMS
The carpometacarpal joint

The configuration of the ligaments and the saddle shape of the CMC joint allow rotation and the four other motions of flexion/extension and abduction/adduction (Fig. 26-8). The trapezium sits palmar of the other carpals, thus allowing the thumb to move in an arc around the fingers. Because of this large range of motion (ROM) and the accompanying normal joint mobility, this joint most frequently requires stabilizing splinting rather than dynamic splinting to gain mobility.

Arthritis. The common deforming force, particularly as seen in osteoarthritis or rheumatoid arthritis, is the strong pull of the adductor pollicis muscle, which originates palmarly on the third metacarpal and inserts on the first metacarpal. The other short intrinsics of the thumb that originate on the carpals and insert primarily on the distal aspect of the first metacarpal provide a deforming force to flex the first metacarpal. With strong intrinsic muscles and the frequent powerful pinching and flexion movements, the dorsal aspect of the CMC joint is stressed, allowing the first metacarpal to sublux dorsally and radially in relationship to the trapezium (Fig. 26-9).

As the base of the first metacarpal subluxes dorsally, there is often an accompanying tilt of the first metacarpal shaft so that the metacarpal shaft becomes flexed. If, radial subluxation also occurs, it allows adduction of the distal part of the first metacarpal. Any splint fitted to stabilize dorsoradial subluxation of the CMC joint must apply a stabilizing extension force to the palmar and ulnar aspect of the distal end of the metacarpal while providing counter pressure to the dorsoradial aspect of the base of the metacarpal (Fig. 26-10). Stabilizing this joint in relationship to the other metacarpals is mandatory to support the CMC joint during pinching.

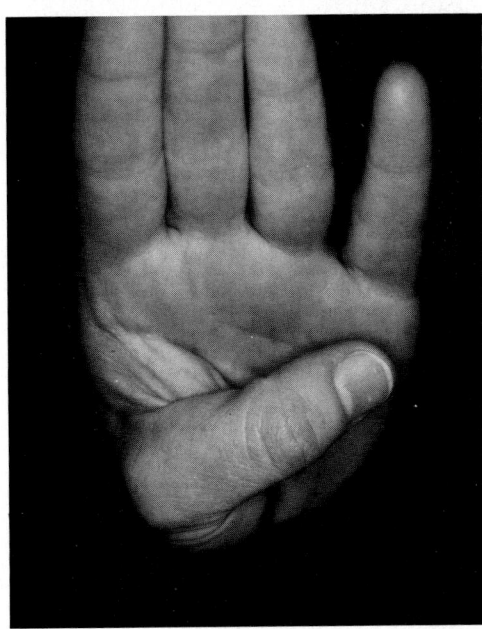

Fig. 26-7 Antepulsion (full flexion and rotation) of the thumb.

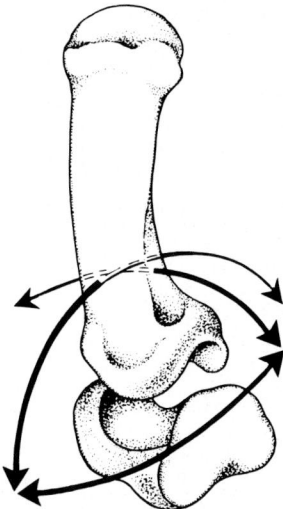

Fig. 26-8 The saddle shape of the carpometacarpal joint allows multiple planes of motion. (From American Society for Surgery of the Hand: The hand: examination and diagnosis, ed 2, New York, 1983, Churchill Livingstone.)

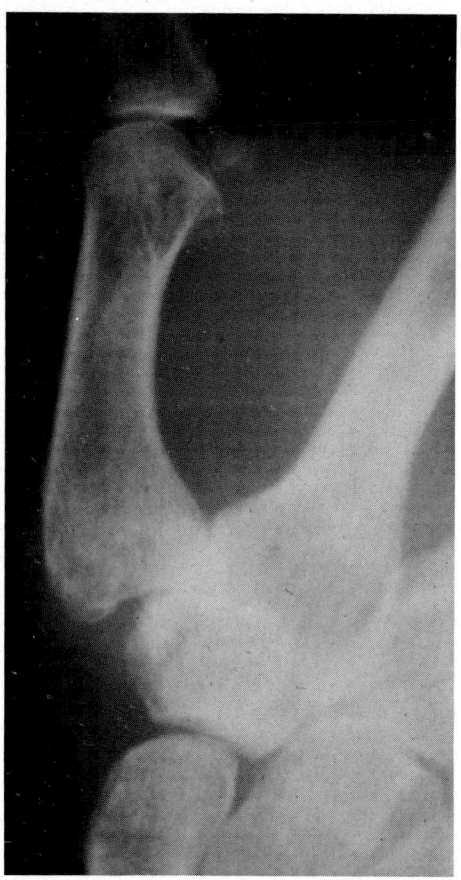

Fig. 26-9 X-ray showing dorsoradial subluxation of the carpometacarpal joint.

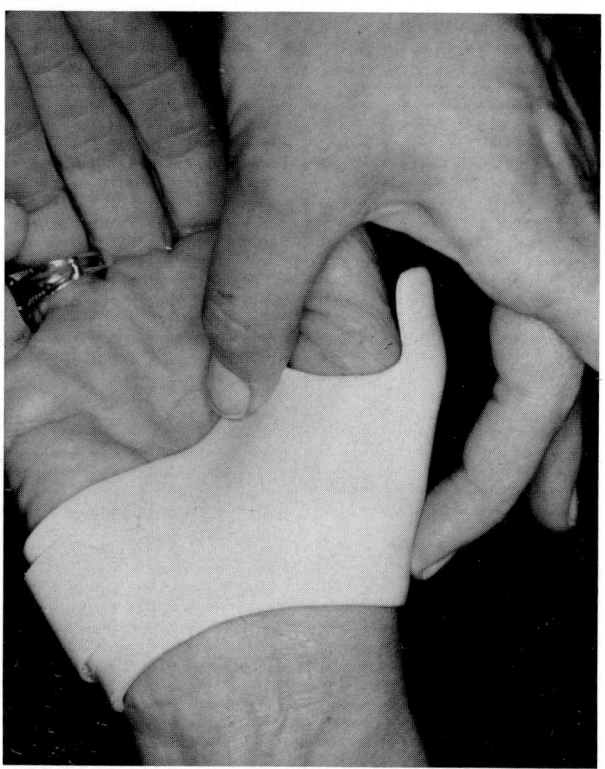

Fig. 26-10 When constructing a carpometacarpal splint, the force must be applied as shown to stabilize the carpometacarpal joint out of its subluxed position.

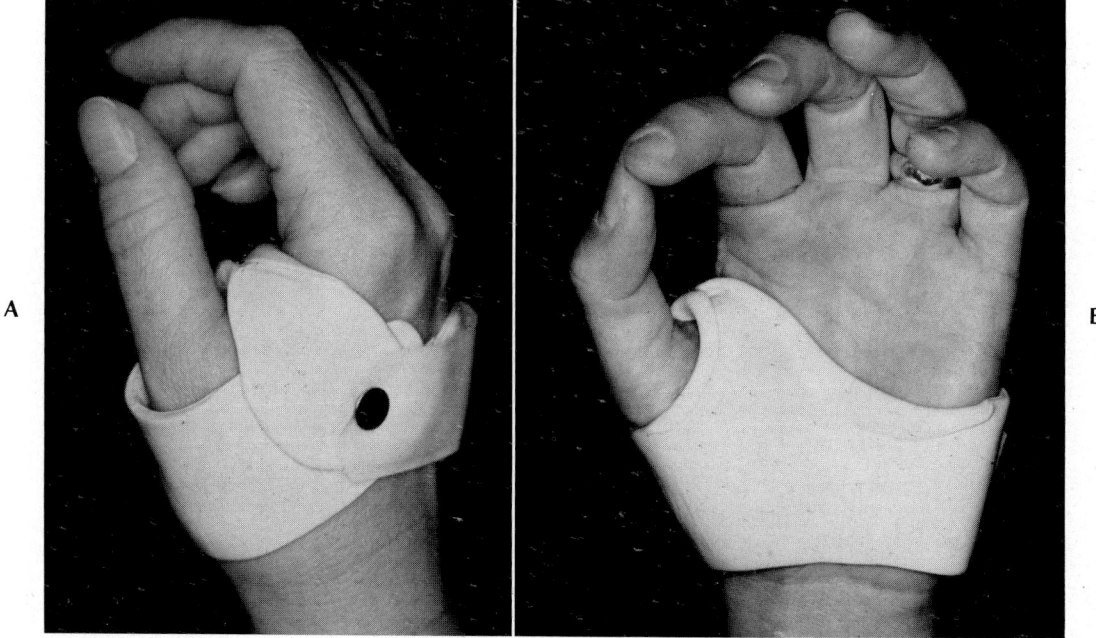

Fig. 26-11 **A** and **B,** Splint that stabilizes carpometacarpal joint during pinching.

Before consideration for arthroplasty, corticosteroid injections, oral anti-inflammatory drugs, and splinting may be used to control the symptoms. Splinting can be effective only to stabilize subluxed joints. If the CMC deformity has progressed to dislocation that is not manually reducible, splinting will be of little value and will likely increase the pain. An ill-fitting splint for this problem will not relieve pain, and the patient will undoubtedly complain that the splint is cumbersome.

Although some clinicians immobilize the wrist for stabilization of this joint, it is my clinical experience that persons with CMC arthritis are greatly relieved of their

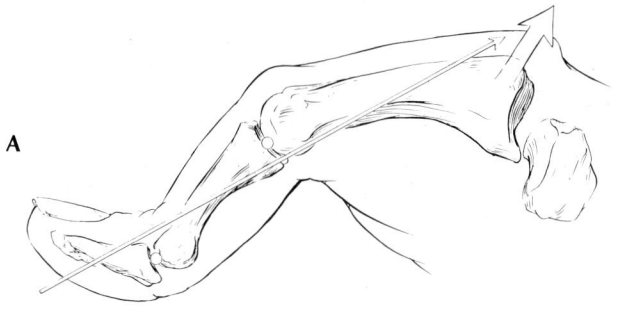

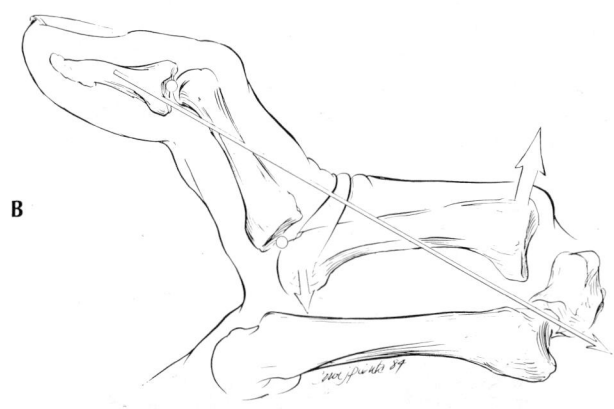

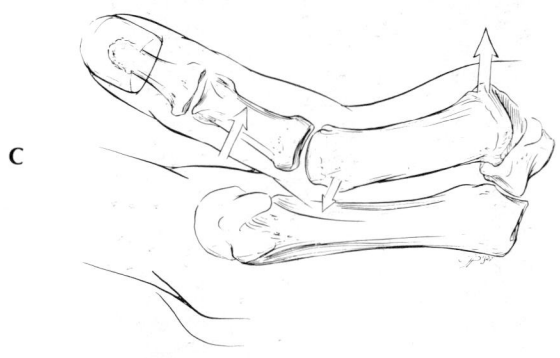

Fig. 26-12 Primary carpometacarpal joint pathology leads to deformities as described by Nalebuff. **A,** Type II, flexion of the metacarpophalangeal joint with extension of the interphalangeal joint. **B,** Type III, hyperextension of the metacarpophalangeal joint with abduction/flexion deformity of the first metacarpal. **C,** Type IV, adduction/flexion deformity of the metacarpal with laxity of the ulnar collateral ligament. (From: Colditz JC; In Malick M and Kasch M, editors: Manual on management of specific hand problems, Pittsburgh, 1984, Harmarville Rehabilitation Center.)

symptoms by using a small splint with no accompanying wrist immobilization (Fig. 26-11). Patients are willing to trade the loss of palmar sensibility for increased comfort and power during pinching and fine motor activity.

Rheumatoid arthritis. In the rheumatoid hand, subluxation of the CMC joint alters the balance throughout the entire thumb. Primary involvement of the CMC joint leads to deformities, types II, III, and IV, as described by Nalebuff[2] (Fig. 26-12).

In the type II deformity, as the CMC joint subluxes, the balance of motion at the MP and interphalangeal joints is altered by the pull of the extrinsic and intrinsic muscles. This may appear to be a boutonniere deformity because hyperextension of the interphalangeal joint and flexion of the MP joint is seen, but the primary deforming force is located at the CMC joint. The progression of the deformity can often be slowed by stabilizing the CMC joint in a slightly extended position, as described above (Fig. 26-11).

In the type III deformity, the primary site of involvement is also the CMC joint, with dorsal and radial subluxation allowing the first metacarpal to become adducted. Laxity of the volar plate of the MP joint allows MP hyperextension to accommodate the loss of abduction at the CMC joint and progresses to a significant swan-neck deformity. It is difficult to appreciate this deformity in the early stages, although it would be appropriate to provide a CMC joint–stabilizing splint with a small block to prevent MP hyperextension (Fig. 26-13). Often this deformity is seen late, and although splinting may be of some value for symptomatic relief, it

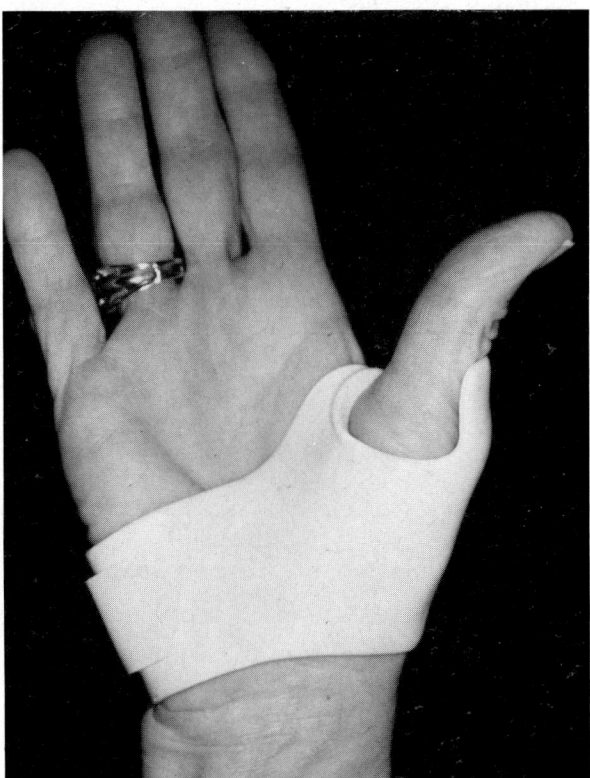

Fig. 26-13 A splint for carpometacarpal subluxation with metacarpophalangeal block to be used when associated metacarpophalangeal joint hyperextension is noted.

can do little to alleviate or prevent further deformity. Surgery is indicated.

The fourth type of deformity described by Nalebuff also shows primary subluxation of the CMC joint. The first metacarpal again subluxes at the CMC joint and becomes adducted. Tasks requiring abduction of the thumb are accomplished by laxity of the ulnar collateral ligament of the MP joint, allowing excessive radial deviation. Once the first metacarpal has become adducted, only surgery can alleviate this imbalance.

The metacarpophalangeal joint

The configuration of the collateral ligaments of the MP joint of the thumb allows stability of the MP joint during both flexion and extension (Fig. 26-14). Although the MP joint is basically a hinge joint, the ligaments allow more radial and ulnar deviation than most other hinge joints in the upper extremity. The normal range of motion at the MP joint is variable. Persons with naturally limited MP joint flexion often tend to have a greater range of interphalangeal flexion than those who have 90 degrees of flexion of the MP joint. For this reason, whenever splinting the MP joint of the thumb for flexion, one must examine and measure the contralateral thumb to determine the normal motion for that individual.

Collateral ligament injury. The most common problem seen at the MP joint is injury to the ulnar collateral ligament. Traditionally it is called a "gamekeeper's thumb" because of the gamekeepers who killed the birds by twisting their necks, constantly stressing this joint.

Though this injury to the MP joint of the thumb can avulse a fragment of bone requiring an open reduction, a grade 1 or grade 2 tear of the collateral ligament can be managed by splinting the joint to prevent radial and ulnar deviation. Traditionally managed in a thumb spica cast, protection of the healing ligament with a properly molded splint that does not immobilize the wrist is possible (Fig. 26-15).

To immobilize the MP joint first construct a CMC joint splint to obtain adequate purchase on the thumb metacarpal. The small extension that is added around the proximal phalanx to prevent motion at the MP joint level can be part of the splint. The patient retains functional use of the thumb and maintains full interphalangeal joint motion without stress to the MP joint. An identical design may be used for a period of continued immobilization following surgical repair of this injury.

Capsular tightness following trauma. Ligamentous injuries to the MP joint or fractures at or near the MP joint will often limit active and passive flexion. It is not adequate to attach a finger loop from a wrist cuff to the thumb because normal motion of the CMC joint will be affected more by this force as it is transmitted across the stiff MP joint. For improvement of motion of the MP joint into flexion, one must first stabilize the CMC joint by holding the thenar eminence area and then provide an outrigger that specifically places a pull at a 90-degree angle to the axis of the proximal phalanx of the thumb (Fig. 26-16). As the thumb MP joint motion increases, this outrigger must be changed to provide a correct line of pull.

The interphalangeal joint

The interphalangeal joint of the thumb is vulnerable to injury because it is involved in all our manipulative tasks. It is a stable hinge joint. Although fusion has been said to be an excellent solution for problems at this joint, loss of interphalangeal joint motion in the dominant hand of someone who handles small objects will prove to be a functional limitation. In many individuals the range of hyperextension available at the interphalangeal joint of the thumb is considerable and those persons establish a pattern of direct pinch onto the pulp of the thumb, which uses this hyperextended position (Fig. 26-17). One should not ignore this normal hyperextension when splinting to regain function.

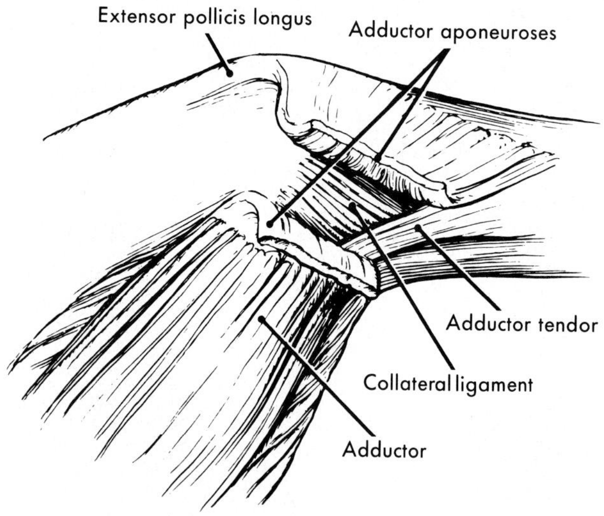

Fig. 26-14 Metacarpophalangeal joint ligament configuration showing the adductor aponeurosis, the collateral ligament, the adductor tendon, the adductor muscle, and the extensor pollicis longus. (From: Palmar A and Louis D: J Hand Surg 3:544, 1978.)

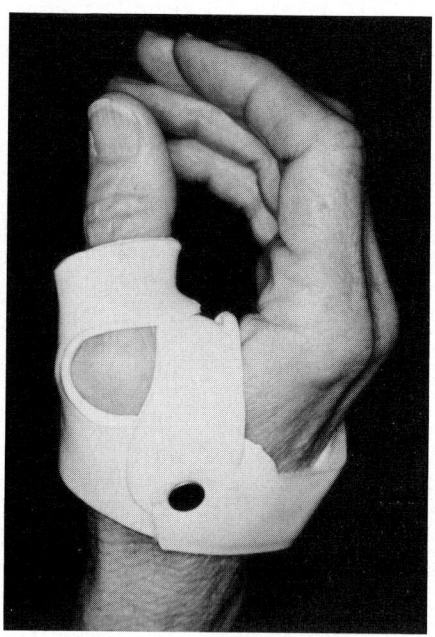

Fig. 26-15 Splint to stabilize the metacarpophalangeal joint following injury and/or surgery to the ulnar collateral ligament.

Capsular tightness of the interphalangeal joint

Dynamic splinting. When interphalangeal joint motion is limited following a fracture, dislocation, or crush injury, the splinting rationale is identical to that of the MP joint because force must be transmitted specifically to the interphalangeal joint and the motion of the MP and CMC joint must be blocked (Fig. 26-18). Just as with the MP joint flexion splint, the line of pull is altered as the ROM improves.

Serial static splinting. Splinting to gain full interphalangeal extension of the thumb is often at the request of the patient to reestablish the normal hyperextended pinch pattern. This may be accomplished with serial splinting, either with a molded palmar thermoplastic shell or a serial plaster cast. At times it may be better to provide a dynamic extension force to this joint if the other alternatives are unrealistic in relation to the patient's life-style, or if alternating flexion and extension are required.

Posttraumatic adduction contractures

Adduction contractures of the thumb are often seen following major trauma or prolonged immobilization of the hand. This may be secondary to muscle imbalance such as median nerve palsy, or following soft tissue injury to the hand where the thumb has been allowed to remain in the adducted and flexed position as soft tissues heal; the CMC joint of the first metacarpal rests in an adducted/flexed po-

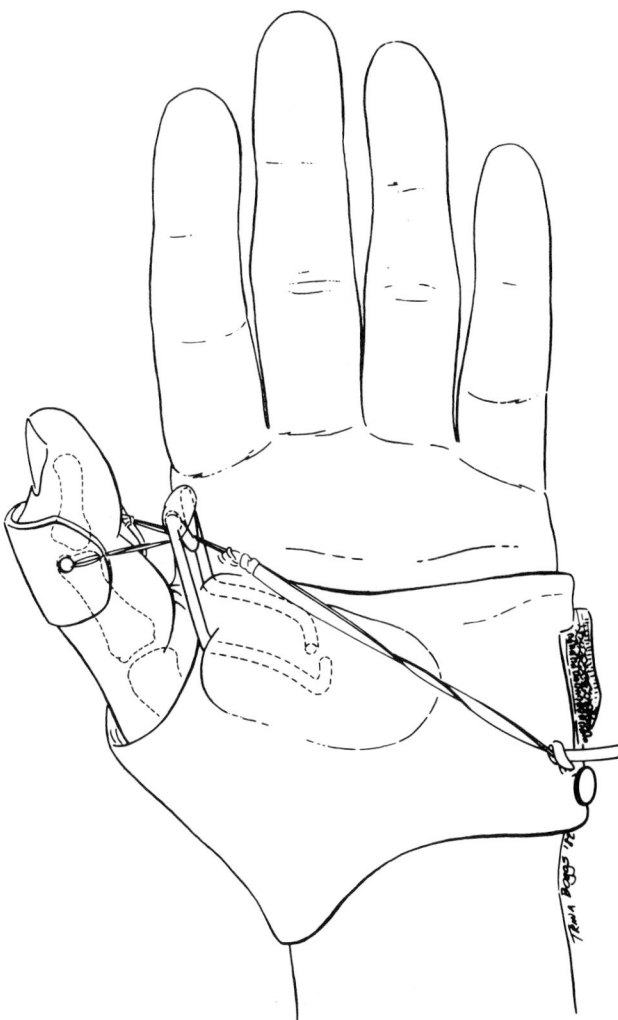

Fig. 26-16 Dynamic thumb metacarpophalangeal flexion splint. (From: Colditz J; Am J Occup Ther 37:184, 1983.)

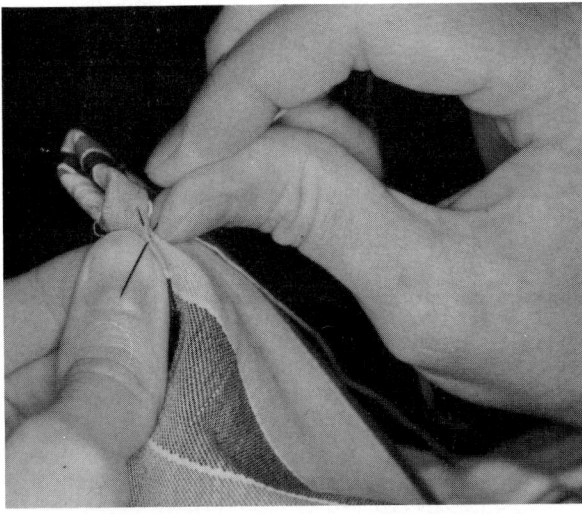

Fig. 26-17 Normal interphalangeal hyperextension is used in many daily tasks.

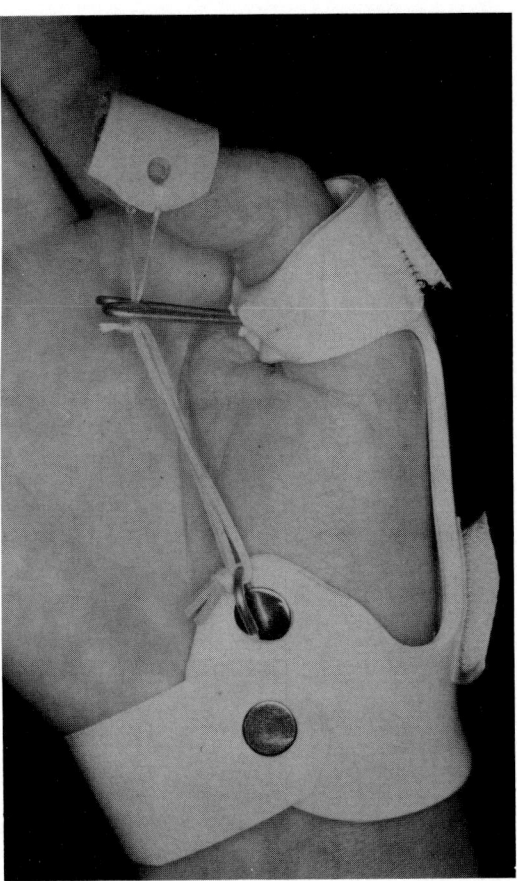

Fig. 26-18 Dynamic interphalangeal flexion splint that stabilizes the metacarpophalangeal and carpometacarpal joints.

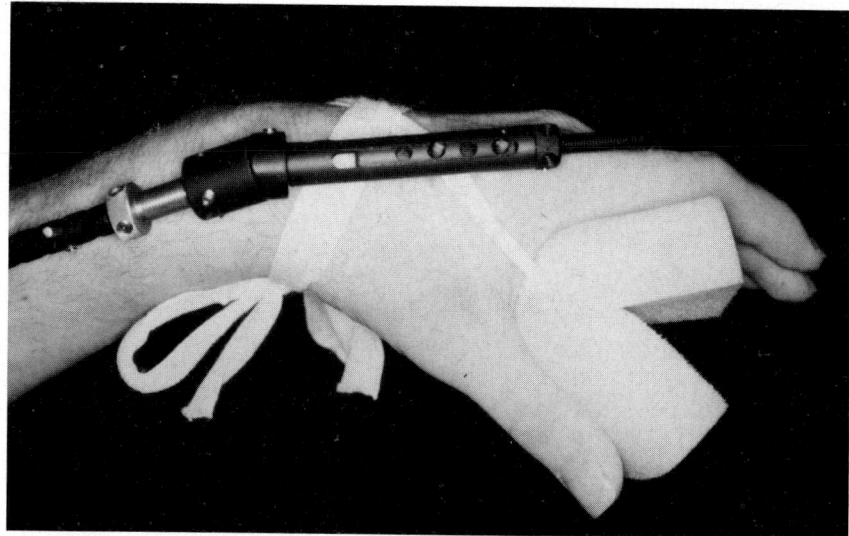

Fig. 26-19   A foam splint that gently maintains abduction of the first web space.

sition. Although specific trauma to the CMC joint can produce an adduction contracture, the usual pathology of this deformity is in the soft tissues of the first web space. The first dorsal interosseous and the adductor muscles along with the accompanying fascia have been allowed to rest in a shortened position.

Functional abduction of the thumb is not simply an index of the angle between the first and second metacarpals. It is also the ability to extend fully all the joints of the index finger and thumb to obtain maximum distance between the two. Theoretically, one could have normal abduction of the first metacarpal in relation to the second metacarpal, but with severe flexion contractures of the thumb and index finger the hand would lack functional abduction of the thumb (the ability to grasp objects in the first web space). Traditional resting splint designs have advocated holding the MP joints of the fingers in full flexion with interphalangeal joint extension and holding the thumb in a palmarly abducted position. The soft tissue, skin, and muscles between the first and second metacarpals are not held in a stretched position when the thumb is in palmar abduction. I therefore recommend that a resting splint should maintain the intrinsic-plus position of the fingers but hold the thumb in a more abducted and extended position to maintain length of the adductor and other intrinsics, as well as the fascia and skin. Since the thumb is more powerful in flexion than extension, this is a better position to help the patient regain balanced motion.

There are a number of splinting approaches that may be helpful in alleviating an adduction contracture of the thumb.

Dynamic splinting. A mild positional contracture secondary to immobilization and disuse may be alleviated simply by using a large piece of foam placed in the first web space and tied in place with a gentle strap going around the wrist in a figure eight (Fig. 26-19). Overnight wear will allow the expansion of the foam to position the thumb in more abduction.

Dynamic splinting of the thumb to gain abduction of the

CMC joint and stretch of the first web space is mechanically difficult, since the soft tissues of the web space leave little surface area on which to apply a force that is not distal to the MP joint (Fig. 26-20). It is important to be aware that the MP joint of the thumb often has some normal radial and ulnar deviation. Functional abduction needed to hold a large object requires full extension of the MP joint and often uses

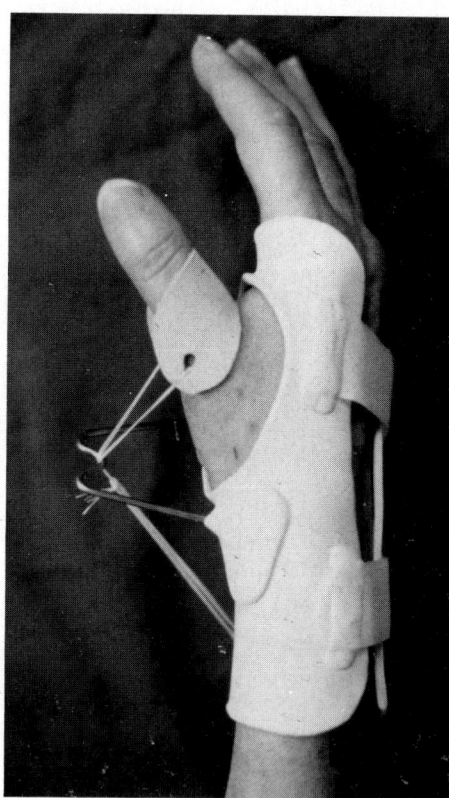

Fig. 26-20   Dynamic splint for thumb abduction.

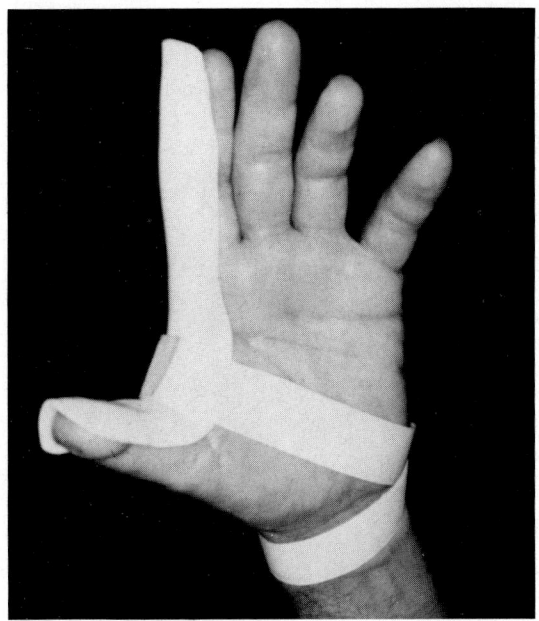

Fig. 26-21   Splint for full abduction of the first web space.

the accompanying full radial deviation, a point of detail worthy of analysis when splinting for an adduction contracture.

In severe injuries the patient may be wearing a dynamic splint for prolonged periods of time during the day to obtain better motion of the fingers. In such cases it is appropriate to add an outrigger to keep the web space of the thumb open since the hand is immobile while in the splint. Care should be taken to apply the force at less than a 90-degree angle so as to pull on the first metacarpal and not the proximal phalanx.

Serial static splinting. To affect the soft tissue problem of an adduction contracture, it is appropriate to provide night splinting, which holds the thumb and index finger in full extension and abducts the first and second metacarpal (Fig. 26-21). If these are molded carefully, one need not apply undo pressure to the MP joint of the thumb, and they can be slowly changed to accommodate elongation of the soft tissues.

THE THUMB IN MEDIAN AND ULNAR PALSY
Median palsy

The kinetic balance of the thumb is significantly altered in median nerve palsy. Median nerve palsy demonstrates the pattern of flexion of the thumb as it lies in the adducted position across the plane of the hand. If left unsplinted, the shortened adductor pollicis and first dorsal interosseous passively limit abduction of the first metacarpal.

Soon after a laceration of the median nerve, a static abduction splint is used to maintain the soft tissue length. A small static abduction splint or the traditional c-bar do not maintain the full stretch of the soft tissues of the first web space. Although these splints may be useful during the day to stabilize the thumb, a full abduction splint at night best maintains full abduction (Fig. 26-21).

As sensibility returns, it is usually concurrent with some reinnervation of the intrinsics of the thumb. To strengthen these intrinsics and reinforce normal use of the thumb it is counterproductive to continue immobilization of the CMC joint. A splint should be used, which allows active use of the returning short abductor and opponens while excluding the strong extrinsic power to the thumb. Either a small leather splint or thermoplastic splint will assist the patient in using the returning musculature (Fig. 26-22).

Ulnar palsy

The thumb in ulnar nerve palsy has a significant disability since part of the balanced stabilizing force at the MP joint

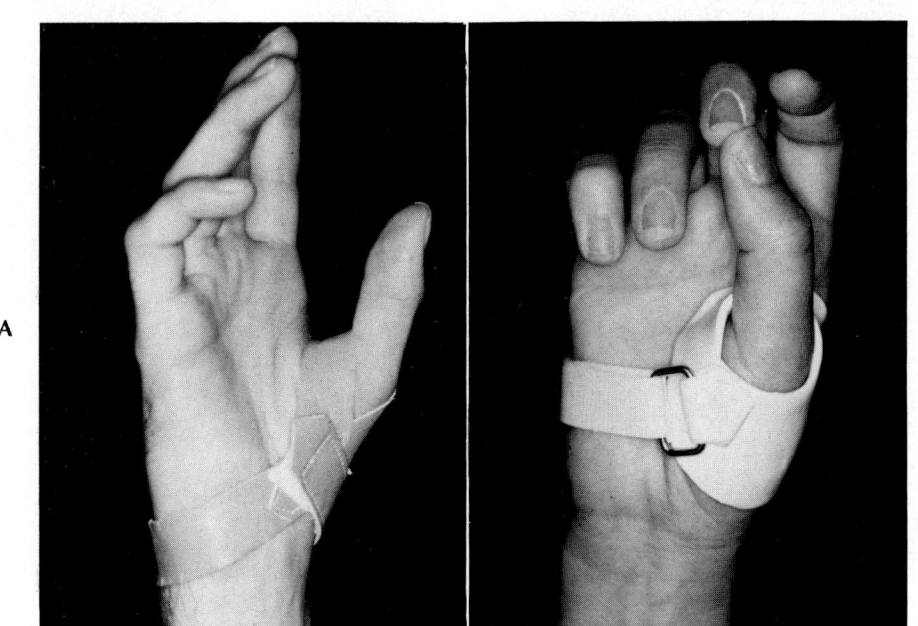

Fig. 26-22   Splints for functional abduction of the thumb. **A,** Leather. **B,** Thermoplastic material.

is lost. Froment's sign (hyperflexion of the interphalangeal joint and hyperextension of the MP joint during forced pinch) is an indication of the weakness of the adductor pollicis and half of the flexor pollicis brevis of the thumb. However, with normal sensibility in the thumb, index, and long fingers and otherwise unimpeded motion, it is difficult to provide a splint for the thumb, which stabilizes in one direction without impeding other function; thus a splint is not usually recommended. Tendon transfers may be recommended.

TENDON LACERATIONS OF THE THUMB
Flexor pollicis longus

The flexor pollicis longus tendon may be managed by dorsal block splinting and rubber band traction after the Kleinert method. A pulley on the palmar bar is recommended to place the line of pull at a right angle to the thumb. Full extension is limited by the wrist being held in flexion and the first metacarpal being positioned in flexion.

After active motion is begun at about 3 weeks, a proximal block is always needed to block the unimpeded motion of the CMC joint and assist in transmitting glide of the flexor pollicis longus at the MP and/or interphalangeal joint distally. This can be done effectively with positional blocking splints that the patient uses as he is returning to normal functional activity (Fig. 26-23). In distal lacerations the strong intrinsics of the thumb flex the MP joint, leaving little available excursion for interphalangeal joint flexion. A longer splint blocking both MP and CMC joint motion may be necessary.

Extensor pollicis longus

Extensor pollicis longus lacerations are best managed by meticulous attention to splinting following the repair. Since the extensor pollicis longus crosses the wrist at an oblique angle, it is important for full excursion of this tendon that the thumb be held in full abduction and extension with concurrent wrist extension (Fig. 26-24). It is advisable to position the interphalangeal joint in maximum extension, so that when initiating a rehabilitation program, the patient does not have a significant active lag in extension and a range of flexion to gain.

Extrinsic flexor or extensor tightness

Any injury to the hand or thumb can result in tightness of the extrinsic muscle-tendon units. Trauma specifically to the thumb will allow part of the extrinsic system to adhere at the level of injury, limiting glide. Movement of proximal and distal joints will alternately affect other joint motion. To effectively splint muscle-tendon unit tightness one must include all joints crossed by the unit and place the unit on maximum stretch. An example is tightness of the flexor pollicis longus, which would require splinting of the wrist in extension concurrent to all joints of the thumb being extended.

Mild tightness can easily be remediated by serial positional night plaster splinting. More specific limitation of excursion caused by adherence of the tendon somewhere along its glide path requires that all joints distal to the level of adherence be splinted. An example is a laceration of the extensor tendon just proximal to the MP joint, which then limits flexion of the MP and interphalangeal joints because it is adherent. A splint to stretch this adherence would flex the MP and interphalangeal joints concurrently, but the po-

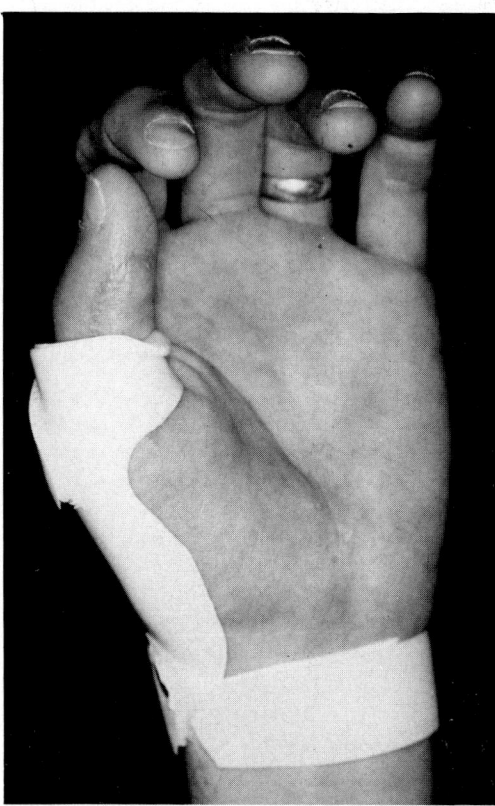

Fig. 26-23 Splint to block carpometacarpal and metacarpophalangeal motion and thus facilitate the isolated glide of the flexor pollicis longus.

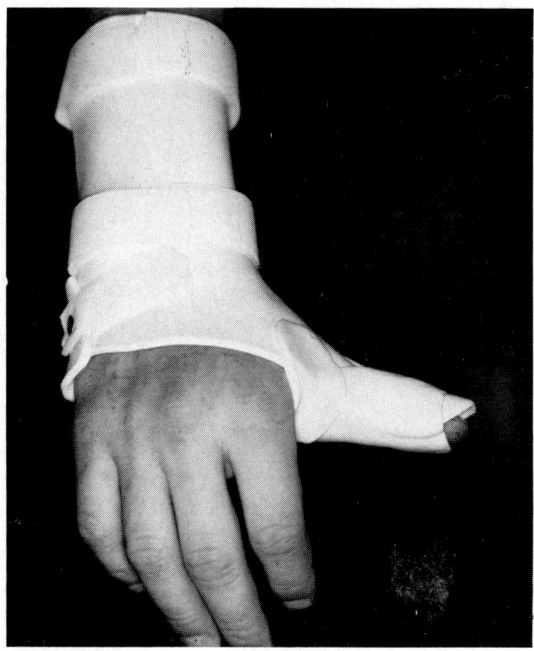

Fig. 26-24 Splint to immobilize lacerated extensor pollicis longus.

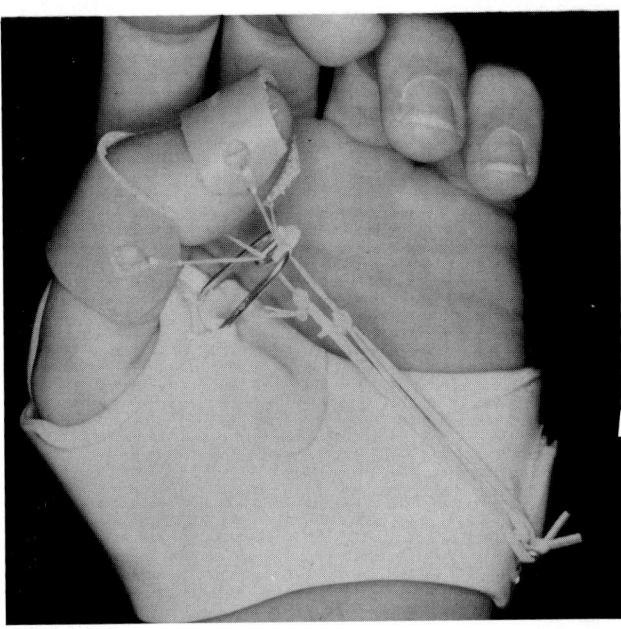

Fig. 26-25   Splint for concurrent dynamic flexion of the thumb metacarpophalangeal and interphalangeal joints.

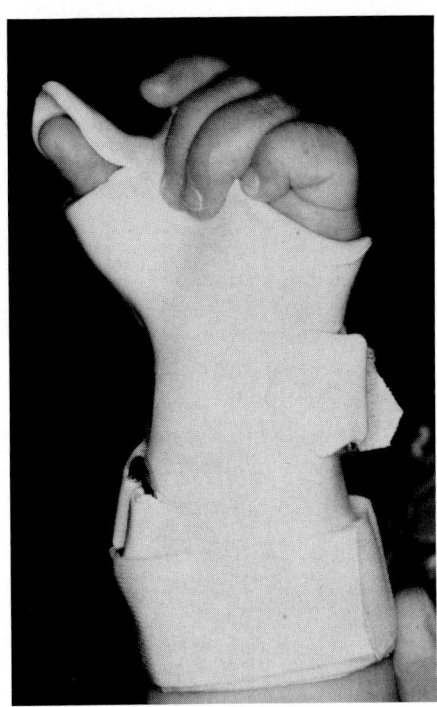

Fig. 26-26   Splint to maintain young child's thumb in abduction.

sition of the CMC and wrist joints are irrelevant since they do not alter the excursion at the site of adherence (Fig. 26-25).

CONGENITAL ADDUCTION OF THE THUMB

Newborn children may exhibit a thumb-in-palm deformity where the thumb is held adducted and flexed against the palm. This may be the result of intrauterine positioning of the thumb allowing the soft tissue to shorten, it may be a manifestation of a central nervous system disorder with spasticity, or it may be a feature of other abnormalities such as arthrogryposis. In children with spasticity this deformity can often be associated with finger or wrist deformities.

Appropriate splinting to hold the soft tissues on stretch is difficult in this population because of the lack of bony prominences and abundant soft tissue. The splint must go proximal to the wrist with numerous straps for adequate purchase (Fig. 26-26). In children with deformities caused by positioning of the soft tissues, the full-time use of these splints is recommended as early as possible so the child can integrate the thumb into normal developmental activities.

CONCLUSION

The thumb has complex movement, making it unique within the hand. To be able to properly evaluate splinting needs and construct a splint with correct stabilizing and mobilizing forces, the therapist must understand the detailed anatomy and kinesiology of the thumb.

REFERENCES
1. Bell C: The hand. Its mechanism and vital endowments as envincing design. The Bridgewater Treatis, London, 1833, Wm Pickering.
2. Nalebuff EA: Diagnosis, classification, and management of rheumatoid thumb deformities, Bull Hosp Joint Dis 29:119, 1968.
3. Zancolli EA: Structural and dynamic bases of hand surgery, ed 2, Philadelphia, 1979, JB Lippincott.

27

Postoperative management of capsulectomies

Georgiann F. Laseter

Capsulectomy of the metacarpophalangeal (MP) and the proximal interphalangeal (PIP) joints is performed to improve motion in stiff joints with normal articular surfaces and is necessitated by the failure of conservative procedures, such as exercises and splinting, to improve motion.

The therapist's role in the management of the postoperative capsulectomy patient begins before the surgery. Many times the patient undergoes therapy before the decision to perform a capsulectomy is made. The result of that therapy program can actually be the determining factor regarding whether the patient needs capsulectomy. Once tissue equilibrium has been reached and the decision has been made to perform the capsulectomy, the therapist's important function before surgery is to educate the patient about what will be expected of him after the capsulectomy and why his postoperative performance is critical in obtaining optimum motion and function.

The therapist must have a good knowledge of hand anatomy and a keen appreciation for the physiology of wound healing and tissue reaction to injury that causes and prolongs stiffness. Multiple variables in the results of capsulectomy are involved, and as more supplementary procedures are added to the capsulectomy, poorer results and even complications may be anticipated.[4] For this reason, it is important that the therapist obtain a copy of the operative report to have information regarding exactly what structures in the capsulectomy procedure were surgically involved.

COMPARISON OF TREATMENT NEEDS IN ACUTE INJURIES AND THOSE AFTER CAPSULECTOMY

The general needs of treatment applicable to the acutely injured patient closely correlate with the needs of treatment applicable to postcapsulectomy patients and include the following:
1. Pain control
2. Edema reduction
3. Exercises
4. Splinting
5. Functional activiteis

Control of pain and reduction of edema postoperatively are of paramount importance in the management of the patient who has undergone a capsulectomy procedure.

Pain

The amount and duration of pain vary considerably among patients with hand injuries. Some patients may have minimal and transient discomfort, whereas in others pain is the major problem with the hand.[13] Many patients who undergo capsulectomies have had significant difficulties with pain and

reflex sympathetic dystrophy (RSD) before the capsulectomy. Gould and Nicholson[6] reported in their series that patients with quiescent RSD who underwent capsulectomy tended to have poor results despite sympathetic blockades performed during and after the operations. In many cases, their RSD symptoms recurred in various degrees after the capsulectomy.

Useful methods of controlling pain after a capsulectomy may be the use of a transcutaneous nerve stimulator and/or elevation to decrease edema. In addition, modalities producing either heat or cold can be interspersed with other treatment techniques to improve circulation and help the hand relax. Massage and the use of goal-directed activities are also useful in assisting the patient to work through his pain.

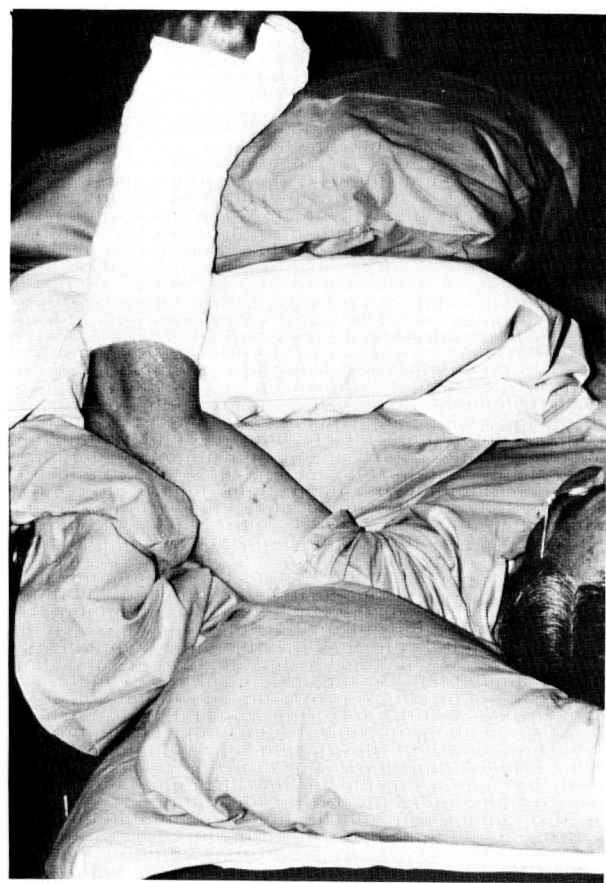

Fig. 27-1   Position of elevation while patient is supine.

Edema

The need to control edema is obvious when the effects of this condition are reviewed. Swelling around a joint causes stretching of the skin and soft tissue in that area, which in turn produces limited motion and ultimately increased scarring about the joint.[13] Elevation is the primary treatment for edema, and the proper position is with the wrist higher than the elbow and the elbow higher than the shoulder at all times, regardless of whether the patient is lying, sitting, or standing. Just exactly what is meant by elevating the hand is subject to broad interpretation by the patient unless it is specifically spelled out and constantly reinforced until the edema is gone.

Lying down, the patient can properly elevate the hand by positioning two to three pillows at his side (Fig. 27-1) or with the use of a commercial arm-elevation device.

When sitting, the patient should sit next to a table and place a stack of magazines or pillows under the elbow (Fig. 27-2).

When standing or walking, the patient should place his hand on top of his head (Fig. 27-3). Doing so will properly elevate the hand and is not so fatiguing for the upper extremity as just attempting to "salute the ceiling" with the hand.

Elevation is of prime importance in decreasing pain, especially in immediate postoperative situations, and this should be stressed to the patient. As healing progresses and

reaction decreases, the hand may still swell intermittently. The patient is instructed that when the hand does swell he should resume strict elevation until this again subsides.

In addition to elevation of the hand during treatment, active exercises,[1,8] massage in a distal-to-proximal direction,[7] and other measures such as the use of elastic compression garments and gloves and an intermittent compression unit[5] may be helpful to eliminate excess fluid in the hand.

Clinically the measurement of edema can be accomplished by the use of a commercially available water-displacement device (Fig. 27-4) or by recording of the circumferential measurements at certain landmarks on the hand and wrist, with care being taken to record the exact way in which the measurements are performed so that they can be repeated consistently on reevaluation.

Exercises

Active exercises are carried out entirely by the patient's own muscle power in the affected limb under varying degrees of encouragement by the therapist. Passive exercises are produced by a force other than normal contraction of the muscle—for example, by the therapist or by the patient using his unaffected hand to exercise his affected hand.

Active range-of-motion exercise is the only therapy of permanent benefit.[1] In active movement, the blood flow in the limb varies directly with the degree of activity in the muscle. Passive range-of-motion exercise produces very lit-

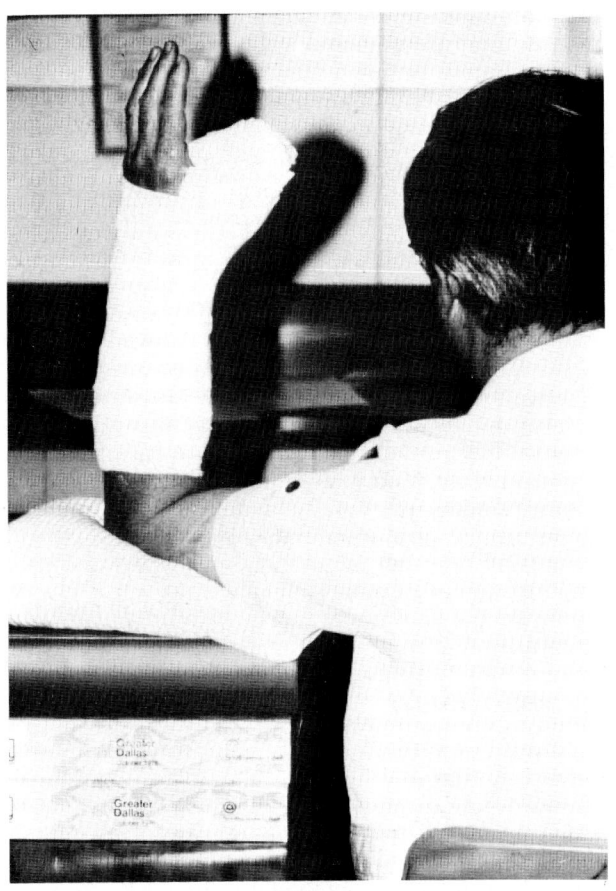

Fig. 27-2   Position of elevation while patient is sitting.

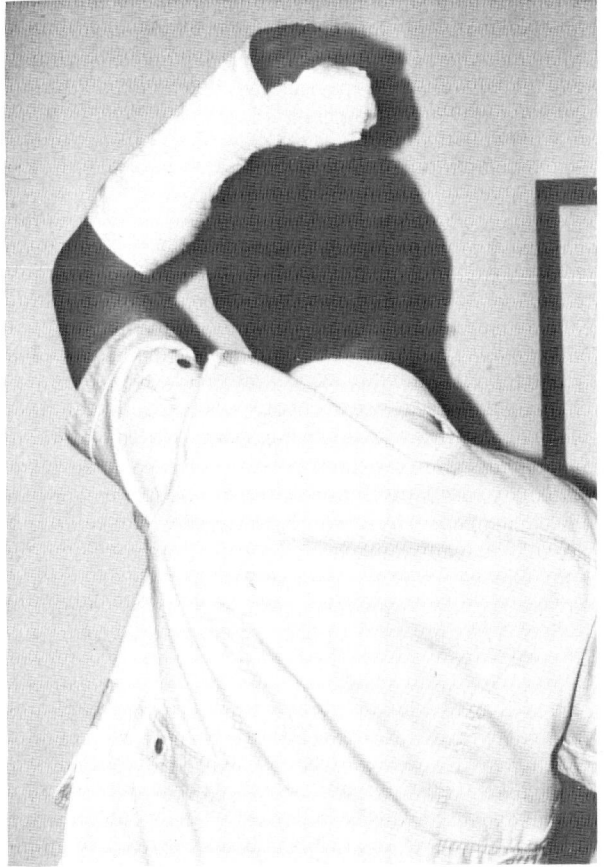

Fig. 27-3   Position of elevation while patient is standing.

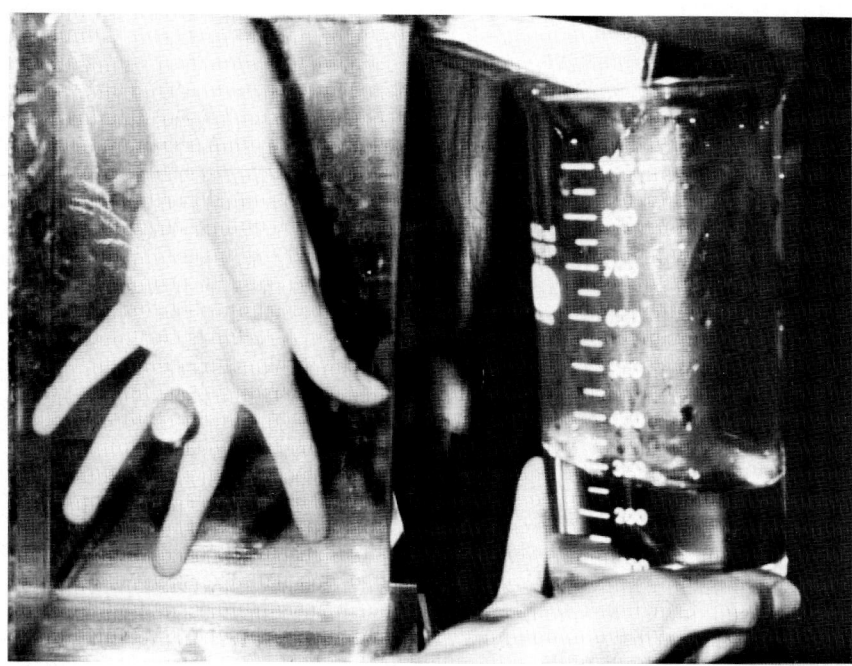

Fig. 27-4 Volumeter. This device calculates the degree of hand edema by measurement of water displacement. Measurements should be made bilaterally as a basis for comparison.

tle change in the blood flow of the limb, but it does tend to prevent adhesions between muscle planes and to maintain range of motion of the joints.[2]

Both passive and active exercises are important in improving motion after a capsulectomy. In attempting to decide what type of exercise program should be emphasized, determine whether passive motion exceeds active motion at a particular joint. If the passive motion exceeds the active motion, an active exercise program to overcome tendon weakness or adherence proximal to that site is necessary. If the passive motion does *not* exceed active motion, passive exercises to assist in overcoming the restriction in joint range of motion should *augment* the active exercise program.

The patient must learn that all active and passive exercises must be gentle enough to avoid tissue reaction, but frequent enough to gently stretch, but not tear, adhesions. The patient can usually be taught to apply the appropriate force for short periods of time, many times per day. The key to such self-treatment is the appreciation of the difference between discomfort and pain. The discomfort of a properly applied force is beneficial and should be tolerated, because the tissues will gradually yield to such treatment. The amount of force and direction of its application must be reduced until the discomfort is tolerable and the tissue reaction is not excessive.

The patient should be instructed in the specific reasons for and the correct way to perform the individual exercise programs. The exercises are best done in small amounts, frequently throughout the day, and for a certain number of repetitions. For example, the patient could be told to sustain each exercise effort for 10 seconds and repeat it five times on the hour while awake.

Splinting

Splinting is an important part of the postoperative rehabilitation of capsulectomies. A static progressive splint fitted while the parts to be splinted are being stretched allows the splint to conform to this forced fixed position and is useful in that the stresses developed in the tissues are transmitted to the offending scar.[13] When the scar matures and loosens, another splint is fitted to progressively increase the position desired. Thus a static progressive splint is helpful for night wear because it helps the patient keep the gains he has made during the day with his exercises. In the early stages after surgery, a static splint is safer for wear at night than a dynamic splint because of the edema and the possibility of circulatory constriction.

The use of dynamic splints is important for daytime wear as an adjunct to the patient's exercise program. When not exercising or performing skin care, the patient's hand must be splinted in the desired position to maintain and improve the surgical correction.

It is extremely important that the patient's splints are very closely monitored, and it may be necessary to change them daily. The patient needs to be given very detailed wearing instructions and precautions, and every step must be taken to ensure that the splints are as comfortable as possible.

Functional activities

Along with the specific exercises and splinting, it is beneficial to involve the patient in performance of some type of functional activity. It is not enough to regain a certain number of degrees in range of motion. This must be combined with the actual functional use of the hand by performance of some type of purposeful activity with tools and

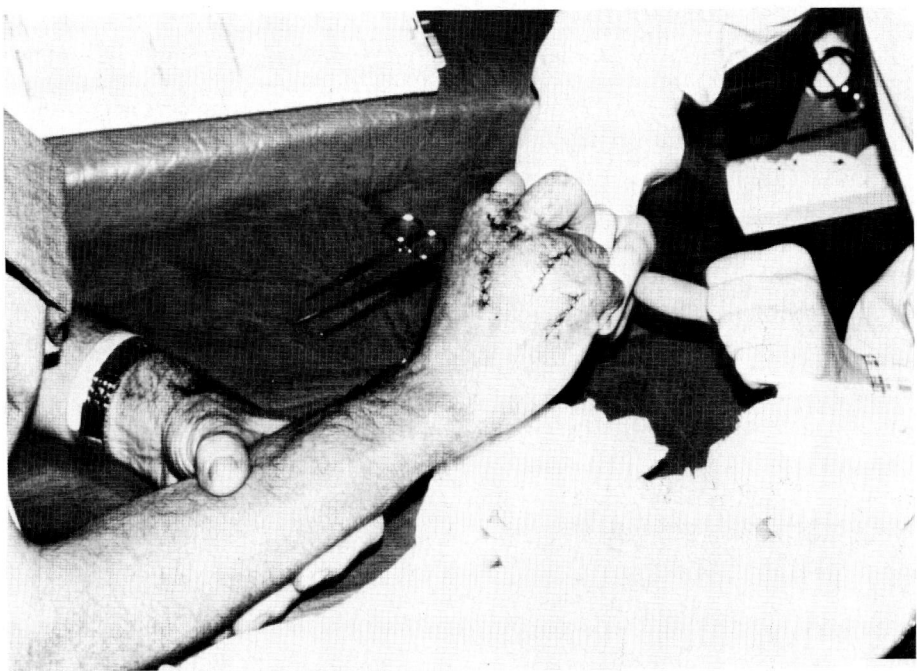

Fig. 27-5   Exercise program is usually started 1 to 3 days postoperatively.

materials.[9] The use of functional activities is also helpful in retraining the patient in the way in which he uses his hands and in showing him that the improvement in motion that he has gained from his capsulectomy has also upgraded the function of his hand.

• • •

Now that the general principles have been discussed, the specifics of treatment for patients who have undergone capsulectomies at the MP joint or at the PIP joint can be detailed. Most capsulectomy patients start their postoperative programs anywhere from the first to the third day after surgery (Fig. 27-5). The sutures remain in place from 14 to 21 days postoperatively. The patient must be taught skin care to avoid reactivity about the sutures or infection. These patients need to be closely monitored for 3 to 6 weeks after surgery. Maximum improvement from a capsulectomy may be expected 3 to 5 months postoperatively.[3]

METACARPOPHALANGEAL JOINTS

MP joint capsulectomies are performed to improve flexion. Exercise and dynamic splinting are the primary means of maintaining and increaasing the MP joint flexion gained through surgery.[13]

The patient should be carefully instructed in the passive and active exercises necessary. The metacarpals should be firmly stablized before force is applied to the proximal phalanx. It is extremely important to observe the patient's response to passive stretching and to be aware of his pain tolerance. Although some degree of discomfort is felt during passive exercise, the patient should be taught that this should

subside shortly after completion of the passive stretching. Active exercises are beneficial in decreasing edema and in preventing the joint surfaces from adhering during this edematous phase. Active exercise is necessary to maintain the gains made by the passive stretching. In general, the patient should perform both passive and active exercises after capsulectomy three to five times every 30 minutes to 1 hour while awake, depending on the edema and tissue reactivity.

Many patients undergoing MP joint capsulectomy have been using their digital extensors to extend their wrists for a long period of time, as is seen in patients who have had a Colles' fracture (Fig. 27-6). This substitution pattern has actually contributed to MP joint stiffness in extension or hyperextension. Preoperatively, it is important to recognize this pattern and attempt to reeducate and strengthen the wrist extensors in extending the wrist without the use of the digital extensors.[12] Patient reeducation and strengthening of the wrist extensors must continue postoperatively because if not watched closely, the patient will again be attempting to extend his wrist with his digital extensors, and so his efforts will be counterproductive to MP joint flexion.

Flexion splints for the MP joints can be fabricated to include either a volar or a dorsal forearm splint. The volar splint covers the forearm and palm to the distal palmar crease to provide stability of the wrist, but unfortunately, when dynamic traction is applied, the splint slips distally and flexion of the MP joints is blocked by the displaced edge of the splint.[13]

The use of a dorsal splint can avoid this problem. The outrigger arises from a volar forearm piece to provide the proper angle of 90 degrees on the proximal phalanges (Fig.

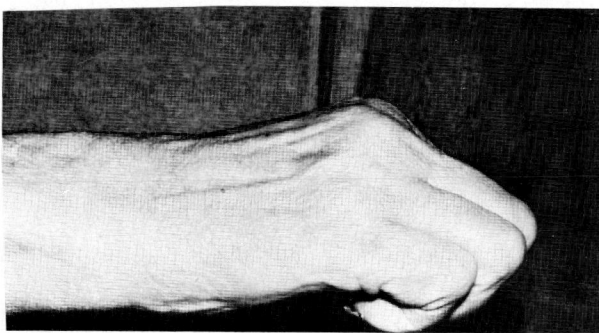

Fig. 27-6 Attempted wrist extension with digital extensors. This substitution pattern is counterproductive to finger flexion and must be overcome to develop range of motion in flexion and to develop grip strength.

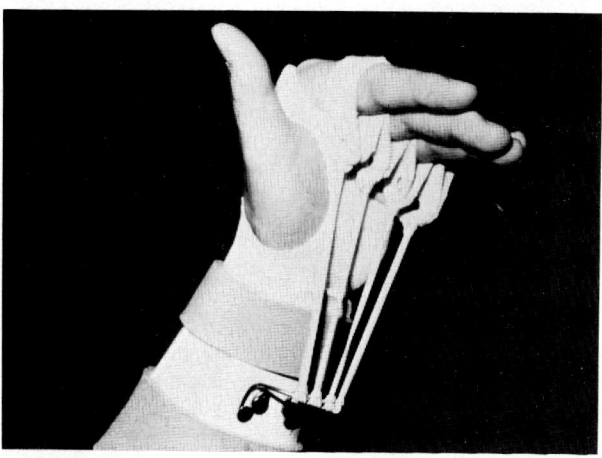

Fig. 27-7 Dorsal splint with dynamic metacarpophalangeal joint flexion slings. This splint, worn during the day after metacarpophalangeal joint capsulectomies, adequately stabilizes the wrist, supports the metacarpal arch, and flexes the metacarpophalangeal joints.

27-7). To ensure stability, this dorsal splint must include a properly fitting metacarpal bar, which should be thin, rounded, and positioned proximally to the distal palmar crease. When the proper force of the splint is established and there is no evidence of decreased circulation or pressure areas, the patient gradually increases the amount of time that the splint is worn during the day.[11]

In the early stages after surgery, when edema is still a problem, the wearing of the patient's dynamic splint may aggravate the edema or produce pressure areas. Therefore a progressive static splint to be worn at night to extend the wrist and flex the MP joints is made, of either plaster or thermoplastic material (Fig. 27-8), and is preferable in assisting the patient in keeping the gains that he has made during the day with his exercises.

PROXIMAL INTERPHALANGEAL JOINTS

The PIP joints more often become fixed in flexion than they do in extension, but a capsulectomy may be required for either condition.

Extension contracture

Initially, the exercise program includes passive flexion and extension of the PIP joint and active blocked flexion and extension exercises. The patient is instructed to do these exercises three to five times on the half-hour or every hour while awake.

The joint is splinted alternately in flexion and extension in a dynamic splint during the day. According to how the patient progresses, it may be necessary to splint the joint alternately each night in flexion and extension or only in flexion.

Alternating the dynamic action can keep the joint mobile during the period of fibrous tissue deposition and organization.

If intrinsic releases are performed with the PIP joint capsulectomy, it is necessary to splint the joint in the position of intrinsic stretch—with the MP joints extended and the

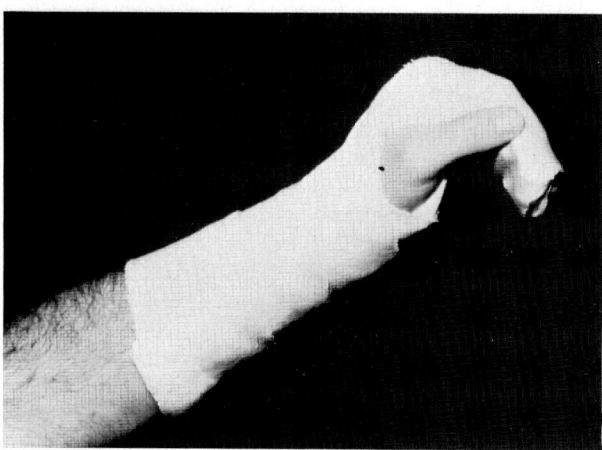

Fig. 27-8 Progressive static splint. For night wear after a metacarpophalangeal joint capsulectomy, this splint keeps the wrist in extension and the metacarpophalangeal joints in maximum flexion. Use of a stockinette to secure the splint in place is preferable to elastic wraps, which have a greater chance of causing edema and circulatory constriction.

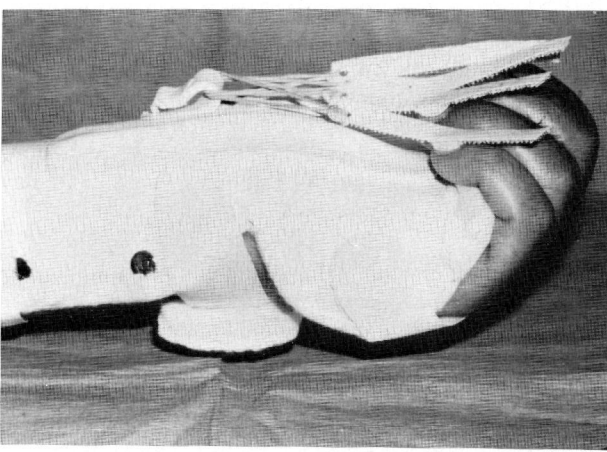

Fig. 27-9 Intrinsic stretch position splinting. When intrinsic releases are carried out with proximal interphalangeal joint capsulectomies, the hand needs to be splinted with the metacarpophalangeal joints extended and the proximal interphalangeal joints flexed.

PIP joints flexed (Fig. 27-9). Intrinsic stretch exercises (Fig. 27-10) should be part of the postoperative exercise regimen.

Flexion contracture

Depending on the severity of the flexion contracture to be corrected and the preferred method of the surgeon, the PIP joint may be pinned in extension after a capsulectomy. PIP joint exercises and splinting for capsulectomies performed to release flexion contractures in the PIP joints are initiated after the pins are removed. The patient is then fitted with a static finger-extension splint after the removal of the pin (Fig. 27-11). Extension is emphasized and maintained by the use of the splint because the extensor tendon has become so stretched as a result of the flexion contracture that it needs to be protected.[10] Failure to splint the finger constantly in extension after this procedure, except during exercise or skin care, will result in a recurrence of the flexion contracture.

The exercise program should include passive and active extension and active flexion exercises. One can encourage extension at the PIP joint by having the patient passively flex the MP joint while he attempts to extend the PIP joint actively (Fig. 27-12). In this manner, the power of the extrinsic extensors is transferred to the PIP joint and enhances the contribution of the intrinsics in extending that joint.

When the swelling diminishes, a dynamic PIP joint extension splint may be introduced and may be alternated with the use of a dynamic flexion splint during the day and a static extension splint at night, depending on the patient's progress.

If the oblique retinacular ligaments at the distal inter-

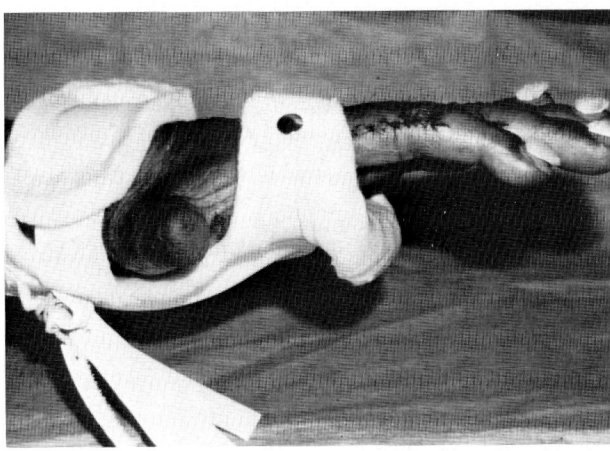

Fig. 27-10 Intrinsic stretch exercise. Holding the metacarpophalangeal joint in maximum extension and then attempting to flex the proximal interphalangeal joint puts the intrinsic muscle on a stretch.

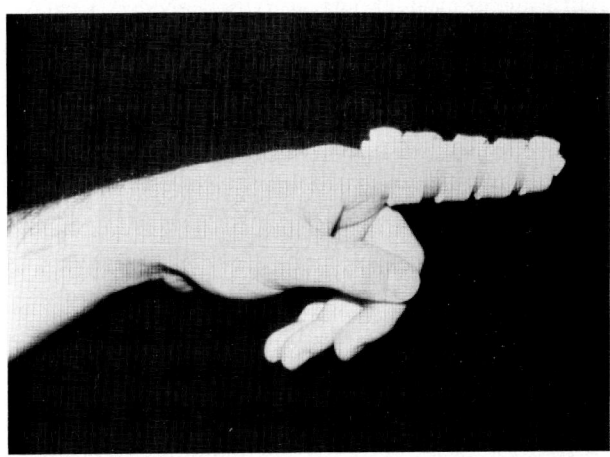

Fig. 27-11 Static finger extension splint. This is used after a proximal interphalangeal joint capsulectomy for a flexion contracture. The splint is padded and has soft strapping for comfort and ease of application and removal for exercises.

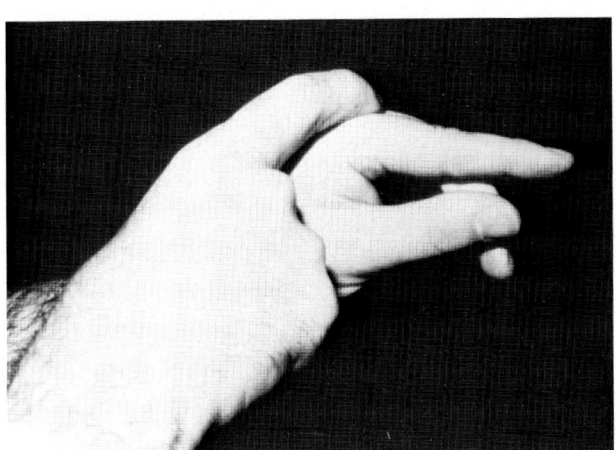

Fig. 27-12 Active extension of the proximal interphalangeal joint can be encouraged by holding the metacarpophalangeal joint in flexion while actively attempting to extend the proximal interphalangeal joint. This technique transfers the power of the extrinsic extensors and enhances the contribution of the intrinsics in extending the proximal interphalangeal joint.

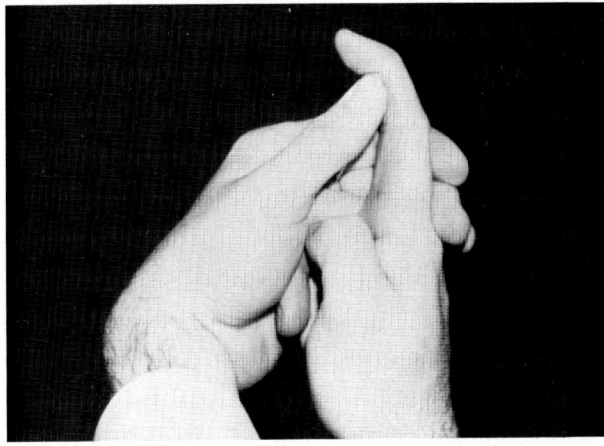

Fig. 27-13 Oblique retinacular ligament stretching is performed by stabilizing the proximal interphalangeal joint in maximum extension and then actively flexing the distal interphalangeal joint.

phalangeal joint have become tight because of a prolonged flexion contacture in the PIP joint, it is necessary to institute oblique retinacular ligament stretching exercises postoperatively (Fig. 27-13). During the finger flexion exercises, it is important for the patient to maintain wrist extension actively or passively so that the flexor tendons are working through their optimal range of motion.

CONCLUSION

The management of patients who have undergone either MP or PIP joint capsulectomy correlates closely with the management of acute hand injuries. Patient education before the surgery and the control of pain and edema after the surgery are critical factors in the success of the exercise and splinting programs in the patient after capsulectomy. The home exercise and splinting programs must be reviewed often and changed as the patient progresses.

Initially, after surgery these patients are encouraged to begin using the hand for light, everyday activities. A patient progresses to more dextrous activities and heavier tasks as the hand function improves. Skillful observation, accurate reevaluation, and adaptation on the part of the therapist in managing the patient's postoperative program, as well as the motivation and follow-through of the patient, are the keys to gaining and retaining improved range of motion and function after a capsulectomy procedure.

REFERENCES

1. Beasley RW: Principles of managing acute hand injureis. In Converse J, McCarthy J, and Littler JW, editors: Reconstructive plastic surgery, ed 2, vol 6, Philadelphia, 1977, WB Saunders Co.
2. Boyes JH: Bunnell's surgery of the hand, ed 5, Philadelphia, 1970, JB Lippincott Co.
3. Carter PR: Personal communication, Dallas, 1983.
4. Curtis RM: Capsulectomy of the interphalangeal joints of the fingers, J Bone Joint Surg 36:1219, 1954.
5. Curtis RM; Management of the stiff hand. In Hunter JM and others, editors: Rehabilitation of the hand, ed 2, St Louis, 1984, The CV Mosby Co.
6. Gould J and Nicholson B: Capsulectomy of the metacarpophalangeal and proximal interphalangeal joints, J Hand Surg 4(5):482, 1979.
7. Knapp ME: Massage. In Kottke F, Stillwell GK, and Lehmann JF, editors: Krusen's handbook of physical medicine and rehabilitation, ed 3, Philadelphia, 1982, WB Saunders Co.
8. Kottke FJ: Therapeutic exercise to maintain mobility. In Kottke FJ, Stillwell GK, and Lehmann JF, editors: Krusen's handbook of physical medicine and rehabilitation, ed 3, Philadelphia, 1982, WB Saunders Co.
9. Lankford LL, Carter PR, and Magnenat GF: The value of a hand therapy unit in rehabilitation of the disabled hand. Unpublished paper, Dallas, 1977.
10. Littler JW: Principles of reconstructive surgery of the hand. In Converse J, McCarthy J, and Littler JW, editors: Reconstructive plastic surgery, ed 2, vol 6, Philadelphia, 1977, WB Saunders Co.
11. Malick MH: Manual on dynamic hand splinting with thermoplastic materials, Pittsburgh, 1974, Harmarville Rehabilitation Center.
12. Rosenthal EA: The extensor tendons. In Hunter JM and others, editors: Rehabilitation of the hand, ed 2, St Louis, 1984, The CV Mosby Co.
13. Weeks PM and Wray RC: Management of the stiff hand. In Management of acute hand injuries, St Louis, 1978, The CV Mosby Co.

VI
TENDONS

28

Nutritional aspects of tendon healing

Peter C. Amadio, Scott H. Jaeger, and James M. Hunter

Controversy over nutritional and healing pathways in tendons has existed since well before the start of the twentieth century. In 1852 Sir James Paget[36] studied the healing of Achilles tendons in rabbits and concluded that the "nucleated blastema" that formed derived from the cut tendon ends rather than the sheath of surrounding soft tissue. William Adams, studying the same animal model 2 years later, came to the opposite conclusion.[1] Over 100 years later there is still discussion about whether tendon as a tissue has the potential to heal an injury; the extent to which such "intrinsic" healing occurs in actual clinical practice is still unknown.

An increasing amount of information is available on tendon nutrition and metabolism. By correlating data from anatomic, biochemical, physiologic, and clinical research conducted over the past decade, a perspective for better

understanding of this crucial problem for the hand surgeon and the hand therapist may be achieved.

ANATOMIC DATA

Injection studies of flexor tendons have delineated the pattern of vascular anatomy by tendon and by digit.[25,29,33] Outside the digital sheath, tendons have an excellent blood supply, arriving through circumferential mesotendineal vessels. An infolding of this mesotendineum allows this type of vascular nutrition to extend into the proximal portion of the digital sheath as well. Within the sheath, blood is carried to the tendon through a series of vincula, whose number varies from digit to digit[33] and which decrease in extent with age.[29] Between the vascular domains of the vincula, relatively avascular watershed zones are seen[25] (Fig. 28-1). These watershed zones vary in size and number by digit

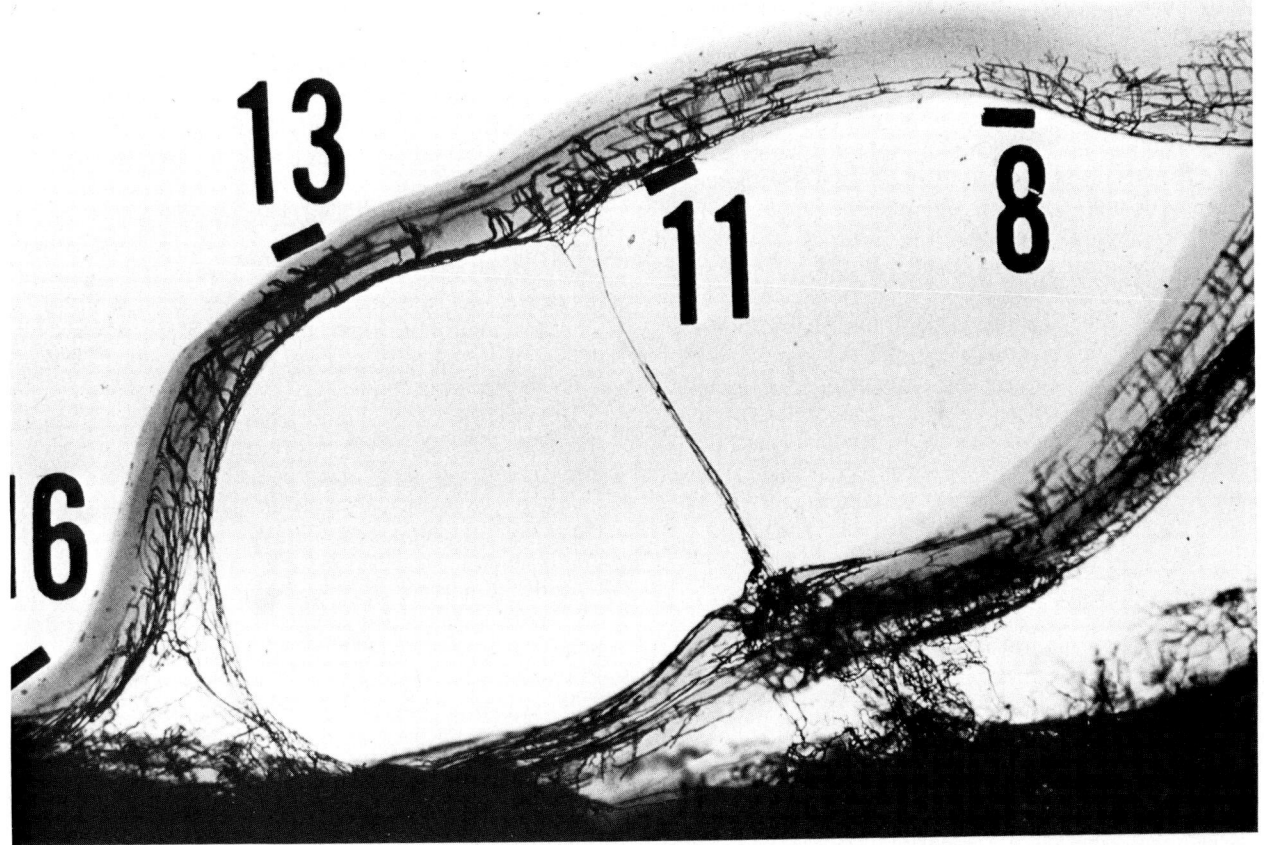

Fig. 28-1 Injection study showing the typical vascular pattern in human flexor tendons. Note the volar avascular area between marker 8 and marker 11.

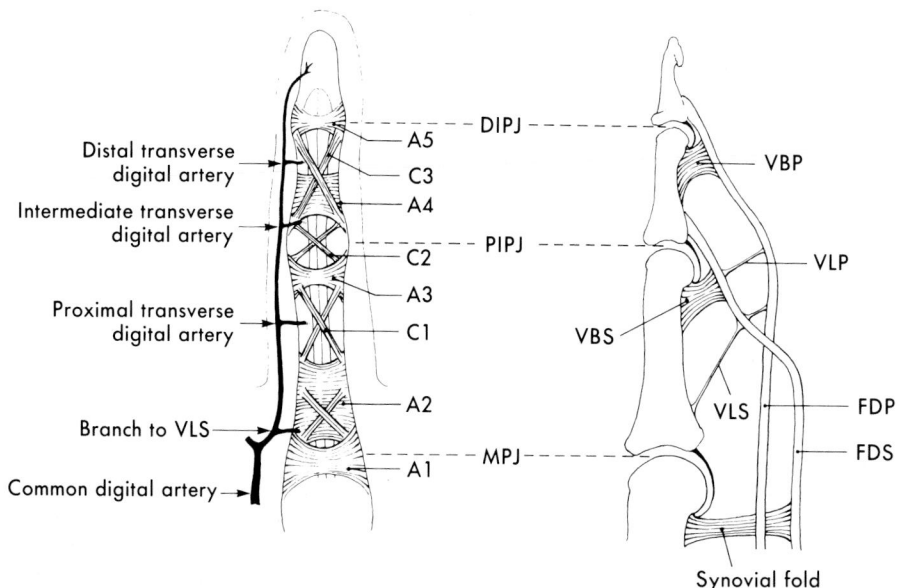

Fig. 28-2 The annular *(A)* and cruciate *(C)* pulleys, along with their relationship to the joints and the transverse branches of the digital artery, which nourish the tendon sheath and the vincula. *VBP*, short vinculum to profundus; *VLP*, long vinculum to profundus; *VBS*, short vinculum to the superficialis; *VLS*, long vinculum to the superficialis; *FDP*, flexor digitorum profundus; *FDS*, flexor digitorum superficialis; *MPJ*, metacarpophalangeal joint; *PIP*, proximal interphalangeal joint; *DIP*, distal interphalangeal joint.

and increase in size with advancing age.[29]

The vincula are known to be fed by constant branches of the digital arteries, which take their origin roughly at the level of the metacarpophalangeal and interphalangeal joints. These branches are in jeopardy during surgical dissection to expose the neurovascular bundles or the lateral margins of the pulley system.

The flexor pulley system has been well described by Doyle,[7] who provided the currently accepted nomenclature of annular and cruciate pulleys (Fig. 28-2). The importance of the fibrous pulleys in controlling active motion by prevention of bowstringing is well known. More recently, Weber[46] has studied the nutritional role the pulleys might play in providing a firm opposing surface to the volar, avascular areas of tendon, allowing for contact lubrication and pumping of nutrients into the interstitium in a manner similar to that seen in articular cartilage. Lundborg[22-24] has shown that tenocytes in the volar avascular areas reside in lacuna-like structures, as chondrocytes do. Recent biochemical and physiologic data suggest that the volar tendon and cartilage analogy extends beyond microscopic appearance, as discussed later in this chapter[11,12,18,34,35] (Table 28-1).

Table 28-1 Tendon

	Compression	Tension
Cells	In lacunae	Along collagen fibers
Blood supply	Avascular	Vascular
GAG	C-6-S	DS
PG	50% HMW	90% LMW
Collagen	Type I	Type I
Fibril size	Small	Large
Fibril orientation	Random	Parallel to tension

BIOCHEMICAL DATA

Research in tendon biochemistry has focused on two areas: intracellular mechanisms and extracellular matrix composition.

Tenocyte systems have been used by biochemists for many years in the study of collagen metabolism and its regulation. These cells have been shown to be very active metabolically, with the ability to divide, migrate, and alter the mechanical properties of tendon in response to a variety of stimuli. In both cell and tissue culture, tenocytes synthesize large amounts of type I collagen and smaller amounts of a number of glycosaminoglycans (GAG).[13,16,19] Although small in absolute amount, these GAGs are important in regulating the size and shape of the collagen fibrils and therefore control the ultimate material properties of the tendon itself.[18] All the respiratory enzymes needed for aerobic and anaerobic metabolism are present in tenocytes.[16]

In the presence of serum, tenocytes, even of mature animals, will divide; recent experiments[13,27,33] have shown that a serum clot encasing a plug of rabbit tendon provides sufficient nutrition for cell division and, if fibrin is added to the system, the tenocytes will migrate out of the plug along the fibrin strands.[5]

Both the number and organization of collagen fibrils in tendon are under tenocyte control. When experimental animals are exercised, the stressed tendons hypertrophy, with increases in both collagen content and tensile strength.[45,47] Cells grown on a pulsating membrane not only synthesize collagen, but also orient the fibers parallel to the lines of tension.[19,44]

In living tendon the collagen fibers are oriented longitudinally and consist of a bimodal population of very large and more numerous small fibrils.[37,38] The large fibrils have great tensile strength and increase in number with exercise.[47] The smaller fibrils, with high surface-to-volume ratios, bind extensively to each other and to the larger fibrils, giving excellent resistance to creep deformation[43] (that is, "stretching out"). A given quantity of collagen then might have very different mechanical properties, depending on the fibrillar organization.

The regulation of fibril size in tendon has been studied in experimental animals. The critical factor appears to be the type of GAG that the cells synthesize.[11] Tenocytes typically secrete dermatan sulfate GAG in the form of low molecular weight, nonaggregating proteoglycan. This low molecular weight proteoglycan appears to bind directly to the collagen fibril, allowing closer packing of large fibrils around a dermatan sulfate proteoglycan core. Tendon cells exposed to compressive stress respond by synthesizing a large molecular weight, chondroitin-sulfate–rich proteoglycan. This large proteoglycan serves to disperse collagen fibrils and inhibit fibril aggregation. The net effect is a network of small, randomly oriented fibrils.[18]

In the absence of tension, collagen organization is significantly disturbed. Beckham[6] treated chick embryos with curare and found that development of tendon and tendon sheath was completely arrested in the absence of movement.

Where tendons pass through a fibro-osseous sheath, the areas of the tendon directly beneath the fibrous pulley experience compressive forces. This area of the tendon has been shown to be rich in chondroitin sulfate, measuring about 3.5% of the dry weight. On the opposite side or the tension surface of the tendon, the GAG is much less, only about 0.5%, and it is almost all dermatan sulfate.[11,18] (GAG is about 9% of the dry weight of articular cartilage.) The compression side has a higher percentage of smaller fibrils than the tension side, consistent with the hypothesis that, with less tensile stress, fewer large "tensile" fibrils would be made. Gillard[11] performed an experiment in which he transposed the tendon away from the pulley, eliminating the "compression side." Biochemical analysis of the transposed tendon showed a decrease in total GAG toward 0.5% and the conversion of GAG type to dermatan sulfate, a trend that was reversed when the tendon was relocated beneath the pulley.

It is interesting to speculate on the possible nutritional relevance of the data just presented. The volar, avascular areas of human tendon are exposed to compressive forces; increased chondroitin sulfate in this area would, by dispersing the collagen fibrils, provide a better milieu for diffusion of nutrients from the synovial fluid into the tendon. Weber[46] has recently demonstrated that this volar area does indeed have increased diffusional capability and that this capacity was increased by tendon motion, suggesting a milking action similar to that seen in articular cartilage. The work of Salter[42] has demonstrated the benefit of early passive movement in the healing of cartilage injury.

Recent studies have begun to investigate the effect of continuous passive motion (CPM) on tendon healing. Preliminary results show that CPM has little effect on reduction of adhesions after tenolysis; studies on the effect of CPM on tendon healing after tendon injury are currently underway. Studies by Gelberman[10] and others have already confirmed the utility of intermittent passive motion on tendon healing; recent work by Hitchcock[15] suggests early active motion, where possible, may be the best of all.

PHYSIOLOGIC DATA

The relative contribution of synovial and vascular nutritional pathways to tendon inside the digital sheath has been the subject of considerable debate. This point has clinical relevance, since frequently tendon injury includes some damage to the vincular system. The resulting avascular areas can be extensive (Fig. 28-3). If synovial nutrition plays a small role, such injuries would be practically doomed to adhesions and a poor result. If synovial nutrition is significant, even avascular tendons might survive to heal without restricting adhesions.

Manske[26,28] has reported a series of experiments comparing the relative contribution of synovial and vascular routes in nutrition in metabolic studies of hydrogen washout and amino acid uptake. His work shows a much greater and more rapid uptake of nutrient by the synovial fluid pathway. Lundborg[14,22] developed an experimental model in which segments of rabbit tendon were encased in dialysis tubing (to prevent cellular migration from synovium) and implanted within the knee joint as a "tissue culture in situ." He showed not only preservation of viability in this system, but also attempts at healing of experimental wounds to the implanted tendon. In this model, the healing cells appeared to rise from both the epitenon and tenocytes themselves. These studies indicate an important role for synovial fluid in tendon nutrition.

No discussion of the physiology of tendon healing would be complete without mention of the classic work of Potenza.[39-41] In his dog model, experimental tendon injuries were repaired within the flexor sheath and treated, in the then-standard way for humans and for uncooperative laboratory animals, by immobilization. This work repeatedly demonstrated a lack of intrinsic response within the tendon, with all healing arriving from the sheath and surrounding soft tissue by way of adhesions. This work also showed that more extensive soft-tissue injury such as resection of sheath, or of superficialis tendon in the case of profundus repair, caused much greater adhesions. Even forceps marks on the tendons stimulated adhesion formation.[40] For many years, the well-documented evidence from this study was used to support the hypothesis that there was no potential for intrinsic healing in any injured tendon within a fibroosseous sheath. Subsequent work by McDowell and Synder,[30] however, demonstrated that even with a dog model this might not be the case. They pointed out that since the vincular system is poorly developed in the dog, the only potential for tendon nutrition within the sheath is by diffusion of synovial fluid. Because the Potenza model calls for complete tendon immobilization, the pumping mechanism is lost, this route is blocked, and the tendon is left with inadequate nutrition. In a partial injury model permitting active motion, adhesion-free healing can occur in the dog tendon system, showing that the postinjury treatment regimen plays an important role in the overall quality of the result after tendon injury.

Salter[42] has shown that avascular cartilage heals experimental wounds much better if motion, and therefore active diffusion, occurs. The same may be true for the analogous avascular areas in tendons. In the McDowell model, the sheath is not disturbed, a partial injury is creased in the tendon, and no immobilization occurs, thus allowing continued free synovial nutrition. Uniformly, these dog tendons

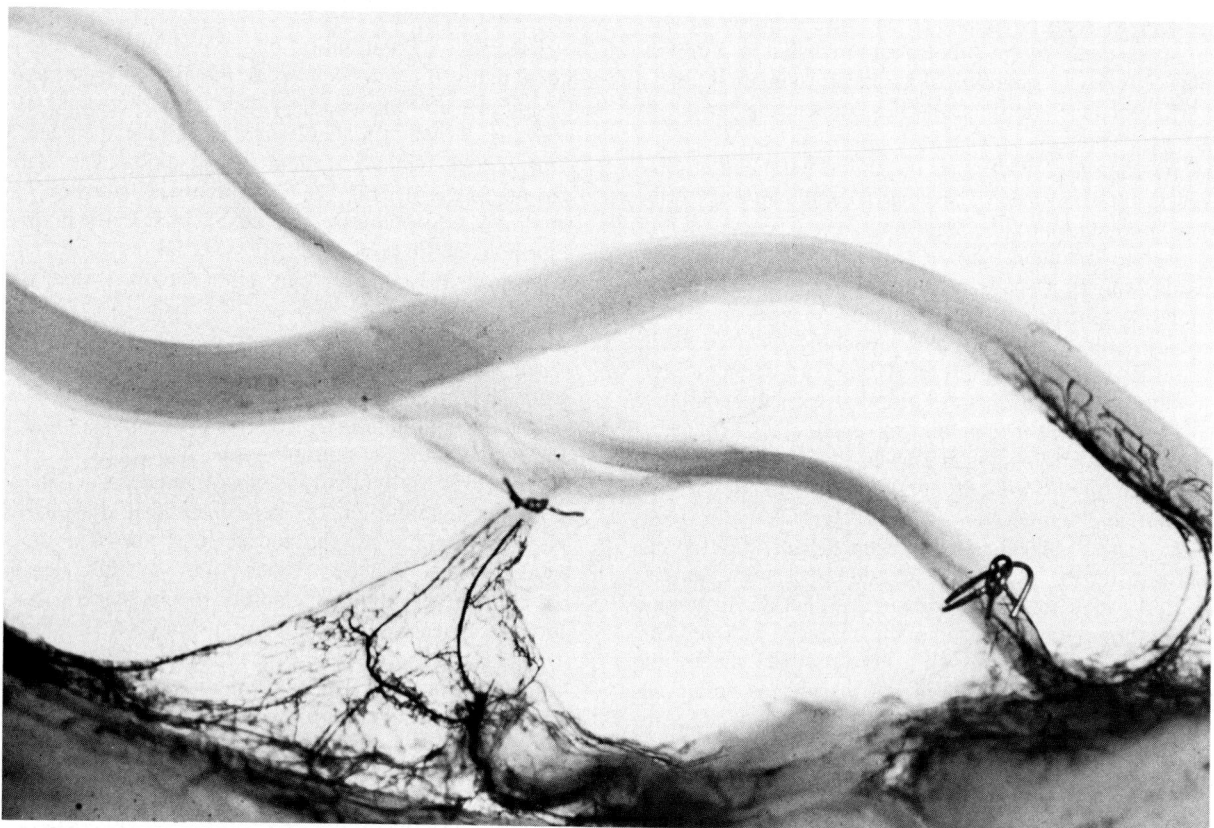

Fig. 28-3 Injection study as in Fig. 28-1, but with the two vincula to the superficialis ligated, showing loss of intratendinous circulation not only in the superficialis but also in the profundus.

were able to heal without adhesions. More recent work by Schepel,[17] in a primate model perhaps more similar to the human case, was again able to demonstrate adhesion-free tendon healing when vincula and synovial relationships were not disturbed.

All this evidence suggests that when experimental conditions that avoid ischemia can be created, adhesion-free tendon healing can apparently occur.

The careful control evident in laboratory experiments unfortunately cannot be brought into the clinical situation completely, not only because of variables related to the type of injury, but also because of patient variables such as number and location of vincula and quality of synovial fluid nutrition. Matthews[31,32] has shown by injection studies that in cases of experimental injury to rabbit flexor tendons, adhesions formed only when the experimental injury had caused a loss of vascularity to the cut tendon end. This varied with the level of injury. This line of evidence would suggest that although synovial nutrition is sufficient for homeostasis and limited healing, in tendon systems in which a vincular system is well developed, both routes may be required for healing of major tendon injury.

Recent clinical studies have also shown that vincular injury is a major determinant of the result after tendon injury. When vincular structures remain uninjured, clinical results are typically good; similar tendon injuries associated with vincular damage do significantly less well.[4]

A clinical demonstration of the importance of blood supply to tendon healing may also exist in the case of the common trigger finger. Histologic examination of trigger tendons shows degenerative changes similar to those found in other collagenous structures where hypovascularity and attrition take their toll, such as the rotator cuff of the shoulder.[2] Light and electron microscopy have shown similar pathologic features, including calcification, in both conditions. When the relative frequency of triggering by digit[9,21] is compared with the known distribution of vincula as calculated by Ochiai and associates,[33] an interesting correspondence is noted (Table 28-2). The anatomic location of tendon swelling and degeneration in trigger fingers is usually in the hypovascular watershed areas of the flexor profundus and superficialis; perhaps it represents a hypertrophy because of a relative lack of nutrient flow.

A COMPOSITE PICTURE

Sufficient data have accumulated over the past decade to confirm that tendon is a vital, dynamic tissue. Tenocytes respond to mechanical stimuli to modify their intercellular matrix strength and permeability. Nutrition arrives through both synovial and vascular sources; where both are present, both are important. Given adequate nutrition, tenocytes can divide and migrate and have been shown now in several different species to be capable of adhesion-free healing.[17,30]

Figure 28-4 outlines our current concept of the self-regulation of tendon structures. Tenocytes respond to changes in mechanical stress by altering the type and amount of glycosaminoglycan synthesized and thereby the spacing and amount of collagen fibrils, thus altering tendon strength.

Table 28-2 Tendon

Finger	Relative frequency of triggering (%)*	Absent vinculum longus superficialis (%)†	Absent vinculum longus profundus (%)†
Index	10	10	0
Middle	39	40	12
Ring	39	55	10
Little	12	10	3

*From Lipscomb PR: Surg Clin North Am 24:780-794, 1944.
†From Ochiai N, Matsui J, Miyaji N and others: J Hand Surg 4:321-330, 1979.

Permeability to nutrients, important in maintaining the higher metabolic level required at increased synthetic rates, is also changed. The changes in matrix strength then modify the perceived stress on the cell, completing the self-regulatory loop. The entire process is modified by tissue age and available base-line vascular nutrition. When the system fails, degenerative changes such as triggering can occur and the response to injury is modified.

CLINICAL APPLICATION

These concepts of tendon healing can be applied in the approach to the patient with flexor tendon injury. The goal is to restore the best possible environment for tendon healing and to maintain it throughout the recovery period.[25] As a first step, it is important to obtain a better understanding of the anatomy of the injury. To this end, a record should be made not only of the level of injury on the skin with relation to the flexion creases, as described by many authors, but also of the level with regard to tendon and vincular anatomy. Bleeding of tendon ends can also be evaluated before repair. All lacerated tendons should be repaired with a volar, non-hemostatic, minimally reactive nonabsorbable suture. Careful handling of the tendon is important, since the work of Potenza has clearly shown that all areas of forcep or clamp violation of epitenon serve as foci for adhesions. A circumferential repair at the tendon juncture may help to invert tendon fibers and present a smooth surface to facilitate rapid reestablishment of epitenon continuity. It may also add strength to the repair.[20] Finally, the tendon sheath is repaired to restore the potential for synovial fluid nutrition. Sheath closure may also help prevent triggering of the tendon juncture as it glides through the pulley system.

Postoperatively, early mobilization techniques are employed to apply controlled tension to the repair site, to stimulate tenocyte synthesis, and to promote the milking action of sheath or synovial fluid penetration of the tendon. We have used a combination of the methods described by Kleinert[17] and by Duran and Houser[8] to provide differential gliding of profundus and superficialis and also the dynamic effects of active extension with passive flexion with positioning of the wrist and metacarpophalangeal joints to further control the maximum possible tensile stress exerted on the repair.

One may plan the duration of the postoperative protection by the type of healing that is occurring. In a patient with more severe vincular or sheath damage or in the older person, more extrinsic adhesions are expected, and earlier release from immobilization and protection might be advised. The reasons are that we believe healing by extrinsic means is quicker than by the intrinsic route and that the adhesions accompanying extrinsic healing need to be "stretched" so that their restrictive effect on motion is minimized as soon as possible.[3] On the other hand, in the younger patient with intact vincula and a well-repaired sheath, a good potential for intrinsic tendon healing is anticipated. These patients might be protected longer, particularly if they rapidly develop a full active range of motion when voluntary flexion is initiated.

THE FUTURE

Increased knowledge of tendon nutrition and tendon biology will further our understanding of the metabolic processes called into play after tendon injury and the cells responsible for them. Whether the healing cells arise from within the tendon or from the surface of the tendon, float freely across the synovial space, or are some combination of the three is ultimately less important than the concern that they do their job without physically binding tendon to sheath with adhesions. We now know that such adhesion-free healing can occur. In the future, it will be necessary for us to use our growing understanding to select more precisely those patients in whom such healing is possible and preserve this fragile capability through appropriate repair and rehabilitation. In those patients in whom such healing is not possible, alternative forms of hand rehabilitation must be pursued. Our ultimate goal is to provide for each patient with flexor tendon injury an individually tailored solution that will result in a predictably successful outcome.

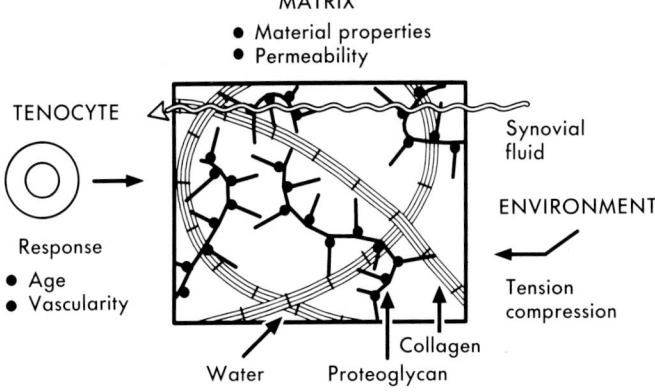

Fig. 28-4 The tenocyte and its environment.

REFERENCES

1. Adams W: On the reparative process in human tendons. 1; also a series of experiments on rabbits, London, 1860, Churchill.

2. Amadio PC, Frasca P, and Hunter JM: Histology and SEM and flexor tendons in trigger fingers, Trans Orthop Res Soc 7:345, 1982.

3. Amadio PC and Hunter JM: Prognostic factors in flexor tendon surgery in zone 2. In Hunter JM and others, editors: Tendon surgery in the hand, St. Louis, 1987, The CV Mosby Co.

4. Amadio PC and others: The effects of vincular injury on the results of flexor tendon surgery in zone 2, J Hand Surg 10A(5):626, 1985.

5. Becker H and others: Intrinsic tendon cell proliferation in tissue culture, J Hand Surg 6(6):616, 1981.

6. Beckham C, Dimond R, and Greenlee TK Jr: The role of movement in the development of a digital flexor tendon, Am J Anat 150:443, 1978.

7. Doyle JR and Blythe W: The finger flexor tendon sheath and pulleys. In American Academy of Orthopaedic Surgeons: Symposium on tendon surgery in the hand, St. Louis, 1975, The CV Mosby Co.

8. Duran RJ and Houser RG: Controlled passive motion following flexor tendon repair in zones 2 and 3. In American Academy of Orthopaedic Surgeons: Symposium on tendon surgery in the hand, St. Louis, 1975, The CV Mosby Co.

9. Fahey JJ and Bollinger JA: Trigger finger in adults and children, J Bone Joint Surg 36A:1200, 1954.

10. Gelberman RH and others: Effects of early intermittent passive mobilization on healing canine flexor tendons, J Hand Surg 7:170, 1982.

11. Gillard GC and others: The influence of mechanical forces on the glycosaminoglycan content of the rabbit flexor digitorum profundus tendon, Connect Tissue Res 7:37, 1979.

12. Gillard GC and others: The proteoglycan content and axial periodicity of collagen in tendon, Biochem J 163:145, 1977.

13. Graham MD and others: Intrinsic tendon healing documentation by vitro studies, J Orthop Res 1:251, 1983.

14. Hansson HA, Lundborg G, and Rydevik B: Restoration of superficially damaged flexor tendons in synovial environment, Scand J Plast Reconstr Surg 14:109, 1980.

15. Hitchcock TF and others: The effect of immediate constrained digital motion on the strength of flexor tendon repairs in chickens, J Hand Surg 12A:590, 1987.

16. Jósza L and others: Histochemical and ultrastructural study of adult human tendon, Acta Histochem 65:250, 1979.

17. Kleinert HE, Schepel S, and Gill T: Flexor tendon injuries, Surg Clinic North Am 61:267, 1981.

18. Koob TJ and Vogel KG: Proteoglycan synthesis in organ cultures from regions of bovine tendon subjected to different mechanical forces, Biochem J 246:589, 1987.

19. Leung DY, Glagov S, and Mathews MB: Cyclic stretching stimulates synthesis of matrix components, Science 191:475, 1979.

20. Lin G-Y and others: Biomechanical studies of running suture for flexor tendon repair in dogs, J Hand Surg 13A:553, 1988.

21. Lipscomb PR: Chronic nonspecific tenosynovitis and peritendinitis, Surg Clin North Am 24:780, 1944.

22. Lundborg G and Rank F: Experimental intrinsic healing of flexor tendons based upon synovial fluid nutrition, J Hand Surg 3:21, 1978.

23. Lundborg G and Rank F: Experimental studies on cellular mechanisms involved in healing of animal and human flexor tendon in synovial environment, Hand 12:3, 1980.

24. Lundborg G, Holm S, and Myrhage R: The role of the synovial fluid and tendon sheath for flexor tendon nutrition, Scand J Plast Reconstr Surg 14:99, 1980.

25. Lundborg G, Myrhage R, and Rydevik B: The vascularization of human flexor tendons within the digital synovial sheath region: structural and functional aspects, J Hand Surg 2:417, 1977.

26. Manske PR and Lesker PA: Comparative nutrient pathways to the flexor profundus tendons in zone II of various experimental animals, J Surg Res 34:83, 1983.

27. Manske PR and Lesker PA: Histologic evidence of intrinsic flexor tendon repair in various experimental animals: an *in vitro* study, CORR 182:297, 1984.

28. Manske PR, Whiteside LA, and Lesker PA: Nutrient pathways to flexor tendons, J Hand Surg 3:32, 1978.

29. Matsui T and others: Vascular anatomy of flexor tendons, part II, J Jpn Orthop Assoc 53:307, 1979.

30. McDowell CL and Synder DM: Tendon healing: an experimental model in the dog, J Hand Surg 2:122, 1977.

31. Matthews P: The pathology of flexor tendon repair, Hand 11:233, 1979.

32. Matthews JP: Vascular changes in flexor tendons after injury and repair: an experimental study, Injury 8:227, 1979.

33. Ochiai N and others: Vascular anatomy of flexor tendons. I. Vincular system and blood supply of the profundus tendon in the digital sheath, J Hand Surg 4:321, 1979.

34. Okuda Y, Gorski JP, and Amadio PC: Effect of postnatal age on the ultrastructure of six anatomical areas of canine flexor digitorum profundus tendon, J Orthop Res 5:231, 1987.

35. Okuda Y and others: Biochemical, histological, and biomechanical analyses of canine tendon, J Orthop Res 5:60, 1987.

36. Paget J: Lectures on surgical pathology, p 266, London, 1853.

37. Parry DAD, Barnes GG, and Craig AS: A comparison of the size distribution of collagen fibrils in connective tissues: a function of age and a possible relation between fibril size distribution and mechanical properties, Proc R Soc Lond 203:305, 1978.

38. Parry DAD, Craig AS, and Barnes GRG: Tendon and ligament from the horse; an ultrastructural study of collagen fibrils and elastic fibers and elastic fibers as a function of age, Proc R Soc Lond [Biol] 203:293, 1978.

39. Potenza AD: Effect of associated trauma on healing of divided tendons, J Trauma 2:173, 1962.

40. Potenza AD: Prevention of adhesions to healing digital flexor tendons, JAMA 187:187, 1964.

41. Potenza AD: Tendon healing with the flexor digital sheath in the dog, J Bone Joint Surg 44A:49, 1962.

42. Salter RB and others: The effect of continuous passive motion on healing of full thickness defects in articular cartilage, J Bone Joint Surg 62A:1232, 1980.

43. Scott JE: Proteoglycan-collagen arrangements in developing rat tail tendon, Biochem J 195:573, 1981.

44. Slack C, Flint MH, and Thompson BM: The effect of tensional load on isolated embryonic chick tendons in organ culture, Conn Tiss Res 12:229, 1984.

45. Videman T, Eronen I, and Candolin T: Effects of motion load changes on tendon tissues and articular cartilage, Scand J Work Environ Health 5(suppl 3):55, 1979.

46. Weber ER, Hardin G, and Haynes D: Synovial fluid nutrition of flexor tendon. In Hunter JM, Schneider LH, and Mackin E, editors: Tendon surgery in the hand, St. Louis, 1987, The CV Mosby Co.

47. Woo SL-Y and others: The biomechanical and biochemical properties of swine tendons: long term effects of exercise on the digital extensors, Connect Tissue Res 7:177, 1980.

29

Primary care of flexor tendon injuries

Stephen L. Cash

Over the past two decades the acute repair of flexor tendon injuries has become the standard of care among the majority of hand surgeons.[8-12,14] Earlier, the frequent complications of scarring and poor tendon gliding led to the abandonment of primary repair in preference for tendon grafting. More recently the development of new surgical techniques, the use of early motion therapy programs, and the increase in knowledge of tendon physiology and healing have improved the results, and primary repair of the acutely injured flexor tendon has become popular again.

However, the problems of scarring, stiffness, and poor function continue to occur frequently enough to demand the attention and respect of the treating physician. This chapter focuses on the treatment of flexor tendon injuries within the flexor tendon sheath, the area in which restoration of function is most difficult.

ANATOMY

In 1980 at the First Congress of International Federation of Societies for Surgery of the Hand, agreement was reached in the nomenclature for the flexor tendon zones in the hand (Fig. 29-1):
- Zone I   Distal to superficialis insertion
- Zone II   From A-1 pulley to insertion of superficialis tendon
- Zone III From distal end of carpal tunnel to A-1 pulley
- Zone IV   Within carpal tunnel
- Zone V   Proximal to carpal tunnel

In the thumb, the zones are as follows:
- Zone T I   Distal to interphalangeal joint
- Zone T II   From A-1 pulley to interphalangeal joint
- Zone T III Thenar eminence
- Zone T IV   Carpal tunnel
- Zone T V   Proximal to carpal tunnel

The flexor tendon canal, or sheath, extends from the metacarpal heads to the insertion of the profundus tendon and is a synovium-lined fibrous tunnel that produces synovial fluid to facilitate tendon gliding as well as to aid in tendon nutrition and healing.

Discrete annular and cruciate thickenings in the sheath constitute the pulley system and improve the mechanical efficiency of tendon excursion by preventing bowstringing[4,5] (Fig. 29-2). The annular pulleys are thick and rigid and are composed of transverse fibers, whereas the cruciate pulleys that overlie the joints are thin and flexible to allow for motion. The A-2 and A-4 pulleys, firmly attached to bone, are generally recognized as the most critical to repair or

reconstruct after injury, although all the annular pulleys should be preserved when possible.

At the entrance to the sheath, the superficialis tendon lies volar to the profundus. As they both proceed distally, the superficialis splits into halves, each of which then rotates 180 degrees, spiraling around and then dorsally to the profundus before rejoining its counterpart and ultimately inserting into the middle phalanx (Figs. 29-3, 29-8, and 29-10). At this point the profundus lies volar to the superficialis and continues distally to insert into the distal phalanx. This fascinating anatomic arrangement of the tendons within the sheath has important implications for the surgeon, because lacerations across the proximal phalanx may injure the profundus alone and/or one or both slips of the superficialis. Restoring the correct orientation of the tendons and especially the correct rotation of the two superficialis slips with

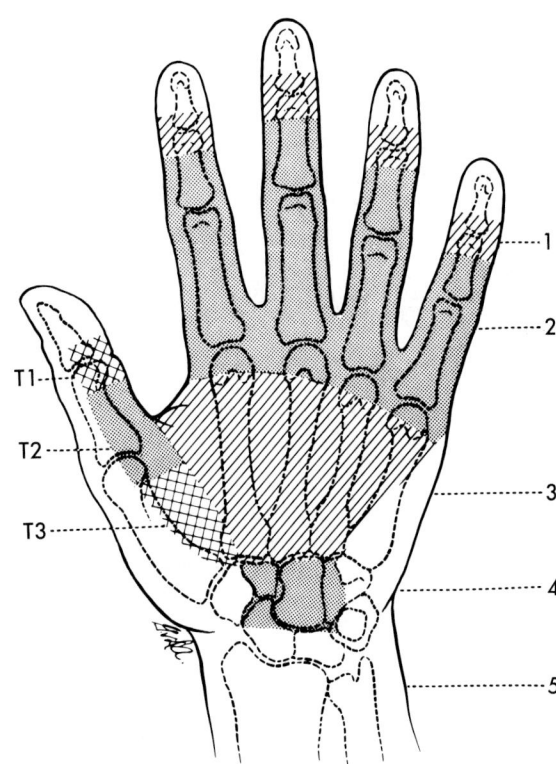

Fig. 29-1 Flexor tendon zones in the hand. (Reproduced by permission from Kleinert HE, Schepel S, and Gill T: Surg Clin North Am 61:267, 1981.)

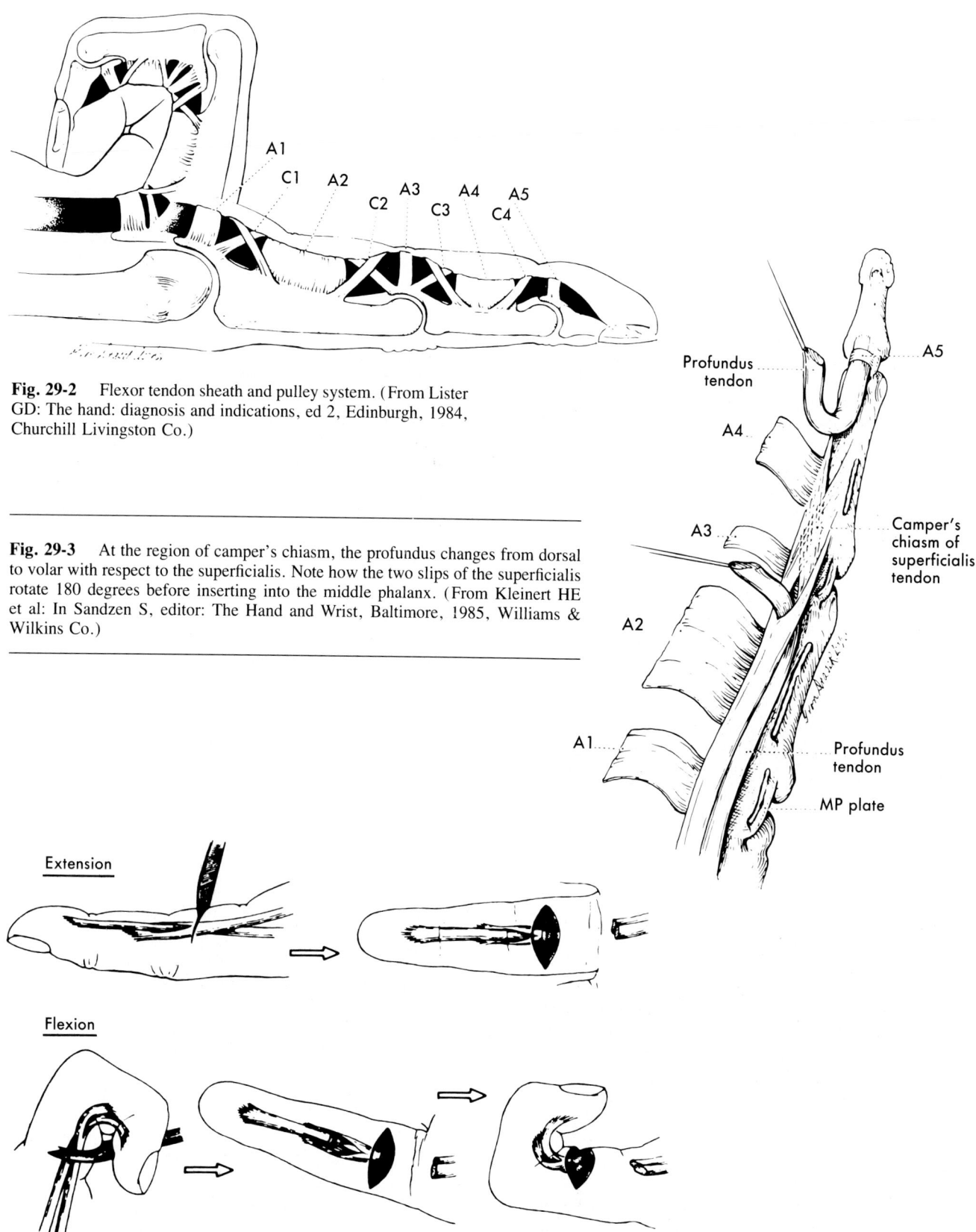

Fig. 29-2   Flexor tendon sheath and pulley system. (From Lister GD: The hand: diagnosis and indications, ed 2, Edinburgh, 1984, Churchill Livingston Co.)

Fig. 29-3   At the region of camper's chiasm, the profundus changes from dorsal to volar with respect to the superficialis. Note how the two slips of the superficialis rotate 180 degrees before inserting into the middle phalanx. (From Kleinert HE et al: In Sandzen S, editor: The Hand and Wrist, Baltimore, 1985, Williams & Wilkins Co.)

Fig. 29-4   When the injury occurs with the finger in extension, the level of skin wound and tendon laceration coincide. When the injury occurs with the finger in flexion, the level of tendon laceration will be distal to the skin wound when the finger is subsequently extended. (Reproduced by permission from Kleinert H, Kutz J, and Cohen M: Primary repair of zone 2 flexion tendon laceration. In AAOS Symposiun on Tendon Surgery in the Hand, St Louis, 1975, The CV Mosby Co.)

respect to the profundus is of paramount importance at the time of repair if unimpeded gliding of the tendons with respect to each other is to be obtained. Furthermore, if the finger is flexed at the time of injury, the level of tendon laceration will be distal to the site of skin laceration, and thus the latter alone is not necessarily a reliable indication of the extent of tendon injury (Figs. 29-4, 29-5, and 29-6). Clearly, a thorough knowledge of the flexor tendon/tendon sheath/pulley anatomy is required at surgery to restore the normal anatomic arrangement and critical tolerances of the intact system.

TENDON NUTRITION AND HEALING

It is believed that tendons receive nutrition through two systems—vascular perfusion and diffusion of nutrients from synovial fluid.

Vascular perfusion is more completely understood.[1,3,18,21,27] The blood supply to flexor tendons is segmented in origin. In extrasynovial areas, the blood supply is from the surrounding vascular paratenon and loose connective tissue. In synovial regions, that is, within the flexor tendon sheath, branches from the digital vessels reach the tendons via the vincula and anastomose with dorsally located

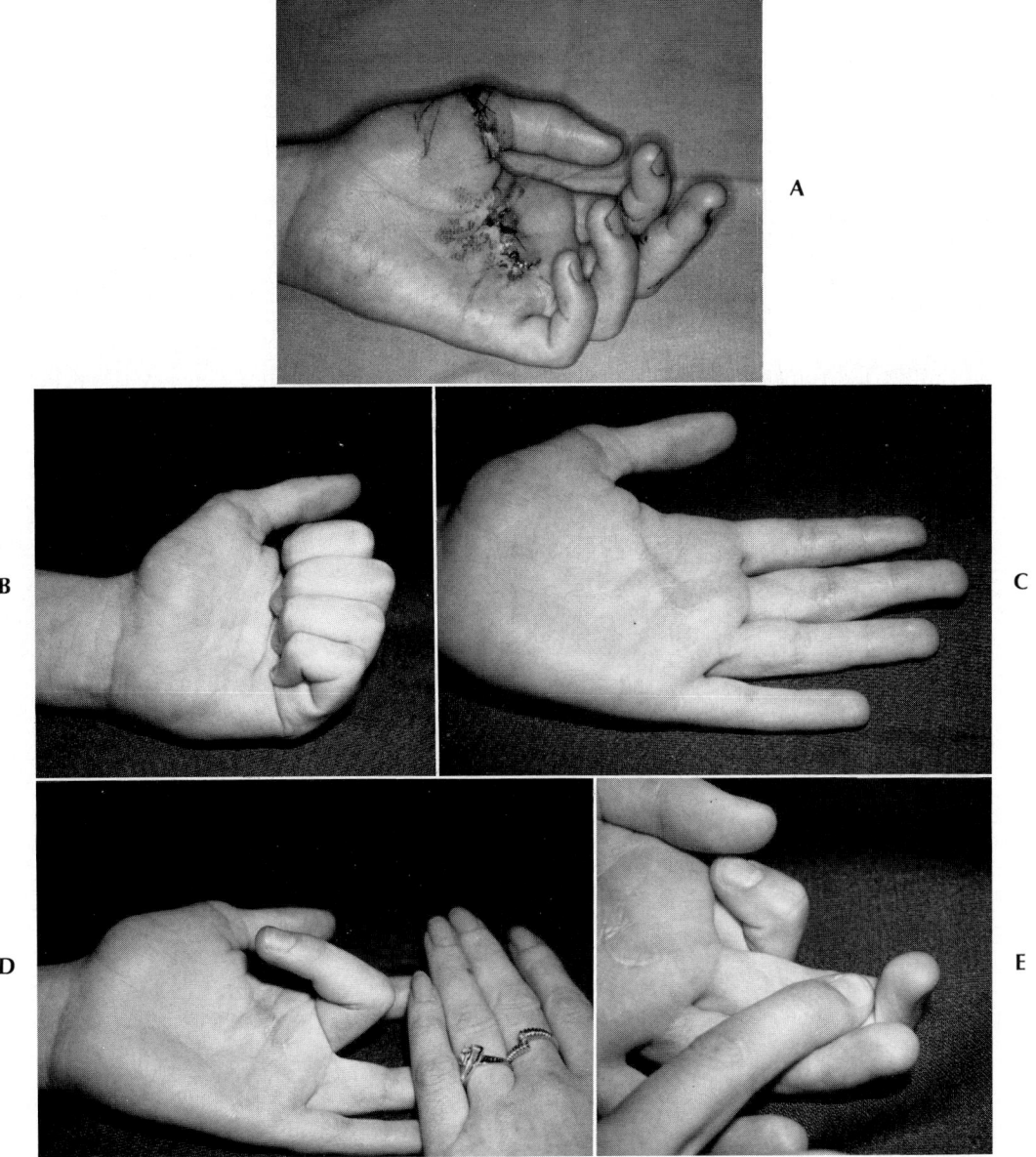

Fig. 29-5 **A,** Eleven-year-old girl with laceration in the palm. Posture of the DIP joint in full extension indicates complete profundus laceration whereas partial flexion at PIP joint suggests incomplete superficialis laceration. Although laceration of the skin is in the palm, the actual level of tendon injury with fingers extended was distal to the A_1 pulley, indicating zone II injury. All of the above were confirmed at surgery. **B** and **C,** Final result at 4 months. Complete flexion and extension. **D** and **E,** Independent function of the profundus and superficialis tendon demonstrated.

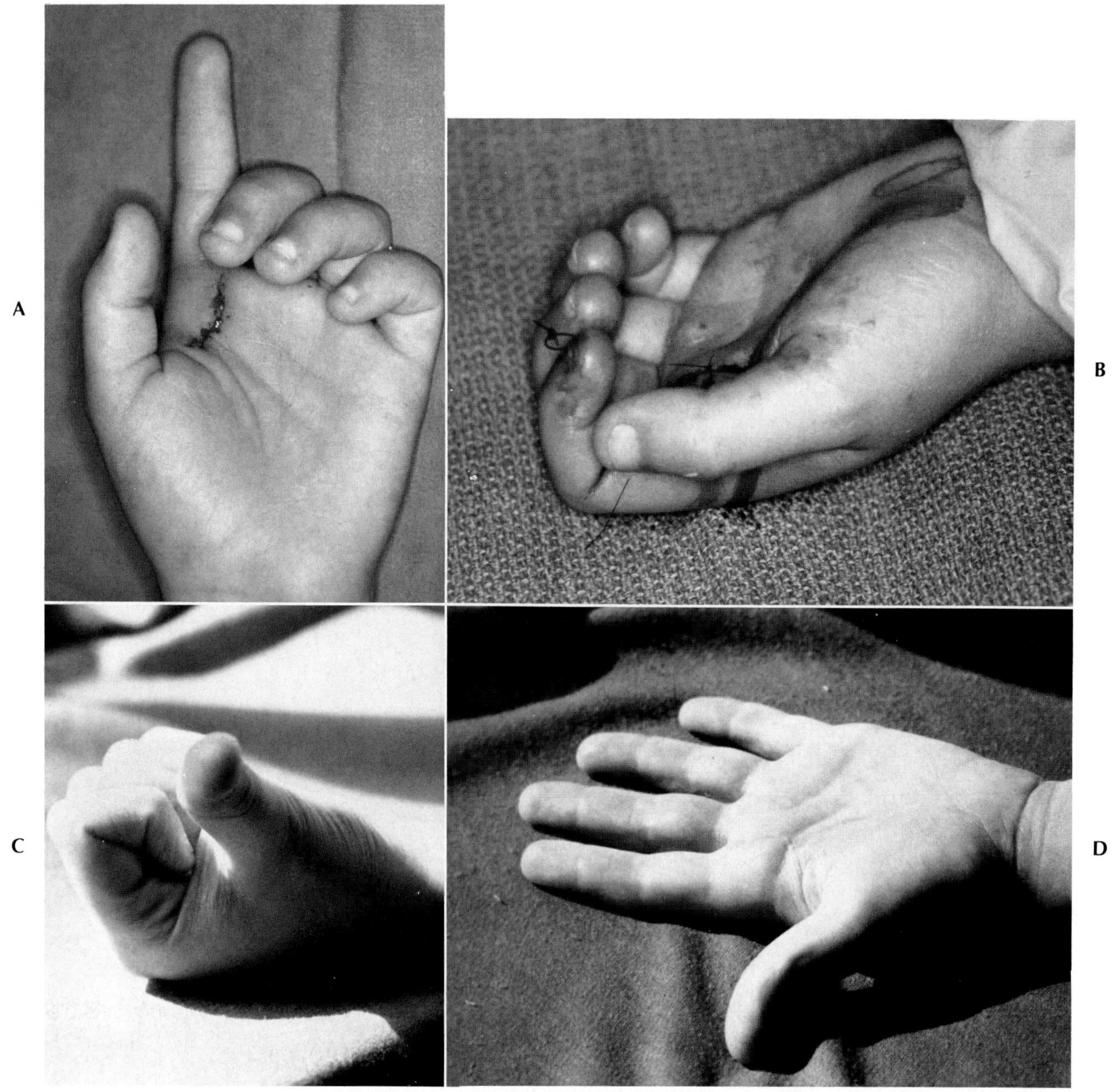

Fig. 29-6   **A,** Six-year-old boy with laceration in the distal palm. Position of the finger indicates complete laceration of both flexor tendons. Although the level of skin laceration suggests zone 3 injury, at exploration when the finger was extended, the level of tendon injury was distal to the A₁ pulley, confirming zone 2 injury. **B,** After repair of both tendons, normal posture of the finger was restored. **C** and **D,** Final result at 5 months. Full flexion and extension achieved.

longitudinal intrinsic vessels within the tendon (Figs. 29-7 and 29-8). In general, each tendon has one vinculum longus and one brevis, although considerable variation is not uncommon. In addition, there are areas of relative avascularity between the vincula and beneath the major pulleys, and the dorsal half of the tendon (where the vincula attach and blood vessels enter) is better perfused than the volar half.

Over the past 15 years, several radioisotope studies have demonstrated that diffusion of nutrients from synovial fluid constitutes an important source of tendon nutrition.[17,21] In contrast to the vascular system, there is no segmental distribution pattern, and the entire tendon can be nourished by diffusion alone. In addition, sequential compression of the tendon against the pulleys during flexion and extension can act as a "pumping" mechanism to increase diffusion of nutrients into the tendon.[33]

As recently as the mid-1970s, it was believed that flexor tendons healed only by an extrinsic process mediated by fibroblasts from surrounding tissues.[6,7,23,29] Although healing per se could occur, the resulting adhesions interfered with smooth tendon gliding. However, since then multiple studies have shown that injured flexor tendons have an intrinsic capacity to heal themselves.[16-18,20-23,25,26,32]

In vivo studies by Lundborg and Rank have shown that

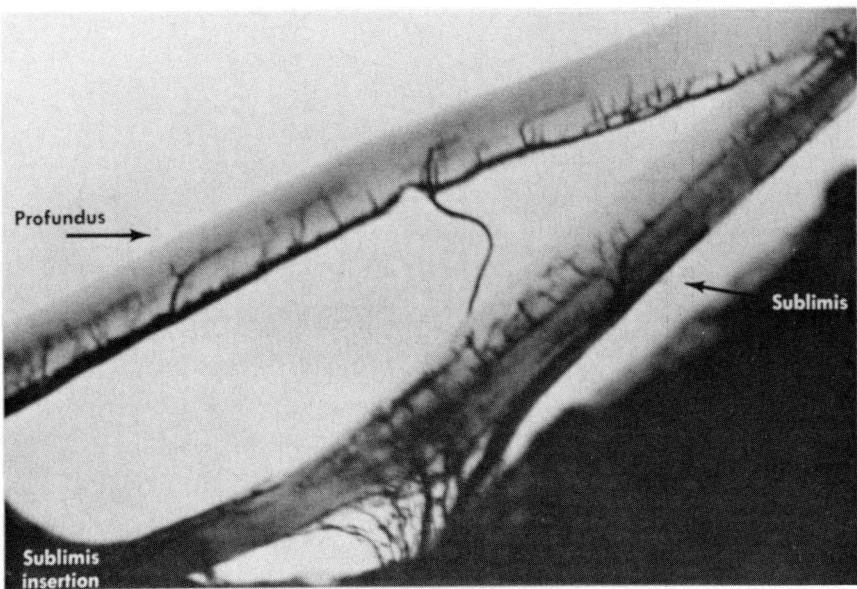

Fig. 29-7   Photomicrograph of an injection study of the intrinsic vascular system. Note the blood vessels traveling in the vincula anastomosing with longitudinally oriented vessels located in the dorsal half of each tendon. (Reproduced by permission from Caplan H, Hunter J, and Merken R: Intrinsic vascularization of flexor tendons. In AAOS Symposium on Tendon Surgery in the Hand, St Louis, 1975, The CV Mosby Co.)

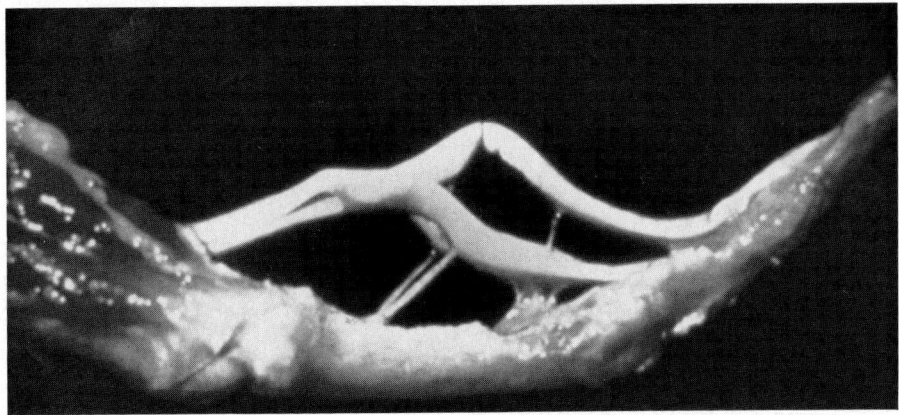

Fig. 29-8   Cadaver dissection demonstrating the vincula longus and brevis. Also note the profundus tendon passing between the two halves of the superficialis tendon. (Reproduced with permission from Johnson MK and Cohen MJ: The Hand Atlas, Springfield, Ill, 1975, Charles C Thomas, Publisher.)

isolated segments of tendon could heal in synovial fluid and tissue fluid environment.[19] In vitro studies by Manske demonstrated healing of tendon segments in tissue culture media devoid of any vascular source.[20,22,23] The conclusion from these studies is that flexor tendons have an intrinsic capacity to heal themselves without ingrowth of fibroblasts (that is, without scarring) in the absence of a vascular supply when nourished solely by synovial fluid.

The clinical significance and application of the foregoing with respect to healing of the injured human flexor tendon is as yet not clearly defined.[15,28,30,31] Theoretically, placement of suture material in the relatively avascular volar half of the tendon and closure of the tendon sheath at surgery should minimize interference with the tendon's intrinsic blood supply and maximize the synovial fluid environment

of the healing tendon. Whether these surgical maneuvers in fact facilitate tendon healing and promote better restoration of function remains to be proven, but most surgeons at this time will probably continue to employ these techniques in the belief that they are beneficial.

INDICATIONS AND TIMING OF TENDON REPAIR

The timing of tendon repairs depends on a number of factors. In general, the acutely impaired flexor tendon should be repaired as soon as possible.[8-12,14] Primary tendon repair is defined as repair usually within 12 hours but occasionally as long as 24 hours after injury. Delayed primary repair occurs between 24 hours and 10 days, early secondary repair between 10 days and 4 weeks, and late secondary repair after 4 weeks. The results of primary, delayed pri-

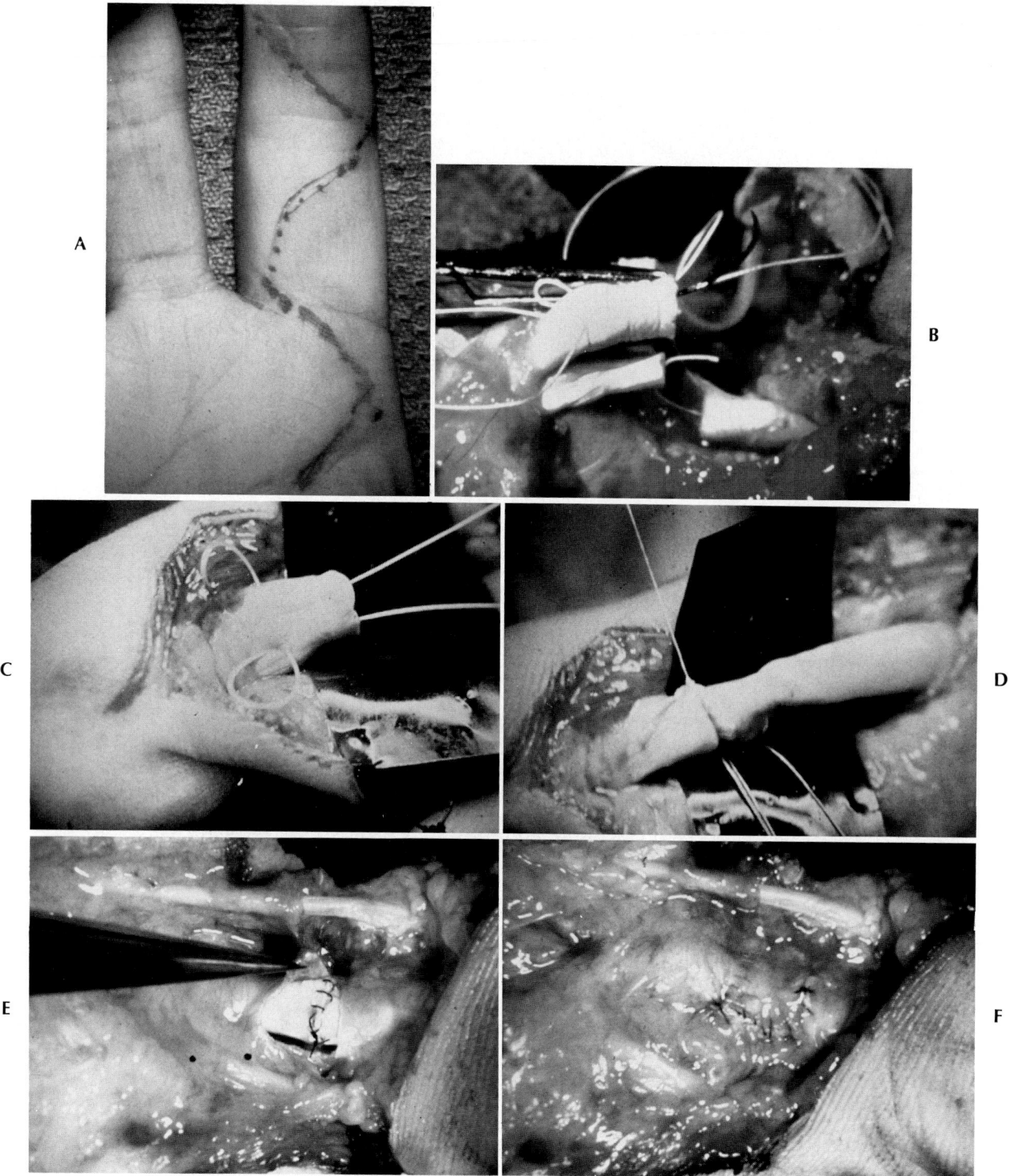

Fig. 29-9 **A,** Zone 2 laceration extended proximally and distally by Bruner zigzag incisions. **B,** Lacerated tendons can be grasped at the cut end with a piece of umbilical tape and hemostat to allow for atraumatic handling while core suture is inserted. **C,** Modified Kessler suture placed in one end of tendon. Loops will be tightened when final tension of repair is adjusted. **D,** Core suture tightened down. Tension must be adjusted accurately to avoid gapping and buckling. **E,** Tendon repair completed by placing a running 6-0 nylon suture in epitenon. **F,** Tendon sheath closed to complete repair. The finger is then taken through flexion and extension to check for unimpeded gliding of the repair tendon. **G,** Diagram of tendon suture technique. (Reproduced with persmission from Kleinert HE, Schepel S, and Gill T: Surg Clin North Am 61:267, 1981.

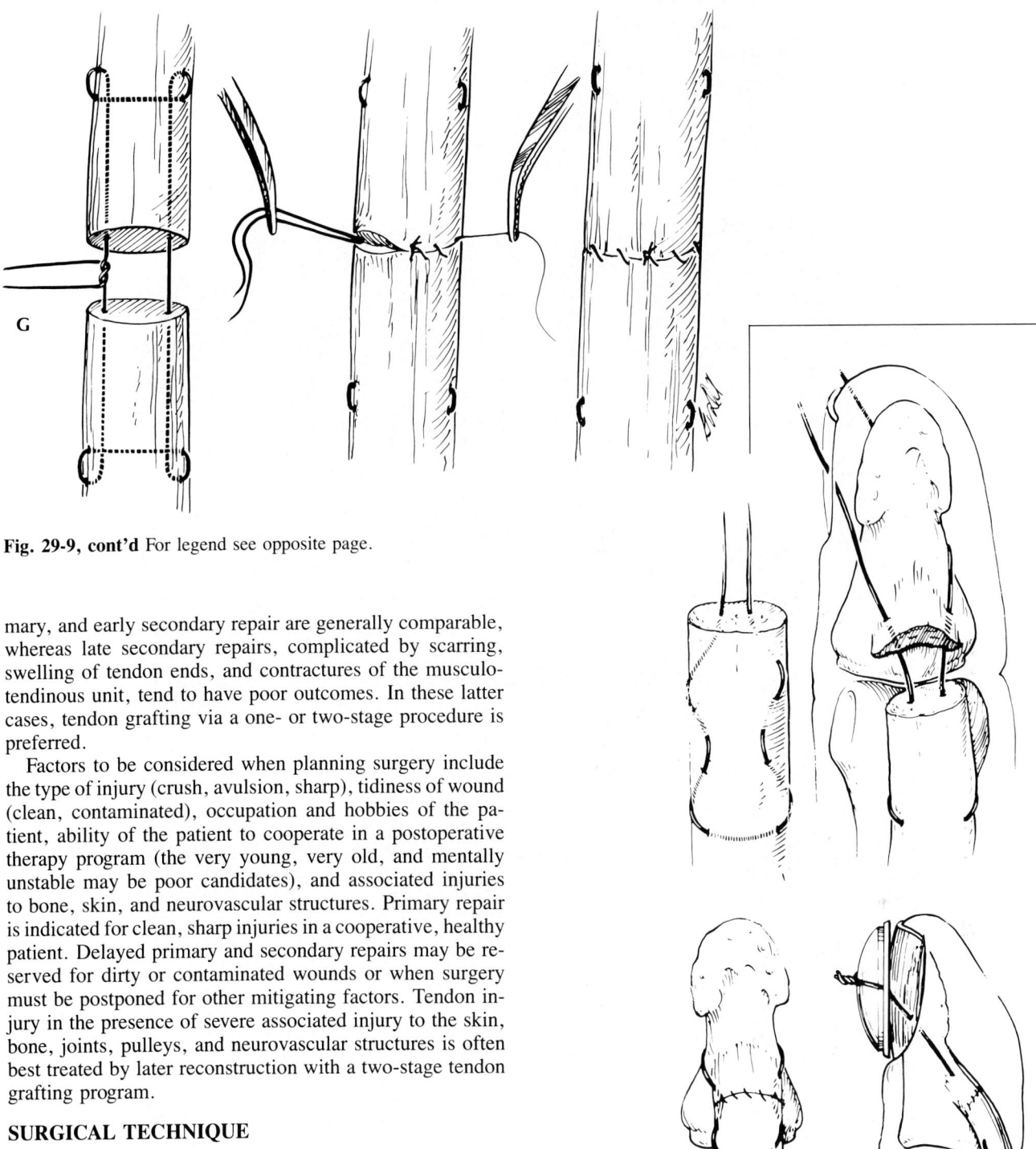

G

Fig. 29-9, cont'd For legend see opposite page.

mary, and early secondary repair are generally comparable, whereas late secondary repairs, complicated by scarring, swelling of tendon ends, and contractures of the musculo-tendinous unit, tend to have poor outcomes. In these latter cases, tendon grafting via a one- or two-stage procedure is preferred.

Factors to be considered when planning surgery include the type of injury (crush, avulsion, sharp), tidiness of wound (clean, contaminated), occupation and hobbies of the patient, ability of the patient to cooperate in a postoperative therapy program (the very young, very old, and mentally unstable may be poor candidates), and associated injuries to bone, skin, and neurovascular structures. Primary repair is indicated for clean, sharp injuries in a cooperative, healthy patient. Delayed primary and secondary repairs may be reserved for dirty or contaminated wounds or when surgery must be postponed for other mitigating factors. Tendon injury in the presence of severe associated injury to the skin, bone, joints, pulleys, and neurovascular structures is often best treated by later reconstruction with a two-stage tendon grafting program.

SURGICAL TECHNIQUE

General or regional block anesthesia is preferred, using a pneumatic tourniquet to provide a bloodless field, as well as loupe magnification to simplify identification of injured structures. The role of prophylactic intravenous antibiotics is controversial in clean injuries; I prefer to give 1 gm of cephalosporin before tourniquet inflation and repeat three to four times over the next 24 hours. In untidy or contaminated wounds this obviously may be continued longer. After a thorough debridement, the wound is best extended by Bruner zigzag incisions to allow identification of and access to all injured structures[2] (Fig. 29-9A). Bone and/or joint injuries are stabilized before actual tendon repair. The relative positions of the laceration through the sheath and ten-

Fig. 29-10 Advancement of profundus tendon into insertion at distal phalanx with pullout wire in zone I injury. (Reproduced with permission from Kleinert HE, Schepel S, and Gill T: Surg Clin North Am 61:267, 1981.)

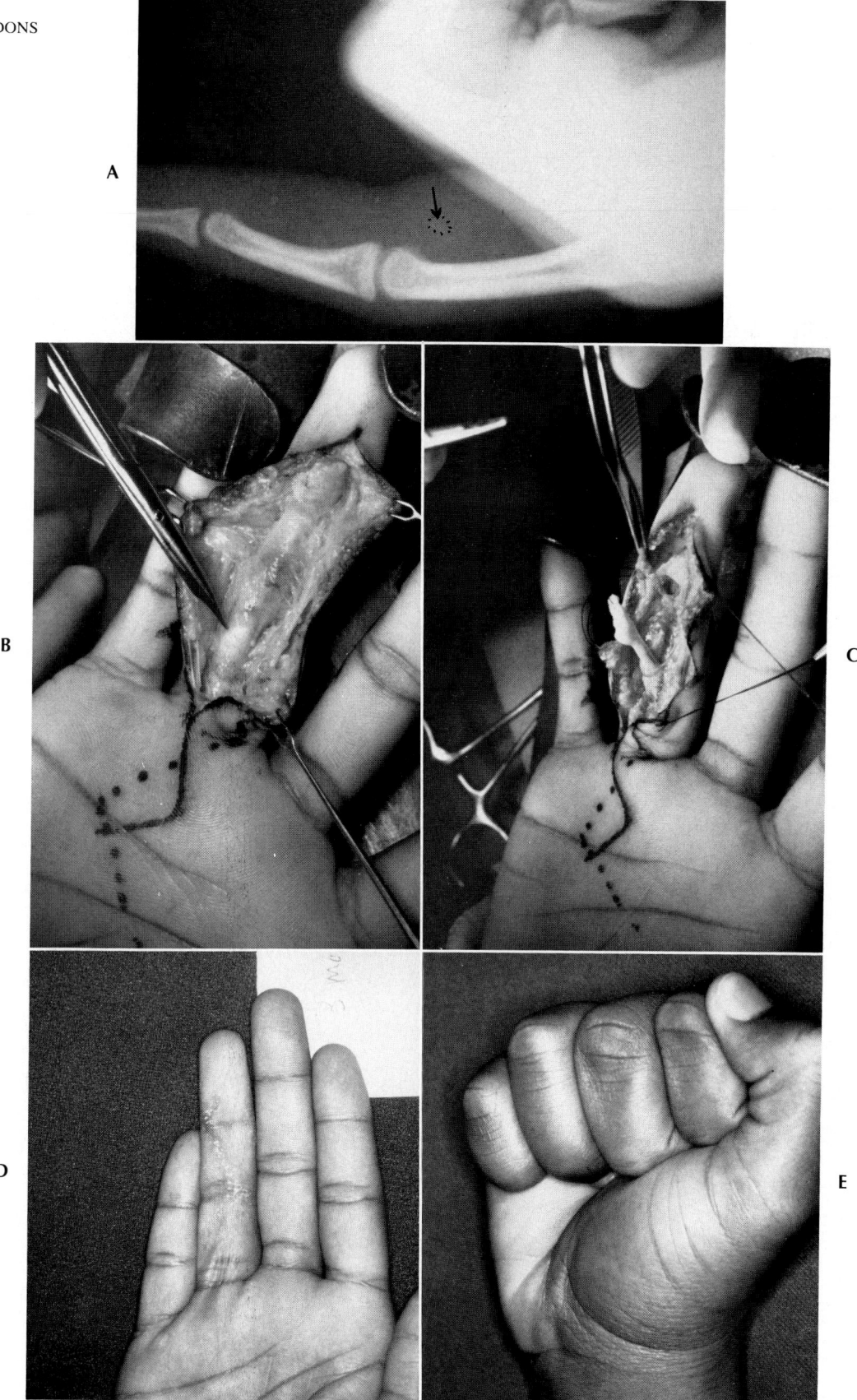

Fig. 29-11 **A,** Fifteen-year-old boy with an inability to flex the DIP joint of the ring finger 5 weeks after a football injury in which he tried to tackle an opponent by grabbing his jersey. The posture of the DIP joint in full extension and the presence of a faint bony spicule on radiograph just proximal to the PIP joint suggests avulsion of the profundus tendon from insertion on the distal phalanx. **B,** At exploration, proximal end of the profundus tendon was found retracted and caught on the distal edge of the A₂ pulley *(tip of scissors).* **C,** Tendon sheath opened, proximal end of profundus retrieved and will be reinserted into distal phalanx with pullout suture. Because the profundus had only retracted to the level of the A₂ pulley, it was possible to readvance it to its normal insertion without undue tension. **D** and **E,** Excellent final result.

don itself are noted. Lister described the technique of making funnel-shaped openings in the cruciate portions of the sheath, sparing the critical A-2 and A-4 pulleys through which the ends of the tendon may be retrieved and repaired; the reader is referred to the original article for specific details.[13]

In distal zone I injuries including tendon lacerations and avulsion from bone, the profundus may be advanced as much as 1 cm and reattached to the base of the distal phalanx with a pullout wire or suture tied over a button on the fingernail (Figs. 29-10 and 29-11).

In zone II injuries, direct tendon repair is performed (Figs. 29-9 and 29-12). After retrieval of the cut tendon ends into the sheath opening, they are transfixed to the sheath with a 25-gauge needle to prevent their retraction during placement of sutures. At all times the tendon is handled delicately, preferably only by its cut end. A 3-0 or 4-0 braided nonabsorbable core suture is placed in the volar lateral aspects of the tendon, using the modified Kessler or Kessler-Tajima techniques. Care is taken to avoid excess tension or gapping at the repair site. In flat tendons, such as the superficialis near its insertion, a simple figure-of-eight suture may be preferable, because a central grasping suture in these tendons may produce buckling. After placement of the core suture, a running, inverted 6-0 nylon suture is placed in the epitenon to smooth out the surface at the repair site. The sheath is then closed with 6-0 nylon to prevent catching of the repair site on the edge of the pulley as well as to restore the synovial fluid environment of the tendon. (This latter point is as yet of unproven benefit in promoting healing of the tendon despite encouraging experimental evidence mentioned earlier.) The finger is then flexed and extended to check for smooth gliding within the sheath. Contrary to earlier teaching, if the sheath cannot be closed directly, it is no longer recommended to "patch" the defect with retinacular grafts from the wrist or foot, because the clinical benefit of this has not been established.[15,30,31] Instead, if the tendon repair catches on the edge of the pulley, the offending edge of the pulley may be resected to allow unimpeded tendon movement, as long as the majority of the pulley is left intact to prevent bowstringing.

In situations in which both the profundus and superficialis (one or both slips) are cut, most surgeons recommend repairing both. However, in some cases the bulkiness of the repairs prevents smooth gliding, and it may be more prudent to repair only one slip of the superficialis or (rarely) not repair it at all, to ensure unimpeded tendon gliding of the profundus tendon. Sacrifice of all or part of the superficialis, although not desirable, is preferable to a mechanically compromised system that will fail.

Finally, in cases in which there is extensive damage or destruction of the A-2 and/or A-4 pulleys, consideration

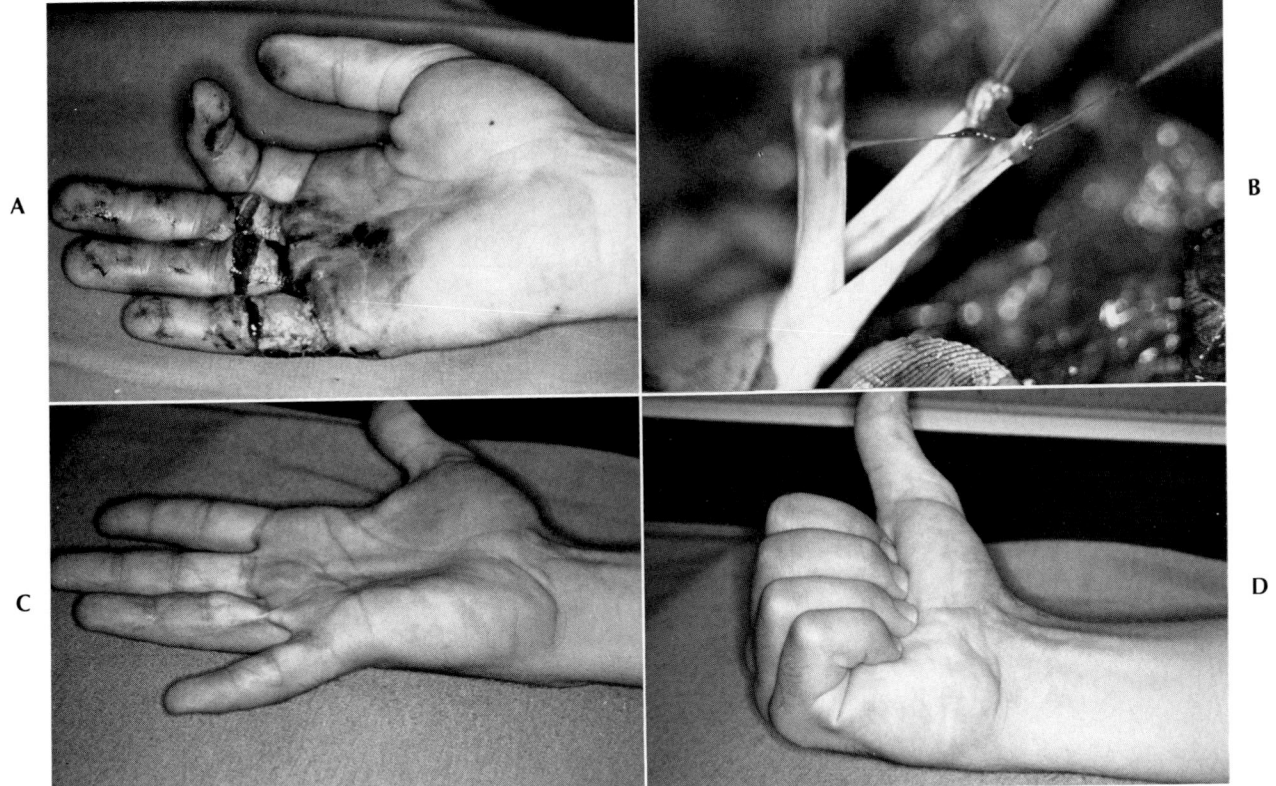

Fig. 29-12   **A,** Twenty-four-year-old man with a knife laceration across the middle, ring, and small fingers. Position of the lacerations and postures of the fingers indicated complete zone II lacerations of the profundus and superficialis tendons in all three fingers. **B,** Exploration revealed complete tendon lacerations as expected. The spiraling relationship of the two superficialis slips with respect to the profundus can be readily appreciated. At this level the two slips need to be repaired separately; thus in effect there will be three tendon repairs. Also note the presence of a vinculum longus running between the profundus and superficilias tendons. **C** and **D,** Final result at 4 months.

should be given to abandonment of primary tendon repair in favor of insertion of a silastic tendon rod with repair or reconstruction of the injured pulley as the first step in two-stage tendon reconstruction procedure. Tendon repair performed simultaneously with repair or reconstruction of an extensively injured pulley system almost always results in extensive adhesion formation with resulting scarring and stiffness. Salvage in this difficult situation inevitably requires a two-stage tendon reconstruction procedure. If wound and other conditions permit, immediate insertion of a silastic rod eliminates one step in the overall process and thereby probably shortens and simplifies the ultimate recovery period.

REPAIR IN OTHER ZONES

Repairs outside the flexor tendon sheath follow the same guidelines previously outlined. The absence of the sheath and pulley systems in these regions is significant in that if scarring occurs to the looser surrounding tissue, there probably will be less restriction of gliding than in zones I and II.

In zone IV injuries, it may be necessary to divide the transverse carpal ligament to obtain exposure for repair, although it is preferable to leave at least a portion of it intact or reconstructed. The ligament functions as a pulley, and bowstringing of the tendons at the wrist, although uncommon, may occur if it remains unrepaired.

POSTSURGICAL MANAGEMENT

This is discussed more fully in other sections, but in brief, I prefer the dynamic traction technique of Kleinert and its modifications[8-12,14,15,31] (Fig. 29-13). In general, the patient is kept in a dorsal dynamic splint with the wrist and MP joints held in flexion. Rubber bands attached to the fingernails passively flex the fingers, whereas the patient is allowed to actively extend them. Full PIP and DIP extension is stressed to minimize flexion contractures. After 3 to 4 weeks, the patient is switched to a wrist cuff, and the dynamic-extension/passive-flexion exercises continue for another 3 to 4 weeks. Then active flexion without resistance is initiated. Gradually, as healing occurs, resistance is added, and the activity level is increased. During this time intermittent splinting may be required to correct flexion contractures. In most cases of uncomplicated healing, unrestricted use of the hand may be allowed at 12 to 16 weeks.

COMPLICATIONS[8,9,12]

Early complications of tendon repair include infection, suture breakage, and mechanical catching of the tendon repair within the sheath.

Late complications include tendon adhesions, tendon ruptures, joint contractures, stretching or attenuation of the repair site, or bowstringing of the tendon caused by incompetent pulleys. The treatment of each complication is individualized for each patient and beyond the scope of this

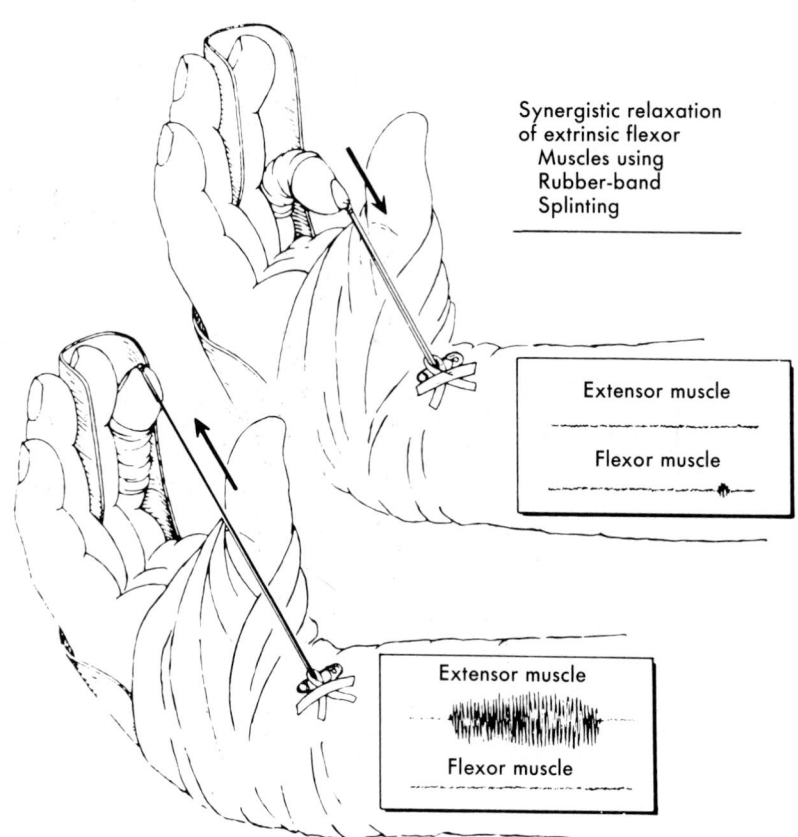

Synergistic relaxation of extrinsic flexor Muscles using Rubber-band Splinting

Extensor muscle

Flexor muscle

Extensor muscle

Flexor muscle

Fig. 29-13 Dynamic-traction exercise system. (Reproduced with permission from Kleinert HE, Kutz J, and Cohen M. In AAOS Symposium on Tendon Surgery in the Hand, St Louis, 1975, The CV Mosby Co.)

chapter. Fortunately, most complications can be minimized by careful attention to detail at surgery and in follow-up care, and nowhere is the old adage "an ounce of prevention is worth a pound of cure" more applicable.

PARTIAL LACERATIONS

Partial tendon lacerations are not uncommon. Small lacerations (less than 25% of the tendon substance) may be treated simply by beveling the cut edges. Lacerations between 25% and 50% may be repaired with a 6-0 nylon running suture in the epitenon, whereas lacerations of greater than 50% probably should be regarded as complete lacerations and repaired with a core suture in addition to epitenon suture. Untreated partial lacerations may cause triggering or catching against the cut edge of the sheath, and thus most volar lacerations in the finger should be carefully explored to ensure the integrity of the tendon and sheath system.

SUMMARY

Flexor tendon injuries continue to pose a challenge to the physician. Successful treatment requires a thorough knowledge of the intricate anatomy of the flexor tendon system, an understanding of tendon nutrition and healing, meticulous and gentle surgical technique, and careful supervision during the postoperative therapy program. Most complications and pitfalls can be avoided by careful attention to details, and a good clinical result may be anticipated in the majority of patients.

REFERENCES

1. Armenta E and Lehrman A: The vincula to the flexor tendons of the hand, J Hand Surg 5:127, 1980.
2. Bruner JM: The Zig-zag volar digital incision for flexor tendon surgery, Plast Reconstr Surg 40:571, 1967.
3. Caplan HS, Hunter JM, and Merklin RJ: Intrinsic vascularization of flexor tendons. In American Academy of Orthopedic Surgeons: Symposium on tendon surgery in the hand, St. Louis, 1975, The CV Mosby Co.
4. Doyle RF and Blythe W: The finger flexor tendon sheath and pulleys: anatomy and reconstruction. In American Academy of Orthopedic Surgeons: Symposium on tendon surgery in the hand, St. Louis, 1975, The CV Mosby Co.
5. Doyle JR and Blythe W: Anatomy of the flexor tendon sheath and pulleys of the thumb, J Hand Surg 2:149, 1977.
6. Gelberman RH and Manske PR: Factors influencing flexor tendon adhesions, Hand Clin 1:35, 1985.
7. Ketchum LD: Primary tendon healing: a review, J Hand Surg 2(6):428, 1977.
8. Kleinert HE and Cash SL: The management of acute flexor tendon injuries in the hand. American Academy of Orthopedic Surgeons. Instructional course lectures 34, 1985.
9. Kleinert HE and Cash SL: Current guidelines for flexor tendon repair within the fibro-osseous tunnel: indications, timing, and techniques. In Hunter JM, Schneider LH, and Mackin EJ, editors: Tendon surgery in the hand, St. Louis, 1987, The CV Mosby Co.
10. Kleinert HE and others: Primary repair of lacerated flexor tendons in no-man's land, J Bone Joint Surg 49A:577, 1967.
11. Kleinert HE and others: Primary repair of flexor tendons, Orthop Clin North Am 4:865, 1973.
12. Kleinert HE, Schepel S, and Gill T: Flexor tendon injuries, Surg Clin North Am 61:267, 1981.
13. Lister GD: Incision and closure of the flexor sheath during primary tendon repair, Hand 15(2):123, 1983.
14. Lister GD and others: Primary flexor tendon repair followed by immediate controlled mobilization, J Hand Surg 2:441, 1977.
15. Lister GD and Tonkin M: The results of primary flexor tendon repair, J Hand Surg 11A:767, 1986.
16. Lundborg G: Experimental flexor tendon healing without adhesion formation: a new concept of tendon nutrition and intrinsic healing mechanisms, Hand 8:235, 1976.
17. Lundborg G, Holm S, and Myrhage R: The role of synovial fluid and tendon sheath for flexor tendon nutrition, Scan J Plast Reconstr Surg 14:99, 1980.
18. Lundborg G, Myrhage R, and Rydevik B: The vascularization of human flexor tendons within the digital synovial sheath region, J Hand Surg 2:417, 1977.
19. Lundborg G and Rank F: Experimental intrinsic healing of flexor tendons based upon synovial fluid nutrition, J Hand Surg 3(1):21, 1978.
20. Manske PR: The flexor tendon, Orthopedics 10:1733, 1987.
21. Manske P, Bridwell K, and Lesker P: Nutrient pathways to flexor tendons of chickens using titrated proline, J Hand Surg 3(4):352, 1978.
22. Manske PR and others: Flexor tendon repair: morphological evidence of intrinsic healing in vitro, J Bone Joint Surg 66A:385, 1984.
23. Manske PR, Gelberman RH, and Lesker PA: Flexor tendon healing, Hand Clinics of North America 1:25, 1985.
24. Manske P, Whiteside L, and Lesker P: Nutrient pathways to flexor tendons using hydrogen washout technique, J Hand Surg 3(1):32, 1978.
25. Matthews P: The pathology of flexor tendon repair, Hand 11:233, 1979.
26. Matthews P and Richard H: Factors in the adherence of flexor tendons after repair, J Bone Joint Surg 58B:230, 1976.
27. Ochiai N and others: Vascular anatomy of flexor tendons I: vincular system and blood supply of the profundus tendon in the digital sheath, J Hand Surg 4:321, 1979.
28. Peterson WW, Manske PR, and Lesker PA: The effect of flexor tendon sheath integrity on nutrient uptake by primate flexor tendons, J Hand Surg 11A:413, 1986.
29. Potenza A: Tendon healing within the flexor digital sheath in the dog, J Bone Joint Surg 44A:49, 1962.
30. Saldana M and others: Flexor tendon repair and rehabilitation in zone II: open sheath technique versus closed sheath technique, J Hand Surg 12A:1110, 1987.
31. Strauch B and others: The fate of tendon healing after restoration of the integrity of tendon sheath with autogenous vein grafts, J Hand Surg 10A:790, 1985.
32. Strickland JW: Flexor tendon injuries. I. Anatomy, physiology, biomechanics, healing and adhesion formation around a repaired tendon, Orthop Rev 15:632, 1986.
33. Weber ER: Nutritional pathways for flexor tendons in the digital theca. In Hunter JM, Schneider LH, and Mackin EJ, editors: Tendon surgery in the hand, St. Louis, 1987, The CV Mosby Co.

30

Postoperative management of flexor tendon injuries

Gwendolyn van Strien

Management of a patient after flexor tendon repair is a challenge for both surgeons and hand therapists. Surgical repairs of flexor tendon lacerations have frequently been unsatisfactory because of fixed adhesions that prevented the tendon from gliding. Researchers have shown that early mobilization can prevent the formation of limiting scar tissue without jeopardizing tendon healing, and surgeons, with hand therapists, have incorporated many different forms of early mobilization into their postoperative treatment programs. Knowledge of flexor tendon anatomy and physiology and understanding the basic principles of tendon healing are essential for hand therapists who are responsible for the postoperative care of patients with primary flexor tendon repairs.

ANATOMY

The anatomy as related to primary flexor tendon repair of the flexor digitorum superficialis (FDS), flexor digitorum profundus (FDP), and flexor pollicis longus (FPL) is reviewed here. The digital flexor tendons and the thumb flexor tendon originate from muscles in the proximal one third of the forearm. In the forearm (zone 5) the tendons are surrounded by a loose connective tissue, the paratenon.[50] In the carpal tunnel (zone 4), in the proximal palm (zone 3), and in the digits and thumb (zones 2 and 1), the flexor tendons are surrounded by a synovial sheath. Many variations of the synovial sheath system exist. Usually the FPL has its own sheath, also called radial bursa, which continues into the thumb, where the tendon enters the fibroosseus canal of the thumb. The synovial sheath that envelops all digital flexor tendons in the carpal tunnel is continuous with the digital sheath of the small finger and is called ulnar bursa, whereas the index, long, and ring fingers have individual digital synovial sheaths, noncontinuous with the ulnar bursa. The thin synovial sheath of the FDS and FDP should not be confused with the flexor retinaculum or fibroosseus tunnel in the finger. The flexor retinaculum, or pulley system, surrounds the flexor tendons and the synovial sheath. The synovial lining of the sheath provides a synovial fluid, which facilitates smooth gliding and provides the tendon with nutrition, supplementing the blood supply to the tendon.[16,40,42,44,46]

As the two tendons enter the proximal end of the fibroosseus tunnel or pulley system, the FDS lies volar to the profundus tendon. At the level of the proximal phalanx, the FDS splits into two slips, which rotate 180 degrees around the FDP, to join dorsally in a chiasm (Camper's chiasm) at the level of the proximal interphalangeal (PIP) joint.[69] Both tendon slips from the FDS continue distally, inserting into the middle phalanx dorsal to the FDP. The FDP continues on in the fibroosseus tunnel inserting into the base of the distal phalanx (Fig. 30-1).

The fibroosseus tunnel, or pulley system, extends from the metacarpal heads of the fingers and thumb, respectively, to the insertion of the profundus tendon and pollicis longus tendon at the distal phalanx. This area also corresponds with flexor tendon zones 1 and 2[35] (Fig. 30-2). The flexor retinaculum consists of a series of transversely oriented fibrous bands, or annular pulleys, between each annular pulley there is a cruciform thickening or cruciate ligament[17,67] (Fig. 30-3).

The flexor retinaculum and sheath are well-vascularized except for the friction surface of the pulleys. The function

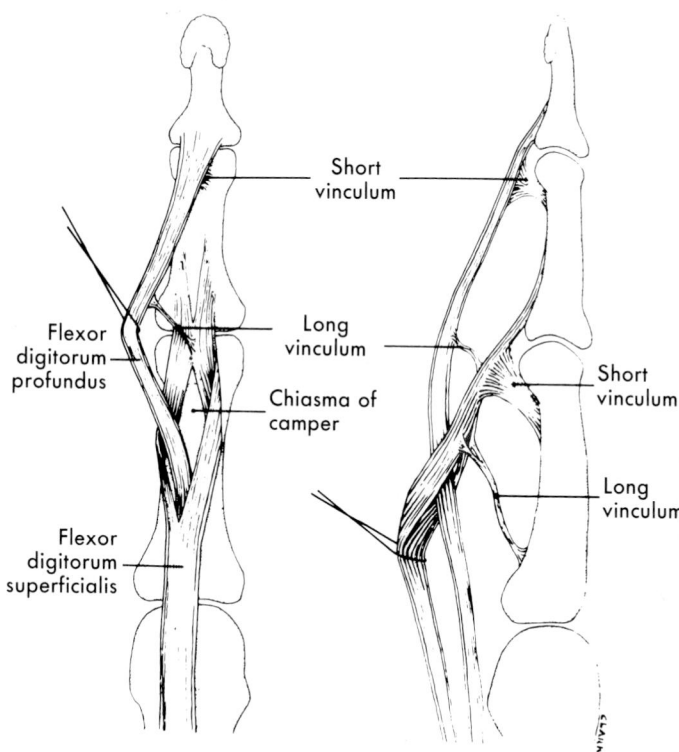

Fig. 30-1 The flexor digitorum superficialis lies volar to the flexor digitorum profundus as the tendons enter the sheath. At the level of the proximal phalanx the superficialis tendon splits and moves around to the dorsal side of the profundus tendon to form Camper's chiasm and insert into the middle phalanx. Both the flexor digitorum superficialis and flexor digitorum profundus have a short and long vinculum. The vinculum longus profundus is a continuation of the vinculum brevis superficialis. (From Schneider LH: Flexor tendon injuries, Boston, 1985, Little, Brown & Co Inc. Reproduced by permission.)

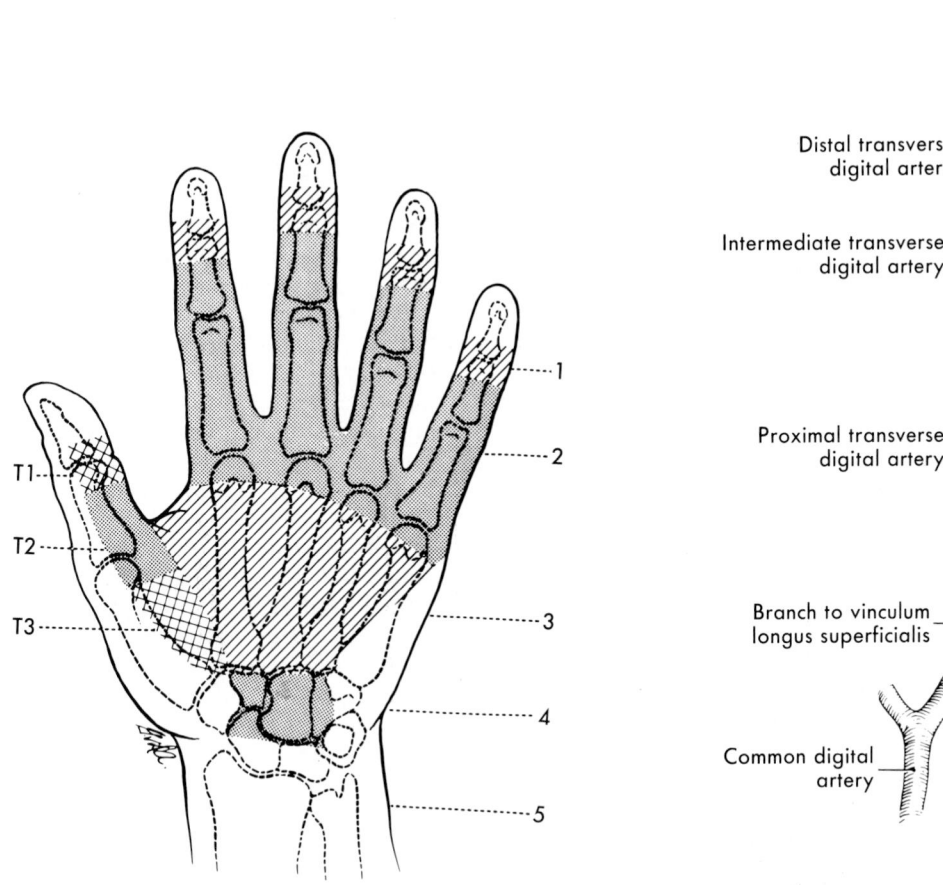

Fig. 30-2 Flexor tendon zones of the hand. (From Kleinert HE, Schepel S, and Gill T: Flexor tendon injuries, Surg Clin North Am 61:267, 1981.)

Fig. 30-3 The fibroosseous tunnel or pulley system, with five annular pulleys *(A1 to A5)*, and three cruciform ligaments *(C1 to C3)*. Note the width of the *A2* and *A4* pulleys. (From Schneider LH: Flexor tendon injuries, Boston, 1985, Little, Brown & Co Inc. Reproduced by permission.)

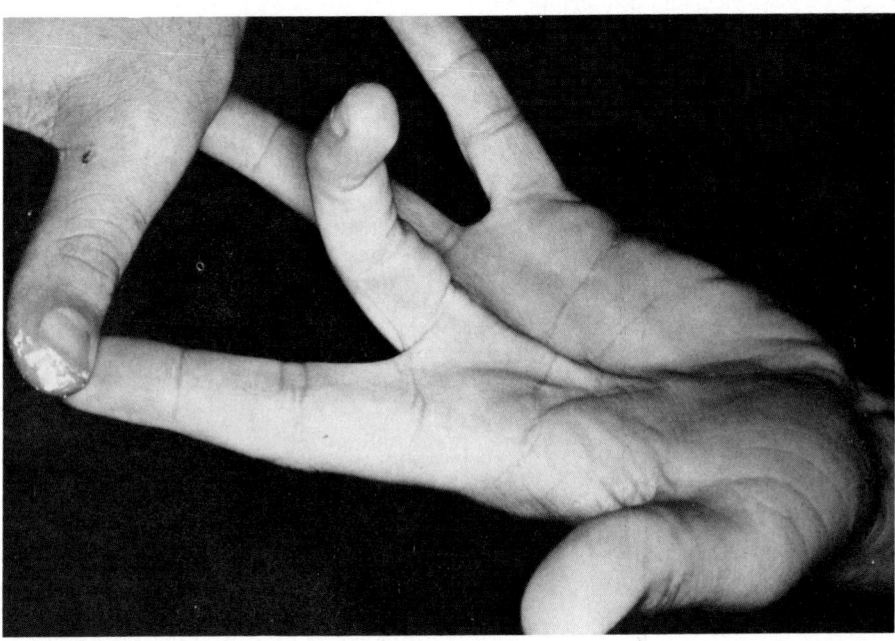

Fig. 30-4 Bowstringing of the flexor tendons is illustrated in this patient with absent pulleys because of a childhood injury.

of the pulley system is to hold the tendons close to the bone, thus preventing bowstringing of the tendons (Fig. 30-4). Doyle and Blythe[17] determined the relative importance of each pulley by serial excision. The effect of pulley resection was measured by the ability to flex the fingertip, the amount of force required to flex the digit, and the tendon excursion needed to touch the palm. The data revealed that the A_2 and A_4 pulleys are most important for achieving normal tendon function.

NUTRITION[34,36,67,78]

It was long believed that tendons were avascular. This belief changed in 1916 when Mayer[50] demonstrated blood supply to the tendons through injection studies on cadavers and animals. Other studies have elaborated on the work by Mayer, and all have confirmed the presence of vascular supply to the tendon.* Peacock[56] measured the metabolic rate of the tenocyte to prove that tendons consist of living tissue, and even though the metabolic rate is extremely low, it indicates the need for tendon blood supply.

Mayer[50] described three main sources of blood supply to a flexor tendon. The two less important sources are the proximal vessels entering at the musculotendinous junction and the distal bony-tendinous insertion. The third and most important source of blood supply comes from vessels in the surrounding tissues.

Two different areas need to be described for the third source of blood supply. In the forearm and proximal palm, where the tendon is not surrounded by a retinaculum, an abundance of vessels enter the tendon at random from the surrounding tissues. Within the pulley system, the small vessels originating from the surrounding tissues enter the tendon through mesotenon extensions called vincula. The vincular anatomy and the points of entry into the flexor tendons can vary from digit to digit. The vincular anatomy and its anomalies have been well documented in the literature.†

Two types of vincula are described for each tendon: the vinculum longus and vinculum brevis (Fig. 30-1). Both superficialis and profundus tendons have a vinculum brevis. The vinculum longus for the profundus tendon is a continuation of the vinculum brevis superficialis. The long vinculum to the FDS is often absent.[53] The small vessels entering the vincula originate from four transverse communicating arteries, which branch from the two digital arteries. The vincular vessels communicate with the intratendinous vessels (one arteriole and one or two venules) that lie longitudinally within the tendon and originate in the palm.[14,19,41,53] These longitudinally oriented vessels are located in the dorsal half of each tendon, leaving the volar side of the tendon relatively avascular.[2,15,41,46,53] Areas of relative avascularity between the segmental vincular blood supply are often described as "watershed," or critical tendon zones.[41,45]

In zone 2, where the tendons are surrounded by the pulley system and areas of relative avascularity exist, tendon nutrition comes from two sources—the blood supply and synovial diffusion.

Investigators have shown that under certain conditions synovial fluid can provide the essential nutrition for tendon viability and even the elements necessary for healing after tendon injury.[20,40-46,51] Manske and associates[44] and Lundborg and Rank[42] showed viability of a tendon segment immersed in synovial fluid, detached from all blood supply. These studies demonstrated the role of synovial diffusion as an important pathway for nutrition.

Tendons will absorb nutrients from the synovial fluid, especially on the volar avascular side and in the areas between vincular blood supply. Synovial fluid is "forced" into the tendon under influence of high pressure against the pulleys during active flexion of the finger.[41,51,77] The pumping mechanism, under influence of pressure of the tendon against the firm resistance of the pulleys, has been compared to the mechanism of synovial diffusion in articular cartilage.[2,40,77] Biochemical and physiologic evidence presented by Amadio and associates[2] supports the suggested analogy between synovial diffusion in cartilage and the synovial diffusion on the volar side of flexor tendons.

A delicate balance between both nutritional pathways (blood supply and synovial diffusion) is found within the flexor tendon sheath. In the fibroosseus tunnel the dorsally located tendon vessels and the segmental vincular arrangement leave large volar parts of the tendon relatively avascular. Nutrition to these "watershed" areas is supplied mostly by diffusion from the synovium. When injury occurs in these relatively avascular areas, the balance is disturbed and excessive adhesion formation is often seen. The adhesions bring the additional blood supply to the tendon necessary for the healing process, yet they limit free tendon glide.

Injury to the vincular system will also affect the nutritional balance and has been shown to have a negative effect on tendon healing and cause adhesion formation.[3,5,39] In a microscopic study on living tendons Schatzker and Branemark[66] demonstrated that additional nutritional pathways are needed when the vincula are severed. Another example of vincular injury can occur when both superficialis and profundus tendons are lacerated. Some surgeons would remove the injured FDS and repair the FDP. Clinically, a better result has been reported when both the superficialis and profundus tendons are repaired.[67] Removal of the superficialis tendon disrupts the blood supply through the vinculum brevis superficialis, which in turn supplies the vinculum longus of the profundus tendon.

BASIC CONCEPTS OF TENDON HEALING

Histologically tendon consists of connective tissue, and its function is to link muscle to bone. It is comprised of collagen bundles (70% of dry weight[29]) with only a small amount of proteoglycans and elastic fibers. The collagen bundles are longitudinally oriented parallel bundles surrounded by epitenon.

After a tendon is lacerated and repaired, the entire wound actually involves more than just the tendon. All surrounding tissues, such as skin, subcutaneous tissues, and underlying tissues are also involved in the wound healing process. In the first few days after repair, the wound is filled with a cicatrix, consisting of ground substance and many types of cells. Scar formed in the first 3 weeks will "glue" all involved tissue layers together, and independent function is

---

*References 12,14,19,41,52,66,70.
†References 12,14,34,36,53,70.

Table 30-1   Tendon healing phases

Phases	Time period	Characteristics
Exudative phase	0-4 days	Inflammatory response, cell migration, wound cavity filled with cicatrix
Fibroblastic phase	5-21 days	Fibroblasts in wound, collagen synthesis, increased tensile strength, intramolecular cross-linking
Remodeling phase	3 wk-6 mo/1 yr	Intermolecular cross-linking, collagen production/lysis, scar remodeling

lost. This was described by Peacock[57] as the one-wound concept.

Three phases are described for wound healing (Table 30-1): the exudative phase, the fibroplasia phase, and the collagen-remodeling phase.[57]

The exudative phase starts immediately after injury. Tensile strength diminishes in the first 3 to 5 days because of softening of the tendons ends.[47,73] Immediately after injury an inflammatory reaction changes the permeability of the vascular system. As a result, there is an influx of leukocytes, and macrophages, among other inflammatory elements, in the wound area. Macrophages are important for stimulating growth and migration of fibroblasts.[30]

During the second phase, fibroblasts migrate to the wound area and start production of tropocollagen approximately 5 days after injury.[57] Tropocollagen is a triple-helix molecule with little tensile strength. After the weak hydrogen bonds of the tropocollagen molecule are replaced by stronger cross-links between the three strands of the helix, collagen fibers are formed and tensile strength starts to develop. The fibroblasts continue to synthesize new collagen until day 21. The collagen molecules form a randomly oriented network, creating a bond between all tissues in the wound. From day 5 to day 21, tensile strength increases rapidly as the collagen matures and the intramolecular cross-linking continues.

Intermolecular cross-linking between other collagen fibrils can start during the second phase of wound healing, but it usually starts approximately 21 days after injury.[57,80] This coincides with the beginning of the third phase of wound healing (the remodeling phase), which starts 3 weeks after injury and continues until 6 months or a year after injury. In the remodeling phase differentiation between the tissues is achieved, and dense, unyielding scar can be changed into more favorable scar.[80] Scar remodeling is characterized by a balance between collagen production and collagen lysis.[30] The randomly oriented collagen between tendon ends, under the influence of stress, is slowly replaced by newly formed collagen oriented along the long axis of the tendon, thus providing increased tensile strength.[11,47] The randomly oriented fibers of the scar between tendon and surrounding tissues, however, must become loose and filmy to regain gliding function.[77]

When an adhesion-bound tendon gains motion, it is usually not because adhesions are broken, but rather lengthened or changed under influence of stress.[4,34] Brand[11] stated that if living tissue is subjected to slight tension for a relatively long period of time,"the living cells will sense the strain and the collagen fibers will be actively and progressively absorbed and laid down again with modified bonding patterns." This model may be the explanation for clinical ob-

servations that repaired tendons, under the influence of gentle stress, regain motion and restore gliding surfaces during the collagen remodeling process.

Attempts have been made by many researchers to influence the quality of tendon healing by influencing quantity and type of adhesion formation. To limit fixed adhesions, weak healing is needed between tendon and surrounding tissues. In contrast, strong healing and tensile strength is needed between the tendon ends to transmit muscle power. This type of differential wound healing seems necessary to recover a free-gliding and functioning tendon after flexor tendon repair.

EXTRINSIC VERSUS INTRINSIC HEALING

Tendon healing has been researched by many authors over the last decades, but the exact mechanism of tendon healing is still unknown. The type of tendon nutrition, but even more the origin of fibroblasts, supplied during wound healing is still disputed. Some researchers believe that the ingrowing adhesions supply the fibroblasts necessary for wound healing.[59,60] Others believe the tendon itself has healing potential.[23,39,42,43,51] The role of the tendon in the healing process was believed to be passive until Mason and Shearon[48] in 1932 showed that beginning the fifth day after injury, tenocytes contribute to the healing process. Three descriptions of possible mechanisms of tendon healing are discussed in the literature, the intrinsic and extrinsic mechanisms of tendon healing, and a combination of these mechanisms.

Extrinsic healing depends on formation of adhesions between tendon and surrounding tissues. These adhesions provide the blood supply and the cells (in particular, fibroblasts) needed for tendon healing. Unfortunately, they also prevent the tendon from gliding. The research supporting this method of healing indicates that the tendon has no active role in the healing process, whereas adhesion formation is vital to tendon healing.[59,60]

Intrinsic healing occurs between the tendon ends only, without formation of limiting adhesions.[23,42,43,51] This type of healing relies on the synovial fluid for nutrition and does not result in restricted motion of the tendon. The cells needed for tendon healing are supplied by the epitenon and endotenon itself.[39] The works of Lundborg and Rank[42,43] clearly demonstrate the intrinsic healing potential of tendons. A divided and repaired segment of rabbit tendon was placed in the synovial cavity of the knee joint. The tendon healed and developed tensile strength without vascular blood supply, demonstrating that the tendon has intrinsic potential to heal. The experiment was repeated with the segment placed in a dialyzing membrane to prevent cell seeding from the synovial fluid. The tendon was still able to heal, showing that collagen must be secreted by the tendon itself.

A third group of investigators believe the tendon probably heals through a combination of both intrinsic and extrinsic processes. Mason and Shearon,[48] in 1932, found evidence of healing by both intrinsic and extrinsic means. Lacerated tendons in dogs showed a fibroblastic healing response triggered by the sheath 5 days after repair. Tenocytes started proliferating 2 to 3 weeks after repair, showing an intrinsic healing response. Flynn and Graham[22] reported similar results in dog tendons. Although the experimental research presented demonstrates that tendon healing is possible by either intrinsic or extrinsic means, in most clinical situations adhesions are seen to a varying degree, and the healing response is probably a balance between intrinsic and extrinsic healing.

FACTORS AFFECTING TENDON HEALING

Several factors have been reported to affect different phases of tendon healing,[1] and these factors may determine the end result of a flexor tendon repair. Some of these factors can be identified during surgery, and it is important that the surgeon communicates this information to the therapist.

Some factors are patient related: age, general health, what type of scar formation is typical for the patient, and patient motivation. Some factors are injury or surgery related: the level or location of the injury, the amount of associated trauma (especially neurovascular injuries), sheath integrity, and finally, surgical techniques and suturing methods.

Patient-related factors

Age. The only documented age-related factor is the number of vincula, which decreases as a person gets older.[1] As a result, larger areas within the tendon will be devoid of blood supply, and this causes decreased healing potential in the injured tendon of an older person. Also, in theory, cell-aging could cause decreased healing capacity of the tenocytes.[2,63]

General health and healing potential. In general, patients in good health can expect to have good healing potential. Certain life-styles or dietary habits can have a negative effect on the healing potential of a patient. For example, a patient who smokes cigarettes can have delayed healing, caused by the constricting effect of tobacco on the circulation. Patients who have a large intake of caffeine can expect similar effects. Patients who have a tendon repair should therefore avoid caffeine products and tobacco during the first few weeks following surgery.

Type of scar formation. Scar formation is different for each person. In the clinic one can observe typical differences between types of scars formed by patients even though injury and postoperative treatment are essentially the same. Generally, two types of patients can be described: the "heavy scar formers" and the "low scar formers." The amount of scarring is directly and inversely related to the effectiveness of the remodeling phase. If there is little scar formation, the remodeling is more rapid and a better functional end result is achieved.

Motivation. The patient's motivation and ability to follow the postoperative program are critical factors in determining the end result of a primary flexor tendon repair. A good understanding by the patient of his role in the rehabilitation process is imperative. Each patient's expectation of the quality of the end result is different and often occupation related.[2] Individual rehabilitation goals should be set for each patient, and job simulation should always be considered in the later stages of postoperative care.

When the surgeon expects a less than perfect result, it is important that this information be communicated not only to the therapist but also to the patient. Patient education can minimize the danger for rupture and prevent overzealous patients from exercising too much or too forcefully and maybe encourage less motivated patients to follow instruction carefully and understand the importance of their own involvement.

Injury and surgery-related factors

Level of the injury. Injuries are categorized in zones as defined by the International Federation of Societies for Surgery of the Hand (IFSSH)[35] (see Fig. 30-2). An injury in zone 2 will often form limiting adhesions between tendon and surrounding tissues. This increase in adhesion formation was explained earlier in this chapter by the relative avascular areas in the tendon at this level. In comparison, injury at the level of the forearm and proximal palm, that is, zones 3 and 5, result in less adhesion formation between the tendon and surrounding soft tissues because of the abundant vascularity of tendons surrounded with paratenon.[15] In addition, in the forearm the adhesions that may form between tendon and the loose connective tissue called paratenon do not usually restrict motion as much as the adhesions that form between tendon and the firm, well-anchored flexor retinaculum. A different problem can occur in zone 4, where the digital flexor tendons lie in close contact with each other in the narrow carpal tunnel. Adhesions do not form as much between tendon and surrounding tissues, but do form between the digital flexor tendons themselves, thereby limiting differential glide of the tendons.

Type of injury and amount of trauma. Much of the results of tendon repair is dependent on the type of injury and the amount of trauma. If the wound was untidy and the patient developed an infection after surgery, then a delay in the healing process can occur.[54] Crushing or blunt injuries usually cause more trauma to the surrounding tissues than sharp injuries and result in more scar formation. Crushing injuries also cause more vascular trauma; trauma to the vincula, especially, can impair postoperative healing.[5]

Associated injuries such as fractures or repaired neurovascular bundles alter postoperative management and can cause a negative effect on the results of tendon repair. Scott and associates[68] reported a significant negative effect on the results of flexor tendon repair in patients after digital replantation with associated neurovascular injuries and fractures.

Another example of the influence of the amount of injury is the isolated FDP injury in zones 1 and 2. The prognosis for isolated profundus injuries is better than that for injuries including the FDS tendon.[1,21,72] Not only is more trauma usually involved when both tendons are injured, there is also more chance of vincular injury. The resulting adhesion formation between FDP and FDS limits the differential glide between both tendons.[1,77]

The prognosis for partial lacerations is also better than that for complete lacerations. A partially lacerated tendon has less vascular compromise than a completely severed tendon. Partial lacerations of 50% or more, however, are generally treated as complete lacerations by the surgeon and the therapist. Triggering may occur when the irregular tendon surface of an untreated partially lacerated tendon catches on the sheath.

Sheath integrity. Repair of the sheath and especially the pulleys is important for restoration of tendon function.[41] Injury to the pulley system affects the mechanical advantage of the tendon. The loss of tendon function resulting from loss of one or more pulleys was demonstrated in a study by Doyle and Blythe.[17]

Sheath and pulley injury also affect tendon nutrition because of the function of the pulleys in synovial diffusion. As described earlier, the pulleys create a firm opposing surface for the volar avascular side of the tendon during flexion. If this "pumping mechanism" between the volar avascular side of the tendon and the pulley indeed resembles the diffusion in articular cartilage, then pulley repair is imperative for optimal tendon healing conditions. Salter[65] demonstrated improved healing in avascular articular cartilage because of the apparent effects of early mobilization on synovial diffusion.

With the exception of the pulleys, synovial sheath repair may not improve the healing of repaired flexor tendons. In a study by Peterson and associates[58] closure of the sheath did not affect the results of flexor tendon repair. It appears that a single cell layer much like a sheath regenerates in the first postoperative days.[59,60] Amadio and Hunter[1] compared one group of 28 patients where the sheath was not repairable and a second group of 29 patients where sheath repair was possible. No statistically significant difference in average range of motion (ROM) between the two groups of patients was reported, and the authors concluded that in the absence of pulley injury, sheath repair does not significantly affect the results of tendon repair.

Repair of the pulley system has been proven to be essential for optimal functional recovery after flexor tendon repairs. The effect of synovial sheath closure is still disputed and surgeons may choose not to repair the sheath. Many surgeons will, however, attempt to repair the sheath to prevent the possibility of triggering of the tendon-repair site on the open sheath.

Surgical techniques. Meticulous surgical techniques can minimize the amount of additional tissue trauma and hematoma and reduce the number of adhesions.[78] Excessive postoperative hematoma causes increased inflammatory and cellular responses. An increase in the amount of hematoma may therefore increase the number of adhesions surrounding repaired tendon.[6]

The delicate handling of the tissues by the surgeon is imperative. Potenza[61] demonstrated that even the marks of the forceps on the epitenon can trigger adhesion formation. The effect of different surgical variables on adhesion formation in repaired tendons was investigated.[49,54] The authors demonstrated an increase in adhesion formation when suture material was added to a gliding tendon. Injury to the sheath and splinting were other variables investigated; they also increased adhesion formation. Other researchers demonstrated an increase in adhesion formation after placing a suture in an uninjured tendon.[39,78] Placement of a "foreign object" such as suture material caused an inflammatory response resulting in adhesion formation.

The strangulating effect on intratendinous vessels with certain suture techniques could also provoke adhesion formation. Decreased circulation to the tendon after placing a suture in intact tendon was demonstrated in studies by Bergljung.[7,8] To avoid the dorsally based intratendinous vessels, sutures are most often placed in the relatively avascular volar aspect of the tendon.[33,67]

EARLY MOBILIZATION

In 1984 Hunter[54] stated that the number one challenge in hand therapy for the next decade will be to change the results of postoperative tendon repairs by controlling factors that could affect the biology of tendon healing.[54] The most important of these factors in the postoperative period seems to be physical stress, applied to the healing tendon anastomosis through early mobilization of the tendon.

Effects of motion on tendon healing

Beneficial effects of early mobilization and stress applied to tendon anastomoses have been demonstrated in a number of laboratory experiments. Mason and Allen,[47] in 1941, reported that motion created a stronger repair. Tensile strength increased rapidly after the seventh day, especially when there was protected mobilization. Birdsell and associates[9] reported that the already relatively inactive tenocyte in mature tendon has even lower activity if the tendon is immobilized.

Gelberman and associates did a series of experimental studies of early passive mobilization of tendons in dogs.[24-27] In 1980 these authors reported that compared to delayed mobilization and immobilized tendons, the tensile strength and excursion of mobilized tendons was superior. In a 1981 study, biochemical and microangiographic evidence showed that early-controlled passive motion improved the quality of the healing response by stimulation of maturation and remodeling of the scar. A third study by this group in 1982 demonstrated that at 12 weeks more excursion of the repaired tendon was achieved as well as an increase in strength, probably as a result of improved intrinsic healing and consequently restored gliding surfaces. Microscopic evidence in a study by Gelberman, Vande Berg, Lundborg, and Akeson[27] showed extrinsic healing by ingrowth of connective tissue from the sheath and intrinsic healing by cellular proliferation of the endotenon in immobilized flexor tendon repairs in dogs. In contrast, in the same study intrinsic healing with no adhesion formation was found in tendons treated with early passive mobilization. The studies by Gelberman and associates support the hypothesis that motion has a beneficial effect on tendon nutrition, tenocyte metabolism, or both.

Early mobilization of the primary flexor tendon repair

The primary repair as a treatment for tendon lacerations was not popular among surgeons in the earlier decades of this century, and delayed tendon grafting was preferred by most surgeons.[10,13,62] Bunnell reported that rest or immobilization was necessary for the repair to heal, yet the resulting adhesions gave an unsatisfactory functional end result.[13] Harmer was probably one of the first surgeons, while experimenting with early motion for tendon repairs to limit adhesion formation, to develop a special suture technique allowing early mobilization of the repaired tendon.[31,32]

After disappointing results with tendon grafting as treatment for tendon repairs had been reported, Verdan sparked new interest in primary flexor tendon repair with results from his own work.[74] In 1975 Verdan[75] presented a review of different treatment techniques for flexor tendon repair. In this review he credited Kleinert especially for developing a technique using dynamic traction in a protective position allowing early motion.

The postoperative technique designed by Kleinert[34] requires a dorsal protective splint holding the wrist and interphalangeal joints in a protected position to avoid tension on the repaired tendon(s). Kleinert originally used a splint that held the wrist at 20 degrees less than full flexion and both the metacarpophalangeal (MP) joint and proximal interphalangeal (PIP) joints at 10 to 20 degrees of flexion. Dynamic traction was applied by attaching a rubber band to the nail of the involved finger through a nail suture and securing the rubber band to the volar side of the splint proximal to the wrist level. Within 2 or 3 days following surgery active extension exercises were started. Finger flexion was achieved by the recoil of the rubber band after the extensors relaxed. The splint was discharged at 21 days and active exercises were begun. Lister,[34] in 1977, provided additional backing for dynamic traction when he demonstrated with electromyographic (EMG) studies the reciprocal relaxation of the FDP during active extensor digitorum communis contraction against the rubber band traction (Fig. 30-5).

In 1975 Duran and Houser[18] reported the results of their technique of passive mobilization for primary tendon repairs in zones 2 and 3. They stated that 3 to 5 mm of passive motion of the tendon anastomosis was sufficient to prevent adhesions. Differential passive gliding exercises for FDP and FDS were initiated under direct vision in the operating room and followed up twice a day after surgery to achieve maximum glide for all tendons repaired. Controlled passive motion to both involved an uninvolved fingers was continued for 4 or 5 weeks. Between exercise periods the hand was placed in a protective position and dynamic traction was applied through a dorsal splint. Duran was inspired by the work of Young and Harmon[81] and Kleinert.[34] Young, as reported by Duran, used passive motion without splinting for tendon repairs since 1941. In 1960 Young and Harmon[81] reported good results with a technique of passive extension followed by rubber-band traction pulling the finger back into flexion. The rubber band was attached to a wrist band, and no additional protective splinting was used.

Both Duran and associates and Kleinert and associates reported 75% to 80% good-to-excellent results with their techniques. Evaluation of the patients and the criteria for good or excellent results were different for both studies; nevertheless, the results from both studies are much better than the results achieved with tendon grafting. Strickland and Golgovac[72] also reported improved results when using Duran's method rather than 3 weeks of immobilization followed by exercises.

There are some possibly detrimental effects of physical stress on tendon repairs. When stress is applied too early or too forcefully, rupture can result. The tensile strength cannot tolerate any more than gentle forces until about the fourth week.[6] Urbaniak and associates[73] measured the tension in milligrams during full active flexion and power grip. The data ranged from 500 to 2600 mg for active flexion and from 4000 to 20,000 mg for power grip. These numbers illustrate the large forces that would be applied to the repair when active flexion is started. Most surgeons will not start active motion of the repaired tendon before 3 to 4 weeks.[18,33,34,67]

Another example of negative effects of motion is the excessive inflammatory reaction that can result from too much stress. This can cause an increase in collagen deposition in the wound, resulting in more scar tissue. Early mobilization, when performed carefully, seems to have a beneficial effect on the quality of tendon healing. Too much stress too early, however, can have adverse effects on the healing process. Exercise programs should therefore be carefully supervised by surgeon and therapist, and the patient should be well instructed in the exercise program and understand his role in the postoperative course of therapy.

POSTOPERATIVE PROTOCOL FOR PRIMARY FLEXOR TENDON REPAIR
General considerations

The two most frequent causes for failure of primary tendon repairs are adhesion formation and ruptures of the repaired tendon.[67] In the following protocol, protective splinting and early protected mobilization are combined in a way meant to encourage optimal healing while limiting adhesion formation, with little chance of rupturing the repaired tendon. The early controlled mobilization program presented in this chapter is the one used at the Hand Rehabilitation Center (HRC) in Philadelphia. The protocol is based on the works of Kleinert and associates[34] and Duran and associ-

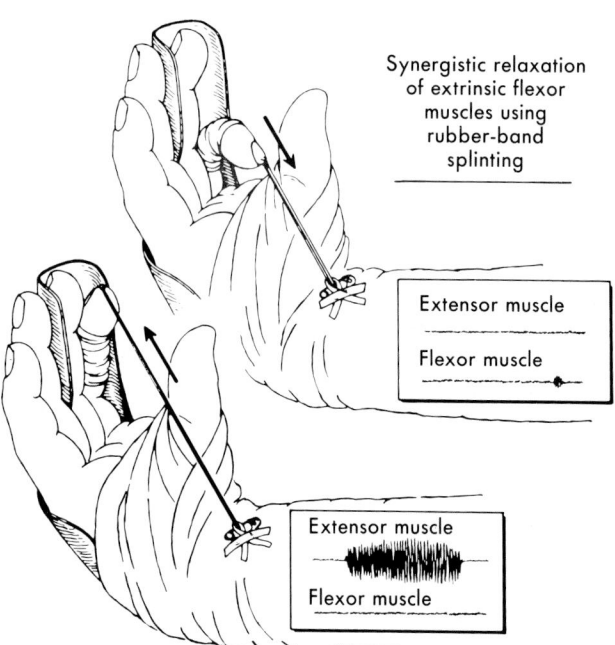

Synergistic relaxation of extrinsic flexor muscles using rubber-band splinting

Extensor muscle

Flexor muscle

Extensor muscle

Flexor muscle

Fig. 30-5 Electromyography showing reciprocal relaxation of the flexor digitorum profundus during active extension against the rubber band. (From Kleinert HE, Kutz JE, and Cohen MJ: Primary repair of zone 2 flexor tendon lacerations. In AAOS: Symposium on Tendon Surgery in the Hand, St. Louis, 1975, The CV Mosby Co.)

ates.[18] The resulting program consists of protective splinting and early active extension against rubber-band traction, combined with controlled passive exercises for the interphalangeal (IP) joints.

Taking a referral

It is important for the therapist to know what factors affect recovery of function after flexor tendon repair. These factors are the type and level of injury, the structures involved (bone, skin, neurovascular bundles), the patient's potential for healing and tendency for scarring, surgical procedures and techniques, and patient motivation.

Therefore, when taking a referral for splinting and therapy for a patient after primary tendon repair, a therapist needs to have information about the following:

1. Mechanism of the injury
2. Level or zone of the injury
3. Which tendons were repaired; which were left unrepaired; and whether injury included partial lacerations
4. Condition of the tendons
5. Amount of tension on the repairs
6. Involvement of other structures (for example, pulley or nerve repairs) and associated injuries (such as fractures) requiring special precautions
7. Position of the splint and any special considerations or precautions concerning the splint program

Postoperative protocol

The HRC protocol for primary repairs is divided into four phases: early phase, early intermediate phase, intermediate phase, and late phase. The rate at which an individual progresses through the phases is determined by the amount of adhesion formation and by how well the tendon is gliding. If the tendon is gliding well, indicating that adhesion formation is limited, the repair will be protected longer and the pace of the patient's program will be slowed. When excessive adhesion formation occurs, the pace of the program will be increased.

Early phase: 1 to 4 weeks. Goals for this phase are (1) to fabricate a splint or alter the postoperative cast to protect the repair but allow early motion, (2) to instruct the patient in the early motion exercise program, and (3) to instruct the patient in edema control and prevention techniques. The prevention of complications, especially the development of PIP flexion contractures, is also important during this phase.

The first therapy visit usually occurs on the first day following surgery. At that time the plaster cast with bulky dressing is modified to allow for motion. The dressing is "debulked" in the palm to allow for passive flexion of the digits (Fig. 30-6). The cast may start slipping distally after debulking; and this should be checked by the therapist. It can be prevented by securing the cast with tape across the palm and around the wrist and forearm. The wrist should be placed at 30 degrees of flexion. The MP joints are placed at 70 degrees flexion, whereas the dorsal part extending to the tips of the fingers allows full extension of the IP joints (Fig. 30-7).

The angle of the MP joints should be 60 degrees of flexion or more to ensure that most of the power for PIP extension is achieved by the relatively stronger long extensors with assistance from the lumbricals. If the splint holds the MP joints in too much extension, or if the splint does not fit

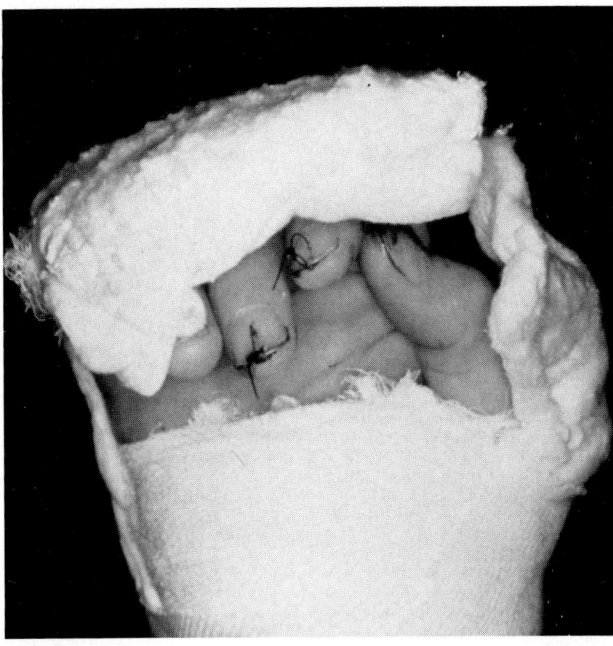

Fig. 30-6   The postoperative bulky dressing is modified to allow for motion.

correctly and allows the hand to slip, the MP joint can buckle out of the splint and the long extensors will extend the MP joint. Then the lumbricals will be less able to assist in extending the PIP joint, and contractures of the PIP joint can result.[36]

The importance of achieving full extension of the PIP and distal interphalangeal (DIP) joints from day one after surgery cannot be stressed enough. Unfortunately, PIP joint contractures sometimes do occur. Most of the time these contractures could have been prevented by meticulous supervision of the splint and a correctly performed exercise program. A more detailed section on the prevention of PIP contractures will follow later in this chapter.

As mentioned earlier, the cast may slip distally after debulking the dressing. This must be checked by the therapist

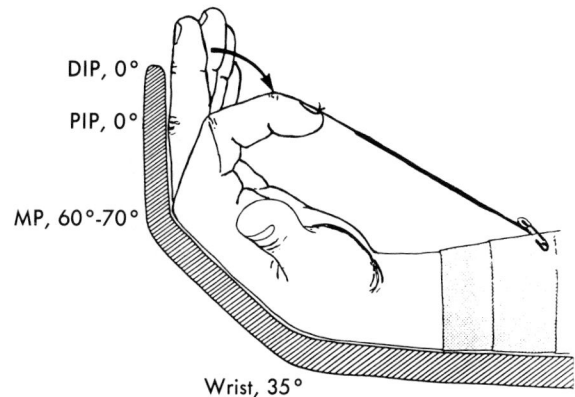

Fig. 30-7   The splint should place the wrist at 30 degrees of flexion, and the metacarpophalangeal joint at 70 degrees of flexion. It is imperative that full extension of the interphalangeal joints is possible within the limits of the splint.

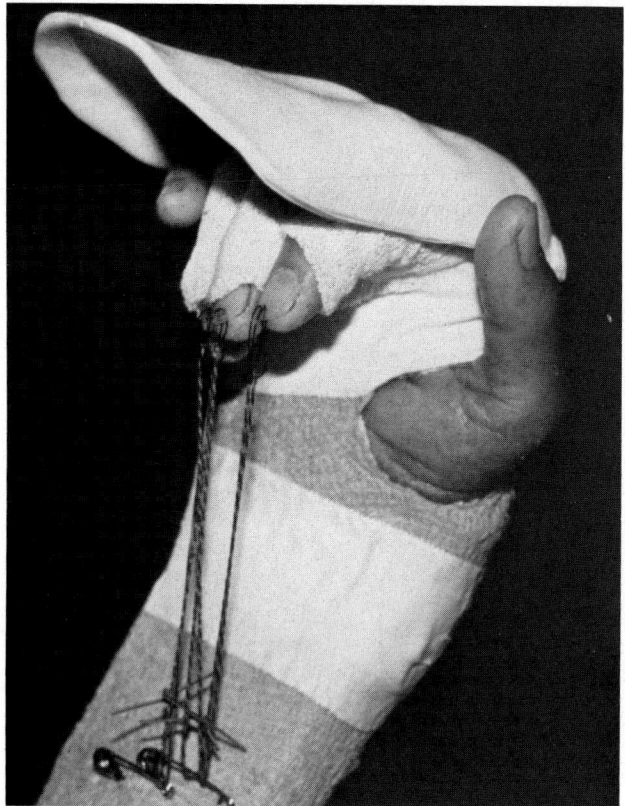

Fig. 30-8 Tape can be used across the palm and at the wrist to prevent the splint from slipping distally.

because it can cause an alteration of the angle at which the digits are to be placed, or it can interfere with the correct execution of the exercise program, and development of contractures is also a threat. If the plaster cast fits well, it is secured with nonelastic tape through the palm and at the wrist to prevent the cast from slipping distally. If the plaster cast is not positioning the hand correctly or is uncomfortable for the patient, a thermoplastic splint is fabricated. Because of possible postoperative edema this splint is secured in the first week with an elastic wrap. Tape may be used at the palm and wrist to prevent the splint from slipping distally (Fig. 30-8). When edema is under control, the splint can be secured with Velcro closures.

Thin elastic thread* is used for dynamic traction. The elastic is placed through a nail suture, applied during surgery. If a nail suture was not used by the surgeon, a dressmaker's hook can be glued to the nail. The thread is doubled and attached to the volar side of the forearm with a safety pin, approximately 3 inches proximal to the wrist crease. The tension should be light enough to allow full active extension of the interphalangeal joints and strong enough to pull the fingers back into flexion (Fig. 30-9). When the fingers are at rest in the position of flexion, there should be minimum or no tension. Sometimes the patient has problems reaching the last degrees of full extension against the rubber band on the first day after surgery, because of general postoperative weakness and pain. In that case the therapist can instruct the patient, for the first few days, to assist the active extension against the rubber band by manually releasing

*North Coast Medical, Inc., Campbell, Calif.

Fig. 30-9 Dynamic traction is achieved by using elastic thread. The thread is attached approximately 3 inches proximal to the wrist crease. The amount of tension should allow for full active extension within the limits of the splint, whereas the elastic thread should pull the finger back into flexion.

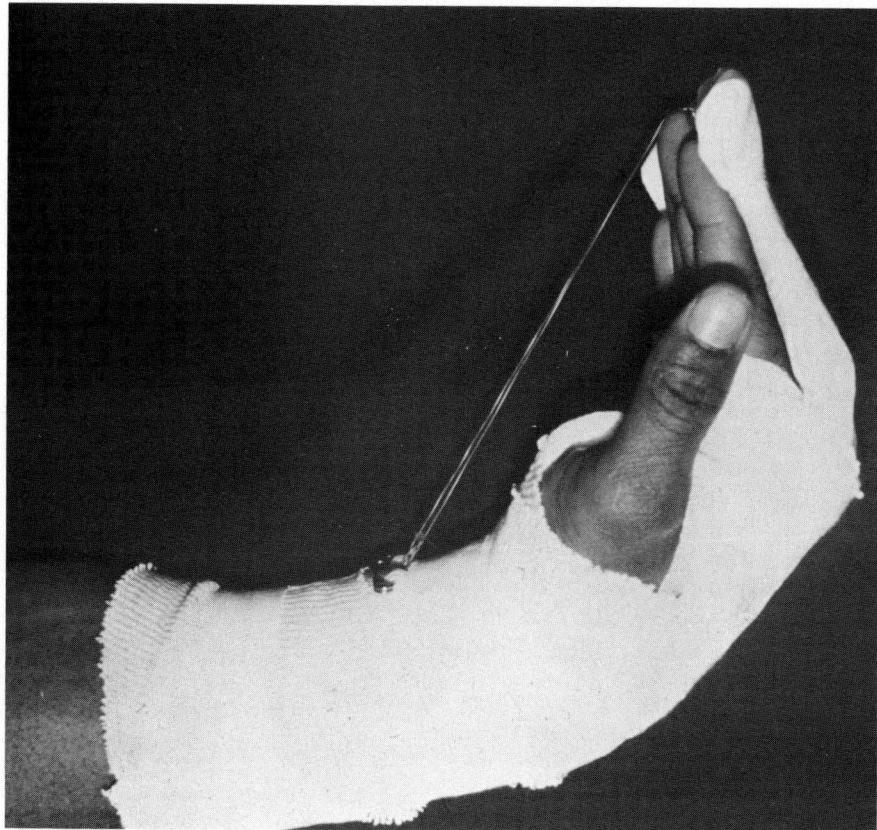

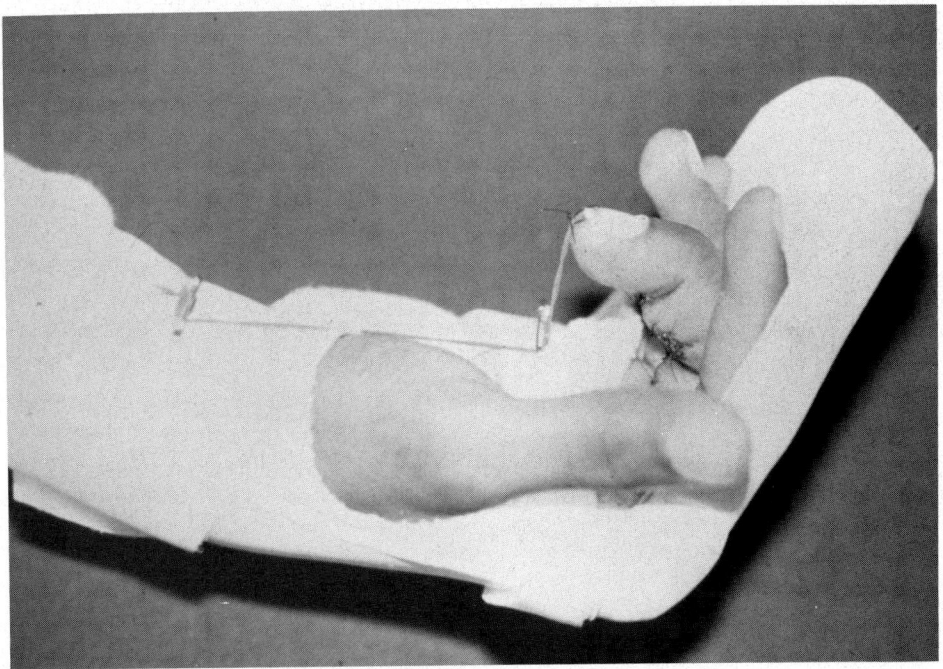

Fig. 30-10   A safety pin can be used to redirect the line of pull.

some of the tension on the rubber band with the uninvolved hand. It is imperative, however, when using this technique, that at the end of active extension the patient relaxes the finger and allows the rubber band to pull the finger back into flexion.

In some cases not enough DIP flexion is achieved with the rubber band. Most of the flexion will occur at the PIP joint because of the position of the rubber-band attachment to the wrist. When more DIP flexion is required, a safety pin can be used to redirect the line of pull into the palm (Fig. 30-10).

Redirecting the line of pull is also used for thumb flexor tendon repairs. Correct positioning of the thumb at rest is achieved, while at the same time optimum length for dynamic traction is obtained by redirecting the line of pull over the ulnar side of the wrist (Fig. 30-11).

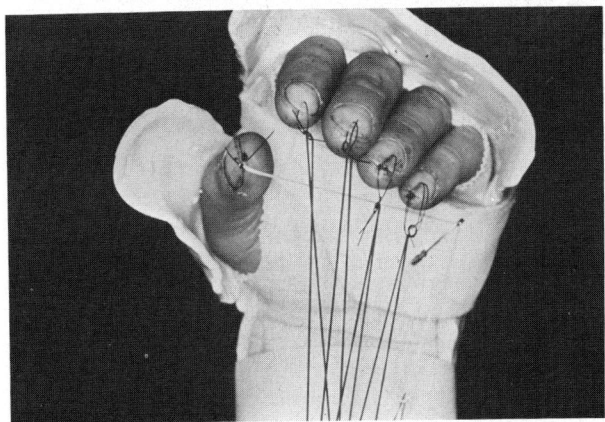

Fig. 30-11   Redirecting the line of pull for flexor tendon repairs of the thumb, using a safety pin.

A special situation needs mentioning: repair of the profundus tendon of one of the ulnar three digits. Many surgeons feel that all three digits should be included in dynamic traction to prevent rupture caused by strong contraction of the common profundus muscle belly.

After dynamic traction is applied, the patient is cautioned that no active flexion of the involved digits is allowed. However, the uninvolved digit(s) can actively flex and extend, if the involved digit(s) is held in passive flexion. The splint cannot be removed by the patient. At this time, the patient is instructed to keep the hand and extremity elevated for edema control. If edema persists, stronger measures of edema control can be used. These measures will be discussed later in this chapter. Patient education or parent education is essential at this point, and reasons for exercises and precautions should be given.

The patient is instructed in a home exercise program consisting of hourly active extension exercises to the limits of the splint, with 10 repetitions each exercise session. These same exercises are used for lacerations in zones 1 to 5. In addition, a passive exercise program is engaged four times daily for all digits including uninvolved digits. Sometimes the passive exercise program is not started until the second visit, so as not to overwhelm the patient on the first postoperative day. Passive flexion exercises are performed for isolated MP, PIP, and DIP flexion followed by full passive flexion to the DPC. Passive PIP extension is performed to prevent PIP flexion contractures. Passive extension is performed with the MP joint held down in 90 degrees of flexion to avoid excessive tension on the repair. Extension pressure with the uninvolved hand is applied at the middle phalanx (Fig. 30-12). Passive DIP extension is done with both the MP and PIP joints flexed, again to prevent tension on the repair (Fig. 30-13). Care is taken to avoid passively extending the PIP and DIP joints simultaneously. All exercises

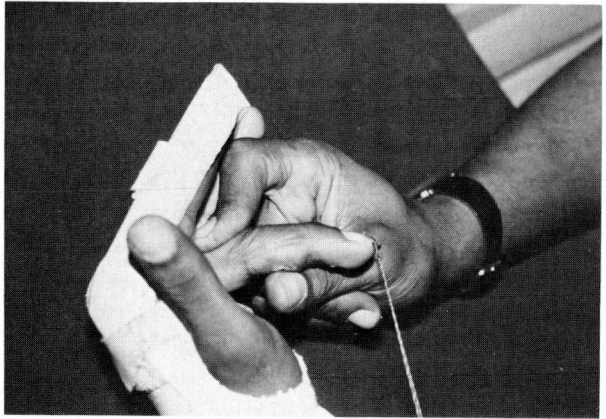

Fig. 30-12 Passive proximal interphalangeal extension exercises are done with the metacarpophalangeal joint held in full flexion. Pressure for extension should be directed at the middle phalanx.

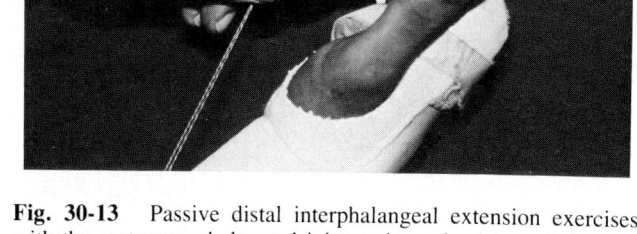

Fig. 30-13 Passive distal interphalangeal extension exercises with the metacarpophalangeal joint and proximal interphalangeal joint held in flexion.

are repeated 10 times, and each position is held for 5 seconds.

All exercises are performed by the patient and checked by the therapist before the patient can go home. If active PIP extension is still a problem, a felt wedge can be placed behind the proximal phalanx to increase MP flexion which, in turn, will facilitate active PIP joint extension. The patient can also use the uninvolved hand and manually hold down the MP joint in more flexion.

During the early phase the patient is seen two or three times a week. It is important to regularly check the tension of the rubber bands to make sure the finger is passively pulled into flexion and allows full extension to the limits of the dorsal splint. As postoperative edema decreases, the correct position of the MP joint in the splint will also need monitoring.

As discussed above, after the first week, if additional edema control is needed, a Coban* wrap tube for each finger, made out of 4-inch wide Coban, can help reduce swelling without interfering with the exercises.

The sutures are usually removed at 10 to 14 days. When the wound permits, massage is initiated. The patient is instructed in retrograde massage, which is a distal to proximal "milking" motion, to aid venous drainage. Scar management is also initiated by instructing the patient in deep massage techniques, again, when the wound permits, thus mobilizing and softening the scar.

At 2 to 3 weeks the scar sometimes seems to harden and the patient may experience a more "sluggish" feeling when performing the exercises. This observation may be explained by the fact that this time period corresponds with the time period in the wound healing process when intermolecular cross-linking of the collagen molecules starts.

Early intermediate phase: 4 to 6 weeks. Goals during this phase are (1) to increase gliding potential by starting active "place-hold" exercises, (2) to discharge the patient from the dorsal protective splint into a wristlet, allowing some wrist motion, and (3) to continue edema control, scar management, and prevention of PIP contractures as needed.

*North Coast Medical, Inc., Campbell, Calif.

Generally, lacerations in zones 3 and 5 have fewer complications than lacerations in zone 2 because of the relatively good vascularity and the type of adhesions formed in zones 3 and 5. Special attention should be given at this time to the assessment of differential tendon glide after tendon lacerations in zone 4.

At 3 weeks the patient is evaluated to decide what course of therapy should be chosen. If at this time the tendon glides easily, the repair is protected for at least another week. If at this time tendon glide is minimal, the patient is started on gentle active exercises in the splint. The dorsal splint is discharged in the fourth week unless a longer protection period is necessary. For example, if tendon repair is combined with nerve repair the hand is held in the protected position for 6 weeks. If the patient shows extremely good gliding of the repaired tendon, the hand is also held in the protective splint up to 6 weeks.

If the dorsal protective splint is removed, dynamic traction is continued. The proximal end of the rubber band is now attached to a wristlet or wrist band (Fig. 30-14). The patient is instructed to avoid simultaneous wrist and finger extension.

The exercise program in the early intermediate phase includes initiation of active flexion through "place-hold" exercises in slight flexion, mid-flexion, and full flexion. Differential glide of the tendons is encouraged by performing these exercises in different positions. Doing the exercises in different positions is especially important for lacerations in zone 4 where isolated tendon glide can be restricted because of adhesions formed between different tendons in the carpal tunnel.

The active hourly extension exercises against the rubber band are continued with the wrist held in neutral. Passive flexion and extension exercises are continued, as in the early phase, four times a day, and special attention is given to possible contracture development. Active wrist exercises are initiated with the fingers passively flexed to avoid tension on the tendon repair. Edema control through elevation and massage and scar management are continued in this period.

The place-hold exercises used at the HRC can sometimes be started as early as 3 weeks if tendon glide is restricted.

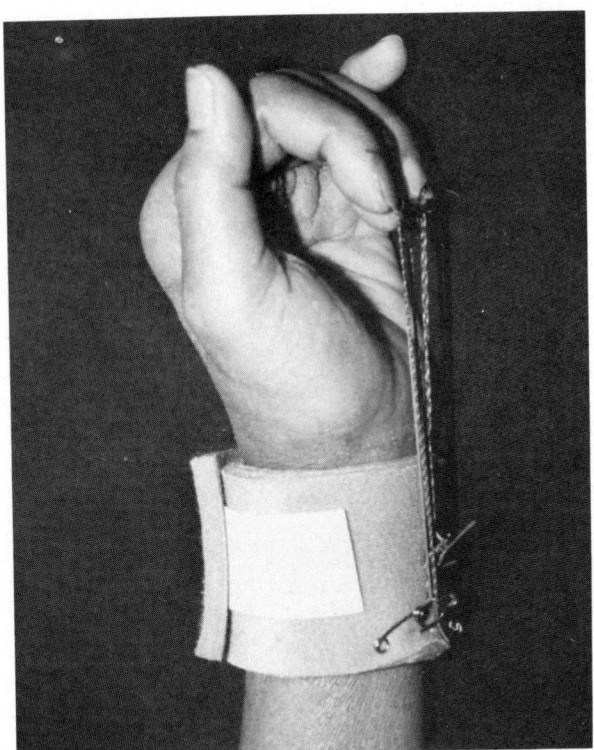

Fig. 30-14 At approximately 4 to 6 weeks dynamic traction is continued in a wristlet, allowing wrist motion.

This exercise achieves the same tendon excursion as does active flexion but requires less force than when the tendon has to pull the finger from an extended position. The patient presses the finger(s) passively into full flexion with the uninvolved hand. Then, on releasing the pressure of the uninvolved hand, the patient attempts to hold the flexed position of the fingers. This exercise can also be done in different fisting positions to encourage differential tendon glide.

Intermediate phase: 6 to 8 weeks. The most important goal during this phase is to achieve full active glide and maximum differential glide of both tendons. All protective splinting should be discontinued; however, if needed, cor-

rective splinting can be initiated at this time. Work therapy can be initiated to increase tendon glide and to start strengthening the hand and upper extremity. Contracture control, edema control, and scar management will continue if necessary.

At 6 weeks the wristlet is discontinued and active motion is initiated using tendon gliding exercises. Differential tendon gliding exercises (TGE) were developed at the HRC based on a study by Wehbe and Hunter.[79] The authors concluded that three different hand positions (hook-fist, straight-fist, and full-fist) (Fig. 30-15) produced maximum differential glide between FDP, FDS, and surrounding tissues. Maximum excursion of profundus tendon in relation to the sheath and bone is achieved when making a full fist, and maximum excursion of the superficialis tendon in relation to the sheath and bone is in the straight fist position. The hook position produces maximum differential glide between profundus and superficialis tendons. These exercises are performed three to four times a day and repeated 10 times for each type of fist. Again, these exercises can be especially important for a zone 4 laceration where differential glide can be a problem.

Blocking exercises of PIP and DIP joints to encourage isolated tendon gliding are initiated and gradually increased during this period, again depending on the progress of the individual patient. When superficialis pull-through is restricted, casts can be fabricated immobilizing the DIP joint in extension, while allowing PIP joint motion (Fig. 30-16). These casts can be worn during exercises and activities if necessary. Removable cylinders of plaster, immobilizing the PIP joint and leaving the DIP joint free, can be fabricated for each individual finger and help the patient to stabilize for isolated FDP exercises. Other blocking devices, such as the Bunnell block, may be used, and sometimes the patient can stabilize the digit with the uninvolved hand. Isolated superficialis exercises are done by flexing one finger at a time at the PIP joint, with the uninvolved hand keeping the other fingers in extension. This exercise is best performed with the hand resting flat on the table (Fig. 30-17).

More aggressive edema control exercises can be started at this point. An extremely effective way of reducing edema in the hand is by flexing and extending all digits at the same time while the hand is held overhead with the arm extended at the elbow. Repeated active fisting, even when done gently,

There are three ways of making a fist:

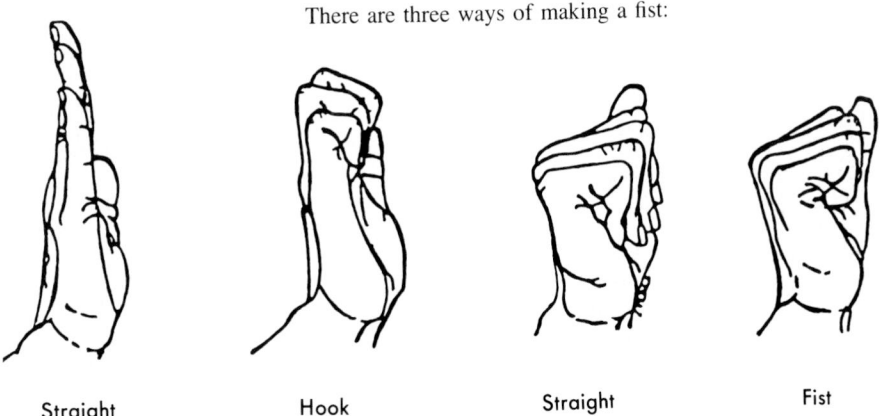

Straight   Hook   Straight   Fist

Fig. 30-15 The three different positions of tendon gliding exercises; hook-fist, straight-fist, and full-fist.

will help "pump" the swelling, with gravity, towards the heart.

Scar management is continued in this period with scar massage and, in some cases, pressure applied with an Elastomere* (Fig. 30-18) held in place with Coban wrap. This can be worn only when not exercising so as not to impede motion.

---

*Dow Corning Corp., Midland, Mich.

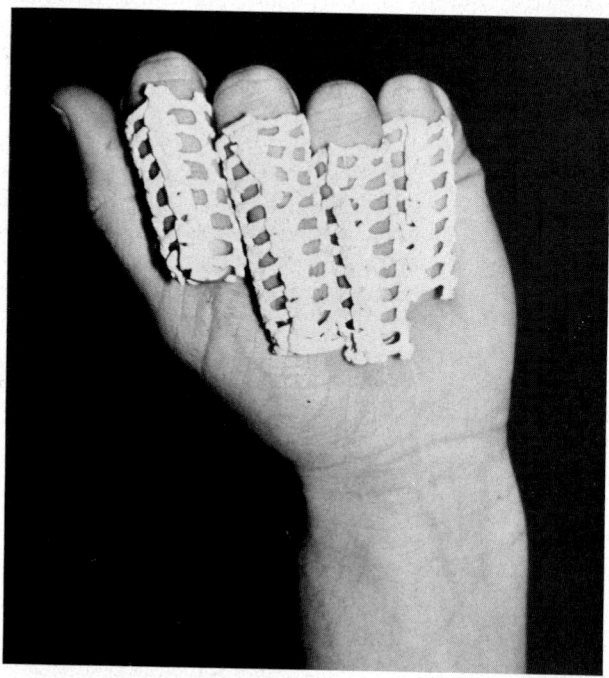

Fig. 30-16 To encourage superficialis pull through, these casts immobilize the distal interphalangeal joint in extension, while allowing active proximal interphalangeal joint motion.

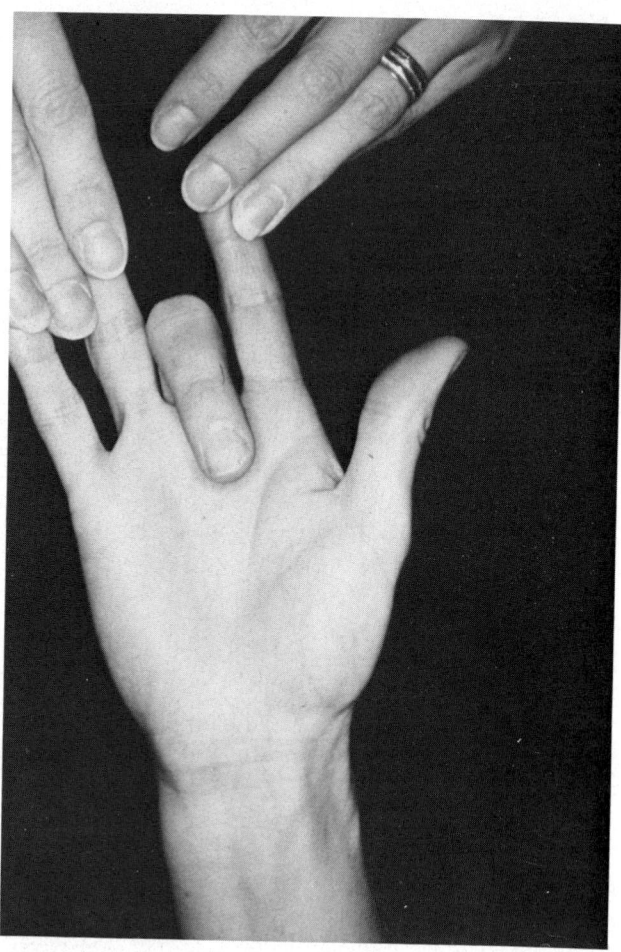

Fig. 30-17 Active isolated superficialis exercise: flexing one finger at a time at the PIP joint while holding the other fingers in extension with the uninvolved hand.

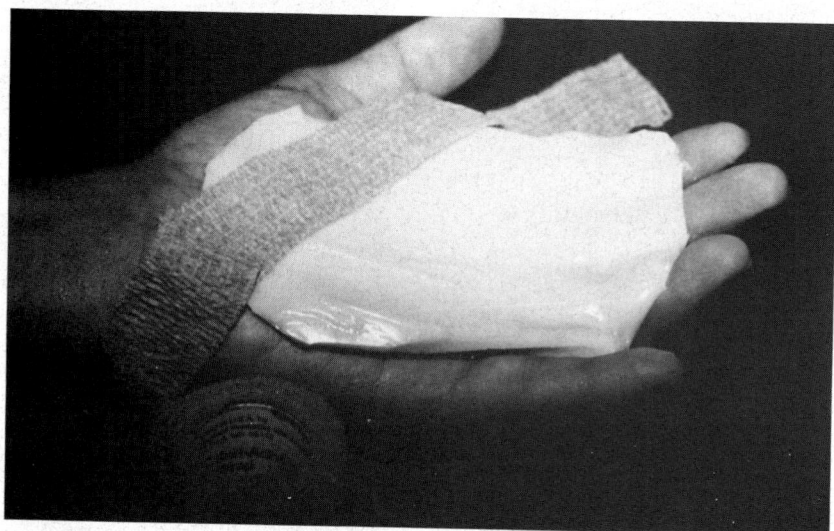

Fig. 30-18 Continuous pressure for scar control can be achieved by using an Elastomer, held in place with Coban tape or an Ace wrap.

Contracture control during this phase can be more aggressive. Gentle passive stretch may be applied. Some patients may require additional splinting at this time. Dynamic splinting may be used for contracture control but can also facilitate pull-through for the tendon. If the contracture is caused by tendon tightness, a plaster stretcher is the choice of treatment (Fig. 30-19)(see Chapter 90). Other splints that might need to be provided at this time are anticlaw splints in the presence of median, ulnar, or combined nerve injury.

At this time use of the involved hand in activities of daily living (ADL) such as writing and eating are encouraged. Built-up handles might be necessary to facilitate functional use of the hand.

Work therapy is usually initiated during the intermediate phase. When moderate amounts of motion of the tendon are achieved and glide is relatively good, the routine protocol is followed with work therapy starting at 6 weeks. When the patient has extremely good glide, work therapy might not be initiated until 8 weeks. In contrast, the patient who has restricted tendon glide because of adhesion formation might start work therapy at 5 weeks after repair. Initially, the work therapy program consists of sustained grip exercises such as woodworking (Fig. 30-20) and isometric exercises for strength. Woodworking is started with two 15-minute sessions and increased to four 15-minute sessions during the first week. The isometric exercises are kept in the 1- to 3-lb range the first 2 weeks. Biofeedback may be used for facilitation of the injured muscle-tendon unit and for relaxation of the antagonist. The home program at this time may include massage, scar control through constant pressure, corrective splinting, TGE and blocking exercises, woodworking exercises and isometrics.

Therapeutic heat modalities are often used when scar remodeling and elongation of limiting adhesions is necessary. The beneficial effect of heat combined with stretch to facilitate lengthening of the tissue has been well documented

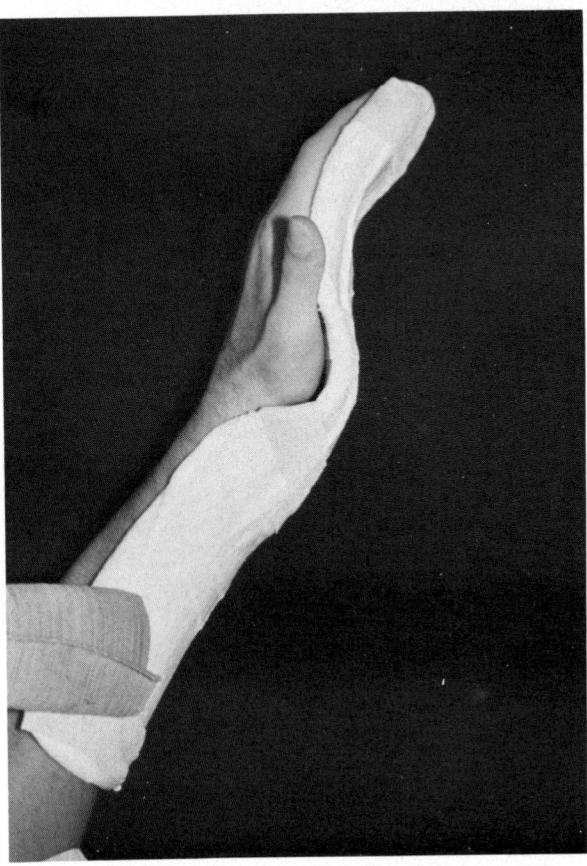

Fig. 30-19   Plaster stretchers are the treatment of choice for flexor tendon tightness.

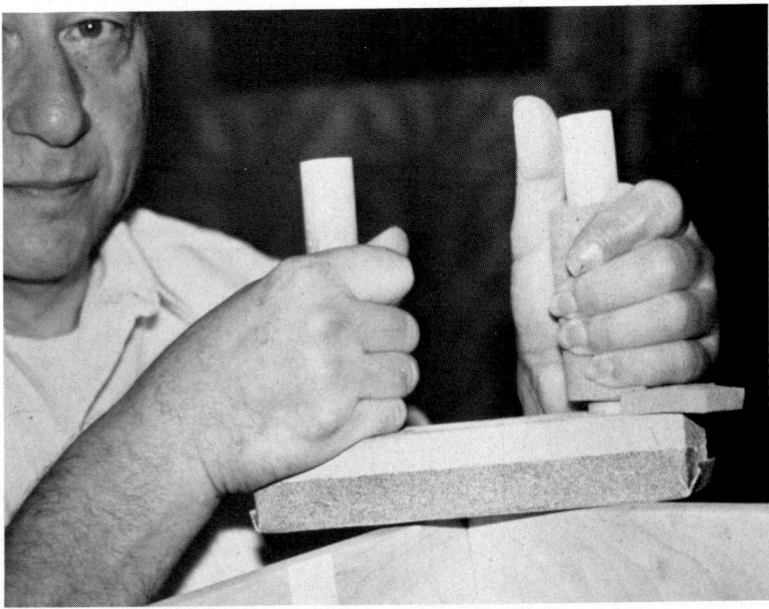

Fig. 30-20   Sustained grip exercises, such as woodworking, can be extremely helpful in achieving tendon pull through when adhesions limit tendon glide.

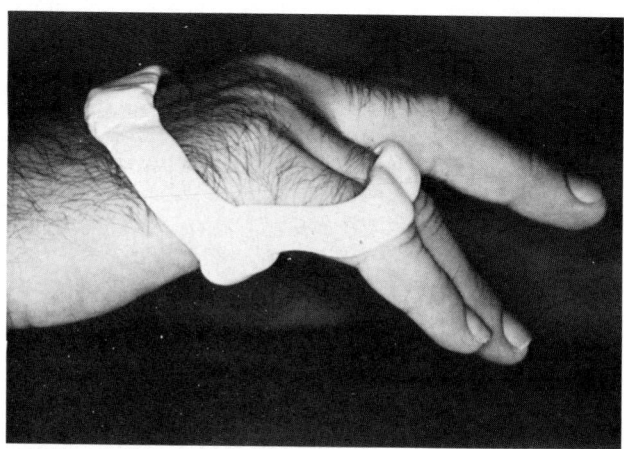

Fig. 30-21 In the presence of ulnar, medium, or combined-nerve injury, continued splinting, such as an anticlaw splint, may be indicated.

in in vitro studies.[37,38,76] Gertsen[28] showed that a temperature rise of 39° to 47° C resulted in an increase in tissue extensibility.

Detrimental effects on tendon healing, however, have been reported with ultrasound therapy applied during the early phases of tendon healing by Roberts and associates.[64] Surgically repaired rabbit tendons were treated with cast immobilization or cast immobilization combined with ultrasound therapy to the repair site for 6 weeks. Ultrasound was applied 5 minutes, 5 days per week, at a dosage of 0.8 W/cm^2. At 6 weeks the group treated with immobilization by casting showed good tensile strength. The group treated with casting and ultrasound showed no evidence of healing and, consequently, less tensile strength.

The possible beneficial effects of ultrasound therapy on tendon healing have more recently been investigated in a study by Stevenson and associates.[71] Chicken tendon healing was observed in different treatment groups for tensile strength and functional recovery. One group of chickens was treated with immobilization for 4 weeks; the other group was treated with immobilization for 4 weeks with daily ultrasound therapy begun at 4 weeks. The results of this study showed a significant improvement of functional recovery, with no effect on tensile strength, for the group treated with ultrasound. The authors further suggest that the mechanism of action of ultrasound therapy on tendon healing may be caused by the nonthermal effects on tissues, possibly the inhibition of maturation of collagen.

Based on the results of the study by Roberts and associates,[64] ultrasound therapy should not be used during the first 6 weeks of tendon healing. The study by Stevenson and associates[71] gives some evidence of the beneficial effect of ultrasound on tendon healing when started in a later phase of healing. However, until more research has been done to investigate the exact mechanism of ultrasound therapy applied to healing tissues, ultrasound should not be begun until the late phase (8 weeks) when the scar has matured.

Late phase: 8 to 12 weeks. The most important goals in this phase are improvement of strength and endurance.

Emphasis during this period is on return to work. The exercise program and home program are directed toward strengthening and functional use of the hand. Grip and pinch measurements are taken weekly to monitor progress. Splinting may continue during the late phase, especially in the presence of median, ulnar, or combined nerve injury and may include anticlaw or C-bar splints to position the thumb (Fig. 30-21).

Work therapy at this time consists of combined grip and wrist motion exercises, such as weight-well exercises, supination/pronation bar, regressive resistive exercises, and upper body strengthening with pulley exercises. Sustained grip exercises are continued with woodworking up to three

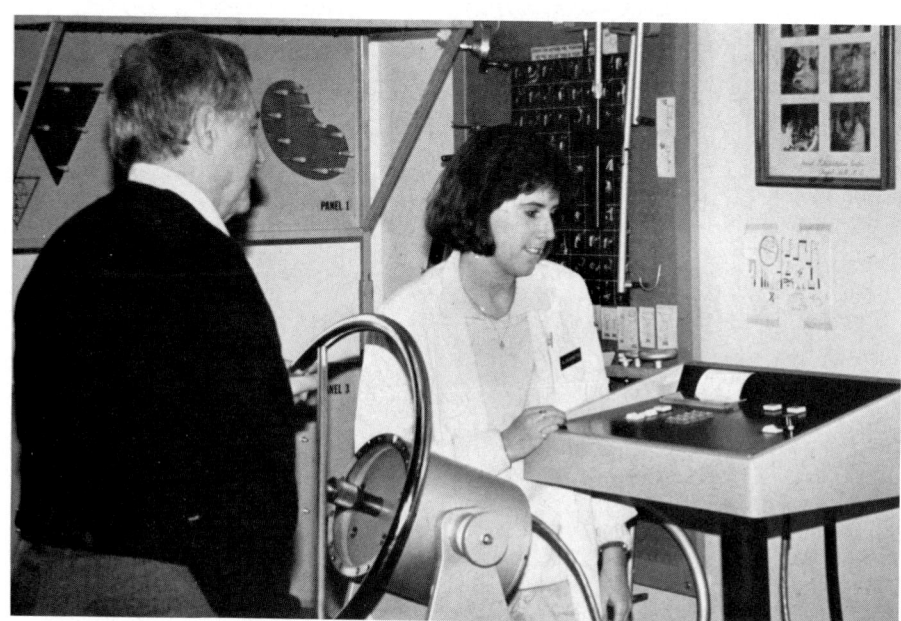

Fig. 30-22 Job simulation is an essential part of the late rehabilitation phase.

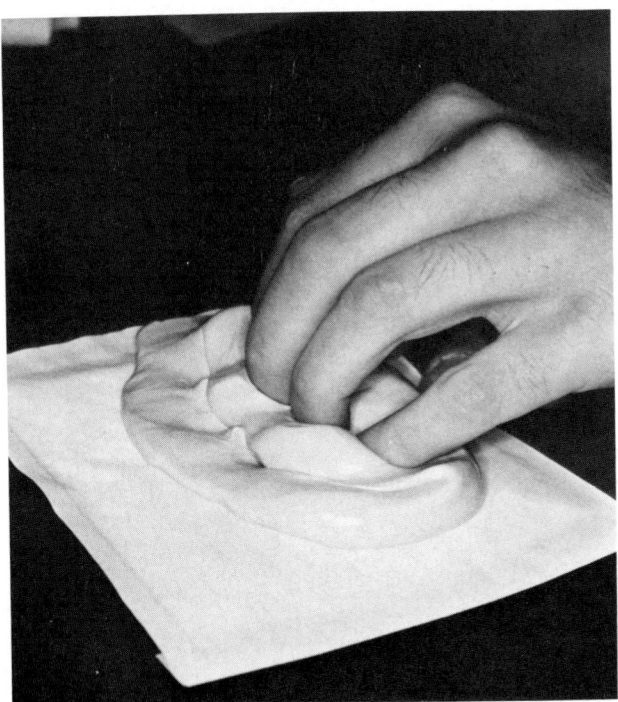

Fig. 30-23 Putty exercises are an important part of the home program in the intermediate and late phases for achieving tendon glide and strength.

30-minute sessions. Job simulation is introduced during this time and work simulator exercises are initiated (Fig 30-22).

The home program at this time will include exercises with putty (Fig. 30-23), the hand helper, regressive resistive exercises, and woodworking. The patient is encouraged to perform job simulation tasks at home such as tool handling (Fig 30-24) and repetitive lifting.

In this late phase the amount of resistance and performance time of job simulation tasks is increased. The patient is usually evaluated for return to work before discharge from therapy.

COMPLICATIONS
PIP contractures

One of the problems often seen in patients with dynamic traction in the protective dorsal splint is PIP contracture. A thorough splint check by the therapist can prevent the development of this complication. The therapist should look for proper positioning of the MP joint in the splint. To prevent the splint from slipping distally the therapist must ensure good fit and proper strapping of the splint, especially through the palm. The therapist should make sure when fabricating a dorsal hood that the patient can fully extend the PIP and DIP joints within the splint (Fig. 30-25). And finally, the therapist should regularly check the tension of the rubber bands. The tension should allow the patient to fully extend the finger. To prevent contractions, the therapist should also carefully instruct the patient on the exercise program and check for correct execution of the program. Patient or parent education is essential for success of this treatment protocol.

Despite all best efforts by therapist and patient, contractures can still develop. If full PIP extension is not reached by the end of the first week, some additional splinting is needed. First, a simple felt block can be placed behind the proximal phalanx during extension exercises to increase MP flexion. The increase in MP flexion makes extension exercises more efficient at the PIP joint. The same effect can also be achieved by having the patient manually hold down the proximal phalanx with the uninvolved hand. If this is not enough, a passive interphalangeal extension splint, made of alumafoam can be fitted within the dorsal splint (Fig. 30-26). This splint slips on and off the distal end of the

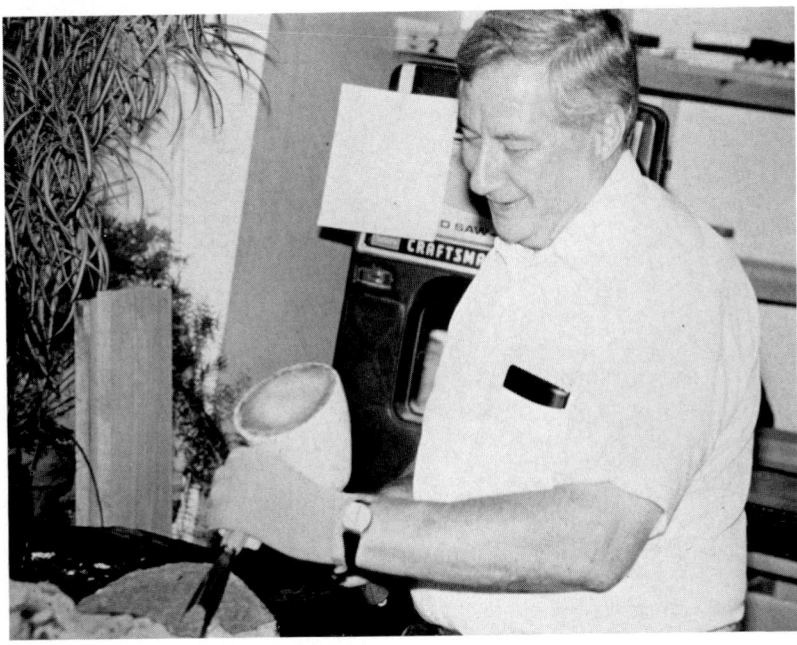

Fig. 30-24 Tool handling will often be part of the job simulation exercises in the late phase.

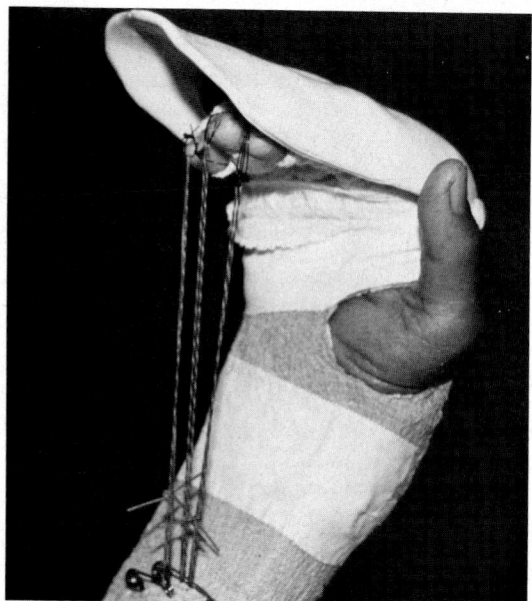

Fig. 30-25 Full active extension of both the proximal interphalangeal and distal interphalangeal joints should be possible in the splint.

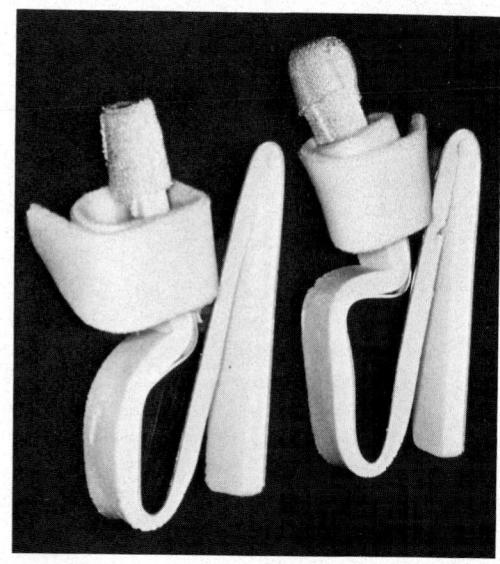

Fig. 30-26 Passive proximal interphalangeal (PIP) extension splint can be fabricated to hold the metacarpophalangeal joint in more flexion to maximize PIP extension exercises. The splint slips on and off the distal end of the dorsal protective splint and is worn intermittently during the day. This splint can also be fabricated for the distal interphalangeal joint.

dorsal protective splint. The splint positions the MP joint in maximum flexion so that tension is taken off the flexor tendons. This makes it possible to then apply a gentle stretch at the PIP joint, rather than on the flexor tendons, by placing a static adjustable strap around the middle phalanx (Fig. 30-27) The splint is worn for half an hour, three to four times a day. The amount of tension applied by the strap and the duration of use can be gradually increased over the first 4 weeks.

After the dorsal protective splint is discontinued, PIP contractures might still require corrective splinting. Most surgeons and therapists follow similar treatment protocols during the first 3 to 4 weeks. Discrepancies exist, however, on when and how to correct PIP contractures after the dorsal splint is removed. Some surgeons and therapists feel comfortable with beginning static serial splinting as early as 4 weeks.[55] Kleinert[54], Duran[54], Hunter[54], and Schneider[67] start dynamic or static splinting at 6 to 8 weeks.

The key to static and dynamic corrective splinting for PIP joint contractures is to provide a gentle passive stretch to the limiting structures of the joint without stressing the repaired tendon too much. If flexion is limited because of flexor tendon tightness, plaster stretchers should be used (see Chapter 90). The decision about when to initiate splinting and what type to use is based on good evaluation skills, knowledge of collagen synthesis, and knowledge of tendon healing.

The amount of force to use for corrective splinting and the decision of when to use dynamic versus static splinting are important. Dynamic traction is usually considered a more aggressive corrective splinting method than static splinting. The therapist should realize that forceful manipulation of tissues can cause an inflammatory response, which could induce more scarring and worsen the contracture. Gentle stretch applied over long periods of time is the

method of choice for most situations. However, each decision should be made based on the status of the patient and the patient's understanding of the use of corrective splints. Most therapists will be familiar with the situation in which a patient, despite careful instructions, proudly tells you he or she could "tolerate" the splint for 3 hours!! The patient

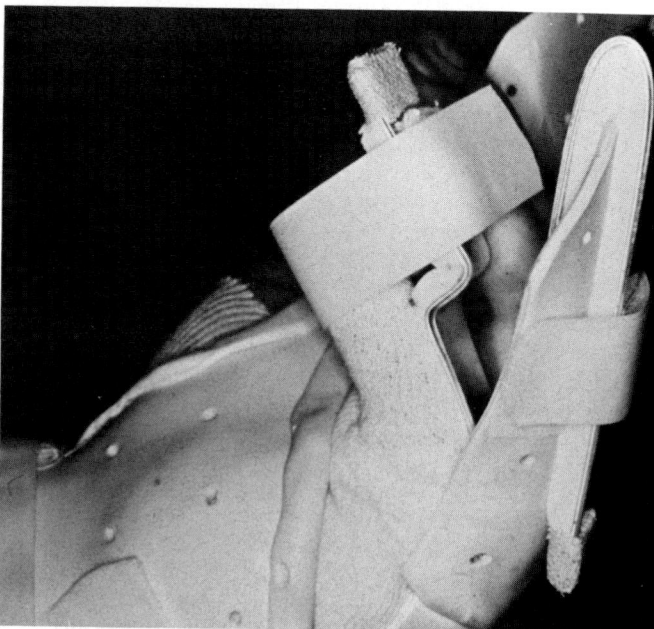

Fig. 30-27 A static adjustable strap can be used in conjunction with the passive proximal interphalangeal (PIP) extension splint to correct PIP contractures.

should be well instructed in the use of the splint, and should also understand the principles of prolonged gentle stretch.

Lack of tendon glide at the DIP joint

Another criticism of the Kleinert technique of dynamic traction is that the rubber band pulls the PIP joint in flexion but the DIP remains in extension. If the DIP joint is not flexed sufficiently during dynamic traction, FDP glide will remain limited beyond the middle phalanx. A method was proposed to include the DIP joint more effectively in dynamic traction by redirecting the line of pull to the palm with a safety pin or manually with the uninvolved hand. This method, however, needs careful supervision. The increased tension needed for flexing the entire finger can cause two problems. A DIP contracture may develop because the patient is not able to achieve full DIP extension during active extension exercises. Another problem that can develop is overstretching of the distal portion of the extensor tendon, resulting in a lack of active extension at the DIP joint.[55] To prevent these complications from occurring, it is suggested that the line of pull be redirected to the palm during the hourly active extension exercises while making sure that full PIP and DIP extension is achieved. Between exercises the standard line of pull to the forearm can be maintained.

Pulley repair and bowstringing

Bowstringing of the tendon can be avoided by surgical repair of the pulley system. When pulleys are repaired they need to be protected throughout the postoperative therapy program. The simplest method for protecting a reconstructed pulley is to ask the patient to apply pressure with the uninvolved hand over the reconstructed pulley during active flexion and extension. A combination of protection with a ring made of thermoplastic material and manual pressure during exercises is also possible.

During the first 3 to 4 weeks when no active flexion is performed, the pulley should still be protected. Because the first week or two postoperative edema might be present and could change circumferential measurements dramatically, an adjustable, soft felt and Velcro ring can be fabricated. When edema is under control, an adjustable thermoplastic ring can be fabricated, still with Velcro closure to allow for adaptation to possible fluctuations in swelling (Fig. 30-28). Eventually the thermoplastic ring can be replaced by a metal ring. The reconstructed pulley should be protected for 4 to 6 months, according to Mackin.[55]

Ruptures

Rupture of a tendon repair is the second most frequent cause for failure of primary flexor tendon repairs. Patient education and adaptation of the postoperative protocol to the individual patient can probably prevent most ruptures. A good example of the need to adapt the protocol to the individual patient would be the patient with extremely good early glide of the tendon. This patient should not be taken out of the protective splint too early because he is more prone to ruptures. If the tendon is healing mostly by intrinsic means, there will be less adhesion formation. One should realize, however, that because extrinsic blood supply by way of scar adhesions is limited, the tendon will have a lower rate of healing and at 4 weeks the juncture might still be weak. The decrease in blood flow to the tendon may increase the need for protective splinting up to 6 or 8 weeks. Initiation of active or resistive exercises should also be delayed for this patient.

Patient education in the above described example will be very effective in preventing ruptures. The patient with good glide of a repaired tendon must understand why he needs to be held in a protective splint longer and, why in his case, the start of active or resistive exercises may be delayed. Sometimes the therapist may decide to keep the overly active patient in a protective splint between exercises, even after the dynamic traction is discontinued, just as a reminder not to simultaneously extend the fingers and wrist.

Heavy resistive flexion exercises are probably not the most frequent cause for ruptures. Based on clinical observations,[55] it seems that a sudden passive stretch with wrist and finger joints in extension simultaneously, or a sudden change of the type of exercises from exercises normally performed in therapy, is a more frequent cause for ruptures. This last example stresses the importance of job simulation as an important part of the last weeks of therapy. If a patient can successfully do regressive resistive exercises with a 5-lb weight, it doesn't necessarily mean he can start playing the drums in a heavy metal rock band without rupturing the tendon.

CONCLUSION

Early protected mobilization as a postoperative treatment of flexor tendon lacerations has been developed based on research demonstrating the beneficial effects of motion on tendon healing. It is still unknown if a tendon heals by intrinsic or extrinsic means or both. Nevertheless, tendons are able to heal with less adhesions, and unyielding scar around tendon can be lengthened or remodeled, allowing the tendon to glide freely.

Many different forms of early protected mobilization exist and have been shown to result in strong, freely gliding tendon repairs. Ideally, the surgeon and therapist will combine their skills and knowledge to create an individualized

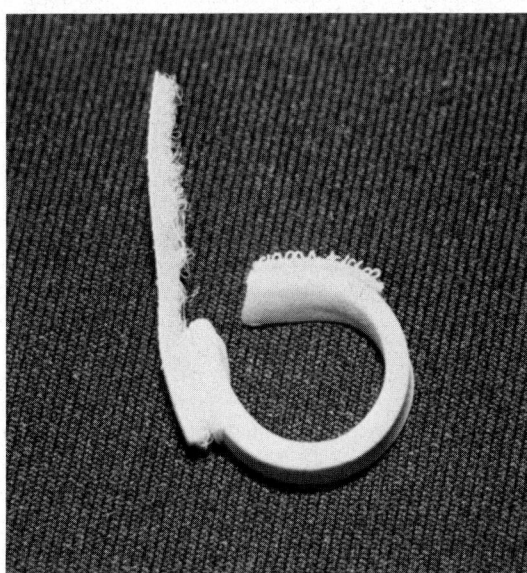

Fig. 30-28 Thermoplastic ring with adjustable Velcro closure to use for pulley protection. The strap allows the splint to be adjusted to accommodate fluctuating edema problems.

postoperative treatment program for each patient. Finally, the role of the patient in the postoperative rehabilitation process is imperative. The team of surgeon, therapist, and patient are ultimately responsible for the end result.

REFERENCES

1. Amadio PC and Hunter JM: Prognostic factors in flexor tendon surgery in zone 2. In Hunter JM, Schneider LH, and Mackin EJ, editors: Tendon surgery in the hand, St. Louis, 1987, The CV Mosby Co.
2. Amadio PC, Jaeger SH and Hunter JM: Nutritional aspects of tendon healing. In Hunter JM and others, editors: Rehabilitation of the hand, ed 2, St. Louis, 1984, The CV Mosby Co.
3. Amadio PC and others: The effect of vincular injury on the results of flexor tendon surgery in zone 2, J Hand Surg 10A(5):626, 1985.
4. Arem A and Madden J: Effects of stress on healing wounds. I. Intermittent noncyclical tension, J Surg Res 20:93, 1976.
5. Banes AJ and others: Effects of trauma and partial devascularization on protein synthesis in the avian flexor profundus tendon, J Trauma 21(7):505, 1981.
6. Beasley RW: Tendon injuries. In Beasley, RW: Injuries to the hand, Philadelphia, 1981, WB Saunders Co.
7. Bergljung L: Vascular reactions after tendon suture and tendon transplantation: a stereomicroangiographic study in the calcaneal tendon of the rabbit, Scand J Plast Reconstr Surg 4 (suppl):7, 1968.
8. Bergljung L: Vascular reactions in tendon healing, Angiology 21:375, 1970.
9. Birdsell DC, Tustanoff ER, and Lindsay WK: Collagen production in regenerating tendon, Plast Reconstr Surg 37:504, 1966.
10. Boyes JH: Discussion. In Cramer LM, and Chase RA, editors: Symposium of the hand, vol 3, St. Louis, 1971, The CV Mosby Co.
11. Brand PW: Clinical mechanics of the hand, St. Louis, 1985, The CV Mosby Co.
12. Brockis JG: The bloodsupply of the flexor and extensor tendons of the fingers in man, J Bone Joint Surg (Br) 35:131, 1953.
13. Bunnell S: Surgery of the hand, ed 4, Philadelphia, 1964, JB Lippincott Co.
14. Caplan HS, Hunter JM, and Merklin RJ: Intrinsic vascularization of flexor tendons. In American Academy of Orthopaedic Surgeons: Symposium on tendon surgery of the hand, St. Louis, 1975, The CV Mosby Co.
15. Chaplin DM: The vascular anatomy within normal tendons, divided tendons, free tendon grafts in rabbits, J Bone Joint Surg (Br) 55:369, 1973.
16. Cohen MJ and Kaplan L: Histology and ultrastructure of the human flexor tendon sheath, J Hand Surg 12-A:25, 1987.
17. Doyle JR and Blythe WF: The finger flexor tendon sheath and pulleys: anatomy and reconstruction. In American Academy of Orthopaedic Surgeons: Symposium on tendon surgery of the hand, St. Louis, 1975, The CV Mosby Co.
18. Duran RJ and Houser RG: Controlled passive motion following flexor tendon repair in zone II and III. In American Academy of Orthopaedic Surgeons: Symposium on tendon surgery of the hand, St. Louis, 1975, The CV Mosby Co.
19. Edwards DAW: The bloodsupply and lymphatic drainage of tendons, J Anat (Br) 80:11, 1946.
20. Eiken O, Lundborg G, and Rank F: The role of the digital synovial sheath in tendon grafting in the digit, Scand J Plast Reconstr Surg 9:182, 1975.
21. Ejeskar A: Flexor tendon repair in no-man's land: results of primary repair with controlled mobilization, J Hand Surg 9A(2):171, 1984.
22. Flynn JE and Graham JH: Healing of tendon wounds, Am J Surg 109:315, 1965.
23. Furlow LT: The role of tendon tissues in tendon healing, Plast Reconstr Surg 57:39, 1976.
24. Gelberman RH and others: The effects of mobilization on the vascularization of healing flexor tendons in dogs, Clin Orthop 153:283, 1980.
25. Gelberman RH and others: The influence of protected passive mobilization on the healing of flexor tendons: a biochemical and microangiographic study, Hand 13:130, 1981.
26. Gelberman RH and others: Effects of early intermittent passive mobilization on healing canine flexor tendons, J Hand Surg 7:170, 1982.
27. Gelberman RH and others: Flexor tendon healing and restoration of the gliding surface. An ultra structural study in dogs, J Bone Joint Surg (Am) 65:70, 1983.

28. Gertsen JW: The effect of ultrasound on tendon extensibility, Am J Phys Med 34:662, 1955.
29. Grant ME and Prockop DJ: the biosynthesis of collagen, New Engl J Med 286:194, 1972.
30. Hardy MA: Preserving function in the inflamed and acutely injured hand. In Moran CA, editor: Hand rehabilitation, New York, 1986, Churchill Livingstone.
31. Harmer TW: Tendon suture, Boston Med Surg J 167:808, 1917.
32. Harmer TW: Tendon surgery, Surg Clin North Am 1(3):809, 1921.
33. Kleinert HE and Cash SL: Current guidelines for flexor tendon repair within the fibro-osseous tunnel: indications, timing, and techniques. In Hunter JM, Schneider LH, and Mackin EJ, editors: Tendon surgery in the hand, St. Louis, 1987, The CV Mosby Co.
34. Kleinert HE, Kutz JE, and Cohen MJ: Primary repair of zone 2 flexor tendon lacerations. In American Academy of Orthopaedic Surgeons: Symposium on tendon surgery of the hand, St. Louis, 1975, The CV Mosby Co.
35. Kleinert HE and Verdan C: Report of the Committee on Tendon Injuries, J Hand Surg 8(5): 794, 1983.
36. Kutz JE and Bennet DL: Tendon injuries. In Watson N, and Smith R, editors: Methods and concepts in hand surgery, St. Louis, 1978, The CV Mosby Co.
37. Laban MM: Collagen tissue: implications of its response to stress in vitro, Arch Phys Med Rehab 43:461, 1962.
38. Lehman JF and others: therapeutic temperature distribution produced by ultrasound as modified by dosage and volume of tissue exposed, Arch Phys Med Rehab 48:662, 1967.
39. Lindsay WK and Thomson HG: Digital flexor tendons: an experimental study, Br J Plast Surg 12:289, 1960.
40. Lundborg G, Holm S, and Myrhage R: The role of synovial fluid and tendon sheath for flexor tendon nutrition, Scand J Plast Reconstr Surg 14:99, 1980.
41. Lundborg G, Myrhage R, and Rydevik B: The vascularization of human flexor tendons within the digital synovial sheath region: structural and functional aspects, J Hand Surg 2:417, 1977.
42. Lundborg G and Rank F: Experimental intrinsic healing of flexor tendons based upon synovial fluid nutrition, J Hand Surg 3:21, 1978.
43. Lundborg G and Rank F: Experimental studies on cellular mechanisms involved in healing of animal and human flexor tendon in synovial environment, Hand 12:3, 1980.
44. Manske PR, Birdwell K, and Lesker PA: Nutrient pathways to flexor tendons of chickens using tritiated proline, J Hand Surg 3:32, 1978.
45. Manske PR and Lesker PA: Nutrient pathways of flexor tendons in primates, J Hand Surg 7:436, 1982.
46. Manske PR, Whiteside AL, and Lesker PA: Nutrient pathways to flexor tendons using hydrogen washout technique, J Hand Surg 3:32, 1978.
47. Mason ML and Allen HS: The rate of healing of tendons, Ann Surg 113:424, 1941.
48. Mason ML and Shearon CG: The process of tendon repair: an experimental study of tendon suture and tendon grafts, Arch Surg 25:615, 1932.
49. Matthews P and Richards H: Factors in the adherence of flexor tendons after repair, J Bone Joint Surg 58B:230, 1976.
50. Mayer L: Tendon transplantations, Surg Gynecol Obstet 22:182, 1916.
51. McDowell CL and Snyder DM: Tendon healing: an experimental model in the dog, J Hand Surg 2:122, 1977.
52. Nichols HM, Lehmann WL, and Meek EC: Alteration of the bloodsupply of flexor tendons following injury, Am J Surg 87:279, 1954.
53. Ochiai N and others: Vascular anatomy of flexor tendons. I. Vincular system and bloodsupply of the profundus tendon in the digital sheath, J Hand Surg 4:321, 1979.
54. Panel Discussion 1, Tendon healing. In Hunter JM, Schneider LH, and Mackin EJ, editors: tendon surgery in the hand, St. Louis, 1987, The CV Mosby Co.
55. Panel Discussion 4, Rehabilitation: fexor and extensor tendons. In Hunter JM, Schneider LH, and Mackin EJ, editors: Tendon surgery in the hand, St. Louis, 1987, The CV Mosby Co.
56. Peacock EE: A study of the circulation in normal tendons and healing grafts, Ann Surg 149:415, 1959.
57. Peacock EE: Biological principles in the healing of long tendons, Surg Clin North Am 45:2, 1965.
58. Peterson WW, Manske PR, and Lesker PA: The effect of flexor sheath integrity on nutrient uptake by primate flexor tendons, J Hand Surg 11A: 413, 1986.
59. Potenza AD: Tendon healing within the flexor digital sheath in the dog. An experimental study, J Bone Joint Surg (Am) 44:49, 1962.

60. Potenza AD: Critical evaluation of flexor tendor healing and adhesion formation within artificial digital sheaths. An experimental study, J Bone Joint Surg (Am) 45:1217, 1963.

61. Potenza AD: Prevention of adhesions to healing digital flexor tendons, JAMA 187(3):99, 1964.

62. Pulvertaft RC: Tendon grafts for flexor tendon injuries in the fingers and thumb: a study of technique and results, J Bone Joint Surg 38B:175, 1956.

63. Richards HJ: Repair and healing of the divided digital flexor tendon, Injuries 12(1):1, 1980.

64. Roberts M, Rutherford JH, and Harris D: The effect of ultrasound on flexor tendon repairs in the rabbit, Hand 14:17, 1982.

65. Salter RB and others: The effect of continuous passive motion on healing of full thickness defects in articular cartilage, J Bone Joint Surg 62A:1232, 1980.

66. Schatzker J and Branemark JP: Intravital observations on the microvascular anatomy and microcirculation of the tendon, Acta Orthop Scand (suppl):126, 1969.

67. Schneider LH: Flexor tendon injuries, Boston, 1985, Little, Brown & Co.

68. Scott RA, Howar JW, and Boswick JA Jr: Recovery of function following replantation and revascularization of amputated hand parts, J Trauma 21(3):204, 1981.

69. Shrewsbury MM and Kuczynski K: Flexor digitorum superficialis tendon in the fingers of the human hand, Am J Surg 109:272, 1965.

70. Smith JW: Blood supply to tendons, Am J Surg 109:272, 1965.

71. Stevenson JH and others: Functional, mechanical, and biochemical assessment of ultrasound therapy on tendon healing in the chicken toe, Plast Reconstr Surg 77:965, 1986.

72. Strickland JW and Glogovac SV: Digital function following flexor tendon repair in zone 2: a comparison of immobilization and controlled passive motion techniques, J Hand Surg 5:537, 1980.

73. Urbaniak JR, Cahill JD, and Mortensen RA: Tendon suturing methods: analysis of tensile strength. In American Academy of Orthopaedic Surgeons: Symposium on tendon surgery of the hand, St. Louis, 1975, The CV Mosby Co.

74. Verdan CE: Primary repair of flexor tendons, J Bone Joint Surg 42A:647, 1960.

75. Verdan CE: The decades of tendon surgery. In American Academy of Orthopaedic Surgeons: Symposium on tendon surgery of the hand, St. Louis, 1975, The CV Mosby Co.

76. Warren CG, Lehmann JF, and Koblanski JN: Elongation of rattail tendon: effect of load and temperature, Arch Phys Med Rehab 57:465, 1971.

77. Weber ER, Hardin G, and Haynes D: Synovial fluid nutrition of flexor tendons. Presented at the thirty sixth Annual Meeting of the American Society for Surgery of the Hand, Las Vegas, Nev, Feb 23-25, 1981.

78. Weeks PM and Wray RC: Tendon gliding and repair. In Management of acute hand injuries: a biological approach, ed 2, St. Louis, 1978, The CV Mosby Co.

79. Wehbe MA and Hunter JM: Flexor tendon gliding in the hand. Part I. differential gliding, J Hand S 10-A:575, 1985.

80. Weiner IJ and Peacock EE: Biologic principles affecting repair of flexor tendons, Adv Surg 5:145, 1971.

81. Young RES and Harmon JM: Repair of tendon injuries of the hand, Ann Surg 151:562, 1960.

31

Management of flexor tendon lacerations in zone 2 using controlled passive motion postoperatively

Robert J. Duran, Carl R. Coleman, James F. Nappi, and Lori A. Klerekoper

The purpose of this chapter is to present the repair and postoperative management and rehabilitation of flexor tendon injuries in zone 2.

It has been determined that 3 to 5 mm of extension motion of the tendon anastomosis in a passive exercise program is sufficient to prevent firm adherence of a repaired flexor tendon in zone 2 of the hand.[1] We have chosen the term *controlled passive motion* to best describe the postoperative exercise program.

SURGICAL TECHNIQUE

It is important to repair both the flexor digitorum superficialis (FDS) and the flexor digitorum profundus (FDP) tendons. If the joint capsule, nerves, and arteries are severed, they are also repaired. The flexor tendons are retrieved as gently as possible. We prefer to control the tendons with traction sutures at the periphery of their cut ends.

Tenorrhaphy is achieved by a modified Kessler suture of 5-0 nonabsorbable synthetic material. This is supported by peripheral 6-0 mattress sutures. Because the FDS becomes thin near its insertion, mattress sutures alone are used in this area.

Considerable attention is given to the flexor tendon sheath. It may be necessary to release the sheath laterally for a few millimeters to permit the tendon anastomosis to move distally for 3 to 5 mm; otherwise the anastomosis may not clear the damaged area and could actually impinge on the annulus distally, increasing the risk of tendon separation. Closing the sheath is desirable if it does not interfere with the extenson of 3 to 5 mm.

After repairs are completed, the wrist is placed in 20 degrees of flexion. The metacarpophalangeal (MP) joint of the finger is maintained in its normal balanced position of flexion throughout the controlled passive motion program. Only the distal interphalangeal (IP) and proximal interphalangeal (PIP) joints are moved during the postoperative passive motion exercises.

In surgery under direct vision, the distal phalanx is moved enough in extension so that one can see the anastomosis of the FDP glide distally 3 to 5 mm (Fig. 31-1, A and B). Motion is only at the distal interphalangeal (DIP) joint during this exercise. To be certain of moving the anastomosis, the movement of the digit *must* be a motion of *extension*. This motion of extension has assured us that the anastomosis of the FDP has been moved, not only away from fixed structures that may have been damaged in the area (sheath, capsule), but also away from the repair of the FDS.

Continuing under direct vision in surgery, one grasps and

extends the middle phalanx until both anastomoses glide distally 3 to 5 mm (Fig. 31-1, C and D). Motion is only at the PIP joint during this exercise. This motion is essential for the FDS anastomosis. Both anastomoses have moved distally away from fixed, damaged structures. Actually measuring the range of the DIP joint and PIP joint may be helpful as a guide later in the passive motion exercises (Fig. 31-2). We suggest using these measurements particularly when the surgeon does not have experience with this technique. This allows precision in the number of degrees required at the DIP and PIP joints to give 3 to 5 mm of motion of the anastomosis.

A dorsal splint extending distally to the level of the PIP joints is used for wrist and MP joint immobilization with the wrist maintained in a flexed position at 20 degrees (Fig. 31-3). A removable inclined sponge wedge beneath the hand may be helpful if only the index finger is involved. The flexed wrist places the index finger in considerable extension at the DIP and PIP joints. This position of extension may create difficulty in getting sufficient tendon excursion. During the exercises, the wedge is removed and the wrist allowed to be in neutral position. This places the index finger in sufficient finger flexion to perform the controlled passive motion exercises. The wedge is then replaced, returning the wrist to 20 degrees of flexion until the next exercise period. This has not been a problem in the long, ring, and little fingers, and the wrist may remain in 20 degrees of flexion during the exercise.

At the end of the procedure, a hole is placed in the free border of the fingernail and a nylon suture is placed through it, tied, and connected to a rubber band. The rubber band is secured with a safety pin to the volar aspect of the forearm dressing under light tension. It is very important that the tension on the elastic band be very light so that PIP joint flexion is not increased. This is helpful in preventing a PIP joint flexion contracture. Alternatively, a corset hook may be glued to the nail and elastic traction applied. The elastic traction acts to return the DIP and PIP joints to their original position after the passive extension exercises are completed.

POSTOPERATIVE MANAGEMENT

Exercises are started *immediately*, the first having been carried out during direct vision of the anastomosis in surgery, as described previously (Fig. 31-1). Our routine is to carry out the exercises twice daily, once in the morning and once in the evening, with six to eight motions for each tendon per session. Between exercises the fingers are covered securely with a stockinette (Fig. 31-4). This prevents

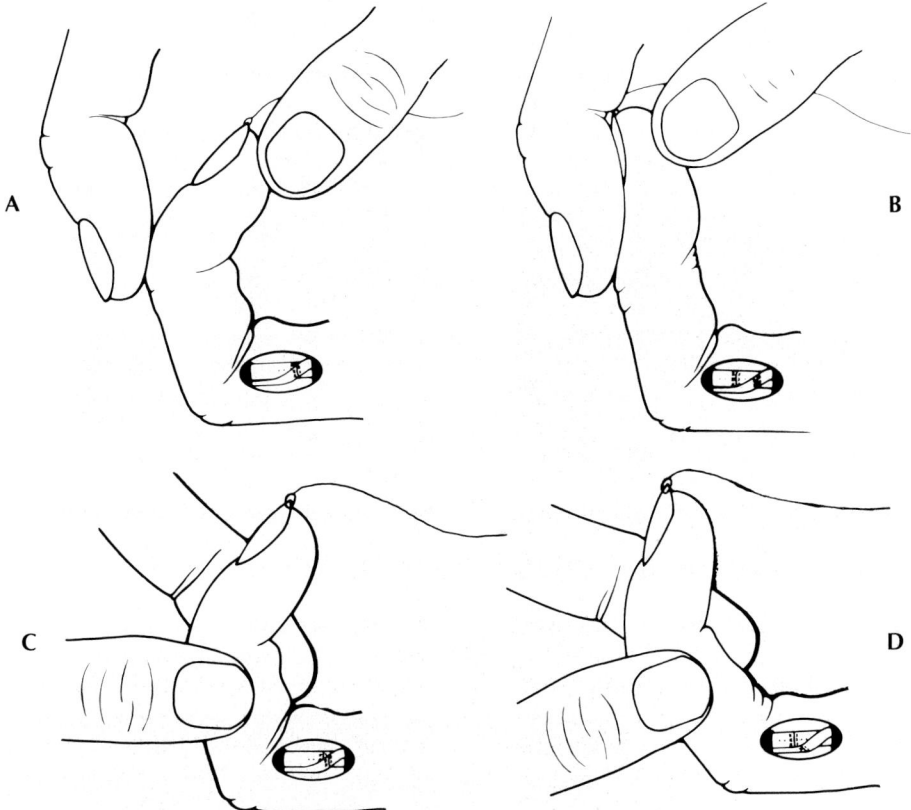

Fig. 31-1   **A,** Diagram of controlled passive motion exercise. Metacarpophalangeal joint should remain in the normal balanced position of flexion. Extension of the distal interphalangeal joint sufficient to move the anastomosis 3 to 5 mm. Only the distal interphalangeal joint moves during this exercise. **B,** Note the distal migration of anastomosis of the flexor digitorum profundus tendon away from that of the flexor digitorum superficialis tendon. **C,** When the middle phalanx is extended, both anastomoses glide distally. Only the proximal interphalangeal joint moves during this exercise. **D,** Anastomoses are thus moved away from the fixed structures that may have been injured. Elastic traction returns the finger to the original position.

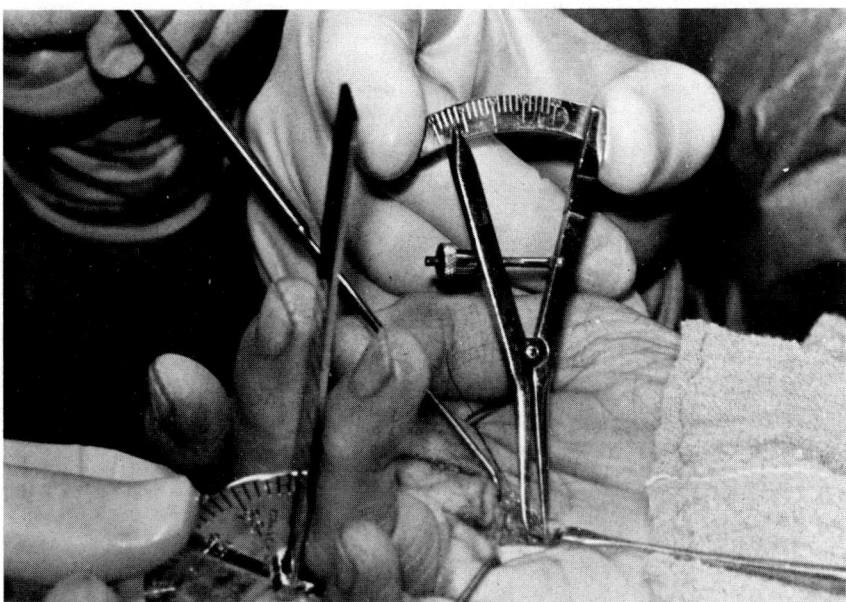

Fig. 31-2   Evaluation of the degrees of extension of the proximal interphalangeal and distal interphalangeal joints is necessary to have 3 to 5 mm of extension motion of anastomoses. This aid is helpful in precise postoperative passive exercises.

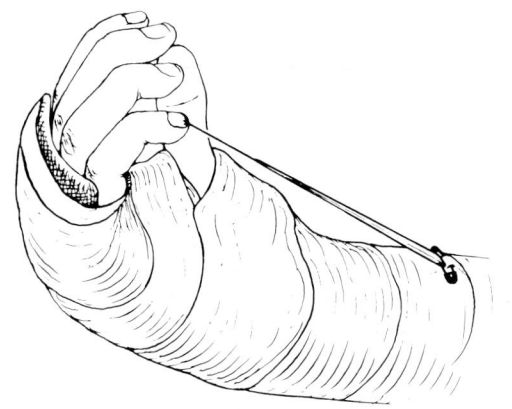

Fig 31-3 Dorsal splint extending to the proximal interphalangeal joints with wrist in approximately 20 degrees of flexion. Metacarpophalangeal joints remain in the normal balanced position of flexion.

impulsive grasping. To prevent stiffness, the uninvolved fingers are passively exercised at each session. Training of the patient or parents is essential for success of the procedure. Instruction is begun immediately, with the patient observing during the first session and then carrying out the exercises when surgeon, hand therapist, and patient are confident.

Controlled passive motion alone is continued for 4½ weeks. The dorsal splint is then removed, and the rubber band traction is attached to a wrist band (Fig. 31-5). Passive motion exercises are continued, along with gentle active extension exercises. One week later the wrist band and nail suture are removed.

Active flexion is initiated at 5½ weeks. The FDP is exercised actively by stabilizing the middle phalanx and gently, actively flexing and extending the distal phalanx 10 to 12 times. The FDS is exercised by holding the uninvolved fingers in extension and actively flexing and extending the PIP joint 10 to 12 times. Finally, all fingers are flexed and extended approximately 10 to 12 times as in normal grasping and extension. Passive stretching for joint mobilization is

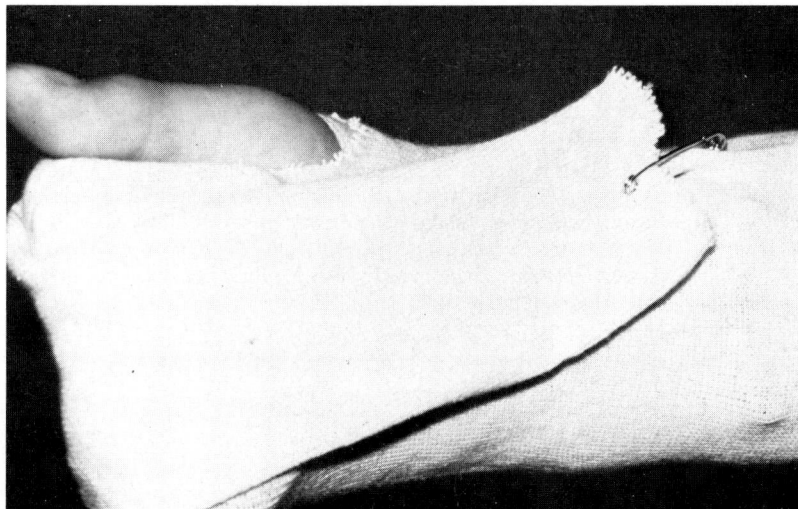

Fig. 31-4 Fingers are covered securely with a stockinette between exercises. This provides additional protection to fingers. In this case flexor tendons in three fingers are involved.

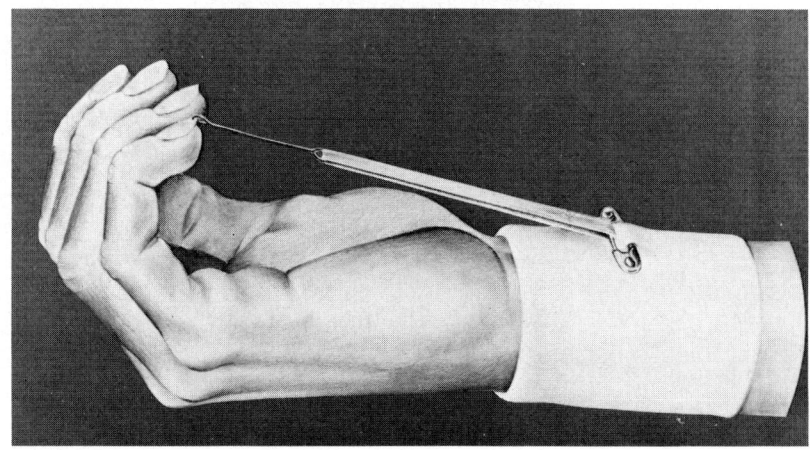

Fig. 31-5 Dorsal splint removed and wrist band applied at 4½ weeks with nail suture and rubber-band traction. Passive motion exercises are continued an additional week along with gentle active extension exercises.

then initiated. Each joint is gently, passively flexed. With the MP joint in full flexion to prevent undue tension on the tendon anastomoses, the PIP joint and the DIP joint are gently, passively extended. These exercises are repeated each hour. The finger is protected from resistive flexion for the next 2 weeks, until 7½ weeks have elapsed from the time of the tendon repair.

It may be necessary to use a dynamic splint to correct a PIP joint flexion contracture whether it is related to primary joint injury or secondary flexion contracture. If a flexion contracture is present at the PIP joint, extension splinting is used 6 weeks after tendon repair. The dynamic splint is hand-based with a long MP joint block of approximately 20 degrees of flexion. The tension is light to begin with, and then for the next 2 weeks, the splint is worn intermittently and the tension is gradually increased as needed.

Approximately 7½ to 8 weeks after tendon repair, gentle resistive flexion exercises are introduced, first using a sponge ball and then advancing to a soft-grade putty. Exercises emphasize composite flexion and isolated joint flexion, asking the patient to whole-hand grasp and then hook the involved finger. Light grasping is allowed, but excessive force to the injured finger is avoided for an additional 2 to 4 weeks. Active flexion and extension mobilization exercises are continued, emphasizing isolated and composite joint actions. Generally, most of the gain in flexion and extension has been achieved 3 months after surgery.

DIGITAL REPLANTATION

Digital replantation, with both flexor and extensor tendon repairs, presents a unique rehabilitative challenge. Three weeks of postoperative immobilization frequently results in the need for subsequent tenolysis. One of us (JFN) has used controlled passive motion in replantation in zone 2 for the past 4 years and has noted significant improvement in the functional results. Avoidance of rubber band traction is the only deviation from the controlled passive motion program. He reports further that he has not had any problems with vascular or neural repairs. A more detailed report of these cases is to be published.

REFERENCE

1. Duran RJ and Houser RG: Controlled passive motion following flexor tendon repair in zones 2 and 3. In American Academy of Orthopaedic Surgeons: Symposium on tendon surgery in the hand, St. Louis, 1975, The CV Mosby Co.

32

Indications for tendon grafting

R. Guy Pulvertaft

A tendon divided by injury, destroyed by disease or infection, or absent through congenital fault may under favorable circumstances be replaced successfully by a tendon taken from elsewhere in the body. A tendon transferred to serve a different purpose may be lengthened by a tendon graft to reach a new attachment.

The use of tendon grafts stems from the teaching of Bunnell, whose first publications on this subject appeared in 1918[3] and 1922.[4] The earliest mention of the successful use of a free tendon graft was by Robson in 1889,[18] who restored an extensor tendon by using a flexor tendon taken from a severely injured finger of the same hand.

Over the years many investigations have been made into the nature of tendon healing. We now know that when the ends of a divided tendon are held in apposition, healing takes place by cells arising from the tendon itself,[9-11] as well as by the proliferation of cells from the surrounding synovium or paratenon.[14] The same process occurs at the junction of tendon and graft. It has been demonstrated that two sections of tendon, isolated within the synovial cavity of a joint and devoid of blood supply, will heal by cells from their epitenon and are nourished by the synovial fluid of the joint.[9,10] Surgical technique needs to be gentle and precise to limit the cellular ingrowth from the surrounding tissue, which is attracted to the tendon-graft junction and to any damaged areas on the graft surface. It is these links that are the precursors of adhesions.

Successful results from tendon grafting depend on (1) a mobile digit with minimal scarring and at least one digital nerve intact, (2) a meticulous surgical technique, (3) a cooperative patient, and (4) carefully graduated mobilization. If the digital unit is not in satisfactory overall condition, consideration should be given to a two-stage procedure.[7] At the first operation, scars are excised, contractures are corrected, the damaged tendons are removed and new pulleys constructed if necessary, and injured nerves are repaired. A flexible silicone rubber rod is placed in the tendon bed; it is attached securely to the distal phalanx, while its proximal end is left free to glide in the tissue planes above the wrist. The digit is exercised by passive motion, causing the development of a sheathlike tunnel into which a tendon graft is inserted to replace the rod a few months later (see Chapter 34).

The most common cause of failure is adhesion between tendon or graft and the surrounding tissues. In an effort to overcome this problem, specialized forms of grafting have been used, including pedicle grafts[12] and homografts of the complete flexor system.[6,13] Permanent artificial "tendons" have also been used.[7,19] The generally accepted practice today is secondary autogenous grafting according to established techniques, with recourse to two-stage grafting when necessary.

There is rarely any lack of autogenous tendons for use as grafts, the most suitable are plantaris, palmaris longus, and extensor digitorum longus. The choice depends on their availability and the nature of the case. The plantaris is the longest tendon and makes an excellent graft. It is my first choice. Its slimness is an advantage, particularly when one is restoring profundus in the presence of a normal superficialis. Palmaris will reach from the distal phalanx to the proximal palm but, except for the thumb, will not reach above the wrist, and this can sometimes be a disadvantage. Plantaris and palmaris, which are occasionally absent, are removed by use of a distal and proximal exposure; the tendon is freed through the distal wound and drawn out through the proximal wound, so that the use of a tendon stripper is avoided. In this manner the tendons are removed with the minimum of paratenon. The toe extensor tendons cannot be slipped out in the same fashion, owing to linkage with the adjacent tendons, which necessitates open dissection. The flexor digitorum superficialis is a convenient tendon, when it is divided, to bridge a gap in the profundus tendon divided in the central and proximal palm and at the wrist.

It has become accepted practice to encourage controlled movements within a day or two of performing a direct suture of flexor tendons injured within the digital theca. My own experience leads me to believe that after grafting operations it is wiser to keep the hand at rest for 3 weeks before allowing movement.[15]

The graft enlarges with the stimulus of work and becomes capable of withstanding normal strains. I have not seen a rupture or detachment later than 10 weeks after operation. There is ample evidence that a graft performed in childhood increases in length with the growth of the hand.

INJURY
Flexor profundus division

Division of the flexor profundus tendon beyond the insertion of the flexor superficialis is normally treated by immediate suture when wound conditions permit. If the profundus is cut more proximally but the superficialis is intact (a not uncommon injury), it has been my practice to ignore the tendon injury with the intention of elective treatment later, because the results of suture were not dependable. However, improved techniques now offer a good prospect of success by direct suture in this difficult zone. If the profundus injury was overlooked or deliberately ignored, the choice of later treatment depends on several factors. Secondary suture may be possible in the distal part of the finger, but if this cannot be done because of retraction and for the proximal divisions, the ideal treatment is the replacement of profundus by a graft, with the superficialis being left intact.[16] This operation is one of some magnitude for a comparatively small defect, and it should be advised only when the patient is determined to seek perfection or when the patient is a child with an unknown future occupation. The possibility of increasing the disability by failed surgery exists, and the surgeon should therefore be experienced in tendon grafting. The choice, which should be fully discussed with the patient, lies between tendon grafting, arthrodesis or tenodesis of the distal joint, or acceptance of the disability.

Flexor profundus and superficialis division

The arguments in favor of primary or secondary suture versus secondary grafting when both tendons are cut in the distal palm or in the finger have strengthened in recent years. The use of magnification and the improvements in technique are leading surgeons to perform direct suture and obtain a high level of success.[8] I believe it is fair comment to say that these results are attributable to the wise selection of cases and superb craftsmanship. There are surgeons called on to treat these difficult injuries who do not have wide experience in hand surgery, and there remains a case for skin suture only to be followed by grafting later by a surgeon qualified to do so. Secondary grafting under favorable circumstances has a success rate of 70% to 80%.[1,15] Minimal requirement for "success" is defined as flexion to within 2.5 cm or less of the distal palmar crease, with extension restricted by less than a sum total of 40 degrees at the interphalangeal joints.

Flexor pollicis longus division

Division of the flexor pollicis longus tendon distal to the metacarpophalangeal joint is normally treated by suture. Division of the tendon deep to the thenar muscles may also be sutured at the emergency operation, but one should not forget that the tendon lies in close relationship to the digital sensory nerves and the motor nerve to the thenar muscles and that these structures are at risk. In replacement of the flexor pollicis longus by a tendon graft it is important that the graft should reach from the distal phalanx to above the wrist. In my experience it is a reliable operation that rarely fails to give an adequate flexion range.

Division of flexor tendons in palm and wrist

The best results are obtained by primary suture. It may prove impossible to perform a secondary suture, owing to retraction of the proximal part, without causing undue tension. This retraction is most pronounced when the injury has been in or proximal to the carpal tunnel. Under these circumstances, continuity can be restored when the gap in the profundus is bridged by a short graft taken from the superficialis. Apart from divisions in the distal palm, which should be regarded as being within the finger, there is rarely any need to perform complete graft replacement for these injuries.

Extensor tendon divisions

Tendon divisions on the dorsal surface of the hand and wrist under suitable conditions of wounding are well treated by primary suture. Secondary end-to-end suture may be possible, but, in late cases, attachment to an adjacent intact tendon or transfer to a tendon such as the extensor indicis proprius may be indicated. Tendon grafting is more likely to be required after severe wounds where there has been extensive skin damage and subsequent scarring. Since free tendon grafts should not be placed in scar tissue, it is necessary to these cases to replace the scar by a skin flap as a preliminary procedure.

Tendon grafting after long delay

A patient may be seen several years after a tendon injury has been sustained, either because treatment has not been given or because previous surgery has failed. These neglected cases are usually encountered after divisions within the digital theca. Tendon grafting can restore function, provided that there is good passive movement of the digit and there is acceptable sensibility. Surprisingly, in my own series of 42 patients suffering from profundus and superficialis divisions with an average delay of 5 years, the overall results were slightly better than those of the regular series.[17] In all the delay cases one of the muscles of the affected digit was used as a motor. On reflection, it would have been wiser in some of the cases to have transferred a superficialis tendon, prolonged if necessary by a free graft, from an adjacent finger.

A stricter selection for operative suitability in the delay series probably accounts for the better results. The lesson I have learned from this experience is that delay does not worsen the prognosis and it is safe and advisable to wait for some months to permit the tissues to make a full recovery from the initial trauma. One should bear this in mind when treating children under 4 years of age, who are unlikely to cooperate well in the aftercare. No harm will come from delaying the operation for a year or two.

Rheumatoid disease

Tendon rupture in rheumatoid disease occurs as a complication in rheumatoid nodules within the tendon, disease of the synovium and the tendon sheaths, and attrition against sharp edges of eroded bone. Tendon suture is usually impossible because of actual loss of tendon substance and retraction. Linkage to an unaffected adjacent tendon or tendon transfer is usually the best method of repair for extensor tendons. Occasionally it is necessary to extend a transferred tendon by a free graft. Standard methods of grafting are sometimes indicated for flexor tendon restoration, but the prognosis is less favorable than in nonrheumatoid patients.

INFECTION

Sometimes one sees a patient in whom the flexor tendons have become adherent or destroyed within the digital sheath after septic tenosynovitis but the finger has retained good passive mobility. A tendon grafting operation offers a chance of restoring function, and a two-stage procedure should be considered.

A guarded prognosis should be given.

CONGENITAL ABSENCE OF TENDONS

Provided that there is an adequate joint motion and a suitable muscle available, a free tendon graft can be used successfully to provide active movement. Pulleys may need to be set up and use made of the two-stage method.

PARALYSIS

Loss of function caused by irreparable lesions of the spinal cord and peripheral nerves can be restored in many instances by transference of expendable active muscles. The tendons of these muscles may need to be lengthened by tendon grafts. Leprosy is the most common cause of peripheral nerve lesions; in the upper limb the effects are seen in the ulnar nerve at the elbow and in the median nerve at the wrist, producing partial or total intrinsic paralysis of the hand. Given suitable conditions and effective aftercare, consistently good results can be obtained from operations for the clawed fingers and thumb of the intrinsic-minus hand, by use of some adaptation of the Stiles-Bunnell principle.[2] The muscle chosen to provide power may be a superficialis, which is divided into four slips to reach the wing tendons of the extensor tendon complex without an intervening graft, or extensor carpi radialis brevis prolonged by grafts taken from plantaris tendon[2] or fascia lata.[5]

SUMMARY

Autogenous tendon grafting is widely used in the restoration of tendon defects and paralysis in the hand. Success depends on careful selection of the case, a gentle and precise surgical technique, and efficient aftercare.

REFERENCES

1. Boyes JH and Stark HH: Flexor-tendon grafts in the fingers and thumb, J Bone Joint Surg 53A:1332, 1971.
2. Brand PW: Tendon transfers in the forearm. In Flynn JE, editor: Hand surgery, ed 3, Baltimore, 1982, Williams & Wilkins.
3. Bunnell S: Repair of tendons in the fingers and description of two new instruments, Surg Gynecol Obstet 26:103, 1918.
4. Bunnell S: Repair of tendons in the fingers, Surg Gynecol Obstet 35:88, 1922.
5. Fritschi EP: Reconstructive surgery in leprosy, Bristol, 1971, John Wright & Sons, Ltd.
6. Hueston JT, Hubble B, and Rigg BR: Homografts of the digital flexor tendon system, Aust NZ J Surg 36:269, 1967.
7. Hunter JM and Aulicino PL: Salvage of the scarred tendon systems, utilizing the Hunter tendon implant. In Flynn JE, editor: Hand surgery, ed 3, Baltimore, 1982, Williams & Wilkins.
8. Lister GD and others: Primary flexor tendon repair followed by immediate controlled mobilization, J Hand Surg 2:441, 1977.
9. Lundborg G and Rank F: Experimental intrinsic healing of flexor tendon based upon synovial fluid nutrition, J Hand Surg 3:21, 1978.
10. Lundborg G and others: Superficial repair of severed flexor tendon in synovial environment, J Hand Surg 5:451, 1980.
11. Matthews P and Richards H: The repair potential of digital flexor tendons, J Bone Joint Surg 56B:618, 1974.
12. Paneva-Holevich E: Two-stage tenoplasty in injury of the flexor tendons of the hand, J Bone Joint Surg 51A:21, 1969.
13. Peacock EE Jr and Madden JW: Human composite flexor tendon allografts, Ann Surg 166:624, 1967.
14. Potenza AD: Concepts of tendon healing and repair. In American Academy of Orthopaedic Surgeons: Symposium on tendon surgery in the hand, St Louis, 1975, The CV Mosby Co.
15. Pulvertaft RG: Tendon grafts for flexor tendon injuries in the fingers and thumb, J Bone Joint Surg 38B:175, 1956.
16. Pulvertaft RG: The treatment of profundus division by free tendon graft, J Bone Joint Surg 42A:1363, 1960.
17. Pulvertaft RG: Flexor tendon grafting after long delay. In Tubiana R, editor: The hand, vol 2, Philadelphia, 1985, WB Saunders Co.
18. Robson AWM: A case of tendon grafting, Trans Clin Soc London 22:289, 1889.
19. Sarkin TL: The plastic replacement of severed flexor tendons of the fingers, Br J Surg 44:232, 1956.

33

Tenolysis: dynamic approach to surgery and therapy

Lawrence H. Schneider and Evelyn J. Mackin

The surgical release of nongliding adhesions that form along the surface of a tendon after injury or repair is a useful procedure in the salvage of tendon function.* Tendon adhesions occur whenever the surface of a tendon is damaged either through the injury itself, be it laceration or crush, or by surgical manipulation.[5,14] At any point on the surface of a tendon where violation occurs an adhesion will form in the healing period.[7,9] Whenever these adhesions cannot be mobilized by therapy techniques, tenolysis should be considered. This procedure is as demanding as tendon repair itself and cannot be undertaken lightly. It represents another surgical onslaught in an area of previous trauma and surgery. If the procedure is unsuccessful, the patient's hand may show no improvement or even be worse. The risk of further decreasing the circulatory supply and innervation to a borderline finger is a real one. Rupture of the lysed tendon, a disastrous complication, is another hazard of tenolysis.

PREOPERATIVE EVALUATION FOR TENOLYSIS

Patient selection is a vital aspect in successful tenolysis. The patient should have been in an adequate therapy program combining active motion techniques with gentle passive motion exercises for approximately 3 months and progress should be at a standstill. This time interval allows for wound healing and maturation while the patient is trying to stretch the adhesions that have formed.[22] The patient's level of cooperation in a postoperative program can also be evaluated during this interval. A patient unable to put himself fully into the program should be rejected for lysis.

At 3 months,[22] if the range of movement attained is regarded by patient and surgeon as inadequate, discussion is entered into regarding the risks and rewards of lysis in view of the functional demands and needs of the patient. A realistic picture must be drawn. A cold, insensate finger will not be improved even if a full range of motion could be regained. The decision to perform tenolysis is often subjective. For example, 50% of a normal range of motion may be reasonable to accept, especially in an aged person or one who has concurrent joint surface injury or degenerative arthritis. The presence of adequate skin cover is another prerequisite for this surgery.

Ideally, the patient who would be best suited would be one whose repaired tendon had a localized adhesion that limited gliding. On release a full range of motion is regained. This, however, is the uncommon situation. More frequently, the adhesions involve a long segment of the involved tendon and require extensive exposure for release. Joint contracture, which can occur secondary to the tendon

fixation, may also require correction and further complicates the surgery and the patient's recovery.[18]

TECHNIQUE

Once the patient meets the criteria established, lysis is performed under local anesthesia to allow full evaluation during the procedure itself.[4] It is through this technique that one can determine whether release of the offending tendon-system adhesions is adequate to restore motion or the patient also requires surgical release of the joints. At times it is necessary to turn the hand over and release the opposing tendon system also. This situation is not uncommon in crushing injuries, especially if there are associated phalangeal fractures. All patients for flexor lysis have been prepared for the possibility of staged tendon reconstruction if a reasonable flexor mechanism cannot be salvaged.[3]

The local anesthesia used is 1% or 2% lidocaine infiltrated locally in the skin or as a digital block at the metacarpal level. Nerve blocks at the wrist can also be used but, with resultant paralysis of the intrinsic muscles, some benefits of this technique are sacrificed.

The administration of intravenous medication relieves anxiety and alleviates tourniquet pain. The use of a fentanyl-droperidol mixture marketed as Innovar* has proved useful. The anesthesia technique has been modified in that less of the combination is now used for induction. First, 0.5 to 1 ml of fentanyl-droperidol is given intravenously, and then a second and third dose of a similar amount of fentanyl alone is added at intervals of 4 to 5 minutes for induction. Only fentanyl is then added as required for the patient's comfort and allowed by the vital signs.

Monitoring of the vital signs by experienced anesthesia personnel in an operating room environment is necessary. Careful titration of the medication is also necessary. Overuse depresses the patient's function and his ability to cooperate. With proper dosage, the tourniquet has been tolerated for as long as 1 hour. The dissection proceeds rapidly and the patient's range of motion is constantly reevaluated until tourniquet paralysis intervenes at between 20 and 25 minutes. If further dissection is needed, it is continued as necessary and evaluation is carried out after the tourniquet is released and hemostasis is obtained. If further surgery is deemed necessary, reinflation can be carried out and dissection continued until completed. The surgeon can directly determine whether the tendon motor actually is effective and flexor pulleys are adequate. He can also tell whether the lysed tendon appears healthy or a tendon graft in one or two stages is advisable. When lysis is successful and the

---

*References 1,10,11,15,16,19,21

*McNeil Co., Ft. Washington, Pa.

range of motion actively attained appears acceptable, the wounds are closed and a dressing is applied, so that an early postoperative motion program is allowed.

Summary of surgical technique

Flexor lysis[12] (Fig. 33-1)
1. Zigzag incision; if necessary, be prepared to expose the entire course of the tendon.
2. Preserve pulleys as possible.
3. Release joints if significant contractures exist.
4. Look carefully at the site of the tendon repair. The surgeon should be wary of a gapped tendon that has filled in with scar tissue. Although one may succeed in creating a tendon out of this scar tissue, if a large gap is present, the tendon will be too long and has an increased chance of rupturing. (See 5.)
5. Prepare patient for possibility of staged tendon reconstruction if lysis by this technique appears unfeasible.[3]

Flexor lysis after failed direct repair has been more successful than after failed tendon graft, a finding that leads us to prefer direct repair, early, in flexor injuries when wound conditions allow.[13]

Extensor lysis (Fig. 33-2)
1. Curvilinear incision over adherent area is used.
2. Joint releases; dorsal capsulotomies are often needed.
3. Try to preserve dorsal retinaculum at wrist.

When both flexor and extensor tendons are involved in adhesions, the prognosis is notably poorer but occasionally finger salvage can be achieved (Fig. 33-3).

POSTOPERATIVE MANAGEMENT

The procedures surrounding the tenolysis operation are as vital as the lysis itself. Complications can develop unless a careful postoperative hand therapy program is initiated. Some of these complications include pain, persistent edema, rupture, and recurrence of adhesions with resulting loss of motion and flexion contracture. The patient must understand that some discomfort is to be expected postoperatively; however, it is vital that he work through the soreness of the

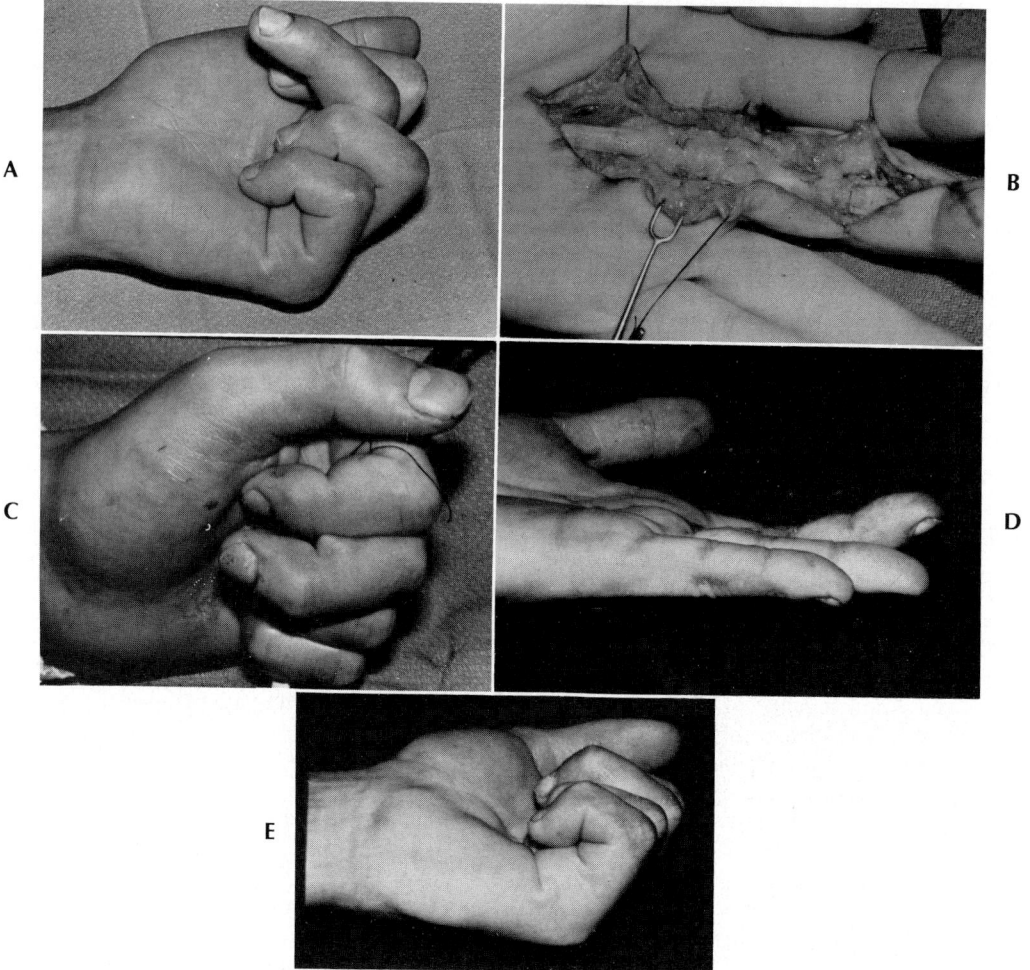

Fig. 33-1   Flexor lysis: a 17-year-old boy severed both flexor tendons in his left long finger. After primary repair of his flexor digitorum profundus, he had minimal pull-through of his flexor system at 4 months after repair. **A,** Attempted flexion of the left long finger. **B,** During tenolysis, massive adhesions were found at the repair site. **C,** After lysis under local-sedation technique, he obtained excellent active flexion with hand lying on a table. **D** and **E,** Through an active therapy program he maintained the gains accomplished through surgery. Photographs of extension and flexion taken at 3 months after surgery.

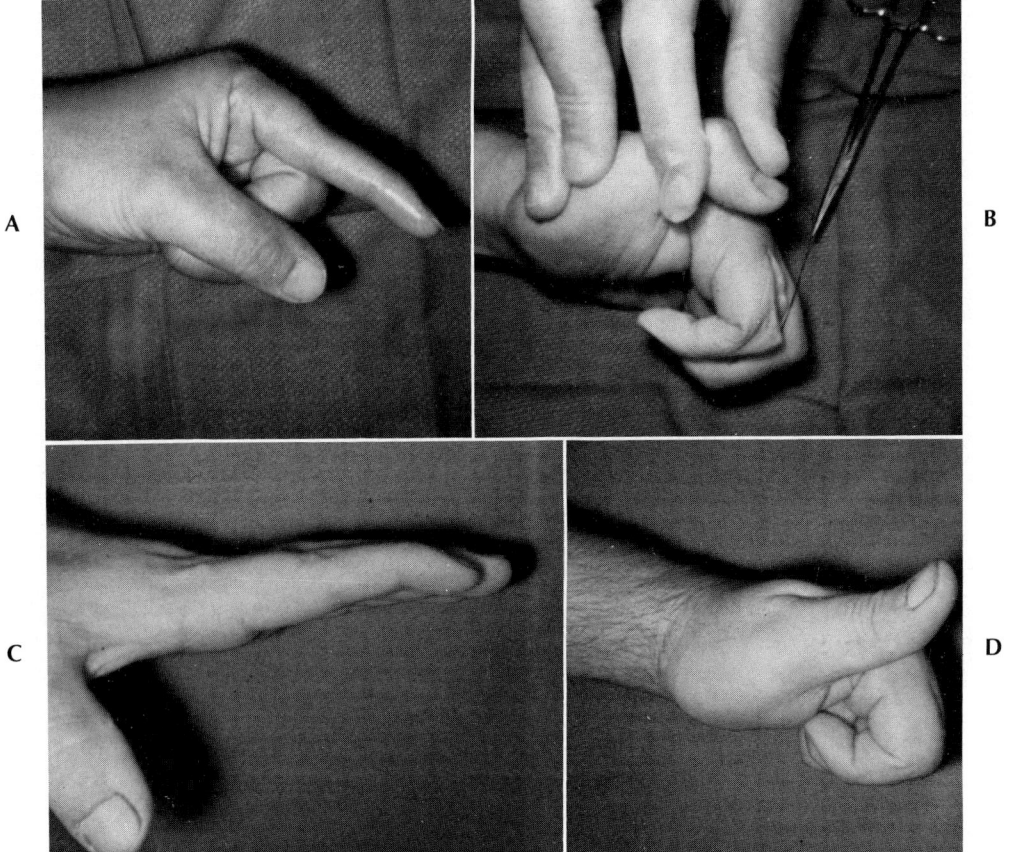

Fig. 33-2 Extensor lysis: a 42-year-old man severed his extensor mechanism over the proximal interphalangeal joint of his left index finger. After repair extension contracture persisted despite active exercise program. **A,** Fixed extension posture of the finger before lysis. **B,** On an operating table, after lysis of tendon adhesions and release of dorsal capsule of the proximal interphalangeal joint, he could flex actively to 90 degrees. **C** and **D,** Range of motion was retained with therapy as shown at 3 months after tenolysis.

early postoperative days if the range of motion attained at surgery is to be maintained.

Successful postoperative management of the lysed tendon depends on close communication between surgeon and therapist, enabling the initiation of an appropriate treatment program. The therapist must be informed of the integrity of the lysed tendon, the intraoperative range of motion (active or passive), and the prognosis. Unless the lysis has been performed with the patient under local anesthesia and demonstrating his active potential intraoperatively, neither surgeon nor therapist can be assured that the motion-limiting adhesions have been completely removed. Postoperative results are therefore compromised. The patient may try extremely hard to gain full motion only to find that the remaining adhesions have made it impossible. When the surgeon can inform the therapist of the intraoperative active range of motion and measurements have been recorded, goals can be set. Furthermore, intraoperatively the patient can see his digits moving through the arc of motion. This will reinforce and encourage his postoperative efforts.

Evaluation

Because in the early postoperative stage of the tenolysis patient can lose the intraoperative gains in motion in as little

as a few days owing to the dynamics of the healing process, careful evaluation must be performed and documented from the initial visit. Evaluation should include wound assessment, edema, pain, active and passive range of motion, and sensibility.

Because the patient is encouraged to move immediately within the postoperative dressing, the dressing is debulked to allow for active exercises 24 hours after surgery. At this time the therapist can inspect the wound for excess swelling or inflammation. As with all open wounds, the therapist should wear sterile gloves to prevent contamination of the wound. As a further precaution, the patient's hand can be rested on a sterile field.

The patient's subjective assessment of his pain provides an insight into his level of pain tolerance and his ability to cooperate with the early active exercise program.

Active and passive range-of-motion exercises are measured initially with a goniometer over a light sterile digital dressing. Measurement of the distance from the finger pulp to the distal palmar crease during active flexion is taken because this measurement relates to the function of grasp.[17] Extension must also be closely monitored. Gentle passive range-of-motion measurements at each joint in both flexion and extension are taken.

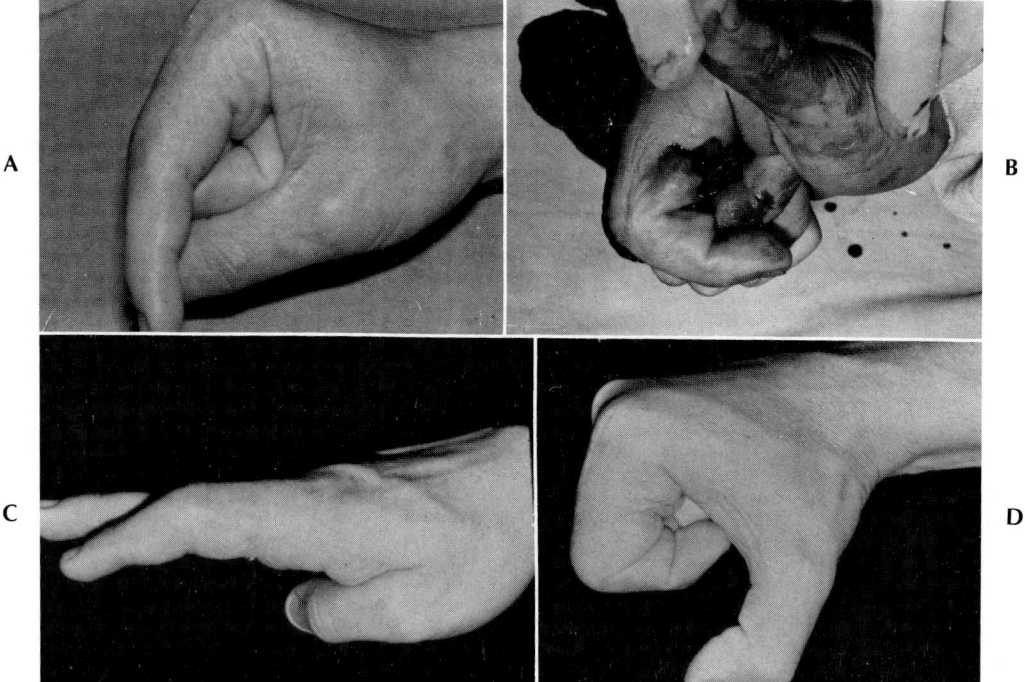

Fig. 33-3   Combined extensor and flexor lysis: a 35-year-old man sustained a crush injury to his right index finger. His extensor system was primarily involved. His finger became contracted in extension and he had only 20 degrees of flexion from a straight position at the proximal interphalangeal joint. **A,** Maximum active flexion at the proximal interphalangeal joint. **B,** Lysis of extensor tendon system with release of proximal interphalangeal joint dorsal capsule returned passive flexion, but active flexion was not regained until volar exposure revealed adhesions of the flexor tendons. With release of these adhesions, he regained active flexion as shown here. **C,** Active extension was maintained at 4 months. **D,** Active flexion was also possible at 4 months.

Lack of sensibility owing to previous trauma to the fingers may affect the patient's ability to exert maximum tendon pull-through and may affect functional recovery.

Treatment

Therapy begins the first postoperative day. It includes wound care, edema control, splinting when necessary, active and passive range-of-motion exercises, and return to functional activities.

Wound care. The dressing applied at surgery is changed. A piece of sterile nonadhering dressing is laid over the incision. A thin, dry dressing is placed over the nonadhering dressing and then covered with a piece of tube bandage. To be effective, the dressing applied to the digits must not restrict the patient's exercise program. If resection into the palm or forearm was necessary, the incision is also bandaged to protect the wound from contamination.

Control of edema. Swelling is a common reaction in the digit disturbed by surgical release of nongliding adhesions. The importance of controlling edema and thereby avoiding complications must be emphasized. The hand is maintained in elevation after surgery to minimize limb dependency and thus assist in edema control.

An effective early exercise that incorporates elevation and active motion is to have the patient elevate both arms over the head and make as firm a fist as possible. The patient can begin by performing 5 repetitions every other hour and, as exercises become easier, increase it to 5 to 10 repetitions hourly.[8]

Coban wraps applied carefully to the digit over the sterile dressings also assist in the reduction of edema. Coban is applied distally to proximally and must be wrapped without tension. Tightly applied Coban will interfere with the circulation of the finger.

Splinting. Splinting is an important part of postoperative care. In those patients with limited flexion and good extension preoperatively, a dorsal resting splint may be worn postoperatively for approximately 2 weeks with the wrist in approximately 30 degrees of flexion and the metacarpophalangeal (MP) joints and interphalangeal (IP) joints in balanced flexion.

Those patients who had joint contractures corrected through lysis require immediate postoperative splinting in extension to maintain the extension achieved intraoperatively. The splint may be applied as early as the first postoperative day depending on the quality of the tendon (Fig. 33-4, *A, B, C,* and *D*). Splints must be carefully fitted to gently hold the digits in extension. Each time the patient is seen in therapy the splint should be reevaluated so that necessary adjustments can be made as changes in motion occur. Initially the splint is removed only for exercise and wound care. As healing and motion progress, daytime splinting is gradually reduced but nighttime extension splinting may be necessary for 6 months.

When the retinacular pulley system is found to be inadequate during lysis of the tendon, reconstruction of the damaged pulley is indicated. The basic anatomy of the flexor pulley system is a precise biomechanical design that permits

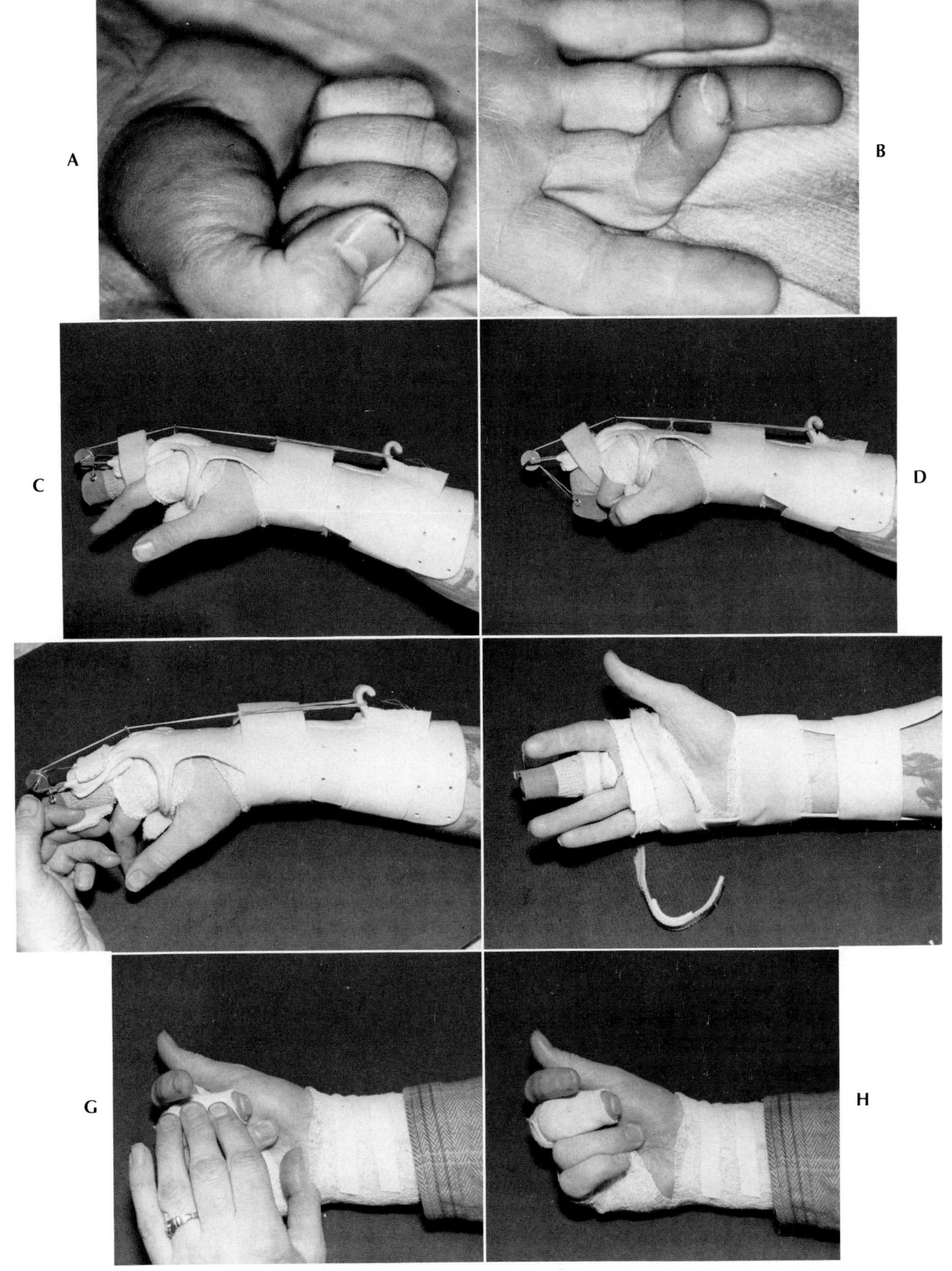

Fig. 33-4   Patient with severe flexion contracture at proximal interphalangeal joint and tendon bowstringing. This finger has systemic tenosynovitis, healed with delayed rupture of the flexor system and failed tendon grafting. Patient underwent tenolysis and A2 pulley reconstruction. **A,** Preoperative active range-of-motion MP 5/90, PIP 75/110, and DIP 30/30. **B,** Preoperative passive extension limited to active extension. **C,** Dorsal outrigger maintaining extension of proximal interphalangeal joint is worn day and night. **D,** Flexion within the dynamic splint. Finger slings assist proximal interphalangeal joint extension. **E,** Pulley ring is fitted with splint in place. **F,** Additional pulley ring carefully fitted without splint on the finger is worn during exercise sessions. **G,** "Passive hold" exercise. Lysed finger is passively flexed with uninvolved hand. **H,** Passively flexed finger is released and held in flexion with its own muscle power with pulley ring support.

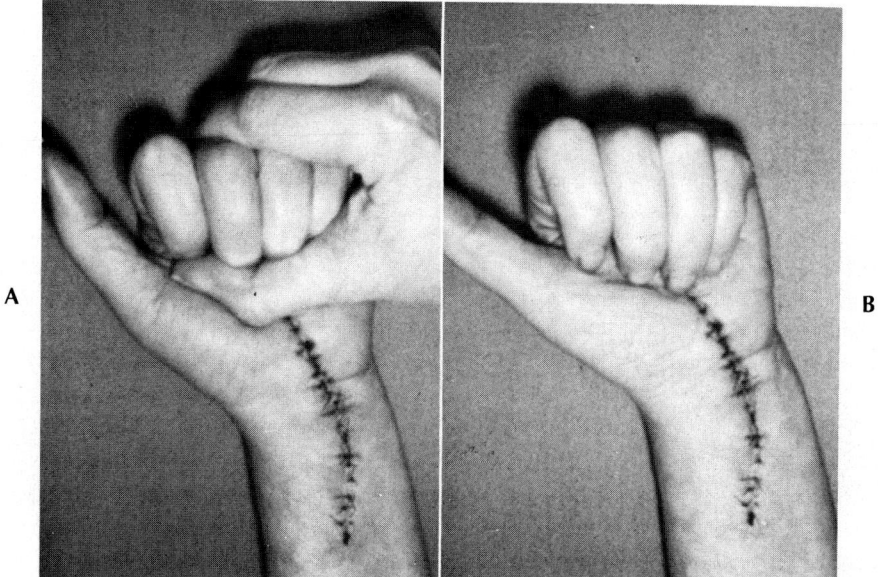

Fig. 33-5   Passive fist-making. **A,** Patient presses his involved hand into a tight fist with his uninvolved hand. **B,** Then the involved hand is released, and the patient tries to retain the fist with his muscle power.

lubricated gliding of the tendon while transmitting the power of the forearm musculature to the bones of the finger. Unless this arrangement can be restored during the tenolysis procedure, the functional arc of motion cannot be restored despite the lysis.

Reconstructed pulleys must be protected. An adjustable pulley ring fabricated from Velcro and felt is used initially until edema subsides (usually during the second postoperative week). Then a molded thermoplastic ring is used and should be worn for 6 months after surgery. Some patients elect to wear a metal ring instead of the thermoplastic ring for greater durability and improved aesthetics.

When an extension splint is required, two pulley rings may be necessary to ensure adequate protection of the repaired pulley. One pulley ring is fitted with the splint in place and acts as a counterforce to the passive extension of the proximal interphalangeal (PIP) joint provided by the extension outrigger. The other pulley ring is fitted without the splint on the hand and is worn during exercise sessions (Fig. 33-4, *E, F, G,* and *H*).

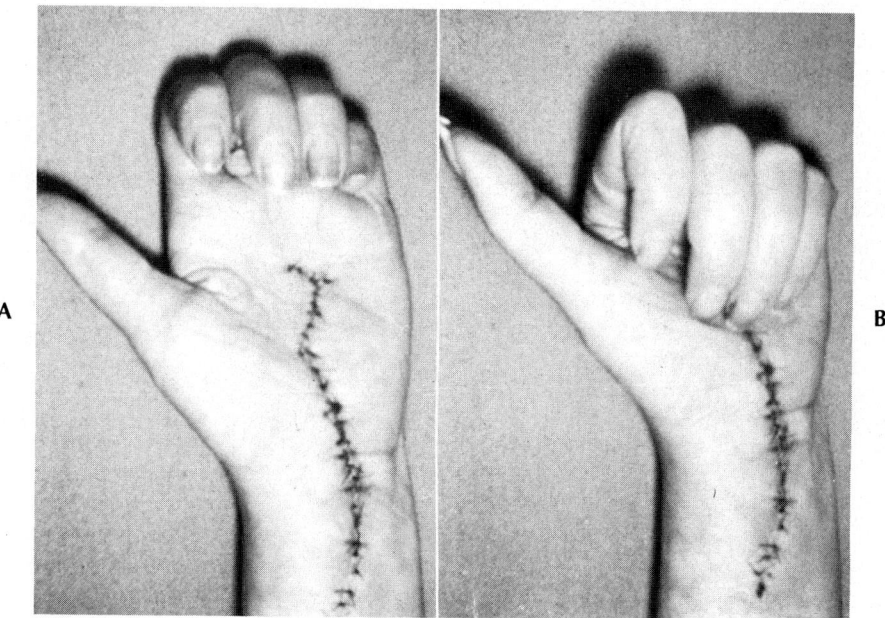

Fig. 33-6   Tendon-gliding exercise. **A,** Full flexion of the interphalangeal joints with the metacarpal joints in full extension. **B,** *Maintain full flexion* of the interphalangeal joints and roll the fingers in to make a tight fist.

Active range of motion. Gentle active finger exercises are begun during the first postoperative visit and include the following:

1. "Place hold" exercise. Patient relaxes his forearm muscles and presses the involved digits into his palm. The uninvolved hand is released, and the patient holds the involved fingers in flexion with his own muscle power (Fig. 33-5).
2. Finger blocking. Distal interphalangeal (DIP) joint flexion with the PIP joint and MP joint held in extension with the uninvolved hand followed by PIP joint flexion with the MP joint held in extension.
3. Finger extension.

Depending on the level of discomfort, 5 to 10 repetitions of each exercise are performed hourly. If no additional discomfort or swelling is felt following the exercises, then the number of the exercises begun at 5 repetitions each hour is gradually increased to 10 repetitions hourly. If, however, the discomfort should increase or last more than 10 to 15 minutes after completion of the exercises, the number of repetitions and frequency of the exercises should be decreased, i.e., 3 repetitions of each exercise every other hour. Assessing the patient's discomfort and pain tolerance can be a valuable guideline to establishing an exercise program. It can prevent the exercise program from being too vigorous and increasing discomfort or pain or too gentle, thus discouraging maximum efforts to pull the tendon through the lysed area.

Although patients have been informed preoperatively of the importance of an early therapy program, they are often reluctant to exercise the so recently operated finger, confusing discomfort with pain. This can be a time when therapist and patient meet on a common platform, for each must put considerable effort into the postoperative program if maximum results are to be attained. Each must feel the other's sincerity. The therapist must tell the patient that he or she understands the discomfort the patient is having. He or she must, however, encourage the patient to move the lysed finger, telling him that despite the discomfort, if he exercises today, the exercises will be easier tomorrow. Gen-

uine concern and encouragement by the therapist will net returns in cooperation as the patient participates in the therapy program.

PIP joint flexion contractures may result in tight intrinsic muscles. When the contracture is released at surgery, holding the involved MP joint in flexion with the uninvolved hand encourages PIP joint extension.

As motion improves, the exercise program is modified. Usually by the second week tendon-gliding exercises can be initiated.[20] (Fig. 33-6).

Passive range of motion. Patients are instructed in gentle passive range of motion of all joints. Five to 10 repetitions are performed three times a day beginning with the first postoperative day.

Forceful passive motion of the joints is not indicated. Such motion is painful and only increases pain and swelling. When pain becomes intolerable, therapy will not succeed.

Functional activities. Light activities of daily living may be begun at 2 to 3 weeks along with an increased exercise program using wood blocks and dowels.

Graded grip-strengthening activities are begun at 3 to 4 weeks, for example, beginning with putty and the Hand Helper and progressing to woodworking, ceramics, progressive resistive exercises, and pulleys. The goal during this phase of therapy is to maintain the active range of motion gained in the early postoperative days and to increase strength within that range. Heavy resistive exercise is generally begun at the eighth postoperative week. The goal is to return the patient to full work at 8 to 12 weeks after tenolysis (depending on the job duties).

POSTOPERATIVE MANAGEMENT USING LOCAL ANESTHESIA

A technique that has been useful in helping a patient get through the difficult first week after lysis employs an indwelling polyethylene catheter[2] inserted after the surgical procedure in the area of the tenolysis (Fig. 33-7). Before closure of the wound the catheter is laid proximally to the site of surgery over the sensory nerve branches. This catheter is used to instill small amounts (1 or 2 ml) of local

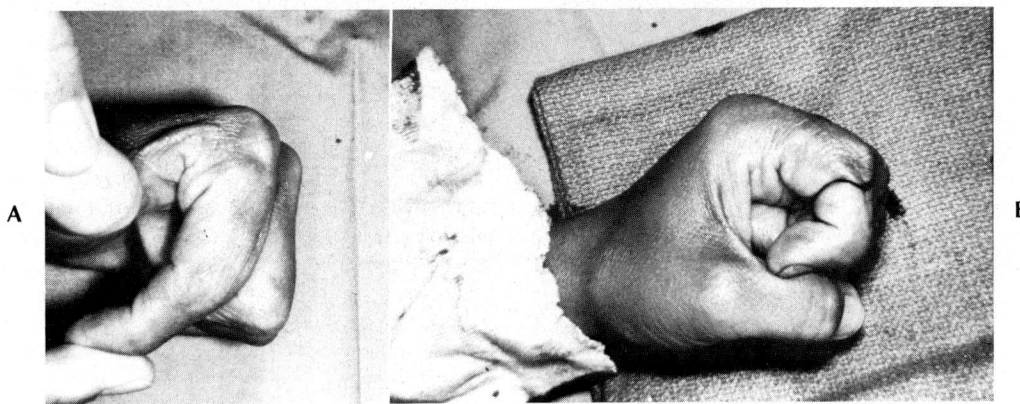

Fig. 33-7 Extensor lysis. Patient lacerated his extensor tendon over dorsum of the proximal phalanx. **A,** Passive flexion of finger 2 years after repair. Preoperative range of motion: MP 0°/90°, PIP 20°/20°, DIP 0°/45°. **B,** After extensor tenolysis and proximal interphalangeal joint capsulectomy under local-sedation technique, patient obtained excellent flexion. Intraoperative active range of motion: MP 0°/90°, PIP 0°/90°, DIP 0°/60°. Flexion 1/2 inch to DPC. *Continued.*

anesthetic into the operated area to allay pain during the exercise periods. The catheter is left in place for 5 to 7 days, during which time the patient is on a regimen of systemic antibiotics.

Postoperative therapy begins a few hours after surgery in the patient's hospital room, assisted by the nursing staff and the surgeon. The patient is shown how to self-administer the anesthesic slowly into the wound. Rapid instillation produces pain. Active assistive exercise in encouraged.

When the patient is seen by the therapist on the first postoperative day, the dressing applied at surgery is removed. The petrolatum gauze covering the incision line is

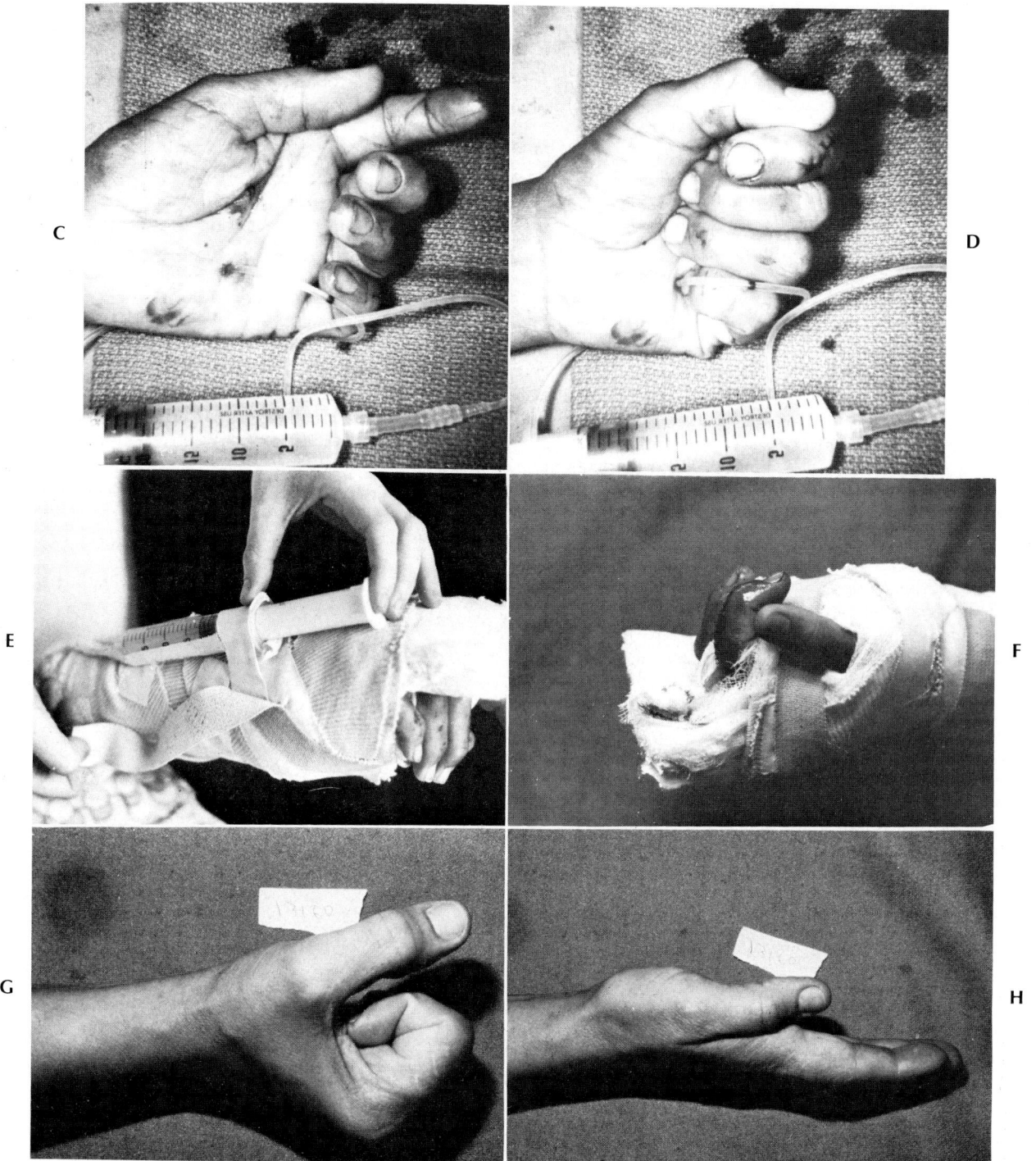

Fig. 33-7 cont'd   C, Before closure of wound a soft Jackson-Pratt catheter is laid proximally to the site of surgery over sensory-nerve branches. **D,** Active flexion. **E,** Syringe (20 ml) containing the local anesthetic is taped to the forearm dressing. **F,** Sterile dressing applied to the wound must not restrict home exercise program, so full active flexion and extension can be carried out within the confines of the splint. **G,** Three months after tenolysis procedure. Patient exceeded range of motion gained intraoperatively: MP 0°/90°, PIP 0°/95°, DIP 0°/60°. Full flexion to the DPC. **H,** Extension.

left on as a protective covering for a few days. To protect the catheter entrance site and surgical incision from contamination, the therapist places the patient's hand on a sterile field during the exercise session (Fig. 33-8, *A* and *B*).

At the end of the exercise session, an antibiotic ointment is applied to the catheter entrance site and along the incision line. Dry sterile dressings are then applied and are not removed until the treatment session on the following day.

The goal is to achieve the active range of motion obtained at surgery by the time the catheter is removed at 5 to 7 days.

The catheter is removed on approximately the fifth postoperative day. The skin suture holding the catheter in place is cut, and the catheter is easily removed (Fig. 33-9). An-

tibiotic ointment is applied to the catheter entrance site. A whirlpool bath is not permitted until the wound has completely healed.

The postoperative exercise program is the same as described eariler.

SUMMARY

Through the judicious use fo tenolysis, a surgical procedure of such magnitude that it should not be underestimated, salvage of tendon function is attainable in patients whose results after tendon injuries are unsatisfactory. Close cooperation among patient, surgeon, and therapist is necessary to make this procedure worthwhile.

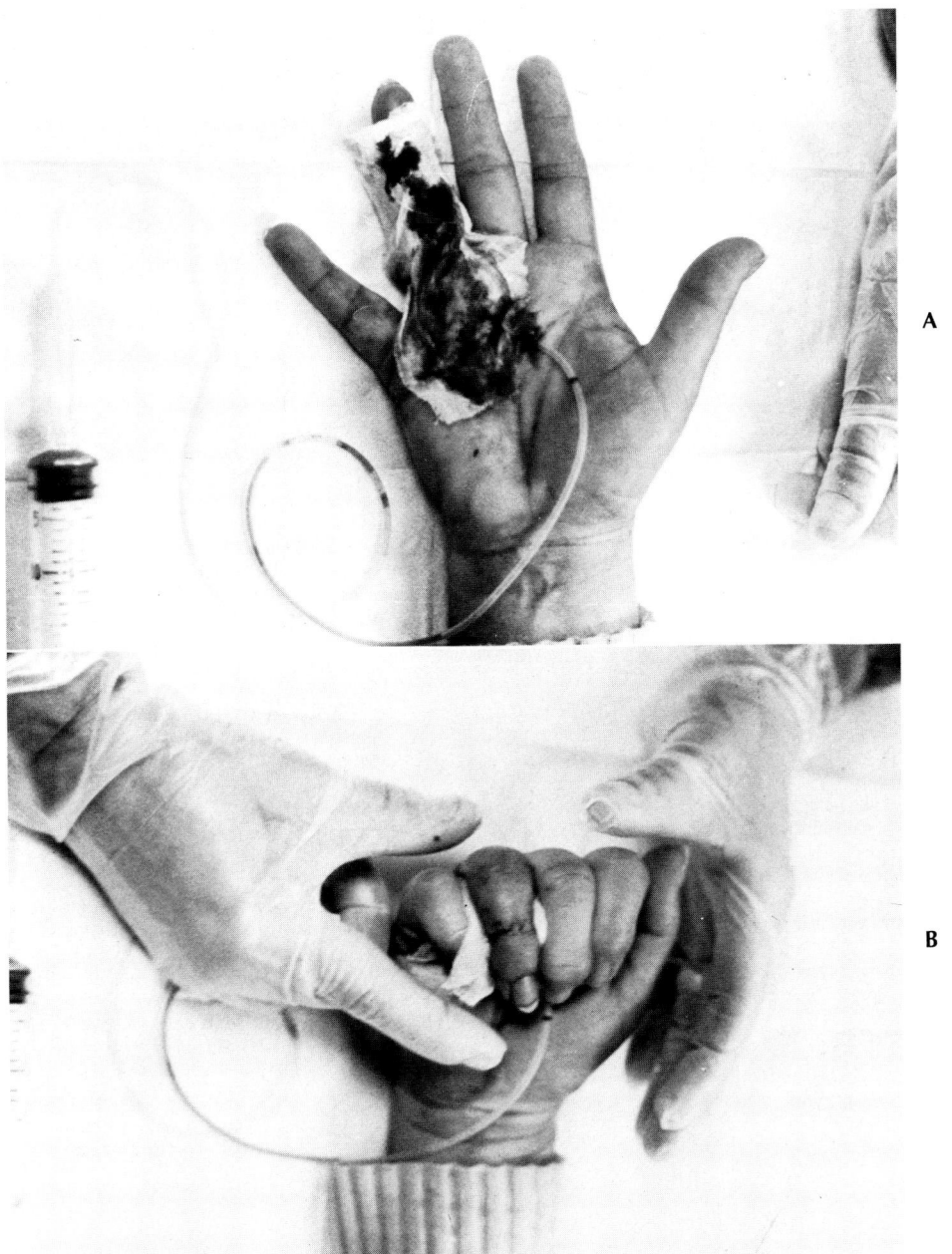

A

B

Fig. 33-8 **A,** Postoperative therapy is carried out in as clean an environment as possible. Patient's hand is placed on a sterile field. Petrolatum gauze covering the incision line is left on as a protective covering for a few days. **B,** Therapist wears sterile gloves during treatment.

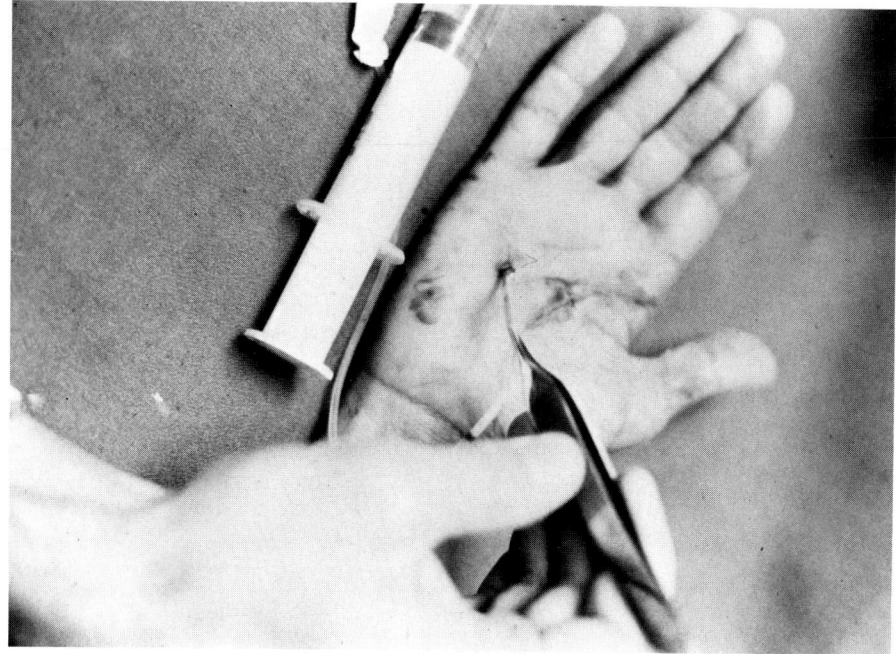

Fig. 33-9 Catheter is removed on approximately the fifth postoperative day. Skin suture holding catheter in place is cut, and catheter is easily removed. Antibiotic ointment is applied to the catheter entrance site.

REFERENCES

1. Fetrow KO: Tenolysis in the hand and wrist, J Bone Joint Surg 49A:667, 1967.
2. Hunter JM, Seinshimer F, and Mackin EJ: Tenolysis: pain control and rehabilitation. In Strickland J and Steichen J, editors: Difficult problems in hand surgery, St Louis, 1982, The CV Mosby Co.
3. Hunter JM and Salisbury RE: Flexor tendon reconstruction in severely damaged hands, J Bone Joint Surg 53A:829, 1971.
4. Hunter JM and others: A dynamic approach to problems of hand function, Clin Orthop 104:112, 1974.
5. Lindsay WK and Thomson HG: Digital flexor tendons: an experimental study, Br J Plast Surg 12:289, 1960.
6. Mackin EJ: Benefits of early gliding after tenolysis. In Hunter JM, Schneider LH, and Mackin EJ; Tendon surgery in the hand, St Louis, 1987, The CV Mosby Co.
7. Matthews P and Richards H: Factors in the adherence of flexor tendons after repair, J Bone Joint Surg, 58-B:230, 1976.
8. Moberg E: Personal communication.
9. Potenza AD: Critical evaluation of flexor tendon healing and adhesion formation within artificial digital sheaths, J Bone Joint Surg 45A:1217, 1963.
10. Schneider LH: Flexor tendon injuries, Boston, 1985, Little, Brown & Co.
11. Schneider LH: Flexor tenolysis. In Hunter JM, Schneider LH, and Mackin EJ: Tendon surgery in the hand, St Louis, 1987, The CV Mosby Co.
12. Schneider LH and Hunter JM: Flexor tenolysis. In American Academy of Orthopaedic Surgeons: Symposium on tendon surgery in the hand, St Louis, 1975, The CV Mosby Co.
13. Schneider LH and Hunter JM: Flexor tendons—late reconstruction. In Green DB, editor: Operative hand surgery, New York, 1988, Churchill Livingstone.
14. Schneider LH and others: Delayed primary flexor tendon repair in no man's land, J Hand Surg 2:452, 1977.
15. Strickland JW: Flexor tenolysis, Hand Clin North Am 1:121, 1985.
16. Strickland JW; Flexor tenolysis: a personal experience. In Hunter JM, Schneider LH, and Mackin EJ: Tendon surgery in the hand, St Louis, 1987, The CV Mosby Co.
17. Tonkin MA, Burke FD, and Vavian JPW: Dupuytren's contracture: a comparative study of fasciectomy and dermofasciectomy in one hundred patients, J Hand Surg 9-B(2):156, 1984.
18. Verdan CE: Tenolysis. In Verdan CE, editor: Tendon surgery of the hand, Edinburgh, 1979, Churchill Livingstone.
19. Verdan CE, Crawford GP, and Martini-Benkeddache Y: The valuable role of tenolysis in the digits. In Cramer LM and Chase RA, editors: Symposium on the hand, vol 3, St Louis, 1971, The CV Mosby Co.
20. Wehbe MA and Hunter JM: Differential tendon gliding in the hand. Paper presented at the annual meeting of the American Society for Surgery of the Hand, Atlanta, 1984.
21. Whitaker JH, Strickland JW, and Ellis RG: The role of tenolysis in the palm and digit, J Hand Surg 2:462, 1977.
22. Wray RC, Moucharafieh B, and Weeks PM: Experimental study of the optimal time for tenolysis, Plast Reconstr Surg 61:184, 1978.

34

Staged flexor tendon reconstruction using passive and active tendon implants

James M. Hunter, Daniel I. Singer, and Evelyn J. Mackin

The objective of the two-staged flexor tendon method is to improve the predictability of final results in difficult problems dealing with tendon reconstruction. The surgeon who is capable of achieving a good result with flexor tendon grafting in the tendon bed with minimal scarring may achieve better results in the poorer grade of cases by using the two-stage method. Patients who are considered suitable candidates for flexor tenolysis should also be considered candidates for reconstruction, because the preoperative assessment may prove inaccurate at the time of surgery. Only at the time of surgery can the surgeon make a true estimate of the extent of scarring and injury to the tendon gliding bed and retinacular pulley system.

The transformation of the stiff, scarred, and functionless tendon complex to its gliding pliable preinjury state can be accomplished by the two-stage tendon graft method using the Hunter silastic tendon implant* at stage I. Restoration of the fibroosseous canal by reconstruction of pulleys and fibrous sheath around the tendon implant has resulted in good gliding biomechanics and a fluid nutrition system that can nourish the subsequent stage II tendon graft free of adhesions.

This chapter highlights the indications and technique of the two-stage tendon graft using the Hunter gliding tendon implant.

INDICATIONS FOR STAGED TENDON RECONSTRUCTION

A tendon implant is indicated in the following situations: (1) as a temporary segmental spacer in selected primary injuries where tendon repair is not possible (when the conditions are favorable, a primary flexor tendon repair is the procedure of choice); (2) scarred tendon beds where a one-stage tendon graft can be predicted to fail; and (3) salvage situations where despite predicted degrees of stiffness, scarred tendon bed, and reduced nutrition, useful function can be returned. This procedure has been successfully used in extensor tendon reconstruction, reconstruction of the severely mutilated hand, and construction of tendon systems in congenital anomalies with deficient tendon systems.[19] Any tendon transfer that would have to traverse a suboptimal bed is also a candidate for this procedure (Fig. 34-1). This procedure may also be indicated for grafting of a profundus tendon through an intact superficialis when the profundus tendon bed is scarred.[20] In a grade V or VI salvage finger, particularly when the adjacent finger has been amputated,

the passive or active tendon may be used to create a "Superficialis Finger." Arthrodesis is performed on the distal joint, and the distal juncture of the implant is to the middle phalanx.[9,15]

In acute trauma the tendon implant may also be used if the wounds have been adequately debrided and rendered surgically clean. When the injury requires simultaneous fracture fixation and flexor and extensor tendon repair, one should consider the use of a tendon implant in the flexor system.

The most recent indication for a two-stage procedure has been in replantation surgery. In multiple digital amputations the use of the implant in the flexor system at the time of replantation may significantly simplify the postoperative rehabilitation. A full-length tendon implant or even a short spacer can maintain the fibroosseous canal and regenerate a flexor sheath in damaged areas after the fracture or fusion has healed and the neurovascular status is stabilized. The passive flexion and active extension have helped rehabilitate both the flexor and extensor systems simultaneously and have significantly improved the function of replanted digits. If the replantation is proximal to zone 2 or at wrist level, it is reasonable to repair the flexor tendons primarily and place extensor implants dorsally, since the wrist is usually flexed to protect the neurovascular repairs. Again the postoperative rehabilitation is simplified.

Acute infection, of course, is an absolute contraindication to this procedure. Appropriate surgical and antimicrobial treatment and subseqent wound healing will allow the procedure to be carried out at a later date without complication. A digit that has borderline nutrition, bilateral digital nerve injuries, and severe joint stiffness may be better treated by amputation rather than reconstruction.

PREOPERATIVE HAND THERAPY

Before tendon surgery, all patients should be placed on a hand therapy program designed to mobilize stiff joints, minimize joint contracture, and improve to the maximum the condition of the soft tissue (Fig. 34-2). Extensor tendon imbalance should be noted.

Motion is encouraged by buddy-taping the involved finger to an adjacent digit to simulate active flexion. Whenever the adjacent finger is used the involved finger must come into play, incorporating it into useful function. A web strap, carefully applied, provides a means to improve passive flexion of the digit.

Splinting to correct flexion contractures begins before stage I surgery and continues through stage I and stage II.

---

*Holter-Hausner, Intl., Bridgeport, Pa.

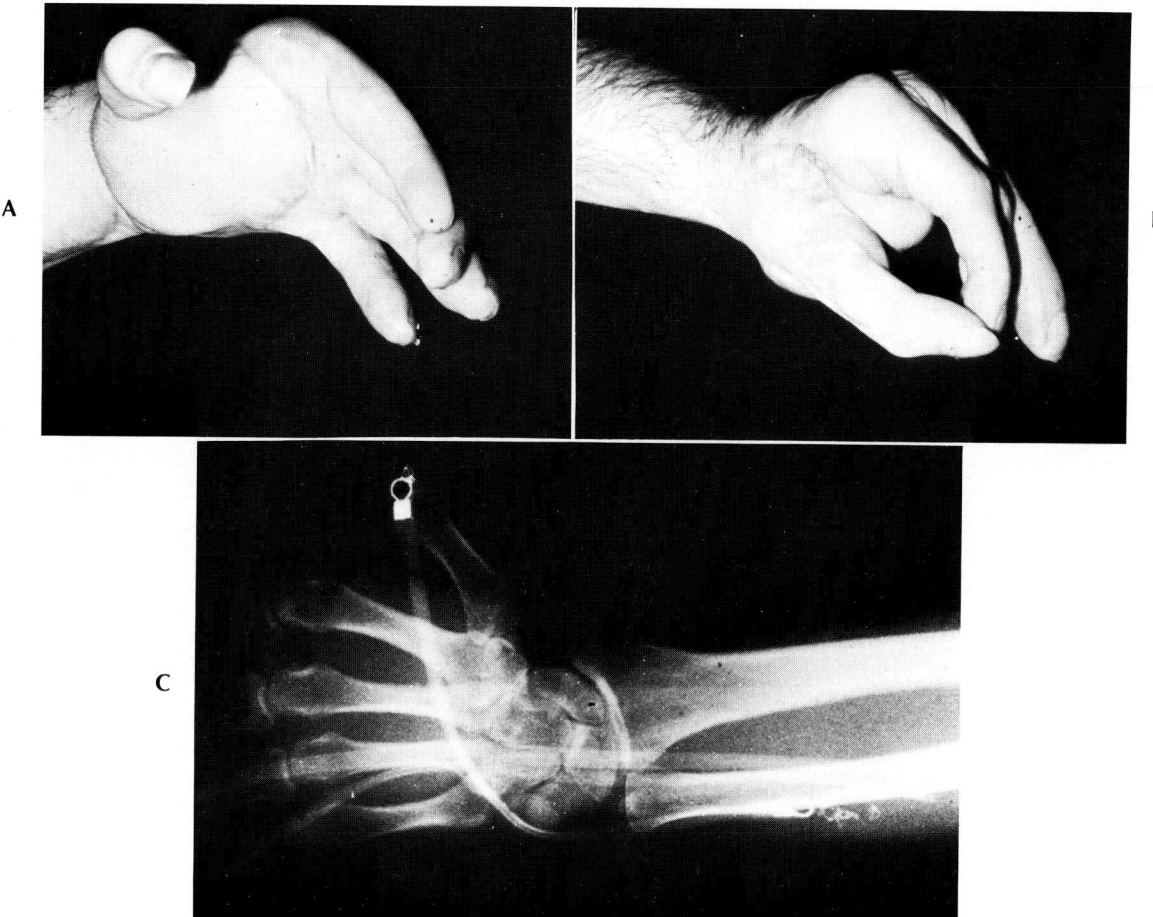

Fig. 34-1   Opponensplasty using an active tendon implant. This can also be performed with a passive implant. The motor is the flexor digitorum superficialis of the long finger. **A,** Thumb extension. This patient lost all thenar muscles and the flexor pollicis longus tendon in a hamburger press. After débridement, metacarpophalangeal arthrodesis, and pedicle skin grafting, first-stage active tendon was used to restore opposition. **B,** Thumb in opposition. **C,** Roentgen-ogram of patient shown in **A** and **B**. Excursion was approximately 2.5 to 3 cm.

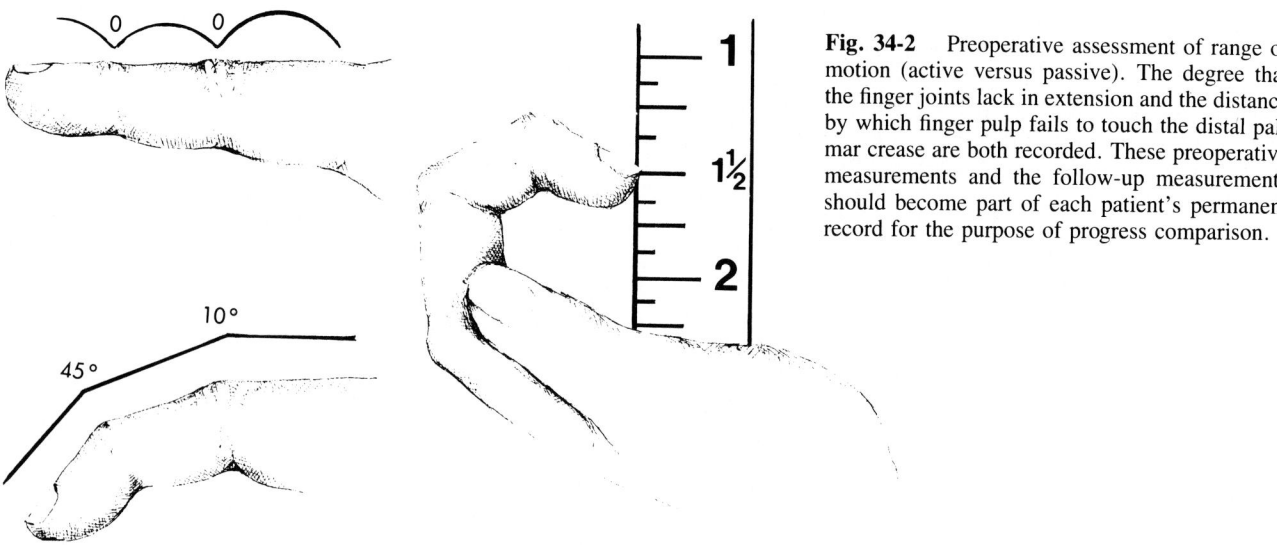

Fig. 34-2   Preoperative assessment of range of motion (active versus passive). The degree that the finger joints lack in extension and the distance by which finger pulp fails to touch the distal palmar crease are both recorded. These preoperative measurements and the follow-up measurements should become part of each patient's permanent record for the purpose of progress comparison.

It must be emphasized that a flexion contracture before stage I can become a worse problem after stage II. Splinting to correct and prevent further contractures must be integrated into the patient's daily regimen during the entire tendon reconstruction procedure. In patients who have a deep cicatrix resulting from previous injury or previous surgery or patients who form scar tissue easily, it may be necessary to continue night-extension splinting for 6 months after stage II.

When passive flexion of the finger is limited and full extension of the proximal interphalangeal (PIP) joint is also limited, the patient should alternate the extension splint with the flexion device; that is, the web strap is worn intermittently during the day, and the extension splint is worn at night. The decision regarding when to proceed with stage I surgery should be based on the combined judgments of the surgeon and hand therapist, judgments based on the success of preoperative splinting and patient motivation.

TYPES OF IMPLANTS

Two basic types of Hunter tendon implants have evolved from the experience gained in experimental and clinical trials during the past 25 years: passive implants and active implants (Fig. 34-3).

The initial concept in 1960 was to design an actively gliding artificial tendon or prosthesis. Limited success was achieved. However, because of terminal juncture separation under stress, the method was later converted to passive gliding until further design and material improvements could produce proximal and distal attachments that were reliable for an extended period.[6, 10-12]

All the implants have a core of woven Dacron that is pressure molded into a radiopaque silicone rubber. The surface finish is smooth and the cross-sectional design is ovoid to aid optimal tendon sheath development (Fig. 34-4).

The passive gliding program implies that the distal end of the implant is fixed securely to bone or tendon while the proximal end glides freely in the proximal palm or forearm. Movement of the implant is produced by active extension and passive flexion of the digit. A new biologic sheath begins to form around the implant during the period of gliding that follows stage I surgery. The new sheath progresses through a 4-week phase of biologic maturity and develops a fluid system that supports gliding and nutrition gliding for the tendon graft after stage II. Usually, 3 to 4 months after stage I surgery the implant can be electively replaced by a tendon graft.

The implant incorporates design characteristics of firmness and flexibility to permit secure distal fixation and minimize the buckling effect during the passive push phase of gliding. The implant is available commercially.

The two passive tendon implants differ only in their distal juncture. One implant has a stainless steel distal metal end plate that is attached to the distal phalanx by a screw (Fig. 34-5). It provides excellent fixation to bone eliminating proximal migration of an implant, the principal cause of sheath synovitis. It also provides the added benefit of shortening the second-stage procedure. The screw hole in the

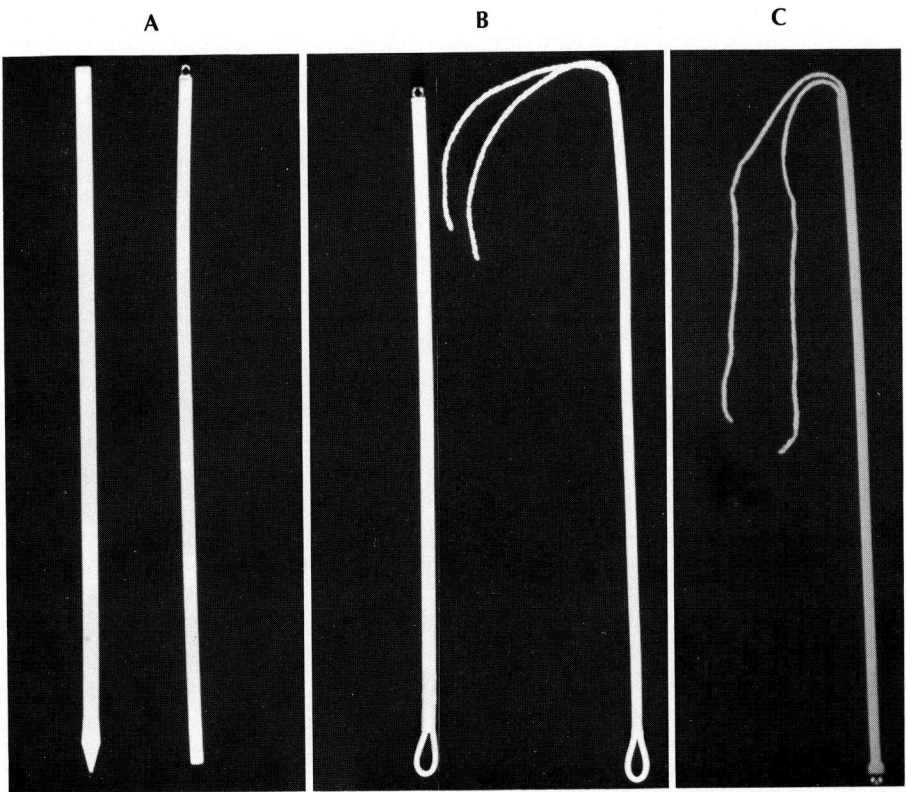

Fig. 34-3   **A,** Passive, gliding tendon implants. **B,** Active, gliding tendon implants. *Left,* Metal end-screw fixation and fixed-length loop system. *Right,* Dacron braid interlacing and loop system with adjustable-length design. **C,** Active, gliding tendon implant. Metal end-screw fixation with two free, porous Dacron cords with adjustable-length design.

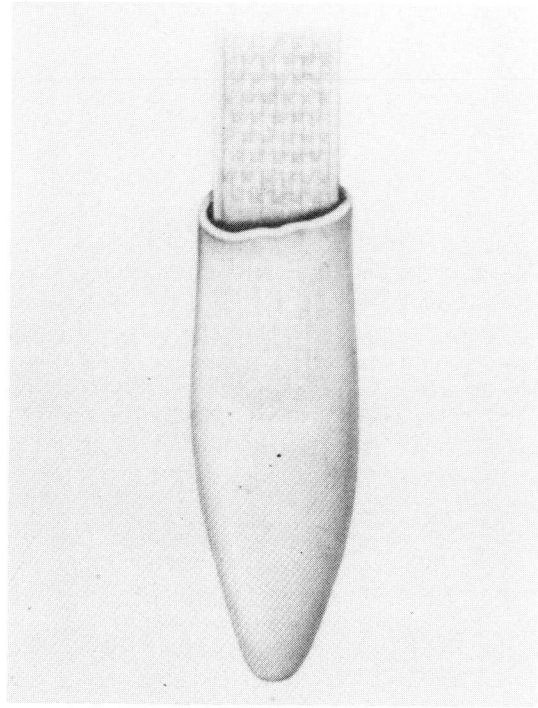

Fig. 34-4 Implant. Silicone rubber has been cut away to show Dacron woven tape added to give body to the implant.

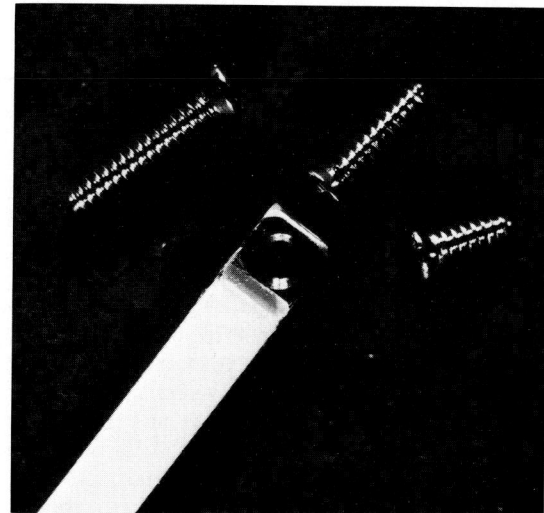

Fig. 34-5 Distal juncture with screw-fixation metal end plate.

distal phalanx acts as a guide hole that is further enlarged in an oblique fashion for the acceptance of the tendon graft. The Woodruff* and the A-O 2 mm bone screws are available in various sizes. The length of the screw is determined from the preoperative roentgenogram. A pilot hole is drilled (Fig. 34-6, *A*) at a 15- to 20-degree angle to the distal interphalangeal (DIP) joint with a 0.035-inch Kirschner wire (K-wire). The length of the screw should be sufficient to engage the dorsal cortex of the phalanx but not pass beyond it because this may result in pain dorsally. The tip of the screw should be proximal to the germinal matrix of the nail so as not to cause a nail deformity. This implant is available in 6, 5, 4, and 3 mm diameters. The lengths are either 23 or 25 cm. These implants can be trimmed proximally to the appropriate length.

The passive tendon implant without a screw fixation terminal device is held in place with a 4-0 nonabsorbable suture that is woven through the distal end of the implant; this distal end is secured under the profundus stump (Fig. 34-6, *B*). Care must be taken to place the suture through the central Dacron core. The distal juncture is also reinforced with two lateral sutures of Dacron. This implant is available in the following sizes: 3mm × 23 cm, 4 mm × 23 cm, 5 mm × 25 cm, and 6 mm × 25 cm. This implant can also be shortened and should be trimmed at the distal end.

The passive tendon implant is indicated for the young patient with an open epiphyseal plate. A 3-mm tendon implant is often used. The digital end is sutured to the stump of the profundus. Once again, the sutures must be placed in the Dacron core because if the sutures are just in silicone

rubber, the distal end will loosen during passive mobilization after the stage I surgery.[7]

Molded radiopaque oval silicone rods (Swanson-Hunter design) are available from the Dow Corning Company in diameters of 6, 5, 4, and 3 mm and may be cut to the appropriate length (Fig. 34-7).

Active tendon implants for temporary replacement are constructed from two cords of high tenacity Dacron especially designed to be compatible with the medical grade of silicone rubber and with human tendon or bone. The Dacron design is woven similar to the collagen helix and permits progressive tissue ingrowth. All the implants have a core of the Dacron cords that is pressure molded into a radiopaque 2-cm silicone rubber shaft. The four types of active tendon implants differ in their distal and proximal junctures: (1) two free porous Dacron cords at each end, (2) stainless steel metal end plate distally for wire or screw fixation and two free porous Dacron cords proximally, (3) two free porous cords of Dacron distally and a preformed Dacron silicone loop proximally, and (4) single-unit tendon implant with stainless steel metal end plate distally and a preformed Dacron silicone loop proximally in four lengths.

Two of the implants terminate proximally in the preformed Dacron silicone loop through which the proximal tendon motor is woven (Fig. 34-8). The implants without loops terminate proximally in the open end with the two free porous Dacron cords with adjustable length design.

The tendon implants also provide two types of distal junctures: the previously described screw-plate juncture or the two free porous Dacron cords that can be placed through drill holes in the bone. The tensile strength of the distal metal juncture to the tendon implant shaft has been rated at more than 100 pounds.

The active tendon implants are to be used as temporary extended tendon prostheses. The benefit of this type of implant has been the ability to select a motor before stage II and to have this motor "tuned," in that it is actively moving the finger. It also serves to test the pulleys that have been reconstructed during the first stage. The proximal motor

---

*Zimmer-Rodewalt, Sewell, NJ. Synthes, Inc., Paoli, Pa.

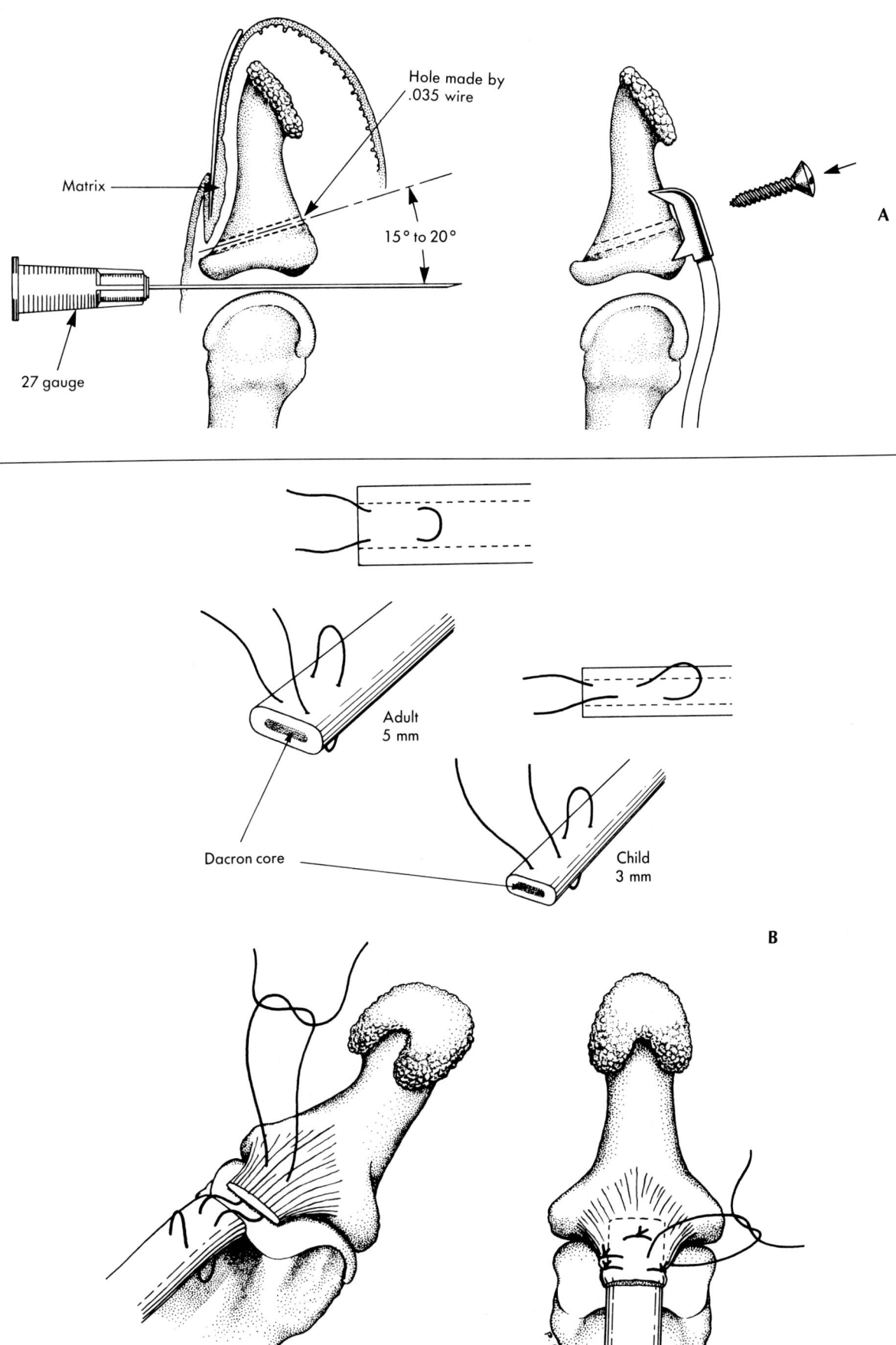

Fig. 34-6   **A,** Distal plate-fixation plan for the Hunter tendon implant. **B,** Fixation of the reinforced tendon implant (rod) without the metal plate.

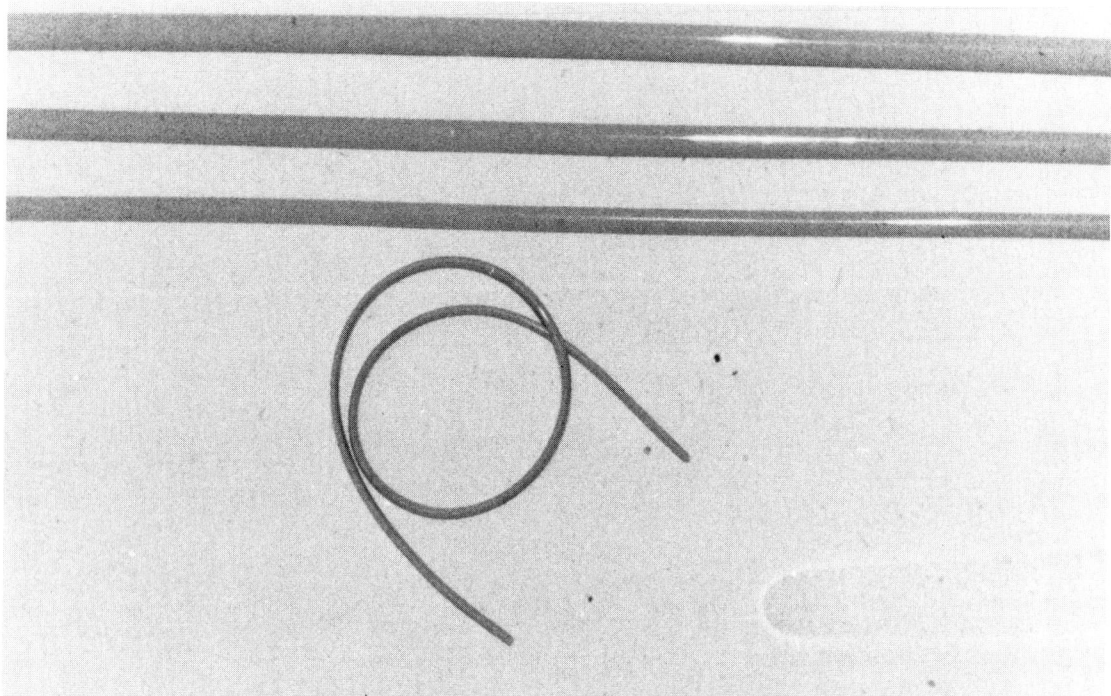

Fig. 34-7 Molded, unreinforced silicone rods. Notice flexibility of the implant without the Dacron core. (Dow Corning Corp, Midland, Mich.)

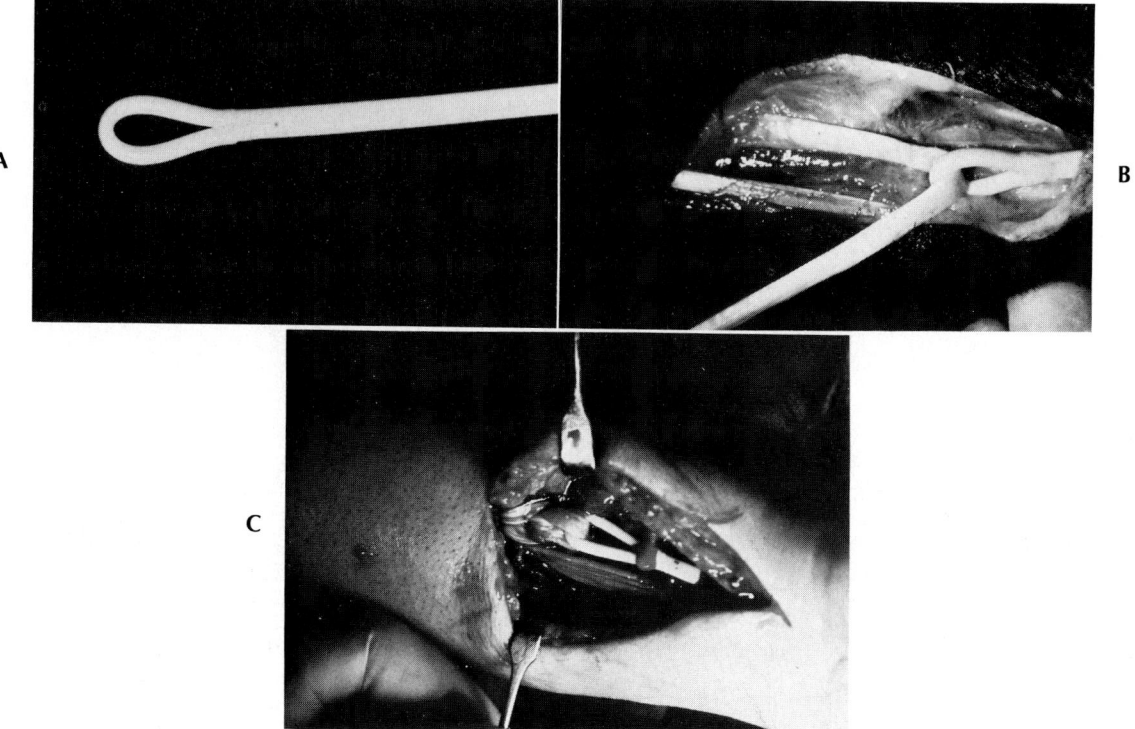

Fig. 34-8 **A,** Active implant, proximal, silicone-coated Dacron loop for motor tendon unit juncture. **B,** Appropriate motor is chosen and pulled through the loop to set tension. **C,** Completed juncture of the active-tendon implant and the proximal motor tendon.

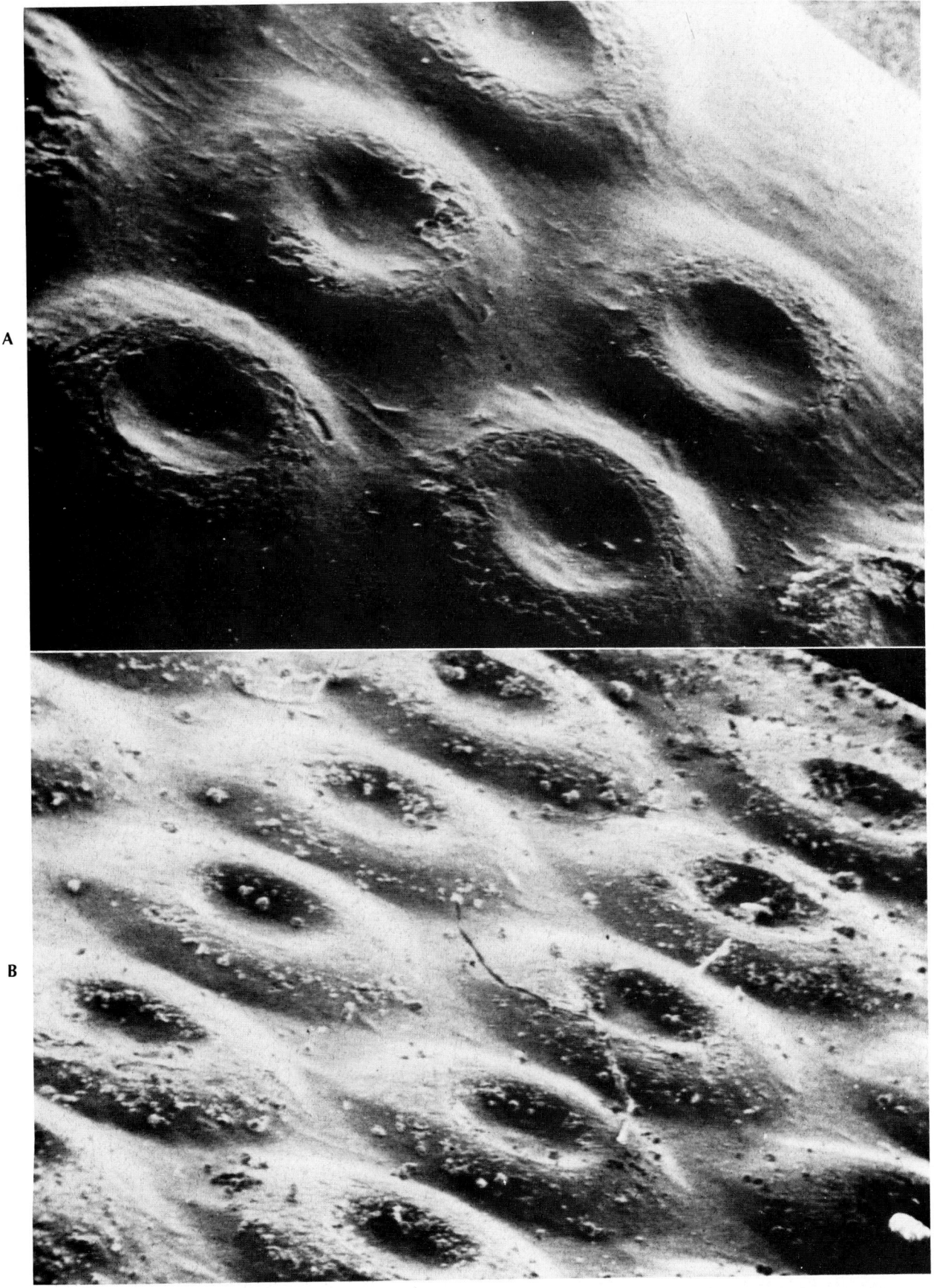

Fig. 34-9 **A,** Scanning electron micrograph of the surface of the clean and sterile implant before handling. (40× .)
B, Scanning electron micrograph of implant after handling with dry gloves. Notice surface contaminants. (40× .)

Continued.

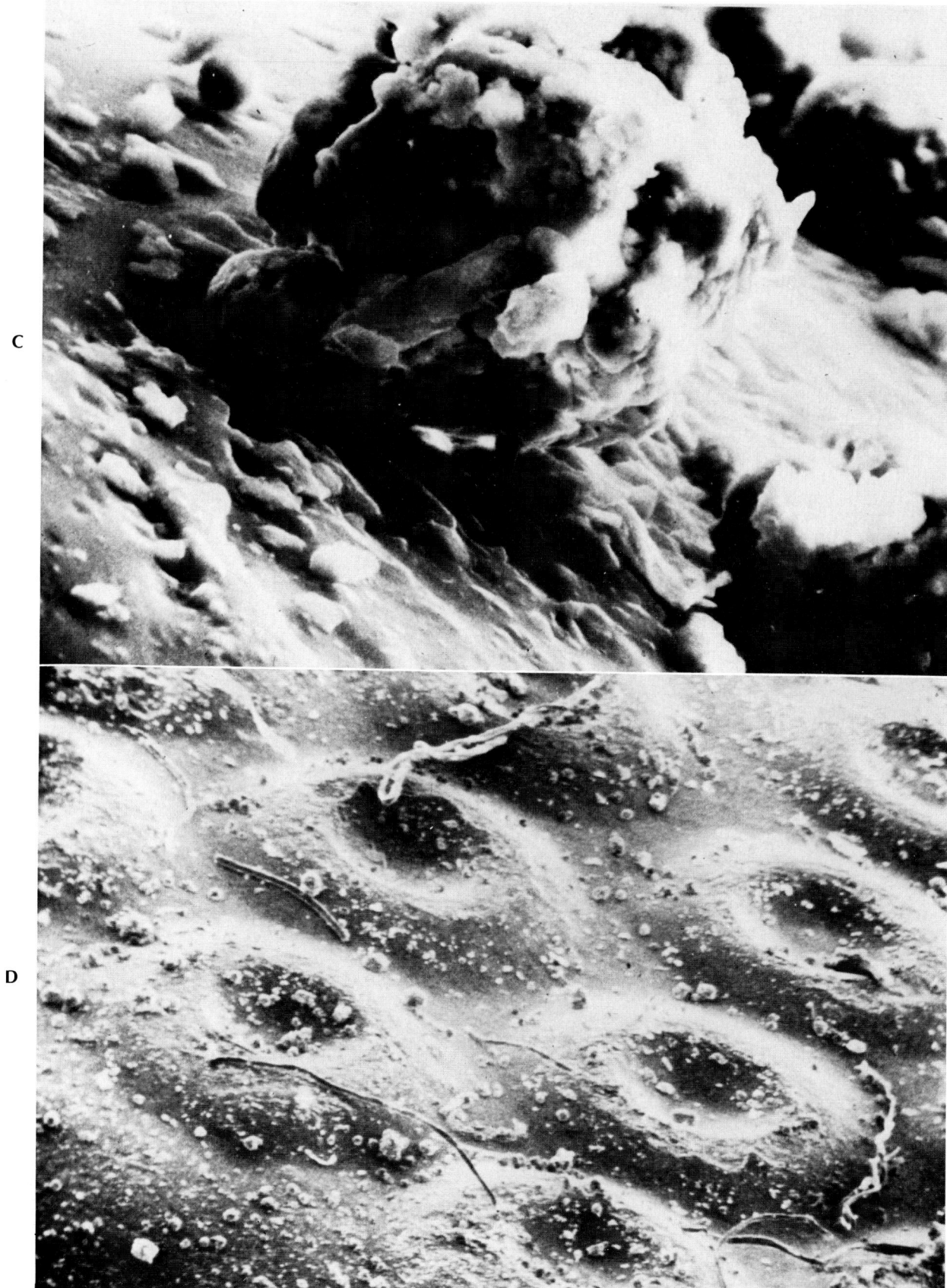

Fig. 34-9, cont'd **C,** One particle from previous illustration. (800× .) **D,** Scanning electron micrograph of implant after handling with dry gloves and placing on a towel. Notice the large increase in surface contaminants. Contamination can be avoided by keeping the implant and gloves moist at all times. (40× .)

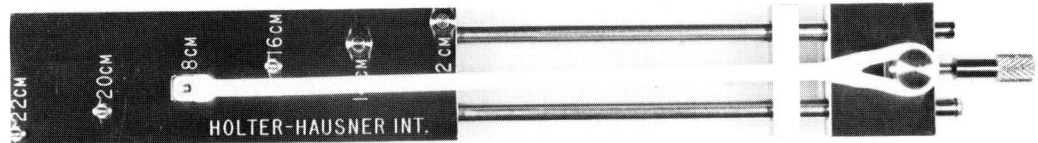

Fig. 34-10   Active tendon autoclave instrument maintains tendon length integrity and permits touch-free handling during surgery.

juncture is easily identified in the second stage, and the fibrous sheath motor tendon unit is kept intact and the graft weaved through the healed tendon complex. The tension is set, and the graft is sutured.

CARE OF SILICONE RUBBER

Silicone rubber is highly electrostatic; as a result, it attracts airborne particles and surface contaminants (Fig. 34-9). Once the implants are removed from the sterile package, they must be kept moist at all times. They should be placed in a sterile solution of saline, Ringer lactate, or triple antibiotic irrigant. Gloves and sponges coming into contact with the tendon implant should always be wet. They should preferably be handled with atraumatic instruments. Attention to these details will prevent the development of a synovitis, which could interfere with the subsequent development of the pseudosheath. Autoclave preparation for surgery requires special care (Fig. 34-10).

ANESTHESIA

If a passive tendon implant is to be performed, this is done with the patient under axillary block or general an-

esthesia. If patient participation is required to determine function—that is, tenolysis versus implant or an active tendon implant—we prefer to use local anesthesia (1% lidocaine infiltration)[5] and tourniquet control augmented by intravenous analgesia such as droperidol and fentanyl (Innovar) or titrated intravenous meperidine (Demerol) and diazepam (Valium). This will allow patient compliance for assessment of function of the tenolysis or help in establishment of the appropriate tension in the active tendon implant. Selected second-stage procedures have also been done in this manner. This allows the setting of appropriate tension of the tendon graft.

For the patient to perform these complicated procedures under local anesthesia, a qualified anesthesiologist is needed to keep the patient sufficiently sedated to allow tolerance of the tourniquet. The patient should, however, be arousable when his compliance is required. Adequate premedication and a good rapport between the anesthesia personnel and the patient are mandatory. Patients have tolerated the tourniquet for consecutive periods up to 1 hour in this manner. The tourniquet is deflated intermittently (approximately every 30 minutes) to avoid tourniquet paralysis, and function is tested. If the patient cannot tolerate this procedure, the anesthesiologist can provide a general anesthetic. Most patients do not recall the surgical procedure postoperatively. This anesthetic technique has been used in some procedures lasting for as long as 4 hours.

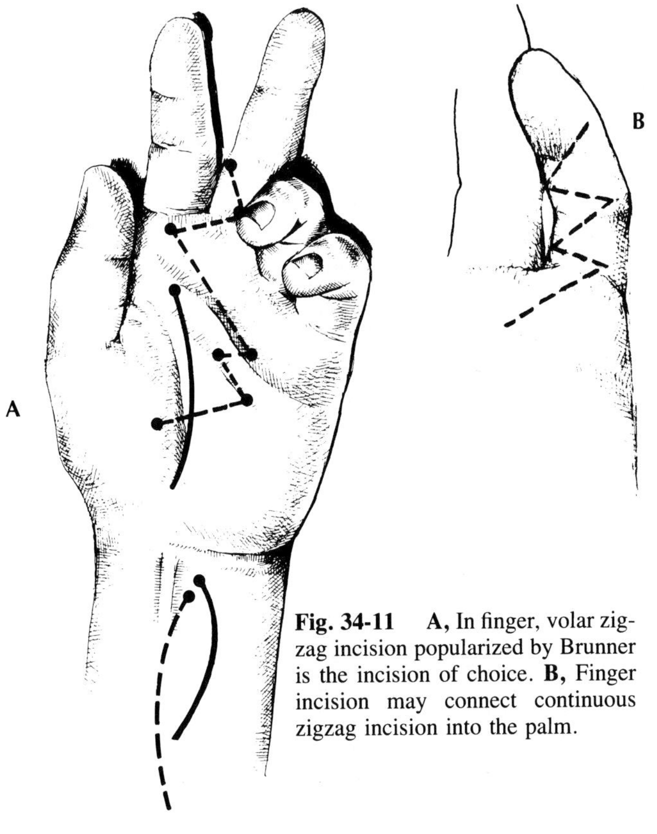

PASSIVE TENDON IMPLANT
Stage I surgery

In the finger the volar zigzag incision popularized by Julian Bruner is the incision of choice (Fig. 34-11). This incision spares the deep vascular connections to the tendon bed and permits a complete exposure of the tendon bed. The incision begins at the tip of the finger and proximally enters the palm. The incision must reach the distal extent of the transverse carpal ligament to facilitate the subsequent passage of the implant. The skin flaps should be of full thickness, with the corners lying over the neurovascular bundles to prevent marginal skin necrosis. The digital neurovascular bundles must be identified and protected. All the undamaged segments of the fibroosseous pulley system are spared. After the entire canal has been exposed, an isolated, curved incision is made proximally to the wrist crease. This incision is usually based on the ulnar aspect of the forearm. The ulnar artery and nerve and median nerve are identified and protected. The plane between the superficialis and profundi is identified and enlarged with blunt finger dissection. By making transverse window incisions in the flexor canal between A_1 and A_2, the cruciates, the mid-A_2 pulley levels, one carefully excises the scarred flexor tendons. At the levels of the cruciate pulleys, the proper digital arteries give four

Fig. 34-11   **A,** In finger, volar zigzag incision popularized by Brunner is the incision of choice. **B,** Finger incision may connect continuous zigzag incision into the palm.

Fig. 34-12 Diagram of pulley system and relationship of the digital artery branches and vinculum system.

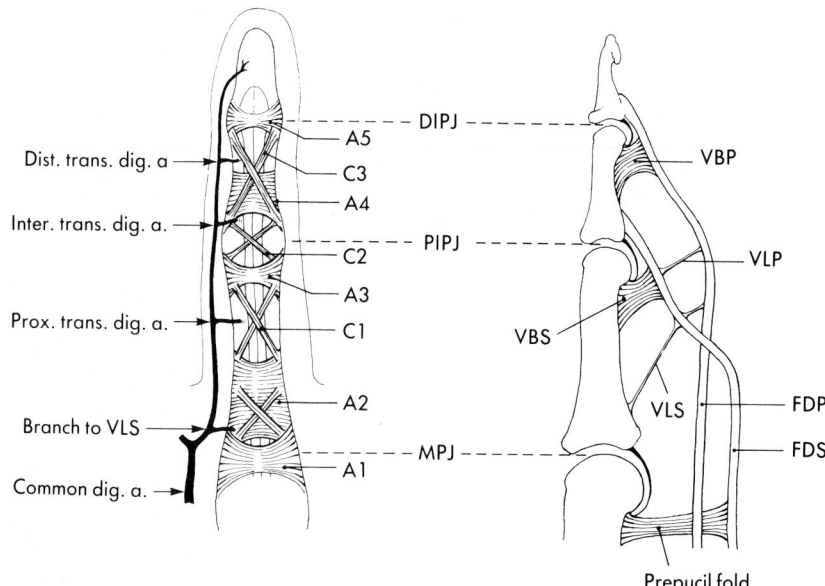

Dist. trans. dig. a
A5
C3
A4
C2
A3
C1
A2
Branch to VLS
A1
Common dig. a.

Inter. trans. dig. a.

Prox. trans. dig. a.

DIPJ
PIPJ
MPJ

VBP
VLP
VBS
VLS
FDP
FDS

Prepucil fold

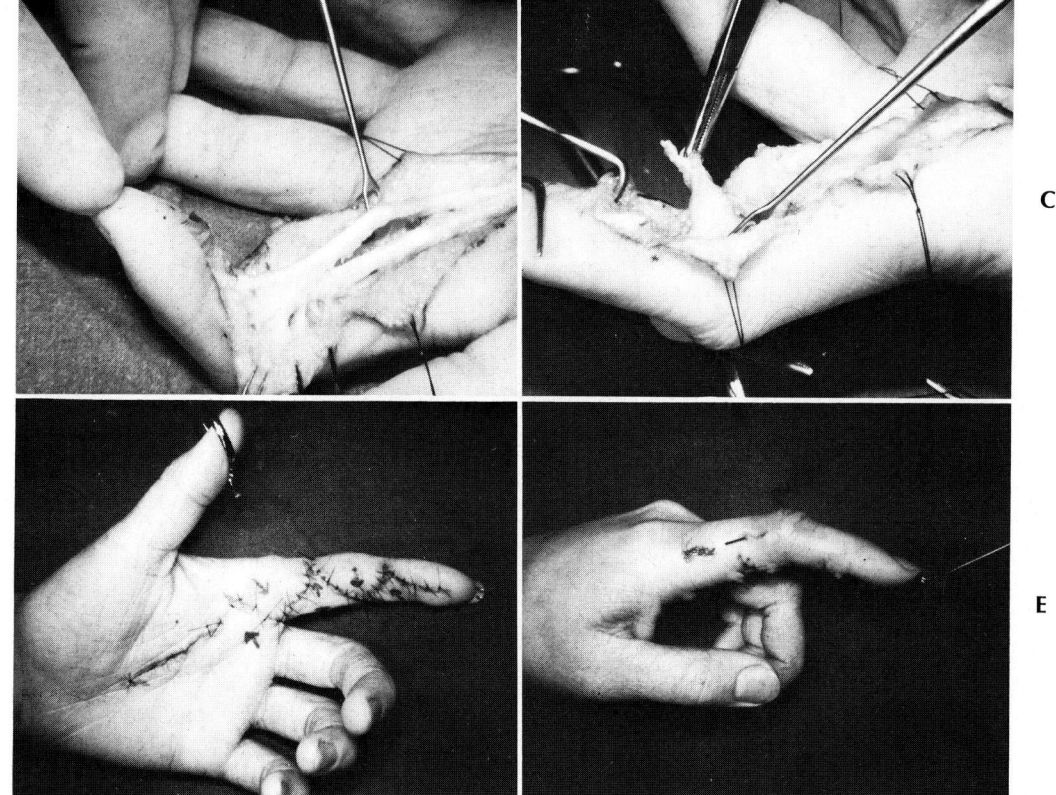

A

B

C

D

E

Fig. 34-13 **A,** Preoperative photograph of patient with a flexion contracture at the proximal interphalangeal joint and bowstringing of tendons caused by absence of pulleys. **B,** Scarred tendons are exposed through the zigzag incision. Note absence of pulley system and the scar underneath the bowed tendons. **C,** Scarred tendons are excised and contractures are released. **D,** After implant has been inserted and pulleys have been reconstructed, V to Y technique is applied to the zigzag incision to gain extension and release skin tension. **E,** Postoperative stage I. Notice the absence of bowing across the proximal interphalangeal joint after contracture release, pulley reconstruction, and skin advancement. Proximal interphalangeal joint is temporarily pinned in extension.

transverse tributaries that supply the synovial bed and the vincular system. If possible, these arterial branches are spared (Fig. 34-12).[7]

The excision of damaged tendons will often be time consuming, The surgeon must carefully excise scarred and adherent tendons while preserving uninjured portions of the sheath retinaculum. A generous segment of the distal profundus tendon, at least 1 cm, is preserved, and the joint capsule is left intact. It will probably be necessary to sacrifice the A_5 pulley to perform this adequately. The metacarpophalangeal (MP), DIP, and PIP joints should be left undisturbed if all contractures can be released by tendon removal and by incision of the contracted cutaneous skin ligaments or the oblique retinacular ligament of Landsmeer. The contracted finger will often require shifting or advancement of local skin flaps. The V-to-Y technique may be applied to gain extension and release skin tension (Fig. 34-13). One may best salvage severe contractures with skin loss by shifting skin flaps proximally in the finger and skin grafting the distal defects. Sometimes in a severely damaged digit a reasonable way to proceed with the restoration of digital motion is to create a Superficialis Finger.[9] The implant covered by viable skin flaps is fixed to the base of the middle phalanx, and arthrodesis is performed on the distal joint. This allows concentration of surgical and postoperative management to obtan PIP motion at the expense of DIP joint.

If the superficialis tendon bed has not been injured, it is left intact over the PIP joint.

Scarring of the tendons at the PIP joint level is often responsible for a flexion contracture. Meticulous dissection of mature scar at this level will permit increased ranges of motion and minimized flexion contracture after stage II. The profundus and superficialis tendons are removed from the proximal pulley and sharply divided into the proximal palm. Scarred or shortened lumbrical muscle is resected to prevent the problem of a "lumbrical-plus" finger. If the palm is uninjured, the lumbrical and profundus complex with surrounding mesotenon is carefully preserved for stage II juncture. If more than one implant is to be used and crowding is observed in the carpal canal, the superficialis may be pulled through the carpal canal and excised in the forearm.[7]

If resection of scarred tendons fails to release the contracture, scarring of the joint capsule or skin ligaments should be suspected. Capsulotomy of the volar plate is often helpful. The cord portion of the collateral ligament is preserved for stability. Scarring of skin and of the ligament complex on either side of the finger, will maintain a contracture and may require opening by V-to-Y or advancement flap and skin grafting. The joint should be immobilized in extension postoperatively with a K-wire for 7 to 10 days and then mobilized by controlled intermittent splinting. These procedures will be most effective if the neurovascular bundle on only one side of the finger is damaged. In all instances of severely damaged digits the tourniquet should be deflated and the vascularity of the finger inspected frequently.[7] In poor situations, arthrodesis or amputation may be indicated.

Retinacular pulley reconstruction. The basic anatomy of the flexor pulley system is a precise biomechanical design that permits lubricated gliding of two tendons while transmitting the power of the forearm musculature to the bones

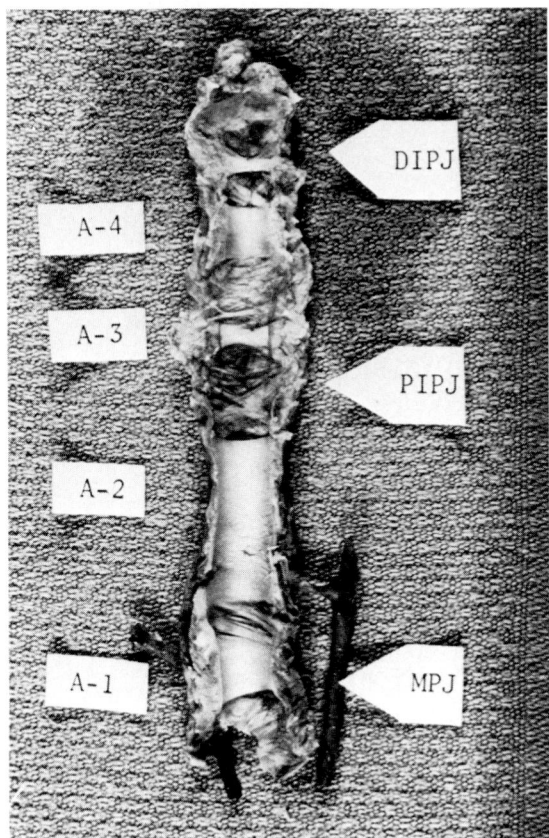

Fig. 34-14 Anatomic dissection of flexor canal viewed from within.

of the fingers (Figs. 34-12 and 34-14). Reconstruction of scarred or injured flexor retinaculum is the key to maximal digital flexion. Unless this arrangement can be restored at stage I surgery, the functional arc of motion cannot be restored despite good postoperative hand therapy.

The pulley retinaculum is preserved when possible, and some collapsed sections may be dilated by instrumentation. If the pulley segments are of insufficient size to carry the implant, they should be excised, with a flap of the base portion in the periosteum being left for suture during tendon graft pulley reconstruction. If the A_1, A_2, and A_4 pulleys appear weak or are absent, they are reconstructed. Four pulleys are preferred: one proximal to each of the three finger joints and one at the base of the proximal phalanx (Fig. 34-15).

Tendon material (flexor digitorum superficialis or profundus) to be discarded is excellent for building pulley. Several techniques may be applied, depending on location of injury and the surgeon's preference. We prefer to wrap the tendons around the phalanx extraperiosteally but under the extensor apparatus proximal to the PIP joint while over the extensor apparatus distal to the PIP joint. It is wrapped twice around the phalanx and sutured to itself or to the rim of the fibroosseous canal (Fig. 34-16). This is performed over a sizer implant to prevent making the pulley too tight. The pulley should be as broad as possible, and an implant should be used that fills the tendon bed but does not bind on glide testing. The average-sized implant generally has been 3 or 4 mm in women and 4 to 5 mm in men (Fig. 34-

A

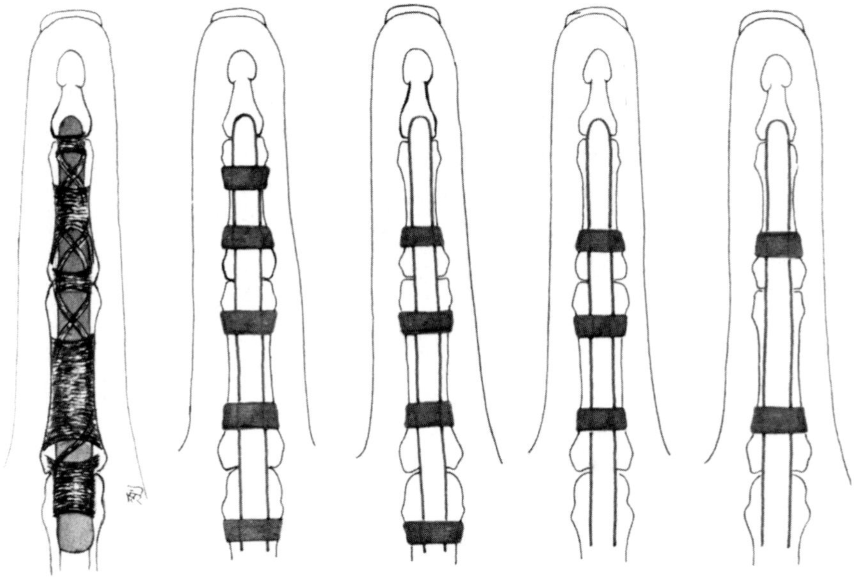

B

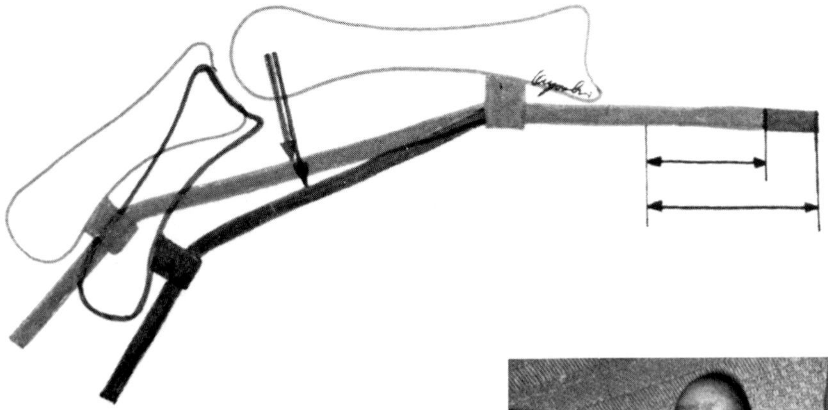

C

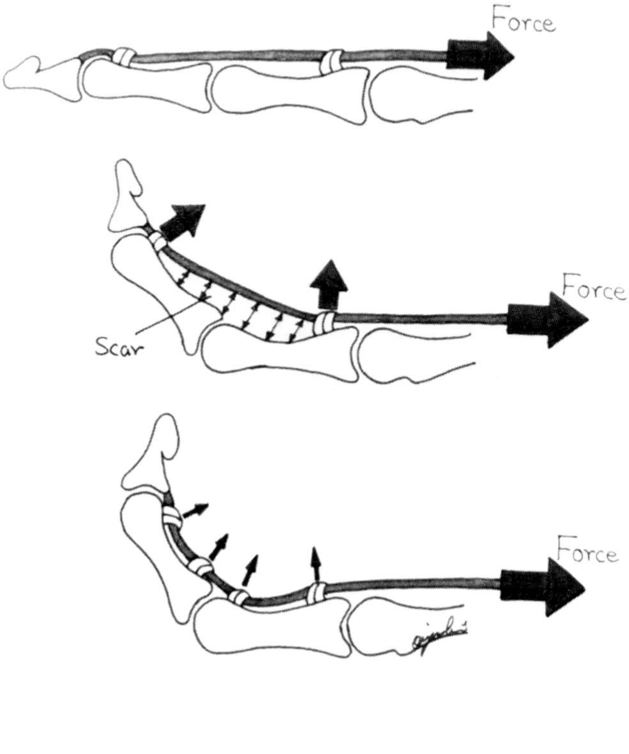

Force

Force

Scar

Force

Force

D

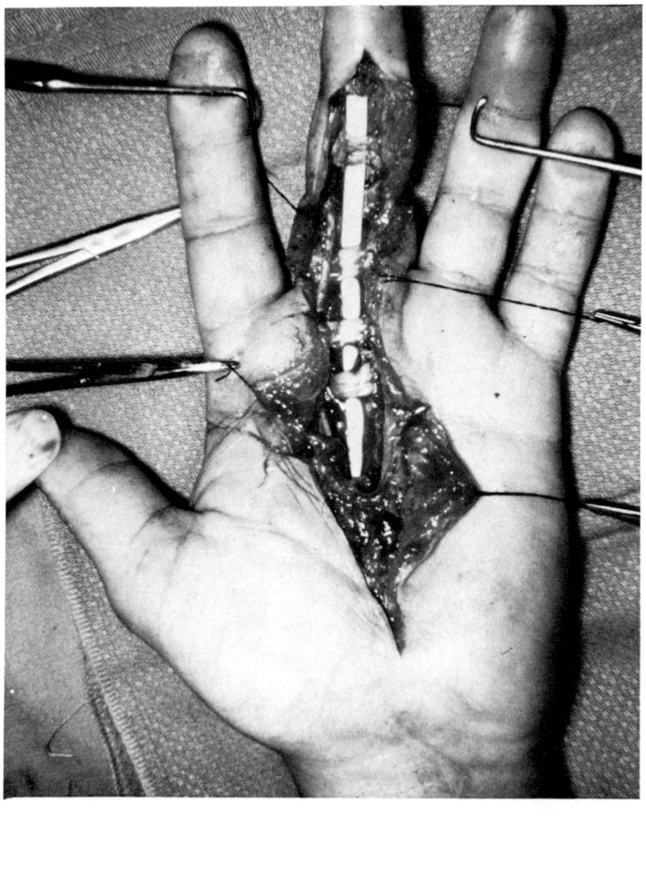

Fig. 34-15 **A,** Normal pulley system on far left. Preference of pulley reconstruction decreases from left to right. Pulley system to far right will provide the least digital flexion per unit of excursion. **B,** Two pulley systems demonstrating decreasing amount of digital flexion per unit of tendon excursion because of the lack of adequate pulleys. **C,** Lack of pulleys not only results in a decrease of digital flexion, but also encourages recurrence of contractures as scar accumulates under bowstring tendons. **D,** Reconstructed four-pulley system.

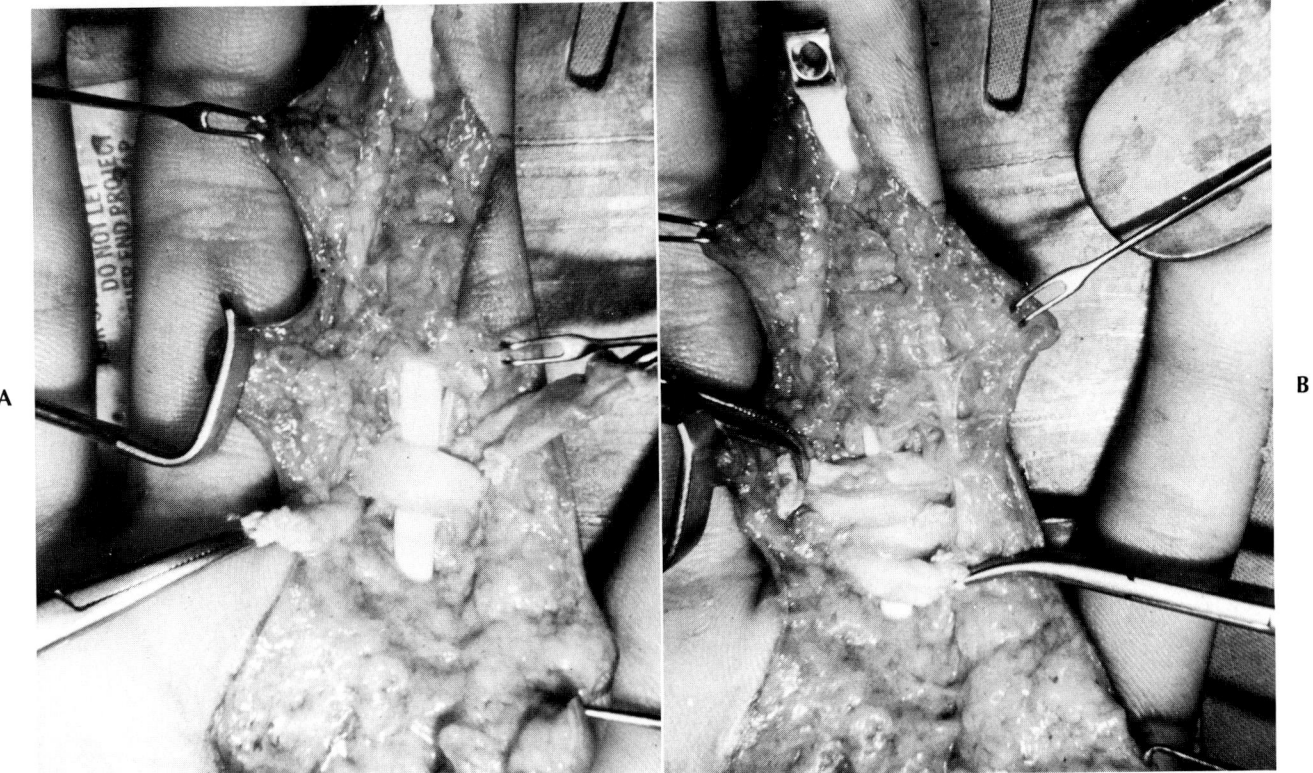

Fig. 34-16   **A,** Sublimis remnant is wrapped under the extensor apparatus and over the implant to reconstruct the A2 pulley. **B,** After tendon is wrapped around twice, it is sewn to itself and the rim of the fibro-osseous canal. Pulley should be as wide as possible without blocking motion itself.

17). The pulleys must not be unduly bulky or too close to the joint, or they may act as a mechanical block to flexion by abutting on one another.

Based on this method of pulley reconstruction, the pulleys are balanced; that is, the reconstructed pulleys are balanced around MP joint and the PIP joint both in tightness and distance from the joint. They should be located just so they are off the widest part of the condyle at the metaphyseal-disphyseal junction. This location offers the dual benefit of

minimizing pulley tension and at the same time maintaining good finger function by restricting bowstringing and thus keeping the tendon excursion for joint motion within physiological range.[5]

Tendon implant sizers are passed through the pulley system. The finger is held flat on the table, and the implant is *moistened* and pulled gently back and forth. A malleable blunt tendon instrument is passed deep through the carpal tunnel to appear in the forearm deep to the superficialis and

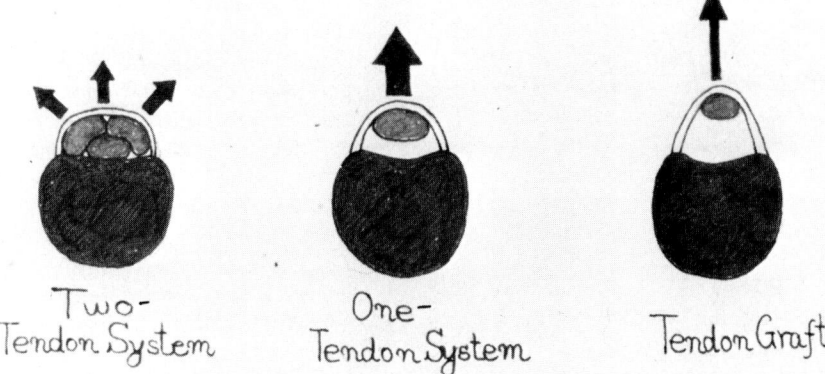

Fig. 34-17   The practice of replacing the anatomical two-tendon system with a small tendon graft causes a basic failure in the biomechanics of gliding. At stage I the pulley should be snug, and at stage II the tendon graft should closely represent the size of the new synovial space to enhance *good* flexion. Normal flexion cannot be achieved; it was lost at injury.

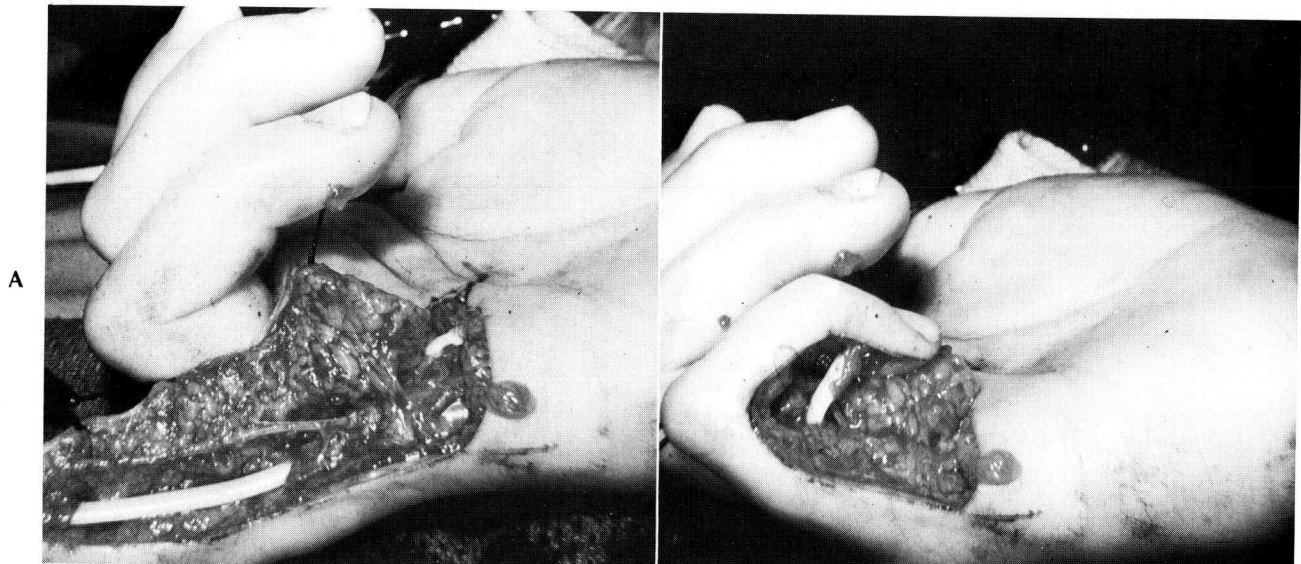

Fig. 34-18 **A,** Digital extension with implant in flexor canal. Notice the lack of pulleys around the proximal interphalangeal joint. **B,** Tension is placed on the implant, and the digital flexion is recorded. Notice deficient flexion because of the lack of pulleys. Pulley reconstruction is indicated to maximize the digital flexion.

volar to the profundus. The instrument is passed gently when one is seeking the soft mesotenon spaces. Implant binding will occur most often at the narrow, flat distal (A₄) annulus requiring tendon-graft pulley reconstruction. The length of the implant is determined so that on full extension of the finger the proximal end can be seen 1 to 2 inches proximal to the wrist crease. The implant is then secured to the distal phalanx as previously described. One tests passive gliding of the implant by moistening the implant bed with saline solution and holding the wrist and digit in neutral flexion while passively flexing and extending the finger. Motion should be free, with a measured range of motion between 3 and 4 cm at the proximal end. Buckling of the implant may occur distally to the tight pulley. If present, this must be corrected by free grafting before closure or synovitis may develop and adversely affect the development of the pseudosheath.

Testing the pulley system. Testing the pulley system and recording range of motion constitute the important last maneuver of stage I before wound closure. The free proximal end of the implant is grasped and pulled, with the finger being brought from extension to maximum flexion. The following are recorded: (1) the predicted active range of motion versus the passive range of motion; (2) the measured distance of the proximal end necessary to produce the active function (this will assist in selection of the stage II motor tendon); (3) the attitude of the finger in relation to the pulley system (if this maneuver does not produce full flexion or produces a pulley rupture, it may be necessary to modify the pulley system) (Fig. 34-18); and (4) the security of the distal end attachment of the tendon implant should be carefully checked. The implant is then placed in the interval between the flexor superficialis and flexor profundus. This interval must allow the implant to glide proximally without kinking when the MP joints and wrist are flexed.

The wound is then closed distally to proximally and,

finally, the soft tissue recess for the implant in the forearm is checked with a moistened gloved finger and passive gliding is reviewed. The hand is positioned with the wrist in 30 degrees of flexion, the MP joints in 60 to 70 degrees of flexion, and the interphalangeal (IP) joints in full extension for final dressing. This position after stage I permits the proximal sheath to form in the long position.

Complications. Complications are rare if the procedure has been performed meticulously with careful handling of the soft tissues and the implant. Proper postoperative therapy and careful monitoring of the patient's progress also help prevent any complications. The reported complication is synovitis from loosening of the distal juncture with proximal migration of the implant.

Synovitis is characterized by discomfort in the operated digit, swelling along the volar aspect of the finger, decreased motion, swelling at the incision site in the forearm, and lack of signs of systemic illness. Synovitis may result from improper handling of the implant at the time of insertion. Silicone rubber attracts free particles of lint or glove powder (see Fig. 34-9). This problem is best treated by prevention. As previously stated, the implant should be kept moist at all times and wet gloves should be used to handle the implant. Buckling of the implant under tight pulleys will also result in a synovitis. This also is easily prevented by attention to detail at the time of pulley reconstruction. Overzealous therapy has also caused synovitis. However, this should resolve with 5 to 7 days of immobilization followed by gradual resumption of activity. Rupture of the distal juncture of the implant and subsequent proximal migration is the commonest cause of synovitis (Fig. 34-19). The surgeon should test the strength of the distal juncture intraoperatively and x-ray films should be obtained at 1 and 6 weeks postoperatively and before stage II. If the prosthesis becomes dislodged after stage I, one should rest the hand and proceed with the second-stage tendon graft.

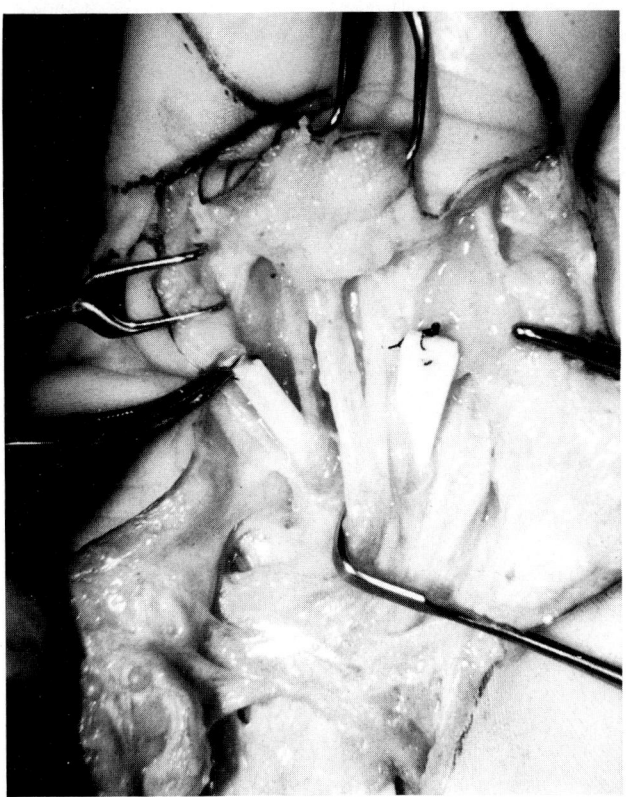

Fig. 34-19 Synovitis caused by rupture of the distal juncture and the proximal migration of implants into the palm. Improper suture technique of the implant to the profundus stump resulted in this avoidable complication.

If synovitis from all the above causes is not remedied by rest and immobilization, the stage II procedure should be performed earlier and the thickened synovium excised in the region of the proximal juncture. Continued mobilization of the digit in the face of a synovitis results in a thickened sheath, and the result will be a recurrence of contractures and loss of motion.

Infection is very rare and will usually manifest itself early in the postoperative period. Pain, fusiform swelling, lymphadenopathy, elevated temperature, and increased white blood count are the classic symptoms. Treatment should be immediate. Removal of the implant, immobilization, adequate irrigation, débridement, and appropriate antibiotics will resolve the problem. After the soft tissue is healed and the infection is resolved, there is no contraindication to performing the stage I procedure again. It is our practice to place the patient on perioperative antibiotics, as is done with most other orthopedic implants.

Stage II surgery

As stated, the compliance of the patient in setting the tension in stage II greatly facilitates the outcome of this procedure. The anesthesia employed is preferably local with intravenous sedation, but routine general anesthesia can be selected as required.

The exposure of the distal juncture should be adequate, however, it does not have to extend across the PIP joint. Care is taken not to injure the pseudosheath. After the distal juncture has been exposed, it is left intact and the proximal juncture is exposed. Proximally the implant is grasped with an instrument (rubber-shod forceps), and the sheath at the site of the juncture is carefully examined. Portions of soft sheath may be retained at the surgeon's discretion. However, if synovitis has been present, the thickened sheath must be completely removed at the proximal juncture site to the wrist flexion crease. The active potential range of motion of the finger and the excursion necessary to produce it are determined by laying the hand and finger flat on the table and then firmly pulling the implant proximally. The surgeon should note (1) the excurson of the implant to produce the range of motion from maximum extension to maximum flexion (Fig. 34-20), (2) the distance the finger pulp rests from the distal palmar crease, and (3) joints with restricted motion. The motor tendon (flexor digitorum superficialis, FDS, or flexor digitorium profundus, FDP) is selected and grasped with a small hemostat. The hand is elevated and the tourniquet released while the lower leg is prepared to remove a plantaris tendon graft.

The plantaris tendon is preferred because it is longer and usually approaches the size of the implant that is being removed, that is, approximately 3 mm. If the plantaris tendon is absent, a long toe extensor is harvested. A Brand tendon stripper is used to harvest the grafts.[1,21]

We have frequently used a long toe extensor tendon when the plantaris is absent. If a toe extensor is used, it is usually necessary to make three or four transverse incisions to prevent injury to the graft. One incision is made at the metatarsophalangeal joint of the toe, the next just distal to the retinaculum of the ankle, and a third just proximal to the retinaculum. The tendon is stripped and passed through each incision until the musculotendinous juncture is reached. The fifth toe should not be used because it usually has only one toe extensor. Shoter tendon grafts, for example, palmaris longus, extensor indicis, extensor digiti minimi, and segments of superficialis are removed by standard technique and may be used for (1) thumb, little finger, and superficialis fingers or (2) index, long, and ring fingers with an attachment to a tendon juncture in the uninjured palm.

Distal juncture. The tendon graft, carefully stripped of all paratenon, is sutured to the proximal end of the implant and pulled through the new tendon bed (Fig. 34-21). The implant is detached from the distal phalanx and discarded. A Bunnell type of weave is placed through the distal end of the graft with monofilament stainless steel or nonabsorbable suture.[2,3] A pull-out wire is no longer used. An oblique hole is made in the distal phalanx under the profundus stump remnant and enlarged with a curette. A Keith needle is drilled through the distal phalanx and exists dorsally in the middle of the nail. The suture is then pulled through the distal phalanx by threading it through the Keith needle. As the Keith needle is advanced through the tip of the finger, one must watch the graft being pulled into the drill hole on the volar side of the finger. This tendon-to-bone juncture is most important and, when healed, will prevent any distal ruptures of the graft. The wire is tied over a button on the dorsum of the fingernail (Fig. 34-22). Reinforcing sutures on either side of the graft will help anchor the distal juncture. After this is completed, the distal juncture is closed. If a Superficialis Finger is being performed, a similar procedure is followed; however, the drill hole is

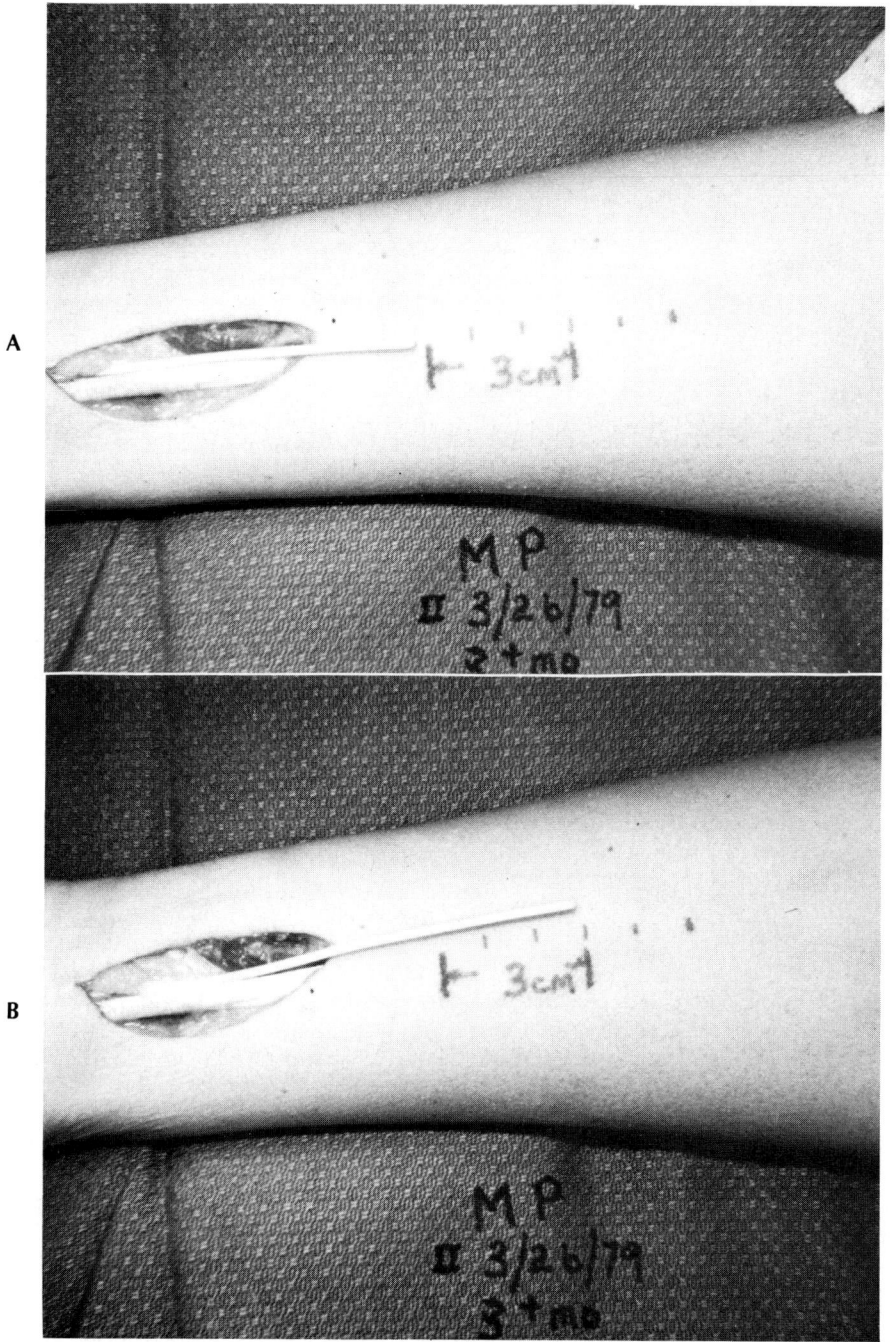

Fig. 34-20 **A,** Implant is exposed in the forearm. **B,** Excursion of the implant is 3 cm.

placed at the base of the middle phalanx (Fig. 34-23). We prefer to tie the suture directly over the middle phalanx dorsally through a small dorsal counter-incision, preventing the complications of a dorsal button directly over skin.

Proximal juncture. The final phase of the stage II technique is directed toward completion of the proximal juncture. The motor is selected, and the graft is placed through the tendon motor temporarily and fixed with either wire or Mersilene suture. The attitude of the finger with the wrist in neutral should be one of slightly more flexion than the adjacent digit (Fig. 34-24). At this point, the patient's com-

pliance is enhanced if the patient is under leptoanalgesia, alleviating the guesswork in setting the tension of the graft.[4] The patient is asked to flex and extend his fingers, and the tension of the graft is then adjusted accordingly. The selected tendon motor must supply the same excursion or better, if a good result is to be achieved. When the tension is correct, the graft is woven through the motor tendon and sutured into place using the technique described by Pulvertaft (Fig. 34-25).[17,18]

The Pulvertaft end-weave technique is preferred for a single tendon juncture, that is profundus of the index, flexor

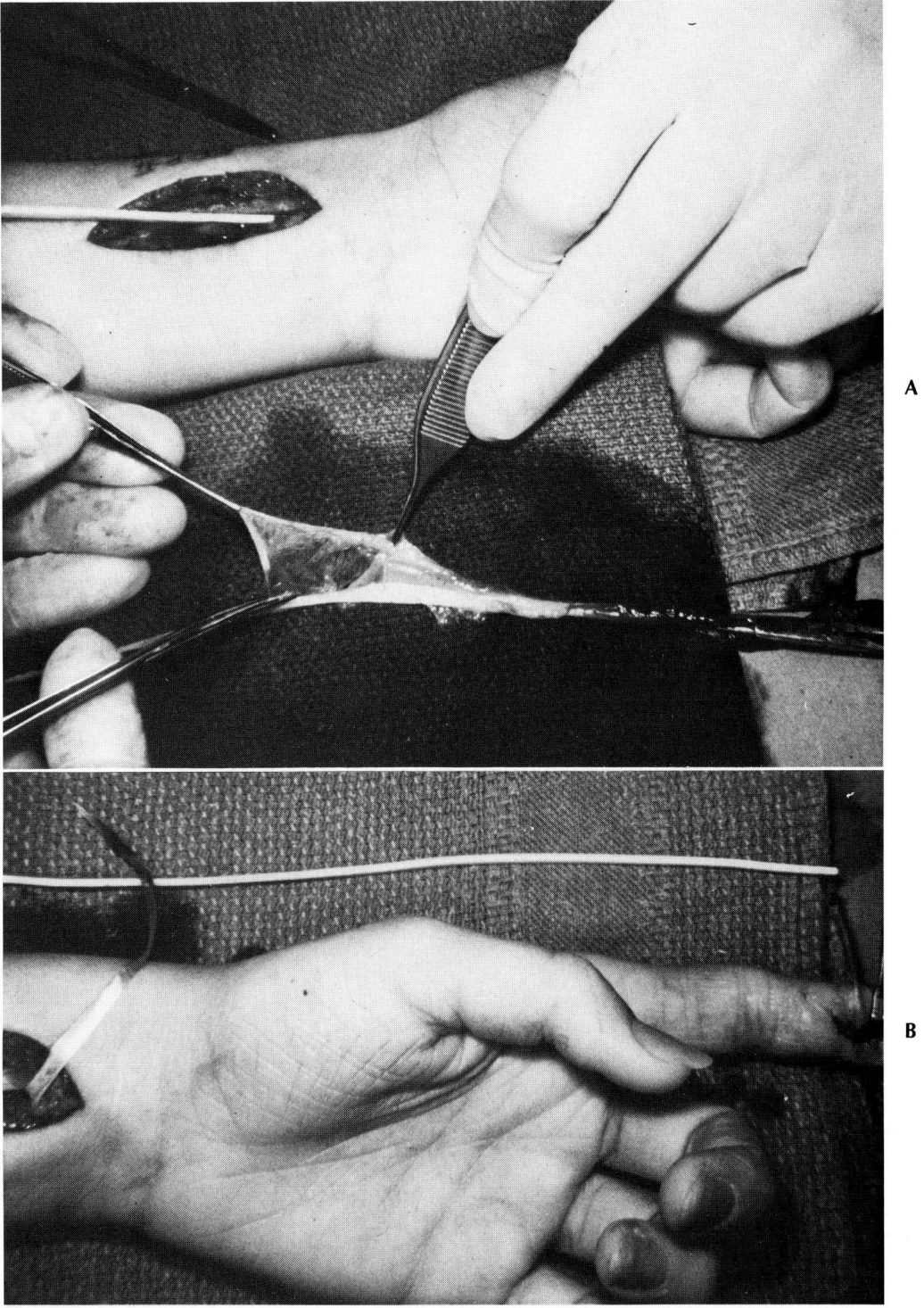

Fig. 34-21   **A,** Peritenon is carefully removed from the tendon graft. **B,** Tendon graft has been sutured to the proximal aspect of the implant and then pulled into the new tendon bed from the proximal to distal position.

pollicis, or superficialis. The multiple end weave is preferred for a profundus, long, ring, or little finger juncture. It is extremely important to make sure that the suture passes through the graft and into the motor to prevent subsequent slipping of the proximal juncture. One must also be sure that the pseudosheath does not impede excursion of the

tendon graft juncture, and, if necessary, more of the proximal sheath should be excised to permit full extension.

After repeated manipulations of the finger, it should remain in slightly more flexion than normal. The juncture is completed by a second interweave and suture fixation, and the wound is closed. The postoperative plaster splint dress-

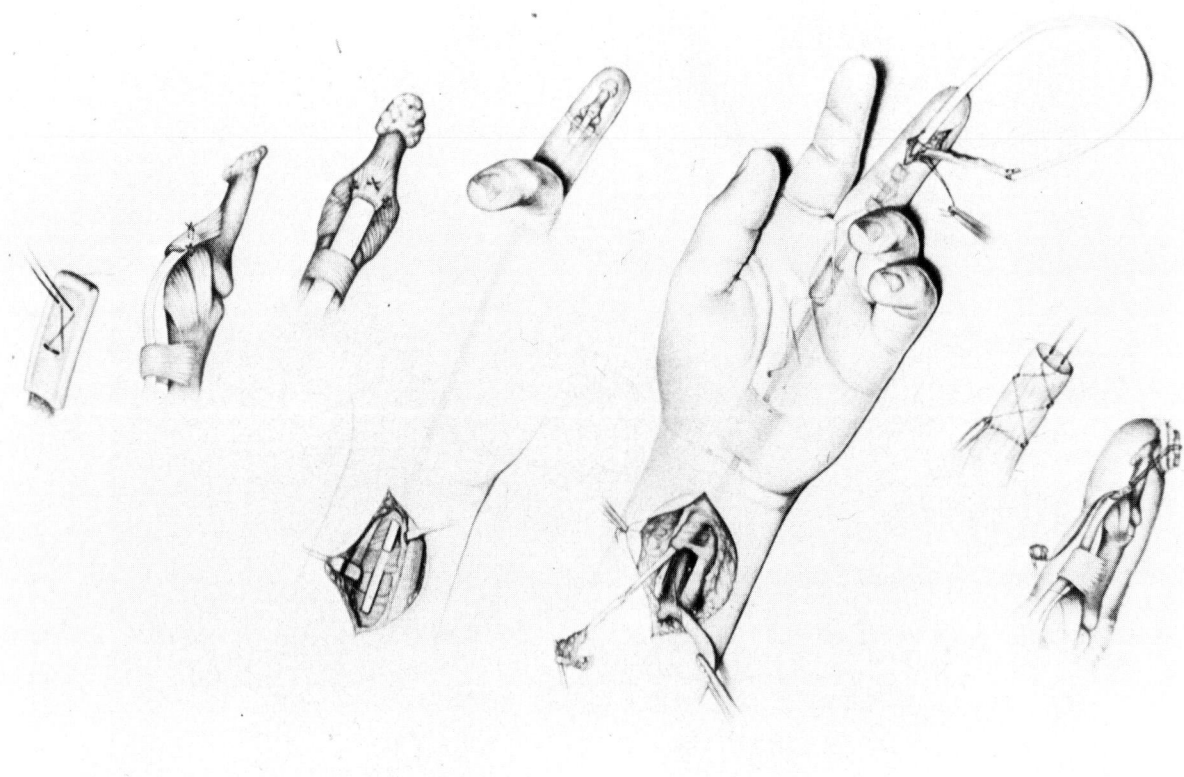

Fig. 34-22 Diagram of stage I procedure, the four figures on left and stage II, the three figures on right. (From Hunter JM and Salisbury RE: J Bone Joint Surg **53A:**836, 1971.)

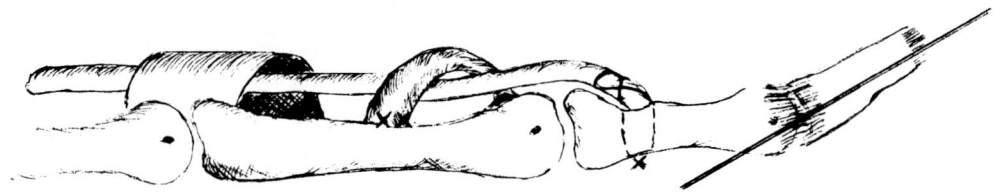

Fig. 34-23 Stage I, superficialis finger. Implant is carried to the base of the middle phalanx and fixed in place by a wire suture passed through two small drill holes. Reinforcing sutures are added. Distal phalanx is either tenodesed or arthrodesed.

ing fits securely with the wrist in 30 degrees of flexon, MP joints in 70 degrees of flexion, and IP joints in full extension.

Complications. Two complications after stage II tendon grafting deserve discussion: (1) adhesions along the tendon graft or at the proximal anastomosis and (2) rupture of the juncture of the tendon graft. Restrictive adhesions may occur anywhere along the course of the graft; however, they are most common at the junctures. They are also prone to occur in areas where there is poor graft gliding and thus an inadequate fluid nutrition system. This may happen in areas where the pulleys are too tight or there has been dense scar. If these adhesions significantly restrict motion, a tenolysis procedure should be performed.

If tenolysis is necessary for adhesions, it is performed 4 to 6 months after stage II using local anesthesia, with intravenous sedation.[4,14] The region of the proximal juncture

should be explored first, with attention directed initially to the junction of the new tendon sheath and the tendon graft, then to the proximal juncture, and last to the tendon graft within the new sheath. Only adhesions that actually restrict motion should be treated.

After surgery, immediate active motion of the lysed tendon graft is necessary to preserve the increased ranges of motion. Many of these patients will return to therapy with an indwelling catheter placed next to the median and/or ulnar nerves. Marcaine is injected every 4 to 6 hours postoperatively to minimize pain and maximize active movement. The catheter can be left in place up to 5 days. All these patients will require a most carefully coordinated management program directed by surgeon and therapist. (Refer to Chapter 33.)

Rupture of the graft can occur at either end and may be

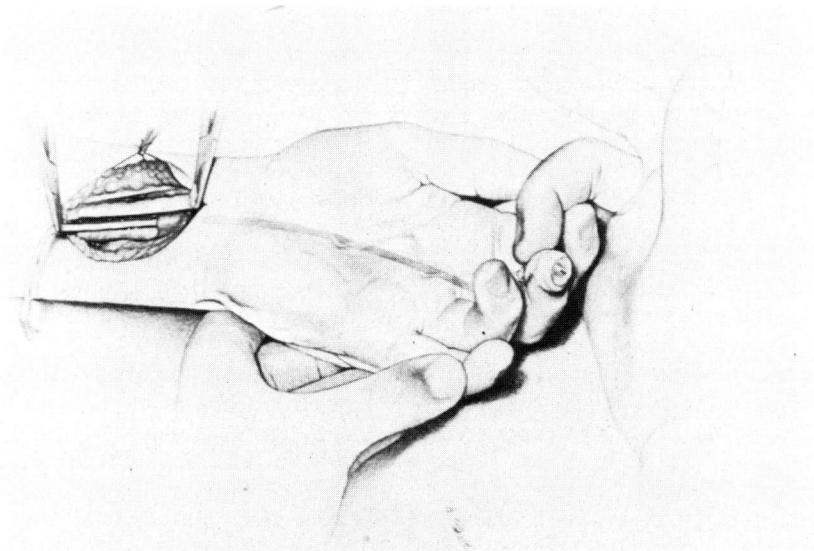

Fig. 34-24   Appropriate tension is set on the tendon graft and it is woven through the motor tendon.

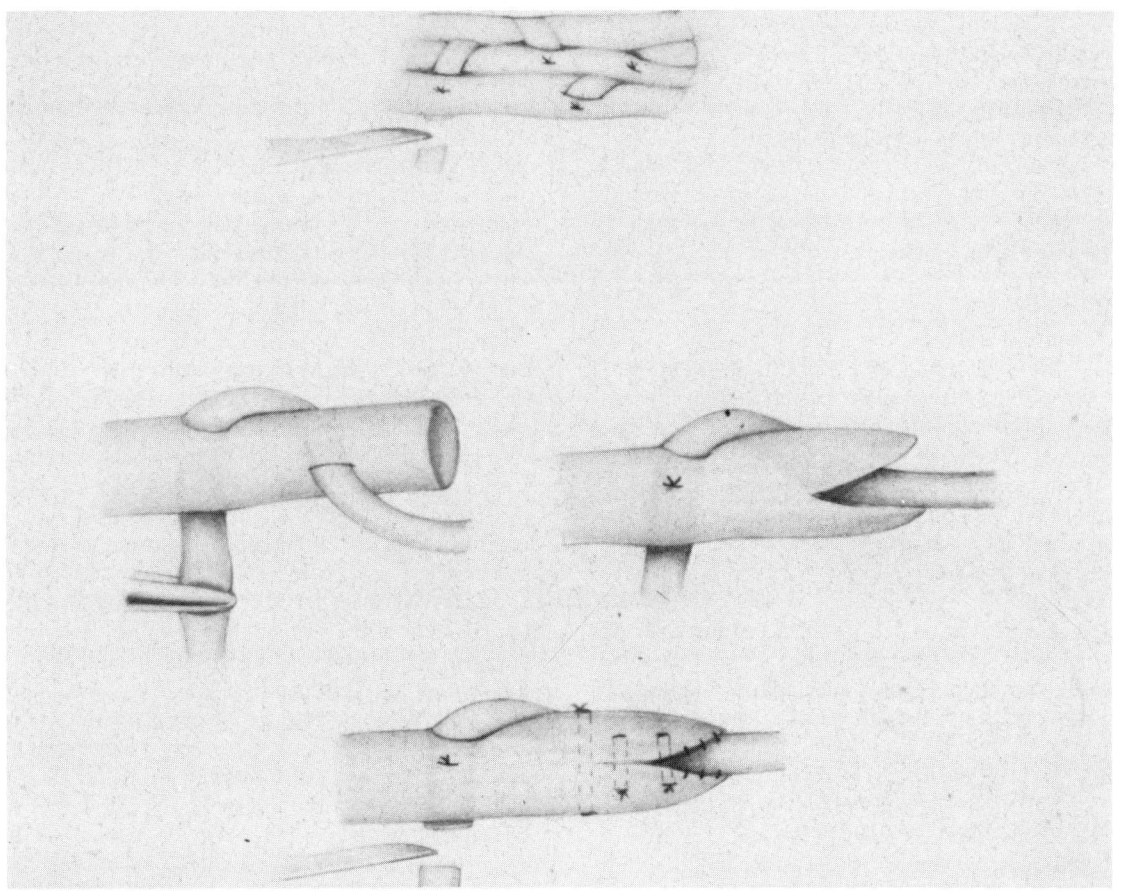

Fig. 34-25   Pulvertaft type of weave of motor tendon graft juncture. Care must be taken to assure passage of the sutures through the donor and recipient tendons to avoid complication of the proximal anastomosis rupture.

attributable to faulty operative technique. One must be sure that the tendon is drawn into the bone at the distal juncture. If there is a good tendon-bone interface, rupture at this area is highly unlikely once healing has occurred. Rupture early at the proximal juncture may result from faulty weaving and suturing of the tendon graft when one is performing the Pulvertaft juncture.[17,18] *Late tendon rupture* is unusual but may occur if extreme force is applied. Immediate exploration is indicated, for it is often possible to reattach the graft, particularly in instances where the patient had a good gliding situation before rupture.

Superficialis finger (Redemption Operation-Osborne)

An alternative technique for the severe salvage situation is a *superficialis finger*.[9,15] This useful technique is indicated in contracted fingers with poor nutrition, multiple-finger reconstructions, and fingers with mallet deformities or poor DIP joint function. By eliminating DIP motion (tenodesis or arthrodesis) the surgery-therapy team can concentrate on MP and PIP motion only. This arc of motion represents approximately 85% of motion of a normal finger.

At stage I the implant is carried to the base of the middle phalanx and fixed in place by suture passed through two small drill holes. Reinforcing sutures are added. The suture is tied directly over the middle phalanx dorsally through a small doral counter incision. This prevents the complications of a dorsal button directly over the skin. The distal phalanx undergoes either tenodesis or arthrodesis to a fixed angle of flexion (see Fig. 34-23). At stage II, reconstruction for the superficialis finger follows the same procedure as described for tendon grafting to the distal phalanx. If the range of motion at the MP and PIP joints is good, the superficialis finger is a very acceptable salvage technique.

A possible complication after stage II tendon grafting is pulley rupture, distal or proximal to the PIP joint, resulting in a bowed finger. A useful result may be salvaged by creating a Superficialis Finger.

Postoperative therapy

Passive tendon implant

Stage I. A 48- to 72-hour course of antibiotic prophylaxis is initiated in the operating room before wound closure. During the first 3 weeks the patient's hand is kept in a protective dorsal splint. Attention to the postoperative dressing is important to permit appropriate early hand therapy. We have preferred less bulky hand dressings so that complete passive digital flexion is possible within the dressing. The protective dorsal splint is applied to extend 2 cm beyond the fingertips with the wrist flexed to 30 degrees, the MP joints flexed to 60 to 70 degrees, and the IP joints in full extension. It is essential that the splint allow full active extension of the IP joints. Light, protected function initiated in the first week consists of gentle passive flexion and light finger trapping, 10 repetitions of each exercise four times a day (Fig. 34-26, *A* and *B*).

If a PIP or DIP joint flexion contracture existed before state I surgery, it is likely to recur postoperatively. If contractures begin to recur, they should be treated immediately with IP joint passive extension splints worn within the dorsal splint and gentle manual passive extension of the contracted joints.

The postoperative splint is removed after 3 weeks, and programmed activity is begun with finger trapping (Fig. 34-26, *C*). Whirlpool baths facilitate motion. Lanolin massage alleviates dryness and softens the tissues. A Velcro trapper is added to the finger exercise (Fig. 34-26, *D* and *E*). Strapping the involved finger to the adjacent normal finger incorporates the involved finger into useful function. At 6 weeks, with the use of the trapper, some patients may be able to return to their employment during the period before stage II tendon grafting.

The goals of hand therapy for the period between stage I and stage II operations are to obtain good mobility of the joints, passive flexion of the digit to the distal palmar crease (or motion equal to that obtained at stage I surgery), correction of flexion contractures, and a viable gliding system. The hand should be in its best possible condition before stage II surgery (Fig. 34-26, *F*).

Stage II. Postoperatively, the patient's hand is kept in a protective dorsal splint: the wrist in 30 degrees of flexion, the MP joints at 70 degrees, and the IP joints in full extension. The therapist must be certain that the patient can *fully extend* the IP joints. The dressings are essentially the same as those used postoperatively in the stage I operation. If the dressings do not permit full passive digital flexion, some of the dressing may have to be removed. When the dressing is removed, the splint may not fit as securely. Additional adhesive tape or Coban should be applied across the forearm, wrist, and palm to ensure that the patient's hand will not slip proximally within the splint, putting tension on the newly sutured junctures.

The concept of early mobilization in primary tendon repair has improved tendon gliding and should be applied to patients undergoing staged tendon grafting. One advantage of elastic band traction is facilitation of tendon and joint movement without requiring active pull on the flexor tendon. Another advantage is that the resting position in passive flexion protects against sudden injury. If the patient jerks the hand during sleep or if he falls, the elastic band protects the juncture from the stress of active flexion.

Although a monofilament suture is placed through the distal fingernail at surgery, we prefer to wait until the patient goes to therapy the first postoperative day before fitting for the elastic band so that the quality, positioning, and tension of the band can be accurately established. The elastic band should be placed approximately 3 inches proximal to the wrist crease on the volar aspect of the forearm dressing with the finger in its normal alignment. The tension of the rubber band is important. It should be adjusted so that the elastic band pulls the finger into flexion at rest and yet permits the antagonist muscles to actively fully extend the finger within the limits of the splint so that flexion contractures do not develop. The patient is instructed to actively extend the finger, then to reciprocally relax as the elastic band flexes the finger. This is repeated 10 times every hour (Fig. 34-26, *G*). We have found that the commercially available graded rubber bands are never quite right. If the elastic band holds the finger in the appropriate flexion at rest, it often does not allow the patient to actively extend his finger fully against the tension of the elastic band. Failure to completely extend the PIP and DIP joints will result in flexion contractures. The elastic that best suits our purpose is elastic thread. It may be used as a single strand, and as the patient becomes stronger the strands may be doubled, increasing the tension.

In addition, gentle passive flexion of each IP joint is carried out, 10 repetitions several times a day. Manual passive flexion of the joints must be done carefully. Previous operations and too much passive cranking may cause attenuation of the extensor tendon; thus as we strive to get passive DIP joint flexion, we also emphasize active DIP joint extension.

Particular attention should be paid to contracture control of the DIP and PIP joints. Salvage fingers may have poor extensor tendon function because of tendon attenuation or adhesions from previous surgeries. These fingers are especially prone to recurrent contractures. Early attention to beginning flexion contractures is of primary importance. Patients who have difficulty with contractures before stage I and stage II surgeries are likely to develop these recurrent contractures. If the dorsal splint does not allow full extension of the PIP joint, the patient must be instructed to passively flex the MP joint of the involved finger into more flexion, thereby facilitating active extension of the IP joints. The therapist can also place a piece of felt behind the proximal phalanx so that when the patient actively extends the involved digit, the MP joint is held in strong flexion at that point so that the patient can fully extend the IP joints.

When the surgeon and the therapist are alerted to the development of PIP or DIP flexion contractures, passive extension of the IP joints may be initiated as early as the first week. No tendon tension passive extension may be initiated. Tension is taken off the tendon juncture by flexion of the adjacent joint; that is, with the dorsal splint supporting the wrist, the MP joint is held in flexion, while the PIP joint is gently extended with the pressure of extension at the middle phalanx. If the DIP joint shows a beginning contracture, the therapist may support the MP and PIP joints in flexion and gently extend the DIP joint (Fig. 34-26, *H*). Passive extension effected by this technique decreases the tension at the tendon juncture. These passive extension ex-

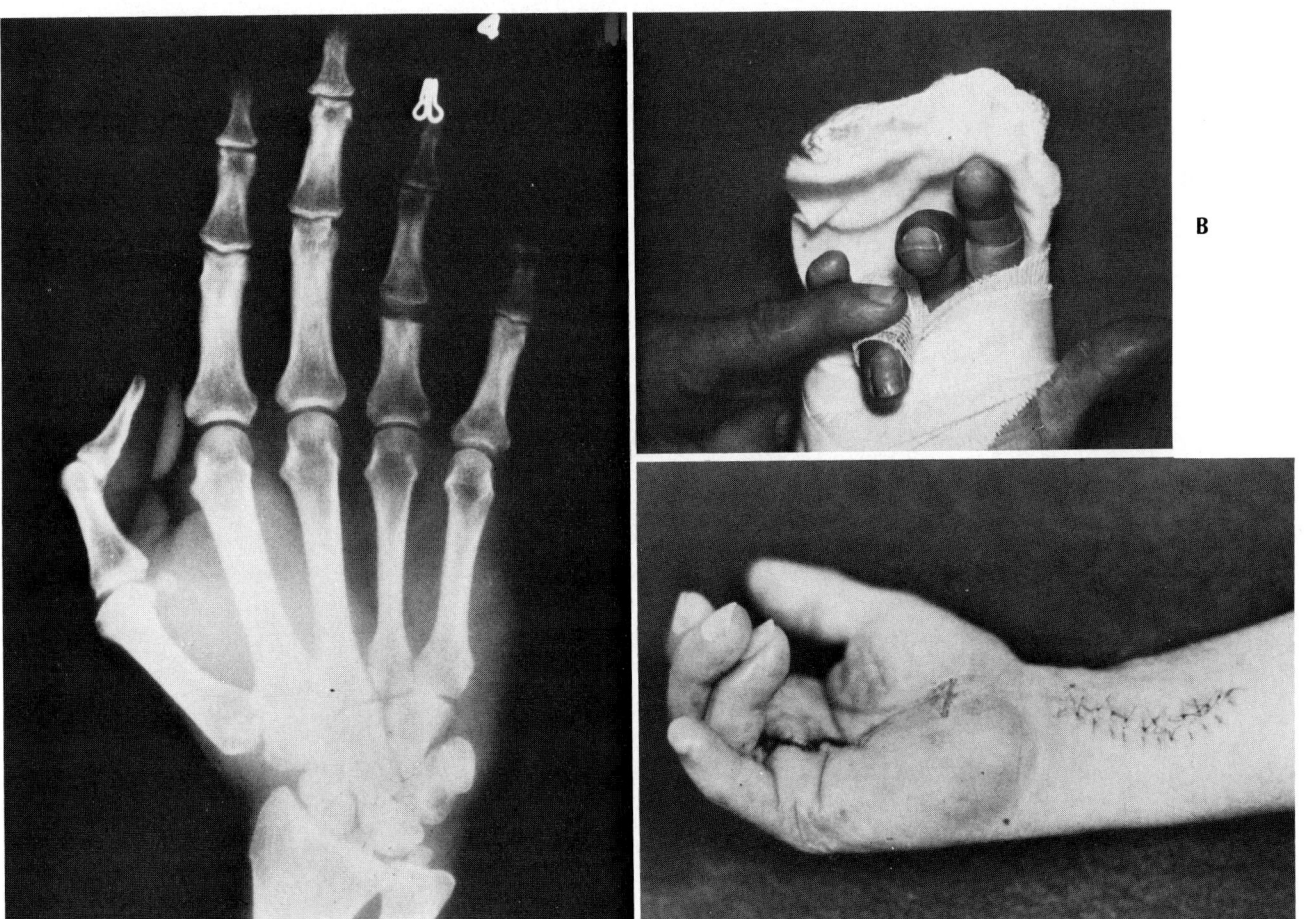

Fig. 34-26   A, Microsurgical replantation of the ring finger with insertion of a Swanson Silastic implant in the proximal interphalangeal joint. The patient, a 49-year-old right-handed welder, had sustained a band saw amputation of the left ring finger at the proximal interphalangeal joint, with partial amputation of the small finger at the distal interphalangeal joint. The patient suffered a myocardial infarction 3 days after discharge from the hospital; there was no previous cardiac history or any indication of cardiac distress while in the hospital. As a result, therapy was not initiated until 7 weeks after replantation. By then the wound had healed; however, the delay in beginning therapy resulted in an adhered flexor tendon system in the ring finger, limiting active flexion. Thus the patient became a candidate for staged tendon reconstruction. **B** to **L** further illustrate this patient's case. **B,** Gentle passive motion was initiated the first week after stage I surgery. **C,** Finger trapping.

Continued.

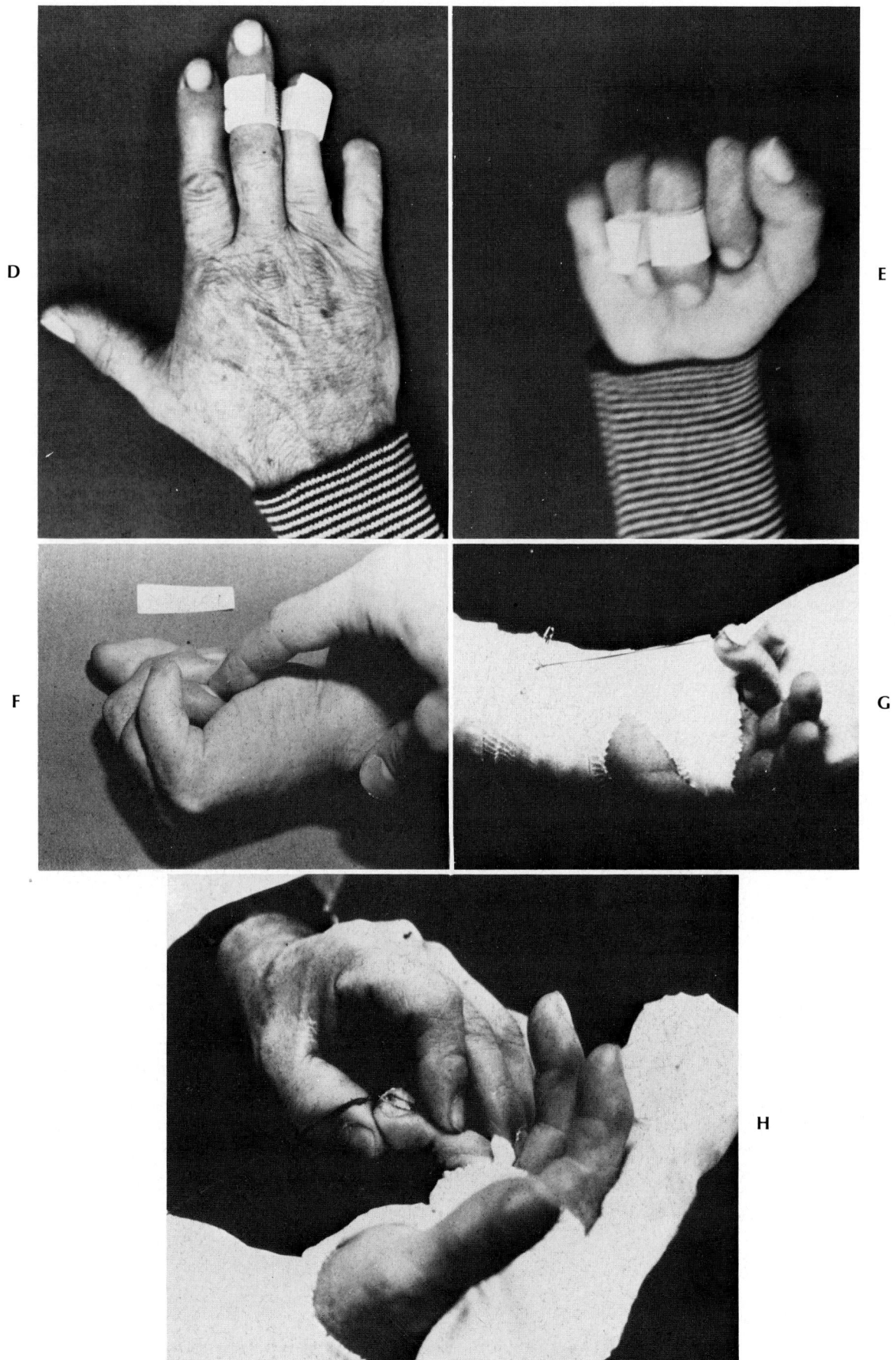

Fig. 34-26, cont'd For legend see opposite page.

ercises should be included in the patient's home program.

Persistent flexion contractures may require a proximal joint wedge or a PIP joint passive extension splint. An AlumaFoam* splint that positions the MP joint in greater flexion and gently pulls the contracted IP joint into extension with a Velcro strap is custom fitted within the dorsal splint. This contracture-control splint should be worn intermittently during the day. The exact schedule depends upon the feel of the contracture, that is, whether it will quickly or slowly respond to stretching. With this technique of passive stretching we have found that problems with flexion contractures can be minimized and overall tendon function enhanced.

Full excursion of the tendon graft occurring within the first 3 to 4 postoperative weeks indicates minimal adhesion

---

*Conco Medical Co., Bridgeport, Conn.

---

formation. In such a case the tendon junctures are at greater risk of rupture if stressed. We have found this to be especially true when active tendon implants have been inserted, in which the flexor system is already geared up for active motion after stage I surgery. Those patients who move exceptionally well (70% of the final goal) during the first 3 weeks are protected longer than 4 weeks to minimize the chance of rupture. Results have steadily improved over the past decade so that 90% of the passive range of motion recorded at stage II should be achieved in the final result. The button is removed at 5 to 6 weeks.

When the dorsal splint is removed, usually at 4 weeks, the patient's hand is maintained in a wristlet with elastic band traction attached to the fingernail suture. The wristlet permits full active extension of the IP and MP joints with the wrist in a neutral position. The elastic band pulls the

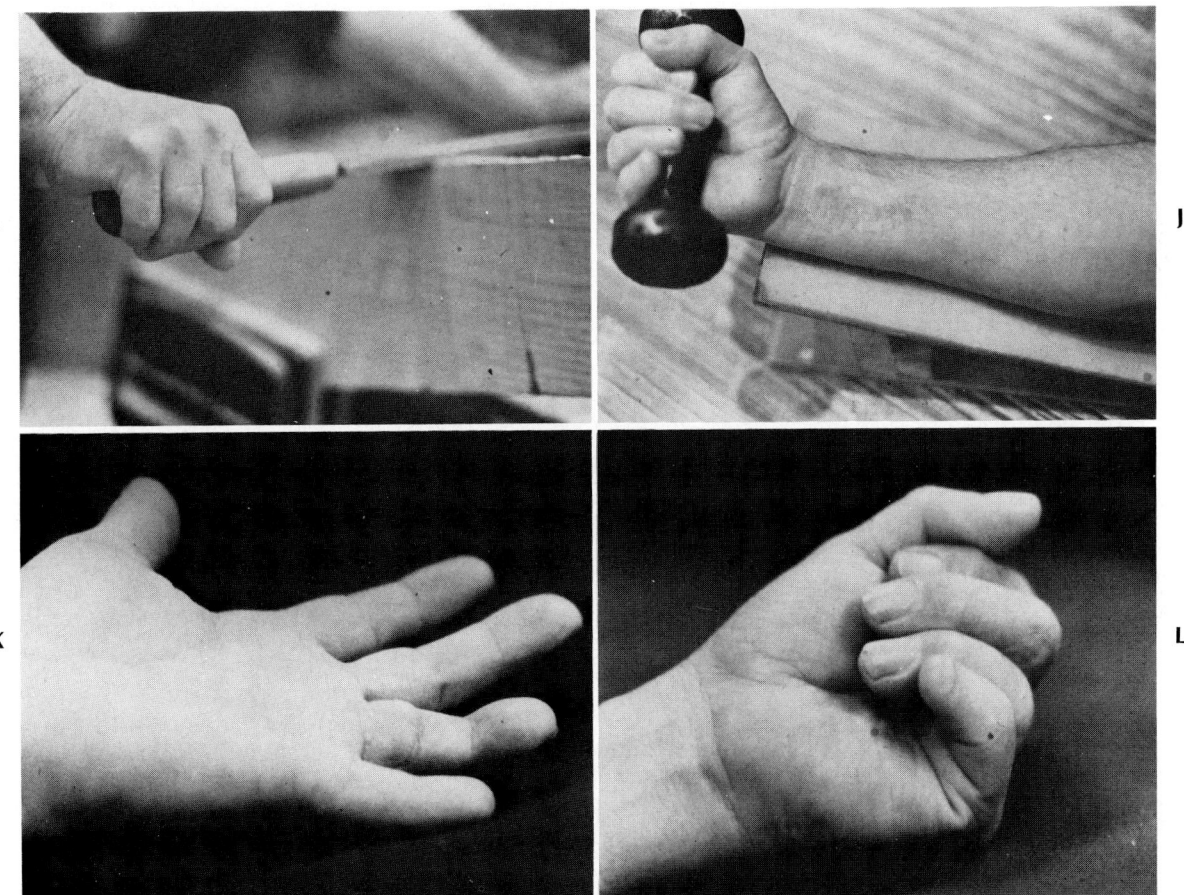

Fig. 34-26, cont'd Strapping the involved finger to the adjacent normal finger incorporates the involved finger into useful function. **D,** Extension. **E,** Flexion. **F,** Condition of the patient's finger improved: finger was supple with good skincondition, active potential of 1.5 cm was achieved (1.5 cm at stage I surgery), Tinel's sign was present at the fingertip, and x-ray film revealed good excursion of the tendon implant. **G,** Dynamic splinting was initiated the first day after stage II surgery. active extension and passive flexion were performed with elastic band attached to the fingernail. **H,** Gentle passive extension of the distal interphalangeal joint. Metacarpophalangeal and proximal interphalangeal joint flexion decreases tension at the tendon juncture. **I,** Tendon and joint reconstruction enables the patient to use his ring finger as a stabilizer when using a tool in a sustained grip activity. **J,** Grip strengthening at 3 months. **K,** Extension, and **L,** flexion at 12 weeks after surgery. Considering the severe nature of this patient's amputation injury, the subsequent tissue ischemia, the unique problems of establishing adequate circulation to the replanted part, the development of a new functionally adapted fibrous capsule for the Swanson Silastic implant and tendon gliding after the two-stage tendon reconstruction using a Hunter passive tendon implant, and the myocardial infarction, this patient had come a long way.

fingers back into flexion at rest. Wrist dorsiflexion may be done with the fingers resting in flexion. Contracture control is continued.

At 6 to 10 weeks, the wristlet is removed and the patient begins active flexion exercises. The initiation of active flexion depends on the restoration of active motion. When adhesions seem to be restricting motion, we begin active flexion earlier and have held the patient back when active flexion is excellent. Finger blocking, tendon gliding exercises, and the use of putty may be initiated at this time. Whirlpool therapy may be started again. Fingers that have been stiff before stage I surgery may require softening with lanolin massage.

At 10 weeks the patient may begin light supervised woodworking (sanding, filing) (Fig. 34-26, *I*). Progressive weight resistance exercises and heavy resistance exercises are not permitted until 3 months after surgery (Fig. 34-26, *J, K,* and *L*).

Early active motion. If at surgery the surgeon judges the tendon bed to be in excellent condition and the graft junctures to be strong, then active flexion may be initiated without the use of an elastic band, even as early as the first postoperative week. We begin with a passive hold exercise within the dorsal splint. The splinting guidelines for this method of early motion are essentially the same as those discussed for early motion using elastic band traction. A protective dorsal splint holds the wrist in 30 degrees of flexion during the exercise.

The passive hold exercise is performed in the following manner. The forearm muscles of the involved extremity must be relaxed. The patient gently presses the fingers into flexion with the uninvolved hand, releases the uninvolved hand, and tries to hold the fingers in flexion with his own muscle power. It takes less force to maintain a flexed finger in flexion than to actively pull the finger into flexion from an extended position, whereas the benefits of tendon excursion is the same as in active flexion. We ask the patient to carry out this exercise in full flexion and at two levels of partial flexion. Three repetitions at each level are performed three to four times a day. In addition, gentle passive flexion of the IP joints is performed several times a day within the

dorsal splint. If the patient begins to glide the tendon very early and excellent tendon pull-through is demonstrated, we slow him down at 2 weeks by applying elastic band traction. The patient can still do the passive hold exercise; however, the elastic band traction program adds protection.

The 6- to 12-week postoperative program is essentially the same as that described earlier. Careful attention is also given to the prevention of flexion contractures.

Special considerations

Moleskin sling. When a nylon suture cannot be attached to the tip of the fingernail at surgery (for example, because of absence of the fingernail), a sling of moleskin may be used to provide elastic band traction around the button and pullout wire. The sling is applied laterally on the finger from the PIP joint to the fingertip. A segment of moleskin about 3 inches long and ½ inch wide is folded in half, and an eyelet is punched through at the folded end. An S hook, made from a paper clip, is hooked through the eyelet opening, and an elastic band is attached from it to a safety pin on the volar surface of the forearm dressing or to a wrist cuff. Tincture of benzoin applied to the finger helps the moleskin adhere (Fig. 34-27, *A* and *B*).

ACTIVE TENDON IMPLANT
Stage I surgery

Active tendon implants follow the same general guidelines for insertion as described earlier for passive tendon implants using the same incisions. The motor tendon unit in the forearm is exposed and tested for excursion. The profundus of the injured digit or digits is the preferred choice, but if excursion is insufficient, another available motor tendon unit is chosen. A superficialis motor unit can be chosen if necessary but its excursion potential is less than that of an intact profundus. However, superficialis muscle power may be used to advantage to motor the finger when the surgeon elects to use only the PIP joint while performing an arthrodesis on the distal joint—the Superficialis Finger (Fig. 34-28, *A to I*). The length of the implant is estimated by measuring the distance from the distal phalanx or middle phalanx to the motor tendon unit in the forearm.

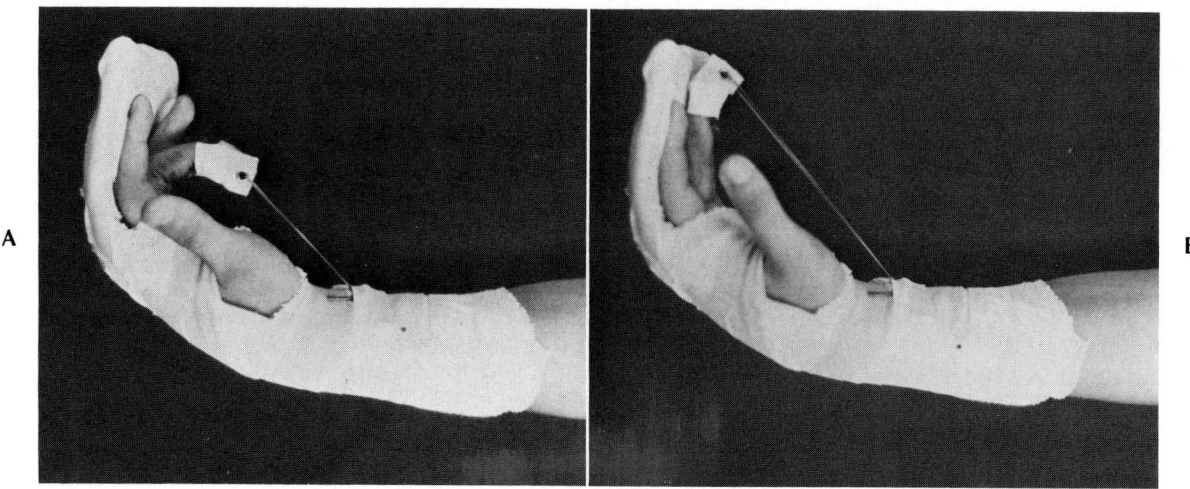

Fig. 34-27 Moleskin sling may be used to provide elastic-band traction. **A,** Passive flexion. **B,** Active extension.

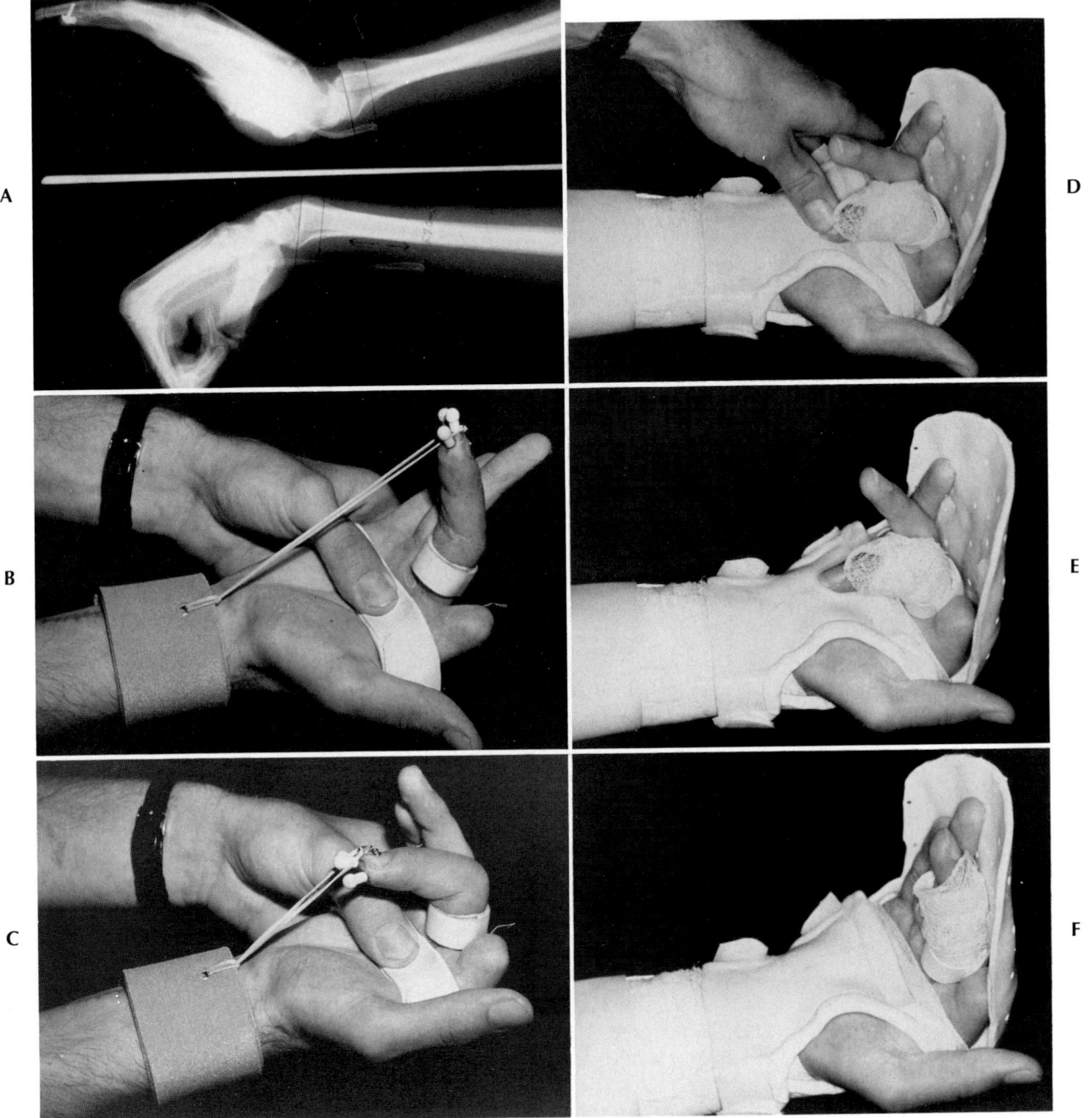

Fig. 34-28   **A,** Superficialis Finger. The patient, a 23-year-old right-dominant surveyor, incurred a severe injury to his right hand with a log splitter. The index finger was shattered and unsalvageable. The long finger was amputated and replanted. Vascularity was reestablished to the long finger, but the tendons were badly damaged and not repaired primarily. Subsequently the patient underwent a tendon graft procedure 8 months after injury. A swan-neck deformity developed, and the patient underwent a secondary revision 8 months later. Approximately 2 years after injury the patient was seen at the Hand Rehabilitation center. He had good neurovascular function in the finger, but lacked active flexion. He had maintained good passive range of motion, which made the finger salvageable for flexor reconstruction. It was felt that the patient could benefit from tendon reconstruction using the active tendon implant and "superficialis finger" reconstruction. The flexor tendon graft was excised. A volar plate advancement tenodesis was performed to prevent hyperextension of the proximal interphalangeal joint. The distal interphalangeal joint was arthrodesed. The active tendon implant was inserted and the A2 and A1 pulleys were reconstructed. A dorsal protective splint was applied at surgery. Elastic-band traction was added in therapy on the first postoperative day. **B,** and **C,** Wristlet and elastic-band traction were applied 6 weeks postoperatively. Reconstructed A1 and A2 pulleys are protected with pulley rings. Direct digital pressure from the uninvolved hand adds additional support to the reconstructed A1 pulley during the early training program. **D, E,** and **F,** Stage II: "passive hold" exercise (described in text).

Continued.

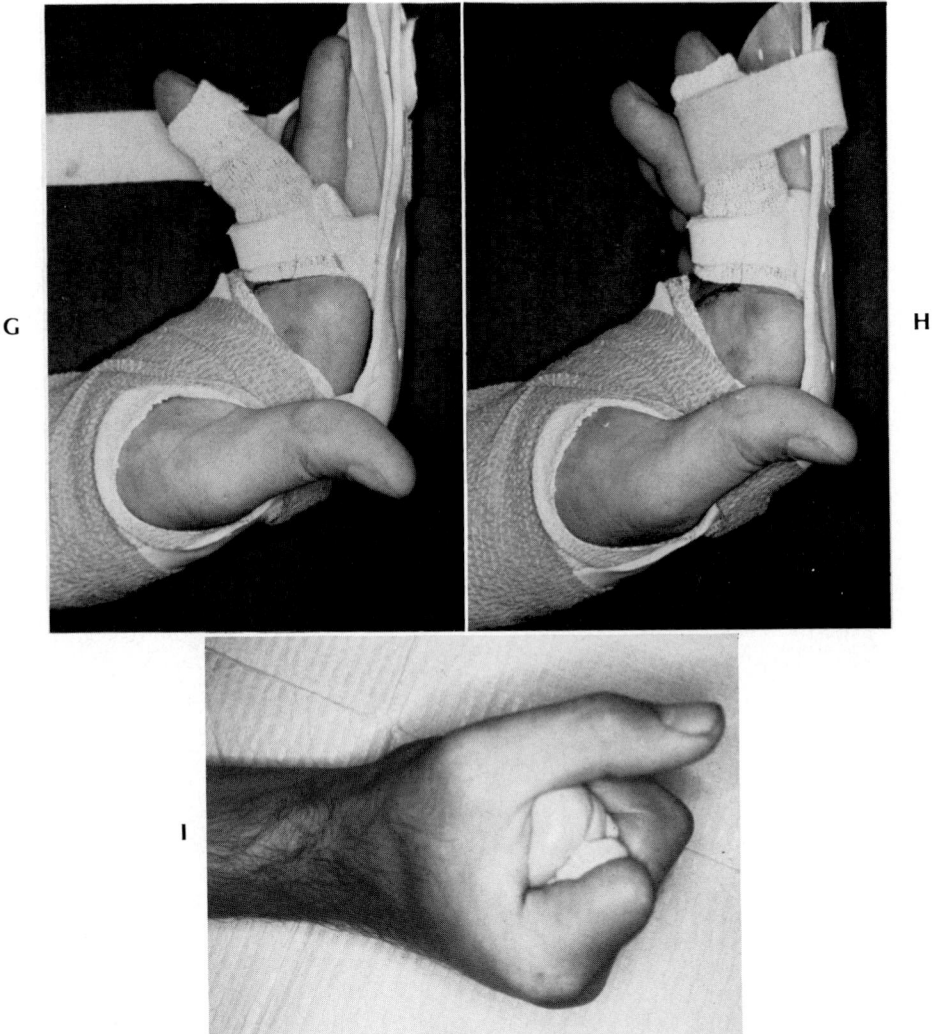

Fig. 34-28 cont'd   **G** and **H,** Passive extension of proximal interphalangeal joint. Felt wedge places the proximal phalanx in more flexion. With the felt wedge in place, the Velcro strap gently pulls the proximal interphalangeal joint into −20° extension. Volar plate reconstruction prohibits further proximal interphalangeal extension at this time in the therapy program. **I,** Resistive exercises were initiated 12 weeks after surgery.

The stainless steel distal component is passed from the palm through the pulleys in the finger using a no-touch technique. Moistening the device with Ringer solution will facilitate this process. The distal component should pass through the normal A_1 and A_2 retinacula with gentle manipulation. Thread a generous length of wet umbilical tape or heavy nonabsorbable, nonmetallic suture through the distal component screw hole. Grasping both ends of the tape or suture, use it to guide the distal component through the A_3 and A_4 pulley. In some cases the normal A_4 retinaculum is not of sufficient diameter to permit passage of the distal component. Consequently, the A_4 retinaculum should be opened for implant placement. Cut the A_4 retinaculum along the periosteal rim on the middle phalanx. Repair exactly and secure the A_4 pulley with multiple Dacron sutures using small drill holes if necessary. The tendon with free porous Dacron cords at the proximal end is passed through the pulley system distal to proximal with ease.

If good retinaculum cannot be salvaged, free tendon graft material is preferred; use either a portion of an excised flexor tendon or the palmaris longus. The preferred technique, as discussed earlier, is to pass the tendon graft around the bone extraperiosteally under the extensor apparatus proximal to the PIP joint while over the extensor apparatus distal to the PIP joint. It is wrapped twice around the phalanx and sutured to itself or to the rim of the fibroosseous canal. To pass the loop to the proximal wrist, manually compress the proximal loop and pass it from palm to forearm through the carpal canal. If necessary, use a tendon passer having a diameter slightly larger than that of the device to carry the implant into the carpal canal. Again, the use of wet umbilical tape looped through the implant proximal loop and carried into the forearm on a tendon passer will facilitate passage of the implant.

Distal fixation. The distal component must be secured to bone in a way that will achieve a strong, durable, immediate juncture. A 27-gauge needle is passed through the lateral space of the distal IP joint and out of the dorsum (see Fig. 34-6, *A*). With the joint identified, the base of the distal phalanx is stripped of volar periosteum. The needle point is used as a reference point in the following steps:

1. Bearing in mind that the ideal position of the distal component is with its proximal edge 2 and 3 mm distal to the joint, with the joint identified, visualize or measure to determine the point where the screw should enter bone. The 2 mm A-O screw system may be used, or take an 0.035 K-wire and, placing one end on the determined point, hold it parallel to the needle. Then tilt the uppermost tip of the K-wire distally approximately 15 degrees.
2. Pass the K-wire externally. Turn the finger for a lateral view. The K-wire should have missed the joint and the base of the nail and be in cortical bone. Wire location should be central.
3. The recommended bone screw is the 2 mm Woodruff or Synthes A-O. Holding the joint securely, carefully remove the K-wire. Secure the distal end of the device by carefully turning the screw into the screw hole made by the K-wire. The screw should appear dorsally. A minimum amount (less than 1 mm) is acceptable, but if in excess of 1 mm, make a small dorsal transverse incision

and trim excess screw. The screw fit should feel firm all the way and final fixation should be secure. If the final screw turns are loose the system may not stand cyclic force. Redo the fitting more distally in bone or go to the alternate technique and twist wire the end piece to bone.

4. The profundus tendon stump may be drawn over the distal component and sutured laterally to provide a soft tissue buffer preventing irritation of the overlying skin.
5. A strip of superficialis tendon may be drawn over the distal component and sutured laterally at the middle phalanx level in the superficialis finger procedure.
6. Release the tourniquet, review all wounds, wash out, and close the distal incision.

The distal component is designed to permit fixation by two *twisted wires through bone,* as well as by screw. If the bone has been fractured or shows osteoporosis, wiring is preferred. Also, if during preparation for screw insertion the bone is deformed, wire fixation by two drill holes is preferred. The distal component *must* be pulled securely to bone to prevent movement and wire fracture.

Proximal juncture: loop method. The length of the motor tendon must be sufficient to pass through the proximal loop and return proximal for at least two 90-degree passes through the tendon. Desired excursion of the motor tendon is 4 cm for the FDP and 3 cm for the FDS. If the patient can be aroused from anesthesia during this last phase of tendon surgery, an accurate assessment of the muscle amplitude is possible. Otherwise, the traditional techniques of flexing the wrist to secure a cascade of balance in the fingers is effective. We generally prefer that the operated finger is slightly more flexed than the adjacent fingers.

The selected tendon is passed through the implant loop and then through a small longitudinal split in the tendon. One suture is placed through the tendon and the tension is tested. Tension is tested by moistening the implant surface, followed by flexion and extension of the wrist. The finger should lay in extension during wrist flexion and show a position of balance with the adjacent fingers on wrist extension. If balance is acceptable, place a second suture and turn the tendon 90 degrees through one or two additional longitudinal splits in the tendon. Retest tendon balance and be sure there has been no loss of tendon tension.

Proximal juncture: porous Dacron weave method. The Dacron within the tendon implant is a woven tubular twill especially prepared with porosity for ingrowth to perform in connective tissue such as tendon or ligament. This technique will be useful when very short or very long tendon defects are encountered. With care the silicone rubber can be peeled away from the Dacron and the silicone part of the tendon can therefore be shortened. Using magnification, care is taken not to damage the Dacron weave during this technique.

The Dacron is woven into the lateral borders of the tendon and fixed with nonabsorbable sutures at points of exit. After three or four passes, the Dacron can be tied securely with a square knot, reinforced with 3-0 dacron sutures and the ends cut with electric cautery. Use taper-cut needles only during all reenforcement procedures. Cutting needles will seriously damage the delicate Dacron weave. In the event of a proximal juncture failure if there is full passive gliding on x-ray film reexamination, stage II surgery can be delayed, providing no signs of synovitis are noted.

Stage II surgery

The interval between stage I and stage II can be quite variable when the functioning active tendon implant is used. The active tendon implant should be retained past 4 months so the patient can derive the full benefit of the implant, especially the maturing of the proximal juncture and the biologic softening of connective tissues. Patients who have returned to work and a normal life-style can benefit beyond 1 year before stage II tendon grafting.

At operation the limits of extension and flexion of the finger are measured and recorded. A short Brunner zigzag incision is made to locate the distal end of the device where it is attached to the phalanx. This attachment is left intact and a secondary ulnarly curved volar incision is made through the previous stage I incision in the forearm so as to expose the proximal end of the device.

Either the plantaris tendon from the forearm or a long toe extensor tendon is obtained from the leg for use as the tendon graft. The palmaris longus tendon or segments of a superficialis tendon will suffice for short tendon grafts, for example, thumb, fifth finger, and superficialis finger reconstruction. The proximal end of the device is extricated from the motor tendon by cutting the Dacron and silicone loop. When the device and tendon have been sufficiently separated, trim proximal end of the device to a straight edge. One end of the tendon graft is sutured to the proximal end of the device with a suture. Leaving the distal end of the device attached to the distal phalanx, the rest of the device with the attached tendon graft is pulled distally through the new sheath. The device is then detached distally, removed, and discarded. The stage II procedure is completed by following established techniques for tendon grafting with one important exception—the connective tissue around the proximal juncture should be carefully preserved and closed around the new tendon graft juncture with fine sutures.

Postoperative therapy

Stage I. Stage I reconstruction requires careful structured postoperative care to facilitate orderly pseudosheath development around the tendon implant and prepare the patient's hand for return to work (Fig. 34-28, *A* to *I*). Therapy begins the first postoperative day and is the same as for a tendon graft, that is, stage II without rubber band, although slightly more rigorous. It begins with the passive hold exercise described earlier. Hand dressings must permit full passive flexion of the digits into the palm. At 2 weeks when the patient demonstrates good tendon gliding, elastic band traction is added. The passive hold exercise is continued, however; the elastic band adds protection.

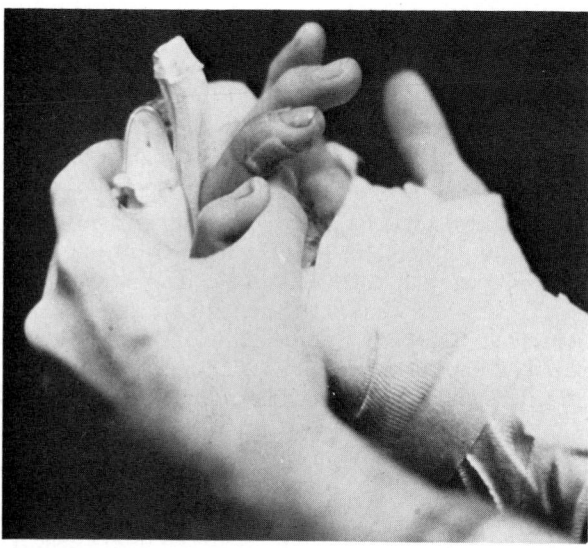

Fig. 34-29   Pulley supported with finger during active flexion.

Pulley reconstruction at stage I surgery using a passive tendon implant attached only distally does not require protection since the patient will be performing passive motion. Reconstructed pulleys in the presence of an active tendon implant must be protected with a pulley ring. Protection during the early postoperative days may be with a Velcro-and-felt pulley ring or support with pressure from a finger of the opposite hand (Fig. 34-29). When postoperative edema decreases, the soft pulley ring can be replaced with a thermoplastic pulley ring and eventually a metal ring in some cases. Pulley reconstruction is as sensitive as tendon repair and should be protected for 6 months (Fig. 34-30, *A* to *F*).

If the patient does not have full active IP joint extension, a contracture control program discussed earlier must be initiated during the first week. The IP joint passive extension splint is fitted within the dorsal splint. As the contracted joint is pulled gently into extension, a counterforce is applied over the reconstructed pulley to prevent attenuation of the pulley.

Squeezing a piece of foam is allowed after 3 weeks and light putty squeezing after 4 weeks, 10 repetitions several times a day. The passive hold exercise is continued. Overzealous use of the digit soon after surgery is to be avoided, as this may result in a synovitis that generally responds to rest and splinting.

Fig. 34-30   **A,** Metallic implant arthroplasty for degenerative arthritis performed on a 54-year-old right-dominant man. Approximately 4 years after surgery he lost motion, and pain developed in the digit. Evaluation at the Hand Rehabilitation Center disclosed that the implant had fractured and perforated the proximal phalanx volarly, with rupture of the flexor digitorum profundus and flexor digitorum superficialis tendons of the long finger. Stage I surgery involved insertion of a Swanson joint implant and a Hunter active-tendon implant. **B,** Stainless steel distal metal end plate is attached to the distal phalanx by screw fixation. The profundus stump is drawn over the distal component and sutured laterally to provide a soft tissue buffer, preventing irritation of the overlying skin. **C,** Preformed silicone-coated Dacron loop for motor tendon unit juncture. **D,** Postoperative dorsal protective splint and elastic-band traction. Velcro and felt pulley ring protects the reconstructed pulley. Active extension/passive flexion. **E,** When postoperative edema decreases, Velcro and felt pulley ring is replaced with a thermoplastic pulley ring. **F,** Metal ring pulley support. Reconstructed pulleys are protected for 6 months. **G,** Stage II, 6 weeks after surgery. Early pain-free tendon gliding may require that protective splinting be extended beyond the 6-week period.

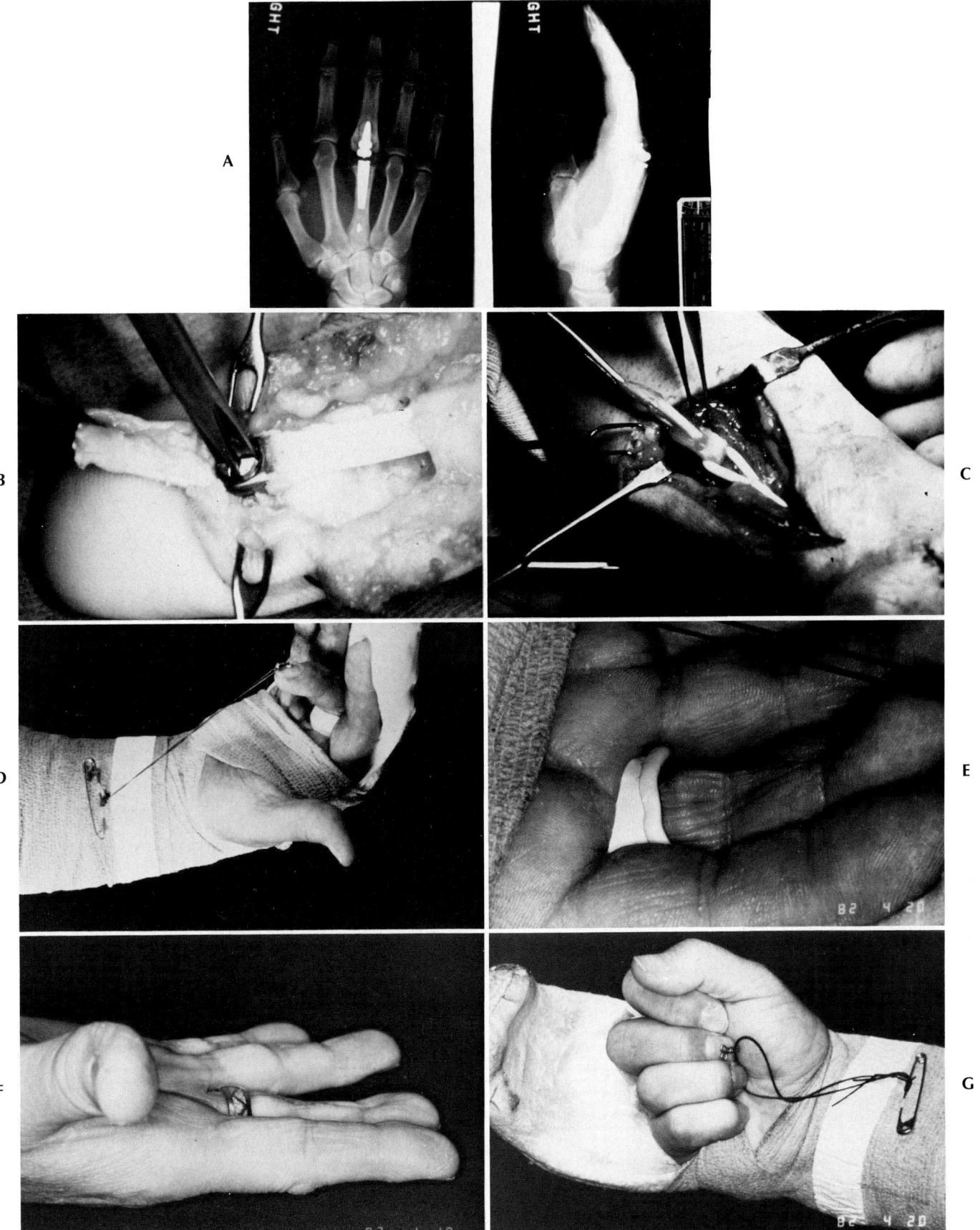

Fig. 34-30   For legend see opposite page.

At 6 weeks the protective dorsal splint may be removed and a wristlet and elastic band traction applied permitting wrist extension to neutral and full extension of the MP and IP joints. An active patient may necessitate the use of the dorsal splint for more than 6 weeks, with freedom from the splint for exercising under supervision.

Usually by 8 weeks patients are permitted full activities with restrictions on full power grip until 12 weeks after surgery.

The immature mesothelial sheath is formed around the tendon implant by 4 weeks and becomes mature by 4 months. Four to 6 months between stage I and stage II are required to facilitate hand reconditioning. When tendon and joint function is satisfactory, stage II is often delayed for up to 2 years or longer. As time passes with the tendon implant in the digit, the motor unit becomes stronger, range of motion is maximized, and soft tissue becomes more pliable. The digit is better prepared for stage II.

Stage II. Stage II surgery consists of removal of the active tendon implant, insertion of a tendon graft through the new psuedosheath, followed by postoperative therapy to facilitate gliding of the tendon graft and achieve maximum digital motion.

Postoperatively the patient's hand is kept in a protective dorsal splint: the wrist in 30 degrees of flexion, the MP joints at 70 degrees and the IP joints in full extension. Early mobilization with elastic band traction begins the first postoperative day. The patient actively extends the finger, then reciprocally relaxes, permitting the elastic band to flex the finger. This is repeated 10 repetitions hourly. Gentle passive motion is carried out 10 repetitions several times a day with care being given to extensor tendon attenuation. Attention is given to contracture control. Postoperative therapy is similar to the stage I period. However, because very early pain free gliding generally occurs, protective splinting may be extended beyond the usual 6-week period, if necessary to protect against excessive force on the tendon junctures. (Fig. 34-30, *G*). Initiation of the wristlet at 6 weeks may be extended to 8 weeks and active exercise at 8 weeks to 10. Timetables should always be adjusted to the patient's progress.

SUMMARY

The two-stage tendon graft technique using the Hunter *passive tendon* implant has been clinically proved to be a consistently reliable technique of salvaging scarred tendon systems.[8,13] The production of a pseudosheath provides the fluid nutrition system for nourishment of the subsequent tendon graft. This fluid nutrition system, combined with early protected gliding of the graft, has resulted in a significant reduction of postoperative adhesions. The release of contractures and the reconstruction of pulleys of the proper size, location, and quantity, combined with a supervised therapy program, result in maximal postoperative digital motion.

The Hunter passive tendon remains a valuable tool in the armamentarium of hand surgery and can be used in all two-stage reconstruction. However, we now see the advantages of having a predictable active tendon implant that will have its most productive result in the working man, allowing him to return to work and use his hand for extended periods of time while building a new sheath. The passive tendon implant will also build a synovial sheath throughout the finger, palm, and forearm; however, the active tendon implant adds the interface between the muscle tendon in the forearm so that while the new sheath is forming, the proximal juncture also matures. Our clinical experience has been that at stage II surgery, which could be a year or 2 later, we have a better finger because the entire system is biologically functioning. We have a better hand, a softer finger, and improved general nutrition and also have overcome the problem of patient morale and motivation. He has had a functional tendon working.

The active tendon implant is not indicated for children with an open epiphyseal plate. A 3 mm passive tendon implant is often used and sutured to the stump of the profundus.

The active tendon implant program shows sufficient clinical predictability to be considered a viable alternative method when dealing with the problems that follow flexor tendon injury or disease.

REFERENCES

1. Brand P: Principles of free tendon grafting, including a new method of tendon suture, J Bone Joint Surg, 41B:208, 1959.
2. Bunnell S, editor: Hand Surgery in World War II, Washington, DC, 1955, Medical Department of the United States Army, Office of the Surgeon General, Department of the Army.
3. Bunnell S: Bunnell's surgery of the hand, ed 4, Philadelphia, 1964, JB Lippincott Co. (revised by JH Boyes).
4. Erickson JC III, Hunter JM, and Schneider LH: Neuroleptanalgesia and local anesthesia for a dynamic approach to surgery of the hand. Videotape narrative description and scientific exhibit for American Academy of Orthopaedic Surgeons, April 11-14, 1976, Philadelphia, Pa.
5. Hume EL: Flexion tendon reconstruction (Panel discussion #10). In Hunter JM, Schneider LH, and Mackin EJ, editors: Tendon surgery in the hand, St Louis, 1987, The CV Mosby Co.
6. Hunter JM: Artificial tendons: early development and application, Am J Surg 109:325, 1965.
7. Hunter JM: Active tendon prosthesis: techniques and clinical experience. In Hunter JM, Schneider LH, and Mackin, EJ, editors: Tendon surgery in the hand, St Louis, 1984, The CV Mosby Co.
8. Hunter JM and Aulicino PL: Salvage of the scarred tendon systems utilizing the Hunter tendon implant. In Flynn JE, editor: Hand surgery, ed 3, Baltimore, 1981, Williams & Wilkins Co.
9. Hunter JM, Blackmore S, and Callahan AD: New concepts in management for the two stage active tendon implant, J Hand Ther 2(2), 1989.
10. Hunter JM and Jaeger SH: The active gliding tendon prosthesis: progress. In American Academy of Orthopaedic Surgeons: Symposium on tendon surgery in the hand, St Louis, 1975, The CV Mosby Co.
11. Hunter JM and Jaeger SH: Tendon implants: primary and secondary usage, Orthop Clin North Am, 8(2):473, 1977.
12. Hunter JM and Jaeger SH: Flexor tendon implants and prostheses. In Rubin LR, editor: Biomaterials in reconstructive surgery, St Louis, 1983, The CV Mosby Co.
13. Hunter JM and Jaeger SH: Staged tendon grafting using tendon implants. In Tubiana R, editor: The hand, vol 3, Philadelphia, WB Saunders Co (in press).
14. Hunter JM and others: A dynamic approach to problems of hand function: using local anesthesia supplemented by intravenous fentanyl-droperidol, Clin Orthop 104:112, 1974.
15. Hunter JM, Schneider LH, and Fietti VG: Reconstruction of the sublimis finger, Orthop Trans 3:321, 1979.
16. Mackin EJ and Hunger JM: Pre- and post-operative hand therapy program for patients with staged gliding tendon implants (Hunter design), Philadelphia, 1989, Hand Rehabilitation Foundation.
17. Pulvertaft RG: Tendon grafts for flexor tendon injuries in the fingers and thumb: a study of technique and results, J Bone Joint Surg 38B:175, 1956.
18. Pulvertaft RG: Experiences in flexor tendon grafting in the hand, J Bone Joint Surg 41B:629, 1959.

19. Tubiana R: Greffes des tendons flechisseurs des doigts et du pouce: technique et resultats, Rev Chir Orthop 46:191, 1960.
20. Verdan CE: Primary and secondary repair of flexor and extensor tendon injuries. In Flynn JE, editor: Hand surgery, Baltimore, 1966, Williams & Wilkins Co.
21. White WL: Secondary restoration of finger flexion by digital tendon grafts: an evaluation of seventy-six cases, Am J Surg 91:662, 1956.

BIBLIOGRAPHY

Brand P: Principles of free tendon grafting, including a new method of tendon suture, J Bone Joint Surg 41B:208, 1959.
Bruner JM: The zig-zag volar digital incision for flexor tendon surgery, Plast Reconstr Surg 40:571, 1967.
Doyle JR and Blythe W: The finger flexor tendon sheath and pulleys: anatomy and reconstruction. In American Academy of Orthopaedic Surgeons: Symposium on tendon surgery in the hand, St Louis, 1975, The CV Mosby Co.
Hunter JM: Artificial tendons: early development and application, Am J Surg 109:325, 1965.
Hunter JM: Two stage tendon reconstruction using gliding tendon implants. In Rob C and Smith R: Operative surgery, Sevenoaks, Kent, 1978, Butterworth & Co (Pubs), Ltd.
Hunter JM and Jaeger SH: The active gliding tendon prosthesis: progress.

In American Academy of Orthopaedic Surgeons: Symposium on tendon surgery in the hand, St Louis, 1975, The CV Mosby Co.
Hunter JM and Jaeger SH: Tendon implants: primary and secondary usage, Orthop Clin North Am 8(2):473, 1977.
Hunter JM and Salisbury RE: Use of gliding artificial implants to produce tendon sheaths: techniques and results in children. Plast Reconstr Surg 45:564, 1970.
Hunter JM and others: The use of gliding artificial tendon implants to form new tendon beds, J Bone Joint Surg 51A:790, 1969.
Hunter JM and others: Sheath formation in response to limited active gliding implants (animals), J Biomed Mater Res 5(1):163, 1974.
Hunter JM and others: Study of early sheath development using static non-gliding implants, J Biomed Mater Res 5(1):155, 1974.
Pulvertaft RG: Tendon grafts for flexor tendon injuries in the fingers and thumb: a study of technique and results, J Bone Joint Surg 38B:175, 1956.
Pulvertaft RG: Experiences in flexor tendon grafting in the hand, J Bone Joint Surg 41B:629, 1959.
Rayner CRW: The origin and nature of pseudo-synovium appearing around implanted Silastic rods: an experimental study, Hand 8:101, 1976.
Urbaniak JR and others: Vascularization and the gliding mechanism of free flexor-tendon grafts inserted by the silicone-rod method, J Bone Surg 56A:473, 1974.

35

The extensor tendons

Erik A. Rosenthal

Normal hand function mirrors the integrity of the extensor tendons. Their contribution to the balance, power, dexterity, and range of hand activities is critical; any restraint on them will be reflected in a proportional loss of function. The impact of an injury on the extensor tendons is often regarded as less serious than a flexor tendon injury. The treatment and rehabilitation of the injury often are believed to be less intricate, less time consuming, and associated with a relatively favorable prognosis compared with flexor tendon injuries. Experience, however, demonstrates that injuries to the extensor tendons can be equally complex, time consuming, frustrating, and disappointing. The extensor muscles to the digits are weaker, and their capacity for work and their amplitude of glide are less than their flexor antagonists, yet they require a latitude of motion that is not necessary for flexor function. The extensor tendons distal to the dorsal carpal ligament are relatively thin, broad structures that present a disproportionately large surface vulnerable to injury and susceptible to the formation of restraining scar. The complex interrelationships within the intricately designed extensor tendons of the digits increase their susceptibility to functional disarray after injury. Any violation of the extensor tendons or their investments introduces the potential for a functional deficiency.

WRIST EXTENSOR TENDONS

The wrist extensor tendons are the key to balanced hand function and to the success of rehabilitation after injury. Positional grip depends on the selective stabilizing forces of the three wrist extensor tendons. The digital extensor tendons, in the absence of the wrist extensor tendons, can secondarily induce wrist extension. Wrist extension is then the obligate follower of finger extension: an unnatural functional sequence. This substitution, however, lacks normal power and is devoid of flexibility in spatial positioning of the hand.

The stations of the extensor carpi radialis longus and brevis and the extensor carpi ulnaris are fixed relative to the axis of wrist motion at the level of the distal radius by the septa that partition the fibroosseous tunnels beneath the dorsal carpal ligament (Fig. 35-1). The dorsal carpal ligament represents the well-developed supratendinous layer of the extensor retinaculum that covers each of the six extensor compartments. The infratendinous layer is well-developed only in the ulnar three compartments; the continuous layer beneath the tendons of the fourth and fifth compartments is distinct from the subsheath that stabilizes the extensor carpi ulnaris (ECU) within the sixth.[84,118]

Each of the three wrist extensors has a different mass

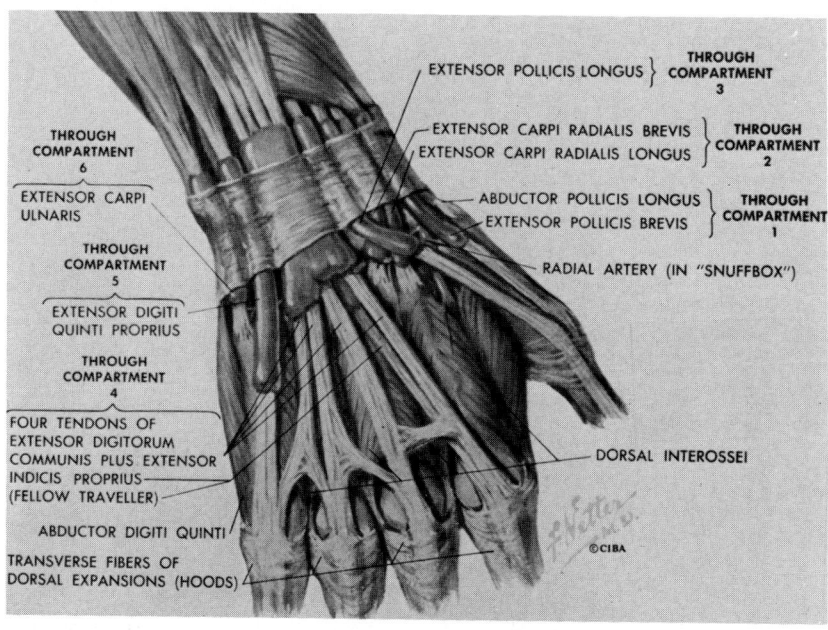

Fig. 35-1 Extensor tendon anatomy. (From Lampe EW: Surgical anatomy of the hand, Summit, NJ, 1969, by permission of CIBA Pharmaceutical Co.)

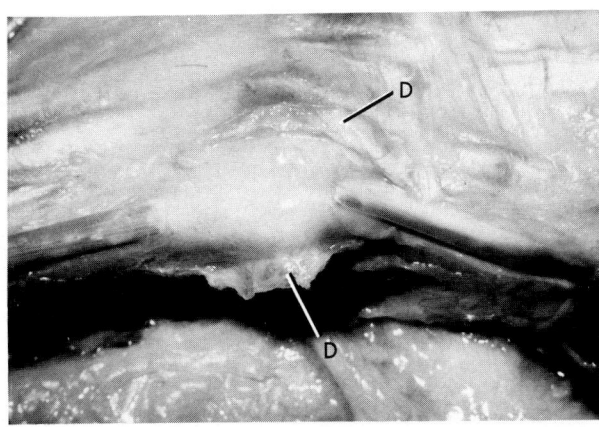

Fig. 35-2 Fascial anatomy of the extensor carpi ulnaris tendon. Dorsal carpal ligament is reflected. Tendon is secured in the groove of the ulnar head by a collar of deep fascia. Angulation of the tendon increases displacement forces during supination. Insertion of tendon on the fifth metacarpal to the right. *D*, Dorsal carpal ligament.

fraction (muscle volume, which reflects capacity for work or repetitive effort), tension fraction (cross-sectional area, which reflects muscle strength), and moment arm (perpendicular distance from the axis of wrist motion).[3,10,51] These differences are manifest in variations of performance and contributions to wrist motion.

The extensor carpi radialis longus (ECRL) has the largest mass fraction; the ECU has the smallest. The ECU has the largest tension fraction; the ECRL has the smallest. The extensor carpi radialis brevis (ECRB) has the longest moment arm relative to the axis of wrist flexion/extension; the ECU has the shortest. The ECU has the longest moment arm for ulnar deviation; the ECRB has the shortest. The radial wrist extensors have an amplitude of 37 mm during wrist flexion/extension; the ECU has 18 mm.[8] In practical terms, the ECRL has the greatest capacity for work; the ECU has the greatest strength. The ECRB occupies the most efficient position for wrist extension, the ECRL for radial deviation, and the ECU for ulnar deviation. These three muscles with different anatomic endowments are cerebrally integrated to balance wrist extension and flexion and ulnar and radial deviation.

The ECU is unique among the wrist extensor tendons. It exhibits some degree of contraction during all phases of wrist motion. Its variable potential for wrist extension depends on the position of forearm rotation. During pronation the normal tendon rests on the medial side of the ulnar head and stabilizes the wrist: it is a strong ulnar deviator, it balances the tension of all tendons radial to the axis of wrist motion, which is in the proximal end of the capitate, but it is a relatively weak wrist extensor. When the forearm is supinated, its moment arm for wrist extension lengthens and the ECU becomes a more efficient wrist extensor.[127]

The tendon of the ECU, which inserts distally on the base of the fifth metacarpal, is firmly stabilized in its groove on

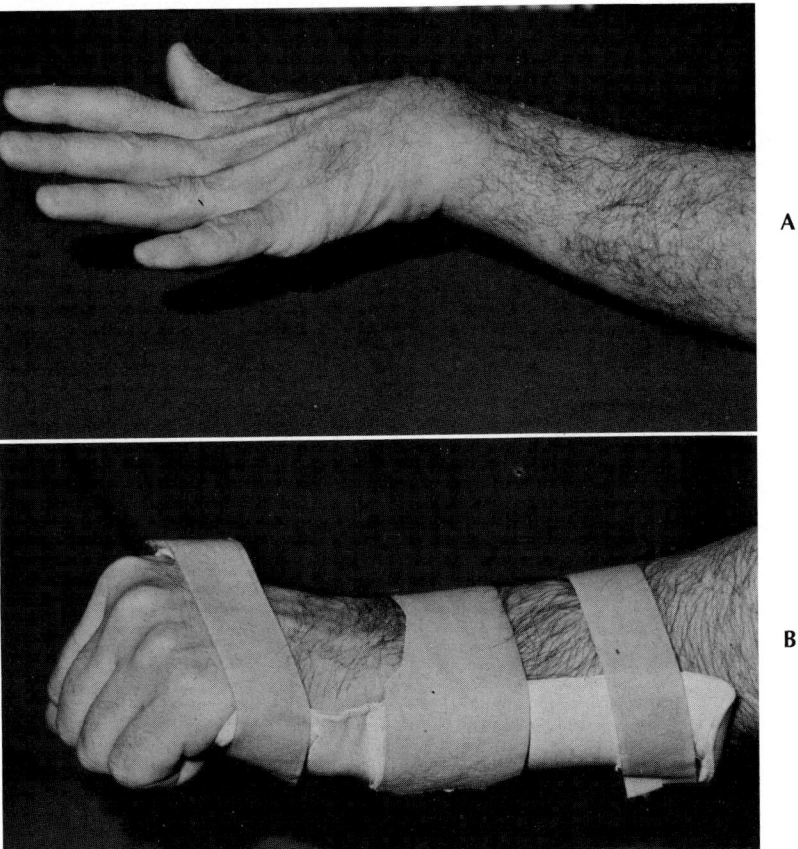

Fig. 35-3 Loss of wrist extensor function after trauma, with no direct insult to wrist extensors. **A,** Substitution pattern employing digital extensors to extend wrist. **B,** Early splinting and reeducation of wrist extensors are necessary.

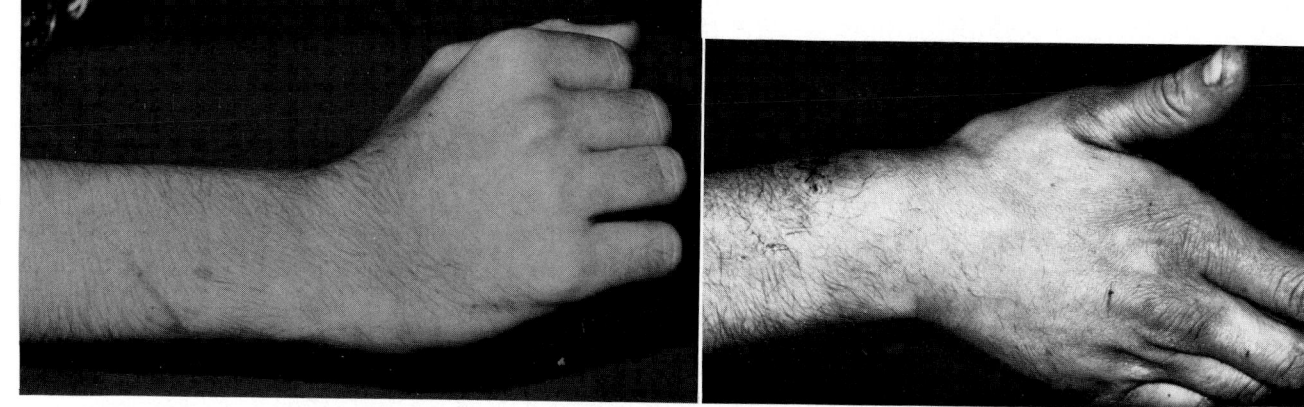

Fig. 35-4 **A,** Interruption of the extensor carpi ulnaris introduces imbalance of wrist extensors. Therapy after repair requires an awareness of the multiple facets of normal extensor carpi ulnaris function. **B,** Laceration of radial wrist extensor tendons. Inability to deviate the wrist radially introduces a major deficiency in spatial positioning of the hand and grip strength.

the ulnar head by a strong collar of synovium-lined deep fascia that is an extension of the infratendinous layer of the extensor retinaculum, distinct from the overlying supratendinous layer that constitutes the dorsal carpal ligament[111] (Fig. 35-2). Ulnar translational forces increase with an obtuse angulation of the tendon during supination. Attrition of the ECU from stress-induced tenosynovitis with partial tendon rupture is a source of chronic ulnar wrist pain.[16] The deep fascial yoke over the ECU may rupture with subluxation of the ECU from its groove during forearm rotation.[22,87] This painful condition reflects a specific anatomic deficiency. Reconstruction with a radially based flap from the dorsal carpal ligament is feasible when symptoms persist despite conservative treatment.[11]

Deterioration of wrist extensor function may occur after an injury to the hand or wrist without direct trauma to the wrist extensor tendons. A wrist drop occurs, and a pattern substituting the digital extensors is adopted to implement extension of the wrist. This centrally mediated inhibition of the wrist extensor tendons should be detected early and supportive wrist splinting initiated. The wrist is supported in slight extension, permitting digital flexion and extension while the wrist extensors are being retrained. Extending the wrist against resistance while the digits are fully flexed is helpful in this pursuit. The natural synergy between the wrist extensors and digital flexors facilitates recovery (Fig. 35-3).

Laceration of the ECU introduces a significant imbalance in some patients. The inability to balance the tension of the radial wrist extensors produces persistent radial deviation of the wrist. Extension in ulnar deviation is precluded, grip is weak, and most functions are performed awkwardly (Fig. 35-4, *A*). Laceration of the radial wrist extensors, too, can interfere significantly with balanced spatial positioning of the hand and dexterity of grip (Fig. 35-4, *B*). All the wrist extensor tendons contribute significantly to normal function, and each should be repaired after injury.

DORSAL FASCIA

An appreciation of the fascial anatomy of the dorsum of the hand is helpful for the design of surgical procedures and

for modification of a hand therapy program after an injury. The skin over the dorsum of the hand is pliable, lacking the fascial septa that stabilize the palmar skin. The skin redundancy associated with digital extension is consumed during grip. This tightening of the dorsal skin compresses the underlying dorsal veins and lymphatics, providing an efficient venous and lymphatic pump.

The superficial fascia is composed of a variable fatty layer and a deeper membranous layer, which contains the large dorsal veins, superficial lymphatics, and sensory branches of the radial and ulnar nerves. The superficial fascia is loosely attached to the deep fascia, with the interface representing a potential space. Dorsal subcutaneous bleeding and lymphedema distend this reservoir, tethering the fingers in extension and the thumb in supination. The pump mechanism is hampered, swelling increases, and grip becomes restrained further. Dorsal cicatrix similarly blocks normal grip mechanics. The penalty for uncontrolled dorsal swelling is secondary joint stiffness with tightness of the metacarpophalangeal (MP) joints and dorsal fascia of the thumb web (Fig. 35-5).

The dressing applied after repair of a wound or operative procedure should contribute to the control of dorsal edema and discourage hematoma formation. Sterile Dacron batting,* immersed in saline solution and applied wet about the wound, provides gentle compression of the hand and diffuses expressed blood away from the wound. This useful technique is comfortable for patients (Fig. 35-6).

The deep fascia of the extensor surface of the forearm is reinforced over the axis of wrist motion as the dorsal carpal ligament and continues distally as the superficial layer of the deep fascia over the dorsum of the hand (Fig. 35-7). Vertical septa beneath the dorsal carpal ligament attach to the radius and ulna, defining fibroosseous tunnels that contain the extensor tendons and their synovial sheaths. These septa position and maintain the extensor tendons relative to the axis of wrist motion in the proximal pole of the capitate. Distal to the dorsal carpal ligament the deep fascia is composed of two layers, a dorsal supratendinous layer and a

---

*Manufactured as Mountain Mist by Stearns & Foster, Cincinnati.

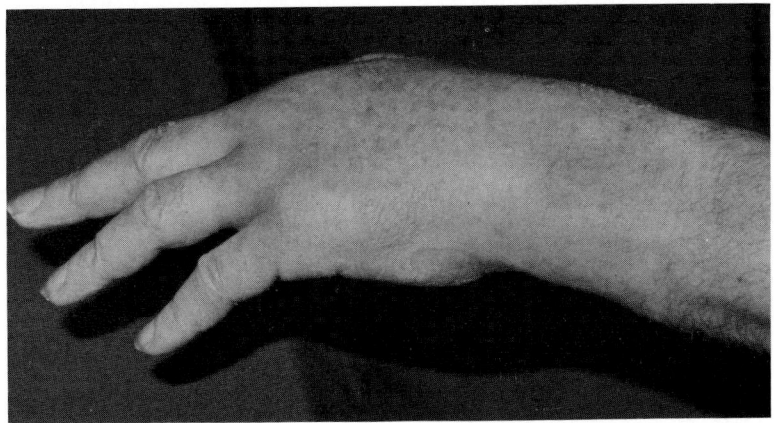

Fig. 35-5   Distention of dorsal skin and fascia reverses transverse metacarpal arch and tethers digits in extension.

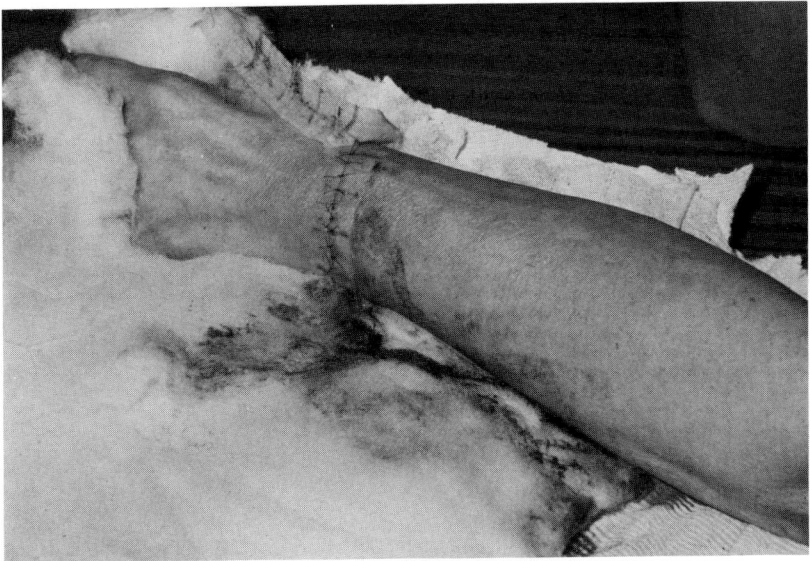

Fig. 35-6   Wet polyester batting makes comfortable, gently compressive dressing and disperses blood away from wound.

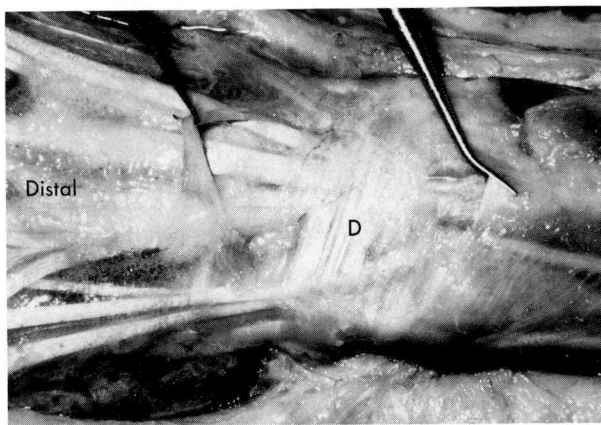

Fig. 35-7   Anatomy of deep dorsal fascia. Probe elevates deep fascia proximally while hook holds deep fascia distally to transverse fibers of dorsal carpal ligament. Areolar peritendinous fascia, the paratenon, envelops extensor tendons beyond the dorsal carpal ligament. Fascia contributes to the efficiency of tendon excursion and intrinsic tendon circulation. *D,* Dorsal carpal ligament.

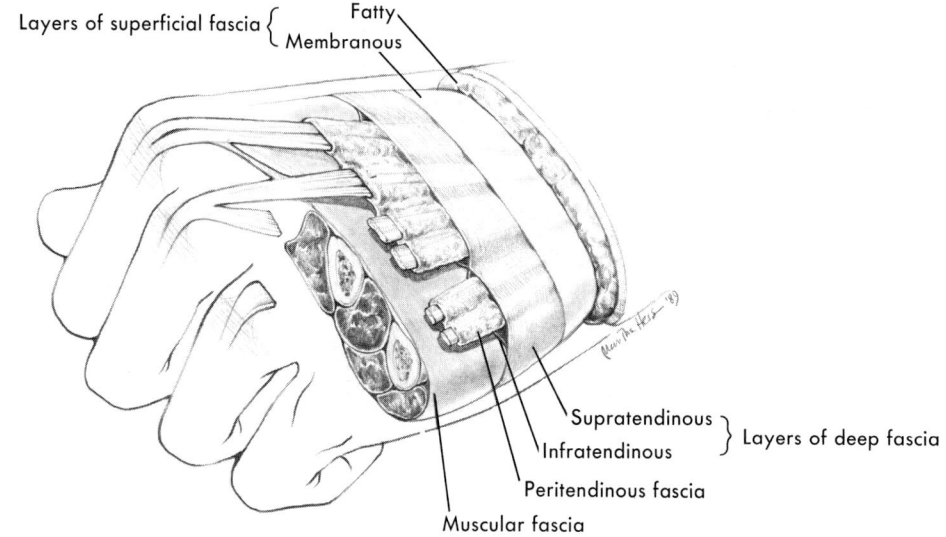

Fig. 35-8 Dorsal fascia of hand. (Redrawn from Anson BJ, et al: Surg Gynecol Obstet 81:327, 1945.)

deep infratendinous layer. They define a closed fascial space bordered by the synovial sheaths of the extensor tendons proximally, the index and fifth metacarpals, and the metacarpal heads distally. The flattened finger extensor tendons course between these two layers of the deep fascia, invested in a vascularized film of peritendinous fascia, the paratenon. The infratendinous layer of the deep fascia rests on the interosseous fascia (Fig. 35-8).

The peritendinous fascia is represented in the embryonic hand and is believed to give rise to the extensor tendons. The numerous anatomic variations in the extensor tendons may reflect developmental variations in the precursor of adult paratenon.[19,43,46,81] This transparent vascular membrane permits gliding of the extensor tendons within the small tolerances of the two layers of the deep fascia. Its response

to certain traumatic conditions demonstrates a prodigious capacity for generating scar tissue and adhesions.

The extensor tendons receive their blood supply through vascular mesenteries—mesotendons. These are analogous to the vincula of the flexor tendons.[130] Branches of the radial and ulnar arteries, perforating dorsal branches of the anterior interosseous artery, and vessels originating in the deep palmar arch are carried to the tendons in these flexible folds of delicate fascia. The mesotendons are longer and adapted to a longer tendon excursion where the extensor tendons are synovial beneath the dorsal carpal ligament and are significantly shorter within the deep fascial pocket over the metacarpals.[129] The intratendinous vascular architecture of the extensor tendons is similar throughout.[120] Synovial diffusion is the major nutritional pathway for the extensor tendons

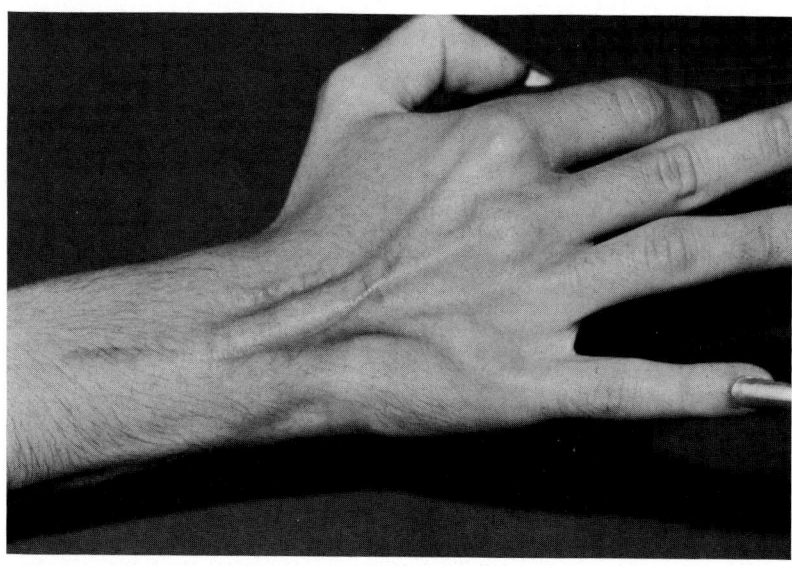

Fig. 35-9 Dorsal bowing and reduced effective extensor excursion as a result of removal of the dorsal retaining layers. Segments must remain to preserve function and avoid disfigurement.

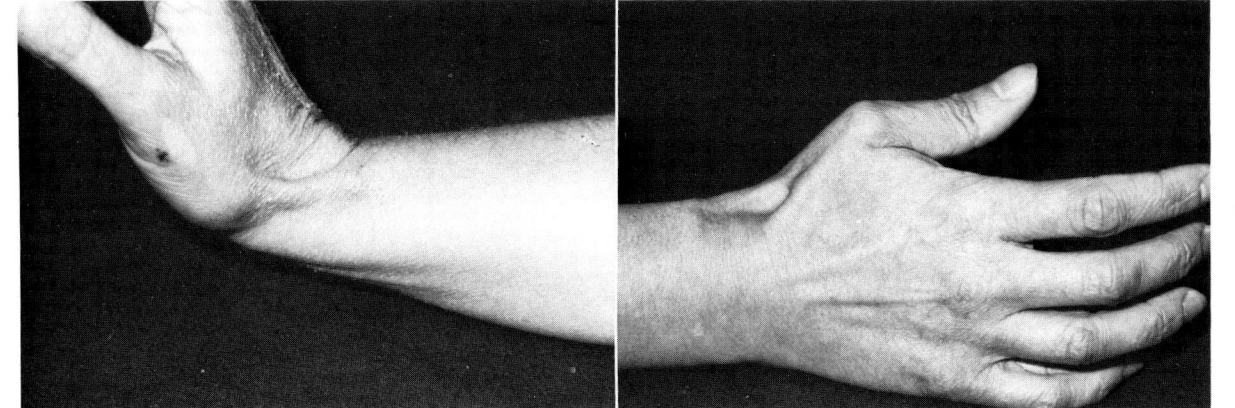

Fig. 35-10   Thumb imbalance reflecting removal of dorsal carpal ligament and deep fascia, retaining abductor pollicis longus and extensor pollicis brevis. **A,** Displacement of tendons and bowing with wrist extension-flexion. **B,** Exaggerated extension of first metacarpal with extension lag at metacarpophalangeal joint resulting from alteration of moment arms and decreased effective excursions of these tendons. Deep fascia distal to dorsal carpal ligament should be retained during surgery.

beneath the dorsal carpal ligament. The vascular contribution through the mesotendons is significantly less; longitudinal intratendinous circulation has no demonstrable input.[68]

The deep layers of the dorsal fascia contribute a dual function to the extensor tendons. The supratendinous layer constitutes a dorsal pulley, essential for an efficient distal transfer of the inherent strength and amplitude of the extensor muscles. Selective removal of portions of the dorsal fascia is compatible with retained function. Excessive removal, however, results in unsightly bowing and altered extensor kinetics (Fig. 35-9). Fasciectomy also can introduce thumb imbalance with extensor tendon deficiencies (Fig. 35-10). The contribution of the deep fascia to the intrinsic nutrition of the extensor tendons may parallel the role of the fibroosseous sheath in synovial diffusion of the flexor tendons.[68,130]

FINGER EXTENSOR TENDONS
Proximal to MP joints

The extensor tendons of the MP joints of the fingers are the extensor digitorum, extensor indicis, and the extensor digiti minimi. The tendons of the extensor digitorum pass beneath the dorsal carpal ligament within synovial sheaths. They flatten distally between the layers of the deep fascia. The extensor digitorum contributes substantial tendons to the index, long, and ring fingers, giving a variable slip to the small finger: extension of the MP joints of the long, ring, and small fingers depends on the position of the adjacent fingers; independent extension is lacking[70] (Fig. 35-11). Extensor autonomy is less in the long finger and least in the ring finger. This reflects fibrous connecting bands within the muscle belly of the extensor digitorum in the forearm and does not depend on the integrity of the juncturae tendinum.[49] A separate muscle belly of the extensor digitorum to the index finger with individual nerve supply from the posterior interosseous nerve can preserve independent index finger extension after the extensor indicis has been transferred.[77]

The extensor indicis and extensor digiti minimi have independent muscles that allow independent function. Extension of the index and small fingers is readily performed, irrespective of the flexed position of the other fingers (Fig. 35-12). The extensor indicis may contribute a tendon to the thumb; the extensor indicis and pollicis communis tendon is a rare variant.[19]

The juncturae tendinum are broad intertendinous connections that diverge from the ring finger extensor tendon. These bands connect with the long, small, and, variably, the index finger extensor tendons. This connection with the index finger extensor tendons is commonly only a vestige (Fig. 35-11). These bands assist extension of adjacent connected fingers by transferring forces during extension. Laceration of an extensor tendon proximally may be obscured by the contribution of these bands. Demonstration of a full

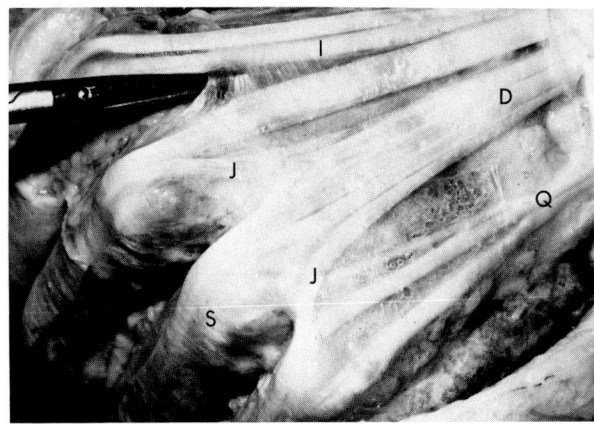

Fig. 35-11   Extensor tendon anatomy. Deep fascia has been removed. Instrument lifts vestige of junctura tendinum to index extensor tendons. *D,* Extensor digitorum; *I,* extensor indicis; *Q,* extensor digiti minimi; *J,* junctura tendinum; *S,* sagittal bands over ring metacarpophalangeal joint. Juncturae tendinum dynamically stabilize extensor tendons during grip.

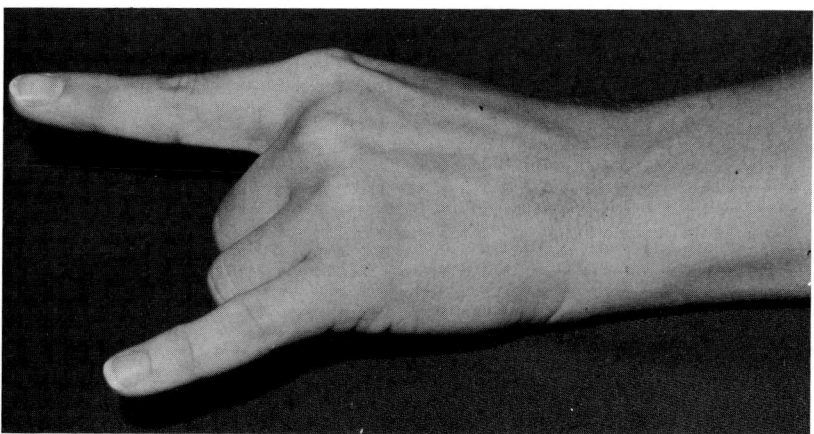

Fig. 35-12 Extensor indicis and extensor digiti minimi have independence of function from separate muscles. No distal tethering exists with flexion of the other fingers. Extensor digitorum to the index finger may have separate muscle belly with an individual nerve supply.

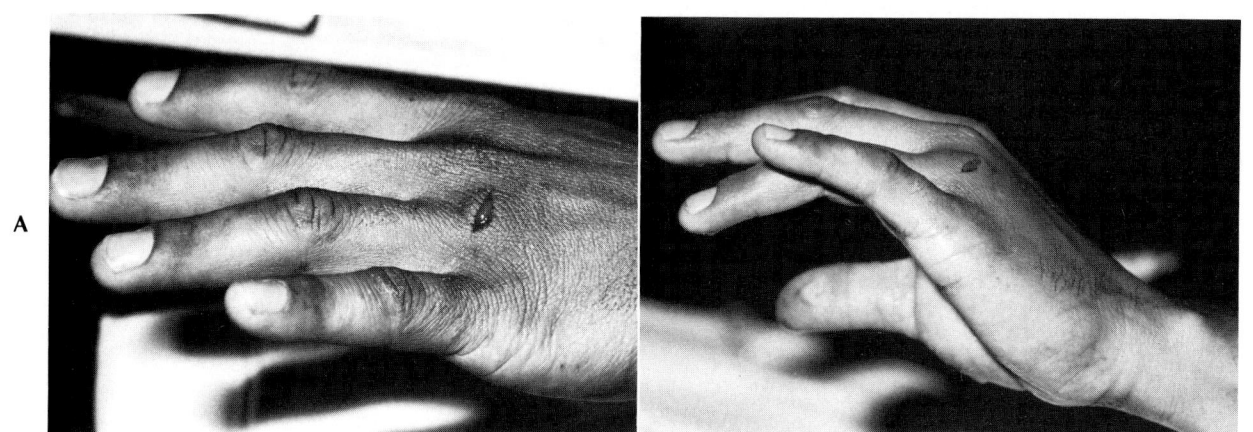

Fig. 35-13 Laceration of extensor tendon to ring finger. **A,** No apparent deficit with wrist in neutral. Metacarpophalangeal joint extension accomplished through fascial connection. **B,** Deficit apparent when function is tested with combined wrist and finger extension.

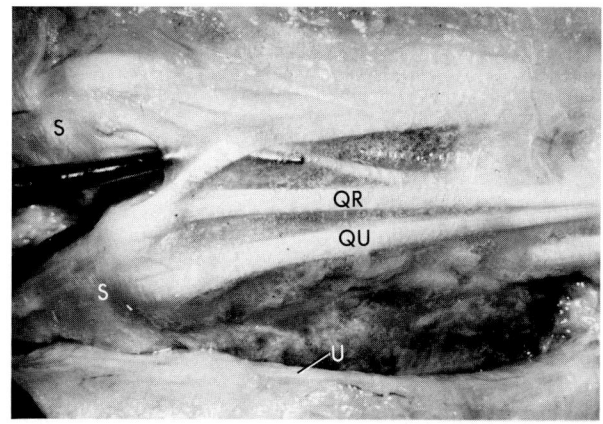

Fig. 35-14 Extensor tendons to the small finger. Deep fascia has been removed. Instrument lifts oblique junctura to small finger. This oblique connection may mask rupture of the extensor digiti minimi proximally. *QR*, Radial tendon extensor digiti minimi; *QU*, ulnar tendon extensor digiti minimi; *S*, sagittal bands; *U*, dorsal sensory branch of ulnar nerve.

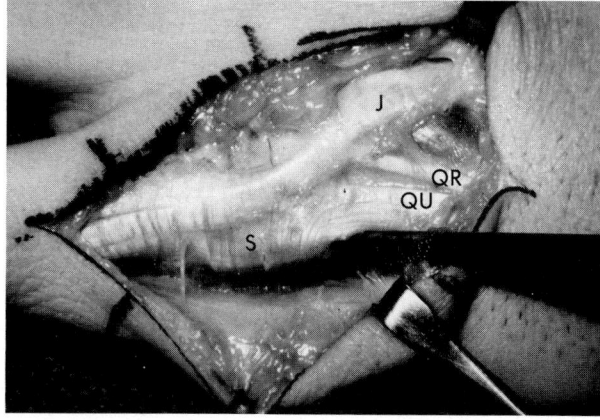

Fig. 35-15 Extensor tendon insertion at metacarpophalangeal joint of the small finger. Extensor digiti minimi gains attachment to the lateral tubercle of the proximal phalanx through insertion of its ulnar tendon into abductor digiti minimi tendon. *J*, Junctura tendinum; *QU*, ulnar tendon extensor digiti minimi; *QR*, radial tendon extensor digiti minimi; *S*, sagittal bands.

range of potential motion with direct visualization of the injured tendon is required before the possibility of a lacerated tendon can be discarded (Fig. 35-13). A junctura between the index extensor digitorum and extensor pollicis longus is an anatomic variant. Thumb interphalangeal joint flexion restrains index finger extension when this variant exists.[116]

The juncturae tendinum develop increased tension with a more transverse orientation as they glide distally during finger flexion. This distal migration with active finger flexion dynamically stabilizes the fingers by transmitting forces to the radial sagittal bands of the index and long fingers and to the ulnar sagittal bands of the ring and small fingers. Active grip thus contributes to the stability of the transverse metacarpal arch and to the centralization of the extensor tendons over the dorsum of the MP joints.[1]

The extensor tendons to the small finger have important anatomic features.[100] An oblique junctura from the ring finger will permit continued extension of the small finger after interruption of the extensor digiti minimi more proximally. The patient is frequently unaware of any deficit until the decreased strength and lost autonomy are demonstrated. This situation is frequently seen in patients with rheumatoid arthritis (Fig. 35-14).

The extensor digiti minimi gains attachment to the abductor tubercle of the base of the proximal phalanx through insertion of its ulnar tendon into the abductor digiti minimi tendon (Fig. 35-15). Some patients with ulnar palsy who are incapable of hyperextension of the MP joint and do not develop a claw deformity acquire an abduction deformity of the small finger (Wartenberg's sign) from paralysis of the third palmar interosseous muscle. The abducted small finger is associated with an oblique junctura from the ring finger, a weak biomechanical link. The extensor digiti minimi is relatively unopposed and abducts the small finger. Patients who do not acquire this deformity have a transverse orientation of the junctura, a biomechanically forceful link that opposes the deformity.[6]

The contributions of the juncturae are respected during reconstruction for extensor tendon ruptures in the rheumatoid patient; distal ends of ruptured tendons are sutured to intact adjacent tendons. Tension at the tendon junction is adjusted with the fingers held slightly less than full flexion. This ensures that the juncturae are sufficiently oblique for transmission of active extension forces and avoids an extensor tenodesis caused by excessive restraint through the juncturae as they tighten transversely during active finger flexion.

Secretan's disease. Hard, brawny edema involving the dorsum of the hand has stimulated controversy since it was described in 1901.[104] The condition follows trauma to the dorsum of the hand, often pursues a protracted course, and has been associated with an unfavorable surgical prognosis.[98] It has been considered synonymous with factitious, or self-induced, edema.[89,110] Monetary gain and compensation award have been considered significant causative factors. The anatomy of the dorsum of the hand and the clinical observations at surgery support the contention that there is a specific pathologic entity involving peritendinous fibrosis about the extensor tendons and juncturae tendinum within the confines of the layers of the deep fascia after trauma, which is different from factitious dorsal edema.[90,92] The form

and distribution of the fibrosis conform to the fascial anatomy previously described.[47] The inelastic peritendinous scar restricts excursion of the finger extensor tendons and their juncturae, blocking longitudinal and transverse tendon glide. Surgical, psychologic, and rehabilitative treatment are necessarily integrated. This condition presents a diverse spectrum of challenges with a cautious prognosis.

Tendon rupture. The wrist and finger extensor tendons are exposed to entrapment by fractures of the distal radius[45,67,78] and dislocations of the distal ulna.[83] Attrition with delayed rupture has been reported from multiple conditions including anomalous extensor brevis manus muscle,[44,93] fixation screws,[72] rheumatoid tenosynovitis, granulomatous tenosynovitis, extraskeletal osteochondroma,[72] Kienböck's disease,[72] and instability of the distal ulna after excessive surgical resection.[79]

Distal to MP joints

The form and complexity of the extensor tendons change at the level of the sagittal bands that shroud the MP joints of the fingers. Distally they consist of a continuous sheet of precisely oriented fibers that transmit tension. This fiber array wraps the finger skeleton in the form of a bisected cone. It is composed of a tendon system, which transmits tension and imparts motion, and a retinacular system, which stabilizes the tendon system. An alteration in the alignment or length of the three phalanges of the fingers changes the normal adjustment of forces within the tendon system and permits the retinacular system to foreshorten.[60] This imbalance within the tendon system establishes deformities; the tightening of the retinacular system fixes these deformities and resists correction.

The broad fibrous dorsal hood of the finger MP joints consists of fibers from the juncturae tendinum, sagittal bands, and extensor tendon. This blend of fibers is strong except in the long finger where the oval-shaped extensor tendon rests on the underlying sagittal bands, attached by a relatively weak fibrous layer. Ulnar displacement forces are greatest with the MP joints in full extension, decrease during the first 60 degrees of flexion, and then progressively increase with greater flexion. Relatively little force is needed to maintain a normally located extensor tendon. Significantly higher restraining forces are required to prevent displacement of a tendon that is displaced ulnarward; an ulnar displaced tendon tends to displace further with increased flexion.[52] Sagittal band rupture can occur during full extension or with grip, is more likely with ulnar wrist deviation, and usually involves the radial sagittal fibers. In the long finger the extensor tendon can separate from the underlying sagittal bands and displace without sagittal band rupture.

The extensor tendons have a variable insertion on the base of the proximal phalanx, which is not significant for extension of the fingers.[48,60,121] This insertion, if present, centralizes the extensor tendon but contributes little to the normal kinematics of finger extension. There is a linear relationship between excursion of the extensor tendons over the dorsum of the hand and the angle of motion of the MP joints.[3,23] Extension of the MP joint is achieved through the sagittal bands, which are vertically oriented fibers that shroud the capsule and collateral ligaments, connecting the extensor tendons with the volar plate and proximal phalanx on both sides of the joint.[41] These broad bands constitute

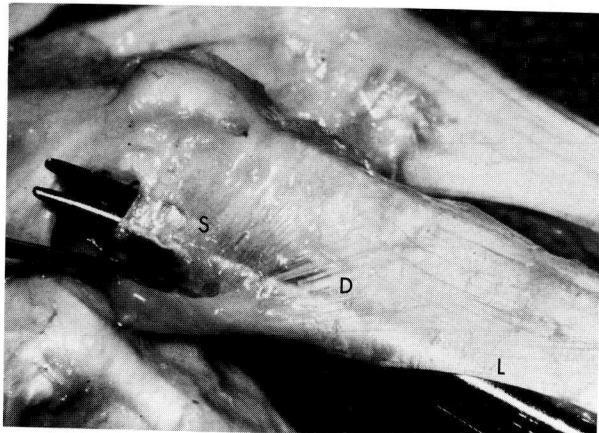

Fig. 35-16 Dorsal apparatus of finger. Hook retracts interosseous muscle. Sagittal bands separate intrinsic muscles from the metacarpophalangeal joint capsule. Sagittal bands and oblique fibers of the intrinsic tendon transmit extension forces. Vertical fibers of intrinsic tendons transmit flexion forces. Delicate fibers are vulnerable to interference by scar. *S,* Sagittal bands; *D,* vertical fibers of intrinsic tendon; *L,* oblique fibers of intrinsic tendon.

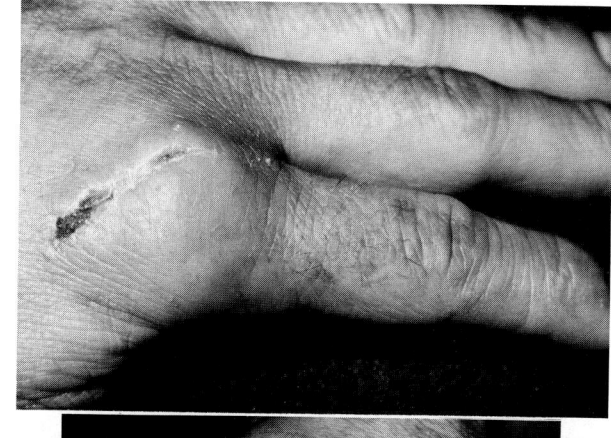

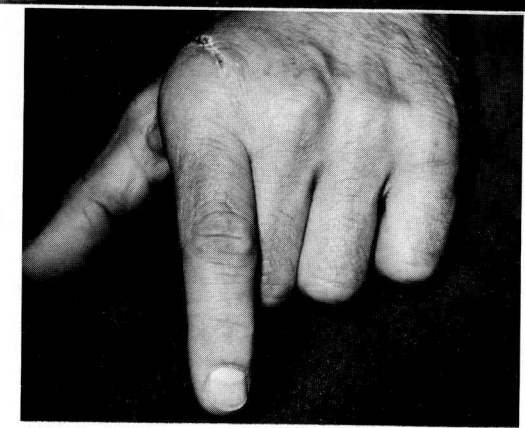

Fig. 35-17 Laceration of radial sagittal bands of index finger without repair. Deformity has developed. **A,** Ulnar displacement with palmar subluxation of extensor digitorum results in palmar subluxation with incomplete extension of metacarpophalangeal joint. **B,** Deformity includes ulnar angulation and supination of injured finger.

functional slings that pass between the joint capsule and the intrinsic muscles (Fig. 35-16). They hood the axis of joint motion during extension and pass distally to the axis of motion during flexion. They stabilize the extensor tendons over the dorsum of the MP joint during flexion, augmenting the juncturae tendinum.[128]

Laceration or closed rupture of the sagittal bands disrupts the stability of the extensor tendons over the MP joints. The extensor tendon displaces ulnarward during flexion. Active extension produces ulnar angulation of the MP joint with supination of the finger (Fig. 35-17). A painful snap may accompany extension as the extensor tendon relocates dorsally. Tightness develops that maintains the ulnar deviation deformity, prevents dorsal relocation of the extensor tendon, and precludes full active extension of the MP joint.

Distal to the sagittal bands the lumbrical and interosseous muscles contribute proximal vertical and distal oblique fibers to the extensor tendon over the proximal phalanx (Fig. 35-18). The vertical fibers transmit flexor forces to the proximal phalanx, which flex the MP joint. The oblique fibers transmit extension forces to the proximal and distal interphalangeal joints. This combined sheet of extrinsic and intrinsic motored fibers over the proximal phalanx is appropriately termed the *dorsal apparatus,* because it contributes both flexion and extension (see Fig. 35-16).[109]

The extensor tendon continues as the central tendon to insert on the dorsal base of the middle phalanx with medial fibers from the intrinsic tendons. The conjoined lateral bands represent the continuation of the oblique fibers of the intrinsic tendons, supplemented by lateral fibers from the central extensor tendon (Fig. 35-19). The lateral bands continue distally, converging over the middle phalanx as a single terminal tendon that inserts on the dorsal base of the distal phalanx (Fig. 35-20, *A*).

The functional composite of extrinsic and intrinsic tendons in the fingers transmits extension and flexion forces. The extrinsic extensor tendons are primarily extensors of the MP joints; they are capable of secondarily extending the interphalangeal joints only if hyperextension of the MP joint

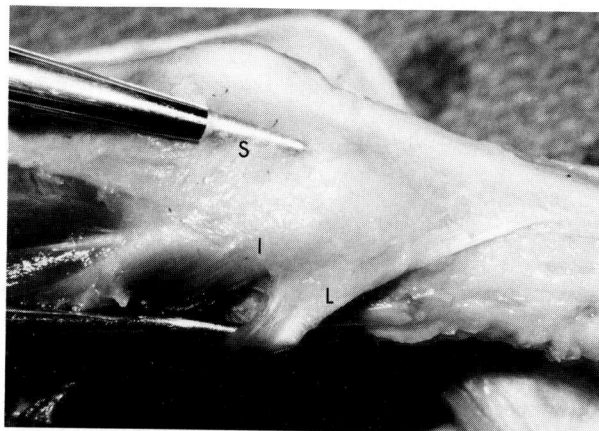

Fig. 35-18 Extrinsic and intrinsic tendons merge about the radial side of the index finger metacarpophalangeal joint. Sagittal bands effect metacarpophalangeal joint extension. Interosseous and lumbrical muscles transmit tension through dorsal apparatus and lateral bands for metacarpophalangeal flexion and interphalangeal extension. *S,* Sagittal bands; *I,* interosseous tendon; *L,* lumbrical tendon.

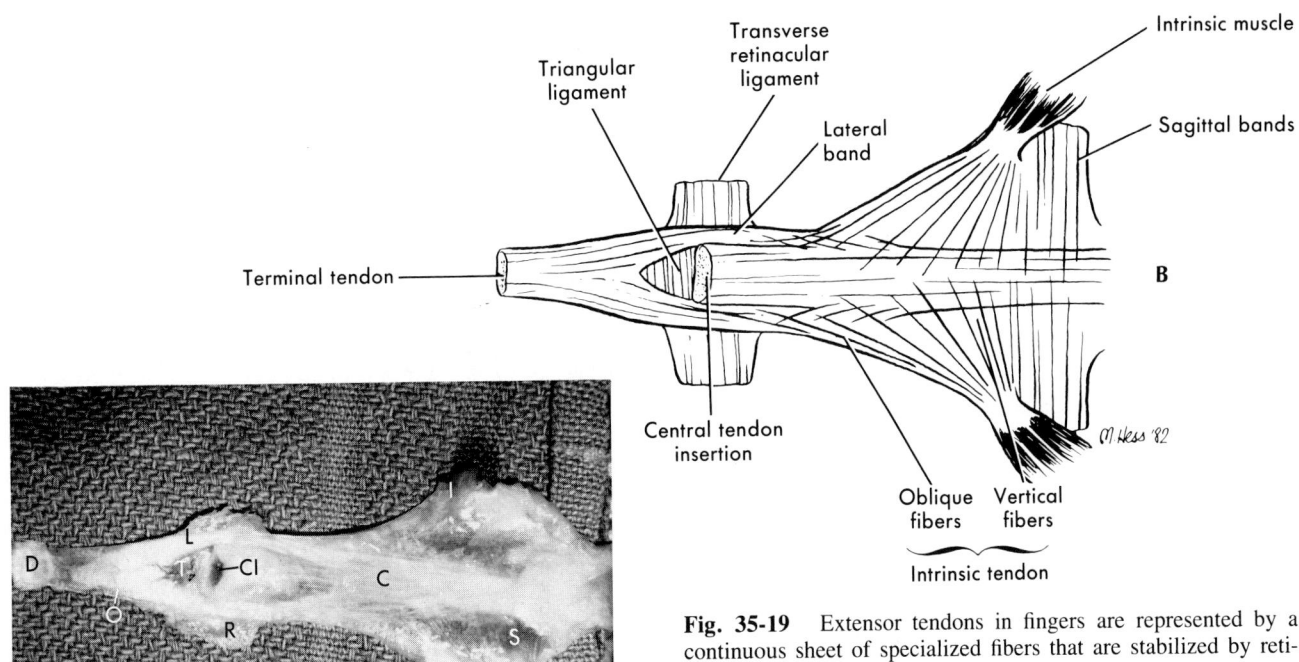

Fig. 35-19   Extensor tendons in fingers are represented by a continuous sheet of specialized fibers that are stabilized by retinacular ligaments. **A,** Deep side of extensor tendon complex. Terminal tendon is at left. **B,** Schematic drawing of **A.** *C,* Central tendon; *CI,* central tendon insertion; *D,* terminal tendon; *I,* intrinsic tendon; *L,* lateral band; *O,* oblique retinacular ligament; *R,* transverse retinacular ligament; *S,* sagittal bands; *T,* triangular ligament.

is prevented. The intrinsic tendons flex the MP joints and extend the interphalangeal joints.[65]

The lateral bands normally lie dorsal to the axis of motion of the proximal interphalangeal (PIP) joints during extension and descend to the axis of joint motion during flexion. This shift of the lateral bands permits synchronized motion of both PIP and DIP joints by compensating for the difference in the radii—or moment arms—of both joints. The smaller DIP joint would extend disproportionately relative

to the PIP joint without the compensation provided by the shifting of the lateral bands.[109,128]

The connection between the central tendon and lateral bands represents a crisscrossing of fibers in separate layers; the fibers from the central tendon pass superficially to those from the intrinsic lateral bands. Descent of the lateral bands during flexion is accompanied by an increase in the longitudinal angle between these fibers. This shift in geometric form is analogous to the expansion of a taut mesh.[103] The

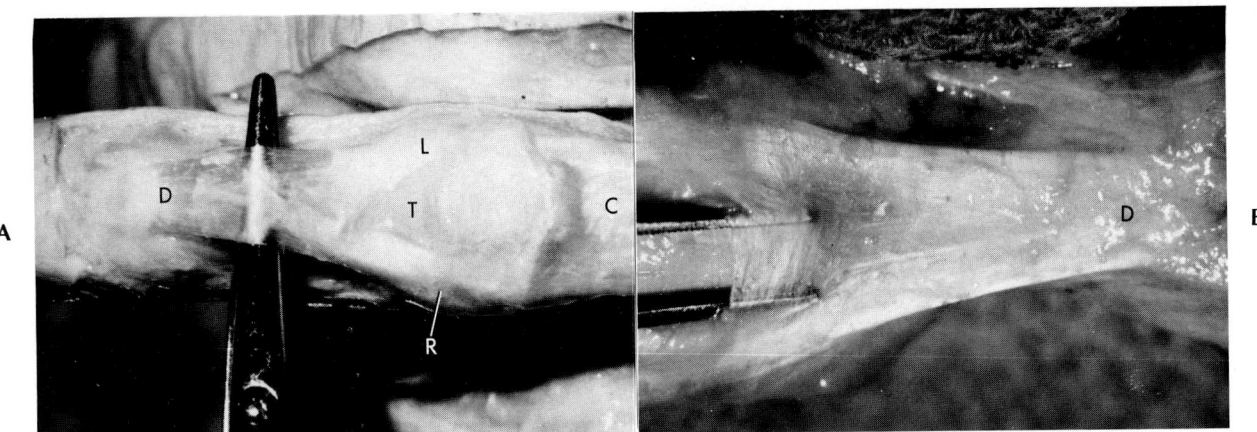

Fig. 35-20   Extensor tendon anatomy about proximal interphalangeal joint and middle phalanx. **A,** Connections between oblique retinacular ligaments and merged lateral bands have been divided to demonstrate tendon anatomy. **B,** Forceps elevate the dorsal fibers of the retinacular ligament, which comprise the triangular ligament. These restrain descent of lateral bands normally; scarring can impair flexion. Dissection of extensor tendon over the middle phalanx during repair of mallet finger injuries invites scarring with restricted distal interphalangeal joint motion. *C,* Central tendon; *D,* terminal tendon; *L,* lateral band; *R,* transverse retinacular ligament; *T,* triangular ligament.

delicacy of this fiber interplay emphasizes the vulnerability of the extensor tendons in the fingers to the restraints of scar.

Retinacular ligaments. The retinacular ligaments consist of fibers that encircle the finger obliquely about the PIP joint. They originate proximally from the flexor fibroosseous sheath and palmar plate and course dorsally and distally about the joint. Their function is analogous to that of the sagittal bands about the MP joints. Fibers palmar to the lateral bands—the transverse retinacular ligaments—contribute to axial stability of the PIP joint, restrain dorsal displacement of the lateral bands, and assist descent of the lateral bands during flexion. Dorsally these fibers connect the lateral bands: proximal fibers roof the insertions of the central tendon and medial fibers of the intrinsic tendons; more distal fibers—the triangular ligament—connect the converging conjoined lateral bands (Fig. 35-20, *B*). Preservation of the triangular ligament after rupture or surgical division of the central tendon retains active extension of the PIP joint without development of a boutonnière deformity. Interruption of the transverse retinacular ligaments fosters dorsal displacement of the lateral bands with development of a swan-neck deformity.

The oblique retinacular ligaments originate from the flexor fibroosseous sheath at the proximal phalanx, pass palmar to the axis of the PIP joint deep to the transverse retinacular ligament, and insert on the dorsal base of the distal phalanx adjacent to the terminal extensor tendon.[37] Distal fibers interdigitate with the terminal tendon before inserting, an important anatomic feature that influences the clinical presentation of the mallet tendon lesion.[112,128]

The oblique retinacular ligaments probably contribute little to extension in the normal finger.[41,105] They may stabilize the loaded fingertip when fully flexed under certain circumstances, such as the intrinsic-plus position with the DIP joint flexed during chuck pinch or fingering the E string of a violin.[4] They can contribute significantly to deformity in the imbalanced finger.

The terminal tendon alone is capable of completely extending the distal phalanx. The dorsal rectangular segment of the collateral ligaments of the DIP joints can support the distal phalanx in 45 degrees flexion. In the absence of the terminal tendon, the fully flexed distal finger joint will passively return to midflexion because of the collateral ligaments assisted by the dorsal capsule and oblique retinacular ligaments. Only the terminal tendon can complete extension of this joint.[106]

EXTENSOR TENDON INJURIES ABOUT THE FINGER MP JOINTS

Closed soft tissue injuries about the MP joints of the fingers jeopardize the extensor tendons, sagittal bands, collateral ligaments, and adjacent intrinsic tendons. Closed fractures of the metacarpal and sprain fractures of the MP joints cause swelling and pain that must be differentiated from soft tissue injuries by careful clinical and radiographic examination. Radiographs for evaluation of swelling and tenderness after injury of the finger MP joints should include posteroanterior (PA), lateral, and Brewerton views* to eliminate the possibility of occult marginal fractures.

Differential diagnosis

Subluxation of the extensor tendon. Subluxation of the extensor tendon at this level was described in 1868.[62] It may result from chronic sustained forces,[9,42,82] tendon attrition, sudden exertion,[5,99] or direct trauma.[117] Rupture of the radial sagittal bands usually occurs,[125] except in the long finger where the extrinsic extensor tendon may dislodge from its weak attachment to the underlying sagittal fibers.[52] A partial arcuate tear in the ulnar sagittal bands with chronic pain and swelling over the MP joint without displacement of the extensor tendon also has been described.[56] Displacement of the tendon in the acute injury is commonly obscured by swelling. Extensor tendon subluxation with ulnar finger angulation of the index, long, or ring finger may not appear immediately and will not develop with a partial rupture of the radial sagittal bands. Ulnar angulation of the small finger

---

*An anteroposterior tangential view of the metacarpal heads, useful for visualizing the fossae of origin of the collateral ligaments. The dorsum of the extended fingers rests on the cassette with the MP joints in 65 degrees of flexion. The x-ray beam is perpendicular to the cassette and directed 15 degrees from the ulnar side.

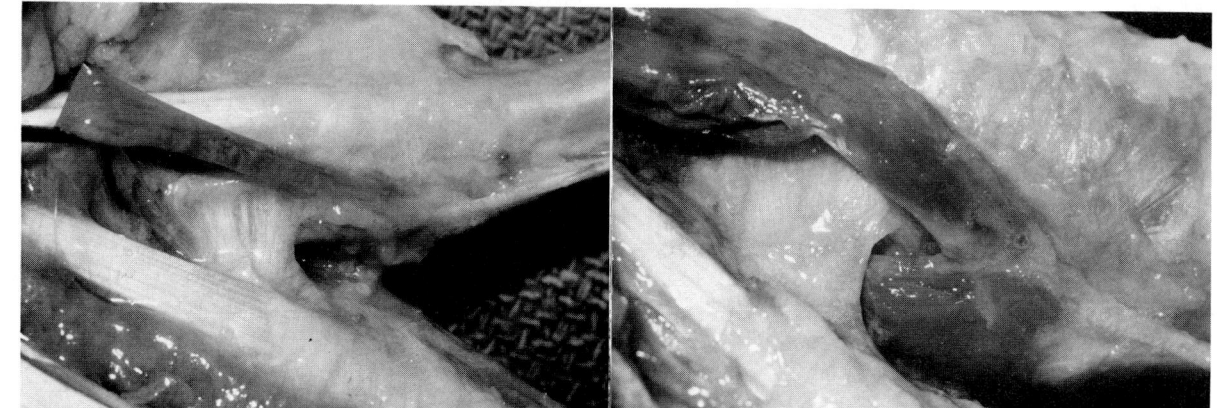

Fig. 35-21 Lumbrical and interosseous muscles merge distally to interpalmar plate ligament: the anatomic basis of saddle syndrome. **A,** Hook lifts third lumbrical palmarward from the ligament connecting the palmar plates of the long and ring finger metacarpophalangeal joints. **B,** Lumbrical merges with second palmar interosseous muscle distally. Adhesions between the ligament and intrinsic tendons may produce painful intrinsic dysfunction.

is opposed by the junctura tendinum. Tenderness, swelling, and ecchymosis are suggestive of fiber rupture in the acute case.

Conservative closed treatment with cast immobilization of the wrist and MP joints in neutral position for 4 to 6 weeks should precede surgical intervention.[95] Primary surgery is indicated in the unusual case when complete rupture of the radial sagittal bands is apparent: the extensor tendon has subluxated, and the finger is angulated.

Surgical repair of a sagittal band defect with extensor subluxation was first described by Haberern.[35] Repair of the radial[52] or ulnar[56] sagittal bands and a variety of surgical tenodeses that maintain the centralized extensor tendon have been described for operative correction of imbalance and dysfunction that persist despite adequate nonoperative treatment.*

*References 14, 21, 25, 53, 69, 71, 125.

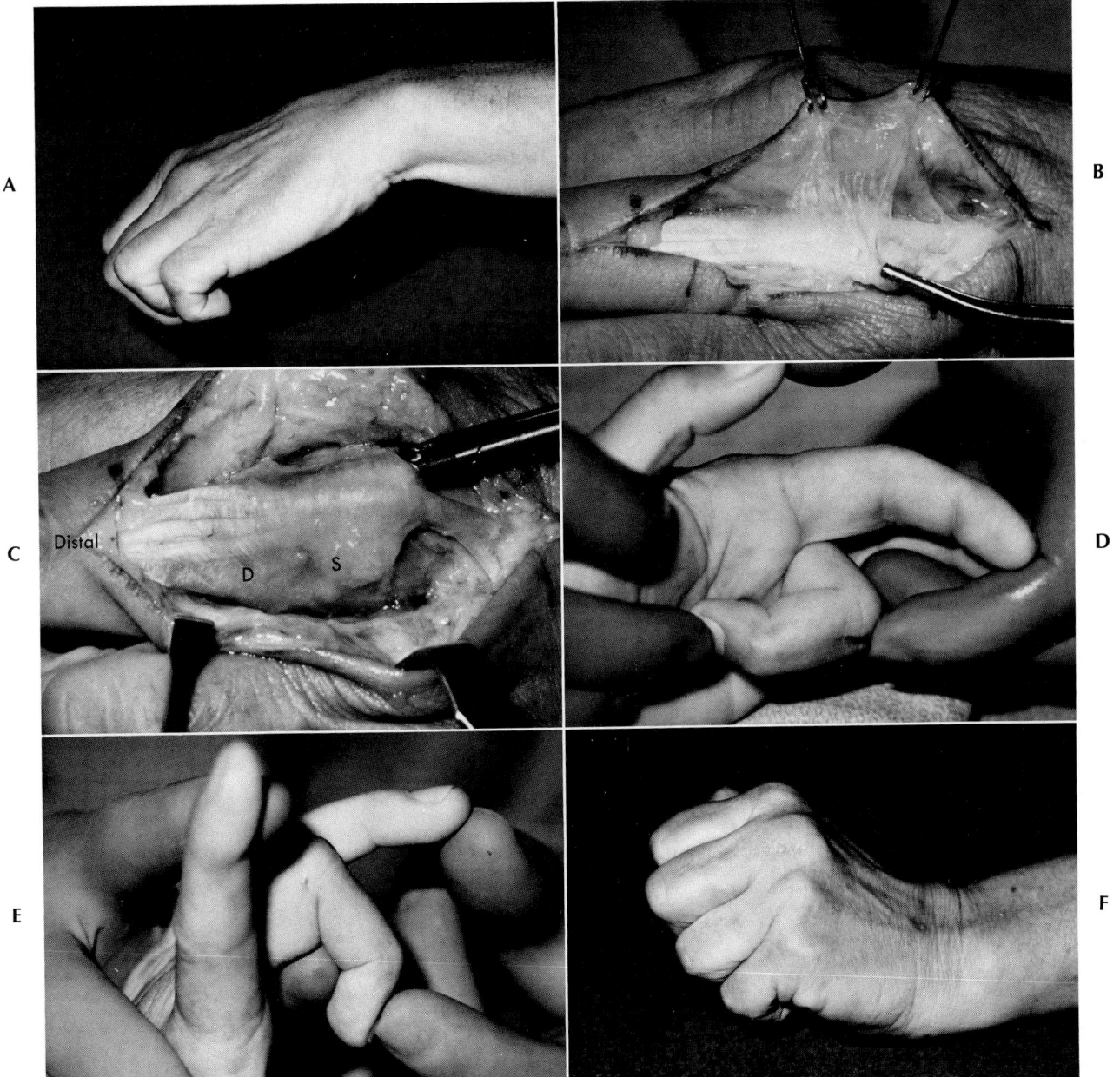

Fig. 35-22   Extrinsic and intrinsic dysfunction from scarring caused by focal crush injury about the long finger metacarpophalangeal joint in a 54-year-old woman. **A,** Limited, painful grip 6 months following injury. Extrinsic tenodesis and positive intrinsic tightness test were elicited. **B,** Dorsal exposure over metacarpophalangeal joint. Adhesions between skin flap and extensor hood are evident. **C,** Anatomic structures are clearly defined following tendolysis. Instrument is beneath radial sagittal bands and dorsal apparatus. **D,** Extrinsic tenodesis has been eliminated. **E,** Intrinsic tightness test is negative. **F,** Voluntary grip following wound healing and rehabilitation. *S,* Ulnar sagittal bands; *D,* dorsal apparatus.

Saddle syndrome. The interosseous and lumbrical tendons converge distally to the interpalmar plate ligament radial to the MP joint of the long, ring, and small fingers (Fig. 35-21). Consolidation of these tendons by restraining adhesions about the interpalmar plate ligament after closed injuries has been descriptively termed the *saddle syndrome*.[15] This chronic condition is characterized by persistent pain with grip. Direct and compression tenderness between the adjacent metacarpal necks, painful active intrinsic function (MP joint flexion with interphalangeal extension) against resistance, and pain with eliciting the intrinsic tightness test (passive flexion of the interphalangeal joints while the MP joints are supported in extension) support this diagnosis (see Fig. 35-48). Intrinsic restraint can be lateralized by deviating the finger away from the side being tested. Intrinsic tendolysis, including resection of the distal margin of the interpalmar plate ligament through a palmar incision, is indicated when symptoms persist.[15,122]

Collateral ligament rupture. Early diagnosis is apparent when the fully flexed MP joint is unstable to lateral deviation. Normally this joint is most stable in full flexion. Partial ruptures are painful when tested but retain stability. X-ray examinations are essential. Closed treatment is indicated initially for soft tissue injuries; significant joint fractures are replaced and internally stabilized. Closed sprains that continue to be painful after immobilization and supportive nonoperative treatment may require surgery.

Chronic tendon adhesions. Inelastic adhesions between the extensor hood, intrinsic tendons, and underlying capsule may be the source of persistent painful swelling with loss of motion. Thickening of the dorsal joint capsule may develop beneath the scarred extensor hood. Chronic thickening of the extensor hood from repeated trauma, reported in karate players, has been termed *hypertrophic infiltrative tendinitis* (the HIT syndrome).[32] Painful active motion, an extrinsic tenodesis—the extensor-plus phenomenon (see Fig. 35-47)—and positive intrinsic tightness test are all possible findings when adhesions consolidate the extrinsic and intrinsic tendons about the finger MP joints.[96] Tendolysis, which selectively defines the extrinsic and intrinsic tendon systems, in combination with a dorsal capsulectomy when necessary, liberates the tethered tendons (Fig. 35-22).

EXTENSOR TENDON INJURIES AT THE PIP JOINT

Interruption of the extensor tendons at the PIP joint may result from lacerations, closed trauma, burns, rheumatoid synovitis, or tightly applied casts and splints. The deformities that develop reflect a distortion of forces that are normally balanced by tendon and retinacular systems. Early deformities are more easily reversed than lasting ones that have developed ligament and tendon tightness. Persistent deformities acquire a resistance to correction that adversely influences the prognosis for treatment.

Functional anatomy

The central tendon is the primary extensor of the PIP joint. The intrinsic tendons contribute medial slips that insert on the dorsal lip of the middle phalanx adjacent to the central tendon and receive lateral slips from the extrinsic tendon to form the conjoined lateral bands. The lateral bands normally descend during flexion and cover the axis of joint motion, where they are incapable of initiating extension. The central tendon alone is capable of initiating extension of the flexed joint. Tension through the lateral bands increases progressively as the bands migrate dorsally during extension; their contribution to PIP joint extension increases with dorsal displacement. Dorsally stationed lateral bands can maintain extension of the PIP joint. Normally the lateral bands are relaxed when the PIP joint is fully flexed, tethered by the central tendon and incapable of extending the DIP joint. In moderate (30 to 40 degrees) PIP joint flexion, there is weak but evident transfer of tension through the lateral bands to the DIP joint. This can be demonstrated clinically by holding the MP joint in neutral and the PIP joint in moderate flexion: a weak active extension of the DIP joint is evident.

The transverse retinacular ligaments and their dorsal fibers connect the lateral bands and have functional similarities to the sagittal bands about the MP joint; they contribute to extension of the PIP joint. Translation of the lateral bands is controlled by the fibers of the retinacular ligaments. Descent is limited by the dorsal fibers of the retinacular ligament (the triangular ligament); dorsal displacement is restrained by the transverse retinacular ligament. The palmar plate and the flexor superficialis tendon resist hyperextension.

Pathologic anatomy

Disruption of the central tendon interferes with normal active extension of the PIP joint. Initiation of extension of the flexed joint is lost. The final 15 to 20 degrees of active extension is also lost. This can be demonstrated by actively extending the fingers while the wrist and MP joints are supported in flexion: it infers disruption of the central tendon with potential for development of a boutonnière deformity.[13] The positioned PIP joint can be maintained in extension by the lateral bands while they remain dorsal.

Release of the central tendon allows the finger extensor mechanism to slide proximally. This increases forces transmitted to the middle phalanx through the transverse retinacular ligaments and to the distal phalanx through the lateral slips, conjoined lateral bands, and terminal tendon. Active extension of the DIP joint can then be demonstrated while the MP joint is held in neutral with the PIP joint in full flexion.[26] Hyperextension of the PIP joint is resisted by the transverse retinacular ligaments that restrain dorsal displacement of the lateral bands during extension, as well as by the flexor superficialis tendon and palmar plate. These observations form the anatomic rationale for surgical tenotomy of the central tendon in selected patients with mallet finger deformity.[74]

The dorsal fibers of the retinacular ligament (triangular ligament) significantly influence the sequence of events after rupture of the central tendon. Partial tears of the triangular ligament retain sufficient control of the lateral bands to ensure dorsal positioning during extension, with a favorable prognosis for return of extensor function after closed treatment. Partial tears, however, extend if unprotected motion continues after an injury.[76] Complete tear of the triangular ligament, combined with interruption of the central tendon, eliminates control of both joint extension and the lateral bands. This situation initiates an imbalance that results in a fixed deformity unless diligent treatment intercedes. Passive extension of the PIP joint implies that the lateral bands

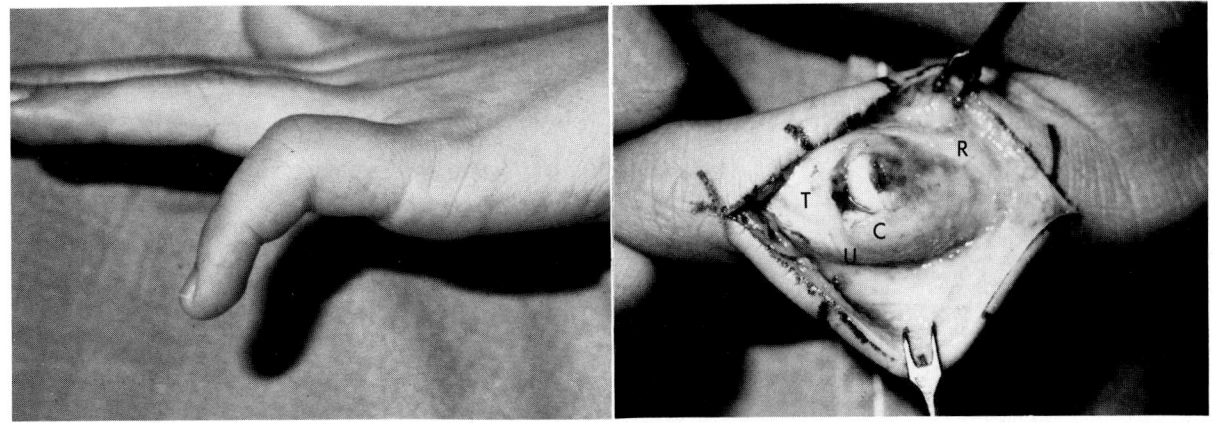

Fig. 35-23   Closed rupture of extensor tendon about proximal interphalangeal joint. Active and passive extension were limited. No resistance to flexion of the distal joint was present. **A,** Clinical posture of injured finger. **B,** Operative findings. Central tendon ruptured with herniation of head of proximal phalanx; triangular ligament was preserved. Radial lateral band trapped beneath condyle of proximal phalanx. Inability to passively extend proximal interphalangeal joint is indication for primary operative repair in extensor tendon injuries at this level. *C,* Central tendon; *R,* radial lateral band; *T,* triangular ligament; *U,* ulnar lateral band.

have relocated dorsally; closed treatment can proceed.

The finger is vulnerable to combined tissue injuries that involve the extensor tendons, collateral ligaments, and palmar plate when the flexed PIP joint is subjected to torsional stress.[33] Axial instability *with* extensor tendon rupture after a closed injury is an indication for primary surgery. Loss of active *and* passive extension of the PIP joint occurs when a lateral band becomes trapped beneath the condylar flare of the proximal phalanx—another indication for primary operative intervention (Fig. 35-23).

Examination of the injured PIP joint

Observation of distribution of swelling and precise localization of tenderness are important during assessment of closed injuries about the PIP joint. Palpation with the finger tip or the eraser tip of a pencil is useful for localizing injury. Active extension of both PIP and DIP joints against gravity and against resistance is assessed. Observe (1) the ability to initiate extension of the fully flexed PIP joint while the MP joint is in neutral,[93] (2) the ability to complete extension of the PIP joint while the wrist and MP joints are flexed,[13] (3) the ability to maintain the PIP joint in full extension, and (4) the ability to extend the DIP joint while the PIP joint is in moderate (30 to 40 degrees) and full flexion.[26] Passive extension of the PIP joint and resistance to passive flexion of the DIP joint while the PIP joint is held in extension are compared with normal fingers. Axial stability for both sides of the joint and hyperextension stability are assessed. Radiographs should include PA, true lateral, and both oblique views.

Some conclusions can be drawn from the systematic examination just described. Palmar tenderness proximal to the PIP joint with normal dorsal examination after a hyperextension injury suggests treatment to prevent a pseudo-boutonnière deformity. Inability to initiate extension of the fully flexed PIP joint or to complete the final 15 to 20 degrees of active extension while the MP joint is flexed implies interruption of the central tendon. The PIP joint can be held in extension by a single lateral band if that tendon rests

dorsally; the other lateral band and the triangular ligament may still be torn. Increased tension—compared with normal fingers—with passive flexion of the DIP joint while the PIP joint is held in extension suggests interruption of the central tendon with proximal slide of the extensor tendons. Weak active extension of the DIP joint with the PIP joint in moderate (30 to 40 degrees) flexion implies continuity of at least one lateral band.[93] Active extension of the DIP joint with the PIP joint in full flexion can be performed only after rupture of the central tendon. Axial instability infers collateral ligament rupture. Axial instability combined with extensor tendon rupture denotes combined tissue injuries and is an indication for primary operative repair.[33]

Boutonnière deformity

The boutonnière deformity develops after an injury to the extensor mechanism and specifically denotes flexion of the PIP joint with hyperextension of the DIP joint. The head of the proximal phalanx herniates through a defect in the extensor mechanism after rupture of the central tendon and dorsal fibers of the retinacular ligament (triangular ligament).[24] An analogous deformity occurs in the thumb with MP flexion and interphalangeal extension. The mechanisms of closed injury include involuntary forceful flexion of an actively extended digit, blunt trauma to the dorsum of the joint, and dislocation of the joint with tearing of the extensor tendons and stabilizing ligaments.

Interruption of the central tendon and triangular ligament permits proximal displacement of the extensor mechanism and palmar shift of the lateral bands. The unopposed flexor digitorum superficialis flexes the PIP joint. The extrinsic extensor tendon, released from the middle phalanx, transfers forces through the sagittal bands that enhance extension of the MP joint. Both extrinsic and intrinsic muscles transmit exaggerated forces through the conjoined lateral bands that extend the DIP joint. The transverse retinacular ligaments, oblique retinacular ligaments, and check ligaments of the palmar plate are loose early in the evolution of the deformity (Fig. 35-24, *A* and *B*). The test for retinacular tightness is

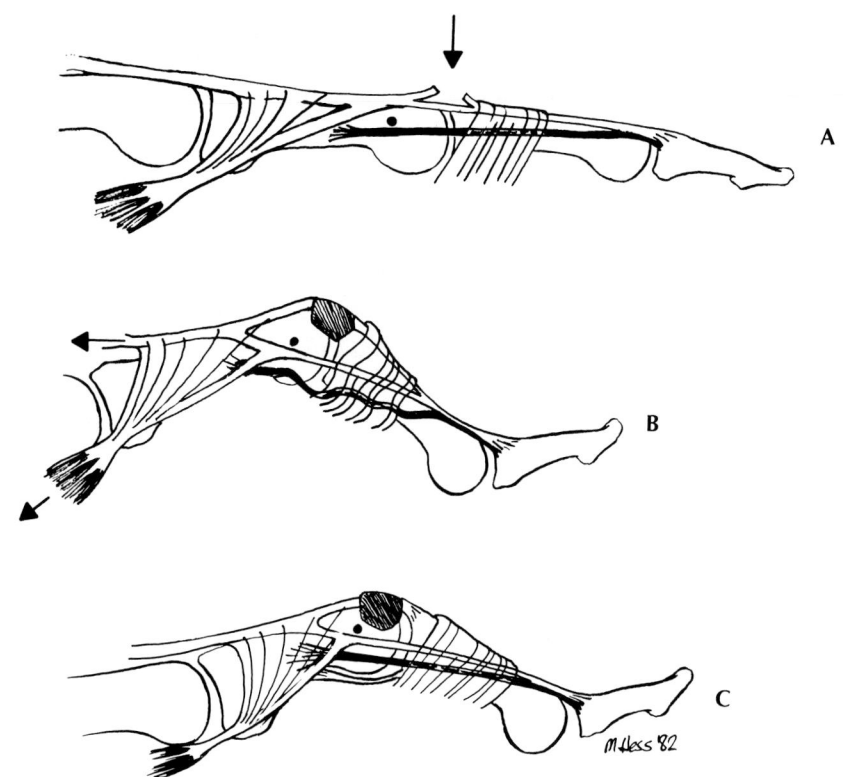

Fig. 35-24 Development of boutonnière deformity. **A,** Injury involves insertion of central extensor tendon at base of the middle phalanx with interruption of the dorsal fibers of the transverse retinacular ligament. **B,** Middle phalanx is pulled into flextion by the flexor digitorum superficialis. Lateral bands displace palmarly over axis of the joint and become flexors of this joint. At this stage, palmar plate ligaments and oblique and transverse retinacular ligaments are loose. The deformity can be reversed with relative ease. **C,** Established deformity with shortening of extensor tendons, tightening of palmar plate ligaments, oblique and transverse retinacular ligaments. Retinacular tightness test is positive. Passive correction of deformity is resisted. Reversal of deformity at this stage is slow and represents a significant commitment by surgeon and therapist.

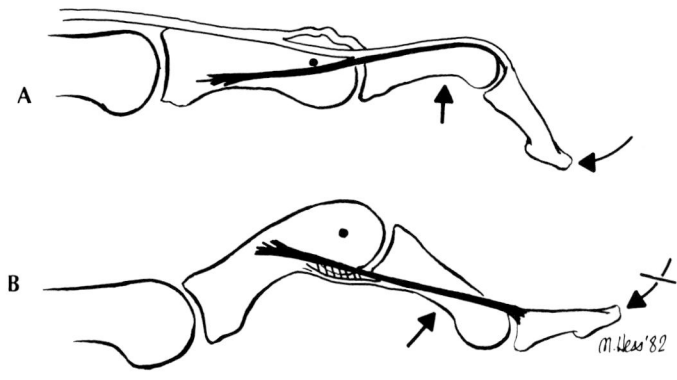

Fig. 35-25 Testing for tightness of oblique retinacular ligament. **A,** Passive extension of middle phalanx with passive flexion of distal phalanx is performed without resistence in normal finger: a negative test. **B,** Contracture of oblique retinacular ligament, with resistant flexion of proximal interphalangeal joint and hyperextension of distal interphalangeal joint. Distal joint cannot be passively flexed when extension of the proximal interphalangeal joint is passively increased: a positive test.

negative, and the deformity is passively reversible (Fig. 35-25, *A*). The lateral bands return to their normal dorsal station and can maintain extension. Prognosis after splinting is most favorable during this early phase.

The lateral bands progressively descend and the PIP joint cannot be maintained in full extension. An active extension lag develops that is passively correctable as long as the transverse and oblique retinacular ligaments and palmar plate remain supple and have not foreshortened (Fig. 35-24, *B*).

The palmarly displaced lateral bands become fixed to the underlying collateral ligaments and joint capsule, as the retinacular ligaments and palmar plate tighten and oppose passive correction (Fig. 35-24, *C*). The DIP joint loses active flexion, develops hyperextension, and progressively loses passive flexion. The retinacular tightness test is then positive (Fig. 35-25, *B*). The deformity is fixed and cannot be reversed without sustained effort. Treatment of the fixed deformity is complicated, and the prognosis is altered (Fig. 35-26).

Nonoperative treatment

Closed extensor tendon injuries about the PIP joint must be accurately appraised and monitored closely (Table 35-1). Prescribed treatment is designed for a specific injury. A

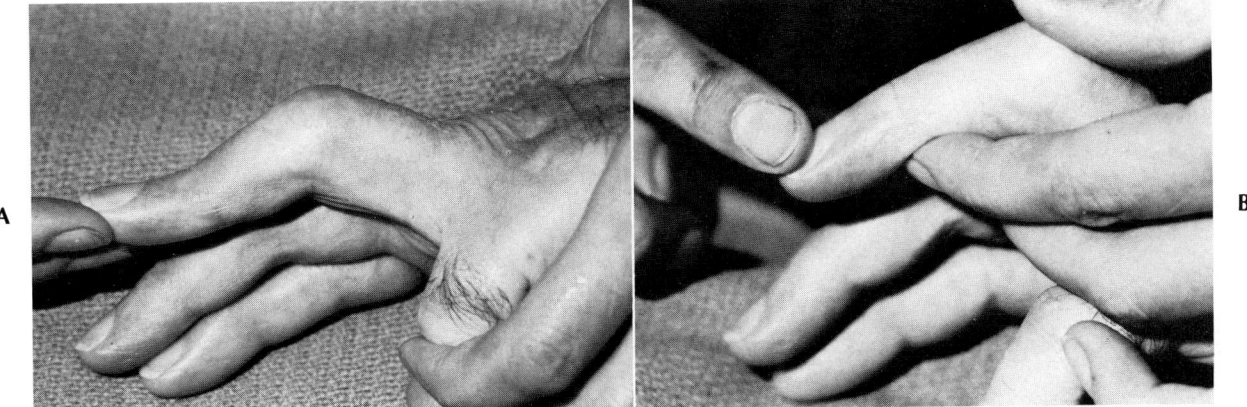

Fig. 35-26   Established boutonnière deformity. **A,** Fixed flexion deformity of proximal interphalangeal joint with hyperextension of the distal interphalangeal joint. **B,** Resistant passive flexion of the distal interphalangeal joint with attempted exension of the proximal interphalangeal joint from tightness of retinacular ligaments augmented by tightness of extensor tendons through displaced lateral bands.

palmar injury with potential for a pseudo-boutonnière deformity is approached differently from a dorsal injury with potential for a classic boutonnière deformity. Swelling and dorsal tenderness should be considered indications of an injury to the extensor tendons even when examination suggests intact structures. Partial ligament and tendon tears may extend unless the injured digit is protected.[76] The PIP joint is splinted in extension, and the digit is reassessed in 1 week. DIP joint motion is permitted during this period. A repeat normal functional examination of the finger implies that complete tendon rupture has not occurred. Splinting is continued for an additional 2 weeks, however, if swelling, tenderness, or ecchymosis is noted during reexamination. Splinting is discontinued after 3 weeks if the patient continues to demonstrate intact extensor tendons and no deformity has developed.

Splint or digital cast for a closed extensor tendon injury about the PIP joint treated without operative intervention immobilizes the PIP joint in neutral. The MP joint and DIP joint are left free. Active distal joint flexion synergistically relaxes the intrinsic and extrinsic extensor tendon muscles. A 3 to 4 mm glide is imparted to the central tendon through the lateral bands while the PIP joint is restrained.[60] The

oblique retinacular ligament is also exercised through continued distal joint motion.

A splinting program recommended for treatment of the established boutonnière deformity should be tailored to fit the tissue requirements of the patient. The physician and therapist should be familiar with the anatomy of the extensor tendons and the pathomechanics of the deformity being treated. Initial splinting supports the PIP joint in neutral while permitting active flexion of the DIP joint. This is continued without interruption for 6 weeks. Carefully monitored flexion of the PIP joint is then initiated. The PIP joint is supported in extension for another 2 to 4 weeks whenever active motion is not being pursued. The requirement for continued support of the PIP joint is determined by the presence or absence of postural stability of the finger. Splinting is reinstituted if an extensor lag or boutonnière deformity recurs. Splinting is recommended only at night when PIP joint extension can be sustained and there has been no deterioration during subsequent visits.

The time required for rehabilitation of the boutonnière deformity by splinting can be prolonged. Resistant cases can require attention and supervision for 6 to 9 months after injury. Tissue maturation with realization of the full poten-

Table 35-1   Treatment of closed injuries of the extensor tendons of the proximal interphalangeal (PIP) joint

Clinical findings		
Suggestive examination	Active extension loss	Active extension loss
Active extension	Passive extension	Passive extension loss
Passive extension	No fracture	? Axial instability
No fracture		? Fracture
Treatment		
Splint PIP joint	Splint PIP joint for 6 weeks	Primary repair
Reassess in 1 week	? Kirschner wire	Open reduction fracture
		? 2nd-stage tendon reconstruction

Modified from Rosenthal EA: Extensor surface injuries at the proximal interphalangeal joint. In Bowers WH, editor: The hand and upper limb, vol 1, The interphalangeal joints, London, UK, 1987, by permission Churchill Livingstone, Inc.

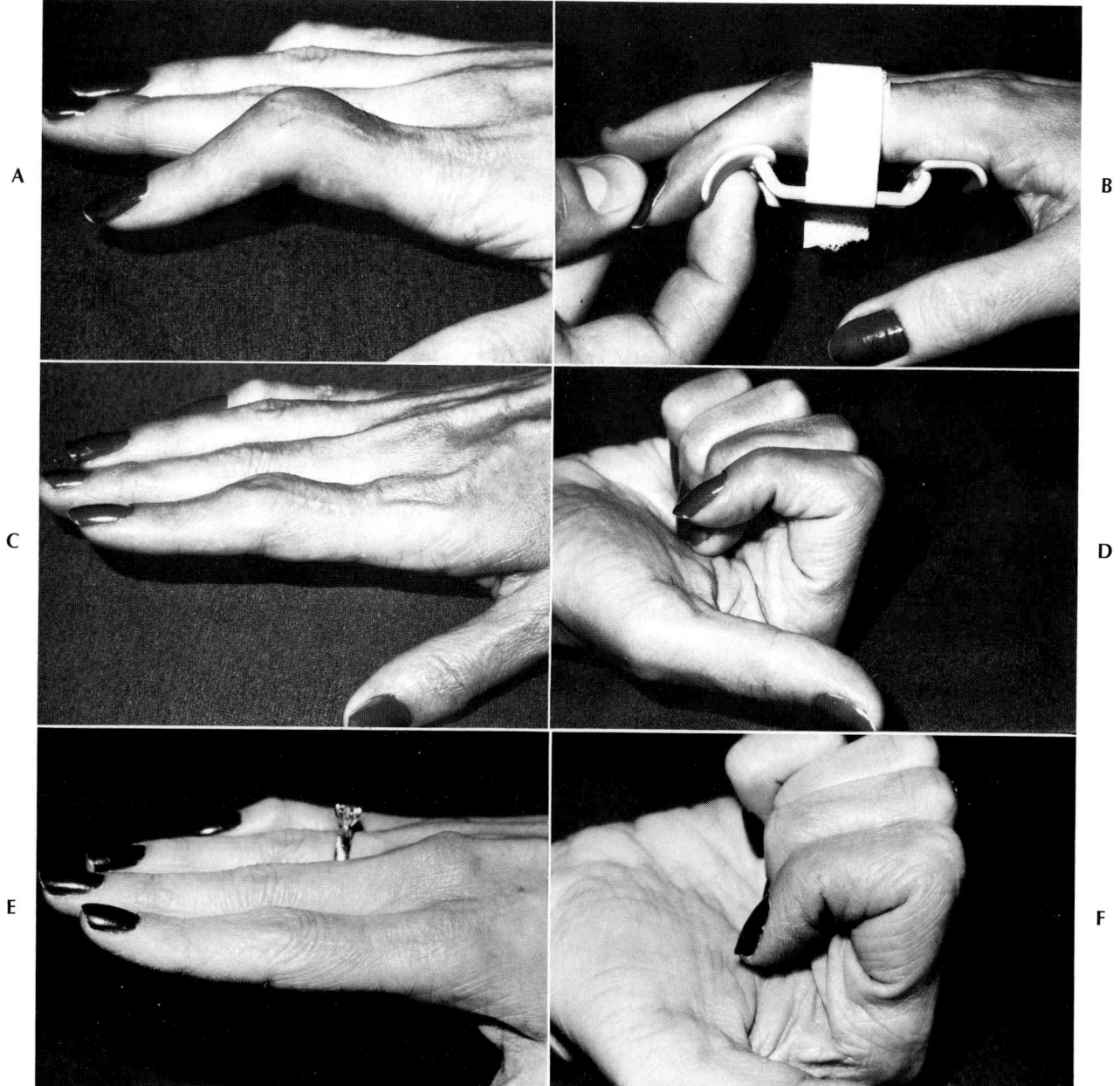

Fig. 35-27 Conservative treatment of boutonnière deformity. Laceration of extensor tendons with delayed primary treatment and wound infection. **A,** Fixed deformity with resistant flexion of proximal interphalangeal joint and extension of distal joint. **B,** Supervised dynamic splinting designed to reestablish extension of the proximal joint and flexion of the distal joint deformities. (Splint marketed as New Extension Finger Splint in six sizes by Christensen Orthopedic Supply Company [COSCO], Hermosa Beach, CA.) **C,** Five months after program instituted, active extension with normal power was present. Tissue softening is progressing. Dorsal bump presents cosmetic disfigurement. **D,** Active flexion after 5 months. **E,** Complete extension with mature soft tissues and reduced disfigurement after 3 years. **F,** Active flexion after 3 years.

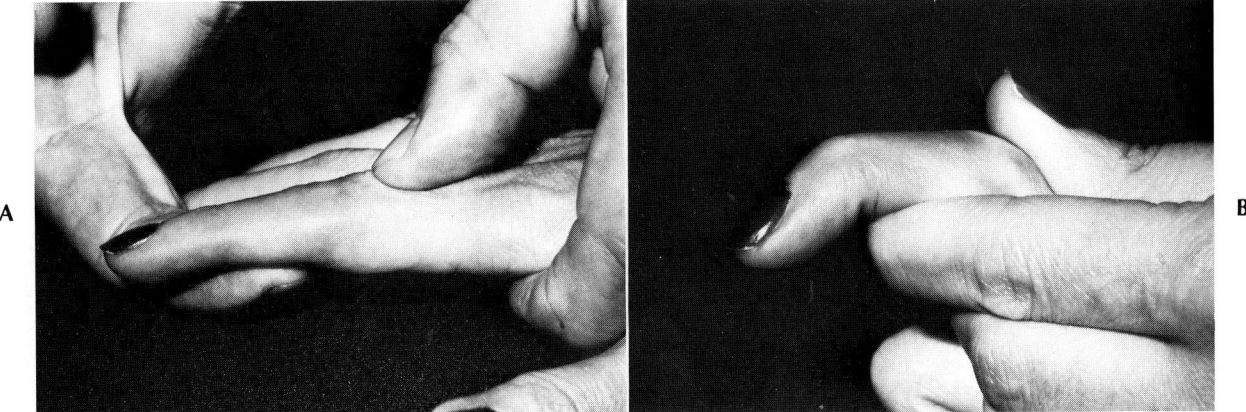

Fig. 35-28   Passive correction of deformity before surgery improves prognosis. **A,** Reversal of flexion deformity of proximal interphalangeal joint. **B,** Active flexion of distal interphalangeal joint with complete passive extension of proximal interphalangeal joint confirms sufficient lengthening of extensor tendons and retinacular ligaments for appropriate consideration of surgery.

tial function of the finger may not be achieved for a full year (Fig. 35-27).

Operative treatment

Surgical repair is indicated for the acute closed injury with loss of passive extension of the PIP joint and in combined tissue injuries when central tendon rupture is associated with joint instability. Severe soft tissue injuries associated with fractures may require staged reconstruction: the fracture is repaired primarily, and tendon restoration is performed as a second-stage procedure after the fractures have healed.

Surgery for the chronic boutonnière deformity is a selective decision. The impact of a mild (less than 30 degrees) flexion deformity of the PIP joint is individually diverse and may not significantly interfere with grasp or finger function. The cosmetic deformity often is disliked by patients but may not be sufficient for them to request surgical reconstruction. A comfortable and useful range of active flexion of both interphalangeal joints provides excellent function despite the persistence of a slight flexion deformity of the PIP joint.

More severe deformities do create functional impairments. A large portion of the handicap with an established boutonnière deformity reflects loss of distal joint flexion. Candidates for surgery should be carefully selected after evaluating their symptoms, deformity, anticipated improvement from treatment, and compliance. Selection as a candidate for surgery implies a willingness to participate in a closely supervised, often prolonged, rehabilitation program after surgery.

Reversal of the PIP joint flexion deformity with active DIP joint flexion should be achieved before surgery (Fig. 35-28). The results from surgery are better when joint deformities are corrected preoperatively.[66] Mature, hard, resistant scar occasionally demonstrates a surprising plasticity when subjected to tension for long periods. Tendon reconstructions alone will not improve the passive correction that preoperative treatment has gained (Fig. 35-29).

Fingers that cannot be corrected by means of splinting

and supervised therapy require extensive surgical releases that introduce new imbalances capable of promoting additional deformity (Fig. 35-30). The works by Burton[12] and Rosenthal[97] provide expanded discussions of operative management of deformities from extensor tendon injuries about the PIP joint.

EXTENSOR TENDON INJURIES AT THE DIP JOINT

Mallet finger is synonymous with interruption of the extensor tendon mechanism at the level of the DIP joint. The term is not descriptive but has gained universal acceptance for the deformity that results (Fig. 35-31).

The terminal extensor tendon represents the distal extension of the merged lateral bands that insert on the dorsal base of the distal phalanx. The more central fibers of the tendon are bordered by the distal extensions of the oblique retinacular ligaments that insert on the lateral base of the distal phalanx adjacent to the terminal tendon.[128] The interweaving of adjacent tendon and ligament fibers before inserting contributes to the success with treatment of central tendon injuries at this level.

Patterns of injury

The patterns of closed injuries depend on the position of the DIP joint at the time of injury and on the direction of the injuring force. The treatment depends on the type of injury.

Passive flexion of the distal phalanx is resisted by tension through the terminal tendon through the initial 45 degrees of DIP joint flexion. The oblique retinacular and collateral ligaments are normally relaxed through this range. Direct trauma to the partially flexed distal phalanx ruptures (frays) the central fibers of the terminal tendon over the trochlea of the middle phalanx.[112] The oblique retinacular ligaments are not under tension and remain intact. The interwoven border fibers of tendon and ligament retain some anatomic continuity with the base of the distal phalanx (Fig. 35-32). The partial extension that these patients appear to retain is

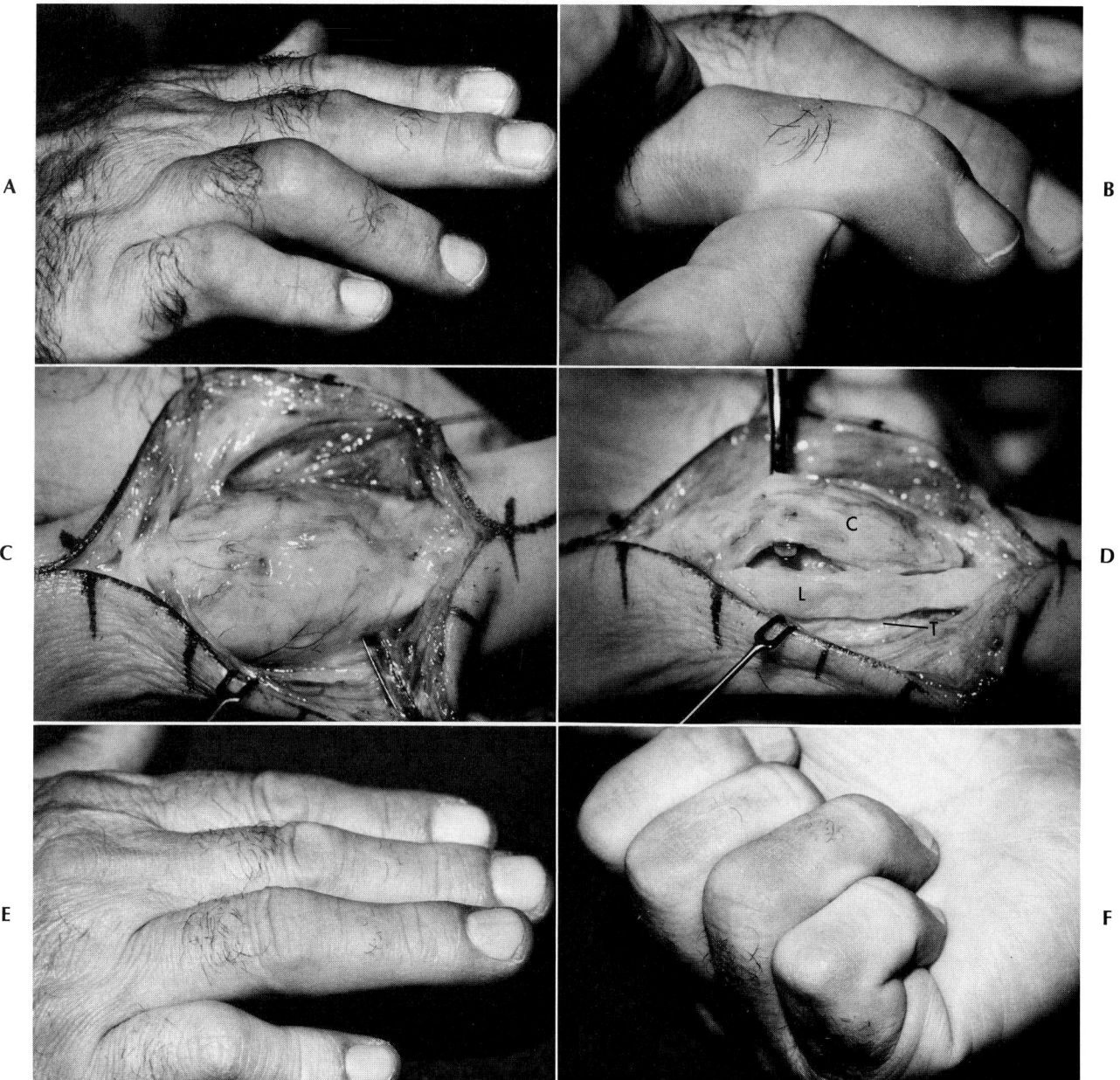

Fig. 35-29 Chronic boutonnière deformity with functional impairment. Closed ring finger injury in 67-year-old man initially treated with 2 weeks splinting. Regression followed removal of splint. **A,** Posture when first evaluated. Passive correction of the proximal interphalangeal joint achieved with splinting. **B,** Active distal joint flexion with proximal interphalangeal joint in neutral confirms reversal of tendon and ligament tightness. **C,** Normal tendon anatomy about the proximal interphalangeal joint transformed by scar; subluxated ulnar lateral band adherent to capsule. **D,** Elevator lifts central tendon created from scarred tissue. Lateral bands surgically defined. Thick transverse retinacular ligaments incised. Proximal and distal joint extensor tendons were functionally rebalanced. **E,** Active extension 7 months after surgery lacks 20 degrees. **F,** Active flexion at 7 months. *C,* Central tendon; *L,* lateral band; *T,* transverse retinacular ligament.

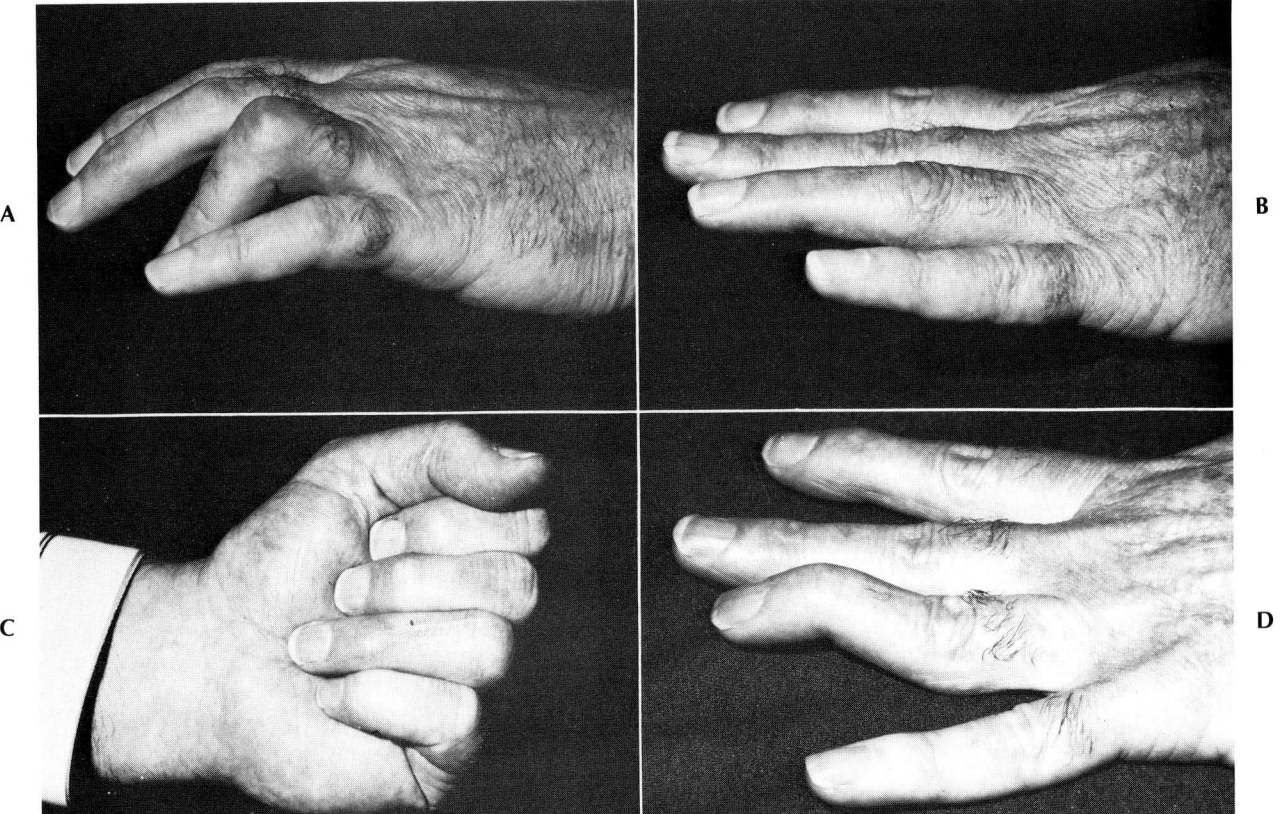

Fig. 35-30   Man, 45 years old, with closed injury of extensor tendons at the proximal interphalangeal joint. Unsuccessful surgery 3 months after injury for uncorrected boutonnière deformity. Surgery included suture of lateral bands dorsally with terminal tendon tenotomy. **A,** Fixed deformity when first seen 4 months after surgery. **B,** Clinical extension 6 months after anatomic reconstruction of the central tendon, palmar plate release, and resection accessory collateral ligaments of the proximal interphalangeal joint. The extensor tendon over the middle phalanx was not disturbed. **C,** Active flexion 6 months after surgery. **D,** Posture 9 years after reconstruction. Swan-neck deformity has developed from hyperextension instability of the proximal interphalangeal joint. The distal interphalangeal joint is actively flexed. Mature scar retains some plasticity when subjected to chronic tensions. Extensive surgical releases introduce a potential for imbalances beyond those in original deformity.

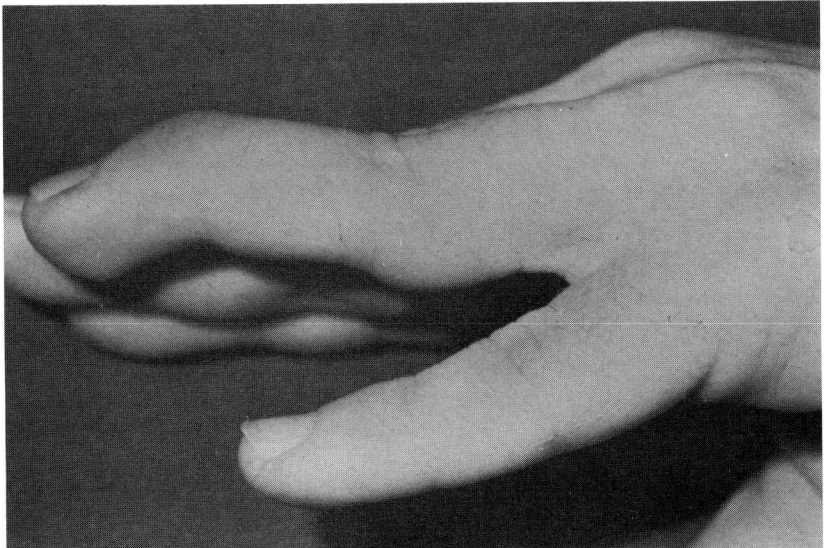

Fig. 35-31   Mallet finger with hyperextension deformity of the proximal interphalangeal joint. Interruption of terminal tendon concentrates extension forces at the middle phalanx. Swan-neck deformity with mallet tendon lesion has a wide range of severity.

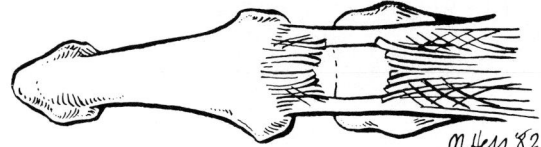

Fig. 35-32 Mallet tendon lesion. Rupture of terminal tendon occurs proximally to its insertion over trochlea of the middle phalanx. Interweaving between the extensor tendon and oblique retinacular ligament may maintain some continuity of the extensor tendon with the distal phalanx.

from the collateral ligamants of the joint and retinacular ligaments.[106] The extensor lag is passively correctable. This is a pure tendon lesion.

The terminal tendon and the oblique retinacular ligaments are both under tension when the DIP joint is flexed beyond 45 degrees. Passive flexion of the distal phalanx while tension is transmitted through the terminal tendon produces a dorsal avulsion fracture with total interruption in the functional continuity of the extensor tendon[115] (Fig. 35-33).

A longitudinal impaction force that hyperextends the DIP joint creates a large articular fracture of the base of the distal phalanx[61] (Fig. 35-34, *A*). This is a significant joint injury. The impact on extensor tendon function is often small, without a mallet deformity. The large dorsal fragment retains collateral ligament attachments to the middle phalanx. Dorsal fractures of more than one third of the base of the distal phalanx may be unstable.[114,124] The degree of instability relates to disruption of collateral ligament attachments to the distal fracture fragment. A stable distal fragment flexes; the unstable distal fragment is pulled proximally by the flexor profundus and subluxates palmarward (Fig. 35-34, *B*). Patients are inclined to dismiss the injury as trivial and may not seek early treatment.

Development of deformity

Interruption of the terminal tendon insertion permits retraction of the extensor tendons proximally. This transfers tension to the central tendon and conjoined lateral bands. The central tendon (via its bony insertion) and the lateral bands (via the transverse retinacular ligaments) concentrate extension forces on the middle phalanx. The palmar plate resists hyperextension of the PIP joint. The retinacular ligaments are initially lax. Hyperextension of the PIP joint develops if the palmar plate is lax. The flexor profundus flexes the DIP joint, and a mild swan neck deformity develops. The severity of the deformity is inversely proportional to the stability of the palmar plate at the PIP joint (Fig. 35-35). The swan neck deformity from a mallet tendon lesion is not usually severe enough to impart difficulties with finger flexion unless hyperextension of the PIP joint is advanced.

Treatment

Open injuries. Lacerations of the terminal tendon should be approximated. Intramedullary Kirschner-wire (K-wire) pinning of the DIP joint in slight hyperextension will coapt the tendon ends in tidy wounds without the need for tendon sutures.[58] Divided tendons that require suture repair are approximated with fine 5-0 or 6-0 braided white synthetic sutures. The DIP joint is still pinned, because security of the repaired tendon depends primarily on the K-wire. Motion is begun after 6 weeks. The distal joint is supported by splinting between active motion sessions for an additional 2 weeks. Development of an extensor lag indicates the need for further supportive splinting.

Closed injuries. The *mallet tendon lesion without fracture* should be treated with uninterrupted immobilization of the DIP joint in slight hyperextension for 6 weeks.[21,115] The PIP joint is not immobilized. The classic treatment proposed by Smillie,[108] which immobilized the PIP joint in flexion and the DIP joint in hyperextension, is no longer advocated.

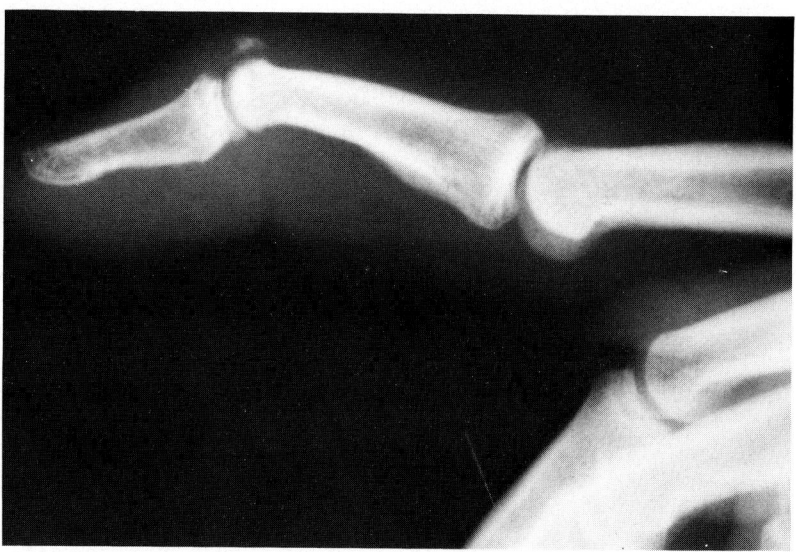

Fig. 35-33 Total interruption of the terminal extensor tendon insertion with the adjacent retinacular ligaments may be associated with a small dorsal avulsion fracture. This produces a mallet deformity. Residual extension of the distal interphalangeal joint caused by collateral ligaments.

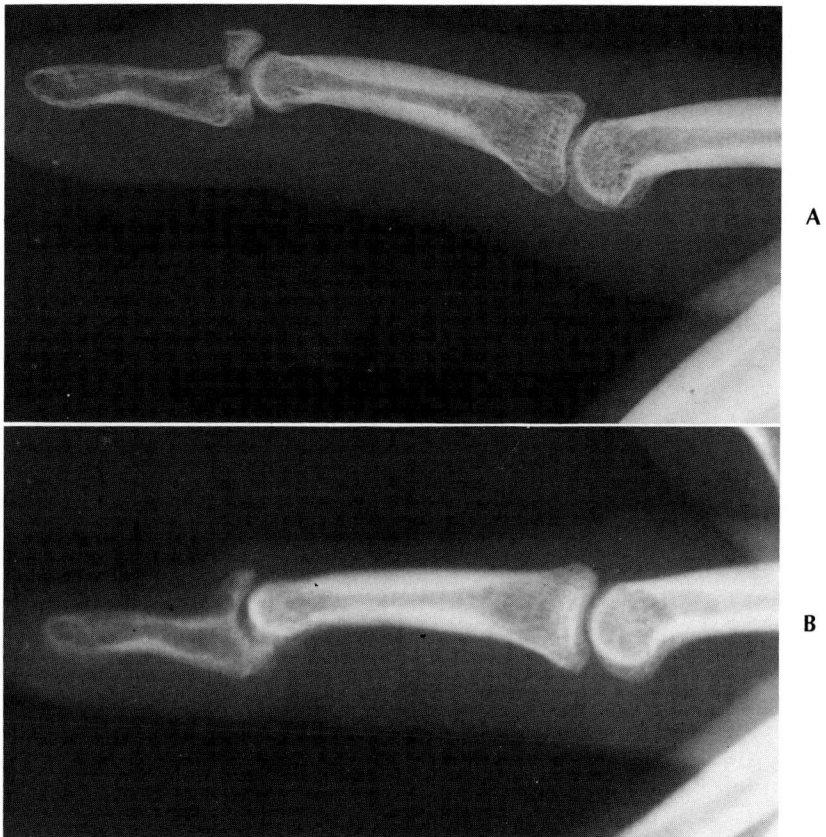

Fig. 35-34 Impaction hyperextension injury produces major articular fracture with potential instability of distal interphalangeal joint, usually without mallet deformity. **A,** Roentgenogram at time of injury. Patient was treated with digital casting for 3 weeks, followed by 3 weeks of splinting. **B,** Three months after injury. Early remodeling with persistent palmar subluxation is evident; traumatic arthritis is established. Major articular distal joint injuries are unstable. Despite significant potential for remodeling, operative reduction with internal stabilization is meritorious.

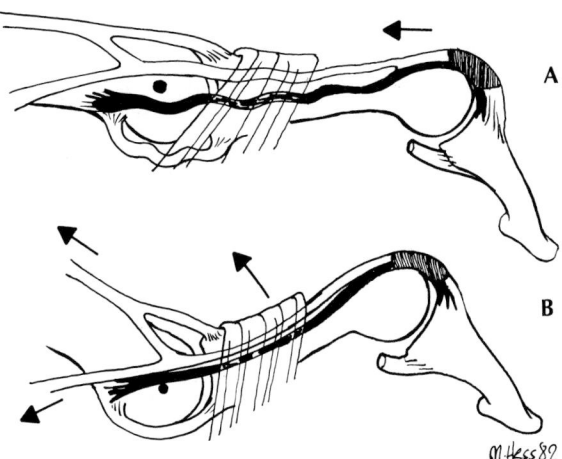

Fig. 35-35 Development of mallet deformity. **A,** Interruption of extensor tendon over distal interphalangeal joint permits unopposed flexion of joint by flexor digitorum profundus tendon. Loss of distal restraint permits proximal slide of extensor tendons. Oblique retinacular ligaments and lateral bands become slack. Palmar plate at the proximal interphalangeal joint resists hyperextension at the proximal interphalangeal joint. **B,** Concentration of the extension forces from extrinsic and intrinsic muscles transmitted through the central tendon, lateral bands, and transverse retinacular ligaments produces hyperextension at the proximal interphalangeal joint. Hyperextension increases as palmar plate yields. Transposed dorsal lateral bands and tight oblique retinacular ligaments resist flexion until forced palmarly over the condylar flares of the proximal phalanx from extreme flexion of the distal joint by flexor profundus.

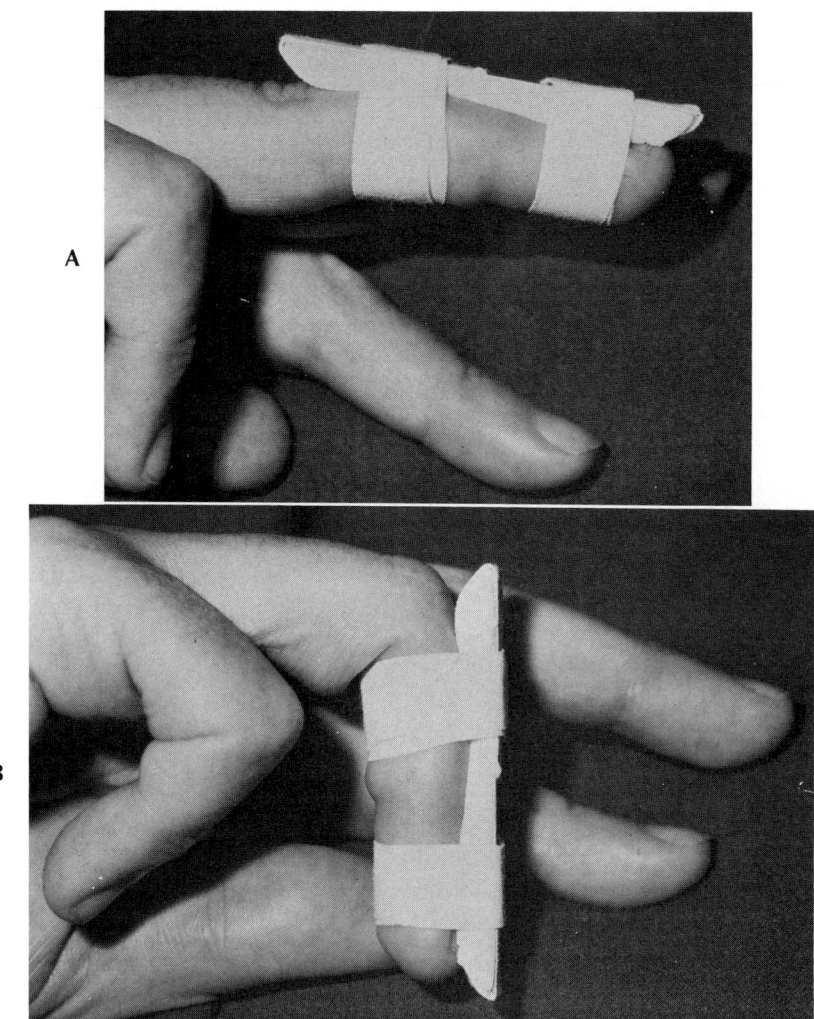

Fig. 35-36 Dorsal splint for mallet finger. **A,** Splint maintains distal joint in slight hyperextension. Hyperextension is an individual determination. **B,** Proximal interphalangeal joint motion is encouraged throughout the 6 weeks of uninterrupted splinting recommended for initial treatment of mallet finger. Proximal interphalangeal joint flexion has little impact on the distal tendon injury with the distal interphalangeal joint in hyperextension in the normal finger.

Hyperextension may produce dorsal skin blanching with cutaneous and terminal tendon ischemia. The safe position for splinting is individualized; dorsal skin should not blanch in the splinted position.[88] Reliable patients can be treated with splinting; others may require K-wire pinning. Some patients require adjusting the attitude of the splinted joint as the swelling of injury subsides and further extension is tolerated.

Numerous designs for prefabricated mallet splints have been marketed. The traditional Stack splint has been windowed to permit evaporation of moisture and pulp contact during splinting.[113] Perforated thermoplastic splints with Velcro straps are also available.[54] The variations in digital contour, joint flexibility, and swelling after injury support use of splints individually crafted for each injured finger. Dorsal splinting of the DIP joint with a foam-padded aluminum splint does not encroach on the tactile palmar surface of the finger and avoids localized pressure over the site of tendon injury (Fig. 35-36). A better-fitting splint is achieved by thinning the foam of commercially available splints. Cloth adhesive tape between the foam and skin reduces maceration. The splint may be changed periodically by the insightful patient; other patients require more frequent visits to the physician or therapist. Active motion of the PIP joint is continued throughout the period of splinting; this flexion reduces tension at the site of injury. Distal joint motion is begun after 6 weeks of continuous splinting. Night splinting of the distal joint is continued for an additional 4 weeks after distal joint motion is begun (Fig. 35-37).

Loss of active extension—an extension lag—and decreased distal joint flexion from terminal tendon scarring both are complications from closed treatment of the mallet tendon lesion.[101] Dorsal skin maceration or necrosis is a complication of improper splinting. Full-time splinting should be reinstituted if clinical regression occurs after active distal joint motion is begun.

Treatment of the *distal tendon avulsion fracture* is the same as that described for a pure tendon lesion. Positioning

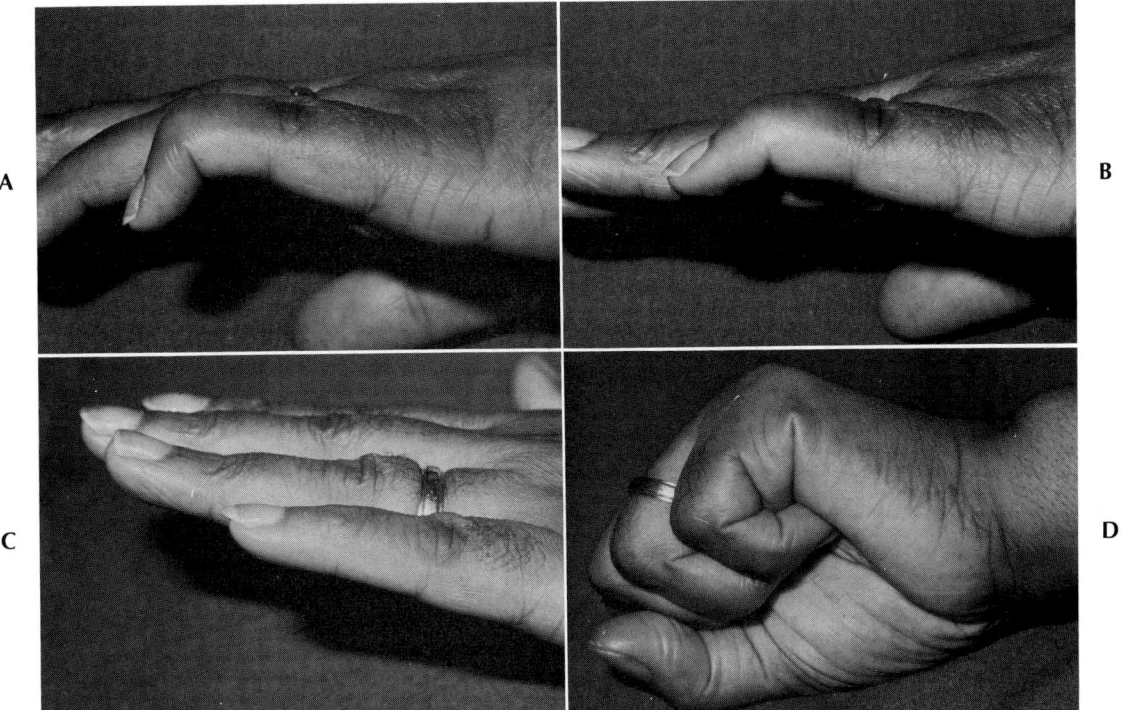

Fig. 35-37 Chronic mallet deformity from blunt injury in 54-year-old woman. **A,** Resting attitude of −70 degrees. **B,** Active extension to −55 degrees, suggesting potential benefit from splinting. **C,** Active extension after 7 weeks of uninterrupted splinting and an additional 4 weeks of night splinting. **D,** Active flexion.

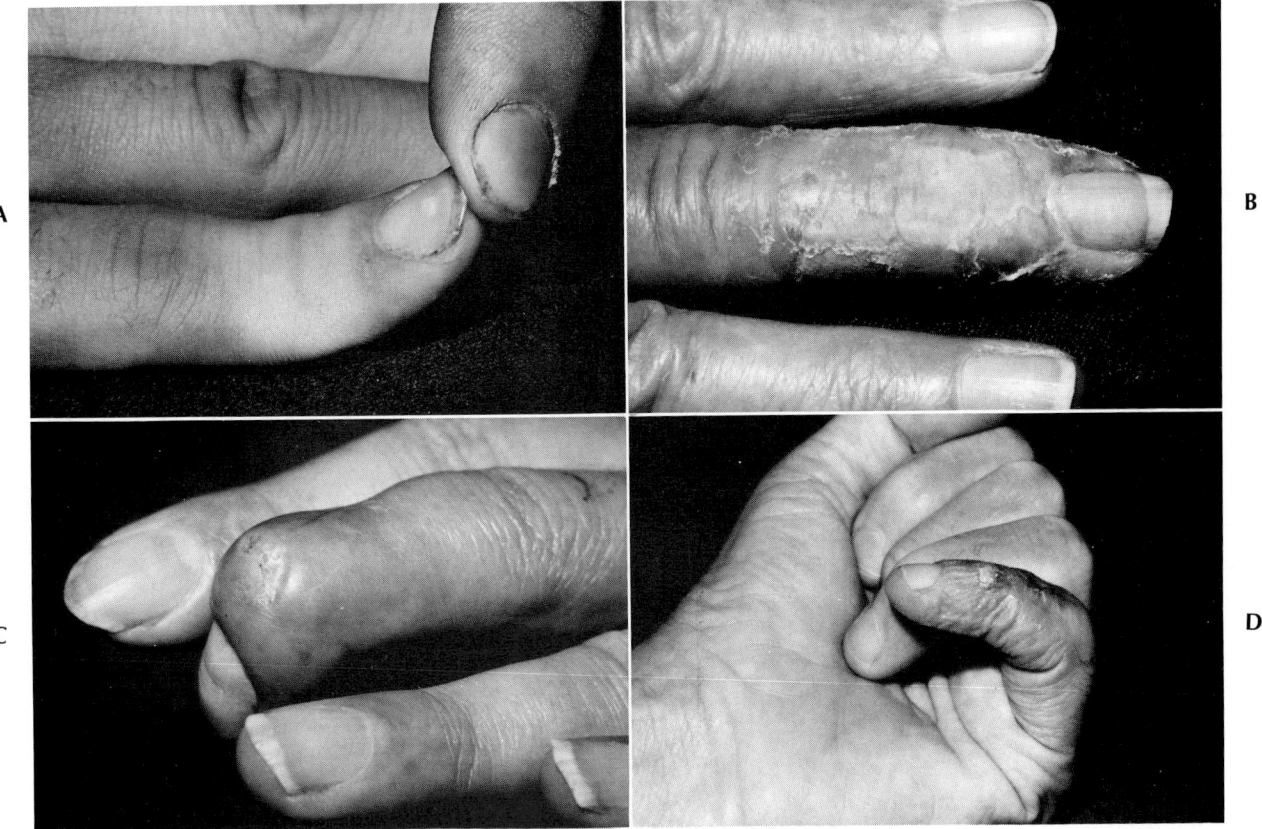

Fig. 35-38 Complications of treatment for mallet finger deformity. **A,** Dorsal skin blanching signifies ischemia of subcutaneous tissues and the terminal tendon. **B,** Maceration of dorsal skin beneath the splint from neglect. Secondary infection can develop. **C,** Chronic pyarthrosis with necrosis of the terminal tendon following surgery. Middle phalanx projects through the scar. **D,** Tenodesis of the extensor tendons with osteomyelitis of the middle phalanx following surgery. Distal joint is subluxated.

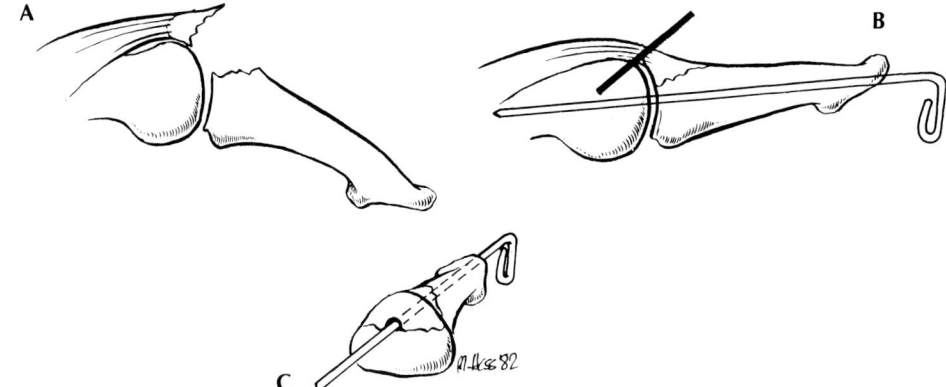

Fig. 35-39 Operative method for major articular fracture of the distal interphalangeal joint. **A,** Injury represents significant interruption of articular surface with potential instability. Impact upon extensor tendons may be small. **B,** Accurate reduction of fracture fragments. Longitudinal wire stabilizes the distal joint in neutral or slight extension. Oblique buttress wire compresses the fracture site and prevents retracation of the proximal fragment by extensor tendon. **C,** Palmar surface of the proximal fragment may be notched to accommodate Kirschner wire.

the distal joint in slight extension returns the distal phalanx to the small proximal fragment. Success can be monitored by comparing lateral x-ray films taken before and after splinting. Calcification of the bridging callus may form a dorsal beak that nonetheless represents functional continuity of the extensor tendon and is not usually symptomatic.

Nonoperative treatment of larger *articular fractures of the distal phalanx* has been recommended because of the significant capacity of the distal phalanx to remodel its articular surface and the incidence of complications after surgery.[124] The most frequent impairment after open reduction of a major articular fracture of the distal phalanx is decreased flexion of the DIP joint from a scar tenodesis over the middle phalanx.[38] Other reported complications from surgery for this injury are wound infection, thinning of the dorsal skin, joint injury, nail bed injury, pulp fibrosis, pain, and dysesthesias[85] (Fig. 35-38). Despite the capacity for these injured joints to remodel with nonoperative treatment,[123] an accurate approximation of the fracture fragments has merit.[80,114] Approximation of the distal phalanx to the retracted proximal fragment can be performed through a transverse incision localized over the fracture site without disturbing the terminal tendon proximal to the joint. The dorsal capsule proximally should not be disturbed. An oblique .028 K-wire compresses the fracture site and prevents proximal retraction of the terminal tendon.[64] The anterior edge of the dorsal fragment can be notched to accommodate the wire that stabilizes the distal joint. This delicate procedure is technically demanding and represents a challenge in precision. The wires are removed after 6 weeks, and active motion is begun. Night splinting is continued for 2 to 4 weeks until absence of an extension lag is assured (Fig. 35-39).

Chronic mallet finger deformity may implicate only the DIP joint or may demonstrate an imbalance collapse of the entire finger, a swan neck deformity. Secondary suture or plication of the terminal tendon scar has been advocated. Results are not uniformly good. The tendon has a small excursion, and a tenodesis that restricts distal joint motion is likely to form. If the distal joint is unsightly or intrusive, an arthrodesis provides a painless, stable, cosmetically improved finger.

The chronic mallet finger with a swan-neck deformity presents a more complex problem. Surgery to rebalance the finger should not be considered unless both joints are healthy and the joint deformities are passively correctable. The finger can be rebalanced by tenotomy of the central tendon insertion at the PIP joint.[7,34,40] The lateral slips to the intrinsic tendons and at least one of the transverse retinacular ligaments must be preserved. The lateral slips retain terminal tendon continuity with the extrinsic extensor tendon. The transverse retinacular ligaments resist PIP joint hyperextension from dorsal displacement of the lateral bands. An extensor tendolysis over the middle phalanx is needed if there is no improvement in distal joint position after the tenotomy (Fig. 35-40).

Swan-neck deformity in a mallet finger with significant hyperextension of the PIP joint may be rebalanced with an oblique retinacular ligament using a free tendon graft.[55,119] The tendon graft passes from the dorsum of the distal phalanx around the digit palmar to the flexor sheath and is attached proximal to the PIP joint. This reverses both distal joint flexion and proximal joint hyperextension.

SWAN-NECK DEFORMITY

The collapse deformity of the fingers that is metaphorically called the swan-neck deformity is a postural deformity with numerous causes. The deformity results from an imbalance of forces within the finger that creates an instability with collapse between the proximal, middle, and distal phalanges. Hyperextension of the PIP joint with flexion of the DIP joint—the swan-neck deformity—is the postural deformity that results.

The swan-neck deformity that follows the mallet finger tendon injury is one example of such an imbalance. The pathomechanics of swan-neck deformity from other causes, however, result in similar distortions of the finger extensor tendons and retinacular and capsular ligaments. The initiating factor may be increased forces through the extensor or intrinsic tendons, PIP joint instability, loss of the flexor superficialis tendon, or release of distal extensor attachment.

The basic mechanism in the swan-neck deformity was discussed relative to the mallet finger. The severity of this deformity increases and is more difficult to reverse with

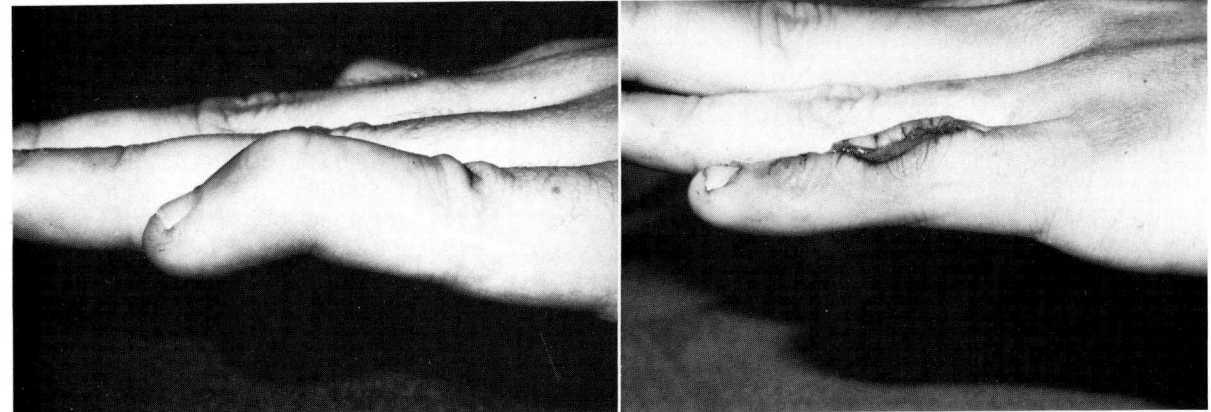

Fig. 35-40   Tenotomy of central tendon insertion on middle phalanx for treatment of selected patients with passively correctable mallet deformity. Tenotomy permits readjustment of tensions through extensor tendons, reversing extensor deficiency at the distal interphalangeal joint and reducing hyperextension forces at the proximal interphalangeal joint. **A,** Preoperative view of patient with a history of three ruptures of the terminal tendon while playing football and two previous surgical attempts at anatomic reconstruction. **B,** Active extension after tenotomy of the central tendon with tendolysis over the middle phalanx. Both transverse retinacular ligaments were preserved.

other etiologies: the transverse retinacular ligaments stretch, triangular ligament fibers shorten, and the lateral bands displace dorsally where they are tethered more securely. The hyperextended PIP joint then resists flexion. A self-sustaining deformity is established as the oblique retinacular ligaments displace dorsally and shorten. Contracted oblique ligaments and lateral bands cannot traverse the condyles of the proximal phalanx during flexion. PIP joint flexion, which normally anticipates flexion of the distal joint, is then preceded by distal joint flexion; synchronized interphalangeal joint flexion is halted. Distal joint flexion proceeds without flexion of the PIP joint until sufficient force develops in the flexor profundus tendon to overcome resistance by the structures dorsal to the PIP joint. An abrupt flexion then occurs as the lateral bands snap over the proximal phalanx. These are the pathomechanics of an established swan-neck deformity. Joint deterioration from rheumatoid synovitis or injury hinder treatment further.

The numerous causes of swan-neck deformity may be grouped anatomically by the pathway through which the deformity is initiated:

- Extrinsic tendon tightness
- Intrinsic tendon tightness
- Articular
- Distal tendon release

Normal variants

People with normally hypermobile interphalangeal joints can produce swan-neck deformities of all fingers voluntarily by contracting their finger intrinsic muscles. Aside from the curiosity they may attract, these hands represent normal variants and do not need treatment.

Extrinsic tendon tightness

Tightness through the central tendon hyperextends the middle phalanx. Cerebral palsy with spasticity of the extensor digitorum is a dynamic cause in this category.

Both flexion deformity of the wrist and subluxation of the finger MP joint tighten the extrinsic extensor tendon by

lengthening the dorsal skeleton. MP joint subluxation can develop from rheumatoid synovitis, intrinsic contracture, or excessive surgical release of the collateral ligaments. In each instance, PIP joint hyperextension (resistance to passive flexion) increases with MP joint flexion. This is an important distinction from intrinsic tightness.

Extensor tendon scarring over the dorsum of the hand that produces an extensor-plus tenodesis increases tension through the central tendon while the MP joint is flexed (see Fig. 35-47).

Treatment of swan-neck deformity caused by conditions in this category is incomplete unless the proximal abnormality is corrected. Hyperextension of the PIP joint is a distal deformity that stems from a more proximal imbalance.

Intrinsic tendon tightness

Increased tension through the intrinsic tendons can produce palmar subluxation of the MP joint as well as hyperextension of the PIP joint in the fingers. Deformity is resisted by the glenoidal segments of the collateral ligaments at the MP joint and the palmar plate and flexor superficialis at the PIP joint. Spasticity in cerebral palsy, rheumatoid arthritis, ischemic intrinsic muscle contracture, and posttraumatic intrinsic tightness all instigate deformity by increasing tightness through the intrinsic tendons. Tendon transfers for weakness or claw deformity in the ulnar-palsied hand can inititate swan-neck deformity by this same pathway. Less severe tightness exhibits a positive distal intrinsic tightness test (see Fig. 35-48). Advanced tightness affects the MP joint in addition to the PIP joint.

Treatment of conditions in this category is directed toward releasing the intrinsic tightness and rebalancing the deformities. The procedures selected depend on the stage of the condition and on which joints are deformed. For example, flexor tenosynovectomy combined with distal intrinsic resections may suffice in rheumatoid disease with stable MP joints. Otherwise, proximal intrinsic tenotomy with MP jont arthroplasty may also be necessary to rebalance the fingers.

Articular

Rupture of the palmar plate of the PIP joint permits hyperextension, which may progress without early protective splinting. The treatment is reattachment of the palmar plate, which has avulsed distally. This is feasible in longstanding ruptures and has been successfully performed as long as 10 years after injury.

Synovitis of the MP or PIP joints can destabilize fingers. Rheumatoid arthritis and psoriatic arthritis are the most commonly seen forms. Lupus arthritis results in joint deformity by a different mechanism but does not develop synovitis with cartilage erosion. Periarticular inflammation stimulates adhesions to the tendons, sagittal bands, and retinacular ligaments. This category of swan neck deformities is difficult to treat, because deteriorated joints are involved with adherent, displaced extensor tendons.

Distal tendon release

Release of the terminal extensor tendon concentrates extensor tension on the middle phalanx through the central tendon after a mallet tendon lesion. Hyperextension deformity with fracture of the middle phalanx has the same result: the distal extensor tendon is functionally lengthened. The deformity that develops includes a tenodesis over the fracture site. Prognosis for distal joint motion after fracture repositioning is guarded in these cases.

Loss of the flexor superficialis tendon eliminates an important stabilizer of the PIP joint. The severity of the deformity that results depends on the inherent stability of the palmar plate. This tendon should be divided as far proximally as possible when used for tendon transfer to preserve maximum tendon attachments within the flexor fibroosseous sheath proximal to the interphalangeal joint.

THUMB EXTENSOR TENDONS

The extensor pollicis longus is the most mobile of the digital extensor tendons. Its 58 mm longitudinal excursion exceeds that of the other digital extensor tendons. A 13 mm medial-lateral translation of the tendon distal to the radius occurs with first metacarpal flexion and extension. The extensor pollicis longus supinates and adducts the thumb, extends the thumb MP joint with the extensor pollicis brevis, extends the thumb interphalangeal joint with the dorsal hood fibers from the thumb intrinsic muscles, and is the only tendon capable of hyperextending the interphalangeal joint. Hyperextension of the interphalangeal joint normally precedes extension of the MP joint when the extensor pollicis longus is activated.[46]

The abductor pollicis longus and extensor pollicis brevis tendons are secured over the lateral border of the distal radius within the first dorsal fibroosseous compartment. Distal to the dorsal carpal ligament, they pass beneath the superficial layer of the deep fascia. Fasciotomy distal to the dorsal carpal ligament when surgery is done for stenosing tenosynovitis of the extensor tendons (de Quervain's disease) may alter the balance of forces about the thumb.[126] Radial bowing of the abductor pollicis longus and extensor brevis tendons produces an exaggerated extension of the first metacarpal with an extension lag of the MP joint (see Fig. 35-10).

Extensor tendon anatomy about the MP joint resembles that of the finger PIP joint. Transverse fibers, similar to the transverse retinacular ligaments, shroud the capsule and attach to the flexor fibroosseous sheath.[73] The adductor pollicis on the ulnar side and the abductor pollicis on the radial side contribute dorsal expansions that stabilize the extensor tendons and transfer extension forces to the interphalangeal joint (Fig. 35-41). The intrinsic muscles of the thumb can thus extend the interphalangeal joint to neutral but are not capable of hyperextension.

The extensor pollicis brevis usually inserts on the dorsal base of the proximal phalanx but commonly has a second insertion into the extensor pollicis longus.[50] It extends the first metacarpal and the MP joint. Interruption of the extensor pollicis brevis introduces extension weakness at the base of the proximal phalanx. As the MP joint flexes, increased tension develops through the extensor pollicis lon-

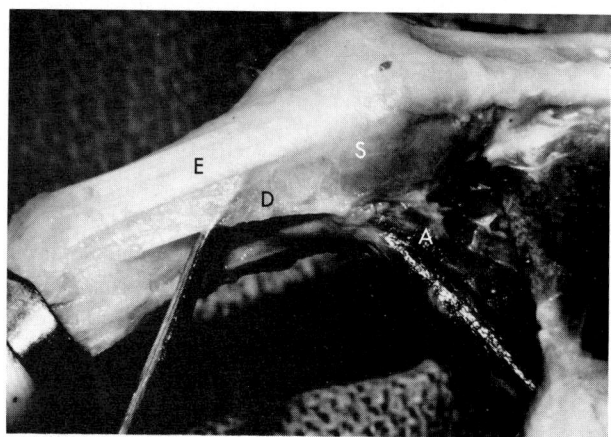

Fig. 35-41 Extensor apparatus of thumb. Adductor pollicis contributes to expansion of the dorsal apparatus and assists extension of the interphalangeal joint. Vertical fibers about the metacarpophalangeal joint resemble the transverse retinacular ligaments of the fingers. *A,* Adductor pollicis muscle; *D,* dorsal apparatus; *E,* extensor pollicis longus tendon over proximal phalanx; *S,* fibers representing homolog of transverse retinacular ligament.

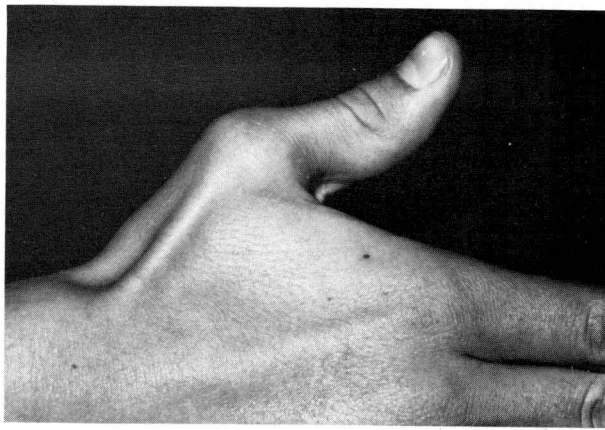

Fig. 35-42 Rupture of extensor pollicis brevis and dorsal fibers of the extensor apparatus produce loss of metacarpophalangeal joint extension. Displacement of the extensor pollicis longus may accentuate flexion of the metacarpophalangeal joint and contributes to hyperextension of the interphalangeal joint. Extensor pollicis longus tendon is clearly identified.

gus, which hyperextends the interphalangeal joint (Fig. 35-42).

The extensor pollicis longus can extend the MP joint through the fibers of the dorsal apparatus. Diastasis or rupture of these fibers permits palmar displacement of the tendon. The tendon flexes the MP joint when displaced below the axis of joint motion, which exaggerates extension forces at the interphalangeal joint. This extrinsic-minus deformity, common with rheumatoid arthritis, is analagous to the boutonnière deformity of the finger.

Closed injuries

Rupture extensor pollicis longus. The extensor pollicis longus is subject to continued stress during performance of normal activities. Tenosynovitis has been attributed to overuse in the classical drummer's palsy. Musicians with impairment of this tendon experience difficulty with dextrous maneuvers. Thumb-under transpositions on the piano keyboard or manipulations of a stringboard are severely hindered with a painful affliction involving the extensor pollicis longus.[18]

The tendon usually ruptures at the level of the distal radius beneath the dorsal carpal ligament. Rheumatoid synovitis and fractures of the distal radius, often undisplaced, are common predisposing conditions; surgery of the distal radius,[107] uremia, diabetes, and local steroid injections are less commonly implicated.[36] The cause of the rupture is believed to be ischemia of a segment of the tendon that normally has poor vascularity. Microangiographic studies suggest that pressure from the effusion that accompanies synovitis or a fracture impedes the intrinsic nutrition in this tendon segment.[27] Oral anabolic steroids have been associated with tendon fiber dissociation with calcification and rupture.[57]

The most disabling impairment after rupture of the extensor pollicis longus is extension lost at the MP joint (Fig. 35-43). The origin of the extensor pollicis longus is long, and the muscle retains some contractility after tendon rupture. The myostatic tightness that develops with attritional rupture can be overcome by strong thenar and thumb flexor antagonsists after reconstruction. Successful rehabilitation with an intercalated free tendon graft that bridges the rup-

tured tendon ends depends on the potential function of the retracted muscle.[39] Extensor indicis tendon transfer—rerouted superficial to the deep fascia distally to the dorsal carpal ligament and sutured to the extensor pollicis longus at the MP joint of the thumb—is technically easier, requires only one tendon repair, and simulates the normal vector of the extensor pollicis longus.[102] The extensor indicis and extensor pollicis longus have comparable mean fiber length and tension fraction.[10,17] The index finger usually retains independent extension from the extensor digitorum after transfer (Fig. 35-44).

Rupture insertion extensor pollicis longus. Closed rupture of the extensor pollicis longus mimics the mallet tendon injury of the finger. Loss of full active extension of the interphalangeal joint with localized dorsal swelling occurs. Incomplete extension after flexion is retained from the collateral ligaments and joint capsule. Treatment is by uninterrupted dorsal splinting with the interphalangeal joint in hyperextension for 6 weeks. Subsequent night splinting for an additional 2 to 4 weeks is usually recommended. The position of splinting should not create skin blanching.[20,75,86]

REHABILITATION

Injured extensor tendons are prone to restraint from scar formation and can be difficult to rehabilitate. Their dis-

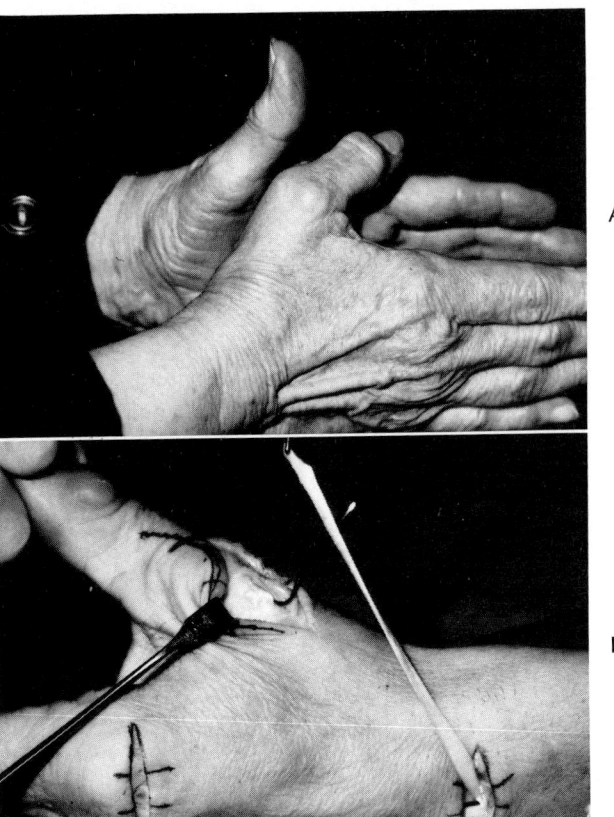

A

B

Fig. 35-44 Ruptured extensor pollicis longus. **A,** Loss of metacarpophalangeal extension and interphalangeal hyperextension. **B,** Reconstruction with extensor indicis transfer. Extensor indicis has an excursion comparable to extensor pollicis longus; course simulates vector of the ruptured tendon.

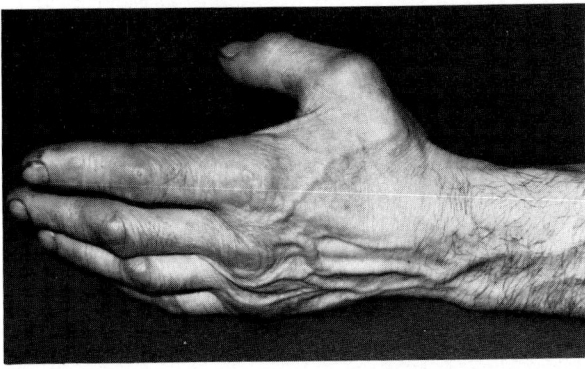

Fig. 35-43 Rupture of extensor pollicis longus at the level of Lister's tubercle. Tendon is not clinically apparent. Loss of metacarpophalangeal extension is the most significant functional loss. Demonstrated extension of the interphalangeal joint is by intrinsic muscles through their contribution to dorsal apparatus.

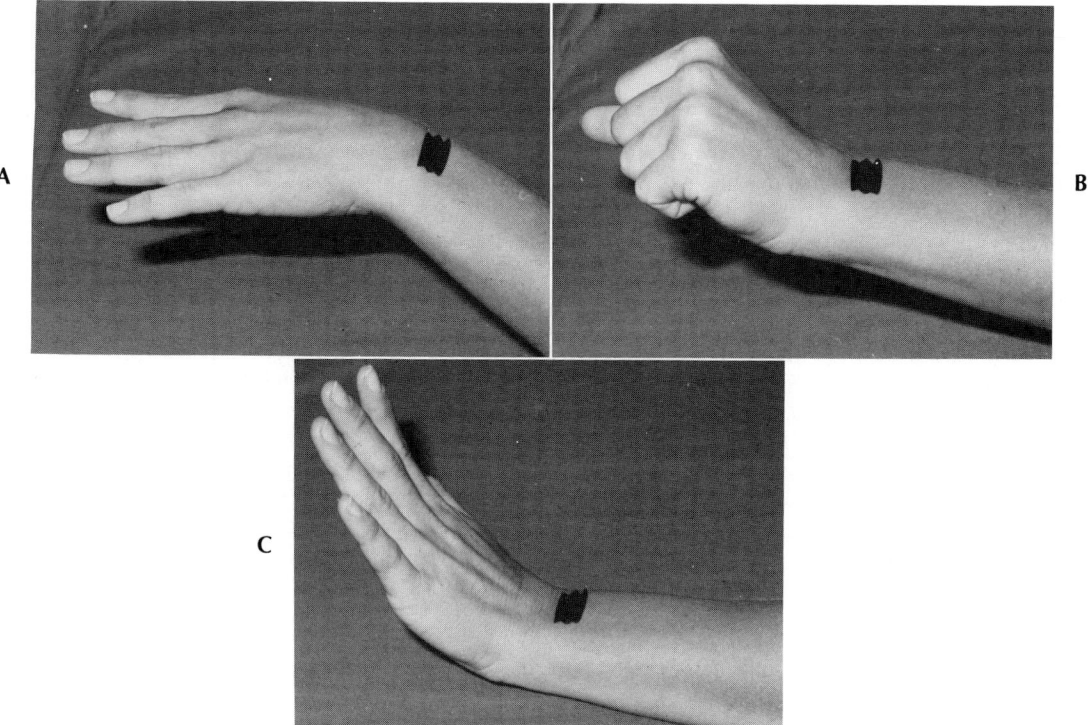

Fig. 35-45 Tendon restraint proximal to dorsal carpal ligament. **A,** Wrist flexion prematurely extends digits because of the extensor tenodesis. **B,** Active digital flexion passively extends the wrist. **C,** Active combined wrist and digital extension may be preserved if glide is not obstructed proximally.

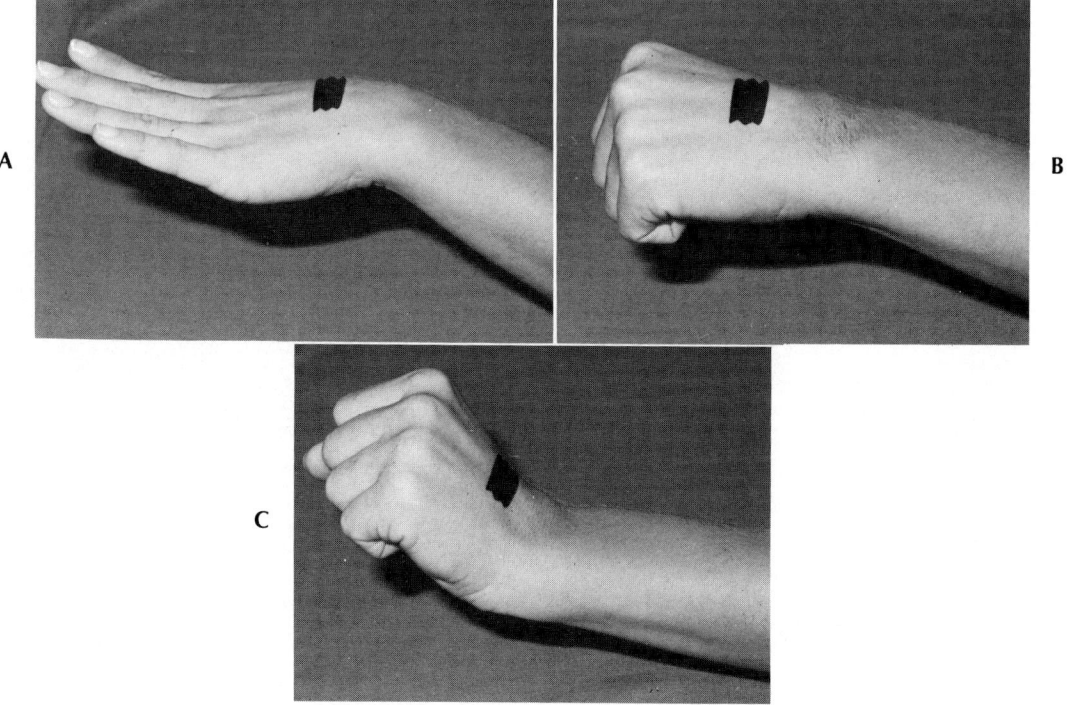

Fig. 35-46 Gliding scar distal to dorsal carpal ligament. **A,** Bulky scar abuts dorsal carpal ligament preventing simultaneous wrist and finger extension. **B,** Finger flexion before wrist extension increases the potential for wrist extension. **C,** Wrist and finger flexion may not be impaired.

proportionately large surface area with comparatively less tendon excursion, strength, and capacity for sustained work compared with flexor tendons, introduces special problems after injury and reparative surgery. The extensor tendons distal to the synovial sheaths beneath the dorsal carpal ligament are wrapped in delicate paratenon, a vascularized membrane with a prodigious capacity for scar formation after injury. Because of success with early protected motion after flexor tendon repairs, this practice has been applied to extensor tendon injuries with encouraging results.[2,28-30,59,63,91] Awareness of the contributions of the superficial layer of the deep fascia and paratenon to the nutrition and function of the extensor tendons over the dorsum of the hand has contributed to modifications of traditional methods for repair of these tendons. Delicate surgical technique with selective fascial closure over repaired tendons, combined with an early protected motion program, has improved the functional gains and lessened some encumbrances from uncontrolled scar about the repair sites. These methods are discussed in greater detail in Chapter 36.

An awareness of the excursions imparted to the extensor tendons by motion of the wrist and the MP and interphalangeal joints is helpful in rehabilitating injured hands. Each wrist extensor tendon has a total excursion of approximately 33 mm. The extrinsic finger extensors have a total excursion of about 50 mm: 31 mm with wrist flexion-extension; 16 mm with MP joint motion; 3 to 4 mm with PIP joint motion; and, 3 to 4 mm with DIP joint motion.* The extensor pollicis longus has a total excursion of 58 mm: 35 mm with wrist motion; 15 mm with MP joint motion; and 8 mm with flexion and extension of the interphalangeal joint.[3]

Sites of blockage from tendon adhesions can be localized by comparing active and passive ranges of motion. Skin adherence, localized induration, and dimpling are reliable indicators of restraining scar. The following discussions relate to the extensor tendons and retinacular systems. These principles cannot be applied unless the joints are passively mobile.

---

*DIP joint motion imparts motion to the extensor tendon over the proximal phalanx only when the PIP joint is restrained. Normally, terminal tendon excursion is dissipated at the level of the PIP joint by the migration of the lateral bands and does not impact on the extensor tendon more proximally.

Patterns of scar restraint

Proximal to dorsal carpal ligament. Scar adhesions of the finger extensor tendons proximal to the dorsal carpal ligament restrain combined wrist and finger flexion; only wrist flexion is impaired when the wrist extensor tendons are involved. A reciprocal wrist extension/finger flexion latitude may be adopted to enhance grip: active finger flexion passively extends the wrist; wrist extension permits the fingers to flex further by reducing the distance between the blockage and the extensor tendon insertions. Passive wrist flexion invokes a tenodesis that passively extends the fingers (Fig. 35-45).

Distal to dorsal carpal ligament. Neither active nor passive wrist motion is impaired. The pattern of scar restraint at this level depends on whether the scar glides—as with a bulky tendon repair—or is anchored to the deep fascia. *Gliding scar* limits motion because of its inability to fit beneath the deep fascia or dorsal carpal ligament proximally. Combined wrist and finger extension is restricted. Wrist extension may be enhanced by flexing the fingers first. This pulls the bulky scar distally, further from the distal edge of the abutting ligament, which allows a greater excursion to occur during wrist extension before the scar is again blocked by the dorsal carpal ligament proximally (Fig. 35-46).

Anchored scar fixing the digital extensor tendons to the deep fascia produces an extensor-plus phenomenon. This tenodesis passively extends the interphalangeal joints of the finger as the MP joint is flexed. Active and passive reciprocity exists between the MP and interphalangeal joints (Fig. 35-47). Combined MP and interphalangeal flexion is prevented: as the interphalangeal joints are flexed, the tenodesis is transferred proximally and the MP joints passively extend.

Intrinsic tightness versus tendon scarring. Both tightness of the intrinsic muscles and adhesions adjacent to the extensor hood about the MP joint that involve the intrinsic tendons can interfere with finger flexion. Active and passive flexion may be painful with either condition. Scar involving the extensor hood can produce a clinical picture that is indistinguishable from an intrinsic contracture by clinical testing. Intrinsic tightness is tested by passively extending the finger MP joint while flexing the interphalangeal

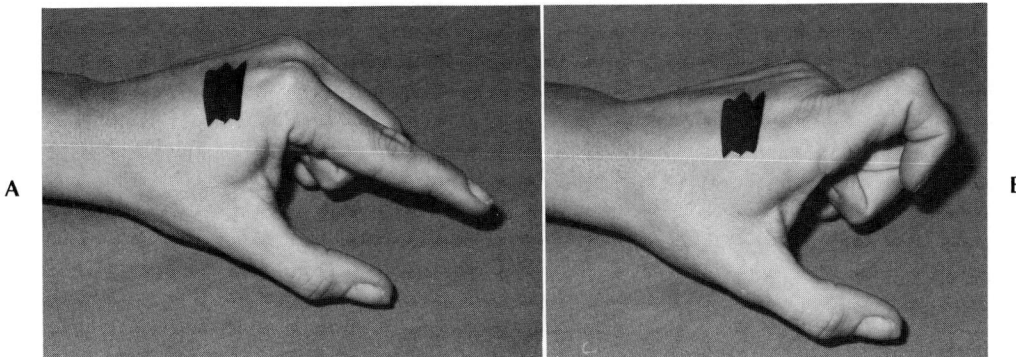

Fig. 35-47   Extensor-plus finger tenodesis caused by restrained extensor tendons proximal to metacarpophalangeal joint. **A,** Active and passive flexion of the metacarpophalangeal joint produces passive tenodesis with extension of the interphalangeal joints. **B,** Active or passive interphalangeal flexion passively extends metacarpophalangeal joints.

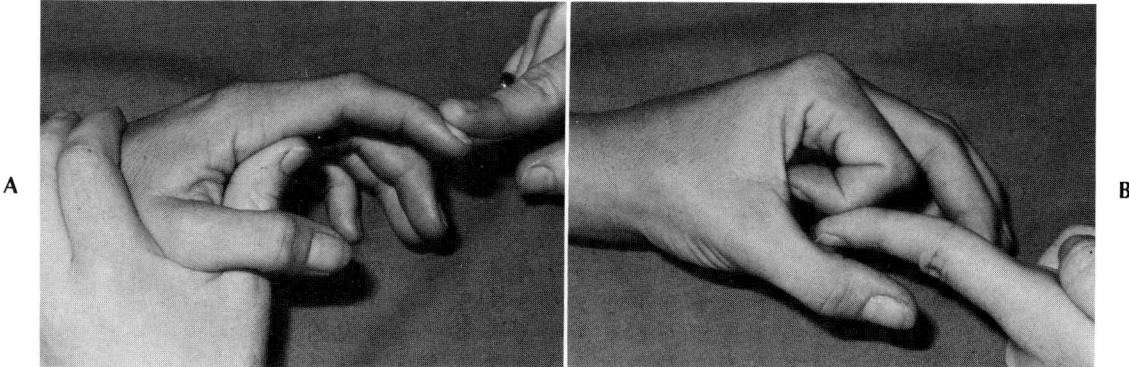

Fig. 35-48 Intrinsic-plus test (Finochietto). **A,** Passive flexion of the interphalangeal joints while the metacarpo-phalangeal joint is supported in neutral tests for tightness through the distal intrinsic tendons. The radial and ulnar intrinsics can be individually tested by deviating the finger away from the side being tested. **B,** Metacarpophalangeal flexion relaxes intrinsic muscles, lessens tension through extensor tendons, and decreases resistance to passive inter-phalangeal joint flexion.

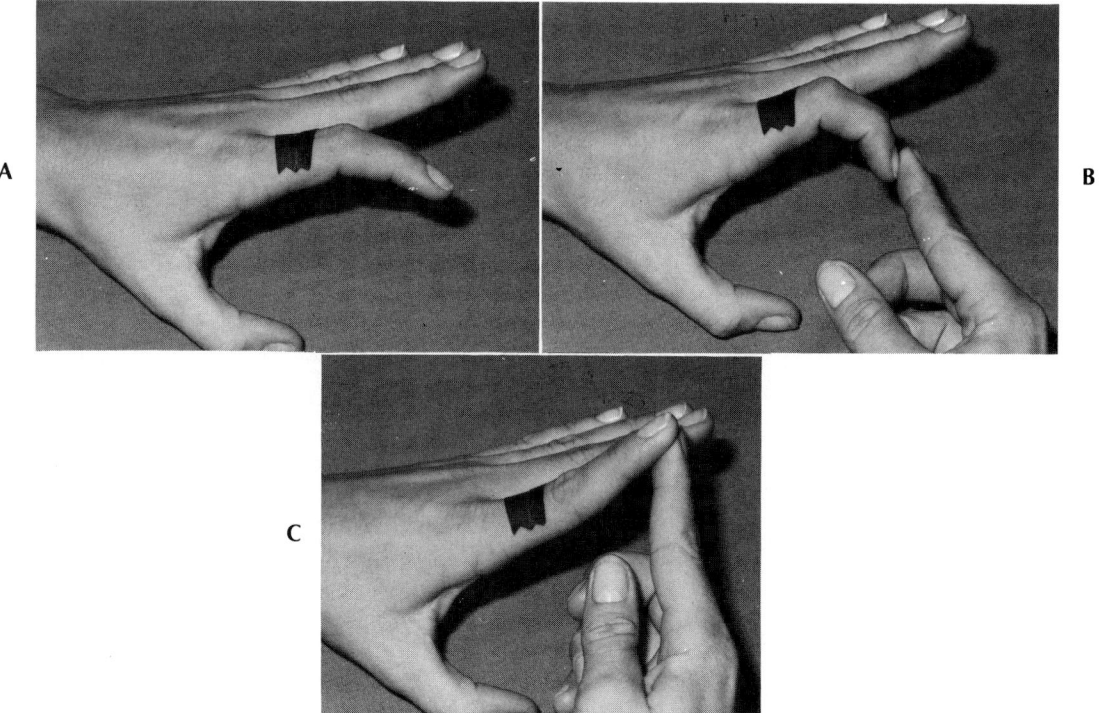

Fig. 35-49 Scar restraint of dorsal apparatus. **A,** Active extension beyond resting position is prevented. **B,** Active and passive flexion is resisted, often feeling "springy." **C,** Passive extension is present if interphalangeal joints are healthy.

joints—the intrinsic tightness test described by Fino-chietto.[31] The radial and ulnar intrinsic muscles of each finger may be evaluated separately by deviating the finger away from the side being tested. Intrinsic restraint suggested by testing may be caused by muscle contracture or adhesions of the intrinsic tendons distally. Careful clinical examination often can differentiate scarring about the intervolar plate ligaments—the saddle syndrome—from scarring about the extensor hood at the MP joint. The location of swelling and tenderness is helpful in differentiating these conditions. The

discernment may not be absolute before surgery; it is then made at the time of tendolysis (Fig. 35-48).

Proximal phalanx. Scarring of the extensor tendons over the proximal phalanx may involve the central tendon, intrinsic expansions, or the entire dorsal apparatus. The resting position of the PIP joint reflects the position of the extensor tendons when motion was arrested. Active extension of the PIP joint beyond the resting position is lacking. Frequently an extension lag is present, and passive correction to neutral is possible. Active and passive flexion of the PIP joint is

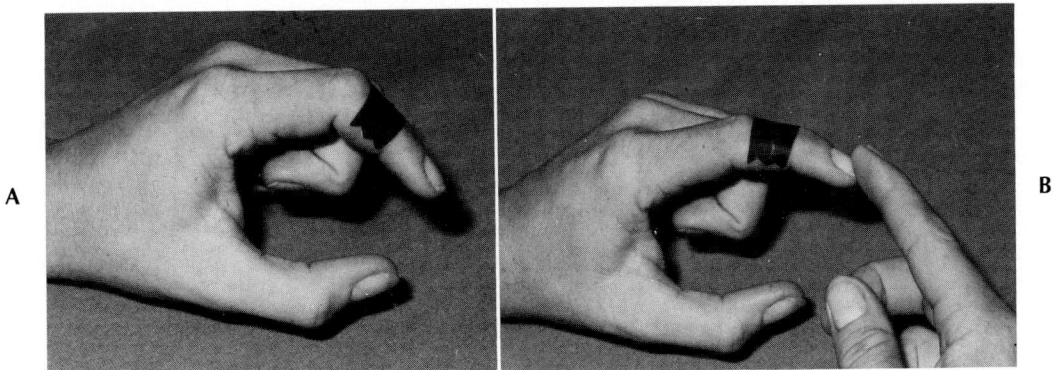

Fig. 35-50 Extensor tendon restraint over middle phalanx. **A,** Active distal joint flexion is lacking. Extension lag may be present. **B,** Passive distal joint flexion is "springy" or blocked. Associated resistance of the proximal interphalangeal joint flexion implies restraint of the lateral bands and triangular ligament.

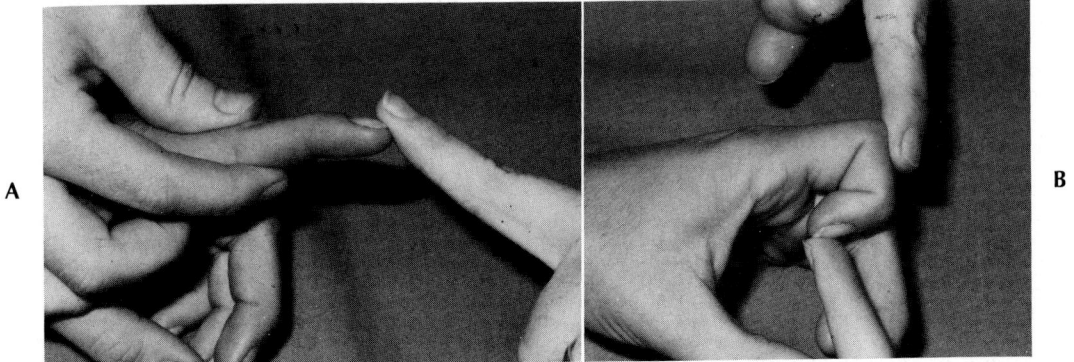

Fig. 35-51 Retinacular tightness test or intrinsic intrinsic-plus phenomenon. **A,** Oblique retinacular ligament tightness tested by passively flexing the distal joint while the proximal interphalangeal joint is supported in neutral. Resistance is relative and should be compared with normal fingers. Relative resistance indicates a positive test. **B,** Combined flexion of both interphalangeal joints is present normally and with mild ligament tightness. Test is dependent on the position of the proximal interphalangeal joint.

blocked; there is often an elastic or springy quality of restricted joint motion during testing (Fig. 35-49).

Flexion of the PIP joint can be blocked also by scarring of the triangular ligament. This restrains the lateral bands dorsally and can consolidate the lateral bands with the central tendon insertion. PIP joint flexion is blocked in both instances: in the first, palmar descent by the lateral bands is prevented; in the second, a tenodesis with the central tendon exists. There is usually restricted flexion of the DIP joint when flexion of the PIP joint is blocked by these conditions.

Middle phalanx. Scarring of the extensor tendon over the middle phalanx restrains flexion of the DIP joint. Active and passive restraint that is unrelated to the position of the PIP joint suggests scarring of the extensor tendon. The retinacular ligaments are usually involved also (Fig. 35-50). These ligaments have little influence on the normal finger but play a significant role in the scarred or imbalanced finger by limiting distal joint motion and fostering deformity. A tight, oblique retinacular ligament produces a positive retinacular tightness test, also called an intrinsic intrinsic-plus phenomenon.[4] Normally there is some passive flexion of the DIP joint while the PIP joint is supported in extension.

Shortening or scarring of the oblique retinacular ligament restrains distal joint flexion. This restraint depends on the position of the PIP joint, which differentiates this from fixation of the extensor tendon (Fig. 35-51).

REFERENCES

1. Agee J and Guidera M: The functional significance of the juncturae tendinum in dynamic stabilization of the metacarpophalangeal joints of the fingers, Personal communication, Sacramento, Calif, 1982.
2. Allieu Y and others: Suture des tendons extensuers de la main avec mobilisation assisteé A propos de 120 cas, Rev Chir Orthop 70 (Suppl. II):69, 1984.
3. An KN and others: Tendon excursion and moment arm of index finger muscles, J Biomech 16:419, 1983.
4. Bendz P: The functional significance of the oblique retinacular ligament of Landsmeer: a review and new proposals, J Hand Surg (Br) 10:25, 1985.
5. Binlftikhar T and others: Spontaneous rupture of the extensor mechanism causing ulnar dislocation of the long extensor tendon of the long finger, J Bone Joint Surg (Am) 66:1108, 1984.
6. Blacker GJ, Lister GD, and Kleinert HE: The abducted little finger in low ulnar palsy, J Hand Surg 1:190, 1976.
7. Bowers HW and Hurst LC: Chronic mallet finger: the use of Fowler's central slip release, J Hand Surg 3:373, 1978.
8. Boyes JH: Bunnell's surgery of the hand, ed 5, Philadelphia, 1970, JB Lippincott Co.

9. Bracey DJ and Jeffreys TE: Habitual extensor tendon dislocation, Hand 11:284, 1979.
10. Brand PW, Beach RB, and Thompson DE: Relative tension and potential excursion of muscles in the forearm and hand, J Hand Surg 6:206, 1981.
11. Burkhart SS, Wood MB, and Linscheid RL: Posttraumatic recurrent subluxation of the extensor carpi ulnaris tendon, J Hand Surg 7:1, 1982.
12. Burton RI: Extensor tendons—late reconstruction. In Green DP, editor: Operative hand surgery, ed 2, New York, 1988, Churchill Livingstone, Inc.
13. Carducci AT: Potential boutonnière deformity: its recognition and treatment, Orthop Rev 10:121, 1981.
14. Carroll C, Moore JR, and Weiland AJ: Posttraumatic ulnar subluxation of the extensor tendons: a reconstructive technique, J Hand Surg 12A:227, 1987.
15. Chicarilli ZN and others: Saddle deformity. Posttraumatic interosseous-lumbrical adhesions: review of eighty-seven cases, J Hand Surg (Am) 11A:210, 1986.
16. Chun S and Palmar AK: Chronic ulnar wrist pain secondary to partial rupture of the extensor carpi ulnaris tendon, J Hand Surg (Am) 12A:1032, 1987.
17. Cooney WP: Tendon transfer for median nerve palsy, Hand Clin 4:155, 1988.
18. Crabb DJ: Hand injuries in professional musicians: a report of six cases, Hand 12:200, 1980.
19. Culver JE Jr: Extensor pollicis and indicis communis tendon: a rare anatomic variation revisited, J Hand Surg (Am) 5:548, 1980.
20. Din KM and Meggitt BF: Mallet thumb, J Bone Joint Surg (Br) 65:606, 1983.
21. Doyle JR: Extensor tendons—acute injuries. In Green DP, editor: Operative hand surgery, ed 2, New York, 1988, Churchill Livingstone, Inc.
22. Eckhardt WA and Palmer AK: Recurrent dislocation of the extensor carpi ulnaris tendon, J Hand Surg 6:629, 1981.
23. Elliot D and McGrouther DA: The excursions of the long extensor tendons of the hand, J Hand Surg (Br) 11:77, 1986.
24. Elliott RA: Boutonnière deformity. In Cramer LM and Chase RA, editors: Symposium of the hand, St. Louis, 1971, The CV Mosby Co.
25. Elson RA: Dislocation of the extensor tendons of the hand, report of a case, J Bone Joint Surg 49B:324, 1967.
26. Elson RA: Rupture of the central slip of the extensor hood of the finger: a test for early diagnosis, J Bone Joint Surg (Br) 68:229, 1986.
27. Engkvist O and Lundborg G: Rupture of the extensor pollicis longus tendon after fractures of the lower end of the radius: a clinical and microangiographic study, Hand 11:76, 1979.
28. Evans RB: Therapeutic management of extensor tendon injuries, Hand Clin 2:157, 1986.
29. Evans RB and Burkhalter WE: Early passive motion in complex extensor tendon injury. Communication: Second International Meeting of American Society of Hand Therapists, Boston, 1983.
30. Evans RB and Burkhalter WE: A study of the dynamic anatomy of extensor tendons and implications for treatment, J Hand Surg (Am) 11:774, 1986.
31. Finochietto R: Retracción de Volkmann de los músculos intrinsecos de las manos, Bol Trab Soc Cir Buenos Aires, 4:31, 1920.
32. Gardner RC: Hypertrophic infiltrative tendinitis (HIT syndrome) of the long extensor: the abused karate hand, JAMA 211:1009, 1970.
33. Garroway RV and others: Complex dislocations of the proximal interphalangeal joint, Orthop Rev 13:21, 1984.
34. Grundberg AB and Reagan DS: Central slip tenotomy for chronic mallet finger deformity, J Hand Surg 12A:545, 1987.
35. Haberern JP: Ueber Sehnenluxationen, Deutsch Zietschrift für Chirurgie, 62:191, 1902.
36. Haher JN and others: Bilateral rupture of extensor pollicis longus, Orthopedics 10:1577, 1987.
37. Haines RW: The extensor apparatus of the finger, J Anat 85:251, 1951.
38. Hamas RS, Horrell ED, and Pierret GP: Treatment of mallet finger due to intra-articular fracture of the distal phalanx, J Hand Surg (Am) 3:361, 1978.
39. Hamlin C and Littler JW: Restoration of the extensor pollicis longus tendon by an intercalated graft, J Bone Joint Surg (Am) 59:412, 1977.
40. Harris C: The Fowler operation for mallet finger deformity, J Bone Joint Surg (Am) 48A:613, 1966.
41. Harris C: The functional anatomy of the extensor mechanism of the finger, J Bone Joint Surg 54A:713, 1972.
42. Harvey FJ and Hume KF: Spontaneous recurrent ulnar dislocation of the long extensor tendons of the fingers, J Hand Surg (Am) 5:492, 1980.
43. Hollinshead WH: Anatomy for surgeons: the back and limbs, ed 2, vol 3, New York, 1969, Harper & Row Publishers, Inc.
44. Ishizuki M, Furuya K, and Kumakura T: Extensor digitorum brevis manus associated with attrition rupture of a common extensor tendon, J Hand Surg (Am) 11:582, 1986.
45. Itoh Y and others: Extensor tendon involvement in Smith's and Galeazzi's fractures, J Hand Surg 12A:535, 1987.
46. Jackson WT and others: Anatomical variations in the first extensor compartment of the wrist: a clinical and anatomical study, J Bone Joint Surg (Am) 68:923, 1986.
47. Johansson SH: Peritendineous fibrosis of the dorsum of the hand, Fifth World Congress of Plastic and Reconstructive Surgery, London, 1971, Butterworth & Co, Ltd.
48. Kaplan EB: Functional significance of the insertion of the extensor digitorum communis in man, Anat Rec 92:293, 1945.
49. Kaplan EB: Anatomy, injuries and treatment of extensor apparatus of the hand and digits, Clin Orthop 13:24, 1959.
50. Kaplan EB: Functional and surgical anatomy of the hand, ed 2, Philadelphia, 1965, JB Lippincott Co.
51. Ketchum LD and others: The determination of moments for extension of the wrist generated by muscles of the forearm, J Hand Surg 3:205, 1978.
52. Kettelkamp DB, Flatt AE, and Moulds R: Traumatic dislocation of the long-finger extensor tendon: a clinical, anatomical and biomechanical study, J Bone Joint Surg 53A:229, 1971.
53. Kilgore ES and others: Correction of ulnar subluxation of the extensor communis, Hand 7:272, 1975.
54. Kinninmonth AW and Holburn F: A comparative controlled trial of a new perforated splint and a traditional splint in the treatment of mallet finger, J Hand Surg (Br) 11:261, 1986.
55. Kleinman WB and Petersen DP: Oblique retinacular ligament reconstruction for chronic mallet finger deformity, J Hand Surg (Am) 9:399, 1984.
56. Koniuch MP and others: Closed crush injury of the metacarpophalangeal joint, J Hand Surg 12A:750, 1987.
57. Kramhøft M and Solgaard DP: Spontaneous rupture of the extensor pollicis longus tendon after anabolic steroids, J Hand Surg (Br) 11:87, 1986.
58. Kus H: Nahtlose Rekonstruktion des Strecksehne bei Hammerfinger (Sutureless reconstruction of the extensor tendon in mallet finger), Handchir Mikrochir Plast Chir 16:231, 1984.
59. Laboureau JP and Renevey A: Utilisation d'un appareil personnel de contention et de rééducation segmentaire élastique de la main type «crabes», Ann Chir 25, 165, 1980.
60. Landsmeer JMF: The anatomy of the dorsal aponeurosis of the human finger and its functional significance, Anat Rec 104:31, 1949.
61. Lange RH and Engber WD: Hyperextension mallet finger, Orthopedics 6:1426, 1983.
62. Legouest L: Sociéte impériale de chirugie. Gazette de hôpitaux 138, 1868.
63. Lemke T, Crayen P, and Maroske D: Funktionelle Behandlung der Strecksehnenverletzung an der Hand, Chirurg 55:264, 1984.
64. Light RR: Buttress pinning techniques, Orthop Rev 10:49, 1981.
65. Littler JW: The finger extensor mechanism, Surg Clin North Am 47:415, 1967.
66. Littler JW and Eaton RG: Redistribution of forces in the correction of the boutonnière deformity, J Bone Joint Surg 49A:1267, 1967.
67. Mackay I and Simpson RG: Closed rupture of extensor digitorum communis tendon following fracture of the radius, Hand 12:214, 1980.
68. Manske PR, Ogata K, and Lesker PA: Nutrient pathways to extensor tendon of primates, J Hand Surg (Br) 10:8, 1985.
69. McCoy FJ and Winski AJ: Lumbrical loop operation for luxation of the extensor tendons of the hand, Plast Reconstr Surg 44:142, 1969.
70. Mestagh H and others: Organization of the extensor complex of the digits, Anat Clin 7:49, 1985.
71. Michon J and Vichard P: Luxation latérales des tendons extenseurs en regard de l'articulation métacarpo-phalangiènne, Rev Med de Nancy 86:595, 1961.

72. Miki T and others: Rupture of the extensor tendons of the fingers: report of three unusual cases, J Bone Joint Surg (Am) 68:610, 1986.

73. Milford LW: Retaining ligaments of the digits of the hand, Philadelphia, 1968, WB Saunders Co.

74. Milford LW: The hand, St. Louis, 1971, The CV Mosby Co.

75. Miura T, Nakamura R, and Shuhei R: Conservative treatment for a ruptured extensor tendon on the dorsum of the proximal phalanges of the thumb (mallet thumb), J Hand Surg (Am) 11A:229, 1986.

76. Montant R and Baumann A: Rupture luxation of the extensor apparatus of the finger of the first interphalangeal articulation, Rev d'Orthop 25:5, 1938.

77. Moore JR, Weiland AJ, and Valdata L: Independent index extension after extensor indicis proprius transfer, J Hand Surg 12A:232, 1987.

78. Murakami Y and Todani K: Traumatic entrapment of the extensor pollicis longus tendon in Smith's fracture of the radius—case report, J Hand Surg (Am) 6:238, 1981.

79. Newmeyer WL and Green DP: Rupture of digital extensor tendons following distal ulnar resection, J Bone Joint Surg (Am) 64:178, 1982.

80. Niechajev IA: Conservative and operative treatment of mallet finger, Plast Reconstr Surg 76:580, 1985.

81. Ogura T, Inoue H, and Tanabe G: Anatomic and clinical studies of the extensor digitorum brevis manus, J Hand Surg 12A:100, 1987.

82. Ovesen OC, Jensen EK and Bertheussen KJ: Dislocation of extensor tendons of the hand caused by focal myoclonic epilepsy, J Hand Surg (Br) 12B:131, 1987.

83. Paley D, McMurty TV, and Murray JF: Dorsal dislocation of the ulnar styloid and extensor carpu ulnaris tendon into the distal radioulnar joint: the empty sulcus sign, J Hand Surg (Am) 12:1029, 1987.

84. Palmer AK and others: The extensor retinaculum of the wrist: an anatomical and biomechanical study, J Hand Surg (Br) 10:11, 1985.

85. Patel MR, Desai SS, and Bassini-Lipson L: Conservative management of chronic mallet finger, J Hand Surg 11A:570, 1986.

86. Primiano GA: Conservative treatment of two cases of mallet thumb, J Hand Surg (Am) 11:233, 1986.

87. Rayan GM: Recurrent dislocation of the extensor carpi ulnaris in athletes, Am J Sports Med 11:183, 1983.

88. Rayan GM and Mullins PT: Skin necrosis complicating mallet finger splinting and vascularity of the distal interphalangeal joint overlying skin, J Hand Surg 12A:549, 1987.

89. Reading G: Secretan's syndrome: hard edema of the dorsum of the hand, Plast Reconstr Surg 65:182, 1980.

90. Redfern AB, Curtis RM, and Shaw Wilgis EF: Experience with peritendinous fibrosis of the dorsum of the hand, J Hand Surg 7:380, 1982.

91. Regnard PJ and others: Extensor tendon injuries: presentation of a series of ninety-nine cases, Ann Chir Main 4:55, 1985.

92. Riordan D: Peritendinous fibrosis of the extensor tendons, J Bone Joint Surg 47A:632, 1965.

93. Riordan DC: In Dobyns JH, Chase RA, and Amadio PC, editors: Year book of hand surgery, Chicago, 1988, Year Book Medical Publishers, Inc, 68.

94. Riordan DC and Stokes HM: Synovitis of the extensor of the finger associated with extensor digitorum brevis manus muscle: a case report, Clin Orthop 95:278, 1973.

95. Ritts GD, Wood MB, and Engber WD: Nonoperative treatment of traumatic dislocations of the extensor digitorum tendons in patients without rheumatoid disorders, J Hand Surg 10A:714, 1985.

96. Rosenthal EA: Tenolysis: AAOS Sound Slide Program No. 719, 1978.

97. Rosenthal EA: Extensor surface injuries at the proximal interphalangeal joint. In Bowers WH, editor: The Hand and Upper Limb, vol 1: The interphalangeal joints, London, 1987, Churchill Livingstone, Inc.

98. Saferin WH: Secretan's disease, Plast Reconstr Surg 58:703, 1976.

99. Saldana MJ and McGuire RA: Chronic painful subluxation of the metacarpal phalangeal jont extensor tendons, J Hand Surg 11A:420, 1986.

100. Schenck RR: Variations of extensor tendons of the fingers, J Bone Joint Surg 46A:103, 1964.

101. Schneider LH: Complications in tendon injury and surgery, Hand Clin 2:361, 1986.

102. Schneider LH and Rosenstein RG: Restoration of extensor pollicis longus function by tendon transfer, Plast Reconstr Surg 71:533, 1983.

103. Schultz RJ, Furlong J II, and Storace A: Detailed anatomy of the extensor mechanism of the proximal aspect of the finger, J Hand Surg 6:493, 1981.

104. Secretan H: Œdéma dur at hyperplasie traumatique du métacarpe dorsal, Rev Med Suisse Romande 21:409, 1901.

105. Shrewsbury MM: A systematic study of the oblique retinacular ligament of the human finger: its structure and function, J Hand Surg 2:194, 1977.

106. Shrewsbury MM and Johnson RK: Ligaments of the distal interphalangeal joint and the mallet position, J Hand Surg 5:214, 1980.

107. Siegel D, Gebhardt M, and Jupiter JB: Spontaneous rupture of the extensor pollicis longus tendon, J Hand Surg (Am) 12:1106, 1987.

108. Smillie IS: Mallet finger, Br J Surg 24:439, 1937.

109. Smith RJ: Balance and kinetics of the fingers under normal and pathological conditions, Clin Orthop 92:104, 1974.

110. Smith RJ: Factitious lymphedema of the hand, J Bone Joint Surg 57A:89, 1975.

111. Spinner M and Kaplan EB: Extensor carpi ulnaris: its relationship to the stability of the distal radioulnar joint, Clin Orthop 68:124, 1970.

112. Stack HG: Mallet finger, Hand 1:83, 1969.

113. Stack HG: A modified splint for mallet finger, J Hand Surg (Br) 11:263, 1986.

114. Stark HH: Troublesome fractures and dislocations of the hand, Instruct Course Lectures, AAOS 19:130, 1970.

115. Stark HH, Bayer JH, and Wilson JN: Mallet finger, J Bone Joint Surg 44A:1061, 1962.

116. Steichen JB and Petersen DP: Junctura tendinum between extensor digitorum communis and extensor pollicis longus, J Hand Surg 9A:674, 1984.

117. Straus FH: Luxation of extensor tendons in the hand, Ann Surg 111:135, 1940.

118. Taleisnik J and others: The extensor retinaculum of the wrist, J Hand Surg 9A:495, 1984.

119. Thompson JS, Littler JW and Upton J: The spiral oblique retinacular ligament, SORL J Hand Surg 3:482, 1978.

120. Tubiana R: The hand, vol 1, Philadelphia, 1981, WB Saunders Co, p 297.

121. Tubiana R and Valentin P: The anatomy of the extensor apparatus of the fingers, Surg Clin North Am 44: 897, 1964.

122. Watson HK, Ritland GD, and Ghung EK: Posttraumatic interosseous lumbrical adhesions, a cause of pain and disability in the hand, J Bone Joint Surg (Am) 56:79, 1974.

123. Weinberg H, Stein HC, and Wexler M: A new method of treatment for mallet finger, Plast Reconstr Surg 58:347, 1976.

124. Wehbé MA and Schneider LH: Mallet fractures, J Bone Joint Surg (Am) 66:658, 1984.

125. Wheeldon FT: Recurrent dislocation of extensor tendons in the hand, J Bone Joint Surg 36B:612, 1954.

126. White GM and Weiland AJ: Symptomatic palmar tendon subluxation after surgical release for de Quervain's disease: a case report, J Hand Surg (Am) 9:704, 1984.

127. Youm Y, Thambyrajah K, and Flatt AE: Tendon excursion of wrist movers, J Hand Surg (Am) 9:202, 1984.

128. Zancolli EA: Structural and dynamic basis of hand surgery, ed 2, Philadelphia, 1979, JB Lippincott Co.

129. Zbrodowski A: Vascularization and anatomical model of the mesotendons of the extensor digitorum and extensor indicis muscles, J Anat 130:697, 1980.

130. Zbrodowski A, Gajisin S, and Grodecki J: Vascularization of the tendons of the extensor pollicis longus, extensor carpi radialis longus and extensor carpi radialis brevis muscles, J Anat 135:235, 1982.

36

Therapeutic management of extensor tendon injuries

Roslyn Brown Evans

Surgical and therapeutic management of the injured extensor system requires the same meticulous care afforded the flexor tendon injury. The experienced hand surgeon and hand therapist appreciate the compromise to hand function that results from poor management of the extensor tendon injury.

The purpose of this chapter is to review current rehabilitation techniques for the treatment of the simple extensor injury at all levels and to describe an early passive motion program for management of the extensor injury with combined lesions. Anatomy and surgical management are described in Chapter 35.

Progressive treatment requires that the therapist have a working knowledge of the dynamic anatomy of the extensor

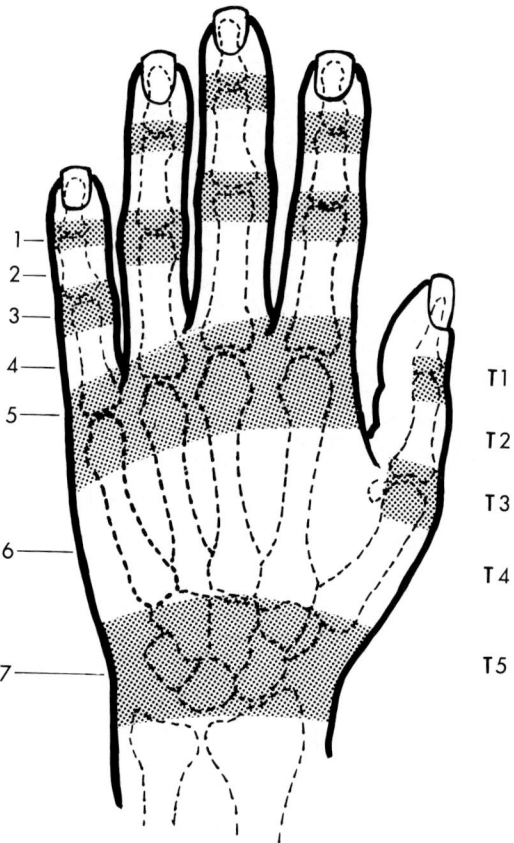

Fig. 36-1 Extensor tendon zones as defined by the committee on tendon injuries for the International Federation of the Society for Surgery of the Hand. (From Kleinert HE, Schepel S, and Gill T: Flexor tendon injuries, Surg Clin North Am 61:267, 1981.)

system. Knowledge of the amount of tendon excursion that occurs relative to joint motion, work capacity requirements of each muscle-tendon unit, and the interrelationship of extrinsic and intrinsic tendon systems is critical in the development of a rehabilitation plan.[7]

Characteristics of the extensor tendon vary at each level affecting treatment. The Committee on Tendon Injuries for the International Federation of the Society for Surgery of the Hand defines extensor tendon injury by delineating seven zones for the extrinsic finger extensors and five zones for the thumb extensors[34] (Fig. 36-1).

Schedules for immobilization, mobilization, and implementation of controlled stress to healing tendons depend on nutrition and excursion of the tendon as it varies at each of these anatomic levels and on tensile strength of the tendon as it develops through the stages of wound healing. Controlled stress is the amount of passive tendon excursion that can be safely and effectively used with early passive motion programs for the healing tendon.

This cumulative knowledge allows us to establish certain guidelines for treatment; however, each case should be considered individually, with treatment altered to accommodate the circumstances of the individual patient and injury. The surgeon should apprise the therapist of the quality of the repair, alterations in tendon length, integrity of the tissue, status of adjacent tissue, and additional pathologic conditions that might alter time schedules for stressing the repaired tendon or mobilizing joints. The patient should be evaluated in terms of anticipated compliance. This information will influence any variation from suggested timing of immobilization and mobilization schedules.

In general, control of edema during the inflammatory phase and precise positions of splint immobilization are significant factors in determining postoperative results and length of rehabilitation for any extensor injury. The importance of wound care, edema control, and patient education is well documented in the literature.*

The purpose of tendon rehabilitation is to apply stress with precision in accordance with tensile strength and excursion throughout the stages of wound healing so that differential tendon gliding is reestablished.

ZONES I AND II

A lesion of the terminal extensor tendon results in a flexion deformity of the distal interphalangeal (DIP) joint, commonly referred to as the "mallet" or "baseball" finger. Treatment and prognosis of the mallet finger depend on associated

---

*References 5, 12, 27, 50, 52, 62.

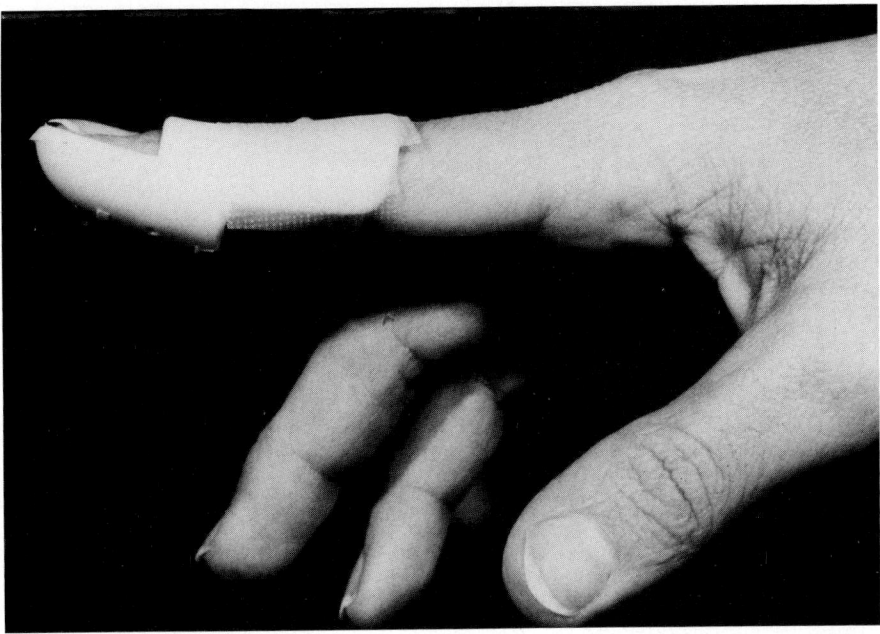

Fig. 36-2   A stack splint for zone I extensor tendon injury immobilizes the distal joint in slight hyperextension. (From Evans RB: Therapeutic management of extensor tendon injuries, Hand Clin 2:157, 1986.)

tissue injury and age of the lesion before treatment.[29,64] These injuries may be open or closed, and with or without associated fracture or fracture dislocation. In many cases, conservative treatment with splint immobilization is sufficient to restore tendon continuity.[29,68] However, open injury, associated fracture, or chronic deformity may require direct repair or Kirschner wire (K-wire) fixation.* (See also Chapter 35.)

Most authors recommend approximately 6 to 8 weeks of continuous extension splinting with both conservative or operative treatment.[3,10,38,68] (See also Chapter 35.) The DIP joint can be immobilized with commercially available Stack splints, aluminum-padded splints, or molded thermoplastic splints (Fig. 36-2). Splint application may be volar or dorsal. However, dorsal immobilization permits more freedom of the proximal interphalangeal (PIP) joint and allows the fingertip its sensory function (Fig. 36-3).

Splint position and skin integrity should be monitored carefully, because vascular nutrition to the skin of the distal digital joint area can be diminished.[42,63,70] The distal joint is immobilized at 0 degrees of extension or slight hyperextension.[3,10] Extreme hyperextension jeopardizes circulation to the dorsal skin by stretching the volar vasculature, which provides nutrition to the area distal to the termination of the dorsal vessels and may create skin necrosis.[42,62] Rayan and Mullins in a study of skin necrosis complications associated with mallet finger splinting suggested a position of hyperextension less than the angle that causes skin blanching, a precursor of skin necrosis. They determined the average total passive hyperextension of the distal joint to be 28.3 degrees and found that circulation to the dorsal skin was compromised when the distal joint was splinted at more

*References 10, 28, 29, 30, 38, 60, 64, 68.

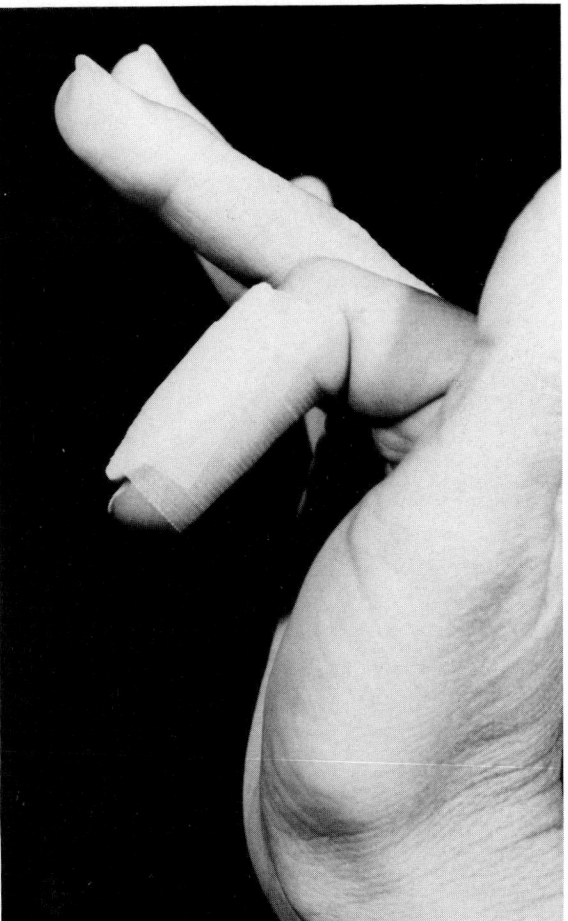

Fig. 36-3   Dorsal immobilization of the distal joint permits more freedom of the proximal interphalangeal joint, and allows the fingertip its sensory function. (From Evans RB: Therapeutic management of extensor tendon injuries, Hand Clin 2:157, 1986.)

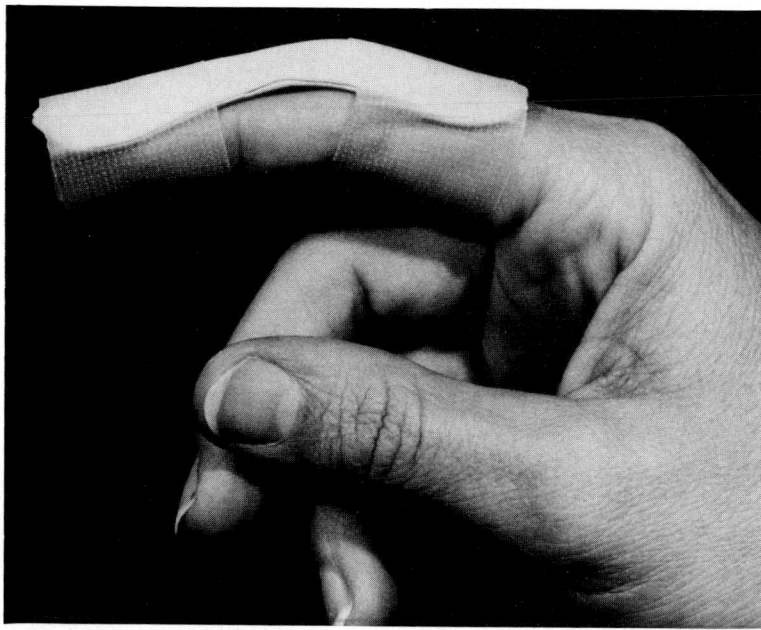

Fig. 36-4   The proximal interphalangeal joint should be splinted in slight flexion in the mallet finger that develops a swan-neck posture, to advance the extensor mechanism distally by virtue of the central slip. (From Evans RB: Therapeutic management of extensor tendon injuries, Hand Clin 2:157, 1986.)

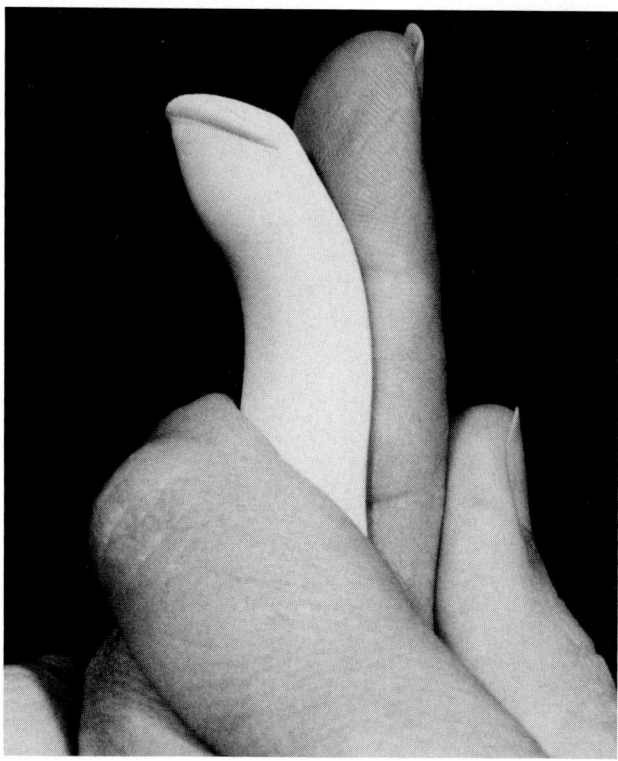

Fig. 36-5   A template exercise splint will set limits for graded flexion and prevent overstretching of the terminal extensor tendon in the overly ambitious patient. (From Evans RB: Therapeutic management of extensor tendon injuries, Hand Clin 2:157, 1986.)

than 50% of its total hyperextension.[54] Splint immobilization that allows even slight flexion will result in extensor lag, because the tendon callus will heal in an elongated position.[29]

Skin maceration can be prevented by lining the splint with moleskin to absorb perspiration and by changing the lining if it becomes damp. The splint must be adjusted as edema decreases, to provide a precise fit.

During the immobilization phase, the patient should be seen weekly for wound care when necessary, for adjusting the fit of the splint and for maintaining motion in unaffected joints. The distal joint must be held in extension continuously during splint adjustments to prevent attentuation of the healing tendon.

If the PIP joint exhibits a posture of slight hyperextension, the proximal joint should be splinted at 30 to 45 degrees of flexion while the distal joint is splinted in full extension to advance the extensor mechanism distally by virtue of the central slip[3,64] (Fig. 36-4). (See also Chapter 35.) This long splint may be exchanged for a shorter distal joint splint after the first 2 weeks.[64]

After 6 weeks of uninterrupted splinting in extension, very gentle flexion exercises are initiated. The opposing flexor digitorum profundus is a powerful musculotendinous unit and will easily overstretch the more fragile terminal extensor tendon. Brand calculated the work capacity of the extensors to be less than one third of the flexors; therefore mobilization should first emphasize full extension with gradual increments of flexion not only for zone I, but for all levels of extensor injury.[7,12] Extensor tendon excursion is minimal at this level.[5,7,33,56,61]

Instructions to the patient should be very specific. During the first week of mobilization, no more than 20 to 25 degrees of flexion of the distal joint should be allowed. During the second week, if no lag has developed, distal joint flexion to 35 degrees is allowed. The overly ambitious patient will benefit from a template exercise splint with specific angles of motion preset to prevent overstretching of the terminal tendon (Fig. 36-5).

If an extensor lag develops, resplinting is indicated and exercises are delayed for several weeks.[10,68] (See also Chapter 35.) Day splinting is recommended during the first 2 weeks of the mobilization phase; night splinting should be continued another 4 weeks.

Prehension and coordination activities should supplement range-of-motion (ROM) exercise. Desensitization of a painful tip may be necessary with crush injuries before the pa-

tient will incorporate the digit into prehension activities (see Chapter 45). Exercise may gradually proceed to resistive grasp and pinch activities, but no attempt to achieve complete function before 3 months should be made.[64]

Therapy to the DIP joint is primarily educational. If the patient understands the nature of his injury and the rationale for treatment, he should be able to perform most of his therapy independently.

ZONES III AND IV

Extensor tendon injuries in zones III and IV may result in a boutonnière deformity.[60] Rupture or attenuation of the extensor tendon over the PIP joint, if the triangular ligament

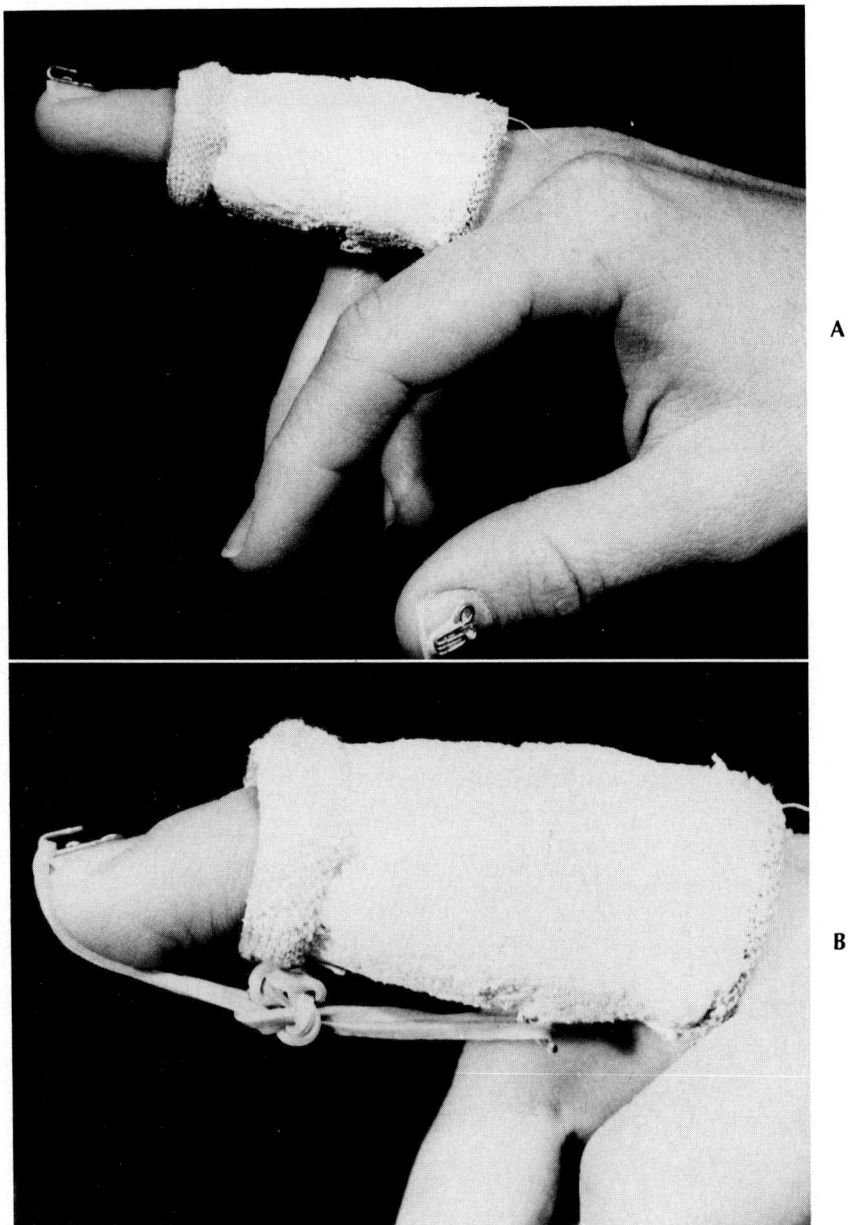

Fig. 36-6   A, A cylinder plaster cast immobilizes the proximal interphalangeal joint at 0 degree extension. The circumferential pressure of the cast will reduce digital edema. **B,** Gentle intermittent traction can be incorporated into the digital cast to stretch the distal joint if the oblique retinacular ligaments are tight. (From Evans RB: Therapeutic management of extensor tendon injuries, Hand Clin 2:157, 1986.)

also is stretched or damaged, creates a gradual progressive volar displacement and shortening of the lateral bands. This alteration of normal biomechanics results in loss of extension at the PIP joint and hyperextension of the distal joint.[64,68]

There are conflicting opinions in the literature concerning direct repair and immobilization with K-wire versus conservative management of the open zone III injury.[10,55,62,68] However, most authors recommend conservative treatment of the acute closed injury at this level with uninterrupted immobilization of the PIP joint at 0-degree extension for 6 weeks.[10,55,64,68]

Both conservative and operative treatment require precise digital splinting and, often, assistance in rebalancing the intrinsic and extrinsic tendon systems if the DIP joint is tight in extension or rests in hyperextension.[10,26]

The PIP joint can be immobilized with a volar-static splint or with a circumferential finger cast (Fig. 36-6, *A*). The finger cast is preferable, because its circumferential pressure will help reduce edema and because it is more difficult to remove, thus reducing the risk of patient noncompliance (see Chapter 91). The PIP joint must be splinted at absolute 0 degrees to prevent tendon healing in an elongated position with a resultant extensor lag.

A light, tubular gauze dressing is applied to the digit to protect the wound and skin. If the wound area is fragile, a small square of Velfoam is placed directly over the PIP joint to disperse pressure before the fast-setting plaster is applied. Care must be taken to ensure good digital circulation during cast application. The cast should be removed several times for wound care, and a new cast should be applied as edema decreases, to ensure proper fit during the first 7 to 10 days.

If the lateral bands require no surgical repair, the distal joint is left free to prevent distal joint tightness and lateral band adherence.[37] Distal joint flexion is encouraged. If the lateral bands are repaired, the DIP joint should also be immobilized for 4 to 6 weeks.[38]

Active distal joint flexion or intermittent traction will provide improved extensibility to the oblique retinacular ligaments for the digit with limited distal joint flexion (Fig. 36-6, *B*).

Mobilization schedules vary slightly between the fourth and sixth weeks, depending on integrity of the tissue and status of the PIP joint. Most authors agree that the central slip will tolerate gentle flexion exercises at 6 weeks, with continued extension splinting another 2 to 4 weeks between exercise sessions.[10,38,68] (See also Chapter 35.)

I initiate isometric extension exercises within the confines of the digital cast at 3 weeks to be done by the patient five or six times per day to provide controlled stress at the repair site, followed by active flexion at 5 to 6 weeks.

Zone III or IV injuries associated with osseous injury or osteoarthritis will not tolerate 6 weeks of immobilization well. Significant joint stiffness may complicate the rehabilitation process. Consideration of controlled passive motion of 25 degrees at 3½ to 4 weeks should be given to these complex injuries. Moving the PIP joint passively from 0 degrees to 25 degrees of flexion will create 3 mm of excursion of the central slip if the moment arm of the extensor tendon is 0.75 cm. This amount of excursion is based on Brand's method of calculating tendon excursion in relation to moment arms and radians.[7] This concept is discussed in detail in the section "on early passive motion." The PIP joint remains splinted in extension between controlled exercise sessions and follows the usual protocol at 6 weeks.

Allieu and others describe an early controlled passive motion program for the extensor system at all levels with

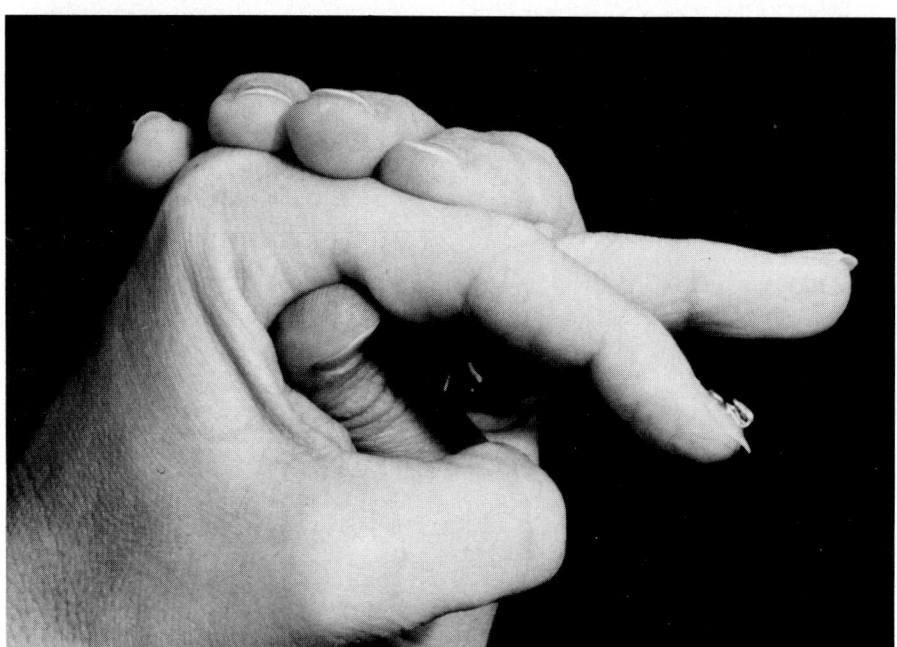

Fig. 36-7   The proximal phalanx of the affected digit is held manually in flexion as the patient extends the proximal interphalangeal joint. This position encourages intrinsic extension while directing the force of the extrinsic extensor tendon more distally.

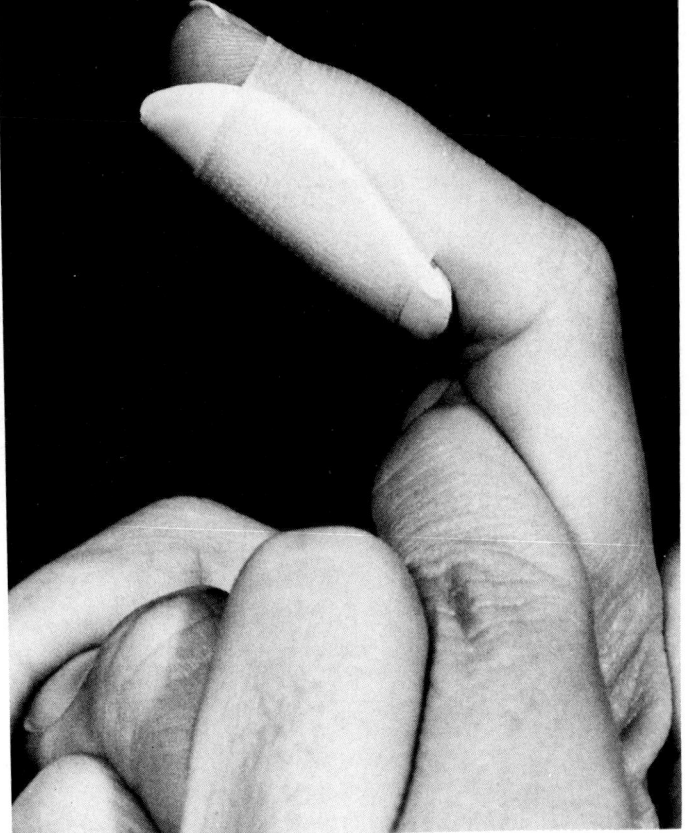

Fig. 36-8 Flexion forces are applied to the proximal interphalangeal joint with **A,** a dynamic splint that blocks the metacarpophalangeal joint in extension and applies traction to the midphalanx level; **B,** a hand-based, static exercise splint that blocks the metacarpophalangeal joint in extension and encourages acute proximal interphalangeal joint flexion in the hook-fist position; and **C,** a distal joint-blocking splint that negates profundus force, manual blocking of the metacarpophalangeal joint, and active flexion of the proximal interphalangeal joint.

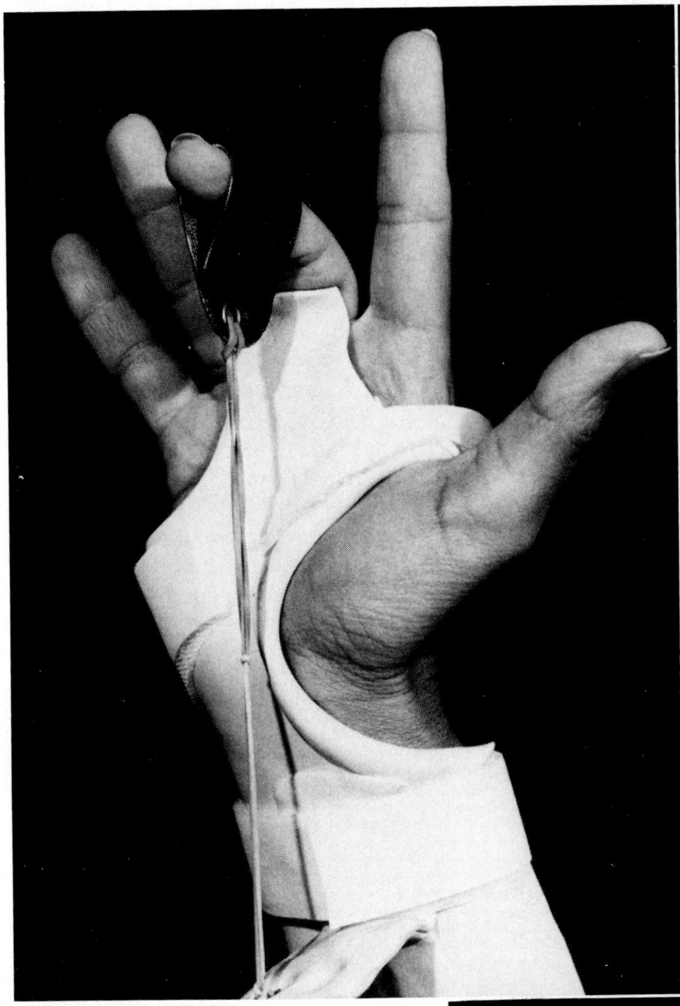

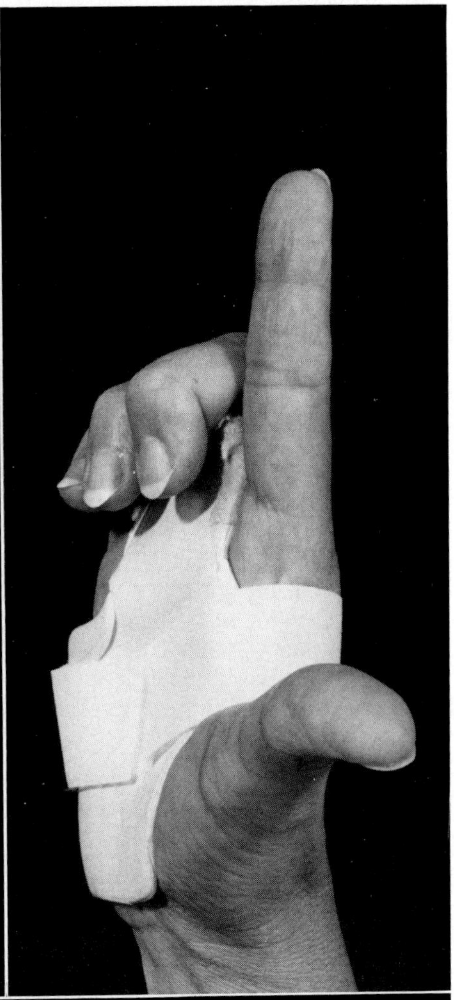

good results. However, their results distal to the metacarpophalangeal (MP) level had the least satisfactory outcome, with only 50% graded as good or excellent.[2]

Exercise at 6 weeks begins with teaching the patient to relax the proximal joint into flexion, followed by extension with moderate force. It is important to teach the patient to support the proximal phalanx in flexion as he extends the PIP joint. The force of the extensor tendon is then more distal, and the finger is in a more effective position for intrinsic extension[65] (Fig. 36-7).

Excursion of the tendon and resistance are gradually increased during the eighth to tenth week, augmented by dynamic splinting into flexion if no extension lag exists. Splinting and exercise forces can be focused at the PIP joint level to improve proximal joint flexion and extensor tendon excursion by (1) applying a forearm-based dynamic splint that blocks the MP joint in extension and applies traction to the midphalanx level, (2) applying a hand-based exercise splint that blocks the MP joint in extension and encourages PIP joint flexion in the hook fist position, or (3) splinting the distal joint, manually supporting the proximal phalanx, and actively flexing the PIP joint (Fig. 36-8).

Digital swelling can be controlled with Coban wraps. Scars can be softened with massage and silicone elastomer molds applied with pressure. Exercises should emphasize blocking of individual joints and grasping activity. Osteoarthritic fingers with inflammation and incomplete interphalangeal (IP) flexion should not engage in repetitive grasping activity, because this may encourage triggering in the flexor system.[15]

The chronic or fixed boutonnière deformity will require splinting and exercise to regain passive motion for both IP joints before surgery.[55] The postoperative result in a chronic deformity is related to the preoperative motion.

Schneider and Smith reviewed a number of surgical approaches and provided a comprehensive bibliography for treatment of the chronic boutonnière deformity.[55]

ZONES V AND VI

Rehabilitation of the simple extensor tendon injury in zones V and VI can be relatively uncomplicated. Atraumatic surgical technique, preservation of the paratenon, and proper postoperative immobilization minimize problems of the rehabilitation phase. Reestablishing tendon glide in this area is facilitated by the abundant and mobile soft tissue that characterizes the dorsum of the hand.[3,50]

The therapist's concern during the first 3 postoperative weeks is for wound care and proper postoperative immobilization to protect the repaired structures. Edema control is important to minimize adhesion formation and joint problems. The acute inflammatory response associated with early wound healing may limit joint motion. The accumulation of protein and fluid in the extravascular space causes shortening and thickening of the periarticular structures.[27] The extensor tendons have 11 to 16 mm of excursion at this level, requiring protection of wrist and digital joints to protect the repair site from rupture.[5]

The wrist is immobilized in surgery at approximately 40 to 45 degrees of extension, MP joints from 0 degrees extension to 20 degrees of flexion, and IP joints at 0 degrees of extension. Many authors recommend splinting the MP joints in mild flexion to retain the integrity of the collateral ligaments.[10,28,46,61] This position often creates an extensor lag and is indication for the early passive motion technique, which is explained later in this chapter.[12-14]

During the first therapy visit, preferably on the third to fifth postoperative day, the patient is seen for wound care, splinting, and assessment of anticipated joint problems. By manually and passively placing the wrist in maximum hyperextension while supporting the digital joints in full extension, the therapist can gently assess the "feel" of each MP joint by gently moving the index and long finger from slight hyperextension to 11 degrees and the ring and little finger from slight hyperextension to 16 degrees (Fig. 36-9). This protected passive motion will create 2 mm of glide and will not jeopardize the repair.[14] These excursions are calculated from Table 36-3. If the MP joints are already becoming stiff, the therapist and surgeon should consider careful controlled passive motion of MP joints by the therapist during dressing changes.[12-14] Tension on the repair and integrity of the tissue should be considered. This is explained in detail in the section on early passive motion.

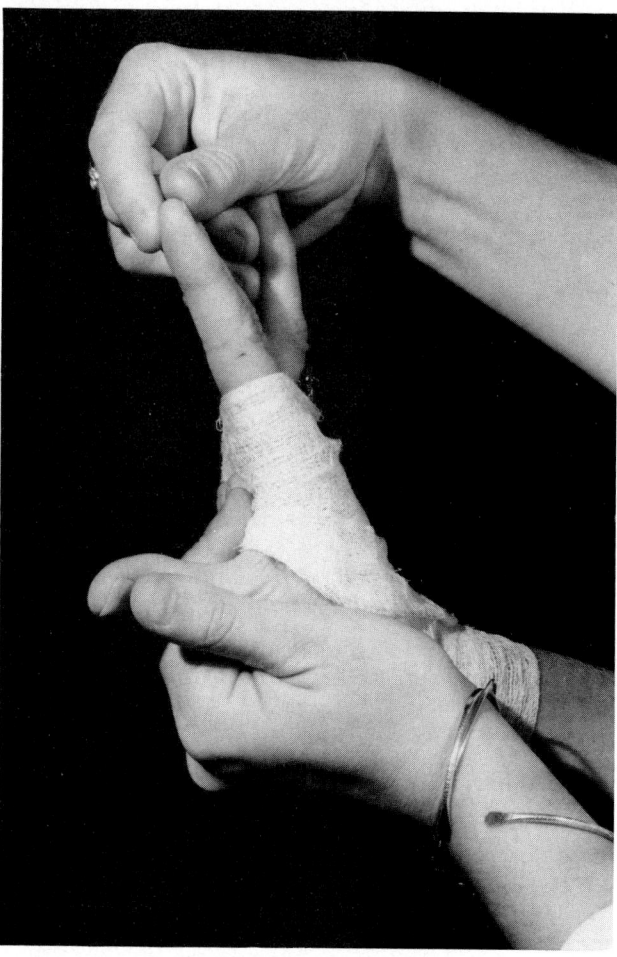

Fig. 36-9 Therapists should assess the status of the periarticular structures of the metacarpophalangeal joint during the initial visits. The wrist and digits are held passively in maximum extension as the therapist passively moves the metacarpophalangeal joints from slight hyperextension to 11 degree flexion for the index and long finger and 16 degree flexion for the ring and small finger. Excessive joint tightness necessitates a change in splint position or consideration of controlled, passive motion.

Anticipated problems of PIP joint tightness, such as are associated with arthritis, should also be addressed at this first therapy visit. There is little tendon excursion created in zones V, VI, or VII with IP joint motion.[5,6] Therefore with the wrist and MP joints completely extended, careful individual passive motion of each PIP and DIP joint can be accomplished for repairs in zone VI.[14] In Zone V, PIP flexion beyond 45 degrees is dependent on the integrity of the repair.

To allow the patient independence with this technique, the immobilizing splint is cut away under each PIP joint to allow motion at this level (Fig. 36-10, *A*). However, resting these proximal joints in flexion, particularly in the edematous hand, may result in flexion contracture and extensor lag. A removable volar component can be applied to the splint to rest the IP joints in extension between exercise periods to prevent these problems (Fig. 36-10, *B*).

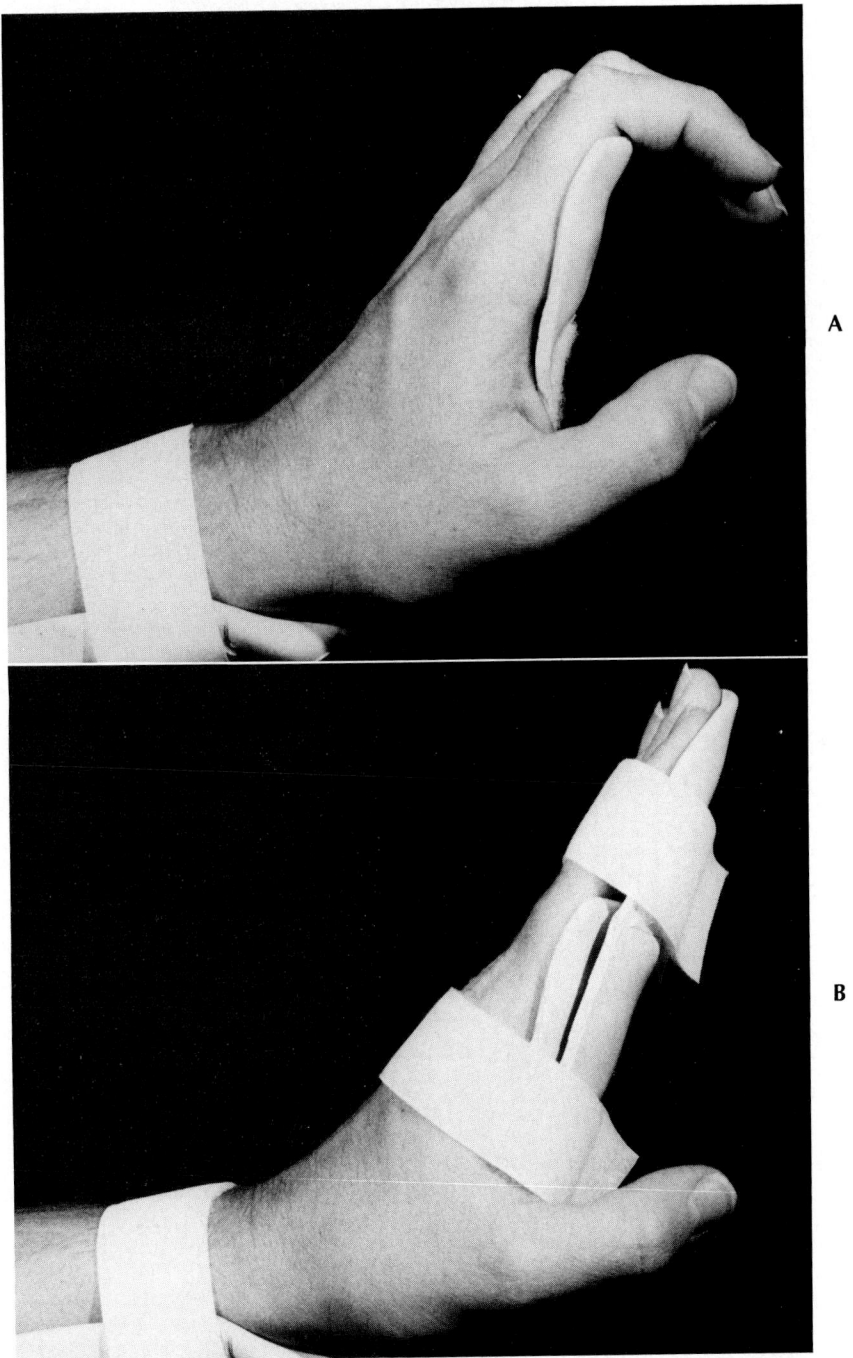

Fig. 36-10   **A,** A static extension splint that immobilizes the wrist and metacarpophalangeal joints in extension allows motion of the proximal and distal interphalangeal joints without jeopardizing the repair in zones V, VI, and VII. **B,** A removable extension component is applied between exercise sessions to prevent volar plate tightness and extension lag. (From Evans RB: Therapeutic management of extensor tendon injuries, Hand Clin 2:157, 1986.)

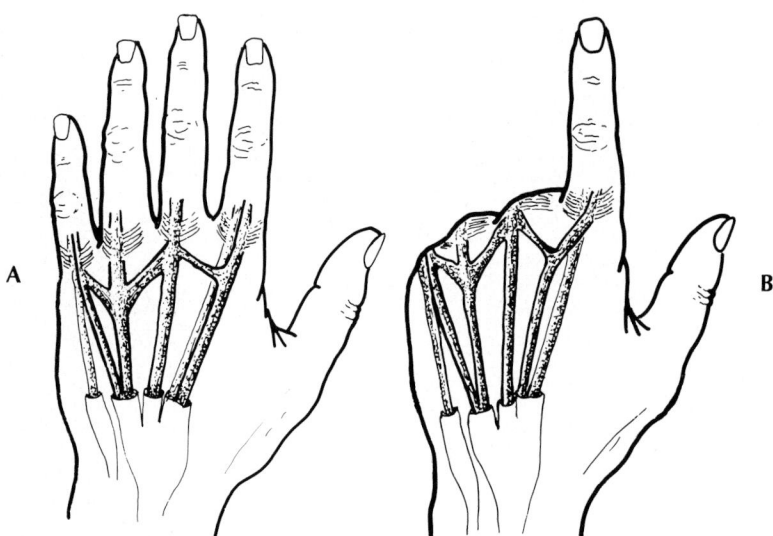

Fig. 36-11 **A,** Repair of the extensor digitorum communis, distal to the juncturae for the middle finger, is splinted with the middle metacarpophalangeal joint resting at 0 degrees, adjacent finger metacarpophalangeal joints at 25 to 30 degree flexion. This position relieves tension at the repair site, while maintaining collateral ligament integrity of the uninvolved fingers. **B,** Tension is reduced on the anastomosis of the extensor digitorum communis when the repair site is distal to the juncturae tendinum if the adjacent fingers are held in slight flexion. This advances the proximal end of the severed tendon by a force of the intertendinous connection. (From Beasley RW: Hand injuries, Philadelphia, 1981, WB Saunders Co.)

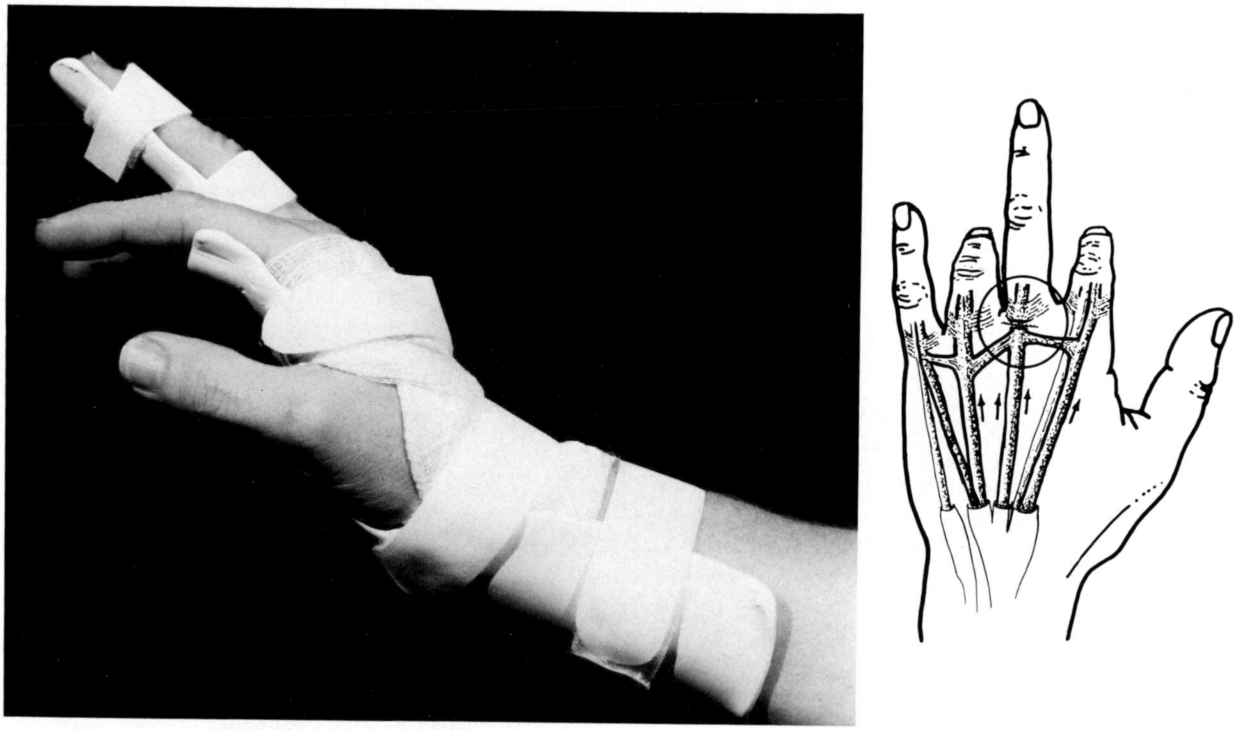

Fig. 36-12 **A,** The extensor digitorum communis to the index lies parallel and lateral to the extensor indicis proprius during rest and simultaneous extension of all digits. **B,** Flexion of the ulnar three digits with the index held in extension creates differential excursion between these two tendons. The extensor digitorum communis to the index finger is pulled superficial and medial to the extensor indicis proprius through a force created by the juncturae as the extensor digitorum communis to the middle finger advances distally with metacarpophalangeal flexion. (Redrawn from Fahrer M: Interdependent actions of the fingers. In Tubiana R, editor: The hand, vol 1, Philadelphia, 1981, WB Saunders Co.)

Simple laceration to the extensor indicis proprius and extensor digiti minimi requires immobilization only of the repaired tendons.[16,65] However, with the extensor digitorum communis one must consider the juncturae tendinum, which, while functioning to dynamically stabilize the MP joints, also limits independent function of these tendons.[1,16] If the repair site is proximal to the interconnecting tendon, all fingers should be splinted in extension. If it is distal to the interconnection, the adjacent fingers can be held in 30-degree flexion (Fig. 36-11, *A*). The latter position permits advancement of the proximal end of the severed tendon by a force of the intertendinous connection, thus actually reducing tension on the anastomosis[3] (Fig. 36-11, *B*).

If both the extensor indicis proprius and extensor digitorum communis to the index are repaired, differential glide between the two tendons during the mobilization phase can be reestablished by actively or passively moving the ulnar three fingers into complete flexion while the index is extended. Fahrer explained this dynamic anatomy.[16] The extensor digitorum communis to the index lies parallel and lateral to the tendon of the extensor indicis proprius during rest and simultaneous extension of all fingers (Fig. 36-12, *A*). The juncturae tendinum between the index and middle digitorum communis is superficial to the extensor indicis proprius. With flexion of the long finger MP joint, the index extension digitorum communis is pulled medially by the intertendinous connection crossing over the extensor indicis, creating differential excursion between these two tendons[16] (Fig. 36-12, *B*).

I prefer to start guarded active motion 3 weeks after repair.

As with any hand injury, treatment begins by cleansing and softening the skin. The hand may be cleansed and debrided in a small portable whirlpool where the wrist and fingers can be supported in extension. The patient is instructed in retrograde massage techniques to reduce edema and to soften adhesions. The patient must understand that the repair does not have normal tensile strength at this stage. He or she should be taught to protect the anastomosis by proper positioning.

Gentle active and active assistive exercise on the third to fourth week should emphasize extension at the MP joint with the wrist extended and relaxation of these joints to 30 to 40 degrees of flexion.

The IP joints may be exercised through a full range with the wrist and MP joints extended. The wrist is actively moved from a relaxed neutral position to extension with the fingers extended. Between exercise sessions, the volar static splint of the immobilization period can be worn. It should be altered to allow motion for the proximal joints. If the MP joints are stiff, a dorsal dynamic extension splint that rests the MP joint at 0 degrees but allows controlled flexion should be worn during the day (Fig. 36-13).

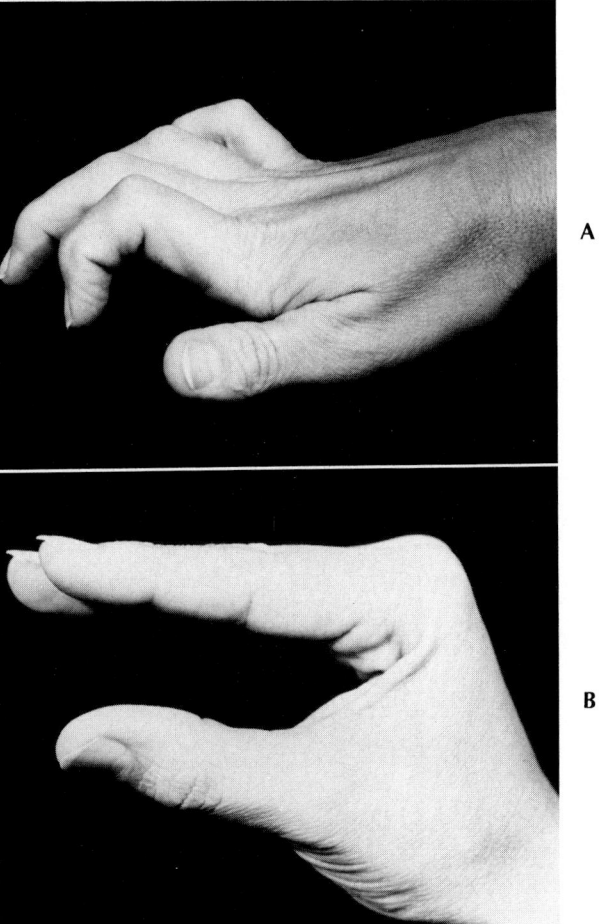

A

B

Fig. 36-14 **A,** The "claw" position isolates extrinsic finger extensors. **B,** The "intrinsic-plus" position will stretch the metacarpophalangeal collateral ligaments respecting tension at the anastomosis. (From Evans RB: Therapeutic management of extensor tendon injuries, Hand Clin 2:157, 1986.)

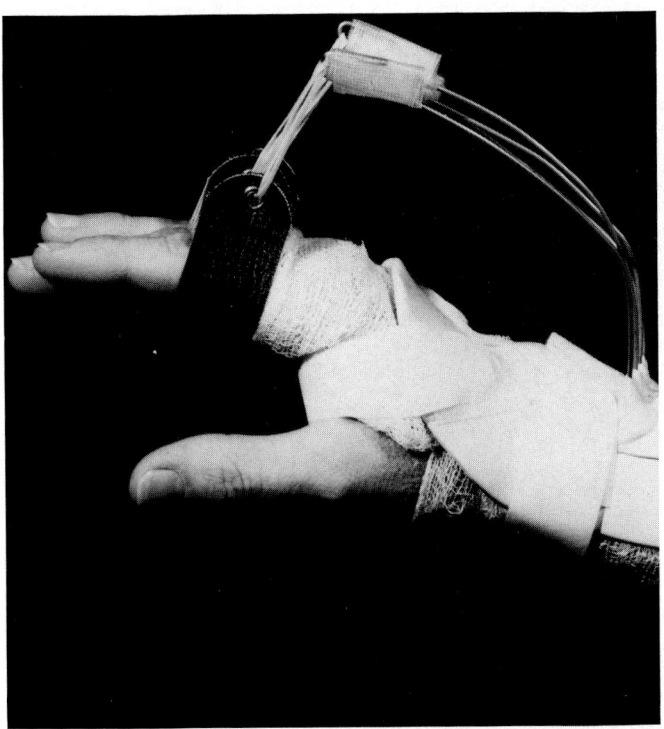

Fig. 36-13 A dorsal dynamic extension splint that rests the metacarpophalangeal joints at 0 degrees and allows controlled flexion will prevent excessive stress on the repair site while encouraging joint motion and increased tendon excursion.

Individual finger extension exercise and the "claw" position will direct controlled stress to the adhesions and is appropriate at 4 to 5 weeks[16,65] (Fig. 36-14, *A*). The "intrinsic-plus" position will improve MP joint flexion while respecting tension at the suture line (Fig. 36-14, *B*). Active wrist flexion is gradually increased with the fingers in a relaxed position. A wrist-control splint is sufficient protection at 5 weeks.

Composite finger flexion is facilitated with the use of graded dowels at 5 to 6 weeks. Simultaneous finger and wrist flexion, functional electrical stimulation, and dynamic flexion splinting are safely incorporated into the treatment plan at 6 to 7 weeks. The therapist may have to consider functional electrical stimulation and dynamic splinting earlier if extrinsic tendon healing has created dense adhesions. Strong resistive exercise should be delayed until the tenth to twelfth week.

ZONE VII

The extensor tendons are synovial at the wrist where they pass through six fibroosseous canals as they gain entrance to the hand.[10] The synovial sheaths and dorsal retinaculum act as pulleys, maintaining the relationship of tendon to bone while allowing for changes of direction. The synovial sheaths may be important to tendon nutrition at this level.* (See also Chapter 35.)

The moment arms and consequently excursions are greatest for the digital extensor tendons at the wrist level.[5,7]

If the finger extensors are involved, the MP joints and

---

*References 4, 5, 10, 44, 58, 61.

wrist must be splinted in extension during the immobilization phase (Fig. 36-15). Multiple repairs of the extensor digitorum communis require differential tendon-gliding exercises in the third to sixth week to reestablish independent finger motion. This is accomplished by moving each digit individually into graded flexion—30 degrees the third week, 45 degrees the fourth week, 60 degrees the fifth week, and 90 degrees the sixth week—while adjacent fingers are held in extension. Combinations of dynamic flexion and extension splinting can be used in the sixth to eighth week to create a shear between these tendons, thus improving differential excursion (Fig. 36-16). Otherwise mobilization and splint schedules are similar to those of zone V.

Inability of the extensor digitorum communis to glide through the retinacular area creates a mechanical disadvantage, increases friction, and can be a factor in dorsal tenosynovitis. Adhesions proximal to the dorsal carpal ligament restrict combined wrist and digital flexion. (See Chapter 35.) Wrist flexion creates an exaggerated tenodesis effect on the long extensors, depriving the patient of power grip.[8]

Scar distal to the retinaculum permits composite wrist and finger flexion. However, combined wrist and finger extension is impaired, because scar will not allow the tendons to glide proximal beneath the dorsal carpal ligament (see Chapter 35). The scar can be treated with transverse friction massage, silicone Elastomer molds applied with pressure, and mechanical stress applied to the tendons in all areas of motion by the sixth week.

Disruption or extensive excision of the dorsal carpal ligament increases the moment arm of the extensor tendons and decreases mechanical efficiency.[4,7,58,61] Bowstringing of the extensor tendons at the wrist level translates to an ex-

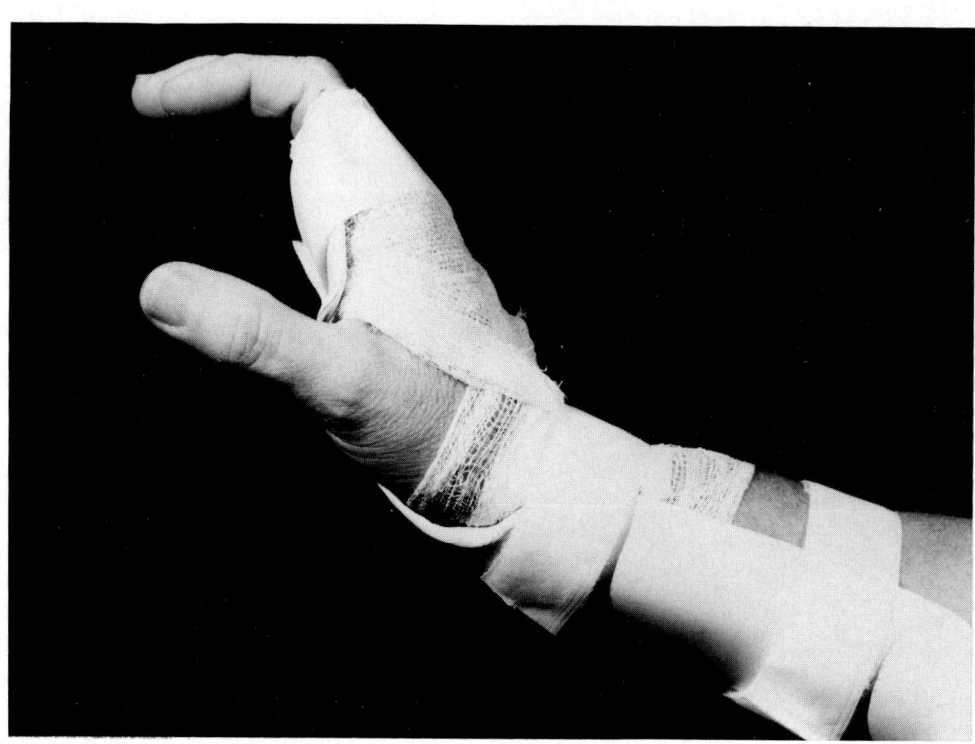

Fig. 36-15   Repair of the digital extensors in zone VII requires immobilization of the wrist and metacarpophalangeal joints.

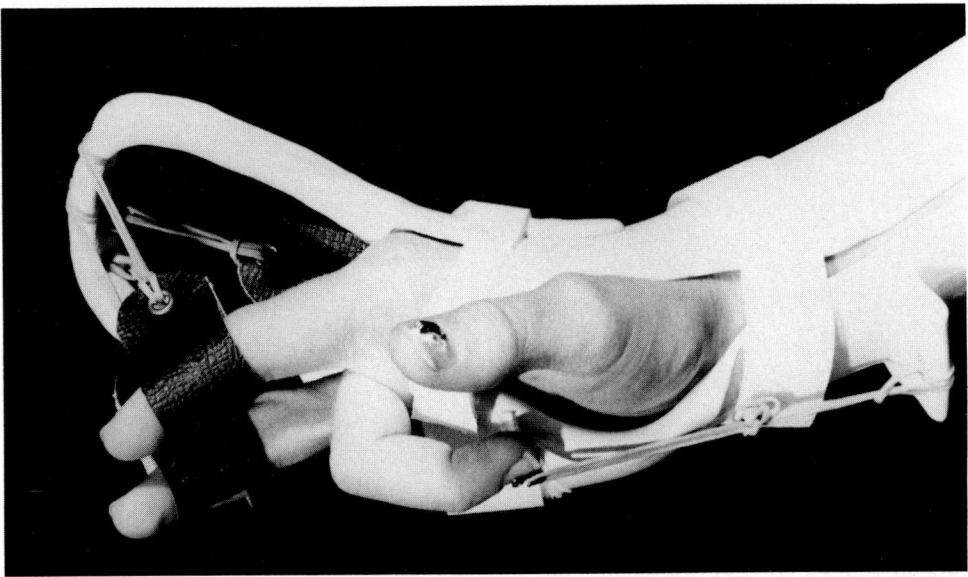

Fig. 36-16 Combination of dynamic flexion and extension splinting will create a shear between the tendons of the extensor digitorum communis in the fourth compartment.

Table 36-1 Excursions for the wrist extensors as reported by Bunnell

	Flexion	Extension	Radial deviation	Ulnar deviation
ECRL*	16 mm	21 mm	8 mm	16 mm
ECRB	16 mm	21 mm	4 mm	12 mm
ECU	14 mm	4 mm	3 mm	22 mm

*ECRL, extensor carpi radialis longus; ECRB, extensor carpi radialis brevis; ECU, extensor carpi ulnaris.

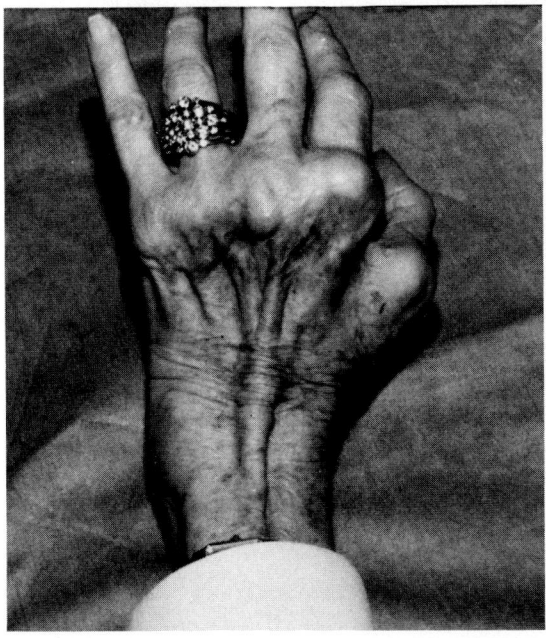

Fig. 36-17 Disruption of the dorsal carpal ligament increases the moment arm of the extensor tendons creating an extensor lag at the metacarpophalangeal joint.

tensor lag at the MP joint (Fig. 36-17). Boland correlated loss of the extensor retinaculum to extensor lag of only 2 to 4 degrees at the wrist level, but as much as 70 degrees at the MP level, depending on the width of retinacular fascia lost.[4] With decreased mechanical efficiency, the workload of the extensor tendons is increased, especially during activities requiring sustained wrist and finger extension. Therefore the therapist should be aware that (1) with an absent or diminished dorsal retinaculum, it may not be possible to correct lag at the MP joint with therapy and (2) altered biomechanics from adhesions or lost pulley may result in cumulative trauma problems. Treatment should be adjusted appropriately.

Work capacity and load requirements for the wrist extensors are great, requiring protective wrist extension splinting for as long as 8 weeks.[7,61] The wrist tendons are stressed with radial and ulnar deviation as well as in the flexion-extension arc. Tendon excursion as it relates to flexion, extension, and radial and ulnar deviation determines exercise programs (Table 36-1).

Protected motion relative to these excursions may begin at 3 to 4 weeks. At that time the wrist may be actively moved from 30 degrees of extension to 60 degrees of extension with gravity eliminated. At 4 to 5 weeks the wrist may be moved to 0 degrees. Complete flexion should not be attempted until the eighth week. Radial and ulnar deviation may be actively moved through 50% of range of motion by the fourth to fifth week, progressing to full motion by the seventh to eighth week. To effect maximum excursion of the extensor carpi ulnaris, the wrist should be exercised into ulnar and radial deviation, with the forearm both supinated and pronated.[5,28,61]

THE RHEUMATOID RUPTURE IN ZONES V, VI, AND VII

Rehabilitation of repaired extensor tendons in zones V, VI, and VII in the rheumatoid hand requires consideration

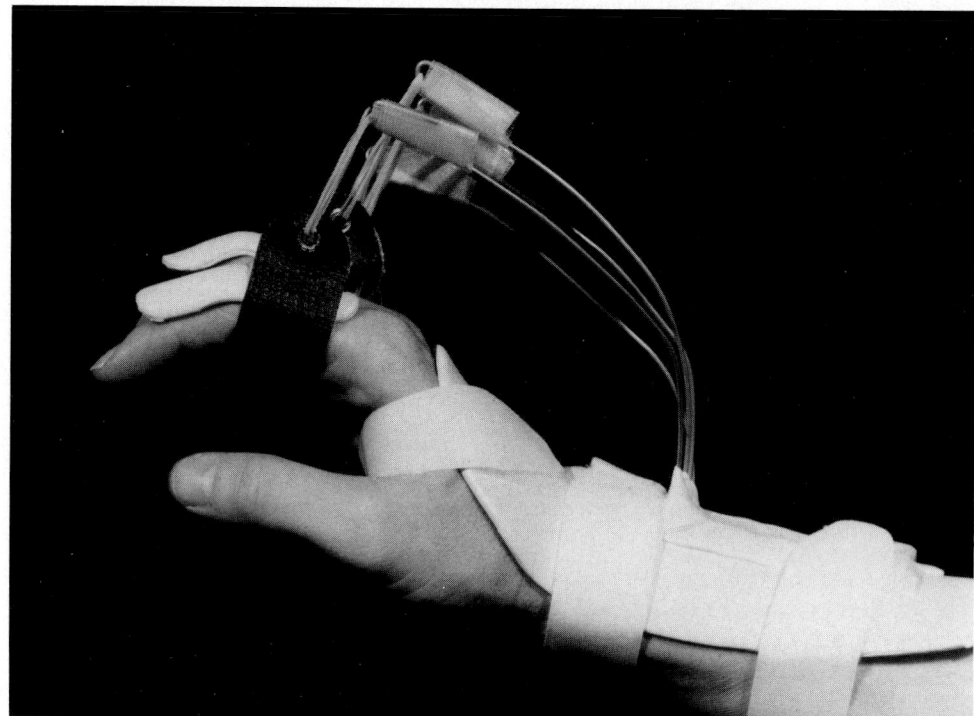

Fig. 36-18   Swan-neck deformities should be counterbalanced with digital splinting to help transmit extensor forces to the zone V and zone VI levels when active extension exercise is initiated.

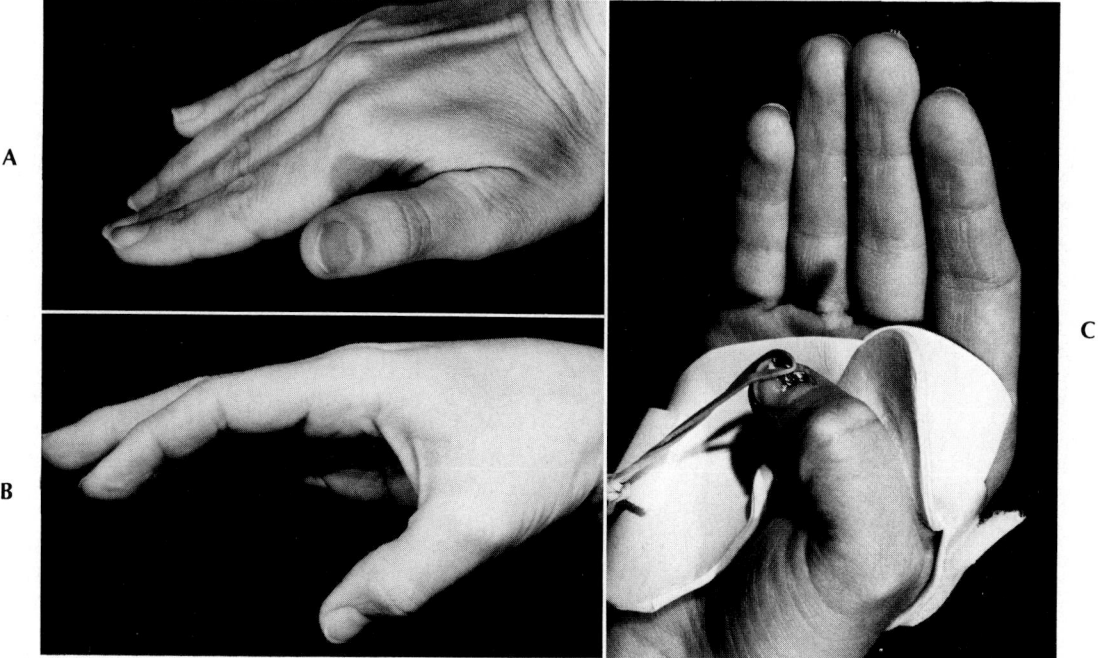

Fig. 36-19   **A,** The thumb should be exercised from complete retropulsion with the wrist extended to **B,** simultaneous abduction and flexion with the wrist flexed to obtain complete excursion by the sixth week. **C,** Combinations of dynamic abduction and flexion splinting will encourage reorganization of peritendinous adhesions. (**C** from Evans RB: Therapeutic management of extensor tendon injuries, Hand Clin 2:157, 1986.)

of altered biomechanics created by the imbalance between the extrinsic and intrinsic systems, the effects of immobilization on rheumatoid joints, and the integrity of the tendons as noted at surgery.[17,47]

The type of repair—end-to-end anastomosis, suture of the distal stump to an adjacent tendon, or tendon transfer—will affect the immobilization schedule. In general, protective splinting should be extended a few extra weeks. Early controlled passive motion to the distal points, done either manually by the therapist or with controlled extension splinting (as will be explained), should be considered to minimize joint problems.

Repairs in zones V, VI, and VII associated with intrinsic tightness should be splinted with MP joints at 0 degrees and the fingers free distal to the PIP joint in the immobilization phase.

At 3 weeks if the dorsal skin is not fragile, a dynamic extension splint holding the wrist extended and MP joint dynamically extended to 0 degrees is applied, with a radial pull if indicated. Swan-neck deformities can be counterbalanced with dorsal, digital, static splints which are taped at the proximal phalanx only and hold the PIP joint at about 30 degrees of flexion. This splint arrangement allows proximal joint flexion, inhibits the swan-neck deformity, and helps transmit extensor forces to zones V and VI levels when active extension exercises begin (Fig. 36-18). The goal with extensor repair combined with swan-neck deformity is to facilitate MP joint extension, PIP joint flexion, and intrinsic stretch.

THE THUMB

The thumb extensor tendons are divided into five zones[34] (see Fig. 36-1). Injuries in TI and TII are treated similarly to injuries of zones I and II of the finger.[68] Reports in the literature on the mallet thumb indicate that the injury is rare and that conflicting opinions exist concerning surgical repair versus conservative splint management.[9,48,51,53] Zone TI injuries require that the IP joint be splinted 8 weeks continuously at 0 degrees of extension or slight hyperextension with conservative management, and 5 to 6 weeks with operative repair. Both approaches require an additional 2 to 4 weeks of splint immobilization between exercise sessions.[9,48,51,53]

Zone II injuries are immobilized with a hand-based static splint that immobilizes the MP and IP joints at 0 degrees and radially extends the thumb. Active motion is initiated at 4 to 5 weeks with several more weeks of splint protection.

Injuries in zones III and IV should be splinted with the thumb MP joint at 0 degrees and slight abduction, the wrist at 30 degrees of extension.

Zone V injuries create difficult rehabilitation problems. Dense adhesions frequently limit excursion of the extensor pollicis longus at the retinacular level.[12-14] Improper immobilization in which the MP joint is hyperextended or insufficient web space is maintained will create extension contracture of the MP joint, first web contracture, and problems regaining excursion.[12,68] Dynamic splinting of the MP joint with the wrist and first metacarpal extended is appropriate at 4 weeks to correct MP joint problems; combinations of abduction and flexion with splinting and exercise are appropriate at 6 weeks for excursion problems (Fig. 36-19).

EARLY PASSIVE MOTION IN THE COMPLEX INJURY

The complex extensor tendon injury creates difficult rehabilitation problems that often result in limited recovery or additional surgical procedures.[12-14] (See also Chapter 15.) A complex extensor tendon injury is identified as one in which the periosteum of bone, extensor retinaculum, or adjacent soft tissues are injured. A proliferative fibroblastic response can be expected with injury to the periosteum with extensive soft tissue damage or at the retinacular level, which will jeopardize tendon glide.[44,49,68] (See also Chapter 12.) Immobilization of extensor injuries in zones V, VI, and VII associated with combined lesions frequently results in adherent tendons, extensor lag, and joint contracture.[12-14]

In response to these problems, a controlled passive motion program for the complex extensor tendon injury in zones V, VI, VII, TIV, and TV was established in 1979 by Dr. William Burkhalter and me. The 9-year study has been reported several times and to date includes 126 cases with an average total active motion of 212 degrees per digit with one reported rupture.[12-14] Precise guidelines for correlating tendon excursion with joint motion for the controlled passive motion program were suggested by Dr. Burkhalter and me based on a study of excursion and biomechanics of the extensor system.[14]

Rationale

The rationale for applying controlled stress to the healing extensor tendon is made on the basis of these assumptions: (1) the controlled stress of protected early motion has a positive effect on tensile strength, tendon excursion, repairsite cellularity, peritendinous vessel density and configuration, intrinsic healing, and increased synovial diffusion to the tendon* (see also Chapters 12 and 28); (2) the technique of early passive motion of flexor tendons as described by Duran, Kleinert, and others may be applicable to extensor tendon injuries when reestablishing extensor tendon excursion is anticipated to be a difficult rehabilitation problem† (see also Chapter 31); and (3) 5 mm of passive tendon glide is sufficient to prevent dense adhesions at extensor tendon repair sites based on Duran's suggestion that 3 to 5 mm of passive glide will safely influence flexor tendon adhesions.[11]

Applying controlled stress to the healing tendon can be done safely and effectively based on the results of our 9-year study. However, the therapist must understand tendon excursion as it relates to joint motion to apply stress with precision. The following calculations on extensor tendon excursions in zones V, VI, VII, TIV, and TV based on literature review, biomechanics, and intraoperative measurement provide the clinician with the technical data necessary to deliver precisely 5 mm of passive tendon glide in these zones.[14]

Literature review of reported excursions were variable but within a consistent range.‡ Differences may exist between the individual extensor digitorum communis (EDC) tendons, as well as from person to person. Bunnell's cadaver studies of excursions provided the most detailed information and correlated closely with those recently described by

---

*References 18, 20-25, 35, 39-41, 43-45, 66, 67, 69.
†References 11, 19, 36, 49, 57, 71, 72.
‡References 5, 7, 33, 56, 60, 65.

Table 36-2   Excursions reported by Bunnell

	TOTAL	Wrist	MP	PIP	DIP
Extensor digitorum communis					
Index	54 mm	38 mm	15 mm	2 mm	0
Long	55 mm*	41 mm	16 mm	3 mm	0
Ring	55 mm	39 mm	11 mm	3 mm	0
Small	35 mm	20 mm	12 mm	2 mm	0

	TOTAL	Wrist	CMC	MP	IP
Extensor pollicis longus					
Thumb	58 mm	33 mm	7 mm	6 mm	8 mm

From Boyes JH: Bunnell's surgery of the hand, Philadelphia, 1970, JB Lippincott Co.

Brand.[5,7] Bunnell assigned values for individual finger tendons at each MP, PIP, and DIP joint, with the wrist in a neutral position[5] (Table 36-2).

Biomechanical considerations

The existence of a constant relationship between MP joint motion and tendon excursion was studied.

Biomechanically, the excursion of the extensor tendon at the MP level is directly proportional to angular changes of the joint.[5] Brand described the existence of a constant extensor tendon moment arm at the MP joint level, which although not precisely constant, does not change dramatically with joint motion.[7]

Considering the existence of this rather constant relationship, I propose a simple equation for determining excursion of the extrinsic finger extensors in zones V, VI, and VII: joint motion divided by tendon excursion for that particular joint is equal to the number of degrees of motion required to effect 1 mm of tendon glide.[14]

$$\frac{\text{Joint motion (degrees)}}{\text{Tendon excursion (mm)}} = \text{Degrees/mm}$$

Application of this equation is contingent on total joint motion and total tendon excursion for each individual finger at the MP level and the amount of excursion considered effective and safe for providing controlled stress to the healing tendon.

The suggested equation is applied with these values for MP joint motion: 85 degrees, index; 88 degrees, long; 90 degrees, ring; and 92 degrees, small finger.[31,59] Excursions used were those described by Bunnell, because he measured each finger separately (see Table 36-2). Controlled stress allowing 5 mm of passive glide, as suggested by Duran and substantiated by the results of the authors' pilot study, was determined to be a safe and effective excursion[11,13] (Table 36-3).

Brand calculated tendon excursion in terms of radians.[7] A radian is a unit of angular motion that defines joint motion and tendon excursion in relation to the moment arm of the joint in question[7] (Fig. 36-20). Brand believes that the radian concept is particularly applicable to the MP joint, because there is a constant axis of joint motion and a rather constant

Table 36-3   Calculation for EDC excursion at the MP level

Index	$\dfrac{85°}{15\text{ mm}}$ = 5.66° per mm × 5 mm = 28.3°
Long	$\dfrac{88°}{16\text{ mm}}$ = 5.5° per mm × 5 mm = 27.5°
Ring	$\dfrac{90°}{11\text{ mm}}$ = 8.18° per mm × 5 mm = 40.9°
Small	$\dfrac{92°}{12\text{ mm}}$ = 7.66° per mm × 5 mm = 38.33°

tendon moment arm throughout the arc of motion.[7] He calculated the mean moment arm for the index MP joint to be 10 mm in cadaver studies.[7] Therefore angular motion of one radian (57.29 degrees) would produce 10 mm of extensor tendon excursion (Fig. 36-21, *A*). To obtain the 5 mm of excursion suggested to prevent dense adhesions, the joint would need to be moved through .05 radian or 28.64 degrees of angular movement (Fig. 36-21, *B*). This compares closely with my suggested equation that calculates that 28.3 degrees of MP motion effects 5 mm of extensor tendon excursion in the index finger.

Because joint size varies, the therapist must consider that it is the constant relationship of tendon excursion to angular

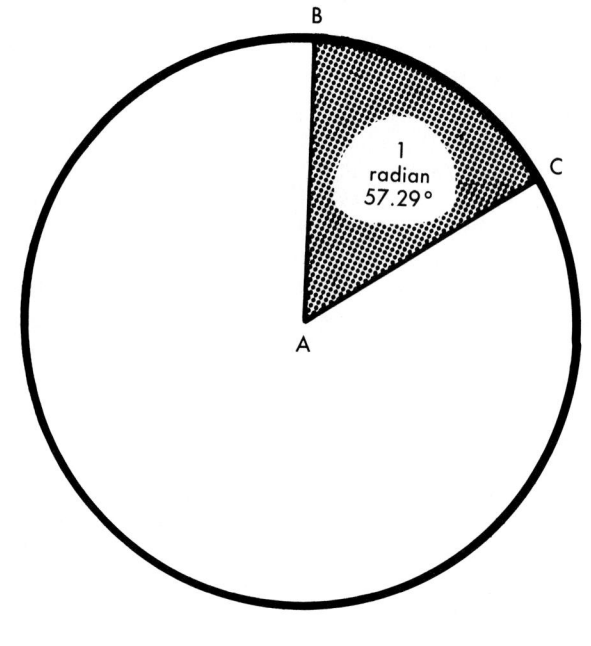

A = Axis

AB = Radius

AB = BC

BAC = 57.29°

Fig. 36-20   A radian is the angle that is created when the radius laid along the circumference of a circle is jointed by a line at each end to the center or axis of the circle. Angle BAC equals one radian, or 57.29 degrees.[9]

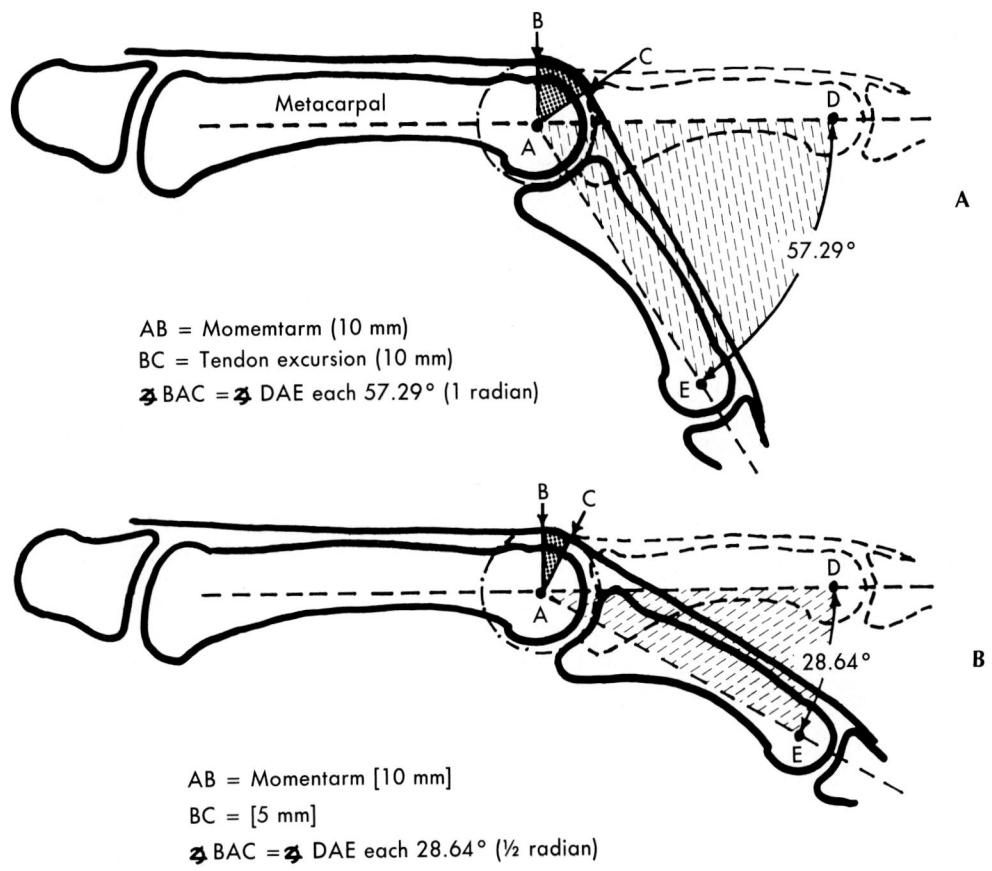

INDEX
E D C Excursion calculated at M P level by radians

AB = Momemtarm (10 mm)
BC = Tendon excursion (10 mm)
∡ BAC = ∡ DAE each 57.29° (1 radian)

A

AB = Momentarm [10 mm]
BC = [5 mm]
∡ BAC = ∡ DAE each 28.64° (½ radian)

B

Fig. 36-21   **A,** If the head of the metacarpal is considered in terms of a circle, the moment arm of the exensor tendon is equal to the radius of that circle. If metacarpophalangeal joint motion equals 57.29 degrees, or one radian, extensor tendon excursion is equal to the moment arm, or AB = BC. If the moment arm equals 10 mm, angular change of 57.29 degrees effects 10 mm of extensor tendon excursion.[9] **B,** Angular changes of 0.5 radians, 28.3 degrees, effects the 5 mm of extensor tendon excursion recommended for the early passive motion program. (**A** from Brand PW: Clinical Mechanics of the hand, St. Louis, 1985, The CV Mosby Co; **B** from Evans RB and Burkhalter W: A study of the dynamic anatomy of extensor tendons and implications for treatment, J Hand Surg 11A:774, 1986.)

change and the length of the moment arm that is important. For example, if the MP joint of the small finger has a moment arm of 7.5 mm, angular change of 0.5 radians, or 28.64 degrees, will produce 3.75 mm of glide. To effect 5 mm of glide, it would be necessary to calculate:

$$\frac{28.64°}{3.75 \text{ mm}} = 7.64° \text{ per each mm glide} \times 5 \text{ mm} = 38.2°$$

The smaller ulnar joints then might need to move through more than 0.5 radians to produce 5 mm of excursion. This correlates to my equation in which the ulnar digits require more MP motion to effect the 5 mm of respective tendon excursion. This is related to relative increased joint motion and decreased extensor excursion for the ulnar digits.[5,33,59,61]

Intraoperative measurements correlated closely with the suggested equation and measurement by radians. Burkhalter found by gross measurement that approximately 30 degrees of MP joint flexion effected 5 mm of extensor tendon glide in zones V, VI, and VII.[13,14]

The extensor pollicis longus tendon

Joint motion was also determined to produce 5 mm of excursion of the extensor pollicis longus tendon (EPL) at the retinacular level where tendon adherence is frequently a problem. Excursions for the EPL vary in the literature from 25 to 60 mm.[5,33,56] The simple angular arrangement of the flexion-extension axis at the MP level of the fingers does not exist for the EPL in zones TIV and TV. Calculating excursion is complicated by the oblique course that the tendon takes at Lister's tubercle, by the moments of adduction and external rotation at the carpometacarpal level, and by the fact that alterations in thumb position alter moment arms at each joint.[7,32] Therefore intraoperative studies determined the joint motion necessary to create 5 mm of EPL excursion in zones TIV and TV. Burkhalter found that with the wrist in neutral and the thumb MP joint extended, 60 degrees of IP joint motion effected 5 mm of tendon excursion at Lister's tubercle.

Postoperative management

The complex extensor tendon injury in zones V, VI, VII, TIV, and TV are splinted 3 days postoperatively.[12-14] Controlled stress is applied to the healing extrinsic finger extensors by allowing the tendons to glide 5 mm within a forearm-based dynamic extension splint. Stress is relieved at the repair site by positioning the wrist in extension, usually 40 to 45 degrees. The MP and IP joints rest in traction at 0 degrees (Fig. 36-22, *A*). An interlocking palmar-blocking splint will permit only the previously determined angular changes at the MP level. The patient actively flexes the MP joints until the fingers touch the volar block, then

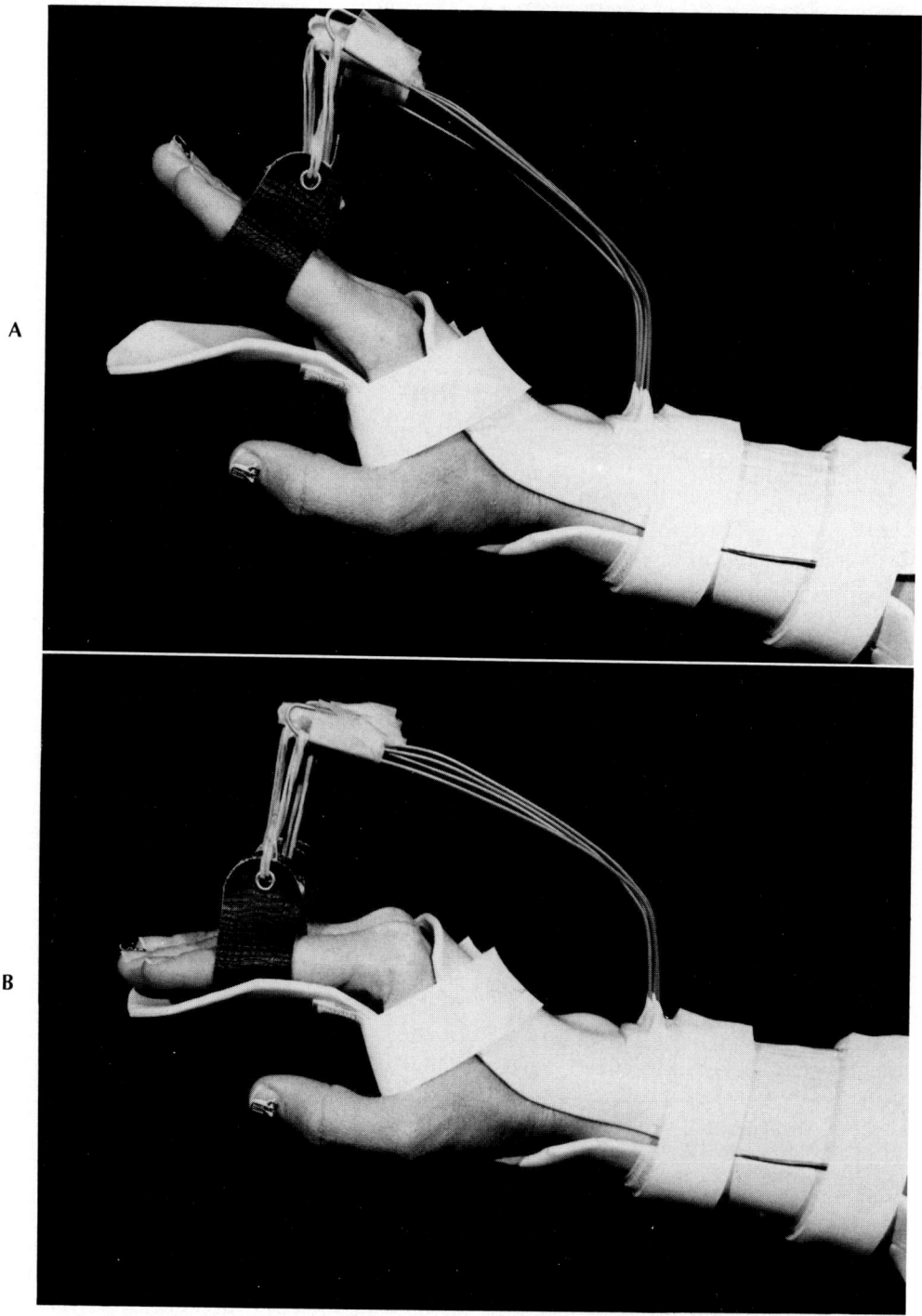

Fig. 36-22 **A,** A dorsal forearm-based, dynamic extension splint immobilizes the wrist at 45 degrees extension and rests all finger joints at 0 degrees to prevent extensor lag. A volar block permits only the predetermined metacarpophalangeal joint flexion, allowing slightly more flexion for the ulnar digits to achieve the necessary tendon excursion. **B,** The patient actively flexes the digits to the volar block 10 repetitions each waking hour to create 5 mm of passive excursion for the extensor tendons. Dynamic tractions return the digits to 0 degrees. (**A** from Evans RB and Burkhalter WE: A study of the dynamic anatomy of extensor tendons and implications for treatment, J Hand Surg 11A:774, 1986.)

relaxes the fingers, allowing the outrigger to bring the digits to 0-degree extension. The patient repeats the exercise ten times each waking hour (Fig. 36-22, *B*). If the PIP joints do not rest at 0 degrees within the extension slings or if the patient has difficulty flexing the MP level, digital extension splints may be taped to the digit to ensure that the motion is occurring at the MP level. The patient is seen in therapy for wound care, splint adjustments, and controlled passive motion to the IP joints to minimize IP joint problems. During dressing changes the therapist may perform passive range of motion to the PIP joints to reduce digital edema and prevent joint stiffness.

The therapist holds the wrist in maximum extension and the MP joints at 0-degree extension and passively moves each PIP joint. I allow 45 degrees of IP motion for zone V, 60 degrees of motion for zone VI, and 80 degrees of motion for zone VIII injuries, based on excursion studies and clinical experience in 126 cases.[14]

The patient follows the active-flexion, passive-extension

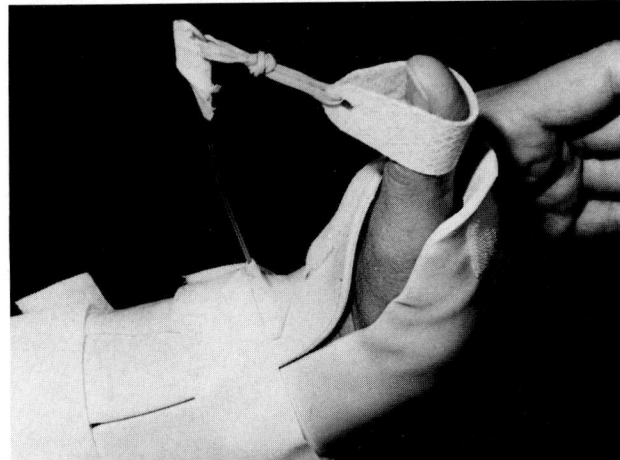

A

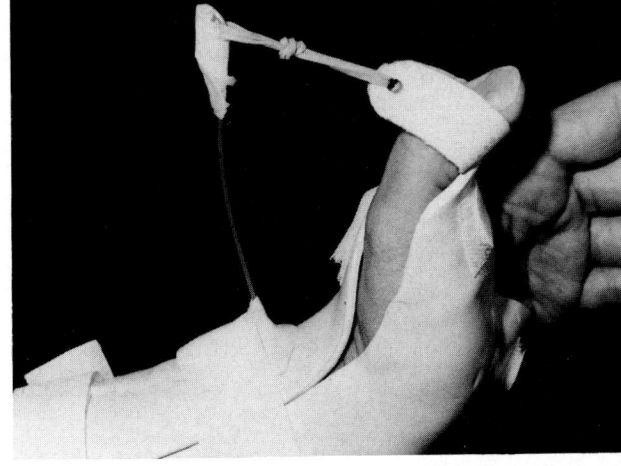

B

Fig. 36-23   **A,** The repaired extensor pollicis longus in zones IV and V is splinted with the wrist extended, carpometacarpal joint neutral, metacarpophalangeal joint at 0 degrees, and interphalangeal joint resting at 0 degrees by dorsal dynamic traction. **B,** The patient flexes the distal joint through its range 10 repetitions each hour to effect 5 mm of glide at the retinacular level. (**B** from Evans RB and Burkhalter WE: A study of the dynamic anatomy of extensor tendons and implications for treatment, J Hand Surg 11A:774, 1986.)

exercise regimen at home within the confines of the dynamic extension splint and volar block.

This regimen is followed for 21 days, at which time the volar block is removed and splint protection is provided during the day by the dynamic extension component for another 3 weeks. The volar component is worn at night during this additional 3-week period. Gradual active motion is initiated at 3 weeks as described in the previous section on zones V and VI. The usual protocol for extensor tendon rehabilitation follows for exercise and splinting.

The EPL is splinted with the wrist extended, carpometacarpal joint in neutral position, and MP joint at 0 degrees (Fig. 36-23, *A*). Dynamic traction rests the IP joint at 0 degrees but allows 60-degree active flexion (Fig. 36-23, *B*).

Resting the digital joints at 0 degrees prevents extensor lag.[12-14] The controlled stress to the tendon is thought to influence intrinsic healing, metabolic activity, tensile strength, and excursion.* (See also Chapters 12 and 28.) The MP joint motion prevents extension contractures and helps maintain collateral ligament integrity. This controlled intrinsic flexion promotes a tightening of the dorsal skin, which helps to create venous and lymphatic return, thus reducing edema and improving local nutrition.[66] (See also Chapter 35.)

The studies on controlled stress to healing tendon and reports of early passive motion for the complex extensor injury indicate that it may also be appropriate to use this technique in some cases with the simple extensor injury in zones V, VI, VII, TIV, and TV with the compliant patient.

SUMMARY

In the simple extensor injury, meticulous care in properly immobilizing each joint, combined with edema control, allows the patient to begin the mobilization phase with rehabilitation problems minimized. In the complex extensor injury in the described zones, early passive motion should be considered to reduce the complications common to crushing injuries or combined lesions of the extensor tendons.

*References 11, 14, 20-25, 34-36, 41, 45, 67, 69, 71.

REFERENCES

1. Agee J and Guidera M: The functional significance of the juncturae tendinae in dynamic stabilization of the metacarpophalangeal joints of the fingers. Presented at the 35th annual meeting of the American Society for Surgery of the Hand, Atlanta, Feb 1980.
2. Allieu Y, Asencio G, & Rouzaud JC: Protected passive mobilization after suturing of the extensor tendons of the hand: a survey of 120 cases. In Hunter JM and others, editors: Tendon surgery in the hand, St. Louis, 1987, The CV Mosby Co.
3. Beasley RW: Hand injuries, Philadelphia, 1981 WB Saunders Co.
4. Boland D: Anatomical and biomechanical observations of the extensor retinaculum. Scientific poster session, 41st annual meeting of the American Society of Hand Surgeons, New Orleans, Feb 1986.
5. Boyes JH: Bunnell's surgery of the hand, Philadelphia, 1970, JB Lippincott Co.
6. Brand PW: Biomechanics of tendon transfer, Orthop Clin North Am, 5:205, 1974.
7. Brand PW: Clinical mechanics of the hand, St. Louis, 1985, The CV Mosby Co.
8. Burkhalter, WE: Personal communications, Jan 1988.
9. Din KM and Maggitt BF: Mallet thumb, J Bone Joint Surg 66(B):606, 1983.

10. Doyle JR: Extensor tendons—acute injuries. In Green DP, editor: Operative hand surgery, New York, 1982, Churchill Livingstone, Inc.
11. Duran RJ and Houser RG: Controlled passive motion following flexor tendon repair in zones II and III. In AAOS symposium on tendon surgery in the hand, St. Louis, 1975, The CV Mosby Co.
12. Evans RB: Therapeutic management of extensor tendon injuries, Hand Clin 2:157, 1986.
13. Evans RB and Burkhalter WE: Early passive motion in the complex extensor tendon injury. Paper presented at the Second International Meeting of the American Society of Hand Therapists, Boston, October 19, 1983.
14. Evans RB and Burkhalter WE: A study of the dynamic anatomy of extensor tendons and implications for treatment, J Hand Surg 11A:774, 1986.
15. Evans RB, Hunter JM and Burkhalter WE: Conservative management of the trigger finger: a new approach, J Hand Ther, 1:59, 1988.
16. Fahrer M: Interdependent and independent actions of the fingers. In Tubiana R editor: The hand, vol 1, Philadelphia, 1981, WB Saunders Co.
17. Flatt AE: Care of the arthritic hand, ed 4, St. Louis, 1983, The CV Mosby Co.
18. Flint MH: Connective tissue organization. In Tubiana R editor: The hand, Philadelphia, 1981 WB Saunders Co.
19. Furlow LT: Early active motion in flexor tendon healing, J Bone Joint Surg 54(A):911, 1972.
20. Gelberman RH and others: The influence of protected passive mobilization on the healing of flexor tendons, Hand 13:120 1981.
21. Gelberman RH & Manske PR: Effects of early motion on the tendon healing process: experimental studies. In Hunter JM and others, editors: Tendon surgery in the hand, St. Louis, 1987, The CV Mosby Co.
22. Gelberman RH and others: The effects of mobilization on the vascularization of healing flexor tendons in dogs, Clin Orthop 153:283, 1980.
23. Gelberman RH and others: Flexor tendon healing and restoration of the gliding surface: an ultrastructural study in dogs, J Bone Joint Surg 65A:583, 1980.
24. Gelberman RH and others: The early stages of flexor tendon healing: a morphological study of the first 14 days, J Hand Surg 10A:776, 1985.
25. Gelberman RH and others: Effects of early intermittent passive mobilization on healing canine flexor tendons, J Hand Surg 7:170, 1982.
26. Harris EC: Intrinsic balance of the extensor system. In Hunter JM and others, editors: Tendon surgery in the hand, St. Louis, 1987, The CV Mosby Co.
27. Hobby J: Postoperative edema. In Tubiana R, editor: The hand, Philadelphia, 1985, WB Saunders Co.
28. Holdeman V: Rehabilitation of extensor tendon injuries. In Hunter JM and others, editors: Rehabilitation of the hand, St. Louis, 1984, The CV Mosby Co.
29. Iselin F: Reconstruction techniques for treating mallet finger. In Hunter JM and others, editors: Tendon surgery in the hand, St. Louis, 1987, The CV Mosby Co.
30. Iselin F, Lerame J and Godoy J: A simplified technique for treating mallet fingers: tenodermodesis, J Hand Surg 2:118, 1977.
31. Joint motion: method of measuring and recording, Am Acad Ortho Surg, p. 27, 1965.
32. Kapandji IA: Biomechanics of the thumb. In Tubiana R editor: The hand, Philadelphia, 1985, WB Saunders Co.
33. Kaplan EB: Functional and surgical anatomy of the hand, ed 2, Philadelphia, 1965.
34. Kleinert HE and Verdan C: Report of the committee on tendon injuries, J Hand Surg 8:795, 1983.
35. Landi A: Oxidative enzyme activity in flexor tendons. In Hunter JM and others, editors: Tendon surgery in the hand, St. Louis, 1987, The CV Mosby Co.
36. Lister GP and others: Primary flexor tendon repair followed by immediate controlled mobilization, J Hand Surg 2:441, 1977.
37. Littler JW: The digital extensor-flexor system. In Converse JM editor: Reconstructive plastic surgery, vol 6, Philadelphia, 1977, WB Saunders Co.
38. Lovett WL and McCalla MA: Management and rehabilitation of extensor tendon injuries: symposium on rehabilitation after reconstructive hand surgery, Philadelphia, 1983, WB Saunders Co.
39. Lundborg G and others: Superficial repair of severed tendon in synovial environment, J Hand Surg 5:451, 1980.
40. Lundborg G and Rank F: Experimental intrinsic healing of flexor tendons based on synovial fluid nutrition, J Hand Surg 3:21, 1978.
41. Lundborg G and Rank F: Tendon healing: intrinsic mechanisms. In Hunter JM and others, editors: Tendon surgery in the hand, St. Louis, 1987, The CV Mosby Co.
42. Macht SD and Watson HK: The Moberg volar advancement flap for digital reconstruction, J Hand Surg 5:372, 1980.
43. Manske PR and Lesker PA: Diffusion as a nutrient pathway to the flexor tendon. In Hunter JM and others, editors: Tendon surgery in the hand, St. Louis, 1987, The CV Mosby Co.
44. Manske PR & Lesker PA: Nutrient pathways to extensor tendons within the extensor retinacular compartments, Clin Orthop 181:234, 1983.
45. Mason ML and Allen HS: The rate of healing of tendons: an experimental study of tensile strength, Ann Surg 113:424, 1941.
46. Milford L: The hand, St. Louis, 1982, The CV Mosby Co.
47. Millender LH, Nalebuff EA, and Feldon PG: Rheumatoid arthritis. In Green DP editor: Operative hand surgery, New York, 1982, Churchill Livingstone, Inc.
48. Miura T, Ryogo N, and Shuhei T: Conservative treatment for a ruptured extensor tendon on the dorsum of the proximal phalanges of the thumb (mallet thumb), J Hand Surg 11A:229, 1986.
49. Nissenbaum M: Early care of flexor tendon injuries: application of principles of tendon healing and early motion. In Hunter JM and others, editors: Rehabilitation of the hand, ed 1, St. Louis, 1978, The CV Mosby Co.
50. Parry CBW: Rehabilitation of the hand, ed 3, London, 1973, Butterworth and Co, Ltd.
51. Patel MR, Desai SS, & Bassini-Lipson L: Conservative management of chronic mallet finger, J Hand Surg 11A:570, 1986.
52. Prendergast K: Therapist's management of the mutilated hand. In Hunter JM and others, editors: Rehabilitation of the hand, ed 2, St. Louis, 1984, The CV Mosby Co.
53. Primiano GA: Conservative treatment of two cases of mallet thumb, J Hand Surg 11A:233, 1986.
54. Rayan GM & Mullins PT: Skin necrosis complicating mallet finger splinting and vascularity of the distal interphalangeal joint overlying skin, J Hand Surg 12A:548, 1987.
55. Schneider LH and Smith KL: Boutonnière deformity. In Hunter JM and others, editors: Tendon surgery in the hand, St. Louis, 1987, The CV Mosby Co.
56. Steindler A: Kinesiology of the human body under normal and pathological condition, Springfield, 1964, Charles C Thomas Publisher.
57. Strickland JW and Glogovac SV: Digital function following flexor tendon repair in zone II: a comparison of immobilization and controlled passive motion techniques, J Hand Surg 5:537, 1980.
58. Taleisnik J and others: The extensor retinaculum of the wrist, J Hand Surg 9A:495, 1984.
59. Thromine JM: The clinical examination of the hand. In Tubiana R, editor: The hand, Philadelphia, 1981, WB Saunders Co.
60. Tubiana R: Injuries to the extensor apparatus on the dorsum of the fingers. In Verdan C, editor: Tendon surgery of the hand, New York, 1979, Churchill Livingstone, Inc.
61. Tubiana R: Architecture and functions of the hand. In Tubiana R, editor: The hand, vol 1, Philadelphia, 1981, WB Saunders Co.
62. Tubiana R: The management of hand wounds. In Tubiana R, editor: The hand, vol 2, Philadelphia, 1985, WB Saunders Co.
63. Tubiana R: Stiffness of the fingers: anatomical, pathological, etiological, and clinical considerations. In Tubiana R, editor: The hand, vol 2, Philadelphia, 1985, WB Saunders Co.
64. Tubiana R: Injuries to the digital extensors, Hand Clin 2, 149, 1986.
65. Valentin P: Physiology of extension of the fingers. In Tubiana R, editor: The hand, vol 1, Philadelphia, 1981, WB Saunders Co.
66. Verdan C: Lymphatic vascularization of tendons. In Tubiana R, editor: The hand, vol 1, Philadelphia, 1981, WB Saunders Co.
67. Weber ER: Nutritional pathways for flexor tendons in the digital theca. In Hunter JM and others, editors: Tendon surgery in the hand, St. Louis, 1987, The CV Mosby Co.
68. Wilson RL: Management of acute extensor tendon injuries. In Hunter JM and others, editors: Tendon surgery in the hand, St. Louis, 1987, The CV Mosby Co.
69. Woo SL-Y and others: The importance of controlled passive mobilization on flexor tendon healing: a biomechanical study, Acta Orthop Scand 52:615, 1981.

70. Woodbourne RT: Essentials of human anatomy, New York, 1965, Oxford University Press.
71. Young RES and Harmon JM: Repair of tendon injuries of the hand, Ann Surg 151:562, 1960.
72. Zbrodowski A, Gajisin S and Grodecki J: Vascularization and anatomical model of the mesotendons of the extensor digitorum and extensor indicis muscles, J Anat 130:697, 1980.

ADDITIONAL READINGS

Elson RA: Rupture of the central slip of the extensor hood of the finger: a test for early diagnosis, J Bone Joint Surg [Br] 68B:229, 1986.
Niechajev IA: Conservative and operative treatment of the mallet finger, Plast Reconstr Surg 76:580, 1985.
Regnard PJ and others: Extensor tendon injuries: presentation of a series of 99 cases, Ann Chir Main 4:55, 1985.
Saldana MJ and McGuire RA: Chronic painful subluxation of the metacarpal phalangeal joint extensor tendons, J Hand Surg IIA:420, 1986.

VII
NERVE INJURIES

37

Nerve response to injury and repair

George E. Omer, Jr.

The peripheral nerves are extensions of the central nervous system and are responsible for integrating the activities of the hand. Interruption of the structural continuity of a peripheral nerve results in derangement of the involved functional units. A functional unit is called a "neuron." The neuron consists of the nerve cell nucleus and cytoplasm (perikaryon) in the anterior column of the spinal cord (motor neurons) or the dorsal root ganglia (sensory neurons), the nerve cell cytoplasm in the peripheral nerve trunk (axon), and the anatomic unit at the synaptic terminal (such as the extrafusal fibers of muscles of Meissner's touch corpuscles) (Fig. 37-1). If the central cell body (perikaryon) were the height of an average man, its axon would be 1 or 2 inches in diameter and would extend more than 2 miles.[17] The number of neurons is constant after birth, and there is no replacement when a nerve cell is destroyed.

The axon may be surrounded by Schwann cells, which form the insulation (myelin) for fast conduction of nerve impulses. External to the Schwann cell layer is a connective tissue sheath termed the "endoneurium" (Fig. 37-2). The endoneurial tube (Schwann tube or Büngner band) may contain only one myelinated axon or several unmyelinated axons. The nerve fiber (axon and sheath) is the smallest structural unit of the peripheral nerve. Nerve fibers are gathered into aggregations called fasciculi, funiculi, or nerve bundles. Each fasciculus is composed usually of a mixture of motor, sensory, and sympathetic fibers. The perineurium is a relatively fine but strong connective tissue sheath that encases each fasciculus. Fasciculi are arranged usually in groups as they proceed peripherally. The groups (bundles) of fasciculi are embedded in epineurium (intraneurial epineurium, intrafascicular epineurium, or epineu-

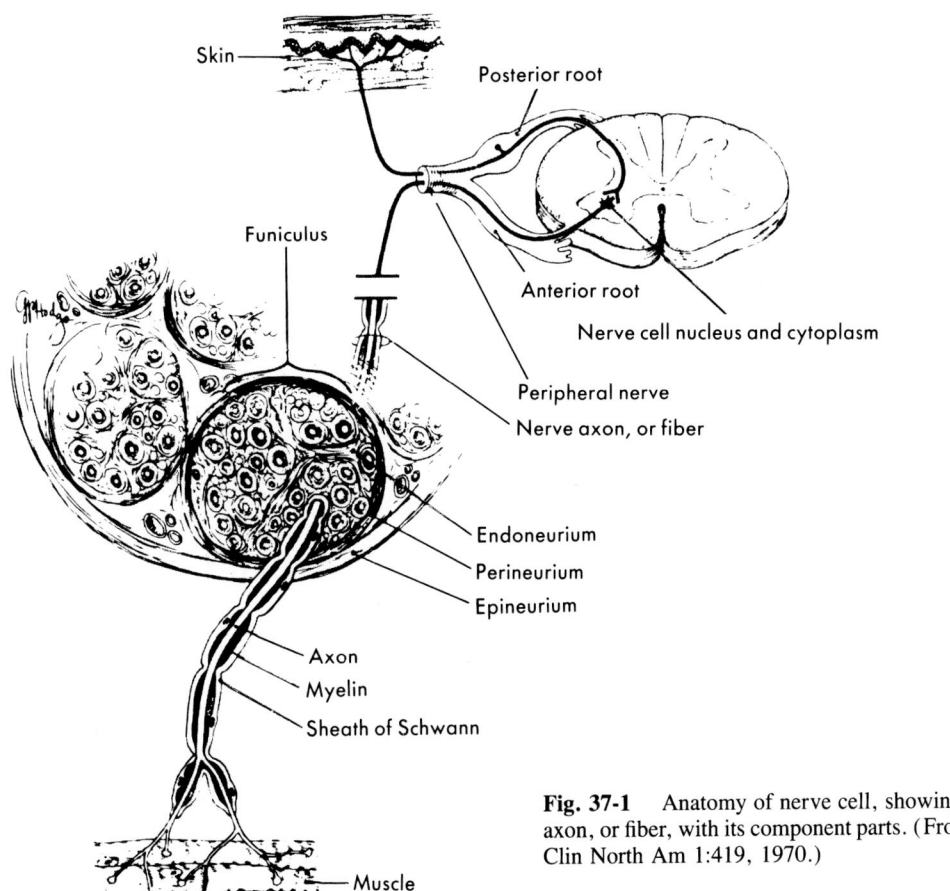

Fig. 37-1 Anatomy of nerve cell, showing cell body and nerve axon, or fiber, with its component parts. (From Grabb WC: Orthop Clin North Am 1:419, 1970.)

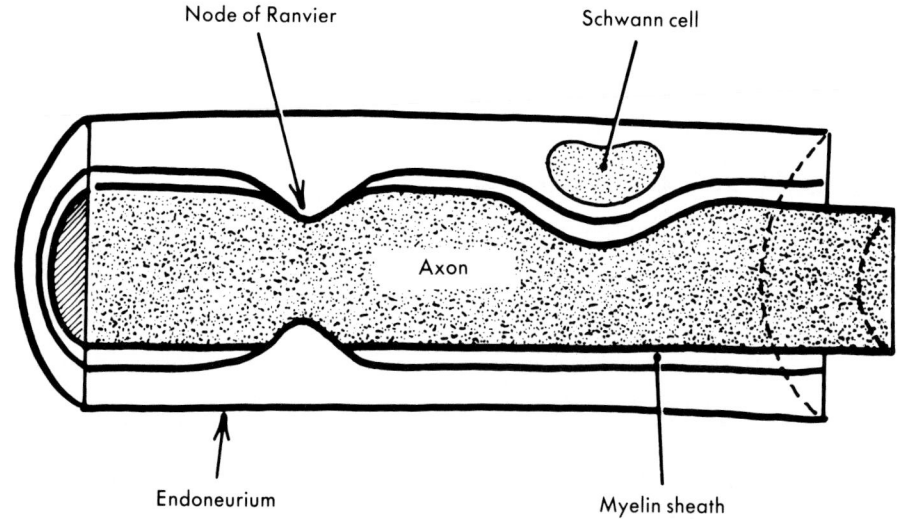

Fig. 37-2 Basic anatomy of a myelinated nerve fiber. (From Urbaniak JR and Warren FH: Application of microsurgical techniques in the care of the injured peripheral nerve. In AAOS Symposium on Microsurgery, St Louis, 1979, The CV Mosby Co.)

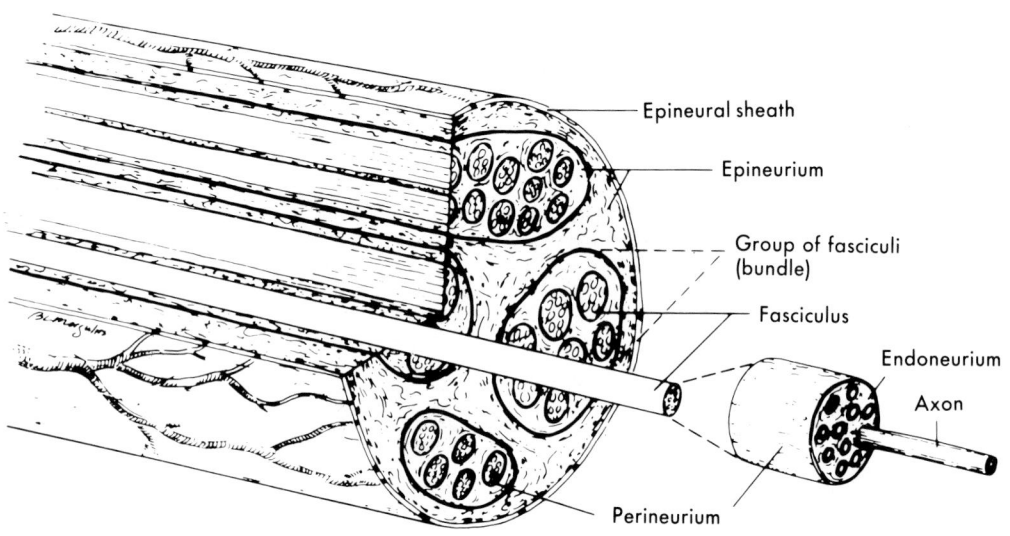

Fig. 37-3 Basic structures of a peripheral nerve. (From Urbaniak JR: Clin Orthop Rel Res 163:57, 1982.)

rial connective tissue). The amount of epineurial tissue within a peripheral nerve trunk may range from 25% to 75% of the cross-sectional area[69] (Fig. 37-3). The epineurium is condensed at the surface of the nerve trunk to form a definite encasing sheath, the epineurial sheath (nerve sheath or circumferential sheath).

INJURY

After injury to the axon there are retrograde reactions involving the central cell body. The more proximal the extremity injury (axonal level) and the greater the violence to the axon (stretch avulsion as opposed to transection), the more severe the reaction to the central cell body. Estimates of neuronal death range from 30% to 75%.[69] Even if the nerve cell survives, the volume (length) of axon that must be regenerated may exceed the metabolic capacity of the central cell body. Retrograde effects will be more serious

in sensory than in motor neurons, and sensory recovery will be slower and less satisfactory than motor recovery.[65] A child has a greater regeneration potential than an adult and a shorter axon distance between the spinal cord and functional end organs.

In the distal nerve stump all the neuronal elements undergo secondary degeneration. Morphologic changes occur within 24 hours after injury, and all unmyelinated axons degenerate within 1 week.[51] Muscles respond to nerve stimulation for 4 or 5 days, and ascending (sensory) nerve action potentials can be recorded for 6 to 8 days after axon division.[71] By 3 weeks after injury most of the axon and myelin have been digested by the Schwann cells, and by 8 weeks the débridement is complete.[16] With subsequent collapse of the individual endoneurial tubes, the reentry of regenerating axons may be difficult. This shrinkage of the distal stump is maximal at approximately 3 months after injury.[71] Endoneurial tubes within the distal segment of a disrupted nerve may wither to 10% of their original diameter,[25] and to what extent the endoneurial tube can expand in response to ingrowing axons is unknown. The conduction velocity in sutured human nerves frequently remains slow (20% to 60% of normal) even with clinical return of function.[25] The prognosis for recovery is better when nerve suture is performed within 3 months after injury.

For nerve regeneration to occur, myelinated axon sprouts must enter a distal endoneurial tube (Schwann tube or Büngner band) and be invaginated by Schwann cells and then remyelinated. Schwann cells of unmyelinated axons do not form compact columns analogous to the bands of Büngner. In a mixed nerve perhaps 50% of the regenerating motor neurons will grow down sensory pathways and the remainder correctly enter motor pathways.[20] However, many neurons in the motor pathway may be inappropriate in that they previously served antagonists of the muscle being reinnervated.[11] In like manner, sympathetic axons regenerating through endoneurial tubes destined for muscle form no functional end-organ connections and deny the entry of motor axons. Only slight rotation of either end of a severed nerve would produce misdirected axons or appose significant numbers of axons to an impervious epineurium and perineurium. The amount of tension, both circumferential and longitudinal, within a sutured nerve is directly related to connective tissue proliferation at the anastomosis.[35] The maturing scar tissue will shrink and constrict the axons. The regenerating axons may fail to achieve myelination, which would then lead to anatomic but not functional innervation of the end organs.

Denervation of skeletal muscle results in progressive shrinkage of muscle fibers and ultimate destruction. After 3 months the motor end plates become increasingly distorted by proliferating connective tissue. Denervated muscle does survive for relatively long periods, as evidenced by biopsy material and the persistence of fibrillations.[66] Muscle fiber viability can be demonstrated up to 3 years after denervation, but atrophy and connective tissue proliferation may preclude functional recovery after reinnervation.[71] The clinical impression that electrical stimulation of denervated muscle delays muscle fiber derangement and motor endplate destruction has not been supported by human microscopic studies or measured work capacity of the muscle before and after denervation.[47,74] However, experimental long-term stimulation of muscle has demonstrated histochemical evidence of fiber-type transformation[56] and the prevention of decreased oxidative enzymes.[41] Muscle regeneration will occur under the stimulus of a functional nerve to supply both afferent and efferent pathways of the neural reflexes controlling muscle contraction.[4]

The extent to which biologic mechanisms are influenced by electrical forces is unknown.[6,7,9] Direct electrical current has been shown to stimulate growth of neurons in vitro[61] similar to the facilitatory effects of nerve growth factor, which has a predominant role only on embryonal neural tissues. There is current research[42] on the effect of minute direct electrical currents to the area of a nerve repair (suture site) after laceration. Insufficient data are available to determine if nerve regeneration will be enhanced by electrical forces.

Sensory receptor end organs that are denervated undergo progressive degeneration over several months, and it is prob-
able that adult mammals lack the ability to form new sensory receptors after nerve transection.[51] After 4 months the Meissner corpuscle is incapable of full response to a regenerating axon.[15] The Meissner corpuscle appears to be about midway in the rate of degeneration between the rapid Merkel cell–neurite complex and the more stable pacinian corpuscle. It is unknown whether a regenerating axon can innervate a different sensory receptor, such as a quickly adapting axon innervating a Merkel cell–neurite complex, nor is the potential functional result known. It would appear that sensory end organs are even more susceptible to degeneration than skeletal muscle is, and a delay longer than 6 months between injury and suture will handicap the recovery of sensation.

The rate at which the axon regenerates has clinical importance. There are three periods of delay: neuronal survival, crossing the area of nerve disruption, and the end-organ connection. The patient's age and the tissue homeostasis of the involved extremity are important factors. The rate of growth gradually slows as the length of the axon increases. For practical use, after suture of a divided peripheral nerve there is a 3- to 4-week latent period, followed by axon advance of approximately 1 mm per day.[59]

In the clinical situation, there are three basic injury-regeneration patterns to consider, as outlined by Seddon[57]: Minimal nerve injury is termed "neurapraxia," in which the nerve is intact but conduction is impaired. Moderate injury, termed "axonotmesis," is characterized by interruption of the axons and their myelin sheaths; however, the endoneurial tubes remain intact and guide the regenerating axons to their appropriate peripheral connections. Severe injury, termed "neurotmesis," describes a nerve that has either been completely severed or is so seriously disorganized that spontaneous regeneration is impossible. Most traumatic accidents, including fractures, dislocations, and gunshot wounds, can result in any one of these three types of injury. Lacerations usually result in neurotmesis. Total loss of nerve function after this injury demands exploration and suture of the affected nerve.

NOCICEPTIVE COMPLICATIONS OF NERVE INJURY

Current investigation indicates that pain may be a specific sensory event and not merely excessive stimulation of other sensory modalities. Current investigation has resulted in better definition of the specific pain receptors in the skin, viscera, and deep somatic structures. All these receptors respond to innocuous stimulation, whether it is mechanical, thermal, electrical, or chemical. A significant portion of the bare nerve endings are termed "nociceptors" and respond only to strong stimulation that is potentially damaging to tissue. In the peripheral nervous system, the small myelinated axons are called "A-delta" (class III) and conduct at 12 to 80 meters per second. Approximately 25% of these axons are nociceptors and are stimulated by temperatures above 45° C or below 10° C and by intense mechanical stimulation. The even smaller unmyelinated axons are termed "C-delta" (class IV) and conduct at 0.4 to 1.0 meters per second. Approximately 50% of these axons are nociceptors. Iggo has defined the characteristics of the nociceptors as follows: very high thresholds to mechanical or thermal stimuli, relatively small receptive fields, and persistent after discharges for any suprathreshold stimulus.[27] There are three groups of nociceptors: high-threshold mechanoreceptors, heat nociceptors, and "polymodal" nociceptors responsive to both noxious mechanical and noxious thermal stimuli.[8] Polymodal and heat nociceptors can be sensitized after repeated or prolonged stimulation, or during regeneration after section of nerve, so that their thresholds for activation can be lowered to levels of stimulus intensity that are ordinarily innocuous. This could account for the pain states occurring after burns or nerve injury.[62]

The sympathetic nervous system of the upper extremity is concentrated in the thoracic portion of the spinal cord. Myelinated sympathetic axons exist through the anterior nerve root and then separate to form the white rami that enter the thoracic ganglia. A synapse occurs, and the postganglionic unmyelinated axons exit from the thoracic ganglia and enter the peripheral nerve. Since preganglionic axons form plexuses and synapses with many different postganglionic axons, a sympathetic discharge may affect several different target organs represented in more than one dermatome. Activation of a sympathetic discharge may elicit either an excitatory or an inhibitory response in different target organs, based on the relative potencies of the various catecholamines released at the neuroeffector junction. During an abnormal process, such as reflex sympathetic dystrophy, there may be great variations in the extremity, such as vasodilatation or vasoconstriction, increased redness or pallor, sweating or dryness, coolness or heat, depending on the severity or the state of involvement of different organs.

Injured nerve axons are excited by norepinephrine, which is the substance released at the neuroeffector junction by efferent impulses in the sympathetic nervous system. In the normal intact sensory nerve, sympathetic transmitters do not evoke obvious injury signals, although they may modulate sensitivity. Partially damaged nerve membrane and the unmyelinated axons (sprouts) within a neuroma are highly sensitive to norepinephrine. Stimulation of myelinated axons releases local endorphins, which dampen or stop the oversensitive spontaneous activity of these unmyelinated axons at the spinal cord level. When tissue is injured, the nociceptors are influenced by sympathetic efferents, the chemical environment, the vasculature, the temperature, and high-frequency antidromic impulses.

The study of peripheral receptors led to an understanding of the relationship between humoral mediators and pain. Acute inflammation invokes an exudative response that results in hydrolysis of extracellular macromolecules and breakdown of intracellular compounds.[60] The immediate mediators include histamine, released from basophils and mast cells, and serotonin, released from platelets. At the same time, plasma precursors are activated to form materials with a low molecular weight that provoke acute vascular inflammation and pain. All injured cells release prostaglandins and thromboxanes. These mediators are also liberated by mechanical pressure, electrical stimulation, radiation, or thermal injury. They induce pain in two ways: (1) direct irritation or stimulation of the nociceptors and (2) sensitizing the nociceptors to the pain-provoking effect of kinins and similar substances. The humoral mediators lower the threshold to pain transmission and increase the intensity of the stimulus.

We would suffer unrelenting pain if there were no endogenous defense against these humoral mediators. The

mechanisms that limit their activity are being identified. For example, histaminase is produced to break down histamine, and peptidases degrade the kinins. Specific drugs can interrupt metabolic reactions such as the injury of cells to form prostaglandins and thromboxanes. The clinical value of nonsteroidal anti-inflammatory agents, such as aspirin or indomethacin, is that they block the metabolic pathway for the formation of prostaglandins and thromboxanes.[72]

The action potential produced by stimulation of the nociceptors passes to the dorsal horn of the spinal cord, which has six laminae of cell networks that both process and transmit the impulses.[54] There appear to be two types of pain-related sensory neurons in the dorsal horn. Class 1 nociceptive neurons are located in the most superficial layer of the dorsal horn (lamina 1). Class 1 neurons are responsive to injurious levels of stimulation.[14] Class 2 nociceptive neurons are located primarily in lamina 5 and respond to low-intensity stimulation, but as the intensity of stimulation is increased these neurons follow with more vigorous and sustained discharge.[73] Class 2 neurons are impinged upon by both somatic and visceral sources and may be involved in visceral referred pain.[24] Melzack and Wall[34] postulated a dynamic interaction (control gate) among large and small afferent neurons, mediated through the small cells of the substantia gelatinosa (lamina 2 and 3). Large afferent neurons excite the cells of the substantia gelantinosa and increase presynaptic inhibition (closing the gate) to noxious impulses incoming on small afferent neurons. Small afferent neurons inhibit the cells of the substantia gelatinosa and thus decrease the presynaptic inhibition (opening the gate). Pain is perceived when a threshold level of nociceptive action potential is attained by the central transmission neurons.

Nociceptive impulses are transmitted from the dorsal horn of the spinal cord to all levels of the central nervous system. The neurons in laminae I, IV, V, and VI of the dorsal horn connect to the spinothalamic system, the neospinothalamic tract, and the paleospinothalamic tract.[13,70] The neospinothalamic tract runs to the thalamus, where it synapses with central neurons that pass to the somatosensory cortex. This tract conveys information for perception of sharp, well-localized pain. The older paleospinothalamic tract projects to the spinal cord and the thalamus, where it synapses with neurons that connect with the limbic forebrain structures. This tract conveys information for the perception of poorly localized, dull, aching, burning pain. Impulses transmitted by this tract provoke suprasegmental reflex responses concerned with circulation, respiration, and endocrine function. In addition, there are multisynaptic afferent systems, including the spinoreticular system, spinocervicothalamic system, dorsal intracornu system, and other complex tracts. In this infinitely duplicated system for the reception, transmission, and perception of pain, there is specificity at the periphery, but in the central nervous system the specificity is lost completely.

Supraspinal descending neural systems modify the nociceptive impulses. The pyramidal tracts, rubrospinal tracts, and retinculospinal tracts influence transmission in the dorsal horn.[22,63] The descending fibers from the cortex of the brain affect transmission in the thalamus, reticular formation, dorsal column of the cord, and other relay stations.

In 1969 Reynolds[55] stimulated cells in the periaqueductal periventricular gray matter and produced profound analgesia at the spinal cord level. This stimulation-produced analgesia can completely inhibit the pain-evoked discharges of class 2 dorsal horn neurons, without affecting their responsiveness to nonpainful stimuli.[43] This appears to be the same descending circuit affected by morphine to produce analgesia.[31] One particular spinal pathway conveying these descending pain-modulatory impulses is the dorsolateral funiculus, which terminates in the dorsal horn of the spinal cord. The neurotransmitter carried by these cells and released in the spinal cord is serotonin.[2,62] Either chemical or dietary depletion of brain serotonin levels increases sensitivity to pain. Tolerance develops to stimulation-produced analgesia, and cross-tolerance is found between morphine and stimulation-induced analgesia.[32] The morphine antagonist naloxone reverses stimulation-produced analgesia[1] when the stimulator is located ventrally within the periaqueductal gray matter, but it does not block analgesia when the stimulator is located dorsally within the periaqueductal gray matter.[3]

There are stereospecific receptors for the alkaloids from the opium poppy in the brain.[19] These receptors are confined to nervous tissue and perhaps the transmission of pain.[52] Hughes and colleagues[26] extracted a peptide of low molecular weight from the brain that acted as an agonist at opiate receptor sites, and its action was prevented by narcotic antagonists. The peptide was named "enkephalin." Others noted that the amino acid sequence of enkephalin was identical to that of beta-lipotropin C-fragment, a pituitary peptide. A higher opiate activity was exhibited by the beta-lipotropin C-fragment peptide than by enkephalin.[10] The C-fragment is now named "beta-endorphin." Beta-endorphin produces analgesic effects three to four times more potent than those of morphine when injected intravenously.[68] Pretreatment with naloxone eliminates the analgesia. A possible neurotransmitter or neuromodulator role for these neuropeptides is suggested by studies showing that they affect the action or release of dopamine and acetylcholine.[29,30,38] Acupuncture analgesia may be mediated by morphine-like hormones or neuropeptides released by the pituitary.[53] Thus it may be possible that the physiologic role of opiates and endogenous opiate-like neuropeptides involves the transmission of pain. The endogenous opiate-like neuropeptides may act on both presynaptic and postsynaptic opiate receptors in the spinal cord and brain. The same substance may be used as a neurotransmitter in one instance, a neuromodulator in another, and a hormone in still another situation.[21,44]

In addition to the endogenous opioid mechanism for analgesia, there may be a nonopioid mechanism. Mayer and colleagues[31] reported that naloxone blocked acupunctural analgesia, but not hypnotic analgesia in humans. Stimulation-produced analgesia is effective when the stimulator is in one portion of the periaqueductal gray matter but is not effective when the stimulator is moved to nearby sites.[3] Mayer and Price[33] have proposed that the descending pain-inhibitory mechanism may involve both a serotonergic and an enkephalin-like neurotransmitter system. Endorphins (enkephalins) may act as hormone-releasing or hormone-inhibiting factors in peripheral target organs such as the adrenal medulla and the pancreas.[5] Electrical or chemical stimulation of either system produces analgesia, whereas chemical or surgical blockade of either prevents analgesia.

TIMING OF NERVE REPAIR

No controlled prospective study comparing clinical function after primary and secondary nerve suture has been reported. Clinical studies in the human show considerable variation because the return of useful function depends as much on the total response of the extremity to the injury as on the regeneration of the injured nerve.[45,46]

Our preference is to suture a severed nerve during the first 24 hours when there is a "clean" laceration and to wait 3 to 5 days when there is an injury to an extremity that is managed best with a delayed primary closure.[48] An extensive extremity wound dictates that nerve suture be delayed until after there is homeostasis of the involved tissues and the correct level of demarcation of the nerve injury can be determined.

Advantages of nerve suture at the time of acute injury include the following: (1) nerve stumps require minimal mobilization and débridement because the cut ends have not retracted and become embedded in scar tissue; (2) extensive dissection of the extremity is not required to remove scar tissue; (3) the axonal bundles at the nerve ends are more likely to correspond; (4) satisfactory suture can be performed without tension; (5) immediate suture reduces the time for which peripheral tissues are denervated and the patient is impaired; and (6) if a second operation is required, it is technically easier because the nerve ends are not retracted and the amount of nerve to be débrided (and therefore the gap to be closed) is reduced. Primary suture should be reserved for those cases in which the conditions of injury justify immediate closure and in which surgery can be done by an adequate operating room staff.

Advantages of delayed primary closure over acute closure include the following: (1) a contaminated wound will have become either clinically infected or safe for reconstructive surgery; (2) the repair is an elective procedure performed by an experienced surgeon; and (3) wound closure can incorporate additional débridement, stabilization of skeletal elements, and distal flap coverage.[12]

Advantages of delayed nerve suture (after 3 weeks) include the following: (1) the total injury to the extremity can be evaluated; nerves are only as functional as their sensory receptors and the viable muscle-tendon motor units; (2) multiple nerve involvement can be approached with incisions clear of the primary scar; (3) the extent of intraneural fibrosis and axonal damage at the nerve ends can be accurately determined, and débridement will offer the potential for less blocking scar; and (4) the epineurium is then thicker and facilitates epineurial sheath suture technique, and the intraneurial epineurium is also thicker for group fascicular (axonal bundles) suture technique.

Closed fractures of long bones with associated nerve injuries present a problem concerning the time for elective exploration and possible nerve suture. Approximately 85% have spontaneous recovery. A poorer prognosis usually involves a fracture adjacent to a joint, a fracture-dislocation with stretching of the nerve, or a severely comminuted fracture. Complete and precise physical examination of peripheral nerve function at the time of injury offers the best baseline for management. Electrodiagnostic studies should be initiated after 1 month and recorded periodically for evaluation of the course of clinical recovery. It is appropriate to explore at 3 to 4 months nerve lesions that result in total functional loss and that are associated with missile and gunshot wounds above the elbow, stretch injuries from dislocation of joints, or fractures that are severely comminuted or adjacent to joint.[49]

NERVE SUTURE

There are only two principles in the techniques for suture of nerves: (1) align the axons (fascicular groups), and (2) avoid tension in all suture lines. The technique of nerve suture is the only factor affecting the return of function that is fully under the control of the surgeon.[35,46]

The controversy of whether epineurial or some type of fascicular (fiber-bundle) repair gives better results is yet to be resolved[50] (Fig. 37-4). Most cleanly severed peripheral nerves should be repaired by the epineurial technique, especially proximal (high) lesions where there are many groups of fascicles (fiber bundles) that cannot be easily identified or matched. Epineurial repair should be selected when a slight amount of tension is necessary at the suture line.[69] Group fascicular (fiber-bundle) repair is indicated for median and ulnar nerves severed at the wrist (Fig. 37-5). The dorsal cutaneous branch of the ulnar nerve and the thenar branch of the median nerve should be separated from the main nerve trunk in these lesions.[37] Group fascicular (fiber-bundle) repair is indicated in nerve-graft anastomoses and is probably responsible for the improved results that can now be expected from that method of repair.[37,66]

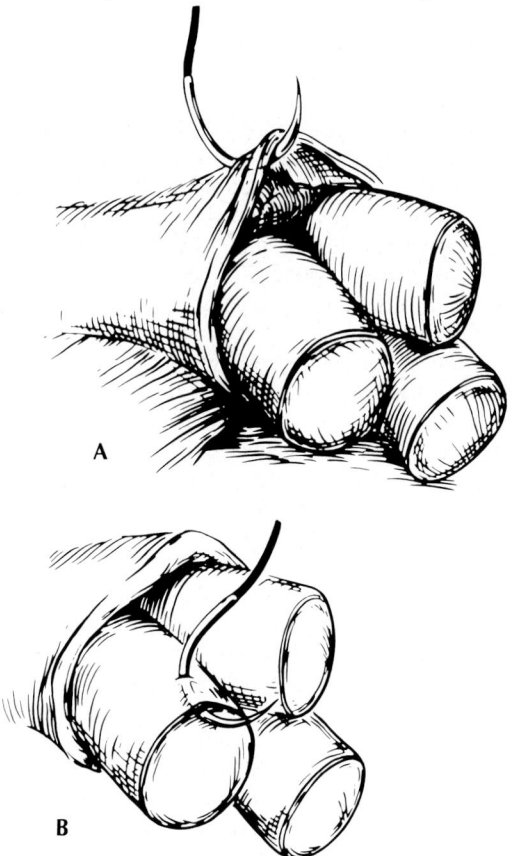

Fig. 37-4 Epineurial and fascicular suturing. **A,** Epineurial repair. Suture is passed through epineurium surrounding three fasciculi. **B,** Fascicular repair. Suture is carefully passed through perineurium of individual fasciculus. Care is taken not to injure intrafascicular contents. (From Urbaniak JR: Clin Orthop Rel Res 163:57, 1982.)

Epineurial suture

The wound must be debrided and the nerve inspected for orientation. The most difficult technical step is the operative transection of the nerve. The goal of transection is to achieve a flat stump for the nerve end and to obtain a flush joint for the anastomosis. The nerve may be wrapped with a slip of paper, or fitted into a neurotome, and then cut with a surgical bladder or microsurgical scissors so that the transverse matched surface between the nerve stumps can be fashioned. If a significant amount of scar is present within the nerve, the transection procedure is repeated until easily identified axonal bundles are seen.

Histologic examination of epineurial repairs done without magnification and fine suture material demonstrate funicular malalignment with gaps, overriding buckling, and straddling.[18] The amount of tension in a sutured nerve is directly related to connective tissue proliferation at the anastomosis.[36] Circumferential tension, with decrease in the cross-sectional area, causes deflection of the funicular alignment with many regenerating axons ending blindly in the endoneurium. Longitudinal tension may result in subepineurial and intrafunicular hemorrhages with fibrosis.

Group fascicular suture

Each fasciculus is usually a mixture of motor, sensory, and sympathetic axons encased by the perineurium. Fasciculi are usually arranged in groups and embedded in epineurium. Epineurium not only is the sheath around the nerve trunk, but also generally comprises 30% to 75% of the cross-sectional area of the nerve.[69] It is important to note that fascicular group repairs have the sutures placed in the deep epineurium and not the perineurium.

Electrophysiologic techniques have been used to aid in fascicular group orientation in acute injuries.[23] It is common to produce motor responses with electrical stimulation of the distal nerve stump for 4 to 5 days after injury. Stimulation of the proximal stump elicits subjective sensations from the patient as long as the cells of origin in the dorsal root ganglia are intact. Studies on the internal structure of nerve trunks are available to indicate the location of motor and sensory fascicular groups.[28,67]

Immobilization periods and methods of mobilization are the same for epineurial and group fascicular suture repairs.

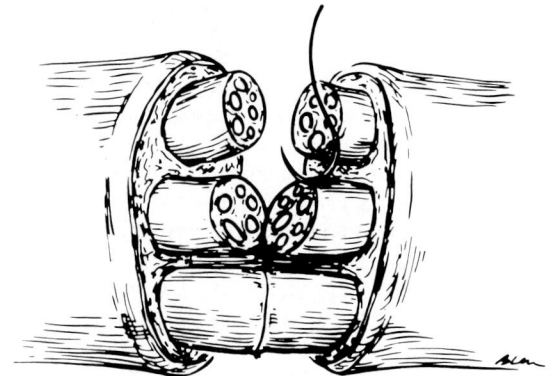

Fig. 37-5 Group fascicular repair. Epineurium has been stripped. Matching groups of fasciculi (bundles) are identified and united by two 10-0 nylon sutures in each bundle of fasciculi. (From Urbaniak JR: Clin Orthop Rel Res 163:57, 1982.)

The extremity should be splinted 3 to 4 weeks for healing of the surgical procedure. Hyperflexion of joints should be avoided and should not be greater than 30 degrees under any immobilization program. After the healing period is complete, joints are mobilized 10 degrees per week.[58,59]

Nerve graft

A nerve graft is indicated to close a gap in a nerve and provides a scaffold that assists the regenerating axons in finding their way into the distal nerve stump and restoring the original pattern of innervation. The nerve graft must be acceptable to the body without producing an inflammatory response or constrictive fibrosis: it should be small enough in diameter to revascularize readily, and it should have a fascicular (funicular) pattern similar to selected fascicular groups in the proximal and distal suture lines.

Seddon popularized the cable graft; his technique involves suturing multiple nerve segments together to equal the diameter of the disrupted nerve, thus forming a multiple-segment cable.[58] The cable graft is superior to grafting of a single large-diameter nerve, because the multiple cables develop an adequate intergraft circulation, whereas a large-diameter nerve will undergo central necrosis. The multiple cable graft is sutured proximally and distally to bridge the gap in the disrupted nerve.

Millesi and associates have improved the multiple cable graft by developing a technique that emphasizes no tension at suture lines, accurate group fascicular alignment, and excision of the epineurium.[36] The healthy epineurium of the nerve trunk is opened longitudinally, both proximally to the neuroma and distally to the fibroma. Groups of fasciculi that have the approximate cross-sectional area of the donor nerve are cut at different levels in both the proximal and distal stumps. The local epineurium, which has been opened, is excised. A sketch of the group fascicular pattern of the nerve ends is made so that one can plan the connecting multiple cable grafts. Each donor nerve graft is sectioned to fit the gap in the disrupted nerve. Each segment of donor nerve graft should be without tension. An operating microscope is most useful, because 10-0 suture material should be used. One suture connects the epifascicular epineurium of the selected fascicular group to the epineurium of the donor nerve graft. Occasionally, as determined under magnification, an additional 10-0 suture is necessary to establish optimal alignment and contact. Natural fibrin clotting provides sufficient tensile strength to prevent disruption, if the graft is long enough to neutralize any tension in the longitudinal direction. If indicated, a tourniquet should be used in nerve grafting, but the pressure is released and meticulous hemostasis is obtained before wound closure. The involved limb is immobilized in comfortable extension for 3 to 4 weeks, and then activity is begun.

After the nerve graft has been performed, the axons cross the proximal suture site and regenerate toward the distal suture site. In a long nerve graft the distal site may scar and block before the axons reach that level. Clinically, this becomes apparent as the Tinel sign stops advancing. After a 45-day delay at this point, the distal suture site should be exposed for evaluation of the neuroma in continuity by electrodiagnostic techniques (nerve-action potentials). If there is not distal electrical conduction, the distal suture site should be resected and a second neurorrhaphy should be performed.

REGENERATION AFTER REPAIR

It has been a clinical assumption that neurons would become degenerated unless peripheral connections are established during regeneration after repair. Recent laboratory studies suggest that neurons do retain the capacity for function for long periods. Sumner[64] allowed the hypoglossal nerve of rats to regenerate after an 84-day delay. Degenerative appearances of perikaryons and dendrites reversed, numbers of synapses per dendrite increased, and somatic bouton frequencies increased slowly.[51]

Morris and associates[39,40] demonstrated two aspects of regeneration with an electron microscopic study in rats. A certain proportion of Schwann cells and their axons are found in "groups." These groups are of two types: one contains a single myelinated axon associated with a variable number of unmyelinated axons; the other type has all axons initially unmyelinated, but by the tenth day possesses at least one myelinated axon. Axons of both groups are believed to be derived from a single transected myelinated axon and are termed "regenerating units."

The second process in regeneration is termed "compartmentation."[40] During the first 6 weeks after division, the original single or dual fascicular configuration of the rat sciatic nerve is replaced by a series of small fascicles, each surrounded by its own perineurium. The change is stimulated by axonal regeneration and is coordinated by changes in Schwann cells and endoneurial fibroblasts, which begin to resemble perineurial cells.

There is extensive reorganization within the regenerating nerve, as demonstrated by "regenerating units" and their "compartmentation." Present surgical concepts that coapt endoneurial tubes in the proximal and distal stumps of the disrupted nerve offer little possibility that appropriate matching will be accomplished. There should be other techniques to promote control between central and peripheral connections.

REFERENCES

1. Adams JE: Naloxone reversal of analgesia produced by brain stimulation in the human, Pain 2:161, 1976.
2. Akil H and Liebeskind JC: Monoaminergic mechanisms of stimulation-produced analgesia, Brain Res 94:279, 1975.
3. Akil H, Mayer DJ, and Leibeskind JC: Antagonism of stimulation-produced analgesia by naloxone, a narcotic antagonist, Science 191:961, 1976.
4. Allbrook D: Skeletal muscle regeneration, Muscle and Nerve 4:234, 1981.
5. Amir S, Brown ZW, and Amit Z: The role of endorphins in stress: evidence and speculations, Neurosci Behav Rev 4:77-86, 1980.
6. Becker RO and Spadaro JA: Electrical stimulation of partial limb regeneration in mammals, Bull NY Acad Med 48:627, 1972.
7. Becker RO: The bioelectric factors in amphibian-limb regeneration, J Bone Joint Surg 43A:643-655, 1961.
8. Bessou P and Perl ER: Response of cutaneous sensory units with unmyelinated fibers to noxious stimuli, J Neurophysiol 32:1025, 1969.
9. Borgens RB, Roederer E, and Cohen MJ: Enhanced spinal cord regeneration in lamprey by applied electric fields, Science 213:611, 1981.
10. Bradbury A and others: Comparison of the analgesic properties of lipotropin C-fragment and stabilized enkephalins in the rat, Biochem Biophys Res Commun 74:478, 1977.
11. Brushart TM and Mesulam MM: Alteration in connections between muscle and anterior horn motorneurons after peripheral nerve repair, Science 208:603, 1980.
12. Burkhalter WE and others: Experiences with delayed primary closure of war wounds of the hand in Viet Nam, J Bone Joint Surg 50A:945, 1968.
13. Casey KL: Pain: a current view of neural mechanisms, Am Sci 61:194, 1973.

14. Christensen BN and Perl ER: Spinal neurons specifically excited by noxious or thermal stimuli: marginal zone of the dorsal horn, J Neurophysiol 33:293, 1970.

15. Dellon AL: Evaluation of sensibility and re-education of sensation in the hand, Baltimore, 1981, Williams & Wilkins.

16. Ducker TB: Metabolic factors in surgery of peripheral nerves, Surg Clin North Am 52:1109, 1972.

17. Ducker TB: Metabolic consequences of axotomy and regrowth. In Jewett DL and McCarroll HR Jr, editors: Nerve repair and regeneration: its clinical and experimental basis, St Louis, 1980, The CV Mosby Co.

18. Edshage S: Peripheral nerve repair: a technique for improved intraneural topography, evaluation of some suture materials, Acta Chir Scand (Suppl) 331, 1964.

19. Goldstein A, Lowney LI, and Pal BK: Stereospecific and nonspecific interactions of the morphine congener levorphanol in subcellular fractions of mouse brain, Proc Natl Acad Sci USA 68:1742, 1971.

20. Grabb WC: Management of nerve injuries in the forearm and hand, Orthop Clin North Am 1:419, 1970.

21. Guillemin R: Discussion in Reichlin S, Baldessarini RJ, and Martin JB, editors: The hypothalamus, New York, 1978, Raven Press.

22. Hagbarth KE and Kerr DIB: Central influences on spinal afferent conduction, J Neurophysiol 17:295, 1954.

23. Hakstian RW: Funicular orientation by direct stimulation, J Bone Joint Surg 50A:1178, 1968.

24. Handwerker HO, Iggo A, and Zimmermann M: Segmental and supraspinal actions on dorsal horn neurons responding to noxious and non-noxious skin stimuli, Pain 1:147, 1975.

25. Hubbard, JH: The quality of nerve regeneration factors independent of the most skillful repair, Surg Clin North Am 52:1099, 1972.

26. Hughes J and others: Purification and properties of enkephalin—the possible endogenous ligand for the morphine receptor, Life Sci 16:1753, 1975.

27. Iggo A: Pain receptors. In Bonica JJ, Procacci P, and Pugni CA, editors: Recent advances on pain: pathophysiology and clinical aspects, Springfield, Ill, 1974, Charles C Thomas, Publisher.

28. Jabaley ME, Wallace WH, and Heckler RH: Internal topography of major nerves of the forearm and hand: a current view, J Hand Surg 5:1, 1980.

29. Jhamandos K, Swaynok J, and Sutak M: Enkephalin effects on release of brain acetylcholine, Nature 269:433, 1977.

30. Loh H and others: Beta-endorphin in vitro inhibition of striatal dopamine release, Nature 264:567, 1976.

31. Mayer DJ and others: Analgesia from electrical stimulation in the brainstem of the rat, Science 174:1351, 1971.

32. Mayer DJ and Hayes R: Stimulation-produced analgesia: development of tolerance and cross-tolerance to morphine, Science 188:941, 1975.

33. Mayer DJ and Price DD: Central nervous system mechanisms of analgesia, Pain 2:379, 1976.

34. Melzack R and Wall PD: Pain mechanisms: a new theory, Science 150:971, 1965.

35. Millesi H, Meissl G, and Berger A: The interfascicular nerve-grafting of the median and ulnar nerves, J Bone Joint Surg 54A:727, 1972.

36. Millesi H: Interfascicular nerve grafting, Orthop Clin North Am 12:287, 1981.

37. Moneim MS: Interfascicular nerve grafting, Clin Orthop 163:65, 1982.

38. Moroni F, Cheney D, and Costa E: Beta-endorphin inhibits ACH turnover in nuclei of rat brain, Nature 267:267, 1977.

39. Morris JH, Hudson AR, and Weddell G: A study of degeneration and regeneration in the divided rat sciatic nerve based on electron microscopy. II. The development of the "regenerating" unit. Z Zellforsch 124:103, 1972.

40. Morris JH, Hudson AR, and Weddell G: A study of degeneration and regeneration in the divided rat sciatic nerve based on electron microscopy. IV. Changes in fascicular microtopography, perineurium and endoneurial fibroblasts, Z Zellforsch 124:165, 1972.

41. Nemeth PM: Electrical stimulation of denervated muscle prevents decreases in oxidative enzymes, Muscle and Nerve 5:134, 1982.

42. O'Brien WJ and Orgel MG: The electrical stimulation of nerve regeneration. Research in progress, July 1979 through May 1982, University of New Mexico, Albuquerque.

43. Oliveras JL, Besson JM, Guilbaud G and others: Behavioral and electrophysiological evidence of pain inhibition from midbrain stimulation in the cat, Exp Brain Res 20:32, 1974.

44. Olson GA and others: The opioid neuropeptides enkephalin and endorphin and their hypothesized relation to pain. In Smith WL, Mersky H, and Gross SC, editors: Pain: meaning and management, New York, 1980, SP Medical and Scientific Books.

45. Omer GE Jr: Injuries to nerves of the upper extremity, J Bone Joint Surg 56A:1615, 1974.

46. Omer GE Jr and Spinner M: Peripheral nerve testing and suture techniques. In American Academy of Orthopaedic Surgeons: Instructional course lectures 24:122, St Louis, 1975, The CV Mosby Co.

47. Omer GE Jr: Complications of treatment of peripheral nerve injuries. In Epps CH Jr, editor: Complications in orthopaedic surgery, Philadelphia, 1978, JB Lippincott Co.

48. Omer GE Jr: The management of traumatic injuries of peripheral nerves in the extremities, Surg Rounds 4:22, 1981.

49. Omer GE Jr: Results of untreated peripheral nerve injuries, Clin Orthop 163:15, 1982.

50. Omer GE Jr: The technical factors influencing the results of the epineurial technique for peripheral nerve repair, Peripheral Nerve, Rep and Reg 3:67, 1986.

51. Orgel MG: Experimental studies with clinical application to peripheral nerve injury: a review of the past decade, Clin Orthop 163:98, 1982.

52. Pert C and Snyder S: Opiate receptor: demonstration in nervous tissue, Science 179:1011, 1973.

53. Pomeranz B, Cheng R, and Law P: Acupuncture reduces electrophysiological and behavioral responses to noxious stimuli: pituitary is implicated, Exp Neurol 54:172, 1977.

54. Rexed B: The cytoarchitecture organization of the spinal cord of the cat, J Comp Neurol 96:415, 1952.

55. Reynolds DV: Surgery in the rat during electrical analgesia induced by focal brain stimulation, Science 164:444, 1969.

56. Salmons S and Henriksson J: The adaptive response of skeletal muscle to increased use, Muscle and Nerve 4:94:105, 1981.

57. Seddon HJ: Three types of nerve injury, Brain 66:237, 1943.

58. Seddon HJ, editor: Peripheral nerve injuries, Medical Research Council Spec Rep Ser 282, London, 1954, Her Majesty's Stationery Office.

59. Seddon HJ: Surgical disorders of the peripheral nerves, ed 2, Edinburgh, 1975, Churchill Livingstone, Inc.

60. Singer SJ: Architecture and topography of biologic membranes. In Weissman G and Claiborne R, editors: Cell membranes: biochemistry, cell biology, and pathology, New York, 1975, Hospital Practice Publishing Co.

61. Sisken BF and Smith SD: The effects of minute direct electrical currents on cultured chick embryo trigeminal ganglia, J Embryol Exp Morphol 33:29, 1975.

62. Sternback RA: Modern concepts of pain. In Dalessio DJ, editor: Wolff's headache and other head pain, ed 4, New York, 1980, Oxford University Press.

63. Stilz RJ, Carron H, and Sanders DB: Reflex sympathetic dystrophy in a 6-year-old: successful treatment by transcutaneous nerve stimulation, Anesth Analg 56:38, 1977.

64. Sumner BEH: Responses in the hypoglossal nucleus to delayed regeneration of the transected hypoglossal nerve: a quantitative ultrastructural study, Exp Brain Res 29:219, 1977.

65. Sunderland S: Nerves and nerve injuries, ed 2, Edinburgh, 1978, Churchill Livingstone, Inc.

66. Sunderland S: Clinical and experimental approaches to nerve repair, in perspective. In Jewett DL and McCarroll HR Jr, editors: Nerve repair and regeneration: its clinical and experimental basis, St Louis, 1980, The CV Mosby Co.

67. Sutherland S: The anatomic foundation of peripheral nerve repair techniques, Orthop Clin North Am 12:245, 1981.

68. Tseng LF, Loh H, and Li C: Beta-endorphin as a potent analgesic by intravenous injection, Nature 263:239, 1976.

69. Urbaniak JR: Fascicular nerve repair, Clin Orthop 163:57, 1982.

70. Webster KE: Somaesthetic pathways, Br Med Bull 33:113, 1977.

71. Weeks PM and Wray RC: Management of acute hand injuries: a biological approach, St Louis, 1978, The CV Mosby Co.

72. Weissman G: Pain mediators and pain receptors. In Bonica JJ, editor: Considerations in management of acute pain, New York, 1977, Hospital Practice Publishing Co.

73. Willis WD, Trevino DL, Coulter JD and others: Responses of primate spinothalamic tract neurons to natural stimulation of hindlimb, J Neurophysiol 37:358, 1974.

74. Wynn Parry CB: Rehabilitation of the hand, ed 3, London, 1973, Butterworths & Co (Publishers), Ltd.

38

Nerve lesions in continuity

Morton Spinner

Nerve compression lesions are a major and significant cause of peripheral neuropathy. Lesions of the upper extremity may potentially involve any nerve. The compressed region usually is localized to a discrete portion of a segment of the nerve, which, because of its anatomic position, is particularly susceptible to entrapment. When a nerve is compressed, it is the peripheral axons within the nerve that suffer the greatest injury. At first, the central fibers may be spared, but as the compression continues or worsens, the central fibers may also become involved. Within the central region, the motor, proprioceptive, light touch, and vibratory sensory axons, which are heavily myelinated, are more vulnerable than the thinly myelinated pain and sympathetic fibers. However, when the compression is of sufficient duration and magnitude, all the fibers are paralyzed.

CLASSIFICATION OF NERVE-COMPRESSION LESIONS

There are two methods of classifying neural compression lesions. Sir Herbert Seddon's method utilizes the three terms "neurapraxia," "axonotmesis," and "neurotmesis." Sir Sidney Sunderland's classification has five degrees of nerve injury. Only the first four apply to nerve lesions in continuity, since the fifth degree refers to an injury in which the nerve is severed and the two ends retract.

Neurapraxia

Sunderland's first-degree lesion corresponds to Seddon's neurapraxia. Neurapraxia is a reversible syndrome. The prognosis for recovery is excellent.

Three types of neuropractic lesions exist: ionic, vascular, and mechanical. The first, ionic, is related to electrolyte-imbalance potassium, sodium, and ATPase disturbance at the node of Ranvier. The second type, vascular, is believed to be attributable to an anoxia at the capillary level within the funiculi, caused by venous obstruction in the epineurium. The third neuropractic lesion, mechanical, has structural changes in the nerve fibers because of compression-shear forces.

There are two basic ultrastructural mechanical lesions of neurapraxia. The first is bulbous myelin lesions with segmental tapering of internodal segments. The second type is paranodal myelin intussusception at the node of Ranvier; in this condition acute local compression produces the myelin invagination. Both lesions occur away from the site of the compression. Initially there is segmental demyelinization, and with healing, there is segmental remyelinization. In neuropractic lesions, there is no wallerian degeneration. The basement membrane of the neural fiber is intact.

Most neuropractic lesions respond to conservative treatment within 3 months. If a patient has a persistent neural compression lesion of spontaneous or traumatic origin that lasts more than 3 months, surgery is indicated, at which time the nerve should be explored at the level of the lesion. When neurolysis is performed, the speed of return of function often suggests the type of neuropractic lesion. If the recovery occurs rapidly, within hours of the procedure, the ionic or anoxic type of lesion is suggested. However, some neuropractic lesions require 30 to 60 days for recovery because a process of demyelinization and remyelinization occurs, indicating a possible structural neuropractic lesion. If a neuropractic lesion is left untreated and the mechanical factors—compression, traction, and friction—persist, the severity may increase.

Axonotmesis

The next level of severity is Seddon's axonotmesis and Sunderland's second-degree lesion. Minor third-degree lesions also fall within this category. With a pure axonotmetic lesion, the axon fiber is damaged at the point of compression. The basement membrane of the axon is maintained, but there is complete wallerian degeneration distal to the level of the compression. The healing process consists in new axonal sprouting and growth, from the point of axon disruption distally. Although the prognosis is good for this degree of injury, the rate of the recovery depends on the distance between the muscle to reinnervate and the site of the lesion. The closer the motor end plates, the earlier the recovery.

Sunderland's third-degree lesion may correspond either to Seddon's classification of axonotmesis or to the next category, neurotmesis, depending on the severity of the injury. In a third-degree lesion, the nerve fibers, including their Schwann tubes, are damaged within intact nerve trunk. The perineurium is basically intact, but internal fibrosis is present, along with damage within the fascicles. Mild lesions, which are reversible, fall within the axonotmetic category. However, in a more severe injury, when the damage may be irreversible as a result of the number of axons involved and the degree of fibrosis within the funiculi, the lesions are classified as neurotmetic.

Neurotmesis

This category is composed of all fourth-degree lesions and the more severe third-degree lesions. A fourth-degree lesion is characterized by extensive or complete fibrosis of a segment of the nerve. The internal structure of the funiculi is severely altered, and neuroma is present. In a complete neurotmetic lesion, there is a nonfunctioning, nonconductive neuroma in continuity.

In the case of a neurotmetic lesion, excision of the neuroma and repair is indicated. It can best be achieved by epineurial repair. If the gap is too great for direct approximation, interfunicular grafting is necessary.

In general, the prognosis for motor recovery after nerve repair is poor if paralysis has been clinically and electrically complete for 10 to 15 months. In such cases, successful recovery after neurorrhaphy depends on the specific nerve involved, the duration of the paralysis, the age of the patient, and the level of the complete lesion. There is little hope for a high ulnar-nerve complete lesion if more than 10 months have elapsed. However, a low median-nerve complete lesion can recover after repair for well beyond 10 months. If the paralysis has extended beyond the critical time, the treatment of choice would be primary muscle transfer.

The prognosis for sensory recovery is much better than for motor recovery. Useful sensory recovery after repair has been achieved with a 25-year-old neurotmetic lesion.

EVALUATION OF NERVE-COMPRESSION LESIONS

To determine the extent of the neural-compression lesion and to decide on the appropriate treatment, one must consider the age of the patient, the complete history, the duration of the paralysis, and the clinical and operative findings. Hereditary factors may also play a part in neural-compression lesions. At this time, however, the role played by any chromosomal-enzymatic factors in the incidence of neural-compression lesions is purely hypothetical. Families and isolated cases in which the patient's nerve were pressure sensitive have been reported. Recurrent episodes and multiple peripheral nerve involvement have also been reported.

It is unusual to have a pure first-, second-, third-, or fourth-degree lesion; most often, they are mixed. Furthermore, when a peripheral nerve can be compressed at more than one level in its passage through the arm, it is known as "double-crush nerve entrapment." Improvement in the symptoms can be achieved with release of one of the site compressions, but it may be necessary to explore additional sites as well.

To predict the lesion mix of a compression syndrome and the extent of each of the degrees, serial clinical examinations may be necessary. Prompt recovery can follow release. The fibers most sensitive to compression are the large myelinated fibers—motor, proprioceptive, light touch, and vibratory. Partial neural-entrapment lesions respond well to surgical release even after 2 to 3 years of sensory and motor symptomatology.

In general, if there has not been progressive improvement in a neural-compression lesion within 3 to 4 months, surgery is indicated.

A number of well-known neural-compression lesions present distinct symptoms. These include the carpal tunnel, Guyon's tunnel, pronator, and cubital tunnel syndromes. The lesion can be confirmed with electroneuromyographic testing. It is essential that the level of the lesion be located accurately, so that decompression is performed at the proper level. For example, if the patient has a high median nerve lesion, intervention at the wrist is no help. Occasionally, anatomic variations or unusual clinical patterns, such as the presence of Sudeck's atrophy in association with a nerve entrapment, can make the problem more difficult to diagnose.

MANAGEMENT OF NERVE-COMPRESSION LESIONS

The extent of the exposure at surgery is always much greater than the site of the lesion would initially suggest. For example, a lesion an inch long would have an incision of at least 5 inches. Indeed, only with careful anatomic exposure of both the gross neural structure and the fine internal structure in normal tissue proximal and distal to the lesion can conversion of the lesion to one of the more advanced degree be avoided. Particular care must be taken to avoid injury to the superficial skin nerves, because postoperative neurotoma of them can be a major postoperative complication.

During the surgery, the neural structure is identified grossly in the normal tissue proximal and distal to its entrapment. The dissection proceeds, separating the epineurium from its scarred bed, from both the proximal and distal sides. If there is a fibrotic band at the area of maximum entrapment, release of the binding structure causes the entire nerve to be liberated. It is possible that there may be a small residual area of indentation in the nerve, but with an intraneural injection of saline solution one can observe the flow. If any obstruction is noted, a localized neurolysis is necessary.

Neurolysis usually separates the epineurium from its scarred bed or removes crossing thrombosed vessels or thickened fascia. At times, however, the funiculi may require internal dissection.

When it is used, internal neurolysis should be adapted to the individual case. For example, in a carpal tunnel syndrome with advanced thenar atrophy and minimal sensory disturbance, after release of the flexor retinaculum, the motor branch is identified and is traced from its departure point from the median nerve distally into the thenar muscles. In the distal course, it frequently penetrates a separate foramen in the flexor retinaculum, which may be the offending obstructive site. The compression can occur at the proximal or distal level of this retinaculum; so the motor funiculus is traced proximally through the main median nerve trunk, including the area distal and proximal to the edges of the flexor retinaculum.

Often with the carpal tunnel syndrome, pain and numbness are the major complaints, with the long finger most involved. In these cases, after opening the epineurium, one separates the medial two or three funiculi as a group, beginning distal or proximal to the transverse carpal ligament in the normal median nerve. The internal neurolysis should include the region of the median nerve compressed by the proximal and distal edges of this ligament. One leaves the adjacent funiculi, which are clinically uninvolved, as they are. In elderly patients, long-finger discomfort and dysesthesias may persist for an extended period after isolated carpal tunnel relase. Since selective internal neurolysis has been added to the procedure for patients with this syndrome, in which long-finger pain predominates preoperatively, this morbidity has been improved significantly.

When internal neurolysis is used, it should be limited to the fasciculi that are clinically involved. Extensive internal neurolysis can induce fibrosis throughout the neural layers. The integrity of the perineurium is crucial for normal neural function. It acts as a supporting structure for maintenance of normal pressure gradient within the funiculus. It maintains the internal environment within the funiculus, and acts

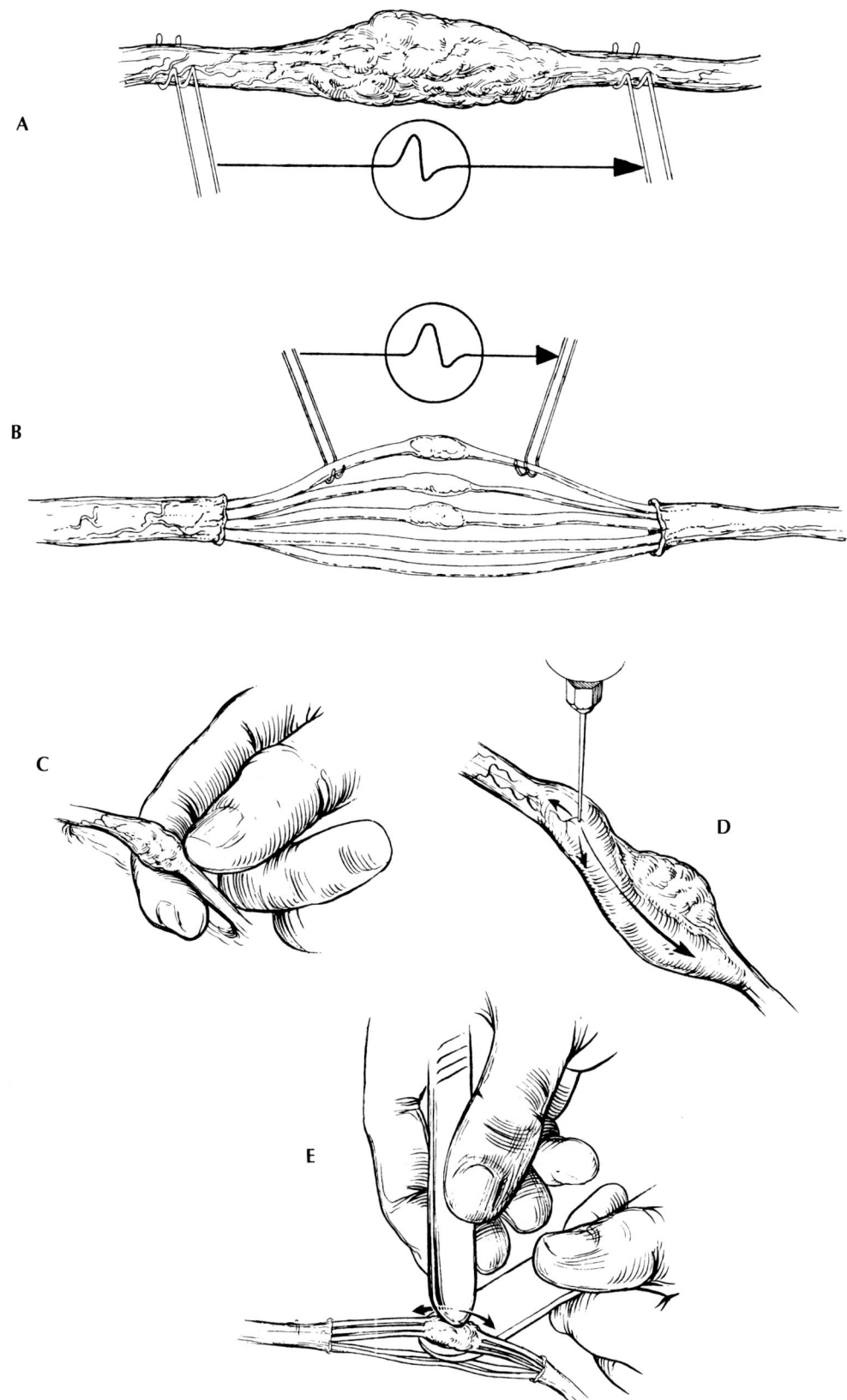

Fig. 38-1 Intraoperative techniques for nerve lesions. **A** and **B,** Intraoperative nerve conduction study across the neuroma may be helpful in evaluation of lesion in continuity. **C,** Palpation of nerve may reveal a rock-hard neuroma with little likelihood of intact fascicles. **D,** Injection of saline deep to the epineurial sheath can help differentiate intact from damaged fascicles. **E,** Intrafascicular dissection separates intact fascicular bundles from those that are involved in a neuroma. Firmness of a funicular neuroma can be evaluated further with the aid of a scalpel handle.

as a barrier for the passage of proteins and other large molecules. Furthermore, the perineurium is a mirror in the peripheral nerve of the central blood-brain barrier. When the perineurium is violated, there is a herniation of axons. The axons that bulge out of the perineurial window undergo pathologic changes. At first, there is segmental demyelinization, followed by localized remyelinization with restoration of the perineurium. In clinical cases for which pain is attributable to a localized lesion, the epineurium is frequently opened, but the perineurium is only opened rarely. However, there are specific indications for violating the perineurium. For example, opening may be necessary when the patient has a third-degree lesion with intraneural fibrosis. The degree of the internal fibrosis and therefore the extent of the third-degree lesion within the nerve may not be clear. Thus on rare occasion it may be necessary to open the perineurium to improve neural function.

EVALUATION OF NEUROMA IN CONTINUITY

Several methods may be used to evaluate a neuroma in continuity (Fig. 38-1). Once it has been determined that surgery is required, certain intraoperative techniques can be used to evaluate the lesion. During surgery, electrical stimulation proximal and distal to the neuroma before one frees it completely is useful, with observation of the peripheral muscle and limb response. Other intraoperative conduction studies may be made across the neuroma, but they require more refined instrumentation. If the neuroma is stony-hard to palpation, the prognosis is poor for neural recovery by neurolysis. However, a soft enlargement of the nerve is a favorable sign for restoration of neural function. Intraneural saline injection followed by external and internal neurolysis, if necessary, with use of the operating microscope or ocular

magnification can be helpful. Magnification is essential in the evaluation of the appearance of the funiculi. The firmness of the funicular neuromas can be evaluated with the aid of the scalpel handle, but the single fascicular electrical recording technique offers the most critical intraoperative evaluation.

When intraoperative evaluation indicates that a complete neuroma in continuity exists, excision of the neural lesion and neurorrhaphy constitute the treatment of choice.

When managing injuries, one must evaluate each on its own merits. After humeral fracture, the radial nerve may have had relatively minor trauma and may recover spontaneously in 3 to 4 months. On other occasions, it may have been lacerated and require prompt repair, or it may be entrapped in scar tissue and require neurolysis. It may also have sustained a fourth-degree neural lesion, necessitating excision of a neuroma in continuity and neurorrhaphy (Fig. 38-2).

CLINICAL HIGHLIGHTS
Median nerve syndromes

The carpal tunnel syndrome is the result of median nerve compression in a narrowed carpal tunnel. It is a fairly common entrapment syndrome, seen most frequently in women between 40 and 60 years of age. Pain and paresthesia in a distal median nerve distribution are the usual complaints,

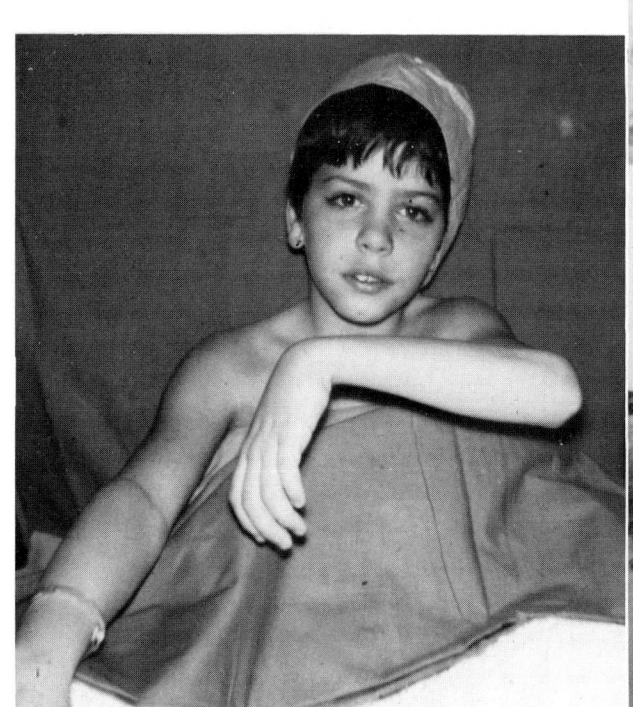

A

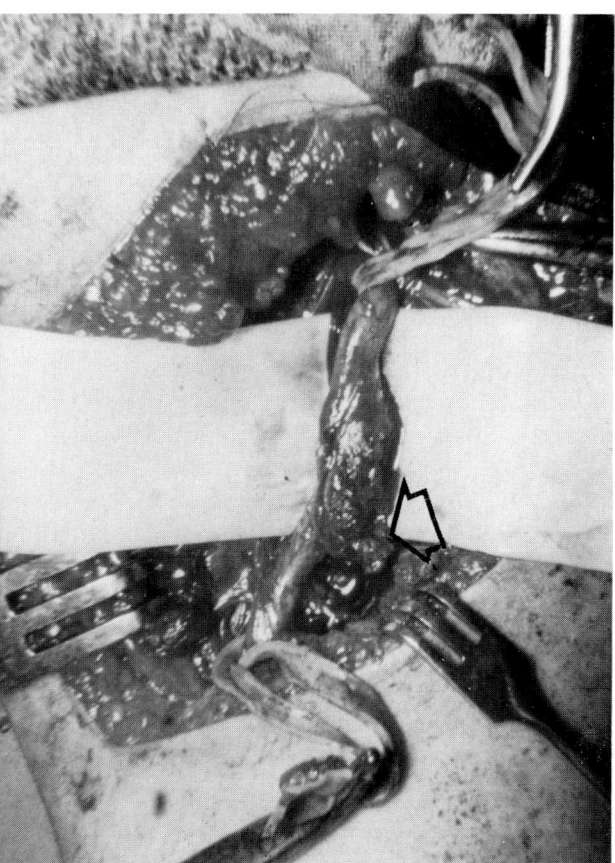

B

Fig. 38-2   Radial nerve injury. **A,** This boy had a healed humeral fracture but no evidence of radial nerve function 6 months after injury. **B,** Surgical exploration revealed a fourth-degree lesion of the radial nerve *(arrow).*

with nocturnal burning pain in the hand often being reported as well.

Carpal tunnel syndrome has many significant symptoms and signs, including numbness of the radial 3½ digits, atrophy of the thenar muscles, a Tinel sign at the wrist, a Phalen sign, increased symptoms on application of an arm tourniquet, and motor and sensory nerve electromyographic abnormalities. Often, however, numbness may be restricted to the long finger, and there may be no atrophy of the thenar muscles, and no Tinel and Phalen signs. In approximately 25% of patients with carpal tunnel syndrome, the electro-myogram may be normal. Sensitivity to cold may be the major presenting symptom. Sympathetic overflow associated with the carpal tunnel syndrome has been observed by Linscheid.

After fractures and dislocations at the wrist, median and ulnar nerve entrapment can be the cause of reflex dystrophy of the hand. It may be necessary to release one or both of these nerves to relieve the pain and stiffness characteristic of reflex dystrophy. The diagnosis of nerve entrapment can be confirmed by electromyographic studies.

Patients with carpal tunnel syndrome respond to conser-

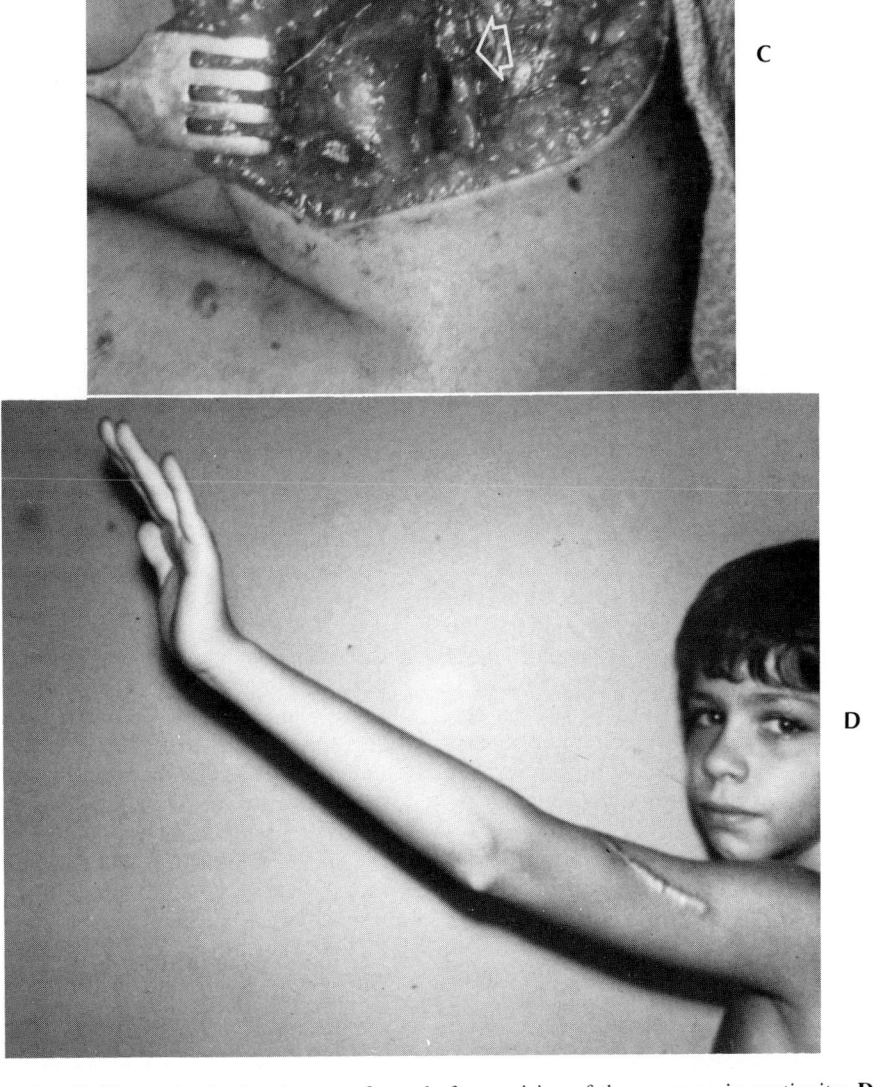

Fig. 38-2, cont'd   **C,** Neurorrhaphy has been performed after excision of the neuroma in continuity. **D,** Excellent recovery of radial nerve function is demonstrated 1 year later.

vative measures of treatment. The combined treatment of splinting the wrist in a neutral position and administering a diuretic is effective in these patients. Vitamin B$_6$ (100 mg twice a day) has also been helpful in some cases. Any underlying systemic disease should be brought under control. If conservative methods do not provide relief, it may be necessary to release the transverse carpal ligament through surgery. The incision is made on the ulnar side of the carpal tunnel, with step-cutting at the distal flexion crease of the wrist and extension of the incision to the ulnar side of the distal forearm if additional exposure is necessary. Care must be taken to preserve the median palmar cutaneous nerve, because injury to it often causes postoperative pain.

The pronator syndrome is caused by entrapment of the median nerve in the proximal part of the forearm. This syndrome is difficult to diagnose with certainty. Usually the patient has a 9-month to 2-year history of nonlocalized forearm pain. The most consistent finding has been reproduction of pain in the proximal part of the forearm on resistance to pronation of the forearm and resistance to flexion of the superficial flexor muscle of the long and ring fingers. Patients may report numbness in some digits innervated by the median nerve. Even though the Tinel sign may aid localization, it may not appear for 4 to 5 months after the initial examination. Electromyographic studies may aid in the diagnosis, particularly when the results of several examinations are compared.

Anatomic abnormalities observed in the pronator syndrome are (1) hypertrophy of the pronator teres, (2) fibrous bands within the pronator teres, (3) a thickening of the lacertus fibrosus, (4) passage of the median nerve deep to both heads of the pronator teres, and (5) a thickening of the flexor superficialis arch. Median nerve thickening at the level of the compression has been observed; the degree of thickening seems to be directly related to the duration of symptoms.

The surgical procedure, when necessary, consists in release of the lacertus fibrosus and all compressing fibrous structures crossing the nerve. Translocation of the median nerve anterior to the pronator teres to a subcutaneous position is occasionally necessary. When this is done, the pronator teres is lengthened at its musculotendinous junction and brought posterior to the median nerve. If the flexor superficialis arch is thickened, it is released to allow the median nerve to be superficial in the middle third of the forearm. The skin incision should be S or chevron shaped, through which the lacertus fibrosus is initially visualized. The median nerve is identified proximal to the lacertus and then traced distally. Continuity of the branches of the medial cutaneous nerve of the forearm must be carefully preserved, since severance may result in a postoperative symptomatic neuroma.

The anterior interosseous nerve syndrome results from the compression of the anterior interosseous branch, usually at a site close to its origin from the median nerve. The paralysis of the long flexor of the thumb and the flexor digitorum profundus to the index and long fingers causes the hand to display a typical pinch attitude. Paralysis of the pronator quadratus muscle is also observed. Sometimes paralysis is limited to the distal phalanx of the thumb or index finger. There are usually no sensory abnormalities. If a Martin-Gruber anastomosis, a connection between the an-

terior interosseous nerve and the ulnar nerve, is present, the entrapment of the anterior interosseous nerve may produce paralysis of some of the intrinsic muscles of the hand. There are anatomic variations in the anastomosis between the ulnar and median nerves within the flexor digitorum profundus, and so the muscle is innervated to variable degrees by both nerves, and flexion of the distal phalanx of the digits may be impaired variably in this neural-entrapment lesion.

Exploration of the anterior interosseous nerve is indicated if the paralysis does not subside spontaneously within 8 to 12 weeks. The median nerve should be identified proximal to the lacertus fibrosus and traced through the region of the pronator teres where the anterior interosseous nerve usually originates. The most common restraining structure is a tendinous origin of the deep head of the pronator teres, which crosses the anterior interosseous nerve at its origin from the median nerve. Other causes of anterior interosseous nerve entrapment are enlarged bicipital bursas, other tendinous structures, thrombosed ulnar collateral vessels, old penetrating local scars, and anomalous passage of the radial artery.

A supracondyloid process is another cause of high median-nerve entrapment. It is an anomalous spur found 3 to 5 cm above the medial epicondyle in 1% of limbs. The connection between the two bony prominences is the ligament of Struthers, which completes the fibro-osseous tunnel. The median nerve passes through the tunnel, usually accompanied by the ulnar artery. This anomaly is usually asymptomatic, but after trauma it may produce median neuritis.

Radial nerve syndromes

Posterior interosseous-nerve syndrome may present in two ways, but there is no sensory deficit in either one. In the first pattern, all the muscles supplied by the posterior interosseous nerve do not function. The patient cannot extend the thumb, long, index, ring, and little fingers at the metacarpophalangeal joints. The wrist can dorsiflex only in a dorsoradial direction, as a result of a muscular imbalance of the wrist extensors because of paralysis of the extensor digitorum communis and the extensor carpi ulnaris.

The second pattern is characterized by a lack of extension of one or more of the digits at the metacarpophalangeal level. Paralysis of the remaining digits often develops when the neural lesion is not recognized or treated. Frequently, posterior interosseous nerve entrapment occurs where the nerve pierces the two heads of the supinator muscle. This area, the arcade of Frohse, is fibrotendinous in 30% of limbs. Other causes for entrapment of the posterior interosseous nerve may be compression by a soft-tissue tumor, synovial proliferation in rheumatoid disease, Volkmann's ischemia, and fractures or dislocations of the head of the radius. The symptom complex known as lateral epicondylitis, or tennis elbow, characterized by pain about the lateral aspect of the elbow, can be attributable to posterior interosseous-nerve compression at the arcade of Frohse. It is confirmed by reproducing the pain at the common extensor origin on resistance to long-finger extension with the elbow extended. Direct pressure along the course of the radial nerve anteriorly is also painful. Electrical conduction studies of the radial nerve across the elbow may reveal motor-latency prolongation. Some patients who have not responded to conservative treatment, to release of the lateral epicondylar soft tissues, or to excision of a portion of the orbicular ligament, have been helped by release of the posterior interosseous nerve as it enters the supinator. If pain persists after the customary surgery for tennis elbow, posterior interosseous nerve compression should be considered as a possibility.

Two surgical approaches can be used in exposing and tracing the entrapped posterior interosseous nerve. Either the radial nerve is identified above the elbow, proximal to its site of division, or the superficial radial nerve is identified under the fascia of the brachioradialis in the forearm and traced proximally to the main radial nerve trunk. Then the posterior interosseous nerve is identified and traced through the two heads of the supinator.

Superficial radial nerve entrapment is a syndrome characterized by pain in the proximal part of the forearm and hypesthesia on the dorsum of the thumb. There is no associated muscle weakness or paralysis, and no motor-conduction abnormalities can be observed by electromyography.

Ulnar nerve syndromes

In the wrist, the ulnar nerve can be involved in Guyon's tunnel. There may be a purely motor or a purely sensory deficit, or a combination of the two. Either the main ulnar nerve or one of its terminal branches may be entrapped, depending on the localization of the compression. In the cubital tunnel syndrome the ulnar nerve can be compressed just distally to the medial epicondyle as it passes through the two heads of the flexor carpi ulnaris.

When one is translocating the ulnar nerve anteriorly, subcutaneous or deep to the flexor-pronator group of muscles, it is important to trace the ulnar nerve 8 cm proximally to the medial epicondyle to the region of the arcade of Struthers, where the ulnar nerve passes from the anterior compartment of the arm to the posterior in the distal third of the arm. Release of this arcade and excision of the adjacent medial intermuscular septum prevent a secondary entrapment of the ulnar nerve at the level of the arcade of Struthers.

In the thoracic outlet syndrome, which occurs at the base of the neck, the ulnar nerve is most frequently compressed at the level of the first rib or at the costoclavicular area. It presents with radicular pain along the medial aspect of the arm to the hand. There are motor and sensory disturbances in the distribution of the ulnar nerve. If appropriate confirmatory tests are positive and conservative treatment is unsuccessful, surgery is indicated.

Cervical arthritis can cause symptoms of numbness in the ring and little fingers with weakness of the digits. On rotation, extension and lateral bending of the neck with reduplication of the radicular complaints are produced. Such clinical findings can help localize the cause of the symptoms. Pain on direct pressure or percussion along the course of the nerve can also help to locate the level of the pathologic condition.

Bowler's thumb

Bowler's thumb is characterized by pain in the thumb, numbness most noticeable on its ulnar aspect, a palpable mass at the base of the thumb, a Tinel sign on percussion of this mass, and a history of bowling. The use of a protective thumb guard and redrilling of the bowling ball so that it is "scythed" at the top are helpful conservative measures for a short period. Surgery is indicated when conservative measures do not relieve the symptoms. Neurolysis, excision of the markedly thickened epineurium, and rerouting of the involved digital nerve into a new soft-tissue bed are indicated.

Similar localized digital compression neuropathy has been seen with baseball batters, and its management is identical in principle.

Multiple entrapment lesions

A nerve can be entrapped simultaneously at two levels; similarly, more than one nerve can be entrapped in a limb. Electromyographic studies are not always sensitive enough to localize a double lesion. It may be necessary to explore a peripheral nerve at two sites. It is also possible that a patient may have two completely separate neurologic conditions, such as syringomyelia of the neck and a compressed peripheral nerve. Furthermore, it is important to avoid a mistaken diagnosis of a localized process that causes a conduction delay, if the problem is instead actually a diffuse peripheral neuropathy. Examination of other peripheral nerves will serve to prevent this error.

39

Thoracic outlet syndrome complex: diagnosis and treatment

Stephan H. Whitenack, James M. Hunter, Scott H. Jaeger, and Richard L. Read

Thoracic outlet syndrome is a term generally used to describe the group of neurovascular compression syndromes about the shoulder. Thoracic outlet syndrome (TOS) remains a confusing and somewhat controversial subject.[33] The syndrome is best viewed as a clinical complex that may include four parts: (1) compression neuropathy of the brachial plexus, (2) compression vasculopathy of the subclavian vessels, (3) reflex sympathetic dystrophy (RSD), and (4) cervical-brachial myofascitis. The purpose of this chapter is to broaden the understanding of the various clinical manifestations of TOS, which should improve both the diagnosis and treatment of this difficult entity.

HISTORICAL BACKGROUND

Many different and distinct entities have been grouped together under the category thoracic outlet syndrome. Rob[52] is generally credited with coining the term *thoracic outlet compression syndrome*. Peet and associates[47] first grouped cervical rib syndrome, scalenus-anticus syndrome, subcoracoid-pectoralis minor syndrome, costoclavicular syndrome, and first thoracic rib syndrome under TOS. Others have added the scalenus medius syndrome, Paget-Schroetter syndrome (effort thrombosis of subclavian vein), rucksack palsy, droopy shoulder syndrome, and hyperabduction syndrome. Although including these separate syndromes under one heading can obscure the important differences in diagnosis and treatment, such a grouping is more likely to aid in understanding TOS.

The history of TOS has been well documented in many earlier excellent reviews.[16,43,73] The first recognition of cervical ribs dates to Galen and Vesalius. Sir Astley Cooper was said to have treated cervical ribs medically with some success. Willshire[74] is generally credited as the first to make the diagnosis of "cervical rib syndrome." Coote reported the first successful cervical rib resection in 1861. W.W. Kean[24] and Halsted[17] wrote extensive reviews and described surgical results.

Ultimately patients were described with similar or identical symptoms in the absence of a cervical rib. Murphy[41] in 1910 was the first to resect a normal first rib with relief of symptoms. In 1927 Brickner[3] was the first to describe resection of the normal first rib in the American literature. In that same year, Adson and Coffee[1] began a shift in thinking with their belief that the symptoms were related to the relationship of the anterior scalene to the cervical rib and not to the rib itself. This belief was based on operative findings, surgical results, and the fact that most cervical ribs were asymptomatic. Adson's operative procedure consisted of section of the anterior scalene, removal of any

tendinous bands, and occasionally removal of the tip of the cervical rib. No attempt to remove the whole rib was made. The well-known Adson test was also described at this time.

The next step in surgical thinking led to the resection of the anterior scalene in the absence of a cervical rib. Scalenus anticus syndrome, as credited to Naffziger[42] by Ochsner,[44] became a relatively common diagnosis and scalenotomy a common procedure. However, over time the failures in treatment in patients with "Naffziger's syndrome" led to disenchantment with scalenotomy. It is important to remember that other upper extremity pain syndromes had not yet been described, and that many failures may have been in diagnosis, rather than procedure. Cervical radiculopathy was described in 1943 by Semmes and Murphy.[58] It was not until 1953 that Kremer[27] properly described carpal tunnel syndrome.

Other etiologic factors were also described to explain the symptoms being attributed to scalenus anticus syndrome. Lewis and Pickering[30] in 1934 and subsequently Eden[12] in 1939 implicated compression of the neurovascular bundle between the clavicle and the first rib as the cause of the symptoms. This was later termed the "costoclavicular compression syndrome" by Falconer and Weddell.[14] Eden also further defined abnormalities of the first rib contributing to the syndrome. Wright[76] in 1945 added the concept of hyperabduction of the arms causing neurovascular compression at two levels. In addition to the similarly described costoclavicular compression, he added the concept of compression by the posterior border of the pectoralis minor against anterior border of the upper ribs. The Wright test was also described at this time.

In 1953 Lord[32] added the concept of resection of the clavicle for relief of the costoclavicular compression syndrome. Scalenotomy remained the preferred procedure, but because of disenchantment with results as described by Raaf,[50] scalenotomy fell into disfavor. Falconer and Li[13] were the first to support direct attack on the first rib in 1962. Later that same year, during the presidential address before the American Association of Thoracic Surgery, O. Theron Claggett[5] solidified the importance of the first rib as the common denominator in the pathophysiology of TOS. His approach was a posterior, thoracoplasty type of resection of the first rib, befitting a thoracic surgeon trained in tuberculosis surgery.

A major advancement in the surgical approach to TOS was reported by Roos[52] in 1966. The transaxillary first rib section that he described rapidly became the standard procedure for patients with TOS. Roos's 93% improvement rate was reaffirmed by others, including Urschel.[71,72] Roos

530

has also been primarily responsible for redirecting attention away from the vascular compression and to the brachial plexus compression. Roos has also carefully classified the many different types of congenital bands that contribute to TOS.[54]

Other techniques for first rib removal have also been described. The supraclavicular technique was first described by Murphy[9] in 1910. Good results have more recently been reconfirmed by Tyson[27] and Thomas.[28] An anterior infra-clavicular approach has also been described by Nelson[29] for rib resection.

The involvement of the upper brachial plexus with the previously described congenital bands was further described by Roos[56] in 1982. This led to the concept of combined first rib resection by means of the transaxillary approach and superior approaxh with scalenectomy.

A supraclavicular approach to the brachial plexus with anterior and middle scalectomy, resection of congenital bands, neurolysis, and, when necessary, first rib resection and sympathectomy became our approach in early 1982.[21]

Without an understanding of the pathophysiology and presentation of patients with TOS, many patients will be misdiagnosed for long periods, and many patients will remain undiagnosed. Proper treatment of all aspects of thoracic outlet syndrome is dependent on such understanding.

PATHOPHYSIOLOGY—GENERAL CONSIDERATIONS

The thoracic outlet is bounded by the anterior scalene muscle anteriorly, medial scalene muscle posteriorly, the clavicle superiorly, and the first rib inferiorly.

A number of structures are at risk of compression in the thoracic outlet; one of these is the brachial plexus. The etiology of the resultant brachial plexus compression neuropathy is multifactorial, and certain risk factors predispose to this syndrome. There are three categories of risk factors: (1) congenital-structural, (2) posttraumatic-structural, and (3) posttraumatic-postural. When an inciting event occurs, a clinically significant compression of the brachial plexus can result jointly. The patient's degree of congenital predisposition and the nature of the inciting event will determine the severity and clinical course of the brachial plexus compression neuropathy. The cause can be extrinsic compression by adjacent structures or the intrinsic compression effect of reactive perineural fibrosis ensuing from repetitive mechanical irritation of the plexus by altered anatomy or posture.

Next to the brain, the hand is considered most responsible for the progress of mankind. Evolution of our ancestors permitted erect posture, freeing their hands for the use of tools. This manual ability gave impetus to the development of civilization. However, the advantages of biped posture did not come without a price. The human body is not structurally designed to tolerate upright posture. A good example of inadequate human anatomic design is the frequent degeneration and pain of the lumbar spine in response to the stresses of standing erect. Postural brachial plexus compression neuropathy is another example of a malady caused by forcing anatomy designed for quadruped ambulation to accommodate erect posture.

During embryologic development, the forelimb buds must rotate 270 degrees to produce the human upper extremity. The rotation occurs at the thoracic outlet level, and the nerves of the brachial plexus are twisted and positioned precariously at the center of the rotation. In addition, the space available in the thoracic outlet is limited by the human requirement for a solid, stable clavicle an unyielding structure. Also, with age the scapula tends to descend, and further alteration of the outlet is possible, especially in females where the descent is normally more rapid and can be accelerated in some cases by increased brassiere strap pressure owing to overtly large breasts. This is a portion of the "droopy shoulder syndrome."[67,68]

In most people, extreme abduction of the shoulder will decrease or obliterate the radial pulse. In fact, during World War I, soldiers used a well-known technique to appear deceased when their trenches were overrun. If the extreme posture is maintained, paresthesias will develop because of compression of the brachial plexus. Nearly all humans can have this nerve compression syndrome because normal human shoulder anatomy is itself a risk factor. The compression syndrome is acute, intermittent, voluntary, and completely reversible.

Therefore even the normal human anatomy is a risk factor in the development of nerve compression syndrome. Ordinarily there is little symptomatology, but if a particular patient has a significant (1) congenital anomaly, (2) traumatic alteration of the size of the thoracic outlet, or (3) traumatic alteration of posture, the probability of a clinically important neurogenic or vascular compression syndrome increases.

Congenital factors

The presence of any congenital intersegmental anomalous structures, such as anomalous muscles, aberrant bands, or extra ribs at the site of nerve root circumvolution, can increase the risk of direct nerve compression.[6,22,40] The most common anomalies are anomalous fibrous bands, anomalous muscles, and cervical ribs. While these anatomic variations may cause little trouble to the patient under normal circumstances, the presence of these anomalies is a risk factor to the development of more serious compression neuropathies, especially after injuries that result in the production of the local and distant trauma factors.

Local trauma factors

Local trauma factors are posttraumatic alterations of the local anatomy that cause direct compression of the brachial plexus. These factors result in alterations of the spatial anatomy of the thoracic outlet. A good example is the exuberant callus that can arise from a malunited fracture of the clavicle. Another less commonly recognized example is fibrotic contraction of scalene muscles torn during whiplash-type injuries.

Traction trauma factors

Mechanism of the trauma can be an important factor in the production of compression neuropathies. Traction injuries can have a twofold effect on the brachial plexus. There can be an immediate, direct-effect nerve injury, and there can be a later, indirect-effect compression injury.

The direct injuries can be severe to mild. The most severe is the brachial plexus tear after a traction injury. This results in a neurotmesis, and the prognosis is poor for complete resolution. A less severe traction force can cause a moderate stretch and result in an axonotmesis. Here the prognosis is much better. Mild stretch injuries cause neuropraxia of the brachial plexus. The prognosis for these injuries is for complete recovery and full resolution as long as no other trauma is associated with the traction injury.

However, significant local trauma can result in a direct brachial plexus compression neuropathy because of scarring of structures near the nerves. The indirect mechanism involves trauma to the arm and hand, which results in considerable pain and can cause guarding. If untreated, the guarding can lead to postural brachial plexus compression neuropathies, associated compression phenomenon such as vasculopathies, and even RSD.

Distant trauma factors

Distant trauma can cause compression of the brachial plexus. The compression results from anatomic alterations associated with the guarding posture adopted by many patients with painful lesions of the upper extremity distal to the thoracic outlet. A good example of a distant factor is a painful lesion of the hand, such as a painful neuroma.* The posture protects the injured part from possible mechanical stimulation, which would evoke pain, but alteration in the carriage of the shoulder girdle decreases the size of the thoracic outlet and alters the path of the neural structures. The decreased size can cause direct compression of the brachial plexus, and the alteration of path can cause deformation of the individual cords by extra ribs and aberrant bands between the normally circumvoluted cords of the plexus. Here a postural abnormality can exacerbate any previously asymptomatic congenital factor.

The site of the compression varies and depends on a number of considerations. The compression can be direct between the clavicle and first rib, and the medial cord is the structure usually involved, because the plexus can be tethered by the first rib and clavicle and the lateral trunk can be compressed against one of the transverse processes.

Scalene muscle spasm is an important factor because it is a component of the original guarding posture, and it increases as pain caused by the compression neuropathy becomes more severe. The scalene muscles elevate the first rib and tighten previously existing bands, causing more compression and more pain; hence a "vicious" cycle ensues.[38,39,48,69]

A single traumatic incident is not required to incite the vicious cycle of compressive neurogenic pain and muscle spasm. Many patients perform vocational and avocational activities that require repetitive above-shoulder-level movements. Because of the aforementioned risk factors of normal human thoracic outlet anatomy, small traumas can occur with each repetitive motion; these can lead to a cumulative trauma that can be of sufficient magnitude to elicit the syndrome. Behavioral and vocational modifications can be of great preventative value.

Essentially, the problem is an involuntary maintenance of an abnormal posture, which is worsened by a vicious cycle of muscle spasm. The compression syndrome is now chronic and involuntary, but it is still reversible if the appropriate treatment is instituted. The treatment considerations involve patient education, behavior modifications, exercises, and treatment of the inciting site of pain.[36,59,66]

One of the most difficult aspects of managing postural brachial plexus compression syndrome is recognizing and treating the associated problems, which are both a cause and a result of the syndrome. In the absence of treatment of nerve compression and the inciting site of pain or cumulative trauma, a number of associated problems can develop. These associated problems can become so severe and chronic that they can surpass the compression syndrome symptomatically, and by increasing the postural alteration they can cause the compression syndrome to worsen.

The most problematic aspect of these associated problems is that, later in the course, they can obscure the true diagnosis by adding more complaints to an already confusing symptom complex. These associated problems are cervical-brachial myofascitis, periscapular trigger points, temporal headache, cervical muscle pain, subacromial bursitis, and biceps tendonitis. Chronic muscle spasm causes the cervical pain. In addition, the muscle spasm results in inflammation at the sites of insertion and origin of the muscles, causing the trigger points, bursitis, and tendonitis. Occipital headaches are examples of referred pain caused by neurogenic irritation near the cervical nerve root level.

The most severe associated problem is a concurrent RSD. In these cases, the progression of the syndrome is especially rapid and difficult to control, and the prognosis is much worse.

Finally, the compression neuropathy syndrome becomes chronic, involuntary, and irreversible to nonoperative measures.

HISTOLOGIC RESPONSE OF THE BRACHIAL PLEXUS

Compression causes a mechanical irritation to the nerves of the brachial plexus, which can lead to an intrinsic compression of the nerves by the effect of the reactive perineural fibrosis.[64,65] In addition, the compression has the effect of decreasing neural flow and blood flow, which can cause ischemic damage and result in more perineural and intraneural fibrosis. Contraction of fibrotic scar can cause further nerve compression and even cause spindle neuromas.

Clinical presentation

A patient suffering from brachial plexus compression neuropathy will usually complain of pain, paresthesias, and weakness in the involved extremity. The distribution of the pain and paresthesias will not be anatomically located as precisely as lesions involving individual peripheral nerves, whose distributions are well known. This is because of the poor understanding of the anatomic variability of the brachial plexus, the sensory overlaps of the nerves emanating from the plexus, and the variability of areas of the plexus compressed.

The most common complaint is symptoms in the ulnar three digits, which corresponds to compression of the medial cord of the plexus. The lateral trunk distribution is the ulnar and a portion of both the median and radial nerves. For example, weakness may be noted in the medial cord distribution, which is those muscles innervated by the ulnar and a portion of the medial nerve. Motor effects are not usually pronounced nor seen as atrophy.

The significant aspects of the history deal with (1) the

*References 5, 8, 9, 20, 21, 28, 34.

preexisting pain syndromes, (2) the mechanism of the trauma, (3) the site of the trauma, (4) the chronology of the symptom onset, (5) the patient's daily activities, and (6) the patient's social environment.

Preexisting pain syndromes are a causative factor by postural alteration, especially chronically painful neuromas. It is important to determine the mechanism of injury, because traction injuries have both direct and postural effects. Questions regarding the site of the trauma must be asked to discover any local injury such as a clavicle fracture, which may have a direct effect.

Symptom onset chronology is important especially when there is a delayed onset of the nerve compression symptoms because some local injuries, such as whiplash caused tears of the scalene muscles. The tears lead to later scar contracture, which causes delayed brachial plexus compression. The patient's daily activities are important because the symptoms of the syndrome are exacerbated by repetitive activities, especially those above shoulder level.

Often the patient will report a sudden increase in overhead activity, such as an ordinarily sedentary person trying to paint the interior of his entire house in one weekend. Other patients will admit trouble with hair hygiene to the point that they have voluntarily changed their hair style for one that requires less maintenance. An assessment of the patient's social environment is necessary to evaluate the psychological factors that may be of importance in the management of the syndrome.

Psychologic considerations

Chronic neurogenic pain syndromes such as the TOS complex can cause severe psychologic disturbances, and preexisting psychologic disturbances can contribute to the cause of chronic neurogenic pain syndromes.[31] Effective treatment of these syndromes requires the physician to be aware of the psychologic factors that often complicate the management of these patients.

Because of lack of reliable objective pain evaluation techniques, difficulty is encountered in determining the relative importance of the psychologic factors and their relationship as either a cause or an effect of the chronic pain syndrome. Therefore our inability to quantitatively assess the importance or degree of psychologic contribution to chronic pain presents an additional obstacle to the treatment of these patients.

The clinical course of the chronic pain syndromes is perplexing and at times extremely unsatisfying. In some cases, physician-patient relationships can be undermined by conflict-of-interest issues that can interfere insidiously with the success of the treatment regimen. Impending workmen's compensation claims and liability litigations can have a significant effect on the patient's response to any therapeutic measures.

However, despite the frustration of not attaining the desired or expected therapeutic result, the physician should not assume too readily that the failure of treatment in one of these patients is caused by the fact that the patient is psychologically ill, malingering, or motivated solely by secondary gain.

Proper consideration of these issues as impediments to successful treatment is important, but care must be taken to ensure that misconceptions not be allowed to interfere with

good medical judgment and the quality of care. An approach must be adopted that will accept and integrate both the neurogenic and psychologic factors, in the management of patients with chronic neurogenic pain.

Since it is apparent that psychologic factors play a role in chronic neurogenic pain syndromes, the physician must then employ techniques that will verify the subjective complaints of the patient. For example, drawing of pain distribution by the patient at each visit can be very helpful in assessing patient subjective reliability. Minnesota Multiphasic Personality Index (MMPI) testing can be helpful in assessing personality factors of the patient that may impact on his subjective reliability and response to treatment.

Formal physical capacity evaluations (see Chapter 7), with special attention paid to inconsistent results, can demonstrate the presence or absence of honest cooperation on the part of the patient. In severe cases successful treatment requires a multidisciplinary approach, including a hand surgeon, hand therapist, neurologist, psychologist, anesthesiologist, thoracic surgeon, and vocational rehabilitator.

Examination

Observation is an essential part of the examination, one must look for unequal shoulder heights and guarding posture. The hand may be cool to the touch, and there may be signs of RSD. Scars on plams and elbows may be seen because of previous unsuccessful carpal tunnel and cubital tunnel releases.

Clinical tests

There are two categories of clinical tests: those with vascular indicators and those with neurologic indicators. The Adson test, the Wright test, and the costoclavicular compression test are examples of vascular tests. The indicator in these tests is the loss of the radial pulse. The tests are designed to compress the subclavian artery by placing the patient in stressful postures They are somewhat helpful in demonstrating the compression vasculopathy syndrome, but a positive test is present in many asymptomatic persons. These tests are of little definitive help in the diagnosis of neurogenic compression. However, there are some helpful guidelines. When either the Adson or Halstead test is positive with only minimal motion of the arm or neck, the compressive band or muscle generally appears to have more involvement with the brachial plexus also. These patients also seem to be more susceptible to brachial plexus injury from the repetitive trauma of arm use.

The neurologic tests are palpation of plexus, the supraclavicular Tinel sign, and the stress abduction test. They have neurologic indicators, which are reproduction of the pain and paresthesias. The tests are provocative maneuvers and postures that will demonstrate nerve irritation and postural nerve compression. While some asymptomatic individuals may have positive findings on these tests, judgment of the clinical significance of a positive result can be made by considering the speed of onset and the severity of the symptomatic indicators during the examination. When used by a therapist with some experience, the neurologic tests can be quite helpful and accurate in making the diagnosis.

We have also discovered a new maneuver that seems to be helpful with some cases of neurogenic thoracic outlet syndrome. The Hunter test is performed similarly to the

Halstead maneuver. The test is begun with the shoulder abducted to 90 degrees and the elbow flexed 90 degrees. The arm is then straightened. Patients with traction and fixation of the plexus to the surrounding tissues describe a painful shooting sensation going down the arm in the distribution of the involved nerves.

OBJECTIVE STUDIES

Once the surgeon suspects TOS from the history and physical examination, a number of objective studies are necessary to confirm the diagnosis and rule out other entities.

Chest roentgenography

Roentgenograms of the chest in the posteroanterior and lateral projections are very important. They can give information regarding the presence of cervical cysts and thoracic masses.

Cervical spine roentgenography

Roentgenograms of the cervical spine are an essential part of the evaluation of TOS. Cervical spondylosis can simulate the syndrome and can be ruled out; however, the presence

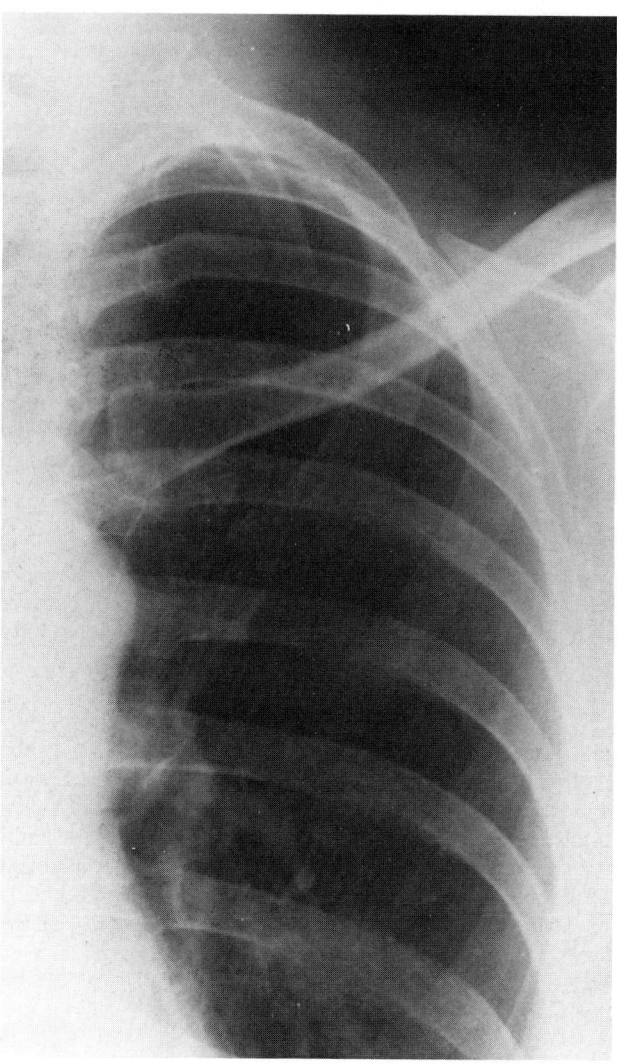

Fig. 39-1   Chest radiograph showing a cervical rib.

of degenerate changes need not exclude the possibility of the presence of TOS. Cervical ribs, malunited fractures of the clavicle, and roentgenographic evidence of compressing masses can be objectively noted by this study (Fig. 39-1). Attention should be paid to the length of the C7 transverse process. A correlation appears to exist between the types of dense musculotendinous bands that cause many of the symptoms and the length of the transverse process.

Angiography

Transfemoral subclavian angiography can be helpful when the vascular expression is severe, but it is rarely indicated when the neurologic expression of the syndrome is dominant. The possible morbidity associated with the study does not usually justify its use in these cases.

Somatosensory evoked potentials

Somatosensory evoked potentials (SSEP) are an effective adjunct test for measuring brachial plexus and more central neurologic conduction parameters. This test is usually performed with digital stimualtion of the median, ulnar, and radial nerves with proximal recording of the ascending sensory responses at the supraclavicular brachial plexus, the C2 level of the cervical spine, and the contralateral somatosensory cortex. Relative conduction times between each of these sites is measured preferably on a bilateral basis, and the results are replicated at least one time for accuracy. This is a relatively painless, noninvasive test that is associated with exceedingly low morbidity.

Electroneuromyographic evaluation

Electromyography and nerve conduction velocity studies have been one of the traditional methods of evaluting TOS. A classic measurement is to calculate the motor conduction velocity of the ulnar nerve across the supraclavicular transaxillary segment of the ulnar nerve component of the medial cord of the brachial plexus. Normal values for conduction velocity for this segment have been calculated at 72 m per second, with a normal and acceptable range being between 60 and 72 m per second. When conduction velocities of less than 60 meters per second were seen, TOS was a possible diagnosis, and surgical resection of the first rib was carried out after conservative therapy failed.

The validity of this technique of assessment has been challenged. Some patients who exhibit many signs and symptoms of TOS would have normal supraclavicular transaxillary ulnar conduction velocities. This seeming paradox may be explained in part because the site of supraclavicular stimulation, which is Erb's point, may be distal to the site of irritation or compression. In this situation, the small area of segmental injury would be proximal to the site of stimulation, and with normal conduction velocity values, a diagnosis of TOS might be erroneously ruled out.

In an attempt to evaluate more accurately the probability of injury to the proximal region of the lower trunk of the brachial plexus, techniques of C8 root level stimulation have been described by McLean and Taylor, later by Johnson, and still later by Pavot and associates.[46] This involves the use of stimulation with intramuscular needle electrodes placed at the C8 root level. When this technique is used in conjunction with traditional methods of supraclavicular ulnar nerve stimulation and distal recording over the ulnar abductor digiti quinti, they present a way of objectively evaluating the entire peripheral and plexus components of the ulnar nerve, including the proximal portion of the lower trunk, where it may be irritated or compressed, as it traverses the proximal region of the first rib.

A protocol for performing electrophysiologic testing for TOS was developed at the Hand Rehabilitation Center using both traditional ulnar nerve conduction parameters and C8 nerve root level stimulation techniques. The C8 root level stimulation technique was futher developed to include testing the patient not only in traditional resting positions, but also in positions of provocation that would impart intermittent stress on the lower trunk of the brachial plexus. These positions included both long axis traction postures and shoulder girdle depression that would stretch the lower trunk and the medial cord over the first rib. Additionally, overhead positions of hyperabduction and vertical flexion that would press the lower trunk and medial cord of the brachial plexus between the clavicle and the first rib and/or stretch the distal plexus nerves under the coracoid process and the pectoralis minor or over the humeral head were employed.

Because evoked motor amplitude is a function of the number of viable motor axons conducting, it is reasonable to consider amplitudinal changes as a sensitive indicator of segmental neuropathy in the brachial plexus. Conduction time or latency is a measure of *internodal* conduction and reflects on the integrity of the myelin sheath of the nerve. As such, slowing of conduction time could reasonably be considered as an additional sensitive indictor of segmental neuropathy in the brachial plexus. Acordingly, we at the Hand Rehabilitation Center hypothesize that changes in evoked amplitude and/or slowed conduction time across the lower trunk of the brachial plexus on the side-to-side comparison, as well as slowing of conduction velocity across the medial cord of the brachial plexus, would be indicators of local neuropathic change within the lower trunk and/or medial cord distributions of the brachial plexus. These recordings were performed with the patient under resting conditions and also following dynamic activity or positions of provocation.

C8 root stimulation technique may show either a local slowing of conduction time across the lower trunk of the brachial plexus or it may show a drop in the evoked motor amplitude measured peak to peak; these may be seen in any one or all of the previously described stress positions. Conduction times greater than 1.0 m per second on a side-to-side basis are considered to be significant, and amplitudinal losses in excess of 25% from that which was observed with supraclavicular level stimulation are considered to be significant as long as the correct stimulating electrode placement has been maintained. Abnormalities seen at this level suggest a proximal lower trunk level lesion.

Major problems of diagnosis

The major problem is a lack of a definitive, objective test to confirm the diagnosis of brachial plexus compression neuropathy. This is important because a great deal of confusion and controversy is associated with the characteristics and even the existence of the syndrome.

A definitive, objective test is needed to improve the appreciation and the general management of this misunder-

stood malady. At this time, work is underway in an attempt to enhance the electrodiagnostic testing techniques. These projects deal with improved interpretation of the somatosensory evoked potentials and improved measurement of impaired nerve conduction across the brachial plexus using C8 nerve root stimulation and stress provocative studies. The provocative stress studies are of great interest because the syndrome's symptoms are often intermittent and related to posture. It is hoped that this research will help elucidate this perplexing disease.

Differential diagnosis

The differential diagnosis must include the consideration of cervical nerve root compression, median nerve compression, ulnar nerve compression, spinal cord lesions, and pure RSD. One must be aware of possible associated multiple sites of nerve compression. This is referred to as a "double crush," which has been a controversial concept; however, recent research has demonstrated the problem in the laboratory.[57,70]

The most important factor in the evaluation of a patient with chronic pain is that awareness is the key to the diagnosis.

TREATMENT
General considerations

Successful treatment requires consideration of both the nerve compression and the associated problems. The approach may demand consecutive management because the two aspects of the syndrome are intimately interrelated.

Treatment of cervical-brachial myofascitis

Tendonitis, shoulder bursitis, and periscapular trigger points are expressions of localized areas of inflammation. They will respond to a coordianted effort of physical therapy modalities and local steroid-anesthetic injections. The modalities include hot packs, ultrasound, phonophoresis, iontophoresis, and deep massage.

Treatment of reflex sympathetic dystrophy

Early diagnosis of RSD is the key to successful treatment, and an intensive treatment regimen must be instituted early.[35] It is necessary to break the cycle when the cycle is reversible. Later the functional limitations are considerably more refractory to treatment. The pathophysiologic cycle and clinical stages of the syndrome should be considered carefully in the choice of the treatment regimen.[25,26,51,60-62]

Nonoperative treatment of reflex sympathetic dystrophy

Physical therapy. Hand therapy has an important role in the treatment of RSD; initial attempts focus on the various modalities of physical therapy. Edema control is accomplished with elevation, wrapping, and intermittent compression. Joint mobilization is essential, but this must be done with great care.

Active exercises are encouraged; they are safe when performed within the limits of pain tolerance. The maintenance of good shoulder posture is especially important. Passive exercises can be detrimental and should not be considered unless supervision and extreme care are ensured. If passive exercises are done improperly, they may lead to increased edema, pain, and subsequent joint stiffness.

Transcutaneous electrical nerve stimulation (TENS) can be helpful in controlling the "C" pain fiber effect on the pain perception gate.[37,63] Multiple treatments are required, but the units can be effective in permitting better patient cooperation during the essential work of active exercise and edema control.

Medications. Various oral medications can be helpful when their use is directed toward the various aspects of the physiologic vicious cycle, but the incidence of harmful side effects is high, especially with long-term therapy. Analgesics, membrane stabilizers, and central nervous system depressants are useful in the control of the pain perception, which can increase sympathetic outflow. In the early stages of the syndrome, antiadrenergics and the recently developed calcium channel blocking agents have use as a method of attaining a medical sympthectomy.

Nonsteroidal, anti-inflammatory drugs will control some of the associated problems that tend to worsen the course of the dystrophy. Steinbrocker and Argyrose have reported favorable responses to oral steroids in conrolling many aspects of the disease, but their use is limited by the severe associated side effects.[36] A method that takes advantage of the beneficial effects of steroids, but avoids the damaging side effects has been introduced by Poplawski.[49] The procedure involves the intravenous instillation of local anesthetics and soluble prednisone in a Bier block technique to localize a concentrated steroid preparation in the affected extremity. The blocks are followed by range-of-motion physical therapy treatments. Significant imporvements have been noted in several cases, but occasionally multiple blocks are required.[4]

Sympathetic blockade. If the theory regarding the pathophysiology of RSD is correct, the treatment most specific for the entity would be sympathetic blockade. The blockade would interrupt the vicious cycle, mediated by the autonomic nervous system, by either temporarily or permanently blocking the sympathetic efferent system. The temporary block can be accomplished by regional sympathetic block or intravenous administration of agents that produce a chemical sympathectomy. Permanent blockade is attained by surgical stellate sympathectomy.

A sympathetic block has both a diagnostic and a therapeutic function. Technically successful blockades that do not relieve the burning pain should alert the clinician to the possibility of an alternative diagnosis. Usually three to five intermittent blocks are necessary to obtain the desired therapeutic benefit. Blockade is followed by a course of physical therapy to improve range of motion and decrease swelling. When a patient responds to an individual block but the effect is short lived, a surgical sympathectomy should be considered after a series of three to five blocks. The result of regional sympathetic blockade is encouraging in reducing pain and improving function in as many as 80% of the patients treated.[15,29]

Other agents have been used in the Bier block technique to produce a sympathetic block. The two drugs in current use are guanethidine and reserpine. Guanethidine functions as a false transmitter displacing epinephrine from the nerve endings.[11] Reserpine blocks prevent reuptake of catecholamines, thereby depleting storage of epinephrine in the nerve endings. Double blind studies have shown guanethidine to significantly reduce pain in comparison to saline controls.[15] Sympathetic blockages may last up to 4 days with guanethidine. Reserpine has also been used successfully.[2]

However, in recent double blind studies in normal volunteers, reserpine had no effect and guanethidine blocked only adrenergic receptors causing peripheral vasodilation and had no affect on cholinergic receptors (they did not decrease sweating).[21] These studies therefore question the efficacy of these drugs. In addition, the Food and Drug Administration (FDA) has not approved guanethidine or reserpine for intravenous use.[18,19]

Operative treatment. Surgical treatment is indicated in the management of RSD in the following instances: (1) correction of exacerbating or precipitating lesions (painful neuromas), (2) surgical excision of the stellate ganglion, and (3) late reconstruction procedures of salvage function.

The indications for the sympathectomy are a chronic syndrome resistant to nonoperative treatment with symptoms that interfere with activities of daily living and employment possibilities. Further support for the surgical sympathectomy includes these factors: (1) narcotics are needed for pain control and (2) stellate glanglion blocks provide good temporary relief from symptoms.[45]

Any surgical procedures planned for a patient with RSD should be considered a significant risk. The cycle may be self-perpetuating to some degree after the initial injury has resolved, and any surgical intervention can reincarnate the full-blown dystrophy. Precautions can minimize this possibility. Perioperative stellate sympathetic blockage, intensive edema control, and early ROM exercises are of great benefit.

A number of serious complications can occur in the operative treatment of RSD. Aside from reactivation of the malady, a serious complication of surgical treatment is Horner syndrome, which can occur after surgical stellate ganglion sympathectomy.

Treatment of vascular compression

Uncomplicated vascular compression is treated surgically as a part of any of the standard approaches to the neurogenic type. In the uncommon instance of subclavian stenosis complicating TOS, surgery is indicated only if symptomatic. Arm claudication or subclavian steal are treated with bypass or endarterectomy techniques no different from those not associated with TOS, but in combination with a standard procedure for TOS. Poststenotic dilation of the subclavian artery requires no specific treatment. True aneurysms must be repaired.

Treatment of nerve compression

Nonoperative treatment. The nonoperative treatment of the nerve compression includes physical therapy, exercises, patient education, and splints. The exercises are useful in both controlling muscle spasms and stretching tight muscles that are adding to the compression. Patient education is also very important.

Patients are taught to avoid activities that cause compression while substituting patterns of behavior and posture that relax the thoracic outlet. Behavioral modification is especially necessary to relieve the symptoms and prevent recurrence. One must beware of recurrence if previous activities are resumed. Airplane splints are indicated for severe, acute cases. See Chapter 40 for a thorough discussion of the therapeutic management of TOS.

Oral agents can be complementary to the physical therapy modalities. When inflammation is suspected as a significant factor, oral anti-inflammatory agents are useful in decreasing pain and improving patient cooperation in physical therapy. Short-term narcotic therapy is occasionally beneficial but may be difficult to discontinue and ultimately be more detrimental than useful. Therefore narcotics should be used very cautiously. High-dose, short-term oral steroids may occasionally be helpful in refractory cases; membrane stabilizers are indicated in cases where neuritis is paramount.

The results of nonoperative treatment can be very satisfying. In our experience, approximately 60% to 80% of patients improve with nonoperative therapy. Although some may not be completely relieved of their symptoms, they are able to resume their work and lives with few limitations. Therefore all aspects of the nonoperative regimen with regard to both nerve compression and associated problems should be exhausted before surgical treatment is considered.

Operative treatment

Indications. Operative treatment is indicated when there is no significant improvement with nonoperative treatment in those patients with severe symptoms. The surgeon should always be sure that a complete therapy program has been properly administered before recommending surgical intervention.

Several types of patients require special consideration; they generally are not responsive to nonoperative therapy. Patients with markedly positive vascular signs, such as complete obliteration of the radial pulse simply with turning the head or elevation to only 30 degrees, do not respond to nonoperative therapy in our experience. Presence of a cervical rib or other structural abnormality makes conservative treatment unlikely to be successful.

Procedures. Since its introduction by Roos in 1966, transaxillary first rib resection has been the most commonly employed procedure for the treatment of TOS. Although less demanding than other approaches to the first rib, it remains a difficult procedure to perform properly. In cases of first rib anomaly, purely vascular expression, or involvement of the lower trunk only, first rib resection by way of the axilla is often the best procedure.

First rib resection by way of an anterior subclavicular or posterior approach has limited application. The posterior approach is most commonly used to remove the posterior portion of an improperly resected first rib.

The most common types of congenital bands that have been described insert on the anterior first rib and sometimes the pleura. Anomalies of the subclavian muscles also usually attach to the first rib. Thus transaxillary rib resection is often successful by removing the fixed point. The majority of patients with a short history and without any history of severe whiplash type of injury will do well with the axillary approach. Most studies and our own results support this approach in these patients, who are by far less common in our practice. This may well be because the more straightforward cases have already been selected out.

The standard approach we use is a supraclavicular approach. The anterior and middle scalene muscles are removed, not divided. This allows for complete visualization of the proximal brachial plexus, which is the site of nearly all compressive lesions. If a careful history is taken, one will find that nearly all cases involve some type of trauma. The operative findings are consistent with this: scarring of the scalenes to the plexus, dense perineural fibrotic tissue at the site of compression by most congenital anomalies, and severe foreshortening of the tissues forming the axillary sheath in those patients with a positive Hunter sign. These problems can best be attacked through the supraclavicular approach.

In addition, the involvement of other branches of the plexus (suprascapular, long thoracic, dorsal scapular, and pectoral, for example) can only be handled with the supraclavicular approach. Cervicothoracic sympathectomy can be easily accomplished if necessary. First rib resection is done selectively when there is any compression by the clavicle and rib or any tenting of the lower trunk over the rib or rib anomalies.

A comment must be made about the controversy that largely exists in the neurology literature about the very existence of TOS. Wilbourn[75] has gone so far as to divide cases into "true neurogenic" and "disputed" types, essentially based on electromyogram (EMG) criteria only. Because consistent EMG criteria are not met in many cases, the existence of the diagnosis is questioned. The "true neurogenic" type is uncommonly seen, but in our experience it represents only the extreme end of the spectrum of compression. In the only cases we have seen that meet Wilbourn's criteria, the compression is so severe that the nerves are edematous and appear partially demyelinated on inspection. It seems quite inappropriate to deny the vast majority of patients the chance for improvement.

POSTOPERATIVE CARE

Postoperative therapy begins on the first postoperative day with gentle, full ROM exercises combined with the same modalities used preoperatively. This is done in an effort to reduce any chances of binding of the brachial plexus by scar tissue. If there is any question of poor compliance or inability to perform the exercises, therapy must be done with supervision, even in the hospital if necessary.

RESULTS

The quality of the operative results are dependent on the accuracy of the diagnosis, the completeness of the nerve release, and the quality of the postoperative care. As expected, the results are much less consistent in operations for recurrent cases. Therefore it is very important to release the nerve completely and begin early gliding exercises to obtain successful results during the initial release.

Over the past 7 years we have performed 300 procedures for TOS. The complications, which have been remarkably few, include one thoracic duct leak, one phrenic nerve paresis requiring postoperative ventilation, one infection leading to ruptured pseudoaneurysm of the subclavian artery, one subclavian vein injury, and two permanent nerve injuries resulting in motor dysfunction. Both nerve injuries occurred in patients who had received radiation for breast cancer and many years later developed TOS as a result of an injury. In both cases the pain complex has been relieved but with significant motor impairment. Thus any procedure in the presence of prior irradiation must be viewed with extreme caution.

The results of surgical treatment must be viewed from the perspective of degree of improvement, rather than complete relief of symptoms. Most patients we have seen have a chronic compression or traction neuropathy. Just as with carpal tunnel syndrome, persons whose injuries result from repetitive trauma and who develop chronic scarring should not necessarily be expected to be able to return to the same level of activity as before injury. We always explain to the patient that the goal is 70% to 80% improvement, and more than this is unrealistic. When viewed in this way, the results have been excellent, with very few poor results. In retrospect, some of these poor results may have been predicted, which explains why the more recent results have improved.

One of the few major difficulties has been delayed recurrence of symptoms. Nearly all of these are the result of either a repeat whiplash type of injury or cessation of exercises early in the postoperative period. It must be emphasized that the patient must perform the stretching program on a daily basis for at least 2 years, because scar contracture can continue for this length of time.

REFERENCES

1. Adson AW and Coffey JR: Cervical rib: a method of anterior approach for relief of symptoms by division of the scalene anticus, Ann Surg 85:839, 1927.
2. Benzon HT, Chomka CM, and Brunner EA: Treatment of reflex sympathetic dystrophy with regional intravenous reserpine, Anesth Analg 59:500, 1980.
3. Brickner WM: Brachial plexus pressure by the normal first rib, Ann Surg 85:858, 1927.
4. Christensen K, Jensen EM and Noer I: The reflex sympathetic dystrophy response to treatment with systemic corticosteroids, Acta Chir Scand 1248:653, 1982.
5. Clagett OT: Research and prosearch (presidential address) J Thorac Cardiovasc Surg 44(2):153, 1962.
6. Dale WA and Lewis MR: Management of thoracic outlet syndrome, Ann Surg 181:575, 1975.
7. Dale WA: Throacic outlet compression syndrome, Arch Surg 117:143, 1982.
8. Decarvalho, Pinto, VA and Junquira LCU: A comparative study of the methods for prevention of amputation neuroma, Surg Gynecol Obstet 99:492, 1954.
9. Dellon AL, Mackinnon SE, and Pestronk AP: Implantation of sensory nerve into muscle: preliminary clinical and experimental observation of neuroma formation, Ann Plast Surg 12:30, 1984.
10. Doupe J, Cullen C, and Chance G: Post traumatic pain and the causalgic syndrome, J Neurol Neurosurg Psychiatry 7:33, 1944.
11. Drucker W and others: Pathogenesis of post traumatic sympathetic dystrophy, Am J Surg 97:454, 1959.
12. Eden KC: The vascular complications of cervical ribs and thoracic rib abnormalities, Brit J Surg 27:111, 1939-1940.
13. Falconer MA and Li FWP: Resection of the first rib in costoclavicular compression of the brachial plexus, Lancet 1:59, 1962.
14. Falconer MA and Weddell G: Costoclavicular compression of the subclavian artery and vein: relation to the scalenus anticus syndrome, Lancet 2:539, 1943.
15. Glynn CJ, Base RW, and Walsh JA: Pain relief following post ganglionic sympathetic blockade with intravenous guanethidine, Br J Anesth 53:1297, 1981.
16. Greep JM and others, editors: Pain in the shoulder and arm, The Hague, 1979, Martinus Nijhoff.
17. Halsted WS: An experimental study of circumscribed dilatation of an artery immediately distal to a partially occluding band, and its bearing on the dilatation of the subclavian artery observed in certain cases of cervical rib, J Exp Med 24:271, 1916.
18. Hanningtonkiff JG: Intravenous regional sympathetic block with guanethidine, Lancet 1:10, 1974.
19. Hanningtonkiff JG: Relief of Sudeck's atrophy by regional intravenous guanethidine, Lancet 1:113, 1977.
20. Herndon JH, Eaton RG, and Littler JW: Management of painful neuromas in the hand, J Bone Joint Surg 58A:369, 1976.
21. Jaeger SH, Whitenack SH, and Singer DI: Nerve injury complications—management of neurogenic pain syndromes, Hand Surg Clin North Am, February 1986, p 217-34.
22. Jaeger SH and others: Thoracic outlet syndrome: diagnosis and treatment, In Hunter JR and others, editors: Rehabilitation of the hand, ed 2, St Louis, 1984, The CV Mosby Co.
23. Jaeger SH and others: Mid-latency somatosensory evoked potential abnormalities in proximal sensory neuropathies, Muscle Nerve, p 618, September 1985.
24. Kean WW: The symptomatology, diagnosis, and surgical treatment of cervical ribs, Am J Med Sci 133:173, 1907.
25. Kleinert HE: Post traumatic sympathetic dystrophy, Orthop Clin North Am 4:917, 1973.
26. Kleinert HE and Southwick GJ: Reflex sympathetic dystrophy. In Difficult problems in hand surgery, St Louis, 1982, The CV Mosby Co.
27. Kremer M and others: Acroparesthesia in the carpal tunnel syndrome, Lancet 2:590, 1953.
28. Laborde KJ and Tsumin T: Results of the surgical treatment of painful neuromas in the hand, J Hand Surg 7:1998, 1982.
29. Lankford L and Thompson J: Reflex sympathetic dystrophy, upper and lower extremity: diagnosis and management, American Academy of Orthopaedic Surgeons Instructional Course Lectures, vol 26, St Louis, 1977, The CV Mosby Co.
30. Lewis T and Pickering G: Observations on maladies in which the blood supply to the digits ceases intermittently or permanently, Clin Sci 9:327, 1934.
31. Livingston WK, Pain mechanism, a psychological interpretation of causalgia and its related states, New York, 1943, Macmillian Inc.
32. Lord JW: Surgical management of shoulder girdle syndromes, Arch Surg 66:69, 1953.
33. Lord JW: Thoracic outlet syndrome: real or imaginary? NY St J Med 45:1488, 1981.
34. Mackinnon SE and Dellon AL: Radial and lateral antebrachial cutaneous nerve overlap, Amer Soc Surg Hand Annual Meeting, Anaheim, January 1985.
35. Mackinnon SE and Holden LE: The use of three-phase radionucleotide bone scanning in the diagnosis of reflex sympathetic dystrophy, J Hand Surg 9:556, 1984.
36. Mass DP: Treatment of painful neuromas by their transfer to bone, Plast Reconst Surg 74:1825, 1984.
37. McKain CW, Urban BJ and Goldner JD: The effecs of intravenous regional guanethidine and reserpine—a controlled study, J Bone Joint Surg 65A:801, 1983.
38. Melzack R and Wall P: Pain mechanisms—a new theory, Science 150:971, 1965.
39. Meyer RA, Campbell JN, and Roger SN: Neuroma activity originating from a neuroma in a baboon, Soc Neuro Science Abst 8:855, 1982.
40. Miller G: Acute vs chronic compressive neuropathy, Muscle Nerve 7:427, 1984.
41. Murphy T: Brachial neuritis caused by pressure of first rib, Aust Med J 15:582, 1910.
42. Naffziger HC and Grant WT: Neuritis of the brachial plexus mechanical in origin: the scalenus syndrome, Surg Gynecol Obstet 67:722, 1938.
43. Nelson RM and Davis RW: Thoracic outlet compression syndrome: collective review, Ann Thorac Surg 8(5):437, 1969.
44. Ochsner A, Gage M, and DeBakey M: Scalenus anticus (Naffziger) syndrome, Am J Surg 28:699, 1935.
45. Paulombo L: Upper dorsal sympathectomies without horner's syndrome, Arch Surg 83:717, 1955.
46. Pavot A, Ignacio D, and Gargour G: Diagnosis of thoracic outlet syndrome by assessment of conduction time from C8 root supraclavicular fossa in the lower trunk of the brachial plexus. Proceedings of American Academy of Physical Medicine and Rehabilitation, 1983.
47. Peet RM and others: Thoracic outlet syndrome: evaluation of a therapeutic exercise program, Staff Meetings Mayo Clin, p 281, 1956.
48. Petropoulos PC and Stefanko S: Experimental observations on the prevention of neuroma formation, J Surg Res 1:241, 1961.
49. Poplawski ZJ, Wiley AM, and Murray JF: Post traumatic dystrophy of the extremities. A clinical review and trial treatment, J Bone Joint Surg 65A:642, 1983.
50. Raaf J: Surgery for cervical rib and scalenus anticus syndrome, JAMA 157:219, 1955.
51. Richards R: Causalgia, a centennial review, Arch Neurol 16:339, 1967.
52. Rob CG and Standeven A: Arterial occlusion complicating thoracic outlet compression syndrome, Brit Med J 2:709. 1958.

53. Roos DB: Transaxillary approach for first rib resecton to relieve thoracic outlet syndrome, Ann Surg 163:354, 1966.
54. Roos DB: Congenital anomalies associated with thoracic outlet syndrome, Am J Surg 132:771, 1976.
55. Roos DB: Recurrent thoracic outlet syndrome after first rib resection, Acta Chir Belg 79:363, 1980.
56. Roos DB: The place for scalenectomy and first rib resection in thoracic outlet syndrome, Surgery 92:1977, 1982.
57. Seiler WA and others: Double cruch syndrome: experimental model in the rat, Surg Forum 34:59, 1983.
58. Semmes RE and Murphy F: The syndrome of unilateral rupture of the sixth cervical intervertebral disc with compression of the seventh cervical nerve root, JAMA 121:1209, 1943.
59. Smith JR and Gomas NH: Focal injection of neuromata of the hand with triamcinolone acetonide. A preliminary study of twenty two patients, J Bone Joint Surg 52A:71, 1970.
60. Steinbrocker O: The shoulder-hand syndrome: present perspective, Arch Phys Med Rehab 49:388. 1968.
61. Steinbrocker O and Argyrose TG: The shoulder hand syndrome: present status as a diagnostic and therapeutic entity, Med Clin North Am 42:1533-1553, 1958.
62. Steinbrocker O, Spitzer N, and Friedman HH: The shoulder hand syndrome in reflex dystrophy of the upper extremity, Ann Intern Med 29:22, 1947.
63. Stilz RJ, Conn H, and Sanders DB: Reflex sympathetic dystrophy in a 6 year old successful treatment by transcutaneous nerve stimulation, Anesth Analg 56:438, 1977.
64. Sunderland S: The connective tissues of peripheral nerves, Brain 88:841, 1965.
65. Sunderland S: Nerve and nerve injuries, ed 2, New York, 1978, Churchill Livingstone.
66. Swanson AB, Bover NR, and Biddulph SL: Silicone rubber capping of amputation neuromas. Investigational and clinical experience, Interclin Info Bull 11:1, 1972.
67. Swift TR and Nichols FT: The droopy shoulder syndrome, Neurology 34:212, 1984.
68. Swift TR and Roos DB: TOS or just droopy shoulders, Aches Pains 6:813, 1984.
69. Tufa JW and Boothe PN: Treatment of painful neuromas of the sensory nerves in the hand for comparison of tradition and newer methods, J Hand Surg 1:44, 1976.
70. Upton ARM and McComas AJ: The double crush syndrome in nerve entrapment syndromes, Lancet 2:359, 1973.
71. Urschel H, Paulson B, and McNamara J: Thoracic outlet syndrome, Ann Surg 6(1):1968. 6
72. Urschel HC and Razzuk MA: Management of thoracic outlet syndrome, N Engl J Med 286:1140, 1972.
73. Urschel HC and Razzuk MA: Thoracic outlet syndrome, Surg Annu 5:229, 1973.
74. Willshire WH: Supernumery first rib: clinical records, Lancet 2:633, 1860.
75. Wilbourn AJ: Thoracic outlet syndrome, AAEE Course D, 1984.
76. Wright IS: The neurovascular syndrome produced by hyperabduction of the arm, Am Heart J 29(1):1, 1945.

40

Therapist's management of thoracic outlet syndrome

John Barbis

Thoracic outlet syndrome (TOS) is not a single pathologic condition that affects a single structure and produces a single pattern of symptoms. It is a term that describes a group of pathologic conditions that compress or restrict mobility of the brachial plexus and produce a highly variable set

---

POTENTIAL CAUSES OR PRECIPITATING FACTORS IN THORACIC OUTLET SYNDROME

Anatomic anomalies

Osseous anomalies of the ribs or clavical
Cervical ribs
Cervicodorsal scoliosis
Anomalous structure of the scalene musculature
Anomalous fibrous bands between the ribs and cervical vertebrae
Vascular anomalies of the subclavian artery or vein

Muscular imbalances

Scalene anticus syndrome
Pectoralis minor syndrome
Subclavius muscle tightness
Omohyoid tightness
Middle scalene syndrome

Postural or environmental causes

Poor posture
Overhead work postures
Heavy lifting
Costoclavicular syndrome
Large breasts
Narrow bra straps

Trauma

Traction or penetration injuries of the brachial plexus
Fractures of the clavicle or ribs
Shoulder fractures or dislocations
Whiplash
Trauma to the upper extremity or spine
Sports injuries

Others

Tumors
Surgery of the thorax or upper extremity
Irritation after the removal of subclavian intravenous catheter
Reflex sympathetic dystrophy
Smoking
Cervical disk disease
Shoulder instability

---

of symptoms. Restriction of the plexus may be caused by connective tissue adhesions or compressions produced by anatomic anomalies,* muscle tightness,† posture,‡ trauma,[1,4,18,41,42] tumors,[17,21,26,42] or other causes[9,30] (see box at left). Because of the location or the extent of the restrictions or compressions, symptoms may vary widely. Pain, paresthesia, numbness, or weakness can exist singly or in combination. Symptoms may occur at rest or only with particular activities or postures. Location of symptoms may also vary widely. Symptoms may be referred to any part of the upper quarter or to the neck, head, or face. The most common referral pattern, however, tends to follow C_8 and T_1 nerve root distributions.[42]

Vascular changes may or may not accompany neurologic symptoms. Changes in pulse pressure and skin temperature or texture may be caused by a direct compression of the subclavian artery or vein by the tissue that also compresses the plexus. Changes in vascular status can also be caused by vasomotor irritation.[54] Reflex sympathetic dystrophy may accompany TOS.[18]

Although Adson's test and the hyperabduction and costoclavicular tests use a change in radial pulse as a positive sign of TOS, recent studies[2,7,42,44] show that vascular compression in these test positions can be physiologic and not necessarily indicative of TOS. Compromise of vascular elements does occur in approximately 10% of TOS patients[17] and if left untreated can result in serious complications.[14,17,46] When vascular compromise is suspected, the therapist should refer the patient back to the physician for further diagnostic tests and vascular studies.

TOS can be difficult to diagnose or evaluate. Because many other problems in the upper quarter or cervical spine may produce the same symptoms as TOS (see box on p. 541), it can be overlooked as a possible cause of pain in the upper quarter. TOS can also be present with one or more problems in the upper quarter.[5] Pain and neurologic symptoms of spinal origin,[16,27,38] pathologic conditions of the shoulder,[8,24,38] tumors, and distal entrapments of the peripheral nerves[5,17,42,50] may produce similar symptom complexes that can make diagnosis difficult. In addition, interaction between TOS and an undiagnosed concomitant problem in the neck, shoulder, or arm can make the development of a rational treatment program frustrating, because the treatment approaches to the two problems may conflict.

Behavioral and psychologic problems of chronic pain add

---

*References 1, 6, 14, 17, 21, 26, 41-43, 53.
†References 1, 6, 20, 21, 32, 49.
‡References 3, 6, 31, 38, 44, 48, 49.

CONDITIONS THAT PRODUCE SYMPTOMS SIMILAR TO THORACIC OUTLET SYNDROME

Pancoast's tumor
Cervical and thoracic pain syndrome
Cervical and thoracic fracture
Cervical and thoracic spine tumors
Spinal disk disease
Reflex sympathetic dystrophy
Blockage of the subclavian artery or vein
Bursitis, tendinitis, or capsulitis of the shoulder
Acromioclavicular joint separation
Carpal tunnel syndrome
Ulnar nerve entrapment
Radial nerve entrapment
Clavicular fractures
Raynaud's syndrome
Subscapular nerve entrapment
Dorsal scapular nerve entrapment
Long thoracic nerve entrapment
Axillary nerve entrapment

COMPONENTS OF THE SUBJECTIVE EVALUATION

Description of symptoms
Behavior of symptoms
History of symptoms
Irritability of condition
Medical history
Relevant family or work history

---

to the difficulties of evaluating and treating the TOS patient.[13,28,29,46,52] Many TOS patients have been symptomatic for many months or years without diagnosis or adequate care. As a result, these patients may amplify or denigrate their symptoms, and it may take several visits to accurately and completely describe their condition. Drug dependencies, depression, and family, employment, or marital problems are common in the chronic pain group[28,29] and make an active, independently oriented treatment program essential for success. Psychologic counseling, biofeedback, and stress management are important components of the care plan when these problems are present. It is essential to develop a coordinated effort between psychologic and physical therapies.

DEVELOPMENT OF THE CARE PLAN

Any treatment program for TOS must begin with a thorough medical evaluation and physical therapy assessment not only to rule out other potential problems that produce similar symptoms, but to discover other problems that may complicate the treatment plan. In addition, any patient with symptoms for longer than 1 year should be evaluated by the psychologic service to determine if counseling would be valuable.

Because the medical aspects of making the differential diagnosis of TOS were discussed in Chapter 39, physical therapy assessment and development of a treatment plan are emphasized here.

Physical therapy evaluation

Because of the variable complex of symptoms and the frequency with which other problems in the neck and upper extremity coexist with TOS, a thorough evaluation must be performed that carefully assesses the cervical spine, thoracic spine, lumbar spine, shoulder girdle, shoulder, and the rest of the arm. A thorough upper quarter evaluation is a necessary prerequisite to development of a treatment plan that

is effective, does not overlook other significant conditions, and will not cause undue discomfort. This extensive evaluation may take 30 to 60 minutes to complete. In addition, if the patient's signs and symptoms do not indicate a clear pattern of care, several visits may be necessary to assess trial treatments. This trial and assessment process is especially important in developing an exercise program. The physical therapy assessment has two components: a subjective and an objective evaluation.[8,15]

Subjective evaluation. The component sections of the subjective evaluation are listed. Careful questioning of the patient and documentation of the answers is important for the following.
1. Planning the extent and vigor of the objective evaluation
2. Planning the treatment program
3. Assessing the effectiveness of the treatment plan
4. Determining the need for additional testing, counseling, or treatment (psychologic, family, occupational, or medical)
4. Providing documentation for insurance reimbursement or legal purposes

The area and extent of symptoms are most easily documented through use of a body chart on which the therapist can indicate the areas of pain, paresthesia, or loss of sensation (Fig. 40-1). Areas of paresthesia or numbness should be clearly marked because these areas will be explored more carefully during the objective evaluation.

Various pain evaluation scales or questionnaires can be used to document the level or extent of pain and disability.[13,19,40] Pain questionnaires other than that shown in Fig. 40-1 can be used to determine behavior of the pain, but there are several questions that are of particular importance and should be included in the evaluation, because they will indicate the pattern of symptoms caused by the pathologic condition and the functional level of the patient.
1. Is the pain constant or intermittent?
2. Is there pain at night, and what is its extent?
3. How does the pain vary in intensity and location as the day progresses?
4. What activities or postures particularly aggravate symptoms?
5. What activities or postures seem to ease or eliminate symptoms?

Of particular importance during this part of the subjective evaluation is the determination of the irritability of the condition. Irritability as stated by Maitland[33] is "determined by relating the vigor of an activity which causes pain, firstly to the degree of pain that ensues, and then to the length of

Date_____

Name_____

Address_____

_____

Date of birth_____

Date of injury_____

Occupation_____

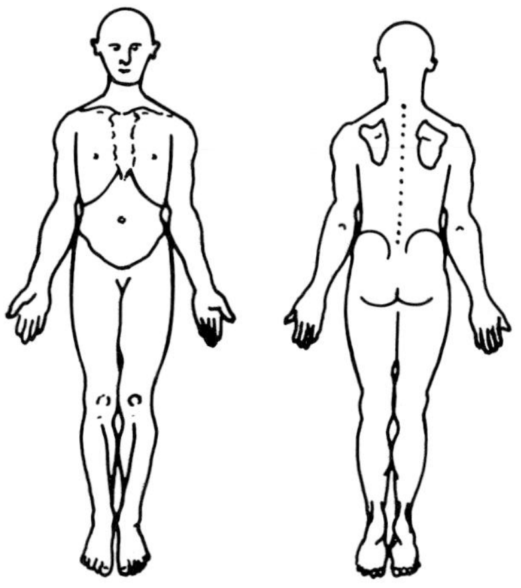

Subjective evaluation   Pain 1 2 3 4 5 6 7 8 9 10

Symptoms now_____

_____

History_____

_____

_____

Previous treatment_____

Constant/Intermittent   Irritability_____

When worse   Moving   Sitting   Lifting   Lying   Working   A.M./P.M.

Other_____

When better   Moving   Sitting   Lifting   Lying   Working   A.M./P.M.

Other_____

Disturbed sleep   Pain on   Coughing/Sneezing

Medical history:

X-rays_____   Medications_____

General health_____

Recent surgeries_____

History of accidents_____

Fig. 40-1   Subjective evaluation and history form.

time taken for this increased pain to subside to its usual level." The determination of irritability involves a series of three questions:

What activity caused the pain?
What was the severity of that pain?
What was the duration of that pain before it subsided?[33]

An accurate determination of the irritability of the condition can be particularly useful in directing the vigor of the objective evaluation: it can prevent the evaluation being (1) too vigorous, thus aggravating the patient's symptoms or (2) too gentle, thus preventing the therapist from accurately determining the extent of the problem. It can also become an important determinant in developing the vigor of the exercise program.[33]

Determining an accurate chronology for the development of the present problem and other relevant medical problems is an essential component of the information-gathering process. Knowing the pattern of onset of symptoms, past care, history of trauma or accidents, past medical conditions, present health, and present treatment (such as medications and counseling) is essential to determine if any specific treatments are contraindicated and to design a comprehensive care plan.

Objective evaluation. The goals of the objective evaluation are as follows:

1. Document the quantity and quality of active and passive motions for the cervical spine, thoracic spine, lumbar spine, shoulder girdle, shoulder, and the rest of the arm
2. Determine the change in symptoms with repeated motions in the cervical and thoracic spines
3. Determine mobility of the brachial plexus
4. Document relevant postural abnormalities
5. Document neurologic status
6. Document muscle strength
7. Document functional status

Objective evaluation of the TOS patient should involve a thorough upper quarter assessment. It is important to evaluate not only all of the possible areas that can produce symptoms, but also areas that are affected by the treatment program. Of particular importance outside the upper quarter is the lumbar spine. The mobility and status of the lumbar spine must be evaluated because many of the activities and postures that are normally a part of the treatment plan depend on normal lumbar motion. Restrictions or pain production

Posture
Sitting____
Standing____
Sleeping____

Movement loss
Cervical spine
Flexion____
Extension____
Rotations____
Side Flexions____

Thoracic spine
Flexion____
Extension____
Rotations____

Test movements
Cervical spine
Protraction____
Rep. protraction____
Retraction____
Rep. retraction____
Extension____
Rep. extension____
Rotation R____
Rep. rotation____
Rotation L____
Rep. rotation____
Side flexion R____
Rep. side flexion____
Side flexion L____
Rep. side flexion____

Thoracic spine
Flexion____
Rep. flexion____
Extension____
Rep. extension____
Rotation R____
Rep. rotation____
Rotation L____
Rep. rotation____
Inspiration____
Exspiration____

Lumbar spine
Flexion____
Side flexion R____
Side flexion L____
Extension____
Rotation R____
Rotation L____

Shoulder	Active	Passive	Static
SCAP adductor			
SCAP abductor			
SCAP elevation			
SCAP depression			
SCAP rotations			
G/H external rotation			
G/H internal rotation			
G/H flexion			
G/H abductor			
G/H ext-adductor (hand behind back)			

Continued.

Fig. 40-2 Objective evaluation form.

in the lumbar area may require significant modifications in the treatment plan. The components of the objective evaluation are assessments of the following:

1. Range of motion of the cervical spine, thoracic spine, lumbar spine, shoulder complex, and chest wall
2. Repeated movements in the cervical and thoracic spines
3. Muscle strength and function in the upper quarter
4. Sensory function in the upper quarter
5. Work, leisure, and resting postures
6. Coordination and endurance in the upper extremity
7. Vascular assessment
8. Brachial plexus mobility tests

An outline of the objective evaluation appears in Fig. 40-2. As seen, the evaluation is extensive. All of these procedures may not be required with each patient. Because of the severity of the patient's symptoms, the therapist may determine that some of the tests may be too vigorous and cause excessive discomfort. With such a patient, the complete evaluation may take several visits to perform and may be performed only as the acute discomfort diminishes. With a patient with minimal symptoms or lack of subjective neurologic complaints (weakness, paresthesia, or numbness), the evaluation can be shortened. As the patient's history and symptoms become more complicated, the evaluation must become more thorough. With all patients, the evaluation should be extensive enough to develop a set of goals, trial treatment plan, and means of measuring progress. Only a brief evaluation may be tolerated by a patient in severe discomfort, and in this case, only a brief evaluation may be needed to determine an appropriate pain management program that identifies the best resting position for the patient.

Elbow	Active	Passive	Static
Flexion			
Extension			
Forearm			
Pronation			
Supination			
Wrist			
Flexion			
Sustained flexion			
Extension			
Hand			
Finger Flexion			
Abduction			
Adduction			
Thumb Flexion			
Extension			
Abduction			
Adduction			
Opposition			

TOS stress tests	Neurological	Vascular
Adson's		
Tinnell's wrist		
Tinnell's TOS		
Costoclavicular		
Stress abduction		
Uett		

Sensory_____

Reflexes_____

Palpation_____

Fig. 40-2, cont'd Objective evaluation form.

For a patient with moderate chronic discomfort, a more extensive evaluation may be needed to determine the treatment goals, because several different structures may be involved and the interaction of the different problem areas may necessitate a change in the normal treatment progression.

Cyriax,[8] Maitland,[33] and others[3,15,19,48] describe effective upper quarter evaluations. All of these sources indicate that it is essential to isolate individual structures during the tests to accurately clear or implicate specific structures in the production of the symptom complex. Referred pain, abnormal function, or poor postures (which can be caused by primary cervical, thoracic, or shoulder problems) must be noted, and a hierarchy of problems must be delineated. The use of selective tension tests, as described by Cyriax,[8] with the symptom reproduction and reduction concepts of Maitland[33] and McKenzie[36,47] can be helpful in isolating the structures that are producing symptoms and in separating primary from secondary problems.

Specific active, passive, and isometric tests, used in a systematic way to determine those movements and postures that accurately reproduce or reduce the symptoms, can help clarify the treatment program for a patient with complex symptoms. McKenzie's evaluation of the cervical and thoracic spines, which uses repeated motions and the concept of the centralization of pain, can be valuable in determining if the syndrome has a spinal origin.

Tinel's, Adson's, the costoclavicular, the stress abduction tests, and Elvey's Upper Extremity Tension Test (UETT) can be used to test the status of the brachial plexus. Tinel's test is a gentle tapping or percussion of the thoracic outlet area to reproduce the symptoms. Adson's test (Fig. 40-3) uses cervical rotation and extension and sustained inspiration to produce a change in the radial pulse or a reproduction of the symptoms. The costoclavicular test (Fig. 40-4) re-

quires the patient to assume and maintain an exaggerated military position (scapulae fully adducted and depressed and head erect). Again, either a reproduction of the symptoms or a change in the radial pulse is considered diagnostic of TOS. During the stress abduction test (Fig. 40-5), the patient assumes and maintains a sitting position with the arms abducted and externally rotated to 90 degrees and the forearm flexed to 90 degrees. The hands are then rapidly opened and closed for 2 to 3 minutes or until the symptoms are provoked. Adson's, the costoclavicular, and the stress abduction tests can be used to test both the vascular and neurologic components of the syndrome (see Chapter 39).

One of the most important tests for a patient suspected of having TOS or in whom the diagnosis has been made, is Elvey's test for the mobility of the brachial plexus and nerve root.[10] Elvey's UETT is analogous to the straight leg raising test for lumbosacral nerve roots and the sacral plexus. The test can determine if any restrictions of the nerve roots or plexus are produced as the neural elements of the upper extremity are placed on stretch by a series of sequential movements at the shoulder, elbow, forearm, and wrist. The test is positive if after careful positioning of the shoulder, elbow, and forearm, wrist extension reproduces the symptoms (Fig. 40-6). The test helps discriminate between either a neural or a glenohumeral source of the symptoms. Kenneally[25] describes the performance of this test as follows:

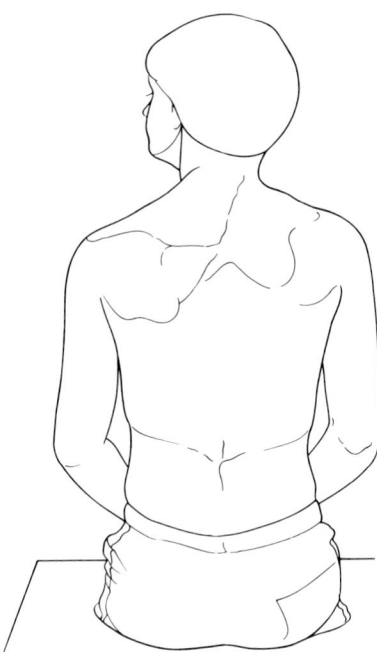

Fig. 40-3 Adson's test. Loss of radial pulse is a vascular indicator.

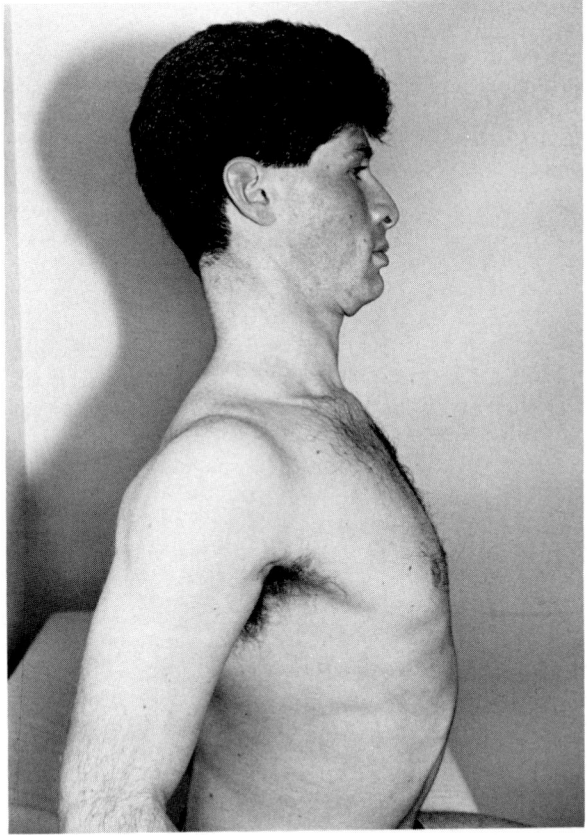

Fig. 40-4 Costoclavicular test. Scapulae are fully adducted and depressed. The head is held erect.

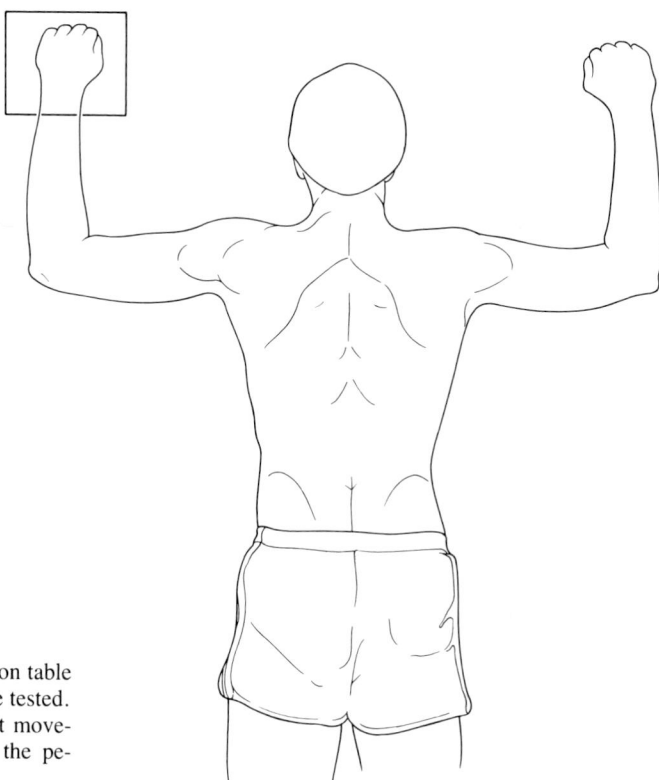

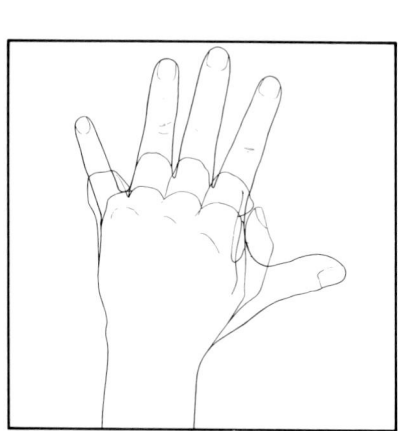

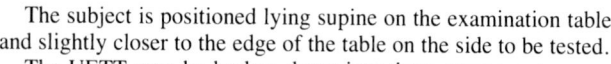

Fig. 40-5   Stress abduction test.

The subject is positioned lying supine on the examination table and slightly closer to the edge of the table on the side to be tested.

The UETT may be broken down into three component movements, each producing progressively greater tension in the peripheral nerve/nerve root system of the upper limb.

The three component movements are

1. Shoulder abduction, lateral rotation, and extension behind the coronal plane
2. Forearm supination and elbow extension
3. Wrist and finger extension[25]

In addition to determining the source of symptoms, this test can be extremely valuable in developing parameters for the exercise program. Through careful performance of the test, a relatively accurate determination can be made of the point at which restriction of the neural elements is encountered and the range in which exercises should be performed.

A functional assessment that identifies those postures and activities that either produce or reduce symptoms is essential to determine how to modify the patient's postures or activities to reduce stress on the plexus. The patient's standing, sitting, sleeping, and working postures should be evaluated to determine if they should be modified to remove the stress or compression from the plexus or to allow the upper quarter to function more efficiently.

The extent of the neurologic evaluation can vary widely depending on the status of the patient. An extensive neurologic evaluation including detailed muscle testing and sensory testing may be necessary for the patient with extensive peripheral deficits. Such testing may be important (1) in determining whether this patient is a candidate for surgery or (2) for documenting change in his condition. For those patients with minimal neurologic complaints, a brief screening evaluation that tests the status of major muscle groups, reflexes, and sensibility is all that is necessary to learn if major deficits are present.

TREATMENT

Because of the complexity of signs, symptoms, and problems that the TOS patient has, the therapist may find it difficult to develop a treatment plan. As a result, treatment programs for the TOS patient can range from complex programs that involve multiple modalities, exercises, and manual techniques to simple, standardized home exercise programs, that are given to every patient. Both of these approaches should be avoided. It is essential for the therapist to keep the treatment program simple, by focusing treatment on only one or two treatment goals at a time, and to adapt the treatment plan to the needs of the individual. This approach allows the therapist to more accurately assess the effectiveness of the program and can prevent excessive patient discomfort. It can also prevent patient and therapist confusion that often develops during TOS treatment. Patient confusion can be caused by the therapist presenting too much information in a short time and exceeding the patient's ability to assimilate it. Patient confusion can also occur by being presented with information or a treatment program that is different from previous treatment programs. Therapist confusion usually develops when the patient does not improve or respond as expected. If the treatment program is too vigorous and procedures have not been added in a sequential manner, it is difficult to determine if the whole program or a single component of that program is inappropriate for that patient. It therefore is difficult to know how to change or adapt the treatment program to the needs of the individual. Although some minor discomfort is expected during the treatment program, excessive discomfort can hinder patient progress and can lead to chronic pain behaviors, poor healing, and most important, poor patient compliance. Excessive discomfort can confuse both the patient and the therapist and lead to poor clinical decisions.

Guidelines to development of a successful TOS treatment program are the same as those of any rehabilitation program. These rules (Fig. 40-7) become even more important as the patient's symptoms and problems become more complex.

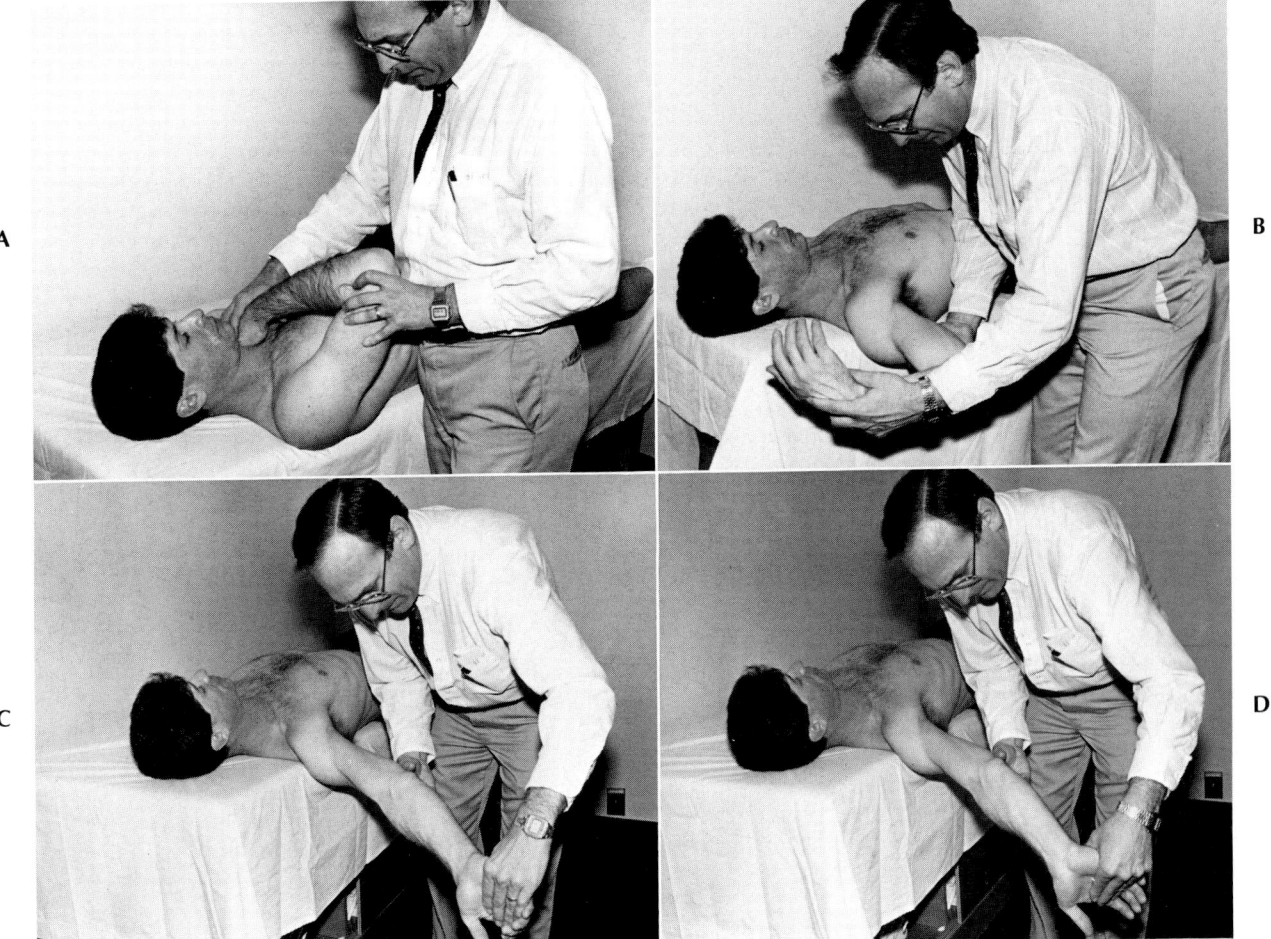

Fig. 40-6   Upper extremity tension test. **A,** First, the arm and scapula are placed in a resting position. **B,** Next, the scapula and shoulder are placed at rest. **C,** Then the elbow and forearm are positioned just short of the onset of the symptoms. **D,** The wrist is then extended to reproduce the symptoms.

Guidelines to the Development of a Successful
TOS Rehabilitation Program

1. Perform and document a disciplined evaluation.
2. Establish and prioritize treatment goals.
3. Keep the treatment plan focused on the primary goal or goals; do not attempt to do too much too soon.
4. Emphasize patient self-reliance and independence in the treatment plan; do not do for the patients what they can do for themselves.
5. Individualize the treatment program to the needs and the resources of the patient.
6. Objectively evaluate the progress of the patient and the effectiveness of individual treatment interventions.
7. Change the treatment plan if progress is not seen.
8. Instruct patients in self care and prophylaxis.

Fig. 40-7   Guidelines for a successful TOS rehabilitation program.

Treatment goals

Any rehabilitation program must have goals. Not only do treatment goals provide a way to communicate expected outcomes for care and establish a yardstick by which effectiveness of care can be evaluated, they also provide a mechanism through which the provider can organize and set priorities in the elements of the care plan. Establishing treatment goals and setting priorities for each patient are the starting points for development of the treatment program. By so doing, the therapist can choose the modalities, procedures, and exercises that best meet the needs of the patient. If the patient does not progress, adjustments can be made without major disruption of the treatment plan.

It can be helpful to use the following general goals to organize and set the priorities of the care plan for the TOS patient:

1. Control symptoms
2. Restore adaptively shortened tissue to normal length
3. Restore muscular balance
4. Develop and maintain improved posture and body mechanics
5. Develop or improve stress-management techniques
6. Prevent recurrence of symptoms

For some patients, not all of these goals may be appropriate or need to be in the treatment plan. For other patients, all goals are appropriate. It is the responsibility of the therapist to establish the most important goal(s) and orient the care plan around it. As treatment progresses, priorities will change and the treatment plan should reflect those changes. The treatment program for TOS should be a dynamic, adaptable plan that recognizes that the syndrome can be complex and requires a well-designed, well-monitored, individualized care plan.

McKenzie's system[36,47] for the diagnosis and treatment of mechanical problems of the cervical and thoracic spines can be valuable in determining if the symptom complex has a cervical component and in developing the treatment plan. If the patient shows signs of a derangement of the cervical or thoracic spines (see box below), those movements or postures that centralize and reduce the derangement should be used for treatment.[36,47] Any derangement of the cervical or thoracic spine should be reduced before treating any compression or restriction of the brachial plexus. The successful reduction of a cervical derangement before the start of a treatment program for TOS can rapidly clarify the extent of the irritation of the plexus and simplify the treatment plan. If the patient shows signs of the dysfunction or the postural syndrome (see box below) along with TOS, both problems can be treated simultaneously.

Symptom control. Symptom control usually requires modalities and maintenance of positions that remove compression or tension from the brachial plexus. Of the two techniques, the latter can be more effective in gaining prolonged control over symptoms, but it is the more difficult to attain. Use of modalities (such as heat, cold, and electrical stimulation) is an important adjuvent to care when the patient is in severe discomfort such that no position, posture, or activity decreases or eliminates pain. Use of moist heat and ice can be effective in modulating or eliminating pain for limited periods. Their use within a home program to manage pain can be important. In addition, the use of ice can be used to control discomfort and inflammation that occur after exercise. One of the first activities of the therapist is to carefully instruct the patient in the safe and effective use of moist heat (such as hot packs and hot baths) and ice. If the plexus appears to be actively inflamed, the patient can place an ice pack over the cervical and shoulder area for 20 minutes every 2 hours. Transcutaneous electrical nerve stimulation (TENS) is also used at home. It can control the intensity of pain. Other modalities, such as ultrasound, diathermy, electroacupuncture, He-Ne laser, and high-frequency electrical stimulation, have been suggested as effective modalities for providing temporary relief from pain.[6,19,45,49] All of these modalities are believed to relieve pain either by providing a stimulus that modulates the incoming sensory information in the Melzack and Wall theory of pain control or stimulating the production of endorphin.[13,34,39,40] Although these modalities are commonly used to control TOS pain, there are no controlled studies that show they are effective in relieving TOS symptoms. Michlovitz,[40] Mannheimer,[34] and others[14,19] are excellent sources for the use of modalities in treatment of TOS pain.

The most effective means of controlling TOS symptoms

McKENZIE'S CLASSIFICATION OF THE MECHANICAL DISORDERS OF THE THORACIC AND CERVICAL SPINE

Postural syndrome

Pain is intermittent

Pain is not referred

No loss of motion or provocation of symptoms with repeated movements

Pain is produced by prolonged maintenance of specific postures

Dysfunction syndrome

Pain is intermittent

Pain is not referred (except in a nerve root adhesion)

Pain is felt at the end of range and not during movement

No centralization or peripheralization of symptoms is seen on repeated movements

Derangement syndrome

Symptoms may change in intensity, character, and location with repeated motions and changes in posture

Spinal motions can show a rapid gain or loss of motion on repeated movements

Symptoms can be referred

Pain can be constant or intermittent

Centralization or peripheralization will be seen on repeated motions

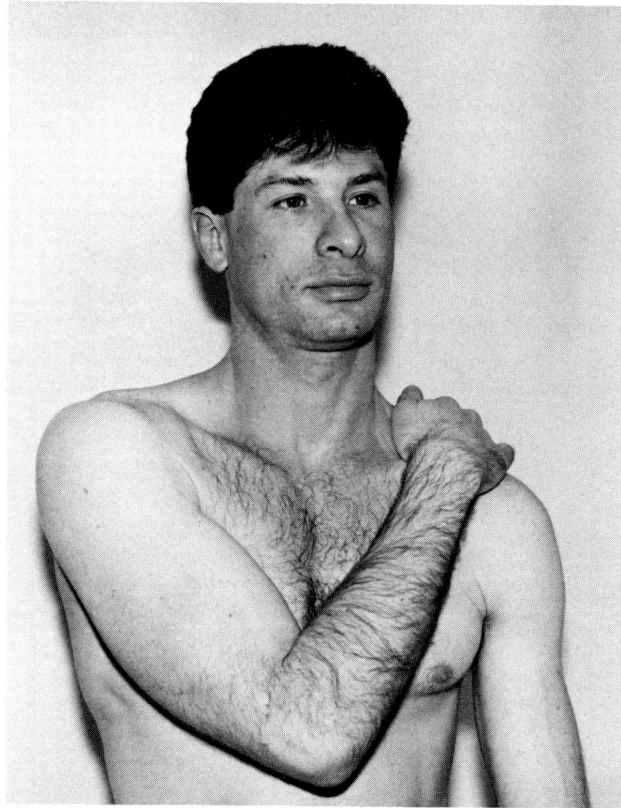

Fig. 40-8 Rest position for T.O.S. The scapula is abducted and elevated and the shoulder is internally rotated and adducted.

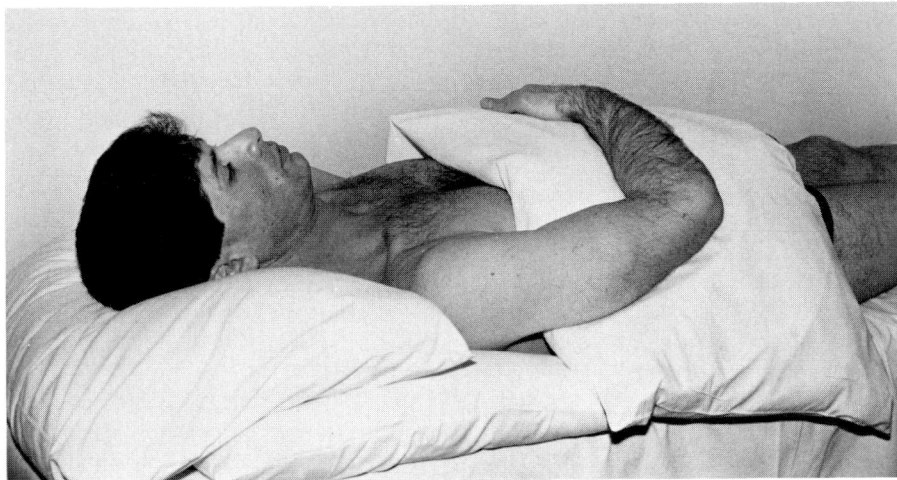

Fig. 40-9 Rest position in supine position. Pillows should be used to support the thoracic spine, scapula, and arm.

is to place the plexus in a position where it cannot be compressed or stretched. Careful positioning of the affected arm or scapula can rapidly decrease or eliminate symptoms. Symptoms usually return once the position or posture is changed, but the position can help relieve pain or decrease inflammation. The rest position is with the scapula in abduction and elevation and the shoulder in internal rotation and adduction (Fig. 40-8). A sling or shoulder immobilizer can be worn continuously for a few days, or it can be used only during activity to provide support and protect the plexus from irritation. The patient should also be instructed how to assume a rest position at night by using pillows to support the arm and scapula (Fig. 40-9) and how to use a pillow or armrest to support the arms while sitting (Fig. 40-10).

Although the position in Fig. 40-8 provides some control over symptoms, the patient should be warned that maintenance of this position for long periods will actually inhibit progress, because the plexus will tend to adhere in that position and further motion will be lost. This rest position will also be important, because it will be the position from which brachial plexus gliding exercises will start.

Restore normal length of adaptively shortened tissue. Adaptively shortened tissues that either compress or prevent normal movement of the brachial plexus are the structures most commonly responsible for symptoms. Lengthening of these tissues therefore becomes one of the primary goals of the treatment program. A vigorous stretching program can be attempted, however, only after inflammation is controlled, if present. If stretching is attempted too soon or too vigorously, the inflammatory response in the area will be maintained or even increased and the patient will be exposed to unacceptable discomfort. If the patient is in significant discomfort and if no position or posture can be found to significantly decrease or eliminate pain, several days of rest, antiinflammatory therapy (ice and antiinflammatory medication), and pain modulation procedures should be used before starting the stretching program. If the patient still does not respond in a few days, a stretching program can be carefully added to the pain modulation procedures. If the patient continues to show no adequate progress in a few days, he should be reevaluated to determine if another prob-

lem is responsible for the discomfort or if the patient is a candidate for surgery.

Once the stretching program is started, the patient should be encouraged to perform the exercises on a regular basis throughout the day. According to the degree of inflammation and the severity of the problem, the patient is encouraged to perform five to ten repetitions every 2 to 4 hours throughout the day. The patient is instructed either to maintain the arm at rest between exercises if it is sore or to use the arm within tolerable limits during later stages of recovery. The goal of the stretching program is to stress the shortened tissue without causing additional inflammation. Performing

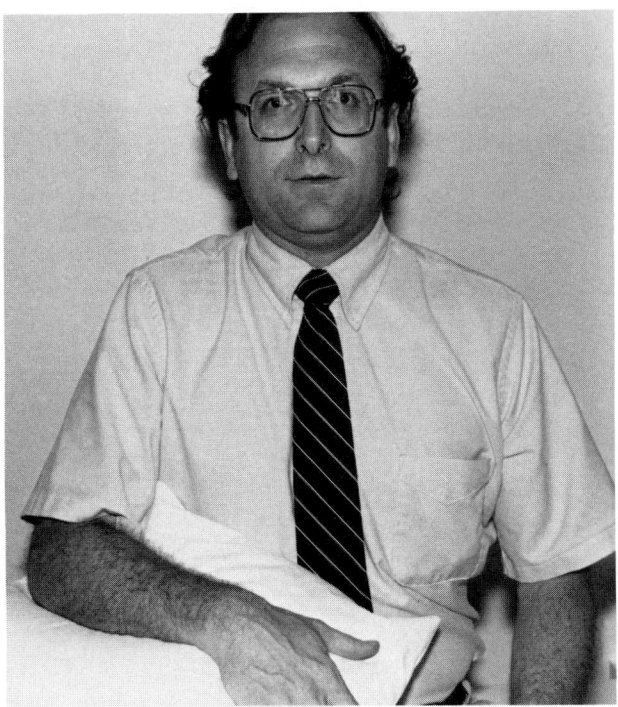

Fig. 40-10 Rest position is sitting using pillows to support the scapula and arm.

a few repetitions several times during the day may be the best way to accomplish that goal without inflaming the plexus. The plexus can be inflamed easily, and there is some evidence that the inflammation can be latent and not express itself for 5 to 6 hours after activity.[31]

For all of the exercises, each of the repetitions should be performed from a position of rest or neutral to the point where pain or strain is felt. The patient is warned not to push through pain, because this can rapidly inflame the area and hinder progress. As treatment progresses, the point at which pain or strain is felt should progress further into the range and the therapist must ensure that the patient continues to stretch the desired structure. It is also important for the therapist to watch for secondary problems at the shoulder or neck. As movement increases, it is not unusual to develop shoulder impingement or cervical derangement. The treatment program may need to be adapted or changed as these secondary problems are exposed. The development of these secondary problems can often be prevented if proper postures and techniques are emphasized during the exercises.

By far the most important form of exercise is self-stretching. Therapist techniques, such as joint mobilization techniques, ultrasound and stretch, spray and stretch,[49] myofacial release techniques, proprioceptive neuromuscular facilitation (PNF),[51] and other manual stretching techniques[11] are valuable when a patient plateaus or in the presence of secondary problems.

Smith[45] and Howell[19] emphasize the need to mobilize the first rib and the acromioclavicular joint to increase the dimensions of the costoclavicular space. Mobilization or manipulative techniques of the first rib can be used over the costovertebral joint or the rib itself. Manual techniques to increase mobility of the acromioclavicular joint are (1) direct pressure over the joint or (2) use of clavicular or scapular motions.

For any of the manual techniques, it is important to remind patients of their responsibilities and to reinforce the home program and concept of self-responsibility.

Brachial plexus gliding exercises. The most effective and adaptable method of applying stress to the plexus is use of UETT for an exercise. Patients with severe restrictions of the plexus may produce a strain or a discomfort solely by depressing or adducting their scapula from the rest position. Each repetition should proceed from an area of min-

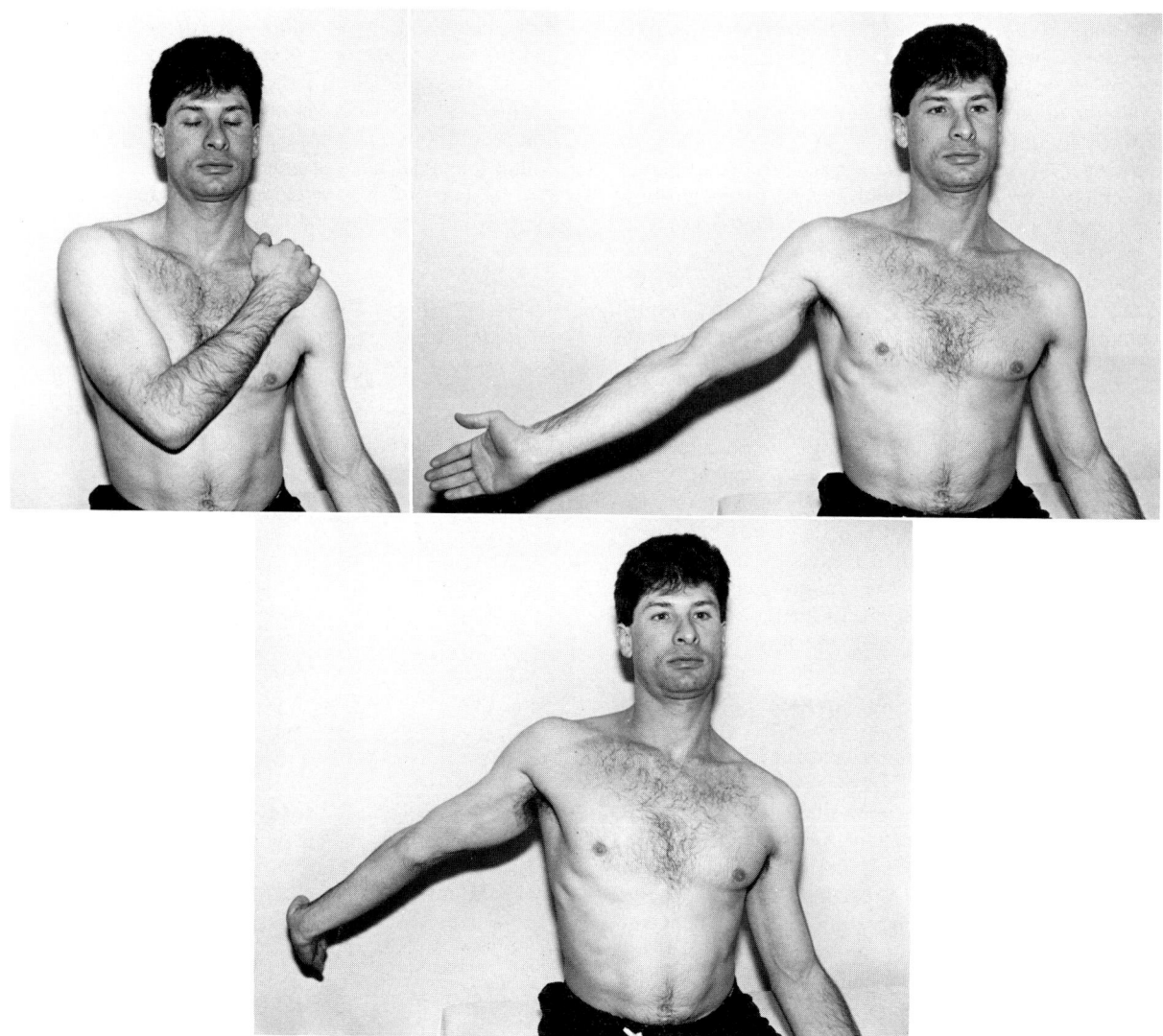

Fig. 40-11 Brachial plexus stretch while sitting.

imal or no discomfort to the point at which the pain or strain starts and back to the rest or pain-free position. As the restriction decreases, more shoulder abduction and external rotation can be incorporated into the exercise. During the later stages of treatment, wrist extension and contralateral cervical sideflexion can be used to produce additional stress. Brachial plexus gliding exercises can be adapted for sitting or standing positions and do not need to be done in supine (Fig. 40-11).

The plexus can also be stretched by performing external rotation in 90 degrees of abduction while lying in supine (Fig. 40-12) or while leaning into a corner (Fig. 40-13). Wrist extension can also be incorporated into these exercises.

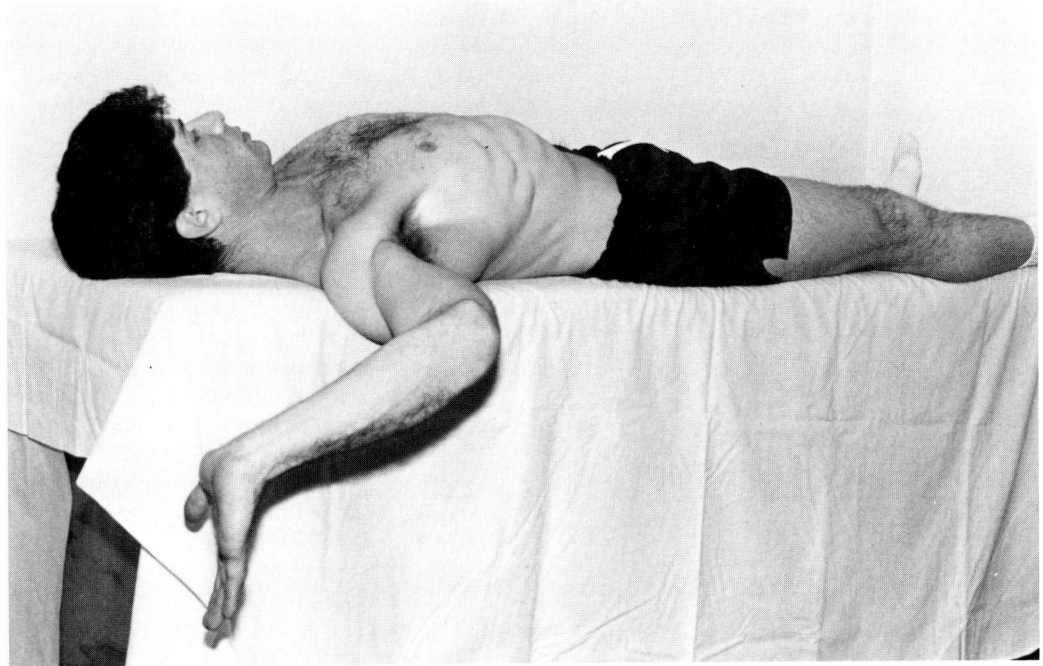

Fig. 40-12 Brachial plexus stretch in supine position using wrist extension and external rotation at 90 degrees of abduction.

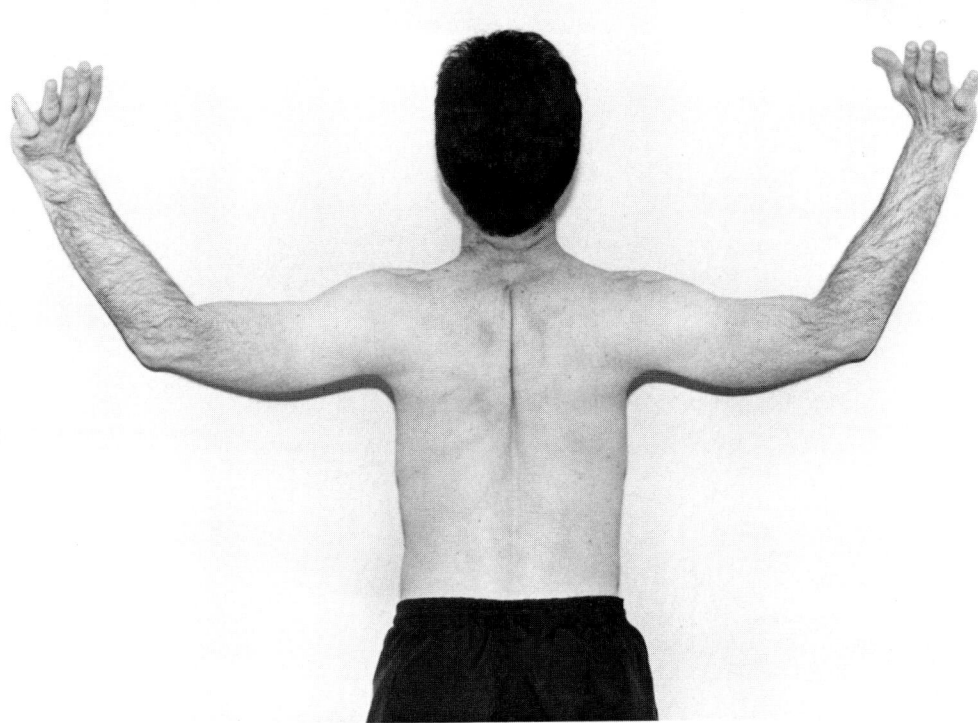

Fig. 40-13 Brachial plexus stretch while leaning into a corner.

These exercises are designed for patients with less restriction of the plexus and those who are not acutely inflamed. In supine, gravity causes the weight of the arm in external rotation to place a stress not only on the plexus, but also on the internal rotators of the shoulder. In the second exercise, the weight of the body as the patient leans into the corner places a stress on the plexus, the internal rotators of the shoulder, the abductors of the scapula, and the thoracic and lumbar spines. Any patient using the corner exercise should be carefully instructed in its use, because it can place significant stress on a number of tissues that can be easily irritated.

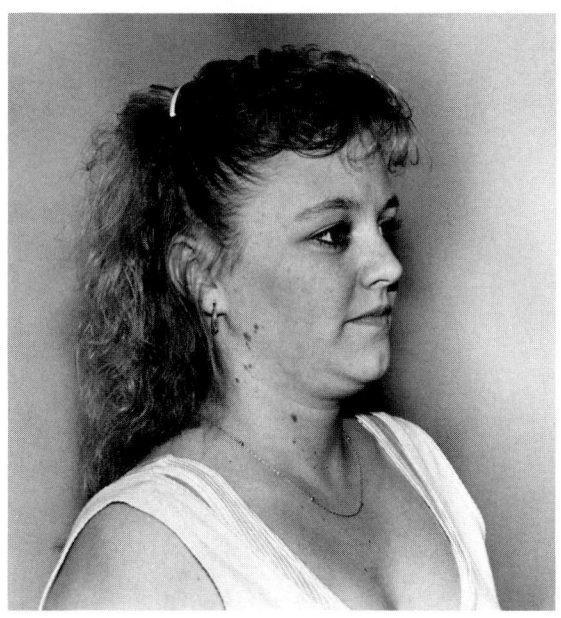

Fig. 40-14 Cervical retraction in sitting position.

Cervical spine exercises. Restoring normal cervical motion is important for restoring normal muscle length to the scalenes, which can entrap the plexus, and also for allowing the patient to achieve normal posture. The loss of normal cervical motion with the maintenance of the forward-head or flexed posture can also place an increased pressure on the disk and musculature of the lower cervical spine, producing secondary problems in those areas.[27,36,37] All cervical motions should be performed carefully, and symptoms should be monitored to ensure that no pathologic condition of a cervical disk is produced or exacerbated during exercises. Three motions that are most commonly lost to adaptive shortening in TOS are cervical retraction, extension, and contralateral sideflexion.

In all cervical exercises, patients should start from either the position of no pain or minimal pain. They should then proceed to the point of strain or pain using active motions. At no time should patients push through pain or should increased discomfort last longer than 5 or 10 minutes after exercise. If no pain or strain is produced during exercise, patients can use their hands to apply overpressure or guide their movement so that the area of restriction is engaged.

Cervical retraction. Cervical retraction can be performed in either the sitting or supine position (Fig. 40-14 and 40-15). For patients with severe restriction of this motion, the head may need support with a pillow while the patient is lying in supine and the exercise is performed into the pillow. During the exercise in both the supine and sitting positions, the head is brought back straight as if the chin were gliding over the surface of a plate. It is sometimes necessary to use the hand to add sufficient pressure or guide the movement. Several treatments may be required before patients with severe restrictions of this movement develop the correct technique. Two common mistakes that decrease the effectiveness of this exercise are slight elevation (Fig. 40-16) or slight dropping (Fig. 40-17) of the chin.

Cervical extension. The exercise starts from a comfort-

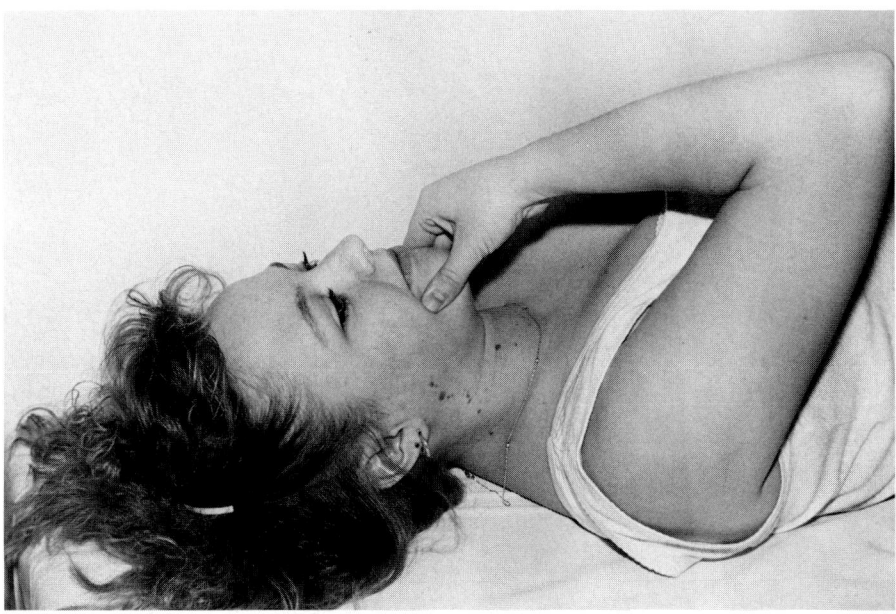

Fig. 40-15 Cervical retraction in supine position using the hand for overpressure.

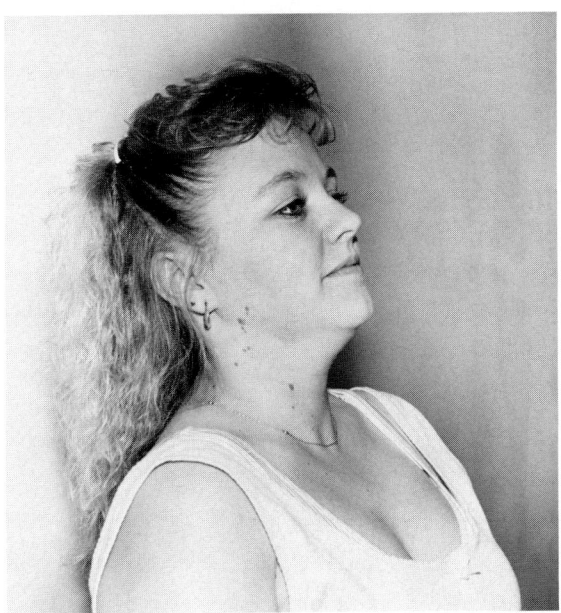

Fig. 40-16 Poor technique—elevated chin—during cervical retraction.

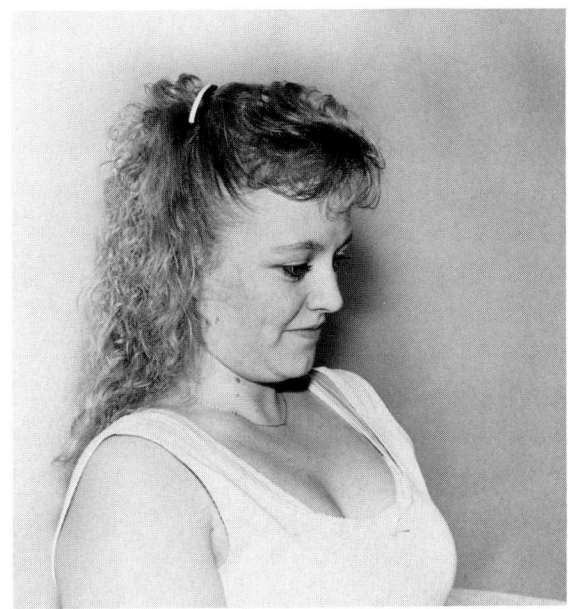

Fig. 40-17 Poor technique—depressed chin—during cervical retraction.

able position where the head is retracted slightly without producing discomfort. The exercise proceeds through the extension of the head and lower cervical spine (Fig. 40-18). It is important to maintain the retracted position as much as possible during the extension movement. Retraction will allow more lower cervical motion during the exercise. The hand can be used to apply overpressure at the end of the movement.

Sideflexions. Sideflexions should be performed bilaterally and can be performed in both the sitting (Fig. 40-19) and supine positions (Fig. 40-20). For patients with significant shortening of the anterior and lateral cervical musculature, the head may need support in the supine position to take the anterior musculature off excessive stretch. The exercise is performed by first retracting the head and then using the ipsilateral arm to pull the ear to the adjacent shoulder while maintaining the retraction. No rotation of the head should occur with this exercise (Fig. 40-21). The exercise is performed similarly in sitting. It is important that this exercise be performed to both sides.

Cervical flexion. Even though most patients are restricted in extension and maintain a forward-head posture, they may show signs of a flexion dysfunction. Many patients will develop transient pain in the rhomboidal areas and down the back as the head is forward-flexed. This motion is stretched by first retracting the head and then gently attempting to bring the chin to the chest (Fig. 40-22). Only three to five repetitions of this exercise should be performed, because it may exacerbate a cervical disk problem if one is present. If no pain or strain is produced during the exercise, the hands may be placed on the head to produce additional pressure.

Thoracic spine. Restrictions of the upper thoracic spine can significantly limit normal cervical extension and can have a significant effect in limiting movement of the upper

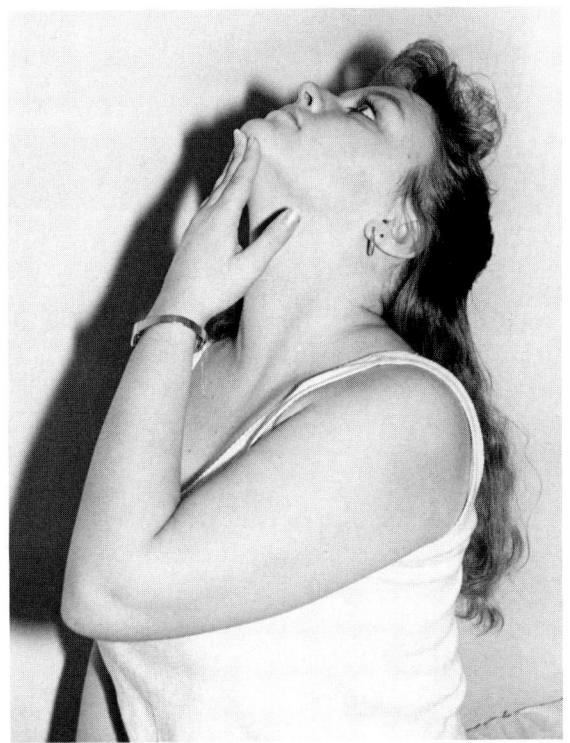

Fig. 40-18 Cervical extension using overpressure.

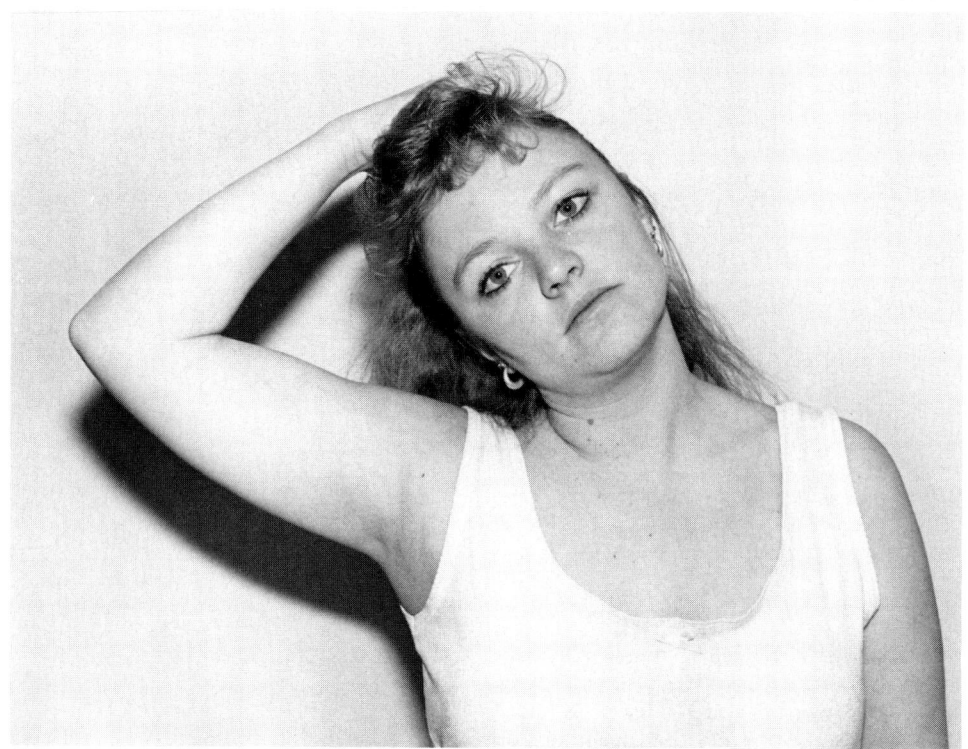

Fig. 40-19   Side flexion of the cervical spine in a sitting position.

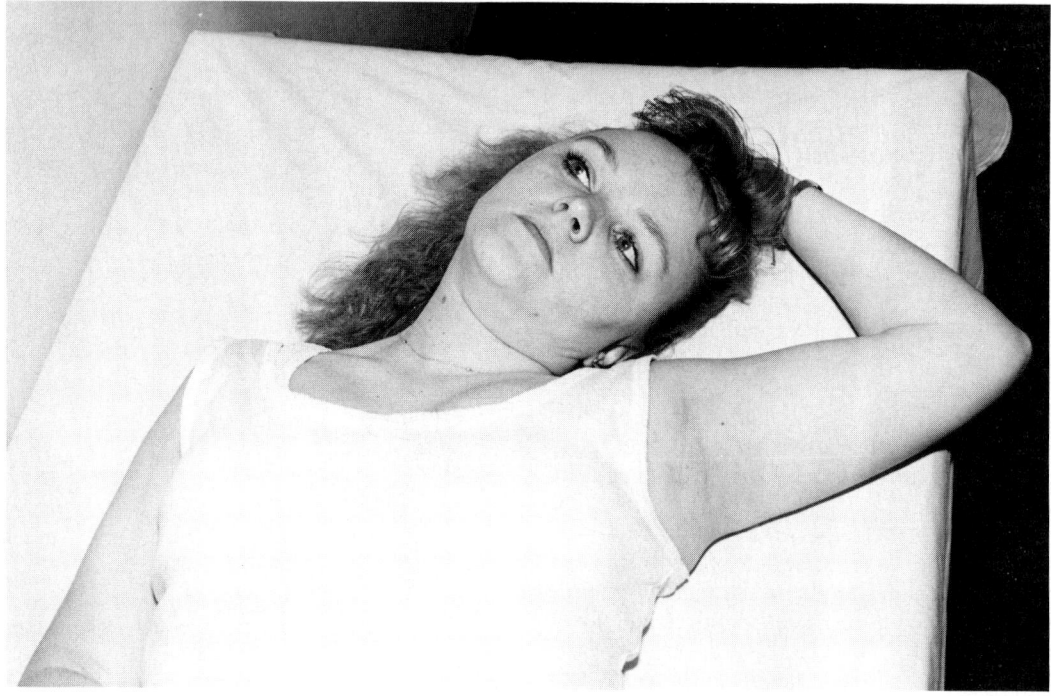

Fig. 40-20   Side flexion of the cervical spine in a supine position.

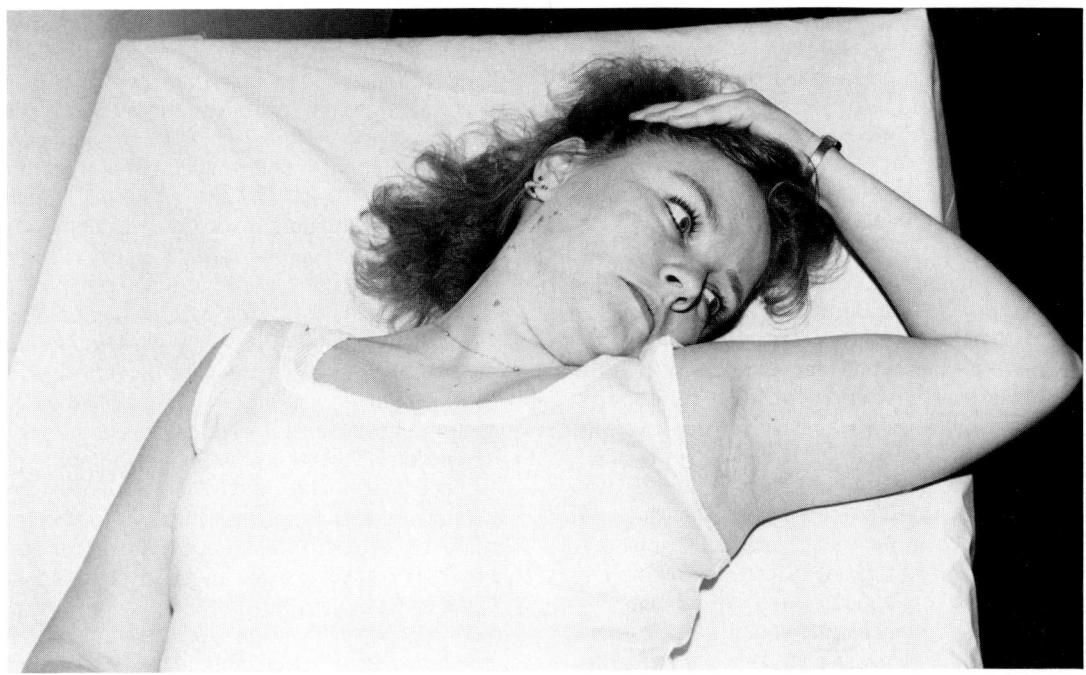

Fig. 40-21   Poor technique—addition of rotation to the side flexion—in side flexion of the cervical spine.

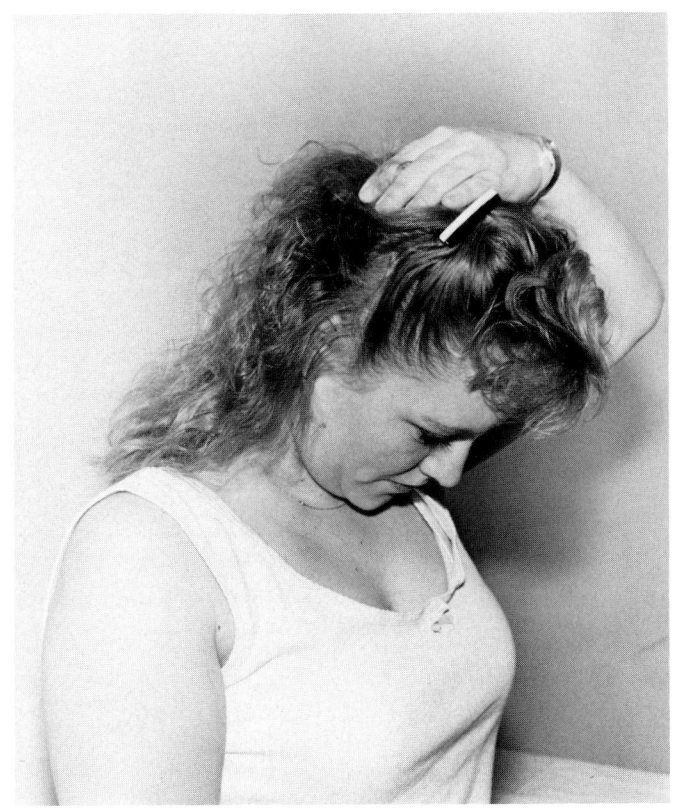

Fig. 40-22   Cervical flexion with overpressure.

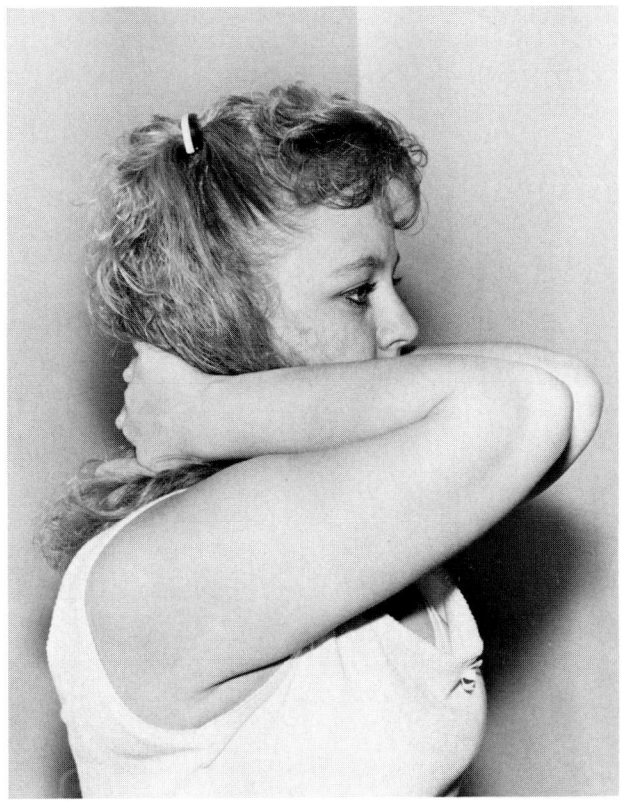

Fig. 40-23   Starting point for the thoracic spine exercises.

ribs. Both flexion and extension exercises are performed while sitting, with the head gently retracted and the hands folded across the cervicothoracic junction and the elbows pointed straight ahead (Fig. 40-23).

Extension. Thoracic extension is then performed by elevating the elbows (Fig. 40-24). Because many patients suffer extension dysfunctions, the starting position for this exercise may be in slight flexion.

Flexion. Thoracic flexion is performed by lowering the elbows toward the chest from the same starting position (Fig. 40-25). Excessive flexion pressure on the cervical spine should be avoided.

Shoulder motions. It is not uncommon for a patient with TOS to also have a shoulder problem or a patient with tendinitis or adhesive capsulitis to have restriction of the plexus. Limited external rotation and abduction of the shoulder because of shortening of the subscapularis muscle, pectoralis major or minor muscles, or the joint capsule can prevent the full ranging of the plexus, and adhesions may form around the plexus as a result of the lack of motion. Pain produced from an entrapped plexus can produce sufficient discomfort to prevent normal shoulder motion and foster a loss of shoulder motion or an adhesive capsulitis. Loss of normal scapular motion caused by tight musculature or weakness can also prevent the normal ranging of the plexus, and adhesions may form around the plexus.

The lack of a functional range of motion at the shoulder (a range of motion that allows the pain-free use of the arms during ADLs, work, and leisure activities) is a significant impediment to a positive long-term prognosis for the TOS patient. Restoring functional range of motion at the shoulder therefore becomes an important objective of the exercise program. Any stretching program for the shoulder must consider both the contractile and noncontractile structures around the shoulder that can prevent normal motion. Tightness of the subscapularis and pectoralis major muscle can prevent normal external rotation, abduction, and flexion. Tightness of the pectoralis major, pectoralis minor, and upper trapezius can prevent the normal motions of the scapulae, which are necessary for normal shoulder motion and normal postures.[3,22,24] In addition, a tight pectoralis minor muscle can directly entrap the plexus as it exits the thoracic outlet. Adhesions of the capsule of the glenohumeral joint or restrictions in movement of the acromioclavicular joint can prevent normal shoulder motions and normal posture.

Eventh,[11] Travell,[49] and Voss[51] developed three different but equally valuable approaches to lengthen shortened or painful muscles. Maitland[33] and Kaltenborn[23] discuss in their texts how to successfully mobilize the glenohumeral, acromioclavicular, scapulothoracic, and costovertebral joints that might be restricted in TOS. Smith[45] and Howell[19] discuss how muscle-stretching and joint-mobilization techniques can be combined into a treatment program. Therapists, however, should not use these techniques until they have received adequate training in their use. The use of manual therapy techniques are valuable but not essential in the treatment of TOS when a pathologic condition of the shoulder is present. The performance of improper or in-

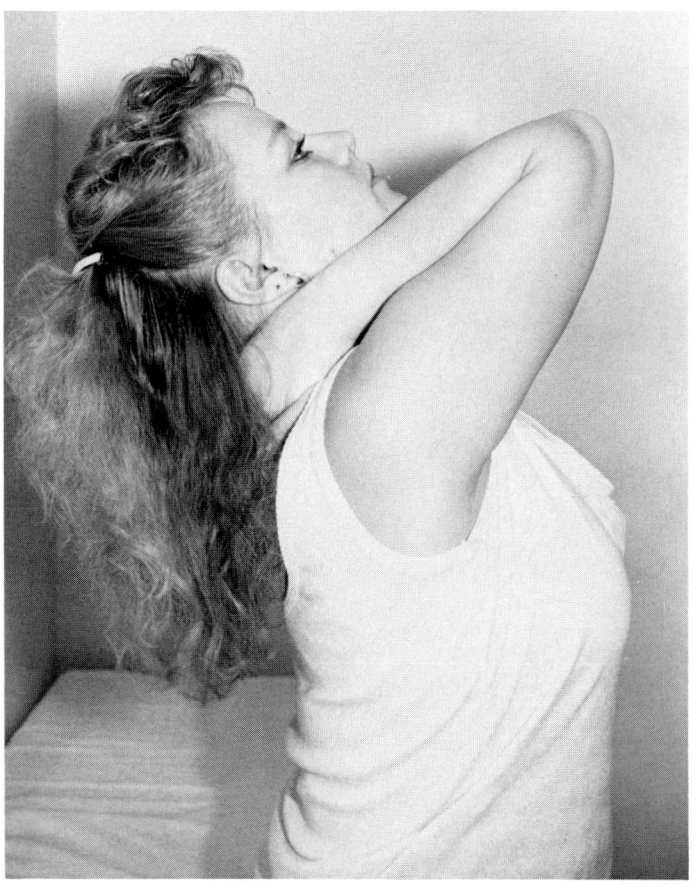

Fig. 40-24 Thoracic extension.

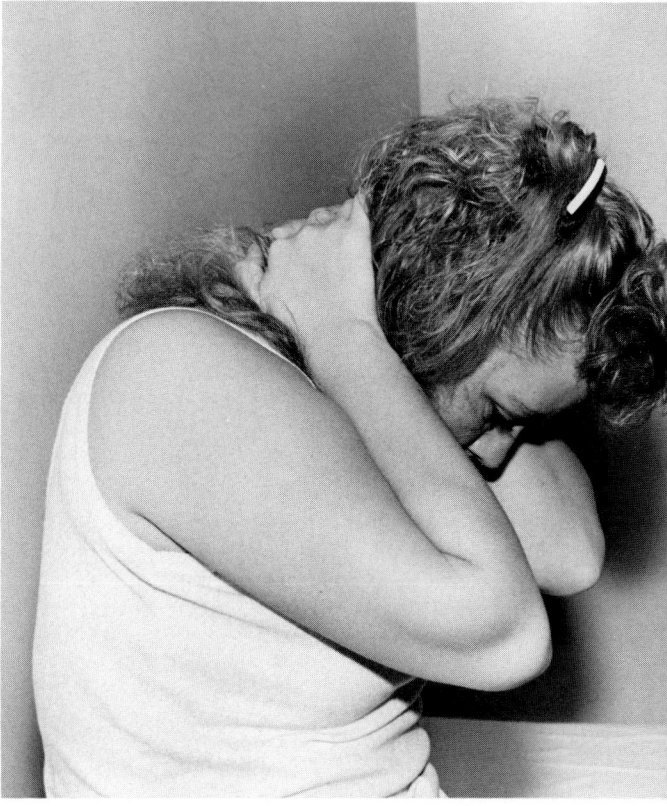

Fig. 40-25 Thoracic flexion.

appropriate techniques can rapidly exacerbate the symptoms, however. If the therapist is not trained in manual techniques, it is important that he or she use self-stretching techniques and other forms of exercise to stretch the adaptively shortened tissue around the shoulder. These forms of treatment can be as effective as manual techniques to improve motion if used carefully and patient compliance is good.

Even when manual techniques are used in the treatment program, it is important to continue to stress the self-stretching program. The self-stretching program for the shoulder is crucial, because any improvement in range created by the manual techniques will be lost unless the patient maintains improvement by stretching between treatments. Any self-stretching program for the shoulder should emphasize external rotation, flexion, and internal rotation at the glenohumeral joint and adduction, elevation, and rotations at the scapulothoracic joint. All motions should be performed actively, starting from a neutral or pain-free position and continuing where pain or strain is felt. The patient should not push through pain or cause repeated impingement at the shoulder. Abduction of more than 120 degrees should be avoided until full painless flexion and external rotation are achieved.

Diaphragmatic breathing. Because of pain, stress, smoking, or learned habits, TOS patients can develop an abnormal breathing pattern that emphasizes upper chest instead of dipaphragmatic breathing. Such a pattern will use the scalenes and sternocleidomastoid muscles during breathing and inhibit attempts to relax and stretch these muscles. As a result, it is important to teach and have the patient practice diaphragmatic breathing. This exercise will also help the patient relax; this breathing pattern is used in most stress-management techniques.

Diaphragmatic breathing emphasizes the use of the diaphragm during relaxed breathing. It can be taught by placing the hand over the abdomen and then having the patient push his abdomen into the hand during relaxed inspiration. Most patients can gain rapid control over this form of breathing. Those who have difficulty developing the proper technique can be aided with biofeedback or other relaxation techniques.[35] The patient should practice the technique for 3 to 5 minutes several times a day. It is also important for the patient to practice the technique while lying, sitting, and standing.

RESTORATION OF NORMAL MUSCULAR BALANCE

Restoring normal muscle balance is important to develop normal movement patterns, maintain motion gained during stretching, and help the patient assume and maintain improved postures. Restoration of normal muscle balance has two components.[22] The first is restoration of normal muscle length. The second is restoration of strength. Normal muscle balance can be successfully achieved only after the length and strength of both the agonist and antagonist muscle groups are returned to functional levels.[22]

Although strengthening is an important component of the treatment process, it can cause unnecessary pain and discomfort if it is not performed carefully. It is important to stress the muscles only within their pain-free arcs of motion. Proceeding outside the pain-free arcs of motion may not only overload the muscle but also overstretch and irritate the plexus or other noncontractile structures. It is also important to avoid impingement of the rotator cuff. The strengthening program should start with isometric exercise and proceed through active and active resistive exercises as the range of motion increases and the condition becomes less irritable. As symptoms resolve, the amount of exercise will also change. During the early stages of the strengthening program, only one or two isometric contractions, held for 6 seconds, will be performed twice a day. As treatment progresses and more stress can be placed on the muscle, frequency of the exercise will decrease but resistance applied to the muscle during the exercise will increase. During the last stages of treatment or prophylaxis, the patient will use heavy resistive exercise only two or three times a week to increase or maintain muscle balance. PNF, free weights, or exercise machines can be used for strengthening. The muscle groups that control external rotation of the shoulder, adduction of the scapula, and extension of the cervical and thoracic spines are commonly weak in relation to their antagonists and become the focus of the strengthening program.

IMPROVEMENT OF POSTURE AND BODY MECHANICS

Poor posture, poor body mechanics, and improper positioning after trauma to the shoulder, neck, or upper extemity can cause, exacerbate, or prevent successful management of thoracic outlet syndrome. As a result, improving the patient's posture and body mechanics are important goals of the treatment program.

The most appropriate postures and body mechanics for management of TOS will vary according to the presentation of the patient during the treatment process. A functional rather than an ideal posture should be emphasized. The functional posture for most TOS patients is one that allows the patient to come as close to the ideal as possible and still remain free of pain. Th erect, square-shoulder posture is ideal (Fig. 40-26), but few TOS patients can maintain this posture at the start of treatment without significant discomfort. Patients can not assume this posture, because the adaptively shortened tissue around the shoulder, neck, or plexus becomes stretched or the neurovascular bundle becomes entrapped as the patient attempts to assume this posture.

The forward-head, round-shoulder posture is believed to be the posture that predisposes the patient to TOS (Fig. 40-27) and other problems.[16,38] Some patients, especially early in care, may have to assume this posture to produce any relief. As treatment progresses and the shortened tissue is lengthened, the patient can begin to assume more of an erect, square-shoulder posture. Trying to progress toward the ideal too fast can be counterproductive, however, because significant pain and discomfort may be produced. Posture must be viewed as the factor that allows the gains from the stretching and strengthening programs to be maintained, but not at the expense of pain and inflammation. The patient must assume postures that rest the irritated tissue between exercises. Posture should not be viewed as a means to lengthen shortened tissue, because the irritation produced by the exercises will not have a chance to subside and will worsen as a result of prolonged stretch created by excessively corrected postures.

It is also important to instruct the patient in proper sleeping or resting postures. Lying supine can produce significant discomfort for a TOS patient. If the abductors of the scapula, the scalenes, and anterior cervical musculature are adaptively shortened and the scapulae and neck are not adequately supported in supine, gravity will retract the shoulders and neck and produce strain and discomfort in both areas. Patients should be instructed to lie supine with their neck and shoulders supported in a pain-free position. At times, two overlapping pillows are needed to support the tightened tissues (Fig. 40-28). Most TOS patients, however, find it more comfortable to sleep on their sides in a modified fetal position, because gravity and the weight of the body will produce scapula abduction (Fig. 40-29). As the patient progresses, it is important to modify his position by decreasing the height of the supports under the shoulders and neck in the supine position and instructing the patient to maintain a more open side-lying position.

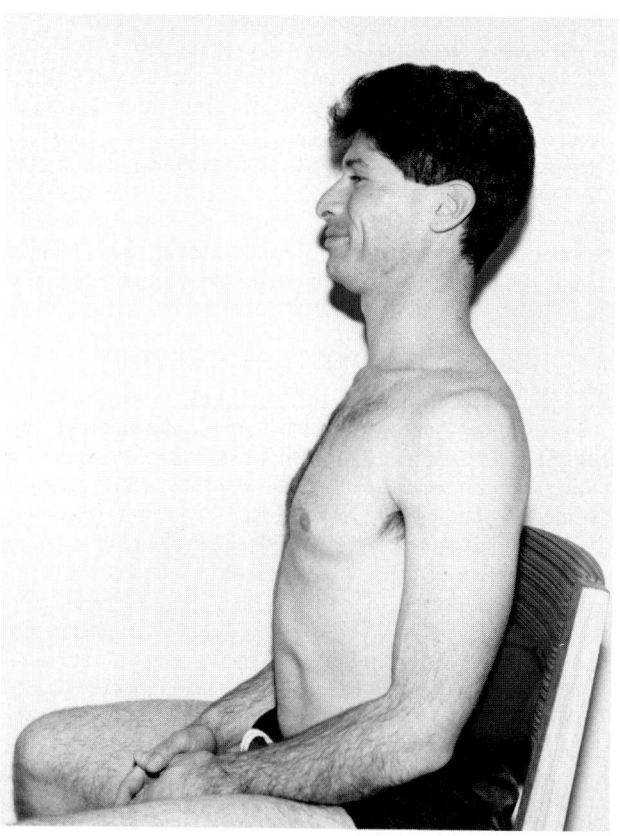

Fig. 40-26 Ideal posture with the head errect and the shoulders squared.

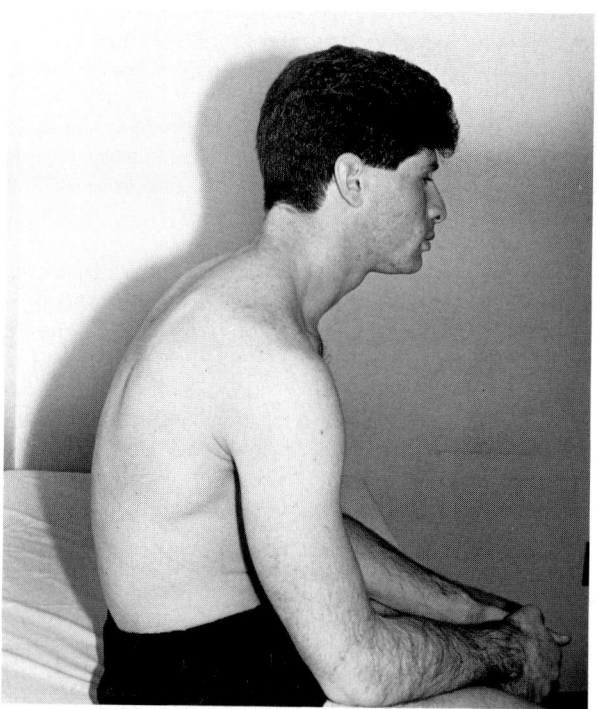

Fig. 40-27 Poor posture.

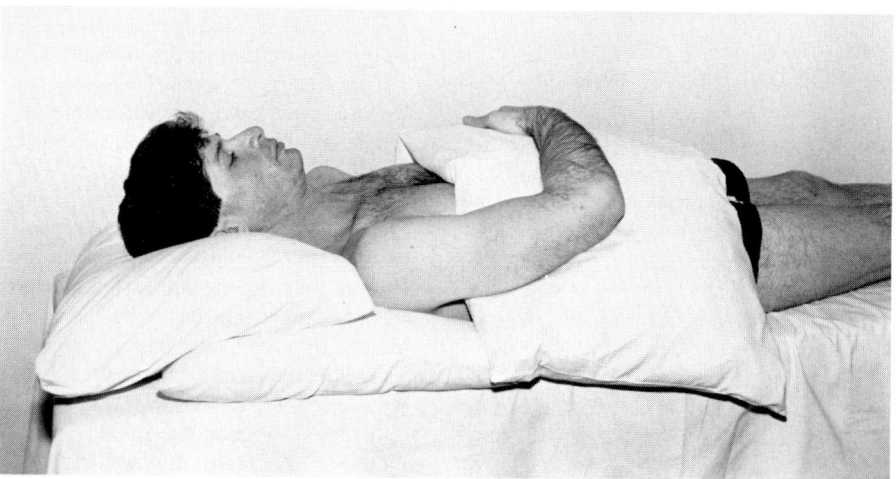

Fig. 40-28 Modified sleeping position in supine position using multiple pillows to prevent onset of symptoms.

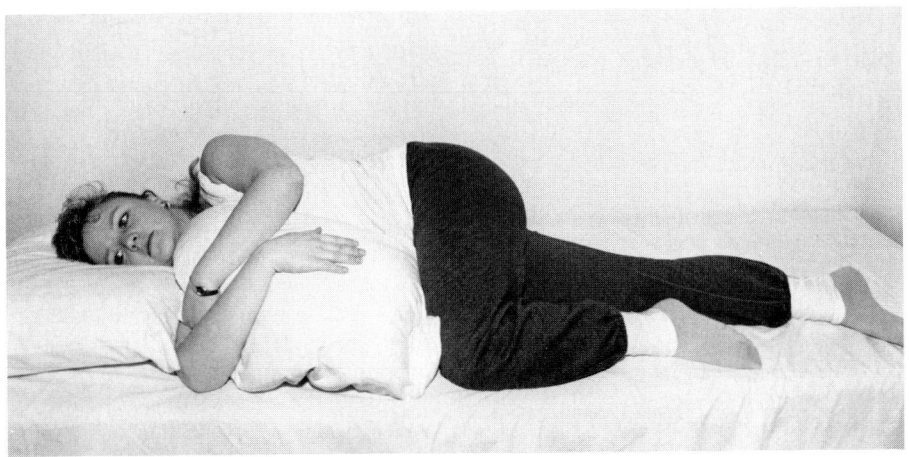

Fig. 40-29 Modified fetal sleeping position.

Patients find compliance with this part of the treatment program difficult, because years of bad habits and learned behaviors must be overcome. If some patients have difficulty maintaining proper posture while sitting or working, it may be necessary to assist them by using a lumbar support during sitting (Fig. 40-30), changing the height of their work areas, or changing their chairs so that they have both lumbar and arm supports. If patients have difficulty maintaining proper sleeping postures, it may be necessary to use restraints or supports to assist them.

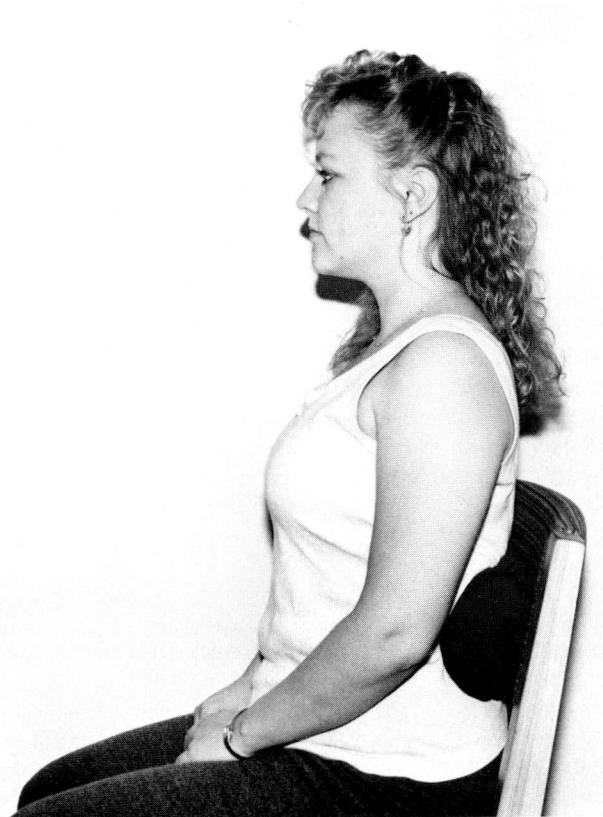

Fig. 40-30 Sitting posture using a lumbar roll to maintain proper posture.

Women with large breasts may be particularly prone to TOS.[9] Many may need to broaden their bra straps to more evenly distribute the pressure of the straps as they cross the shoulder. It may even be necessary for some women to wear a strapless bra to relieve the pressure on the shoulders and allow better posture.[9]

Just as improper postures can irritate symptoms, poor body mechanics can produce many of the same stresses. If patients continue to perform motions that place tension on the plexus or compress the neurovascular bundle, symptoms will be exacerbated. Carrying heavy objects, driving an automobile, working with the arms above shoulder level, and reaching to the side or behind the back are motions that can compress or traction the plexus. Patients should be taught through the use of symptom production and reduction where their functional limits are. If a patient cannot remain within his functional limits, it may be necessary to use a restraint or support to prevent irritation of the plexus. Changes may be needed in the workplace, automobile, and home to prevent the irritation.

DEVELOPMENT OF PATIENT SELF-RELIANCE AND INDEPENDENCE

Developing patient self-reliance and independence is an important goal of the TOS treatment program. Patients must take an active role in their care, because maintenance of proper postures, body mechanics, and consistent exercise are critical to success. Patients can best assume an active role when they understand the rationale for the treatment plan and they feel confident in performing it.[12] The components of a TOS education program are listed in the box on p. 560.

Although there is much material to cover, it can usually be handled easily in the treatment sessions. Skeletons and diagrams of the anatomic relationship of the neck, plexus, and shoulder can help most patients understand how the plexus becomes entrapped by the surrounding structures or how adhesions or scar tissue around the plexus can restrict its movement and cause discomfort. These aids are also valuable in helping the patient develop a model for the effect of the treatment program. Studies have indicated that the outcome of a treatment program can be positively influenced if the patient has an effective understanding of the problem

---

COMPONENTS OF THE EDUCATION PROGRAM FOR TOS

Anatomy of the area
Mechanics of symptom production
Potential causes of TOS
Influence of posture and body mechanics on TOS
Use of superficial heat and cold in the control of pain and inflammation
Structure and rationale for the treatment plan
Type and intensity of the symptoms that are and are not expected during the treatment program
Methods to adapt the exercises and treatment program to change in symptoms
Methods to monitor and adapt posture and body mechanics to home, work, and leisure to foster correct body mechanics and posture

---

and a model that effectively illustrates the treatment program.[12]

Another effective teaching technique is the use of symptom reproduction. By (1) placing the patient in postures or having the patient perform activities (exercises, ADLs, or working activities) while using poor mechanics that reproduce the symptoms and then (2) changing the postures or the mechanics to proper positions or movements that eliminate or improve the symptoms, the therapist uses a powerful tool to teach and reinforce the influence and importance of proper technique and posture on control of symptoms. After the therapist shows the patient how to modify symptoms by changing posture or mechanics, it is important that the patient show the therapist that he can perform the movements or assume the postures that reproduce or reduce his symptoms. Not only is this a powerful teaching tool, it also increases the patient's confidence in his ability to manage the problem.

Other ways to build confidence of a patient are to teach him to differentiate the expected from unexpected symptoms and to manage unexpected symptoms if they appear. Most patients will experience an increase or at least a change in the location of their symptoms as they perform the exercises. If a patient knows what to expect and how to adapt his program to changes in his symptoms, much of the anxiety that occurs when an exercise program is started can be lessened and the patient can assume a more independent role in therapy. Patients should be instructed that an increase in symptoms lasting a few minutes after the exercises are completed should be expected. If no discomfort or strain is felt during the exercises, the exercises are being done incorrectly. If the symptoms last more than 10 or 15 minutes after completion of the exercises, the intensity or the frequency of the exercises should be decreased. The patient should also be advised that the location of the discomfort may change during the exercises or as treatment progresses. If the pain continues, moves more distal, and peripheralizes, the patient should either contact the therapist or not perform more exercises until he is evaluated by the therapist. Peripheralization of pain can indicate exacerbation of a cervical disk problem, and the patient should be evaluated before continuing with the exercise program.[36,37]

Improvement of stress-management techniques

Most TOS patients have experienced the discomfort and disability of the condition or other problems for several months to several years. As a result, many patients have coped with discomfort for a long time, and many exhibit the behavioral characteristics of the chronic pain patient.[17,28,46,52] Many patients are emotionally labile, depressed, passively aggressive, and show inconsistent responses to tests or questions. If patients have had symptoms for longer than 1 year or do not respond as expected to treatment, referral to a psychologic or counseling service should be made. Because of the strains placed on their home lives, careers, and self-images by pain or disability, many TOS patients become overwhelmed by the problems and their normal coping mechanisms are inadequate. Some patients may need only a few sessions of counseling or therapy to restore or develop their means of coping with pain, dysfunction, and strained interpersonal relationships. Reassurance or instruction and practice of relaxation techniques or stress-management techniques may be all that are necessary for the patient to be more responsive to physical interventions. Some patients may, however, have more serious problems that may take extensive counseling or psychotherapy. For these patients, it is important that communication between physical therapy and psychologic services remain close so that a coordinated treatment plan can be developed and the services can reinforce each others goals and objectives.

Prevention

On completion of the treatment program, the patient should have an excellent understanding of those factors that cause or promote return of symptoms. They should also have an excellent understanding of how to treat any minor symptoms that may indicate recurrence of the problem. As a result, most information needed to delineate the preventive program is presented during the treatment program.

Factors that are believed to promote TOS are poor posture and poor body mechanics. If the patients return to their old postures, habits, and activities, the chances of a successful prophylactic program are low. At the end of treatment, it is important to impress on the patient that the new postures, improved body mechanics, and exercises must become permanent parts of his lifestyle. Although the maintenance of proper postures and body mechanics and performance of exercises need not be as rigorous as during treatment, postural awareness and efficient body mechanics must become a part of the patient's consciousness. In addition, the brachial plexus gliding and other postural and stretching exercises should be performed at least once every day. Patients must be taught how to detect early signs of the onset of TOS and how to treat those early signs. They should be taught how to use Elvey's UETT to determine if restrictions in the movement of the plexus are appearing and how to stretch those restrictions. They should be taught how to look for early signs of restriction in the movement of the scapulae, neck, and shoulders and how to treat those restrictions. They should be encouraged to become involved in a regular exercise program that not only stretches and strengthens the upper extremity and spine, but also improves their cardiovascular capacity. Swimming, aerobic dancing, or jogging plus a stretching/strengthening program are all excellent.

MANAGEMENT OF THE PATIENT WHO DOES NOT RESPOND

Some patients do not respond to conservative care. Some patients who do not respond will be candidates for surgery. Others will not. It is difficult to determine what will prevent some patients from responding to conservative care, but there are some factors that will lower the probability of successful management. These factors follow:

1. Symptom duration of longer than 1 year
2. Multiple problems that accompany TOS including pain of spinal origin, severe neuropathy, carpal tunnel syndrome, ulnar nerve entrapment, rotator cuff tear, frozen shoulder, and reflex sympathetic dystrophy (RSD)
3. Severe depression
4. Significant vascular compression
5. Dependencies on analgesics
6. Secondary gain

All of these factors pose significant management problems when combined with TOS, because the treatment plans to deal with them may conflict with the activities involved in the TOS treatment plan. As a result, as one problem is addressed, the other exacerbates, and the patient complains of an unacceptable increase in discomfort. These emotional or behavioral factors pose particular problems, because it is difficult for these patients to comply with the demands of the exercise program. If after 6 to 8 weeks of care with no significant progress when different treatment procedures are attempted, the patient should be reevaluated by the physician or a specialist. A psychologic consultation should also be recommended if one has not already been performed. After the evaluations, the physician, psychologist, and physical therapist should discuss treatment alternatives and the future course of care. Possible alternatives for care are surgery, another trial of conservative care, a period of psychologic counseling or therapy, discharge, or referral to a chronic pain management program. The patient's dependence on physical therapy should be avoided. Many patients depend on therapy for social contact, attention, emotional support, and secondary gain and are difficult to discharge. Every 4 to 6 weeks the patient's progress should be objectively evaluated. If insufficient progress is seen, a team management meeting should be held and the treatment program for the patient should be evaluated. Patients should not remain in therapy if adequate progress is not made.

MANAGEMENT OF THE SURGICAL PATIENT

Management of the surgical patient is similar to the conservative management of the TOS patient except that the patient must be vigorously ranged every 1 to 2 hours to maintain freedom of the plexus. Ranging of the plexus must start as soon after surgery as possible, and the patient should try to move through pain to the end of range. Elvey's UETT, when used as an exercise, is valuable, because the patient can use foream supination and wrist and finger extension to glide the plexus without stressing the surgical wound. Because of the surgical wound in the axillary or supraclavicular areas and the presence of a drain in the wound, scapular motions may be limited immediately after surgery but cervical and other motions can still be performed.

Pain management is also a primary focus after surgery. The irritation produced by the surgery plus the vigorous ranging of plexus can produce significant discomfort. As a result, a comprehensive pain management program that uses medication, modalities, hypnosis, or relaxation exercises, and positioning and support to maintain the irritated tissue at rest between the exercises is necessary. The goal of therapy at this time is to maintain motion of the plexus while inflammation and irritation from surgery resolve. As inflammation resolves, the treatment program can expand to include strengthening and conditioning activities. Care should be exercised at all times to maintain maximum movement of the plexus with minimum irritation and inflammation.

A common occurrence after TOS surgery is a transient loss of sensation in an area or a transient motor weakness to one or more groups of muscles. Patients should be evaluated for these areas of lost sensation and motor weakness. Patients should be informed of their presence to prevent injuries from burns, cuts, or overexertion. The patient should also be reassured that the losses are transient and normal sensation and muscle function should return in a few weeks.

CONCLUSION

Fifty to ninety percent of patients with TOS will respond rapidly and favorably to a conservative treatment program[21,20,42] Most patients after a program of education, exercise, and training in postural correction and body mechanics can regain normal, pain-free function of the upper extremity. The remainder may require surgery or a more extensive program that requires psychologic counseling and more intervention by the therapist through use of modalities and manual therapies. Eighty percent of surgical candidates will respond favorably and rapidly after surgery and a period of rehabilitation that emphasizes maintenance of movement of the plexus and postural correction.[17] Of the patients who do not respond to either conservative or surgical intervention, most suffer from multiple physical or psychologic problems that do not respond to treatment within normal therapy practice. These patients should be referred to chronic pain centers that are designed to deal with these problems.

REFERENCES

1. Adson A: Surgical treatment for symptoms produced by cervical ribs and the scalenus anticus muscle, Surg Gynecol Obstet 85:687, 1947.
2. Aranjo J and others: Reciprocal compression between the axillary artery and brachial plexus, J Cardiovasc Surg 29:172, 1988.
3. Ayub E: Posture and the upper quarter. In Donatelli R, editor: Physical therapy of the shoulder, New York, 1987, Churchill Livingstone, Inc.
4. Bargar W and others: Late thoracic outlet syndrome secondary to pseudoarthroses of the clavicle, J Trauma 24: 857, 1984.
5. Blair S: Avoiding complications of surgery for nerve compression syndromes, Orthop Clin North Am 19:125, 1988.
6. Caillet R: Soft tissue pain and disability, Philadelphia, 1988, FA Davis Co.
7. Colon E and Westdrop R: Age dependent normative values in non-invasive testing, J Cardiovasc Surg 29:166, 1988.
8. Cyriax, J: Textbook of orthopedic medicine: vol I and II, London, 1982, Bailliere Tindall.
9. DeSilva M: The costoclavicular syndrome: a new cause, Ann Rheum Dis 45:916, 1986.
10. Elvey R: Brachial plexus tension tests and the pathanatomical origin of arm pain. In Glasgow E and others, editors: Aspects of manipulative therapy, ed 2, New York, 1985, Churchill Livingstone, Inc.
11. Evjenth O and Hamberg J: Muscle stretching in manual therapy: the extremities. Ailta, Sweden, 1984, Alfta Rehab Forlag.

12. Falvo D: Effective patient education: a guide to increased compliance, Rockville, Md, 1985, Aspen Publishers, Inc.
13. Fields H: Pain, New York, 1987, McGraw-Hill, Inc.
14. Fields W and others: Thoracic outlet syndrome: review and reference to stroke in a major league pitcher, AJR 146:809, 1986.
15. Grant R and others: Clinical decision making in upper quarter dysfunction. In Grant R, editor: Physical therapy of the cervical and thoracic spine, New York, 1988, Churchill Livingstone, Inc.
16. Harms-Ringdahl K and Ekholm J: Intensity and character of pain and muscular activity levels by maintained extreme flexion position of the lower cervical-upper thoracic spine, Scan Rehabil Med 18: 117, 1986.
17. Hawkes C: Neurosurgical considerations in thoracic outlet syndrome, Clin Orthop 207:24, 1986.
18. Horowitz S: Brachial plexus injuries with causalgia resulting from transaxillary rib resection, Arch Surg 120:1189, 1985.
19. Howell J: Evaluation and management of thoracic outlet syndrome. In Donatelli R, editor: Physical therapy of the shoulder, New York, 1987, Churchill Livingstone, Inc.
20. Huffman J: Electrodiagnostic techniques for and conservative treatment of thoracic outlet syndrome, Clin Orthop 207:21, 1986.
21. Jaeger S and others: Thoracic outlet diagnosis and treatment. In Hunter, JM and others, editors: Rehabilitation of the hand, St. Louis, 1984, The CV Mosby Co.
22. Janda V: Muscles and cervicogenic pain syndromes. In Grant R, editor: Physical therapy of the cervical and thoracic spine, New York, 1988, Churchill Livingstone, Inc.
23. Kaltenborn F: Mobilization of the extremity joints. Oslo, 1980, Olaf Norlis Bokandle.
24. Kaput M: Anatomy and biomechanics of the shoulder. In Donatelli R, editor: Physical therapy of the shoulder, New York, 1987, Churchill Livingstone, Inc.
25. Kenneally M and others: The upper limb tension test: the SLR of the arm. In Grant R, editor: Physical therapy of the cervical and thoracic spine, New York, 1988, Churchill Livingstone, Inc.
26. Kline D and others: Surgery for lesions of the brachial plexus, Arch Neurol 43: 170, 1986.
27. Kraemer J: Intervertebral disc diseases, Chicago, 1981, Year Book Medical Publishers, Inc.
28. Kramlinger K and others: Are patients with chronic pain depressed? Pyschol Bull 97:18, 1983.
29. Krueger D: Rehabilitative psychology, Rockville, Md, 1984, Aspen Publishers, Inc.
30. Leffert R: The relationship between deadarm syndrome and thoracic outlet syndrome, Clin Orthop 223:20, 1987.
31. Lishman W and others: The brachial neuropathies. Lancet II: 941, 1961.
32. Machleder H and others: The anterior scalene muscle in thoracic outlet compression syndrome: histochemical and morphometric studies, Arch Surg 121:1141, 1986.
33. Maitland G: Peripheral mobilization, Boston, 1977, Butterworth Publishers.
34. Mannheimer J and Lampe G: Clinical transcutaneous electrical nerve stimulation, Philadelphia, 1984, FA Davis Co.
35. Margolis C and Shrier L: Manual of stress reduction. Philadelphia, 1982, The Franklin Institute Press.
36. McKenzie R: Treat your own back, Lower Hutt, New Zealand, 1981, Spinal Publications.
37. McKenzie R: Treat your own neck, Lower Hutt, New Zealand, 1987, Spinal Publications.
38. McPhee B and Worth D: Neck and upper extremity pain in the workplace. In Grant R, editor: Physical therapy of the cervical and thoracic spine, New York, 1988, Churchill Livingstone, Inc.
39. Melzack R and Wall P: The challenge of pain, New York, 1982, Basic Books, Inc Publishers.
40. Michlovitz S: Thermal agents in rehabilitation, Philadelphia, 1986, FA Davis Co.
41. Moore M: Thoracic outlet experience in a metropolitan hospital, Clin Orthop 207:29, 1986.
42. Pang D and Wessel H: Thoracic outlet syndrome, Neurosurgery 22:105, 1988.
43. Pratt N: Neurovascular entrapment in the regions of the shoulder and posterior triangle of the neck, Phys Ther 66:1894, 1986.
44. Riddell D and Smith B: Thoracic and vascular aspects of thoracic outlet syndrome: 1986 update, Clin Orthop 207:31, 1986.
45. Smith K: TOS: a protocol of treatment, J Orthop Sports Phys Ther 1:89, 1979.
46. Snider H: Minnesota multiphasic personality inventory as a predictor of operative results in thoracic outlet syndrome, South Med J 79:1527, 1986.
47. Stevens B and McKenzie R: Mechanical diagnosis and self treatment of the cervical spine. In Grant R, editor: Physical therapy of the cervical and thoracic spine, New York, 1988, Churchill Livingstone, Inc.
48. Swift T and Nichols F: The droopy shoulder syndrome, Neurology 34:212, 1984.
49. Travell J and Simons D: Myofascial pain and dysfunction: the trigger point manual. Baltimore, 1983, Williams & Wilkins.
50. Urschel H and Razzuk M: The failed operation for thoracic outlet syndrome: the difficulty of diagnosis and management. Ann Thorac Surg 42:523, 1986.
51. Voss D and others: Proprioceptive neuromuscular facilitation, ed 3, Philadelphia, 1985, Harper & Row, Publishers, Inc.
52. Williams A and Schutz R: Association of pain and physical dependency with depression in middle aged and elderly persons, Phys Ther 68:1226, 1988.
53. Wood V: The results of first rib resections in 100 patients. Orthop Clin North Am 19:131, 1988.
54. Yamaga M and others: Quantitative evaluation of autonomic nervous dysfunction in patients with thoracic outlet syndrome, Neuro Orthopedics 5:83, 1988.

41

Prevention of shoulder and neck pain in the rehabilitation of the hand

John Barbis

The development of proximal pain and dysfunction after trauma or surgery to the hand is common. A significant number of patients will develop symptoms in the neck and shoulder even when there has been little or no history of a pathologic condition or trauma to these areas. Prevention of such problems should be addressed when a patient with a pathologic condition of the forearm and hand is treated. Too often such concern is lost in the complexities of treatment of the distal pathologic condition, and the prevention of proximal pain becomes a concern only after symptoms and a new problem develop. Then the delayed intervention shows alleviation of symptoms, and the patient may develop multiple complications that are difficult for the therapist to resolve.

PRESENTATION OF SYMPTOMS

The primary problem in most hand patients who develop resultant neck and shoulder problems is pain. The three areas

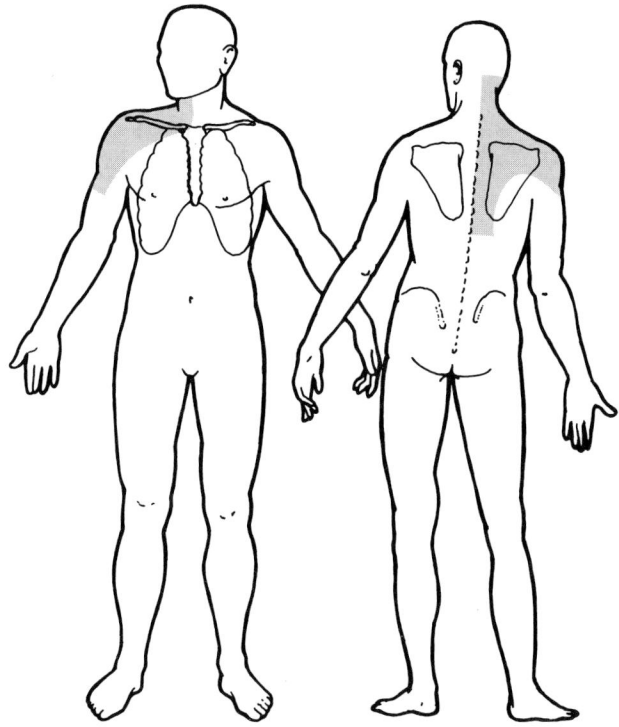

Fig. 41-1 Common locations of cervical pain and shoulder pain caused by trauma or surgery of the hand.

where this pain appears (Fig. 41-1) are the lateral cervical area (commonly extending into the upper trapezius), the parascapular area, and the shoulder (commonly extending to the deltoid tubercle). Although pain is usually the primary symptom, stiffness, weakness, paresthesia, and loss of function may be present. Even more tragic, many of these patients exhibit many of the behavioral characteristics of the chronic pain patient. Treatment after these symptoms develop can be lengthy, expensive, and frustrating for both the therapist and the patient. Preventing the onset of proximal pain and dysfunction, consistently evaluating the patient for the appearance of these problems, and rapidly intervening when the symptoms initially appear may save the therapist and the patient many frustrating weeks of care.

ORIGIN OF SYMPTOMS

The three common locations for these resultant pathologic conditions are the cervical spine, the brachial plexus, and the shoulder joint. The pathologic conditions in these areas could be dysfunctions or derangements of the soft tissues around or joints of the cervical spine, restrictions in the movement of the brachial plexus, and impingements or inflammations of the structures surrounding the glenohumeral joint. The primary etiology for the development of these pathologic conditions is poor posture[7,8,18] or absence of normal movement in these proximal areas.[3,5,12]

EFFECT OF POSTURE ON THE DEVELOPMENT OF THE PROXIMAL PAIN SYNDROMES

As shown by Harm-Ringdahl,[7,8] most important in the development of these symptoms is the forward-head, round-shoulder posture (Fig. 41-2). In her study, Harm-Ringdahl had volunteers with no history of cervical pain or pathologic condition maintain the extreme of that posture for as long as 57 minutes. Each of the subjects developed significant discomfort during the test, and some subjects experienced radiating pain into the hand. In the majority, the proximal and distal symptoms lasted for several days after the test. She concluded, "Maintained extreme position (forward-head posture) in work or leisure postures might be a possible reason for prolonged cervicobrachial pain if provocation is repeated daily and the effect thus accumulates." The maintenance of such a posture for prolonged periods may have a significant impact on the development of symptoms in this area by the following:

1. Creating a compressive force on the posterior portions of the upper cervical joints
2. Creating a strain on the passive connective tissue,[7,8]

563

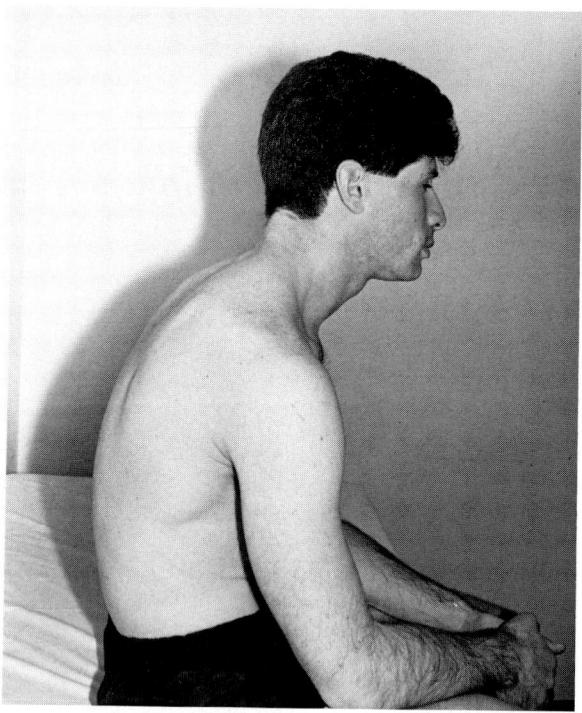

Fig. 41-2 Forward head–round shouldered posture.

the posterior musculature, or the disks[10,14] of the lower cervical spine

3. Creating an environment where adaptive shortening can occur not only to the soft tissues surrounding the spine, but also to the soft tissues around the brachial plexus, restricting its movements

4. Placing the musculature of the shoulder girdle and spine in a position where increased muscular activity is needed for normal activities[2,16,17]

5. Placing the scapula in a position that restricts full active shoulder motion and creating an environment conducive to developing multiple microtraumas from repeated impingements[1,3]

Although the actual pathologic conditions produced by improper posture can vary, the pain referral patterns for these conditions can be similar and the actual cause of the symptoms can be discovered only after a careful evaluation of the entire upper quarter. The lower cervical articulations tend to be most affected by poor postures, and the C5, C6, and C7 pain referral patterns can produce significant shoulder pain and confuse the clinician.[4] In addition, the acutely inflamed shoulder can refer pain into the neck and down the arm, imitating a cervical lesion. When symptoms occur in the cervical and shoulder areas, it is important to evaluate the entire upper quarter before starting a care plan.

Posture

Because of minor anatomic anomalies or large masses of muscle, normal posture may vary slightly within the population. When the external auditory meatus is more than 1 inch anterior to the point of the acromion, most authorities consider the head to be excessively forward.[13] (See Fig. 41-2.) This posture, if it is maintained for extended time, can produce the symptoms seen in Harm-Ringdahl's study.

The forward-head posture is commonly facilitated by the furniture or work spaces in the patient's home or the clinic, by excessively high headrests or pillows, and by casts or slings that the patient must wear. Although these environmental factors and devices may facilitate this posture and in some instances force the patient into this posture, he need not be a helpless victim of this environment. If patients are made aware of the furniture and work spaces that facilitate poor posture and if they are properly instructed and constantly encouraged to (1) use lumbar and cervical rolls to help them maintain good postures and (2) frequently monitor and correct their posture, they can avoid these symptoms.[10,11,18]

When most therapists consider the forward-head posture, they automatically assume such postures occur in sitting and standing and they fail to instruct the patient in sleeping postures. When sleeping supine with one or two large pillows under the head (Fig. 41-3) or lying in the fetal position (Fig. 41-4), the patient is again assuming the round-shoulder, forward-head posture. Instruction in proper sleeping

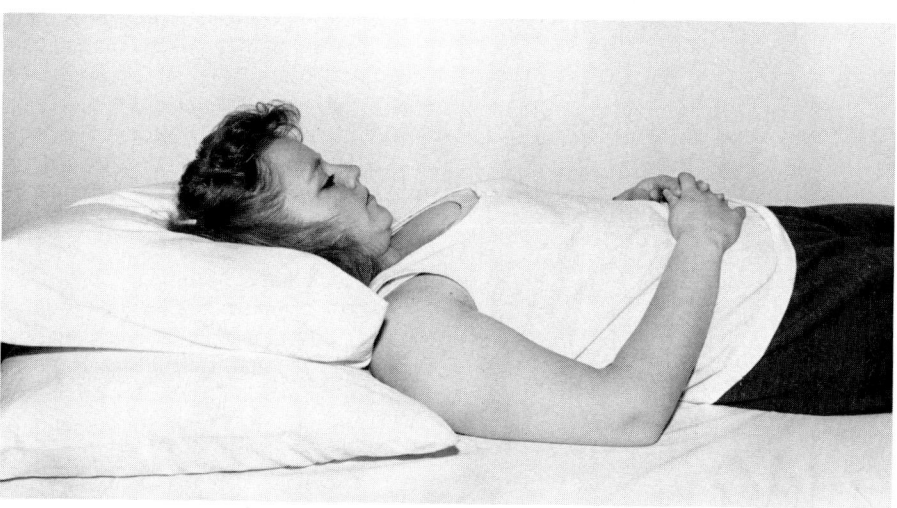

Fig. 41-3 Poor sleeping posture using two pillows under the head.

postures is critical not only to prevent these symptoms, but also to manage and eliminate symptoms if they develop. The hand patient poses a particular problem to the therapist who tries to help him develop a comfortable sleeping posture, because significant limitations in positioning may be placed on the patient by casts, splints, slings, or maintenance of elevation of the hand. A comfortable position that places minimum stress on the cervical or brachial region is im-portant prophylaxis and essential treatment if symptoms occur.

ABNORMALITIES OF OR LACK OF MOVEMENT

Because of (1) the weight of casts or splints, (2) the limitations of movement imposed by the location of casts, splints, or slings, (3) abnormal postures, or (4) the presence of a painful or stiff hand, excessive stress can be placed on

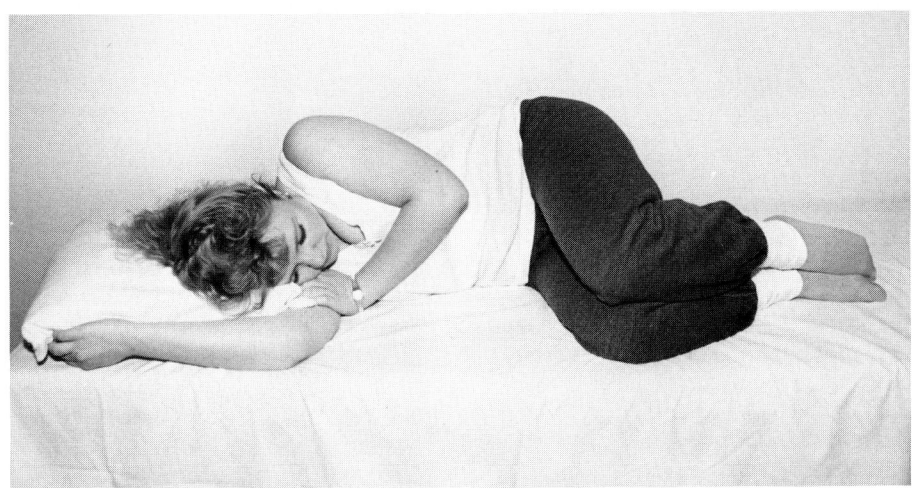

Fig. 41-4   Poor sleeping posture caused by assuming the fetal position.

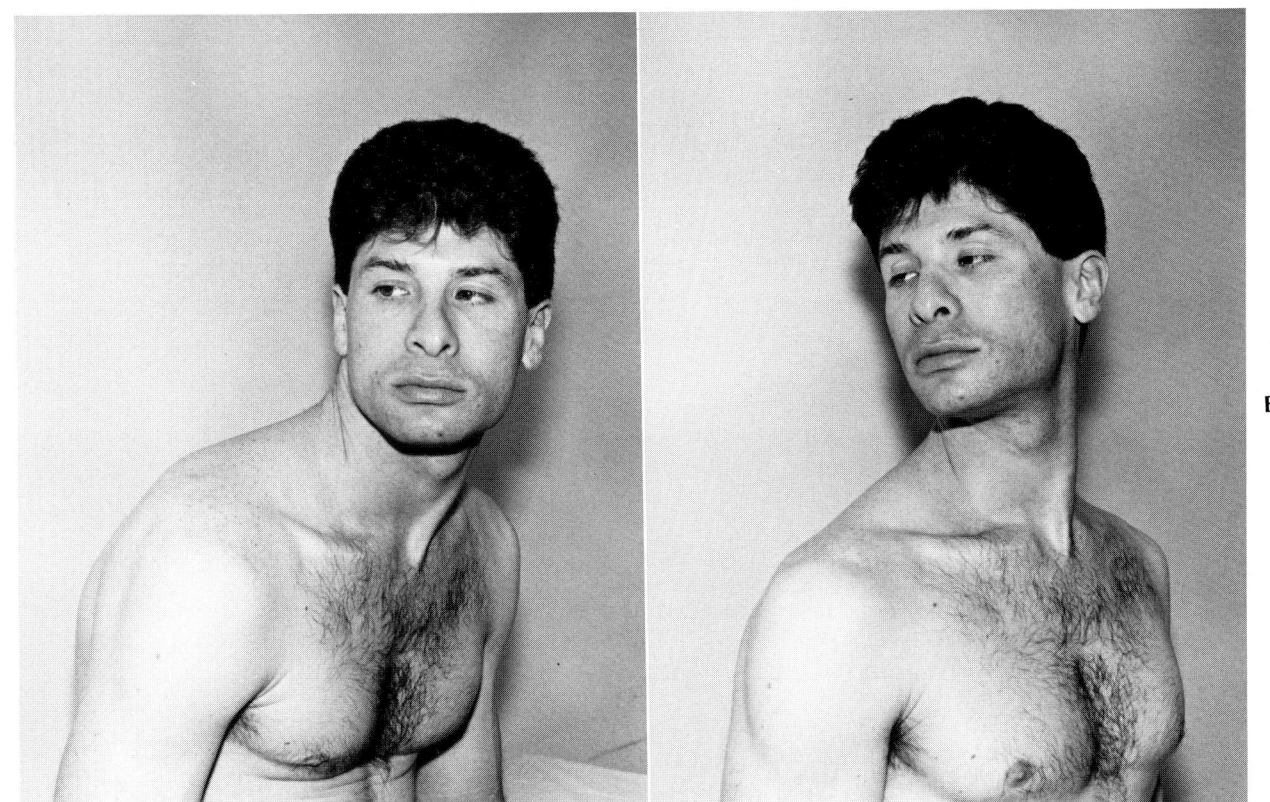

Fig. 41-5   Loss of cervical rotation in the forward head posture. **A,** Rotation in normal posture. **B,** Rotation in poor posture.

the muscles of the shoulder girdle[2] and normal scapulohumeral motion and normal cervical motions may be compromised.

When normal scapulohumeral rhythm is lost (especially through the maintenance of internal rotation with the resultant loss of external rotation and humeral depression by prolonged use of a sling or shoulder restraint), there is opportunity for repeated microtrauma through impingement on flexion and abduction.[9] Decreased mobility after immobilization is most profound and most rapidly develops in patients older than 40 years.[5] Such repeated microtrauma can lead to an inflammatory response at the shoulder that could result in an adhesive capsulitis, chronic rotator cuff syndrome, or osteoarthritis.[5] In the cervical spine, forward-head posture can lead to loss of normal rotation and lateral flexion. In forward-head posture, significant cervical rotation and side flexion are prevented (Fig. 41-5). Such continued inability to move into full rotation or side flexion could again lead to (1) adaptive shortening of the soft tissue around the spine and (2) pain on movement.

The brachial plexus also can be significantly affected by lack of motion at the shoulder and neck. During normal cervical and shoulder motions, the brachial plexus moves.[6,8] When normal motion is prevented at the shoulder or neck, the soft tissue surrounding the plexus (muscle and connective tissue) can adaptively shorten, preventing the normal excursion of the plexus during shoulder movement. This type of pathologic condition could be classified as a form of thoracic outlet syndrome (TOS), and clinically it could produce many of the nonvascular symptoms associated with TOS. Such a limitation could produce significant symptoms in the neck, shoulder, and the entire arm.[6] (See also Chapter 39.)

PREVENTION

The prevention of cervicobrachial problems involves the consistent and persistent coaching of good posture and maintenance of normal motion. The therapist must counterbalance years of possible poor posture and the negative influence of casts, braces, slings, and pain. In addition, the therapist must facilitate the patient's active participation in this process.

Application of these postural sets and normal mechanics must occur not only during therapy but at all times. The therapist must instruct the patient not only on the correct postures and exercises, but also on the early signs of the syndrome. Some of the early signs commonly seen follow:

1. Stiffness of the cervical spine or shoulder
2. Loss of movement in one or more directions in the neck or shoulder (usually without pain or pain only at the end of motion)
3. Intermittent pain or stiffness in the neck or shoulder either on rising in the morning or on repetitive activities
4. Pain or stiffness on driving, reading, or watching television
5. Discomfort or pain in the interscapular area

If the therapist could regularly review the patient's symptoms and provide an awareness to the patient of the significance of his symptoms, developing problems at the neck or shoulder could be identified early, and intervention to prevent spread of or increase in severity of symptoms could

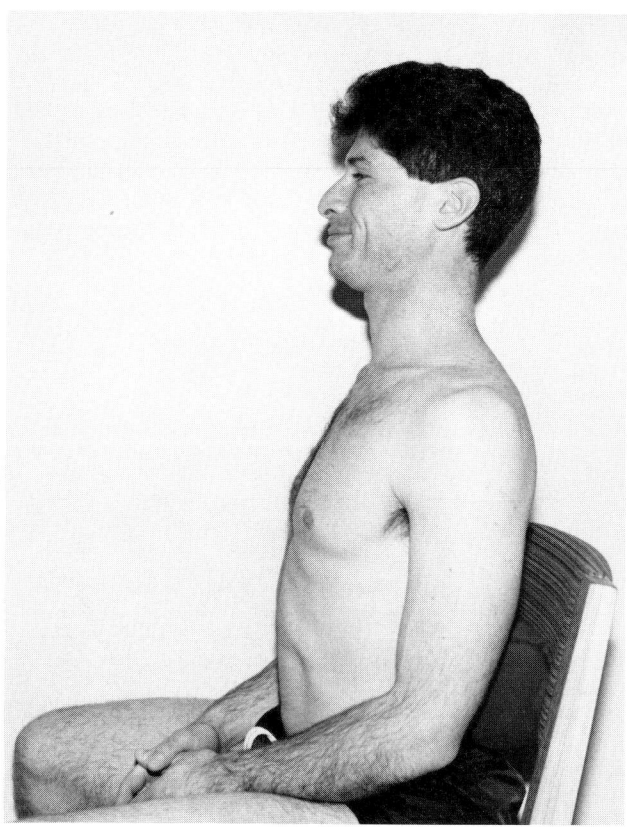

Fig. 41-6 Proper sitting posture.

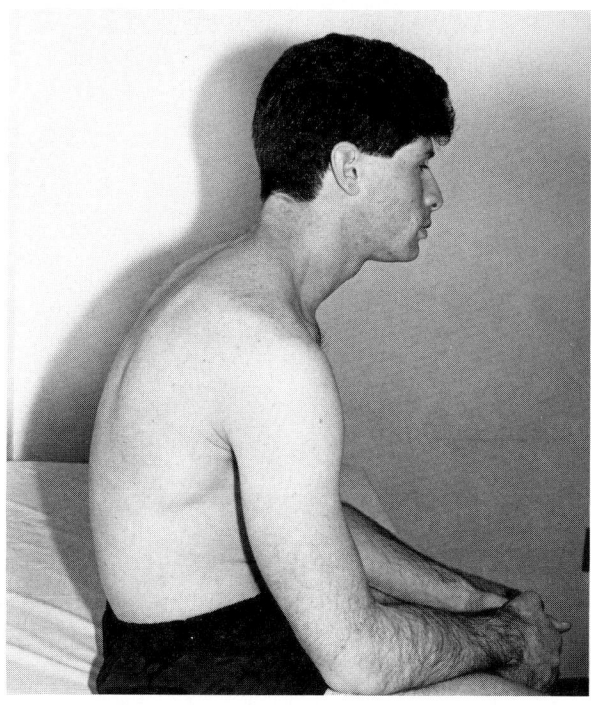

Fig. 41-7 Loss of lumbar lordosis and creation of forward head posture.

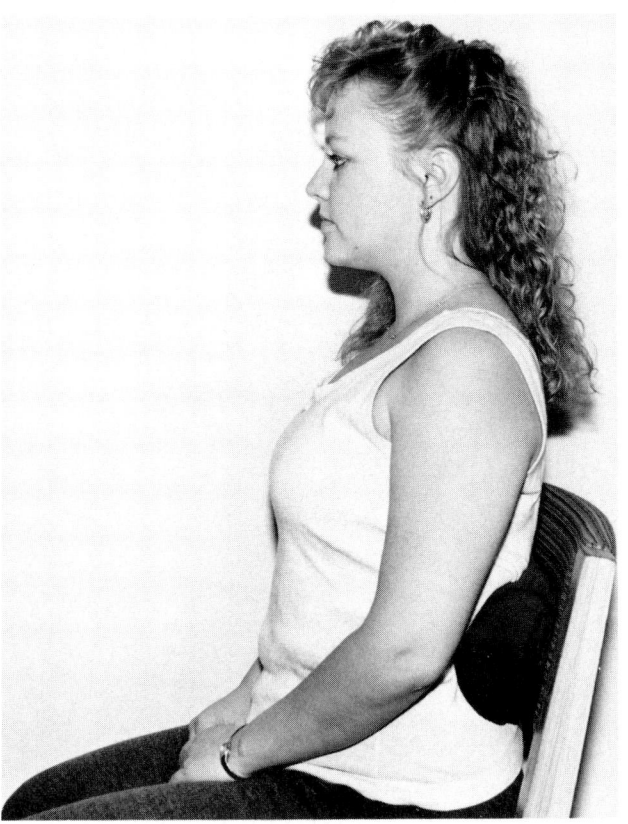

Fig. 41-8   Proper sitting posture with lumbar support.

be started. At this stage, reinforcement of many of the prophylactic concepts may be sufficient to resolve the symptoms.

SITTING POSTURE

Proper sitting posture begins at the lumbar spine (Fig. 41-6). Maintenance of a gentle lordosis in the lumbar spine is essential for a proper relationship between the neck, head, and shoulders. As the lordosis is lost, the head begins to move forward and the shoulders become round (Fig. 41-7). It is difficult to maintain proper posture for longer than 20 minutes unless some passive support is provided to the lumbar spine. The use of a lumbar roll is crucial in such cases (Fig. 41-8). In addition, proper instruction of the patient to avoid poor posture is as follows:

1. Work close to the desk and, if possible, elevate or slant any writing or working surfaces (Fig. 41-9).
2. Avoid reading in bed or watching television in bed (Fig. 41-10).
3. Avoid sitting on soft couches or softly cushioned chairs (Fig. 41-11).[10,11,12]

Also, it is important to explain to the patient that the occasional occurrence of stiffness or minor discomfort that he feels in the neck could be a warning sign of irritation produced in the structures surrounding the cervical spine by postural stresses and that these symptoms should not be ignored. The patient must be instructed that when these symptoms are felt, he should change his posture or begin exercise. If symptoms can be controlled at this stage, the

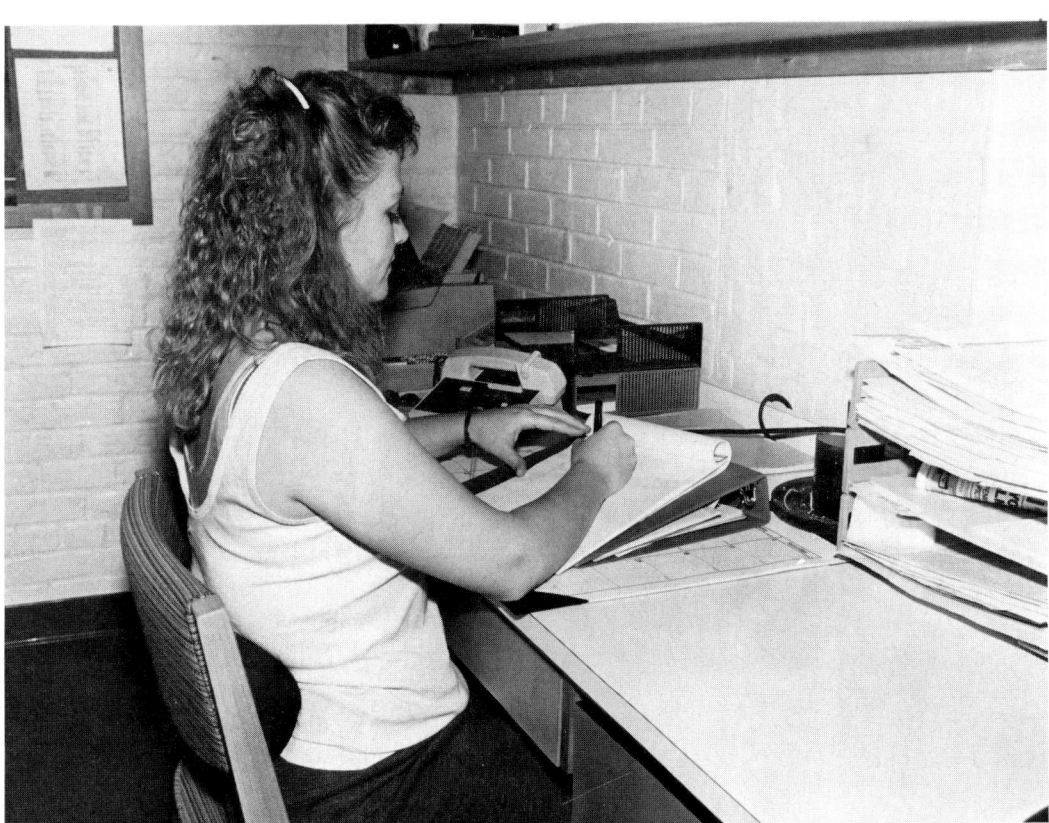

Fig. 41-9   Proper working posture in sitting. A large three-ring notebook can be used to raise and slant the working surface.

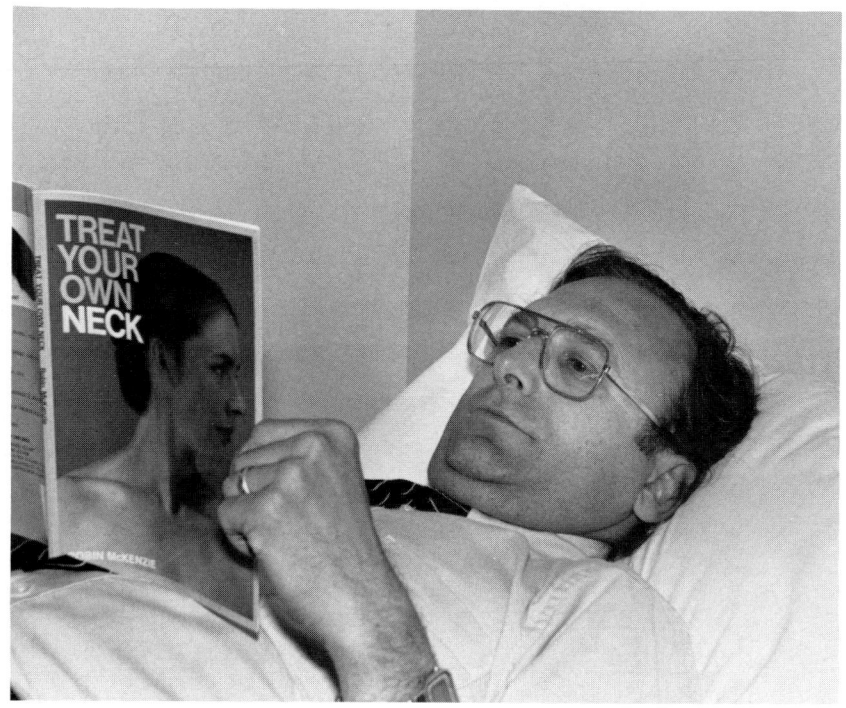

Fig. 41-10 Poor posture caused by reading in bed.

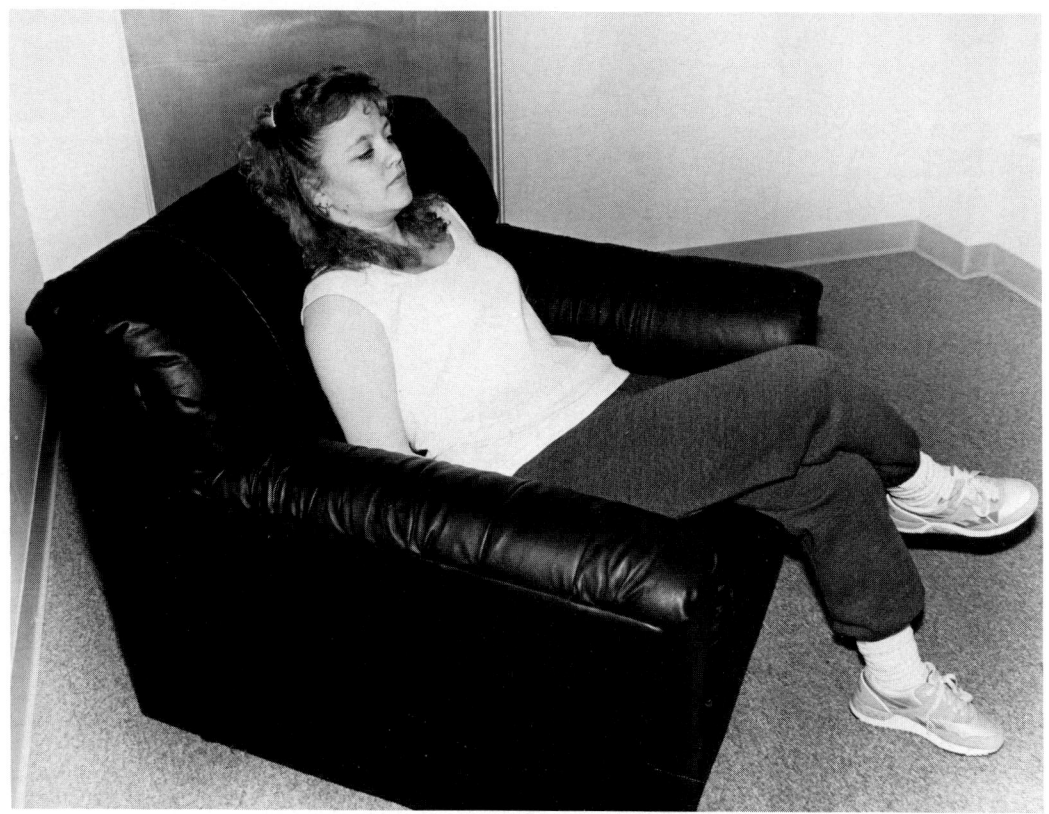

Fig. 41-11 Poor posture caused by sitting in soft chairs.

probability of their progression to more serious problems decreases significantly.[10,11,18]

STANDING POSTURE

Proper standing posture also requires the patient to maintain a gentle lordosis. Either loss of lordosis or excessive lordosis can compromise the relationship between the head, neck, and shoulder (Fig. 41-12).

SLEEPING POSTURES

Movement during the night is essential for normal sleep, but many patients feel that they cannot change their sleeping habits or present postures. A few cannot, but most find that they can successfully change in a few weeks. The optimum sleeping position for most hand patients is on the back with a low pillow or no pillow. In either position, it is essential to have some support for the cervical lordosis.

Such support can be maintained either through the use of the pillow or a cervical roll (Fig. 41-13). Some patients can sleep on their side. While sleeping on the side, the patient should maintain an open, head-up position and avoid the fetal position (Fig. 41-14).

MAINTENANCE OF NORMAL MOTION

Maintaining normal motion does not require much effort, but it does require persistence and consistency. Each exercise should be performed about five to ten times, three to four times per day. It is important to emphasize that the motions must be performed consistently throughout the day and every day. When the exercise is performed, the patient should attempt to move through the entire range. If pain occurs, the patient should be instructed to note where in the range it occurred, whether it increased or decreased as the exercise was performed, and how long it continued after exercise. The goal of the program is to maintain range of motion, and some discomfort, especially strain, is expected. Pain that continues for longer than a few minutes is, however, not an expected effect, and the patient should be evaluated to determine the cause of the discomfort.

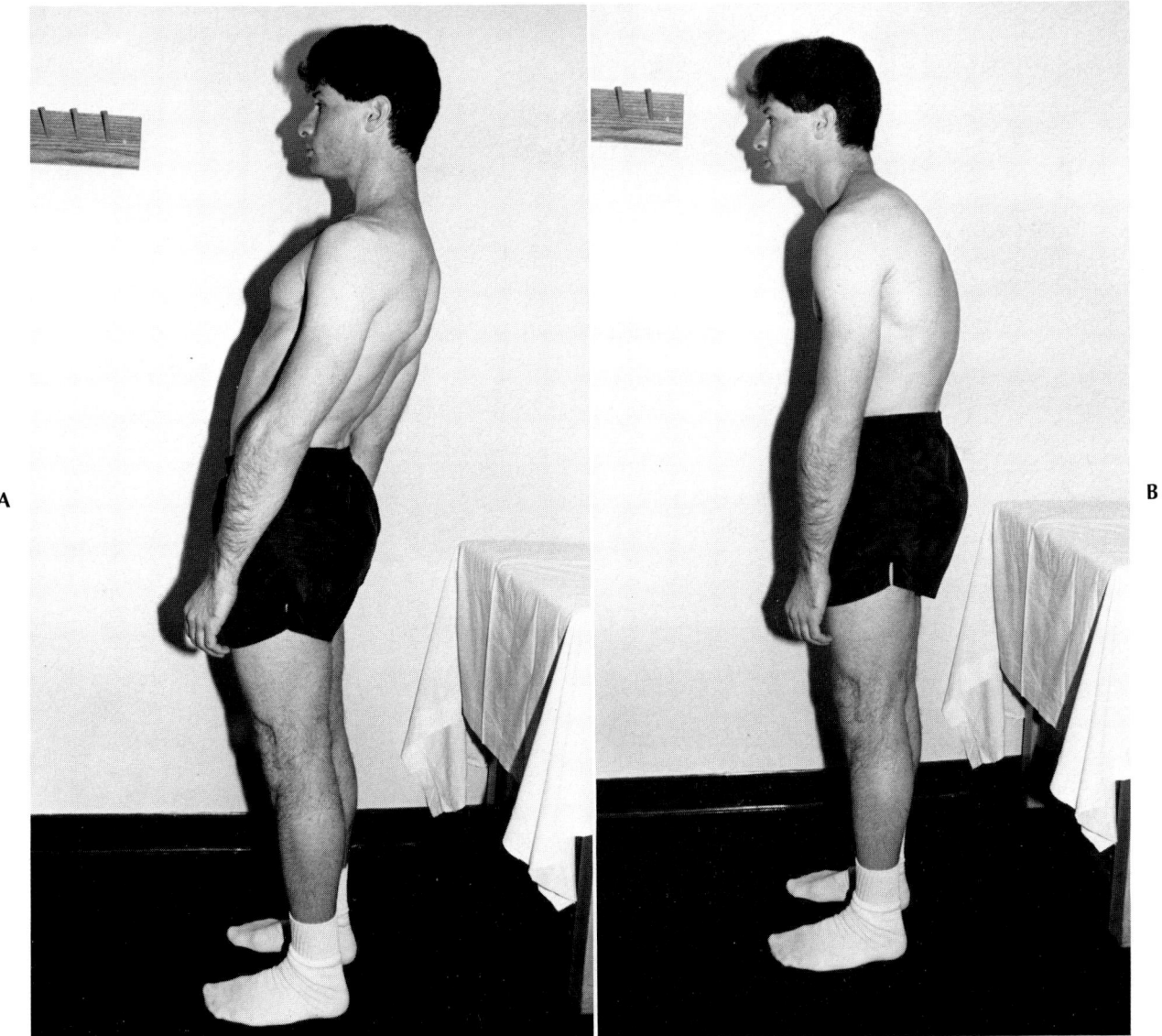

Fig. 41-12 Poor standing postures. **A,** Excessive lordosis. **B,** Loss of lordosis.

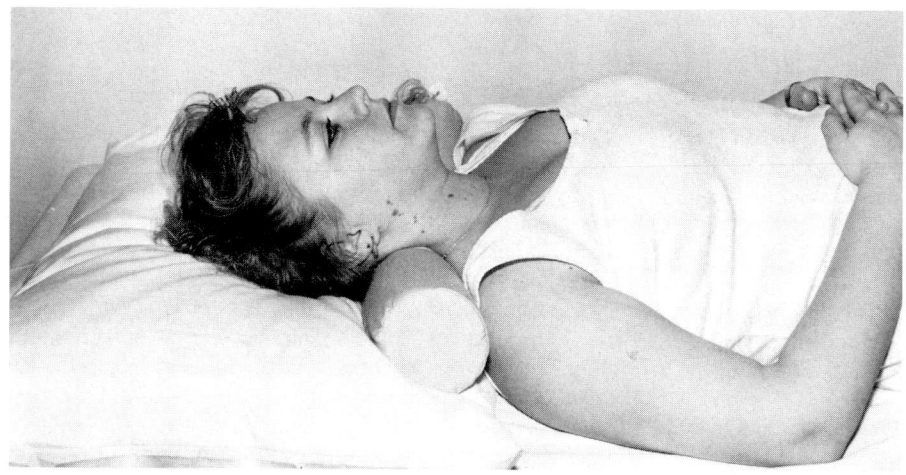

Fig. 41-13   Proper sleeping position with a cervical roll.

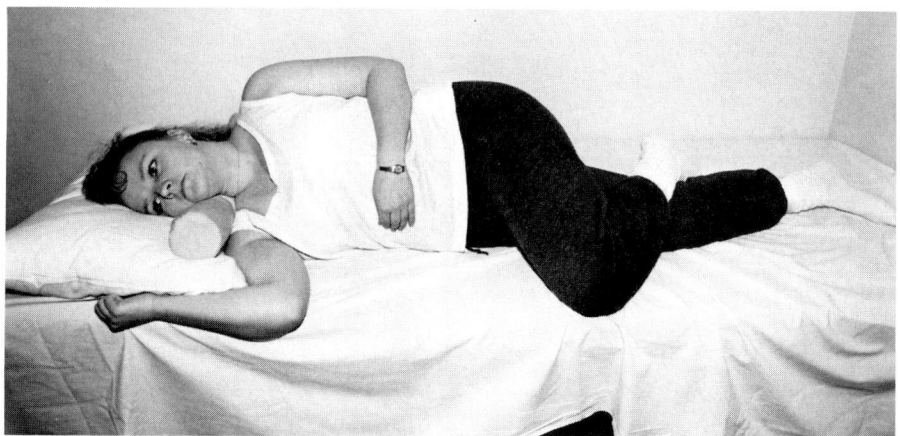

Fig. 41-14   Proper sleeping position when lying on the side.

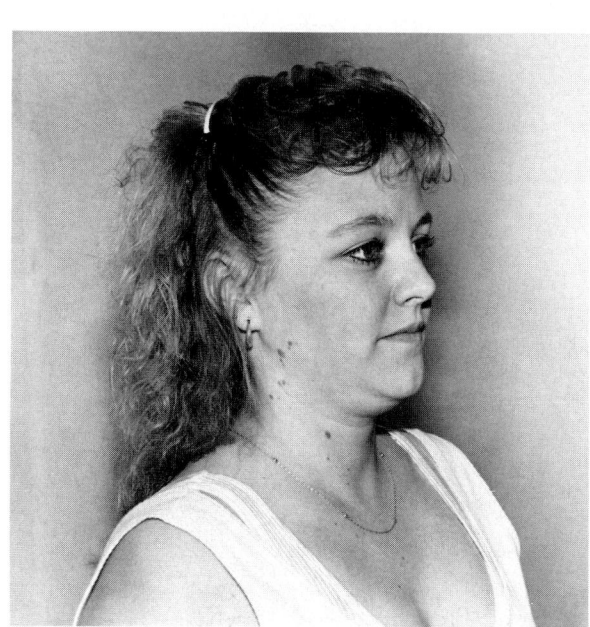

Fig. 41-15   Cervical retraction.

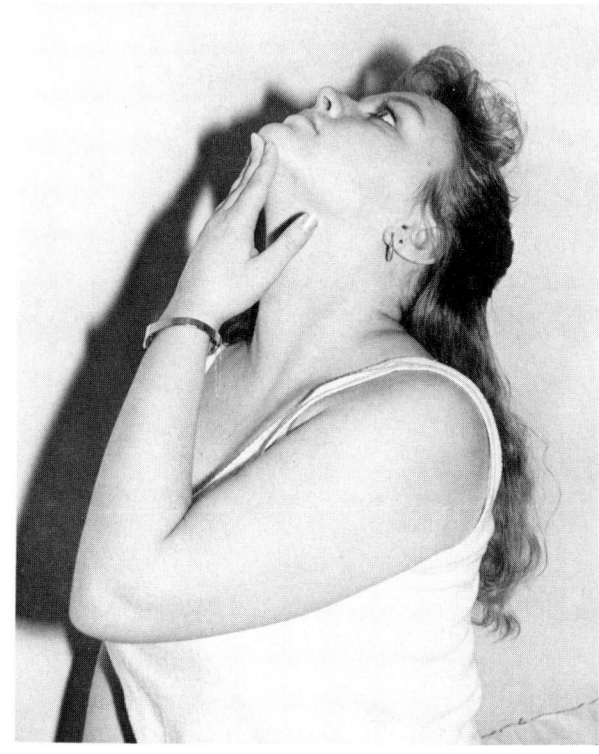

Fig. 41-16   Cervical extension.

CERVICAL RETRACTION (Fig. 41-15)

This motion involves the posterior movement of the head and neck on the shoulders and is an important motion for proper posture. It is commonly referred to as the "chin tuck" position. The retracted position is also very important, because it is the starting position for all of the other cervical exercises. Cervical motion is the greatest when the patient assumes a slightly retracted position. All other cervical exercises will be performed from this starting position. When

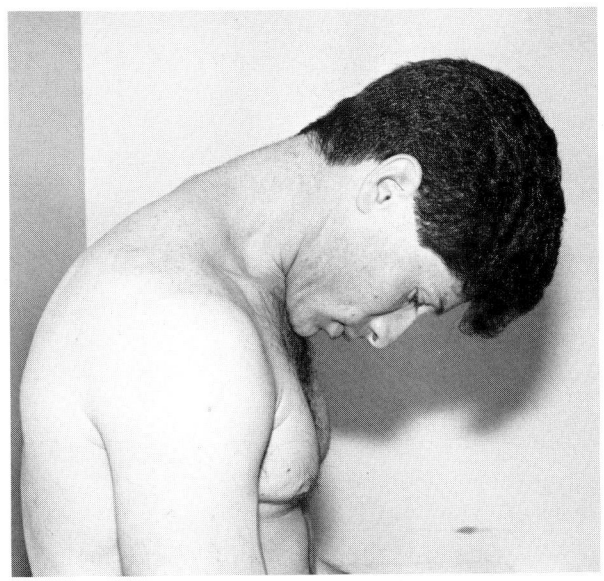

Fig. 41-17   Cervical flexion.

performing the exercise, the patient should proceed slowly and smoothly, either to the start of pain or to the end of the range of motion. It is important to instruct the patient to proceed as far as he can without pushing through the pain. If the patient experiences pain with a movement, he should proceed to where the pain or discomfort starts and should possibly vary the number of repetitions of the exercise. Changing the repetitions, however, should occur only after the therapist carefully evaluates the potential problem.

CERVICAL EXTENSION (Fig. 41-16)

The movement into full extension should start from the retracted starting position and emphasize lower cervical extension (or posterior glide) during the first portion of the motion. Upper cervical extension (extension of the head on the neck) should occur at the end of motion. Using excessive upper cervical motion at the beginning of extension can limit the amount of motion in the lower cervical spine and can cause discomfort. The hand can be used to give gentle overpressure.

CERVICAL FLEXION (Fig. 41-17)

Flexion should start from the slightly retracted starting position. The first part of the movement should emphasize the flexion of the head on the neck, and lower cervical flexion should occur later in the movement. The hand can be used to give gentle overpressure.

Cervical side flexion (Fig. 41-18)

Side flexions should start from the slightly retracted starting position. If possible, the ipsilateral hand should be used to assist with the motion and provide gentle overpressure. This exercise should be performed to both sides.

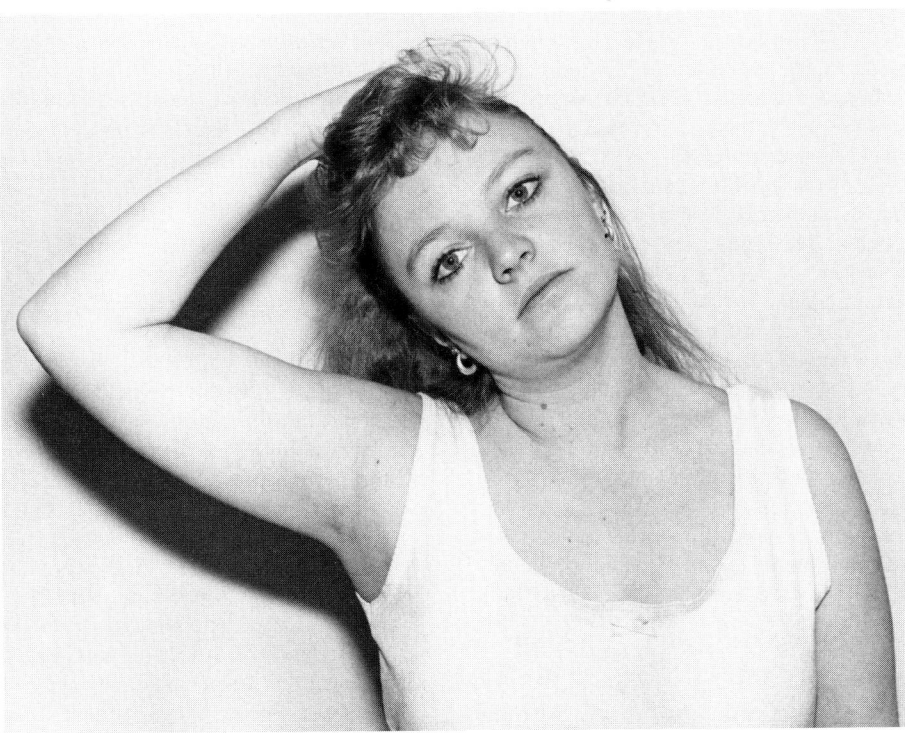

Fig. 41-18   Cervical side flexion.

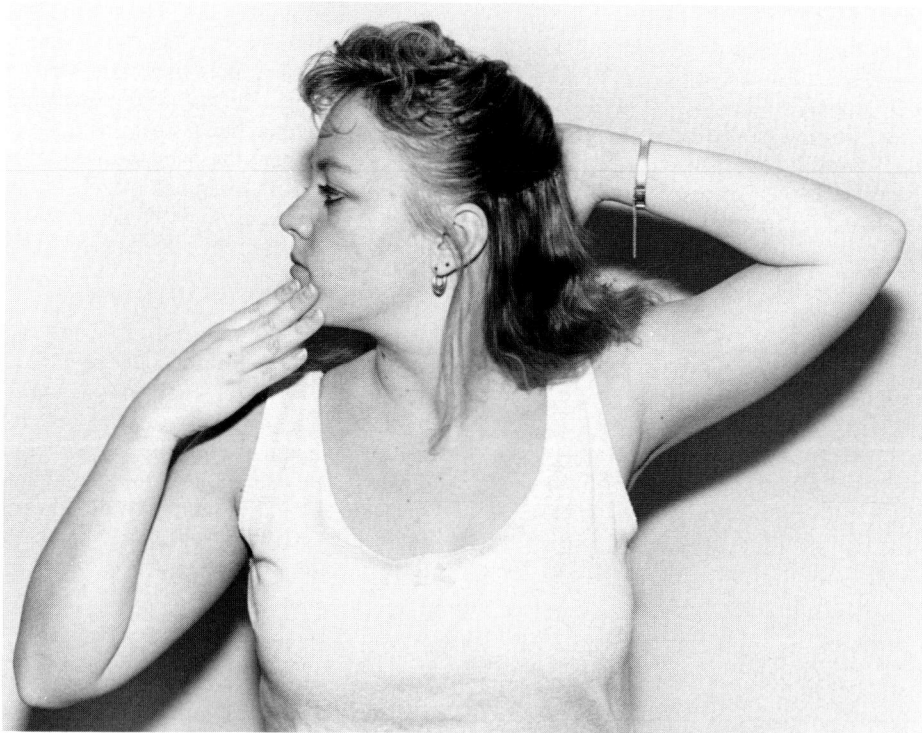

Fig. 41-19 Cervical rotation.

Cervical rotation (Fig. 41-19)

Rotations should start from the slightly retracted starting position. If possible, the hands should be used to assist with the motion and provide gentle overpressure. This exercise should be performed to both sides.

SHOULDER MOTIONS

All shoulder motions should be performed on a regular basis. However, because of the limitations of the individual patient, it may not be possible to complete all of the motions. In such cases it is important to emphasize that the three motions listed here be performed either passively or actively on a regular basis. All of the exercises must be performed in proper posture and should stress normal scapulohumeral rhythm where applicable. Performance of these exercises when the patient is in poor posture can cause discomfort, and full range of motion cannot be attained. Active abduction above 90 degrees is usually the motion that causes the most discomfort at the shoulder. If pain, discomfort, or limitations in the freedom of movement occur on abduction, a careful evaluation should be done. Special attention should be paid to the status of the rotator cuff musculature, limitations of external rotation or humeral depression, and deviations in normal scapulohumeral rhythm. Abduction should not be forced through pain or discomfort, because the potential for the impingement of the cuff musculature and resultant inflammation is too great.

SCAPULAR CIRCLES EMPHASIZING RETRACTION OF THE SCAPULAE (Fig. 41-20)

During this exercise, adduction or retraction of the scapulae must be emphasized. Ten repetitions should occur in one direction and then ten in the other.

Full flexion (Fig. 41-21)

Full flexion should be performed actively or, if necessary, passively, using the other arm for assistance. Often this motion is most comfortably performed in supine.

Full external rotation at 90 degrees of abduction (Fig. 41-22)

This exercise is usually most effectively performed in supine, because gravity can add slight overpressure at the end of range. This exercise is pivotal, because it maintains external rotation, which is necessary for full abduction of the shoulder, and it also allows the plexus to be stretched and mobilized.

TREATMENT OF SHOULDER AND NECK PAIN

As mentioned, if symptoms develop, it is important to perform an upper quarter evaluation to determine the possible source of the symptoms. During the early stages of neck and shoulder pain where poor posture, poor mechanics, or lack of adequate movement or activity may produce a mechanical deformation of tissue, it is important to seek a mechanical answer to the problem by changing the patient's posture, mechanics, or activity level—not to seek a palliative answer by applying modalities that modulate pain (heat, cold, electrical stimulation). Using palliative treatment at this early stage may mask the primary causes of the problem and prevent the therapist finding the cause of the pain. Such passive forms of care do not foster patient independence and may reinforce nonproductive pain behaviors. The passive modalities (especially ice and electrical stimulation) may play a role in the treatment of an acutely inflamed shoulder, but their use in neck pain should be limited.[15] Postural instruction and selected active and passive exercises

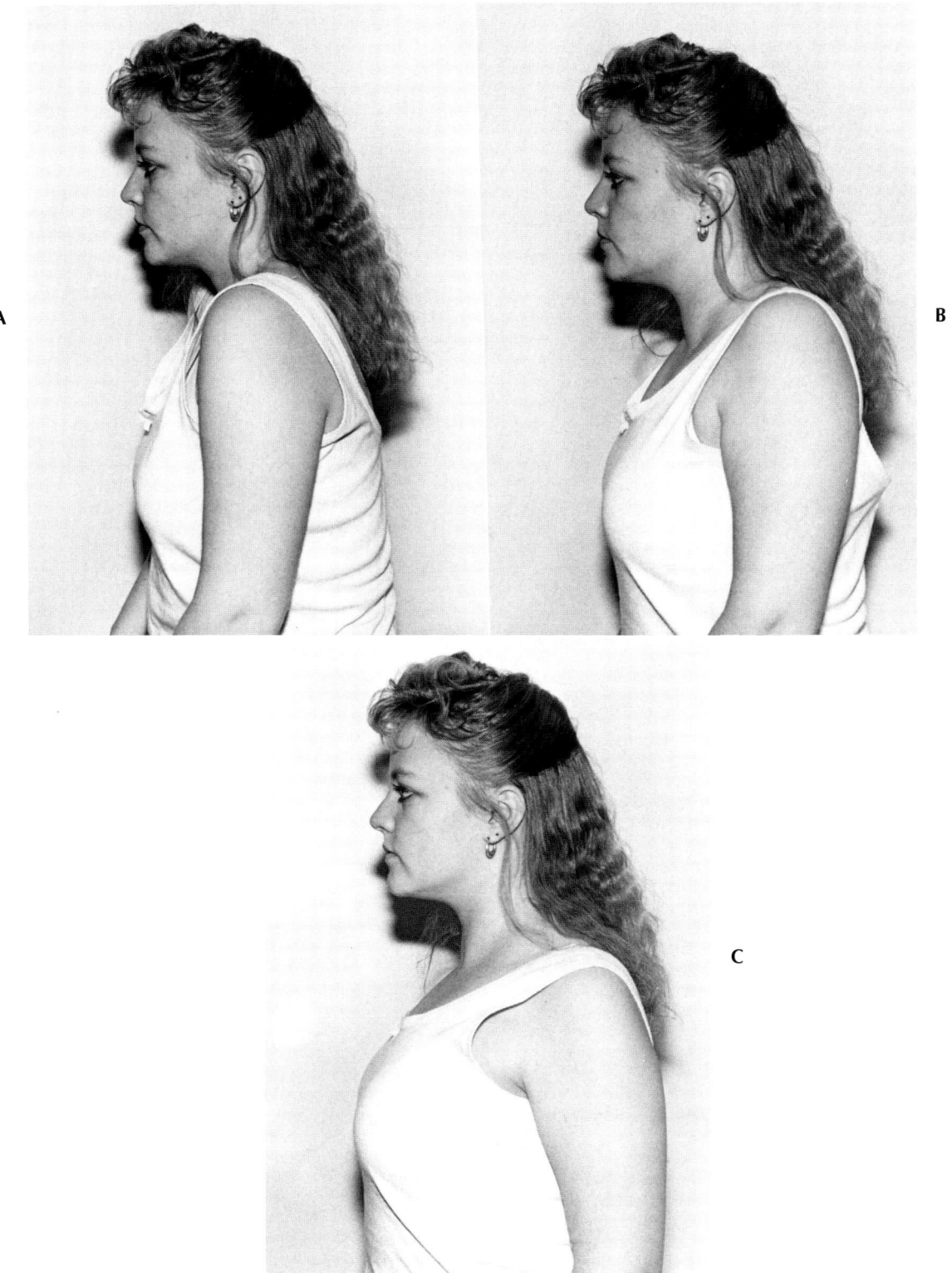

Fig. 41-20   Scapula circles. **A,** Protraction. **B,** Elevation. **C,** Retraction and depression.

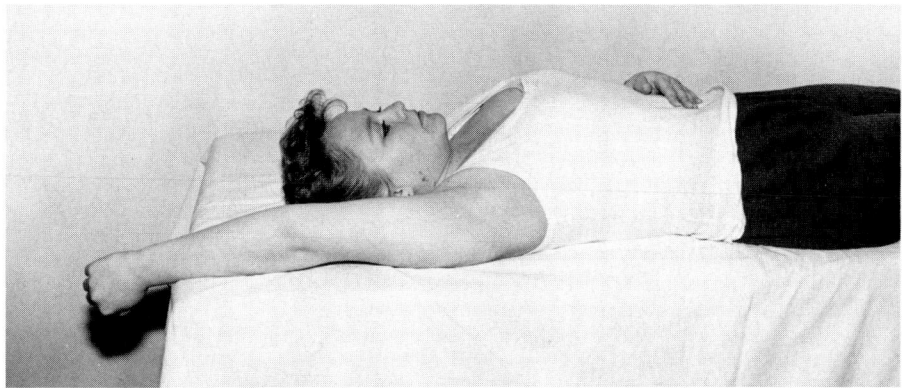

Fig. 41-21   Shoulder flexion in the supine position.

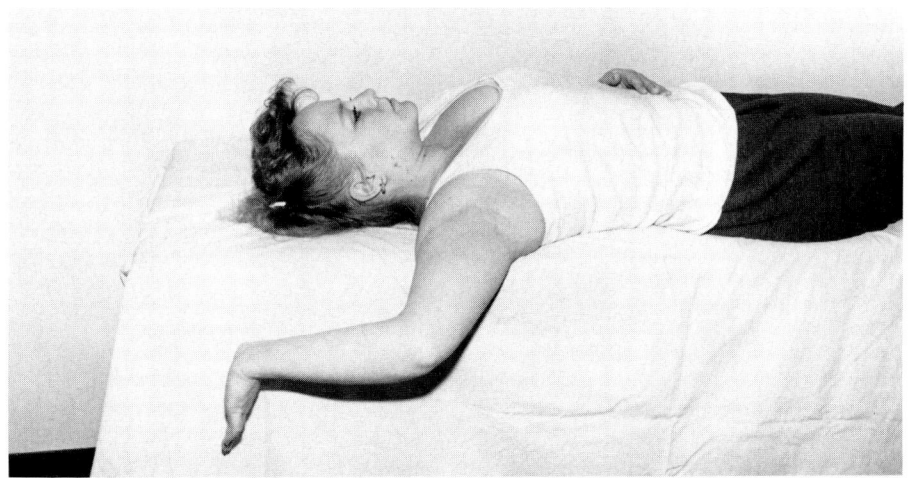

Fig. 41-22   External rotation at 90 degrees of abduction.

may play a more important role in the successful care of this neck pain.[10,11,15,18]

SUMMARY

The development of neck, scapular, and shoulder pain after trauma or surgery to the hand is common even in patients with no history of cervical or shoulder problems. The suspected causes of these problems are the poor postures assumed by patients and the limitations of shoulder and cervical motions imposed by the poor posture and the therapeutic apparatus worn by the patient. Instituting a program of postural instruction and exercise may have a significant effect in preventing proximal pain and dysfunction in the hand patient.

REFERENCES

1. Ayub E: Posture and the upper quarter. In Donatelli R, editor: Physical therapy of the shoulder, New York, 1987, Churchill Livingstone, Inc.
2. Bendix T and Jessen F: Wrist support during typing: a controlled electromyographic study, Appl Ergonom 17:162, 1986.
3. Caillet R: Shoulder pain, ed 2, Philadelphia, 1981, FA Davis Co.
4. Cyriax J: Textbook of orthopedic medicine, vol I and II. London, 1982, Bailliere Tindall.
5. DePalma A: Surgery of the shoulder, ed 3, Philadelphia, 1983, JB Lippincott Co.
6. Elvey R: Brachial plexus tension tests and the pathanatomical origin of arm pain. In Glasgow E and others, editors: Aspects of manipulative therapy, ed 2, New York, 1985, Churchill Livingstone, Inc.
7. Harms-Ringdahl K and Ekholm J: Intensity and character of pain and muscular activity levels elicited by maintained extreme flexion position of the lower cervical-upper thoracic spine, Scan J Rehabil Med 18:117, 1986.
8. Harms-Ringdahl K: On assessment of shoulder exercise and load elicited pain in the cervical spine, Scan J Rehabil Med 1, 1986.
9. Kaput M: Anatomy and biomechanics of the shoulder. In Donatelli R, editor: Physical therapy of the shoulder, New York, 1987, Churchill Livingstone, Inc.
10. McKenzie R: The lumbar spine, Lower Hutt, New Zealand, 1981, Spinal Publications.
11. McKenzie R: Treat your own neck, Lower Hutt, New Zealand, 1987, Spinal Publications.
12. McLaughlin H: The frozen shoulder, Clin Orthop 20:126, 1961.
13. Kendall H and others: Muscle testing and function, Baltimore, 1971, Williams & Wilkins.
14. Kraemer J: Intervertebral disc diseases, Chicago, 1981, Year Book Medical Publishers, Inc.
15. Quebec Task Force on Spinal Disorders: Report of the Quebec Task Force on Spinal Disorders, Spine 12:1, 1987.
16. Schuldt K and others: Effects of changes in sitting work posture on static neck and shoulder muscle activity, Ergonomics 29:1525, 1986.
17. Schuldt K and others: Influence of sitting posture on neck and shoulder EMG during arm-hand movements, Clin Biomech 2:126, 1987.
18. Stevens B and McKenzie R: Mechanical diagnosis and self treatment of the cervical spine. In Grant R, editor: Physical therapy of the cervical and thoracic spine, New York, 1988, Churchill Livingstone, Inc.

42

Sensibility testing: state of the art

Judith A. Bell-Krotoski

The true design and function of cutaneous sensibility have defied simple description. Compared with available knowledge of vision, hearing, and other sensory processes, there is much to be learned of this important sensory function.

Many tests have been popularized for measurement of cutaneous sensibility. These, in fact, represent a multitude of thought processes and perspectives. They are of value in attesting to the complexities involved in measuring a system that is as yet incompletely defined.

One finds in the literature conflicting opinions that are often perpetuated by repetition. There exists an inability to directly compare one testing method with another[17,32] and an apparent limited communication of one discipline with another. If these are confusing to the novice, they are confusing as well to the initiated.

The differing opinions and problems in testing would be simplified if objective tests were available. Some tests are more objective than others. *Tests that were considered objective in the past can be demonstrated to be subjective in application[3,5,8,15] and are further dependent on the technique of the examiner or the individual response of the patient.*

The examiner of cutaneous sensory function is cautioned against placing too much weight on a particular measurement or test. An examiner would be better counseled to remain open to developments in testing, taking all tests and measurements only as samples of the function he or she is trying to measure. As with all samples, they can be misleading when viewed out of context with the whole and are likely to represent only a part of the whole picture. *It is always possible that additional samples will describe a totally different picture.*

What has to be weighed and balanced in sensibility testing is the need for a simple test versus the need for detailed testing (Fig. 42-1). In clinical testing one begins early to feel that to do justice to the patient needing sensory evaluation one would have to devote a professional lifetime to the sorting of information, justification of testing procedure, and documentation of testing results. Most examiners do not have the time for such detailed investigation. There has long been a search for a simple, objective, easy-to-perform sensory test of neural status and hand function. It is recognized that there is a need for a simple test that would be readily available and of little cost for use in a wide variety of clinical settings. It may be that in time there will be such a test. Within the confines of one's own practice, one has to do the best that can be done with what is available. But when possible, it may be wise for the cautious examiner to trade the idea of a simple test for that of thorough testing. *The patient is our real concern. Do we do him justice if we tell him that he does not have a problem on the basis of a simple test?* Can it be determined how one patient functions much better than another with what appears to be an identical injury? How do we really know if one type of surgical repair is better than another in restoring sensory function, or if sensory reeducation is worth the time and effort? These and other questions are as yet unanswered and may not be able to be answered by a simple test.

WHERE DO THE ANSWERS COME FROM?
Literature

There is much to be learned from the literature if one accepts as fact only those things that can be demonstrated as fact, and as theory all else. Many fascinating studies of cutaneous sensibility have been executed since the age of Aristotle. Each study offers insight into the concepts of sensory function and into what has and has not been at-

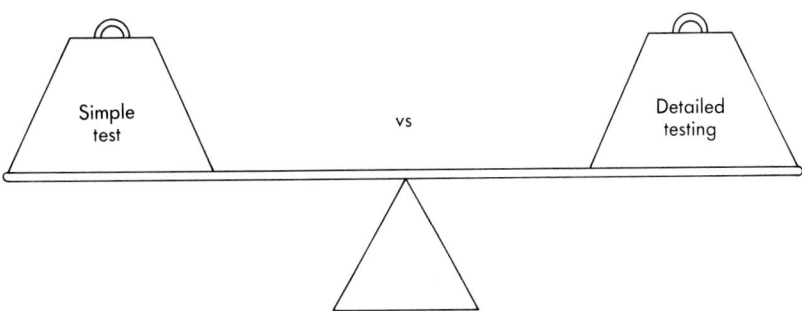

Fig. 42-1 Examiner of cutaneous sensibility must weigh and balance need for simple test versus need for thorough testing. Examiner needs a simple test for use in office and in field situations. He or she also needs information that is not forthcoming from a simple test.

575

tempted in measurement. One need not review every paper that has ever been written on the subject, but it is important that the serious examiner search for original sources of information that might otherwise be taken for granted.

All papers list a bibliography of their information sources referenced. By reading these references, and the studies they in turn reference, one comes into contact directly with the original sources of information. It is often a surprise to find that one's own interpretation of the original study is quite different from the interpretation of the study by another author. For instance, it was in this way that I discovered that von Frey,[37,38] credited as one of the earliest experimental investigators of cutaneous sensation, actually had a better test in the 1890s than presently available renditions of his test. Through the translation of von Frey's original German articles, one discovers that von Frey has a lot to say to us one century later.[39,40] He had anticipated many problems we are now describing with our modern instruments, and modern technology with which to measure them. Much of his original work has been lost through various translations and interpretation. The same is true of other authors.

A standardized test

Beyond consideration of a simple versus detailed test, the question remains, What test could be utilized to provide information internally in a clinic and externally from clinic to clinic? So many tests are available, each with its own respected advocate, that it is difficult for the clinician to decide which to use. The danger herein is that many clinicians are likely to use the most popular method advocated by the strongest examiner. The "most popular method" is not necessarily the most objective or reliable test. Other examiners choose to determine for themselves which test they believe to be optimum. Still others abstain from judgment completely, seeking alternative ways of solving their patient's problems.

One solution to the many varied tests and testing techniques presently utilized in clinical testing might be for examiners to adopt one test in common for reporting results and so on. This sounds reasonable enough, but still another problem remains: one cannot standardize a test until there is one to standardize. So long as clinical tests can be demonstrated to be subjective, the clinician is left "at risk" in making decisions as to neural status based on any test.

There seems to be no escaping the homework required for either finding an objective test or finding ways in which present tests can be made more objective. *It is not enough to identify a single test or to say subjectivity does matter when one cannot know the effect of subjective variables on the interpretation of test results.* The subjective nature of our tests in a day of modern technology where better tests are possible dictates that we first seek an objective test and then seek to standardize it.

One might argue that it is impossible to control all variables in a test situation. Psychologists face this problem in their work even more than examiners of sensibility. In their test design, they first make the test as objective as possible, dealing with variables that can be eliminated. Then when faced with variables that cannot be eliminated such as a test requiring the subjective response of a patient, they minimize the error by finding ways to deal statistically with the subjective element. In sensibility testing, a forced-choice test

that would deal with guessing statistically has been suggested by Dyck and LaMotte.[16,22] In a forced-choice procedure of testing a patient is given a series of stimulations, and the patient must decide on which number of the series he felt the stimulation. According to LaMotte, in a forced-choice procedure of testing, the response bias plays a relatively minor role because a subject can get no better than 50% correct by guessing.

Test battery

Other considerations make it disadvantageous at this time to decide only on one clinical test, even an objective test. Were every clinic to choose only one method of obtaining information, the result might be that of inhibiting the development of other needed information. Suppose the technique chosen contained an unknown variable that eventually rendered all clinical testing invalid? Depending so heavily on one test is comparable to investing all of one's money on one horse in a race. There are ways of predicting which methods might be more advantageous than another in sensibility testing, but the final champion is only proved once when it has made its way to the finish. Efforts to use a single test in the past have had to be abandoned by changes in thought and evidence leading in another direction.[9] There does have to be some common base of communication. If every clinic could use perhaps one or two tests in common, along with their own particular test they believe provides them with the most reliable information, there would be at least some common ground for communication. In addition, clinicians then would be more likely to use at least one clinical test that would later prove reliable and could serve as a basis for comparison with other tests.[7]

Another consideration is that a test battery may in fact be required to provide clinicians with a complete picture of the patient's problem. Many test designs are directed only at one aspect of sensory function. It has become almost universal in thinking recently for examiners to seek a test that not only provides information about neural status, but also includes an indication of the patient's actual ability to function with his present or absent sensibility. Although such a test would be convenient, it may be impossible for only one test to supply this much information. In testing we are asking many questions. As with any investigation, to be assured of clear answers, we may need to break down our questions into their simplest components.

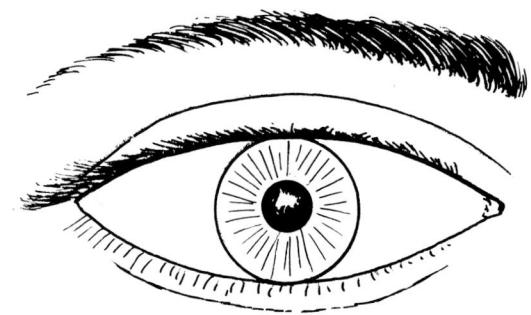

Fig. 42-2 In testing vision of eye, one tests first for visual acuity and then for astigmatism and color blindness. Attempts to measure these three functions together would complicate efforts toward obtaining clear and useful information.

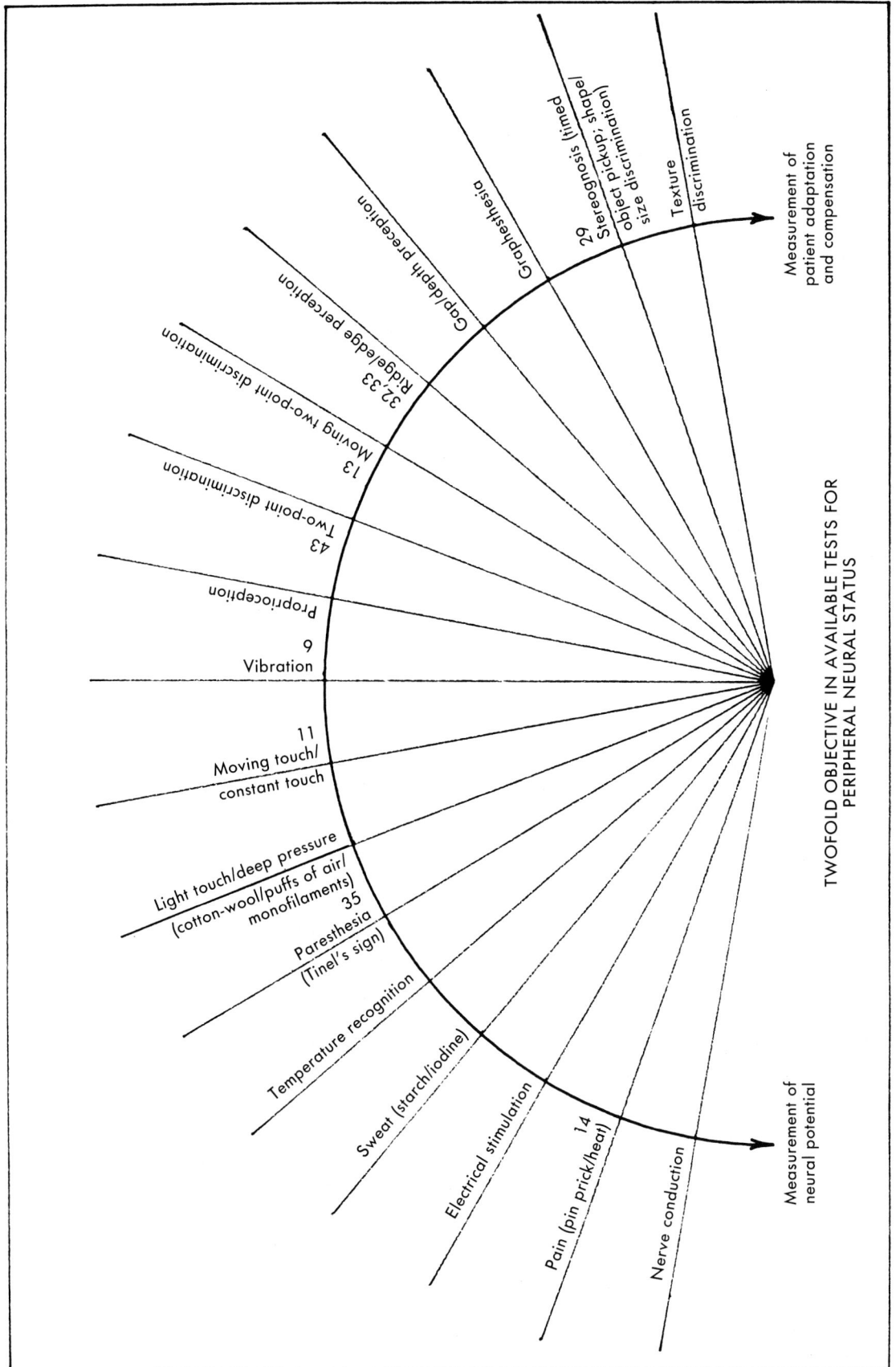

Fig. 42-3   In testing for peripheral nerve status, there exists a twofold objective: determining a patient's neural potential and determining adaptation or compensation for neural diminution. Most tests of neural status can be said to fall in a range between these two ends.

Take, for example, testing of the vision of the eye. In testing the eye, we surely want to know how the eye preceives its environment with whatever vision is present or absent. In our testing we might wish to include the ability to distinguish colors and the ability to visualize objects without perceptual distortion, as well as the visual acuity with which the eyes focus. We would not, however, attempt to test all of the above together by only one test. To do so would complicate our efforts to obtain clear and useful information. We would test first for acuity and then for these other functions (Fig. 42-2).

In cutaneous sensibility testing there exists at least a two-fold objective: that of determining sensory acuity and that of determining the patient's function with his acuity. The first is the patient's potential to function; the second depends on the patient's actual ability to function. Most of our tests for peripheral nerve function can be said to fall in a spectrum between these two ends (Fig. 42-3).

In sensibility testing it may be very important to make a difference in the patient's potential and actual ability. An optimum test for peripheral nerve acuity might be independent of the patient's ability to retain or compensate for his injury. If our question about a nerve after it was repaired is whether it has improved to an acceptable level or will require corrective intervention, we wish to know the specific status of the nerve repair, not if the patient has been able to compensate for the injury by clues and intelligence. Tests such as nerve-conduction velocity, pinprick, and Tinel's sign[35] would fall on the acuity end of the spectrum.

An optimum test for function might depend heavily on the patient's ability to compensate for his injury. The blind can be taught to see with their hands. The "blind hand" may also be taught to see through reeducation and compensation,[10,12,28] and Moberg's timed object pickup[29] would fall on the adaptation-compensation end of the spectrum.

It is possible that there will be a test designed that will meet these two ends: both the patient's potential and his ability to function through adaptation and compensation. It is probable that more than one test will be needed to provide a clear picture.

Neurophysiology

Contrary to what might be conceived by a literature review, neurophysiologists are still trying to isolate the components of "normal" sensibility. Quite naturally, the neurophysiologist is interested in "normal" sensory function, and his test requirements are adjusted accordingly for normal thresholds.[23-25,30,31] The clinician is interested in abnormal thresholds and his tests are focused accordingly. Measurements of both normal thresholds and abnormality contribute to the understanding of sensory neurophysiology. Collaboration of the neurophysiologist and the clinical examiner could prove productive. Such collaboration may in fact be required for resolution of problems inherent in clinical testing and for an accurate description of normal physiology versus abnormality. *If our understanding of neurophysiology is as yet incomplete and measurement tests are subjective, the clinician finds himself in the situation of trying to use an unknown test to define an unknown system.* Either an objective test will have to be used to shed light on the neurophysiology, or the neurophysiology will have to be identified to shed light on an objective test (Fig. 42-4).

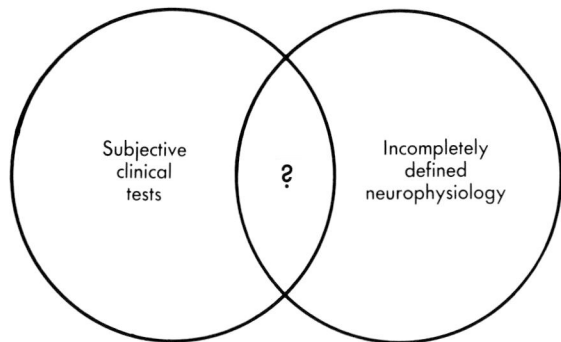

Fig. 42-4 If our understanding of neurophysiology is as yet incomplete and our measurement tests are subjective, we are left with an unknown test trying to define an unknown system. Either an objective test will have to be used to shed light on neurophysiology, or the neurophysiology will have to be identified to shed light on an objective test.

Future objective tests

Because there can be no agreement on the optimum test or tests for sensibility until more is learned about the actual physical properties of the tests and the exact nature and function of cutaneous end organs, there is much to be said both about cooperative studies in general among testing clinics and for the idea of test batteries. There will be no one person who will find the solution to our problems in cutaneous sensibility testing. The answers will come from a composite of information from many investigators representing many disciplines. If ways could be found to compare information, it is believed that so doing could advance testing by several years.

LABORATORY FINDINGS VERSUS CLINICAL TESTING

In the cutaneous layers of the skin are found billions of end organs, which represent the receptive end of the human nervous system. Many advances have been made in laboratory measurements of end-organ function in controlled settings.[20,25,31,45] However, what is found to be true in test conditions in a laboratory cannot always be applied directly to a clinical situation. As with trying to study the internal structure of the atom, were we able to introduce something into the atom with which to measure its physical characteristics, we would have created an artificial situation. Likewise, with end organs, once we have introduced something into an end organ with which to measure it, we have created an artificial situation.

Even when end-organ response can be isolated individually, the response of an end organ to a stimulus individually tells us very little about how that end organ works in concert with the others to produce what we know as cutaneous sensibility. For example, in some instances it is conceivable that some end organ or organs may have to be stimulated to a certain threshold before another can react. It is also conceivable that the response of quickly adapting end organs in some instances give to slowly adapting end organs or vice versa clues or signals that are not measurable by changes in electrical conduction as is commonly done in the lab.[14,17,23,25]

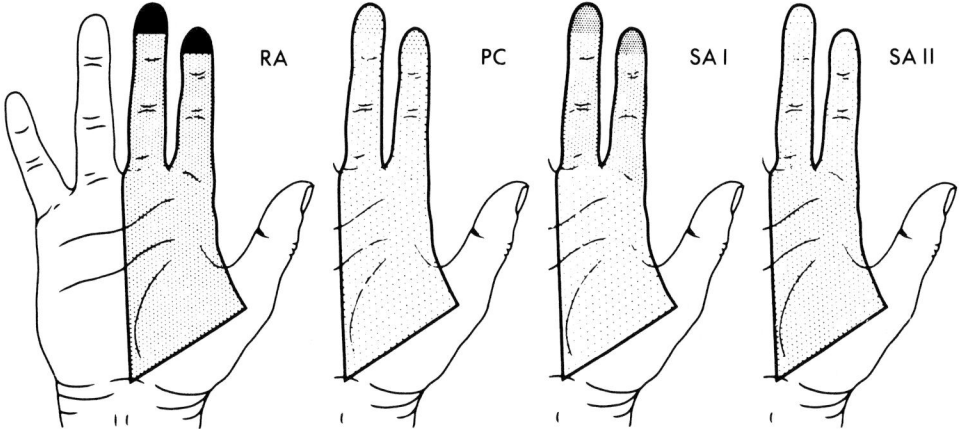

Fig. 42-5   Estimated absolute densities of four types of tactile sensory units in glabrous skin. Each dot represents a single sensory unit innervating skin area. This figure illustrates only the average unit density within a region, whereas dot size and exact location of an individual dot in relation to neighbors has no relevance with regard to receptive field size and spatial distribution of fields. (From Vallbo AB and Johansen RS: The tactile sensory innervation of the glabrous skin of the human hand. In Gordon G, editor: Active touch, Oxford, 1978, Pergamon Press Ltd.)

Organ-specific tests

Attempts have been made by some examiners to divide clinical testing instruments into those that test the slowly adapting end organs and those that test the quickly adapting end organs. Although this at first appears to be a sophisticated approach to testing, it is believed that such efforts are premature at this time. In any given skin area 10 mm^2 there are close to 3000 end organs.[29] Any stimulation of the skin is quite likely to bombard these end organs with stimuli. It would be surprising if any stimulation of an area so densely populated with end organs (both slowly and rapidly adapting) (Fig. 42-5) could select out only quickly adapting fibers or only slowly adapting fibers at the total exclusion of the others.

Although some end organs can be shown in a laboratory situation to be rapidly adapting in response to a stimulus and other end organs to be slowly adapting, there are still others that respond in between and are possibly moderators of the other two types. What would be their role in response to a stimulus? And still further, how is all this interpreted at the central cortex level?

Even if our clinical instruments did not stimulate a broad area of end organs in comparison with isolation of a single end organ in the lab, there are other reasons to believe that our current instruments cannot yet be divided into specific organs for which they test. Our testing instruments provide signals to the end organs in the form of energy produced when the instrument is applied to the skin. This energy can be measured as to its frequency content on a spectrum ranging from low to high frequency. We are more familiar with the frequency spectrum of audible sound waves and of visual light waves. The sound waves in particular are a good analogy because they not only range from low to high frequency, but also stimulate delicate end organs in the ear at specific frequencies to provide one with the sense of hearing. Measurements of cutaneous end organs in the lab have shown slowly adapting fibers to be responsive to low-frequency signals, and rapidly adapting fibers to be responsive to high-frequency signals. *This does not mean, of course, that they do not respond to other frequencies!* It might seem plausible to test differentially the slowly adapting end organs against the rapidly adapting end organs if our testing instruments provide a pure low-frequency or high-frequency signal. However, this is not the case. In a test analysis of the signal produced by the application of test instruments to a strain gauge, currently available clinical test instruments were found to produce signals throughout a broad frequency spectrum.[8] Although providing strong signals at their reported measured frequency, they also produce signals at both low and high frequencies, which would, in fact, stimulate both slowly and rapidly adapting end organs.[4]

Much has been made of the roll of the response to end organs to different frequencies in the lab. Such analysis may eventually decode the response of the end organs to stimuli. But even in the lab, the end organs have been measured mostly in a frequency range from 0 to 300 Hz because of instrumentation limited in the measurement of stimuli at these frequencies. It is possible that end organs are even more sensitive at higher frequencies. The fact that the stimulus signal on instrumentation can be measured only for a certain portion of an energy spectrum does not mean that other portions of the spectrum do not exist or that end organs are not more sensitive at frequencies higher than 300 Hz. Thus information that has been gathered about end organs in the lab is reflective of only part of the spectrum. Newer instrumentation is being designed to measure end-organ function in greater detail at higher frequencies.

Neurophysiology incompletely defined

One of the most interesting studies of end-organ function up to now is a study by Arrington on the sensation of the cornea of the eye.[1] To the cornea of the eye can be attributed the sensations of pain, touch and pressure, heat, and cold. Yet the cornea of the eye is reported to contain mostly unmyelinated c fibers, which are believed to be pain receptors. If an area populated mostly by c fibers can respond to all these stimuli, what then is the role of the other receptors? A touch-pressure test of the sensibility of the eye patterned after the touch-pressure testing of von Frey has been developed.

Both von Frey and Weber attempted, as later Head did, to establish a direct relationship between a specific sensory perception and a specific cutaneous end organ.[6] After exhaustive attempts to do so, they began to believe that little evidence existed for organ-specific function and that the receptors must work in some concert with each other to provide what we identify as distinct sensory perceptions.

Von Frey established the doctrine of four energies in the form of pressure, warmth, cold, and pain. The other senses he believed to be perceptual interactions of pressure and sensations of pain. Von Frey succeeded in demonstrating that there are end organs and that these end organs play a definite but specifically undetermined role in the recognition of pressure, warmth, cold, and pain.

Weber[42,43] described his two-point discrimination test in his paper "De Tactu," in 1834. He intended in his test to show only that a touch on the skin can be distinguished as to the pressure, temperature, and position. Weber was reportedly at great pains not to separate these functions but to show that they do go together and are interdependent.

Consider Weber's example of a recumbent man who has two coins placed on his forehead, for example, a nickel and a quarter. If the nickel and the quarter were of the same temperature, the quarter would be perceived as heavier in weight. If the nickel were cold, however, and the quarter warm, the nickel would be perceived as the same weight or even heavier than the quarter. Weber concluded that if temperature affects perceived pressure, the cutaneous "senses" cannot be separate.

In the years since these early studies, many investigators have continued attempts to identify specific functions of the end organs and to assign them a name. The end organs have been identified according to their size, shape, location, depth from the skin surface, myelination or lack of it, and response in the laboratory to a specific controlled stimulus, but they have not been identified according to their specific function. They have been classified as encapsulated, expanded, and free; as nociceptors (pain), thermoreceptors (heat), and mechanoreceptors (mechanical deformation); and most recently as quickly adapting fibers, slowly adapting fibers type I and type II, and pacinian corpuscles.[36] That the receptors can be measured in some way in response to a given stimulus and can be given a name is somewhat misleading. Even with the best of studies, much of what is believed to be the function of the end organs is theoretical at this time and is subject to change with new information, as it has been in the past. The pacinian corpuscle, a rapid adapter, has been the most studied because it is more easily tested and is the largest in size. Much of what has been found in its response in testing has sometimes been assumed to apply to other tactile receptors. Such assumption may be incorrect, or may be only partially correct.

Two-point discrimination test: a closer look

The Weber two-point discrimination test[13,26,42] was in most common use when I first began testing patients in 1969. This test undoubtedly supplies useful information to examiners of sensibility. However, it is believed significant that many authors became interested in other sensibility tests solely because the two-point discrimination test did not supply answers to many of the problems of patients presenting themselves for evaluation. I sadly watched as many patients were told they had normal "feeling" by earnest physicians who believed two-point discrimination testing to make a definitive diagnosis. History and an examination of probing the affected area belied a normal tactile cutaneous sensibility in some patients who would often repeatedly return for evaluation because their problems had not been resolved. It was found that blindfolding these patients and having them identify an area that changed in feeling as a probe was drawn across their hand would result in a repeatable mapping (the examiner would have to recognize a delay in response in an affected area to obtain a clear line between areas easily felt by the probe and areas of diminution). When this type of testing was repeated on successive visits of the patient and the test results proved identical to those previously mapped, it was deemed that these patients must have discernible areas of diminution or loss of sensibility that were not measured by two-point discrimination testing.

Von Prince had believed more was needed in addition to two-point discrimination testing for peripheral nerve injuries when she began to use the Semmes-Weinstein monofilaments in the 1960s.[41] This was found by the author in later tests of patients with nerve compressions.[2] Werner and Omer[46] noted in a review of 4000 tests with the filaments that the presence of light touch does not necessarily indicate that two-point discrimination is present. Specific examples cited were in such conditions as radiculitis, causalgia, and entrapment syndromes.

It has recently been reported that patients with experimentally induced nerve compressions have been shown to have a normal two-point discrimination test when there was a considerable decrease in nerve-conduction sensory fiber amplitude.[18] In one subject two-point discrimination was still normal at a point when sensory fiber amplitude approached zero. In rephrasing of the discussion of testing with any one test, I wonder how one would have discovered that some patients with a nerve compression may have a normal two-point discrimination examination if only the two-point discrimination test had been used as a measure?[2,19] Patients with nerve lacerations may also have injuries with

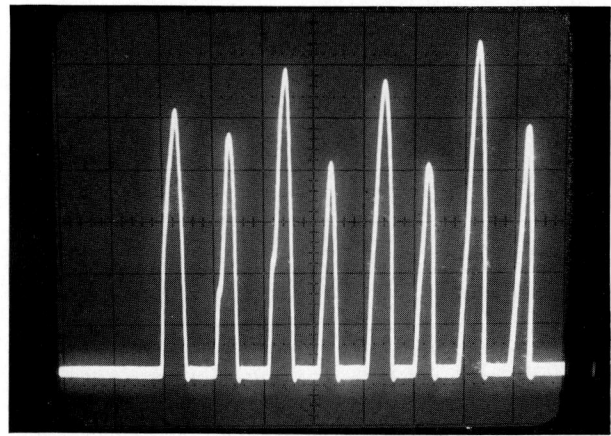

Fig. 42-6 Oscilliscope screen showing application force of one and two points of the Discriminator Testing Instrument.[12] Variation in force in this measurement is at least 500 mg (250 mg/division).

Table 42-1 Stimulus force of a paper clip applied to blanching*

| Tester | Two points in contact | | One point in contact | |
	Mean (gm)	Standard deviation (gm)	Mean (gm)	Standard deviation (gm)
1	**19.16**	7.27	**13.49**	2.83
2	28.32	5.55	16.08	3.95
3	20.53	5.87	14.83	4.79
4	19.39	6.01	17.01	4.81
5	32.15	8.61	17.24	4.04
6	**36.49**	4.94	**17.09**	5.47
Overall	26.01	6.38	17.09	4.32

*Six testers, 20 applications each, alternating between two points in contact and one point in contact.

nerve-compression components attributable to postinjury swelling. How can we determine to what extent patients with nerve lacerations and other injuries have nerve compression as opposed to swelling internal or external to the nerve that may render the two-point discrimination test less accurate? The common use of the two-point discrimination test as a primary measure in the past has most likely delayed recognition of exceptions in testing. The same may be true of other tests. There is no way of knowing until objective testing is routine and the tests can be directly compared.

In the past the two-point discrimination test has frequently been assumed to be objective because it can be reported on in numerical terms. In clinical practice, there is considerable variation in the force and velocity of application among clinicians, a situation that renders the test subjective (Fig. 42-6).[5] For instance, it would be expected to be easier for a patient to distinguish the difference between one and two

points applied at 37 gm of force than to distinguish between one and two points applied at only 19 gm of force (Table 42-1). This was measured in our lab (Paul W. Brand Research Lab) by instrumentation sensitive enough to measure force changes from one application to another. The reproducibility of a consistent application force by an examiner applying two points to the same spot on the same patient was found to vary widely, even when blanching of the skin was used as a control.[5] In the same study it was found that blanching of the fingers occurs at different forces on separate fingers; thus this difference brought into question the use of blanching as a control of application force.

The lack of control on application force is even more pronounced when the stimulus is moved, such as in the recently popularized test of moving two-point discrimination.[11] Here the force applied by the examiner is made to vary even greater by the "hills" and "valleys" of the skin topography as the examiner draws the testing instrument

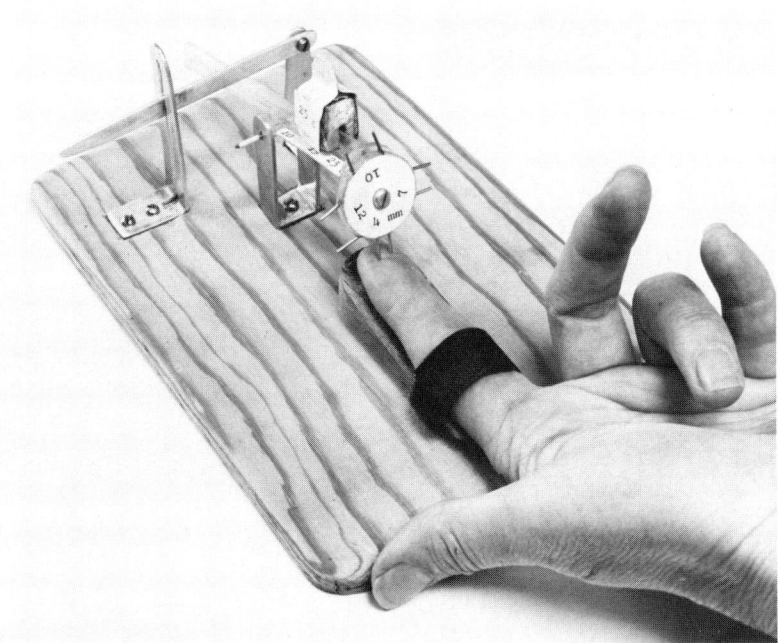

Fig. 42-7 Moberg prototype instrument for a force-controlled, two-point discrimination tester. A 25 g weight can be moved along the scale to vary the force applied. A hand-controlled lever arm lifts and applies the instrument arm with a two-point discrimination testing disk to the tested finger at a controlled force.

against the finger. This does not, of course, mean that the two-point discrimination tests are meaningless, but only that the effect of variations in application force on the accuracy of the tests needs to be further studied. Otherwise, how can the examiner determine if a patient is responding to a difference in recognition of one or two points, or of a heavier or lighter application force? Moberg has developed an experimental two-point discrimination instrument with a controlled application force (Fig. 42-7).[29]

The energy signal of one application of a two-point instrument can be measured on a spectrum analyzer, which has a display similar to an oscilliscope (Fig. 42-8). The energy signal is seen as a scatter of dots that occur at frequencies from 1 to 256 Hz, at various force amplitudes.

Static two-point discrimination has been considered by some examiners of sensibility to be mainly a low-frequency stimulus, mostly stimulating slowly adapting end organs.[13] Rapidly adapting end organs do not respond as well at low frequency (signal dies out). There is a tendency to think slowly adapting end organs also die out at higher frequencies; however, just the opposite may be true. LaMotte tells us slowly adapting end organs may be quite sensitive to higher frequency and rapidly adapting end organs may have low-frequency response. In any case, the energy signal from a two-point testing instrument can be shown to occur throughout a broad frequency spectrum (both low and high frequency). The test then must stimulate both slowly and quickly adapting end organs.

Similarly, in spectral analysis the energy content produced by the Semmes-Weinstein monofilament instrument on application can be shown to occur at both low and high frequencies, sufficient in strength to stimulate both slowly and rapidly adapting end organs (Fig. 42-9). Previously, it was suggested that the Semmes-Weinstein monofilaments test only slowly adapting end organs. The instrument must stimulate both slowly and rapidly adapting end organs.

Semmes-Weinstein monofilaments

Only the monofilament design of testing[5,21,34,40] attempts to control the force of application. This test is not without its problems, which are discussed in Chapter 43,[34,44] but it does approach an objective test of cutaneous sensibility, and the test has been found to be repeatable if the monofilament lengths and diameters are correct[4] (Fig. 42-10).

Vibratory tests

Vibration tests have recently been reviewed as sensibility tests. Most current physiologic studies indicate that vibration as a separate sense does not exist. They indicate that each sensory end organ has its own particular stimulus-response relationship that varies with frequency.[23] The instrument stimuli for the vibration tests are usually hand applied, particularly the tuning fork instruments, and have the same problem of lack of control on force of instrument application. In addition, most commercially available vibration instruments are fixed-frequency instruments that vary only the intensity of a given frequency; they do not provide variable frequencies at fixed intensities.[18] Newer, more costly instruments are being developed to provide selectable controlled frequencies.[27] To be repeatable objective instruments, these instruments must also control the force at which the stimulus is applied.

Nerve conduction velocity

Tests of nerve conduction velocity have been thought to be largely objective tests. Nerve conduction tests depend greatly on technique of the examiner and other variables. The test can vary according to the time of day, temperature

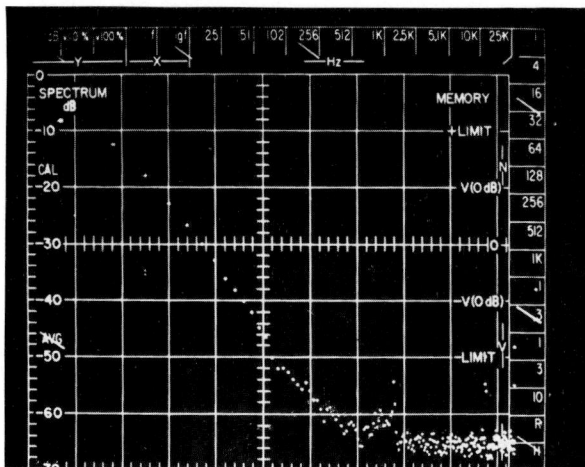

Fig. 42-8 Force spectral content of paper clip two-point discrimination instrument stimuli applied 16 times and averaged (by a spectrum analyzer). The horizontal axis is a logarithmic scale of frequency in Hertz (cycles per second). The horizontal scale spans 1 to 256 Hertz (from left to right). The vertical axis is in decibels referenced to 42.66 g (OdB) on the left. The energy from the instrument application occurs throughout a broad frequency spectrum (both low and high), sufficient enough to stimulate both slowly and rapidly adapting end organs.

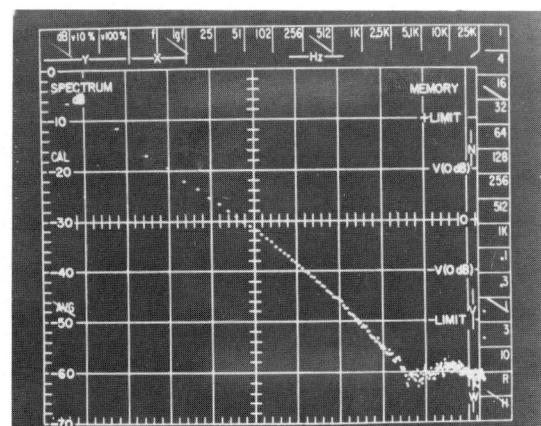

Fig. 42-9 On an expanded scale is shown the force spectral content of a 4.17 (marking number) Semmes-Weinstein Monofilament applied 16 times and averaged. The horizontal axis spans 1-512 Hz (cycles per second). The vertical axis is in decibels referenced to 5 g (OdB) on the left (at 100 Hz the signal is 50 dB below 5 g, which is 15.8 mg). The energy from the instrument application occurs throughout a broad frequency spectrum (both low and high) sufficient enough to stimulate both slowly and rapidly adapting end organs.

of the extremity, size of the electrodes, placement of the electrodes, and individual testing instrument. Used with other tests of sensibility, the test can be of great help in determining the location of nerve injury and in numerically quantifying and documenting nerve problems. It is important to realize that the test in no way can determine what a patient does and does not feel. Attempts to directly correlate nerve conduction with diminished functional cutaneous sensation have been largely unsuccessful. Both nerve conduction tests and cutaneous sensibility tests appear to be needed to adequately clinically classify and monitor peripheral nerve function. Usually the tests will correlate for evidence of involvement or noninvolvement of a nerve. However, exceptions are found. I have found cases in which nerve conduction was "absent" when some Semmes-Weinstein monofilaments could still be felt. In less frequent instances, cases have been seen in which the monofilaments have been "within normal limits" and a nerve shows a "slowed" nerve conduction response.

Other tests

The problems with control of application force and velocity are not limited to the two-point discrimination and vibration tests, but apply to any of our tests that are hand applied.

It is possible that the two-point discrimination tests, the monofilaments, vibration, and other frequently used tests of cutaneous sensibility could be made objective by instrument design that would control the force of application and the velocity of application. The force and velocity of application are foremost in the minds of neurophysiologists and others who are developing controlled laboratory testing of end-organ function. A few prototype instruments are available, some expensive and complicated and others not quite so complicated. When these instruments are available to the clinician, it may then be possible for direct comparison of our clinical tests.

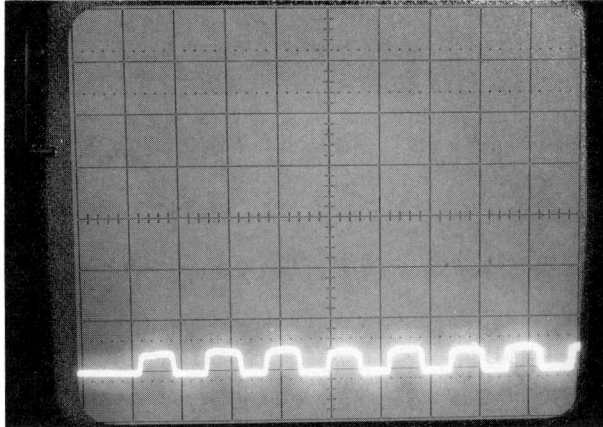

Fig. 42-10 Oscilliscope screen showing force on repeat application of the 2.83 (marking number) Semmes-Weinstein Monofilament. For comparison purposes, this instrument measurement has been made at the same sensitivity as that of the two-point discrimination instrument in Fig. 42-6 (250 mg/division). The instrument application force is repeatable within a small range if the lengths and diameters of the monofilament are correct.

SUMMARY

Cutaneous tactile sensation is no simple perception. It may be that in the end there will be some simple tests to measure it, but one must always appreciate the intricacies and sensitivity of the system. No one person will find the solution to our problems in sensory testing. The answers will come from a composite of information obtained by many investigators over time. It is important for the examiner to realize that although much useful information can be derived from current clinical tests and instruments, there are no "cookbooks." He or she must keep a critical eye toward factors that render tests subjective and carefully integrate test results with the needs and problems of the patient.

REFERENCES

1. Arrington J: Corneal sensation measurement. Presented at the fourteenth annual meeting of the United States Public Health Service Professional Association, Phoenix, Ariz, April 1977.
2. Bell JA: Sensibility evaluation. In Hunter J and others, editors: Rehabilitation of the hand, St Louis, 1978, The CV Mosby Co.
3. Bell JA and Buford WL Jr: Assessment of levels of cutaneous sensibility. Presented at the sixteenth annual meeting of the United States Public Health Professional Association, Houston, Tex, 1979.
4. Bell JA and Tomancik E: Repeatability of testing with Semmes-Weinstein monofilaments, J Hand Surg 12A:155, 1987.
5. Bell-Krotoski J and Buford W Jr: The force/time relationship of clinically used sensory testing instruments, J Hand Ther 1(2):76, 1988.
6. Boring EG: Sensation and perception in the history of experimental psychology, New York, 1942, Appleton-Century-Crofts.
7. Brand PW: Symposium, Assessment of cutaneous sensibility, Comments of chairman, National Hansen's Disease Center, Carville, La, 1980.
8. Buford WL and Bell JA: Dynamic properties of hand held tactile assessment stimuli. Proceedings of the thirty-fourth annual conference of Engineering in Medicine and Biology, 23:307, 1981.
9. Caine DB and Pallis CA: Vibratory sense: a critical review, Brain 89:723, 1966.
10. Curtis RM: Sensory reeducation after peripheral nerve injury. In Fredricks S and Brody GS, editors: Symposium on the neurologic aspects of plastic surgery, vol 17, St Louis, 1978, The CV Mosby Co.
11. Dellon AL: The moving two-point discrimination test: clinical evaluation of the quickly adapting fiber/receptor system, J Hand Surg 3(5):474, 1978.
12. Dellon AL, Curtis RM, and Edgerton MT: Reeducation of sensation of the hand after nerve injury and repair, Plast Reconst Surg 53:297, 1974.
13. Dellon AL, Mackinnon SE, and Crosby PM: Reliability of two-point discrimination measurements, J Hand Surg 12A:5, 1987.
14. Demichelis F and others: Biomedical instrumentation for the measurements of skin sensitivity, Trans Biomed Eng BMR-26(6):326, 1979.
15. Dyck PJ: Quantitation of cutaneous sensations in man. In Dyck PJ and Thomas PK, editors: Peripheral neuropathy, Philadelphia, 1975, WB Saunders Co.
16. Dyck PJ: Assessment of cutaneous sensibility. Symposium presented at National Hansen's Disease Center, Carville, La, 1980.
17. Dyck PJ, O'Brien PC, Bushek W, and others: Clinical vs quantitative evaluation of cutaneous sensation, Arch Neurol 33(9):651-656, 1976.
18. Gelberman RH and others: Sensibility testing in peripheral nerve compression syndromes: an experimental study in humans, J Bone Joint Surg 65A:632, 1983.
19. Gelberman RH and others: Results of treatment of severe carpal tunnel syndrome without internal neurolysis of the median nerve, J Bone Joint Surg 69(6):896. 1987.
20. Gray JAB and Malcom JL: The initiation of nerve impulses by mesenteric pacinian corpuscles, Proc R Soc Lond (Biol) 137:96, 1950.
21. Jamison DG: Sensitivity testing as a means of differentiating the various forms of leprosy found in Nigeria, Int J Lepr 39(2):504, 1972.
22. LaMotte RH: Assessment of cutaneous sensibility, sensory discrimination and neural correlation. Symposium presented at National Hansen's Disease Center, Carville, La, 1980.

23. LaMotte RH and Mountcastle VB: Capacities of humans and monkeys to discriminate between vibratory stimuli of different frequency and amplitude: a correlation between neural events and psychophysical measurements, J Neurophysiol 38:539, 1979.

24. LaMotte RH and Srinivasan MA: Tactile discrimination of shape: responses of quickly adapting mechanoreceptive afferents to a step stroked across the monkey fingerpad, J Neurosci 7(6):1672, 1987.

25. Looft FJ and Williams WJ: One-line receptive field mapping of cutaneous receptors, Trans Biomed Eng BME-26(6):350, 1979.

26. Louis DS and others: Evaluation of normal values for stationary and moving two-point discrimination in the hand, J Hand Surg 9(4):552, 1984.

27. Lundborg G and others: Digital Vibrogram: a new diagnostic tool for sensory testing in compression neuropathy, J Hand Surg 11A:5, 1986.

28. Millesi H and Renderer D: A method of training and testing sensibility of the fingertips, from the Department of Plastic and Reconstructive Surgery, Surgical University Clinic of Vienna and Ludwig-Boltzmann Institute for Experimental Plastic Surgery, Vienna, Austria, 1978.

29. Moberg E: Fingertip function and evaluation of its sensibility. In Fouchett G: Fingertip injuries, New York, Churchill Livingstone, Inc (in press).

30. Mountcastle VB: Medical physiology, ed 12, vol 2, p 1345, St Louis, 1968, The CV Mosby Co.

31. Paul RL, Merzesich M, and Goodman H: Representations of slowly and rapidly adapting mechanoreceptors of the hand in Broadmann's areas 3 and 1 of *Macaca mulatta*, Brain Res 36:229, 1972.

32. Poppen NK: Sensibility evaluation following peripheral nerve suture: critical assessment of the von Frey, two-point discrimination, and ridge tests. In Jewett DL and McCarroll HK Jr, editors: Symposium on nerve repair: its clinical and experimental basis, St Louis, 1979, The CV Mosby Co.

33. Renfrew S: Fingertip sensation: a routine neurological test, Lancet, 1:396, 1969.

34. Semmes J and others: Somatosensory changes after penetrating brain wounds in man, Cambridge, Mass, 1960, Harvard University Press.

35. Tinel J: The "tingling" sign in peripheral nerve lesions, Presse Med 47:388, 1915 (translated by B Kaplan).

36. Vallbo AB and Johansson RS: The tactile sensory innervation of the glabrous skin of the human hand. In Gordon G, editor: Active touch, Oxford, Eng, 1978, Pergamon Press Ltd.

37. von Frey M: Berichte der Sachlichen Gesellschaften der Wissenschaften, Leipzig 46:185, 1894.

38. von Frey M: Physiologie des Sinnesorgane der menschlichen Haut, Ergebn Physiol 9:351, 1910.

39. von Frey M: Zur Physiologie der Juckempfindung, Arch Neurol Physiol 7:142, 1922.

40. von Frey M: Gibt es tiefe Druckempfindungen (?) Dtsch Med Wochenschr 51:113, 1925.

41. von Prince K: Personal communication, 1978.

42. Weber EH: Data cited by Sherrington CS, in Shafer's textbook of physiology, Edinburgh, 1900, Young, J. Pentland.

43. Weber EH: Ueber den Tastsinn, Müller Archiv, 1935, p 152-159.

44. Weinstein S: Tactile sensitivity of the phalanges, Percept Motor Skills 14:351, 1962.

45. Werner G and Mountcastle VB: Neural activity in mechanoreceptive cutaneous afferents: stimulus-response relations, Weber functions and information transmission, J Neurophysiol 28:359, 1965.

46. Werner JL and Omer GE: Evaluating cutaneous pressure sensation of the hand, Am J Occup Ther 24:5, 1970.

BIBLIOGRAPHY

Chochinov RH, Ullyot LE, and Moorehouse JA: Sensory perception thresholds in patients with juvenile diabetes and their close relatives, N Engl J Med 286(23):1233, 1969.

Conomy JP, Barnes KL, and Cruse RP: Quantitative cutaneous sensory testing in children and adolescents, Cleve Clin Q 45(2):197, 1978.

Gelbermann R, Urbaniak J, Bright D and others: Digital sensibility following replantation, J Hand Surg 3:313, 1978.

Jabaley ME: Recovery of sensation following peripheral nerve repair. In Fredricks S and Brody GS, editors: Symposium on the neurologic aspects of plastic surgery, vol 17, St Louis, 1978, The CV Mosby Co.

Jabaley ME and Bryant MW: The effect of denervation and reinnervation of encapsulated receptors in digital skin. In Marchac C and Hueston JT, editors: Transactions of the Sixth International Congress of Plastic and Reconstructive Surgery, Paris, 1976, Masson.

Moberg E: Criticism and study of methods for examining sensibility of the hand, Neurology 12:8, 1962.

Moberg E: Diagnostic and prognostic value of the two-point discrimination test in reconstructive hand-arm surgery, Brain, 1988 (in press).

Naafs B and Dagne T: Sensory testing: a sensitive method in the follow-up of nerve involvement, Int J Lepr 45(4):364, 1978.

Omer GE Jr: Evaluation and reconstruction of the forearm and hand after acute traumatic peripheral nerve injuries. In American Academy of Orthopaedic Surgeons: Instructional course lectures 18:1454, St Louis, 1973, The CV Mosby Co.

Omer GE and Spinner M: Management of peripheral nerve problems, Philadelphia, 1980, WB Saunders Co.

Terzis J: Metabolism of peripheral nerve injuries. In Fredricks S and Brody GS, editors: Symposium on the neurologic aspects of plastic surgery, vol 17, St Louis, 1978, The CV Mosby Co.

43

Light touch–deep pressure testing using Semmes-Weinstein monofilaments

Judith A. Bell-Krotoski

ADVANTAGES OF MONOFILAMENT TESTING

Light touch–deep pressure testing with monofilaments of increasing forces has been described as one of the most objective tests for measuring cutaneous sensibility.[1-5,7,15] The filaments bend when the peak-force threshold has been achieved. A relatively consistent force is continued by the filaments until they are either removed from the skin contact or are severely curved. When they are severely curved, the force on the skin is less than the desired threshold. In addition to controlling the force of application, the filament design attempts to control the velocity of application. If applied too quickly, the filament force will exceed the desired threshold. Otherwise, the bending of the filament minimizes the vibration of the examiner's hand.

The currently available testing instrument is the Semmes-Weinstein[9] Aesthesiometer monofilament testing set (Fig. 43-1). This testing set contains 20 filaments. Smaller sets containing fewer filaments are available on request from the manufacturer.* Although not a perfect testing intrument because of variations in the tip geometry of the filaments, the Semmes-Weinstein monofilament set produces results that

*Available through North Coast Medical, Campbell, Calif. or Research Designs, Inc., Houston.

are repeatable within a certain force range, usually in milligrams.[4] The instrument set succeeds in demonstrating gradients of sensibility diminution.

Color coding of the filament force produces a mapping that provides the examiner with differential thresholds of touch in areas of normal or relatively normal sensibility and areas of diminution (Fig. 43-2). If the application technique is consistent, the mappings produced can be serially compared for changes in neural status (Fig. 43-3). The mappings can be predictors of the rate of neural return or diminution. They can be predictors as well of the quality of neural return, or severity of diminution (Fig. 43-4). Attempts to correlate increasing or decreasing touch thresholds with levels of patient function at this time appear promising, and correlation is perhaps superior to that associated with many other forms of testing.

The monofilament testing is not recommended as an "only" test at this time, for reasons explained in Chapter 42. Used in combination with other clinical tests of sensory function, particularly a test of sensory nerve conduction, the test can lead to the resolution of patient problems that are not resolved by other forms of testing and can clarify other test results. The monofilaments are often used by neurophysiologists in studies to determine end-organ re-

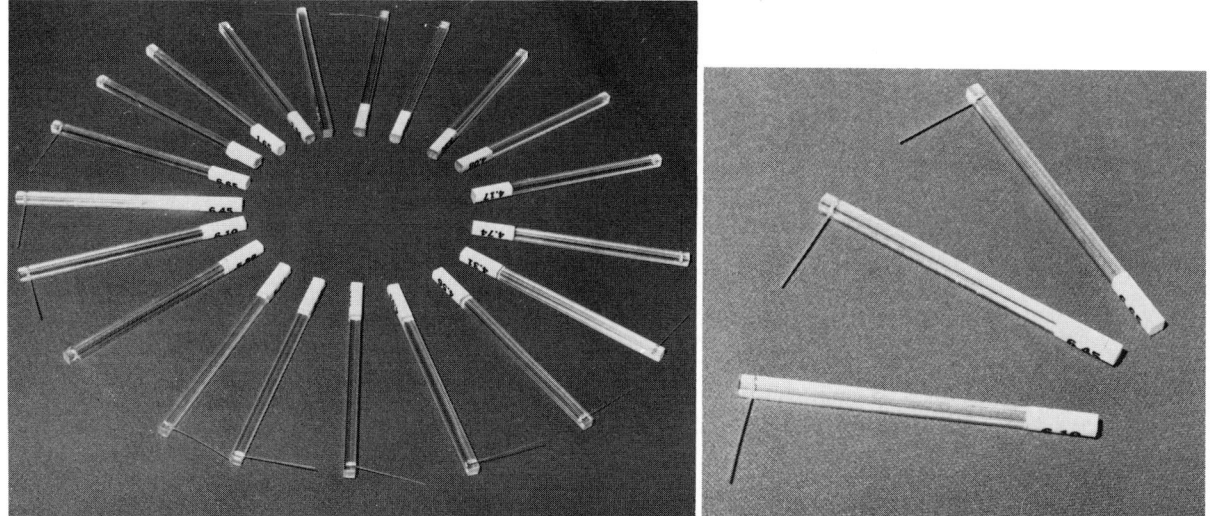

Fig. 43-1   **A,** Semmes-Weinstein Anesthesiometer monofilament testing set. **B,** Close-up view of filaments.

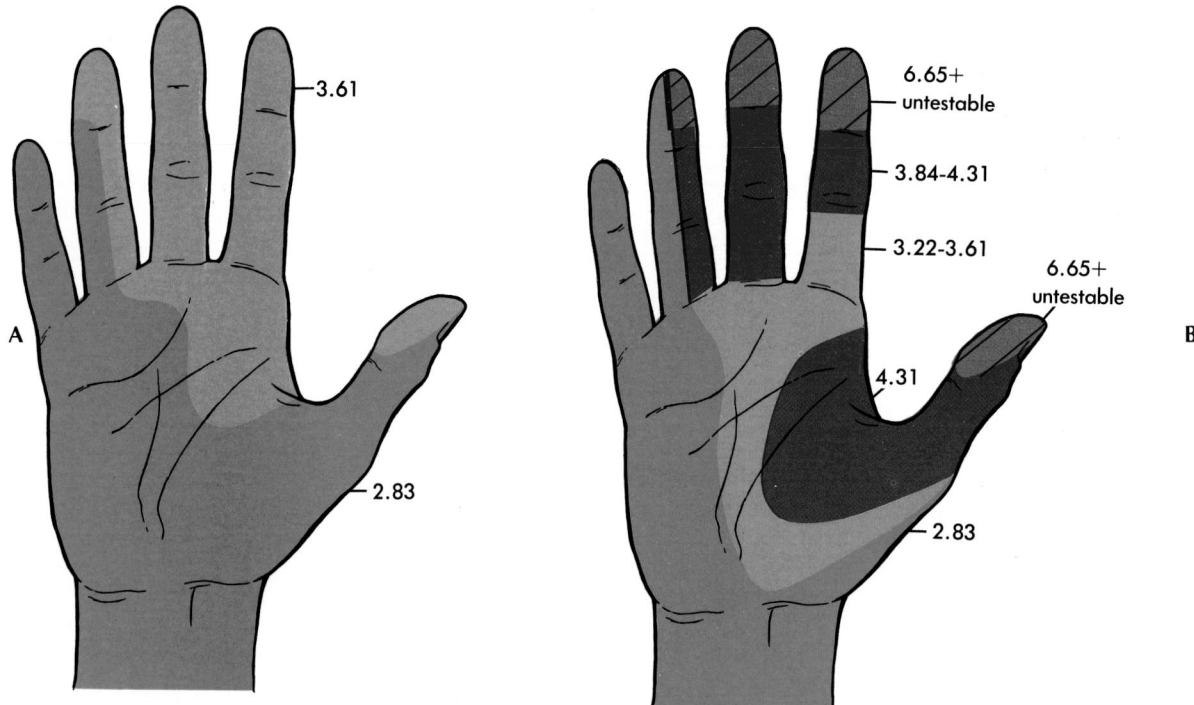

Fig. 43-2 **A,** Monofilament mapping showing a median nerve compression as measured in a woman with a history of numbness for 2 years and no corrective intervention. **B,** Same patient as measured 4 months later. Touch pressure recognition has become worse from diminished light touch to untestable with monofilaments.

sponse. Like the other tests of sensibility, they could be made more objective through careful consideration of their physical properties.

HISTORY OF THE INSTRUMENT

Although von Frey[10] was the inventor of the monofilament form of testing, the currently available testing sets are not identical to the test instrument he described. Von Frey was at pains to put a consistent tip on the ends of each of his filaments. The consistent tip allows that portion of the tip of the filament coming into contact with the skin while the filament is bent, to be held constant in size; it allows only the force to vary from one filament to another. This simplifies and makes more accurate calculations of pressures produced when the filaments are applied to the skin. A consistent tip, in addition, makes the effect of increasing diameters of the filaments inconsequential.

The current testing instrument was developed by Semmes and Weinstein and is described in their book *Somatosensory Changes After Penetrating Brain Wounds in Man.*[9] Semmes and Weinstein desired a measure that would be applicable over a wider range of intensities than von Frey's and one that would provide a progressive force scale. The investigators attempted to show that with their filaments, which increase in diameter to exert increased forces, the common logarithm of the force increases in an approximately linear fashion with the ordinal rank of the filaments. The force increments between filaments are not equal.

The unequal increment in the forces has presented problems when testing scales have been adjusted for believed differences in sensitivities of the thumb, finger, and palm. A close examination of interpretation scales reveals that the filaments have been adjusted by a change to the next heaviest filament. The next heaviest filament in some instances represents an increment of 18.5 mg and in other instances an increment of 165.5 gm of force (Table 43-1). Thus such adjustments in the scale are rendered disproportionate and confusing and should not be used.

Semmes and Weinstein,[9,14] using the currently available monofilaments, established a threshold below which stimuli are never (or rarely) perceived and above which they are always (or nearly always) perceived. In their studies of 20 normal subjects, each with two hands, they found the left hand only slightly more sensitive than the right, with only the left thumb reaching a significant level of difference. The left hand exhibited a more pronounced gradient of sensitivity between parts (thumb and palm) than the right hand, in which there was *no* significant difference in parts (thumb and palm). Thus, even if the monofilaments were ordered with equal force increments between filaments, there are few clear lines, if any, in threshold differences between fingers, thumbs, and palms for adjustments in the testing scales. Testing scales then cannot be arbitrarily altered for fingers, thumb, and palm areas without invalidation of data from areas altered.

I recommend that the examiner use one consistent scale and allow for slight diminutions in sensibility in areas of the skin believed to be slightly less sensitive in touch pressure thresholds, such as callused skin.. An example would be with testing of the plantar surface of the foot. One would not be concerned if this surface reflects a diminished light touch, because one knows the keratin layer of the plantar cutaneous skin to be relatively thick. One would, however, be quite concerned if the plantar surface reflected a dimin-

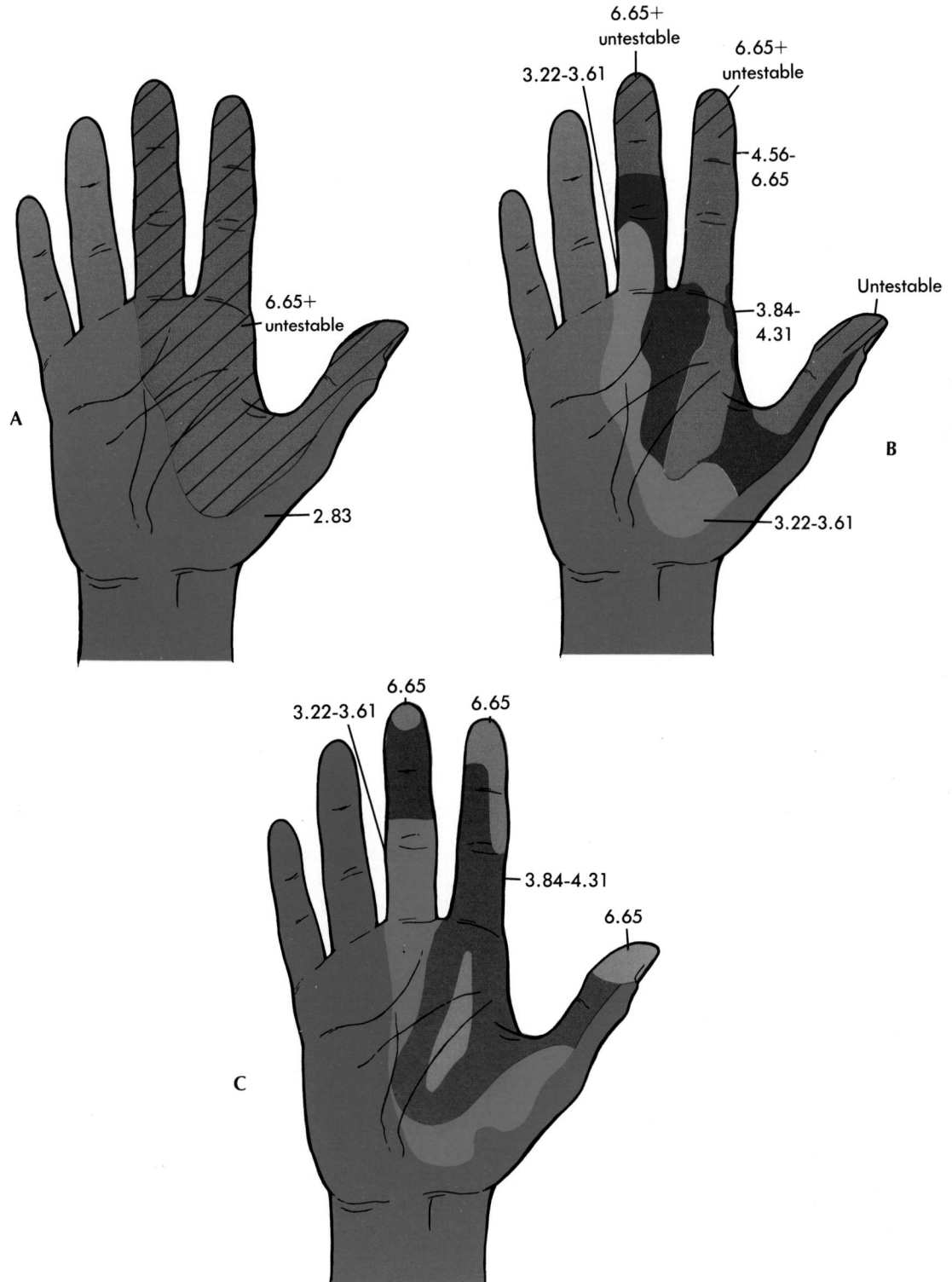

Fig. 43-3   **A,** Monofilament mapping showing a median nerve laceration before surgery. Two-point untestable. **B,** Same patient 3 months after surgery. Two-point untestable. **C,** Same patient 7 months after surgery. Two-point untestable, fingertips now testable with monofilaments.

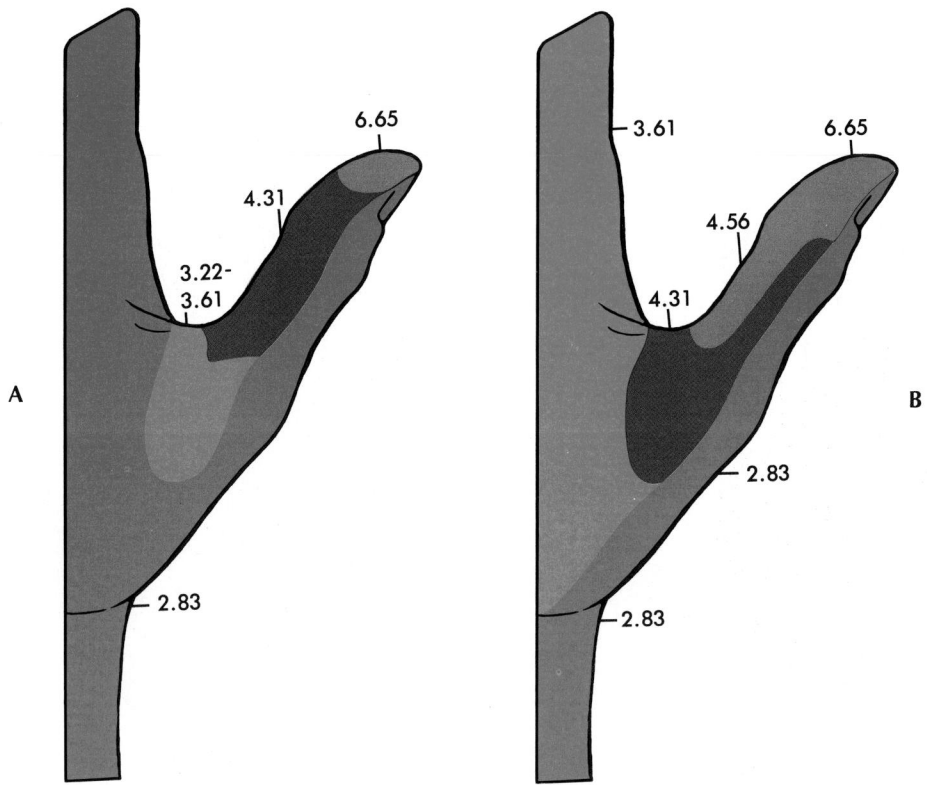

Fig. 43-4 **A,** Two years after incomplete amputation of right thumb. Digital nerves were not resutured. Small centimeter pedicle of dorsal skin was intact. **B,** Same patient after injection of lidocaine around median nerve to determine if innervation was radial nerve or median. Notice that although the volar thumb sensation was downgraded, it and the palmar area of the median nerve did not become asensory. This finding brings into question the blocking of the contralateral nerve in testing. Such blocks may be incomplete and lead to false conclusions.

ished protective sensation because even with callus, the normal patient will have "protective sensation." It is emphasized that variations in normal cutaneous sensitivity thresholds can be measured in milligrams. The force range of the monofilaments is from 4.5 mg, the lightest, to 447 gm, the heaviest, measuring rudimentary residual sensibility.

Although the early investigators using the filaments did succeed in standardizing the filaments with normal subjects and referenced the filaments of increasing and decreasing forces to "normal" thresholds, the filaments were not standardized to functional levels of diminution in the manner they are utilized today. Their greatest value at present is their sensitivity, which allows testing of normal thresholds of sensibility and answers the question, "Is potential sensibility normal or not?" Once an area of normal sensibility has been established, the other filaments of increasing forces can be referenced to this area of normal sensibility to establish a light touch–deep pressure differential in sensory areas, as between the ulnar and median nerves or between the median nerves of the right and left hands.

The credit for equating increasing levels of forces required by the monofilaments to levels of diminution in sensory function goes to Kilulu von Prince.[11,12] Von Prince began grouping the filaments into levels that could be equated with expected levels of function on the part of the patient. Von Prince was greatly influence by the work of Napier[8] and of Moberg.[7] Concurrently with studies being done by Semmes

in sensory losses arising from central origin, von Prince began to investigate the residual function of patients who had received a multiple variety of peripheral nerve injuries from war wounds. Von Prince realized that although some patients would have injuries similar to those of other patients, there was a considerable difference in the level of function of the patients. For example, of two patients who could not tell a difference in testing between one and two points, one could feel a match that would burn his finger and the other could not. Thus she perceived that there must be a protective level of sensation that was not measured by the other test. Of two patients who would have a response to a pinprick, one would have the ability to discriminate textures and one would not. Thus she perceived that there must be a light touch level of sensation that would be equated with the patient's ability to discriminate textures.

Von Prince may have been one of the earliest hand therapists. She was considered rather radical in ideas at the time she developed her concepts of sensory testing. She broke with what was then tradition for therapists in the armed services to develop a common base of training. Considering the development of testing to measure the level of function of peripheral nerve injuries so important, she requested 6 months in which to investigate this area and develop testing scales.

In her early scales, von Prince attempted to equate levels of diminished sensory function with levels of two-point discrimination testing. This was a logical assumption, since

Table 43-1   Rod markings versus calculated force in gram increments from filament to filament

Rod markings (Log 10 force, 0.1 mg)	Calculated force (gm)*		
	Force between filaments	Force between filaments	Force between filaments
Loss of protective* sensation			
6.65†	165.5	447.0	154.5
6.45		281.5	
6.10	52	127.0	46
5.88		75.00	
5.46	14	29.00	3.3
5.18		15.00	
5.07	3.05	11.70	3.15
4.94		8.650	
4.74	1.868	5.500	
4.56†		3.632	
Diminished protective sensation			1.57
4.31†	0.568	2.052	
4.17		1.494	0.3746
4.08	0.4972	1.194	
3.84		0.6958	
Diminished light touch			0.2886
3.61†	0.2422	0.4082	
3.22		0.1660	
Normal			0.0983
2.83†	0.0402	0.0677	
2.44		0.0275	0.0045
2.36	0.0185	0.0230	
1.65		0.0045	

*Scale is linear but does not occur at regular force increments.
†Minikit monofilaments (monofilaments used in short version of test).

the Weber[13] two-point discrimination test was frequently used in practice. This would be changed in later scales when it would be found that although there appears to be a relationship between diminishing levels of two-point discrimination and increasing levels of force required by the monofilaments, the two tests cannot be directly equated.[6]

Omer in particular realized the value of von Prince's work and was instrumental in assuring that her work would continue by other investigators when von Prince was sent to other assignments. He published a paper with Werner in 1970[15] that would add to the "classic" publications in sensibility testing. The testing scale of von Prince was changed in the article by Werner and Omer to omit two-point discrimination as a consideration in the filament testing and treat it as a separate test.

Werner and Omer, who were concerned with point localization of a touch stimulus, developed two interpretation scales, one for point localization and one for area localization. They also described a level of diminished epicritic sensation (diminished light touch).

The interpretation scales of von Prince and of Werner and Omer were frequently used and additional variations de-

veloped for sensory testing in the ensuing years. In 1976 the Bicentennial year, so many scales were available with limited history about their origin that a person using the filaments was unsure of their accuracy and unable to justify this form of testing as a sensitive monitor of peripheral nerve function for presurgical and postsurgical hand cases. An attempt was launched to identify and develop the most accurate scale.

After much comparison, a scale was chosen for interpretation of the filaments (Table 43-2) (other scales were eliminated through clinical trials). This scale was used and reviewed in more than 200 tests of patients with nerve compressions and lacerations. Later it was discovered to be identical to that of the "area-localization" scale described by Werner and Omer. If their level of diminished light touch is further divided into two levels and the full range of filaments are included, this comparison can be seen.[2,15] (Werner and Omer chose to leave out a few filaments.) The chances that two independent investigators would settle on the same interpretation scale for clinical use are quite small unless there are indeed differences in the patient's level of sensory function—that is, light touch and protective sen-

Table 43-2 Scale of interpretation of monofilaments

		Filament markings	Calculated force (gm)*
Green	Normal	1.65-2.83	0.0045-0.068
Blue	Diminished light touch	3.22-3.61	0.166-0.408
Purple	Diminished protective sensation	3.84-4.31	0.697-2.06
Red	Loss of protective sensation	4.56-6.65	3.63-447
Red-lined	Untestable	Greater than 6.65	Greater than 447

*Data from Semmes J and Weinstein S: Somatosensory changes after penetrating brain wounds in man, Cambridge, Mass, 1980, Harvard University Press.

sation—that are measurable at specific forces in a spectrum from light touch to deep pressure.

An area localizaton scale was chosen over scales for point localization because nerves after laceration very often have referred touch, and the maturation of referred touch after nerve injuries in our measurements improved independently of light touch–deep pressure thresholds.

James M. Hunter, at the Hand Rehabilitation Center in Philadelphia, realized the value of the filament mapping in producing information on the patient's neural status that was not forthcoming from other sensory examinations. He encouraged this form of testing with his surgical patients, many of whom came to him with long-standing unresolved peripheral nerve problems.

The monofilaments have more recently been used to map sensibility diminutions and losses in patients with Hansen's disease. These patients can have diminution or loss of feeling in one of three ways—through end-organ invasion by bacilli, through nerve trunk invasion by bacilli, or through nerve compression secondary to swelling. The involvement of peripheral nerves can mimic a peripheral nerve lesion or compression from other causes. Much can be learned of neural function in these patients, and they are a challenge to any of our present tests. The filaments are being used as a sensitive monitor of early changes in sensory status in these patients, who can have reversal or improvement of their neural damage through timely use of steroids and other medications.

PRESENT TECHNIQUE

Testing with the monofilaments begins with filaments in the normal threshold level and progresses to filaments of increasing pressure until touch is identified by the patient (Table 43-2). The filaments 1.65 to 4.08 are applied three times to the same spot. This was found necessary in measurements of the filament forces.[3] One touch may not reach the required threshold of these light filaments. All the filaments are applied in a perpendicular fashion in 1 to 1.5 seconds, continued in pressure in 1 to 1.5 seconds, and lifted in 1 to 1.5 seconds. The filaments 1.65 to 6.45 should bend to exert the specific pressure. Filaments 4.17 to 6.65 are applied only one time. All sensibility testing is performed with careful attention to the normal distribution of the sensory nerves and common variations. A detailed history is taken from the patient and charted as an aid in close examination of the nerve distribution of suspected involvement and the screening of other areas. Unless a higher lesion is suspected from the history, it is often necessary to examine only the hands with the filaments, though *it is possible to test the entire body with the filaments*. For the plantar surface of the foot and areas of callus monofilament 3.61 (marking number) is considered within normal limits in addition to the 2.83 monofilament.

As nerve return progresses proximally to distally, except for cases such as syringomyelia and localized partial lesions, the fingertip in the median and ulnar nerve distribtuions will be the first area to lose sensibility and the last area for return of sensibility. Testing of the fingertips can serve as a limited monitor of corresponding nerve status.

It is more accurate for the same examiners to repeat successive evaluation, but because this is not always possible, the testing can be repeated by other examiners using the same technique.[4] Testing by other examiners is possible when a double-blind situation is desired for studies.

What is mandatory is a quiet testing area; unfortunately this makes the use of the filaments questionable in an open clinic. It is sometimes very difficult for the patient to attend the filaments in a diminished sensory area. As one patient described the problem, it is like asking him to read a technical journal when he does not recognize all the words. Any sound is distracting, and sounds such as people walking by or typing can make it impossible for some patients to feel filaments they may feel in a quiet area. To assure an accurate examination it is most critical for the examiner to be quite certain the patient can and is attending the filaments.

The testing technique described is in contrast to that of other authors who have required area and point localization when testing with the monofilaments. In area localization, after being touched, the patient responds by indicating the *area* that was touched. In point localization, the patient responds by covering the *point* touched with a wooden dowel within a centimeter. Testing by the latter method is more time consuming and is sometimes confusing to patients who have referred touch. It is believed that point localization may reflect the cognitive ability of a patient to adapt to new sensory pathways more than the actual level of return of the nerve and its response to touch. If what we are actually attempting to test is threshold of touch, it is believed that it can be more simply and aptly measured by having the patient respond to stimulation by the monofilament by saying the word "touch." An argument to this effect is that under nerve retraining we can effect an improvement in a patient's point localization and discrimination of sensory input, but few examiners would believe we are actually effecting a change in the physiologic status of the nerve. Point localization is tested in the sensory evaluation but is treated as a tactile discrimination requiring cortical participation. It can be quickly tested, and a note made of the direction and distance in centimeters into another point, area, or finger where the touch is referred.

Consistent colors from cool to warm are used to correspond with the diminishing sensibility levels. These allow a quickly read, consistent, easily comparable mapping of sensibility.

Procedure

1. Draw a probe (a Boley gauge) across the area to be tested in a radial-to-ulnar and proximal-to-distal manner. Ask the patient to describe where and if his feeling changes. *Do not ask for numbness, because the patient's interpretation of numbness varies.*

Dot the area described as "different" with an ink pen. The examination is easier if the patient can identify the gross area of involvement as a reference; if he cannot, proceed the same way on testing but allow more testing time.

2. Establish an area of *normal sensibility* as a reference. Familiarize the patient with the filament to be used, and demonstrate it in the proximal area believed to be normal. Then, with the patient's eyes occluded, demonstrate the filament until the patient can easily identify the filament on the low side of normal (2.83). (The filaments lighter than 2.83 are not necessary unless the examiner is attempting to obtain a differential in a normal range of touch.)

If possible, test the volar surface of the uninvolved hand first, applying the monofilaments to the fingertips and proceeding proximally. If testing is within normal limits, proceed to the dorsum of the hand and then to the involved hand.

Test the involved hand (volar surface) by applying the same filament (2.83) to the fingertips first and working proximally. Dot the spots correctly identified with a *green* felt-tip pen. (Explain to the patient that the second touch he feels is a marking of the pen.) In general, the patient is tested distally to proximally, but a consistent pattern is not used to avoid patient anticipation of the area to be touched. When all the area on the volar surface of the hand that can be identified as within normal limits is marked in green, proceed to the dorsum of the hand and test in the same fashion. Since the sensibility on the dorsum of the hand is not always so well defined as the volar surface, it is easier to establish areas of decreased sensibility on the volar surface first. *Now the gross areas of normal and decreased sensibility have been defined* (Fig. 43-2, *B*).

3. Return to the volar surface of the hand. Proceed to the filaments within the level of *diminished light touch* (Table 43-2), but change the color of the marking pen for this level to *blue*. Test as above in the unidentified areas remaining, working again first on the volar surface and then on the dorsum (Fig. 43-2, *B*).

4. If areas remain unidentified, proceed to the filaments in the *diminished protective sensation* level (*purple*) and then *loss of protective sensation* level (red) and continue testing until all the areas have been identified (Fig. 43-2, *B*).

5. Record the colors and filament numbers on the report form to produce a sensory mapping. (Color and mark hands on form.) Note any variations and unusual responses, especially delayed responses. Delayed responses (more than

3 seconds) are considered abnormal. Note the presence and direction of referred touch with arrows. Note and draw on the form any unusual appearances on the hands, including sweat patterns, blisters, dry or shiny skin, calluses, cuts, blanching of the skin, and so on.

Minikit

Testing of the monofilament instrument application forces indicates that all 20 monofilaments may not be necessary. The variation in force range of one monofilament may sometimes overlap with its neighbor. The monofilaments may therefore be reduced in number without significant loss in sensitivity of the test. A minikit is now available and is considered to be sufficient for most testing. The minikit greatly reduces time required for testing. The minikit filaments represent the cut off forces for each functional level of sensibility—normal, diminished light touch, diminished protective sensation, and loss of protective sensation. Two filaments are included for the loss of protective sensation level. For returning nerve function, the heaviest monofilament is important to signal rudimentary deep pressure sensation. The lightest monofilament of the loss of protective sensation level is also important to define loss of protective sensation versus diminished protective sensation (marking number 4.56).

INTERPRETATION

Turning the data from testing into levels of sensibility and levels of expected patient function, as when one initially tests sensibility, can appear an impossible task at first. With a little experience, however, and some sensitivity to the needs of the patients, it not only can be done, but it also becomes easier.

The following interpretation of monofilament force levels was based on the review I made of 150 cases and 200 tests of patients with peripheral nerve problems at the Hand Rehabilitation Center, Ltd, Philadelphia, from 1976 to 1978. Subsequent discussion of the data with von Prince and experience in use of the interpretation in patients with peripheral nerve problems over the last 10 years has continued to support the relationship of force thresholds to functional sensibility. Comparisons were made between the Semmes-Weinstein monofilaments and other tests of sensibility routinely given to patients as a test battery. The results are summarized in Fig. 43-5.

Normal touch is a recognition of light touch, and therefore deep pressure, that is within normal limits. This level is the most significant of all levels because it allows the examiner to distinguish between areas of normal sensibility and areas of sensory diminution.

Diminished light touch is diminished recognition of light touch. If a patient has diminished light touch, provided that his motor status and cognitive abilities are in play, he has fair use of his hand, his graphesthesia and stereognosis are both close to normal and adaptable, he has good temperature appreciation, he definitely has good protective sensation, he most often will have fair to good two-point discrimination, and he may not even realize he has had a sensory loss.

Diminished protective sensation is just that. If a patient has diminished protective sensation, he will have diminished use of his hands, he will have difficulty manipulating some objects, he will have a tendency to drop some objects, and

Comparison of touch/pressure threshold testing
with other sensibility tests

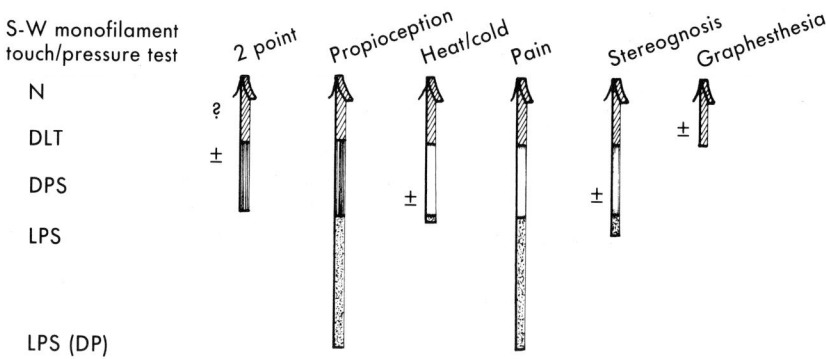

Fig. 43-5   Results of comparison review of 150 cases, 200 tests of patients with nerve compressions or lacerations, and other tests given in a 1976-1978 test battery. Semmes-Weinstein Monofilament functional levels (*N*, normal; *DLT*, diminished light touch; *DPS*, diminished protective sensation; *LPS*, loss of protective sensation; *DP*, deep pressure), can be read vertically. The relationship of the monofilament levels to other sensibility tests can be read horizontally. Although the tests did in general correlate with respect to involvement or noninvolvement, no direct correlation could be made in level results from two-point discrimination testing and monofilament testing. Several cases with nerve compressions measured two-point discrimination within normal limits (3 to 5 mm or 6 mm at fingertips), whereas light touch–deep pressure thresholds were decreased to as low as the diminished protective sensation level. In four patients two-point discrimination testing was abnormal, whereas monofilament light touch–deep pressure testing was within normal limits (two old burns, one cerebrovascular accident, and one partial thumb amputation).

he may complain of weakness of his hand, but he will have an appreciation of the pain and temperature that should help keep him from injury, and he will have some manipulative skill. Sensory reeducation can begin at this level. It is possible for a patient to have a gross appreciation of two-point discrimination at this level (7 to 10 mm).

Loss of protective sensation is again what it says. If a patient has loss of protective sensation he will have little use of his hand, he will have a diminished, if not absent, temperature appreciation, he will not be able to manipulate objects outside his line of vision, he will have a tendency to injure himself easily, and it may even be dangerous for him to be around machinery. He will, however, be able to feel a pinprick and have deep pressure sensation, which does not make him totally asensory. Instructions on protective care are helpful to prevent injury.

If a patient is *untestable*, he may or may not feel a pinprick but will have no other discrimination of levels of feeling. If a patient feels a pinprick in an area otherwise untestable, it is important to note this during the mapping. Instructions on protective care of the hand are mandatory at this level to prevent the normally occurring problems associated with the asensory hand.

Further interpretation of the effect the decrease or loss of sensibility has on patient function depends on the area and extent of loss and whether musculature is diminished.

FUTURE CONSIDERATIONS

A few cases of suspected nerve compression have been found in which all the testing of neural status described is within normal limits, and a patient history is the only indicative finding. A review of the literature quickly shows similar cases. It is suspected that in these cases the patient is not always being tested at the time of his symptoms. He

comes in for testing after he has slept late, had a good breakfast, and had a more quietly paced and lighter duty morning than his normal routine, while in reality he complains of problems only after heavy-duty work of a few hours' duration. Hunter has termed this condition "transient stress neuropathy." It is a challenge to our future testing.

The recognition of threshold levels of light touch–deep pressure is invaluable in peripheral nerve evaluation. Mappings of such thresholds enable the examiner to "see" what is otherwise invisible. I believe this testing method will clearly be validated by improved testing technique and instruments.

ACKNOWLEDGMENT

The author gratefully acknowledges Bill Buford, Bioengineer at the Paul W. Brand Research Laboratory, Gillis W. Long Hansen's Disease Center, Carville, Louisiana, for his help in reviewing the monofilament calculations in developing instrument measurements and collaborating on sensibility test design.

REFERENCES

1. Bell JA: Semmes-Weinstein Monofilament testing for determining cutaneous light touch/deep pressure sensation, Star 44(2),1984.
2. Bell JA and Buford W: Comparison of forces and interpretation scales as used with the von Frey Aesthesiometer. Paper presented at Hand Surgery Correlated with Hand Therapy meeting, Philadelphia, 1978.
3. Bell JA and Buford WL: The force/time relationship of clinically used sensory testing instruments. J Hand Ther 1:76, 1988.
4. Bell JA and Tomancik E: Repeatability of testing with Semmes-Weinstein monofilaments, J Hand Surg 12A:155, 1987.
5. Buford WL Jr and Bell JA: Dynamic properties of hand held tactile assessment stimuli. Proceedings of the thirty-fourth annual conference of Engineering in Medicine and Biology 23:307, 1981.
6. Gelberman RH and others: Sensibility testing in peripheral nerve compression syndromes: an experimental study in humans, J Bone Joint Surg 65A:632, 1983.
7. Moberg E: Objective methods of determining the fucntional value of sensibility of the hand, J Bone Jont Surg 40B:454, 1958.

8. Napier JR: Hands, New York, 1980, Pantheon Press.
9. Semmes J and others: Somatosensory changes after penetrating brain wounds in man, Cambridge, Mass, 1960, Harvard University Press.
10. von Frey M: Zur Physiologie der Juckempfindung, Arch Neurol Physiol 7:142, 1922.
11. von Prince K: Occupational therapy's interest in sensory function following peripheral nerve injury, Med Bull, US Army Europe 23:143, 1966.
12. von Prince K and Butler B: Measuring sensory function of the hand in peripheral nerve injuries, Am J Occup Ther 21:385, 1967.
13. Weber EH: Data cited by Sherrington, CS, in Shafer's textbook of physiology, Edinburgh, 1900, Young, J Pentland.
14. Weinstein S: Tactile sensitivity of the phalanges, Percept Motor Skills 14:351, 1962.
15. Werner JL and Omer GE: Evaluating cutaneous pressure sensation of the hand, Am J Occup Ther 24:5, 1970.

BIBLIOGRAPHY

Arrington J: Corneal sensation measurement. Paper presented to the fourteenth annual meeting of the US Public Health Service Professional Association, Phoenix, Ariz, April 1977.

Chochinov RH, Ullyot LE, and Moorehouse JA: Sensory perception thresholds in patients with juvenile diabetes and their close relatives, N Engl J Med 286(23):1233, 1969.

Demichelis F and others: Biomedical instrumentation for the measurements of skin sensitivity, Trans Biomed Eng BMR-26(6):326, 1979.

Jamison DG: Sensitivity testing as a means of differentiating the various forms of leprosy found in Nigeria, Int J Lepr 39(2):504, 1972.

Naafs B and Dagne T: Sensory testing: a sensitive method in the followup of nerve involvement, Int J Lepro 45(4):364, 1978.

44

Sensibility testing: clinical methods

Anne D. Callahan

Evaluation of the hand with diminished sensibility presents a challenge to the hand therapist. The challenge arises from the complexity of sensibility. It affords the skin protection and provides an exquisitely refined means of exploring and interacting with the environment. How then can the busy clinician accurately assess the scope of sensibility? Cottonwool and the safety pin, traditional tools of the neurologist, are recognized as inadequate for the task. Many additional tests* have been devised in an effort to find a quick, reliable means of evaluation. The challenge to the clinician has therefore expanded to include deciding which tests of the many available should be used to assess sensibility. The purpose of this chapter is to discuss general considerations in sensibility testing, consider the components of a comprehensive sensibility evaluation, and offer guidelines for selection of tests. Special note will be made where differences exist between evaluation after nerve laceration versus evaluation of nerve compression.

GENERAL CONSIDERATIONS IN SENSIBILITY TESTING
Relevant definitions

Sensation versus sensibility. Seemingly opposite definitions of these two terms can be found in current literature.[12,33] For the purpose of this chapter, sensation is defined as "an impression conveyed by an afferent nerve to the sensorium," whereas sensibility is "susceptibility of feeling; ability to feel or perceive."[16]

Academic versus functional sensibility. A distinction is made between return of sensibility as evidenced by the ability to perceive pinprick, touch, and temperature ("academic") and the return of sensibility sufficient to enable the hand to engage in full activities of daily living, including those activities in which vision is essentially occluded while the hand manipulates an object ("functional"). Seddon[43] and Bowden[6] were among the first to make this distinction in assessing recovery of sensibility. Moberg[30,32] has been the most influential in emphasizing the importance of testing functional sensibility.

Tactile gnosis. Tactile gnosis (*gnōsis*, Greek, "knowledge") is a term popularized by Moberg[8] to denote the capacity of the hand to "see" while gripping or manipulating an object even when the eyes are closed, that is, functional sensibility. A distinction is made between tactile gnosis and the central nervous system function described as stereognosis.

Candidates for evaluation

Patients may be referred for sensibility evaluation for any of the following reasons: (1) to aid in diagnosis (e.g., partial versus complete nerve injury, and assessment of sensory changes in carpal tunnel syndrome); (2) to aid in serial follow-up after nerve repair; (3) to aid in disability assessment in compensation cases; and (4) to determine the need or readiness for sensory reeducation.

Components of a sensibility evaluation

A thorough assessment includes the following: a careful history; examination of sympathetic function; appropriate selection of tests; administration of the tests in a standard manner so that as many testing variables as possible can be minimized and so that follow-up evaluation can be reliably compared; and knowledgeable interpretation of information gathered. These components of evaluation will be discussed in this chapter.

OBTAINING THE HISTORY

A careful history, based on medical chart information and skillful interviewing of the patient, will provide the examiner with information that cannot be gained by any specific clinical test. Such information will aid in shortening the time required for testing and will help determine the prognosis for recovery.

A history should include name, age, sex, dominance, and occupation. Age will influence prognosis for recovery. Occupation and whether the dominant or nondominant extremity was injured will help in estimating degree of sensibility recovery required for functional use of the extremity in work and leisure activities.

The date, nature, and level of injury should also be recorded. The time elapsed since the date of injury or repair helps in proper assessment of Tinel's sign and in better interpretation of the presence or absence of sympathetic function. The nature of the injury (such as laceration, crush, traction, compression, or infection) will influence the amount of scarring that occurs, in turn influencing the quality of regeneration. Prognosis for recovery of distal sensory function is partially dependent on the level of the injury; injuries at or proximal to the wrist level rarely result in good functional sensation in the adult.[15,32,33]

The medical chart will frequently document a patient's involvement in litigation. This is important information for the examiner because litigation might influence the level of cooperation of the patient. The best candidate for sensibility evaluation is one who has nothing to gain by positive test results.

---

*References 8, 11, 38, 40, 41, 52.

Skillful interviewing is important. Questions should be phrased in such a way as to avoid leading or suggesting to the patient. Thus an appropriately worded initial question would be, "Please tell me what problems you have in this hand." The patient will then tend to rank his nerve-related complaints without artificial emphasis on sensory disturbances. For example, a patient with carpal tunnel syndrome may not describe any sensory-related problems, limiting his complaint to a weakness in grip strength. In this case one could expect that he would probably test with normal or only slightly diminished sensibility. On the other hand, if he states, "It feels like there is a veil on my fingertips when I try to pick up something," he could be expected to test with slight to moderate loss of sensibility. Terms such as "numbness," "dead," "asleep," and "pins and needles" may refer to hypesthesia, anesthesia, or parasthesia depending on that particular patient's meaning of the term and should be clarified.

Once the patient has described his dysfunction in his own words, the examiner can ask more leading questions to elicit greater detail about the current status of sensibility. Such questioning will help the nonsophisticated or nonobservant patient to articulate his problems. The examiner will want to know if sensibility is improving, getting worse, or staying the same. Are symptoms aggravated by certain positions or activities, and are they relieved by certain positions or motions (such as "shaking of the arm")? Does the sensibility deficit affect performance of activities of daily living?

At this time in the examination it is convenient to assess briefly motor function, including grip and pinch strength, and, in selected cases, individual muscle strength because motor function will affect performance on certain sensibility tests that may be used. The patient's performance during these motor tests can suggest to the examiner his general level of cooperation, as evidence by the shape of his strength curve on the Jamar Dynamometer (refer to Chapter 4) and exertion of maximal effort during muscle testing.

EXAMINATION OF SYMPATHETIC FUNCTION IN THE HAND

Sympathetic fibers subserve vasomotor (*vas*, Latin "vessel"), sudomotor (*sudor*, Latin "sweat"), and pilomotor (*pilus*, Latin "hair") functions in the extremity. After nerve injury the area of loss of sympathetic function closely corresponds to the area of loss of sensory function because the cutaneous sympathetic fibers follow essentially the same pathway to the periphery as the cutaneous sensory fibers.[47] The actual autonomous area of sympathetic function may be smaller than the corresponding autonomous area of cutaneous sensory function because there is more overlap between sympathetic fibers of different nerves than between sensory fibers.[23] The combination of sympathetic and sensory dysfunction results in characteristic trophic (*trophē*, Greek "nourishment") changes in all tissues of the involved area.[47] Examination of the sympathetic function and trophic changes in the hand (Table 44-1) will provide definite information on the nutritional state of the part and suggestive information on sensory function in the part.

The correlation between presence of sympathetic function and sensibility is greatest immediately after nerve laceration and in long-term cases where little or no regeneration has occurred. However, if the original injury were partial or the nerve undergoes incomplete regeneration, there may be return of sympathetic function without significant return of sensation.[34,36,46,47]

Vasomotor changes

Vasomotor function is reflected in temperature, color, and edema. For 2 to 3 weeks after complete denervation, or longer in some incomplete lesions, the skin feels warm to the touch because of vasodilatation secondary to paralysis of the vasoconstrictors.[44] This warm phase is gradually superseded, for reasons not completely understood, by a phase in which the skin feels cool to the touch. During the cold phase the patient may complain of cold intolerance. The skin temperature is abnormally influenced by environmental temperature, particularly cold, and when exposed to cold, the part becomes cold and rewarms slowly.[47] Cold intolerance may extend beyond the denervated part to include the entire hand and will recover only as reinnervation restores normal circulation.[44,47] According to Richards,[42] normal warmth of the skin does not occur until there is a high degree of sensory recovery.

Skin temperature is quickly assessed by use of the dorsum of the examiner's hand to compare the involved cutaneous area with the contralateral normal area. The dorsum is used because it is rich in temperature receptors and is less likely than the warm, moist volar skin to result in a false reading.

During the warm phase, the skin is flushed or rosy. During the cold phase it is usually mottled (a combination of pallor

Table 44-1 Sympathetic changes after nerve injury

Sympathetic function		Early changes	Late changes
Vasomotor	Skin color	Rosy	Mottled or cyanotic
	Skin temperature	Warm	Cool
Sudomotor	Sweat	Dry skin	Dry or overly moist
Pilomotor	Gooseflesh response	Absent	Absent
Trophic	Skin texture	Soft; smooth	Smooth; nonelastic
	Soft-tissue atrophy	Slight	More pronounced, especially in finger pulps
	Nail changes	Blemishes	Curved in longitudinal and horizontal planes; "talonlike"
	Hair growth	May fall out or become longer and finer	May fall out or become longer and finer
	Rate of healing	Slowed	Slowed

and cyanosis) or, in severe cases, reddish blue from stasis.[9] Color is assessed by comparison with the uninvolved hand.

Edema may occur as a result of decreased circulatory function and is more likely after brachial plexus injuries than distal injuries.[44]

Sudomotor changes

Lack of sweating occurs in the autonomous area of the sympathetic fibers immediately after denervation. Abnormally increased sweating, such that beads of sweat are clearly visible, may occur after partial nerve injury, especially when the nerve is irritated and pain is present, or during regeneration of a lacerated nerve.[23]

The presence of sweating does not imply the return of sensory function.[28,34,36] However, the absence of sweating in a recent nerve laceration or in a long-term injury does strongly correlate with a lack of discrimination sensation.[17,30]

Pilomotor changes

Absence of the "gooseflesh" response occurs when there is complete interruption of sympathetic supply to an area.[23] This phenomenon is not regularly included in a sensibility evaluation.

Trophic changes

Interruption of normal nerve supply results in interruption of the normal nutritive process of the tissues, thereby causing some atrophy of all tissues from skin to bone.[9] Decreased nutrition will be evident in skin texture, the soft tissue of the finger pulps, nail changes, hair growth, increased susceptibility to injury, and slowed healing.

Trophic changes are reversible as regeneration occurs. Persistent changes are associated with failure of regeneration or chronic irritation of a partial nerve lesion. Some nerves carry more sympathetic fibers than others; thus median nerve lesions result in more trophic changes (particularly noticeable in the index finger) than ulnar nerve lesions, which result in more changes than the radial nerve. Trophic changes will be more pronounced in causalgic states and in brachial plexus lesions than in simple nerve lacerations.[9,47]

Skin texture. Early on, the skin is thin and smooth, almost "velvety" because atrophy of the epidermis has caused the papillary ridges and finger creases to become less distinct. In long-term cases, the skin becomes shiny, smooth, and inelastic.[47] Examination is by visual observation and by palpation with the dorsum of the examining hand.

Atrophy of finger pulps. The generalized atrophy that follows denervation is most obvious in the pulps of the fingers, which may take on a tapered appearance. In fact, the entire digit may appear noticeably smaller than its corresponding digit on the other hand. This change occurs with long-term denervation because of irreparable injury or failure of regeneration; therefore it is not generally observed to reverse itself.[47]

Nail changes. Changes within the first few months include striations, ridges and similar blemishes, slowed growth, and increased hardness.[47] Later, in response to atrophy of the soft tissue of the digits, the nails conform to the shape of the atrophied pulp. They become smaller than the corresponding nail on the opposite hand and curve in the

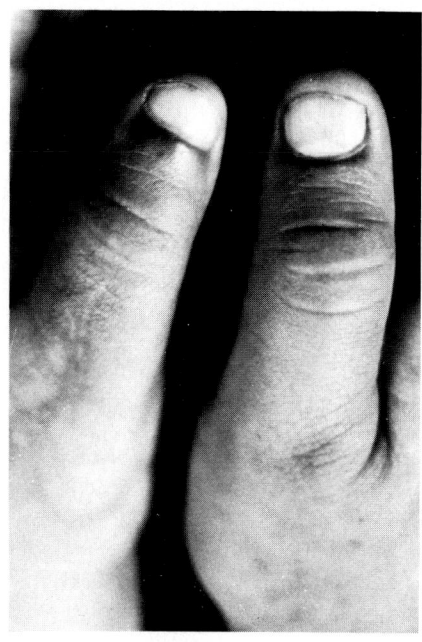

Fig. 44-1 Thumbnail changes in a case of chronic median nerve denervation. Notice that the nail on the left is smaller than the one on the right and has no visible lunula. The thumb has atrophied, and the nail has curved to conform to tapered tip.

longitudinal and horizontal planes. They may become talonlike in appearance. The lunula is diminished or absent (Fig. 44-1). Severe nail changes are signs of long-term denervation and therefore are not likely to improve with time.[47]

Hair growth. Hair may fall out in the region of denervation or may become longer and finer.[9] Occasionally it may demonstrate increased growth, termed "hypertrichosis," which state is most frequently noted on the forearm in radial nerve and median nerve injuries and occasionally in injuries of the brachial plexus.[23] Seddon[44] states that the apparent increase in growth of hair on the forearm is often attributable to atrophy of the denervated part. In causalgia, there is loss of hair where the skin is atrophic and shiny.[47]

Susceptibility to injury and slowed healing. Atrophy of the epidermis and underlying tissue causes the skin to become more delicate and therefore more susceptible to injury from noxious stimuli, including pressure, temperature, and sharp objects. This is clearly exemplified during the pinprick test when atrophic skin is penetrated by a sharp pin and responds with a minute spot of blood whereas normal skin on the same extremity does not. Healing takes longer than in normal skin because of decreased nutrition and vascularity, a condition that reverses itself as reinnervation occurs.[47] The patient who does not compensate for increased susceptibility to injury will frequently present with blisters and ulcers on the denervated skin (Fig. 44-2), whereas the presence of "wear" marks,[30] such as dirt stains and calluses, indicates functional use of the hand and is a sign of useful sensibility. Absence of "wear" marks on skin that has undergone reinnervation and has adequate motor function while other parts of the same hand demonstrate them indicates lack of use and useful sensibility of the unmarked parts (Fig. 44-3).

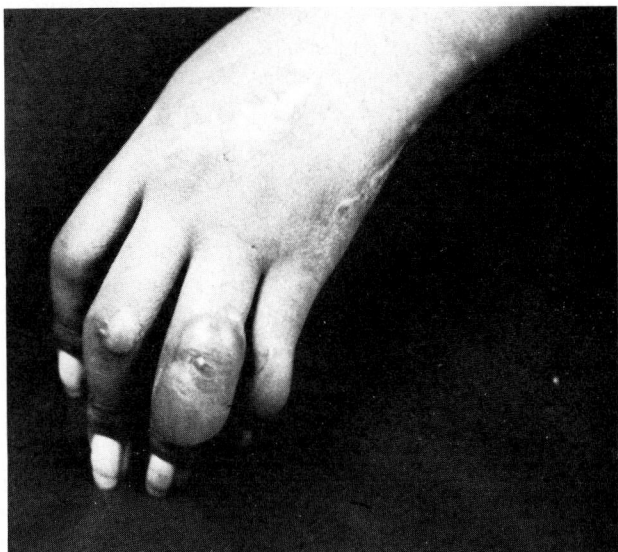

Fig. 44-2 This hand with median and ulnar nerve injury was allowed to rest against a hot radiator, resulting in second-degree burns to ulnar three digits.

A thorough history and examination of the hand will clue the experienced examiner to the status of sensibility in the hand. However, the details of sensory dysfunction and the progress of regeneration can only be determined through the administration of specific clinical tests designed to assess sensibility.

PATTERNS OF SENSIBILITY LOSS AND RECOVERY
Denervation

Pattern of loss. Immediately after denervation the autonomous area of nerve supply is anesthetic. Overlapping areas of supply with neighboring cutaneous nerves are hypesthetic. Therefore careful testing should elicit a borderline transition area between the zones of normal and absent sensibility. The transition area is smaller for touch sensibility than for pain sensibility.[44]

During the early weeks after denervation, some ingrowth of nerve supply from normal nerves occurs along the borders of the anesthetic area, thereby causing apparent shrinkage of the anesthetic zone. The exact mechanism for initiation of this phenomenon is not known.[44,47]

Pattern of recovery. The rate of regeneration of sensory fibers in humans generally falls within an average range of 1 to 2 mm per day, with wider ranges reported by some investigators.[43,47] An initial recovery rate of 3 mm per day is not unusual, with slowing of the rate over time.[43] Factors affecting the rate of regeneration within an individual include the nature and level of the lesion and the age of the patient.[53]

Pain elicited by pinch is a very early sign of sensory recovery and may precede a positive Tinel's sign.[47] Tenderness to pressure and to pinprick precede sensitivity to moving touch, which precedes light touch and discriminative touch.[9,44,47] At first, perceptions are poorly localized and may radiate proximally or distally. Accurate localization is among the last sensory functions to recover.[51]

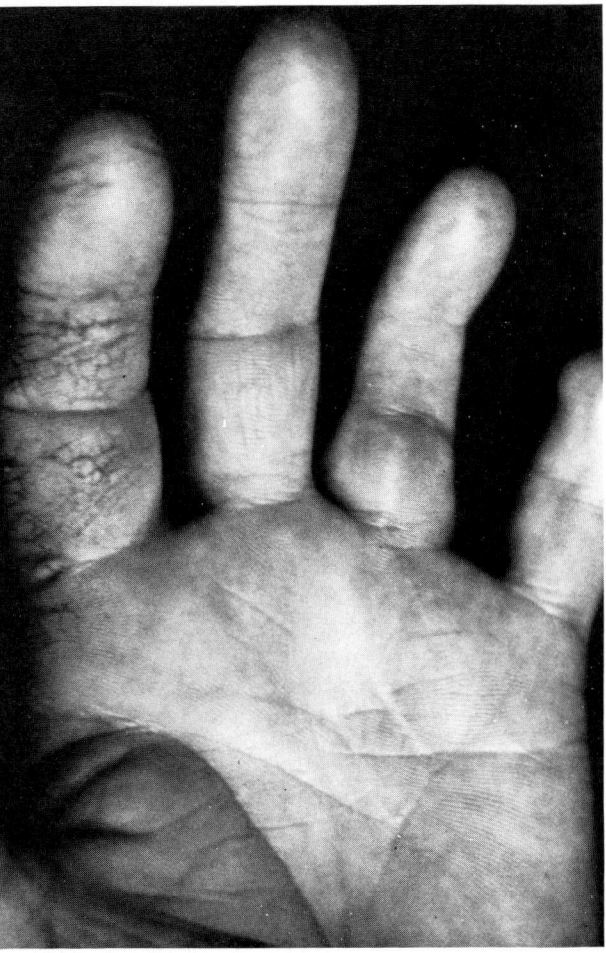

Fig. 44-3 "Wear marks" on this hand of a mechanic indicate that index finger is used for functional activities, but ulnar three digits, which had sustained digital nerve injury 1 year previously, are not. Testing revealed presence of light touch but poor discriminative sensation in involved digits.

Determination and interpretation of Tinel's sign. Tinel's sign[50] is assessed by gentle percussion from distal to proximal along the nerve trunk. The most distal point at which the patient experiences a tingling sensation that radiates distally in the cutaneous distribution of the nerve is the point of positive Tinel's sign. This sign is said to represent the advancing terminations of the regenerating sensory axons. Progress in regeneration can be documented by recording the level of Tinel's sign in successive examinations, using an anatomic landmark as a point of reference.

Seddon[44] states that a positive sign can occur in the presence of a partial, unrepaired nerve lesion, thereby falsely indicating regeneration. He credits Henderson[24] with making the sign more informative by his repeated observations on 400 cases of nerve injury in prisoner-of-war hospitals in World War II. Seddon states, "Henderson found that Tinel's sign became important about 4 months after the time of injury. If it was strongly positive at the level of the lesion but persistently absent below, spontaneous regeneration could not be expected. If the sign was strongly positive at the site of damage and also appeared weakly distal to it, the quality of regeneration would be poor. But a strongly positive sign at the level of the lesion that gradually faded as the response moved peripherally and became stronger in the distal part of the nerve indicated that satisfactory regeneration was in progress."

One must always assess the meaning of Tinel's sign in the context of other information gathered about sensory function. The sign may be absent where too much muscle lies over the nerve to allow adequate percussion of it.[44]

Mapping the area of dysfunction. Assessment of sensibility is made faster and more precise when one maps out the area of sensibility dysfunction before the administration of specific tests. This can be done in two ways.

MAPPING BY EXAMINER. The examiner draws a probe, such as the blunt end of a pen, lightly over the skin, starting from an area of normal sensibility and proceeding to the area of suspected abnormal sensibility. The patient, whose vision is occluded, is asked to immediately say "now" when the sensation produced by the probe is suddenly "different." Using a felt-tip pen, the examiner marks the skin at the spot where the patient said "now" and then proceeds to approach the area of dysfunction from another starting point. The area is thus approached from all directions—proximal, distal, radial, and ulnar—until all boundaries are marked (Fig. 44-4). (Note that in later stages of regeneration, when light touch is only slightly diminished, the patient may not experience a "suddenly different" sensation during application of the probe and so a map of sensory dysfunction is not obtained. This sign is interpreted as excellent progression in recovery of light touch.)

MAPPING BY PATIENT. Some examiners prefer to have the patient map the area of dysfunction. With vision unoccluded, the patient draws the probe across his skin as described above and marks on the skin where the sensation produced by the probe suddenly feels different. This method may allow for a more precise mapping.

With either method of mapping, the probe should be drawn fairly slowly across the skin with a light touch so that no drag is produced. Each time the probe passes over

the same path, a reliable patient will say "now" at the same location. Progress in reinnervation will be reflected in a progressively diminishing "map" size over time. The results of mapping should be transferred to an outline of the hand or photographed to provide a permanent record.

Compression

Pattern of loss. In early or mild cases, the patient might complain of intermittent numbness and paresthesia, especially nocturnal paresthesia, in the cutaneous distribution of the involved nerve. In more advanced cases, the symptoms are more constant and include positive sensibility test findings. In chronic, severe cases motor abnormalities are present.

Sensory fibers are more susceptible to early compression than motor fibers, and the large (touch) fibers are more susceptible than the smaller (pain) fibers. A specific pattern of sensory loss in nerve compression, specifically carpal tunnel syndrome, has been demonstrated by the work of Dellon,[13] Lundborg,[28] Gelberman,[19] and Szabo.[48,49]

Dellon[13] studied a group of 45 patients with 61 compressed nerves, using vibration (256 cps and 30 cps tuning forks), static and moving two-point discrimination, electrodiagnostic studies, Tinel's sign, and Phalen's sign. Among these seven tests, he found that diminished vibratory perception was the earliest detectable clinical abnormality in compression syndromes of insidious onset.

Lundborg and others[28] studied the effects of controlled acute external compression to the median nerves of 16 volunteer subjects. They compared motor nerve conduction, sensory nerve conduction, and two-point discrimination findings at three different levels of compression. Among these three tests, the researchers found a decrease in sensory potential amplitude to be the first detectable abnormality. In several cases, even when sensory potential amplitude was severely reduced, two-point discrimination tested within normal limits.

In another study using the same model of controlled compression on 12 volunteer subjects, Gelberman and others[19] compared findings from the following tests: vibration (256 cps), Semmes-Weinstein Pressure Aesthesiometer (monofilament test), static two-point discrimination, and moving two-point discrimination. They also monitored sensory and motor nerve conduction, subjective findings, and muscle strength. They found the following results:

1. A decrease in sensory amplitude was the earliest electrodiagnostic indication of impaired nerve function.
2. A high correlation was present between the Semmes-Weinstein monofilament test, vibratory testing, and sensory amplitude.
3. Changes in static and moving two-point discrimination consistently occurred together and occurred significantly later than abnormalities on the threshold test (that is, Semmes-Weinstein and vibration tests).
4. Regarding the two threshold tests, they noted a problem with the quantitation of vibratory stimulus and response using the tuning fork, and they described the Semmes-Weinstein monofilament test as the most accurate quantitative test in their model of acute compression.

In the next study in the series, Szabo, Gelberman, and Dimick[48] evaluated 20 patients with idiopathic carpal tunnel

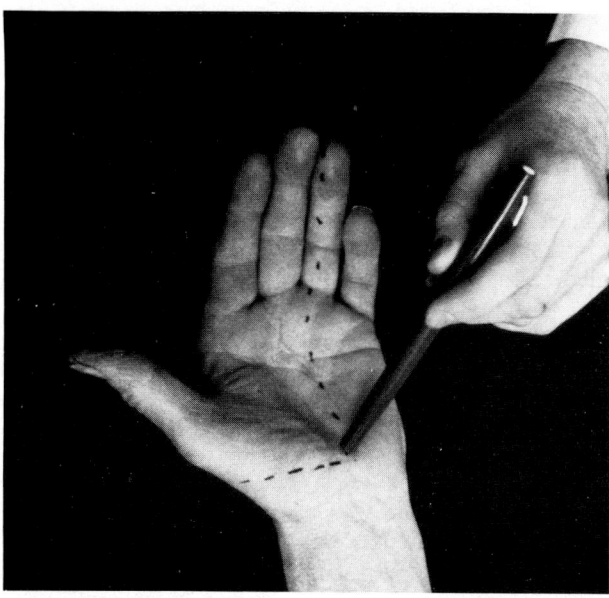

Fig. 44-4 Mapping area of dysfunction helps make subsequent testing faster and more accurate.

syndrome. All patients had objective abnormalities in median nerve conduction at the wrist level. Sensibility tests were administered before and after surgery. The researchers used a fixed frequency (120 Hz), variable amplitude vibrometer (Bio-Thesiometer*), and a 256 cps tuning fork to test vibration. The other tests were Semmes-Weinstein Pressure Aesthesiometer, two-point discrimination, Phalen's test, Tinel's test, and the tourniquet test. Their study confirmed that the threshold tests (that is, vibrometry and Semmes-Weinstein monofilaments) are more sensitive than two-point discrimination in assessing sensibility in chronic compression neuropathies.

In the next study, Szabo and others[49] returned to the model of controlled acute compression in 12 volunteer subjects. Because of the previously noted problem with quantitation of the tuning fork, they sought to compare findings from the vibrometer with findings from the 256 cps tuning fork, Semmes-Weinstein Pressure Aesthesiometer, static and moving two-point discrimination, and electrodiagnostic tests. They used the same vibrometer (Bio-Thesiometer) as in the previously cited study. They found that vibrometer abnormalities were the earliest clinical findings and had a high correlation with the less quantifiable tuning fork and slightly less sensitive Semmes-Weinstein Pressure Aesthesiometer. All three threshold tests were significantly more sensitive than two-point discrimination (p<0.01). They concluded that the vibrometer has significant potential as a clinical and research instrument in nerve compression syndromes.

To summarize, the conclusions to be drawn from these studies of acute and chronic compression neuropathies are the following:

1. The earliest objective finding is decreased sensory amplitude in electrodiagnostic testing.
2. The threshold tests, vibration and Semmes-Weinstein pressure test, are the most sensitive indicators of clinical abnormality in compression neuropathies.
3. A vibrometer offers the advantage of quantification over a tuning fork.
4. Abnormalities in moving and static two-point discrimination are late findings in compression neuropathy.

Pattern of recovery. The degree of recovery depends on the severity of compression. Mild compressions can undergo spontaneous recovery if the initiating cause is removed. Moderate-to-severe cases that require surgical intervention might respond in one of several ways including immediate full recovery; gradual full recovery; a period of postoperative hypersensitivity and nerve irritability followed by gradual full recovery; and partial recovery, with or without accompanying hypersensitivity and nerve irritability. Gelberman has classified carpal tunnel syndrome into four stages (early, intermediate, advanced, and acute) and has described the response to treatment of patients in each category.[18]

CATEGORIES OF SENSIBILITY TESTS

Sensibility tests can be divided into three main categories: threshold (or modality) tests, functional tests, and objective tests.

Threshold tests

Threshold tests seek to determine the minimum stimulus (within the limitations of the test instrument) that can be perceived by the subject. Threshold tests include those for the four classic cutaneous functions (pain, heat, cold, and touch—pressure) and for vibration.[14]

Functional tests

Functional tests allow one to assess the quality of sensibility. For example, is sensibility present on a gross level only, or on a fine discriminative level? Is it useful for fine-prehension tasks? Is it sufficient for daily activities and work tasks where vision is occluded during manipulation of objects? It is these qualities that Moberg has termed "tactile gnosis." These tests might also be considered as integrative tests because they require a higher level of sensory processing than the modality tests do.

Functional tests include static two-point discrimination, moving two-point discrimination, localization, Moberg pickup test, and others.[8,38,40] Some of these require active manipulation of an object rather than simply passive recognition of a stimulus. The requirement for active manipulation is based on recognition that touch is an active, exploratory process of the hand, not merely a passive receptive sense, and therefore touch can be more accurately assessed if the hand is permitted to actively explore and "scan" the object presented.[20]

Objective tests

This category includes the Ninhydrin sweat test and other tests of sudomotor function, nerve-conduction studies, and the wrinkle test.[35] These are termed "objective" because they require only passive cooperation of the patient and not his subjective interpretation of a stimulus. They do not directly correlate with functional sensation after nerve repair.[1,34,36,46] However, the sudomotor and wrinkle tests can be useful in obtaining information about the function of a nerve in children and malingerers, and nerve-conduction tests provide useful information about conduction parameters in a nerve (see Chapter 55).

CONTROL OF VARIABLES IN TESTING

Regardless of which tests are used, one must keep in mind that many variables contribute to the subjective nature of sensibility testing. Some variables can be controlled by the careful tester; others are not yet under our control but are being studied (see Chapter 42). The examiner's knowledge of the nature of these variables and attempt to control them will help make testing more accurate and reliable.

Environment-related variables

Background noise is distracting to the patient and the tester. A test administered in a noisy environment is not the same as one administered in a quiet environment. To minimize the effect of noise, all testing should be done in a quiet room. The examiner must be alert for sound made by a testing instrument before or during the application of a stimulus, which will cue the patient to a change in stimulus. Similarly, the sound of a starched coat sleeve as the examiner moves about will cue the patient to the arrival of a stimulus. These extraneous noises, and other sources of noise, must be eliminated from the sensibility examination.

---

*Bio-Medical Instrument Company, Newbury, Ohio.

Patient-related variables

Patient-related variables have to do with patient attitude, level of concentration, and possibly anxiety level. Each patient will bring his own agenda to a sensibility test. Some will want to test well; others will not. Some are suggestible and may imagine a stimulus when there is none; others admit a sensation only if they are absolutely positive it was felt. Methods are being sought to control for some of these patient-related psychologic variables.[10]

Normal callused skin has a higher sensory threshold than normal uncallused skin in the hand because a given stimulus will deform callused skin less than soft, supple skin. Therefore areas of callosity should be noted so that test results can be more validly assessed. Because sensitivity varies within the normal population, the uninvolved hand is always the best control in the determination of sensibility dysfunction.

Instrument-related variables

Instrument-related variables include quality control in the manufacturing of instruments and variations in the same instrument over time.[27] Instruments that can be calibrated should be regularly. The examiner should be aware of the idiosyncrasies of each instrument that he uses. For example, certain two-point discrimination instruments are heavier than others; so the examiner must be careful not to exert a heavier pressure when testing with a heavier instrument.

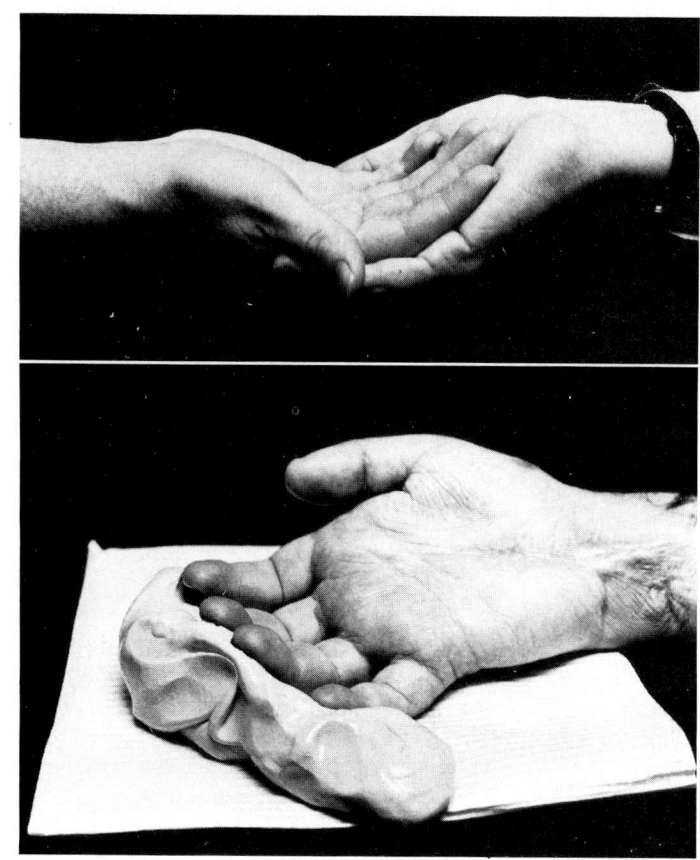

Fig. 44-5 **A,** Hand to be tested should be fully supported in examiner's hand or, **B,** fully supported in putty or a similar medium.

Method-related variables

The same test instrument, even a cotton ball, in two different examiner's hands can produce different results because of differences in the methods of administration. For example, one examiner may use more pressure than the other or may stimulate with a moving instead of a constant touch. Control of method-related variables can be assisted by the following:
1. Standard instructions to the patient before each test.
2. Use a standard method of supporting the hand during threshold testing and certain functional tests. Brand[7] has recommended that the hand be fully supported in the examiner's hand so that inadvertent stretch of tissues and movement of joints can be avoided (Fig. 44-5, *A*). He has further suggested that a better method of support would be to rest the hand in putty or similar medium that would provide full support (Fig. 44-5, *B*). Use of such a medium would have the advantage of eliminating transmission of random vibration in the supporting hand to the hand being tested.[5,7]
3. Parameters of stimulus application must remain the same within a test and between tests. Important parameters include speed of stimulus application, which is known to affect perception,[21] the amount of pressure exerted on the skin, and whether the stimulus is moving or constant.
4. The time interval between applications of the stimulus and the spacing of stimuli must be varied so that the patient cannot anticipate the timing or location of the next stimulus.
5. Results should be carefully documented for better comparison between successive tests.

Bell and Buford[5] demonstrated that when a stimulus is applied with a hand-held instrument, the examiner is unable to control for force of application. In part this is caused by vibration of the hand holding the instrument. An exception is the Semmes-Weinstein Pressure Aesthesiometer. Bell and Tomancik[4] showed that if the lengths and diameters of the filaments are correct, the application forces that they produce are repeatable within a predictable range.

Examiner-related variables

Experience, attention to detail, and concern for adherence to methods of administration will affect test results, as will the examiner's level of concentration and fatigue. To minimize the former variables, the same examiner should perform successive tests on a given patient.

ADMINISTRATION OF SPECIFIC TESTS
Threshold tests

Threshold tests of pain and touch-pressure are particularly useful for monitoring return of sensibility in the early months after nerve laceration.

Threshold tests of vibration and touch-pressure are used to assess early changes in sensibility caused by nerve compression.[13,18,48,49]

A goal in threshold testing is to record information in a way that allows for more reliable comparison with follow-up reports. When testing for pain, temperature, or touch-pressure, one can make testing more systematic and documentation more accurate by use of a work sheet that has a grid superimposed on an outline of the hand (Fig. 44-6). The grid is divided into zones, whose longitudinal lines

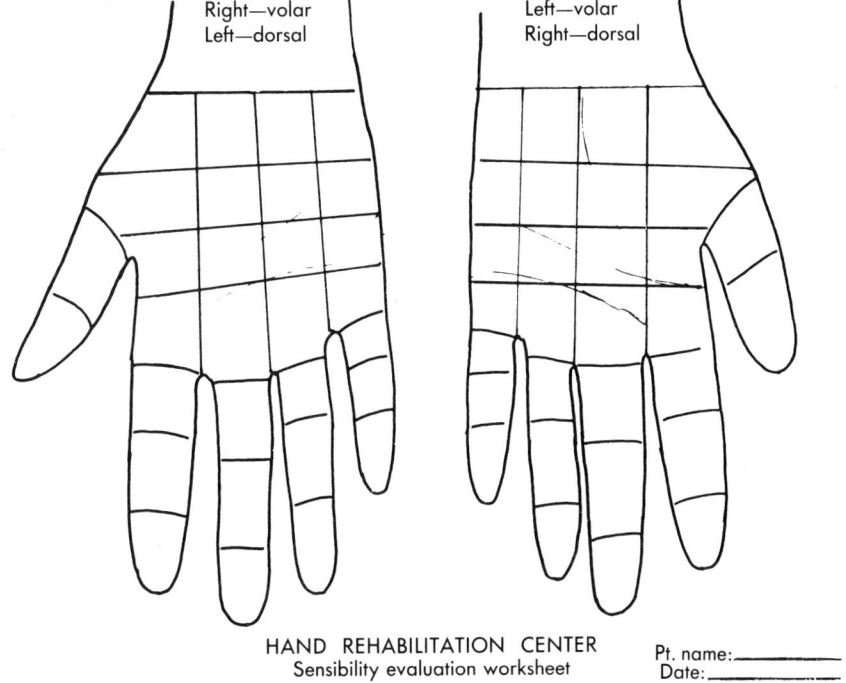

Right—volar
Left—dorsal

Left—volar
Right—dorsal

HAND REHABILITATION CENTER
Sensibility evaluation worksheet

Pt. name:_____
Date:_____

Fig. 44-6   Grid work sheet is recommended during threshold testing to make testing and documentation more systematic.

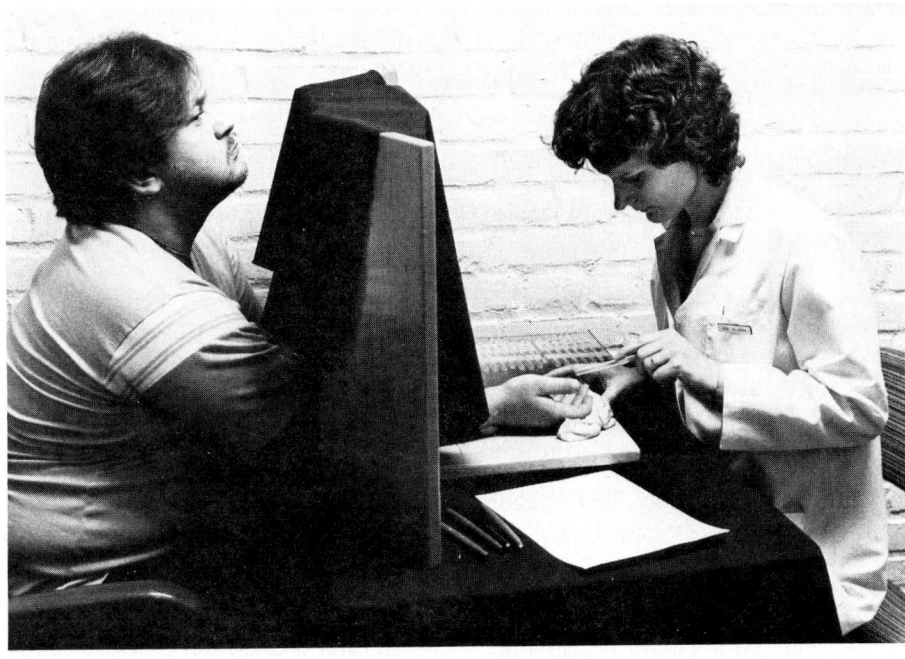

Fig. 44-7   Screen used for sensibility testing allows test instruments and work sheets to be hidden from patient's view.

parallel the rays of the hand and whose horizontal lines correspond to the flexion creases of the digits and palm. This grid was devised by von Prince[51] for use in her studies of light-touch dysfunction in nerve-injured patients in the 1960s, but the grid is useful for other tests as well. During testing, the examiner visualizes the grid on the patient's hand and applies the test stimulus to a particular zone. Correct and incorrect responses are recorded in the corresponding zone on the work sheet. A different work sheet can be used for each test, and the work sheets can be filed for permanent records or the information on the work sheet can be transferred to a more formal report. The use of this grid will be elaborated on below in the description of methodology for the threshold tests.

During all threshold tests the hand is fully supported in the examiner's hand or in putty (Fig. 44-5). Vision is occluded by use of a blindfold, by the patient simply closing his eyes, or by a screen (Fig. 44-7). The last method is ideal because it allows test instruments and recording sheets to be hidden from view even between tests when vision might not otherwise be occluded.

Pinprick. Protective sensation is defined as the ability to perceive painful or potentially harmful stimuli on the skin and in the subcutaneous tissue. Heat, cold, deep pressure, low-grade repetitive pressure, and superficial pain are examples of such stimuli. Of these, the most commonly tested and the one regarded as the best test of protective sensation is superficial pain tested with a safety pin. It is not sufficient simply to require the patient to say "now" when touched with the sharp end of the pin because he may respond simply to pressure of the stimulus and not sharpness of the stimulus. A more accurate assessment of protective sensation requires that he discriminate between the sharp and dull sides of the pin.

When testing with a pin, the examiner should keep in mind that during nerve regeneration a period of hypersensitivity to pinprick will occur. In the area of hyperanalgesia, the response to pinprick will be hyperacute, that is, abnormally unpleasant. Therefore testing should proceed in such a way that the number of applications of the stimulus in one "zone" of the hand are minimized.

The amount of pressure necessary to elicit correct responses on the uninvolved hand is used as a guide for pressure to be used on the involved hand. It is not unusual to observe minute spots of blood where the pin has penetrated the fragile outer layer of skin in a denervated hand, even though only light pressure has been used.

The grid is used as a work sheet during testing. The examiner alternates randomly between the sharp and dull sides of the pin, being sure that each zone has been stimulated at least once by each end of the pin so that true discrimination within an area has been ascertained. A code is used to mark each zone tested on the work sheet, as follows: $+S$ (correct response to sharp), $-S$ (no response to sharp), $+D$ (correct response to dull), $-D$ (no response to dull), "S" (reported dull stimulus as "sharp"), and "D" (reported sharp stimulus as "dull"). The entire area of dysfunction, as determined previously by mapping, is tested.

Results within a zone are interpreted as follows: correct response to both sharp and dull, intact protective sensation; incorrect response to both sharp and dull, absent protective sensation; "S," hyperanalgesic; "D," pressure awareness.

Sunderland notes that the perception of pinprick ranges along a hierarchy that includes absence of awareness, pressure sensation without distinguishing between sharp and dull, hyperanalgesia with radiation, sharp sensation with some radiation and gross localization, sensation of sharpness with or without slight stinging or radiation and fair localization, and, finally, normal perception.[47] Seddon likewise grades the response to pinprick along several parameters.[44]

It should be noted that Kirk and Denny-Brown[26] found pin scratch to be a more reliable stimulus than pinprick in their studies of dorsal-root lesions in monkeys; however, pin scratch has not been generally adopted clinically.

Moberg[32] and Dellon,[14] among others, have stated that they do not test for pinprick because of the discomfort involved to the patient and because the information gained does not correlate directly with functional sensation. However, one can argue for testing pinprick after nerve laceration if other indications of sensibility return are absent. In these instances it becomes important to know if this parameter of protective sensation is intact.

Temperature. Test tubes or metal cylinders filled with hot and cold fluids are the usual instruments used for clinical testing of temperature perception. The limitation of these instruments is that the information obtained is gross if the temperatures are not carefully controlled. The clinician can determine if the patient can distinguish between hot and cold, but not if he can distinguish between temperatures 1° to 5° C apart, as in the normal hand, or if he can distinguish between temperatures along the entire range of very cold to very hot. Therefore the tester must be cautious about reporting that the patient has normal temperature sensation, which implies good discriminative ability, if he has simply tested hot and cold at one interval in the range.

Because of the difficulties in controlling test conditions within a test and between tests and the lack of correlation with functional sensation, many clinicians do not test for temperature discrimination.[14,31,44,47] Some clinicians satisfy themselves with testing simply for the perception of hot and cold on a gross level; others do not test for temperature at all, preferring to allow the presence of pinprick perception to be sufficient evidence of protective sensation.

Light touch–deep pressure. Light touch sensibility and deep pressure sensibility are considered to represent two ends of a continuum of cutaneous sensibility, with light touch being perceived by receptors in the superficial skin layers and pressure being perceived by receptors in the subcutaneous and deeper tissue.[47] Pressure sensibility is a form of protective sensation, because it warns of deep pressure or of low-grade repetitive pressure, which might result in injury to the skin. Light touch sensibility is a necessary component of fine discrimination.

Many have sought to improve the testing of light touch by using an instrument that could grade the amount of pressure applied to the skin from light to deep.[25,44,51] Such instruments have been developed to enable more precise monitoring and documentation of progress in return of light touch and the quality of that touch. These test instruments are all variations on the graded stimulus developed by von Frey in 1895 in his classic studies of touch threshold.

In 1960 Semmes and Weinstein[45] developed a graded light touch testing instrument for use in a study of somatosensory changes in brain-injured adults. The instrument is now

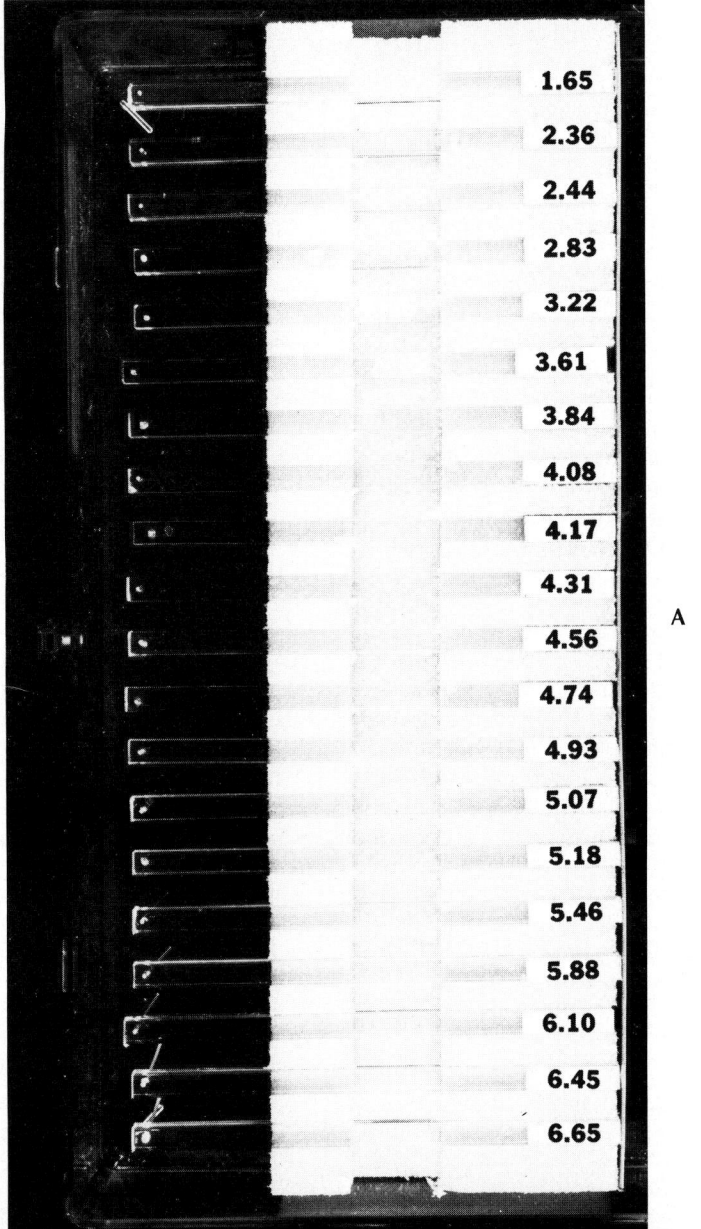

1.65
2.36
2.44
2.83
3.22
3.61
3.84
4.08
4.17
4.31
4.56
4.74
4.93
5.07
5.18
5.46
5.88
6.10
6.45
6.65

A

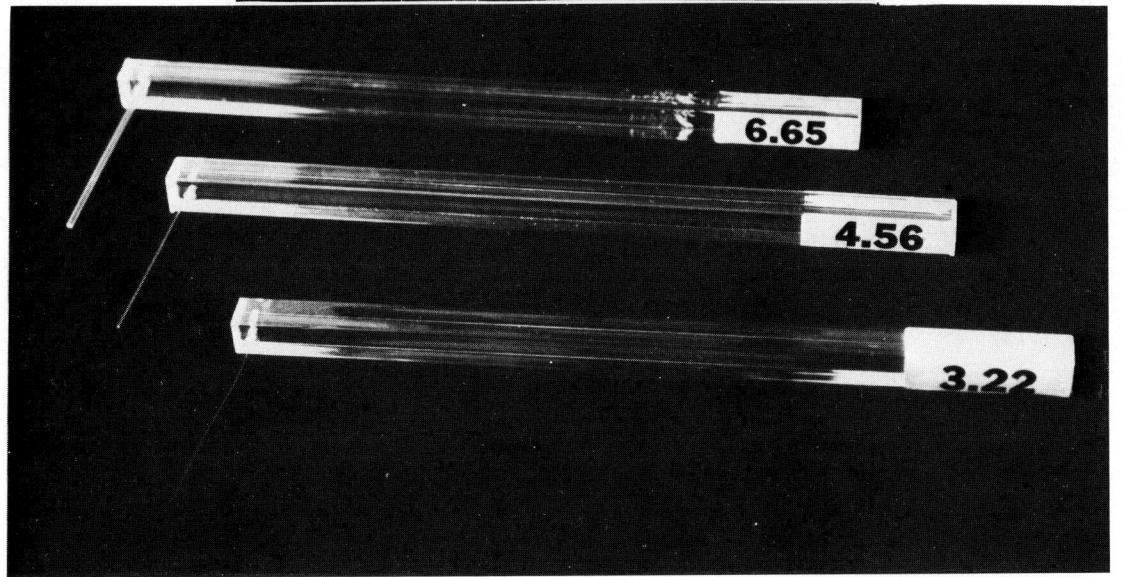

6.65
4.56
3.22

B

Fig. 44-8 **A,** Semmes-Weinstein Pressure Aesthesiometer. **B,** Each probe consists of a nylon monofilament attached to a Lucite rod.

known as the Semmes-Weinstein Pressure Aesthesiometer* and includes a kit of 20 probes (Fig. 44-8, *A*), each probe consisting of a nylon monofilament attached to a polymethylmethacrylate (Lucite) rod (Fig. 44-8, *B*). Each probe is marked with a number ranging from 1.65 to 6.65 that represents the logarithm of 10 times the force in milligrams required to bow the monofilament (log 10 F_{mg}).[27] Thus the finest filament, labeled 1.65, will "bow" when it is applied at a perpendicular angle to the skin with a force of 0.0045 gm, and the thickest filament, labeled 6.65, will bow at 448 gm.

In 1967 von Prince[52] introduced this instrument into the clinic for use in testing light touch–deep pressure sensibility in the nerve-injured hand. Her pioneering efforts were taken up by Werner and Omer[54] and Bell.[3] The methods of administration and interpretation of this test are described in detail in Chapter 43.

Vibration

Tuning fork. According to the methods of Dellon,[14] testing with a 256 cps tuning fork in nerve compression syndromes is done as follows. The tuning fork is first struck against a surface and then one of the prong ends is applied tangential to the surface being tested. (Bell and Buford[5] found that force amplitude is more controllable when the base of the tuning fork is applied.) The examiner attempts to control intensity of amplitude by trying to maintain the same striking force with each application of the tuning fork. The fingertips of the thumb and index fingers are the test sites in median nerve compression, the tip of the small finger in ulnar nerve compression. The patient closes his eyes during the test. The vibrating tuning fork is applied to the test site and to two control sites: the contralateral fingertip and an ipsilateral noninvolved fingertip.

---

*North Coast Medical, Campbell, Calif.

a test site and a control site, he is asked, "How did they feel different?" Responses such as "didn't feel anything," "softer," "louder," "quieter," and others are recorded as "abnormal" perception. Dellon also requires that the vibration be localized, to rule out perception by a neighboring nerve.

Vibrometer. The vibrometer (Bio-Thesiometer) consists of a hand-held, variable-amplitude, fixed-frequency vibrator and a voltage meter (which measures increasing voltage as vibration amplitude is increased). Instructions for operation and administration accompany the instrument. The stimulus is first demonstrated to the patient on an uninvolved area of the hand, starting at an amplitude below threshold and continuing up to and past threshold. The patient is instructed to close his eyes during the test and to say "now" as soon as he feels the first sensation of vibration. The examiner supports the finger being tested and applies the stimulus through a button-shaped vibrating head held against the finger. The suspected involved fingertips are tested, as well as ipsilateral and contralateral fingertips.

The threshold level is recorded in volts from the voltage meter. This reading can be converted to absolute amplitude (measured in microns) through a calibration table furnished with the instrument. Although the vibrometer has limitations in common with other hand-held testing instruments[5] (see Chapter 42), it provides a more quantitative assessment of vibration than does the tuning fork and allows for more reliable comparison of preoperative and postoperative thresholds.

Functional tests

The presence of fine discriminative sensation determines the usefulness of sensibility in daily activities. Therefore selection of tests and interpretation of results must be done carefully before one declares that a patient has normal discriminative sensibility.

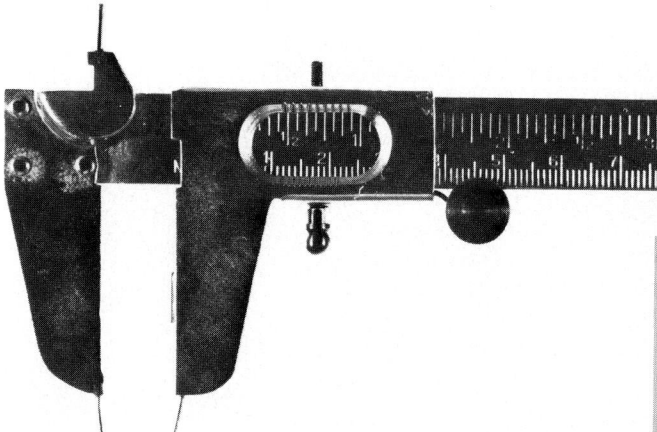

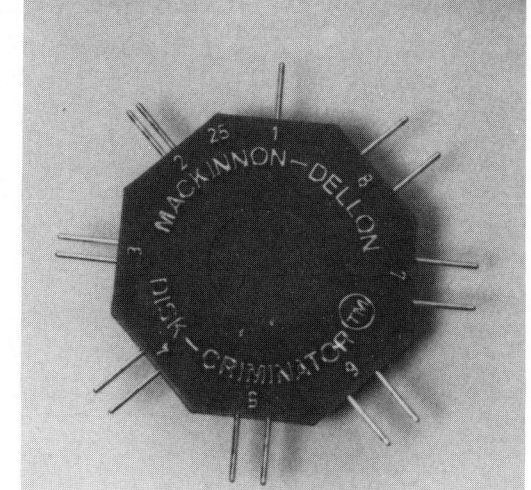

Fig. 44-9 Recommended instruments for testing two-point discrimination include: **A,** Boley Gauge and **B,** the Disk-Criminator.

Static two-point discrimination. Two-point discrimination is the classic test of functional sensibility because it is generally acknowledged to relate to the ability to use the hand for fine tasks.[30,34] (However, Dellon[14] has summarized several studies that refute this correlation.) Moberg has stated that 6 mm of two-point discrimination is required for winding a watch, 6 to 8 mm for sewing, and 12 mm for handling precision tools, and that above 15 mm gross tool handling may be possible, but only with decreased speed and skill.

The test instrument should be light and have blunt testing ends. The Disk-Criminator*[30] and the Boley Gauge† are two such instruments.

During the test, the patient's hand should be fully supported. Vision is occluded. Only the fingertips need be tested because it is the fingertips that are the most important in active exploration and tactile scanning of an object. Testing is begun with 5 mm distance between the two points. One or two points are applied lightly to the fingertip in a random sequence in a longitudinal orientation to avoid crossover from overlapping digital nerves (Fig. 44-10). A common error is to apply too much pressure. Since it is light touch discrimination that is being tested and the patient is to be compared to the normal population, the pressure applied should be very light and stop just at the point of blanching.[7]

---

*Disk-Criminator, PO Box 16392, Baltimore 21210.
†Boley Gauge, Research Designs, Inc., Houston.

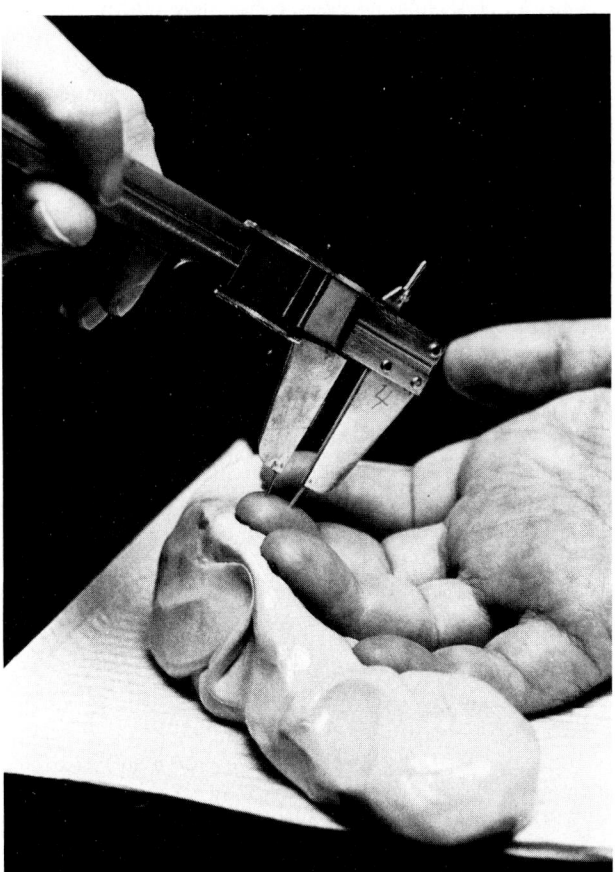

Fig. 44-10 The two-point discrimination instrument is applied lightly to fingertip in a longitudinal orientation.

Seven out of 10 responses must be accurate for scoring. If the responses are inaccurate, the distance between the ends is increased by increments of 1, 2, or 5 mm, depending on the suspected severity of the dysfunction, until the required accurate responses are elicited. Testing is stopped at 15 mm (or less, if the pulp is not of sufficient length) if responses are inaccurate at that level.

Interpretation of scores is based on the guidelines set by the American Society for Surgery of the Hand[2] (Table 44-2).

Localization of touch. None of the tests described thus far have required localization of a stimulus. Localization represents a more integrated level of perception than simple recognition of a stimulus; therefore it should be tested as a separate function. The ability to localize was found by Weinstein[53] in a study of 48 normal adults to have a high correlation with two-point discrimination (.92), while neither two-point discrimination nor localization was found to have a high correlation with light touch threshold (.17 and .28, respectively). Because of its high correlation with two-point discrimination, localization is considered to be a test of functional sensation.

Localization is most appropriate for testing after nerve repair because the poor localization that typically occurs after repair can seriously limit function. The stimulus used is the finest diameter Semmes-Weinstein monofilament that could be perceived throughout the area of dysfunction. Localization is tested over the entire area of dysfunction.

The grid is quite useful for recording the results of this test.[54] With the patient's vision occluded and the hand fully supported, the selected monofilament is applied to the center of a zone. (Similarly, moving touch localization can be tested by applying a moving touch stimulus along the longitudinal midline of a selected zone.) The patient is instructed to open his eyes each time he feels a touch and point to the exact spot touched. His responses will be more accurate if he uses his vision to help localize than if he attempts to localize with his eyes closed.[22] If the stimulus is correctly localized, a dot is marked in the corresponding zone on the work sheet. If the stimulus is incorrectly localized, an arrow is drawn on the work sheet from the site of stimulation to the site of referral (Fig. 44-11). Each zone is stimulated only once. The resulting data on the work sheet are used as the permanent record. The work sheet gives the examiner and the patient a graphic representation of the quality of localization and points out patterns of referral that might be amenable to sensory reeducation. With improvement in localization over time, the localization work sheets should demonstrate fewer and shorter arrows.

Moving two-point discrimination. The rationale for this test, devised by Dellon,[11,12] is that because fingertip sensibility is highly dependent on motion, the stimulus for discrimination testing should be moving. As when testing static

Table 44-2 Two-point discrimination norms

Normal:	Less than 6 mm
Fair:	6 to 10 mm
Poor:	11 to 15 mm
Protective:	One point perceived
Anesthetic:	No points perceived

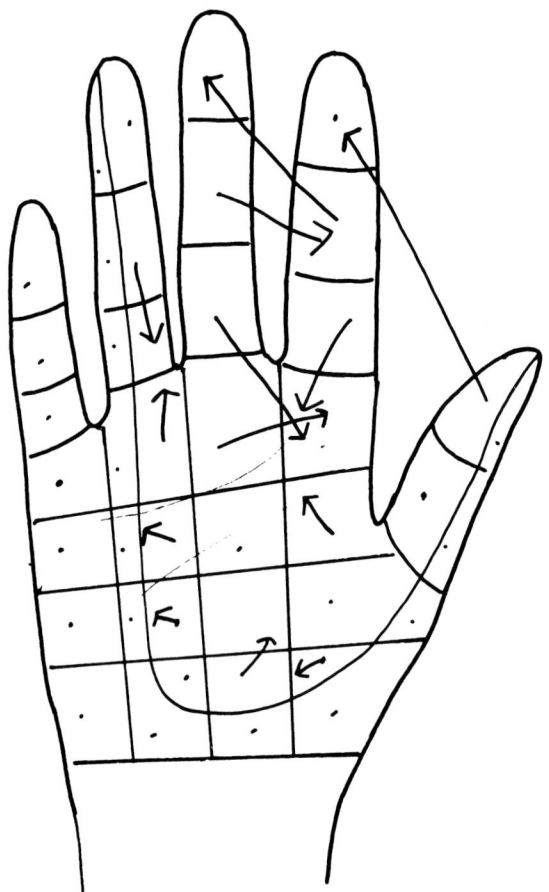

Fig. 44-11 Mapping of localization. *Dot,* Stimulus that was accurately perceived; *arrow,* referred stimulus; *arrowhead,* point to which stimulus was referred.

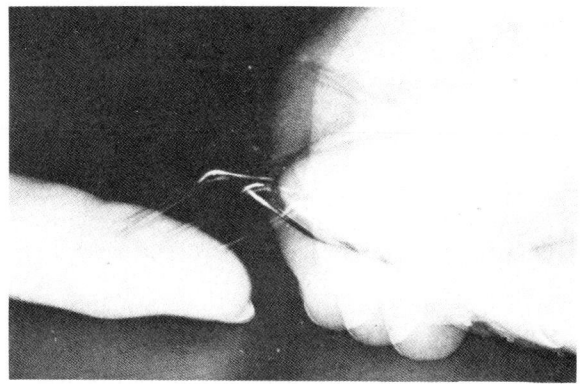

Fig. 44-12 The m2PD instrument is moved lightly across fingertip from proximal to distal position. (From Dellon AL: J Hand Surg 3:474, 1978.)

two-point discrimination, the test instrument for moving two-point discrimination should be light and have blunt testing ends. In accordance with the methods described by Dellon,[11] testing is begun with the instrument set at an 8 mm distance between the two points. The instrument is moved proximally to distally on the fingertip parallel to the long axis of the finger, with the testing ends side by side (Fig. 44-12). The pressure used is just light enough so that the subject can appreciate the stimulus. Once the patient is inaccurate or hesitant in responding, he is required to respond accurately to 7 out of 10 stimuli before the distance is narrowed. Testing is stopped at 2 mm, which represents normal moving two-point discrimination.

Dellon has reported that moving two-point discrimination always returns earlier than two-point discrimination after nerve laceration and approaches normal 2 to 6 months before two-point discrimination reaches normal. Therefore he advocates this test as a more valid assessment of discrimination and as an earlier means of assessing return of discrimination than the classic two-point test.

Moberg pickup test. The Moberg pickup test[30,31] requires motor participation and is most appropriate for median or combined medioulnar lesions. An assortment of everyday objects, the number and nature of which are selected by the examiner, is placed on a table in front of the patient. He is instructed to pick them up one at a time, as fast as he can,

and place them into a box using his involved hand (Fig. 44-13, *A*). The examiner times him and notes which digits are used for prehension. The patient repeats the task with his uninvolved hand. Finally, he is asked to pick up objects again, but this time with eyes closed. Again, time required and manner of prehension are noted. When locating and picking up objects with vision occluded, the patient will tend not to use sensory surfaces that have poor sensibility (Fig. 44-13, *B*).

Norms have not been established for this test. Its value lies in the observations that can be made during the brief time it requires to administer. Taking into account motor deficits, the best comparison for the involved hand is the performance by the uninvolved hand. The test can be made more difficult by requiring the patient to identify the objects as he picks them up.

Dellon modification of Moberg pickup test. Dellon has modified the pickup test by standardizing the items used and requiring identification of them. He chose objects of similar material to avoid giving cues by texture or temperature and objects graded to require increasing ability to discriminate (Fig. 44-14).[12]

In cases in which the ulnar nerve is not involved, the ulnar digits are taped to the palm. The patient is timed as he picks up the objects and places them into a box. If the motor deficit is judged too severe during this sighted part of the test, the test is discontinued. If the deficit is not too severe, vision is occluded and the examiner places one item at a time into the median three digits for patient identification. The time required for identification is recorded; no more than 30 seconds is permitted per object. Each object is presented twice.

Objective tests

Two objective tests, the Ninhydrin sweat test and the wrinkle test, are described below because of their occasional usefulness in testing, especially for children and suspected malingerers. As stated previously, they can give suggestive evidence of sensory function early after nerve laceration and in long-term cases where regeneration has failed, but they do not correlate directly with the presence or absence of sensibility during regeneration.[36,37,47]

Ninhydrin sweat test. The method of administration has

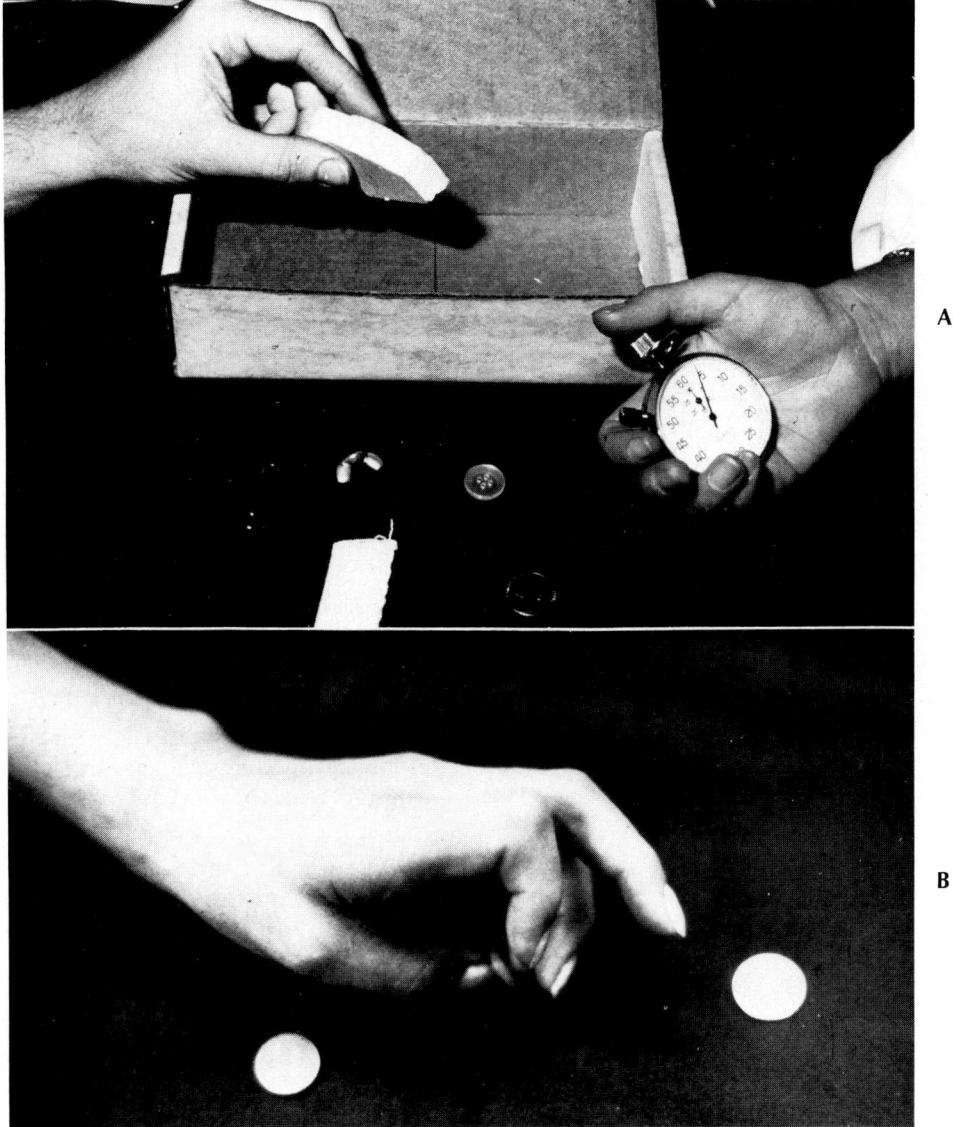

Fig. 44-13 **A,** Moberg pickup test. **B,** When locating and picking up objects with vision occluded, patient will tend not to use sensory surfaces that have poor sensibility.

been described by several authors,[17,30,36,37,46] but those described by Perry[36] and Phelps[37] are the easiest to follow since they make use of commercially available Ninhydrin developer and fixer (Fig. 44-15). The essentials of their techniques are presented below.

The patient's hand is cleansed thoroughly with soap and warm water, rinsed thoroughly, and then wiped with ether, alcohol, or acetone. Perry recommends a 5-minute waiting period to allow the normal sweating process to ensue, whereas Phelps requires a 20- to 30-minute period to elapse before proceeding with the test. During the waiting period, the patient's fingertips must not come into contact with any surface.

At the end of the waiting period, the fingertips are pressed with a moderate amount of pressure against a good quality bond paper (no. 20) that has previously been untouched. The fingertips are traced with a pencil and held in place for 15 seconds. During this time the examiner must be careful not to touch any part of the paper and the patient's fingertips

must not slide on the paper to avoid contamination of the results.

The paper is then sprayed with Ninhydrin spray reagent (N-0507)* and allowed to dry for 24 hours or heated in an oven for 5 to 10 minutes at 200° F (93° C). During the development period the Ninhydrin stains purple the amino acids and lower peptide components of sweat that have penetrated the paper. After development, the prints are sprayed with Ninhydrin fixer reagent (N-0757)* for a permanent record of the results.

According to Perry, a good normal print is one in which dots can be clearly visualized representing discrete sweat gland orifices. A blank print indicates that no sweating has occurred. A smudged print may represent a finger that moved during testing, or hyperhidrosis that has stained beyond its boundaries and may be masking an area of anhidrosis.[36]

---

*Sigma Chemical Company, St. Louis.

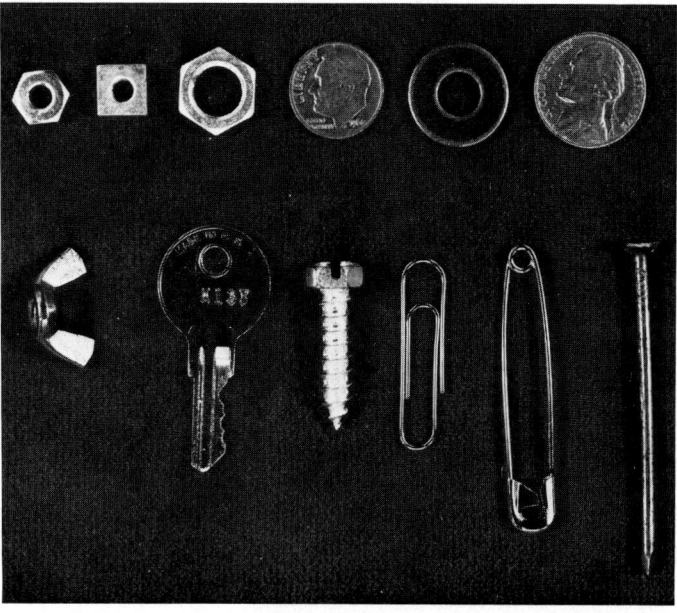

Fig. 44-14 Items used in Dellon modification of Moberg pickup test.

Moberg has scored Ninhydrin test results on a 0 to 3 scale, with 0 representing absent sweating and 3 representing normal sweating.[30]

Wrinkle test. The wrinkle test was described by O-Riain[35] in 1973. He observed that a denervated hand placed in warm water (40° C; 104° F) for 30 minutes does not wrinkle in the denervated area as normal skin does. He associated this phenomenon with an absence of sensory function and the return of wrinkling with a return of sensory function.

In a study of 41 nerve-injured patients, using the same finger-wrinkling method, Phelps[37] found that only after recent complete laceration did an absence of finger wrinkling always correlate with an absence of sensibility. In patients with nerve compression, the presence of wrinkling does not indicate intact sensibility. Therefore the wrinkle test appears to be of most use after recent nerve laceration, particularly in children and others unable or unwilling to cooperate with a sensibility examination.

Phelps noted that the results of finger wrinkling are difficult to document, even photographically. She used the same 0 to 3 scoring system to rate the amount of wrinkling that Moberg used for scoring the Ninhydrin test.

SENSIBILITY EVALUATION BATTERY

Because no single test can adequately assess the complexity of sensibility, evaluation is best approached by a battery of tests. Presented here are recommendations for test

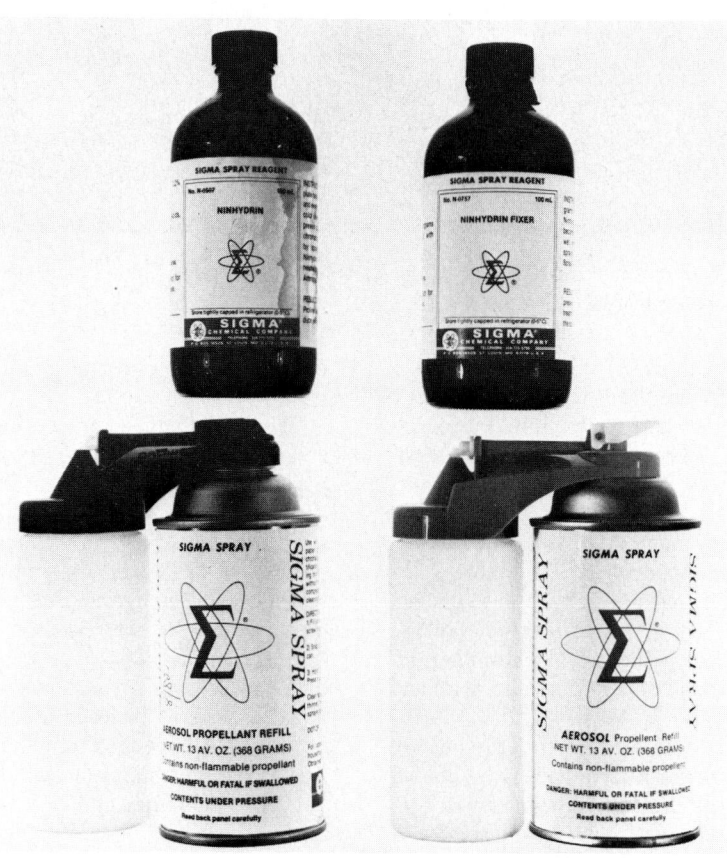

Fig. 44-15 Materials required for ninhydrin sweat test.

selection after laceration, crush, or traction injuries and for compression syndromes.

Laceration, crush, or traction injury

Recommended components of a sensibility battery are the following:
1. History
2. Examination of the hand for evidence of sympathetic dysfunction
3. Tinel's test to determine level of regenerating axons
4. Serial mapping to determine shrinkage or lack of shrinkage of the area of dysfunction
5. Semmes-Weinstein monofilament testing to assess level of touch return. In areas of the hand that are unresponsive to the thickest diameter filaments, the pinprick test is recommended
6. If there is return of touch to the fingertips, static and moving two-point discrimination tests on the fingertips and localization of touch tested on the entire area of dysfunction will provide information on the level of functional return
7. The Moberg pickup test and Dellon modification of the pickup test integrate motor and sensory function and are quickly administered. Either is appropriate for median or combined medioulnar nerve dysfunction. Inspection of the hand for "wear marks" and the patient's report of functional use of the hand in activities of daily living will provide further evidence of functional sensibility

For those suspected of malingering, the Semmes-Weinstein Pressure Aesthesiometer can be especially useful in documenting inconsistencies in responses. For the child, the wrinkle test, possibly the ninhydrin sweat test, and the Moberg pickup test may provide the information desired regarding function.

Compression syndrome

Recommended components of a sensibility battery are these:
1. History
2. Tinel's test at the suspected compression site(s) (though it should be noted that a negative test does not rule out compression at that site)
3. Nerve conduction testing to detect early decrease in sensory nerve potential amplitude
4. Vibratory testing to detect early sensory changes
5. Semmes-Weinstein monofilament testing to detect early changes in touch-pressure perception
6. Static and moving two-point discrimination testing to detect advanced sensory changes

Test selection will be influenced by time available for testing, examiner familiarity with a particular test, and age and concentration level of the patient. In all cases, however, the selected battery must be administered in a manner designed to minimize variables, and the results must be interpreted knowledgeably.

SUMMARY

A thorough and accurate sensibility evaluation requires a careful history, knowledgeable examination of sympathetic function in the hand, skillful interviewing of the patient, and knowledge of available tests and their correct administration. Additionally, the examiner must strive to control the variables associated with testing and select a battery of tests designed to answer specific questions based on the patient's history. The careful examiner who criticizes his methods and who listens to his patients will learn from each patient and will become a skilled examiner. The skilled examiner will accept the challenge of sensibility as an always interesting and at times fascinating task.

REFERENCES

1. Almquist E and Eeg-Olofsson O: Sensory nerve conduction velocity and two-point discrimination in sutured nerves, J Bone Joint Surg 52A:791, 1970.
2. American Society for Surgery of the Hand: The hand: examination and diagnosis, Aurora, Colo, 1978, The Society.
3. Bell JA: Sensibility evaluation. In Hunter JM and others, editors: Rehabilitation of the hand, St. Louis, 1978, The CV Mosby Co.
4. Bell J and Tomancik E: Repeatability of testing with Semmes-Weinstein monofilaments, J Hand Surg 12A:155, 1987.
5. Bell-Krotoski JA and Buford WL: The force/time relationship of clinically used sensory testing instruments, J Hand Ther 1:76, 1988.
6. Bowden REM: Factors influencing functional recovery. In Seddon HJ, editor: Peripheral nerve injuries, London, 1954, Her Majesty's Stationery Office.
7. Brand PW: Functional manifestations of sensory loss. Presented at symposium, Assessment of levels of cutaneous sensibility, US Public Health Service Hospital, Carville, La, Sept 1980.
8. Brunelli SG: Gnostic rings for assessment of tactile gnosis, American Society for Surgery of the Hand Newsletter, no. 53, 1981.
9. Bunnell S: Surgery of the hand, ed 5, revised by Boyes JH, Philadelphia, 1970, JB Lippincott Co.
10. Clark WC: Pain sensitivity and the report of pain: an introduction to sensory decision theory, Anesthesiology 40:272, 1974.
11. Dellon AL: The moving two-point discrimination test: clinical evaluation of the quickly-adapting fiber/receptor system, J Hand Surg 3:474, 1978.
12. Dellon AL: The paper clip: light hardware to evaluate sensibility in the hand, Contemp Orthop 1(3):39, 1979.
13. Dellon AL: Clinical use of vibratory stimuli to evaluate peripheral nerve injury and compression neuropathy, Plast Reconstr Surg 65:466, 1980.
14. Dellon AL: Evaluation of sensibility and reeducation of sensation in the hand, Baltimore, 1981, Williams & Wilkins.
15. Dellon AL, Curtis RM, and Edgerton MT: Reeducation of sensation in the hand after nerve injury and repair, Plast Reconstr Surg 53:297, 1974.
16. Dorland's illustrated medical dictionary, ed 26, Philadelphia, 1981, WB Saunders Co.
17. Flynn JE and Flynn WF: Median and ulnar nerve injuries: a long range study with evaluation of the Ninhydrin test, sensory and motor return, Ann Surg 156:1002, 1962.
18. Gelberman RH and others: Carpal tunnel syndrome: scientific basis for clinical care, Orthop Clin North Am 19:115, 1988.
19. Gelberman RH and others: Sensibility testing in peripheral-nerve compression syndromes, J Bone Joint Surg 65-A:632, 1983.
20. Gibson J: Observations on active touch, Psychol Rev 69:477, 1962.
21. Grindley GC: The variation of sensory thresholds with the rate of application of the stimulus, Br J Psychol 27:86, 1936.
22. Halnan CRE and Wright GH: Tactile localization, Brain 83:677, 1960.
23. Haymaker W and Woodhall B: Peripheral nerve injuries: principles of diagnosis, ed 2, Philadelphia, 1953, WB Saunders Co.
24. Henderson WR: Clinical assessment of peripheral nerve injuries: Tinel's test, Lancet 2:801, 1948.
25. Kanatani FN: A steel wire aesthesiometer. Presented at symposium, Assessment of levels of cutaneous sensibility, US Public Health Service Hospital, Carville, La, Sept 1980.
26. Kirk EJ and Denny-Brown D: Functional variation in dermatomes in the macaque monkey following dorsal root lesions, J Comp Neurol 139:307, 1970.
27. Levin S, Pearsall G, and Ruderman RJ: Von Frey's method of measuring pressure sensibility in the hand: an engineering analysis of the Weinstein-Semmes Pressure Aesthesiometer, J Hand Surg 3:211, 1978.
28. Lundborg G and others: Median nerve compression in the carpal

tunnel—functional response to experimentally induced controlled pressure, J Hand Surg 7:252, 1982.

29. MacKinnon SE and Dellon AL: Two-point discrimination tester, J Hand Surg 10A:906, 1985.

30. Moberg E: Objective methods for determining the functional value of sensibility in the hand, J Bone Joint Surg 40B:454, 1958.

31. Moberg E: Criticism and study of methods for examining sensibility in the hand, Neurology 12:8, 1962.

32. Moberg E: Nerve repair in hand surgery: an analysis, Surg Clin North Am 48:985, 1968.

33. Omer GE: Sensation and sensibility in the upper extremity, Clin Orthop Rel Res 104:30, 1974.

34. Onne L: Recovery of sensibility and sudomotor activity in the hand after nerve suture, Acta Chir Scand (Suppl) 300:1, 1962.

35. O'Riain S: New and simple test of nerve function in the hand, Br Med J 22:615, 1973.

36. Perry JF, Hamilton GF, Lachenbruch PA and others: Protective sensation in the hand and its correlation to the Ninhydrin sweat test following nerve laceration, Am J Phys Med 53:113, 1974.

37. Phelps P and Walker E: Comparison of the finger wrinkling test results to established sensory tests in peripheral nerve injury, Am J Occup Ther 31:9, 1977.

38. Poppen NK: Clinical evaluation of the von Frey and two-point discrimination tests and correlation with a dynamic test of sensibility. In Jewett DL and McCarroll HK, editors: Symposium on nerve repair: its clinical and experimental basis, St. Louis, 1979, The CV Mosby Co.

39. Poppen NK, McCarroll HR, Doyle JR and others: Recovery of sensibility after suture of digital nerves, J Hand Surg 4:212, 1979.

40. Porter RW: New test for fingertip sensation, Br Med J 2:927, 1966.

41. Renfrew, S: Fingertip sensation: a routine neurological test, Lancet 1:396, 1969.

42. Richards RL: Vasomotor and nutritional disturbances following injuries to peripheral nerves. In Seddon HJ, editor: Peripheral nerve injuries, London, 1954, Her Majesty's Stationery Office.

43. Seddon HJ, editor: Peripheral nerve injuries, London, 1954, Her Majesty's Printing Office.

44. Seddon HJ: Surgical disorders of the peripheral nerves, ed 2, New York, 1975, Churchill Livingstone.

45. Semmes J, and others: Somatosensory changes after penetrating brain wounds in man, Cambridge, Mass, 1960, Harvard University Press.

46. Stromberg WB, and others: Injury of the median and ulnar nerves: one hundred and fifty cases with an evaluation of Moberg's Ninhydrin test, J Bone Joint Surg 43A:717, 1961.

47. Sunderland S: Nerves and nerve injuries, ed 2, New York, 1978, Churchill Livingstone.

48. Szabo RM, Gelberman RH, and Dimick MP: Sensibility testing in patients with carpal tunnel syndrome, J Bone Joint Surg 66A:60, 1984.

49. Szabo RM and others: Vibratory sensory testing in acute peripheral nerve compression, J Hand Surg 9A:104, 1984.

50. Tinel J: The "tingling" sign in peripheral nerve lesions (Translated by Emanual B. Kaplan). In Spinner M: Injuries to the major branches of peripheral nerves of the forearm, ed 2, Philadelphia, 1978, WB Saunders Co.

51. Trotter W and Davies HM: Experimental studies in the innervation of the skin, J Physiol 38:134, 1909.

52. von Prince K and Butler B: Measuring sensory function of the hand in peripheral nerve injuries, Am J Occup Ther 21:385, 1967.

53. Weinstein S: Intensive and extensive aspects of tactile sensitivity as a function of body part, sex and laterality. In Kenshalo DR, editor: The skin senses, Springfield, Ill, 1968, Charles C Thomas, Publisher.

54. Werner JL and Omer GE: Evaluating cutaneous pressure sensation of the hand, Am J Occup Ther 24:347, 1970.

45

Methods of compensation and reeducation for sensory dysfunction

Anne D. Callahan

The quality of sensibility that returns to the hand after nerve repair in the adult is well documented in the literature: results are poor, as measured by localization, two-point discrimination, tactile gnosis, and other tests of functional sensation. Numerous investigators* have noted the poor localization that occurs after nerve repair even when there has been good return of pain, temperature, and touch perception. Regarding two-point discrimination Stromberg[23] found that in 150 cases of nerve repair, of which half were at least 2 years after repair, normal or near-normal two-point discrimination was recovered in all children less than 10 years old—but in only three adults. In Onne's[19] classic study of results after "ideal" nerve suture, two-point discrimination was found to correspond with the patient's age up to 20 years. Between the ages of 20 and 30, results varied but were mainly poor. After 30 to 35 years, two-point discrimination was poor in all cases of median or ulnar nerve repair. Similarly, Almquist and Eeg-Olofsson[1] found a linear relationship between two-point discrimination and age until the time of puberty, with adults demonstrating poor clinical results. The universal conclusion is that the prognosis for return of normal sensibility after nerve repair is good in the child but poor in the adult.

WHY THE RETURN OF FUNCTIONAL SENSATION IS POOR

Functional sensation is poor after nerve repair because regeneration of sensory fibers is imperfect. Sunderland[26] has clearly described several of the factors that contribute to imperfect regeneration, as follows.

1. Injury to nerve axons causes injury to the parent neurons. The higher the level of the initial injury, the greater the retrograde damage to the parent cells. The health of the parent cell, in turn, influences the quantity and diameter of the regenerating axons.

2. Regenerating axons must successfully cross the suture site and enter a funiculus (bundle of axons protectively ensheathed by perineurium) in the distal nerve stump. However, the amount and nature of the scar tissue at the suture site will affect the ability of the axons to cross the site. Clean lacerations result in less scarring and better regeneration than either missle or stretch injuries. The denser the scar tissue, the more likely that a regenerating axon will "dead-end" and turn back in its path, thereby contributing to formation of a neuroma at the suture site.

Those axons that successfully bridge the suture site will come upon a distal stump that has atrophied and has a cross-sectional pattern of funiculi that does not exactly match that found in the proximal stump. The result is that axons may fail to enter the distal stump at all or, if they do, may fail to enter a funiculus, terminating instead either in connective tissue outside the nerve or in connective tissue between the funiculi (Fig. 45-1).

3. Successful entry of a regenerating axon into a funiculus still does not ensure successful reinnervation of an end organ. Each funiculus is usually comprised of motor, sensory, and sympathetic fibers in varying proportions, and each fiber is housed in an endoneurial sheath. The regenerating sensory axon must therefore find its way into an

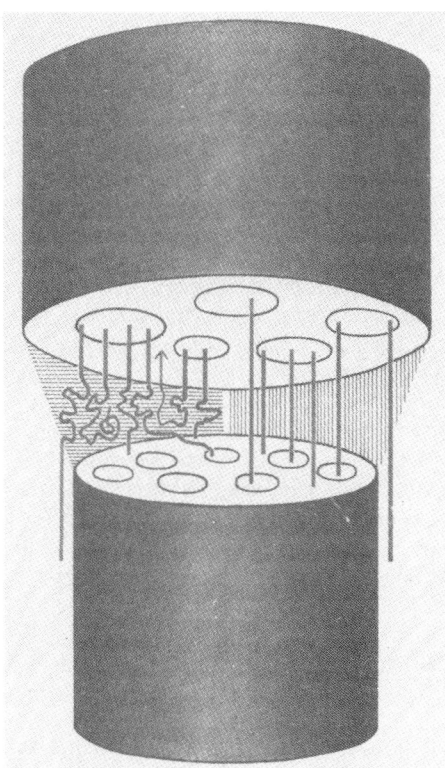

Fig. 45-1 Factors influencing nerve regeneration at suture site include amount and nature of scar tissue, atrophy of distal stump, and a cross-sectional pattern of funiculi that differs from that in proximal stump. (From Sunderland S: Nerves and nerve injuries, ed 2, New York, 1978, Churchill Livingstone.)

---

*See references 2, 14, 17, 23, 24, 26, 27.

611

endoneurial sheath that formerly housed a sensory axon. Even if an axon does enter a functionally similar sheath, chances are that it will not enter the same sheath as previously, and therefore the spatial (somatotopic) organization of the nerve will be altered. This explains why functional results are better after a crush injury to a nerve than after a laceration. In a crush injury where the endoneurial tubes have not been interrupted the regenerating axons will be better able to follow their original endoneurial sheath all the way to the same end organ as before the injury.

4. The final challenge to the regenerating axon is that of successfully reinnervating a sensory end organ. The state of atrophy of the end organ and the degree of myelinization of the regenerated axon are additional factors that will influence quality of regeneration.

It is clear from Sunderland's explanation of factors contributing to imperfect regeneration that the result of regeneration is fewer and smaller nerve fibers and receptors and a pattern of reinnervation that differs from the preinjury pattern. The effect on function of fewer and smaller fibers and receptors is not clear. According to Horch,[15] that particular deficit after nerve repair in a cleanly transected nerve may be less than what naturally occurs in man in the normal process of aging and so may be of less significance than has previously been believed. On the other hand, the effect of the disturbed somatotopic pattern of organizatioan is undisputed. Such a distrubance will result in functional deficits in localization, two-point discrimination, and tactile gnosis, even when there is normal or near-normal perception of pain, temperature, and touch.

IS IT POSSIBLE TO IMPROVE THE LEVEL OF FUNCTIONAL SENSATION AFTER NERVE REPAIR?

At this time it is not clear to what degree it is possible to improve the level of functional sensation that typically occurs after nerve repair. Clinicians have observed for many years that two people with the same level of "academic" sensory recovery after nerve repair may have considerably different levels of function in their nerve-injured hands. Stopford attributed this higher functioning level in some people to "educability" of a "capable patient."[24] Davis[6] reviewed 82 patients after peripheral nerve injury and found that functional recovery was significantly better in those who were motivated to incorporate their injured hand into their occupational and leisure activities, especially if the involved hand was their dominant hand. Bowden[2] was in agreement with Davis' findings and stated that constant use of an involved extremity can lead to greater function in the extremity. Onne[19] also observed the capacity to adapt to sensibility deficits in the hand, depending on the extent to which the hand was consciously used in daily activities and the motivation of the patient. What these investigators and others[15,26] have in common is the notion that a sensibility deficit can be compensated for, and therefore sensibility function improved, by such factors as attitude, persistence, and trainability (that is, motivation) and attention, storage, and recall (that is, learning). Thus, given a certain motivation and opportunity for learning, one person may overcome a sensibility deficit whereas another of lesser motivation and trainability will not.

Given that it is possible to improve overall function in a

hand with a sensibility deficit, is it possible to relearn specific sensory skills, such as two-point discrimination, localization, and tactile gnosis? Opinions and findings vary on this quesion. Ford,[12] Sperry,[23] Hawkins,[14] Bowden,[2] and Horch[15] all opposed the concept of actual relearning of sensory skills after nerve injury, with special emphasis on repeated observation of patients' inability to accurately localize touch several years after nerve repair. Omer[18] noted that patients with poor sensibility could learn to recognize objects used in a daily test over several months, but this skill could not be generalized to other objects. He also pointed out that patients with neurovascular-cutaneous island pedicle transfer could learn to localize correctly at the site of the transfer but that under stress this ability was lost.[17]

In contrast, Parry[20,21] and Dellon[7-10] hold that sensory reeducation as measured by long-term improvements in localization, tactile gnosis, and two-point discrimination is possible in the adult after nerve repair. Parry has incorporated formal sensory reeducation into his rehabilitation program since 1966.[20] In 1976 he reported on the results of his program for the previous 9 years.[21] Patients who had undergone median or medioulnar nerve repair and who had some return of sensation in the fingers were candidates for sensory reeducation. Training was divided into localization exercises and stereognosis tasks. All patients underwent four 10-minute training sessions daily on an in-patient basis. Assessment of results was based on improvements in localization, time and accuracy in recognition of textures, and time and accuracy in recognition of objects. Parry did not use improvement in two-point discrimination as a criterion for success because he believes that it cannot provide a measure of dynamic function after nerve repair. Individual results were not given in his report, but he states that 22 out of 23 patients achieved normal ability to localize within 3 months of training and that in his experience localization almost invariably returns to normal with training.[21] On the whole, the patients also improved in their ability to recognize textures and objects different from the training objects, and the time required for such identification lessened. The length of followup is not clear, but Parry states that improvements were exceeded in those who conscientiously incorporaetd their involved hand into daily activities and were decreased, but still significantly better than previously, in those who did not require use of their hands in daily activities.

In 1974 Dellon, Curtis, and Edgerton[9] reported the results of their sensory reeducation program. Nine patients participated in the program on an out-patient basis, including five who underwent median or ulnar nerve repair, one who underwent ulnar neurolysis, and three who had sustained a compression or crush to the median and ulnar nerves. The program was divided into early-phase and late-phase reeducation. Patients entered the program when their sensory return appeared to have plateaued for at least 3 weeks. Early-phase reeducation was focused on training in the perception of moving and light touch and localization of those perceptions. Training was initiated when the patient could perceive a 30-cps vibration administered through a tuning fork but not moving touch to the same distal point, or could perceive a 256-cps vibration but not constant touch to the same distal point. Use of vibratory perception as a guideline for initiating early reeducation was based on a sequence of sensory recovery observed by Dellon and co-workers in an earlier study.[8] Late-phase reeducation was initiated when moving and constant touch could be perceived at the fingertips with good localization. Late-phase exercises focused on size and shape discrimination and object recognition with use of familiar household objects.[7] Late-phase reeducation continued until two-point discrimination reached normal or had plateaued. Using two-point discrimination as the measure of success, Dellon determined that all six adults who entered the late-phase program recovered normal or nearly normal functional sensation within 2 to 6 weeks of training.[9]

Why were Parry and Dellon successful when others have been so pessimistic? Each made use of higher cortical functions—that is, attention, learning, and memory—to maximize sensory function. Typically, the patient was given a sensory stimulus or task while his vision was occluded, then allowed to open his eyes to integrate the tactile experience with his vision, and finally instructed to repeat the task with his eyes closed for reinforcement of what he had just learned. Attention was maximized by training in a quiet room for short intervals. Daily practice sessions over several weeks reinforced the learning. Thus all the factors noted by earlier observers as important in maximizing function were incorporated into their formal training programs. Their training techniques are similar to those used with success earlier by Forster and Shields[13] and Vinograd[28] in their studies of sensory retraining after insult to the central nervous system.

Thus, although the full potential for sensory reeducation is not known at this time, it appears that the motivated patient can learn to compensate for sensory deficits and, in a structured program that makes use of learning principles, can improve specific sensory skills that contribute to functional sensation.

CANDIDATES FOR SENSORY REEDUCATION

Two groups of patients are considered to be candidates for sensory reeducation after peripheral nerve injury:

1. Those in whom protective sensation is lacking or severely decreased as evidenced by inability to perceive stimuli that are potentially or overtly damaging to the tissues, including pinprick, deep pressure, hot and cold, and repetitive low-grade friction that can result in bruises or blisters. These patients are candidates for protective sensory reeducation.
2. Those who have the ability to perceive pinprick, temperature, and touch, but who lack discriminative sensation (that is, localization, two-point discrimination, and tactile gnosis). These are candidates for discriminative sensory reeducation.

PROTECTIVE SENSORY REEDUCATION

The purpose of protective sensory reeducation is to teach the patient to compensate for the lack of protective sensory input. Because the hand that lacks protective sensation does not experience pain under the same conditions that normally innervated skin does, it is more likely to be subjected to forces and stimuli that a normally innervated hand would withdraw from. The danger from inadvertently subjecting the hand to excessively hot or cold objects or sharp objects is obvious; however, other dangers are more subtle. In his work with patients with Hansen's disease and other neuropathies, Dr. Paul Brand[3] has observed other ways in which the hand without protective sensation is vulnerable to tissue damage because of, in his word, "uninhibited" use.

The first of these dangers occurs from using excessive force when gripping or manipulating objects. A hand that has decreased proprioceptive and pressure feedback will have a tendency to be used with too much force even in simple familiar activities such as turning a key in a door. The unaware person will unconsciously exert too much force in an effort to achieve some sensory feedback from the hand. The result in such activity will be lacerations, abrasions, and other forms of damage to underlying tissues.[5]

A second source of danger lies in subjecting the hand to low-grade repetitive pressure when the hand is engaged in a grip or pinch activity. The hand with normal motor and sensory innervation will accommodate itself to tissue stress for subtle changes in grip or pinch when holding an object for a period of time. These accommodations will occur because the person will experience discomfort or pain from prolonged pressure or shear forces applied by an object on the skin. The hand with decreased sensibility will not experience the discomfort or pain and so will not make the necessary accommodations or will lack the motor ability to change the grip or pinch position to ward off tissue damage. The result is the formation of blisters and bruises. Adapted grips are especially prone to result in damage to tissue from

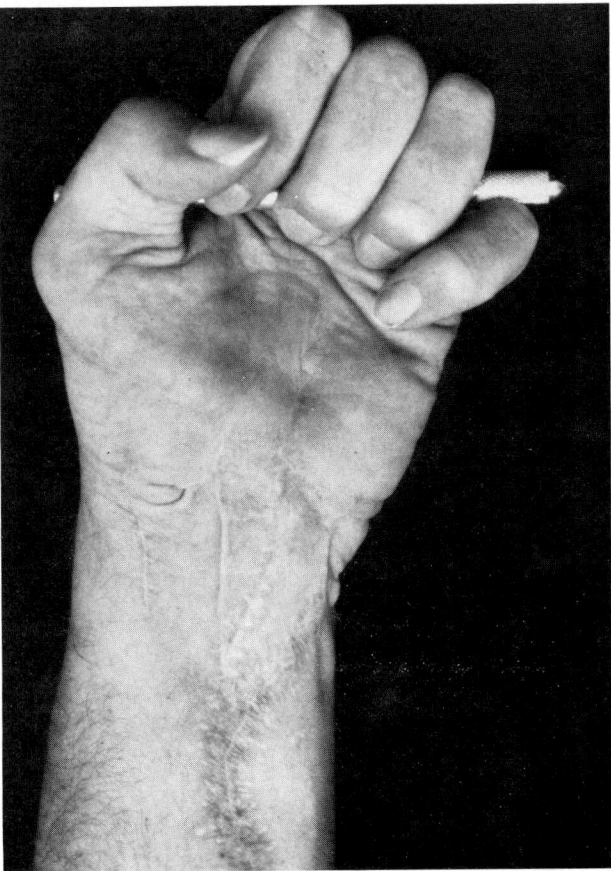

Fig. 45-2 Adapted grips, such as that demonstrated in this replanted hand with reduced sensibility and motor function, are especially prone to tissue damage from stress to areas that do not normally contact an object during grip or pinch.

local stress because areas normally not involved in grip or pinch may be subject to prolonged or repetitive pressure.[3] (Fig. 45-2).

A third source of danger in the hand that lacks protective sensation is a result of the lack of sweating that frequently characterizes such a hand. The skin is dry and smooth and prone to become inelastic and crack from lack of moisture. Dry, cracked skin is more likely to be damaged from daily use than soft, pliant skin and has the further disadvantage of making pinch and grip more difficult because of the lack of friction that moisture adds to the skin.

Methods of compensation for lack of protective sensation

A patient who lacks protective sensation should be instructed in the guidelines advocated by Brand[3-5] and listed below. He should be observed in follow-through during functional activities in occupational therapy.

1. Avoid exposure of the involved area to heat, cold, and sharp objects.
2. When gripping a tool or object, be conscious of not applying more force than necessary.
3. Beware that the smaller the handle, the less distribution of pressure over the gripping surfaces. Avoid small handles by building up the handle or by using a different tool whenever possible.
4. Avoid tasks that require use of one tool for long periods of time, especially if the hand is unable to adapt by changing the manner of grip.
5. Change tools frequently at work to rest tissue areas.
6. Observe the skin for signs of stress, that is, redness, edema, and warmth, from excessive force or repetitive pressure, and rest the hand if these signs occur.
7. If blisters, lacerations, or other wounds occur, treat them with the utmost care to avoid further injury to the skin and possible infection.
8. To keep skin soft and pliant, follow a daily routine of skin care, including soaking and oil massage to lock in moisture.

At the Hand Rehabilitation Center in Philadelphia, patients who lack protective sensation are monitored by visual observation and volumetric readings for signs of stress in the hand after active use that requires gripping or tool handling. Tool handles are built up to accommodate grips and distribute pressure. Patients are instructed in proper skin care and taught to inspect their skin frequently for signs of damage. By following the steps outlined above, one can compensate for a lack of protective sensation and the hand can be successfully reincorporated into gainful activity.

DISCRIMINATIVE SENSORY REEDUCATION

The purpose of discriminative sensory reeducation is to teach the patient to better attend to residual sensory cues so that the brain can better interpret sensory messages transmitted by an altered somatotopic organization at the periphery.

Prerequisites for training

For optimum results from discrimination training certain requirements must be met. The level of return must be such that protective sensation is present and there is return of touch perception out to the fingertips within the range mea-

sured by the Semmes-Weinstein monofilaments* numbered 4.31 or lower. In my experience, the better the return of touch perception, the better the prognosis for retraining in fine discrimination. If the level of return to the fingertips has plateaued in the loss of protective sensation range (that is, touch perception with the Semmes-Weinstein monofilaments is limited to those numbered 4.56 to 6.65), the patient is not ready for and will not benefit from discrimination retraining at this time. The level of touch return at the fingertips, rather than elsewhere in the hand, is used as the criterion, because the fingertips are the most important sensory surface areas for discrimination. The retraining program incorporates the entire hand but puts special emphasis on the fingertips.

The patient must be motivated, intelligent, and able to concentrate. He must be willing to devote time daily to achieve a goal that is not so tangible as motor reeducation. He must be willing to incorporate the hand conscientiously into daily activities that may at first seem easier to perform without use of the involved area.

I have found that the most motivated patient is the one who has diminished sensibility in the median nerve distribution in the dominant hand and whose occupation requires good discriminative sensation. Quite reasonably, if a patient can return to work and otherwise adapt to diminished sensibility in the hand, he is not likely to be motivated to engage in an intensive sensory retraining program.

The patient and therapist must be patient and work to achieve successive short-term goals. Neither should hope for or expect normal sensibility but should work for noticeably increased function from training.

Successful retraining requires appropriate activities. Those that are too easy do not result in learning and those that are too hard will frustrate. Sensory discrimination demands active exploration by the digits, but often the hand with sensory impairment also has motor impairment. Therefore early tasks may involve movement of a stimulus over the digits rather than active exploration by the digits. Tactile cues to uninvolved sensory surfaces on either hand must be avoided at certain times in the training to maximize learning.

At the Hand Rehabilitation Center in Philadelphia, the discriminative reeducation program is divided into tasks that require localization and those that require graded discrimination. Localization training is performed because a high correlation between localization and two-point discrimination (.92) has been found.[30] Therefore it is assumed, though not proven, that training in localization will carry over to discrimination and vice-versa. The two avenues of training, localization and discrimination, are traveled simultaneously with an ultimate goal of successful incorporation of the hand into daily tasks.

Training in localization

Even though a candidate for discriminative sensory reeducation can perceive the touch of a Semmes-Weinstein monofilament marked 4.31 or lower, he may not be able to localize that touch. Therefore retraining is necessary.

Return of moving touch perception precedes constant touch perception.[26] In my experience, moving touch localization precedes constant touch localization, given that both

---

*North Coast Medical, Campbell, Calif.

the moving and constant stimulus are close in application of pressure. Retraining then is carried out for both moving touch localization and constant touch localization, with the expectation being that the former will improve ahead of the latter.

Training procedes in this manner:

1. Ability to localize constant touch and moving touch is tested and recorded to establish a baseline for training (see Chapter 44 for a description of the technique).

2. During training, the therapist (or trainer) visualizes on the involved hand the grid work sheet described in Chapter 44. The touch stimulus, whether moving or constant, is applied to only one arbitrary zone at a time. Limiting the stimulus, especially moving touch, to only one zone at a time helps make the training more systematic and the documentation of responses easier.

3. The stimulus used initially for training is the therapist's fingertip or the eraser end of a pencil applied with a moving touch along the transverse or longitudinal midline of a zone or a constant touch at the center of a zone.

4. With his eyes closed, the patient concentrates on the stimulus as it is applied to a selected zone. He is asked to open his eyes and point to the area stimulated. If he is incorrect, the stimulus is reapplied while he watches so that he can integrate the visual image with the tactile perception. The stimulus is then repeated with the eyes closed, so that he can integrate the tactile experience with his memory of what he just observed when his eyes were open. The entire process is then repeated with a touch stimulus to a different area. Through this process of concentration, immediate feedback, integration of visual and sensory information and memory, and reinforcement by repetition, the higher centers of the cortex can begin to compensate for impaired localization. Through further practice and reinforcement, learning, that is, reeducation, is achieved. The learning principles involved in this training are common to other formal programs.*

5. Twice a month, localization is reevaluated, and changes are documented. As the patient improves in his ability to localize the relatively widespread and heavy pressure applied by a fingertip or pencil eraser, the training stimulus becomes smaller and lighter. Our ideal goal is that the patient be able to localize the touch of a stimulus (as from a Semmes-Weinstein monofilament) that is close to the level of his touch threshold. Therefore our program training in localization tends to continue throughout the reeducation program. This differs from the programs described by Parry[20,21] and Dellon[7,9] in which "normal localization" is reached early in training but appears to be measured by the ability to localize a blunt and fairly widespread stimulus.

Training in discrimination

Activities used at the Hand Rehabilitation Center to encourage discrimination are designed as much as possible to be carried out by the patient without assistance from the therapist or another party at home, thereby reducing therapist time and patient dependence on another person to assist in frequent training sessions. The activities are graded to

require gross to fine discrimination and can be presented to the patient on one of three levels of difficulty:

1. Are these (stimuli) the same or different?
2. In what way are they the same or different?
3. Identify the texture, object, and so on.

Choice of difficulty level within an activity depends on assessment of the patient's present skills in that activity.

Early discrimination tasks do not require active motor function because sensory dysfunction is usually accompanied by motor dysfunction. When a stimulus is to be applied to different areas of the skin for training, the examiner or trainer uses the grid work sheet (see Fig. 44-6) for selection of a zone for stimulating and recording of results. The patient is also familiarized with the grid work sheet and, when working by himself, is instructed to apply a selected stimulus to only a small area of skin at a time. In this way, training is made more systematic.

Texture and shape discrimination tasks. The following activities do not require advanced motor skills. They are heavily relied on for early retraining when coordination is still severely impaired. Each task uses the eyes-closed, eyes-open, eyes-closed sequence with appropriate feedback as described above.

Texture discrimination with sandpaper or other textures on dowels. A coarse grade of sandpaper is attached to one end of several dowels. At the opposite end is attached either the same grade or a different grade, varying from coarse to extra fine (Fig. 45-3, *A*). Both ends of a selected dowel are lightly moved over a zone of dysfunction while the patient's eyes are closed. He is asked to state whether the two ends are the same or different. If he is incorrect, he watches while the same stimuli are reapplied to the same area and then closes his eyes for further reinforcement while they are applied once again. He will require further practice in this area of involved skin. If he is correct, he is given the appropriate feedback, and training proceeds to other areas of the hand. As discrimination improves, the grades of sandpaper chosen for practice become more similar.

The sandpaper is attached to dowels so that the patient can engage in this task without assistance from another person and without inadvertently receiving tactile cues on uninvolved sensory surfaces (Fig. 45-3, *B*). After appropriate evaluation, the therapist selects certain dowels for practice, that is, dowels on which the two sandpaper ends are either far apart or close together in grade. The patient can then apply the reeducation technique to himself at home or in the therapy department. That is, with eyes closed he can pick up any dowel at the center, apply first one end and then the other to an involved sensory area to test himself, and then open his eyes and check the accuracy of his response without having received any cues to uninvolved skin areas. Because the dowel is moved over the involved surface, motor function can be impaired and still allow for reeducation, but the fingers can also be moved over the dowel, if preferred.

Similarly, other textures or substances can be applied to dowel ends and applied in the same way. The patient can make his own reeducation kit for home use.

Texture discrimination using fabrics. At first, a sample fabric is placed in front of the patient whose eyes are closed, and he is asked to match that fabric with one of three fabric choices (Fig. 45-4, *A*). When matching from a small group

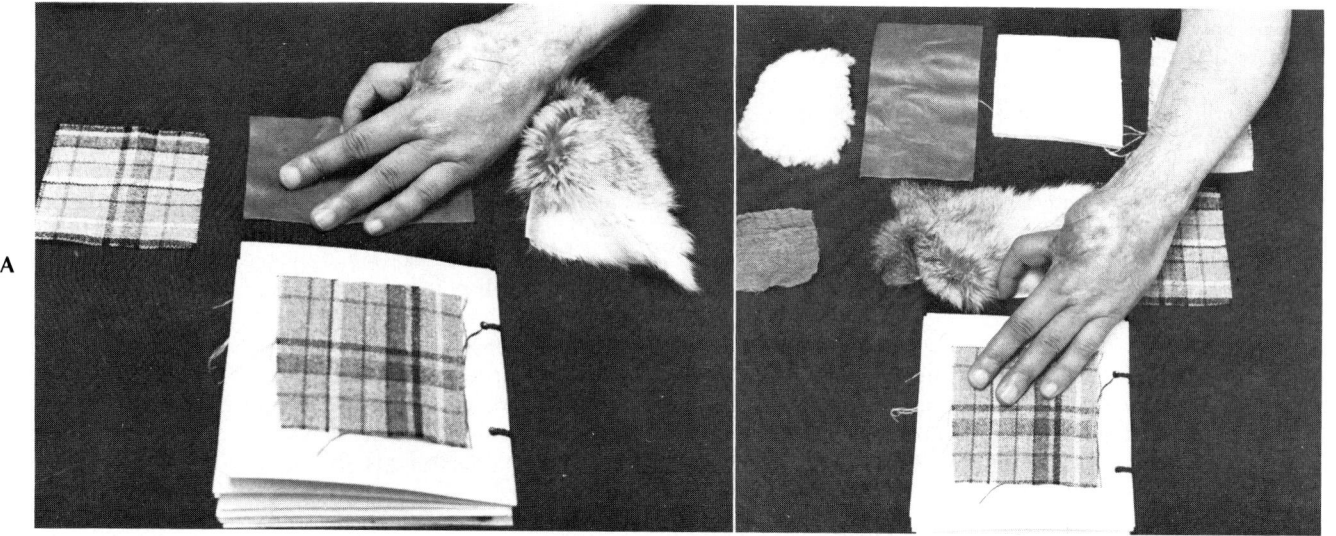

Fig. 45-3 **A,** Early reeducation task requires identification of two identical or different grades of sandpaper attached to either end of a dowel. **B,** Dowels are used to allow patient to self-administer the task without receiving cues on uninvolved sensory surfaces.

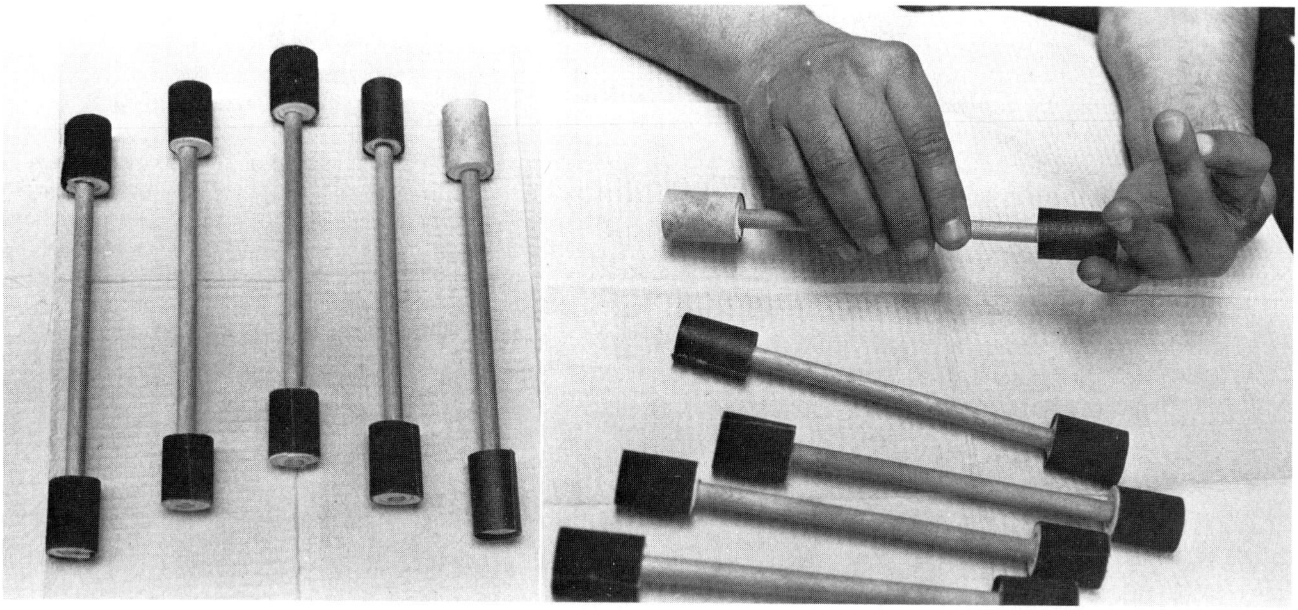

Fig. 45-4 Texture discrimination using fabrics. **A,** Early task requires matching test fabric with one of three choices. **B,** Later task requires matching test fabric with one from a group of possibilities. If properly set up, this task can be carried out independently by patient.

is no longer challenging, matching from a larger group is required, and the patient may be asked to describe the quality of the fabrics.

One can also carry out this activity independently at home by attaching the sample fabrics to cards in a book that has a circular binding so that the patient can flip the book open to any page, with eyes closed, and match the fabric on that page with one from a group of possibilities (Fig. 45-4, *B*).

Differentiation of roughness and smoothness. Differentiation of the rough and smooth edges of coins, nuts, bolts,

and washers is a discrimination task described by Dellon,[9] who has recommended that these objects be carried in the patient's pocket for frequent home training sessions. However, if the patient lacks the motor ability to manipulate such small items, or if tactile cues to a normally innervated thumb are not desired during the manipulation process, the activity can be carried out with the objects seated in putty (Fig. 45-5). With eyes closed, the patient rotates the putty before attempting to locate and identify objects in it using involved sensory surfaces.

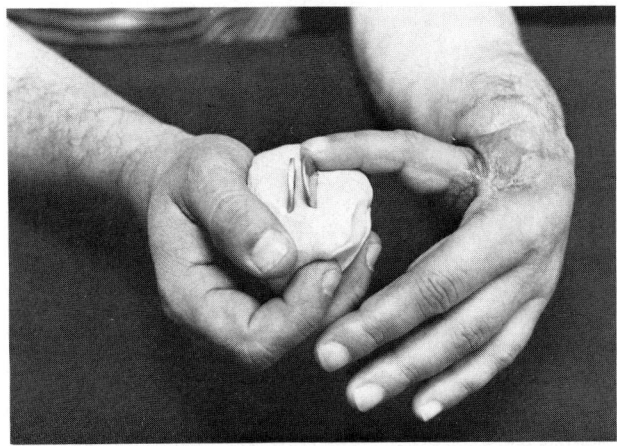

Fig. 45-5 Discrimination of coins, nuts, bolts, and washers. If patient lacks motor ability to manipulate these small objects, or tactile cues to a normally innervated thumb are not desired, task can be carried out independently by seating the objects in putty.

Graphesthesia. The therapist or a third person traces a number or a geometric figure on an involved fingertip or other small area, using a fingertip or blunt instrument, and asks the patient to identify the figure.

Games and puzzles. Discrimination activities that have a game or puzzle quality are generally more enjoyable and challenging to the patient. The more he is mentally involved in the activity, the more he will be able to benefit from it. Three types of activities have been useful in training.

Identification of letters. Block letters formed from adhesive-backed Velcro are superimposed on square blocks of wood (Fig. 45-6, *A*). The blocks are laid facedown. Each one is notched at the top so that the patient can pick it up with his eyes closed and orient it correctly in his uninvolved hand while he tries to identify the letter using his involved fingers. When he believes he has identified the letter, he opens his eyes to check his accuracy. If incorrect, he retraces the letter with his eyes closed to try to determine why he was incorrect. If he is correct, he immediately proceeds to another block. A time limit makes this activity more challenging. As described, the letters are two dimensional. If the patient has sufficient motor function for manipulation, three-dimensional letters cut out of wood are recommended to make the task more difficult.

Braille designs. Millesi[16] has described the use of braille geometric figures for sensory training, and Walsh[29] has described the use of braille designs for training. With use of Walsh's approach, a braille design, such as a house, is imprinted on braille paper (Fig. 45-6, *B*). The design is placed in front of the patient, whose eyes are closed, and he is given a particular task, for example, outline the frame of the house, determine the number of windows, and locate the door. One can grade this task in difficulty depending on how closely spaced the different components of the design are. Patients with a severe problem in localization find this task easier to do with one digit than with several digits because the information from several cross-reinnervated digits can be very confusing when the eyes are closed.

Finger mazes. Finger mazes are devised by use of a col-

ored epoxy* to form a raised design on cardboard (Fig. 45-6, *C*). The patient's fingertip is then placed at the starting point, and he is asked to find his way through the maze to the ending point (indicated by a circle or other sign). Variations of this activity are limited only by the ingenuity of the therapist and patient. The latter will frequently suggest ways to make training easier or more difficult.

Tasks that require motor function. The following tasks are considered to be more difficult because they require greater integration of motor and sensory function and require object recognition. However, these too can be graded from gross to fine and, as long as sufficient motor function is present, can be prescribed concurrently with the above tasks.

Picking out objects from a bowl of sand, wool, styrofoam, rice, etc. (Fig. 45-7). This activity requries differentiation of an object from its background medium. At first, large geometric shapes can be used; later, smaller objects can be used.

Identification of common objects. The patient is asked to select and identify an object from a box of objects. The objects in the box have been chosen either because they are dissimilar to make the task easier or similar to make the task more difficult (Fig. 45-8).

Activities of daily living with vision occluded. Many of our daily grooming and work tasks require manipulation of objects without the assistance of vision. As motor skills improve, activities in occupational therapy should include activities of daily living and work tasks that require use of the involved part without the assistance of vision (Fig. 45-9).

Structure of training session

The exact choice of activity for each patient is based on evaluation of his baseline discrimination skills by use of tests of functional sensation including two-point discrimination, localization, and test of tactile gnosis. Each treatment session should be brief, approximately 10 to 15 minutes, because concentration must remain high for maximum learning. A minimum of one session per day is recommended, though two or three sessions are ideal. Each session should include practice and training from each category of tasks: localization, texture and shape discrimination, puzzles or games, and incorporation of the involved part into activities of daily living. The relationship between the therapist and the patient is dynamic in that the therapist designs the content of the program and gives feedback to the patient, while the patient gives feedback to the therapist regarding relative difficulty of specific tasks and the cues used to discriminate and identify objects.

ASSESSMENT OF RESULTS

The results of training for the patient who requires protective sensory reeducation are measured by a lack of inflammation, blisters, ulcers, and other signs of tissue breakdown over time. The person who has truly learned to protect his hyposensitive hand will not develop these signs of abuse of the hand.

Results in the patient who requires training in discriminative sensation are more difficult to assess and cannot be

---

*Hi-Marks, Mark-Tex Corp., Englewood, NJ.

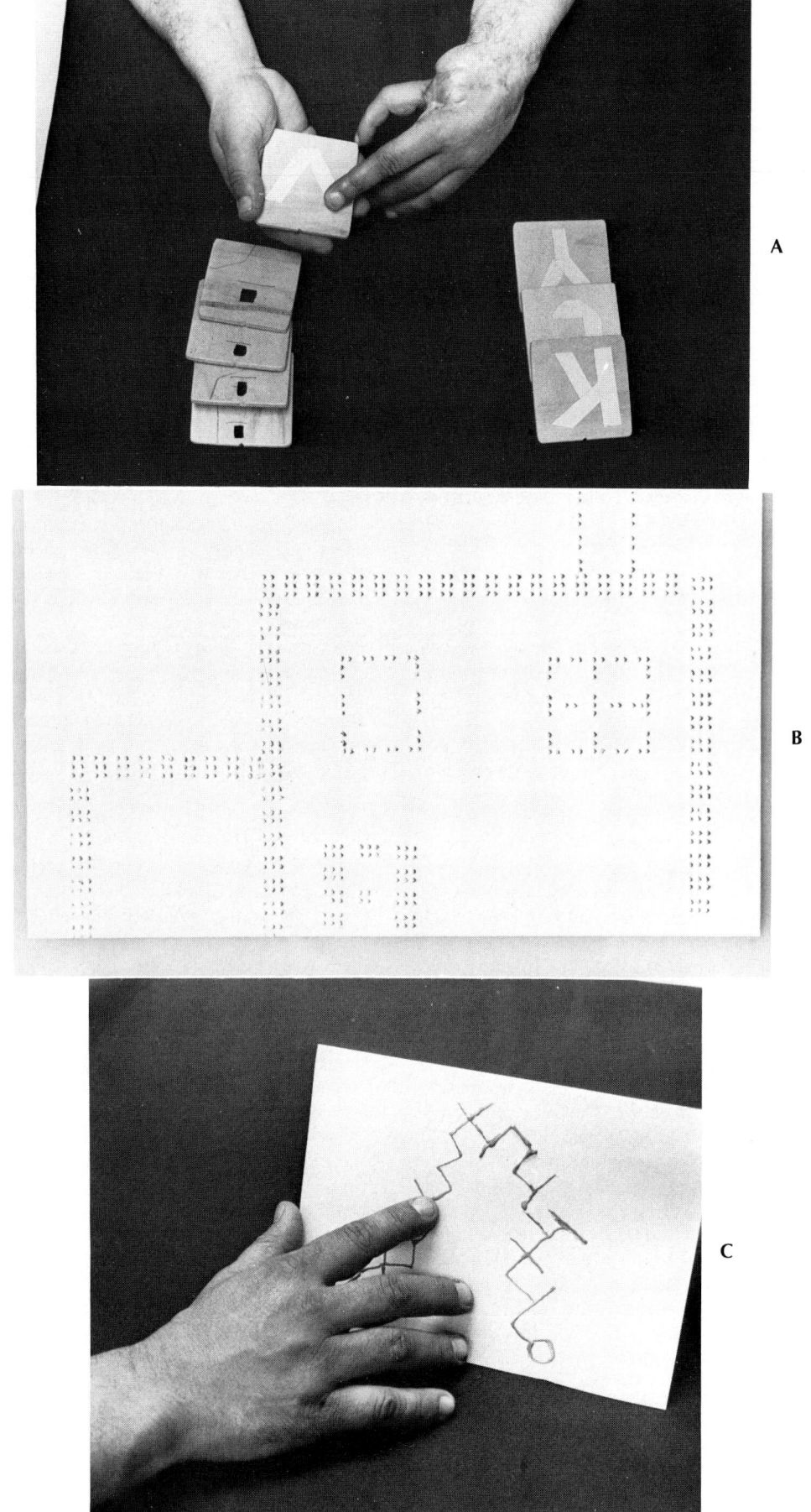

Fig. 45-6 Games and puzzles used to train sensory discrimination. **A,** Velcro letters superimposed on blocks of wood. **B,** Braille designs. **C,** Finger maze.

precisely measured. The following are some of the parameters that are clinically useful for periodic assessment:

1. Mapping. An example of mapping is the use of an outline of the hand to record progress in the ability to localize a stimulus (see Chapter 44).
2. Number of accurate responses. How many objects or textures are identified or matched in a given time period?

3. Time required to complete a task. How long does it take to locate and remove 15 objects from a bowl of rice? How long does it take to complete a finger maze?
4. Improvement in two-point discrimination. Two-point discrimination is a commonly used measure of improvement in sensory reeducation,[9,22] however, some clinicians state that this test is not a valid measurement of functional sensation after nerve repair.[11,20]

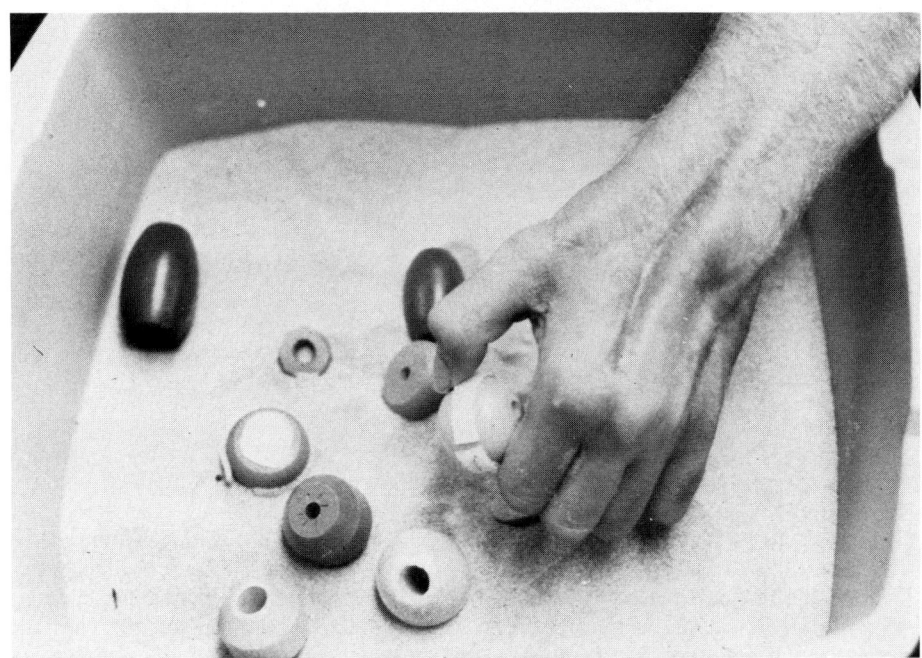

Fig. 45-7 Early reeducation task dependent on motor function requires picking out objects from a background medium, such as sand. Grading is achieved by using smaller, similar objects and requiring identification.

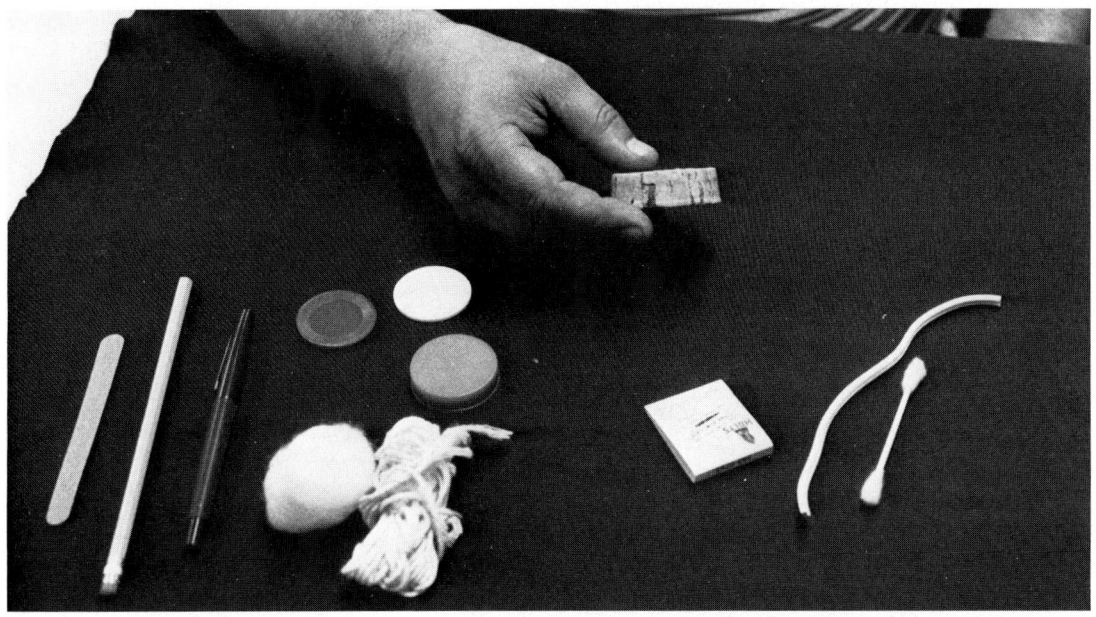

Fig. 45-8 Identification of everyday objects requires manipulation and discrimination.

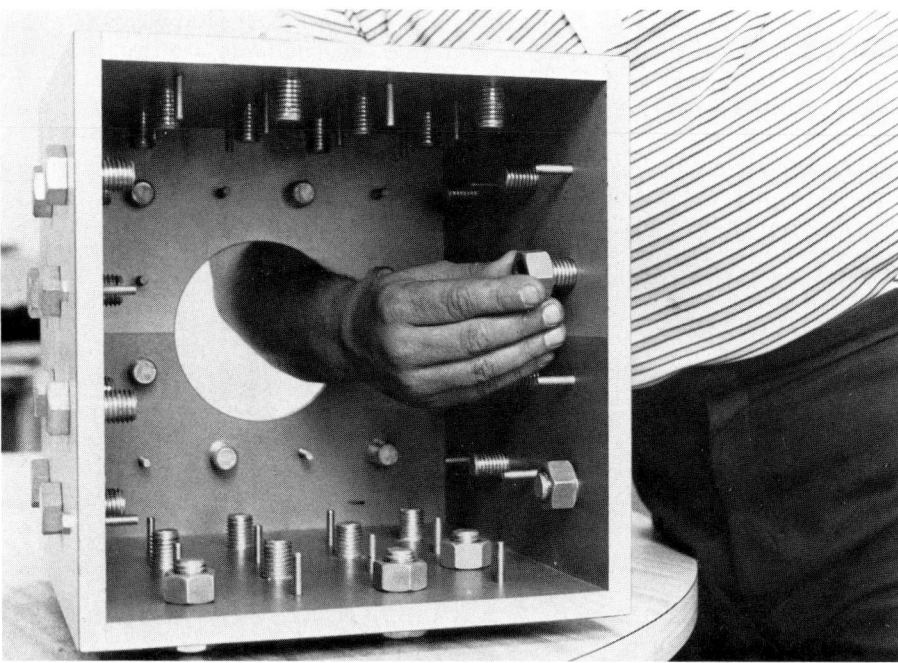

Fig. 45-9   As motor skills improve, appropriate sensory-training activities include work-simulated tasks that require use of involved sensory surfaces without the assistance of vision.

5. Patient's report of increased function in activities of daily living. This, after all, is the most important measure of success. If sensory reeducation results in a person's increased ability to perform activities of daily living, or to handle his tools better on the job, or to better enjoy the tactile sensations of everyday living, then reeducation has been meaningful and successful.

LONG-TERM EFFECTS OF SENSORY REEDUCATION

Patients who have been followed for several years after sensory reeducation have been observed to maintain and increase their functional gains if they continued to use the hand actively for fine activities after discharge from therapy. Some function was lost in those whose work did not require a high degree of sensory function.[21] The finding that maintenance depends on continued use of the hand has been supported by other clinicians.[6,18,19]

SUMMARY

Patients who lack protective sensory function are candidates for training in compensation for lack of protective sensation. Patients who have protective sensation out to the fingertips but lack discriminative sensation are candidates for training in discriminative sensation. The rationale for reeducation programs is that the higher cortical levels of the brain can compensate through attention, integration, and recall for sensory dysfunction. Reeducation requires a patient who is intelligent, motivated, and willing to make a conscious effort to incorporate the involved hand into daily activities and to carry out a structured program on a daily basis. The success of sensory reeducation can be measured along several parameters, the most important of which is

improvement in function in activities of daily living, including work activities. Long-term maintenance of gains will depend on the patient's persistence in using the hand in work and other daily activities that challenge its sensory function. Important gains have been made in reeducation, but studies are still needed to determine the best approach in reeducation and to better define its capabilities.

REFERENCES

1. Almquist E and Eeg-Olofssom O: Sensory nerve conduction velocity and two-point discrimination in sutured nerves, J Bone Joint Surg 52A:791, 1970.
2. Bowden REM: Factors influencing functional recovery. In Seddon HJ, editor: Peripheral nerve injuries, London, 1954, Her Majesty's Stationery Office.
3. Brand PW: Rehabilitation of the hand with motor and sensory impairment, Orthop Clin North Am 4:1135, 1973.
4. Brand PW: Management of sensory loss in the extremities. In Omer, GE and Spinner M, editors: Management of peripheral nerve problems, Philadelphia, 1980, WB Saunders Co.
5. Brand PW and Ebner JD: A pain substitute: pressure assessment in the insensitive limb, Am J Occup Ther 23:479, 1969.
6. Davis DR: Some factors affecting the results of treatment of peripheral nerve injuries, Lancet 1:877, 1949.
7. Dellon AL: Evaluation of sensibility and reeducation of sensation in the hand, Baltimore, 1981, Williams & Wilkins.
8. Dellon AL, Curtis RM, and Edgerton MT: Evaluating recovery of sensation in the hand following nerve injury, Hopkins Med J 130:225, 1972.
9. Dellon AL, Curtis RM, and Edgerton MT: Reeducation of sensation in the hand after nerve injury and repair, Plast Reconstr Surg 53:297, 1974.
10. Dellon AL and Jabaley ME: Reeducation of sensation in the hand following nerve suture, Clin Orthop 163:75, 1982.
11. Edshage S: Experience with clinical methods of testing sensation after peripheral nerve surgery. In Jewett DL, McCarroll HK Jr, and Relton H, editors: Nerve repair and regeneration: its clinical and experiemntal basis, St Louis, 1979, The CV Mosby Co.
12. Ford FR and Woodhall B: Phenomena due to misdirection of regen-

erating fibers of cranial, spinal and autonomic nerves, Arch Surg 36:480, 1938.

13. Foster FM and Shields CD: Cortical sensory deficits causing disability, Arch Phys Med Rehabil 40:56, 1959.

14. Hawkins GE: Faulty sensory localization in nerve regeneration, J Neurosurg 5:11, 1948.

15. Horch KW and Burgess PR: Functional specificity and somatotopic organization during peripheral nerve regeneration. In Jewett DL, McCarroll HK Jr, and Relton H, editors: Nerve repair and regeneration: its clinical and experimental basis, St Louis, 1979, The CV Mosby Co.

16. Millesi H and Rinderer D: A method for training and testing sensibility of the fingertips, Department of Plastic and Reconstructive Surgery, Surgical University Clinic of Vienna and Ludwig-Boltzmann Institute for Experimental Plastic Surgery, Vienna, Austria, 1978.

17. Omer GE: Sensation and sensibility in the upper extremity, Clin Orthop Rel Res 104:30, 1974.

18. Omer GE: Sensory evaluation by the pickup test. In Jewett DL, McCarroll HK Jr, and Relton H, editors: Nerve repair and regeneration: its clinical and experimental basis, St Louis, 1979, The CV Mosby Co.

19. Önne L: Recovery of sensibility and sudomotor activity in the hand after nerve suture, Axta Chir Scand (Suppl) 300:1, 1962.

20. Parry CBW: Rehabilitation of the hand, ed 4, London, 1981, Butterworth & Co (Publishers), Ltd.

21. Parry CBW and Salter M: Sensory reeducation after median nerve lesion, Hand 8:250, 1976.

22. Reid RL: Preliminary results of sensibility reeducation following repair of median nerve, American Society for Surgery of the Hand, Newsletter 15, 1977.

23. Sperry RW: The problem of central nervous reorganization after nerve regeneration and muscle transposition, Q Rev Biol 20:311, 1945.

24. Stopford JSB: An explanation of the two-stage recovery of sensation during regeneration of a peripheral nerve, Brain 49:372, 1926.

25. Stromberg WB, McFarlane RM, Bell JL and others: Injury of the median and ulnar nerves: one hundred and fifty cases with an evaluation of Moberg's Ninhydrin test, J Bone Joint Surg 43A:717, 1961.

26. Sunderland S: Nerves and nerve injuries, ed 2, New York, 1978, Churchill Livingstone.

27. Trotter W and Davies HM: Experimental studies in the innervation of the skin, J Physiol 38:134, 1909.

28. Vinograd A, Taylor E, and Grossman S: Sensory retraining of the hemiplegic hand, Am J Occup Ther 5:246, 1962.

29. Walsh WW: Sensory modalities vs. functional use approach to reeducation, Symposium, Assessment of levels of cutaneous sensibility, US Public Health Service Hospital, Carville, La, Sept 1980.

30. Weinstein S: Intensive and extensive aspects of tactile sensitity as a function of body part, sex and laterality. In Kenshalo DR, editor: The skin senses, Springfield, Ill, 1968, Charles C Thomas, Publisher.

46

Rehabilitation of the patient with an injury to the brachial plexus

Robert D. Leffert

The problem of rehabilitation of a patient with an injury to the brachial plexus is difficult, not only for the patient, to whom it may assume enormous proportions,[7] but in a different way to those who participate in his care. The anatomy of the nerves is complex and difficult to remember, and the infrequency of such cases in most individual practitioners' experience makes the lack of familiarity a significant handicap. The time intervals required for spontaneous resolution of those lesions that heal, as well as the results of central or peripheral reconstruction, involve long-term commitment to patients.

Since patients and their problems present as a series of questions, this chapter will be similarly arranged.

Who are the patients, and what are the mechanisms of injury?

The majority of brachial plexus injuries are caused by traction, which generally results from high-velocity motorcycle accidents or occasionally bicycle or automobile trauma. Far fewer result from falls or industrial injuries in which the weight falls on the shoulder or traction on the arm. The common mechanism is a forceful separation of the head and shoulder during a fall. This stretching of the nerves causes a variety of distributions and degrees of injury, which are the clinically observed deficits. Patients are usually young males in their late teens or early twenties, often unskilled or beginning manual occupations. A considerably smaller number of patients sustain open injuries to the brachial plexus, and these, as well as postanaesthetic palsies, will be briefly discussed.

What are the pertinent clinico-anatomic correlations?

The anatomy is fascinating, complex, and frustrating because, although one could memorize a textbook diagram of how the plexus is arranged, it would not be adequate for application to a significant percentage of clinical situations. A detailed discussion of the anatomy is beyond the scope of this chapter, but fortunately a number of references are available.* Suffice it to say that the classic brachial plexus is formed by the anterior primary rami of C5, C6, C7, C8, and T1 and their terminal outflow (Fig. 46-1). If C4 contributes a significant branch to C5, and it does so in a high percentage of patients, then the term "prefixed" is used. If T2 contributes significantly to T1, then the plexus is said to be "postfixed." This occurs in a significantly smaller group of patients. The importance of these particular variations is that in our dealings with the brachial plexus we

will rely heavily on indirect methods of neurologic diagnosis. Therefore one must be prepared to anticipate variations by at least one spinal level in determining the location of the lesion. Furthermore, in traction lesions, actual avulsion of the nerve roots from the spinal cord may occur. Hence, knowledge of the location of branches known to be given off immediately after the spinal nerve exits from the intervertebral foramen allows for identification of such supraganglionic lesions, which have no potential for useful spontaneous recovery or successful surgical manipulation at present. For example, if a patient has a traction lesion involving C5, C6, or C7 and the scapula is clinically winged, this indicates denervation of the serratus anterior muscle, the nerves for which are root collaterals arising at the spinal canal. On the other hand, an intact serratus in a patient who has paralysis of the lateral rotators of the humerus would indicate a lesion located farther distally. All grades of nerve injury are possible distally, from nondegenerative neurapraxias to frank rupture of the nerves within the substance of the plexus itself. Finally, the presence of an ipsilateral Horner's syndrome in a patient with a traction lesion of the brachial plexus indicates a supraganglionic lesion involving the T1 nerve root and a poor prognosis for that particular root, although in a few cases, some recovery may occur.[46]

What are the clinically observed patterns of injury?

Among patients who have sustained traction injury to the brachial plexus by means of the mechanism described above, there are four commonly observed patterns: (1) the C5-6 lesion, (2) the C5, C6, C7 lesion, (3) the (C7), C8, T1 lesion, and (4) the whole-plexus lesion.

The C5-6 lesion is a common type of injury; it results in paralysis of the deltoid, the lateral rotators of the humerus, and the elbow flexors. The wrist extensors may or may not be paralyzed as well, and if they are, the patient still may be able to dorsiflex the wrist if the finger extensors are intact. The functional deficit is the inability to control the shoulder, which can be neither abducted nor forward flexed, and although the elbow can be extended, it cannot be actively flexed. The sensory loss involves the thumb and the index finger. The incidence of nondegenerative lesions that recover spontaneously is highest in this group, and avulsion of the roots from the cord does not occur frequently. Isolated injuries to the upper trunk have the best prognosis.[4,48]

The C5, C6, C7 lesion includes all of the deficits in the previous group, with the addition of a loss of active wrist and elbow extension and finger extension. It is as if a radial nerve palsy were superimposed upon the C5-6 lesion. There is slightly more sensory loss, which involves the middle

---

*References 6, 15, 18, 21, 22, 23, 27, 30, 53.

finger. The prognosis for spontaneous recovery is less favorable.[4]

The (C7), C8, and T1 lesion represents only a small portion of the adult traction lesions, being considerably more common in obstetrical palsies, in which the term "Klumpke's palsy" identifies it. Although the shoulder and elbow control and wrist extension are preserved, there is loss of active finger flexion and extension, as well as all intrinsic function of the hand. The sensory loss is usually confined to the little and ring fingers, although if C7 is involved, the middle finger will lose sensation as well.

The whole-plexus lesion is the most disastrous of the traction lesions of the brachial plexus, not only in terms of the extent of the lesion, but also in terms of severity and prognosis.[5] Whereas the three former categories can be significantly benefited by peripheral reconstructive surgery, the whole-plexus lesion must be thought of and treated differently, because not only is there profound motor weakness, but total loss of sensibility in the limb as well. This is the "flail-anesthetic limb," which has an extremely poor prognosis for spontaneous recovery.

Before I proceed, I should take note of three other types of injury to the brachial plexus. These are (1) closed infraclavicular injury, (2) postanesthetic palsy, and (3) open injury to the brachial plexus.

Closed infraclavicular injury to the brachial plexus occurs as a result of skeletal injury in the region of the shoulder, usually fractures or fracture-dislocations of the glenohumeral joint or the scapula.[32,34] The nerves are injured by the stretch or compression of the humeral head or the fracture fragments, and usually the prognosis for recovery is considerably better than for the closed supraclavicular injuries. It should be noted, however, that nerves may actually be cut by sharp fracture fragments, which can also produce significant vascular injury. It is important to make sure that a supraclavicular injury does not exist in a patient who has had a shoulder girdle injury, since it will be the supraclavicular injury that determines the prognosis in that case.

Postanesthetic palsy may occur in patients who are under general anesthesia in the operating room.[25,29] This is a preventable type of nerve injury resulting from malposition of the head, neck, or arm at surgery. In almost all cases, even though the paralysis may be widespread, it is usually not permanent and it is less severe than would be seen with a high-velocity injury. The prognosis for full recovery is excellent.

Open injuries to the brachial plexus[8,47] fortunately occur infrequently in civilian practice. If they are the result of gunshot wounds without either vascular or pulmonary complications, they should be treated expectantly, since many of them will recover spontaneously. For patients who have sharp wounds of the plexus involving the upper or intermediate trunk, microsurgical techniques have improved the possibility of functional recovery following direct surgery. Nevertheless, such a case should not be considered an emergency unless, of course, there is a concomitant vascular lesion. In the past I have surgically explored two patients who had had their brachial plexuses severed by chain saws that they had been operating. The damage was extensive in both patients, although in one we were able to do limited neurologic reconstruction, which restored useful elbow function and some shoulder control.

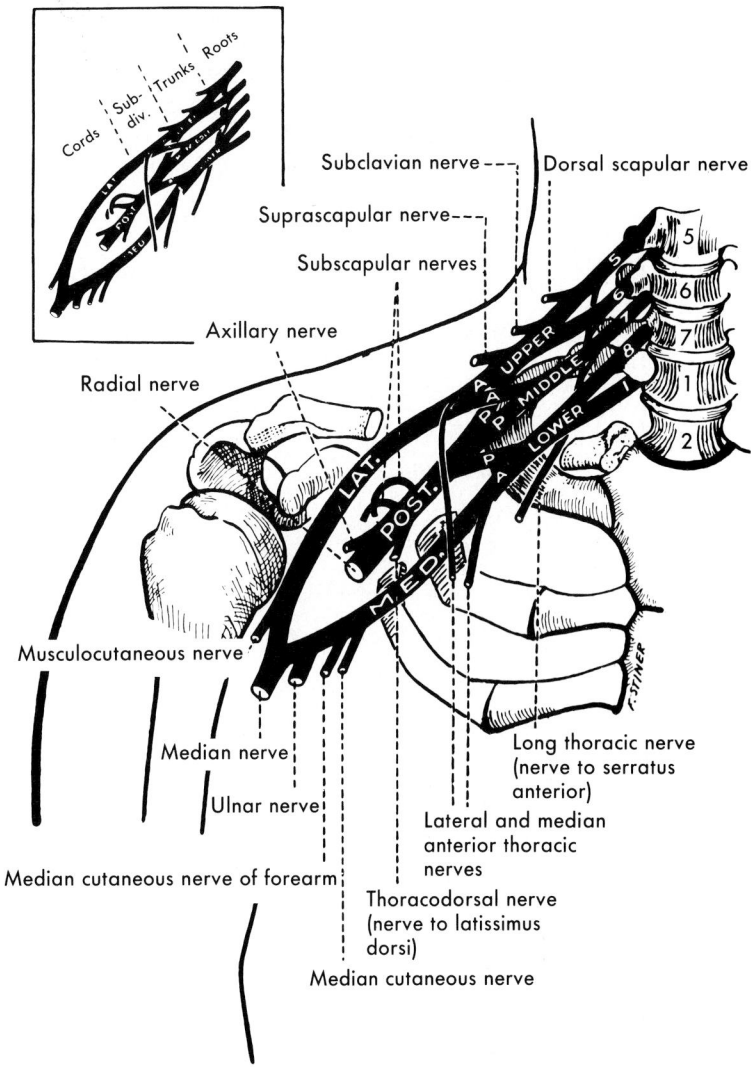

Fig. 46-1 Anatomy of brachial plexus.

What methods of documentation and evaluation are available?

The clinical history is of extreme importance, although sometimes the patient will have sustained a head injury at the time he injures the brachial plexus and so will be amnesic in regard to the event. Nevertheless, it is important to know the date and the circumstances of the injury, whether there was a head injury, and what the initial neurologic deficit in the limb was. The presence of concomitant fractures should be ascertained. Obviously one should know such things as the hand dominance of the patient, his occupation, and whether he has a history of neurologic deficit or injury to the limb. Only then will it be possible to ascertain whether there has been a change since the injury, if the patient was not seen immediately thereafter. Patients who are seen remote from the time of injury should be encouraged to obtain all medical records, including their prior workups. Finally, since many patients with brachial plexus injuries have pain, a history regarding its presence, its course, factors influencing it, and so on will be important.

The physical examination must be conducted in a systematic fashion and recorded so that nothing is omitted. For this purpose, a number of schemes and charts have been devised. I use one that is adapted from Professor Merle d'Aubigne (Fig. 46-2). It includes space not only for the historical data but also for range of motion of all joints in the shoulder girdle and upper limb, manual muscle testing, and sensibility. Each muscle in the limb must be tested and its strength recorded. Sensibility is evaluated by pin and touch. The face should be examined for the presence of Horner's syndrome, and the supraclavicular fossa should be palpated and percussed. If Tinel's sign can be elicited in the supraclavicular fossa of a patient with a flail-anesthetic

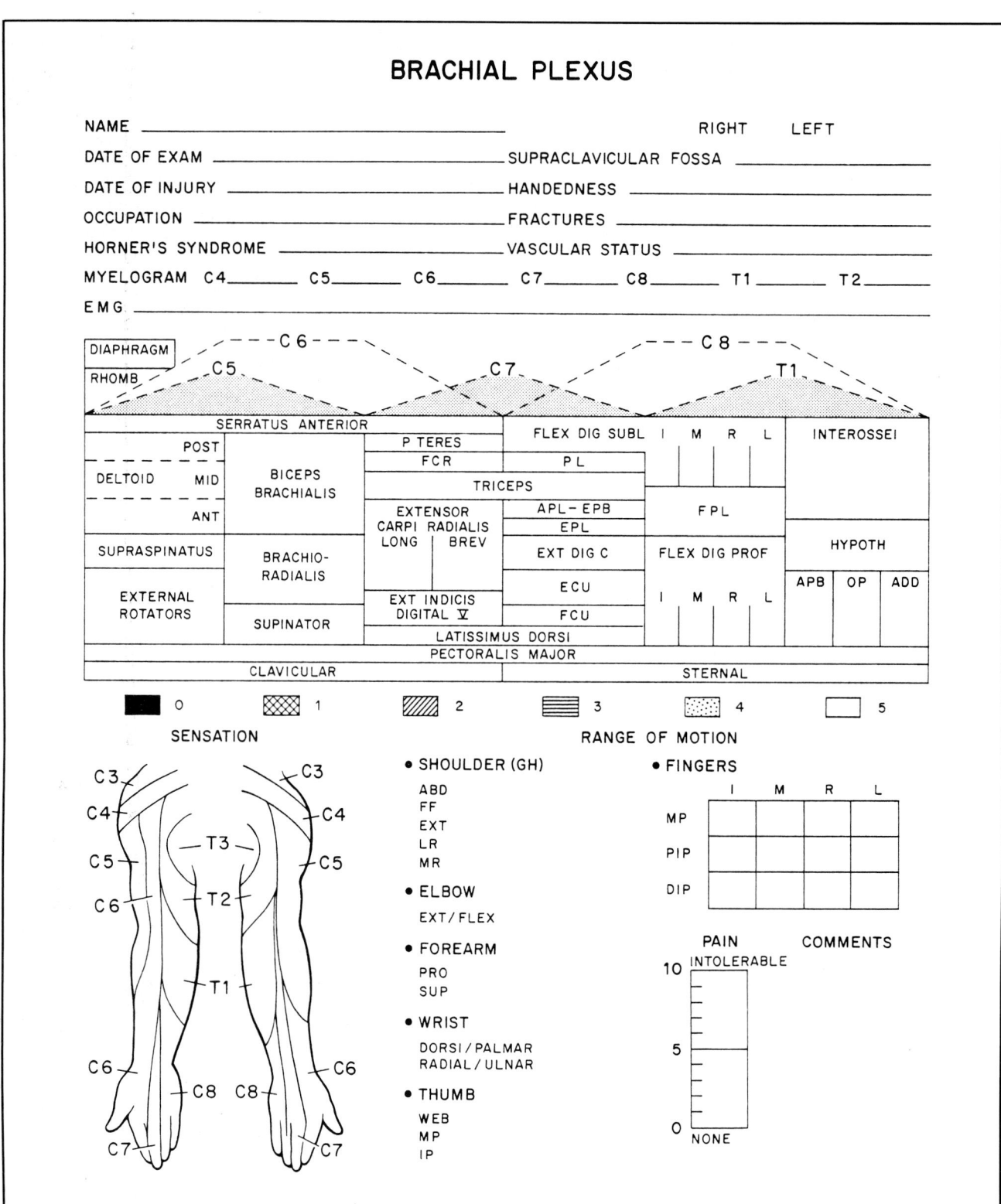

Fig. 46-2   Chart for recording results of physical examination for brachial plexus injury.

arm following a traction injury, then it is extremely likely that at least one root is ruptured distally in the neck rather than avulsed centrally at the spinal cord.

For all patients, it is important to perform a general neurologic examination that includes the lower extremities. The presence of "long tract signs" would indicate spinal cord injury.

Plain radiographs of the cervical spine, ipsilateral shoulder girdle, and any fractures that might be reported or found to be present are taken at the original evaluation.

Myelography is a useful adjunct to clinical evaluation[41,42] but should be delayed in most cases until 1 month after injury to avoid injecting the contrast material into a possibly bloody spinal fluid, since not only may the pertinent details be obscured by blood clot, but also there is a possibility of producing arachnoiditis. Although in the past Pantopaque has been the contrast material used, we have recently used water-soluble materials such as Metrizamide, with computed tomography follow-up so that greater definition at each spinal level can be achieved. The roots themselves can be studied by this method. When a myelogram in a patient with a root avulsion is done several months after the injury, the retracted and scarred meninges will form a traumatic pseudomeningocele, which will appear as a pouch at the level of the root avulsion. It should be emphasized that although myelography offers good presumptive evidence of root avulsion, it is by no means completely reliable,[20,26] and some surgeons have discarded its use altogether. I continue to use myelography, with knowledge of its limitations. Thus far, magnetic resonance imaging has not proved superior to the previously mentioned imaging techniques but may evolve in the future evaluation of the brachial plexus lesions.

Both electromyography and nerve conduction velocity determinations can be used to provide important additional information in the evaluation of a patient with a traction injury to the brachial plexus. Bufalini and Pescatori[9] have shown that since the deep layers of the posterior cervical musculature are serially innervated by the posterior primary rami of the same spinal nerves that provide the anterior primary rami that form the brachial plexus, needle electromyography of these muscles will identify and differentiate root avulsions from distal ruptures. If, for example, the limb musculature is denervated and the erector spinae muscles are not, then the posterior primary rami are intact, and since they are given off immediately after the spinal nerves exist the intervertebral foramina, the lesion must be further distally in the plexus and therefore be a rupture rather than an avulsion. If, on the other hand, both sets of musculature are denervated, an avulsion is present. The electromyogram may be used on serial examination to identify evidences of reinnervation in appendicular musculature that appears to be clinically paralyzed. The test can be done anytime after 3 weeks in a patient who is clinically paralyzed, since that interval is necessary for the development of wallerian degeneration and the appearance of fibrillations on the electromyogram.

Nerve conduction velocity determinations can also be used to distinguish avulsions from distal ruptures. In patients who have root avulsions with paralysis and sensory loss, although motor nerve conduction velocity determination will be impossible since the axon would have been separated from the anterior horn cell in the spinal cord, sensory conduction will be preserved because the dorsal root ganglion is in continuity with the axon or dendrite. Hence, intact sensory conduction in the anesthetic limb is a poor prognostic sign.

The sequence of steps in the evaluation of a brachial plexus injury can be recapitulated as follows: One would perform a detailed history and physical examination initially, whether the patient has just been injured or is being seen after time has elapsed. If electrodiagnostic studies have not been done, they should be and duly recorded. If, for example, electromyograms are done on a patient with a fresh brachial plexus injury and there is evidence of degeneration, there must have been before injury, because it normally takes 3 weeks for this phenomenon to develop. Plain radiographs are taken initially, and if there are any fractures, updated films are obtained. As stated, myelography is usually delayed for 1 month after injury. With the clinical and ancillary studies having been completed, one is ready to formulate the plan for therapy.

How is the treatment plan formulated?[32,33]

In addition to the physician's evaluation, patients should be seen by the occupational therapist and the physical therapist for evaluation and input. Arrangements should be made for detailed and thorough follow-up, which provides increased observation and the possibility of further explanations or ventilating of the patient's concerns. All information compiled from these evaluations is explained to the patients in detail, by means of diagrams and models. Several explanatory sessions may be required because of the technical nature of what is being discussed or anxiety on the part of the patients. It is most important that this information be shared with the patients as soon as it is solidly established, so that as little time as possible is lost in planning the therapy and whatever modifications will be necessary in life-style or ultimate goals.

What operative techniques are available for central neurological reconstruction of the traumatized brachial plexus?

Although the early years of the twentieth century witnessed brave and imaginative attempts to reconstruct the traumatized brachial plexus, enthusiasm gradually waned with the passage of time and more rigorous scrutiny of end results. Notwithstanding some spectacular results, by the time of World War II and for the next two decades, brachial plexus exploration was done largely for the establishment of the extent of the lesions and for formulation of a prognosis.[51] The advent of microsurgery stimulated a new group of surgeons in various parts of the world to reexamine the possibility of reconstructing the injured nerves. The work of Millesi,[38-40] Narakas,[43-45] Allieu,[1] Alnot,[2,3] Lusskin, Campbell and Thompson,[34] and Sedel[50] should be consulted for their specific results. However, it is difficult and sometimes impossible to compare the various reported series in terms of their ultimate functional results. Furthermore, in those patients in whom partial lesions exist and who have the possibility of peripheral reconstruction by means of conventional techniques of arthrodesis and tendon transfer, the lack of a standardized approach to evaluation has thus far made comparison difficult. For those patients with flail anesthetic arms and no possibility of peripheral reconstruction, central neurologic reconstruction remains the only possibility for enhancing neurologic and, ultimately, functional improvement. The general consensus seems to be that the adult traction injuries are best explored within the first 6 months after injury[40] (optimally after 3 months, to allow for whatever diagnostic workup is to be done and the possibility of spontaneous recovery). Although useful results have been reported after the 6-month period and as long as 18 months after injury, the low probability of significant benefit from surgery done after the 6-month period makes it often not worthwhile. Although in our present state of technology, it is impossible to replant a spinal nerve that has been avulsed from the cord, if there is sufficient length of nerve available distal to the intervertebral foramen to serve as a source of axons, then surgical manipulation may be attempted. Because most traction injuries involve extensive longitudinal damage to the nerves, it is highly unlikely that direct suture will be successful in these situations, and some type of nerve graft will be necessary. The sural nerves are often used as donors, and occasionally the medial cutaneous nerve of the forearm taken in the arm. If the ipsilateral ulnar nerve has been defunctionalized by avulsion of the C_8 or T_1 roots, it, too, may serve as a donor for a nerve graft. The prognosis for recovery after grafts of the lower trunk, even in situations in which avulsion has not taken place, is so poor that grafting is hardly worthwhile. The best prognosis is for grafts of the upper and intermediate trunks with the possibility of some shoulder control, as well as recovery of elbow flexion and some wrist motors.[40,45] Occasionally finger flexion can be restored. The restoration of sensibility is, of course, of primary importance, and there have been some successes, particularly with reference to the radial side of the hand. Needless to say, the results obtained from direct neurologic reconstruction are far from normal, but compared to the absolutely hopeless prognosis for the patient with a flail-anesthetic arm that is not operated on, they are sufficiently worthwhile to be recommended, as long as the patient realizes that the objectives are limited.

For the patient with partial function in the limb, there is considerably more controversy about what should be done. The surgeon must be prepared to employ either neurologic reconstruction, peripheral reconstruction in the limb,[31] or a combination of these techniques as required by the patient's needs. Suffice it to say that further documentation of results of these techniques is needed, and I hope it will be forthcoming in the near future.

What are the important nonoperative considerations in patient management during the periods spent waiting either for spontaneous recovery or the results of surgery?

As has been previously noted, patients with brachial plexus injuries have multiple problems resulting not only from the often extensive motor and sensory deficits in the limb, but also from contractures, edema, subluxations, and the possibility of further injury of insensate parts. These patients require careful monitoring by all concerned with their management and continued education so that they can contribute to their care. The control of anxiety and the provision of psychologic support during this difficult time are necessary and ongoing areas of concern. The management of pain will be discussed in a later section.

The shoulder, normally the most mobile joint in the body, not only can become very stiff in a relatively short period of time because of failure to move it passively when active control has been lost, but also is subject to painful subluxation because of the weight of the arm unsupported by the paralyzed muscles. Sometimes the patient will take to unrelenting use of slings to prevent or correct subluxation, with the result that the shoulder loses passive range, particularly in abduction and lateral rotation. Many varieties of orthosis have been designed to offset this problem. Unfortunately, there is no universally applicable orthosis, and each case must be dealt with individually.

The elbow, which may have been injured at the same time the brachial plexus palsy occurred, may become stiff because of continual use of a sling or failure to put it through a full range of motion every day. The hand tends to conform to the contour of the abdomen, against which it rests, with the result that very quickly the metacarpophalangeal joints are ankylosed in full extension and a thumb is in the plane of the palm and therefore useless even if motor control were reestablished. The judicious use of physiologic orthoses and passive range-of-motion exercise, as well as scrupulous attention to the integrity of the skin, is mandatory if the hand is to be returned to a functional status. The patient must be educated to protect his insensate skin from trauma and to avoid persistent edema, since it too will sometimes prove devastatingly permanent once it is established.

Whether to attempt to supply a patient with a functional orthosis to accommodate his flail-anesthetic limb has been a subject of some controversy. Wynn-Parry in England has been particularly successful in providing his patients with functional splints.[54]

What can be obtained from peripheral reconstruction of the shoulder?

The complexity of the motions of the shoulder and the number of muscle couples that are required for normal function make the criteria for evaluation of results of neurologic reconstruction for the paralyzed shoulder particularly demanding. Even if the deltoid can be reinnervated, it is also necessary to have a functioning rotator cuff. Sometimes the cuff can be substituted for by means of tendon transfer.[17] However, with extensive paralysis, even that option is not available, and usually the flail shoulder must either be accepted as such or be fused. It is important to understand the concept of arthrodesis of the shoulder and to realize that it does not mean a shoulder that is completely stiff. The operation makes use of the fact that in normal shoulder motion, the scapula accounts for significant elevation and forward flexion of the arm. If the trapezius and serratus anterior muscles are intact, even in the presence of significant plexus injury, it may well be possible by means of an arthodesis of the glenohumeral joint in a functional position to significantly aid the control of the limb.[49] Specifically, with the glenohumeral joint fused, the patient may forward flex to the horizontal and may be able to reach the other shoulder, the front trousers pocket, and the rear. A number of techniques are available, but the one that I now use involves internal fixation with compression plates and screws. This usually eliminates the need for long-term immobilization in a spica cast. The result is usually significant enhancement of the limb in its role as an assistive member.

Tendon transfer about the shoulder has been practiced in the past, particularly in the treatment of patients with poliomyelitis.[17] Unfortunately, the techniques are not directly applicable to the brachial plexus population, because the number of available muscles in the latter group is usually considerably less than in the former. Nevertheless, for patients with partial lesions, multiple tendon transfers may be quite useful. One of the most successful is that described by L'Episcopo[35] for the restoration of shoulder control in patients who have some deltoid function but lack active lateral rotation control. In these patients, the latissimus dorsi and teres major may be transferred posterolaterally with significant benefit. The important concept in regard to the patient who is considered for tendon transfer about the shoulder is that no single muscle transfer will restore function, and multiple transfers must always be done. It is obvious that a shoulder that has important contractures cannot be expected to benefit from tendon transfer unless those contractures are overcome by means of either physical therapy or direct surgical release.

What techniques are available for the restoration of control to the paralyzed elbow?

Although few would argue about the importance of elbow extension power in normal activities of daily living, the focus of reconstruction in the paralyzed elbow has been flexion. Numerous techniques have, again, been adapted from the experience in poliomyelitis, and the same cautions exist as for the shoulder. Although one can restore active elbow flexion by means of a transfer of the sternocleidomastoid,[10] few use that technique today. The major thrust of surgical reconstruction has been toward the use of the pectoralis and the flexor-pronator muscles at the elbow. Latissimus may sometimes be available and useful.

The flexor-pronator muscles of the forearm and wrist are auxillary elbow flexors. In 1918 Arthur Steindler reported their use in the "flexorplasty," which was the standard treatment of the elbow paralyzed by poliomyelitis.[52] The operation involves transposition of the muscle origins from the medial epicondyle proximally to either the medial intermuscular septum or directly to the bone anteriorly a distance of about 7 cm.[37] This imparts a greater flexion moment to the elbow and may allow the hand to be brought to the mouth or to assist the normal other side. The power attained is usually not more than the ability to lift a few pounds.[28] The elbow is immobilized postoperatively for 4 to 6 weeks, and then a long period of postoperative muscle reeducation is required. If the shoulder is either under good control or fused, the ability to forward flex it and thereby eliminate gravity will enhance the power of elbow flexion by eliminating the weight of the limb. The pectoral transfer, originally described by Clark[13] in 1946, and its modifications,[12] can provide excellent and powerful elbow flexion to the paralyzed elbow if the shoulder is either strong or fused. Failure to recognize this requirement results in loss of power because of the uncontrolled joint and subsequent medial rotation and arm adduction rather than elbow flexion. Although the operative exposure is an extensive one, the postoperative morbidity is not great, and the therapy program is similar to that for the Steindler flexorplasty. In both of these procedures, it is desirable to maintain a permanent flexion contracture of approximately 30 degrees because it

adds to the mechanical advantage of the transfer. It is for this reason that I encourage the use of a sling for 2 to 3 months after either operation.

Transfer of the latissimus dorsi for elbow flexion may be employed in the brachial plexus patient if the muscle is of good quality and power preoperatively.[24,58] Unfortunately, in extensive paralysis, as is often the case, it is not available.

Triceps transfer, again adapted from the polio literature, is available for use to restore active elbow flexion.[10,11] The advantages may be outweighed, however, by the functional loss that forfeiture of active extension implies. Obviously, one would not want to do the operation in a patient who walks on crutches, and certainly not bilaterally. Fortunately, bilateral brachial plexus injuries are rare. Furthermore, the loss of the stabilization and positioning of the forearm and hand that are conveyed by an intact triceps is a significant consideration in use of this transfer. Postoperative phase conversion has not been a significant problem in my experience. However, either preceding or as a substitute for a surgical reconstruction, one might consider the use of a static or dynamic orthosis, with the power for the latter being provided by cable or external power sources.

The timing of these reconstructive procedures must obviously depend on the needs of the patient. In general, when a chronic state has been reached and no further spontaneous recovery has occurred or is deemed likely to occur, then surgical reconstruction may begin. Because of technical considerations, it is wise to begin distally in the limb and work proximally, although the Clark pectoral transfer will have to be preceded by the arthrodesis of the shoulder. If shoulder fusion is done before a Steindler flexorplasty, it becomes very awkward to perform the surgery. Ordinarily I do not advocate arthrodesis of the shoulder before 9 months after injury, but surgery around the elbow distally may be done at 6 months or so, as long as the neurologic status of the limb has been clarified.

What are the problems with the wrist of the brachial plexus–injured patient?

As has already been described, there is a very real danger of development of flexion contracture in the wrist of a patient with major paralysis who is allowed to remain unsplinted and uses a sling. Obviously, the kinesiologic benefits of a mobile wrist need not be justified. However, it should be emphasized that the ability to utilize the tenodesis mechanism of either flexors or extensors by maintenance of wrist mobility is of significant benefit. For the patient who is expected to regain function, the judicious use of long wrist supports, with due regard being given to the possibility of skin breakdown, will maximize the ultimate functional result. For patients with lesions of the lower and intermediate trunk, if active voluntary control of the fingers and thumb is to be even partially restored, it will be necessary to arthrodese the wrist to allow for liberation of the wrist motors and their subsequent use to power the fingers and thumb. The technique of Haddad and Riordan,[16] in which an iliac crest bone graft is inserted from the radial side, is of advantage because it does not produce scarring on the dorsum of the wrist, which might interfere with the gliding of the extensor tendons at a later date. The normal postoperative healing time after that procedure is 8 weeks, during which time it is necessary to maintain the mobility of the joints of the fingers and thumb. Certainly, special situations will sometimes dictate the use of other techniques.

How does the management of the hand of a patient with a brachial plexus injury differ from the management of the hands of patients with other nerve injuries?

The answer to this question is a highly individualized one, depending on the degree of loss in a particular limb. Sometimes, all of the considerations in regard to tendon transfer and arthrodesis that are applicable to patients with more simple, peripheral nerve injuries are entirely transferable to the patient with a brachial plexus injury. It is really a matter of degree, in that the plexus injury patient usually has a more complicated problem that will impose additional restrictions because of involvement of adjacent joints. For these patients, as has been previously stated, the reconstruction of the hand, if it is to be salvaged, should precede consideration of the other joints, for several reasons. The first is that the remainder of the limb has as its purpose the placement of the hand, or terminal device, and if that fails, there is less pressure to reconstruct the other joints. Nevertheless, sometimes the more proximal joints may be all that is potentially salvageable in a limb. If the patient is demonstrated to be uncooperative in the conduct of the reconstruction of the hand, the situation may merit serious reconsideration before the physician proceeds proximally. Then, since the ease of the surgical technique may depend on the placement of the hand on a "hand table," it is certainly easier to do that if the remainder of the limb is mobile.

All of the techniques that are available to maintain mobility, prevent or treat edema, and protect the hand from further injury must be systematically applied to the hand of a patient with a brachial plexus injury. Because these are discussed in great detail in the other chapters of this book, they will not be repeated here.

However, we have recently summarized the use of tendon transfers in our brachial plexus population, and the reader is directed to the review of that experience.[31]

How is pain managed in the brachial plexus injury patient?

A high percentage of patients with traction injuries to the brachial plexus have pain that may initially be very severe. Fortunately, the discomfort usually diminishes with time, and although it may persist, the patient's reaction to it may improve. It is particularly important to identify and deal with anxiety and depression; they may have been present in the premorbid state, but if they are present as a result of injury they may seriously worsen the reaction of the patient to his pain. The treatment of the pain with narcotics on a long-term basis is contraindicated, since this is chronic, "benign" pain. Unfortunately, many patients are started by well-meaning physicians on narcotic medications, and some patients are drug abusers before they are injured. Both classes of patient may be very difficult to wean from their narcotics, and in some cases, which fortunately are rare, it may be impossible. The use of phenytoin (Dilantin) is usually suggested but in my experience is rarely predictively successful. Carbamazepine (Tegretol) has been helpful in some of my patients, but because it has potentially serious side effects, its use must be closely monitored. Some pa-

tients will respond positively to the transcutaneous nerve stimulator, and some maintain that acupuncture has been helpful. I have seen very few patients whose pain has been significantly benefited by hypnosis or psychotherapy, although the latter may be helpful in the management of anxiety or depression.

The surgery for pain of brachial plexus injury has had a long and difficult history. Although at one time it was thought that resection of the traumatic pseudomeningoceles might favorably influence the pain, this procedure does not enjoy popular support today, nor is there great enthusiasm for cordotomy, rhizotomy, or sympathectomy. The question of whether neurolysis is of value in the treatment of pain in brachial plexus injury is still unresolved. Several workers have the impression that reconstructing the plexus itself and augmenting input in a sensory-deprived situation may improve pain. Further work needs to be done in this area. There are some favorable preliminary reports on the use of selective surgical lesions of the substantia gelantinosa of the spinal cord by Dr. Nashold at Duke University.[46] Suffice it to say that the problem of the pain of brachial plexus injury continues to be a difficult one for which no clearly dependable solution exists.

How are the permanently flail-anesthetic arm and hand managed?

Until the recent resurgence of interest in microsurgical reconstruction of the brachial plexus, the standard option for treatment of the flail-anesthetic limb was ablation. Actually, there were three choices, the first of which was to do nothing and to have the patient keep the arm in a sling or his hand in a pocket. For some patients whose life-styles or occupations were not significantly prejudiced by this approach, it could suffice. As long as the limb was not injured, it would be possible for many patients to live relatively unencumbered. Some, however, found that the limb was heavy, annoying, and in the way, and so opted to have it amputated. Often there was no consideration of functional restoration by means of prosthetic fitting, and so the standard treatment was a high humeral amputation. If the patient was not to be fitted with a prosthesis, there really was no time constraint. However, if prosthetic fitting was to be done and the patient was to use the prosthesis, it was best done before 2 years had elapsed since the time of injury.[55] This particular approach, combined with an arthrodesis of the shoulder, did result in some minimal use of the limb, and in some patients, use of the limb in the course of gainful employment. The experience was well documented by Yeoman and Seddon.[54]

Although a flail-anesthetic arm could technically be reconstructed by a series of tenodeses and arthodeses, as documented by Hendry,[19] this particular approach has not been appealing because of the vulnerability of the limb to injury of the insensate skin in the course of normal use.

For patients who may by some combination of central and peripheral reconstruction regain the proximal control of the limb but not have a useful hand, there may be benefit from the performance of a forearm amputation and fitting of a prosthesis. Even in those patients who do not have active control of the elbow or sensation over the proposed forearm stump, if there is proprioception in the elbow, a forearm amputation may be done with the fitting of a prosthesis. We have used this approach for 10 years and have been gratified both by the use of the prosthesis and by the lack of stump complications.

Finally, the question arises as to whether a patient with a painful flail-anesthetic limb can be relieved of his pain by amputation of the limb. Fletcher[14] has objected to amputation in such a situation, as has Seddon,[49] and our experience has been similar.

REFERENCES

1. Allieu Y: Exploration et traitement direct des lesions nerveuses dans les paralysies traumatiques par élongation du plexus brachial chez l'adulte, Rev Chir Orthop 63:107, 1977.
2. Alnot JY: Technique chirgicale dans les paralysies du plexus brachial, Rev Chir Orthop 63:75, 1977.
3. Alnot JY, Augereau B, and Frot B: Traitement direct des lesions nerveuses dans les paralysies traumatiques par élongation du plexus brachial chez l'adulte, Chirurgie 103:935, 1977.
4. Barnes R: Traction injuries of the brachial plexus in adults, J Bone Joint Surg 31B:10, 1949.
5. Bonney G: Prognosis in traction lesions of the brachial plexus, J Bone Joint Surg 41B:4, 1959.
6. Bowden REM: The applied anatomy of the cervical spine and brachial plexus, Proc R Soc Med 59:1141, 1966.
7. Brewerton DA and Daniel JW: Factors influencing return to work, Br Med J 4:277, 1971.
8. Brooks DM: Open wounds of the brachial plexus, J Bone Joint Surg 31B:17, 1949.
9. Bufalini C and Pescatori G: Posterior cervical electromyography in the diagnosis and prognosis of brachial plexus injuries, J Bone Joint Surg 51B:627, 1969.
10. Bunnell S: Restoring flexion to the paralytic elbow, J Bone Joint Surg 33A:56, 1951.
11. Carroll RE: Restoration of flexor power to the flail elbow by transplantation of the triceps tendon, Surg Gynecol Obstet 95:685, 1952.
12. Carroll RE and Kleinman WB: Pectoralis major transplantation to restore elbow flexion to the paralytic limb, J Hand Surg 4:501, 1979.
13. Clark JMP: Reconstruction of biceps brachii by pectoral muscle transplantation, Br J Surg 34:180, 1946.
14. Fletcher I: Management of severe traction lesions of the brachial plexus, J Bone Joint Surg 48B:178, 1966.
15. Goss CH: Gray's anatomy, ed 28, Philadelphia, 1966, Lea & Febiger.
16. Haddad RJ Jr and Riordan DC: Arthrodesis of the wrist: a surgical technique, J Bone Joint Surg 49A:950, 1967.
17. Harmon PH: Surgical reconstruction of the paralytic shoulder by multiple muscle transplantations, J Bone Joint Surg 32A:583, 1950.
18. Harris W: The true form of the brachial plexus and its motor distribution, J Anat Physiol 38:399, 1904.
19. Hendry AM: The treatment of residual paralysis after brachial plexus injuries, J Bone Joint Surg 31B:42, 1949.
20. Heon M: Myelogram: a questionable aid in diagnosis and prognosis in avulsion of brachial plexus components by traction injuries, Conn Med 29:260, 1965.
21. Herringham WP: The minute anatomy of the brachial plexus, Proc R Soc Lond 41:423, 1886.
22. Hollinshead WH: The back and limbs. In Anatomy for surgeons, vol 3, New York, 1969, Harper & Row, Publishers, Inc.
23. Hovelacque A: Anatomie des nerfs craniens et rachidiens et du système grand sympathique, Paris, 1927, Gaston, Dion, p. 385.
24. Hovnanian AP: Latissimus dorsi transplantation for loss of flexion or extension at the elbow: a preliminary report on technique, Ann Surg 143:493, 1956.
25. Jackson L and Keats AS: Mechanism of brachial plexus palsy following anesthesia, Anaesthesia 26:190, 1965.
26. Jelasic F and Piepgres U: Functional restitution after cervical avulsion injury with "typical" myelographic findings, Eur Neurol 11:158, 1974.
27. Kerr AT: The brachial plexus of nerves in man, the variations in its formation and branches, Am J Anat 23:285, 1918.
28. Kettlekemp DB and Larson CB: Evaluation of the Steindler flexorplasty, J Bone Joint Surg 45A:513, 1963.
29. Kwaan JHM and Rappaport I: Postoperative brachial plexus palsy— a study on the mechanism, Arch Surg 101:612, 1970.
30. Leffert RD: Brachial plexus injuries, Ch 1, New York, 1985, Churchill Livingstone, Inc.
31. Leffert RD and Pess GM: Tendon transfers for brachial plexus injury, Hand Clin 4(2):273, 1988.
32. Leffert RD: Brachial plexus injuries, N Engl J Med 291:1059, 1974.
33. Leffert RD: Lesions of the brachial plexus, including thoracic outlet syndrome. In American Academy of Orthopaedic Surgeons: Instructional course lectures, vol. 26, St Louis, 1977, The CV Mosby Co.
34. Leffert RD and Seddon H: Infraclavicular brachial plexus injuries, J Bone Joint Surg 47B:9, 1965.
35. L'Episcopo JB: Restoration of muscle balance in the treatment of obstetrical paralysis, NY State J Med 39:357, 1939.
36. Lusskin R, Campbell JB, and Thompson WAL: Post-traumatic lesions of the brachial plexus: treatment by transclavicular exploration and neurolysis or autograft reconstruction, J Bone Joint Surg 55A:1159, 1973.
37. Mayer L and Green W: Experiences with the Steindler flexorplasty at the elbow, J Bone Joint Surg 36A:775, 1954.
38. Millesi H: Microsurgery of peripheral nerves, Hand 5:157, 1973.
39. Millesi H: Indications et resultats des interventions direct, Rev Chir Orthop 63:82, 1977.
40. Millesi H: Surgical management of brachial plexus injuries, J Hand Surg 2:367, 1977.
41. Murphy F, Hartung W, and Kirklin JW: Myelographic demonstration of avulsing injury of the brachial plexus, Am J Roentgenol Radium Ther Nucl Med 58:102, 1947.
42. Murphy F and Kirkin J: Myelographic demonstration of avulsing injuries of the nerve roots of the brachial plexus—a method of determining the point of injury and the possibility of repair, Clin Neurosurg 20:18, 1972.
43. Narakas A: Indications et resultats du traitement chirurgical direct dans les lesions par élongation du plexus brachial, Rev Chir Orthop 63:88, 1977.
44. Narakas A: The surgical management of brachial plexus injuries. In Daniel RK and Terzis JK, editors: Reconstructive micro-surgery, Boston, 1977, Little, Brown & Co.
45. Narakas A: Surgical treatment of traction injuries of the brachial plexus, Clin Orthop 133:71, 1978.
46. Nashold BS Jr and Ostdahl RH: Dorsal root entry zone lesions for pain relief, J Neurosurg 51:59, 1979.
47. Nelson KG, Jolly PC, and Thomas PA: Brachial plexus injuries associated with missile wounds of the chest: a report of 9 cases from Vietnam, J Trauma 8:268, 1968.
48. Rorabeck CH and Harris WR: Factors affecting the prognosis of brachial plexus injuries, J Bone Joint Surg 63B:404, 1981.
49. Rowe CR: Reevaluation of the position of the arm in arthrodesis of the shoulder in the adult, J Bone Joint Surg 56A:913, 1974.
50. Sedel L: The results of surgical repair of brachial plexus injuries, J Bone Joint Surg 64B:54, 1982.
51. Seddon HJ: Surgical disorders of the peripheral nerves, Edinburgh, 1972, Churchill Livingstone, Inc.
52. Steindler A: Reconstruction work on hand and forearm, NY State Med J 108:117, 1918.
53. Stevens JH: Brachial plexus paralysis. In Codman EA: The shoulder, Brooklyn, NY, 1934, G Miller & Co.
54. Wynn-Parry CB: Rehabilitation of the hand, ed 4, London, 1981, Butterworth & Co (Publishers), Ltd.
55. Yeoman PM: Cervical myelopathy in traction injuries of the brachial plexus, J Bone Joint Surg 50B:253, 1968.
56. Yeoman PM and Seddon HJ: Brachial plexus injuries: treatment of the flail arm, J Bone Joint Surg 43B:493, 1961.
57. Zancolli E and Mitre H: Latissimus dorsi transfer to restore elbow flexion: an appraisal of eight cases, J Bone Joint Surg 55A:1265, 1973.

47

Therapist's management of brachial plexus injuries

Victoria M. Frampton

Successful management of the patient with a brachial plexus injury relies on a well-integrated team approach with careful and accurate monitoring enabling implementation of appropriate treatment programs at all stages of recovery.[3,4] The sudden loss of function in an arm and the subsequent long period of recovery is a very traumatic concept for the patient to absorb and can best be approached by a comprehensive rehabilitation approach. The difficulties outlined in Chapter 46 in reaching a definitive diagnosis can be counterproductive to the patient's rehabilitation. The patient avoids facing the reality of his injury by "waiting" for recovery to occur. This may be misguidedly reinforced by the physiotherapist providing long-term continuous physiotherapy. It is therefore imperative that the correct philosophy of rehabilitation is promoted, that is, the need for the patient to reintegrate into his community as quickly as possible and continue with his life as before instead of sitting at home waiting for the arm to recover.

The physiotherapist's involvement in the management of the patient with a brachial plexus injury falls into three stages: the early stage, the middle stage, and the late stage.

The **early stage** consists of the following:

Assessment—Formulation of a baseline of data on joint range and movement and the motor and sensory function, which assists in diagnosis of the lesion.

Treatment—This includes patient education in maintaining a full range of motion by performing passive movements to the arm, patient education in caring for the anesthetized limb, and relief of pain in avulsion lesions.

Splinting—Provision of a flail arm splint may occur at this stage. Patient motivation, together with comprehensive training in occupational therapy in the use of the splint, is essential if the patient is to make the best use of the orthosis. Late fitting of the splint may lead to failure in the use of the flail arm splint because the patient may have already become one-armed and may have ceased to perform tasks bilaterally.

The **middle stage** consists of the following:

Reassessment—At this stage significant recovery may be occurring. If so, an intensive period of rehabilitation is indicated. Range of movement can be monitored and compared with admission measurements, and pain relief can be reevaluated.

Splinting—Selective return of power to the arm may allow the flail arm splint to be reduced and simplified.

The **late stage** consists of the following:

Assessment—Of the residual loss of function and disability. Full motor and sensory assessment is essential so that suitability for reconstructive surgery can be determined.

EARLY STAGE OF REHABILITATION
Diagnosis

As discussed in Chapter 46, lesions of the brachial plexus may result from direct or traction injuries. It is the latter injury that is the most difficult to diagnose because the extent of the damage caused by the traction to the nerve is not known. Careful assessment by the physician of the signs and symptoms can indicate a preganglionic or postganglionic lesion. Clinical patterns of injury also vary, making diagnosis more difficult.[14] In my experience, the clinical investigations need not always be read before the therapist embarks on a full assessment of the motor and sensory function of the patient with a brachial plexus injury. In this way a purely objective and unbiased assessment is provided and can then be compared afterward with the clinical findings.

Assessment

Records at all stages of recovery are invaluable both as a baseline for comparative information and as an ongoing record to monitor recovery. While working at the Royal National Orthopaedic Hospital, Stanmore, I devised some standardized charts that made assessment easier. These consisted of a summary chart or checklist, a passive range-of-motion (PROM) chart, muscle charts, and a sensory evaluation chart (Fig. 47-1). These are helpful to the therapist managing several brachial plexus patients, as was the case at Stanmore; however, most physiotherapy departments may see only one brachial plexus patient in 1 year. These forms are available from the physiotherapy department at the Royal National Orthopaedic Hospital, Stanmore.

Preganglionic lesions versus postganglionic lesions. The following signs and symptoms characterize many preganglionic lesions.

1. A high-speed, large-impact accident
2. A period of loss of consciousness
3. Associated injuries such as multiple fracture, head injury, and vascular injuries
4. A positive Horner sign, which is present only when an avulsion of the first thoracic root has occurred
5. Presence of sensory action potentials
6. Presence of meningoceles on myelogram, which indicates avulsion
7. Pain in the anesthetic limb

Avulsion pain is of a characteristic nature[13] and frequently misinterpreted by the patient as a sign of recovery. Patients describe the pain as a constant, burning, crushing sensation (some liken it to the hand being crushed in a vice). In addition, they suffer paroxysms of pain, sudden sharp, shooting pain often described as an electric shock in nature.

ASSESSMENT CHART
Brachial Plexus Lesion

Name_____   Date_____

Chart number_____

Dominant limb

History

Lesion

Associated injuries

Date of accident

Description of injury

Mechanism of injury

Speed of injury

Length of loss of consciousness

Treatment to date

Exploration of Brachial Plexus

Findings

Repair

Examination

General appearance and posture

Horner's

Neuroma

Tinel

Passive joint range

Muscle power

Sensory evaluation

Other tests

Splintage

Occupation and domestic situation

A

Fig. 47-1   Evaluation forms for brachial plexus injury. **A,** Summary chart.

Continued.

A

Onset   Pain

Increasing/static/decreasing

Nature

Distribution

Frequency of pain in 1 day

Daily pattern

Aggravates

Eases

Drugs

Sleep disturbance

                                              Comments

Fig. 47-1, cont'd   Summary chart.

B

PASSIVE RANGE OF MOVEMENT CHART
Brachial Plexus Lesions

Name_____

Age_____

Chart number_____

Date_____

		Adm	Dis			Adm	Dis
Shoulder girdle	Elev Retr Protr Depr			Elbow	Flex Ext		
Shoulder	Elev Flex Ext Abd Add I.R. E.R.			Wrist	Flex Ext Pro Sup Abd Add		

Hand   Deformity: Thumb web

                              Intrinsics

Fig. 47-1, cont'd   **B,** Passive range of motion chart.

		Adm	CMC	Dis	Adm	MCP	Dis	Adm	DIP	Dis
Thumb	Flex Ext Abd Add Opp									
		Adm	MCP	Dis	Adm	PIP	Dis	Adm	DIP	Dis
Index	Ext-Flex									
Middle	Ext-Flex									
Ring	Ext-Flex									
Little	Ext-Flex									
Posture:										

B

Fig. 47-1, cont'd **B,** Passive range of motion chart.

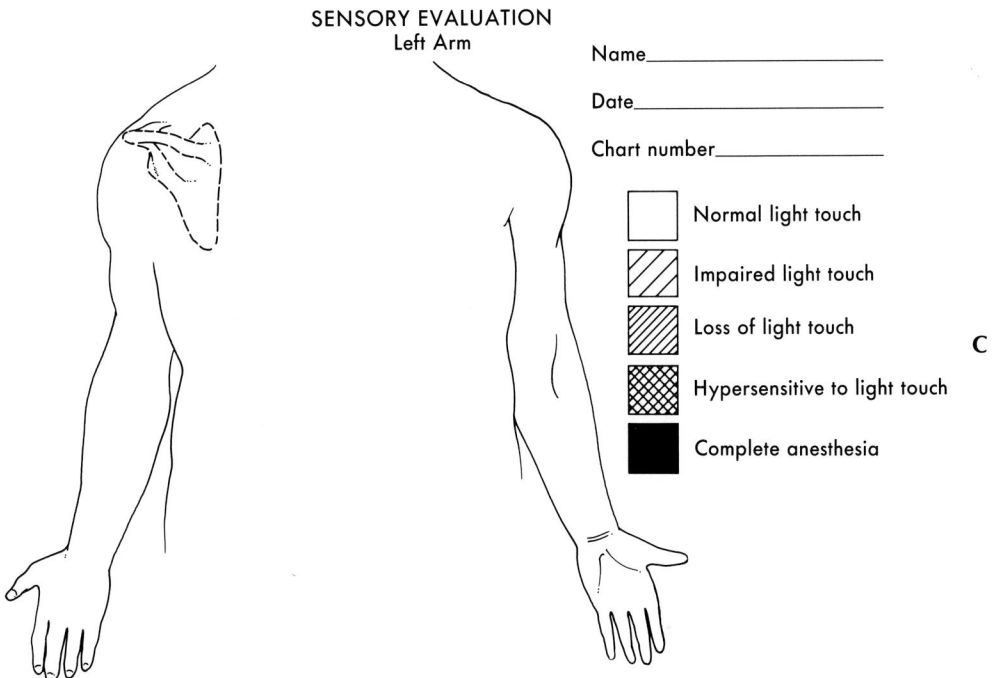

Fig. 47-1, cont'd **C,** Sensory evaluation form.

Although constant, the pain comes in waves; it gradually builds up to a peak or crescendo of pain lasting from a few seconds to a minute and then gradually fades back down to the original constant burning pain. This pain is easily distinguished from causalgic pain[12] and is from a different cause. Patients may stop talking or interrupt an activity to grip the arm during a paroxysm of pain, flexing the head toward the affected arm until the paroxysm of pain has passed. The pain has no pattern and does not vary with external stimulus. Patients may have difficulty getting to sleep, but once asleep, they are not usually awakened by the pain.

It is difficult for the patient to understand why he should feel pain in an anesthetic limb when no pathway is left between the arm and the spinal cord. Interestingly, preganglionic pain is not usually immediate but occurs up to 2 to 3 weeks after injury.[13] Previous experimental work by Loeser and Ward in 1976,[6] demonstrated that following severance of the trigeminal nerve of the cat, the cells in the dorsal horn fired spontaneously. The frequency of this abnormal firing increased over a 3-week period until the cells were firing almost continually. This barrage of abnormal firing could result from the loss of normal afferent input from the nerve that had been divided. Much of the input to the spinal cord results in central inhibition, and its loss leads to the unsuppressed firing of cells in the dorsal horn.[11] The clinical observation of preganglionic pain occurring a few weeks after injury is compatible with these experimental findings. The sudden deafferentation of the spinal cord leads to the lack of central inhibition, which results in the severe pain the patients feel. Interestingly, pain is frequently felt in the dermatome of the root that has been avulsed.

The following signs and symptoms characterize many postganglionic lesions.
1. Slow-speed, small-impact accident
2. No loss of consciousness
3. No associated injuries
4. No Horner sign
5. Negative sensory action potentials
6. Normal myelogram
7. Positive Tinel or neuroma sign
8. No pain

Obviously these signs and symptoms are intended as a guideline to indicate diagnosis and are not definitive.

The presence of a neuroma sign will indicate a rupture as distinguished from a Tinel sign. When tapping over the level of the lesion it will be acutely tender, and the patient will tend to flinch and move away from the stimulus. Paresthesias will be felt in the distribution of that root. There will also be no distal Tinel sign. The presence of a proximal Tinel sign and a distal Tinel sign gives a guideline for the rate of growth of the nerve recovery. The significance of the neuroma sign is that a rupture has most likely occurred, and if it is consistent with other signs and symptoms, no further recovery will occur unless a neurovascular repair is performed. However, repair is rarely performed in the lower trunk of the plexus because nerve growth is slow and intrinsic muscle fibrosis in the hand will have occurred by the time nerve growth is complete.

Motor function. Assessment of motor function in a flail arm has to be approached in a different manner than that of muscle charting in the normal way. The therapist is trying to identify flickers of movement in individual muscles that relate to individual nerve roots. Conventional muscle charting has to be modified in an attempt to produce isolated activity in muscles being tested. In a complete lesion of the brachial plexus, recovery will take place proximally, so a detailed knowledge of the shoulder girdle and its muscles is essential. Detection of a flicker in the rhomboids, for example, indicates recovery in the C5 root. It is important to point out that the extraordinary variation of specific root supplies must be borne in mind when a particular pattern is emerging that is not consistent with the clinical findings. However, there are some consistencies, and activity in the following muscle fibers can generally be relied on.

Upper fibers of pectoralis major (clavicular fibers)—recovery of C5, 6, and 7 (upper trunk)

Lower fibers of pectoralis major (sternal fibers)—recovery of C7 and 8 and T1 (lower trunk)

The technique of muscle charting in a flail arm should adhere to the following guidelines: When testing for pectoralis major clavicular fibers, the therapist supports the patient's whole arm, which should be above the horizontal line of the shoulder joint, and asks the patient to bring his arm across his body.[1a] Obviously the patient would be unable to do that, but with the arm fully supported in the therapist's arms, any activity in the pectoralis major clavicular fibers can be palpated by the therapist's other hand. Similarly, to test for the sternal fibers of pectoralis major, the patient's arm is supported below the horizontal line of the shoulder girdle, and the patient is asked to draw his elbow and arm down into his waist.

Sensory function. As with motor assessment, an accurate sensory assessment can greatly assist in a clinical diagnosis. The anomalies that occur in sensory innervation are well known. The patient with a total avulsion of the plexus will have a virtually anesthetic arm; however, invariably some intact sensation occurs on the inside of the upper arm and over the shoulder girdle, which is presumably from T2 and C4, respectively. This innervation may vary to a greater or lesser degree. More often, in a mixed lesion of the brachial plexus and also when recovery is occurring, the sensory pattern may vary, and it is therefore necessary to have a detailed sensory map showing different qualities of sensation.

Sensory evaluation is not particularly specialized in the brachial plexus patient, and sensory mapping is performed by light fingertip touch only because the arm is paralyzed and one has the value of other sophisticated tests such as sensory action potentials. As the examination is prolonged, it is felt unnecessary to employ other sensory evaluation tests (this, of course, does not apply to the late stage if regeneration has occurred, allowing active movement and a more specific sensory picture is required).

Joint range of motion. Immediately following injury, brachial plexus patients have full range of movement. However, invariably these patients are seen first in physiotherapy departments some time after the initial injury when joint limitation of range of movement has already occurred. Patients develop characteristic limitation of motion as a result of the arm resting in a sling across the body, and this limitation is generally consistent in all patients. A summary of this limitation is as follows:

Shoulder—loss of elevation, abduction and external rotation

Elbow—reduced extension and supination

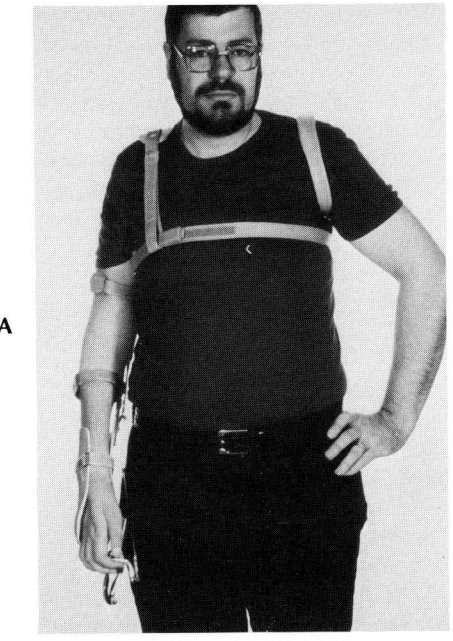
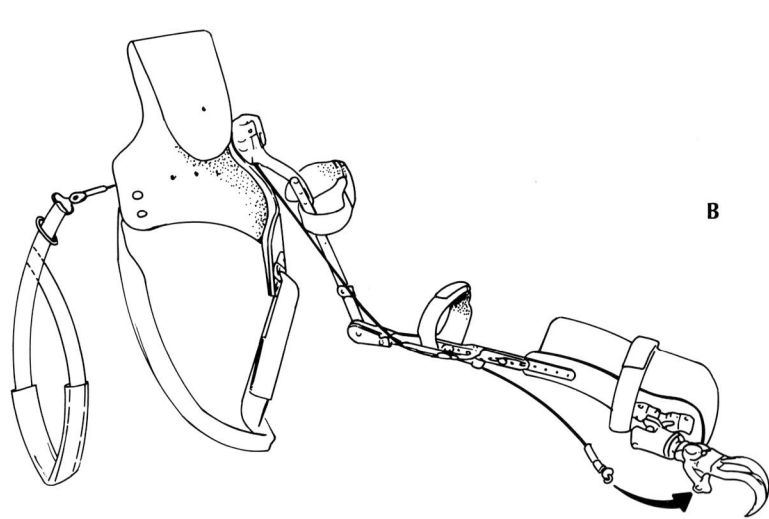

Fig. 47-2 **A,** Functional full-arm splint. **B,** Flail arm splint. (Redrawn from Robinson C: Brit J Occ Therapy 49(10): 331, 1986.)

Wrist—reduced dorsiflexion
Metacarpophalangeal (MP) joint—reduced flexion
Interphalangeal (IP) joints—reduced extension
Soft tissue contracture also commonly occurs. A summary of these follows:

1. Shortening of the long flexor tendons—results in loss of full extension of the fingers
2. Fibrosis of the long extensors and intrinsic complex—results in loss of IP joint flexion when the MP joints are at 90 degrees of flexion
3. Contracture of adductor pollicis—results in loss of thumb web space

Splinting. A patient with a flail arm should never be splinted, because contractures will quickly follow. However, use of the functional flail arm splint* (Fig. 47-2)[9] may provide the patient with bilateral function while he is waiting for recovery to occur. The option of the flail arm splint must be discussed in depth and in detail with the patient. The concept of the splint as a useful tool during the wait for recovery must be emphasized. As with many aspects of rehabilitation, the motivation of the patient is the driving force in the successful application of the flail arm splint. The therapist's judgment is therefore vital when selecting a patient for the use of the flail arm splint. A patient who is not truly motivated or suitable for a flail arm splint may well cause a lot of time to be wasted by the therapist and the patient.

Rehabilitation program

Goals, both general and specific, must be clearly set if the aims of treatment are to be met. The rehabilitation of the patient can best be managed collectively by a team approach of the physician, physiotherapist, occupational therapist, social worker, resettlement officer, and psychol-

ogist all working closely together. The patient's expectations and what he hopes to achieve at this stage of his rehabilitation must be clearly defined. Specific aims of treatment arrived at from careful assessment are as follows:

1. Restore or maintain full passive range of motion in the arm
2. Maintain full extensibility of the soft tissue structures
3. Relieve pain
4. Assess function and suitability for fitting of the flail arm splint and subsequent training in its use
5. Care of the anesthetic arm
6. Restoration of social skills and integration back into life
7. Assessment of work situation with a view to resettlement or alternative work opportunities

Passive movement exercises. The patient is encouraged to take responsibility for his own treatment program at the outset of physiotherapy.[3,4] Patients are expected to do their own passive movements as soon as possible. The movements should be simple, few, and effective (the more complex and numerous, the less likely the patient is to perform them regularly). Movements should be directed at gaining full range of motion and stretching soft tissues at the same time. Table 47-1 lists appropriate exercises. A comparison of the equivalent movement performed by the uninjured arm gives a good guide to the patient of the full range of motion possible and enables him to work towards a specific goal with the flail arm.

If the patient has existing soft tissue and joint contracture, then obviously traditional physiotherapeutic techniques can be employed to mobilize stiff joints and improve extensibility of soft tissue contracture. This treatment, however, should be aimed at active methods, such as soft tissue stretching, massage, and Maitland mobilization techniques[7] because serial splinting has proved to be ineffective in these cases in general. This is probably owing to the fact that

*Hugh Steepers, Ltd., London, U.K.

Table 47-1 Passive movements to the flail arm

Patient's position	Joint	Movement
Lying	Shoulder	Flexion, elevation
Lying	Shoulder	Elevation, external rotation
Lying	Elbow	Support upper arm with opposite hand and use weight of forearm and hand to extend flail elbow
Sitting	Elbow	Grip forearm between knees and extend elbow with the other arm
Sitting	Wrist	Flex, extend, rotate
Sitting	MP and IP joints	Flex all joints simultaneously to make a full fist
Sitting	MP and IP joints	Extend all joints simultaneously
Sitting	Thumb web	Grip hand between knees, gently stretch thumb away from palm

Frampton VM: Management of brachial plexus lesions, J Hand Ther 1(3):118, 1988.

gaining one movement is usually at the expense of the opposite movement and because no active movement is present, achieves no functional objective.

Pain relief. The use of the transcutaneous electrical nerve stimulator (TENS) has proved one of the most effective means in relieving avulsion pain.[11] As discussed earlier, the resulting deafferentation of the spinal cord after an avulsion injury leads to changes in the firing of the dorsal horn cells in the spinal cord. One might argue that application of TENS might artificially restore an afferent input to the spinal cord. Obviously this would necessitate application of the electrodes proximal to the level of the lesion. An illustration of different electrode placements can be seen in Fig. 47-3. In general, in the brachial plexus injured patient one large pad should be placed over the appropriate damaged dermatome (providing there is some residual afferent input) and the other pad may be placed over the nerve trunk of the appropriate root level of damage. Where there is some residual sensation in the arm electrodes can be placed more distally. Pads can also be placed over the area of sensation that is impaired, providing it is not anesthetic, because this would provide no afferent pathway along which the electrical stimulus could pass to the spinal cord. To provide as large an afferent input as possible large electrode pads are recommended in preference to the small pads that are usually issued as standard items with most units.[11] A scrupulous technique and application of electrodes is essential to successful treatments, because poor results can often be attributed to basic trivial technical faults. Single-channel units are usually adequate and the least complicated for the patient to operate. In our experience, one of the most frequent reasons for poor or unsustained pain relief with TENS has been shown to result from inadequate periods of stimulation.[2] A minimum duration of treatment of 8 hours a day for 3 weeks is recommended.

After 3 weeks of treatment the stimulation can be reduced gradually by an hour a day. If the pain returns, the period of stimulation of the reduced hours, for example 4 hours, should be maintained for a few more weeks. It must be emphasized that the nature of this pain is central in essence,

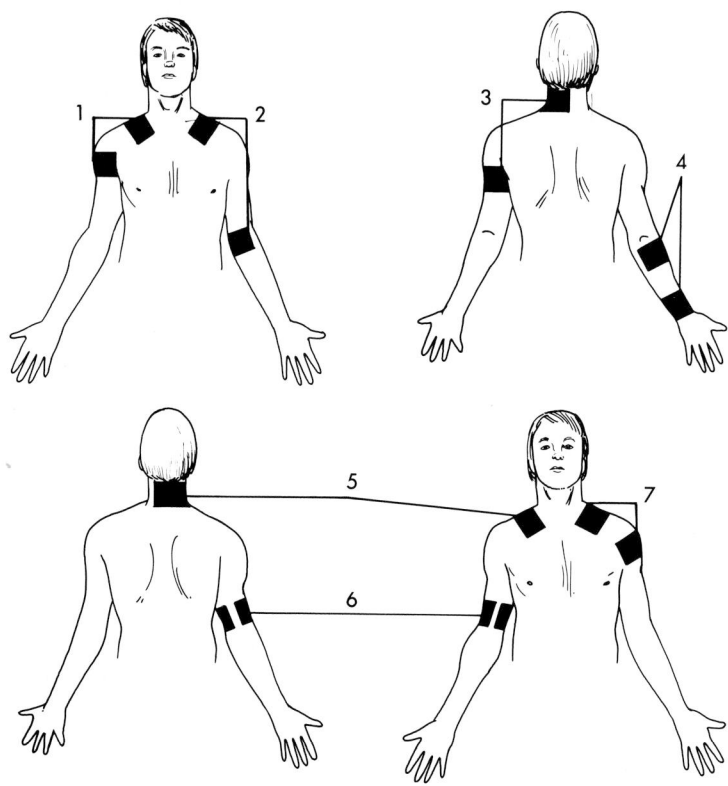

Fig. 47-3 TENS electrode placements 1 to 7 for brachial plexus patients with avulsion pain.

and the hypothesis that is being employed is that TENS is restoring an artificial input to the spinal cord and thus exercising some inhibition centrally. It must be emphasized to the patient that the TENS should not limit functional activities at all; indeed, distraction provides one of the best forms of pain relief for patients suffering with this avulsion pain.

Flail arm splint. The flail arm splint is a modular splint that is, in effect, a skeleton of an upper limb prosthesis that fits over the paralyzed arm[9,14] (see also Fig. 47-2). This splint provides a shoulder support (allowing some abduction and preventing glenohumeral subluxation), an elbow lock device (allowing five alternative positions of flexion of the elbow), and a forearm-to-wrist support trough, which has a platform on the flexor aspect, onto which standard artificial limb appliances can be fitted. These are operated in the same manner as a prosthesis by a cable running from the terminal appliance to a shoulder strap on the opposite shoulder. For partial lesions of the brachial plexus, for example, a lower trunk injury of C8, T1, a gauntlet splint is available that provides just a forearm trough with the standard artificial limb appliances on the platform together with the cable. An elbow lock together with a shoulder support only for upper trunk lesions of the brachial plexus is also available; it may have a wrist drop appliance if required. The flail arm splint is a lightweight modular splint and can be fitted in 1½ to 2 hours. The advantage that it has over a prosthetic arm is the cosmetic advantage of allowing the patient to retain his limb. The alternative of amputation and fitting of a prosthesis is not to be recommended, because paralysis of the shoulder girdle muscles in most brachial plexus lesions prevents good operation of an artificial limb. As mentioned in the introductory discussion, the flail arm splint functions as a tool for use at work and for hobbies. It can be taken off when not in use, leaving the patient's own arm, and thus is cosmetically quite acceptable.

Social and occupational status. Support and counseling must be given from the onset of injury. Most of these patients are young men at the beginning of their careers, who have young families to support. Evaluation of the patient's work must take place at an early stage, and the following pertinent questions must be asked:

1. Can the patient return to his existing employment?
2. Can the patient return to his existing employer in a different occupation?
3. Is retraining in alternative skills the only option?

Traditional methods of training the patient to perform daily living activities with one arm must be taught.

Summary of early stage rehabilitation

At the end of this episode of care at the early stage of rehabilitation, the patient should have achieved and received the following:

1. Possible prognosis of his injury
2. A home exercise program
3. Provision of and training in the flail arm splint
4. If present, control of pain
5. Reestablished his social links
6. Vocational advice and direction
7. A follow-up appointment for review at the middle stage

MIDDLE STAGE OF REHABILITATION

The degree of recovery will vary according to the severity of the original injury. As described earlier, because of the complexity of the injury and the difficulty in defining the exact extent of injury, it is impossible to predict individual prognoses. A lesion that at the beginning was defined as a lesion in continuity may not necessarily produce a good outcome. Reevaluation of the motor and sensory functions will determine when the next episode of treatment should commence. It is important for the patient to attend for an intensive but relatively short period of reeducation and active physiotherapy so that the patient's life and employment status are disrupted as little as possible. Long-term attendance at physiotherapy departments prevents full integration back into the community and slows down ultimate rehabilitation. Aims of treatment at this middle stage are these:

1. Reeducate and strengthen reinnervating muscles
2. Mobilize stiff joints and soft tissue contractures and reinforce home exercise programs
3. Reevaluate pain behavior and modify TENS application if indicated
4. Reevaluate the flail arm splinting with a view to reducing sections if sufficient recovery has occurred

All conventional techniques of reeducation can be employed. The use of proprioceptive neuromuscular facilitation (PNF), brushing, and progressive resisted exercises can all be employed. Techniques of icing can also be used but with caution depending on the state of the sensory function.

Occupational and social situation should also be reevaluated.

LATE STAGE OF REHABILITATION

The last stage of management of patients with brachial plexus injuries is certainly the most critical for the patient. Assessment of the residual disability and evaluation of the functional loss is essential before consideration of reconstructive surgery. In most cases reconstructive surgery is not considered before 2 years after injury. By this time maximum recovery will have occurred. However, on some occasions recovery can continue to a lesser extent for several more years.

Reconstructive surgery in brachial plexus lesions is more complicated than in single peripheral nerve injuries because of the complex nature of the injury.[5] Poor proprioception and reduced range of movement are more widespread. Because muscles derive their power from more than one nerve root, muscles for transfer may not have full power, may lack independent action, and are effective only in a mass pattern of movement. Pain may still be present, causing significant dysfunction on attempted active movement. In many cases a series of operations needs to be planned.[8] For this and all the other reasons already mentioned, consideration for surgery and the subsequent rehabilitation is made more difficult. However, tendon transfers can often be performed earlier in brachial plexus lesions when the definitive diagnosis is known[5]; for example, following exploration and repair of a nerve root rupture, a nerve root avulsion may be identified. In this case, tendon transfer to restore the function of those muscles supplied by the avulsed root may take place earlier. Above all, the degree of sensory function may dictate the success or failure of reconstructive surgery, and therefore preoperative assessment must include a full sensory evaluation.[10,15] Identifying the factors that lead to loss of function may result in a conclusion of sensory impairment being the predominant limiting factor and the motor loss being a minor contributing one. If a sequence of procedures is being planned, it is necessary that the first procedure is maximized before attempting the next. For example, for the patient who has loss of elbow flexion and wrist and finger extension, a decision has to be made regarding which function to restore first. If hand function is restored first, then the provision of an elbow-lock splint to stabilize elbow flexion would assist function in the hand. When a second procedure of restoring elbow flexion is performed, a good functioning hand is already present and would aid recovery by providing a good functioning arm. An in-depth functional assessment is essential. Three fundamental questions must be asked:

1. What is the patient able to do at present?
2. What is he unable to do?
3. What does he want to be able to do?

Finally, after 2 years of rehabilitation the patient might have adopted unusual patterns of movement employing what muscle power he has to effect some activity. It is therefore essential to evaluate what the patient might lose, as well as what he might gain. The classic example is one of a brachial plexus injured patient who also has a lumbar spinal cord injury. The transference of pectoralis major into biceps would restore elbow flexion, but the patient would lose the ability to transfer out of his wheelchair.

Preoperative assessment and treatment

Preoperative treatment may be indicated if any of the above problems have been identified. This might include the following:

1. An intensive period of muscle strengthening to increase a grade of power in a weak motor to be transferred may be indicated, because muscles functionally lose a grade of power on transfer.
2. Reeducation of individual muscle action. If a motor to be transferred is effective only in a mass pattern of movement, reeducation techniques may be required to improve its independent action.
3. Mobilization and soft tissue stretching of any contracture present is essential before transferring a motor around that joint. Serial splinting may be indicated at this stage. For example, a patient requiring an opposition tendon transfer for his thumb may require stretching of the adductor pollicis muscle to allow full excursion of the movement of the thumb.
4. Pain may still be a problem and can seriously jeopardize results if not treated.
5. Reevaluation of sensory function may indicate a need for an intensive period of sensory reeducation[10,15] or pain relief from hypersensitivity.[12] For example, an opposition transfer to the thumb would restore pinch and precision grip, but it may do little to restore function if the sensory function is poor or painful.

Selection of muscles for transfer. Selection of muscles for reconstruction can be helped by writing down the movement lost, the muscle or motor available to restore the loss, its power, and what is left to balance the loss of that transferred muscle.[8] For example, in an upper trunk lesion of the brachial plexus the residual functional loss may be loss of wrist and finger extension. Wrist extension is restored by transferring pronator teres, finger extension by flexor carpi ulnaris (FCU) transfer, and thumb abduction by palmaris longus. In this example, pronator teres is 0, leaving FCU at 3 + the only motor available for transfer. However, the weakness of a muscle for transfer is not always a contraindication to surgery as it might be in the case of peripheral nerve injuries. It may be that two of the three motors are sufficient to restore some function.

Limitation of joint range, soft tissue contracture, lack of power of the transferred muscle, lack of independent action of a transferred muscle and its cocontraction with antagonist muscles, and poor sensory function and pain, result in different goals being set for patients with brachial plexus lesions than for those with peripheral nerve injuries. The principals of tendon transfers learned from single peripheral nerve injuries sometimes have to be modified in brachial plexus lesions in an attempt to improve function. Patients' expectations must be clearly defined, and the goals of the operation explained to them precisely. A clear understanding of the procedure and what is required from the patient greatly assists rehabilitation and reeducation.

Postoperative rehabilitation. Lack of proprioceptive feedback, weakness of a transferred muscle, and one muscle powering two movements may result in different goals of rehabilitation being set for patients with brachial plexus lesions. One might expect in 1 week to have achieved smooth, coordinated wrist and finger extension in a tendon transfer performed for a radial nerve lesion, so that activities requiring coordinated control of wrist extension, while allowing the fingers to perform a more intricate task such as typing, are possible. In a brachial plexus lesion, if one motor is powering two movements, one might concentrate on finger extension while supporting the wrist in a wrist support splint; then work on the wrist extension could be done separately. Trying to activate both movements may cause the motor transfer to fatigue quickly; then trick movements will result. The basic principals of rehabilitation after tendon transfer follows these guidelines:

1. Support the transfer and avoid undue strain and tension.
2. Remembering the old action of a transferred muscle in an attempt to facilitate the new action of the tendon transfer may be effective.
3. Placement of the therapist's hands is vital to encourage correct sensory feedback while at the same time supporting the transfer and palpating to feel the new action of a muscle.
4. Guided resistance to a movement can sometimes reinforce its new action.
5. Accessory joint movements can improve proprioception and joint awareness, while at the same time mobilizing gently any stiff joints involved. This also avoids undue strain on the transfer.
6. Correct commands facilitate reeducation and should be directed at asking for the new action and resisting the old action.
7. In some cases, icing, brushing, and biofeedback can be used to facilitate the new action of a muscle.

Trick movements should be discouraged in the early stages of rehabilitation but may have to be accepted eventually to restore some function. For example, a tenodesis effect by using the tension of a tendon transfer can be employed to effect an action such as release of grip by palmar flexing the wrist, which applies tension on the FCU transfer into the extensor digitorum tendons. Splinting can be helpful and should be used until the patient can use the tendon transfer with good control and coordination of the new action. However, close monitoring of range of movement is essential because this can be lost quickly in the patient with brachial plexus injuries if he is immobilized for any period of time. Apart from reeducation of normal functional activities, it is important to encourage general activities such as swimming and other bilateral activities. The use of a video can be helpful if a sequence of procedures is planned and an ongoing record of functional activities can be kept.

CASE STUDY

Twenty-one year old male student sustained a right brachial plexus lesion and an avulsion of C5 and 6 root. One year following his accident infraspinatus and biceps were 0. He could flex his elbow to 90 degrees by means of Steindler action; this was not functional, however, because he could not use the hand. Also, lack of external rotation of the shoulder meant the forearm came across the body on elbow flexion. As the sequence of procedures was planned, it was decided to restore elbow flexion first, and a Steindler flexorplasty[1] was performed. This was immobilized in 100 degrees of flexion at the elbow for 4 weeks. Reeducation commenced but was restricted by pain as a result of the avulsion lesion. TENS was applied with success, and reeducation was continued for 3 weeks.

Five months later a Zachary transfer[16] was performed to restore some external rotation of the shoulder so that placement of the arm with elbow flexion could be improved. After 6 weeks of immobilization in external rotation and abduction, reeducation commenced, and he had 3 weeks of treatment. Range of movement had to be restored gradually over 7 to 10 days. Foam wedges were effective as temporary splints to gradually reduce the angle of abduction. At a 2-year follow-up he had good elbow flexion to 100 degrees, and the Zachary tendon transfer enabled him to place his hand in a functional plane. Despite the fact that the sequence of operations was well planned, the results were jeopardized by the return of pain, which had to be treated before the next operation could proceed.

In summary, the need for careful, if time-consuming, assessment before reconstructive surgery with emphasis on expected functional improvement is essential. The need to understand surgical procedure is vital. The physiotherapist must establish his or her role within the team as a knowledgeable and enthusiastic member. That role must lie largely in a comprehensive assessment of the patient with complete understanding of his problems, and in the ability to administer appropriate preoperative and postoperative treatment and treatment at all stages of recovery.

REFERENCES

1. Aids to the Examination of the Peripheral Nervous System, London, 1986, Balliere Tindall.
1a. Brooks D: Poliomyelitis: reconstructive techniques. Steindler flexorplasty. In Furlong R, editor: Operative surgery: Rob and Smith, ed 2, vol 8, London, 1969, Butterworths.
2. Erickson, SB: The influence of Naloxone on analgesia produced by peripheral conditioning stimulation, Brain Res 173: 295, 1979.
3. Frampton VM: Management of brachial plexus lesions, Hand Ther 1(3):115, 1988.
4. Frampton VM: Management of brachial plexus lesions, Physiotherapy 70:389, 1984.
5. Frampton VM: Problems in managing reconstructive surgery for brachial plexus lesions contrasted with peripheral nerve lesions, J Hand Surg 11(B): 3, 1986.
6. Loeser JD and Ward AA: Some effects of deafferentation on neurons of the cat spinal cord, Arch Neurol 17:629, 1967.
7. Maitland GD: Peripheral manipulation, ed 2, London, 1987, Butterworths.
8. Omer GE: The technique and timing of tendon transfers, Orthop Clin North Am 5(2):377, 1974.
9. Robinson C: Brachial plexus lesion. Functional splintage, Part 2. Br J Occup Ther 49(10):331, 1986.
10. Salter MI: Hand injuries: a therapeutic approach, Edinburgh, 1987, Churchill Livingstone.
11. Wells PE, Frampton VM, and Bawsher D: Pain management in physical therapy, vol 1, Calif, 1988, Appleton & Lange.
12. Withrington RH and Wynn-Parry CB: The management of painful peripheral nerve disorders, J Hand Surg 9B(1):24, 1984.
13. Wynn-Parry CB: Pain in avulsion lesions of the brachial plexus, Pain 9:41, 1980.
14. Wynn-Parry CB: Rehabilitation of the hand, ed 4, London, 1981, Butterworth & Co (Publishers) Ltd.
15. Wynn-Parry CB and Salter M: Sensory re-education after median nerve lesions, Hand 8:250, 1976.
16. Zachary RB: Transplantation of the teres major and latissimus dorsi for loss of external rotation at the shoulder, Lancet 2:757, 1947.

48

Therapist's management of carpal tunnel syndrome

Patricia L. Baxter-Petralia

Carpal tunnel syndrome is compression of the median nerve at the level of the carpal tunnel (Fig. 48-1). The purpose of this chapter is to provide guidelines for the therapist's management of carpal tunnel syndrome during the nonoperative and the postoperative phases. For approximately 60% of patients with mild carpal tunnel syndrome, Thompson found conservative treatment was sufficient.[21]

PATHOLOGY

Compression of the median nerve within the carpal tunnel can be attributed to an alteration in the osseous margins of the carpus caused by fractures, dislocations, or arthritic joint changes; an increase in volume of tunnel contents secondary to tenosynovitis; or thickening of the transverse carpal ligament (Fig. 48-2).[3,14,16-18,20]

Phelan reported that the most common cause of carpal tunnel syndrome was fibrosis or thickening of the flexor synovium secondary to a chronic, nonspecific tenosynovitis of the flexor tendons in the carpal tunnel.[15] Other cases result from trauma, tumor, or systemic disease.[12]

Sunderland differentiated acute compression of the median nerve from chronic progressive compression.[19] In acute compression a severe deforming force, such as traumatic dislocation of the carpal bones, causes mechanical deformation of the carpal tunnel and ischemic changes of the median nerve. Immediate surgery is necessary to relieve an acute compression and thus prevent permanent nerve dam-

age. Rapid improvement of sensory conduction within 30 minutes follows decompression.[5]

Sunderland outlined the stages of degeneration in chronic progressive compression. In stage I progressive obstruction of the venous return occurs, causing circulatory slowing in the epineurial and intrafunicular tissues. This disturbance leads to pathologic changes inside the funiculi. The intrafunicular capillaries increase the intrafunicular pressure. The combination of intrafunicular pressure and the slowing of the intrafunicular circulation impairs the nutrition of the nerve fibers.[6]

The hypoxic nerve fibers become hyperexcitable and discharge spontaneously. The mylinated fibers are more affected than the thin, finely myelinated or nonmyelinated fibers.[7] Pain and paresthesia result from the imbalance of fiber activity and fiber dissociation.

Nocturnal paresthesia and pain are caused by impeded venous return from the distal part of the limb. At this stage, the structural changes may be corrected by treatment that eliminates or reduces pressure in the carpal tunnel.

In stage II, Sunderland stated that capillary circulation slows so severely that anoxia damages the endoneurium. Edema occurs as protein leaks into the surrounding tissues. Within funiculi, endoneurial tissue accumulates protein, which interferes with the nutrition and metabolism of the nerve fibers. Protein exudate promotes the proliferation of the fibroblasts and the formation of constrictive endoneurial

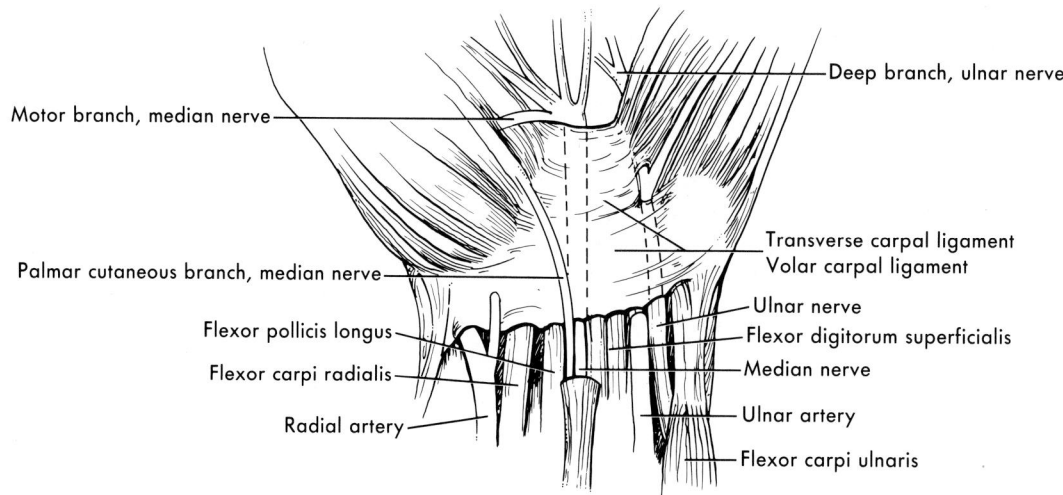

Fig. 48-1 The median nerve passes through the carpal tunnel, along with nine flexor tendons. The transverse carpal ligament supports the median nerve and flexor tendons volarly. (Redrawn from The American Society for Surgery of the Hand: Regional review course in hand surgery, 1985).

640

connective tissues. Segmental demyelination, axon thinning, and destruction of axons are found in individual nerve fibers. The severity of the lesion increases, resulting in greater damage to the sensory and motor fibers unless decompression occurs.

In stage III, nerve fibers can undergo wallerian degeneration with loss of axons, which results in a reduction in the number of axons available for regeneration. The compressed nerve becomes a fibrous cord, and in some cases the few surviving nerve fibers are contained within fibrosed funiculi in a dense avascular epineurium (Fig. 48-3).

Common patient complaints include pain (initially at night) weakness, clumsiness, and occasional burning shoulder pain. With chronic progressive compression, nocturnal pain and diminished sensation in the median nerve distribution may occur gradually and indicate a stage I compression. Burning pain and referred shoulder pain may indicate a stage II compression neuropathy. However, by the time the nerve compression has reached a stage III level, the pain complaints of the patient may have subsided or become more severe.[6] With an acute compression secondary to a traumatic injury, the patient may complain of numbness or severe pain.

Patients may be referred for therapy at any stage of compression. Patients with mild signs of chronic progressive carpal tunnel syndrome may be referred only for a static

wrist extension splint. Patients with acute compression following trauma and others with moderate to severe chronic progressive carpal tunnel syndrome are treated by both the surgeon and therapist.

The surgeon can project the length of treatment and the prognosis based on the extent of nerve degeneration identified through diagnostic tests. Patients should be educated when extensive nerve damage has occured that normal nerve function may not be fully recovered even after surgery and recovery may take place slowly.

EVALUATION OF CARPAL TUNNEL SYNDROME

Clinical signs of carpal tunnel syndrome can include diminished sensation in the thumb, index, long and radial aspect of the ring finger, which are innervated by the median nerve: atrophy of thenar muscles; a positive Tinel's sign at the wrist; and a positive Phalen's sign (Fig. 48-4).[7]

Physical examination by the surgeon may include visual inspection of the hand for pseudomotor changes in the skin area innervated by the median nerve, roentgenographic views of the carpal tunnel, and evaluation of the patient's subjective report of sensory disturbance following the Phalen's test and the Tinel's sign (Fig. 48-5).[3]

Gelberman and others found that the use of the Semmes-

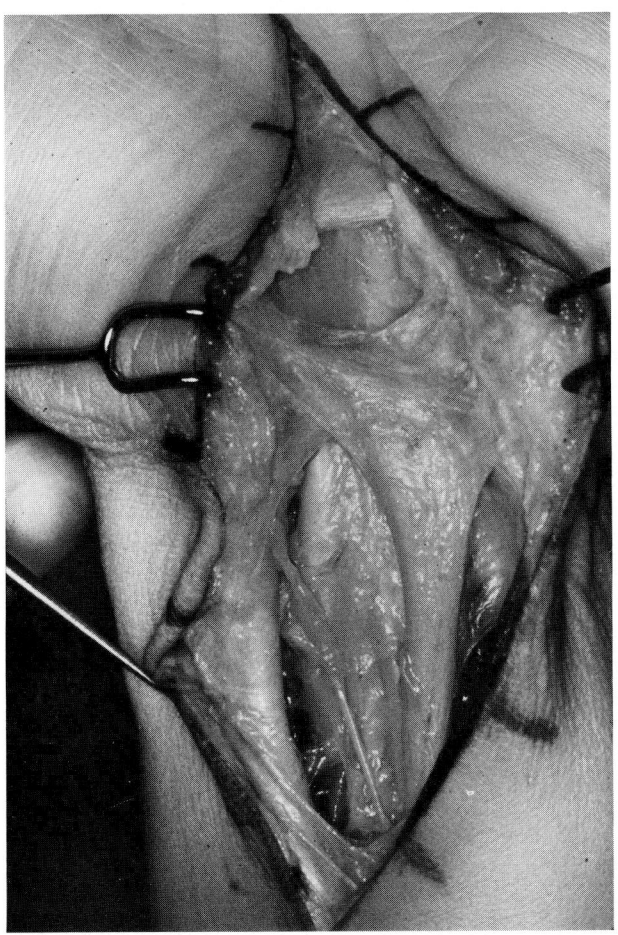

Fig. 48-2 Thickening of the flexor synovium is one cause of compression of the median nerve within the carpal tunnel.

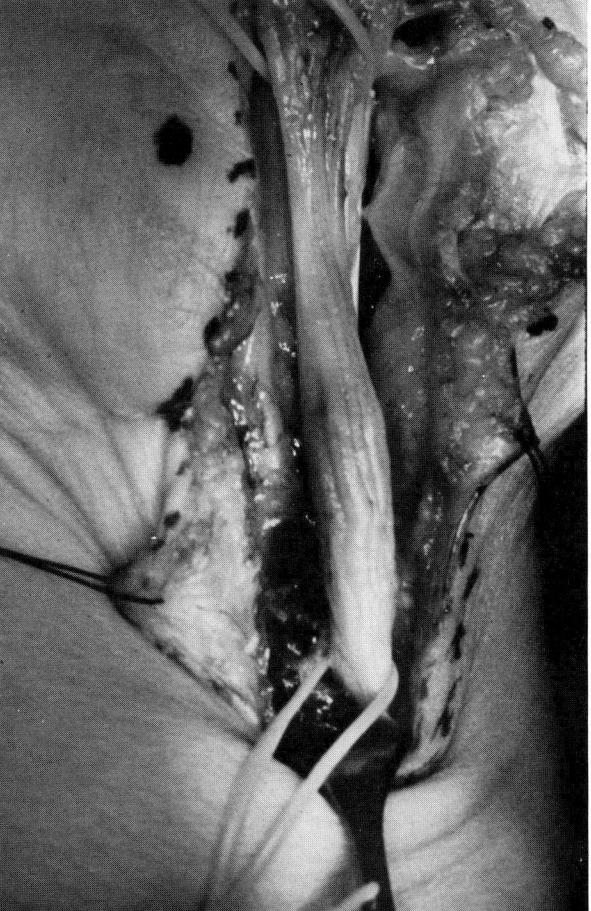

Fig. 48-3 In stage III compression of the median nerve, the compressed nerve undergoes fibrosis.

Weinstein Pressure Asthesiometer,* vibrometry, and nerve conduction studies identify early sensory deficits in the median nerve distribution before abnormalities are detected with two-point discrimination testing.[2] At the Hand Rehabilitation Center of Philadelphia, sensibility studies (including vibrometry, Semmes-Weinstein Presssure Asthesiometer, and two-point discrimination) are performed in

addition to nerve conduction studies and electromyographic studies.

Strength is tested with the Jamar dynamometer* and the Pinch Gauge.† Coordination testing may include evaluation of prehension through the use of the Jebson-Taylor hand function test or the Nine Hole Peg Test.[8,10] Several standardized coordination tests such as the Valpar Work Sam-

---

*North Coast Medical, Inc., Campbell, Calif.

*Asimow Engineering Co., Santa Monica, Calif.
†B&L Engineering, Sante Fe Springs, Calif.

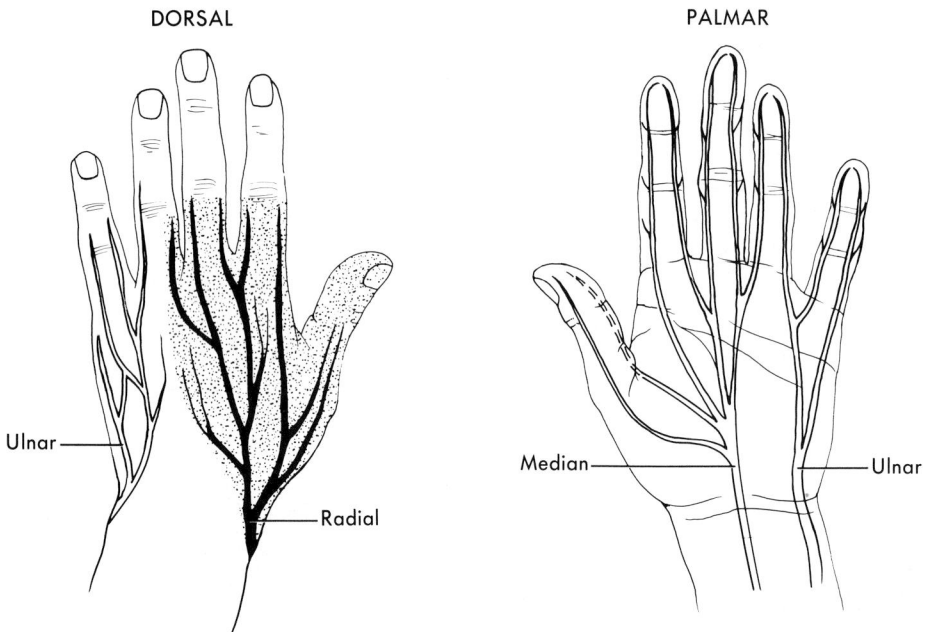

Fig. 48-4 The patient complains of sensory disturbances in the thumb, index, and long fingers and the radial half of the ring finger. (Redrawn from The American Society for Surgery of the Hand: The hand examination and diagnosis, New York, 1983, Churchill Livingstone, Inc.

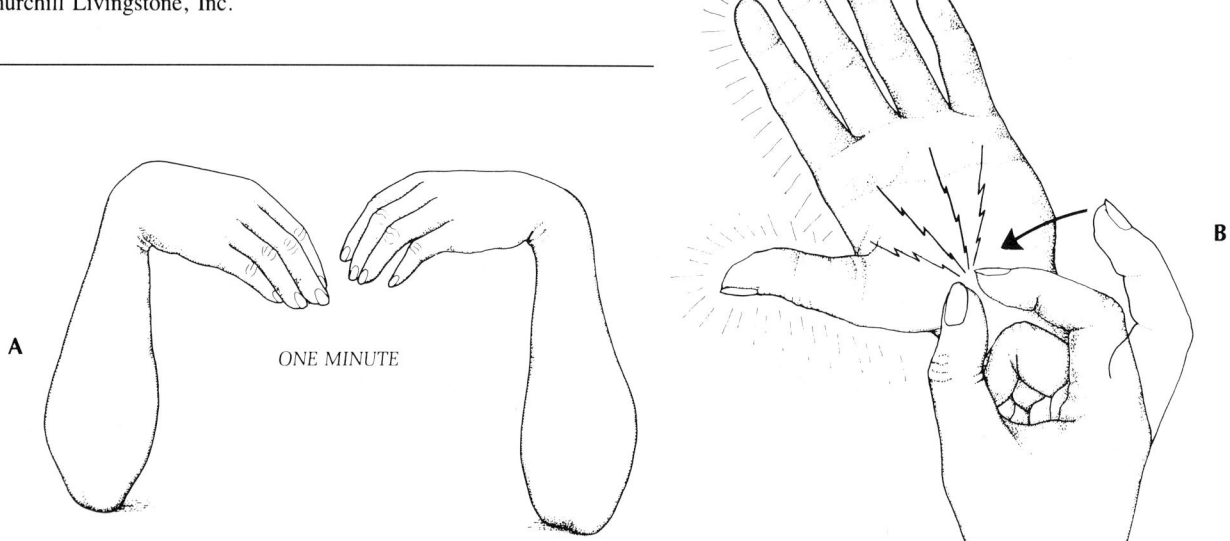

Fig. 48-5 **A,** The patient is asked to report any sensory changes in the median nerve innervated area after holding his wrists flexed for 1 minute. **B,** The examiner taps the hand from the fingertips proximally to the palm. The patient is asked to report any "electric shocks" or tingling when percussed. (Reprinted with permission from The American Society for Surgery of the Hand: The hand examination and diagnosis, New York, 1983, Churchill Livingstone, Inc.)

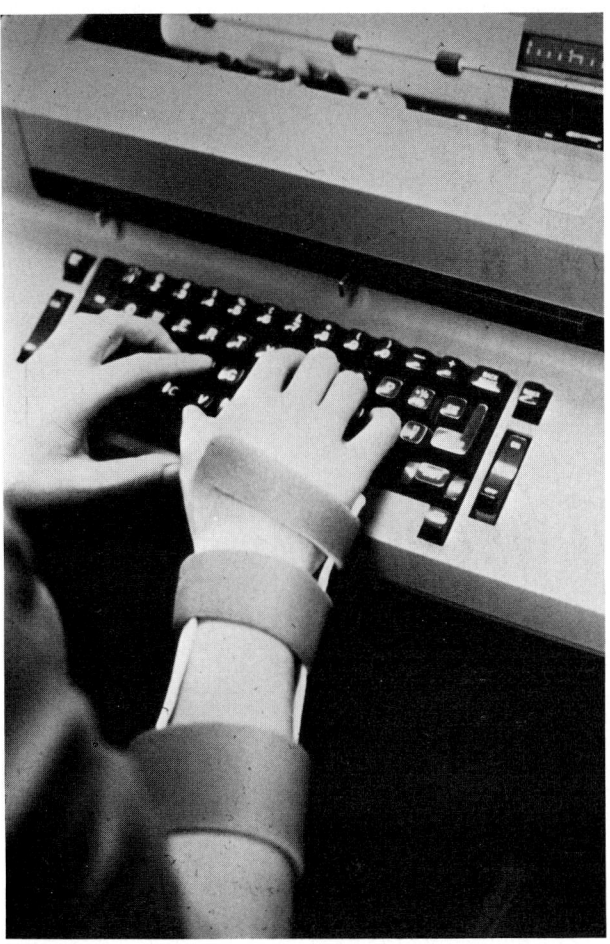

Fig. 48-6 The custom-designed volar wrist-extension splint can be used during work activities. The patient is taught how to maintain flexor muscle relaxation while wearing the splint.

ples* can be used to evaluate endurance for prolonged manipulation.

NONOPERATIVE MANAGEMENT

An individual may seek medical treatment because of symptoms of intermittent paresthesia, clumsiness, and nocturnal pain. Initial treatment by a physician may include a local steroid injection in the carpal tunnel, oral anti-inflammatory medication, and/or a volar wrist splint.[19,21] The therapist may fit the patient with a prefabricated volar wrist splint or fabricate a thermoplastic volar wrist extension splint with the wrist in 10 to 20 degrees of extension. The patient is instructed to wear this splint continually 4 to 6 weeks and to decrease splint use gradually over the subsequent 4 weeks. Instructions in the wear and care of the splint are provided. The patient should understand that the splint is necessary to eliminate the pressure on the median nerve when the wrist flexes (Fig. 48-6).

In addition to splint use, the patient is instructed to avoid certain wrist and hand postures and repetitive wrist motions that can contribute to carpal tunnel syndrome. These include gripping or pinching objects while flexing the wrist and performing repetitive wrist flexion-extension motions (Fig. 48-7).

If the patient must use wrist and hand postures at work that aggravate the carpal tunnel syndrome, he is instructed to perform the job task in a modified method. For example, instead of lifting a box by gripping the handle with the involved hand, the patient is instructed to use an extended palm of the involved hand to assist his other hand in lifting the box. The therapist also instructs the patient to control inflammation through the use of ice packs, tendon-gliding exercises, and elevated activities.[23]

Tendon-gliding exercises facilitate isolated excursion of each of the two flexor tendons to each finger that pass through the carpal tunnel. Each exercise is initiated from a postion of full finger and wrist extension. To obtain maximum differential gliding of profundus with respect to su-

---

*Valpar Work Samples, Tucson.

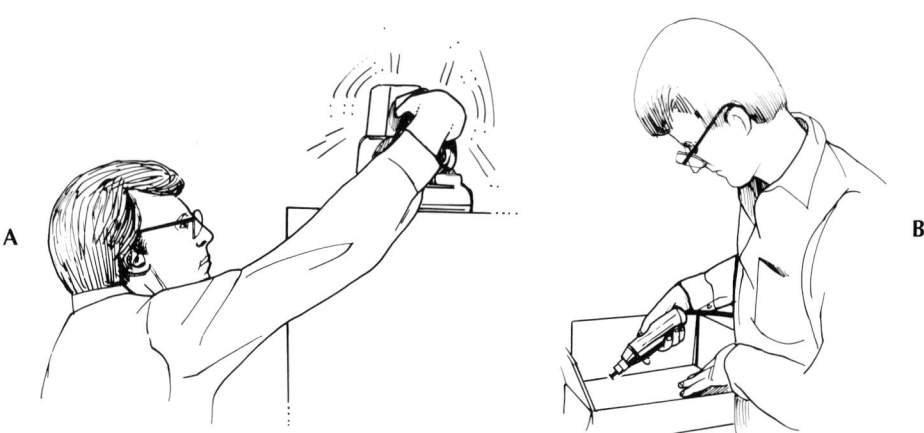

Fig. 48-7 **A,** Flexing the wrist, prolonged reaching, and working with vibrating tools can result in compression of the median nerve. **B,** Gripping a tool by ulnarly deviating the wrist can aggravate the median nerve within the carpal tunnel. (Redrawn from of the Travelers Insurance Companies: A management guide to work place design, The Indusrial Engineering Unit of the Travelers Insurance Companies.)

perficialis excursion, the patient assumes a "hook" fist position. To obtain maximum flexor digitorum superficialis excursion, the patient is instructed to flex the metacarpophalangeal (MP) joints and the proximal interphalangeal (PIP) joints while maintaining the distal interphalangeal (DIP) joints in extension. A full-fist exercise completes the series of tendon-gliding exercises and provides maximum profundus tendon excursion. These exercises are performed five times each, five times daily.

For some patients conservative management results in relief of symptoms, and further intervention is not necessary. Some, however, do not obtain relief from symptoms and may go on to require surgery. Decompression of the median nerve may also be necessary after acute injury. The surgical procedure varies but usually includes a release of the transverse carpal ligament. In selected cases, an external neurolysis or an internal neurolysis may be performed.[19]

Because pressure on the median nerve increases with wrist motion, the patient's hand should be immobilized in a volar wrist cast for 1 week after surgery. If the patient is allowed to remove the cast before 1 week, wrist motion may result in prolonged hypersensitivity.[22]

POSTSURGICAL MANAGEMENT

Goals of therapy during weeks one to three after surgery are control of edema, maintenance of range of motion, restriction of adhesion formation by differential gliding of the flexor tendons of the digits, and protected use of the hand. During the initial 3 weeks after surgery, the patient is instructed to control edema through constant elevation of the

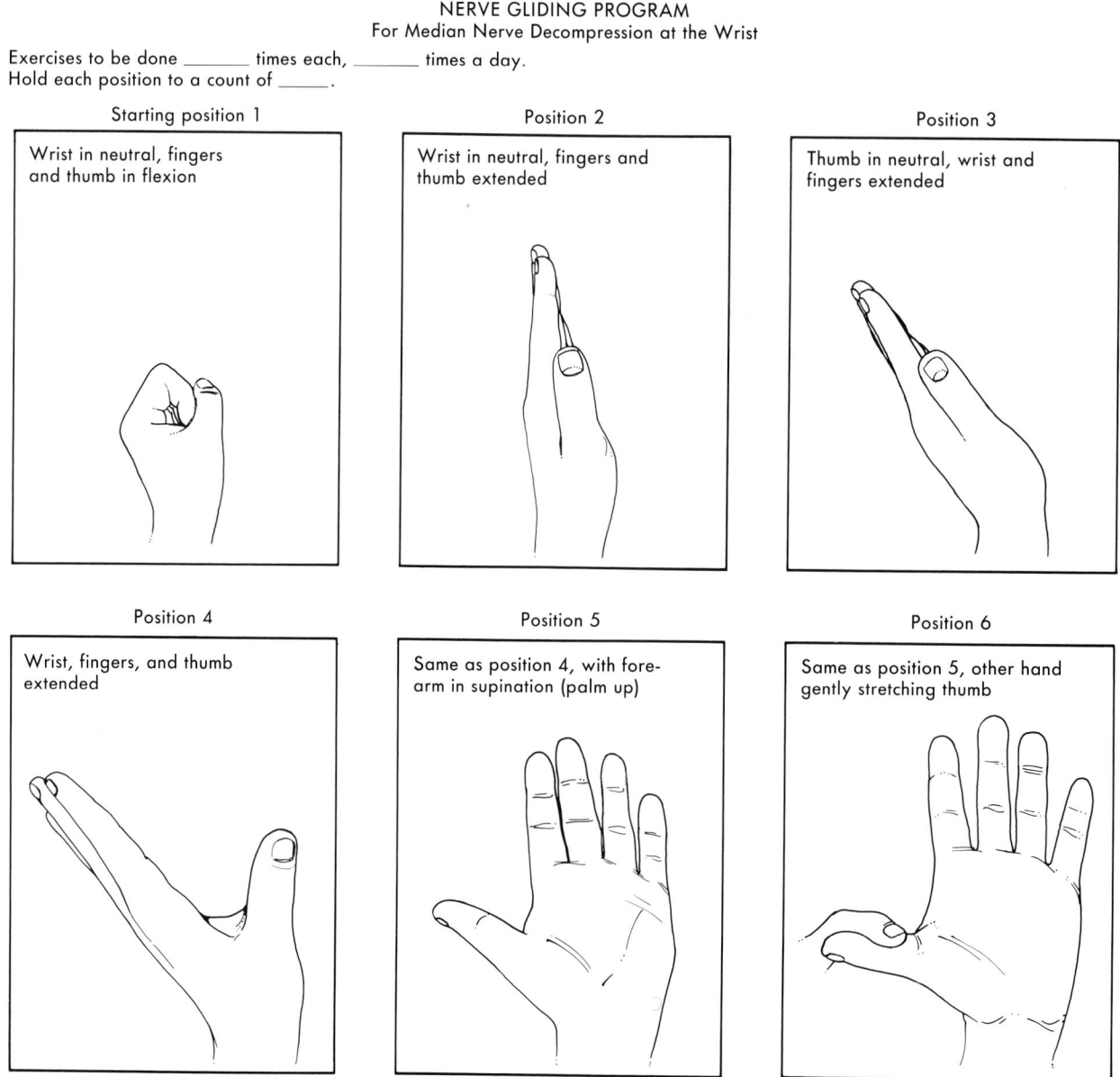

NERVE GLIDING PROGRAM
For Median Nerve Decompression at the Wrist

Exercises to be done _____ times each, _____ times a day.
Hold each position to a count of _____ .

Starting position 1	Position 2	Position 3
Wrist in neutral, fingers and thumb in flexion	Wrist in neutral, fingers and thumb extended	Thumb in neutral, wrist and fingers extended

Position 4	Position 5	Position 6
Wrist, fingers, and thumb extended	Same as position 4, with forearm in supination (palm up)	Same as position 5, other hand gently stretching thumb

Fig. 48-8 Nerve gliding exercises are initiated to facilitate mobilization of the median nerve. James Hunter, M.D., developed the exercises, and Julie Belkin, OTR, designed the home program.

involved hand and retrograde massage. Ten repetitions of tendon-gliding exercises and thumb flexion, extension, and opposition exercises are performed three times daily. Shoulder exercises are performed three times daily to maintain range of motion. Exercises include 10 repetitions of shoulder flexion, extension, and internal and external rotation.

One week after surgery, the volar cast is removed. A volar wrist extension splint is fabricated, positioning the wrist in 10 to 20 degrees of extension; this splint is worn by the patient during sleep and during strenuous activities to provide continued support during the healing phase.

Depending on preoperative severity of symptoms and response to surgery some patients may require few or no therapy sessions, some require moderate intervention (3 to 8 weeks), and some require a comprehensive program (8 to 16 weeks). For those patients requiring further treatment, the goals of therapy 3 to 8 weeks after surgery include reducing edema, modeling the scar, reducing hypersensitivity, and increasing strength and functional use.

At this point, if the patient lacks full range of motion, active and passive exercises are initiated for the digits and wrist. Nerve-gliding exercises are initiated to ensure that the median nerve glides through the carpal tunnel and adjacent thenar and hypothenar eminences. A passive stretch of the thumb into extension is used to prevent adhesion formation along the palmar cutaneous and motor branch of the median nerve (Fig. 48-8). These exercises are performed three times daily for 10 repetitions.

The patient is instructed to continue tendon-gliding exercises and edema control efforts. If edema persists, the patient may be instructed to perform overhead bilateral fisting exercises, 20 repetitions each hour. String wrapping (see Chapter 13) and massage may also be prescribed for edema control.

Elevated prehension activities, such as macramé, can be included in the patient's clinic and home programs to permit gravity to assist in edema reduction. If thick hypertrophic scar is developing at the site of the incision, Elastomer is applied to the palmar scar to model it.

Following surgical decompression, if sensory disturbances result in prolonged paresthesia or hypersensitivity, the patient is instructed in a desensitization program[4] (see Chapter 56).

By the eighth week following surgery, graded isometric and isotonic strengthening exercises for the hand and wrist are initiated. The patient is cautioned against overexercise, which could result in tenosynovitis.

At 8 to 12 weeks after surgery, work hardening is initiated. The patient is instructed to increase use of his hand for light house repair, housecleaning chores, and light work tasks. Patients with sedentary jobs requiring less than 10 pounds of lifting may return to work by the eighth to tenth week.

If a patient's job requires a high frequency of repetitive handling and manipulation or his work requires heavy lifting of more than 10 pounds, it is recommended that he participate in a work tolerance program. His work tolerance is evaluated in therapy as he performs repetitive resistive exercises and job simulation. If swelling or symptoms occur with job simulation, then the length of treatment is prolonged 4 additional weeks.

By the sixteenth postoperative week, the patient's phys-ical capacity to perform his regular job is assessed. (Refer to the chapter on physical capacity evaluation.) Some patients return to their regular jobs; others return to the same place of employment and perform modified work. For example, a packer who worked on a food packing line may be transferred to a light maintenance job and an inspecting job.

The therapist communicates with the employer to explain the patient's limitations and abilities. If the employer cannot offer modified work, the therapist works closely with the rehabilitation specialist, who may present several alternative jobs and their physical demands to the therapist in a written evaluation. Based on the patient's performance in therapy and performance in the physical capacity evaluation, the therapist reviews each job's physical demands to determine the probability of the patient's physical ability to work in each job.

The therapist reports his/her findings to the surgeon who approves or disapproves the patient's release to a specific job.

Patients with long histories of chronic progressive compression may need further treatment for pain control. These patients may have returned to work but continue to have severe sensory disturbances such as sharp pain that radiates into the shoulder and neck. Some patients have their most severe pain at night. Electrical modalities may be helpful. High voltage galvanic stimulation (HVGS) appears to improve circulation and decrease muscle tightness in the neck and shoulder girdle.[11]

For some patients, a transcutaneous electrical nerve stimulator successfully blocks pain signals from entering the spinal cord level.[9] The placement of the electrodes is crucial. Trials at several different locations might be necessary to secure optimum pain relief. Both of these modalities can be rented for home use.

Other techniques have been helpful to patients with severe pain. Contrast baths increase circulation.[12] The patient dips his involved hand alternately in cool water (66° F) for 30 seconds and in warm water (96° F) for 30 seconds, for 15 to 30 minutes. Continuation of massage, splint use, and Elastomer or dermal palmar pads may diminish the patient's discomfort.

Psychological counseling is suggested if the patient or his family appears emotionally drained or depressed. Participation in a pain center program may teach the patient to cope with the chronic pain and learn to live a productive life.

SUMMARY

Therapeutic management of patients with carpal tunnel syndrome varies in the type of treatment and length of treatment. The level of compression of the median nerve and the patient's reaction to the resulting physical changes influence the prognosis of recovery and the length of treatment required. Fabrication of a volar wrist splint and instructions in techniques to minimize pressure on the median nerve may be sufficient for patients with mild carpal tunnel syndrome.

Some patients with moderate carpal tunnel syndrome require 8 to 12 weeks of therapy following surgical decompression. Techniques are used to control edema, promote tendon gliding, model scar, increase range of motion, desensitize hypersensitive skin, and strengthen muscles of the involved hand. Job simulation is used to evaluate the patient's physical capacity to perform regular work duties or a modified job.

Patients with severe carpal tunnel syndrome may require placement in a modified job. Also, pain control techniques have been helpful in teaching the patient to cope with the presence of chronic pain.

REFERENCES

1. Chaffin DB and Anderson GBJ: Occupational biomechanics, New York, 1984, John Wiley & Sons.
2. Gelberman RH and others: Sensibility testing in peripheral nerve syndromes, J Bone Joint Surg 65(A):632, 1983.
3. Gelmers HJ: The significance of Tinel's sign in the diagnosis of carpal tunnel syndrome, Acta Neurochir 49:255, 1979.
4. Hardy MA, Moran CA, and Merritt WH: Desensitization of the traumatized hand, Va Med 109:134, 1982.
5. Hongel A and Mattson HS: Neurographic studies before, after and during operation for median nerve compression in the carpal tunnel, Scand J Plast Reconstr Surg 5:103, 1971.
6. Hybbinette CH and Mannerfelt L: The carpal tunnel syndrome, Acta Orthop Scand 46:610, 1975.
7. Inglis AE, Straub LR, and Williams CS: Median nerve neuropathy at the wrist, Clin Orthop 83:48, 1972.
8. Jebson RH and others: An objective and standardized test of hand function, Arch Phys Med Rehabil 50:311, 1969.
9. Mannheimer JS and Lampe GL: Clinical transcutaneous electrical nerve stimualtion, Philadelphia, 1984, FA Davis Co.
10. Mathiowetz and others: Adult norms for the nine hole peg test of finger dexterity, Occup Ther J Res 5:1, 1984.
11. Michlovitz SL: Thermal agents, Philadelphia, 1986, FA Davis Co.
12. Paget J: Lectures on surgical pathology, Philadelphia, Lindsay & Blakiston, 1854.
13. Parry CB: Rehabilitation of the hand, ed 3, Butterworths, England, 1973.
14. Phalen GS: The carpal tunnel syndrome: seventeen years experience in diagnosis and treatment of six hundred and fifty-four hands, J Bone Joint Surg 48A:211, 1966.
15. Phalen GS: The carpal tunnel syndrome: clinical evaluation of 598 hands, Clin Orthop 83:29, 1972.
16. Phalen GS, Gardner WJ, LaLonde AA: Neuropathy of median nerve due to compression beneath transverse carpal ligament, J Bone Joint Surg (Am) 32:109, 1950.
17. Robbins H: Anatomical study of the median nerve in the carpal tunnel and etiologies of the carpal tunnel syndrome, J Bone Joint Surg 45A:953, 1963.
18. Stack RE: Carpal tunnel syndrome, Am Fam Physician 8:88, 1973.
19. Sunderland S: Nerves and nerve injuries, Baltimore, 1968, Williams & Wilkins.
20. Taylor N: Carpal tunnel syndrome, Am J Phys Med 4:192, 1971.
21. Thompson WAL and Koppell HP: Peripheral entrapment neuropathies of the upper extremity, New Engl J Med 260:1261, 1959.
22. Trombly C and Scott A: Occupational therapy for physical dysfunction, Baltimore, 1977, Williams & Wilkins Co.
23. Weeks P: Lecture on peripheral nerve anatomy, Core concept in hand therapy, St Louis, 1988.
24. Wehbe M and Hunter JM: Flexor tendon gliding in the hand. Part II. Differential gliding, J Hand Surg 10A:575, 1985.

49

Splinting peripheral nerve injuries

Judy C. Colditz

Splinting deformities that are the result of isolated peripheral nerve injuries is both easy and difficult. The ease of splinting is a result of the readily recognizable, frequently identical deformities and, unlike many other hand injuries, standard splinting approaches may be used. The difficulty arises because it is impossible to build a static external device that will substitute for the intricately balanced live muscles that the splint attempts to replace. Although early restoration of balanced motion is the goal, no static device can restore the normal dynamic ability.

The severe sensory loss in the palm resulting from median and ulnar palsies prevents normal use of the hand, even if the motor components of the nerve are totally intact.

The traditional splints designed for use after polio or spinal cord injuries are not appropriate for the peripheral nerve injury. The materials and designs used for permanent deficits are not applicable to the changing dynamics of the injured hand undergoing reinnervation.

PRINCIPLES OF SPLINTS

The purposes common to all splints used for peripheral nerve injuries follow:

1. To keep denervated muscles from remaining in an overstretched position
2. To prevent joint contractures
3. To prevent development of strong substitution patterns
4. To maximize functional use of the hand

Overstretching of muscles

In all cases of isolated peripheral nerve injury, the denervated muscle group will have normal unopposed antagonist muscles still present, which will continuously overpower the denervated musculature, maintaining it on constant stretch. A muscle undergoing reinnervation must overcome this stretched position and achieve a normal resting length before it is able to contract enough to effect joint motion. Short periods during which the unopposed muscles overpower the denervated muscles will not cause harm, but a constantly stretched position will decrease the potential for early return of normal muscle activity. A denervated muscle constrained by appropriate splinting will allow one to perceive the earliest flicker of returning motion, and a properly executed design will enhance returning muscle function instead of strengthening substitution patterns.

Joint contractures

Joints constantly in a deformed position cannot experience the natural glide and stretch of the capsular structures. Even without direct trauma, prolonged immobility will limit the capsular elasticity. The joint must be taken through the full range of motion frequently. It is not adequate to immobilize these joints at one extreme at night and the other extreme during the day. Although positional splinting at night can be useful, the intervention of blocking forces during the day, so that the joints are actively ranged, maintains joint movement while facilitating normal pumping dynamics.

Substitution patterns

In a peripheral nerve injury, there is no opposing balancing force to the intact active muscle group. The patient learns to adapt to the imbalance. Without external constraints applied, the patient reinforces the strength of the

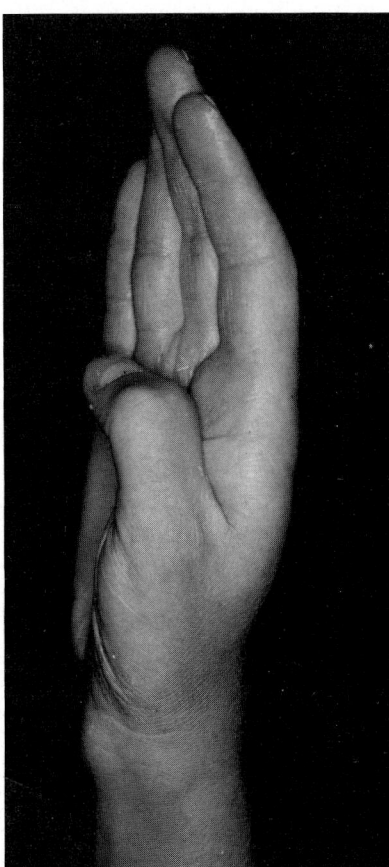

Fig. 49-1 In low median palsy the thumb is carried back and forth across the palm by extrinsic muscles in an adducted position caused by absence of the opponens pollicis and abductor pollicis brevis.

remaining muscles and constantly overpowers the denervated muscles. An excellent example of this is in low median palsy where the intact flexor pollicis longus and extensor pollicis longus carry the thumb back and forth across the palm (Fig. 49-1). As the opponens pollicis and the abductor pollicis brevis begin to function, they have difficulty participating in thumb motion, because the extrinsic muscles have flexed and extended the thumb in an adducted position, overpowering the small muscles. If the extremes of these substitution patterns are prevented, the patient is able to isolate and strengthen returning musculature earlier.

Functional use of hand

The combination of sensory loss and motor imbalance in peripheral nerve lesions makes it impossible to use the hand normally. A splint that effectively substitutes for muscle action and allows repatterning of the hand as sensibility returns and is retrained assists in the ultimate goal of maximizing function.

Cold intolerance is common with nerve injuries, particularly during reinnervation. Protective neoprene mittens or finger sleeves are helpful for patients in colder climates or for those who work in cold environments (Fig. 49-2).

SPLINT REQUIREMENTS
Design

Splints should be kept as simple as possible to accomplish muscle substitution. Bulky splints may be worn by the patient, but they will impede function of the hand rather than reinforce it.

Early after the nerve injury, it is acceptable to cover a denervated area with the splint, but in cases of partial laceration or returning sensation, the tactile surfaces should be left free.

Splints for peripheral nerve injuries should not totally immobilize any joint. For example, splinting of the wrist in radial palsy with a static wrist support prevents the returning wrist extensor muscles from gaining strength or excursion while in the splint.

When to splint

Many peripheral nerve injuries are associated with other trauma to skin, tendon, bone, or vascular structures. Immediately after injury, one must prevent tension on the healing nerve tissues to allow for adequate healing. Thereafter, glide of tendons and joints takes precedence over splinting for the peripheral nerve deformity, because often the splint for the peripheral nerve injury will restrict full movement.

For example, in a laceration at the level of the wrist involving the median and ulnar nerves and wrist and finger flexors, the wrist must be held in flexion during the early stages to prevent tension at the repair sites. Only as wrist motion is gained and excursion of the flexor tendons is achieved will the claw deformity of the fingers be evident. The adherence of the flexors at the wrist will tenodese the finger extensors, providing a built-in splint. Only when the deformity becomes clinically evident should one splint for it.

In long-standing denervation where joint contractures have already developed, one must splint to mobilize the joints before splinting the dynamic deformity.

SPECIFIC NERVE LESIONS

It is easiest to understand the deformity of a pure lesion of the three large peripheral nerves: median, ulnar, and radial. Combinations of nerve injuries, especially when associated with other injuries, require more skill of the therapist to determine treatment priorities, but the principles remain unchanged.

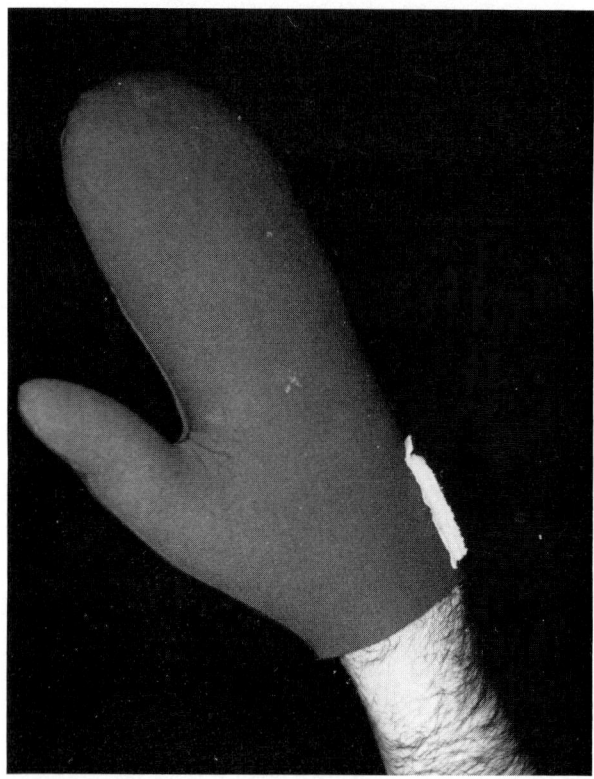

Fig. 49-2 A neoprene mitten may be constructed for the nerve-injured patient to assist with tolerance to cold.

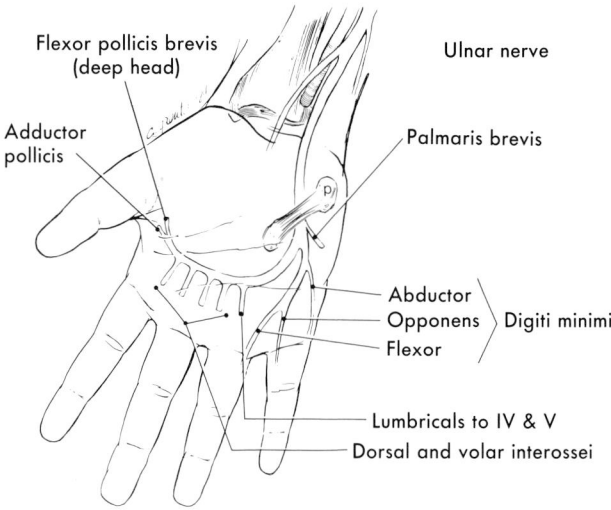

Fig. 49-3 The path of the ulnar nerve in the hand and muscles involved in low ulnar palsy.

Claw deformity

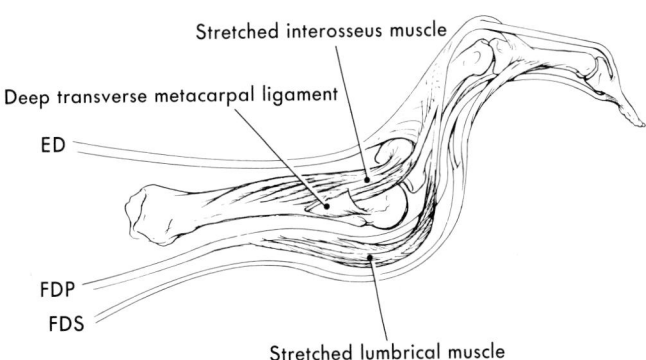

Stretched interosseus muscle

Deep transverse metacarpal ligament

ED

FDP

FDS

Stretched lumbrical muscle

Fig. 49-4 The loss of intrinsic control in the ring and little fingers with ulnar palsy allows the extensor digitorum to hyperextend the metacarpophalangeal joints during active extension of the fingers. The denervated intrinsics are stretched in this claw position.

Ulnar nerve

Low lesion. Laceration of the ulnar nerve at the level of the wrist (low ulnar palsy) results in denervation of the majority of the intrinsic muscles of the hand (Fig. 49-3). The ulnar nerve innervates all of the hypothenar muscles: abductor digiti minimi, flexor digiti minimi, and the opponens digiti minimi, and thus the ulnar border of the transverse metacarpal arch is lost. Loss of the dorsal and volar interossei creates the inability to abduct and adduct the fingers, causing loss of the fine manipulative power of the hand. In addition to the loss of the interossei, the ring and little finger also lose the function of the lumbricals, removing any intrinsic balancing force to the normal extrinsics in these two digits.

The resulting functional deformity is clawing of the ring and little fingers. Because there is no intrinsic control in these digits, the tension of the long flexors is opposed only by the extrinsic extensors, which primarily extend the MP joints (Fig. 49-4). The intrinsic muscles normally flex the MP joint and extend the interphalangeal joints, and when they are absent, there are no prime flexors of the MP joint. In this unopposed position, one can clearly see that both the lumbricals and the interossei are held in a stretched position when the fingers are clawed. In making a full fist, the patient can flex the MP joint actively but only after the interphalangeal joints are fully flexed. The greatest functional loss is the inability to open the hand in a large span to handle objects.

The loss of the powerful adductor of the thumb and the deep head of the flexor pollicis brevis removes one of the supporting forces of the MP joint during pinching, demonstrating Froment's sign: extension or hyperextension of the MP joint with hyperflexion of the interphalangeal joint.[10] This is rarely a deformity that can be assisted by splinting, because stabilizing the thumb is difficult without restricting other essential mobility.

The goal in splinting ulnar palsy is to prevent overstretching of the denervated intrinsic muscles of the ring and little fingers. The MP joints must be prevented from fully extending (Fig. 49-5). Any splint that blocks the MP joint in slight flexion prevents the claw deformity by forcing the extrinsic extensors to transmit force into the dorsal hood mechanism of the finger, extending the interphalangeal joints in the absence of the intrinsic pull (Fig. 49-6). The problem is that a bulky splint that attempts to block the MP joints will definitely impede function of the hand. Because two thirds of the palmar surface of the hand still has normal sensibility, it is mandatory that ulnar palsy splints cover a minimal surface of the palm. Total finger flexion range must also remain unimpeded. In the early stages, blocking the MP joints can be incorporated into the immobilization splint: a dorsal protective splint that prevents wrist extension pre-

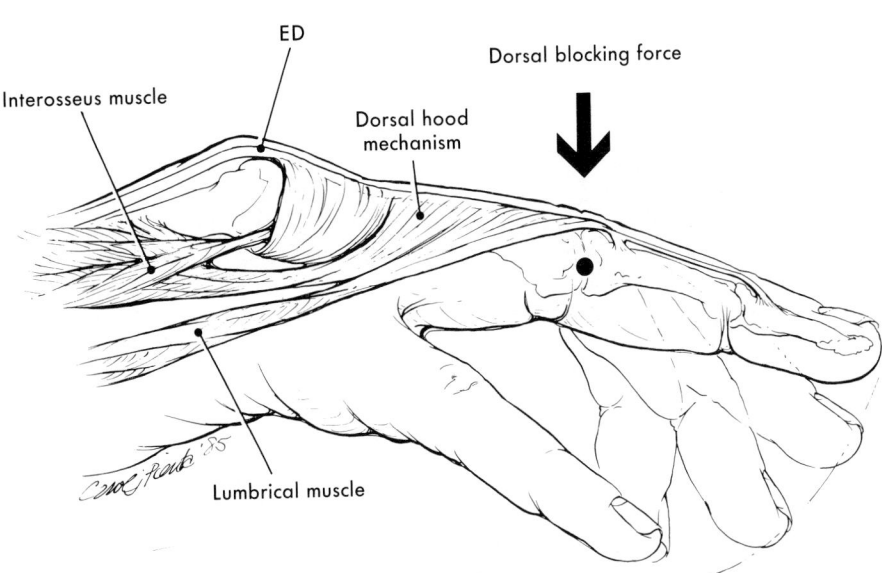

ED

Dorsal blocking force

Interosseus muscle

Dorsal hood mechanism

Lumbrical muscle

Fig. 49-5 A blocking force over the dorsum of the proximal phalanx preventing metacarpophalangeal hyperextension will allow the extrinsic extensor to transmit to the interphalangeal joints in the absence of intrinsic power.

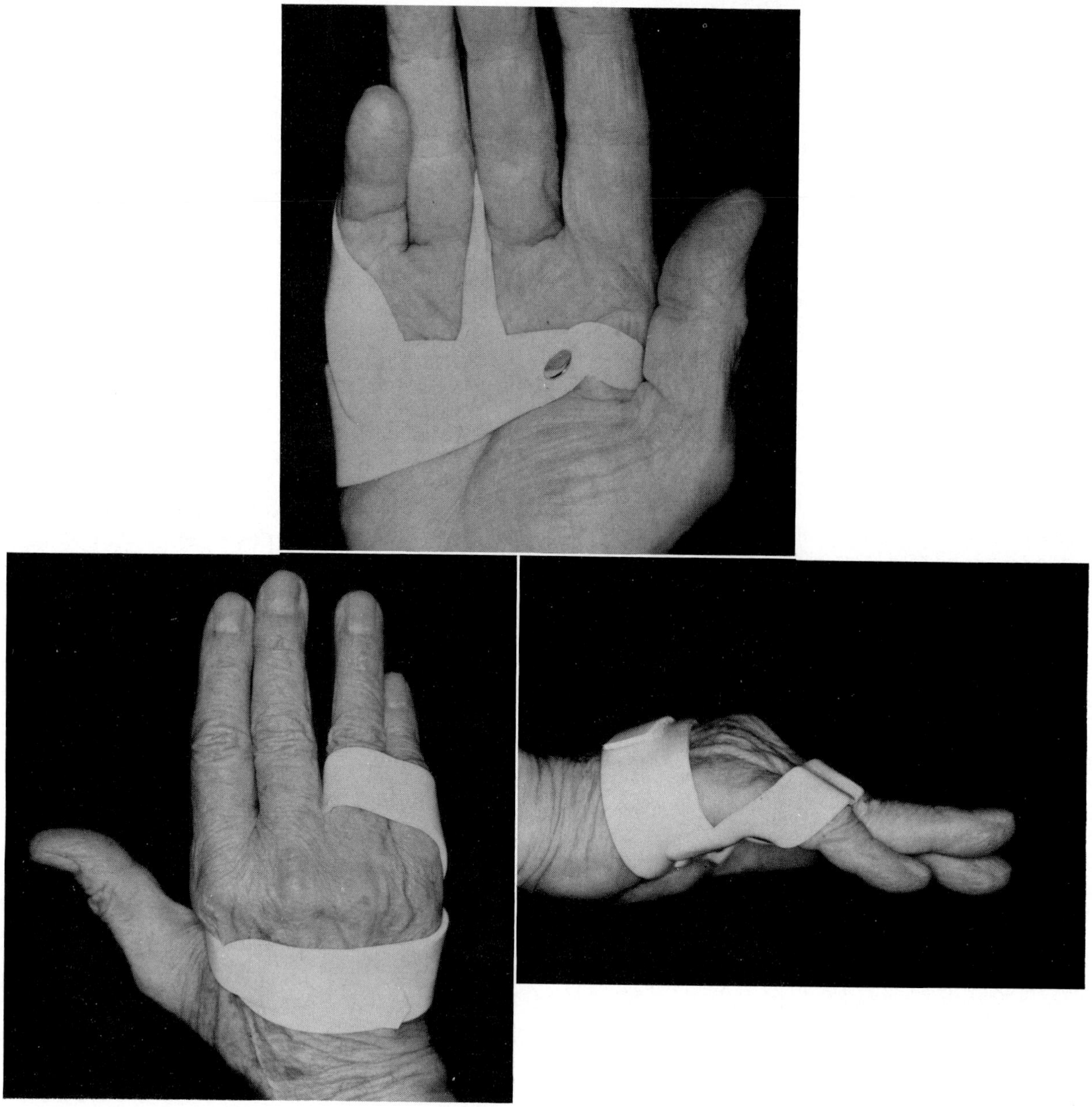

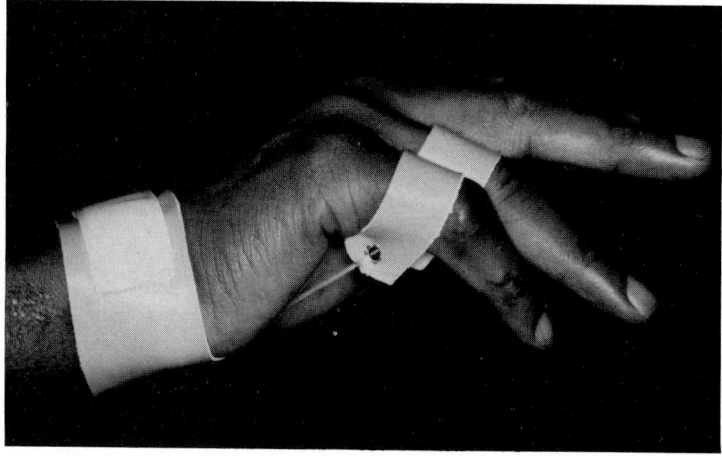

Fig. 49-6 Ulnar palsy splint that blocks hyperextension of the metacarpophalangeal joints but allows full flexion of all finger joints.

Fig. 49-7 An ulnar-palsy splint that uses leather wrist and finger cuffs with a static line to block metacarpophalangeal hyperextension.

vents tension on the nerve and tendon repairs at the level of the wrist. When the wrist is allowed free, a small, molded splint (Fig. 49-6) or leather splint can substitute (Fig. 49-7). Capener advocated a spring wire splint with a coil at the axis of the MP joint, allowing full extension and following the digit through the full range of MP flexion.[6] This splint is somewhat difficult to construct, because the tension of the spring must be exact to be strong enough to actually block MP extension when the patient attempts finger extension. Many therapists who apply a dynamic force for MP flexion, such as the Bunnell knuckle-bender splint,[4] may be misled in their concept, because the patient can then hyperextend actively against the force of the rubber band, actually giving strong proprioceptive input to the extrinsic extensors and thus strengthening them. It is strongly recommended that some means of static splinting be utilized that prevents the MP joint from hyperextending. Flexion contractures of the MP joint caused by blocking splinting are not common; every time the splint is removed for skin care, the extrinsic extensor will still hyperextend the MP joint.

Ulnar palsy

High lesion. High ulnar palsy lesions are commonly associated with trauma at or above the elbow. In addition to the muscles previously mentioned in low ulnar palsy, the profundi of the ring and little fingers and the flexor carpi ulnaris are absent (Fig. 49-8). With absence of tension of the profundi and all the intrinsics of the ring and little fingers, the clawing in the high ulnar nerve lesion is not as obvious. As reinnervation of the profundi occurs, clawing becomes more and more evident, and splinting becomes mandatory rather than optional. There is no difference between the splint designs for the different levels of lesions. In a high lesion, one must instruct the patient to maintain full passive interphalangeal flexion of the ring and little fingers when the profundi are absent.

Median nerve

Low lesion. A laceration at the wrist level creates the devastating injury of low median palsy. It makes up a large portion of the motor of the thumb as well as providing sensibility to the radial three and one-half digits. Motor loss is present in only the radial portion of the hand with this lesion (Fig. 49-9). Loss of the opponens pollicis and abductor pollicis brevis renders it impossible to pull the thumb away from the palm. The thumb is carried across the palm in an adducted position (see Fig. 49-1). Frequently the deformity is not this obvious, because the nerve injury may be partial or one may be observing the not uncommon cross innervation from the ulnar nerve. The lumbricals of the index and long fingers are also absent, but because the ulnarly innervated palmar and dorsal interossei are still present, clawing is usually absent in these two digits. Only in combined median and ulnar palsy does one see clawing of the index and long fingers.

Adduction contractures of the thumb are the most common deformity after a low lesion of the median nerve, and therefore some means of holding the first metacarpal abducted from the hand is necessary (Fig. 49-10). Splinting not only prevents the opponens and abductor pollicis brevis from resting in a stretched position, reinforcing earlier return of their action, but also maintains the soft tissue length of the first web space and provides a force to balance the pull of the normal adductor pollicis. A C-bar design has been traditionally recommended to hold the first metacarpal abducted from the other metacarpals.[4] However, it is difficult to maintain the soft tissue of the first web space fully open while still allowing MP flexion of the index finger. Much

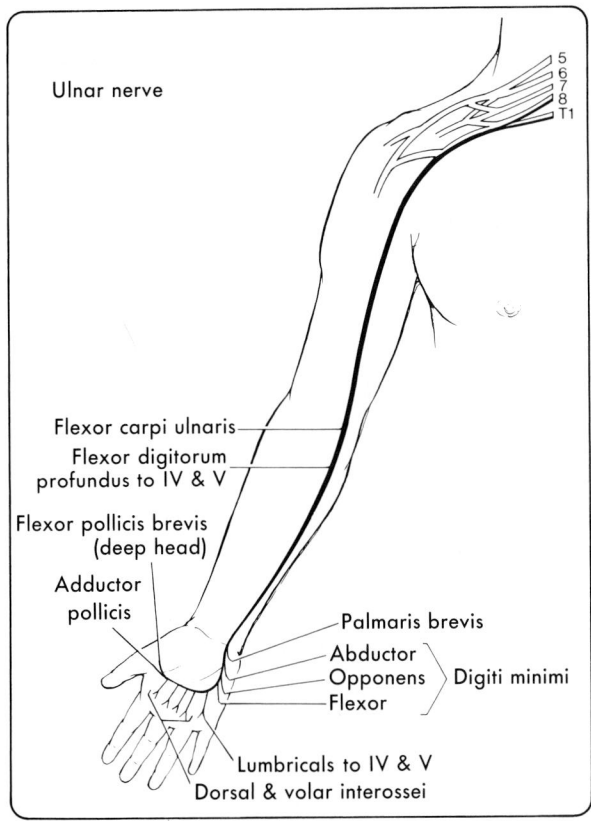

Fig. 49-8 The path of the ulnar nerve and muscles involved in high ulnar palsy.

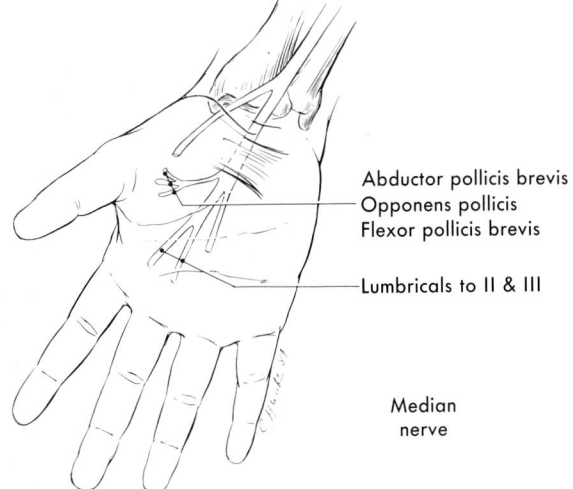

Fig. 49-9 Low median palsy involves intrinsic muscles of the thumb, index, and long fingers.

of the functional abduction of the thumb is the stretch of the soft tissue of the entire web area. The use of a night splint that holds the index finger extended and the thumb abducted is helpful in maintaining all the joint motion necessary for functional abduction of the thumb (Fig. 49-11). A small splint, either of leather or thermoplastic material, for use during the day to hold the thumb in a stabile opposed position (but less than fully abducted) may be the most useful approach (Fig. 49-12). If a daytime splint prevents

full flexion of the MP joint of the index finger, it can lead to an unnecessary extension contracture of this joint.

Because the thumb, index, and long fingers are the prime digits for manipulating objects and sensibility is absent in these digits in the median nerve lesion, it is extremely difficult for the patient to reintegrate the use of the hand into normal activity until the sensory return gives useful feedback. Because reinnervation proceeds proximally to distally, it is common that the motor return precedes full sensory

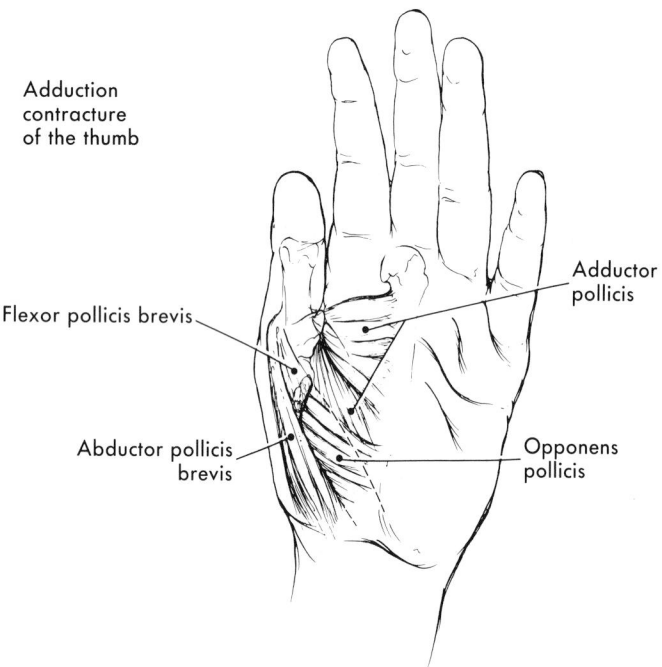

Adduction contracture of the thumb

Flexor pollicis brevis

Abductor pollicis brevis

Adductor pollicis

Opponens pollicis

Fig. 49-10   Adduction contracture of the thumb in median palsy caused by unopposed adductor pollicis.

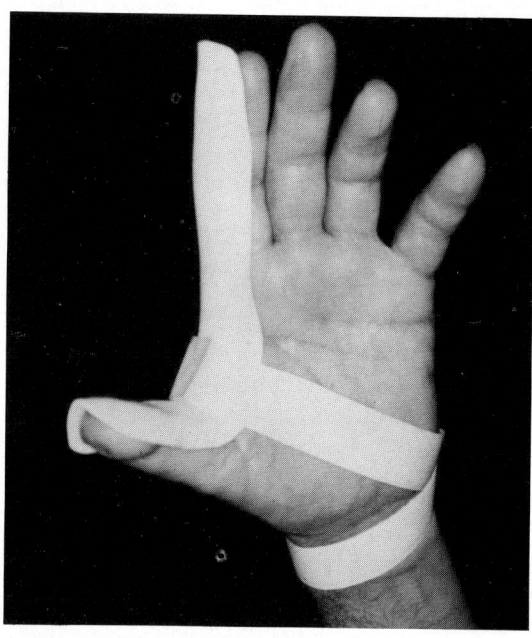

Fig. 49-11   Night splint for full abduction of first web space.

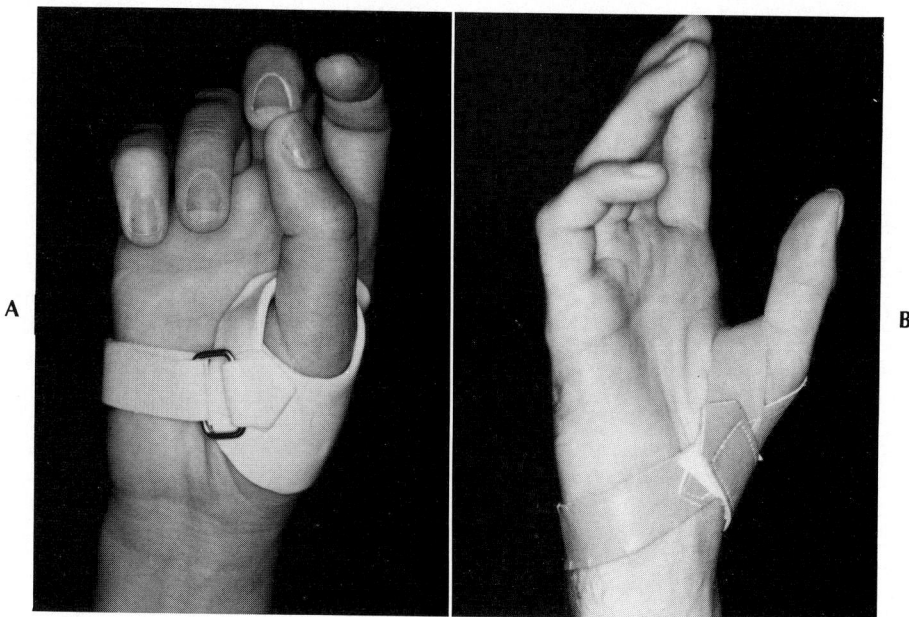

A

B

Fig. 49-12   A small thermoplastic, **A,** or leather, **B,** splint for maintaining functional abduction of first metacarpal while awaiting median nerve return.

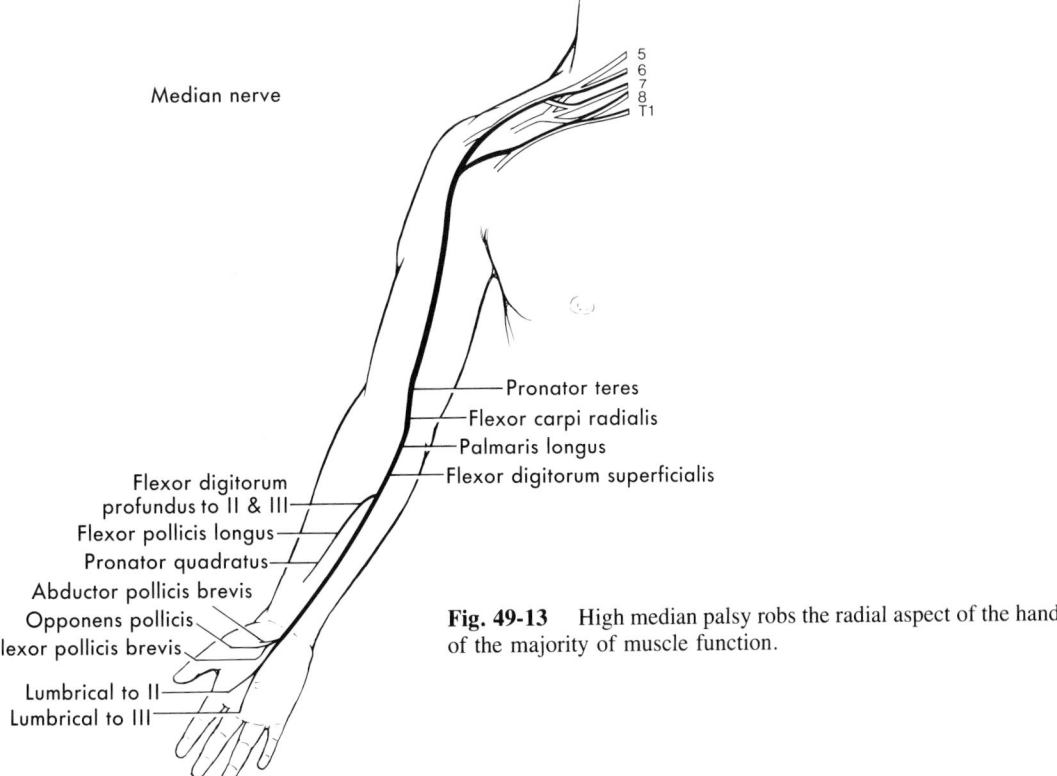

Median nerve

5
6
7
8
T1

Pronator teres
Flexor carpi radialis
Palmaris longus
Flexor digitorum superficialis

Flexor digitorum
profundus to II & III
Flexor pollicis longus
Pronator quadratus
Abductor pollicis brevis
Opponens pollicis
Flexor pollicis brevis
Lumbrical to II
Lumbrical to III

Fig. 49-13   High median palsy robs the radial aspect of the hand of the majority of muscle function.

return, and the splint may be discontinued before one expects more normal use of the hand as a result of some sensory return. For this reason, one should not hesitate to cover the palmar surface during the early stages after nerve laceration, to position the thumb. In many adults, however, and especially with the high nerve lesion, the sensibility may return to a protective level, but the opponens pollicis often does not return to a functional level, thus requiring an opponens transfer.

In the early stages the patient must always demand visual assistance to use the fingertips. As the nerve continues to regenerate, the small leather splint (Fig. 49-12) may assist positioning the thumb in slight abduction and opposition so that the strong extensor pollicis longus does not continue to overpower the returning intrinsics.

Median nerve

High lesion. High median nerve injuries are also seen at or near the elbow. In these lesions the loss of the profundi of the index and long fingers, as well as the superficialis to all fingers, robs the hand of all except gross function (Fig. 49-13). Active pronation is also lost with denervation of the pronator teres and quadratus, but slight abduction of the arm allows gravity to assist with pronation. It is often difficult to maintain passive flexion of the index finger, because buddy taping it to the long finger does not provide adequate passive motion. Even though the long finger appears to flex actively, it is actually being "carried along" into flexion, because it is part of the common muscle belly of the profundi of the long, ring, and little fingers (Fig. 49-14).

In the adult patient with a high median or ulnar nerve lesion, full motor and sensory return never occurs. Splinting these high-level deformities to maintain passive range of

motion is appropriate in preparation for tendon transfers. Some authors suggest very early tendon transfers as an internal splint to prevent the need for cumbersome external devices. No splint need be cumbersome.

Radial nerve

High lesion. Unlike the median and ulnar nerve, the radial nerve is more commonly injured at the high level where it spirals around the humerus (Fig. 49-15). The injury in the spiral groove of the humerus is most commonly as-

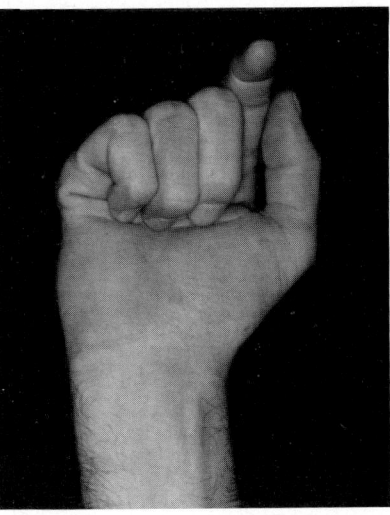

Fig. 49-14   In high median palsy the long finger is carried to flexion because of the common muscle belly, but when tested in an isolated manner will be absent in most cases.

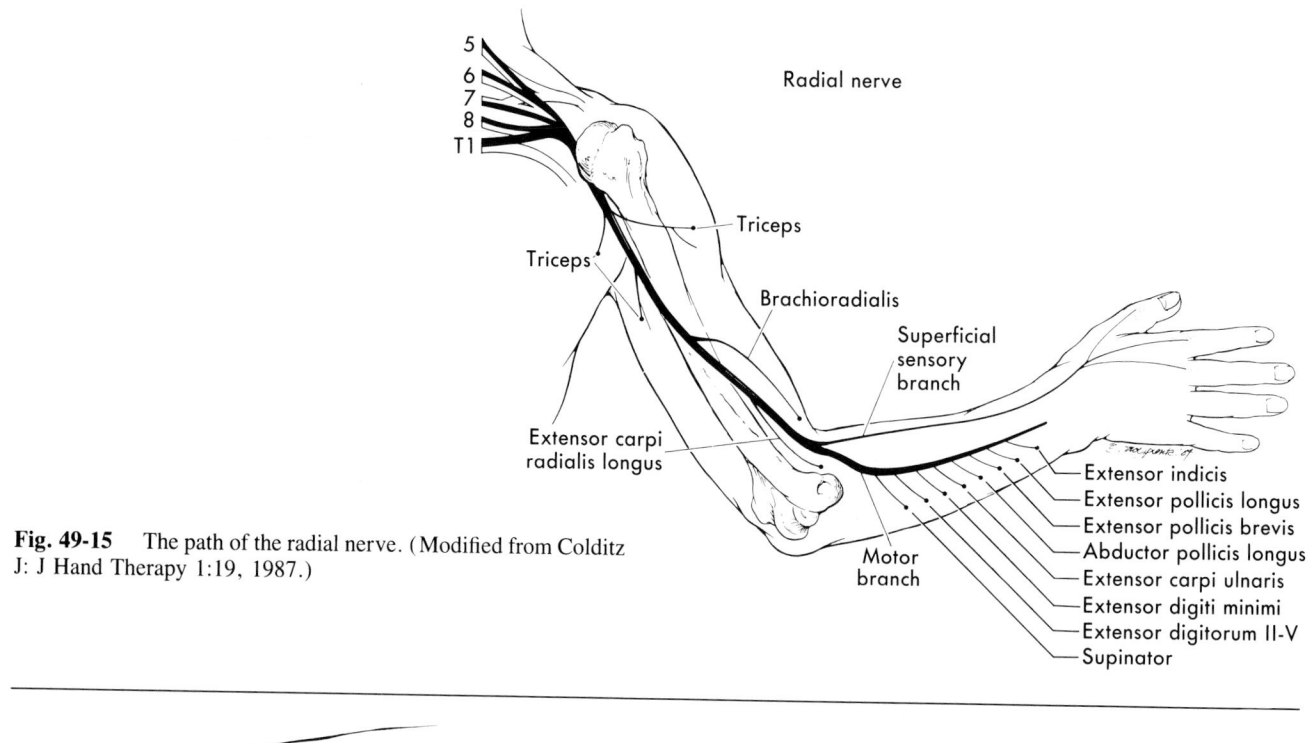

Fig. 49-15 The path of the radial nerve. (Modified from Colditz J: J Hand Therapy 1:19, 1987.)

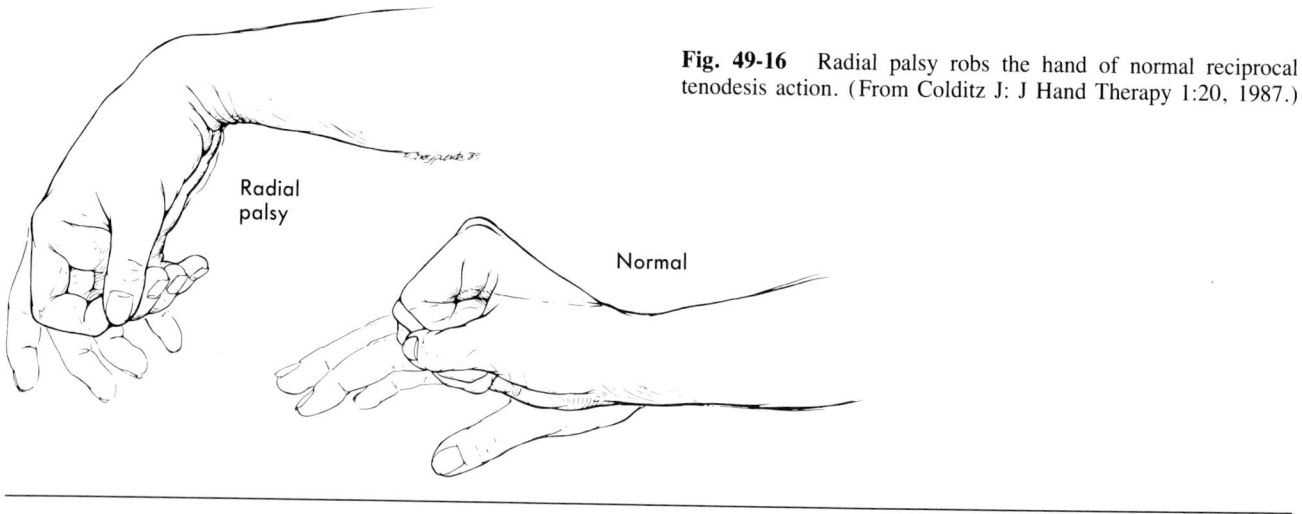

Fig. 49-16 Radial palsy robs the hand of normal reciprocal tenodesis action. (From Colditz J: J Hand Therapy 1:20, 1987.)

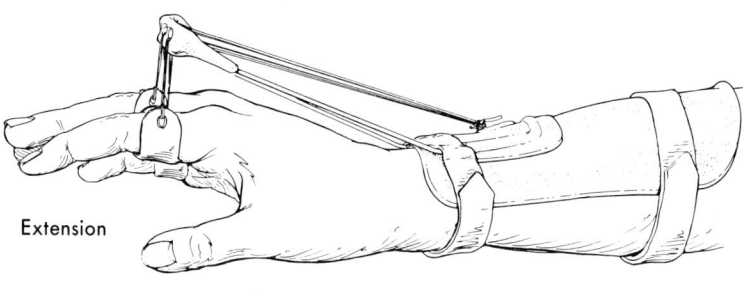

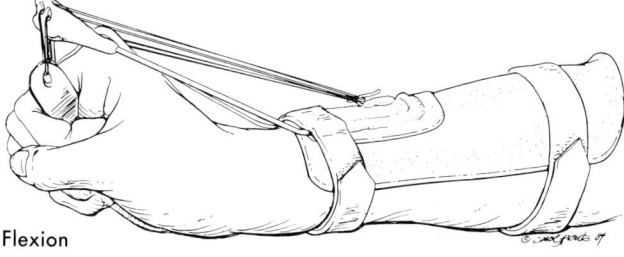

Fig. 49-17 Radial palsy splint, which recreates normal tenodesis action by use of a static suspension line. (From Colditz J: J Hand Therapy 1:21, 1987.)

sociated with humeral fractures and compression syndromes. The sensory loss associated with radial nerve palsy is of less functional loss, because it lies over the dorsoradial aspect of the hand, leaving the entire palmar surface intact. The injury at or below the spiral groove spares the innervation of the triceps, leaving elbow function intact. There is absence of all wrist and finger extensors as well as the supinator.

Unlike the patients who have median and ulnar nerve lesions where sensory loss impedes the functional loss of the hand, the patient with radial palsy caused by a radial nerve lesion has the potential for relatively normal use of the hand, using an appropriately designed splint that harnesses the wrist to allow the finger flexors to function. Although some authors advocate early tendon transfers to eliminate the need for external splinting, this is not the norm in management of radial palsy.[2,5] Barton states that radial nerve palsy usually recovers spontaneously, and therefore effective splinting may be needed for months during regeneration.[1]

The primary functional loss is inability to stabilize the wrist in extension so that one can use the finger flexors normally. The loss of power of the wrist and finger extensors destroys the essential reciprocal tenodesis action vital to the normal grasp and release pattern of the hand (Fig. 49-16). The ideal splint recreates this natural harmony of tenodesis action: finger extension with wrist flexion and wrist extension with finger flexion. Many authors suggest the use of a static wrist support splint, which stabilizes the wrist but does not remedy the problem of lack of finger and thumb extension.[1,3,5,8,9] Thus any grasp/release activity must be aided by the assistance of the uninvolved hand. These splints also frequently cover the valuable area of palmar sensibility.

A splint designed at the Hand Rehabilitation Center in Chapel Hill, North Carolina, and illustrated in 1978 by Hollis provides a static rather than dynamic line to suspend the proximal phalangeal area[7] (Fig. 49-17). This splint allows full finger flexion. Because the wrist never drops below neutral, the powerful flexors can, as they tighten, bring the wrist into a position of extension. During relaxation, as gravity drops the wrist, extension of the MP joints is achieved as a blocking force is transmitted to the loops on the proximal phalangeal area. Full finger extension is accomplished by the intrinsics acting in concert with the blocking action of the splint. Because the patient receives a facsimile of the normal tenodesis effect, training is rarely required to adapt to the splint. The thumb is not always included with an outrigger, but because the wrist has been harnessed by the splint and the thumb extensor and abductors lie on the dorsoulnar surface of the forearm, these muscles have been taken off maximum stretch. The additional cumbersomeness of a thumb outrigger, which must project radially to hold the thumb, and the limitations it imposes on the intrinsic action of the thumb do not, in my opinion, enhance the function of the thumb. It is useful to remember that often the intrinsic muscles still can extend the interphalangeal joint in the absence of the extrinsic extensors.

The advantages of this splint design are numerous. The suspension design allows partial wrist motion and full finger motion (Fig. 49-18). It facilitates maintenance of the normal hand arches, because the CMC joints of the ring and little fingers are unimpeded. This free motion is impossible in static splints or when rigid bars hold either the metacarpal or proximal phalangeal area. Most strikingly, this splint has an absence of splinting material on the palmar surface, allowing normal use of the palm. The greatest advantage of

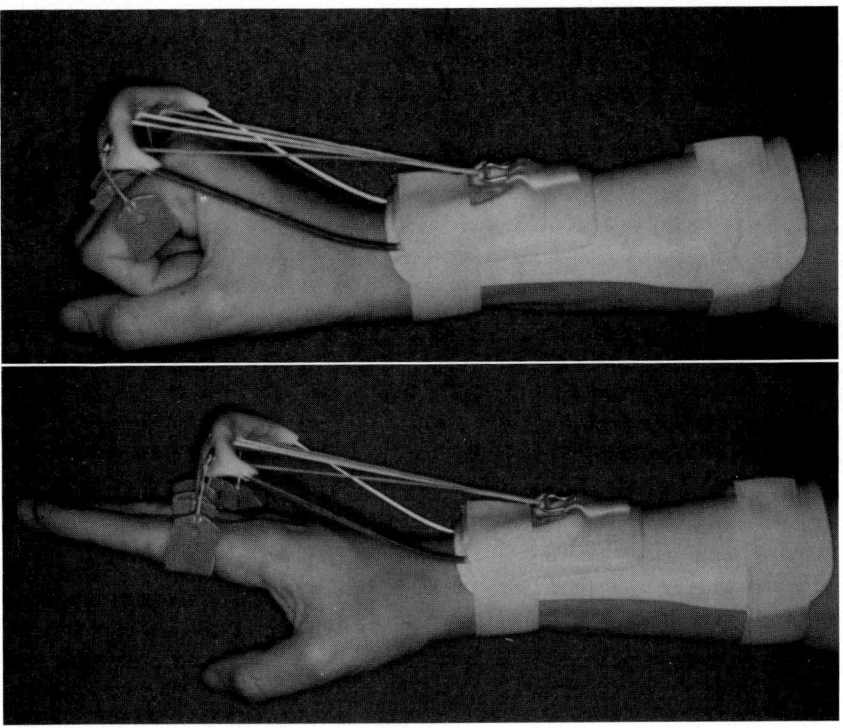

Fig. 49-18 Radial palsy splint allows full flexion and extension of fingers.

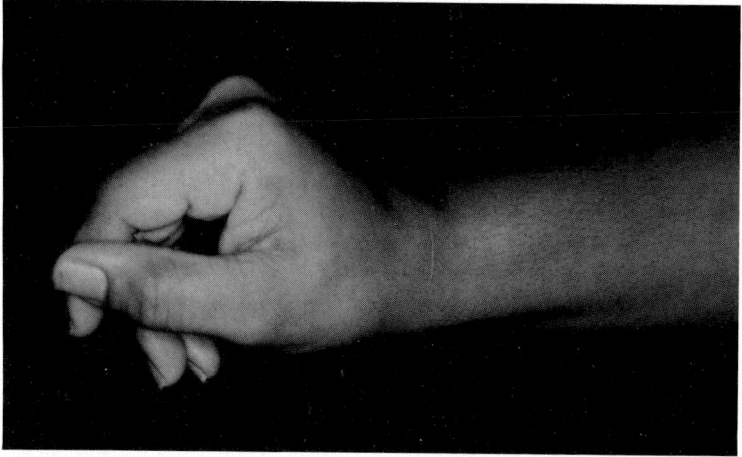

Fig. 49-19 Posture of hand with posterior interosseous palsy showing radial wrist extension.

this splint is its comparatively low profile, which allows it to be used effectively by the patient in the daily routine. As return of function begins, the splint facilitates strengthening of the wrist extensors instead of impeding them. One should be cautioned against designs for dynamic wrist and finger extension, because the powerful unopposed flexors often overcome the force of the dynamic splint during finger flexion.

Radial nerve

Low lesion. After the radial nerve crosses the elbow and plunges below the supinator, it divides, forming the pos-

terior interosseous branch (deep motor) and the superficial sensory branch (see Fig. 49-15). When there is isolated involvement of the deep motor branch, this lesion is called posterior interosseous palsy. In posterior interosseous palsy, radial wrist extension is nearly always spared, and the brachioradialis function will always be present (Fig. 49-19). Clinical presentation of the hand will be one of strong radial deviation of the wrist during attempted wrist extension. Attempted finger extension will demonstrate an intrinsic plus pattern of MP flexion and interphalangeal extension, because the extensor digitorum muscle is not innervated.

Although the clinical picture differs from the high radial

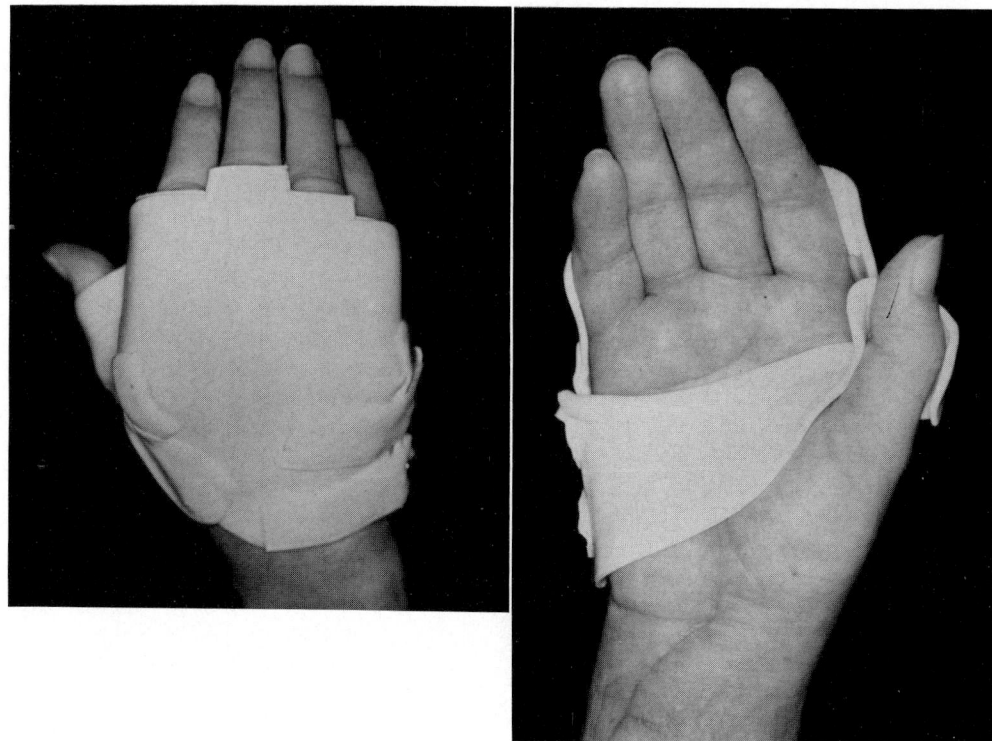

Fig. 49-20 Median and ulnar palsy splint, which blocks all metacarpophalangeal joints and holds thumb abducted.

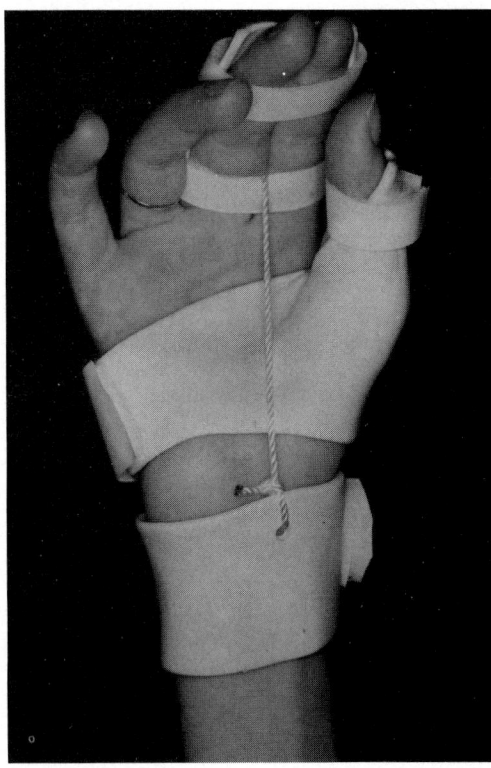

Fig. 49-21 Tenodesis splint, which harnesses the power of wrist extension into a functional pinch.

nerve lesion, the same mechanics for splinting apply. The splint design described previously allows the radial wrist extensors to function normally to stabilize the wrist during finger flexion. Finger extension is achieved by the patient allowing the wrist to drop into flexion as the statically suspended proximal phalangeal area pulls the MP joints into the extension. No joint has been unnecessarily immobilized, and the more normal tenodesis pattern of the hand has been reestablished.

In the unusual circumstance where the posterior interosseous lesion is partial and one sees isolated absence of a finger extensor with adjacent normal finger extension, a simple buddy splint can be of functional value to the patient.

MIXED LESIONS

Mixed nerve lesions provide the ultimate splinting challenge for the therapist, because multiple nerve involvement nearly always accompanies trauma to many other structures, requiring a balance between increasing glide of soft tissues and constraining splinting for the denervated muscles. Monitoring of kinesiologic balance is the guidepost for splinting.

The most common mixed lesion is injury to the median and ulnar nerves, because they both lie on the palmar aspect of the wrist. Division of both of these nerves at the wrist robs the hand of all intrinsic muscles, and therefore clawing

of all four digits must be splinted by blocking the MP joints. Likewise, there are no muscles stabilizing the thumb, and the thumb should be held in an abducted position (Fig. 49-20).

In combined lesions where muscle loss requires static splinting, it is essential that the patient remove the splint and carry out passive ranging of the joints frequently. In isolated nerve injuries, it is usually one muscle group denervated with the antagonist still working. In combined lesions, the imbalance may not be so simple, and as nerve return brings about a change of muscle balance, splinting needs will change.

In cases where only the radial nerve is functioning, one may harness that power into finger flexion by fitting the RIC splint, designed at the Rehabilitation Institute of Chicago. It can be applicable to the occasional nerve palsy patient to both provide a minimal grasp function and maintain some range of finger flexion (Fig. 49-21).

The possible combinations of mixed nerve lesions are endless, because often nerve injuries are partial or of differing severity. A complete manual muscle test and a clear clinical picture of the balance of motion will be the only guides for the therapist to determine the splinting regime.

CONCLUSION

Splinting the deformities that result from isolated nerve injuries in the upper extremity requires a knowledge of normal and pathologic kinesiology to understand the correct design and mechanics of splints. The therapist must have a thorough knowledge of anatomy and the expected course of reinnervation and must have good skills of manual muscle testing to evaluate the nerve-injured hand. The external constraints of splinting should maximize the balance of motion while awaiting return. Changes in splinting must occur in response to kinesiologic and functional changes in the hand to assist in maximum rehabilitation.

REFERENCES

1. Barton NJ: Radial nerve lesions, Hand 5:200, 1973.
2. Bevin AG: Early tendon transfer for radial nerve transection, Hand 8:134, 1976.
3. Bowden R and Napier EM Jr: The assessment of hand function after peripheral nerve injury, J Bone Joint Surg 43B:481, 1961.
4. Bunnell S: Splinting the hand. In American Academy of Orthopaedic Surgeons: Instructional Course Lectures, Vol IX, St. Louis, 1952, The CV Mosby Co.
5. Burkhalter WE: Early tendon transfer in upper extremity peripheral nerve injury, Clin Orthop 104:68, 1974.
6. Capener N: Lively splints, Physiotherapy 53:371, 1967.
7. Colditz JC: Splinting for radial nerve palsy, J Hand Ther 1, 1987.
8. Ellis M: Orthoses for the hand. In Lamb DW and Kuczynski K, editors: The practice of hand surgery, London, 1981, Blackwell Scientific Publications, Inc.
9. Fess EE and Phillips CA: Hand splinting principles and methods, ed 2, St. Louis, 1987, The CV Mosby Co.
10. Froment J: La prehension dans les paralysies, du nerf cubital et le signe du pouce, Presse med 23:409, 1915.
11. Nickel VL, Perry J, and Garrett A: Development of useful function in the severely paralyzed hand, J Bone Joint Surg 45-A:933, 1963.

50

Mechanics of tendon transfers

Paul W. Brand

The whole object of tendon transfer operations is to restore balance to a hand after one or more of its muscles have been paralyzed or destroyed. In so doing the surgeon must compare the usefulness of the action of the lost muscle with that of the muscle that will have to be transferred, leaving a defect in the place where it was before.

It is not enough to consider the function and usefulness of these muscles in a qualitative sense. One has also to make an attempt to quantify the gains and losses at each joint, so that one does not *overbalance* a hand in an attempt to restore balance.

In this process of planning tendon transfers it is useful to think about those mechanical qualities that are transferred with a tendon and those that remain in the distal part of the limb as passive structures that have to be moved and that sometimes resist movement.

FACTORS TRANSFERRED WITH A MUSCLE

When a muscle-tendon unit is transferred, it carries with it some but not all of the qualities it had in its original situation.

Strength

In this context, by strength I mean ability to generate tension in the tendon. The tension capability of a muscle depends on the number of muscle fibers that it has and on the total cross-sectional area of all its fibers. Its ability to sustain its tension over a period of time and over a number of repeated contractions depends also on the adequacy of its blood supply; but the act of transferring a tendon should not change the vascular supply or the nerve supply of its muscle. There used to be a widely quoted rule that said when a muscle-tendon unit was transferred, its strength dropped one level in the scale of 0 to 5 by which muscles were graded.[4,7,9,10,13] This rule was worked out in the days when polio was the most common cause of paralysis demanding tendon transfers, and surgeons had to grade muscles carefully, not just as "paralyzed" and "unparalyzed" but in various grades of paralysis. We were warned not to use a grade 3 muscle without realizing that after transfer it would only work as grade 2. Any truth in this generalization must have resulted from factors other than muscle strength, such as "drag," which we shall discuss later. The actual strength of a muscle is unchanged by transfer.

Just within the last few years surgeons have started to transplant muscles by microvascular and nerve anastomosis. This is quite a different thing from simple transfer; it involves removing a muscle from another limb, with its major artery, vein, and nerve, and placing it in a new situation, using locally available vessels and the motor nerve of the muscle that it is to replace. This is a new challenge, and one for which some of the rules have not yet been worked out. The fascicular patterns of the grafted nerve and the recipient stump may be very different, and even with the highest skill there is no chance that every nerve fiber will get through to a muscle unit. The published reports[3,8] have so far indicated that the successful cases are those in which the transplanted muscles are bigger and bulkier than the muscles they are to replace, presumably to allow for considerable loss of muscle units and yet allow for adequate survival. How much discrepancy to allow between the strength of the donor and the required strength after transplant has not yet been estimated. I would suspect that a ratio of two to one would be a conservative estimate.

For transfer, however, the task is simpler. Here the muscle keeps its nerve supply. The muscle is only redirected, or "transferred." We choose one that is about the right size to restore the balance of the hand that has been disturbed by paralysis. This is not the same as choosing a muscle of the same size as the one it is to replace. In most cases of paralysis the sum of the strengths of all the muscles that remain will be substantially less than the original total. Therefore, to obtain a new balance for the hand, the surgeon should be content to replace only part of the strength of the muscles that have been paralyzed.

Fortunately, there is a good deal of flexibility in this choice because muscles fairly quickly adapt their tension output to the demand. A strong muscle will become weaker if it is not used, and a weak muscle will become stronger, up to a point, so long as it is used to its maximum tension capability. However, it will become stronger only if it is used, and used in phase. A muscle will not become stronger just by being placed in a situation that demands strength. It must be daily and hourly used to its maximum by active contraction. Passive lengthening may occur from the activity of other muscles, but active contraction results from the recognition by the patient of the new function of the muscle. Here the therapist may be a great help. As an aid in the selection of a muscle of the right strength, the tables published by Brand, Beach, and Thompson may be used. At operation the relative diameters of exposed tendons serve as a good approximation. If one muscle is twice as strong as another, then the cross-sectional area of all its muscle fibers will be double that of the other, and the cross-sectional area of its tendon will also be about double that of the other tendon.[2] This is true only of the preparalysis strength. The extent to which tendon diameters change after periods of paralysis or of hypertrophy of the muscle is not known.

Excursion

Another feature of a muscle that is transferred with it is its potential range of excursion. However, this statement needs to be qualified by defining terms. We may recognize three kinds of excursion: *potential, required,* and *available*. If a muscle is freed from all its connective tissue attachments, and the naked muscle is stimulated from its fully stretched position, it should contract through a distance that is about equal to the resting length of its individual muscle fibers. This is a basic quality of muscle fibers, depending on the number of sarcomeres they contain. We have called this the *potential* excursion of the muscle. However, in the intact limb, very few muscles are able to achieve their full potential range of excursion, either because of restrictions imposed by surrounding connective tissue or because the joints they control do not have the range of motion that requires that much excursion. *Required* excursion is determined more by joints than by muscles. It is the excursion that is needed to put the joints through their whole range of motion. The extensor carpi radialis brevis, for example, has fibers that are about 6 cm long and, therefore, could potentially contract through 6 cm. However, the full range of motion of the average wrist can be accomplished with about 3.5 cm. Thus in the average hand this muscle never uses more than 3.5 cm of excursion. Previously published lists of tendon excursions have been mostly estimates of what we now call required excursion.[2] Perhaps the most significant information needed by the surgeon is the *available* excursion, as Freehafer[5] calls it, which he measures at operation after cutting the tendon distally, and which we think is that excursion permitted by the investing connective tissue. This available excursion varies from case to case and probably is largely dependent on the extent to which the patient has actually used the joints and muscles during the previous months. Connective tissue is responsive to the pattern of use. For example, people who have not previously done jogging or ballet dancing find that they cannot stretch their calf muscles far enough to run or dance effectively. By persistent stretching exercises they finally obtain a larger range. Probably they have not actually lengthened their muscle fibers; they have merely lengthened the connective tissue of the paratenon and perimysium. After such activity their available excursion would have increased.

Available excursion may be measured at operation after the tendon to be transferred has been divided. It may be held at its end by a hemostat or stitch and pulled out to its full stretch. At this point the muscle is stimulated by a tetanizing current while the movement of the tendon is measured. If the patient is awake, he may make the contraction voluntarily. The figure should be recorded for reference after surgery. Available excursion is transferred to the new site at operation only if the transfer involves minimal change of position and minimal dissection. Sometimes a long-fibered (long potential excursion) muscle is transferred from a site where it had a short required excursion to a site where it has a long required excursion. In such a case it will take time and active use to lengthen the connective tissue in and around the muscle and tendon so that the available excursion increases to match the new required excursion. If a tendon is to be widely rerouted and if the transfer is done through open wounds, then the normal compliant connective tissue and paratenon are divided and will be replaced by scar. In many operations for tendon transfer the final success or failure is determined more by the mechanical qualities of the paratendinous scar than by any other single factor. It is difficult enough for the patient to have to learn to use a muscle for a new action in an unfamiliar situation, but if that action cannot be accomplished until scar has been mobilized and lengthened, it may never be accomplished at all.

There is wide variation in the mechanical qualities of various types of connective tissue. Paratenon typically is easily stretchable. It has a long, low length-tension curve. This means that a great deal of lengthening results from a very little tension. This situation permits nearly free tendon movement over a wide range of excursion. The common fatty areolar connective tissue that serves to fill spaces between structures in the body is not quite so compliant, but it also will lengthen with moderate tension and then, with repeated movement, will become modified into a kind of paratenon.

Fascia and retinaculum, fibrous septa, and scar all tend to have steep length-tension curves, lengthening only about 10% even under considerable tension. Thus if a tendon comes to lie on a ligament that has been cut or scarified at surgery, the tendon may become united to the ligament through a collagen scar whose short fibers become parallel oriented by the pull of the tendon. Such fibers, only 1 or 2 mm long, would allow almost no tendon movement. If, instead, the transferred tendon is passed through a tunnel in loose fat and connective tissue, then the scar that forms around the tendon will attach it only to the soft and compliant tissues through which the tendon tunneler has found its way. When traction is applied to that tendon, the new scar may not stretch, but the surrounding fat and areolar tissue will stretch and move with the tendon through several millimeters. This early movement will allow the patient to sense the new action and use it. Thus he will continue to stimulate further muscle contraction and movement and further stretch and then lengthening and remodeling of the new paratendinous tissue.

Thus the concept of excursion of a tendon is complex and involves many factors. The true potential excursion, dependent only on the number of sarcomeres in each fiber, is not responsive to movement or active use; it is responsive to the tension in the resting fiber. Tarbary and others[11,12] have shown in experimental animals that if a muscle fiber is immobilized in a slack position it becomes shorter by loss of sarcomeres, and if it is immobilized in a stretched position it becomes longer by the addition of sarcomeres, until neutral tension is achieved.

Thus there is no way that a patient or a therapist can make a permanent change in the length of a muscle fiber. If a hand is kept at rest (splinted) in a posture that keeps some muscles slack and others stretched, every muscle fiber will undergo cell activity, with whole sarcomeres being added to the stretched fibers and removed from the slack fibers until all are returned to their normal tension. When the hand is released and allowed movement again, the patient will find that it is difficult to return to the normal position of rest. It will take time until a reverse process of sarcomere adjustment restores fiber lengths back to what they were.

If a surgeon, while transferring a tendon, makes the new attachment at a high tension, he or she may assume that the result will be a stronger muscle action. This is not so. As soon as the muscle is at a high resting tension, more sarcomeres will be added in series to each fiber until the tension is the same as all other muscles. The fibers will be longer but not stronger.

MECHANICAL FACTORS AT DISTAL END OF TRANSFER
Leverage

All that a muscle can give to a joint is tension and excursion of the tendon. At the joint this is turned into action according to the leverage. The actual movement of a joint around an axis is accomplished by "torque," or "moment." These two terms mean the same thing and are the product of force times leverage, or tension times moment arm. We all know that a lever enables a small force to move heavy objects (Fig. 50-1). We also know that a heavy weight can be moved most easily by a small force if the force is applied far up the lever, away from the axis, or if the load is close to the axis. This increases the *mechanical advantage*. (Mechanical advantage is equal to the moment arm of the force divided by the moment arm of the load.) What we often forget is that the force has to move farther if its lever arm is long and that the load will move very little if its lever arm is short.

Now this concept must be translated into the terminology of tendons and joints. The leverage that a tendon has at a joint is the perpendicular distance between the joint axis and the tendon as it crosses the joint. The lever arm beyond that is the length of the bone or digit distal to the joint axis. Thus it must be obvious at once that in the body almost all levers work with the force at the short end of the lever and the load at the long end. We are using a system of muscles that can produce enormous forces over rather short distances. The lever and pulley systems around joints are designed to take big forces with short ranges and make them effective over bigger ranges, with reduced force. There is no way to beat this system. The price of increased power is reduced range. I often hear surgeons say that they have found a way to increase the "strength" of a transfer at a joint. I rarely hear them mention the amount of excursion that has been used up, leaving less "strength" for other joints in the same sequence, or the fact that the transfer will now be effective over a smaller range.

One reason that surgeons usually do not try to work out the moments or leverages of the tendons they transfer is that they know it is so difficult to identify exactly where the axis of a joint is located. Therefore it is not possible at surgery to measure the perpendicular distance between the axis and the tendon.

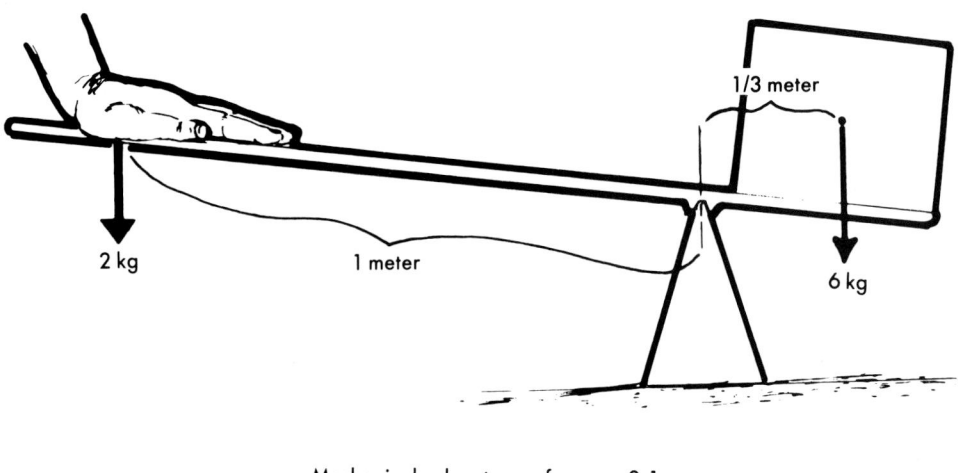

Mechanical advantage of arm = 3:1
Moment of hand = 2 kg-m
Moment of weight = 2 kg-m

Fig. 50-1 Equilibrium in lever system.

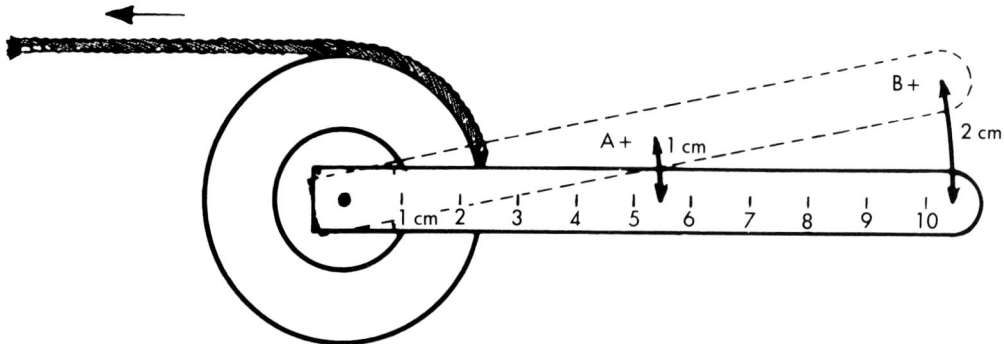

Fig. 50-2 Pulley-wheel axis and lever (tendon and bone at joint). Every point on lever (bone) moves through distance proportional to distance from axis.

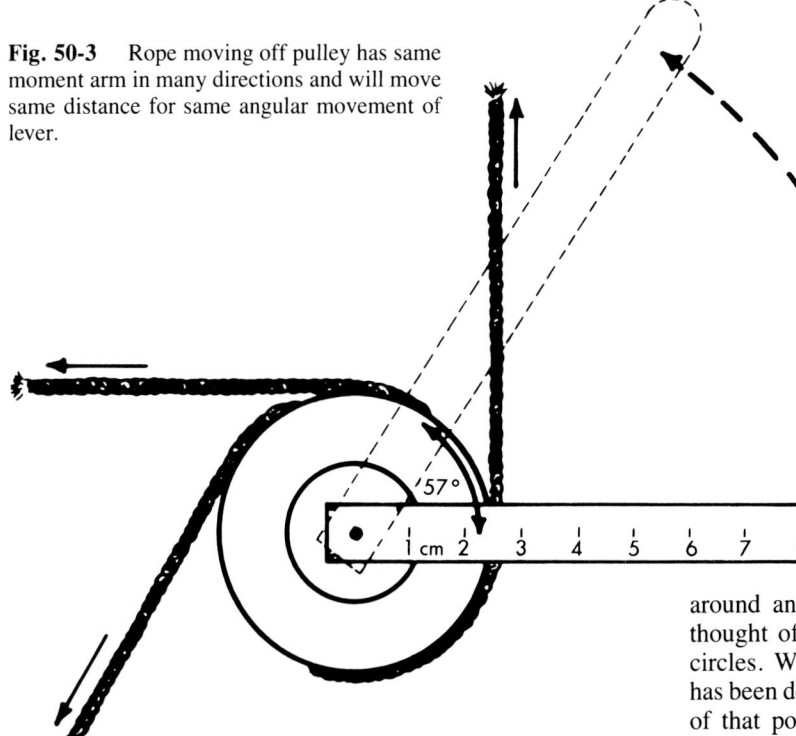

Fig. 50-3 Rope moving off pulley has same moment arm in many directions and will move same distance for same angular movement of lever.

There is, however, a simple and practical method of estimating the moment arms of tendons at joints that will enable surgeons to know exactly how effective each tendon will be at each joint it crosses. The method is based on two rules of geometry (Fig. 50-2). The first is that when a lever (bone) moves around an axis (joint), every point on the lever moves through a distance proportional to its own distance from the axis. The second rule grows out of the first and is an example of it (Fig. 50-3). If a lever moves around an axis through an angle of 57.29 degrees, then every point on the lever moves a distance *equal* to its own distance from the axis. If a length of a radius is marked on the circumference of a circle, and the two ends of that radius are joined to the center, the angle between them is called a radian and measures about 57.29 degrees (Fig. 50-4). As a lever moves

around an axis a number of points on its length may be thought of as marking out a number of arcs of concentric circles. When the lever has moved a radian, every arc that has been described is the same length as the distance (radius) of that point on the lever from the axis. This becomes a way to relate angles to distances; angles of joint movement can be related to excursions of the tendons that cause the movement or are affected by it.

In the stressful, time-dominated atmosphere of the operating room, nobody is going to measure tenths of a degree, or even single degrees. I find it useful to have in the operating room a metal triangle with angles of 30, 60, and 90 degrees (Fig. 50-5). I also have a metal millimeter scale. Keeping

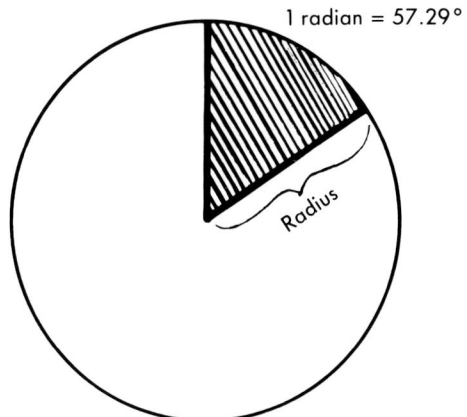

Fig. 50-4 Radius along circumference of circle subtends radian at center.

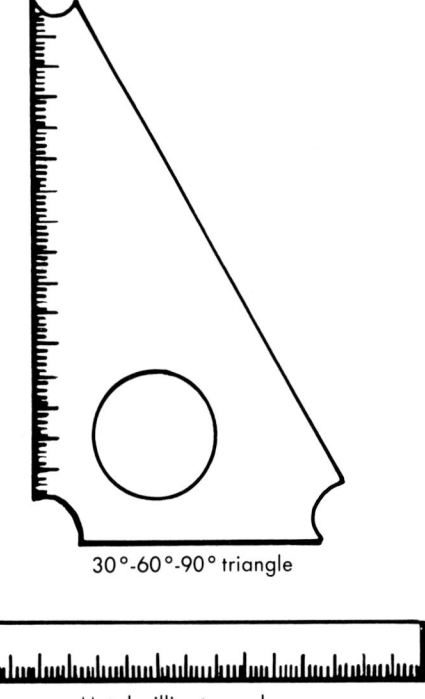

30°-60°-90° triangle

Metal millimeter scale

Fig. 50-5 Corners of triangle are cut out to allow it to fit between fingers over webs with edges intersecting at metacarpophalangeal joint axis.

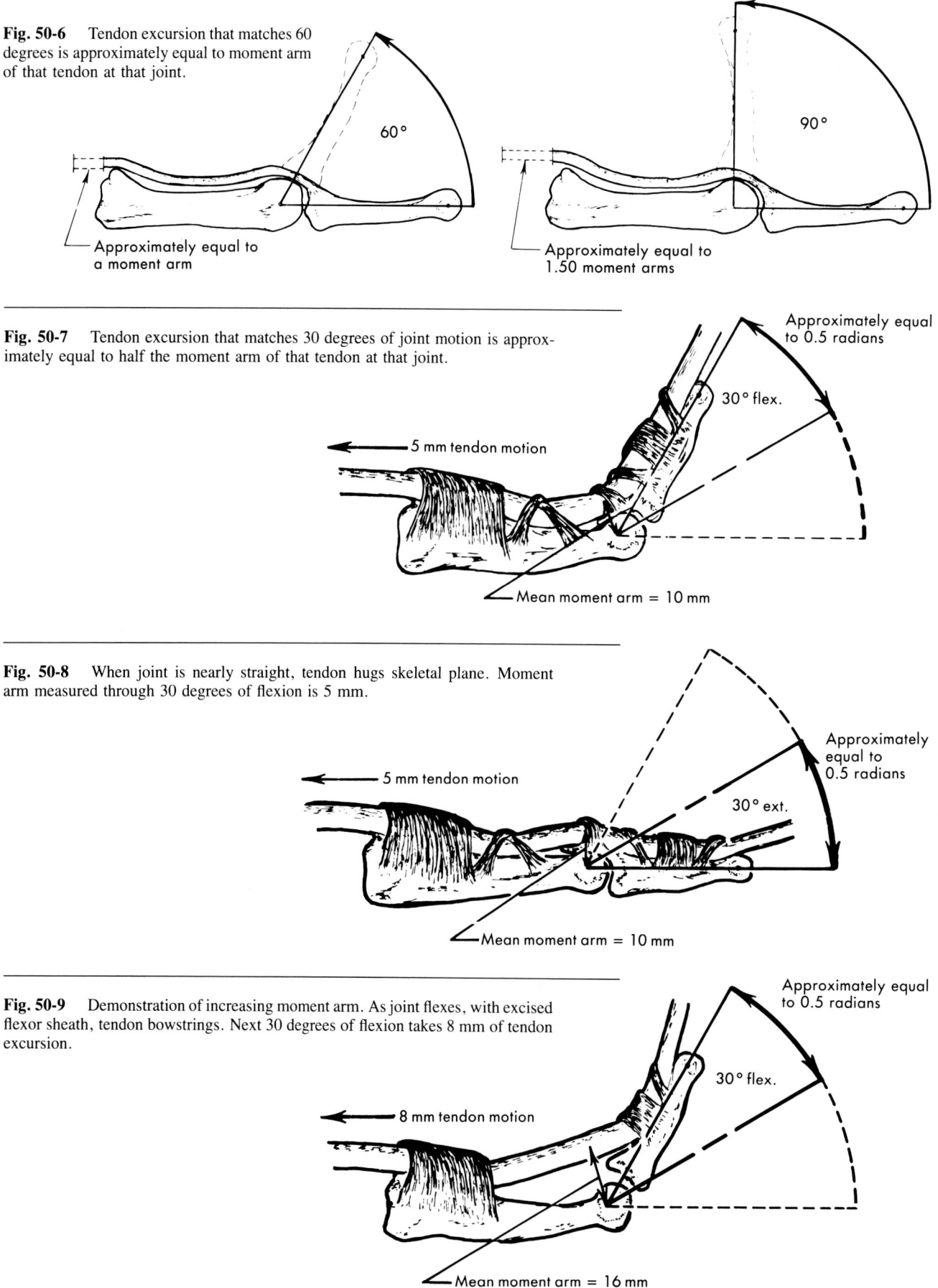

Fig. 50-6 Tendon excursion that matches 60 degrees is approximately equal to moment arm of that tendon at that joint.

Approximately equal to a moment arm

Approximately equal to 1.50 moment arms

Fig. 50-7 Tendon excursion that matches 30 degrees of joint motion is approximately equal to half the moment arm of that tendon at that joint.

Approximately equal to 0.5 radians

30° flex.

5 mm tendon motion

Mean moment arm = 10 mm

Fig. 50-8 When joint is nearly straight, tendon hugs skeletal plane. Moment arm measured through 30 degrees of flexion is 5 mm.

Approximately equal to 0.5 radians

30° ext.

5 mm tendon motion

Mean moment arm = 10 mm

Fig. 50-9 Demonstration of increasing moment arm. As joint flexes, with excised flexor sheath, tendon bowstrings. Next 30 degrees of flexion takes 8 mm of tendon excursion.

Approximately equal to 0.5 radians

30° flex.

8 mm tendon motion

Mean moment arm = 16 mm

a little tension on a tendon, I move a joint through 60 degrees, while my assistant measures exactly how far the tendon has moved. *The excursion of the tendon that matches 60 degrees of joint movement is the same as the moment arm or leverage of that tendon at that joint.* I often use 90 degrees of joint movement, because I find it is easier to guess a right angle. In that case the tendon excursion will be one-and-a-half times the moment arm (Fig. 50-6). If I use only 30 degrees of joint motion, the tendon will move half the moment arm.

Engineers have objected that this becomes imprecise when there is a variable axis (instant center) or when the bowstringing of a tendon results in a changing moment arm. It is in just these situations that this system is so valuable. What is the use of knowing the exact moment arm at which a tendon *ought* to be? I need to know just how effective my tendon is going to be in the place I have put it, even if it is wrong—in fact, *especially* if it is wrong. In the case of a bowstringing tendon the measured tendon excursion will give the *mean* moment arm. In such a case it is useful to take two readings (Figs. 50-7 and 50-8), one of the first 30 degrees of motion and the other of the last 30 degrees of motion. In the case of a flexor tendon graft that has no sheath at the MP joint and that has had a new pulley reconstruction, the surgeon may measure the tendon excursion that matches 0 to 30 degrees, and then 60 to 90 degrees, of MP joint motion (Fig. 50-9). A normal finger might give readings of 5 mm and 6 mm, indicating a moment arm of 10 mm (near extension) and 12 mm (near flexion). The measured excursion has been doubled to obtain the moment arm, because the joint has been moved only 30 degrees at a time rather than 60 degrees. With a well-reconstructed pulley a surgeon might find readings of 5 mm and 7 mm, showing just a little increase in bowstringing. However, if the surgeon gets readings of 5 mm and 10 mm, he or she will know that there is severe bowstringing. The new pulley is either too loose or too far up the finger away from the axis. If the surgeon accepts that result, some poor patient will struggle vainly to obtain flexion of the PIP joint while the MP joint flexes too strongly, using up the best of the available excursion.

Two axes

In placing a tendon transfer the surgeon must consider all the possible directions in which the joint may move in response to the transferred tendon. In many cases there will be an axis for flexion and extension, and another axis for abduction and adduction. The tendon may cross the joint in an oblique direction so that the surgeon may be uncertain exactly how the joint will respond. Here I suggest a quick test. Keep tension on the tendon by a stitch marker while the joint is moved first through 60 degrees of flexion-extension and then through 30 degrees of abduction-adduction. I suggest 30 degrees, because few joints can do a full 60 degrees of lateral movement. Do not forget to double the 30-degree reading to obtain the abduction-adduction moment arm. Now the two vector moment arms can be plotted on a graph to give the real or resultant moment arm as the diagonal of the rectangle so formed (Fig. 50-10).

The third axis—rotation

The third movement is rotation and the axis is longitudinal, at right angles to both the other axes. Many joints, such as MP joints, do not have much active rotation in normal strong hands but may develop significant rotation if the finger either is hypermobile or has damaged stabilizing ligaments as in rheumatoid arthritis. This becomes a more severe problem if a tendon transfer is added that is unopposed in a rotational sense.

Joints in series

In severe paralysis a single tendon is sometimes placed across a series of joints, without the support of other muscles at the proximal joints. This might be satisfactory if each segment of a digit were always supported by external opposing forces as it is when one grasps a cylinder. However, if the distal segment alone is opposed by a force, as in pinch, the proximal segments may buckle. The surgeon must remember the following: (1) A tendon crossing several joints exerts equal force at each. There is no way a person can instruct his muscle to apply more force at one joint than at another. The actual moment or torque that is exerted at each joint varies only according to the moment arms of that tendon at each joint. (2) The distal external force or load at the tip of the digit exerts an opposing moment or torque at each joint, and this also varies according to the moment arm of the external force, at that joint. The moment arms of tendons in the hand are usually small, because tendons are held close to the skeleton and are only a little larger at proximal joints as the skeleton becomes thicker. However, the moment arms of the external force or load are based on the length of the bones and the length of the digit and thus become enormously greater at proximal joints. Thus an unopposed digit may be flexed by a single muscle-tendon unit acting on all of the joints. The flexor profundus, unaided

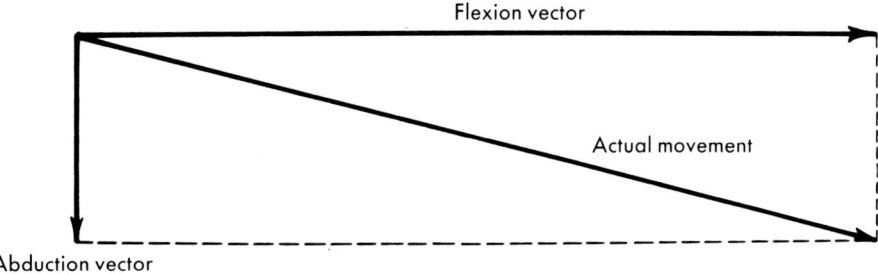

Fig. 50-10   Vector diagram of motion at joint in two planes. There is also a rotational vector, with axis at right angles to the plane of this page.

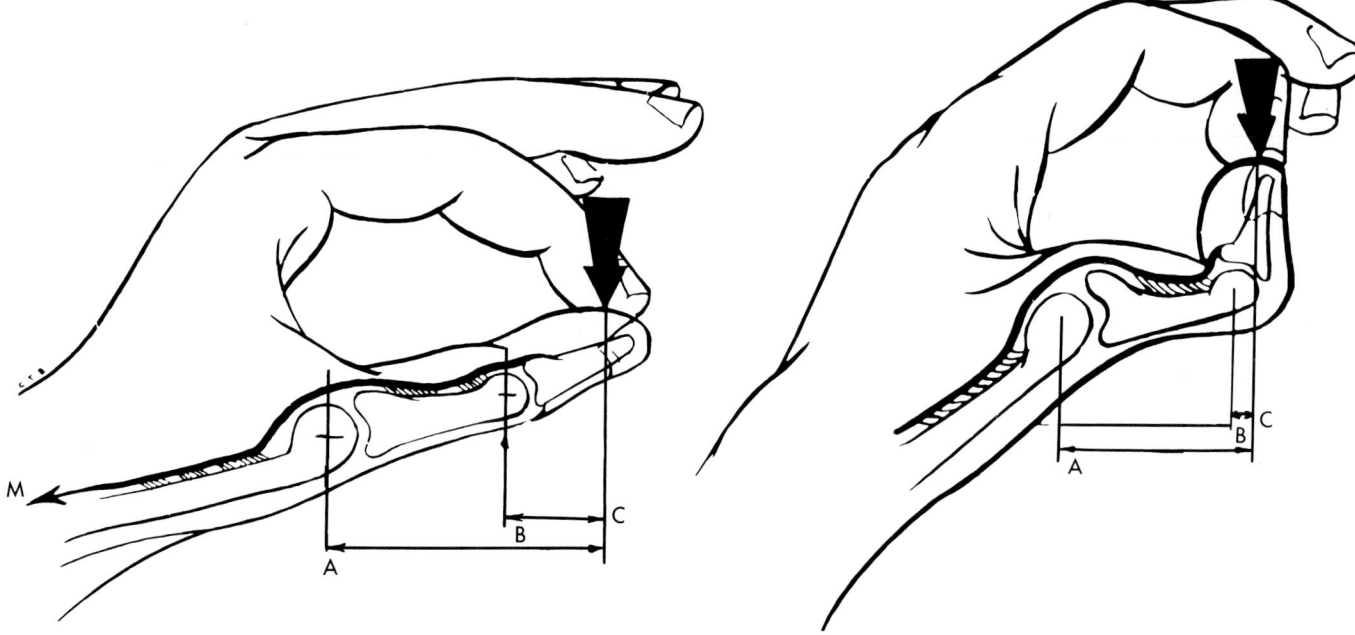

Fig. 50-11   Diagram of a tendon that crosses more than one joint. External force of pinch, *arrow at C,* has a tendency to force joints *A* and *B* into extension. Turning moment at *A* is proportional to *A-C,* whereas that at *B* is proportional to *B-C.* (From Brand PW: Tendon transfers in the forearm. In Flynn JE: Hand surgery, ed 3, Baltimore, 1982, Williams & Wilkins.)

Fig. 50-12   Deformity that results from having only one flexor tendon crossing two joints. (From Brand PW: Tendon transfers in the forearm. In Flynn JE: Hand surgery, ed 3, Baltimore, 1982, Williams & Wilkins.)

by other muscles, produces a full sweep from extended finger to clenched fist. As soon as the finger tip is opposed by a load or external force, it becomes necessary to recruit the flexor superficialis for the PIP and MP joints plus the intrinsic muscles for the MP joints, or the fingers will flex distally and hyperextend proximally.[1]

Consider the mechanism of the well-known Froment sign in the thumb. When the short flexors and adductor muscles are paralyzed, the long flexor will have equal tension along its length and will exert flexion moment at the MP and interphalangeal joints in proportion to the moment arms at each joint, which are only marginally different from each other. When a firm pinch is used, the index finger (Fig. 50-11) may push the thumb toward extension. The long flexor, though, immediately increases its tension to oppose the index finger and stabilize the pinch. However, the *extension* moment resulting from the index finger is far greater at the MP joint of the thumb, where it has more than double the moment arm that it has at the interphalangeal joint.

The long flexor increases its tension to prevent hyperextension at the MP joint and thereby unavoidably flexes the interphalangeal joint, at which less moment is needed. In flexing the interphalangeal joint, the terminal phalanx is brought to a position end-on to the index finger, so that the force from the index is applied still closer to the axis, or even at the axis (Fig. 50-12). Thus the Z-shaped buckling of the thumb becomes irreversible. Many surgeons, noting the flexed tip of the thumb, have assumed that it can be corrected by adding extra power to the extensor. *Not so.* The problem can be corrected only by adding an extra *flexor* to the MP joint so that the long flexor can relax at this joint

and avoid overflexing the interphalangeal joint. Because it is so difficult to balance a series of joints against a distal load, it is often wise to arthrodese one or more joints in the chain so that the few remaining muscles may effectively control the joints that remain. In the example above, arthrodesis of the MP joint of the thumb will allow a strong pinch without the Froment flexion of the tip.

Drag

In any operation for tendon transfer, we consider first the capability of the motor, the muscle-tendon unit that we transfer. Then we consider the geometry and mechanics by which the tension of the motor is transformed into the torque at each joint, and thus into effective movement of segments of limbs. Finally we have to realize that at each stage of this process we shall encounter internal resistance in the form of friction and the need to stretch passive soft tissues. This we may collectively call "drag," which we must recognize as an obstacle that may frustrate all of our endeavors, unless we plan a way to minimize its effect and work to overcome its unavoidable residue.

Friction.   Friction occurs whenever two objects move against each other. It is minimized when their surfaces are congruous and smooth and when the materials have a low coefficient of friction. I am not going to discuss this very much because true independent movement of surfaces over each other occurs only in joints and in synovial tendon sheaths. All the features of the architecture, the selection of low-friction materials for joint surfaces, and the lubrication systems involved are so amazingly well designed and work so efficiently that it is hard to imitate or match them.

There is little we can do to restore them if they are lost. In the case of transferred tendons, true gliding may occur in a sheath if it was there before we interfered and if the transferred tendon has a blood supply. If true gliding is needed after transfer in a place where it was not present before, the only thing we can do is to restore movement of the tendon, which is accomplished by stretching and relaxing the investing connective tissue, and wait for the synovial space to open up in its own good time. Such synovial spaces usually develop on the concave side of a curving tendon, but it takes months to happen.

Lengthening of soft tissue. Except in the limited areas where synovial spaces occur, all movement within limbs is permitted by the lengthening and shortening of connective tissue. We often use the word "gliding" in referring to tendon movement, but it is not real gliding in most cases. A tendon does not move over the tissue next to it. It is attached to the paratenon that surrounds it. That tissue is usually relaxed when the tendon is at its midpoint of motion. It stretches and lengthens when the tendon needs to move. Peritendinous tissues are made of collagen and elastin and of some interesting structureless ground substance that is semifluid and that has gel-like qualities. When this composite soft tissue is subjected to tension, it becomes longer. When relaxed, it shortens back to where it was before. When the tissue is pulled, it takes energy to make it longer. When it is allowed to shorten, it gives up energy.

The application of this simple concept is very straightforward. Every time a tendon is placed in a new situation, it becomes attached there by soft tissue. Therefore every time it moves it takes energy to lengthen that soft tissue, and it tends to get pulled back to its original position of

attachment when it is no longer under tension. The amount of force that it takes to lengthen that soft tissue and the distance through which it has to be lengthened are absolutely critical to the success of any tendon transfer. Yet they are the least studied aspect of tendon transfer. I have made it sound very simple in order that you may be willing to follow me into a step or two of complexity so that we may be in a position to understand and control this most important aspect of tendon transfer operations and postoperative rehabilitation.

Most studies on the mechanical qualities of soft tissues have been done on excised tissue.[6,14] A piece of skin, ligament, tendon, or connective tissue is removed, placed in a machine, and tested under various levels of stress and varying rates of stretch. From these studies we are able to identify the elasticity of a tissue and its viscosity. We may note that there is a hysteresis, in that when a tissue is stretched it lengthens, but when it is relaxed it comes back to its resting state by a different curve and takes longer in the process. We also may note a "creep," which means that when it is overstretched it does not come back to its first length, but remains a little longer (Figs. 50-13, 50-14). This type of study gives a good background for understanding soft-tissue mechanics, but it may give a false impression of what happens in living tissue. For example, if living soft tissue is overstretched, it also will exhibit creep, but this may be accompanied by an inflammatory reaction that occurs in response to the violence that has been done to some elements of the tissue fabric. That inflammation may result in the exudation of some tissue fluid containing fibrinogen, and there may be an incursion of inflammatory cells. The final result may be the laying down of some new interstitial

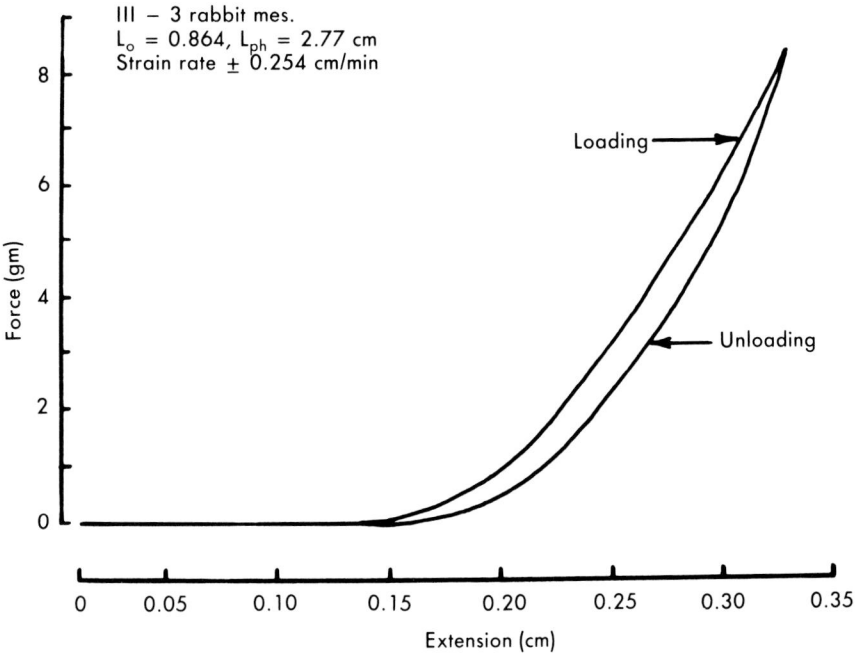

Fig. 50-13 Hysteresis curve. Rabbit mesentery. Loading and unloading curves after Y.C.B. Fung. Note that the stretched length of this tissue is more than three times the relaxed length. This curve shows only the end part of the length-tension curve of a piece of mesentery. The full curve is five times as long and is all flat; that is, the tension needed to lengthen or stretch the mesentery is so small that it is not measurable until the mesentery is nearly fully stretched. This is very much like the behavior of paratenon tissue, for which we do not yet have a precise curve. (From Fung YCB: Am J Physiol 213:1532, 1967.)

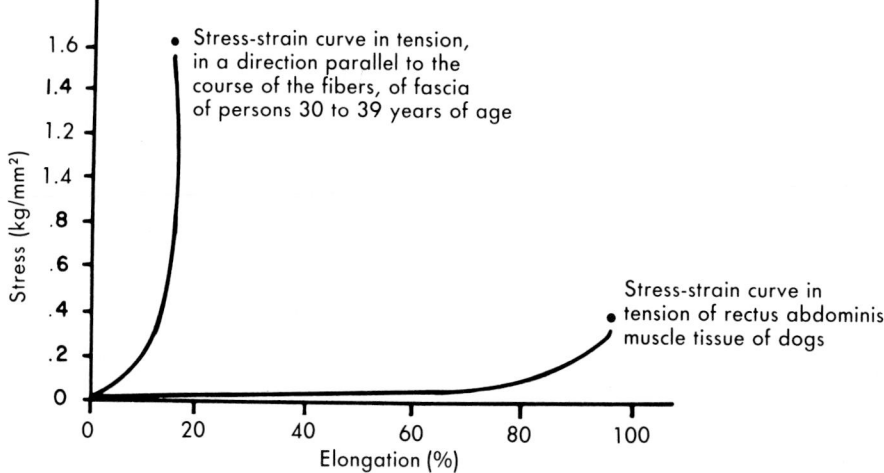

Fig. 50-14 Length-tension curves for fascia (*left*) and muscle (passive stretch only). Note that even fascia and tendon are lengthened 10% to 20% under tension and that muscle fiber is lengthened nearly 60% to 80% before it offers increasing resistance. This is from the fully relaxed length, not the physiologic resting length in situ. (Composite of curves after Yamada H. In Evans FG, editor: Strength of biological materials, Baltimore, 1970, Williams & Wilkins.)

collagen scar that will make the tissue more contracted and less compliant in the future.

We have to study the qualities of *living* soft tissue in response to mechanical force. This must include its ability to *remodel* or to be remodeled. It is this remodeling that is the basis for the gradual increase in range of motion at a joint that is limited by a soft-tissue contracture. It does not improve simply by passive stretching or by creep but by *growing* in length, or remodeling of the shortened tissue. This is the basis by which a transferred tendon gradually becomes free to move. The adhesions have not just been stretched; they have been remodeled, or have grown to accommodate to new requirements. Now some of this remodeling may be just a change in the bonding of collagen, but it is accomplished by living cells, by fibroblasts that act in response to mechanical and biomechanical orders that they understand. Our duty is to learn the type of mechanical stimulus to which these cells respond, and to use these stimuli as our instruments to change the pattern of adhesions and scar.

It is very difficult to study the behavior of collagen and elastin and connective tissue complexes in the intact hand because, as we open the tissues to look, it ceases to be an intact hand. However, even without knowing exactly how these tissues respond, at a molecular level, we may study total tissue response to a known input of mechanical stress. This involves the discipline of the measurement of stress input, recorded against range-of-motion output. Our present methods of prescribing the forces that are intended to lengthen adhesions are usually completely nonquantitative ("use *gentle* passive movement"), and even our measurements of range of motion are partly subjective in that we tend to pull or press a little harder when we measure the range of passive motion if we are expecting or hoping that it has improved.

I suggest, therefore, that all serious hand surgeons and therapists adopt a "torque–range of motion" (T-ROM) principle in monitoring the progress of tendon movement or joint stiffness preoperatively and postoperatively.

The principle of T-ROM is based on the recognition that although we can rarely measure the actual lengthening of any tissue or any adhesion without cutting the skin, their lengthening can be monitored by measuring the angular movement of the joint against the torque applied to it, because all the tissues that concern us have an effect on a joint. Thus we need to have a repeatable way to apply known force at a known distance from the axis while we measure the range of joint motion in response to it.

The key word, for most of us, is *repeatable*. For research workers the actual moment arms and exact forces are very important, but for understanding a given case and for following the progress of scar lengthening it is enough if we use repeatable criteria.

For the measurement of torque I suggest that we apply a known force—say 1 kg—at a standard position, such as at a skin crease, at right angles to a segment of the digit. We measure the joint angle while the torque is being applied. A day later, or a week later, the same force is applied at the same skin crease so that the torque is the same, and then we know for sure that any change in angle represents a change in the tissue restraints at the joint (or around the tendon).

There are three ways to increase the usefulness (and the complexity) of this measurement, each of which will teach us something different.

1. Use a series of forces, to vary the torque. This results in a T-ROM curve (Fig. 50-15). We often use 200, 400, 600, 800, and 1000 gm, applied by a spring scale at the same distance from the joint axis. We measure the joint angle at each level of torque. In general, we find that the *shape* of the curve gives some idea of the quality of the restricting adhesions. A shallow curve shows a compliant tissue. A steep curve means a more rigid tissue, or a tissue with shorter fibers and therefore poor prognosis for great increase in length.
2. Repeat the T-ROM measurement on the finger joint with different positions of the proximal joints (wrist). This gives a good idea of the relative role played by

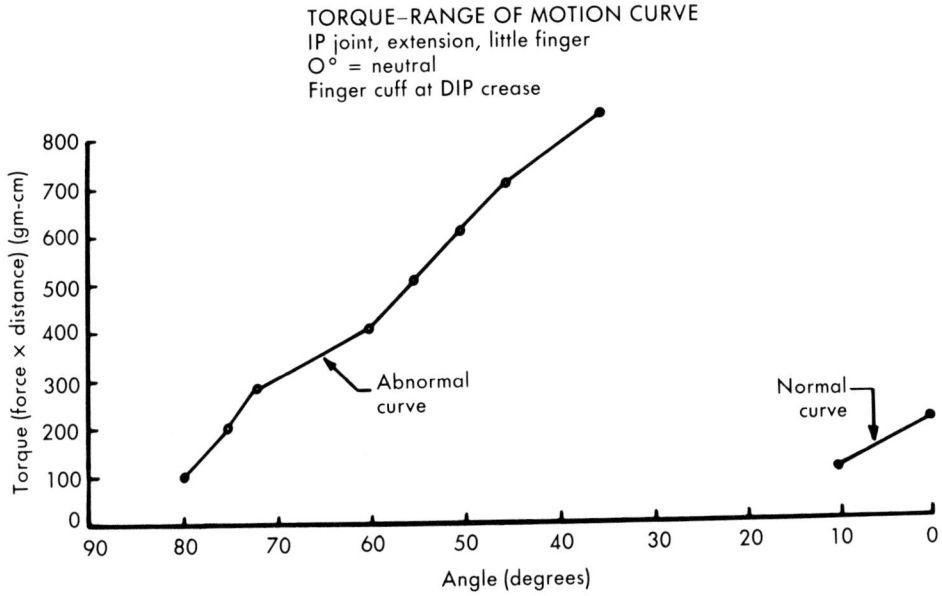

TORQUE–RANGE OF MOTION CURVE
IP joint, extension, little finger
O° = neutral
Finger cuff at DIP crease

Fig. 50-15 Torque-angle curve of a stiff interphalangeal joint moving into extension. The segment of curve on the right shows that a normal proximal interphalangeal joint would need only a small torque to achieve 0 degrees (full extension). The curve of a stiff finger shows a gradually increasing angle with gradually increasing torque. This indicates that the stiffness is "soft"; that is, the resistance is caused by tissues that can be progressively stretched and that therefore may be expected to grow longer with sustained therapy.

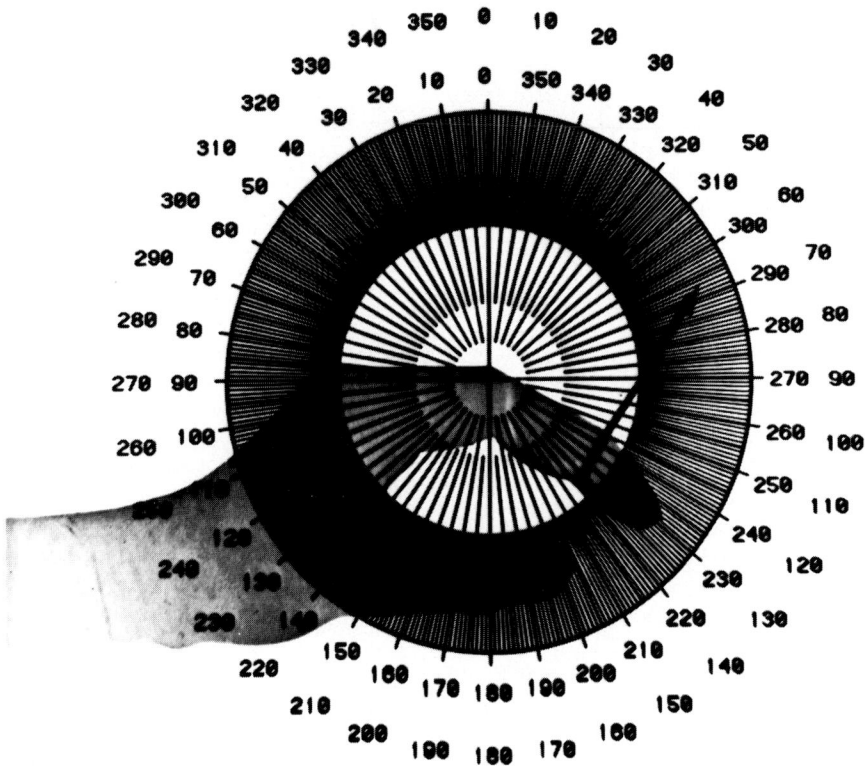

Fig. 50-16 Sunburst protractor. One way to measure torque angles is to have an overhead lamp with a parallel beam (an old slide projector will do). The operator holds the patient's finger level, over the sunburst protractor, and applies tension to a segment of the digit. By moving the hand so that the back of each segment is parallel to rays of the sunburst, the angle can be read without the need to hold a protractor.

proximal tendon and muscle restrictions as compared to distal joint stiffness.

3. Repeat the T-ROM measurement in a time sequence, such as early morning, before exercise, after exercise, or, if the hand is swollen, before and after hand elevation.

Although a T-ROM curve is based on a sequence of angles, it may be interpreted in terms of the length of the soft-tissue restraints that cross the joint and those that limit the excursion of the tendon that crosses the joint.

I recognize that surgeons and therapists will find, at first, that these measurements are time consuming, and that it requires manual dexterity to manipulate a joint, a protractor, and a spring at the same time with only one pair of hands. This will become easier with practice, and there are a couple of tricks that make it simple.

One is to have a voice-activated tape recorder and to speak out the angles and the figures for tension (for torque). This eliminates the need to release the hand and protractor to record the readings. When all measurements are finished, the angle readings and tension readings are plotted on graph paper while the tape is played back. It is a waste of time to record numbers and then make a graph. Record the graph directly with dots or crosses. It is the graph that gets looked at—nobody reads numbers!

With such a monitoring system, it will be possible to be quite precise about relating the therapy program to the changes that result from it. For example, it will be possible to compare the results of intermittent high-torque exercises with the results of continuous immobilization in low-torque extension (or flexion).

In general it will be found that where restraints to joint movement have a viscous element to them, it is best to prescribe a great deal of movement and exercise. Where the restraint is mainly elastic, there may be more benefit from continuous low-torque stretching (for a digit this torque may be as low as 250 gm-cm). To distinguish viscous from elastic resistance, one needs only to measure range of motion before and after a short period of active movement. Since viscous damping of range of motion is mostly caused by movement of fluids in tissues, there would be marked changes in range of motion at the same torque after just minutes of exercise.

• • •

In this chapter on mechanics of tendon transfers I have written mostly about methods of measurement and methods of monitoring change rather than giving instructions about methods of treatment. This is because there is very little available quantitative information on the relative merits of different types of transfer and of different methods of mobilizing stiff joints or adherent tendons. Rather than giving my opinions to rival opinions of others, I want to stress the fact that we need to develop disciplines of measurement so that we can each find out for ourselves whether procedure A is more effective than procedure B. It is numbers that we need, not more theories.

Finally, we have to keep in mind that whenever we direct therapy with the object of changing just one tissue, we will always have some effect on the whole hand and often on the whole person. If we want to lengthen a contracture on the flexor side of a hand, and if we use long-term low-torque extension, by splinting, we may achieve that goal. At the same time we may produce loss of length in dorsal structures and limit flexion. Other fingers in the same hand may lose range of motion just by disuse. Any form of immobilization will tend to cause loss of compliance in capsular tissues and loss of fluid components of hyaline cartilage. Thus, whenever possible, we should avoid single-minded mechanical approaches to any deformity. If long-term tension is called for, at least 1 hour per day should be reserved for free, active exercise and purposeful movement to keep tissue fluids moving, to move collagen fiber on collagen fiber, and to encourage the restoration of normal balance between the fluids and gels in cartilage and in paratenon tissues. Then with restored homeostasis, relaxed fibroblasts, and contented fat cells, we may return to the discipline of tension and torque to accomplish a specific objective.

REFERENCES

1. Brand PW: Tendon transfers in the forearm. In Flynn JE, editor: Hand surgery, ed 2, Baltimore, 1975, Williams & Wilkins.
2. Brand PW, Beach RB, and Thompson DE: Relative tension and potential excursion of muscles in the forearm and hand, J Hand Surg 6:209, 1981.
3. Buncke HJ: The role of microsurgery in hand surgery (presidential address, American Society for Surgery of the Hand), J Hand Surg 6:533, 1981.
4. Daniels L, Williams M, and Worthingham C: Muscle testing: techniques of manual examination, ed 2, Philadelphia, 1956, WB Saunders Co.
5. Freehafer AA, Peckham H, and Keith MW: Determination of muscle-tendon unit properties during tendon transfer, J Hand Surg 4:331, 1979.
6. Fung YCB: Elasticity of soft tissues in simple elongation, Am J Physiol 213:1532, 1967.
7. Legg AT and Merrill JB: Physical therapy in infantile paralysis. Reprinted from Mock HE, Pemberton R, and Coulter JS, editors: Principles and practices of physical therapy, Hagerstown, Md, 1932, WF Prior Co, Inc.
8. Manktelow RT, Zuker RM, and McKee NH: Functioning free muscle transplantation. Presented at the thirty-seventh annual meeting of the American Society for Surgery of the Hand, New Orleans, Jan 18-20, 1982. In J Hand Surg 9A(1):32, 1984.
9. Nelson N: Factors to be considered in evaluating effect of treatment in anterior poliomyelitis, Arch Phys Med 28:358-363, 1947.
10. Sharrard WJW: Muscle recovery in poliomyelitis, J Bone Joint Surg [Br] 37B:63, 1955.
11. Tabary JC and others: Physiological and structural changes in the cat's soleus muscle due to immobilization at different lengths by plaster casts, J Physiol 224:231, 1972.
12. Tabary JC and others: Functional adaptation of sarcomere number of normal cat muscle, J Physiol (Paris) 72:277, 1976.
13. Wright WG: Muscle training in the treatment of infantile paralysis, Boston Med Surg 167:567, 1912.
14. Yamada H: Strength of biological materials, Baltimore, 1970, Williams & Willkins (Edited by FG Evans).

51

Tendon transfers in the upper extremity

Lawrence H. Schneider

The application of the motor power of one muscle to another weaker or paralyzed muscle by the transfer of its tendinous insertion is now well established. This technique, "tendon transfer," was originally referred to as "tendon transplantation," a differentiation that is subtle. "Transplant" implies complete removal of the muscle and "replanting" it in a new location, whereas the term "transfer" seems to describe better the act of redirecting the insertion. "Tendon grafting," quite a different procedure, was a term used interchangeably in the early literature to describe this technique, further adding to the confusion of terminology.

HISTORY

Study of the evolution of the techniques that are now widely accepted takes one through an exciting period in the history of reconstructive extremity surgery. Excellent reviews have been written by Waterman[38] and Adamson and Wilson.[1]

Carl Nicoladoni is given credit by most historians for the first tendon transfer performed in 1880. He took the peroneal tendons and sutured them into the tendo Achillis for talipes calcaneus deformity secondary to infantile paralysis. Soon after the operation, which was carried out in Vienna, he moved to Innsbruck leaving the aftercare to an associate who reported, according to Waterman,[38] that the "anastomosis separated and the procedure was a failure." Interestingly, although he became a great contributor to surgical knowledge, Nicoladoni never performed his procedure again.

What is not commonly acknowledged is that authors for about 100 years had been advocating the repair of severed tendons by "grafting" the distal segment onto adjacent intact tendons. Missa in 1770 sutured the lacerated extensor tendon of the long finger into that of the intact ring finger. Nicoladoni's case probably rates then only as the first reported use of the technique in infantile paralysis but certainly an ingenious contribution nonetheless.[38]

After 1880 there were scattered reports of tendon transfers, but because of technical failures interest generally waned. Then in 1896 Drobnik published 16 cases with follow-up and overall had a successful experience. Included in his list was case number 5, the first tendon transfer for paralysis in the upper extremity. In a patient with partial finger extensor paralysis, Drobnik transferred the extensor carpi radialis longus into the extensor digitorum communis. He also took one half of the extensor carpi radialis brevis and put it into the extensor pollicis longus.[38]

Franke was the first to transfer the wrist flexors for paralysis of the finger extensors, a technique widely used today

after radial nerve injury (Fig. 51-1). He also first performed tendon transfers for infantile spastic paralysis of cerebral origin.[38]

In the 1890s Parrish and Milliken in New York and Goldthwait in Boston established the technique in the United States. Apparently they were not familiar with each other's work or that of Nicoladoni.[38] In 1897 Bradford of Boston published 27 personal examples of what he called "tenoplastic operations."[3] This further popularized the procedure in the United States.

Meanwhile in Germany, Vulpius in Heidelberg, Lange in Munich, and Biesalski in Berlin developed the procedures further.[16] There were disagreements, usually on technical points, among the world leaders. For example, Vulpius believed that the transfer should be fixed to the tendon of the recipient muscle, while Codovilla[13] of Bologna and Jones in England believed that periosteal fixation was superior. Codovilla, an innovator, introduced the concept of transfer through the sheath of the paralyzed tendon. He also lengthened tendons too short to reach the periosteal insertion by fascial strips. Lange approached the length problem with silk thread prolongation of the motor tendon. The problem of fixation of the transferred tendons by adhesions was a serious one, and Mayer of New York worked on this aspect in Lange's clinic, later continuing his work in Berlin under Biesalski. It was Mayer who published, with his mentor, the monograph *The Physiology of Tendon Transplantation*. This work, subsequently published in English in three articles in *Surgery, Gynecology, and Obstetrics*[24] in 1916, renewed interest in tendon surgery in the United States. In this work the need for gentle tissue handling was stressed, along with the importance of clean-gliding tissue planes for successful tendon transfer. Mayer returned to the United States and established himself as a leading orthopedic surgeon.[25] Working in Iowa City, Steindler[37] contributed and perfected many surgical techniques in tendon transfer. Bunnell,[10] the father of American hand surgery, refined much of the work and added a large clinical experience in the upper extremity. He was influenced by his long friendship with Mayer.

Based on the work of these men are the principles of tendon transfer in the upper extremity. Although many of the original procedures were developed in patients with poliomyelitis, in present day surgery most tendon transfers are carried out on patients afflicted with peripheral nerve damage or traumatic muscle loss. Patients with central nervous system disorders are probably the third most frequent group aided by tendon transfer.

The more recent refiners of the work of the masters are

669

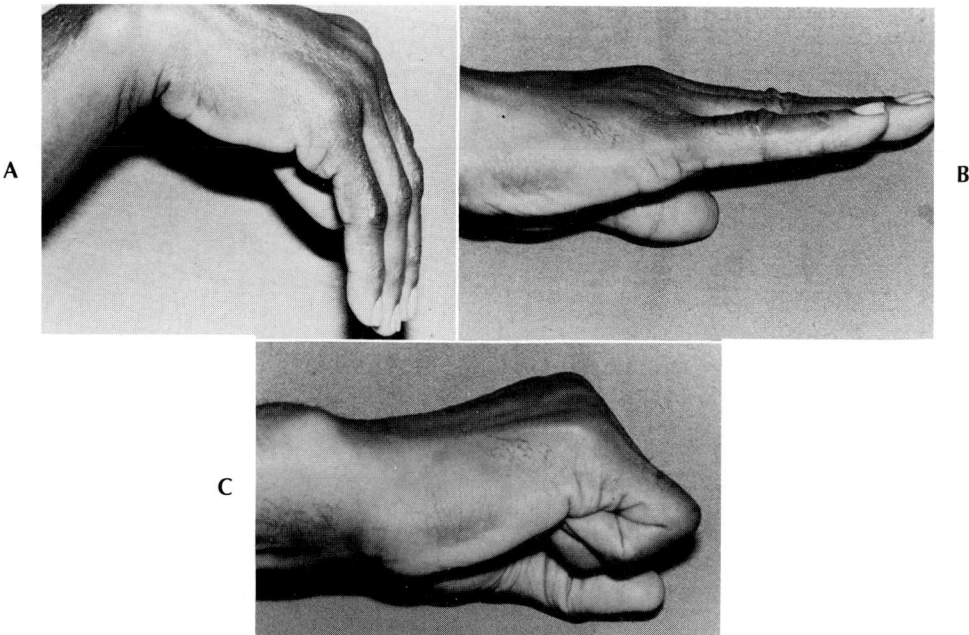

Fig. 51-1   Transfer of the wrist flexor (flexor carpi ulnaris) to extensor digitorum communis in radial nerve paralysis. **A,** Wristdrop and loss of metacarpophalangeal joint extension seen after high radial nerve injury. **B** and **C,** Range of extension and flexion seen 6 months after transfer.

many. Leading these would be Brand,[7] Boyes,[4-6] Curtis,[15] Fowler, Littler,[20,22] Omer,[29,30] Riordan,[31] White,[39] and Zancolli.[40]

INDICATIONS FOR TENDON TRANSFER

The absence of a particular needed function after irreparable nerve injury, nerve disease, or muscle loss should bring up a consideration for tendon transfer. Time should be allowed for wound healing to occur and for recovery of function, either spontaneously in the case of neuropraxia or axonotmesis or for reinnervation after a nerve repair. This usually requires a delay of 4 to 6 months. During this period it is the obligation of the treating physician and therapist to maintain passive mobility in the involved joints. This would be achieved through passive motion exercises and by the use of dynamic splints where indicated. Nerve loss in itself is not always an indication for tendon surgery, since patients can at times perform unexpectedly through substitutive or adaptive methods or can function because of dual innervated musculature and/or variations in innervation. For example, median nerve injury at the wrist may not result in loss of true thumb opposition in many patients, because this action may be performed by use of thenar eminence muscles partially or completely ulnar nerve innervated.[32] The point here is that each problem must be individualized in terms of the loss of function, its severity, the reconstructive possibilities, and the patient's needs and desires. Also to be stressed is the fact that tendon transfer is a palliative procedure that usually does not restore full and normal function. It is a redistribution of available power in an attempt to improve functional impairment.[2]

Once it is decided that tendon transfer has a place in the solution of a particular patient's problem, certain basic conditions must be satisfied.

Joint mobility

The participating joints in the function in question must be capable of passive motion if the transfer is to succeed. Hand therapy using physical modalities, including dynamic splinting, is needed to keep the joints mobile. This therapy can be carried out by the patient himself or through the supervision and guidance of trained therapists. At times, if joints have stiffened and do not respond to therapy, one must do preliminary surgical releases to restore passive mobility.

Adequate soft-tissue coverage

Well-healed and pliable soft tissues must be present to provide gliding planes through which the transfer can function. This may require the preliminary shifting of skin and the use of local or distant skin flaps.

Available motor tendons

A donor muscle must be available in the extremity. In single motor nerve injury in the upper extremity several motor tendons may be available. If two of the three major nerves in the extremity are irreparably damaged, choices are limited and prognosis in terms of function will be greatly reduced. Tendons available in the upper extremity vary with the injury and include wrist flexors, wrist extensors, flexor digitorum superficialis, proprius extensors, and brachioradialis.

SELECTION OF A MOTOR TENDON FOR TRANSFER

Boyes in 1962[5] discussed the factors involved in selection of a motor tendon. Amplitude of the donor tendon and power are the prime factors in tendon selection.

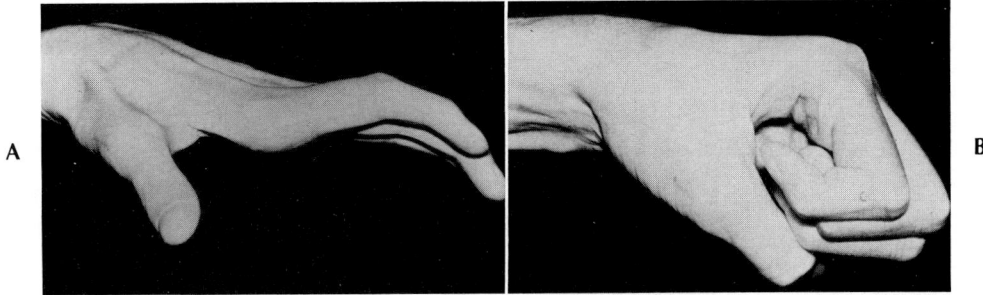

Fig. 51-2   Postoperative photos of patient with severe injury to median and ulnar nerves in proximal forearm, who had undergone transfer of extensor carpi radialis longus into flexor profundi in attempt to restore finger flexion. **A,** Extension of fingers. **B,** Flexion through transfer is surprisingly good.

Amplitude

The distance that a muscle can shorten from its maximum length is the excursion or amplitude. Average amplitude of the wrist flexors and extensors is about 3.5 cm. Full finger extension at the metacarpophalangeal (MP) joints requires 5 cm and the flexor digitorum profundus group an amplitude of 7 cm for full function. As motor tendons, the flexor digitorum superficialis group, which provide an amplitude of about 6 cm, are the only available tendons that can approach the necessary amplitude to replace the profundus. (Obviously when the extensor carpi radialis longus is used to power the flexor digitorum profundus, some sacrifice in range of motion must be accepted [Fig. 51-2]). This deficit is partially overcome by the additional amplitude provided the system by the tenodesis effect of the mobile wrist joint. Restoration of the long extensor system by transfer of a wrist flexor is a better matched situation as far as their respective amplitudes of motion are concerned.

Power

The ability of a muscle to perform work, power, is directly proportional to its cross-sectional diameter. Examples of the relative power of muscles in the forearm are as follows:

Pronator teres, 1.2 m/kg
Brachioradialis, 1.9
Flexor carpi ulnaris, 2.0
Flexor carpi radialis, 0.8
Extensor carpi radialis longus, 1.1
Extensor carpi ulnaris, 1.1

In the preoperative period accurate muscle testing is essential in the evaluation of a potential motor tendon. Each available muscle must be graded to assure adequate strength for transfer. The rating system 0 to 5 is used:

0—Total paralysis
1—Flicker of muscle action
2—Muscle contracts and moves joint with gravity eliminated
3—Muscle moves joint through a full range of motion against gravity
4—Muscle moves joint through a full range of motion against resistance
5—Normal muscle

Because the procedure of tendon transfer weakens the donor muscle by at least one grade, a four-power muscle may be inadequate for transfer.

Direction (Fig. 51-3)

The pathway of the transferred muscle should be as straight as possible to its new insertion. This may require extensive proximal mobilization of the muscle. Care must be taken to avoid injury to the nerve and vascular supply of the muscle.

Phase

Wrist extensors and digital flexors perform synergistically and are said to function in phase. The same applies for the activities of wrist flexors and digital extensors. Although it may be true that transfers within the phasic groupings are easier to train, the phasic action of a transfer is no longer regarded as a major factor in the selection of a motor tendon for transfer. In fact, muscles 180 degrees out of phase are not uncommonly used, an example being the use of the flexor superficialis as a motor for the extensor digitorum communis in radial nerve paralysis.

TECHNICAL ASPECTS OF TENDON TRANSFERS

When one is setting up a transfer procedure, it is helpful to have a plan of action in which available assets are listed against functional needs. Then an attempt is made to rebalance the situation providing power for lost functions while only minimally affecting present function. The importance of a stable functioning wrist is important for success in many transfers, and wrist fusion is contraindicated except in extreme situations. For the same reason, it is necessary to preserve at least one wrist extensor and one wrist flexor when these tendons are used as transfers.

The general rules of tendon surgery have to be observed. Gentle handling of the tendon to avoid damage to its surface is recommended. Wherever possible the tendon is passed through soft gliding planes. Appropriate incisions are planned that cross transversely to the planned direction of the transfer, thereby reducing the area of potential adhesion formation.

Tendon junctures can be carried out end to end, side to side, or by interweaving techniques. The junctures should be strong when nonabsorbable low-reactive 2-0 or 3-0 suture material is used. As a general rule, the transfers are put in so as to err on the tight side. This especially applies when transfers are done into the extensor system, where failures are likely to occur if the transfer is too loose.

Plaster immobilization is used for 3 to 4 weeks before

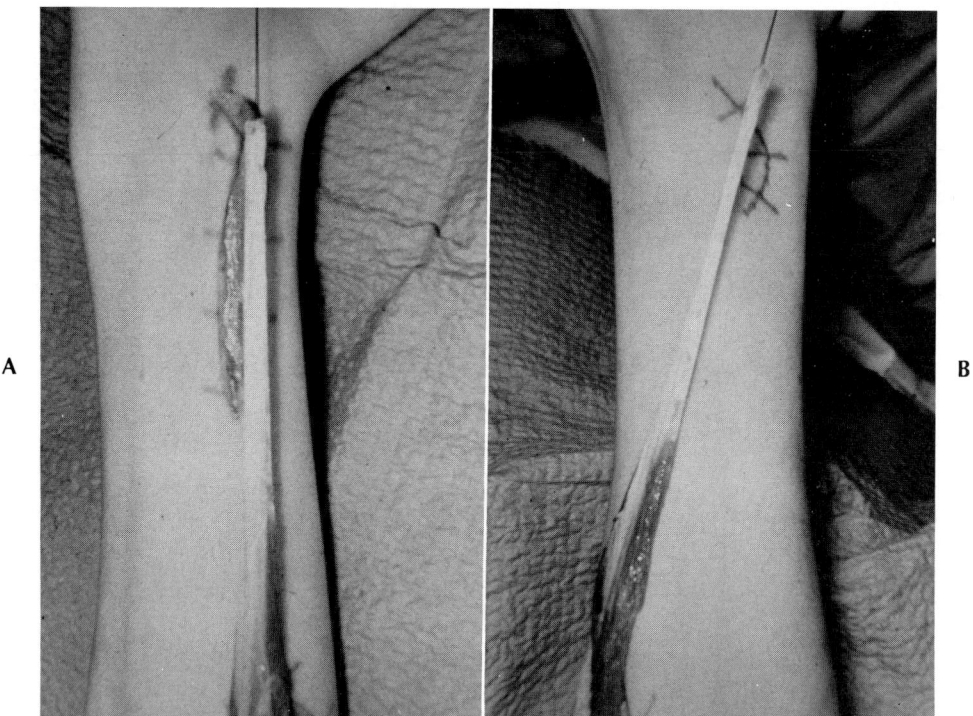

Fig. 51-3 Direction of tendon transfer should be as straight as possible in its route to its new insertion. **A,** Flexor carpi ulnaris is freed from its insertion and taken back into proximal forearm. **B,** Tendon is as straight as possible in its route to its new insertion at the radial wrist extensors in this patient with spastic paralysis.

removal for exercises. Splint protection is usually added for an additional 3 weeks while the muscle is educated in its new role. If the rules are obeyed, this usually is a rapid relearning process but may at times tax the ingenuity of both surgeon and therapist.

RESTORATION OF OPPOSITION TO THE PARALYZED THUMB

Tendon transfers have proven useful in different paralytic conditions. Many of these procedures were developed in the era of poliomyelitis. With the elimination of this once wide-spread source of paralyzed patients, these same transfers now serve in the treatment of those with peripheral nerve injury. At this time patients with irremediable injuries to the peripheral nerves serve as the largest group to benefit from the application of these same techniques. Other conditions for which these procedures are helpful in the upper extremity include tetraplegia,[27] rheumatoid arthritis,[17,23,28] traumatic muscle loss,[34,35] and cerebral palsy.[18] To study these techniques one very common indication for tendon transfer will be illustrated.

Opposition transfer. The application of the tip of our thumb to our fingers is essential for the performance of many fine manipulative functions and even in heavy grip-ping.[8,9,14,36] When the thumb is in true opposition, its pad is opposite the pad of the finger.[11] This complex positioning action is accomplished with the thenar muscles, mainly the abductor pollicis brevis but the opponens as well. The flexor pollicis brevis also contributes. As power is added, the flexor pollicis longus and the abductor pollicis come into play. The motion, occurring mainly at the basilar joint of the

thumb, the trapezial-metacarpal joint, starts with abduction, then pronation and finally flexion in a complex maneuver. It should be stressed that this transfer is palliative, and in severe problems the transfer of one motor cannot restore all elements of this complex action.

Loss of ability to oppose the thumb to the fingers is a devastating loss to the hand. The patients with this deficiency have median nerve injuries at some level, which has led to the paralysis of the thenar group muscles. It is important to note that not all patients with median nerve damage need surgery to restore opposition because some hands function quite well through ulnar innervated muscles in the thenar eminence.[32] Careful preoperative evaluation is therefore essential. In cases where both the median and the ulnar nerves are irretrievably injured, the need for opposition plasty is more clear cut.

General principles. Bunnell[9,10] told us that any tendon pulled subcutaneously from the general area of the pisiform bone and inserted into the dorsal ulnar corner of the base of the proximal phalanx of the thumb would help restore lost opposition. This means that many different tendons could be used in the restoration of this function.[11,12,21,33,36] Minkow[26] and Herrick and Lister[19] undertook review of the literature on this subject and came up with many different techniques and scores of references on this topic.

Preoperative evaluation. The therapist and surgeon should try to learn what the patient needs and expects from the procedure. Since most patients with loss of opposition also have decreased sensation in the thumb, this may, in fact, be the primary functional problem. The preoperative period should be occupied with restoration and maintenance of passive opposition and loosening the basilar joint using hand therapy measures. Pretransfer surgery, such as joint release, may be necessary if therapy cannot return a useful range of passive motion. At times surgical manipulation of the skin in the form of skin grafts and scar revisions may be necessary to provide a satisfactory gliding bed for the tendon transfer. To demonstrate the application of the tendon transfer to the restoration of opposition two cases will be illustrated (Figs. 51-4 and 51-5).

CAUSES FOR DISAPPOINTMENT IN TENDON TRANSFERS

Suboptimal results do occur in tendon transfer, and this is a more likely event where an overly ambitious program is attempted in severe functional loss. This can be avoided if realistic attainable goals are established. Although the reinstitution of active motion is desirable, the treating surgeon should not lose sight of the place for tenodeses and arthrodeses in the reconstructive program.

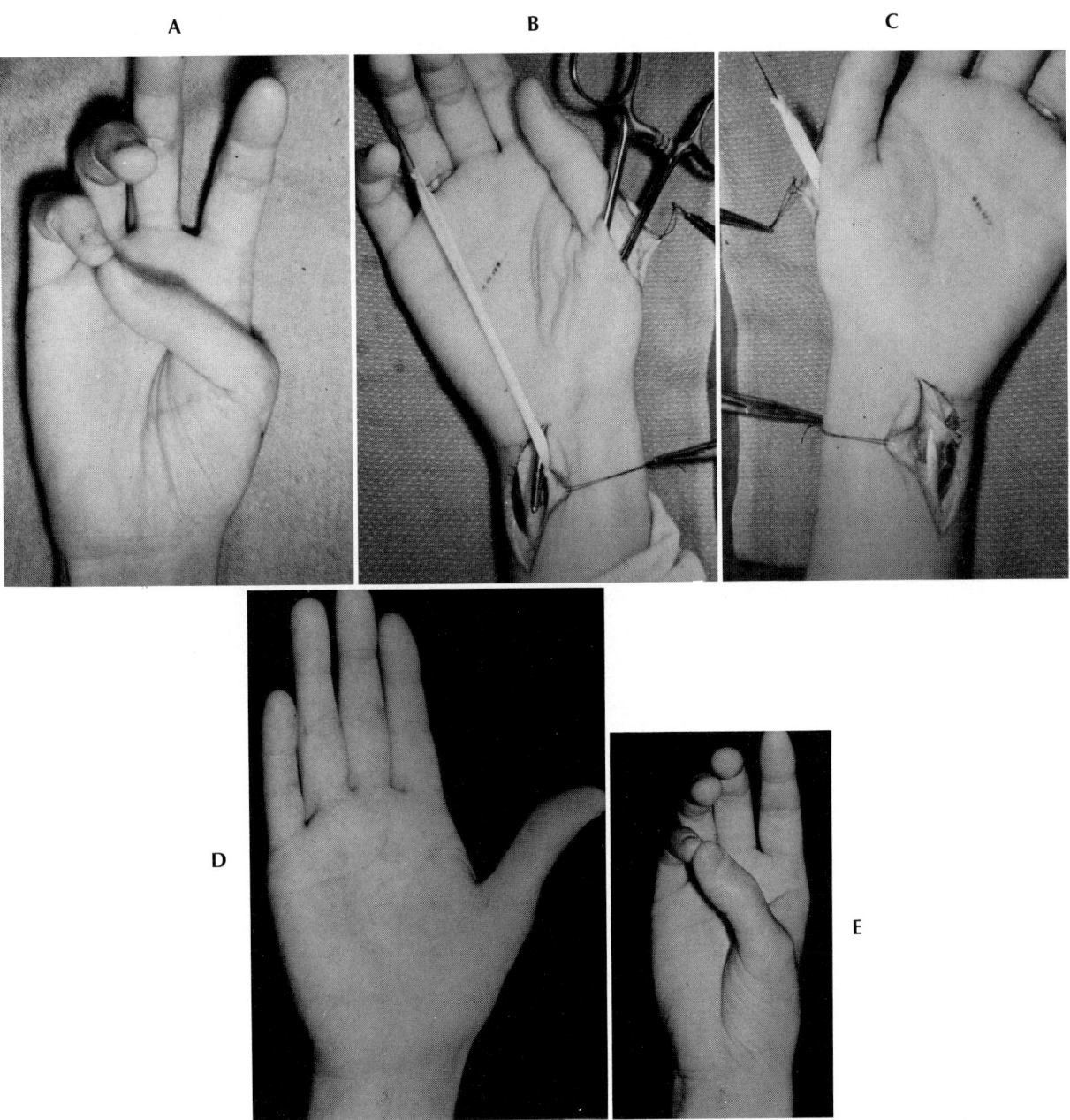

Fig. 51-4   Flexor digitorum superficialis transferred to thumb to restore opposition. **A,** True opposition has been lost because of irreparable injury to median motor nerve branch in thenar eminence. **B** and **C,** Flexor superficialis of ring finger has been removed to wrist level and passed around flexor carpi ulnaris at wrist and then subcutaneously to metacarpophalangeal joint region of thumb. **D** and **E,** Extension of thumb and opposition performed, photographs taken 2 years later.

A   B   C

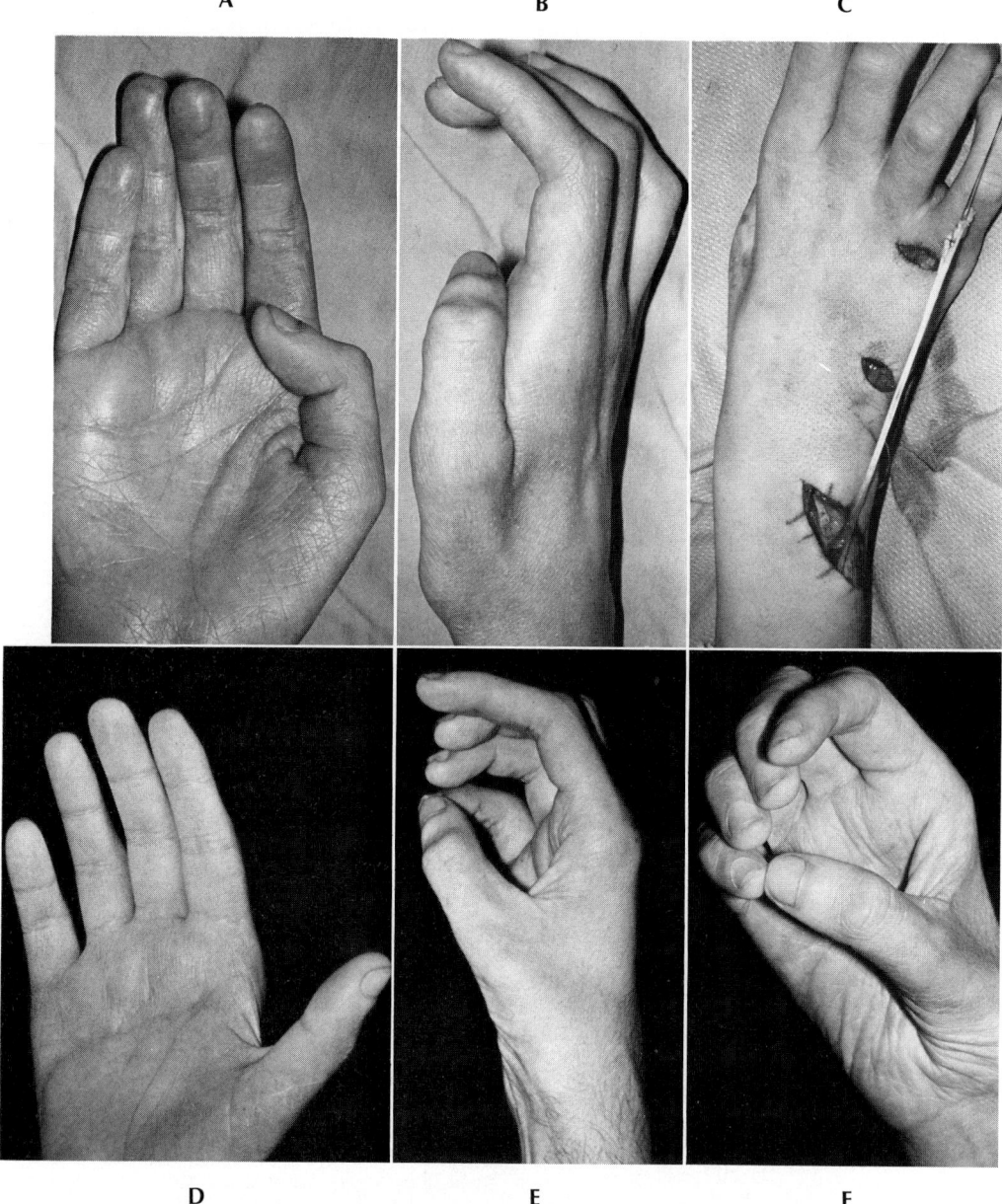

D   E   F

Fig. 51-5 Restoration of opposition using the extensor digiti minimi.[33] Brachial plexus injury had left this 20-year-old man with loss of opposition and a shortage of transferable motors for opponensplasty. The extensor digiti minimi was normal and available. **A,** Preoperative attempt at opposition shows the thumb to be ineffective. **B,** Preoperative radial view. The thumb cannot be brought out of the plane of the palm. **C,** The extensor digiti minimi is mobilized through three incisions and then will be passed subcutaneously around the border of the ulna to be inserted into the abductor pollicis brevis. **D, E** and **F** Result of transfer at 6 months. Excellent opposition has been restored.

When patients whose results were found to be less than expected were analyzed, the following pitfalls were seen to be prominent:

1. Acceptance of less than full passive range of motion before transfer
2. Overestimation of the strength of the donor muscle—careful here especially when transferring a reinnervated muscle
3. Adhesions along the course of transfer
4. Technical failures
    a. Breakdown of the juncture
    b. Transfer put in too loose

The solutions to the above problems are obvious—careful attention to the details of evaluation and surgery.

SUMMARY

The dynamic procedure of the transfer of the action of a muscle from its usual function to a widely different one is still an exciting and challenging area of reconstructive extremity surgery. Careful planning and preoperative patient evaluation, along with strict attention to the rules and details of the procedure, can reward patient, therapist, and surgeon.

REFERENCES

1. Adamson JE and Wilson JN: The history of flexor tendon grafting, J Bone Joint Surg 43A:709, 1961.
2. Beasley RW: Basic considerations for tendon transfer operations in the upper extremity. In American Academy of Orthopaedic Surgeons: Symposium on tendon surgery in the hand, St Louis, 1985, The CV Mosby Co.
3. Bick EM: Source book of orthopaedics, ed 2, New York, 1968, Hafner Publishing Co.
4. Boyes JH: Tendon transfers for radial palsy, Bull Hosp Joint Dis 21:97, 1961.
5. Boyes JH: Selection of a donor motor for tendon transfer, Bull Hosp Joint Dis 23:1, 1962.
6. Boyes JH: Bunnell's surgery of the hand, ed 4, Philadelphia, 1964, JB Lippincott Co.
7. Brand PW: Biomechanics of tendon transfer, Orthop Clin North Am 5:205, 1974.
8. Brand PW: Clinical mechanics of the hand, St Louis, 1985, The CV Mosby Co.
9. Bunnell S: Opposition of the thumb, J Bone Joint Surg 20:269, 1938.
10. Bunnell S: Tendon transfer in the hand and forearm. In American Academy of Orthopaedic Surgeons: Instructional course lectures 6:106, Ann Arbor, Mich, 1949, JW Edwards Co.
11. Braun RM: Palmaris longus tendon transfer for augmentation of the thenar musculature in low median nerve palsy, J Hand Surg 3:488, 1978.
12. Burkhalter WE: Median nerve palsy. In Green DP, editor: Operative hand surgery, New York, 1988, Churchill Livingstone.
13. Codovilla A: Tendon transplants in orthopaedic practice, 1899, translated in Clin Orthop 118:2, 1976.
14. Cooney WP, Linscheid RL, and An KN: Opposition of the thumb: an anatomic and biomechanical study of tendon transfers, J Hand Surg 9:777, 1984.
15. Curtis RM: Fundamental principles of tendon transfer, Orthop Clin North Am 5:231, 1974.
16. Erlacher PJ: The development of tendon surgery in Germany. In American Academy of Orthopaedic Surgeons: Instructional course lectures 13:110, Ann Arbor, Mich, 1956, JW Edwards Co.
17. Ertel AN and Millender LH: Flexor tendon involvement in rheumatoid arthritis. In Hunter JM, Schneider LH, and Mackin EJ, editors: Tendon surgery in the hand, St Louis, 1987, The CV Mosby Co.
18. Goldner JL: Upper extremity reconstruction in cerebral palsy. In Hunter JM, Schneider LH, and Mackin EJ, editors: Tendon surgery in the hand, St Louis, 1987, The CV Mosby Co.
19. Herrick RT and Lister GD: Control of first web space contracture, The Hand 9:253, 1977.
20. Littler JW: Tendon transfers and arthrodeses in combined median and ulnar palsies, J Bone Joint Surg 31A:225, 1949.
21. Littler JW: Restoration of power and stability in the partially paralyzed hand. In Converse JM: Reconstructive plastic surgery, vol 4, Philadelphia, 1964, WB Saunders Co.
22. Littler JW and Li CS: Primary restoration of thumb opposition with median nerve decompression, Plast Reconstr Surg 39:74, 1967.
23. Mannerfelt LG: Tendon transfers in surgery of the rheumatoid hand, Hand Clin North Am 4:309, 1988.
24. Mayer L: The physiological method of tendon transplantation, Surg Gynecol Obstet 22:182, 1916.
25. Mayer L: The physiological method of tendon transplants renewed after forty years. In American Academy of Orthopaedic Surgeons: Instructional course lectures 12:116, Ann Arbor, Mich, 1955, JW Edwards Co.
26. Minkow FV: Operations to restore thumb opposition: an historical review. In AAOS symposium on tendon surgery in the hand, St Louis, 1975, The CV Mosby Co.
27. Moberg E: Current treatment program using tendon surgery in tetraplegia. In Hunter JM, Schneider LH, and Mackin EJ, editors: Tendon surgery in the hand, St Louis, 1987, The CV Mosby Co.
28. Nalebuff EA: Flexor tendon involvement in rheumatoid arthritis. In Hunter JM, Schneider LH, and Mackin EJ, editors: Tendon surgery in the hand, St Louis, 1987, The CV Mosby Co.
29. Omer GE: Evaluation and reconstruction of the forearm and hand after acute traumatic peripheral nerve injuries, J Bone Surg 50A:1454, 1968.
30. Omer GE: The technique and timing of tendon transfers, Orthop Clin North Am 5:243, 1974.
31. Riordan DC: Surgery of the paralytic hand. In American Academy of Orthopaedic Surgeons: Instructional course lectures 16:79, St Louis, 1959, The CV Mosby Co.
32. Rowntree T: Anomalous innervations of the hand muscles, J Bone Joint Surg 44:260, 1949.
33. Schneider LH: Opponensplasty using the extensor digiti minimi, J Bone Joint Surg 51-A:1297, 1969.
34. Schneider LH: Tendon transfers in muscle and tendon loss, Hand Clin North Am 4:267, 1988.
35. Schneider LH and Wehbe MA: Delayed repair of flexor profundus tendon in the palm (zone 3) with superficialis transfer, J Hand Surg 13-A:227, 1988.
36. Smith RJ: Tendon transfers of the hand and forearm, Boston, 1987, Little, Brown & Co.
37. Steindler A: Tendon transplantation in the upper extremity, Am J Surg 44:260, 1939.
38. Waterman JH: Tendon transplantation: its history, indications and technique, Med News 12:54, 1902.
39. White WL: Restoration of function and balance of the wrist and hand by tendon transfers, Surg Clin North Am 40:427, 1960.
40. Zancolli E: Structural and dynamic bases of hand surgery, Philadelphia, 1968, JB Lippincott Co.

52

Preoperative and postoperative management of tendon transfers after ulnar nerve injury

Judith A. Bell-Krotoski

THE ROLE OF THERAPY IN TENDON TRANSFER SURGERY

If surgical repairs were perfect and tissue healing occurred in predictable and precise order and timing, little might be required of therapists in the preoperative and postoperative management of tendon transfers. The surgeon would have only to concentrate on his surgical technique, and the patient would need only to cooperate with immobilization for the necessary healing period. In the imperfect world of reality, surgery is sometimes an art more than a science. Results of tendon transfers depend in large part on the deft hands of skilled surgeons, and anticipated healing can follow any course.

Results of surgery can be greatly enhanced either by the surgeon extending his fingers and becoming a therapist or by his developing a close interactive relationship with a therapist who works in concert with him and the patient. Therapy cannot improve every surgical case, and in some cases it is not needed or warranted in view of cost versus potential benefits. But therapy often can make the difference between a marginal result and a good one, and therapy intervention at appropriate points in patient treatment can ward off potential disasters. Although therapy may add significantly to surgical results, there are no cookbook recipes. Regardless of who assumes the role, the therapist must know specific guidelines and, even more important, must be able to determine when those guidelines apply and when exceptions are appropriate and safely made.

The first rule of therapists, as with surgeons, is to do no harm. The therapist is often in a position to augment or improve surgical results but is also in a position to affect adversely the surgical results. A therapist will never gain the confidence of the surgeon that is necessary to allow early and innovative hand therapy unless it is established that the therapist knows when to consult about problems and changes in treatment. The surgeon/therapist/patient interaction is different with different surgeons, and the treating therapist is well advised to exercise frequently the old adage "when in doubt, check it out."

When an interactive relationship is established between the surgeon and therapist (surgery and therapy), the background is set for a program of postoperative follow-up that is determined by the needs of the patient. In an uncomplicated postoperative period, for example, (1) there is absence of significant swelling or adhesion formation that could limit excursion of tendons and (2) new transfers can be identified and mobilized throughout most range of motion (ROM). The therapist's job is simplified to one of overseeing, pro-

tecting, and implementing the patient's return to hand function in a safe and timely manner.

Not all postoperative hand cases progress so smoothly, and the therapist frequently finds it necessary to become more aggressive in treatment and in implementation of treatment changes. If, for example, a patient is developing abnormal postoperative swelling, it immediately becomes necessary to monitor that swelling and implement remediation techniques.

Elevation of the surgical hand, patient education of the need to elevate the surgical hand, and a plan to check postoperative swelling exemplify the first type of protective/ educational therapy. The therapist's consulting the surgeon and releasing a constricting area of the cast or finding a way to ensure that a noncompliant patient will elevate the hand exemplify the second type, or interventive therapy. Both types of therapy are within the domain of the experienced hand therapist and are routine in the well-developed hand treatment clinic.

THERAPIST IN THE OPERATING ROOM

The importance of the therapist's understanding of the surgical procedure cannot be overstated. The therapist should know the specific muscle-tendon units transferred,[23,32,35,36] including their origin and insertion (normal and transferred insertions), through what route, to what surface, through what pulley (or other structure), and into what structure for attachment.[10,40] The site or level of tendon suture is also important. If tendon grafts are used, the donor tendon, type of graft, and site or level of attachment should be known also. The timing of the surgery or stage of surgery is important to the projection of expected results. Fortunately, this information is usually on the operative report in the patient's medical record. A copy of this report can be included in therapy records.

What is not readily available is subtle information not found in the medical chart. This information includes the surgeon's "feeling" about the success or failure of the surgery, his opinion of the appearance or feel of a tendon, the strength of the anastomosis, his intended tension for the tendon, or the potential he sees for a tendon scarring down or rupturing. These things can be gained only by communication between surgeon and therapist. To foster this communication, the therapist's initial presence in the operating room is advantageous. The therapist's observation of surgery, as normal and poor quality tendons are found, problems are encountered, solutions are worked out, alternate plans are made, and results are anticipated, gives the therapist an understanding difficult to obtain otherwise. For example, the therapist develops an understanding of how much force can safely be used in mobilizing a newly transferred tendon by watching the surgeon retract on the tendon in surgery to check the strength of the anastomosis.

Perhaps most important, the therapist's presence in the operating room gives the surgeon an appreciation of the depth of understanding of the surgical procedure the therapist is willing to seek. The therapist's presence provides opportunity for the surgeon to teach his specific techniques and idiosyncrasies to the therapist. The surgeon then views his therapist as "hand taught." This interaction pays tenfold as the surgeon entrusts to the therapist his cases, in all of whom he has made an investment, has ultimate responsibility, and has the highest hopes for success. The surgeon then appreciates and considers the therapist's comments and suggestions regarding possible surgical procedures, alternate ways of treatment, and new approaches.

Also, the therapist in the operating room has an opportunity to take photographs. Many therapists, while observing surgery, photograph difficult or unusual cases. The photographs are most appreciated after a particularly good result from a difficult case. They become invaluable records for teaching and training and in the monitoring of results from the surgery/therapy program.

TENDON TRANSFERS AS REBALANCING PROCEDURES

Bunnell[3] first described tendon transfers as "rebalancing procedures." Time has only added to the understanding of this approach. The hand is in a delicate but durable balance of flexors and extensors, stabilizers and positioners that quickly interchange in balance and on command for performing 72 operational tasks.[12] With few arguable exceptions, all of the muscles of the hand are needed for operational balance, and one cannot be transferred without having a direct biomechanical effect on others.[6,16,37,41] Thus tendon transfer surgery is the attempt to rebalance internally what has become imbalanced as a result of disease or injury that causes the loss of certain muscles in the system. Tendon transfers therefore must be considered within their functional relationship with other muscle-tendon units.[8]

The therapist can best appreciate and augment the balance that has been restored to a hand that has undergone tendon rebalancing surgery by seeing and measuring the hand before surgery. At that time, the hand exhibits its biomechanical imbalance in a number of ways that can be recorded and with which postoperative balance can be compared.

BIOMECHANICS OF DEFORMITY

In ulnar nerve injuries, the power grip functions of the hand are diminished or lost (the more so, the higher the level of injury). This loss compromises hand function.[11,24] Normally the ulnarmost two fingers, the ring and little, supply the power flexion aspect of the hand, whereas the most radial two fingers, the index and middle, are freed for manipulation with the thumb. When the power function of the ulnar two fingers is lost because of nerve injury, the radial two fingers must assume this function on hand grasp, and freedom for manipulation during grasp is lost. Power grasp is further weakened by the selective loss of intrinsic muscles of the thumb and hypothenar eminence, reducing

hand grasp and the thumb's mechanical stabilization against the fingers during hand use. The lack of intrinsic stabilization of the hypothenar muscles leads to a flattened or reversed metacarpal arch, changing the whole structural arrangement of the thumb and the fourth, and fifth metacarpals, which normally rotate around the keystone second, and third metacarpals during grasp.

Low nerve injury

Fingers. Power grip is specifically diminished in low nerve injuries by the inability of the fingers (most ulnar two and sometimes middle and index) to assume lumbrical positions and gradations of lumbrical positions. The fingers biomechanically collapse on attempts at extension and flexion.[13,17] On attempts at finger extension, the MP joints that have lost their intrinsic support in flexion hyperextend by unopposed overpull of the extrinsic finger extensor (extensor digitorum communis), mechanically limiting full gliding and extension of the dorsal hood and thus full extension of the fingers at the interphalangeal joints[22] (Fig. 52-1). In cases where the PIP joints can fully extend, they do not until the MP joints are fully extended.[19] On patient attempts at finger flexion, the absence of the intrinsics as primary flexors at the MP joint and extenders on the opposite surface at the interphalangeal finger joint results in the unopposed out-of-sequence overpull of the extrinsic finger flexors (flexor superficialis and flexor digitorum profundus) into flexion. The DIP and PIP joints must fully flex before excursion of the extrinsic finger flexors can flex the MP joints.

The intrinsic muscles then supply the balance to the flexor and extensor systems, without which the fingers lose their selective positioning and support in selective positions. The power that would normally be available from the extrinsic

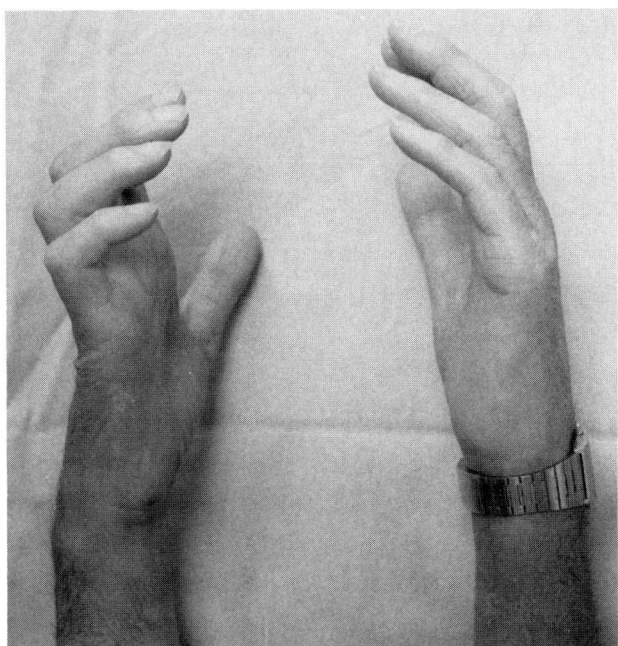

Fig. 52-1 Patient with bilateral nerve loss. Hand on the left is uncorrected; hand on the right has been surgically corrected by intrinsic replacement transfers. Intrinsic muscles of the hand supply balance to the finger flexor and extensor systems, without which the fingers collapse on use.

finger flexors and extensors is lost, because their power is wasted either fully flexing or fully extending their specific finger joints, beginning with the points of their insertions; there is no in-between. This imbalance and collapse of the fingers is seen as the fingers attempt to assume full flexion, extension, and lumbrical positions. The collapse is demonstrated even more markedly by any load that is applied to the fingers, such as when the patient attempts to pick up objects. Objects cannot be held by the involved fingers unless the fingers are fully flexed at the interphalangeal joints (to the size limits of the object).

Although the median nerve usually innervates the lumbricals to the radial two fingers, the index and middle, and the ulnar nerve innervates the dorsal and palmar interossei to all the fingers, there can be overlap of intrinsic innervation between the ulnar and median nerve. The ulnar nerve sometimes innervates all of the intrinsic muscles to the index and middle fingers. The variations in ulnar nerve innervation must be considered in tendon transfer rebalancing. If the intrinsics to the index and middle fingers are only partially innervated or are only weak versus absent, these fingers may not show as much imbalance as the ulnar two fingers and may sometimes be considered normal. The fingers may appear normal only until loaded with external force, such as when the patient begins to pick up a moderately heavy object. It is important that the fingers be loaded with some force resistance for testing. They can be tested in the lumbrical position with resistance at the proximal phalanx. If

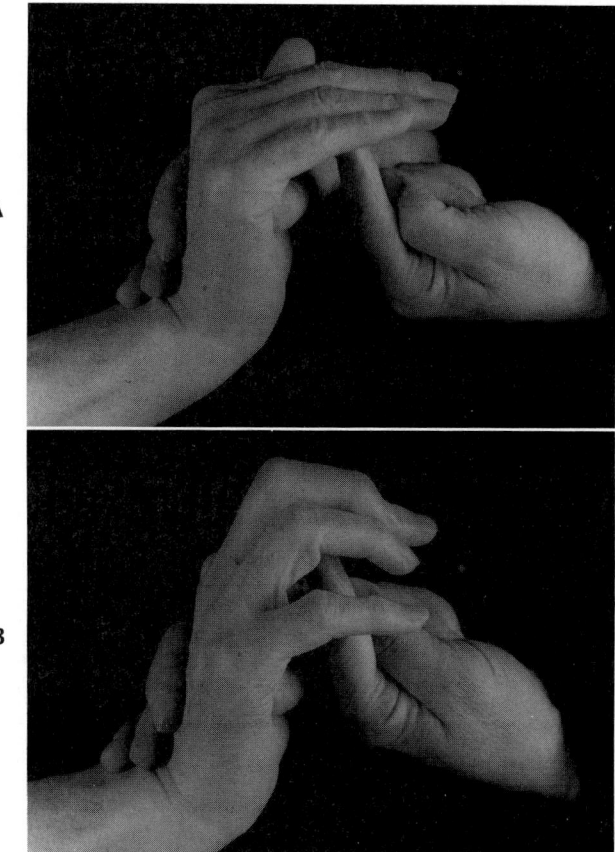

Fig. 52-2 **A,** Intrinsic balance of fingers may appear normal and the patient able to assume a lumbrical position, until loaded with external force. **B,** If the fingers collapse on resistance, they are imbalanced.

they collapse with resistance, as in Fig. 52-2, they too are imbalanced for hand use and should be included in surgical rebalancing procedures.

The hypothenar muscle mass, and in particular the opponens digiti quinti, flexes, stabilizes, and brings into opposition the fourth and fifth metacarpals and ulnar two fingers and, with the thumb, enable the hand to cup the palm securely and grasp around objects. Loss of the intrinsic hypothenar muscles and resultant flattened or reversed metacarpal arch disrupts the grasping and securing power functions of the hand, leaving the patient to experience weakness and clumsiness in handling large objects.

As indicated, the amount of imbalance is sometimes deceptive and can be hidden; that is, some hands with intrinsic losses from nerve injuries may appear "not to claw enough to warrant surgery." Surgery may not be indicated when cosmesis of the hand is the major consideration or in a few instances when the structure of the hand permits the patient to compensate without deforming imbalance. Biomechanically, the ulnar nerve–injured hand is imbalanced and greatly limited in function in the described ways. Even when cosmesis is the major concern, the appearance of the hand may be deceptive, as the imbalance usually becomes more exaggerated over time. Thus appearance of the hand worsens over time, and cosmetic improvement is more difficult.

In the imbalanced hand caused by ulnar nerve weakness or loss, remodeling of the skin and joints usually occurs as the hand is used in abnormal patterns with abnormal forces. The MP joints lose their soft tissue retention and overstretch into hyperextension, sometimes even rupturing volar plates and elongating other soft tissue restraints at this joint by the enormous overpower of the imbalanced extrinsic finger extensor as the patient tries unsuccessfully to fully extend his or her fingers. As the interphalangeal joints remodel, the skin over their dorsal surface grows, whereas skin is lost on the volar surface. Joint stiffness occurs when the joints do not operate in their full range of motion. The extensor tendons eventually become attenuated. All in all, the imbalance is progressive into deformity,[5] and when these changes have occurred, tendon transfer–surgery results are progressively compromised. The amount the surgery is compromised is directly proportional to the extent and duration of secondary changes and tissue remodeling. Tendon transfer surgery therefore is best done while the hands appear not to claw enough to warrant surgery, before secondary remodeling changes have become established and worsened.

Remodeling and progressive deformity take time but are accelerated by the force with which the patient uses the hand and the patient's lack of passive extension of the involved joints. Abnormal forces on joints can add to or cause joint stiffness. The muscle imbalance that occurs when the fingers collapse into flexion causes abnormal force concentrated at the tips of the involved fingers and distal palm as the hand grips and manipulates objects in abnormal positions. In addition to soft tissue damage caused by excessive concentration of force, abnormal forces on joints can add to or cause joint stiffness and cause joint structural damage.[4,38]

Remodeling and progressive deformity are also accelerated by reduced or absent sensory feedback. The sensory portion of the ulnar nerve is often involved if the motor portion is involved. If the sensory portion of the nerve is compromised in addition to the motor part of the ulnar nerve, the patient has lost his feedback system of how much force he is using with his fingers, and enormous force can be concentrated in small areas of skin, such as at the tips of the fingers. The skin was never intended to be subjected to such force on a repetitive basis,[26,39] and the result is injury, scarring, and callus formation, with compromised skin nutrition. In imbalanced hands that are heavily used, bony and soft tissue reabsorption can occur, leading to deformity and shortening of the fingers.

Disuse of the hand does not prevent deformity. Remodeling of the hand will occur in the biomechanically imbalanced hand that is used or in one that is not. In some cases, the greatest tendon attenuation, skin contractures, and joint stiffness will occur in the hand that is not used in preference to a good "other" extremity. This is because some mechanical stress (force × area) on the skin in moderate amounts, as produced in a balanced hand, is normal and is beneficial in maintaining healthy skin. Skin of hands that either can not be or are not used becomes thin and shiny and tears easily. Joints that are not used lose their normal synovial gliding surfaces.[34]

Attenuation of the finger extensor tendons from remodeling can be shown by the examiner fully flexing the patient's MP joints, blocking these in flexion, and asking the patient to extend the interphalangeal joints with the extrinsic finger extensor (extensor digitorum communis) (Fig. 52-3). The intrinsic-minus hand with no tendon attenuation can extend the interphalangeal joints fully when the MP joints are flexed, because the extrinsic finger extensor is positioned where it can extend the interphalangeal joints. If extension of the joints is limited or absent (and the joints will otherwise passively extend), attenuation of the extensor tendons is probable. In checking for attenuation, one must ascertain that the extrinsic extensor has the strength to extend the fingers; for example, no radial nerve involvement is present.

Another remodeling problem can limit or reduce active extension of the interphalangeal joints. Once a hand has been positioned and used in an intrinsic-minus position, that is, "claw hand position," the short extrinsic flexor (flexor digitorum superficialis) muscle-tendon units often become shortened through loss of muscle sarcomeres. The short extrinsic flexor tends to become shortened more than the long extrinsic flexor (flexor digitorum profundus) because of the usually more severe flexion contracture of the fingers at the PIP joint. The long extrinsic flexor can contract also. The initiating cause is the intrinsic-minus imbalance: the muscle-tendon units of the extrinsic flexors respond by readjusting to their reduced tension requirement when the fingers are maintained in a claw position.[27] This contracture can be checked by first passively extending the fingers fully with the wrist flexed, then passively extending the fingers fully with the wrist in extension. Tightness of the extrinsic superficialis will limit the full passive or active extension of the interphalangeal joints with the wrist in extension much more than with the wrist in flexion.

Thumb. The thumb in the ulnar nerve–injured hand similarly becomes imbalanced. In the low ulnar nerve injury, some of the intrinsics of the thumb are disrupted, whereas the extrinsic muscles acting on the thumb remain intact. Usually lost are the lateral half of the intrinsic flexor of the thumb (flexor pollicis brevis), the first dorsal interosseous, and the adductor (adductor pollicis brevis). Some overlap of innervation with the median nerve can occur, particularly in an anatomic Martin-Gruber anastomosis of the nerves.[9] Any disruption of a muscle around the thumb or finger metacarpals causes an instability (flexible torque tube of Agee[1]). The thumb, unlike the fingers, which can be supported by each other, must operate in space by itself.[20] The partial weakness or loss of the thumb intrinsics in the ulnar injured hand causes a collapsing instability of the thumb and a weakened pinch in normal positions (Fig. 52-4).

Without all or part of the intrinsic flexor of the thumb (flexor pollicis brevis), its stabilization, and the stabilization provided by the adductor at the thumb MP joint, the extrinsic flexor (flexor pollicis longus) overpulls into hyperflexion at the interphalangeal joint, as in Fig. 52-5 (Froment's sign).[5] As with the fingers, the thumb must fully flex before full strength of the extrinsic flexor can be used to pick up objects.

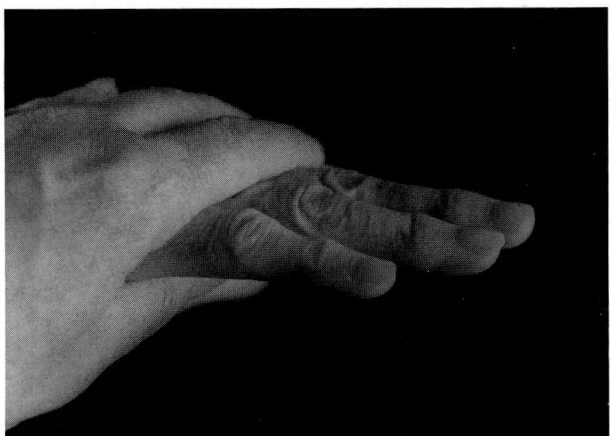

Fig. 52-3 Unless the extensor tendons are attenuated, the ulnar nerve–injured fingers should extend fully at the interphalangeal joint by the extrinsic finger extensor (extensor digitorum communis), when the metacarpophalangeal joint is supported in flexion or kept from hyperextending.

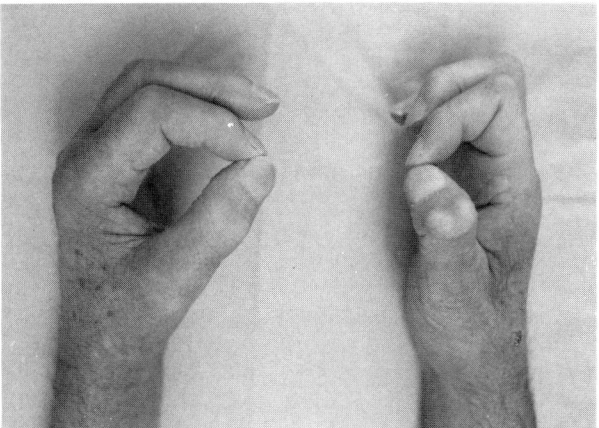

Fig. 52-4 Partial weakness or loss of thumb intrinsic muscles in the ulnar nerve–injured hand also results in a collapsing instability and weakened pinch in normal positions. Hand on the left has been surgically corrected by a ring superficialis transfer to the thumb; on the right, contralateral hand with ulnar nerve injury is uncorrected.

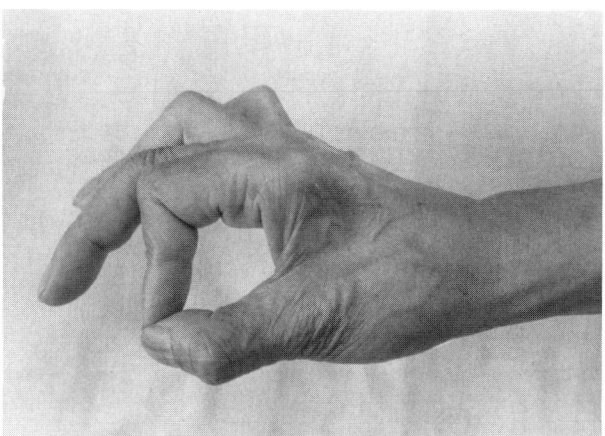

Fig. 52-5 Froment's sign. When used in this position, the thumb must flex at the interphalangeal joint before the strength of the extrinsic flexor (flexor pollicis longus) can be used to pick up objects. The skin and tendons at the interphalangeal joint eventually become attenuated. Note hyperextension of index distal interphalangeal in thumb pinch.

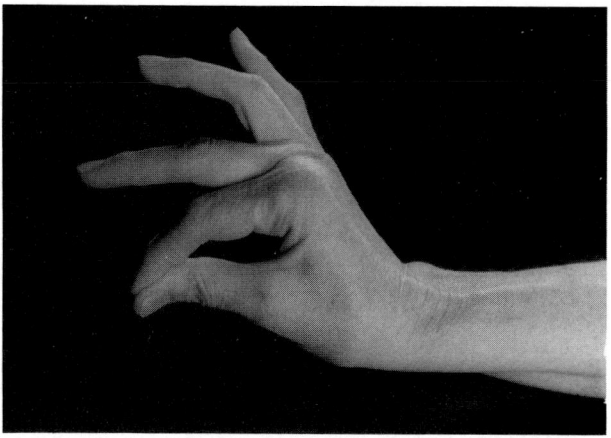

Fig. 52-6 Reverse Froment's sign. The patient attempts to stabilize the thumb by extending the thumb interphalangeal joint, positioning the thumb so the force of the index finger will fully extend the interphalangeal joint and fully flex the metacarpophalangeal joint. In addition to loss of selective thumb positioning except at extremes of joint range, excessive stress produced in joints can be deforming.

Thus the thumb, when used, collapses into flexion.

The patient may attempt to stabilize the thumb also by extending the thumb interphalangeal joint (positioning the thumb so the force of the index against the thumb on pinch will fully extend the thumb interphalangeal joint) and flexing the MP joint as in Fig. 52-6 (reverse Froment's sign).[5] In this case the patient uses the soft tissue restraint of the dorsal MP joint to block further flexion and the volar interphalangeal joint to block further interphalangeal joint extension.

Either way the thumb is used, it is unstable and usually progresses into deformity as the soft tissue restraints tend to remodel and elongate from excessive stress. Abnormal excessive force, which can be deforming, is concentrated in the MP and interphalangeal joints of the thumb and at the tip of the thumb. Secondary joint stiffness and contracture are common, particularly in flexion of the thumb at the interphalangeal joint.

Mechanically, because the thumb must operate by itself in space unsupported by any other digit, it depends on at least three muscles in proper alignment to support its position. To translate directional force across joints, it depends on at least one muscle to hold a joint position and another muscle to supply force in that position. The extrinsic and intrinsic muscles position the thumb. Then the intrinsic muscles supply the power to hold that position for force to be translated by the extrinsic muscles for use. (The whole system is like a fishing rod: the wrist holding the rod is supplying the intrinsic power to stabilize the line, and the winding of the reel is supplying the extrinsic power to bring in the fish. If the intrinsic wrist support is lost, so is the extrinsic power. The hand that was supplying the external power by winding the reel must now support and stabilize the rod, thus the reel cannot be wound.)

The loss of the first dorsal interosseous muscle adds an additional problem to the thumb and also to the index finger, because this muscle is in large part responsible for stabilizing the thumb metacarpal and providing stability for lateral pinch against the index. One head of the muscle originates from the thumb metacarpal and inserts on the base of the index proximal phalanx, and one head originates from the index metacarpal and inserts on the base of the index proximal phalanx. Both provide adduction of the index against the thumb and index stability against ulnar rotation. The first dorsal interosseous has a larger tension fraction than most of the flexor profundus and flexor superficialis muscles.[5] Without this muscle, the thumb loses stability against the index finger, and with the additional adductor muscle loss, the thumb and index tend to rotate in opposite directions on pinch, further adding to instability of the thumb and pinch.

The patient may substitute for loss of the adductor and first dorsal interosseous by pinching to the radial side of the thumb, using the restraints of the thumb radial collateral ligaments (MP and interphalangeal) and the thumb web to limit abduction and external rotation of the thumb. (The extensor pollicis longus muscle also has a small moment for adduction at the MP joint and a large moment for adduction of the metacarpal, but this is combined with external rotation of the thumb.[5]) The ligamentous soft tissue restraints can be abnormally stressed by lack of their normal muscle support. The radial collateral ligament at the MP joint is the most frequently deformed by excessive force. Once this has begun and remains uncorrected, a "crank action thumb" can result[5] and is similar to the mechanics of any mechanical crank, in that any further pinch (force) at the tip or side of the thumb rotates its entire length into external rotation as in Fig. 52-7.

Occasionally the web of the thumb will increase, either with or without the crank action thumb, to the point where any pinch is ineffective, because the index can no longer meet against any restraint of the thumb. Alternatively, the patient may use his extensor pollicis longus to adduct and externally rotate the thumb where it can be used for pinch on the back of the index finger. In Fig. 52-8, thumb abduction, extension, and external rotation moments of the extensor pollicis longus are shown.

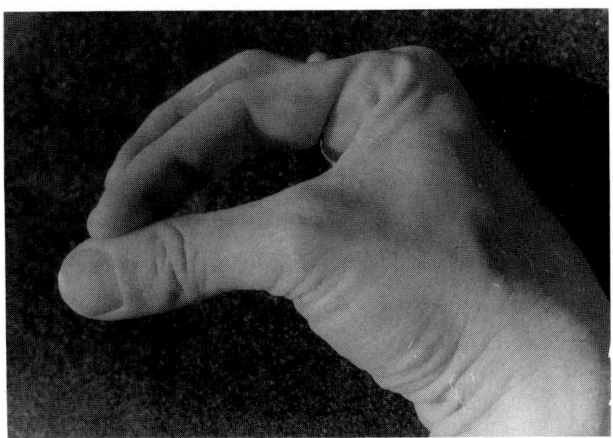

Fig. 52-7 Crank-action thumb. The patient pinches the thumb from the radial side and uses the limits of soft tissue restraints to stabilize the thumb in pinch. Once the radial collateral ligaments have become deformed by excessive stress, or the thumb joints are used in flexion, any additional external force on the tip of the thumb rotates the thumb and progressively increases the deformity.

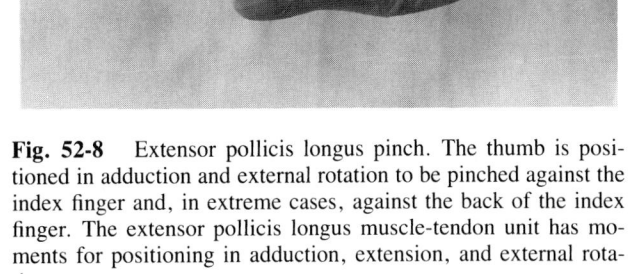

Fig. 52-8 Extensor pollicis longus pinch. The thumb is positioned in adduction and external rotation to be pinched against the index finger and, in extreme cases, against the back of the index finger. The extensor pollicis longus muscle-tendon unit has moments for positioning in adduction, extension, and external rotation.

The patient may attempt to substitute for the first dorsal interosseous at the index finger and stabilize index ulnar rotation on pinch against the thumb by hyperextending the index DIP joint, thus supporting this finger by bracing it along the side of the other fingers. This abnormal positioning of the joint to translate force for prehension also causes progressive deformity in that the DIP extension tends to increase over time. In Fig. 52-4, hyperextension of the index can be seen as the patient pinches against the thumb.

These considerations make it clear that if the hand is to be functional and useful, tendon transfer surgery to rebalance the hand is not a luxury but a necessity, and tendon transfer surgery, although not an emergency, should be planned early before joint stiffness and remodeling occur.

High nerve injury

A high ulnar nerve injury takes the same course as the low ulnar nerve injury in intrinsic muscle involvement and imbalance. In addition to the long extrinsic finger flexor (flexor digitorum profundus) to the little finger, usually the ring is involved (and sometimes other fingers) as well as the ulnar wrist flexor (flexor carpi ulnaris).

As in the low nerve injuries, if the hand is not used, the skin becomes thin, shiny, or macerated where joints are contracted and can tear easily. If the hand is used, the skin becomes thickened and callused anywhere it must assume abnormal contact pressure stemming from mechanically imbalanced muscle-tendon units on use. In Fig. 52-9, callus can be seen on the ring finger of a patient who has lost the flexor digitorum profundus and the ulnar intrinsic muscles. The area of pressure results from the unaided use of the flexor digitorum superficialis. The distal tip of the finger is unable to flex because of the loss of the flexor digitorum profundus. The area of skin taking the pressure on hand use was never intended to sustain such repetitive pressure, and it will probably break down with continual use. The problem in this case can be corrected by suture of the profundus tendon of the little finger to the profundus tendon of the

middle finger, which has a working flexor digitorum profundus muscle-tendon unit.[5]

In high ulnar nerve injury, the patient has even less finger function for power grip than in the low nerve injury and cannot support the wrist in flexion on the ulnar side. The flexor carpi ulnaris is a powerful muscle and is the strongest muscle that crosses the wrist. Its loss to hand function greatly limits use of the hand, because architecturally the more proximal wrist needs stability for force to be translated to the digits.

OBJECTIVE MEASUREMENT AND PREOPERATIVE TREATMENT
Need for objective measurement

Objective measurements that quantify the type and extent of involvement and imbalance are important in preoperative and postoperative records. In this way, changes by surgery

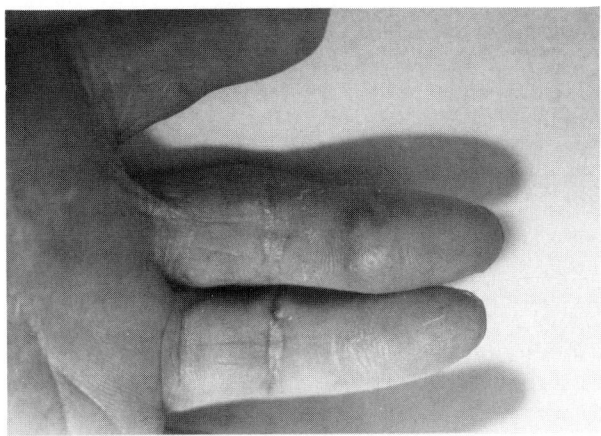

Fig. 52-9 Callus on the ring finger of a patient who has lost the flexor digitorum profundus in a high-ulnar injury. The area of callus results from the use of the short extrinsic flexor in the absence of the long extrinsic flexor.

and changes by therapy can be demonstrated and documented. Adjustments can be made that will improve the overall surgical and therapeutic program.

The postoperative treatment can be dictated by the preoperative measurements. For example, if a hand is hypermobile, a reversing of the metacarpal arch can be much more of a problem after tendon transfers. A wrist extensor transferred in a Brand many-tailed procedure[5] to flex the MP joint and extend the interphalangeal joint of the fingers may unavoidably become an active extender of the fifth metacarpal and lose any ability to function effectively, as intended at the other joints. For such a hypermobile hand, the time the hand is casted or splinted to support the metacarpal arch and the time of limitation of full extension of the metacarpal joints may be extended several weeks. As an alternative, an additional transfer may be included in the surgical rebalancing plan to stabilize the fifth metacarpal in supination, such as a transfer of the extensor digiti minimi in a radial route to the fifth metacarpal.[31]

Need for preoperative treatment

Preoperative recommendations can be made at the time of measurement for therapy that can upgrade the hand status before surgery and increase the chance for success postoperatively. The most obvious treatment indicated is cylinder casting of interphalangeal joints to reduce contractures and mobilize these joints before surgery. Joint contractures that remain uncorrected before surgery can seriously compromise surgical results by mechanically limiting joint extension and reducing intended tension of transferred tendons. If one interphalangeal joint is stiff and the others supple, tendon transfers from the same motor to all fingers can result in the excursion of the transfer taken up differentially by different fingers. Most of the transferred tendon excursion can be taken up by the finger with a stiff joint, rendering ineffective the transfer slips to the other joints.[5]

Any scar decreases the chances of mobility for small joints, and because excessive or unwanted scar formation after tendon transfer is already a potential problem, surgical correction for joint contractures before tendon transfers is usually contraindicated if the contractures can be reduced in any other way. (An exception is when correction cannot be achieved by therapy, such as a superficialis "check-rein" contracture that has developed at the scarred ends from where the superficialis tendon slips have been transferred. Once this contracture has become longstanding, no or little improvement in joint angle is achieved with progressive increases in force, and contracture remodeling attempts usually fail.)

Other therapy may be indicated if it can improve the presurgical hand and increase possibilities of successful surgical outcome. Contracted web spaces may respond to massage and serial splinting. Stiff fingers may be exercised to reduce the amount of viscoelastic tissue resistance they will give to newly transferred tendons. Contracted scar tissue may be softened and relaxed by gentle massage and positive-pressure bandaging and splinting. Mobilization and strengthening of the intended transfers may be desirable before surgery, especially when the donor muscle for tendon transfers has had limited or no use.

A not so obvious recommendation for therapy before tendon transfer surgery is correction of a hand that has developed superficialis tightness (flexor digitorum superficialis). Failures have been encountered in tendon transfer surgeries where these muscle-tendon units have been tight, because the tension provided by intrinsic transfers to the fingers to flex the MP joints and extend the interphalangeal joints is rendered ineffective by the abnormal flexion tension on the interphalangeal joints by the superficialis muscle-tendon units.

The amount of superficialis tightness can be deceiving, because the fingers often will extend fully when the wrist is in degrees of flexion. The extent of tightness is often made apparent by a patient's intolerance to attempts to correct the tightness by splinting the wrist in neutral and fingers fully extended. If the splint is left on overnight, patients insist on removing the splint or, in the presence of insensitivity, develop distal fingertip skin blisters. Therapists find they must begin by splinting the fingers in extension with the wrist in some flexion or by cylinder casting the interphalangeal joints and gradually including the wrist. Gradually, about every other day, the splint can be remolded progressively into extension, as the hand remodels and allows more extension of the muscle-tendon units. It is important to realize that superficialis tightness cannot be corrected after surgery by therapy, because the necessary position to reduce the superficialis tightness is the exact position to affect adversely the desired tension of the new intrinsic transfers.

Another serious consideration is the tendon transfer selection in a hand with superficialis tightness. If a superficialis tendon is transferred from the ring or middle finger to the thumb and the remaining superficialis muscle-tendon units are tight, a marked finger imbalance can occur. The fingers will flex out of phase with the donor finger lagging behind. If the interphalangeal joint from the donor tendon is in any way hypermobile, the reduced tension at the volar interphalangeal joint results in the finger hyperextending on extension while the other finger interphalangeal joints remain in flexion. If intrinsic transfers are made to the fingers the out-of-phase extension of the donor tendon becomes exaggerated and can become progressively deformed in hyperextenson. Therapy can do little or nothing to assist or correct this amount of imbalance after surgery, and further corrective surgery is needed. With care, this problem can be handled by reducing the muscle-tendon unit contractures before surgery or perhaps by routing the intrinsic transfers to all except the sublimis donor finger. This will increase interphalangeal extension tension at the other fingers to counterbalance the flexor muscle-tendon tightness and will result in less extension tension translated to the extension of the donor finger.

The profundus muscle-tendon units may also become shortened, and when this is combined with superficialis tightness, it is sometimes hard to tell how much is profundus and how much is superficialis. The profundus also can affect the tendon transfer tension but is not as critical to the individual finger balance, because it is not usually a donor for transfer. The profundus responds to preoperative remodeling therapy.

Psychologic aspects of therapy are sometimes important in the successful outcome of surgery. It is necessary to enlist a patient's trust and cooperation with the specific and timely follow-up program to mobilize his tendon transfers and minimize complications. The patient is more trusting of a therapist who sees his hand before surgery, because he sees this therapist as one he knows and one who is familiar with his hand and particular problems.

A therapist who sees a hand before surgery thus has opportunities to augment and improve the postoperative treatment. If possible, the therapist should at least "see" the hand. Therapists can work with patients who have had hand surgery, referred postoperatively, but often not as effectively or without guesswork. There is benefit to the therapist's first becoming familiar with the patient, his hand, and the extent of mechanical imbalance that the surgeon is attempting to improve. Therapists often attend, refer to, or are available for medical/surgical hand clinics to make therapy recommendations and become familiar with planned surgical cases.

Where to begin

When the patient is first seen for objective measurements, his proposed surgery can be reviewed with him and it can be made certain that he understands what outcome is expected from surgery. Any misconceptions are best resolved at this point. Often patients feel confined and pressed for time in surgical clinic situations. They later explain to the therapist considerations that may affect their surgical and rehabilitation plans, such as a death in the family or a need to return to work in a time frame that is insufficient for follow-up care such as therapy. Most surgeons appreciate feedback about patient problems.

The patient is told by surgeon and therapist what he should anticipate as a result of the surgery and that, although the surgeon has had much experience, surgery is different in each case and is not 100% predictable. He is told the length of time for immobilization, the anticipated length of time for therapy if no complications develop, and the length of time that might be necessary if problems develop, such as infection or tendon adhesions. Possible complications are explained from the standpoint that they usually do not occur or are normally anticipated and routinely handled. It is explained that if complications occur, the team is prepared to resolve them early, so that they are minimized and results maximized. In this way the patient develops the understanding that although surgery is not always 100% successful, every effort is made for him, and that he will be watched and counseled through the surgery to maximize his benefit. This helps minimize his fear of pain and surprises. Sometimes the patient's greatest discomfort comes from (1) fear of the unknown, (2) concern that having surgery is not in his best interest, or (3) that he will be in a dependent role without assistance.

History taking and initial examination

During the history intake, the therapist has opportunity to observe the patient's use of hands while he or she is not under obvious scrutiny. Much of the examination can be accomplished while shaking the patient's hand, asking for a signature, and watching the patient remove a piece of paper from a wallet or purse to take notes. A functional observation of the patient using the hand sometimes is better made in this way before focus is turned to the hands.

The therapist first specifically examines the hand by noting anything abnormal. Often the patient has a normal

"other" extremity with which range of motion and general appearance of the hand can be compared. All skin contractures, joint contractures, wounds, scars, and general condition of the skin should be noted. These can be recorded easily on a form that has a drawing of the hands to point out locations and problems (Fig. 52-10).

Previous surgeries and dates should be recorded briefly for easy reference, or copies of operative reports and referrals can be attached to therapy forms.

Routine measurements

A voluntary muscle examination is performed using standard muscle grading procedures, noting absences and weaknesses. Particular attention is given to muscles found in specific nerve groups—ulnar, median, and radial—so the extent of nerve involvement is well recognized. Often nerve problems are bilateral and can involve more than one nerve.

A sensory examination is performed using standard measurement technique. Sensory function is measured with regard to function of different nerve groups (ulnar, median, and radial). Screening or mapping with Semmes-Weinstein monofilaments is recommended (see Chapter 43) and at least one other sensory examination. For example, two-point discrimination testing can be done also, because this test is often used for reporting sensory status in the literature. More than one test of sensibility often can provide a better picture of the patient's overall neural status than only a single one.

Special measurements

ROM measurements for the nerve-injured hand require special attention. Particular attention is given the extension of the interphalangeal joints with flexion of the MP joints. The patient is asked to assume a lumbrical position (MP joints flexed and interphalangeal joints extended) as in Fig. 52-2, A. In this position, measurements are taken for joint passive, active, and active-assistive extension angles at the interphalangeal joints. For the active-assistive joint angles, the examiner flexes the MP joint for the patient and blocks extension of this joint while allowing extension of the interphalangeal joints as in Fig. 52-3. The difference between this measurement and the passive joint measurement determines the amount of extension lag that would be present at the interphalangeal joint were intrinsic replacement surgery done. (Unless attenuated, the extensor digitorum communis will fully extend the interphalangeal joints of the fingers in this position, provided the joint is not limited by stiffness, volar skin contracture, or muscle-tendon unit contracture.)

Because the joint angle measurements of the fingers may change when the hand is placed in different wrist positions, the extension measurements at the interphalangeal joints are taken first with the wrist in 45 degrees of extension, then again with the wrist in 45 degrees of flexion. The difference in these two measurements represents the limitation introduced by the extrinsic muscle-tendon units. If extrinsic tightness is present, a difference in the measurements with wrist flexion and extension will occur. Interphalangeal joint extension measurements are taken with the MP joints in neutral position.

Torque range of motion has been described by Brand[2] and is used in some hand treatment programs to objectively assess the balance of joint and muscle-tendon tension before and after tendon transfers. It is particularly useful in as-

HAND SURGERY ASSESSMENT—PREOPERATIVE

Date_____   Patient no._____
Hand: Right or Left   Hand dominance_____
Name_____Birth date_____Sex_____
HD class_____Date dx'd_____Physician_____
Occupation_____Last time reaction/Neuritis_____
Condition of other hand_____
Other information_____

A. Related Problems

Arch reversal angle_____					Superficial tightness	I ____	M ____	R ____	L ____
Scar/callous	I	M	R	L	Cont ret lig	I	M	R	L
Bone absorption	I	M	R	L	PIP Hyperextension	I	M	R	L
Guttered ext mech	I	M	R	L	Attenuated ext mech	I	M	R	L

Sensory loss: Median_____ Ulnar_____ Radial_____
    (3.61 MN [.21 g] or below)
Wrist flexion pattern (describe)_____

B. Muscle Status (5-4-3-2-1)

	Right	Left		Right	Left		Right	Left		Right	Left
ADM			APB			FDS M/R	/	/	ECRL-B		
1st DI			OP			FCR			EPL		
Intr pos I/M	/	/	FPB			FCU			ECU		
Intr pos R/L	/	/	FPL			Pr T			Br Rad		
FDP R/L	/	/				PL					

C. Grip & Pinch

Grip strength	Jamar	Right	Left		Pinch strength	Right	Left
Level_____	A	/	/		Pulp to pulp		
Level_____	B	/	/		Key (lat)		
Level_____	C	/	/		Three-point		
Level_____	D	/	/				
Level_____	E	/	/				

Describe: Grip_____Pinch_____

Finger closure sequence_____

Grip contact holding cylinder   Th   I   M   R   L = T

	Th	I	M	R	L	T
1						
2						
3						

Comments_____

D. Preoperative therapy

Hand exercise _____weeks   Casting_____weeks   Overall duration_____weeks

Type: Wound care   Casting   Splinting
      I M R L   I M R L   I M R L

Fig. 52-10 Sample surgical evaluation form.

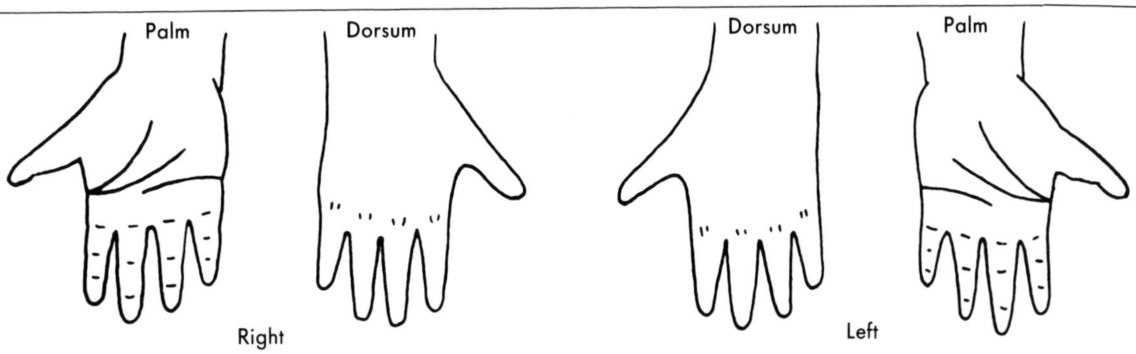

Palm   Dorsum   Dorsum   Palm

Right   Left

E. ROM Measurements

Pretherapy: Date_____

	Right					Left				
	I	M	R	L	Th	I	M	R	L	Th
MP ext/flex										
PIP Extension Active/MP flexed (intrinsic plus)										
Active-Assistive										
Passive										

Thumb web_____   _____

Comments _____

Preoperative: Date_____

	Right					Left				
	I	M	R	L	Th	I	M	R	L	Th
MP ext/flex										
PIP Extension Active/MP flexed (intrinsic plus)										
Active-Assistive										
Passive										

Thumb web_____   _____

F. Functional Assessment

Jebsen Hand Function Test Results: (Normal/Abnormal)_____

G. Other Assessment Information (Y/N)

Torque range of motion_____
Loading of fingers_____
Photographs, video tapes_____
Sphygomanometer_____
Nerve Conduction Tests_____
Harris Mat_____

Comments _____
_____
_____

_____
                                    Therapist

sessing the amount of flexor digitorum superficialis tightness when present. The torque (force × distance from the joint) necessary to achieve full interphalangeal joint extension with the wrist in 45 degrees extension and MP joints in neutral gives an understanding of the amount of resistance the tendon transfers must overcome to be successful. Torque measurements of the force necessary to extend MP joints before surgery give an understanding of the amount of tension that is provided by the transfers when measurements are repeated at the MP joint after surgery (Fig. 52-11). It is important that the therapist recognize the postoperative tension of transfers, because the therapist can optimize or reduce the tension as need be by the soft tissue mobilization or restricted mobilization around the tendon in the eary postoperative phase.

In the thumb the web space should be measured, because this often changes after ulnar nerve injury. The web often contracts or elongates. If contracted, the web greatly limits the grasp of the hand around objects. Thumb web space contractures can require special releases and/or grafts to restore function for successful tendon transfers. Range of motion of the thumb should include abduction out of the

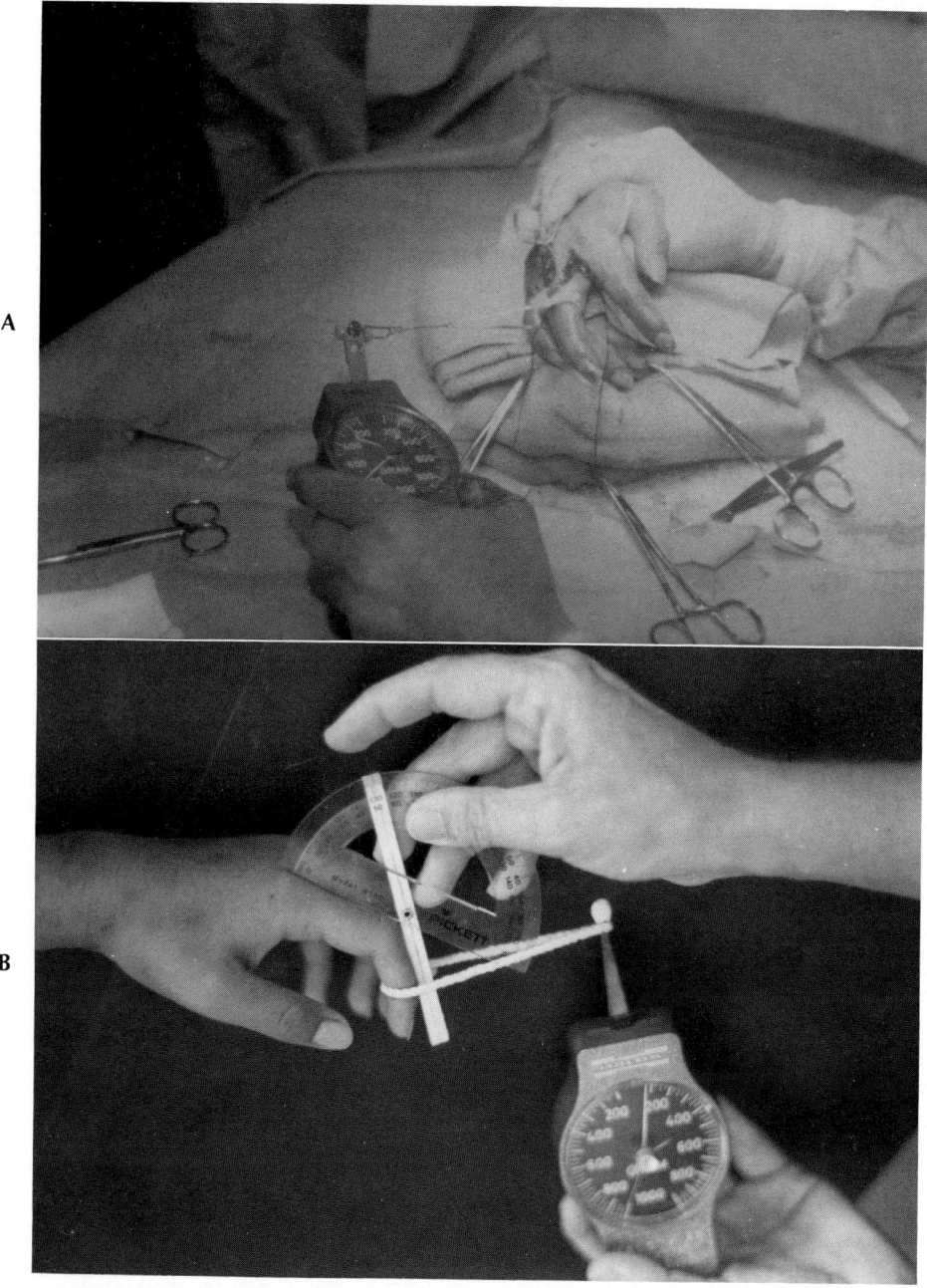

Fig. 52-11 Torque range of motion (TROM), described by Brand, can help assess objectively the balance of joint and muscle-tendon unit tension before and after tendon transfers. **A,** Surgeon measurement of passive resistance to metacarpophalangeal extension before and after tendon transfer surgery to assess transfer-tendon tension. **B,** Therapist measurement of resistance to finger interphalangeal joint extension before and after surgery (once resistance is possible) to assess superficialis tightness before and after surgery.

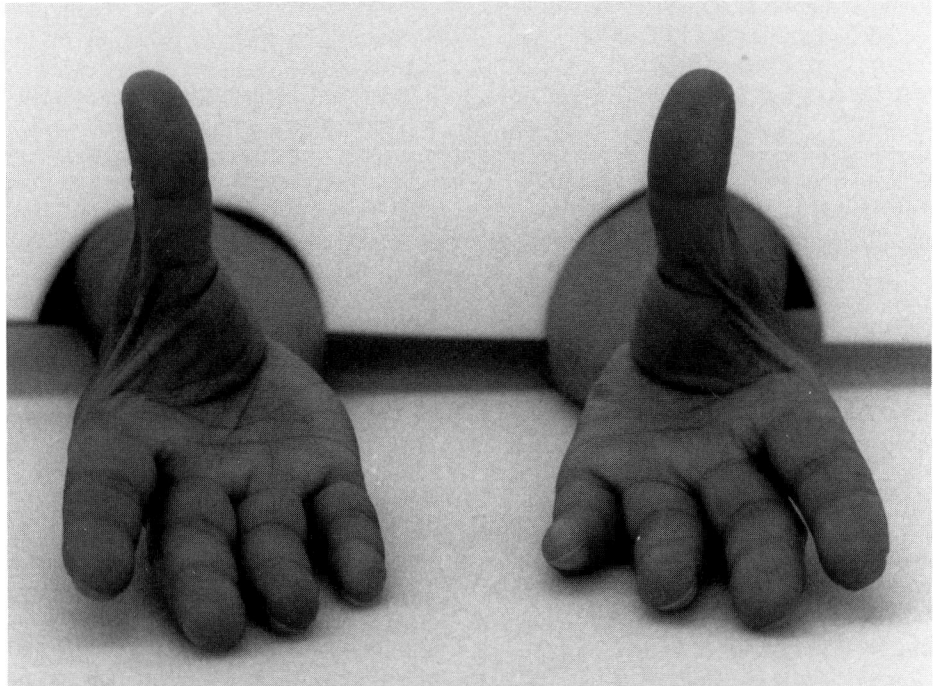

Fig. 52-12   Photographic view from fingertips taken with thumb in abduction and adduction to show muscle imbalance.

palm (Fig. 52-12) as well as active and passive flexion and extension angles of its joints. An active assistive measurement can be made of the interphalangeal joint of the thumb by the examiner's flexing and supporting the MP joint while the patient extends the interphalangeal joint.

From the measurements and examination above, specific problems should be noted if present including: superficialis tightness, Froment's sign, reverse Froment, ligament tightness, hypermobility, arch reversal, guttered extension mechanism (ulnarly decentralized extensor mechanism toward or into interosseous space), ligament laxity, attenuated extensor mechanism, bone absorption, bone deformity, pulley disruption, abnormal sequence of finger flexion/extension, collapse of lumbrical position on resistance at the proximal phalanx, and necessity of wrist to flex for successful finger extension.

Photographic positions

As indicated in the measurements above, the positioning of the fingers and joints is critical in producing the balance of the hand. For this reason photographic records of the most important positions are useful to augment the descriptive information. These photographs should reproduce the ROM measurement positions and should be repeated after surgical correction. The following positions are suggested:

I. Ulnar view (elbows on table)
   A. Lumbrical position
   B. Full finger extension
   C. Active-assistive extension (see Fig. 52-3)
   D. Full finger flexion
   E. Pinch
II. Radial view
   A. Tip pinch
     1. Soft

     2. Hard
   B. Key pinch
     1. Soft
     2. Hard
III. Front midline view (palm up)
   A. Thumb
     1. Adduction
     2. Abduction
     3. Pinch
       a. Index
       b. Middle
       c. Ring
       d. Little

Note in particular the front midline view taken from the fingertips (Fig. 52-12). This view allows record of thumb abduction and adduction. Other views as desired can be taken, but it is important to have standard views that are repeated for every patient.

Functional test

Many functional hand skill tests are available. The optimum functional test is one suited to the requirements of individual patients for work or leisure, because the real disability of the injury is a combination of its physical and psychologic impairment parameters. Most functional tests depend on elements that are repeatable for measurements of change. Of available tests, only a few are standardized,[14] leaving the therapist to select tests and test elements that are best suited to individual patients and programs.

For the ulnar nerve–injured hand, functional tests should include those that will otherwise demonstrate normal pinch, and grasp and release patterns. In this way, mechanical imbalances can be seen and measured in severity, and substitution patterns can be identified. The Moberg pickup test,[28] or a similar one, is a good beginning. This test was originally designed to demonstrate altered sensibility, but it is good for demonstrating prehension patterns of small objects, and the objects are commonly found in any clinic or office. The same series of objects can be used on all patients, and other small objects can be added to those available. How patients pick up the objects with thumb and fingers collectively and individually can be observed and timed. Omer has suggested adding soft chalk to the objects, because the chalk will rub off on the fingers and show contact areas.[29] Normally the fingers should not show any collapse, such as clawing of the fingers or thumb, when picking up the objects. Graded fishing weights (50 to 200 g) are important objects to add, because, often, imbalanced fingers will not collapse or show imbalance until loaded with some force. Small blocks attached to a board with velcro are helpful additions, because these give resistance to patients' fingers and thumb when they are pinched and lifted. The turning of a key in a lock or doorknob can demonstrate key pinch: first positional, as the patient picks up the key; then resistive, as the patient turns the key.

Clear plastic cylinders of three sizes (1½-, 2-, and 3-inch diameters) are useful to demonstrate abnormal grasp patterns. Because the normal fingers and thumb will make total contact on a cylinder, they can be graded as to which segments make contact on the test cylinders.[21] In the event of clawing of the ulnar two fingers and Froment's sign of the thumb, as often happens in ulnar nerve injuries, only the tips of the fingers and thumb will show contact on one or another of the cylinders.

Other large objects can be included to demonstrate gross grasp and manipulaton, such as turning the lid of a jar and picking up a glass one-handed. Writing a name with a pencil can be used to demonstrate dexterity.

Splinting

Splints can be used to restore balance externally for what has become imbalanced internally in the hand. If the hand is not to undergo surgery for a while, an intrinsic splint is recommended for the fingers to help prevent remodeling of tissue into deformity. Just as the examiner can allow the patient to fully extend the interphalangeal joints of an intrinsic-minus hand by flexing the MP joint, a splint can be made to support the MP joints in flexion. This splint is relatively difficult to fit without pressure points and must be checked carefully. The patient can use the strong power of the extrinsic extensor (extensor digitorum communis) to overcome the splint and can receive damaging pressure on the dorsum of the interphalangeal joints at the proximal phalanx. The patient should be taught to extend the fingers with only the minimum extension force necessary. If the patient has developed a pattern of dropping the wrist to achieve finger extension, this problem should be corrected either by instruction or splint immobilization.

The splint should always be padded where it supplies a "lumbrical bar" to hold the finger MP joints in flexion. It has been calculated that, as the patient extends his fingers, for every gram of force that is used to extend the fingers, there is at least twice that force exerted on the dorsum of the finger proximal phalanges.[5] It is no wonder that the skin can easily break down over the dorsum of the phalanx with the lumbrical bar. To allow for this high concentration of pressure, padding of the splint and securing of the hand in the splint by a palmar support that will curve and support the metacarpal arch is important. Usually the lumbrical bar extends across all of the fingers at the proximal phalanx to help disperse force that would concentrate more in the ring and little fingers if splinted separately. Occasionally the ring and little fingers can be splinted alone if pressure problems are controlled. The thumb should be free to move where it does not press against the splint on pinch and cause shear stress. Fig. 52-13 is an example of one such splint. Other designs are available.[15]

The thumb is harder to support externally than the fingers and thus is often left unsplinted. The patient is given corrective exercise instructions, such as therapist or patient blocking of extension of the MP joint with patient active extension of the interphalangeal joint. Splints also can be

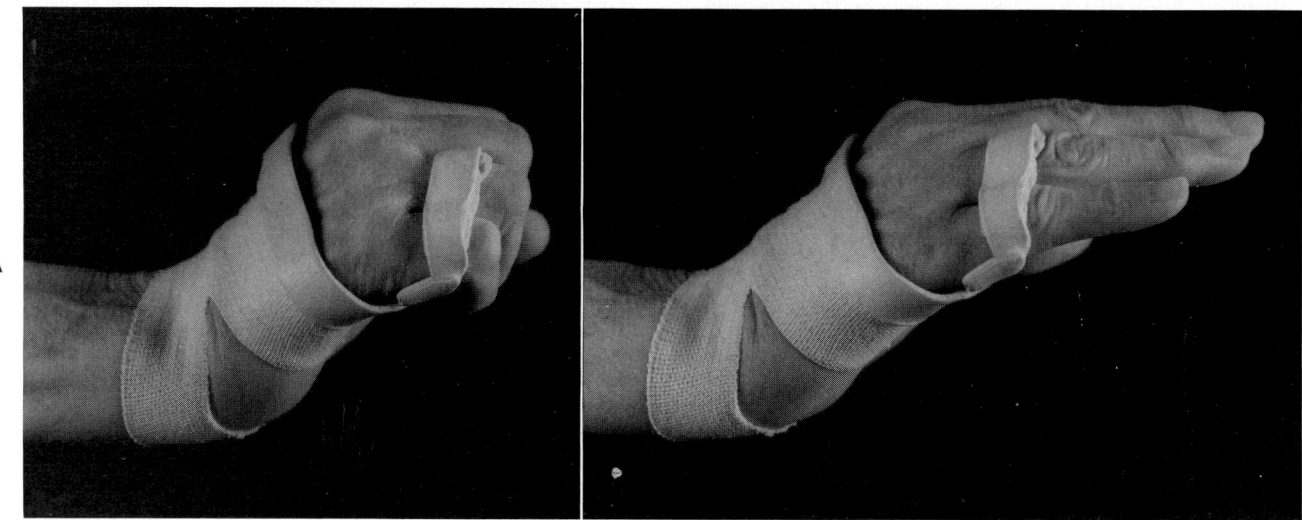

A   B

Fig. 52-13   Splinting to provide external support of finger metacarpophalangeal joints to facilitate interphalangeal extension. **A,** Interphalangeal flexion. **B,** Interphalangeal extension.

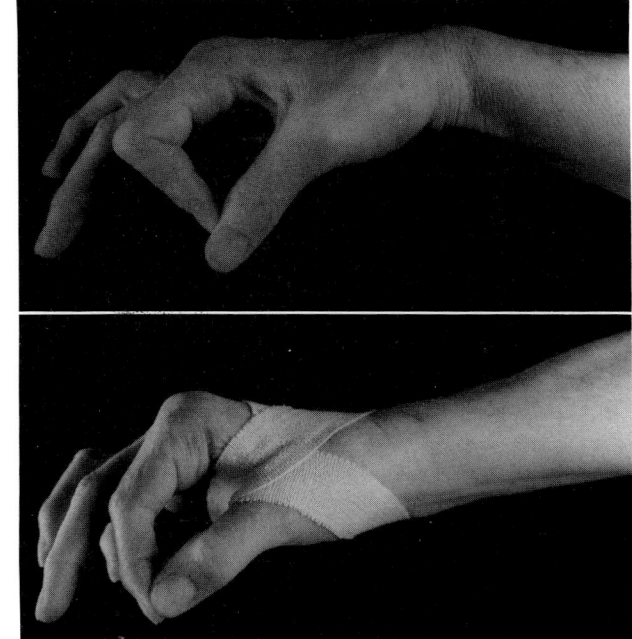

Fig. 52-14 Thumb strapping of thumb with adhesive elastic to support thumb in position for functional pulp pinch. Active wrist extension increases strap support tension and pinch stability. Strapping can be used in conjunction with other splinting. **A,** Pinch without thumb support. **B,** Pinch with thumb support.

made to accomplish this purpose if blocking of the MP joint results in extension of the thumb interphalangeal joint.

Additional splinting is possible to improve thumb positioning and encourage pulp rather than deforming side pinch. The thumb can be strapped in a 1½- to 2-inch—wide figure-of-eight strap made of adhesive stockinette that is wrapped from the forearm around the thumb to supply positioning support,[7] as in Fig. 52-14. Care should be taken that the strapping is proximal to the MP joint and does not therefore increase stress on radial collateral ligaments. One advantage of this type of strapping to achieve thumb positioning is that the support on the thumb will be increased when the patient extends the wrist for pinch and will be decreased as the wrist is flexed.

Serial cylinder casting is used for progressively remodeling the soft tissue of contracted joints (see Chapter 90). The casting technique is indicated when specific range of motion and exercise are not enough to maintain or restore joint range of motion and skin pliability.

Cylinder casting can be used to support the interphalangeal joints of the fingers and transfer the force of the extrinsic flexors to the MP joints as in Fig. 52-15. This allows active flexion of the MP joints in those fingers that are intrinsic-minus. The cast fabrication is the same as that used for cylinder casts for joint remodeling. The casts can be removed, for example, for handwashing, and then replaced.

The thumb can also be cylinder casted at the interphalangeal joints, but like fusion of this joint, casting must be done with caution. A stabilized thumb interphalangeal joint can increase rotation of a crank action thumb[5] as well as provide increased strain on the thumb metacarpal radial collateral ligament.

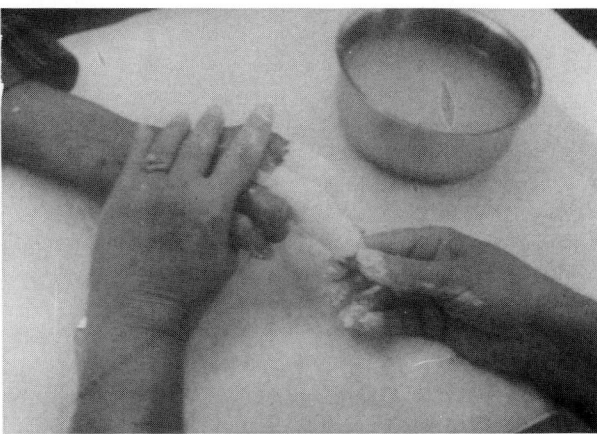

Fig. 52-15 Plaster cylinder casting of the fingers or thumb can be used several ways: (1) to serially correct contractures by progressive remodeling or (2) as an alternate ulnar-nerve splint to support the interphalangeal joints of the fingers or thumb in extension and transfer the force of the extrinsic flexors to the metacarpophalangeal joints. (The fingers usually will not continue to hyperextend at the metacarpophalangeal joints when interphalangeal joints are casted; but if they do, a dorsal block splint to prevent the metacarpophalangeal joints from hyperextending must also be used.)

POSTOPERATIVE MANAGEMENT

Finishing additions and changes are made to the treatment plan in the operating room when the final intricacies of the surgery have unveiled. The surgeon has at this point formulated how he or she perceives the surgery and is developing a plan of follow-up. The therapist should talk with the surgeon soon after surgery while the details of the surgery are still fresh. If the therapist routinely talks with the surgeon after surgery, the surgeon is prepared to offer quick, precise reports of successes and difficulties in the operating room that may affect the course of patient treatment, and he or she conveys clear concerns and specific requests.

In contrast with this surgeon/therapist interaction is the therapist who waits for therapy referrals. The success of the surgery is the surgeon's first concern, after which mobilization and patient return to work are desired. If surgeons must contact therapists and details have become colder, the surgeons are much more likely to do early movement themselves or let the patients do so with instructions, and refer when problems occur or late in follow-up when chances for successful therapy are reduced.

First days after surgery

The hand should be elevated after surgery or otherwise kept from a dependent position, which encourages swelling. The therapist can check the patient's compliance with elevation and, if necessary, fashion one of many possible elevation devices. It is helpful to tell the patient his hand must always be higher than his heart. A sling of stockinette with side cut for the cast and hand and the remaining part tied to an IV tree works satisfactorily. Other methods are available.

When the hand is checked postsurgically, the therapist can examine the hand for areas of constricting cast, friction areas causing abrasion, poor circulation of the hand, or evidence of infection. The conversation with the patient sets the stage for the patient's trust and cooperation in early stages of the treatment program.

The success of the mechanical rebalancing by tendon transfers is often in direct relationship to the maintenance of correct positioning of the hand during healing. The tension of an otherwise successful surgery can be ruined by inadvertent changes in positioning or unsatisfactory positions. It is not uncommon after a long surgical procedure for positioning in the surgical cast to be less than desired. For example, it is not uncommon for the MP joints after intrinsic replacement of the fingers to be in less flexion than desired, or the thumb after an adductor replacement to be in too much extension. The position should be readjusted at first opportunity, which is usually at the first cast change.

One week after surgery

The postoperative cast is often guardedly removed by the surgeon 1 week after surgery and the hand recast to improve position and to accommodate the loss of postoperative swelling; resolution of swelling can allow too much hand movement in the cast and cause the digits to shift into positions that may adversely affect tendon tension. Removal of the cast at this time also allows the hand to be checked for infection, sutures to be removed, and the hand otherwise inspected for healing of surgical wounds. Tendon transfers can be examined for continuity, and the patient is occasionally asked to move them slightly to check their operation. Much movement of the tendons is risky at this point, because too much force could result in elongation of a tendon anastomosis or rupture at the site of suture. The hand is usually recast for a period of 2 more weeks.

Early movement is not as necessary for tendon transfers as for tendon repairs, because transfers are not usually routed through areas of massive scar or at the time of accompanying injury. The routing of tendon transfers is often specifically chosen to avoid areas of previous scar. The advantages of early movement versus later movement of tendon repairs have been debated in surgical lectures and literature.[18] Far more repairs seem to scar down and have limited movement than to rupture, and strong arguments can be made for early movement of any tendon that is sutured, to maintain tendon gliding while limiting the amount of adhesions through which a newly repaired tendon must glide. But scar adhesions in ulnar nerve tendon transfers do not often limit the transferred tendon's function if the hand is held for 3 weeks in a cast. And the cast provides less opportunity for tendon rupture. In addition, tendon grafts may be a part of the transfer surgery, and grafts are believed to require more immobilization for nutrition for healing, although this too has been debated. Some studies indicate that the tendon, while gliding, will be able to derive enough nutrition from surrounding synovial tissue rather than depend on intrinsic tendon healing alone.[25]

More important determinants for late or early movement may be the strength of the tendon suture, the quality of the transfer including graft, and the strength of the tendon attachment during different stages of healing.[30] In any case, it is the surgeon who is in the best position to determine any possibility of early movement. The therapist must work closely with the surgeon and receive his or her concurrence if attempts at early movement are made. Many hands with ulnar nerve transfers will also have sensory involvements,

and the patient, because of impaired sensory feedback, is in danger of pulling too hard on the transfers too soon, particularly in low ulnar nerve injuries where ulnar nerve extrinsic muscle function remains intact. The patient may even rupture in the cast if he attempts to use the hand while casted, and specific instructions for the patient to not use the hand even though it is casted are prudent.

Exceptions do occur that necessitate the early movement of tendon transfers when the transfer must be routed through an area of old scar, and occasionally surgeons simply elect to move the tendon transfer earlier than 3 weeks. This certainly can be done, but risks are obvious and early movement requires the availability, supervision, and close interaction of the surgery/therapy team in a controlled environment with patient cooperation. Therapists in programs where patients may not return as instructed for follow-up or are unavailable for follow-up are advised to leave the cast for 3 weeks.

Early mobilization period

When the postoperative cast is removed, it is weaned away, not totally removed. Frequently, removal of the cast will result in a little swelling of the hand over the next day, because of the release of soft compression that the cast has provided to the hand. This swelling should be minimal and is more controlled if the hand is removed from the cast for a relatively short period (15 to 30 minutes) and then replaced. A half cast secured with a circular plaster or elastic bandage can be used as a splint for this purpose, or a new one can be made, as in Fig. 52-16. The surgeon, therapist, or technician who removes the cast can do so in such a way that the volar portion (or dorsal if desired) can be used as a holding splint. Brand would be quick to say a new cast is desirable, because the hand does not always fit into the cast in quite the same position. To disturb the hand as little as possible, however, when it is first removed from the cast for mobilization of transfers, a half cast can be safely used if the therapist will carefully check and relieve any pressure points of the cast that might cause local skin damage. If functioning well, the half cast can continue to be used as the hand is taken out for progressively more time for mobilization of transfers and restoration of hand function, or a new plaster cast or thermoplastic splint can be made at any desirable point.

Plaster serves as a good material for postoperative cast splints, because the material is inexpensive, allows air access to wounds, can be quickly made, and frequently can be remade as needed for optimum positioning and changes as the hand recovers function. The therapist is not so likely to discard an ill-fitting thermoplastic splint as plaster because of the time and cost involved. (The splint should be fitted to the hand, not the hand to the splint.)

The position maintained during tendon transfer mobilization is at first the same as in the postsurgical cast. Any movement of the hand and new tendons adds to the amount of swelling the patient will have in the first few days. This is because any movement causes rupture of adhesions that have been formed around the entire length of the transferred tendons, in particular at sites of their anastomosis, at incision and dissection sites, and anywhere else proteinaceous fibrinous material has been formed. As adhesion ruptures occur, more protein material is released, encouraging more

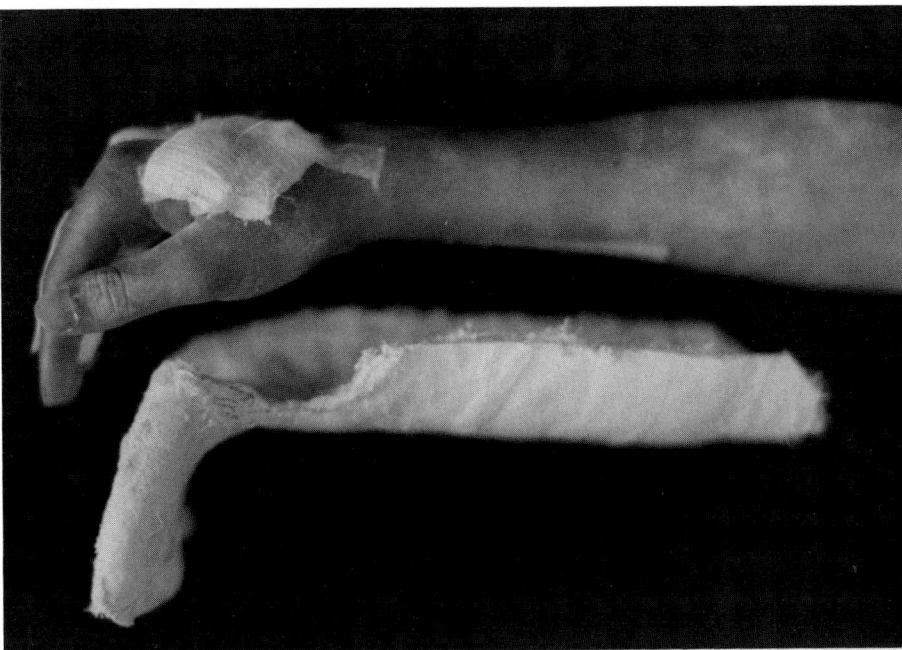

Fig. 52-16 Early postoperative cast splint. A half cast secured with a circular plaster or elastic bandage can be used as a first postoperative early mobilization-period splint. Areas of cast likely to cause pressure should be relieved, not just padded.

scar to be formed. The objective on day one is therefore one of only beginning to mobilize the tendon transfers with a gentle loosening that will cause minimal swelling and additional scar formation. On the first postsurgical day, it is usually sufficient to ask the patient to attempt flexion and extension of the fingers, thumb, and wrist gently through possible range of motion without undue stress. Attempts can be made to identify the tendon transfers by eliciting their slight active pull by the patient. Then the hand is wrapped for another day.

The first day out of the cast is the most exciting for the surgeon, therapist, and patient. Here one sees the evidence of the success or failure of the tendon transfer surgery, and the treatment plan unfolds accordingly. If the transfers can be identified and can support their intended joint(s) and if they appear to glide freely even within a small range of motion, the therapist's job is easy. The treatment plan becomes one of protection for further healing while progressively mobilizing the transfers over the next 3 weeks until moderate resistance can be given to the transferred muscles and other muscles of the hand for strengthening and augmentation of rebalancing.

Positioning is again critical, and the therapist must be sure the desired position is maintained at all joints during the patient's hand use by whatever means are necessary (supervision, splinting) until the tendon transfers are strong enough to support their intended function. The patient cannot just be released to use his hand, because he will quickly return to former disuse habits and by doing so can render the transfers ineffective. For example, a patient who has had an intrinsic-minus hand becomes used to the habitus of wrist flexion and of depending on his extrinsic finger extensor (extensor digitorum communis) to extend his fingers. This muscle can be powerful. If after intrinsic replacement

surgery, the patient is not protected from using this extrinsic finger extensor, the muscle can overcome any tension in the intrinsic transfers and continue to pull the MP joints into hyperextension. By repetitively doing so, he remodels the healing tissue to adjust to this position. The intrinsic transfers may actually rupture. But even if they do not rupture, the overpull of the extrinsic extensor causes a loosening of the fibrous adhesions and soft tissue around and throughout the length of the transferred tendons, which has the effect of reducing their mechanical tension for correction (of the MP joints in flexion and the interphalangeal joints in extension).

Scar tissue is necessary for healing and is not always bad. It becomes bad only when it inhibits function, such as intended tendon gliding. That scar will form along the bed of the transferred tendon can be used to advantage, such as in augmenting the support of the intrinsic transfers in the case cited above. If the positioning of the fingers is supported and maintained throughout tendon healing, some of the adhesions around the tendon and within the surrounding soft tissue will actually aid in supporting the tendons in their new position and in maintaining desired tissue remodeling. Brand[7] often uses the example of the overcorrected intrinsic-minus hand that is now in an intrinsic-plus position with limitation of extension at the finger MP joints and progressive hyperextension (because of mechanical imbalance and tension overpull) at the interphalangeal joints. He maintains that the transferred tendons can actually be released in these cases, and the MP joints will never return to hyperextension. This is because the tissue surrounding the tendon transfers and along the length of the tendon transfers has scarred and remodeled in a position to support the MP joints in flexion and can continue to do so even without the transferred tendons. The tension exhibited by the transfers and their corrective positions of the fingers is very important when the hand begins to move and gives clear evidence of where the correction balance is falling. If the tension of intrinsic transfers is a little less than desired, the MP joint can be protected from full extension by a splint or supervised instruction, and, it is hoped, the forming adhesions will help adjust for the minimal tension.

In the reverse then, if the tension is a little too tight, more freedom is given for full flexion and extension of the transferred tendons so they will be freed as much as necessary from their surrounding tissue restraints.

Most of the balance that results from surgery will be seen in the first 3 weeks of therapy. The patient first learns to identify the transfers on command. The tendon tension can change drastically during this period and should be watched closely. Use of the hand for activities other than identifying

the transfers and finger positioning can markedly affect the tendon balance as the patient reverts to his old habitus. This should be controlled, and the surgical and immobilization period used to break old use patterns. The patient can be told he will never use the hand the same way he did before surgery, because this could waste his surgery. The patient is told that he must first move the hand by assuming the positions requested and that when he masters these, he will progress to other movements.

For intrinsic transfers the position of movement is the lumbrical position. The patient flexes the fingers at the MP joints and then extends at the MP joints to three-fourths extension as in Fig. 52-17. Full extension at the MP joints is avoided, particularly in the first 3 weeks. If exercised to three-fourths extension, the fingers with the transfers will loosen naturally later as the hand is used, and it is far better

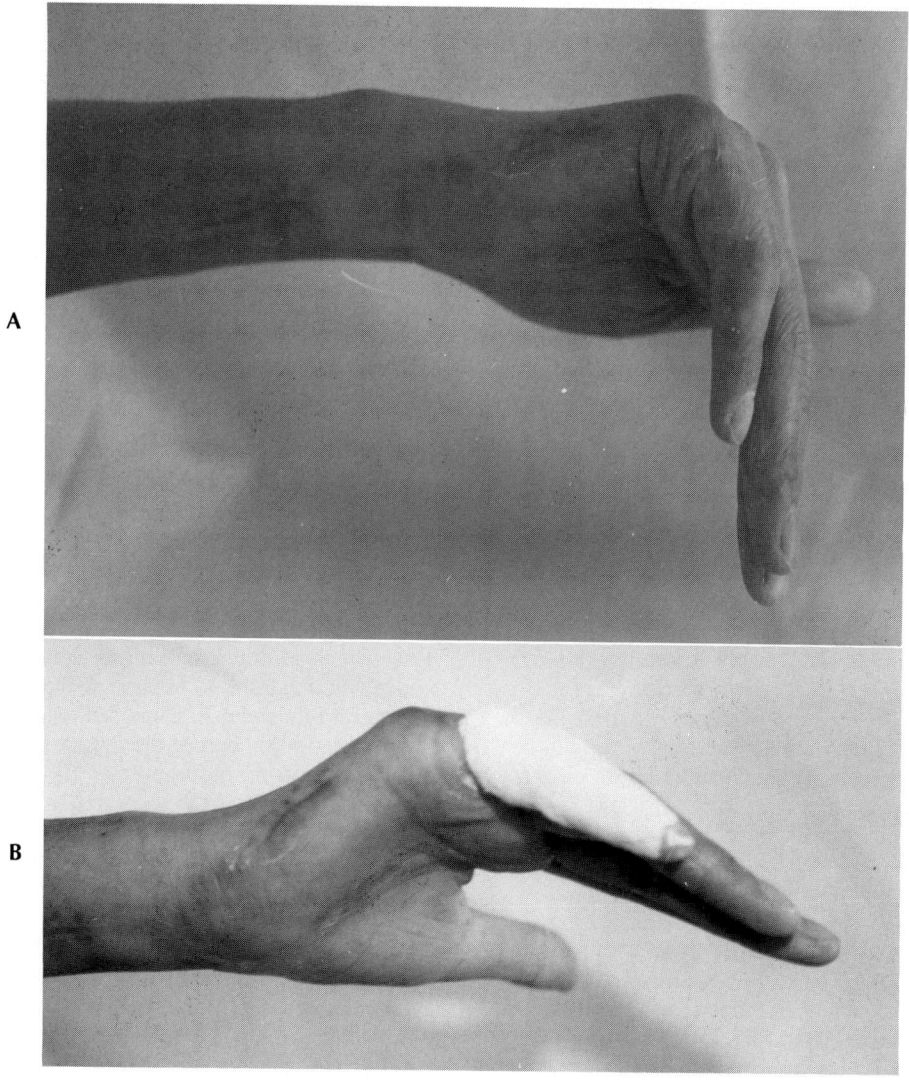

Fig. 52-17   Early postoperative mobilization of intrinsic replacement transfers. **A,** The patient is asked to keep the interphalangeal joints in extension and flex the fingers at the metacarpophalangeal joints. **B,** The patient is asked to keep the interphalangeal joints in extension and extend the metacarpophalangeal joints. The tension of the transferred tendons should be apparent in the amount of metacarpophalangeal flexion maintained. Extension at the metacarpophalangeal joints is increased gradually, but never past neutral or to hyperextension. A full fist is avoided for several weeks.

that the transfers remain somewhat tight than eventually become too loose. If too tight, increased exercises and splinting slightly into the opposite direction 3 to 6 weeks after beginning movement can achieve the required tension. If the transfers become too loose, attempts can be made to splint the fingers at the MP joints into flexion for extended periods and to limit greatly extension of the finger MP joints in extension. But if not successful, the therapist can do nothing more, and the tension can be readjusted only by another surgery.

The balance is checked immediately upon cast removal, and sometimes the patient can move the fingers with the transfer only 15 to 20 degrees. This is gently increased over the first week with the hand out of the splint once daily. The range of motion of the fingers with the transfer should loosen to 75 to 80 degrees of flexion actively at the MP joint to minus 30 degrees extension with the interphalangeal joints of the fingers straight in a neutral position. Then the patient can be asked to flex the interphalangeal joints slightly and move the thumb to restore joint gliding.

The patient is instructed to avoid making a full fist in the first few weeks, because this puts undue stress on the new intrinsic replacement tendon transfers. The flexors of the hand are mechanically stronger than the extensors and will rarely have a problem eventually returning the fingers to a full fist. The patient will appear to be limited in flexion for the first few weeks he moves, because the tension of the transfers initially limits full finger flexion. This is acceptable and even good. If desired, after about 2 weeks when the transfers can be easily identified and the patient can move the fingers in lumbrical positioning, he can flex his fingers slightly from the fingertips after his other exercises.

Once the patient correctly identifies the transfers on command and can assume the lumbrical positioning, he is transferred to light pickup activities with cotton balls. He must continue to exhibit lumbrical positioning upon grasp and release of the cotton and should be supervised. This is when he is most likely to assume old patterns and needs counseling. If he is unable to pick up in a lumbrical position, splinting to assist this should be considered or he should spend more time extending and flexing the finger in a lumbrical position on command.

At the beginning of the 3-week early mobilization period, the hand should be removed from the cast for supervised activity and then replaced in the cast that maintains its lumbrical position of the fingers and abduction of the thumb. Gradually the time out of the cast is increased until the hand is out most of the day but the retainer cast or splint is worn overnight. Range of motion is gradually increased, but unsupervised full range of motion is not allowed, nor is motion against resistance. Any overloading of the tendon junctures before 8 weeks (postsurgery) can result in stretching or rupture/avulsion.[33]

Accessory splinting can be done to help support positioning and achieve a little more correction. If flexion contractures persist at the interphalangeal joints, cylinder casts can be placed on the fingers to encourage interphalangeal extension. Cylinder casts can be placed on the fingers while the fingers are either in or out of the retainer splint, to encourage more MP flexion. In most cases, when cylinder casts are placed on the fingers, the fingers will not extend into hyperextension at the MP joints. If the fingers do completely straighten or hyperextend at the MP joint, they should be protected from hyperextension.

Other pickup activities are introduced, omitting those that require resistive exercise, such as turning a key or opening a jar. Small objects of various shapes are helpful, particularly those that can be stacked and thus encourage shoulder movement. In all cases of pickup activities, the patient should use lumbrical positioning, extending to less than full range of motion at the MP joints. Graded fishing weights are helpful, as are Velcro checkers.

The procedure for mobilization of adductor replacements follows the same principles as for intrinsic replacement surgery except that the thumb is maintained in an abducted position in the postsurgical cast. If the thumb rests in too much extension, it is harder for the patient to identify the transfer and to use it in sequence of prehension with the fingers. If it rests in too much flexion, the transfer can become a little too tight and the skin at the thenar crease may macerate at the suture site. Optimal is abduction out of the palm in a position where the patient will place a little tension on the transfer when the thumb is extended. This helps give him or her some internal feedback from the new transfer.

Sometimes an adductor replacement is done before finger intrinsic replacement, sometimes vice versa, and sometimes both surgeries are done together. For retraining, it is easier if both surgeries are done together. For rebalancing, it is better if one surgery is done first so the second can be adjusted slightly to the first surgery to provide optimum contact surfaces and pinch of the thumb to the fingers.

Late mobilization period

At the end of the first 3-week mobilization period, unless the transfers have become looser in tension than desired, the cast should be removed for the day and be worn at night for another 3 weeks or longer. MP flexion splint can be made to continue to support the fingers and help the patient maintain this position if necessary. The splint can be of the same design as the ulnar nerve splint worn before surgery but is best made to include all of the fingers to minimize pressure points, as in Fig. 52-18. One caution is needed, however, because the interphalangeal joints will extend by the extrinsic extensor when the MP joints are supported in flexion. The therapist must be sure the patient is actually using the transfers. This can be accomplished by frequent removal of the splint for exercise. A splint that prevents only full extension of the MP joints but allows almost full movement otherwise is preferred, to allow full use of the transfers and a gradual return of full finger flexion.

The patient is gradually encouraged to resume normal skill activities (Fig. 52-19), omitting those that offer heavy resistance to the tendons. Gradually full range of motion is encouraged, and mild resistance is allowed. The transferred tendons are protected from heavy use for as long as 3 months. Ruptures have been noted as late as 3 months, when the patient feels it is possible to use the hand normally and falls, grabs a steering wheel, or pulls on a refrigerator. It is explained to the patient that if balance of the hand is achieved, strength will come later and he will have function of the hand for a long time, but if the tendons rupture or if deformity recurs, the hand can be corrected only by another surgery and recovery period.

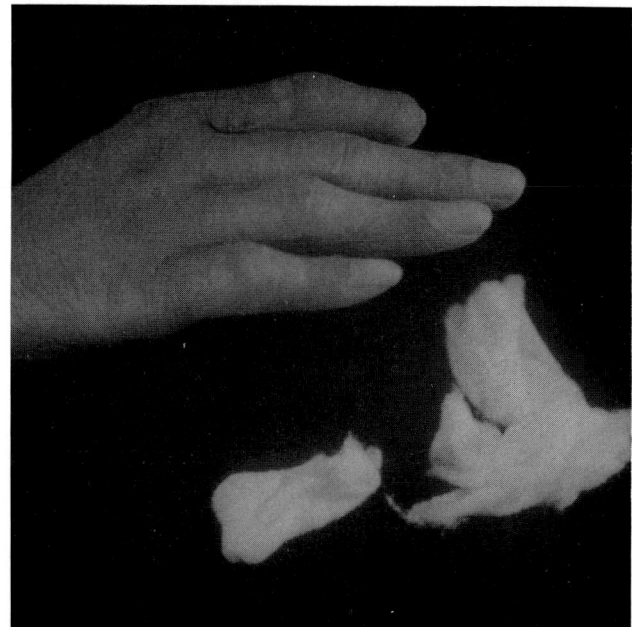

Fig. 52-18 Postoperative late mobilization-period ulnar splint that is padded liberally and includes all of the fingers to minimize point pressure. **A,** Gentle interphalangeal flexion. **B,** Interphalangeal extension with support of the metacarpophalangeal joints in flexion to augment new intrinsic tendon transfers while the hand is used and to prevent inadvertent metacarpophalangeal hyperextension.

Other surgical needs

Not all tendon tension can be readjusted or augmented by positioning of the fingers and mobilization of tendon transfers. Sometimes adjustments must be made in surgery. This is particularly true when one muscle is made to go to more than one finger by more than one tendon slip. The muscle will pull hardest on the tendon with the shortest excursion. All or most of the tension of the muscle may be translated to this shortest tendon, rendering further pull of the other tendon ineffective or impossible. For example, if the superficialis of the ring finger has been transferred as an intrinsic replacement of the little and ring fingers, the flexion tension on one is likely to be tighter than on the other. Sometimes this is not enough to cause a problem, and in fact, the tension to the little finger is often made a little tighter, because it seems often to have the least tension after surgery (possibly because of the hyperextension of the fifth metacarpal). For the appearance and function of the hand, it is even desirable for the little finger to be a little tighter than the ring. But in the instance the tension to the little finger is such that most of the transferred motor power acts on the little finger, the unsupported ring finger may return to clawing (with the MP joint in hyperextension and the interphalangeal joint in flexion). This can easily result in a progressive deformity of both fingers, because not only will the ring finger continue to claw, but the little finger, if it has a very mobile interphalangeal joint, will begin to

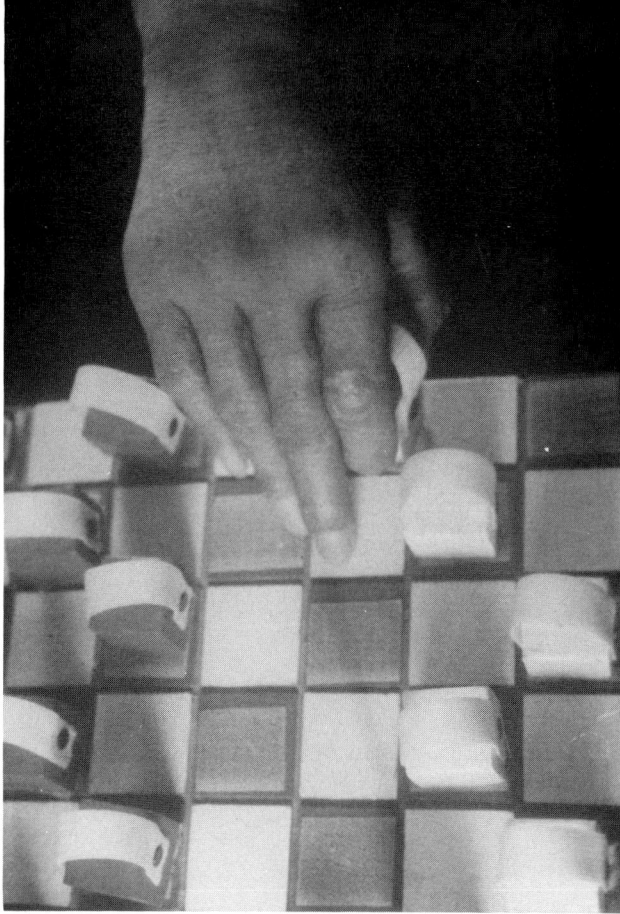

Fig. 52-19 Supervised functional hand use. Essential in early hand use is the transfer to use of corrected positioning. Old habit patterns (e.g., wrist drop to achieve finger extension, forceful extension of the fingers into metacarpophalangeal extension, or full fist too early) are hard to break and can ruin tendon transfer correction. As patients are able to maintain correct positioning and resistance to tendon transfers is safe, they are allowed to assume normal hand skills. Assistive splinting may be necessary to achieve maximum results. Retainer splints can be helpful until no longer necessary. **A,** Light pickup exercise with cotton. **B,** Velcro resistive checkers.

hyperextend at the interphalangeal joint and possibly progressively "swan-neck" from the mechanical overpull of the tendon transfer force.

SUMMARY

Tendon transfer procedures are muscle rebalancing procedures and biomechanically serve to rebalance what has become imbalanced in the hand from disease or injury. The therapeutic management of tendon transfers after ulnar nerve injuries, then, must (1) necessarily replace externally by splinting and/or exercising the imbalance caused by weak or missing muscles, (2) correct secondary problems that have occurred, such as skin and joint contractures, or (3) augment what has been corrected through surgical transfers by corrective positioning and by mobilizing surgical hands in a way that maintains, increases, or decreases transferred tendon tension.

REFERENCES

1. Agee JA and Guidern M: The functional significance of the juncturae tendinae in dynamic stabilization of the metacarpophalangeal joints of the fingers. Paper presented at the Annual Conference of the American Society for Surgery of the Hand, Atlanta, 1980.
2. Bell JA: Rehabilitation: tendon transfers panel discussion, Richard Smith, Moderator. In Hunter JM, Schneider LH, and Mackin EJ, editors: Tendon surgery in the hand, St. Louis, 1987, The CV Mosby Co.
3. Boyes JH: Bunnell's surgery of the hand, ed 5 Philadelphia, 1970, JB Lippincott Co.
4. Brand PW: Paralytic claw hand, J Bone Joint Surg 40B:618, 1958.
5. Brand PW: Clinical mechanics of the hand, St. Louis, 1985, The CV Mosby Co.
6. Brand PW: Biomechanics of tendon transfers. In Hunter JM, Schneider LH, and Mackin EJ, editors: Tendon surgery in the hand, St. Louis, 1987, The CV Mosby Co.
7. Brand PW: Personal communications, 1978.
8. Brand PW and others: Relative tension and potential excursion of muscles in the forearm and hand, J Hand Surg 6:209, 1981.
9. Brandsma JW, Birke JA, and Sims D Jr: The Martin-Gruber innervated hand, J Hand Surg 11A:536, 1986.
10. Brooks AL: A new intrinsic tendon transfer for the paralytic hand, J Bone Joint Surg 57A:730, 1975.
11. Burkhalter WE: Restoration of power grip in ulnar nerve paralysis, Orthop Clin North Am 2:289, 1974.
12. Casanova JS and Grunert BK: Adult prehension: patterns and nomenclature, ASHT Annual Conference Sept. 13, 1987.
13. Cochran GVB: A primer of orthopedic biomechanics, New York, 1982, Churchill Livingston, Inc.
14. Fess EE: The need for reliability and validity in hand assessment instruments, J Hand Surg 11A:621, 1986.
15. Fess EE and Phillips C: Hand splinting principles and methods, ed 2, St. Louis, 1987, The CV Mosby Co.
16. Flatt AE: The care of the rheumatoid hand, ed 4, St. Louis, 1983, The CV Mosby Co.
17. Frost HM: An introduction to biomechanics, Springfield, Ill, 1967, Charles C Thomas Publisher.
18. Gelberman RH and Manske PR: Effects of early motion on the tendon healing process: experimental studies. In Hunter JM, Schneider LH, and Mackin EJ, editors: Tendon surgery in the hand, St. Louis, 1987, The CV Mosby Co.
19. Harris EC Jr: Intrinsic balance of the extensor system. In Hunter JM, Schneider LH, and Mackin EJ, editors: Tendon surgery in the hand, St. Louis, 1987, The CV Mosby Co.
20. Kapandji IA: Biomechanics of the thumb. In Tubiana R, editor: The hand, Philadelphia, 1981, WB Saunders Co.
21. Kumar RP and Brandsma JW: A method to determine pressure distribution of the hand, Lepr Rev 57:39, 1986.
22. Landsmeer JMF: The anatomy of the dorsal aponeurosis of the human finger and its functional significance, Anat Rec 104:31, 1949.
23. Littler JW: Tendon transfers and arthrodeses in combined median and ulnar nerve paralysis, J Bone Joint Surg 31A:225, 1949.
24. Long C and others: Intrinsic-extrinsic muscle control of the hand in power grip and precision handling: an electromyographic study, J Bone Joint Surg 52A:853, 1970.
25. Manske PR and Lesker PA: Diffusion as a nutrient pathway to the flexor tendon. In Hunter JM, Schneider LH, and Mackin EJ, editors: Tendon surgery in the hand, St. Louis, 1987, The CV Mosby Co.
26. Marks R and Payne PA: Bioengineering and the skin, MTP Press United International Medical Publishers, 1979.
27. Mathews R: Personal communications, Rat studies, 1979.
28. Moberg E: Objective methods for determining the functional value of sensibility of the hand, J Bone Joint Surg 40B:454, 1958.
29. Omer GE Jr: Tendon transfers as early internal splints following peripheral nerve injury in the upper extremity. In Hunter JM, Schneider LH, and Mackin EJ, editors: Tendon surgery in the hand, St. Louis, 1987, The CV Mosby Co.
30. Peacock EE Jr: Collagen metabolism during healing of long tendons. In Hunter JM, Schneider LH, and Mackin EJ, editors: Tendon surgery in the hand, St. Louis, 1987, The CV Mosby Co.
31. Ranney DA: Reconstruction of the transverse metacarpal arc in ulnar palsy by transfer of the extensor digiti minimi, Plast Reconstr Surg 52:406, 1973.
32. Riordan DC: Tendon transplantations in median-nerve and ulnar-nerve paralysis, J Bone Joint Surg 35A:312, 1953.
33. Riordan DC: Principles of tendon transfers. In Hunter JM, Schneider LH, and Mackin EJ, editors: Tendon surgery in the hand, St. Louis, 1987, The CV Mosby Co.
34. Salter RB and others: The biological effect of continuous passive motion on the healing of full-thickness defects in articular cartilage: an experimental investigation in the rabbit, J Bone Joint Surg 62A:1232, 1980.
35. Stiles HJ and Forrester-Brown MF: Treatment of injuries of the peripheral spinal nerves, London, 1922, Henry Frowde Hudder and Stoughten.
36. Thompson TC: Modified operation for oppones paralysis, J Bone Joint Surg 24:623, 1972.
37. Van der Meulen JC: Causes of prolapse and collapse of the proximal interphalangeal joint of the hand, Hand 4:147, 1972.
38. Wright V: Stiffness: a review of its measurement and physiological importance, Physiotherapy 59(4):107, 1973.
39. Yamada H: Strength of biological materials, Baltimore, 1970, Williams & Wilkins (Edited by FG Evans).
40. Zancolli EA: Claw hand caused by paralysis of the intrinsic muscles: a simplified surgical procedure for its correction, J Bone Joint Surg 39A:1076, 1957.
41. Zancolli EA: Structural and dynamic bases of hand surgery, ed 2, Philadelphia, 1979, JB Lippincott Co.

53

Preoperative and postoperative management of tendon transfers after radial nerve injury

C. Christopher Reynolds

Peripheral nerve injuries in the upper extremity are caused by laceration, compression, perforation, traction, and occasionally the toxic effects of injected drugs. The radial nerve is particularly susceptible to damage as it courses along the shaft of the humerus. Perforating injuries are common from fragments of fractured bone, though typically the nerve is injured by direct external compression. Sustained pressure under the axilla from crutches may result in significant damage to nerve fibers. Prolonged pressure at the midhumeral level results in paralysis of muscles innervated by the radial nerve; this paralysis is often referred to as "Saturday night palsy" or "drunkard's palsy."[1,2,4]

A familiar clinical picture emerges with radial nerve paralysis. The forearm is pronated and the classic "wrist drop" position is assumed (Fig. 53-1). Grip strength is substantially reduced, because inactive wrist extensors create an unstable wrist and minimize the power of the long finger flexors. The inability to extend the fingers at the metacarpophalangeal (MP) joints prevents satisfactory grasp and release of large objects. Paralysis of the forearm supinator does not pose an additional problem. Supination is still possible through the action of the musculocutaneous innervated biceps brachii.[11,12]

Several tendon transfer procedures are used to restore function after radial nerve injuries.[9,10,13] Muscles commonly used for the radial nerve transfers include the pronator teres for wrist extension, flexor carpi ulnaris or flexor digitorum sublimus for finger extension, and flexor digitorum sublimus

Table 53-1 Commonly used tendon transfers for radial nerve paralysis

Muscle	Action
Pronator teres	Wrist extension (Extensor carpi radialis brevis, longus)
Flexor carpi ulnaris or flexor digitorum sublimus	Finger extension (Extensor digitorum communis)
Palmaris longus or flexor digitorum sublimus	Thumb extension (Extensor pollicis longus)

or palmaris longus for thumb extension (Table 53-1). Procedures affecting wrist and digital extension are among the most favorable and predictable in hand surgery. However, without a comprehensive preoperative and postoperative hand therapy program, success is much more difficult to obtain.

PREOPERATIVE HAND THERAPY PROGRAM

Preoperatively the goals of the hand therapist are to obtain a baseline motor evaluation, maintain function, prevent contractures of the hand and forearm, and strengthen muscles that are to be used for transfer.[8]

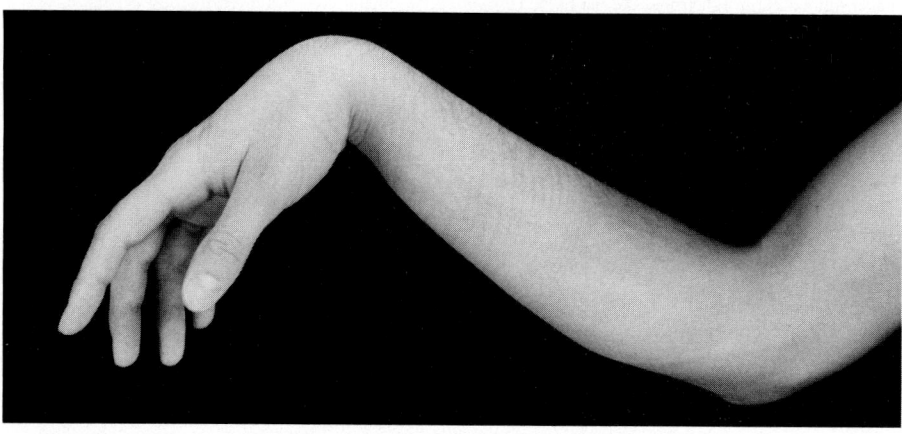

Fig. 53-1 Paralysis of the supinator muscle and all wrist and digital extensors creates the classic wrist-drop posture of the hand and forearm.

Motor evaluation

An early motor evaluation helps determine the level of injury as well as to define a baseline from which progress can be measured if regeneration occurs. Typically, with a high radial nerve palsy the muscles innervated distal to the branches of the triceps are involved. These include the brachioradialis, supinator, and all wrist and long digital extensors. The radial nerve divides into two branches distal to the brachioradialis. The superficial radial nerve, a sensory branch, provides sensation to the dorsal radial aspect of the hand. Because sensory distribution is usually confined to a small dorsal area, sensory loss will have little effect on patient function. The posterior interosseous nerve, the motor branch, has variable innervation. Characteristically, the posterior interosseous nerve innervates at least one radial wrist extensor, the supinator, the extensor carpi ulnaris, and the digital extensors. Wrist drop does not occur with injury to this branch, but wrist extension is radially deviated because of the absence of the extensor carpi ulnaris.[11,12]

A baseline muscle test evaluates the power of individual muscles innervated by the radial nerve. Several methods of manual muscle testing are currently used.[5,7] In addition to these tests, a comparison can be made between the injured and uninjured sides. The brachioradialis, an elbow flexor, is a superficial muscle that stands out readily with resistance to the flexed elbow. To observe a contraction, the forearm is positioned in neutral and resistance is applied at the wrist (Fig. 53-2). If the muscle is weak, the contraction will not be as prominent as the muscle on the contralateral side. Elbow flexion is rarely affected by the absence of the brachioradialis because of the strength of the biceps brachii. Careful observation and palpation of the contraction of the brachioradialis indicate functional regeneration or return.

Wrist extension in a radial direction is accomplished by the extensor carpi radialis longus and brevis. The muscles are tested with the forearm pronated and the wrist positioned over the edge of a table or towel roll. Finger and thumb extensors may substitute for the action of the wrist extensor

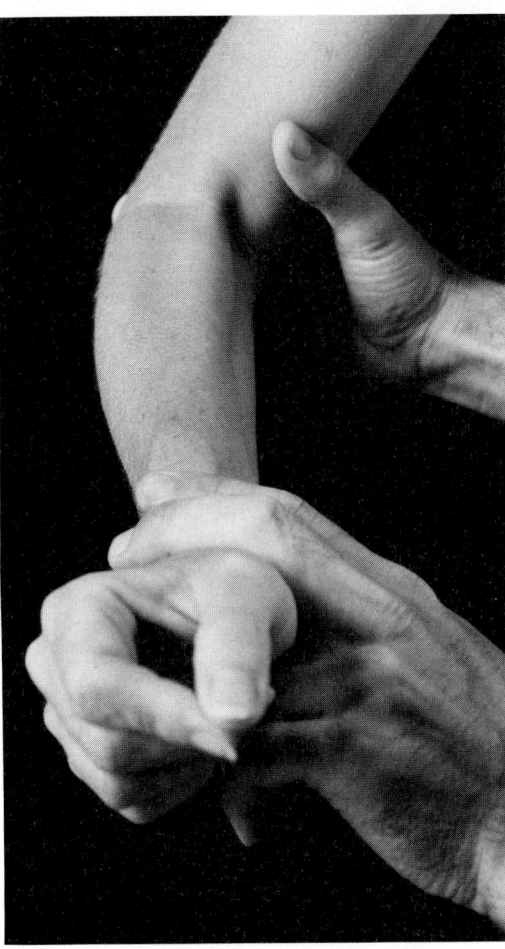

Fig. 53-2   An intact branchioradialis stands out readily when resistance is applied to the flexed elbow.

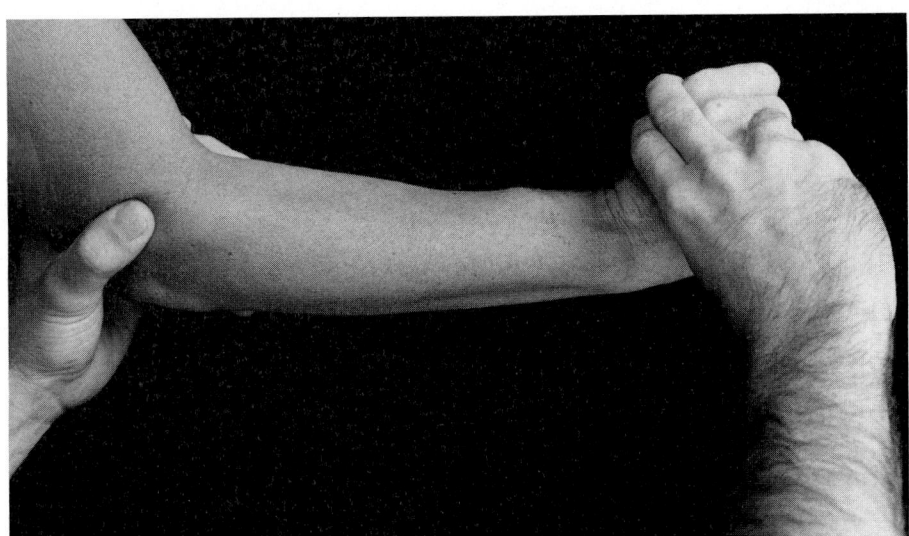

Fig. 53-3   To test the extensor carpi radialis longus and brevis, resistance is applied to the dorsoradial aspect of the hand in the direction of flexion and ulnar deviation.

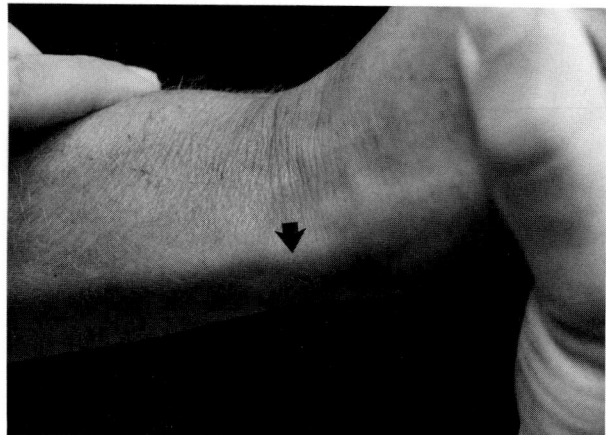

Fig. 53-4   The extensor carpi ulnaris tendon is visible and palpable distal to the ulnar styloid.

muscles. Flexing the fingers and the thumb in the palm helps prevent substitution and isolate wrist extensor power. Resistance is applied to the radial side of the hand as the patient holds the position of extension and radial deviation (Fig. 53-3). A second wrist position is used if the patient cannot extend the wrist against gravity. The forearm is supinated to midline or neutral while the ulnar side of the hand is resting on the table.

The extensor carpi ulnaris (ECU) extends the wrist in an ulnar direction. The muscle is tested in the same fashion as the radial wrist extensors. However, resistance is applied to the dorsum of the fifth metacarpal in the direction of flexion and radial deviation. Careful palpation of the prominent ECU tendon, distal to the ulnar head, is helpful in determining the activity of the muscle when there is significant weakness (Fig. 53-4).

Supination of the forearm is possible through the action of both the biceps brachii and the supinator muscles. The biceps muscle is not the primary supinator of the forearm; however, its influence is significant. As the biceps flexes the elbow, supination occurs. To eliminate biceps activity, the elbow is extended completely, and supination power can be measured. As the patient pronates and then supinates the forearm, resistance is applied at the extreme of supination and then compared with the opposite side (Fig. 53-5).

The extensor digitorum communis, indicis proprius, and digiti minimi extend the fingers at the MP joints of the second through fifth digits. The proper muscle test position is with the wrist in neutral and interphalangeal (IP) joints flexed (Fig. 53-6). A neutral wrist prevents extensor tenodesis of the fingers, and the IP joints are flexed to inhibit the activity of the lumbricales and interossei. In this test position the patient attempts to extend the MP joints against gravity while resistance is applied to the proximal phalanges. If the patient is unable to extend the MP joints against gravity, the hand is repositioned to eliminate gravity's effects. The forearm is placed in neutral while the ulnar side of the hand rests on the table, and the patient is retested. With extreme weakness, observing and palpating tendon movement over the metacarpals is helpful. The extensor indicis proprius and digiti minimi can be isolated by having

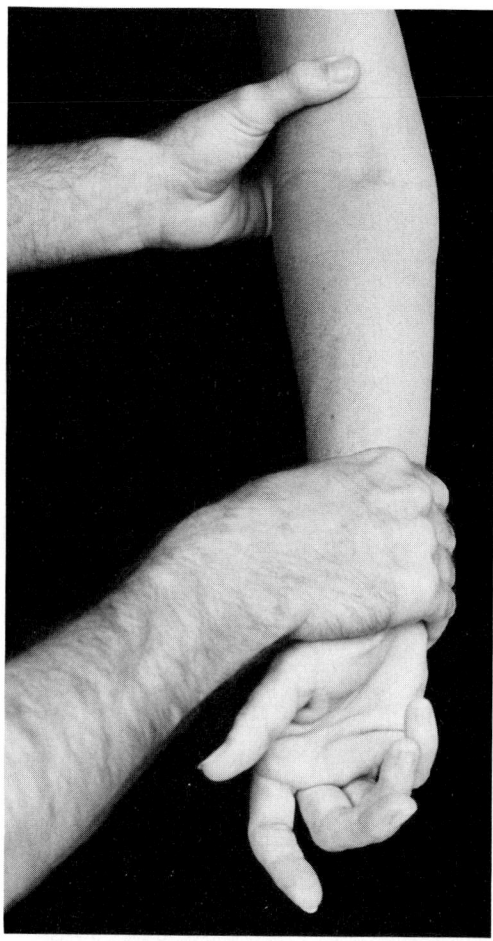

Fig. 53-5   Resisted supination is tested with the elbow extended to eliminate biceps brachia activity.

the patient extend the MP joint of the index finger for the proprius and the little finger MP joint for the digiti minimi.

Muscles of the first extensor compartment, abductor pollicis longus and extensor pollicis brevis, are true radial abductors of the thumb.[12] The abductor pollicis longus is the primary radial abductor of the first metacarpal. The extensor pollicis brevis performs the same task in addition to extending the MP joint of the thumb. These muscles are the most difficult of the radial nerve muscles to isolate and measure. The extensor pollicis longus can substitute for the action of both muscles. Its function can be minimized during testing by flexing the IP joint of the thumb (Fig. 53-7). Careful palpation of the tendons of the first extensor compartment is necessary as the patient radially abducts the thumb and extends the MP joint.

Extension of the distal phalanx of the thumb is accomplished by three muscles. The primary extensor is the extensor pollicis longus. The accessory pull from slips of the abductor pollicis brevis and flexor pollicis brevis, which are innervated by the median nerve, assist in extending the IP joint of the thumb. To prevent abductor pollicis brevis and flexor pollicis brevis activity, the thumb is placed in extreme passive extension. In this position the extensor pollicis longus can extend the IP joint of the thumb. A strong extensor pollicis longus maintains the IP joint in hyperextension against maximum resistance. If the extensor pollicis longus

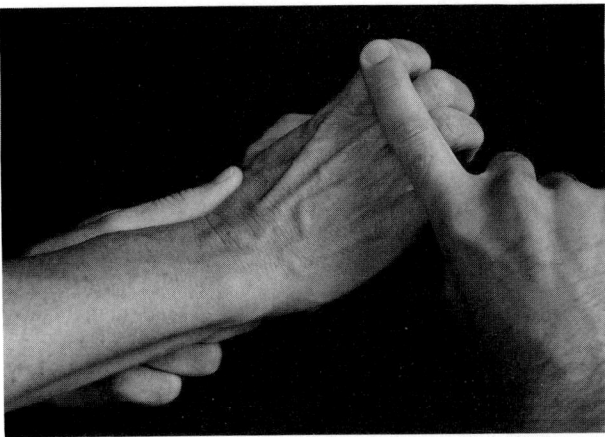

Fig. 53-6 To test extensor digitorum, resistance is applied to the proximal phalanges while the patient maintains the fingers in a claw position.

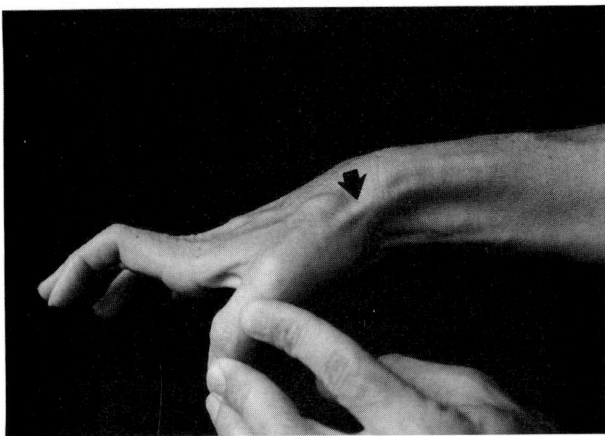

Fig. 53-7 Palpation of the first extensor compartment tendons is necessary to determine their level of activity.

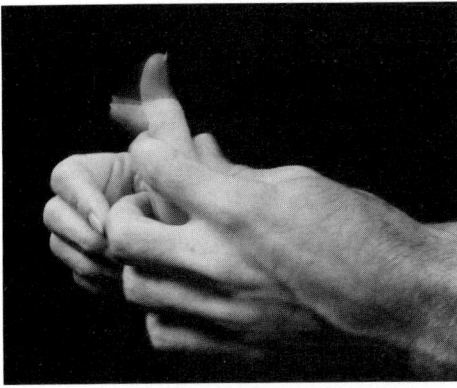

Fig. 53-8 The extensor pollicis longus is the sole extensor of the interphalangeal joint of the thumb when abductor pollicis longus and flexor pollicis brevis activity is eliminated.

is weak, hyperextension of the joint will not occur and palpation or observation of the tendon on the dorsal radial aspect of the wrist is necessary (Fig. 53-8).

Prevention of contractures and maintenance of function

Preventing or avoiding contractures is the second goal of the preoperative program. Maintaining a supple wrist and hand is generally not difficult after radial nerve injuries. If, however, the wrist and digits remain flexed for a prolonged period, the long flexors of the fingers become tight, whereas the long extensors stretch out. Tight finger flexors prevent simultaneous wrist and finger extension. Serial splinting is helpful in overcoming tightness of the long finger flexors. Anterior-posterior plaster splints that are changed frequently will gradually stretch the tight tendons and allow simultaneous wrist and finger extension (see Chapter 90).

More common, bad habits occur that lead to functional problems after tendon transfer surgery. For instance, if the patient allows the wrist to flex during functional activities preoperatively, even after wrist extensor transfers, he may habitually flex the wrist during grasp and release activities. Similarly, habitual finger extension using intrinsic muscles preoperatively continues after tendon transfers. The patient may "forget" how to extend the fingers at the MP joints even after transfers. For these reasons, preoperative splinting and reeducation exercises are necessary.

To maintain function and prevent the establishment of bad habits, the wrist and digits are splinted to support the wrist in neutral or slight extension and recreate extensor power of the digits. One splint option is based on a design illustrated by Hollis in 1978[1,3,6,14] (Fig. 53-9). It allows finger flexion with wrist extension and finger extension with wrist flexion. Slings or loops placed at the proximal phalanges are attached to the forearm by a static, taut line. As the wrist flexes to neutral, the loops support the MP joints in extension permitting intrinsic muscles to extend the IP joints. As the patient flexes the fingers, support at the proximal phalanges through the loops maintains the wrist in extension. A second splint option statically supports the wrist in neutral or slight extension while rubber bands attached to the proximal phalanges dynamically extend the MP joints (Fig. 53-10, *A*). Flexion of the fingers occurs against the rubber band traction while the wrist is maintained in an extended position (Fig. 53-10, *B*).

There are advantages to both splint designs. The Hollis splint has less bulk and enhances function by allowing wrist motion. However, many patients prefer the wrist support afforded by the more rigid and distally based dynamic splint. Both designs offer an effective preoperative tool to improve function while preventing the development of undesirable patterns of movement.

Most patients with radial nerve palsy prefer either of these splints in addition to one that supports the wrist only, such as a custom-made or prefabricated wrist cock-up. These splints provide simple wrist support when finger extension is not necessary. The wrist cock-up is useful when the patient is sleeping or engaged in activities requiring sustained grip.

Strengthening muscles selected for transfers

The final preoperative therapy goal is to strengthen muscles that will be used for transfer.[8] Because a transferred

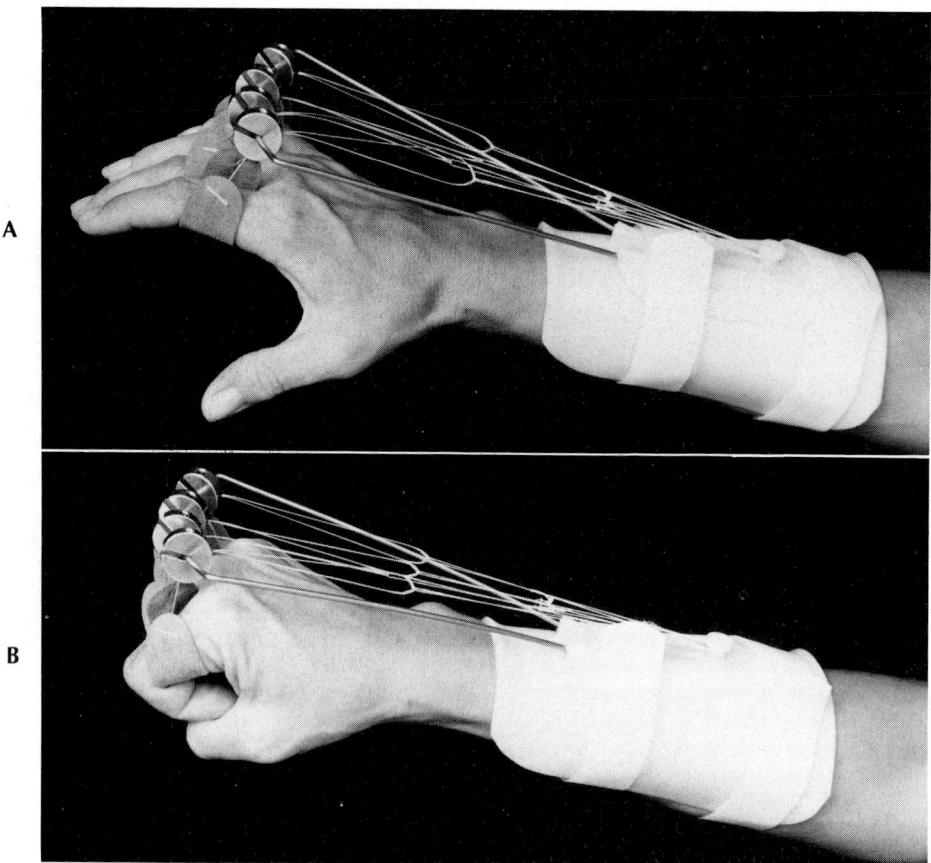

Fig. 53-9   The improved Hollis-type splint prevents wrist drop while allowing finger extension, **A,** and flexion, **B.**

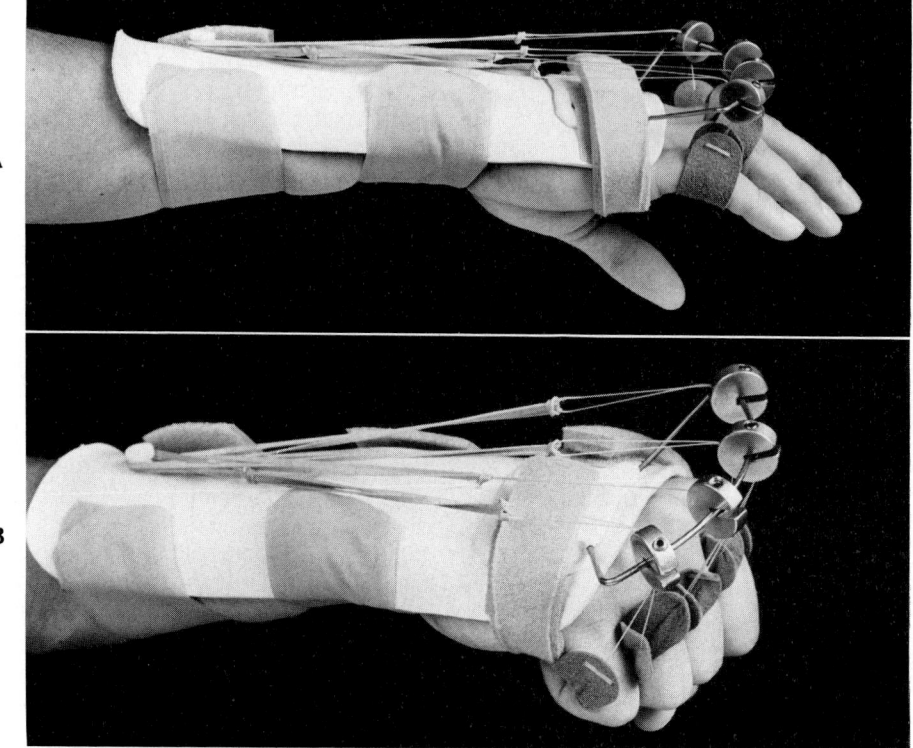

Fig. 53-10   **A,** Another radial nerve splint supports the wrist while rubber-band tension extends the metacarpophalangeal joints. **B,** The wrist is maintained in an extended position with flexion of the fingers.

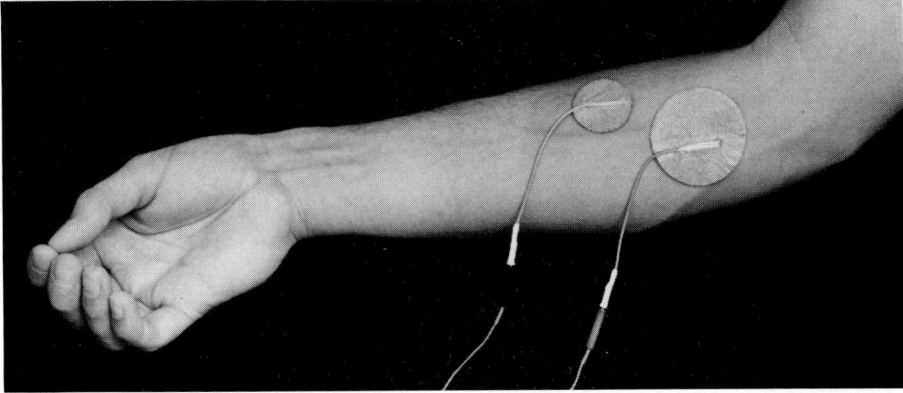

Fig. 53-11   Electrical stimulation is used in conjunction with exercise to increase the strength of muscles to be used for transfer. The pronator teres muscle is stimulated before transfer to the wrist extensors.

muscle loses one grade of strength, it is helpful to increase the tone and cross-sectional diameter of the muscle before transfer. Strengthening can be accomplished by a graded, progressive resistive exercise program and may include electrical stimulation (Fig. 53-11). Isolating muscles for strengthening preoperatively facilitates a postoperative program as well. The patient is more inclined to know how to use the tendon transfer after surgery if the muscle has been isolated and activated preoperatively.

POSTOPERATIVE HAND THERAPY PROGRAM

After tendon transfer surgery for wrist and digital extension, the arm is immobilized in a plaster cast for 4 weeks. The position of immobilization is with the elbow flexed to 90 degrees, forearm pronated maximally, and the wrist extended from 30 to 45 degrees. The MP joints of the fingers are extended to neutral. If transfers are completed for thumb

extension and/or abduction, the thumb is immobilized as well. The IP and MP joints are extended completely, and the thumb is abducted and extended at the carpometacarpal (CMC) joint. Only the IP joints of the fingers remain free. The long arm cast is necessary to prevent supination of the forearm and to protect the pronator transfer. In this position of immobilization, tension is taken off the tendon transfer junctions, and healing takes place without overstretching or rupturing the transfers. During the immobilization period, shoulder motion is maintained with flexion/extension, abduction/adduction, and rotation exercises. IP joint flexion and extension exercises also are done for each of the fingers.

Mobilization and reeducation

Mobilization and tendon transfer reeducation exercises begin 4 weeks after surgery. At this time a removable thermoplastic splint is fabricated to protect the transfers from

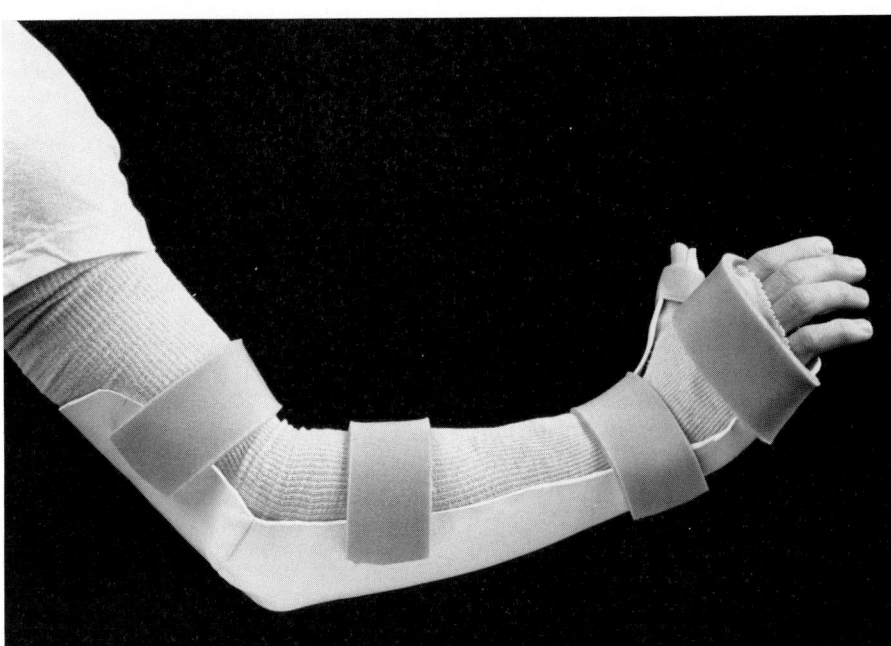

Fig. 53-12   A thermoplastic splint is constructed at 4 weeks after surgery to protect the transfers but can be removed for exercises.

overstretching (Fig. 53-12). Protective splinting is necessary for another 3 to 4 weeks for a total of 7 to 8 weeks after surgery. The thermoplastic splint is fashioned after the postsurgical cast. It protects the patient when he is sleeping or riding in a car or during situations when the arm may be forced into an overstretched position. Initially the splint is removed during the exercise periods and when the patient is bathing or dressing. It is removed more frequently as light activities are incorporated into the exercise and therapy program.

Individual joint range-of-motion exercises are done in the first week of mobilization (Fig. 53-13). Exercising individual joints that were immobilized for 4 weeks will not overstretch tendon transfers. Attention is focused at the MP joints of the fingers. These joints are most susceptible to debilitating extension contractures after postoperative immobilization. The MP joints are exercised with the wrist and the IP joints of the fingers extended. In this manner, flexion and extension of the MP joints are maximized with the least amount of tension on the tendon transfers. In addition to the MP joint exercises, other joints are isolated and range-of-motion exercises are carried out. For example, elbow flexion and extension exercises are done while the forearm is maintained in pronation and the wrist and fingers are held in extension. Exercises for forearm rotation are performed with the elbow flexed and the wrist and fingers maintained in extension. Gentle, active-assisted wrist flexion and extension exercises are done while the elbow is held flexed, forearm pronated, and the fingers positioned in extension. Assistance is needed with extension of the wrist, because the tendon transfer does not function well at this early stage of the mobilization process. Other exercises include gentle, active-assisted range-of-motion for thumb IP, MP, and CMC joints. Care is taken to mobilize individual joints of the thumb and avoid composite IP and MP flexion and abduction to the fifth metacarpal head. Composite motion stretches the thumb transfers too vigorously.

Exercises are performed in the clinic by the therapist, and by the patient at home as well. A home exercise program is outlined in both written and verbal form. The patient is told to remove the splint six to eight times daily and to practice the individual joint range-of-motion exercises ten times.

During the first week of mobilization, attention is also given to the various forearm and hand scars, which may be hypersensitive but most often are just thick and attenuated to the skin and deeper soft tissue structures. Friction massages with a lubricating cream or lotion are done to soften the scar and mobilize adjacent skin and subcutaneous tissues. Hypersensitive scars are desensitized by rubbing progressively coarser fabrics and materials over the scars (see Chapter 56). Transcutaneous electrical nerve stimulation (TENS) is necessary if conventional desensitization techniques are not effective.

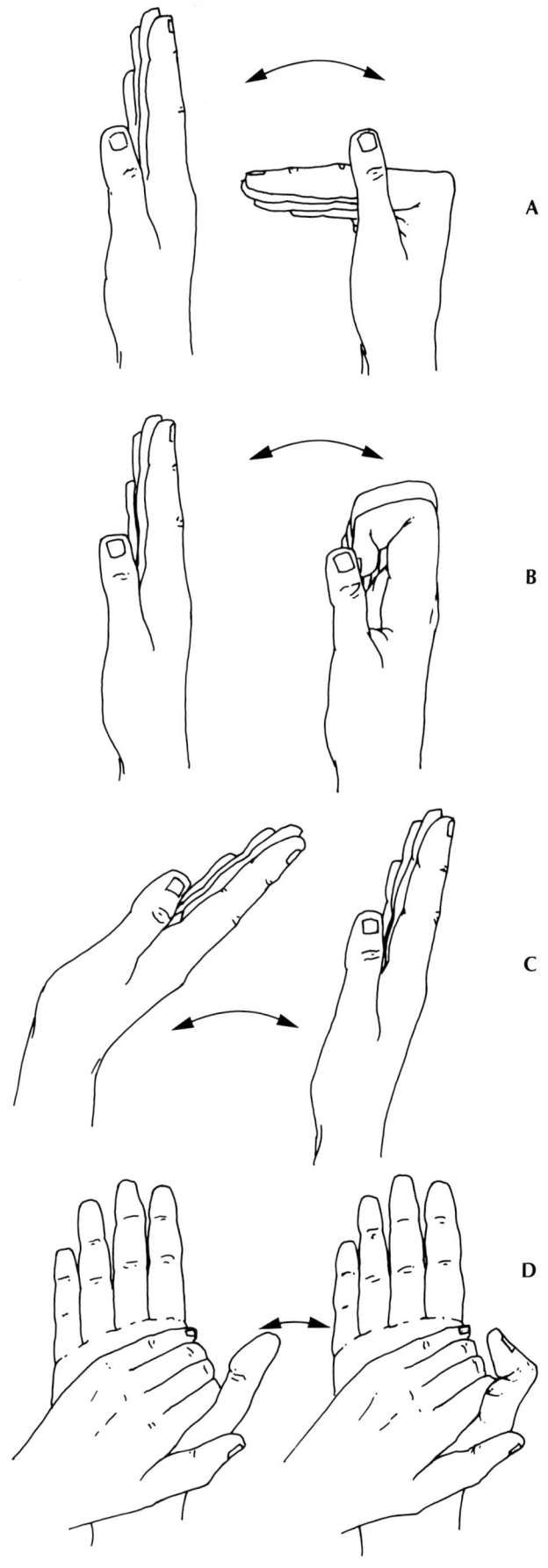

Fig. 53-13 Gentle exercises are performed initially to improve range of motion of individual joints. The metacarpophalangeal joints of the fingers are most susceptible to contracture following tendon transfer surgery. **A,** Gentle metacarpophalangeal flexion and extension with the interphalangeals extended. **B,** Interphalangeal joint flexion and extension with the metacarpophalangeals extended as much as possible. **C,** Gentle wrist flexion to neutral position. **D,** Thumb interphalangeal joint flexion and extension.

Gentle therapeutic heat (from 40° to 45° C) applied in the form of hot packs, paraffin, or fluidotherapy is helpful in increasing elasticity to the tissue as well as reducing joint stiffness and improving blood flow. The patient is instructed to use moist heat at home two or three times daily for 20 minutes.

In the second week of mobilization or the sixth postoperative week, attention is turned to the tendon transfers themselves. Activating the appropriate muscle for a certain task is difficult or easy, depending on the muscles used for transfer and the preoperative training used. Muscles used for normal tenodesing patterns of wrist flexion with digital extension are fairly easy to reeducate. For example, if the flexor carpi ulnaris is used for finger extension, the patient is asked to gently flex the wrist in an ulnar direction while extending the fingers. Performing this motion on the uninjured hand first helps the patient visualize and understand what the therapist is trying to accomplish. Once the patient understands the concept, the motion is attempted on the reconstructed hand. As the patient slowly flexes the wrist, extension of the fingers occurs at the MP joints. The tendons of the extensor digitorum communis muscle across the metacarpals standout slightly, indicating activation of the transfer. Care is taken to avoid wrist flexion past neutral, because this promotes extensor tendon tightness or tenodesis, not pure tendon transfer activity. Therefore the patient should maintain some wrist extension position while attempting to extend the MP joints. Early training attempts result in rapid muscle fatigue. It is not uncommon for the patient to perform only a few repetitions before the transfer tires. The patient must be encouraged to stop exercising when this happens and to not force the muscles to perform. Slow, controlled, and precise contractions are practiced to promote and develop good patterns of motion.

When the palmaris longus is used for thumb extension, the same tenodesing pattern of wrist flexion with digital extension is practiced. The patient palpates and observes contraction of the extensor pollicis longus tendon above the anatomic snuff box when the appropriate muscle is activated.

A reeducation challenge occurs when the finger flexors are transferred to digital extensors. Flexor digitorum sublimus to the extensor digitorum communis or the extensor pollicis longus transfers are prime examples. Greater patient concentration and cooperation are required to achieve extension of the digits with the sublimus transfer.

For MP joint extension of the fingers, the patient is taught to extend these joints while flexing the IP joints of the fingers. In this "claw" position, all long flexors are activated, including the one used for the extensor transfer. For the thumb the patient can perform the same claw movement with the fingers while attempting to abduct and extend the thumb.

A tendon transfer that has excellent reeducation potential is the pronator teres to extensor carpi radialis brevis. The pronator teres is a strong muscle and is the primary pronator of the forearm. Therefore substitution patterns do not threaten the reeducation process. The patient is asked to pronate the forearm while the elbow is extended to achieve wrist extension. Extension occurs in a radial direction only because of the absence of the ulnar wrist extensors but nonetheless is adequate for functional grasp.

During the retraining sessions special care must be taken to keep the wrist and digital extension transfers from overstretching. Simultaneous wrist flexion and composite finger flexion are avoided for 7 weeks after surgery. Wrist flexion is limited to 10 to 30 degrees past neutral until this time.

In addition to specific muscle retraining exercises, other light activities are incorporated into the treatment and exercise program as the patient begins to activate transfers more effectively. This usually takes place late in the second week of mobilization. Light pickup activities, such as the Minnesota Rate of Manipulation, offer excellent training techniques for normal tenodesing. Other repetitive grasp and release exercises are included to provide visual feedback and ensure normal patterns of motion. For thumb transfers, twisting activities, such as nut and bolt assembly, promote extension and abduction.

Mechanical facilitation techniques using faradic stimulation, vibration, or tapping provide additional feedback to help the patient identify the appropriate muscles for the new task. Biofeedback exercises are an integral part of the ther-

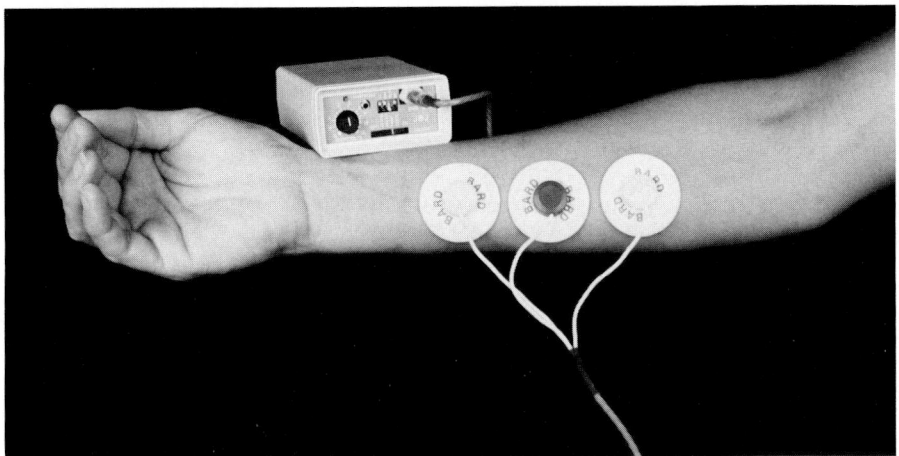

Fig. 53-14 Visual and auditory biofeedback techniques help patients become aware of muscles used for transfer procedures.

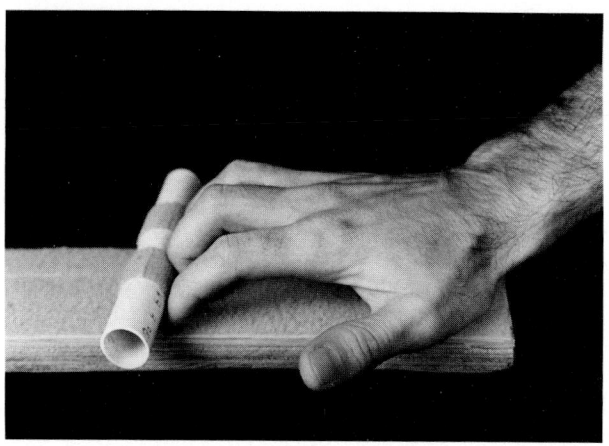

Fig. 53-15 Pushing Velcro dowels on a board exercises the extensor mechanism and strengthens transferred muscle.

apy program especially when antagonistic muscles are used for tendon transfers. A biofeedback machine with auditory or visual signals helps the patient relax or contract the appropriate muscles during reeducation (Fig. 53-14). For example, if the flexor digitorum sublimus of the middle finger is used for extension of the fingers, an electrode is placed over its muscle belly in the forearm. A loud tone indicates contraction of the correct muscle on attempted extension of the fingers. Auditory feedback is especially helpful in the early phases of training when there is little visual evidence of the transfer working. Similarly, biofeedback can be used to relax antagonistic flexors that may be cocontracting as the patient tries to extend the fingers too vigorously. Electrodes are placed on adjacent flexor muscle bellies, and the patient attempts to keep the auditory tone to a minimum.

At 7 weeks after surgery, dynamic splinting is initiated if extrinsic extensor tightness is apparent, but even with dynamic splinting, it is rarely possible to get full composite wrist and digital flexion. If the patient can flex the wrist to 20 degrees past neutral with the fingers fully flexed, functional problems are not significant.

A proximal interphalangeal joint flexion contracture may develop in a finger if its sublimus is used for transfer. Exercises and dynamic splints are incorporated at this time to return the joint to its supple nature.

Strengthening

Resistive exercises are introduced at 8 weeks and protective splinting discontinued. By this time the patient should be capable of using the transfer unconsciously. Manual resistance for wrist and finger extension begins by applying gentle resistance to the dorsum of the wrist and fingers, progressing to light weights for wrist extension and a Velcro dowel board for finger extension (Fig. 53-15).

Resistance can be increased by using various tools on the BTE work simulator for forearm rotation, wrist extension, and grip strengthening. A hand gripper is issued for home exercises along with Theraputty for resistive finger and thumb extension.

SUMMARY

The results of tendon transfer for radial nerve injuries are generally very good. With a conscientious preoperative and postoperative therapy program, maximum potential can be achieved.

REFERENCES

1. Boyes JH: Bunnell's surgery of the hand, ed 4, Philadelphia, 1964, JB Lippincott Co.
2. Burkhalter WF: Tendon transfers as internal splints. In Omer GE and Spinner M, editors: Management of peripheral nerve problems, Philadelphia, 1980, WB Saunders Co.
3. Colditz JC: Splinting for radial nerve palsy, Hand Ther 1:1, 1987.
4. Green DP: Radial nerve palsy. In Green DP, editor: Operative hand surgery. New York, 1988, Churchill Livingstone, Inc.
5. Daniels L and Worthingham C: Muscle testing: techniques of manual examination, ed 3, Philadelphia, 1972, WB Saunders Co.
6. Hollis I: Innovative splinting ideas. In Hunter JM and others, editors: Rehabilitation of the hand. St. Louis, 1978, The CV Mosby Co.
7. Kendall H, Kendall F, and Wadsworth G: Muscles: testing and function, ed 2, Baltimore, 1971, Williams & Wilkins.
8. Laseter GF and others: Rehabilitation: tendon transfers. In Hunter JM, Schneider LH, and Mackin EJ, editors: Tendon surgery in the hand, St. Louis, 1987, The CV Mosby Co.
9. Omer GE: Tendon transfers in radial paralysis. In Hunter JM, Schneider LH, and Mackin EJ, editors: Tendon surgery in the hand, St. Louis, 1987, The CV Mosby Co.
10. Riordon DC: Radial nerve paralysis, Orthopedic Clinics of North Am, April 1974.
11. Spinner M: Injuries to the major branches of the peripheral nerves of the forearm, Philadelphia, 1978, WB Saunders Co.
12. Sunderland S: Nerves and nerve injuries, ed 2, London, 1978, Churchill Livingstone, Inc.
13. Tajima T: Tendon transfers in radial nerve palsy: recommended choices based on retrospective analysis of methods used and their follow-up results. In Hunter JM, Schneider LK, and Mackin EJ, editors: Tendon surgery in the hand, St. Louis, 1987, The CV Mosby Co.
14. Thomas FB: An improved splint for radial (musculospiral) nerve paralysis, J Bone Joint Surg 33B:272, 1957.

54

Preoperative and postoperative management of tendon transfers after median nerve injury

Barbara Goodwyn Stanley

The median nerve plays a vital role in normal hand function by controlling precision pinch, contributing to power grip, and providing sensation to a major portion of the volar surface of the hand. When the median nerve is injured, the resultant functional loss can be substantial. Tendon transfer, a surgical procedure in which a tendon is moved from one insertion to another, can offer the successful restoration of function when motor return is no longer possible.

This chapter will discuss the rehabilitation of tendon transfers following median nerve injury, including preoperative and postoperative evaluation and treatment. Surgical procedures will be highlighted when they apply to the development of the preoperative and postoperative programs. Emphasis will be placed on the opponensplasty, a tendon transfer to restore thumb opposition, since it is the most frequently performed transfer in the upper extremity.

INDICATIONS FOR TENDON TRANSFER

Injury to the median nerve can result from nerve laceration, disease, or compression. Injuries that occur at or above the elbow are referred to as high-level injuries; they affect the extrinsic and the intrinsic median innervated musculature. High-level injuries result in the functional loss of pronation, radial deviation of the wrist, and flexion of the thumb, index, and middle fingers, as well as loss of thumb opposition. The basic requirement for restoration of motor function is the recovery of finger and thumb flexion, as well as thumb opposition. Low-level injuries are more common, generally resulting from glass lacerations or knife wounds at the wrist and are usually associated with injury to other structures in the hand. They affect only the median innervated intrinsic muscles of the hand and result in the functional loss of opposition (Fig. 54-1, *A*). The loss of sensibility in the thumb, index, and middle fingers may prove more disabling to the patient than the significant motor loss from either a high- or low-level injury.

The indications for tendon transfers following median nerve injury vary according to the level of the injury, the quality of motor return that has occurred, the functional requirements of the patient, and the preference of the surgeon. For example, variations in innervation by the median and ulnar nerves may allow satisfactory positioning of the thumb, eliminating the need for an opponensplasty in 30% to 40% of the patients with complete median nerve lacerations.[17] With high-level injuries, extrinsic flexor return generally occurs, making tendon transfers for finger flexion rarely necessary.[5] Unfortunately, reinnervation of the in-

trinsic muscles is less likely with a high-level injury, resulting in the need for an opponensplasty to restore opposition. Concerned that joint stiffness will result from disuse, some surgeons prefer not to wait the many months necessary to determine if reinnervation of the intrinsic muscles will occur.[5] They may elect to perform tendon transfers soon after the neurorrhaphy, especially when thumb opposition is needed, so that the transfer can work as a substitute during regrowth of the nerve, while at the same time preventing contractures and eliminating the need for external splinting. Still other surgeons prefer to wait until they are certain that reinnervation will not occur before performing tendon transfers.

PREOPERATIVE EVALUATION

The initial evaluation establishes baseline information from which to plan a preoperative therapy program and to compare postoperative results. The information provided may also help the surgeon select the appropriate muscle-tendon unit to be transferred and the distal attachment site. The preoperative evaluation should include the following.

Sensibility

Sensibility testing should include assessment of light touch–deep pressure using the monofilaments from the Semmes-Weinstein pressure aesthesiometer, as well as two-point discrimination testing to assess the functional sensibility necessary for fine motor tasks.[18,19] Retesting should be performed on a bimonthly basis to monitor sensibility return.

Skin condition

When evaluating the quality of the skin, the therapist should note sympathetic changes such as dryness, skin non-elasticity, and soft tissue atrophy. Subdermal scarring resulting from the initial injury or from subsequent surgery should be noted, particularly when it lies in the path of a potential tendon transfer.

Range of motion/deformity

A complete range-of-motion (ROM) examination is performed. Special attention is given to the following motions, which may be limited because of median nerve paralysis: forearm pronation, wrist flexion and extension, full passive mobility of the thumb web space, and circumduction of the carpometacarpal (CMC) joint of the thumb.

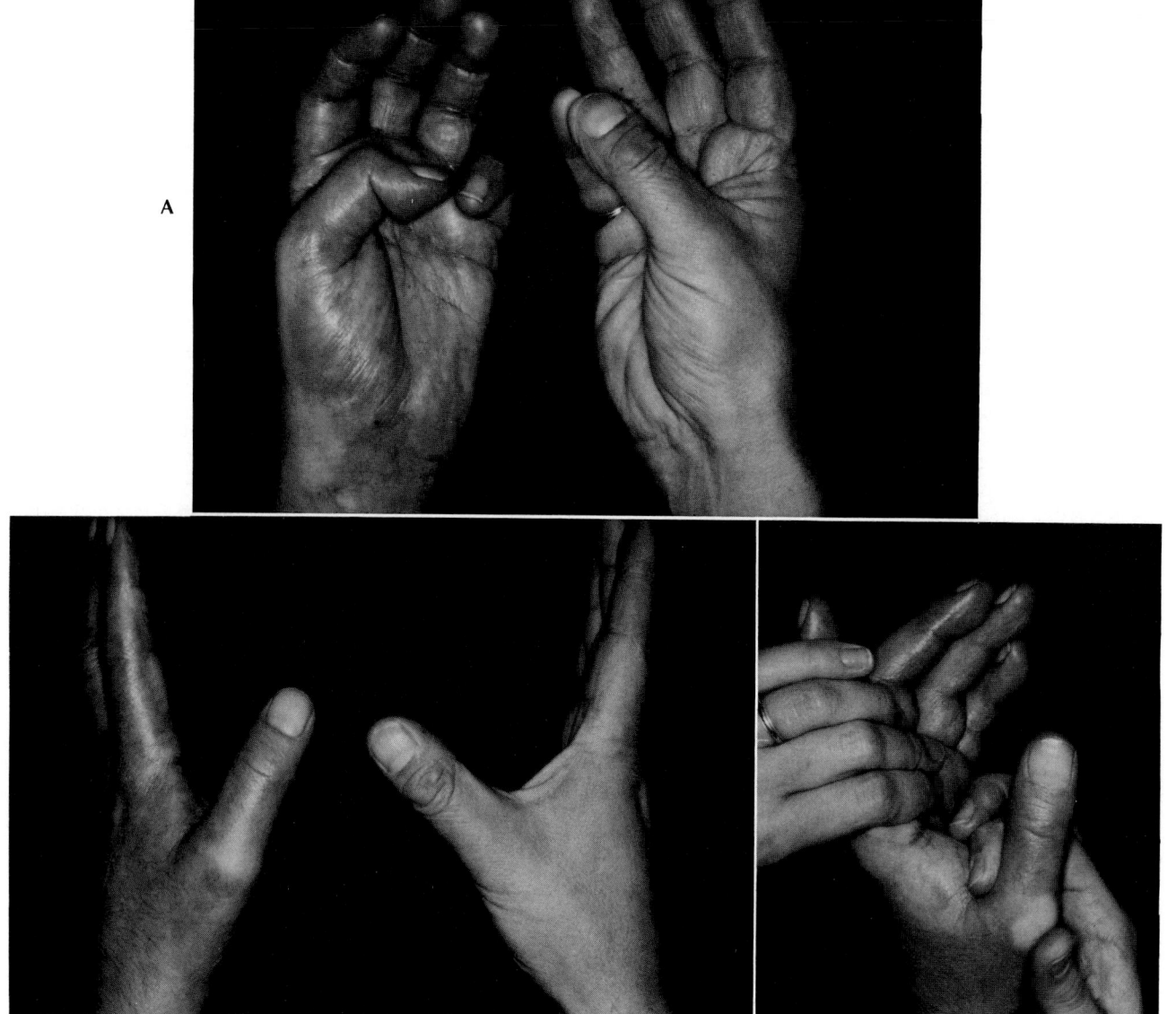

Fig. 54-1   A, With low-level median nerve injuries, attempts at oppostion result in adduction, supination, and flexion of the thumb. **B** and **C,** Shortening of the dorsal skin and fascia of the web prevent both active and passive opposition of the thumb.

Strength

A manual muscle test is performed to assess the progress of returning muscle strength and to test for potential muscle donors. Gross grip and pinch measurements are recorded.

Trick movements are frequently seen with median nerve injuries because of the frequency of anomalous innervations. Discussed below are some of the more frequently seen trick movements associated with median nerve injury.

Forearm pronation. It is important to palpate the pronator teres during active forearm pronation or when maintaining the pronated position against resistance. The therapist should be aware that substitution by the brachioradialis can pronate the forearm from full supination to a neutral position from which gravity can complete full pronation. If the elbow is kept positioned by the patient's side, the pro-

nating effect of shoulder internal rotation can be eliminated.

Wrist flexion. Palpation of the flexor carpi radialis (FCR) during forced wrist flexion is necessary because functional wrist flexion can still be produced by the flexor carpi ulnaris (FCU) or the abductor pollicis longus, even in the absence of the FCR.

Interphalangeal joint flexion of the thumb. The flexor pollicis longus is evaluated with the thumb adducted along the radial aspect of the index finger. This positioning prevents the trick distal interphalangeal (DIP) joint flexion that results by radially abducting the thumb and extending the wrist, thereby pulling on the inert flexor tendon.[20]

Palmar abduction of the thumb. Palmar abduction is tested in a plane at right angles to the palm with the first metacarpal of the thumb held over the metacarpal of the index finger. This position tests the intrinsic abductor pollicis brevis, flexor pollicis brevis, and the opponens muscle. If the thumb deviates toward the radial side of the hand, the patient is substituting with the abductor pollicis longus. Weakened palmar abduction can still be seen in the presence of complete median nerve lesions. This is attributed to an unusually large deep portion of the flexor pollicis brevis, which is normally supplied by the ulnar nerve and the presence of an anomalous or double innervation of the intrinsic thenar innervated muscles.[20]

Opposition of the thumb. Opposition is tested by having the patient touch the tip of the thumb to the tip of the little finger. If done correctly, the thumbnail should be parallel to the nail of the little finger.

Flexion of the DIP joints of the fingers. When testing for flexor digitorum profundus (FDP) function, the wrist is held in neutral, the index metacarpophalangeal (MP) and proximal interphalangeal (PIP) joints stabilized in extension and the DIP joint actively flexed. The same procedure is repeated for the middle finger.

Flexion of the PIP joints of the fingers. When testing for the flexor digitorum superficialis (FDS), the therapist should hold all the fingers in extension except for the finger being tested. The patient is asked to bend the tested finger at the PIP joint. Any tension felt at the distal phalanx indicates substitution by the flexor digitorum longus (FDL) muscle.

Hand function

Functional testing is helpful in quantifying the degree of disability resulting from the median nerve deficit. The Moberg Pickup Test is appropriate for testing median or combined medioulnar lesions.[15] The value of the test lies in the examiner's observations of prehension and substitution patterns when vision is occluded. The Jebson-Taylor hand function test is a timed, unilateral functional hand skills test that focuses on everyday activities such as writing and eating.[9] Even though the test has standardized norms, the patient's results cannot be accurately correlated with these norms because they are based on speed of performance and do not take into account altered prehensile patterns.[1]

Patient's attitude and expectations

The patient must have realistic expectations regarding the outcome of the surgery. Disappointment will inevitably occur if the patient anticipates the restoration of normal function. Educating the patient regarding the importance of his cooperation in the preoperative and postoperative therapy phases will facilitate the rehabilitation process.

Photographic documentation

Photographs or videotapes of the patient taken before surgery are an excellent tool for comparing postoperative results, especially pictures of the patient attempting thumb opposition, abduction, and finger flexion or a videotape of the patient performing the Moberg Pickup Test or Jebson-Taylor hand function test.

PREOPERATIVE THERAPY

Once it is determined that the patient is a candidate for tendon transfers following median nerve injury, the following preoperative factors should be addressed.

Improve skin condition

The preoperative program should strive to improve skin condition so that soft tissue contractures and subdermal scarring do not limit motion following the tendon transfer. This is especially true if the scarring is located in the path of the potential tendon transfer. Lanolin or oil massages should be initiated by the therapist and continued by the patient at home. Compression in the form of Elastomer* or Otoform-K† can be used to minimize established scar.

Restore passive range of motion

Restoring joint ROM before surgery helps eliminate postoperative complications. Any limitation in joint motion that is present before surgery, or is not resolved at the time of surgery, will become more difficult to treat following the postoperative period of immobilization. The preoperative program can use passive manual stretching, active ROM, joint mobilization, continuous passive motion, and splinting to reduce limitations in passive motion. Even though the goal is to obtain full passive motion of all joints in the hand and wrist, the motion of thumb opposition and pronation, as well as wrist flexion and extension, deserves special consideration and will be discussed further in detail.

Thumb opposition and pronation. The primary reason for failure following opponensplasty is contracture of the first web space (Fig. 54-1, *B* and *C*).[2,3,12,14] In the median nerve–injured hand, the unopposed adductor and extensor pollicus longus muscles cause the thumb to assume a position of adduction and supination. With time, this may result in shortening of the dorsal skin and fascia of the web, contracture of the adductor muscle, and limitations of the carpometacarpal (CMC) joint of the thumb. If the problem is not resolved before surgery, the tight web will limit the thumb in abduction and pronation, regardless of the type of transfer performed. Any attempts at pinch between the thumb and index finger with incomplete thumb pronation will only result in further supination of the thumb, overpowering the transfer and reinforcing the old pattern of thumb supination and adduction.

Splints such as an opponens splint or C-bar splint are effective in stretching out the tight web into abduction. It is important to mold the splint with the thumb in palmar abduction rather than radial abduction because more skin and tissue are necessary to achieve palmar abduction than radial abduction. Care should be taken when molding the splints so as not to stretch the thumb distal to the MP joint, inadvertently applying stress to the ulnar collateral ligament (Fig. 54-2). The splint should be remolded when the patient's thumb can be passively stretched into more abduction than the splint maintains. Unfortunately, the opponens splint is ineffective in promoting the pronation component of opposition. Effective splinting for the motion of pronation is difficult at best and is usually so involved that it is discarded by the patient. Awareness of the problem and early prevention through regular passive manual ROM is the therapist's best defense against formation of this frustrating contracture. The patient should be instructed to stretch the thumb into opposition by applying force at the thumb metacarpal, not the phalanges (Fig. 54-2). If limitations cannot be

*Dow Corning Corp., Midland, Mich.
†Dreze, Inc., Unna, West Germany.

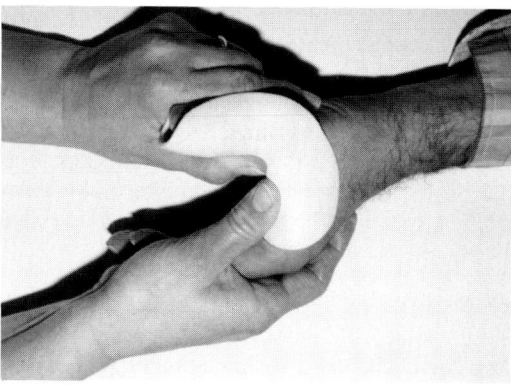

Fig. 54-2 When a thumb web-stretching splint is fabricated, forces should be applied below the metacarpophalangeal joints of the thumb and index finger to prevent strain on the collateral ligaments.

Table 54-1 Possible transfers following median nerve injury

Needed function	Possible motor
Flexion of index and middle finger	Flexor digitorum profundus tenodesis Extensor carpi ulnaris
Thumb flexion	Brachiolradialis
Thumb opposition	Extensor indicis proprius Flexor digitorum superficialis (3,4) Extensor carpi radialis longus Abductor digiti minimi Extensor digiti minimi Extensor carpi ulnaris Palmaris longus

worked out conservatively, a Z-plasty or extensive excision of the deep fascia in the thumb-web space must be done surgically.

Wrist flexion and extension. When the surgical plan involves transfers for the restoration of extrinsic flexor function, full wrist motion is essential. When the extensor carpi radialis longus is transferred to the profundi tendons of the index and middle fingers, a mechanical problem arises because the excursion of the profundus muscle is 50 mm, whereas the excursion of the wrist extensor is only 30 mm.[4] The surgeon may need to place the transfer under excessive tension to accommodate for this difference in excursion. The resultant limited excursion may prevent full extension of the index and long finger, reducing hand function and eventually leading to the formation of flexion contractures. This problem can be adjusted by the patient if full wrist motion is available. By using a dynamic tenodesis approach, wrist flexion will allow full finger extension, and wrist extension will produce full, strong flexion of the involved fingers. The same situation applies when the brachioradialis is considered for restoring flexion of the distal phalanx of the thumb. In this case, obtaining full thumb interphalangeal flexion and extension before surgery is just as important as obtaining full wrist motion.

Isolate potential transfer/maximize strength

Once the muscle to be transferred has been selected by the surgeon, preoperative training should include instructing the patient to isolate the action of the muscle (Table 54-1). This can be accomplished by teaching the patient to palpate the muscle and tendon, or through the use of biofeedback training. Once the patient is able to contract the muscle without assistance, a resistive exercise program for that particular muscle should be performed daily. Brand is a firm believer that it is possible to increase muscle strength before and after transfer with sustained exercise.[3] Because of the 4- to 5-week immobilization period that follows surgery, a generalized preoperative strengthening program will minimize the effects of muscle atrophy in the upper extremity.

SURGICAL CONSIDERATIONS

It is important for the therapist to understand the surgical procedure performed in order to plan and implement an effective therapy program. The therapist must know which motor was used, the direction of pull, and the type and location of the distal insertion. For example, not every surgical procedure for the opponensplasty transfer will give the same result; some will produce more thumb abduction, whereas others may stress thumb flexion. The most frequently used transfer for restoration of opposition uses the superficialis tendon of either the long or the ring finger that is rerouted through a pulley near the pisiform and inserts on the thumb at the insertion of the abductor pollicis brevis. The FDS is second only to the extensor carpi radialis longus in best approximating the force and motion required for full thumb opposition.[6] The Camitz procedure, which uses the palmaris longus tendon lengthened by a strip of palmar fascia and attached at the insertion of the abductor pollicus brevis, will provide excellent abduction but very limited pronation. A therapy program that focuses on thumb pronation following this transfer will only result in frustration for the therapist and the patient.[19] On the other hand, the Royle-Thompson opponensplasty offers good MP flexion and thenar stability, as well as thumb pronation, but it is limited in producing thumb abduction. This is because the transfer uses the FDS motor/tendon through a pulley in the volarcarpal ligament, aligning the transplant with the course of the short flexor.[21] This particular transfer is best suited for combination median/ulnar lesions, when a compromise must be made between restoring thumb opposition and thumb adduction.[5,7,16]

The type of distal attachment will also affect the subsequent therapy program. Some surgical procedures call for a bony attachment of the distal tendon, whereas others may advocate weaving the tendon into another tendon. Active motion may be started earlier with bony distal attachments because they tend to be more secure than tendon-to-tendon attachments.

Postoperative motion will be influenced by the location of the distal attachment. With a transfer of the FDS, Brand recommends attaching one slip of the tendon to the abductor pollicis brevis and one slip to the adductor insertion to increase the pronation effect. With low-level median nerve injuries, especially combined median and ulnar nerve injuries, flexion of the thumb across the palm is achieved by the use of the flexor pollicis longus, which provides the patient's only form of pinch. Once the opponensplasty is performed, this chronic pattern of pinch using the flexor pollicis longus may override the transfer. To compensate for this, the Riordan method attaches the transferred tendon to the abductor pollicis brevis tendon, but continues distally to insert on the hood of the thumb MP joint and to the extensor pollicis longus tendon over the proximal phalanx. By increasing the power of extension at the interphalangeal joint of the thumb, the opponens transfer is allowed to work without the overpowering pull of the flexor pollicis longus. Unfortunately, this transfer also produces 30% to 40% less thumb pronation than other transfers.[6] This particular transfer will be mentioned again in the discussion on immobilization and transfer retraining.

POSTOPERATIVE THERAPY

The postoperative rehabilitation will be approached in three phases: phase I corresponds to the period of immobilization, phase II is the initiation of active motion, and phase III focuses on strengthening and coordination training. These phases of therapy correspond to the stages of internal healing that occurs within the hand. During phase I, complete immobilization of the transfer is required to protect the tendon juncture from external stress while the healing process begins. By the third or fourth week, the tensile strength of the new collagen is sufficient to allow gentle active ROM but resistance exercises should not be initiated until the sixth postoperative week.

PHASE I: IMMOBILIZATION (1 to 3, 4 weeks)

Immobilization allows the transfer to heal in the desired position with a minimal amount of tension on the juncture site. It is possible to stretch a transfer that is too tight, but it is very difficult, if not impossible, to tighten a transfer that has been stretched and is too loose. For this reason, immobilization in the proper position for the required amount of time is essential for a good result. Jacobs and Thompson attributed insufficient postoperative immobilization with being a major cause of failure after opponensplasty and recommended a full 6 weeks of immobilization after surgery.[8] During this time the therapist should monitor the fit of the cast, begin edema control, and initiate active mobilization of the uninvolved joints. The original surgical plaster may be used for the entire immobilization period, or it may be replaced with a lightweight thermoplastic splint to increase comfort and accommodate for decreased edema.

Position of immobilization

Immobilization following transfers for low-level median nerve injuries. When an extensor tendon is used as a motor, such as the extensor indicis proprius, the wrist is held in 30 degrees of volar flexion and the thumb is held in opposition.[5] Because the extensor muscles are weaker than the flexors, extensor tendon transfers may be immobilized for 4 to 5 weeks and then protected for 2 additional weeks during which time the patient can remove the splint for exercise.[13,19] When a flexor tendon, such as the FDP, is transferred, the wrist is held in neutral and the thumb in opposition.[5] Immobilization should last for 3 to 4 weeks with additional protection for 1 to 2 weeks.[19]

If a flexion tenodesis of the PIP joint is performed to avoid formation of a secondary hyperextension deformity following transfer of the FDS, the PIP joint should be splinted in approximately 45 degrees of flexion for 3 weeks.[7] The tenodesis will eventually stretch out to allow full extension while preventing hyperextension of the PIP joint.

When the distal attachment of the transferred tendon is into the extensor pollicis longus, the thumb interphalangeal joint may need to be immobilized in full extension.[5]

Immobilization for transfers following high-level median nerve injuries. Immobilization following transfers for restoration of extrinsic flexor function requires the wrist and fingers to be held in flexion. Some surgeons prefer to treat the transfers to the fingers as they would a primary tendon repair. When extrinsic flexor transfers are done in combination with an opponensplasty, a compromise must be made in determining the best position for postoperative immobilization. It is important to remember that these are just guidelines. Because each case is different, the position of immobilization is best determined by the surgeon.

PHASE II: ACTIVE EXERCISE/TRANSFER RETRAINING (4 to 6 weeks)

By the fourth postoperative week the juncture site is strong enough to allow gentle active motion. Unfortunately, the same collagen formation that is uniting the juncture site may be producing adhesions between the tendon and the surrounding soft tissue. As the scar matures and strengthens over the next few months, it may limit the motion of the transferred tendon. The goal during this phase is to establish a therapy program that minimizes scar formation and uses active motion to facilitate a gliding tendon system without placing unnecessary stress on the juncture site.

Minimize scar

With removal of the splint, lanoline massage is initiated along the incision. Not only does the lanolin moisturize the skin, but the use of deep circular pressure while massaging softens the subcutaneous scar. The patient should be instructed to continue massaging four to five times each day at home. Some form of compression should also be incorporated in the home program.

Facilitate active motion

The goal of early transfer retraining is to achieve the best quality motion possible. For some patients excellent motion may occur with the first attempt, whereas other patients may require a period of transfer retraining. When establishing a transfer retraining program in the clinic and at home, some key principles should be remembered. Initial exercise sessions should be short, so as not to fatigue the transferred muscle. For example, 5 to 10 minutes of exercise, four to five times a day should be adequate in the beginning. The atmosphere should be quiet and the patient relaxed. The patient should avoid straining to move the transfer because this will cause cocontraction of surrounding muscles, which will only impede motion. For continued protection during the first week or two, the patient's hand should remain in the splint when not exercising. When not wearing the splint, the patient should be cautioned against any type of passive motion that may stretch the transfer.

Several techniques are available to assist motion. The initial exercise program should be simple so as not to overwhelm the patient. A good starting place is to ask the patient to perform a task that unconsciously uses the desired motion. For example, following an opponensplasty, the patient is requested to touch the thumb to the fifth finger rather than swinging the thumb out, up, and over. The movement will be easier if the hand is placed in a gravity-eliminated po-

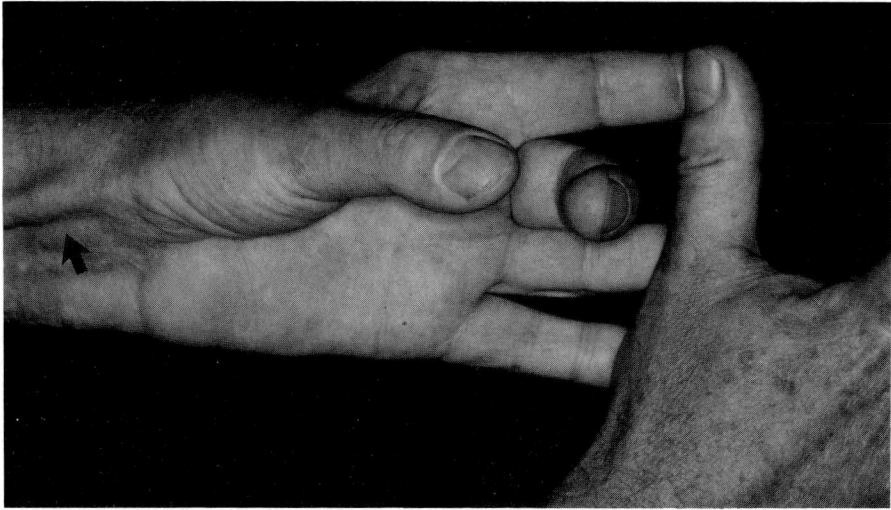

Fig. 54-3   Following a transfer of the flexor digitorum superficialis of the third finger for thumb opposition, active opposition is facilitated by asking the patient to perform the original motion of the transferred muscle, which in this case is isolated proximal interphalangeal joint flexion of the third digit. Note the visibility of the transferred tendon with this exercise.

sition. Some patients find it helpful to perform the desired motion on the uninvolved hand, as well as the involved hand. Once the patient is comfortable moving the transfer, the quality of the motion becomes the focus. In the case of an opponensplasty, emphasis is placed on full thumb pronation and pulp-to-pulp pinch. Even a small amount of motion using the correct pattern of movement is preferable to the old pattern of thumb flexion and adduction.

If the patient continues to have difficulty producing quality motion of the transfer, the following techniques can be evaluated and incorporated into the patient's program.

Facilitative techniques. Several facilitative techniques can be considered. Tapping over the tendon insertion or stroking and pressure over the muscle belly of the transferred tendon may encourage active motion. The therapist may also ask the patient to perform the original motion of the transferred tendon. For example, when the FDS of the third finger has been transferred for thumb opposition, the patient is asked to flex the PIP joint of the third finger while holding the remaining fingers in extension (Fig. 54-3). With transfer of the extensor carpi radialis longus to the profundus tendons of the index and middle fingers, attempts at active wrist extension will contract the transferred tendon, resulting in active flexion of the index and middle fingers. This should not be a difficult transfer to retrain because wrist extension and finger flexion are synergistic motions that occur naturally together. Because of the length-tension relationship of a muscle, active motion can be facilitated by placing the transferred tendon/muscle unit on *gentle* stretch at the time of contraction. For example, active thumb opposition may be facilitated by having the patient actively adduct the thumb before initiating the movement.

Functional activities. Activities that unconsciously use the desired motion can be incorporated so long as they do not provide resistance. Following an opponensplasty, suggested activities would be to have the patient cut with scissors or manipulate a washer between the thumb and each finger while maintaining contact of the thumb pad with the

center hole.[19] Light pickup activities not only promote opposition but also finger and thumb flexion following transfers for restoration of extrinsic flexor function. Toward the sixth postoperative week the patient can begin paper-crumpling activities to promote finger flexion. Lay a single sheet of newspaper or a paper towel on a flat surface and ask the patient to use his fingers, particularly the second and third fingers, to crumple the paper into a ball in his palm. Once the patient progresses to resistance activities he can then end the activity by making a tight fist around the crumpled paper.

Training splints. Following an opponensplasty, if the patient is having difficulty achieving thumb abduction and pronation during opposition, a piece of flexible material, such as an AlumaFoam* splint, can be bent into a U shape and placed between the thumb and fifth finger (Fig. 54-4). The patient should then attempt active opposition using the splint as a guide to align the thumb in proper abduction and pronation. Occasionally a dominating flexor pollicis longus will override a weak opponensplasty and will pull the thumb into its old pattern of flexion and adduction. Splinting or casting of the thumb interphalangeal joint into extension will counteract the flexor pollicis longus, allowing easier transfer motion (Fig. 54-5, *A* and *B*). This should be used as a training tool rather than a permanent functional splint. If the patient is still unable to overcome the flexion force of the flexor pollicis longus after a few weeks of training with the splint, the patient can be taught to thrust pinch during functional use of the hand. With thrust pinching the opposing finger pushes the interphalangeal (IP) joint of the thumb into hyperextension, allowing the MP joint to flex.[12]

Patients with tendon transfers for high-level injuries may have difficulty obtaining pull-through of the tendons transferred for finger and thumb flexion, especially when the MP joint is flexed. When this occurs, the therapist should instruct the patient to bend the PIP and DIP joints while the

---

*Conco Medical Co., Bridgeport, Conn.

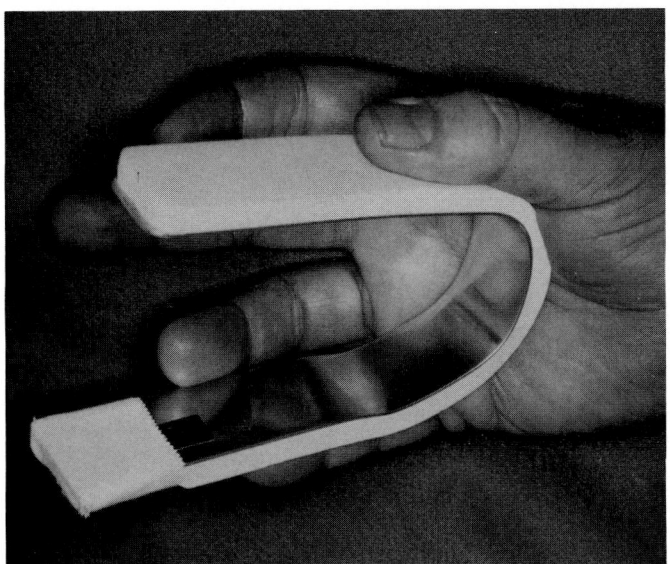

Fig. 54-4   Abduction and pronation is facilitated by using this "U-shaped" splint as a guide to properly align the thumb following an opponensplasty.

MP joint is blocked in extension. A Bunnel block is an excellent tool to assist the patient with this exercise. Or an exercise splint that holds the MP joints in extension yet allows full finger flexion can be fabricated for use during functional activities. As IP joint flexion improves, gradually adjust the splint to allow more MP joint flexion until the patient is able to make a full fist. A similar splint can also be fabricated for the thumb, which blocks the MP joint in extension, isolating the excursion of the transfer to work on the thumb IP joint.

Modalities. If motion continues to be limited, modalities such as biofeedback can be incorporated. This is particularly true when the lack of motion appears to be caused by muscular cocontraction. To test for cocontraction following

transfer of the brachioradialis to the flexor pollicis longus, ask the patient to actively bend the IP joint of the thumb. While the patient is actively bending the thumb, gently push the thumb into further flexion. If resistance is felt when pushing into flexion—resistance that is not caused by passive joint restriction—it is because cocontraction is present as the thumb extensors oppose the transfer. In a situation such as this, biofeedback can be used to relax the antagonist, in this case the extensor pollicis longus, allowing unopposed motion of the brachioradialis transfer. The biofeedback sensors can also be placed on the transferred muscle, such as the brachioradialis, to facilitate active motion. If motion is still limited, electrical stimulation can be used to refine the motion, giving the patient a sense of how the muscle works and what its action is. When using electrical stimulation, a faradic current that produces a tetanic-type contraction should be selected.[11] Electrical stimulation should not be used before the fifth postoperative week unless there is doubt about the continuity of the transfer.[22]

PHASE III: INCREASE STRENGTH/IMPROVE DEXTERITY (6+ weeks)

By the sixth week the tendon juncture sites are strong enough to withstand resistance. Passive stretching and splinting may be initiated to promote full passive ROM. Because the median nerve plays such an important role in pinch and grip, emphasis should then be placed on improving the patient's strength and coordination.

Restore passive range of motion

Limitations in ROM may be present because of joint restrictions, adhesions, excessive tension being placed on the transferred tendon at the time of surgery, or tendon/muscle shortening that occurred during the immobilization period. Gentle passive stretching exercises can be incorporated into the patient's home program four to five times a day. The use of modalities, such as a hot moist pack placed on the volar surface of the forearm and hand, will provide a combination of heat and stretch when extrinsic

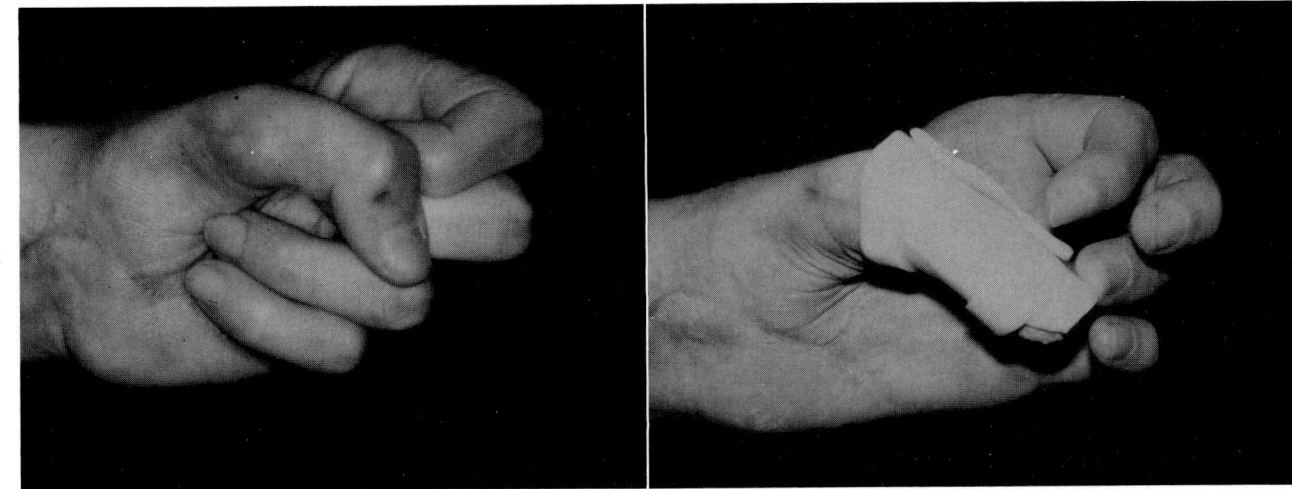

A   B

Fig. 54-5   **A,** In this median and ulnar nerve–injured hand, attempts at opposition following an opponensplasty result in thumb adduction and interphalangeal joint flexion because of the overpowering force of the flexor pollicis longus. **B,** Splinting the thumb interphalangeal joint in extension counteracts the pull of the flexor pollicis longus, improving opposition.

flexor tendon tightness is present following a transfer of the extensor carpi radialis longus to the finger flexors. For patients who have limited active motion of the transfer and appear to be developing excessive scar formation at the incision site, a more aggressive program can be initiated. Serially adjusted volar splints can be fabricated to gradually stretch the wrist and fingers into extension following transfers for restoration of extrinsic finger flexion. The splints can be made of either plaster or a thermoplastic material and should incorporate both the wrist and fingers (see Chapter 90). Most stretching splints are best worn at night so they can provide a prolonged gentle stretch without interfering with functional use of the hand.

Increase strength

Strengthening should progress gradually, with emphasis on the quality of motion of the transfer. If resistance exercises are initiated too rapidly, the patient will use stronger muscles to substitute for the transferred muscle in attempting to perform the desired motion.

Resistance exercises that isolate the transferred muscle can be developed with putty. For example, the patient can do a pinch pot for strengthening an opponensplasty, or do isolated finger flexion with putty to strengthen extrinsic flexor transfers to the index and middle fingers. The patient should start with a putty consistency that offers just enough resistance to allow completion of the motion and then progress to a more resistive putty as his strength improves. Because the transfer was performed to restore function, resistive exercises can be presented in the form of functional activities. Macramé, opening jars, and manipulating clothespins are a few resistive activities suitable for an opponensplasty and for strengthening extrinsic flexors following tendon transfers for high-level injuries.

A weight program should be initiated that strengthens not only the transferred muscle but also the entire upper extremity. Progressive resistive exercises using free weights is an excellent way to strengthen the wrist musculature. Strengthening of the extrinsic flexors is important following high-level injuries, especially when restoration of finger flexion is obtained by suturing the index and middle profundi tendons to the tendons of the ring and little profundi. This is because the ulnar innervated portion of the profundus muscle is now responsible for providing all of the power of finger flexion that was once provided by the profundus and superficialis muscles. Woodworking, or other functional activities that promote sustained grip are very effective in increasing strength and endurance of the extrinsic flexor muscles. Despite a strong transfer that results in excellent motion, wheel chair use, push-ups, and transfers are not allowed for 3 months following high-level median nerve transfers in spinal cord injuries.[10]

Improve coordination

Focusing on the functional use of the hand is a key element in the rehabilitation of the patient with median nerve tendon transfers. Initially the patient is instructed to perform gross prehensile activities, such as buttoning a shirt, tying a shoelace, or manipulating a coin. Emphasis should be placed on performing the task accurately rather than quickly. As the patient improves, more specific tasks, such as writing, knit-

ting, or dealing cards, can be incorporated into the therapy program.

The next phase of coordination training introduces speed as well as accuracy. The therapist should select a task that the patient is comfortable performing but also focuses on the speed with which the task is completed. Initially the practice sessions should be short. As the patient improves, increase the time that the activity is performed. The therapist should observe the patient's pattern of prehension closely and look for patterns of substitution.

The Moberg Pickup Test, the Purdue Pegboard Test, the Minnesota Rate of Manipulation Test, and the Jebson hand function test all offer excellent ways of measuring dexterity. The Purdue Pegboard Test is particularly helpful in evaluating fine prehensile ability and offering the examiner an opportunity to observe problems that may result from median sensory deficits.[1] If diminished sensibility is present, the functional result of the tendon transfer will be limited, even after successful surgery.

COMPLICATIONS

Problems of muscle/tendon imbalance can arise after tendon transfers, because the transferred muscle can no longer perform its original motion. For example, persistent flexion contractures of the PIP joint or swan-neck deformities have been reported in as many as 8% of cases where the superficialis tendon of the ring finger was used for a tendon transfer.[8] Usually the surgeon will try to prevent swan-neck deformities by reinforcing the volar plate during surgery. On the other hand, when excessive scarring results in flexion contractures of the PIP joint, the therapist must use passive stretching and splinting as early as the immobilization phase to prevent deformity. An extensor lag may also occur at the MP joint of the index finger after transfer of the extensor indicis proprius for an opponensplasty. Strengthening of the remaining extrinsic extensor should be encouraged to avoid this deficit.

Most authors agree that the primary reason for failure after opponensplasty is insufficient preoperative thumb motion.[2,3,8] Other common reasons for failure include adhesion formation[3] and technical failure[9] (see also Chapter 51). These findings reinforce the importance of a detailed therapy program to prevent adduction/supination contractures of the thumb and to minimize motion-limiting adhesion during the postoperative program.

SUMMARY

Rehabilitation of median nerve tendon transfer starts preoperatively by reducing joint contractures, increasing skin softness and mobility, and improving strength. The postoperative program will vary depending on the type of transfer that was performed. The period of immobilization will last from 3 to 4 weeks, allowing time for the juncture site to gain strength. Transfer retraining starts with gentle active motion and focuses on the quality of motion. Six weeks after surgery, strengthening exercises and coordination training are introduced. The return of functional sensibility is as important, if not more important, than the successful restoration of motion after median innervated tendon transfers.

REFERENCES

1. Baxter PL and Ballard MS: Evaluation of the hand by functional tests. In Hunter JM and others, editors: Rehabilitation of the hand, St Louis, 1984, The CV Mosby Company.
2. Brand PW: Clinical mechanics of the hand. St Louis, 1985, The CV Mosby Co.
3. Brand PW: Biomechanics of tendon transfers. In Hunter JM, Schneider LH, and Mackin EJ, editors: Tendon surgery in the hand, St Louis, 1987, The CV Mosby Co.
4. Burkhalter WE: Tendon transfers in median nerve palsy, Orthop Clin North Am 5:271, 1974.
5. Burkhalter WE: Median nerve palsy. In Green DP, editor: Operative hand surgery, vol 2, New York, 1982, Churchill Livingstone, Inc.
6. Cooney WP, Linsheid RL, and An K-N: Opposition of the thumb: an anatomical and biomechanical study of tendon transfers, J Hand Surg 9A:777, 1984.
7. Hill NA: Restoration of opposition for the paralysed thumb, Clin Orthop 61:234, 1968.
8. Jacobs B and Thompson TC: Opposition of the thumb and its restoration, J Bone Joint Surg 42:1015, 1960.
9. Jebson RH and others: An objective and standardized test of hand function, Arch Phys Med Rehabil 50:311, 1969.
10. Kelly CM and others: Postoperative results of opponensplasty and flexor tendon transfer in patients with spinal cord injury, J Hand Surg 10A:890, 1985.
11. Kolumban SL: Postoperative physical therapy of the hand, Surg Rehab in Leprosy, from the Schieffelin Leprosy Research Sanatorium.
12. Kolumban SL: Preoperative and postoperative management of tendon transfers. In Hunter JM and others, editors: Rehabilitation of the hand, St Louis, 1984, The CV Mosby Co.
13. Mackin EJ: Therapist's management of tendon transfers. Presented at the symposium and workshop, Rehabilitation of the Hand, Philadelphia, 1984.
14. Mayer L: Operative reconstruction of the paralyzed upper extremity, J Bone Joint Surg 21:377, 1939.
15. Moberg E: Objective measurement for determining the functional value of sensibility in the hand, J Bone Joint Surg 40B:454, 1958.
16. Riordan RC: Tendon transfers in hand surgery, J Hand Surg 8:748, 1983.
17. Rowntree T: Anomalous innervation of the hand muscles, J Bone Joint Surg 31B:505, 1949.
18. Semmes J and others: Somatosensory changes after penetrating brain wounds in man, Cambridge, Mass, 1960, Harvard University Press.
19. Smith RJ and others: Rehabilitation: tendon transfers. In Hunter JM, Schneider LH, and Mackin EJ, editors: Tendon surgery in the hand, St Louis, 1987, The CV Mosby Co.
20. Sunderland S: Nerves and nerve lesions, ed 2, New York, 1978, Churchill Livingstone.
21. Thompson TC: A modified operation for opponens paralysis, J Bone Joint Surg 24:632, 1942.
22. Toth S: Therapist's management of tendon transfers, Hand Clin 2:239, 1986.

BIBLIOGRAPHY

Brand PW: Functional aspects of tendon transfers. Presented at the meeting of the American Occupational Therapy Association, Milwaukee, Wis, 1976.
Littler JW: Dynamic splinting and immobilization. In Converse JM, editor: Reconstructive plastic surgery, vol 4, Philadelphia, 1964, WB Saunders Co.
Omer GE: Evaluation and reconstruction of the forearm and hand after acute traumatic peripheral nerve injuries, J Bone Joint Surg 50A:1454, 1968.
Riordan DC: Tendon transfers in median and ulnar nerve paralyses, J Bone Joint Surg 35A:312, 1953.
Riordan DC: Surgery of the paralytic hand. In American Academy of Orthopaedic Surgeons: Instructional course lectures 16:79, St Louis, 1959, The CV Mosby Co.
Riordan DC: Tendon transfers for nerve paralysis of the hand and wrist, Curr Pract Orthop Surg 2:17, 1964.
Schneider LH: Opponensplasty using the extensor digiti minimi, J Bone Joint Surg 51A:1297, 1969.
Tubiana R: Tendon transfers for restoration or opposition. In Hunter JM, Schneider LH, and Mackin EJ, editors: Tendon surgery in the hand, St Louis, 1987, The CV Mosby Co.

55

Implications of electroneuromyographic examinations for hand therapy

Arthur J. Nelson

The electroneuromyographic (ENMG) examination may be helpful to the practitioner by determining: (1) if lack of movement is mechanical or neurologic, (2) if atrophy is caused by disuse or denervation, (3) if pain is from nerves within the hand or outside the hand, (4) if the current lesion is superimposed on other lesions, and (5) where the nerve lesion is located.

THE ELECTRONEUROMYOGRAPHIC EXAMINATION

The ENMG examination usually consists of two parts, the nerve conduction studies and the electromyographic portion. The nerve conduction studies (NCS) include the study of the conduction velocity of segments of peripheral nerves, the distal latency of motor and sensory components of peripheral nerves, the amplitude and rate of rise of the evoked response wave, and the change in amplitude from one site of stimulation to another. The electromyographic (EMG) studies are needle electrode studies conducted on selected skeletal muscles under the circumstances of rest and various degrees of contraction.

A typical examination of the hand should involve NCS of the median and ulnar nerves, both motor and sensory components, bilaterally. Depending on the hand deficits encountered, the radial nerve may also be included. The muscles of the hand typically used when performing NCS are the abductor pollicus brevis as a distal muscle of the median nerve, the abductor digiti minimi manus of the ulnar nerve and the extensor indicus (proprius) muscle of the radial nerve. These same muscles would also be examined with a needle electrode to identify the EMG action potentials from them at rest and when contracting moderately and maximally. In addition, EMG examination is conducted on intrinsic hand muscles if their deficiency is questionable. Extrinsic forearm muscles of importance to hand function that might be studied are the flexor carpi ulnaris, flexor carpi radialis, flexor pollicus longus, extensor pollicus longus, abductor pollicus longus, flexor digitorum sublimus (FDS), and extensor carpi radialis longus and brevis. The principle involved in selection is examination of a distal muscle and comparison with a more proximal muscle of the same nerve to identify the status of the nerve through its regional segment. For example, if the abductor pollicis brevis reveals neuropathic EMG findings, but a more proximal muscle innervated by the median nerve, such as the FCR, reveals no neuropathic EMG discharge, it becomes additional evidence of the lesion being distal to the latter muscle. Anomalous innervation patterns must be considered always in the interpretation of studies. Overconfidence in conventional innervation should be avoided, and when patterns appear outside the expected pattern, deductive reasoning coupled with sufficient muscle exploration should provide a logical outcome.

Similarly, when denervation of the median nerve occurs, the entire thenar muscle mass is not lost, but some innervation is provided by way of the ulnar nerve. Thus, if one is not precise in localization of the needle electrode, it is possible to misinterpret active innervation in muscles as being supplied by the median nerve when in actuality the apparent action is eminating from deeper muscles innervated by the ulnar nerve.

The proximal and distal principle is also applied when evaluating hand function that may be affected by more proximal neural elements such as the plexus or nerve roots (see Fig. 55-6). Clearly, muscles that are innervated by the posterior primary ramus must be included to differentiate between cervical nerve root and more distal problems such as the brachial plexus.

For clarification of the electrophysiologic report it is helpful to review the neuropathology of the peripheral nerve. The clinical problems that may be encountered in hand care can be subdivided into disorders of the nerve trunk, the axon, its myelin sheath, the motor neuron, the myoneural junction, and the skeletal muscle.

MOTOR UNIT

The anterior horn cell, its axon, and all the muscle fibers supplied by that one neuron are called the "motor unit." The number of muscle fibers supplied may vary from 5 or 6 to 1000 or more. Because the all-or-none law ensures complete firing of the whole motor unit, the smaller the ratio of axon to muscle fibers, the more refined the motor control possible. The smaller motor units are recruited first in progressively more intense contractions, followed by the larger ones in an orderly progression according to the size-order principle of Henneman.

The EMG appearance of a motor unit has a biphasic or triphasic pattern with a duration of 6 to 12 msec and an amplitude of 300 μV to 5 mV or more. The duration of the motor unit is dependent on the spread of the end plate zone as it relates to the total length of the muscle fibers. For example, the abductor pollicis brevis muscle has an end plate zone that represents 50% of the total length of the muscle fibers, resulting in a longer duration than the biceps brachii muscle, which has an end plate zone of approximately 10% of the total length of the muscle, which results

714

in a shorter duration of the motor unit action potential (MAP).

The amplitude of the motor unit potential is the result of the relative size of the muscle fiber membranes that are active within the same time frame. The EMG potential visualized on the screen is a compound one resulting from an amalgamation of all the individualized muscle fiber discharges. The size of the muscle fibers (membranes) coupled with the total conductive area available within the muscle contributes toward the amplitude of the MAP. Amplitude comparisons are difficult to use for assessment of strength, but large differences from one side to the other can have value in making clinical judgments about the relative strength of a given muscle.

Skeletal muscle is structured in such a way that the motor units are in a somewhat checkerboard configuration. According to Buchthal,[1] a motor unit occupies approximately 5 to 11 mm^2 within a given muscle. If the electrical discharges are to be effectively displayed on the electromyogram, the needle electrode must be within the vicinity of the motor unit that is active. Movement of the electrode even a few millimeters away from the active motor unit will decrease the amplitude of the response by 90%. This factor explains why surface electrodes are not employed for the accurate delineation of the motor unit potentials and are used for the determination of gross electrical discharge from a whole muscle.

The nerve trunk contains thousands of axons with varying diameters organized in bundles with connective tissue sheaths. These bundles are then enveloped in an overall sheath called the "epineurium." The speed of conduction along the nerve trunk is a reflection on the collective diameters plus the amount of myelin coating of the axons contained therein. Because the fibers are in a braided configuration, it is necessary to provide a more than maximum (supramaximal) stimulation to ensure that all the fibers are stimulated.

NEUROPATHOLOGIC CORRELATES OF ELECTROMYOGRAPHIC FINDINGS

Disorders of the motor neuron, its axon, the nerve trunk or any of its components, the myoneural junction, or the muscle itself may be involved in hand problems. To rank neural disorders affecting the hand from the most frequently encountered to the least frequently encountered, one would start with entrapment of the peripheral nerve, which is quite commonly encountered. Then come peripheral nerve injuries, followed by axonal or motor neuron disease, which is not a commonly encountered problem, and, finally, myoneural junction and myopathic disorders, which are rarely encountered.

Entrapment syndromes

There are many sites of entrapment or compromise of peripheral nerves, but a common site is the *median nerve at the wrist*. It is believed that the median nerve is compromised by either lack of space in the carpal tunnel or inflammation of the tendons, blood vessels, or other contents of the tunnel.[2] The compression affects the fibers that are more metabolically dependent, the thickest fibers. Many sensory fibers are in the thicker category, except for those involved with pain and temperature, which thereby results

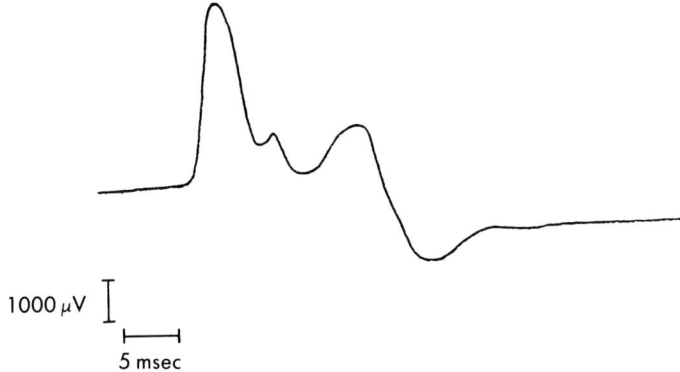

Fig. 55-1   Evoked motor response of ulnar nerve at the wrist.

1000 μV

5 msec

in a loss of light touch sensibility but a retention of pinprick and crude touch sensibility. The thicker motor axons may also be affected early in the course of this disorder. Because the evoked electrical stimulation of the nerve trunk will activate all the fibers capable of conduction, the ones that conduct the fastest will be observed as the first component of the response wave (Fig. 55-1). In some patients the sensory component will reveal a prolonged latency, but the motor component may be within normal limits (that is, 3.7 ± 0.3 msec for the median nerve at 8 cm from stimulating to pickup electrode). When the distal latencies are near the borders of normal, it usually proves helpful to compare the two limbs and to compare the findings with the distal latency of the ulnar nerve because there should be no more than a 1 msec difference with distance held constant.

Another feature of the evoked response to note is the amplitude of the evoked response. If loss of the amplitude is more than 50% when compared with the opposite side and the recording technique has been completed with care on both sides, it is to be noted and may be of clinical significance if other electrical findings correlate with this change.

The EMG may reveal MAP changes such as increased amounts of polyphasic MAP in muscles innervated by the median nerve distal to the wrist where the nerve has been compromised for several months (Fig. 55-2). It is essential to survey muscles from each of the major peripheral nerves and the cervical nerve roots to assure that the complaints are not from other neuronal disorders.

Many patients with carpal tunnel syndrome reveal bilateral changes in their median nerves. When this occurs, it is important to determine if the other peripheral nerves, such as the ulnar nerve, also manifest distal delays or evidence or neuronal disorder that might suggest a peripheral neuropathy multiplex. Persons suffering from generalized peripheral nerve disease are typically more vulnerable to nerve compression. The therapist should know if the compression lesion is superimposed on a generalized peripheral neuropathy because the therapist must exercise care when providing splinting that will avoid compression of other peripheral nerves while keeping the median nerve from being compressed against the carpal tunnel's superior surface when in extension. A neutral wrist position provides the least compromise of the nerve.

The case that presents a mild distal delay of the motor

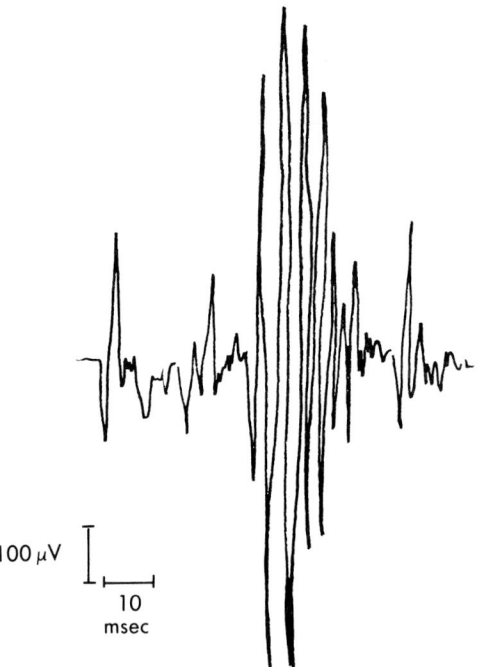

100 µV

10
msec

Fig. 55-2 Chronic neuropathic motor unit potential and normal motor units.

or sensory component of the median nerve is typically treated with neutral wrist support coupled with steroid infiltration of the carpal tunnel. No exact boundaries of the test results determine surgical intervention or conservative care. Operative intervention is considered most effective in those suffering from more prolonged latencies that are the result of mechanical disruption of the nerve without other neuropathic disease present.

Tardy ulnar palsy

Another compressive disorder of somewhat frequent occurrence is compromise of the ulnar nerve at the region of the elbow. One should flex the elbow while recording to avoid a false-positive determination of slowing of conduction across the elbow. A significant slowing of conduction of the ulnar nerve across the elbow may or may not result in any motor impairment of the intrinsic hand muscles innervated by the ulnar nerve, because slowing does not necessarily impair function.

In addition to a local change in the conduction velocity across the elbow, as the compression of the ulnar nerve continues there will be a reduction in the amplitude of the sensory nerve action potential (SNAP). At this stage the MAP may be of normal amplitude. There may be concomitant EMG changes consisting of complex, polyphasic MAPs that result from collateral sprouting from the noncompressed intact axons to the denervated muscle fibers. The muscles affected will extend from the elbow distally to the forearm muscles and to the intrinsic hand muscles innervated by the ulnar nerve. When there is motor affectation, it is helpful to determine by means of the electrophysiologic data if there is axonal degeneration. The use of electrical stimulation would be influenced by the presence of axonal degeneration. In a recent study by Pachter and

others[6] they noted that electrical stimulation performed when fibrillation had decreased resulted in greater muscle bulk and strength than a nontreated sample of rats with peripheral nerve lesions. Vrbová indicates that stimulation of a fibrillating muscle tends to decrease the fibrillation, and she suggests that too early stimulation may retard reinnervation.

What type of stimulation is best? The duration of the pulse of direct current applied by the negative pole should be as close to the optimal chronaxie value (minimal duration) as possible. Also, it appears that the more the pattern of stimulation simulates functional motion or is actually involved in performance of some activity, the more effective the reinnervation. This would mean placing the electrical stimulation on muscles during the time they are needed to carry out an activity.

As soon as the muscle is fully reinnervated, conventional strengthening through active and resistive exercise should begin. The relative intensity of muscle contraction may be monitored with a surface electrode EMG. Training with an EMG should use the information to predict the muscle's needed output. This is best done if the activity is performed rhythmically and with a regular, predictable pattern to it. To simply confirm muscle action with EMG feedback is of some help, but more gains can be obtained by using this information for prediction of outcome.

Patients should be instructed to keep their forearm in supination if they have to rest on the affected elbow, because this will draw the ulnar nerve away from the site of pressure.

Deep branch of the ulnar nerve

The deep branch of the ulnar nerve, which sweeps into the palm of the hand, is subject to entrapment in the canal de Guyon. This involvement is tested by stimulation of the ulnar nerve at the wrist and placement of pick-up electrodes over the abductor digiti minimi muscle and over the first dorsal interosseous muscle. One might expect that a latency difference between the two pickup points will be less than 0.7 msec. Additionally, one might expect to find normal EMG findings in the hypothenar musculature, but the other intrinsic musculature innervated by the ulnar nerve may reveal neuropathic EMG changes, such as polyphasic MAPs, or spontaneous activity at rest, such as positive sharp waves or fibrillation potentials, as well as reduction in the recruitment of MAPs.[3]

Electrical stimulation would be instituted when fibrillation had subsided. After a 6- to 8-week interval, the evoked response should be repeated for comparison with the previous study to determine changes in latency or amplitude to determine the prognosis.

Deep interosseous branch of the radial nerve

Protracted compression of the upper arm is most frequently a part of the history of patients' suffering from radial nerve palsy, but lead poisoning may also affect the radial nerve selectively. The deep interosseous branch departs from the main radial trunk in the region of the spiral groove of the humerus, and stimulation applied there is directed distally to pickup electrodes placed over an outcropping muscle on the dorsum of the forearm (such as the extensor pollicis longus). Another point of stimulation of this branch would be the anterolateral cubital fossa. If the nerve has a simple blockade of conduction (neuropraxia), typically there will be no response proximal to the area of the block but a normal response distal to it. The EMG findings in distal muscles will not reveal any evidence of denervation (such as fibrillation or positive sharp waves) in a neuropractic lesion. It is important to recall that if the distal portion of the nerve degenerates (as occurs in the Wallerian type) it could take 7 to 14 days; therefore the EMG taken during that interval will probably reveal an absence of MAPs but not a specific indication of axonal degeneration. If no EMG evidence of axonal degeneration occurs after 14 days, it is quite probable that the defect is one of blockade. Recovery may be expected spontaneously within the next 2 weeks if the lesion is a local block (neuropraxia).

Median nerve entrapped in pronator teres

The median nerve may be compromised in the region of the elbow, possibly where it pierces the pronator teres or where it passes beneath the ligament of Struthers. When this is the area of encroachment, it may be recognized by a loss of conduction of evoked responses from above the elbow through the forearm area. This is usually coupled with good conduction below the elbow (antecubital fossa). If the EMG detects evidence of axonal degeneration, such as fibrillation, positive sharp waves at rest, or increased polyphasicity with moderate contraction in the long flexor of the thumb and other muscles below the pronator teres, such evidence would implicate this proximal area. As the thenar muscles innervated by the median nerve should also reveal neuropathic EMG findings, a complete study must include muscles proximal to the wrist so that this identification of the lesion is ensured.

Deep interosseous branch of median nerve

The deep interosseous branch of the median nerve splits from the main trunk soon after it leaves the pronator teres and innervates the flexor pollicis longus and the pronator quadratus.[5] The electrodiagnostic findings will be confined to prolonged conduction time over this branch to the flexor pollicis longus or to the pronator quadratus, and if axonal degeneration has taken place only to these muscles, the EMG findings associated with denervation (such as fibrillation and positive sharp waves) will be localizing. The most obvious deficit functionally will be loss of flexion strength of the distal phalanx of the thumb. This lesion may easily be confused with the carpal tunnel syndrome. To distinguish between them, sampling from the flexor pollicis longus and the thenar musculature distal to the wrist as well must be conducted.

Peripheral nerve injuries of median and ulnar nerves

Traumatic lesions of the median and ulnar nerves induced by lacerations at the wrist are frequently encountered by the hand therapist. The electromyographer provides clarification of the extent of neural impairment. When tendons have been severed, it is sometimes difficult to determine if lack of motion is the result of pain and restriction or of denervation.[3]

During the denervation phase, fibrillation potentials of short duration (1 to 3 msec) and of relatively low amplitude (100 to 300 μV) and positive sharp waves (Fig. 55-3) may be seen 7 to 14 days from the time of the injury. When several months have passed, the fibrillation and positive sharp waves found at rest usually decrease. For monitoring

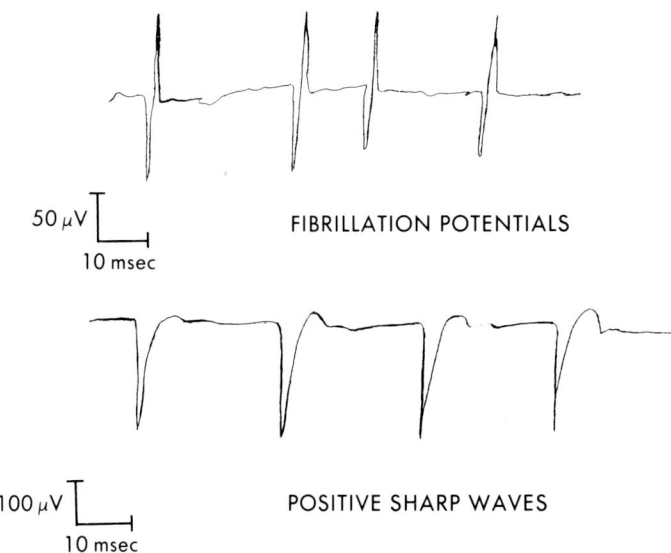

50 μV ⌐ 10 msec   FIBRILLATION POTENTIALS

100 μV ⌐ 10 msec   POSITIVE SHARP WAVES

Fig. 55-3   Denervation potentials at rest.

of the amount of spontaneous activity (fibrillation and positive sharp waves) the following four categories have been established:

1. Few scattered fibrillation potentials
2. Consistently found fibrillation potentials for brief periods
3. Relatively prolonged periods of fibrillation and trains of positive sharp waves
4. Prolonged periods of fibrillation potentials and sustained trains of positive sharp waves (Fig. 55-3)

The appearance of brief-duration, low-amplitude, polyphasic motor unit potentials (BLAP) (sometimes called "nascent" potentials) are indicative of reinnervation and typically precede the onset of clinical return of movement. At this stage, electrical stimulation and exercise are indicated, because the muscle has lost some of its denervation sensitivity and is physiologically capable of receiving electrical stimulation without detracting from reinnervation. As the muscle responds to activity and if resistance is added, the fibers hypertrophy and subsequently an increased amplitude of the MAP results. Possibly because of collateral sprouting (spreading of an endplate zone), the MAP increases its duration (to 20 msec or more). The combination of these two factors results in higher amplitude potentials and longer duration (15 to 20 msec) (HALD) (Fig. 55-2).

The intensity of exercise should be increased with graduated stress on the effected musculature so that the muscle will become capable of sustaining activity for the period of time required for accomplishing specified activities of daily living. For example, one should consider the duration of palmar prehension needed for bringing the utensil to the mouth and also for the repetition needed for feeding oneself a meal. What is the duration of total activity? How may rest be obtained and at what intervals? If the exercise program may be enhanced by use of EMG (integrated) information, the patient not only will get augmented sensory feedback but also will be provided with information about the efficiency of the muscle. When the EMG tracing line falls off, it can be the result of fatigue or it could also be caused by lack of effort. Sometimes a very highly motivated person may synchronize motor units in such a manner that the integrated EMG line becomes slightly increased over a previously maximum effort.[4]

FUNCTIONAL ELECTRICAL STIMULATION

The EMG findings also provide the therapist with information that is useful for initiation of functional electrical stimulation (FES). Stimulating weakened, denervated muscles can be more effective if included within a functional pattern of motion. The pattern of stimulation must take into consideration the rate of tension development, the amplitude or intensity of the contraction, and its duration. The number of repetitions is determined by the needs of the activity under usual circumstances. Most intrinsic hand muscle activity appears to involve rapid, mild-intensity contractions that are alternately sustained for several seconds, giving way to a low-grade activity that might be sustained for several minutes. This sequence should then be repeated for the usual duration of the activity (for example, from 6 to 10 minutes for feeding).

Radial nerve injury in spiral groove of humerus

Injury to the deep interosseous branch of the radial nerve results in loss of wrist and finger extension along with the extension and abduction movements of the thumb.

The evoked responses of this branch of the radial nerve result in amplitudes of approximately 4 to 7 mV. If axons are lost, that loss will be reflected in a proportional reduction of amplitude of the evoked response. The preinjury amplitude may be estimated by reference to the evoked response of the opposite nonaffected side.

The functional implication of reduced amplitude in the response wave would be a corresponding loss of strength in the early stages of the problem. As the intact axons sprout to the affected ones, the number of active muscle fibers increases proportionately. As they are exercised, the strength will be expected to increase progressively even if there may be no further reinnervation by the original axons that were damaged. If the percentage of damaged axons is considerable, the compensatory hypertrophy of the remaining intact fibers may not be adequate to bring the muscle tension to a functional level.

The EMG findings can be of further assistance by showing the relative number of motor units available, which is evidenced by the recruitment pattern during maximum effort. The smoother the progression of the recruitment of motor units from smaller to larger, the more refined the control will be. Where the larger motor units are available, the movements become tremendous and have an all-or-nothing quality.

Proximal peripheral nervous disorders

The hand may be affected by any number of problems affecting the peripheral nervous system. Electromyography can be helpful in delineating where the lesion may be located. In addition to the distal sites noted previously, there are some proximal lesions to consider, such as the brachial plexus or the cervical nerve roots or spinal cord.

Brachial plexus

Some typical electrophysiologic findings from a relatively acute brachial plexus lesion would typically include EMG findings consisting of fibrillation and positive sharp waves at rest, with diminished recruitment of motor units proportional to the compromise of the components of the brachial plexus. The anatomic pattern is of greatest importance for identification of the site of involvement. For example, if the hypothenar muscles and the extensors of the thumb are involved, it is evident that the problem is not confined to the ulnar nerve. It is possible that the disorder could result from involvement of two peripheral nerves, but as a general rule one should seek out a single source such as the lower trunk of the brachial plexus or the eighth cervical and first thoracic nerve roots.[7]

To further distinguish involvement between the lower trunk (brachial plexus) and the cervical nerve root, the evoked responses (conduction studies) can be instructive. The motor conduction studies will be normal because conduction does not change in axonal degeneration unless more than 80% of the fibers are degenerated. If a significant number of axons are lost, the amplitude of the evoked response will be reduced (especially when compared to the opposite side). If the problem is distal to the dorsal root ganglion, the sensory evoked response will be reduced proportional to the degree of affectation.

In compromise of the lower trunk, the sensory action potential (SAP) can frequently be reduced to 50% of the nonaffected side, whereas in cervical radiculopathies there is no reduction in the SAP (Fig. 55-4).

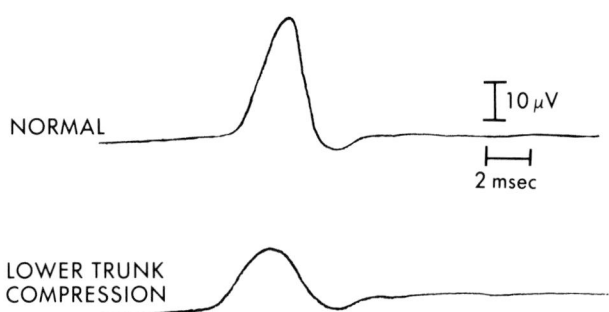

Fig. 55-4 Sensory action potential. Normal versus brachial plexus compression.

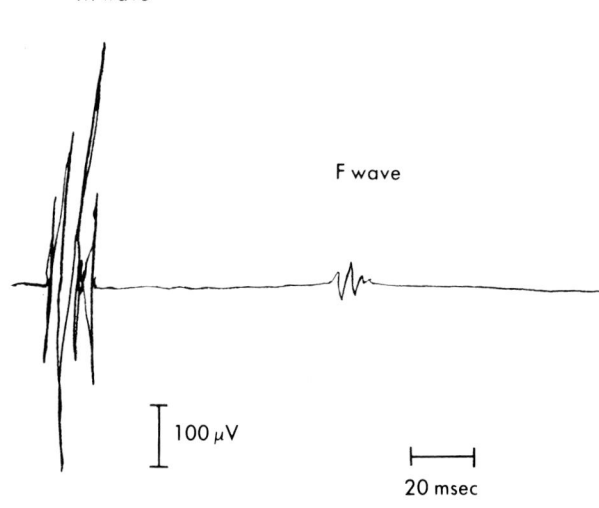

Fig. 55-5 Motor-evoked responses—M wave and F wave.

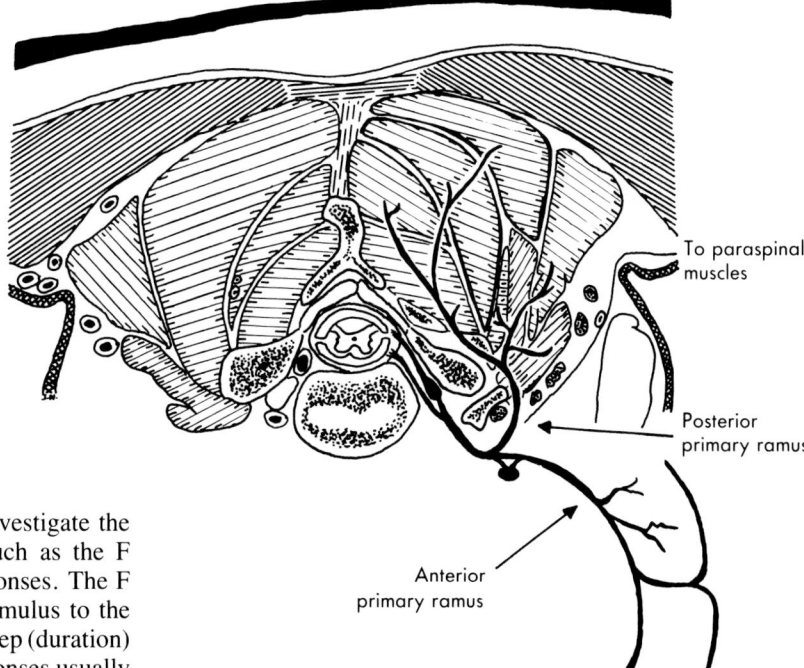

Fig. 55-6 Anterior and posterior primary rami.

Some conduction studies may be used to investigate the proximal portions of the involved nerves, such as the F wave or somatosensory cortically evoked responses. The F wave involves the delivery of an electrical stimulus to the median or ulnar nerve, and with a sufficient sweep (duration) available on the oscilloscope, two distinct responses usually are obtained (Fig. 55-5). The first, or larger, amplitude is the M response (the response obtained during conventional conduction studies), and the second, or smaller, amplitude (50 to 100 μV) will appear somewhere between 24 and 29 msec delay (latency). The longer the arm, the longer the latency will be; therefore the involved arm should be compared with that of the opposite side and measurements of each arm length be taken.

With pick-up electrodes affixed to the hand area of the somatosensory cortex opposite the stimulated median nerve, one may study the evoked responses elicited by a train of 500 stimuli to determine if there is any delay between Erb's point to the spinal cord. This type of study requires special instrumentation but can be an added valuable resource in differentiating between radiculopathies and distal peripheral nerve disorders.

The differentiation between a cervical radiculopathy and a brachial plexus lesion is furthered by EMG examination of the paraspinal muscles in the cervical area. If there are neuropathic EMG findings in the erector spinae muscles corresponding to the same segmental distribution through the anterior ramus, the lesion will be proximal to the division of anterior and posterior rami (Fig. 55-6).

A further distinction between ventral root and dorsal root involvement in cervical radiculopathies may be made on the basis of EMG studies and clinical symptomatology. In ventral root affectation, there will be more EMG findings associated with axonal degeneration (such as fibrillation, positive sharp waves, and complex MAPs). Deep throbbing or aching pain within the myotome is more typical of ventral root compression. The dorsal root symptom is characterized by lancinating or shocklike pain that follows the dermatome or sclerotome, reaching a maximum in the fingers or palm of the hand. These symptoms may also be correlated with disturbances in vasomotor tone. Dorsal root affectation will reveal neither peripheral loss of sensory response in conduction studies nor any positive EMG findings. Extensive disk protrusions may compromise both ventral and dorsal components, resulting in both sets of symptoms.

NEURONOPATHIES

ENMG is essential to the delineation of anterior horn cell disease in patients who demonstrate atrophy and wasting of intrinsic hand musculature plus difficulty chewing and swallowing or spasticity. In disorders such as amyotrophic lateral sclerosis, the intrinsic hand muscles frequently demonstrate EMG signs of denervation, such as fibrillation potentials at rest and diminution of motor unit recruitment. The conduction studies are usually within normal limits except for some loss of amplitude in the response wave. Because the reduced amplitude can also result from the more benign disuse atrophy, it must be correlated with EMG evidence of denervation, such as fibrillation at rest, to be indicative of anterior horn cell disease.

MYELOPATHIES

Myelopathies (spinal cord disorders) do not manifest specific EMG or conduction changes. Somatosensory evoked responses will be helpful in delineating spinal cord disturbances by monitoring conduction along the spinal cord. However, the detection of minor or early myelopathy may not be readily made with any certainty using current technology.

MYONEURAL JUNCTIONAL DISORDERS

The myasthenic syndrome and myasthenia gravis generally do not produce changes specific to the hand. When a patient manifests a generalized lack of endurance or weakness, one should conduct repetitive stimulation (Jolly test) studies to look for a decrement in the motor-response wave. Generally, in myasthenia gravis there is a decrement in the response to repetitive stimulation, whereas in the myasthenic syndrome there is a potentiated response after a brief

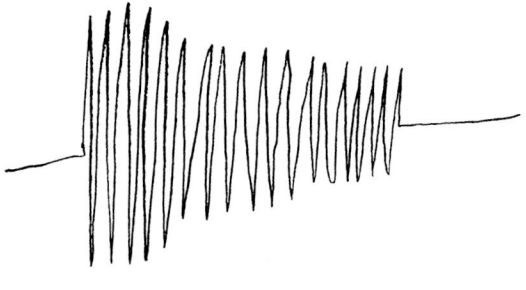

MYASTHENIA GRAVIS

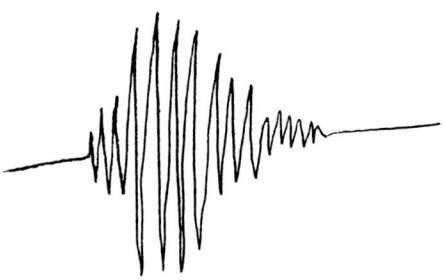

MYASTHENIC SYNDROME

Fig. 55-7 Response to repetitive stimulation in myasthenia gravis and in myasthenic syndrome.

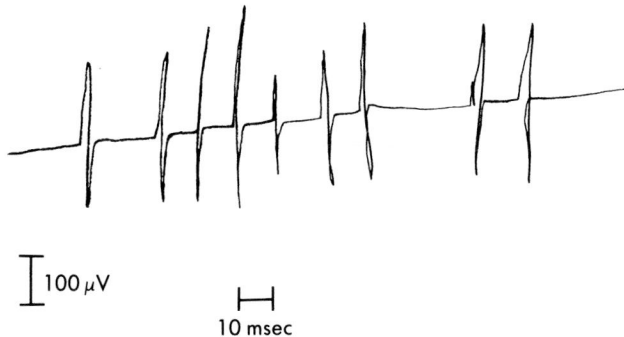

$$\mathbin{\text{I}} 100\,\mu V \qquad \vdash\!\dashv$$
$$\qquad\qquad\quad 10\ \text{msec}$$

Fig. 55-8   Myopathic motor unit potentials.

exercise bout, followed by a decrement of the response (Fig. 55-7).

MYOPATHIES

Many myopathic disorders are made manifest through weakness of the proximal muscles, and only relatively few myopathies manifest themselves with distal weakness. The majority of myopathies reveal EMG MAPs that are of brief duration and relatively low amplitude (BLAP potentials) with voluntary contractions. Another characteristic finding would be good recruitment (complete interference pattern) of motor units with relatively minor exertions (Fig. 55-8).

Some myopathies may manifest EMG changes that are more typically associated with neuropathic disorders. It is sometimes difficult to discern with electrophysiologic methods alone which type of disorder is involved. From the viewpoint of developing therapeutic strategies, the type of EMG findings are not specific, but fatigue is to be avoided for optimal care of persons with primary muscle disease. Exercise of myopathic muscle is indicated but not to the point of exhaustion.

SUMMARY

Conduction studies and EMG studies for the care of patients with hand disorders are mainly concerned with the identification of the site and nature of the lesion and its magnitude. Slowing of the conduction will not result in any significant loss of strength but rather a loss of motor control. Presence of conduction of evoked stimuli and a decrease in fibrillation after a peripheral nerve injury would signal the time to start electrical stimulation and eventually exercise. When weakness is present, the recruitment of motor units visualized on the EMG can assist in determining the optimal exercise or other treatment recommended.

Hand symptoms associated with neuropathies may be traced to lesions of the brachial plexus or cervical nerve roots, as well as to local lesions of peripheral nerves. The EMG can assist in localizing the lesion and therefore directing treatment at the correct area. EMG can also help determine when electrical stimulation may be most effective.

Differentiation between motor neuron disorder, muscle disease, myoneural junctional disorders, and neurologic problems is of importance to direct treatment to the source of the disorder.

REFERENCES

1. Buchthal F and Rosenfalck P: Action potential parameters in different human muscles, Acta Psychiatr Neurol Scand 30:125, 1955.
2. Eliasson SG, Prensky AL, and Hardin WB: Neurological pathophysiology, London, 1975, Oxford University Press.
3. Liveson J and Spielholz NI: Peripheral neurology, Philadelphia, 1979, FA Davis Co.
4. Nelson AJ, Moffroid M, and Whipple R: Relationship of integrated EMG to isokinetic contractions of ankle dorsi and plantar flexors. In Desmedt JE, editor: Recent advances in EMG and clinical neurology, vol 3, Basel, 1973, S Karger, AG.
5. Nelson RM and Currier DP: Anterior interosseous syndrome, Phys Ther 60:194, 1980.
6. Pachter BR, Eberstein A, and Goodgold JG: Electrical stimulation effect on denervated skeletal myofibers in rats, Arch Phys Med Rehabil 63(9):427, 1982.
7. Waylonis GW: Electromyographic findings in chronic cervical radicular syndromes, Arch Phys Med Rehabil 49:407, 1968.

56

Desensitization of the traumatized hand

Lois M. Barber

The patient with hypersensitivity occurring after hand trauma presents the physician and the therapist with a unique challenge, both in evaluation and in treatment of the problem. The lack of an objective assessment of both the complaint and the improvement, as well as the deficiency of published formalized treatment procedures, has made hand hypersensitivity particularly thought provoking.

The purposes of this chapter are to discuss the development of and indications for a method of desensitization treatment, to describe the Downey Hand Center Hand Sensitivity Test (DHCHST), an instrument for measuring the status and improvement of hypersensitivity, and to outline the progress of 124 patients who completed the desensitization test and treatment at the Downey Hand Center (DHC).*

LITERATURE REVIEW

Methods for decreasing hypersensitivity of the injured hand are just now appearing in the literature.[1,3,7,18] Several earlier approaches to the desensitization of painful scars and amputation stumps have been documented.[2,6,9,10,12-15] Rubin recorded complete relief of pain and tenderness caused by phantom limb, neuroma, and scar origin, in 23 of 37 areas of hypersensitivity, with the use of ultrasound treatment.[12] Vibration has historically been used in the treatment of hypersensitive scars. Russell and Wall theorized that the nerve fibers concerned with firing hyperpathic sensations are very easily traumatized into inactivity by a vibrator.[14,17] Hochreiter, in her study of the effect of vibration of 80 Hz on tactile sensitivity, stated that vibration results in an elevated tactile threshold and that the increase lasts for at least 10 minutes but not as long as 15 minutes, a duration indicating that vibration actually reduces tactile sensitivity.[8] Brown hypothesized that in dropping particles from a height over the involved area one can elicit a response similar to vibration.[3] Melzak relates that vibration is also able to modify the amount of pain produced by noxious stimulation of the skin in normal subjects.[10]

Russell theorized about the use of percussion to treat painful amputation stumps and phantom limbs. He posited that conduction in a mixed nerve is easily interrupted by repeated pressure without causing pain and that the regenerating nerve fibers, which form neuromas in an amputation stump, might well be even more vulnerable to minor trauma than normal nerves and nerve endings are. It was considered likely, therefore, that if painful neuromas are repeatedly percussed, their nerve fibers would gradually degenerate and be replaced by fibrous tissue.[15] A survey of phantom limb treatment lists a number of approaches to the problem of painful stumps in phantom limb, only one of which is stump conditioning or desensitization.[16]

Hardy described a sequential method of desensitizing the traumatized hand. Five levels of desensitization included use of paraffin, vibration, massage, constant touch-pressure, textures, object identification, and specific tools to simulate common job activities. Work simulation was included as a final level of the desensitization program.[7] Brown stated that desensitization techniques aided in the physiologic and psychological change toward normalcy and advocated the use of textural stimulation and the judicious use of vibration as well as the performance of functional activities as means of desensitization.[3]

A survey of 32 surgeons and therapists by me in 1982 indicated that desensitization is included as part of the treatment regimen of a number of therapists and physicians and that the majority of them would like to see a proved method of desensitization developed.

DEFINITIONS

Hypersensitivity, as used in this chapter, is defined as a condition of extreme discomfort or irritability in response to normally nonnoxious tactile stimulation.[20] It is important to point out that the hypersensitivity referred to throughout this chapter occurs at or near the injury site and is not to be confused with the general manifestations of pain, as seen in causalgia or the shoulder-hand syndrome.

Two relevant dictionary definitions of "desensitize" are as follows: "to lessen the sensitiveness of, to eliminate the native or acquired reactivity or sensitivity of an animal, organ, tissue, etc., to an external stimulus such as an allergen" (Random House Dictionary) and "to render less sensitive or insensitive as to light or pain" (American Heritage Dictionary).

Treatment in this chapter is defined as the use of modalities and procedures designed to diminish or reduce symptoms. Desensitization treatment as described here is specifically designed to reduce the symptom of hypersensitivity in the injured hand. Although a connection may be theorized, it is not to be confused with that used for sensibility reeducation.

DEVELOPMENT OF TREATMENT

After working with a significant number of patients at the Downey Hand Center, it became evident to the staff that the natural tendency for many patients was to protect the sensitive areas after injury or surgery. Use of parts of the hand commonly involved in pinch and grasp was avoided, a situation that resulted in awkward pinch patterns, such as

---

*Downey Community Hospital Hand Center, Downey, Calif.

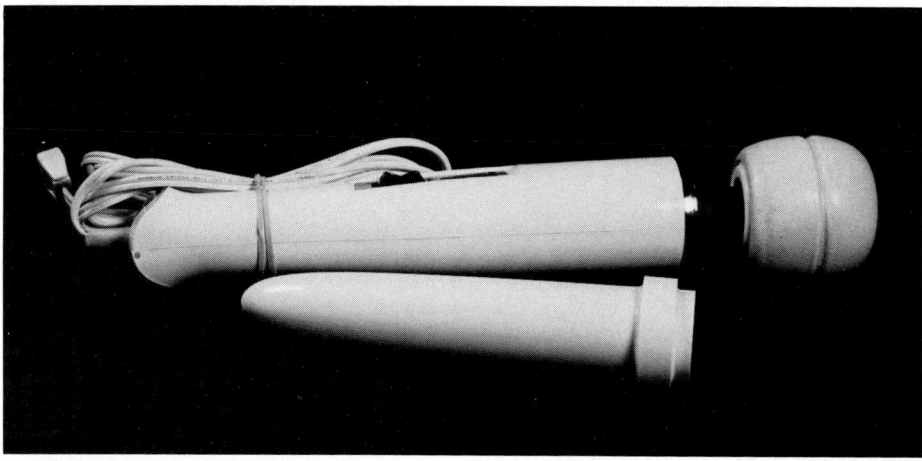

Fig. 56-1 Vibrators. Electric vibrator with speeds of 83 cycles and 100 cyles used for clinic treatment *(top).* Battery-operated vibrator with speeds of 100 cycles and 125 cycles used for home treatment *(bottom).* (Vibrators available from Fred Sammons, Inc, 145 Tower Drive, Burr Ridge, Ill 60521, BK 5207 and BK 5203.)

extensor habitus. Patients found use of the hand with areas of hypersensitivity dangerous in that when they were touched inadvertently they might withdraw and drop whatever they were working on, possibly hurting themselves or others. This condition was a definite deterrent to returning to work. Part of the therapist's role became to inform the patient that it was not only all right but actually beneficial to touch the hypersensitive areas.

In 1976, as a first step in organizing our program, a hierarchical method of treatment of the hypersensitive hand injury was begun at the Downey Hand Center. Our staff arbitrarily picked 10 different textures and 10 different particles and lined them up in what was considered a logical hierarchy of least irritating to most irritating. I published a general description of this method in 1978.[1] Three types of modalities were used: dowel textures, with use of materials glued onto ½-inch dowel sticks; contact, with use of particles such as rice and beans; and vibration, with use of battery-operated and electric plug-in vibrators (Fig. 56-1). These first two modalities were then divided into 10 subcategories each, four in the case of vibration, and organized in what was considered a logical hierarchy of least irritating to most irritating.

These textures and particles were chosen on the basis of how tactilely stimulating they seemed to be, from giving very little tactile sensation to giving a significant amount. We can only speculate about whether subjects are sensitive to the textures or to the pressure exerted by the modalities employed.[20] Another consideration was availability of the materials so that the treatment could be standardized if desired.

After this method was used over a period of several months, it was determined that the predetermined hierarchy was not a sound basis for treatment. Many patients found some particles and textures irritating that were not irritating to the normal, and vice versa. It was therefore decided to have the patient determine his own hierarchy of hypersensitivity for the contact and immersion textures and base his treatment on this. This method of treatment proved effective, in that most patients improved and progressed in their treatment hierarchy. In many cases, for comparison, we also

recorded the patient's hierarchy on the normal side, the results of which will be the subject of a future article.

In the process of researching the subject, it was noted that a type of hierarchical desensitization was also used with phobias and in the art of karate. Anxiety hierarchies consisting of sequentially more threatening situations were introduced in the late 1950s to treat phobias. The therapy was terminated when the final item on the hierarchy could be tolerated by the patient.[19] The rationale of having a patient touch progressively irritating textures, in theory, is not unlike any progressive exercises that we do from gross to fine and from light to heavy. Progressing from nonirritating to irritating seemed the logical way to proceed. This process is also based on a fundamental tenet of occupational therapy, in that it is "given in increasing doses as the patient's condition improves."[11]

DOWNEY HAND CENTER HAND SENSITIVITY TEST

The staff was gratified by the patients' improvement with this method and felt a need to validate the procedure so that it could be more confidently used and shared with others. Therefore, in 1980, a new instrument, the Downey Hand Center Hand Sensitivity Test, was developed to measure the effects of desensitization treatment.[20] First, detailed instructions were written for administration of the test so that use of the tool could be consistent. In the case of the dowel textures, the tester randomly selected one of the 10, instructing the patient to rub, roll, or tap the texture over the hypersensitive area. Then a random dowel was selected and the patient was asked, "Which of these is the most irritating?" Dowel textures ranged from moleskin to Velcro hooks, as follows:

1. Moleskin
2. Felt
3. Quickstick
4. Velvet
5. Semirough cloth
6. Velcro loops*

---

*Velcro USA, Inc., New York, NY.

7. Hard T-Foam
8. Burlap
9. Rug back
10. Velcro hooks

The contact or immersion particles were contained in 3-pound coffee cans into which the patient was instructed to immerse the hand. The 10 particles ranged from cotton to plastic squares and were numbered for recording purposes as follows:

1. Cotton
2. Terry cloth pieces
3. Dry rice
4. Popcorn
5. Pinto beans
6. Macaroni (salad)
7. Plastic wire insulation pieces
8. Small beebees or buckshot
9. Large beebees or buckshot
10. Plastic squares

The tester randomly selected one of the 10, instructing the patient to repeatedly immerse his hand in it. Then another random texture was selected and the patient was asked, "Which of these is the most irritating?" This procedure was repeated until a sequence was established of all 10, ranging from the least irritating to the most.

To keep a consistent number of 10 with all three modalities, a hierarchy of 10 was also established for vibration, based both on speed of vibration and on amount of contact. The 83- and 100-cycle vibrator was used only in the clinic, and the 23- and 53-cycle vibrator was used at home. The patient continued the vibration step for 10 minutes a session. The hierarchy is as follows:

1. 83 cycles, near but no actual contact on the area
2. 83 cycles, near but no actual contact; 23 cycles, near but no actual contact
3. 83 cycles, no contact; 23 cycles, intermittent contact
4. 83 cycles, intermittent contact; 23 cycles, intermittent contact
5. 83 cycles, intermittent contact; 23 cycles, continuous contact
6. 83 cycles, continuous contact; 23 cycles, intermittent contact
7. 100 cycles, intermittent contact; 53 cycles, intermittent contact
8. 100 cycles, intermittent contact; 53 cycles, continuous contact
9. 100 cycles, continuous contact; 53 cycles, continuous contact
10. No problem with vibration

The method was the same as that used for the dowel and contact modalities.

To determine how reliable the tool was for normal persons and whether differences in reliability existed because of ethnicity, sex, or the hand being tested, a standardization sample of 40 volunteers with normal hands, 20 to 40 years of age, consisting of 10 male and 10 female Anglo-Americans and 10 male and 10 female Mexican-Americans were selected. A normal hand was defined as a hand presenting without pain, neurologic deficit, or skin abnormality. Each subject's hierarchy of sensitivity of both hands was determined as described above. The subjects were retested in 2 weeks. The test-retest reliability figures were as follows:

dowel textures—right hand .77, left hand, .79; contact particles—right hand .74, left hand, .80; vibration—right hand .82, left hand .82. There were no statistically significant differences in reliability because of sex, ethnicity, or which hand was being tested. Therefore it was concluded that the HCHST could be used as both a research and a clinical tool.[20]

Because the same modalities were used in both testing and clinical practice, which might be confusing, it was important to differentiate the use of the DHCHST, the actual testing tool, from the desensitization treatment, which is described next. Because its function is to measure change, the DHCHST could be used to test the effectiveness of other forms of treatment in addition to the regimen described in this paper. Despite the fact that the DHCHST was validated on normal hands, the experience gained using the instrument in the study described in this paper demonstrated its value as a tool in assessing change in the injured hand.

DESENSITIZATION TREATMENT AND DOCUMENTATION

Any patient referred to the Downey Hand Center who had an area of hypersensitivity on the hand that exhibited extreme irritability to the touch was a candidate for desensitization treatment. How disabling the hypersensitivity was to him was determined by administration of the DHCHST and observation of the patient's use of the hand. Before initiation of treatment, the results of the DHCHST and other information were recorded on the desensitization treatment form (Fig. 56-2).

After documentation and testing, treatment was begun with the texture, particle, and vibration level the patient could use; the treatment was done for 10 minutes, three or four times a day. In the case of the dowel textures (Fig. 56-3), he was instructed to use one that was slightly irritating but that he could tolerate rubbing, rolling, or tapping on the sensitive area for a 10-minute period (Fig. 56-4). Dowel textures were convenient in that they could be carried with the patient and used during the day.

Contact particles (Fig. 56-5) were generally used in the clinic; however, when indicated, the patient was given a home program as well. The patient was instructed to put his hand in the particles and either move the hand about in the particles or drop them onto the area, such as the back of the hand or other parts not involved in grasp. Again, the patient was asked to choose the particle that was slightly irritating but tolerable for 10 minutes (Fig. 56-6). This was indicated by writing the date next to the number of the particle on the record form.

In the case of vibration, the patient chose where he was on the predetermined vibration hierarchy by going through as much of the sequence as possible with the therapist. He was then started on the level of the hierarchy that he could tolerate for 10 minutes, two or three times a day. The vibration hierarchy was based on the cycles per second of the two vibrators plus the amount of contact on or near the area. In the beginning stages the vibrator might not touch the scar or wound site at all but touched as close to the periphery as possible. The predetermined vibration hierarchy has not been foolproof in that more cycles per second were not necessarily more irritating to the injured hand than less. For instance, in a few cases the home-vibrator speed of 23 cycles

THE DOWNEY HAND CENTER HAND SENSITIVITY TEST (DHCHST)
DOWNEY COMMUNITY HOSPITAL - HAND REHABILITATION CENTER

1. Name _____ Age _____ Sex _____ Language Barrier Yes _____ No _____ Hispanic Yes _____ No _____
2. Diagnosis _____
3. Source of pain: Amputation _____ Scar _____ Crush _____ Neuroma _____ Burn _____ Other _____
4. Description of painful area: Initial: _____
5. Dominance: Right _____ Left _____ Discharge _____
6. How injury occurred _____
7. Date(s) of injury _____ Date(s) of Surgery _____ Date of 1st Rx after surgery _____
8. No. of weeks from DOI to 1st Des. Rx: _____ No. of weeks from surgery to 1st Des. Rx: _____
9. No. of weeks between 1st and last Rx: _____ No. of treatments _____ Referring M.D. _____
10. Occupation _____ Return to Work: Yes _____ No _____ Previous Job? Yes _____ No _____

11. Dowel Textures - Date | Contact Textures - Date | Vibration - Date

12.	1		1		1
13.	2		2		2
14.	3		3		3
15.	4		4		4
16.	5		5		5
17.	6		6		6
18.	7		7		7
19.	8		8		8
20.	9		9		9
21.	10		10		10
22.	Init	N	DC		N	DC

23. Int. Did the Desensitization Treatment affect your sensitivity today? Yes _____ No _____
24. How? Increased it? Yes _____ No _____ Decreased it? Yes _____ No _____
25. How much? A Lot _____ Some _____ Very Little _____ How much? A Lot _____ Some _____ Very Little _____
26. 2 Wks Has the Desensitization Treatment affected your sensitivity? Yes _____ No _____
27. How? Increased it? Yes _____ No _____ Decreased it? Yes _____ No _____
28. How much? A Lot _____ Some _____ Very Little _____ How much? A Lot _____ Some _____ Very Little _____
29. DC Did the Desensitization Treatment affect your sensitivity? Yes _____ No _____
30. How? Increased it? Yes _____ No _____ Decreased it? Yes _____ No _____
31. How much? A Lot _____ Some _____ Very Little _____ How much? A Lot _____ Some _____ Very Little _____
32. DC Which Treatment affected your sensitivity the most? _____ Comments _____
INSTRUMENT USED: DOWNEY HAND CENTER HAND SENSITIVITY TEST

Fig. 56-2 Desensitization form.

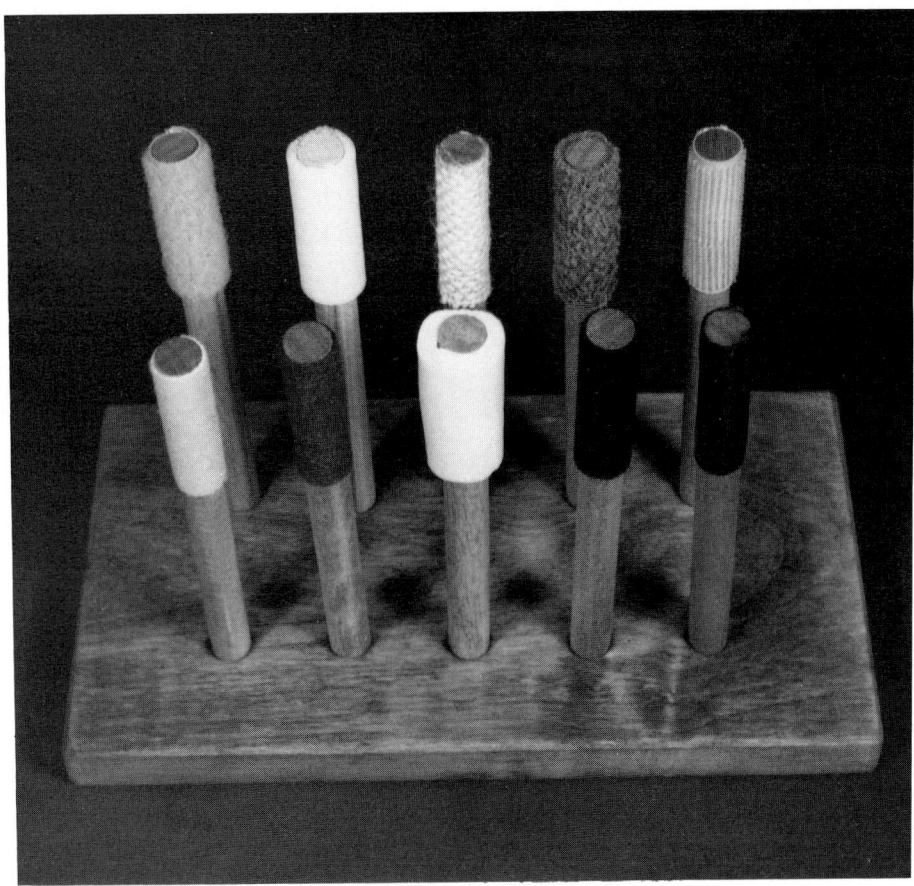

Fig. 56-3   Dowel textures used in Downey Hand Center Sensitivity Test to determine treatment hierarchy and for clinic and home treatment. Range from smooth fabric to Velcro Hook.

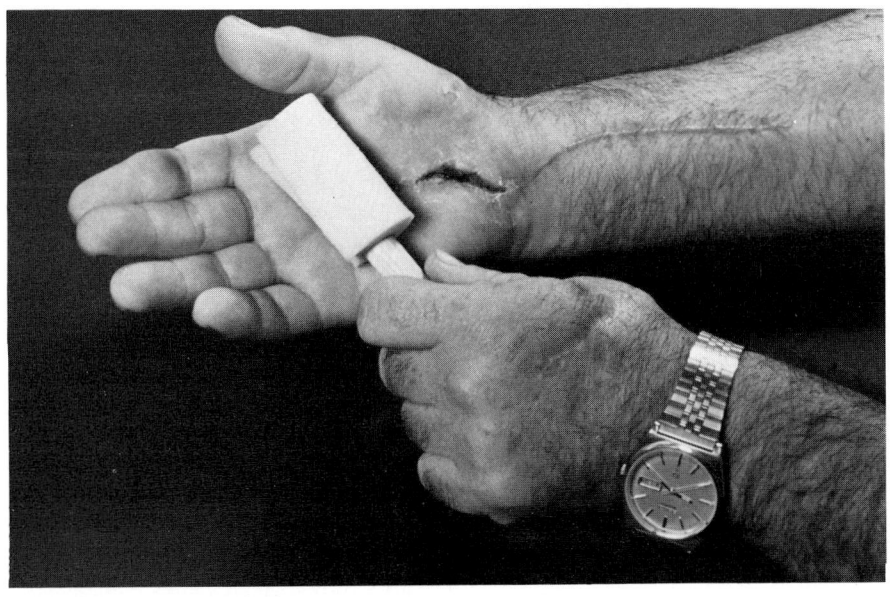

Fig. 56-4   Patient using dowel texture near healing wound and over healed area.

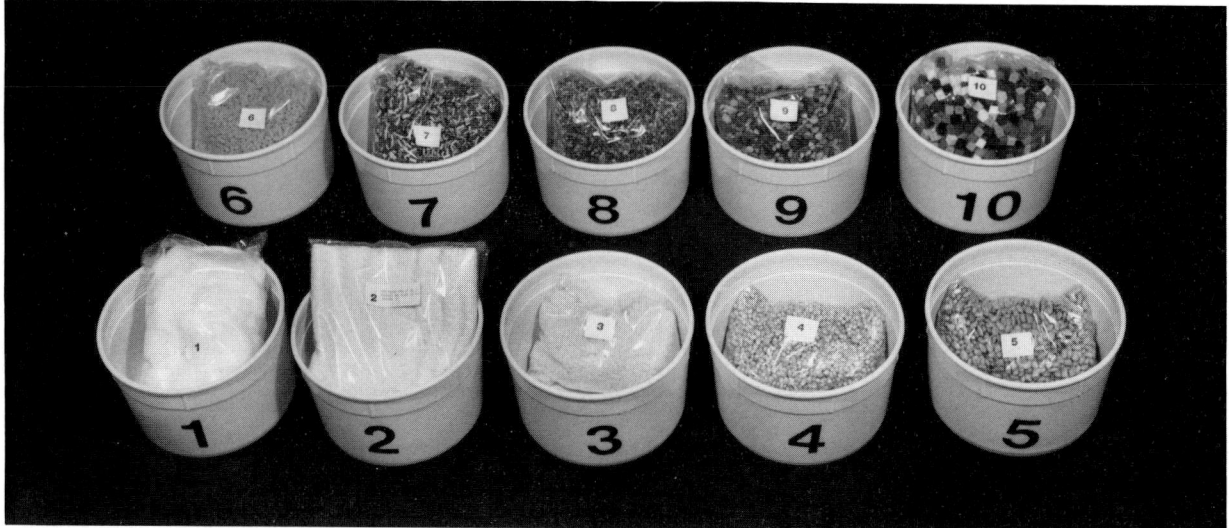

Fig. 56-5   Contact particles in plastic containers used to determine treatment hierarchy and for treatment. Range from soft cotton to hard pebbles.

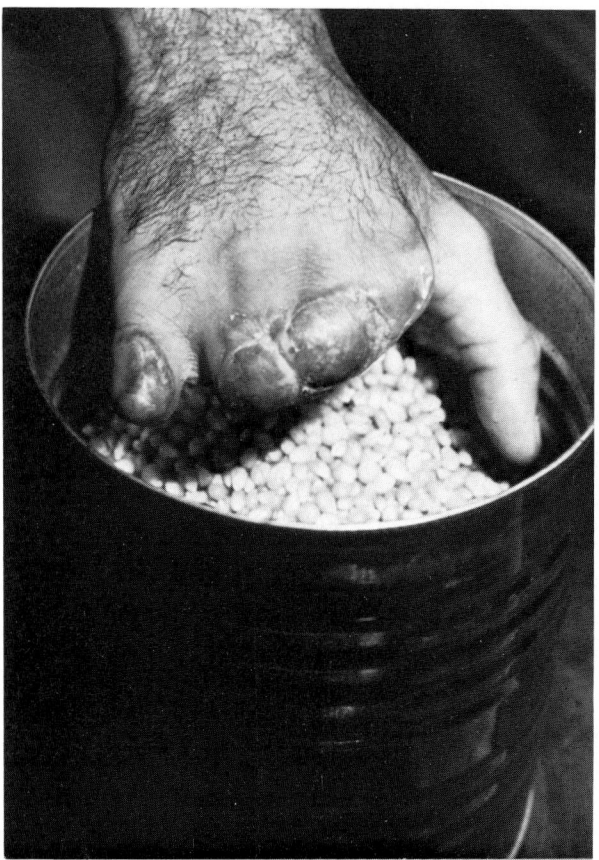

Fig. 56-6   Patient with amputated fingers immersing hand repeatedly in popcorn as step in desensitization treatment.

per second was more irritating than when set at 53 cycles. Since few patients reached 9 or 10 on the hierarchy, it appeared that the highest levels were the most irritating.

The patient's treatment regimen included other therapeutic activities such as exercises and therapeutic handicrafts. Use of the hypersensitive part was encouraged (Fig. 56-7). The actual desensitization treatment was done by the patient, took approximately 20 minutes of the 2- to 3-hour treatment session, and was done any time during the treatment session, depending on the availability of equipment and the patient's preference. Part of the desensitization treatment, such as use of the battery-operated vibrator and the dowel textures, was done by the patients at home. These modalities were also kept by the patient after discharge.

PSYCHOLOGICAL IMPLICATIONS

The major effect of the motivation and the psychological status of the patient must be acknowledged. In the case of neuromas occurring after amputation, Grant[6] stated that in the majority of patients these symptoms gradually faded and use of shortened members resumed with little or no disability. Of the two major reasons for persistence of pain after amputation, one was infection, with resulting excessive scar, and the other was a greater or lesser instability of the psyche of the patient. Of course, the psychological implications are great when one is dealing with the subject of hypersensitivity. Russell[14] stated that the physician should at all times be prepared to embark on what might be termed "a game of bluff with the patient's higher cerebral mechanisms." Clark[4] reported that suggestion directed toward increasing the tolerance of thermal pain decreased the probability of withdrawal response.

The power of suggestion, no doubt, has some influence. The therapists supervising the desensitization treatment at the Downey Hand Center had a positive attitude regarding the potential benefits to the patient, based primarily on positive experience with its use. They estimated that 75% to 80% of the patients were significantly helped by the desensitization treatment.

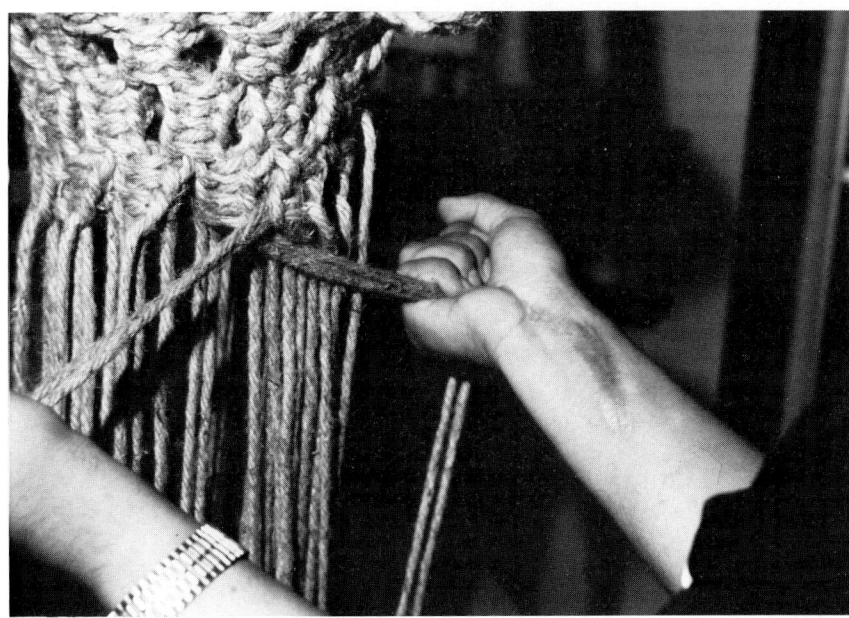

Fig. 56-7 Patient using therapeutic craft (macramé knotting) to repeatedly stimulate sensitive palmar scar and provide stretch to scar over distal part of forearm.

In responding to the aforementioned survey, one physician who works with farmers who sustained hand injuries stated, "I treat mostly well-motivated, self-employed farmers and ranchers who don't complain about neuromas, etc., except under dire circumstances. Because of the mechanized nature of farms these days, we get quite a few crush amputations, yet the percentage that get problems is quite small. Perhaps it has something to do with the motivation aspect. The patients just don't seem worried."[5]

Looking at groups and generalizing conclusions does not necessarily demonstrate the impact that reduction in hypersensitivity may have on a person. The clinician needs to be alert to each person's needs.

J.E. was a 25-year old Mexican-American male machine operator who suffered a degloving injury to the ulnar aspect of his right, dominant hand 2 years before referral to the Downey Hand Center. He had been unemployed since injury. He had had a number of surgical procedures in attempts to gain function in the small finger and reduce hypersensitivity in the ulnar aspect of his hand. On first interview at the DHC, he was unable to hold anything in the hand that might touch this hypersensitive area and was unable to touch this part to any surface, as would be required for writing. He was referred specifically for transfer of dominance. Because of the generally healthy status of his right hand, which demonstrated good range of motion except in the little and ring fingers and exhibited a 25-pound palmar pinch and a 30-pound lateral pinch, the patient was begun on a treatment program with emphasis on desensitization. Hypersensitivity was unquestionably the patient's most limiting problem. He was extremely apprehensive about even lightly touching the sensitive area and incredulous when he was told it was beneficial for him to do so. After a couple of days of therapy he began to feel a change and participated maximally in his program.

At discharge, after participating in 32 therapy sessions over a period of 6 weeks, each including desensitization treatment, he complained of only a small area of hypersensitivity about the size of a dime on the ulnar aspect of his palm. He was able to use the hand for all functional activities, including writing, and could handle such things as macramé cord and a hammer without difficulty. He reached 10 on both the dowel and contact textures and 9 on the vibration hierarchy, having started on level 6 dowels, 4 contact, and 3 vibration. He felt that vibration was the most beneficial modality. At discharge he was scheduled to begin training as a mechanical draftsman. The rehabilitation counselor and the therapist were optimistic about his future vocational potential. The patient expressed sincere gratitude and had an optimistic outlook on his future.

This is a dramatic example of someone who, prior to the initiation of a desensitization program, believed "If it hurts, you should not touch it," and had not been instructed otherwise. It is an example of how beneficial desensitization treatment can be.

DESCRIPTION OF GROUPS STUDIED

The patient group described in this chapter participated in treatment as described above at the Downey Hand Center between March 1980 and March 1982. During this time approximately 400 patients participated in desensitization treatment, approximately 40% of the total population of patients seen at the DHC. Of the 400 who participated to some extent in desensitization treatment, 124 patients had complete records of their DHCHST and the treatment and were used in the following conclusions. The majority of the patients were manual laborers; 67 had hypersensitive scars, 44 amputations, and 13 crush injuries. Other diagnoses such as grafts, burns, and neuromas were also treated, but the numbers were too small for comparisons and the records were incomplete. Seventy-four (60%) of the total were Mex-

DESCRIPTION OF GROUP STUDIED (n = 124)		
Hypersensitive scars 67	Amputations 44	Crush injuries 13
Male 90	Female 34	
Mexican-Americans 74	Anglo-Americans 50	

ican and 50 (40%) Anglo-Americans; only 34 (28%) were females (see boxed material above).

The term "hypersensitive scars" referred to scars caused by surgical procedures, lacerations, or other injuries and included digital nerve lacerations and neuromas. These patients were started with the desensitization program as soon as healing had occurred or as soon as the patient could touch the vibrator or the dowel texture near the scar.

Amputations were divided into tip amputations, phalangeal amputations, and a mixture of these. The total group of 44 amputations included 23 with tip amputations of one or two fingers, 16 who had amputations of one phalanx and tip or two of each of these, and five who had amputations of more than two sites.

The term "crush injuries" referred to those patients who had a hand injury primarily involving a crush. The injury might also have involved fractures and minor lacerations as well.

SUMMARY OF FINDINGS

The patient's hypersensitivity was considered improved each time he progressed a step in his hierarchy. Maximum improvement was assumed when the patient had reached step 10 in all three modalities.

I will not speculate regarding the physiologic reasons for the improvement made. Since all patients participated in a variety of treatment tasks, many including touching the hypersensitive area, along with desensitization treatment, caution must be exercised when one concludes that the improvement demonstrated was attributable to desensitization treatment by itself.

The end of treatment came when the patient had made improvement in hand function and was no longer vocationally limited by his hypersensitivity. In many patients other factors, such as loss of strength, limited range of motion,

or loss of digits, were the most disabling factors. Maximum improvement (level 10 on the three modalities) in hypersensitivity was not imperative to return to work. How disabling hypersensitivity was depended on many factors, such as hand affected, severity of injury, and location and extent of hypersensitivity. All patients were given the option to continue desensitization after discharge and were provided with dowel sticks and a home vibrator.

In our analysis of the number of weeks between the first treatment and the first change within the three major categories of patients and the categories of treatment modalities (Table 56-1), we found that within 2 to 3 weeks almost all patients had made one change in their hierarchy in at least one modality.

In looking at how many subjects reached the highest level (10) on any of the hierarchies, we found that anywhere from 60% to 75% in all three groups reached that level on the dowel hierarchy. The patients with amputations seemed significantly more sensitive to the vibration hierarchy. Although only 7% of amputation patients whose vibration responses were recorded reached 10 on the vibration hierarchy, 35% believed that vibration was the modality that helped the most. It is also interesting to note that when we look at the patients' responses regarding which modality they believed affected sensitivity the most, the smallest percentage of people in each of the three categories believed that the dowel textures were the most effective. However, the greatest percentage in each category reached 10 on the dowel hierarchies (Table 56-2).

The length of treatment averaged about 7 weeks and was initiated an average of 8½ to 13 weeks after injury. Amputations, on the average, required a longer healing period before treatment could be begun (Table 56-3).

The logical next question when one looks at results is, "How many of those patients returned to gainful employment?" Olivia Diaz, M.S., C.R.C., consultant to the Downey Hand Center between April 1981 and May 1982, interviewed a randomly selected group of 24 patients at least 6 weeks after discharge. Diaz found that 18 of them were working, all at their previous jobs. Two, not currently working, had returned to their previous jobs after discharge but were later laid off because of lack of work. The other four of those not working had physical problems other than hypersensitivity that prevented their return to work. The jobs they returned to were machine operator, machinist, warehouseman, butcher, hand assembler, general steel worker, wood assembler, welding technician, and press-brake operator in a sheet-metal shop, all of which require heavy and constant use of the hands. Twenty-two of the 24 said that they continued to experience sensitivity but not to a degree that prevented their return to work.

Table 56-1 Number of weeks between first treatment and first change (rounded to nearest 0.5 week)

	Scar (n = 67)		Amputation (n = 44)		Crush (n = 13)	
	Range	Average	Range	Average	Range	Average
Dowel textures	0.5 to 10	2	0.5 to 14	3	0.5 to 3	1.5
Contact particles	0.5 to 10	2	0.5 to 8	2	0.5 to 20	3.5
Vibration	0.5 to 24	3	0.5 to 9	2.5	0.5 to 4	2

Table 56-2   Patients reaching level 10 and patients' responses

	Dowel textures	Contact particles	Vibration	Unknown
Patients reaching level 10 on modality				
Scar	76%	63%	21%	
Amputation	61%	23%	7%	
Crush	62%	54%	22%	
Patients' responses: which treatment affected sensitivity the most				
Scar	11%	21%	60%	8%
Amputation	9%	49%	35%	7%
Crush	16½%	37½%	46%	0

CONCLUSION

A method of desensitizing the traumatized hand that has hypersensitivity attributable to scar, crush injuries, or amputation was presented. The 124 patients included in the Downey Hand Center study improved to the extent that they were discharged from treatment without hypersensitivity severe enough to prevent them from returning to work. Objectively, they all showed improvement in some aspect of the Downey Hand Center Hand Sensitivity Test. In retrospect, a major value of this study may have been in the questions it raised. Would it be just as effective to have a hierarchy of five steps in each modality? Are there some contact particles and textures that could be eliminated? Which would be the best to maintain? Is the value mainly in the fact that the patient is in a somewhat elaborate manner guided in merely touching the sensitive area? It is also interesting to speculate if the patient might progress in his hierarchies in the DHCHST by doing other activities, such as crafts alone or exercises not necessarily so finely graded as those presented. The subject, indeed, remains mysterious. Although many patients, one can legitimately argue, can do very well without direction, there are those who definitely need it, as the case study illustrated. A case study such as this also invalidates the philosophy "Leave him alone and he will get better on his own," which is claimed by some. In the case of the motivated farmers, this may often be true. However, it is also hard to quantify the importance of a casual bit of encouragement, like "Touch it a lot; it will make it better," by a trusted physician.

Future analyses of these procedures could perhaps deal with such interesting factors as location of hypersensitivity, effect of handedness, occupation, and time after onset in relation to level of improvement, all questions that were not thoroughly dealt with in this analysis.

Although the subject is complex and the questions are endless, there was significant evidence presented to suggest strongly that stimulating hypersensitive areas helped reduce hypersensitivity. The systematic approach described gave the therapist and the patient a guide and focused attention on the problem. This method gave the patient the necessary guidelines to do his own desensitization treatment. It also had the element of gratification in that progress could be periodically assessed and documented.

Although the subject is complex and many questions remain unanswered, I hope this information is both stimulating and helpful, and even more I hope that the clinician will continue to pursue the unanswered questions.

TESTING AND TREATMENT MATERIALS AVAILABLE

Because of inaccessibility, the battery-operated vibrator is now 100 and 125 cycles per second. The Hard T-foam dowel texture is now Hard T-foam–like material, and the BBs and buckshot immersion particles are now pebbles. The effect of these changes, if any, on testing or treatment is unknown to the author.

ACKNOWLEDGMENTS

I wish to acknowledge Dr. Elizabeth J. Yerxa for her assistance in compiling and editing the manuscript; Andres Rosales, C.O.T.A., and Wendy Black, C.O.T.A., for compiling data; Dr. Garry Brody, Laurie Meadows, O.T.R., and the Downey Hand Center staff and patients for their support of the desensitization project; and Frances Robertson for invaluable assistance in typing, editing, and data organization. Photographs were taken by Susie Lee and Larry Coolidge.

Desensitization testing and treatment materials are available from LMB Hand Rehab Products, Inc., San Luis Obispo, Calif., and North Coast Medical, Campbell, Calif.

Table 56-3   Time to first treatment and length of treatment (average, nearest 0.5 week)

	Time between onset and first treatment	Length of treatment
Scar (n = 67)	11	6.5
Amputation (n = 44)	13	7
Crush (n = 13)	8.5	7.5

REFERENCES

1. Barber LM: Occupation therapy for the treatment of reflex sympathetic dystrophy and post-traumatic hypersensitivity of the injured hand. In Fredericks S and Brody GS, editors: Symposium on the neurologic aspects of plastic surgery, St. Louis, 1978, The CV Mosby Co.
2. Blitz B, Dinnerstein AJ, and Lowenthal M: Attenuation of experimental pain by tactile stimulation: effect of vibration at different levels of noxious stimulus intensity, Percept Mot Skills 19:311, 1964.
3. Brown DM and Ellis RA: A physiological basis for desensitization of the hypersensitive upper extremity, Unpublished manuscript, 1982.
4. Clark WC: Pain sensitivity and the report of pain: an introduction to sensory decision theory, Anesthesiology 40:272, 1974.
5. Collins P: Personal communication, 1982.

6. Grant GH: Methods of treatment of neuromata of the hand, J Bone Joint Surg 33A:841, 1951.
7. Hardy MA, Moran CA, and Merritt WH: Desensitization of the traumatized hand, Va Med 109:134, 1982.
8. Hochreiter NW: Effect of vibration on tactile sensitivity, Phys Ther 63(6):934, 1983.
9. Mathews GJ and Osterholm JL: Painful traumatic neuromas, Surg Clin North Am 51:1313, 1972.
10. Melzack R: The puzzle of pain, New York, 1973, Basic Books, Inc.
11. Mock HE and Abbey ML: Occupational therapy, JAMA 91:797, 1928.
12. Rubin D and Kuitert JH: Use of ultrasonic vibration in the treatment of pain arising from phantom limbs, scars and neuromas: a preliminary report, Arch Phys Med Rehabil 36:445, 1955.
13. Russell WR: Painful amputation stumps and phantom limbs, Br Med J 1:1024, 1949; Treat Serv Bull 4:48, 1949.
14. Russell WR, Espir MLE, and Morgenstern, F: Treatment of postherpetic neuralgia, Lancet 1:242, 1957.
15. Russell WR and Spalding JMK: Treatment of painful amputation stumps, Br Med J 2:68, 1950.
16. Sherman RA, Sherman CJ, and Gall NG: A survey of current phantom limb pain treatment in the United States, Pain 8:85, 1980.
17. Wall PD and Cronly-Dillon JR: Pain, itch and vibration, Arch Neurol 2:365, 1960.
18. Wilson RL: Management of pain following peripheral nerve injuries, Orthop Clin North Am 12:343, 1981.
19. Wolpe J: Systematic desensitization, J Nerv Ment Dis 132:189, 1961.
20. Yerxa EJ and others: Development of a hand sensitivity test for use in desensitization of the hypersensitive hand, Am J Occup Ther 37(3):176, 1983.

57

Myofascial pain in the upper extremity

Christine A. Moran, Sandra Richards Saunders, and Susan M. Tribuzi

Forty million Americans suffer from various forms of pain, for which an estimated one billion over-the-counter pain medications are sold each year.[34] Pain is typically classified according to cause, severity, or structure involved. Despite the classification, the treatments are consistently similar. If the patient with pain does not respond to conventional treatment techniques, he is told to "live with it."

Myofascial pain (MFP) is a syndrome recognized, described, and treated since the 1930s. By definition, MFP is a local irritation in muscle, fascia, tendon, or ligament that exhibits local tenderness, specific pain patterns, and autonomic symptoms that are easily reproducible and specific to that tissue.[83] Patients with myofascial pain must be treated according to the locus of their pain and not necessarily the presentation site of their pain.

In this chapter a complete profile of myofascial pain is offered. First, a historical review of MFP is presented. Next, a detailed presentation of MFP evaluation will acquaint the reader with the necessity of clearly identifying the *locus* of the patient's pain. Finally, various treatment techniques are outlined. Several case studies supplement the areas of evaluation and treatment for clearer illustration.

HISTORICAL REVIEW

Descriptions of specific musculoskeletal syndromes date back to 1592, when the term *rheumatism* was first used by Guillame de Baillou.[63,64] By the eighteenth century, the term muscular rheumatism was used to label disorders manifested by pain and stiffness in the muscles and soft tissues.

In 1843 Froriep, a German physician, was credited with first describing painful hard places in the muscles of patients diagnosed with rheumatism.[2,63,67,83] Froriep used the term *Muskelshwiele*, "muscle callus" to describe palpable exudations or callus or hardening located in subcutaneous tissue, skin, muscle, and periosteum. Following Froriep's work, these palpable hard nodules in muscles were more frequently recognized by physicians, along with an increase in use of massage for treatment.

Some 50 years later in 1898, Strauss reported his theory that these muscle hardenings were caused by excess connective tissue.[67] He described these "hardenings" as commonly found in the muscle and adjacent subcutaneous tissue, in the entire muscle, and running parallel to the muscle fiber where multiple hardenings or knots were seen. Strauss emphasized the necessity to develop skill in palpation techniques and advocated treatment of heat and massage to these areas.

Early twentieth century (1900-1935)

By the early twentieth century the confusion started. The term *muscular rheumatism* (or just *rheumatism*) had been commonly used to describe generalized musculoskeletal pain with unknown cause. The term was criticized as being a "diagnostic scrap box in which one is accustomed to throw promiscuously all those ailments accompanied by pain which cannot conveniently be otherwise classified."[2] In 1904 Sir William Gowers, a French physician, reclaimed the idea that inflammation in fibrous or connective tissue was the cause of muscular rheumatism and introduced the term *fibrositis*.[23] The term was intended to describe the "supposed pathophysiology of muscular rheumatism."[62]

Gowers's original article made no mention of palpable findings nor did it favor massage or electricity as treatment in the early stages. He did, however, advocate treatment of rest, diaphoresis, aspirin, and daily local hypodermic injections of cocaine or eucaine for 2 to 3 weeks.[23] The term *fibrositis* gradually became associated with other conditions involving soft tissue pain with negative laboratory test or x-ray examination findings.[40]

Late in 1912 Muller described detailed features of muscular rheumatism or fibrositis, which he believed occurred in three stages: the actue, subacute, and chronic stage.[56] In the acute stage, symptoms included severe pain, pressure sensitive areas in the muscle, multiple muscle involvement, spasms, impaired mobility, swelling, and an increase in temperature. The subacute stage was marked with a decrease in pain, stiffness, and secondary spasms with an increased palpable tension in the primary musculature. And finally, in the chronic stage, the symptoms found in stages one and two disappeared or persisted, with variable hypertonias, fiber hardening, and swelling. Muller used the term *insertion nodules* to describe these fiber hardenings. He felt most physicians denied the existence of these insertion nodules, whereas masseurs looked for them and successfully treated them.

Llewellyn and Jones authored a book titled *Fibrositis*, which further promoted the use of the term.[50,67] In their text they distinguished between articular fibrositis, neurofibrositis, and myofibrositis. Myofibrositis was defined as an "acute or chronic inflammatory change in the interstitial fibrous tissues of striated and voluntary muscle, the parenchymatous elements of which are secondarily implicated." Llewellyn and Jones also distinguished between acute and chronic myofibrositis and provided readers with detailed examination techniques.

During World War I Schade took advantage of his hospital experience and patient exposure to more closely examine these muscle hardenings.[36,42,67] He examined the upper trapezius and pectoralis major muscles during and after anesthesia and, in some cases, rigor mortis. Schade postulated that these muscle hardenings were a result of increased viscosity of muscle colloid; he proposed the term *myogelose,* "muscle gelling."

Two years later another German physician, Fritz Lange, added yet another term to the growing list, *Muskelharten,* referring to muscle hardening or indurations.[42,67,83] Lange described five causes of muscle hardening: overexertion, chronic fatigue, chilling, decreased circulation, and metabolic disturbances. He employed a special technique of palpation in which the skin was lubricated and a rolling motion performed with the fingers positioned in a transverse direction to the muscle fibers. Lange also introduced the use of a blunt instrument to perform a forceful massage to these muscle hardenings. The massage became known as gelotripsie and was considered an operative procedure.

Max Lange, a student of Fritz Lange, shared his instructor's interest in muscle hardening and authored a book on the subject in 1931.[42,67,83] The text described the distribution, origin, and pathology of muscle hardening from an orthopedic view. Max Lange advocated treatment of gelotripsie massage, with acute cases frequently only needing one treatment, whereas chronic cases required daily treatment for 2 to 3 weeks and as long as 4 to 6 weeks for persistent cases. Follow-up treatment often included exercise programs, self massage, activity moderation, and diathermy. When Max Lange published his book *Die Muskel-Haerten* in 1931, he predicted that 20 years would pass before the medical profession recognized the significance of these muscle hardenings.[46] Little did he know that more than 50 years would pass before their significance was recognized and appreciated.

Mid-twentieth century (1935-1965)

In the mid-twentieth century, new approaches to the treatment of muscle hardening evolved but not without the addition of new terminology. During this time the attention was focused on the tendency of these muscle hardenings, tender points, or nodules to produce pain at a distant site. In 1936 Edeiken and Wolferth introduced the term *trigger zone* into the literature.[14] They used the term to describe the area in which pain was felt from palpation of a tender spot over the scapula. The use of similar terms—trigger area, trigger point, and trigger spot—were soon to follow.

In 1937 Hans Kraus, an Austrian-born physician, introduced a new concept of muscle hardening treatment.* A friend of Kraus's described a technique used by a circus gymnast to keep injured performers working despite the most severe sprains and strains. The injured performer would soak a towel in alcohol, then wrap it around the injured area and expose it to a steady cloud of steam. This could result in a numbness in the painful areas so that the performer could begin to move the injured extremity. This procedure was performed two to three times a day, and after a day or 2 the performer was back to full strength and mobility. Kraus was impressed by this technique and tried it in his office. But he found the preparation of towels, alcohol, and steam to be too cumbersome. He experimented with different chemicals before introducing the use of ethyl chloride, a topical anesthetic. Kraus sprayed ethyl chloride in parallel rows over the painful area, exercising the muscle between applications. He used the term *MECE* to describe

his treatment of movement, ethyl chloride, and elevation. Kraus's treatment by MECE was a new approach from the traditional treatment of rest, ice, compression, and elevation (RICE) practiced by the majority of physicians.[35,42] In chronic or stubborn cases that did not respond to ethyl chloride therapy, Kraus advocated a treatment technique of novocaine injection into the muscle. Kraus believed that ethyl chloride or injection therapy disrupted the pain-reflex-pain cycle.[35] The following year, a German paper authored by Reichert further identified clinical features of painful muscles, which included point tenderness associated with muscular hardening with referred pain.[67] In the same year, Kellegren published his observation of referred pain arising from muscle.[37] He concluded that whereas fascia and tendon sheath gave rise to localized pain, muscle gave rise to diffuse pain, which is referred and predictable. Kellegren was credited as the first to identify and diagram the referral patterns of pain from muscle. Few authors before his work recognized that pain radiating from individual muscles followed a particular pattern.

The work of three more authors followed. The first was Gutstein, who published first under the name Gutstein, then Gutstein-Good, and later as Good. In his publications, he used various terms to describe basically the same condition. Terms used by Good included *muscular rheumatism, nonarticular rheumatism, myalgia spots, idiopathic myalgia, fibrositis, rheumatic myalgia,* and *rheumatic myopathy.*[20,21,25,83,84] It was Good who called attention to the patient's pain reaction when a tender spot was palpated. This later became known as the jump sign.

The second author was Kelly, an Australian who published numerous scientific papers between 1941 and 1963 on the topic of fibrositis.[38,39] Kelly believed that "fibrositis was a functional neurological disturbance originating at the myalgic lesion which was due to a local rheumatic process."[90] Kelly noted that injection of the primary myalgic spot provided pain relief, whereas injection in the area of referred pain only aggravated the condition.

The third contributor was Janet Travell, M.D. She has published more than 38 scientific papers on the topic of myofascial pain. Travell was the first female physician for the White House, serving as President Kennedy's personal physician and friend.[77] She treated Kennedy's trigger points in his back and prescribed the famous rocking chair as part of his treatment program.

In her early papers, Travell used the terms *idiopathic myalgia* and *myalgia,* but later she referred to trigger areas and trigger points.[83] In 1952 Travell began promoting the terminology *myofascial pain* and *myofascial syndrome* to "include both the red contractile and white fibrous elements of skeletal muscle."[77] Travell further redefined trigger points as having circumscribed deep tenderness, a localized twitch, or fasciculation that, when stimulated, caused referred pain.[68]

Travell, inspired by Kraus's writing on the use of ethyl chloride spray, also advocated its use in trigger point treatment.[76] However, ethyl chloride spray had its drawbacks, as it was highly flammable, explosive, and potentially dangerous if inhaled. Travell worked closely with the Gebauer Chemical Company,* current manufacturers of Fluori-

---

*References 10, 11, 35, 41, 67, 83.

*Gebauer Chemical Company, Cleveland.

Methane spray, researching alternative chemical sprays for treatment use.[76,78]

Fluori-Methane spray, selected by Travell, eventually was marketed in a bottle with a calibrated nozzle. This nozzle was designed to deliver a jet stream, which was more effective for spot cooling than the previously used diffuse mist.[76,77,78]

While Good, Kelly, and Travell had their own theories on the cause of myofascial pain, they all advocated the treatment of myalgic spots, tender spots, or trigger points by injection with procaine. Other individuals researching and publishing on myofascial pain syndromes and trigger points during this time included Sola, Kutert, Long, Bonica, Cooper, Gorral, Bates, and Grunwaldt.[68]

Late twentieth century (1965-present)

In the late twentieth century, questions were raised regarding the similarities between trigger points and acupuncture points.[43,54] Melzack, Stillwell, and Fox reported that 71% of trigger points have identical locations to acupuncture points.[55] This could be coincidental because there are approximately 1000 different acupuncture points identified in the literature.[70]

Fibrositis also continued as a controversial topic and was considered a "wastebasket term in need of redefinition."[83] In 1968 Kraft, Johnson, and LaBan established four criteria for improving current diagnostic standards and for distinguishing the fibrositis syndrome from other conditions causing muscle pain.[40] Their four criteria included a positive "jump sign," a "ropy" muscle consistency, dermographia, and a characteristic relief of pain by ethyl chloride spray. In 1981 fibrositis was once again redefined by Smythe as a "generalized musculoskeletal syndrome" characterized by widespread aching of more than 3 months' duration, local tenderness at 12 to 14 specific spots, skin rolling tenderness over the upper scapular region, and disturbed sleep with morning fatigue and stiffness.[71,85] At the 1986 Symposium on Fibrositis/Fibromyalgia debate, the need for further clarification continued.[5,26,30,69]

Kraus and Travell continued as key researchers and authors on the topic of myofascial pain during this time period. Kraus published *Clinical Treatment of Back and Neck Pain* (1970) and *Sports Injuries* (1981), both emphasizing trigger points as a source of referred pain.[42,44] Travell and Simon published the first of two volumes, *Myofascial Pain and Dysfunction: the Trigger Point Manual* in 1983. This text is one of the most current and comprehensive resources on the topic of myofascial pain.

With this historical perspective, one can see that myofascial pain is not a new concept (see box below). Rather the understanding of clinical symptoms and clinical presentation have evolved. Not to be confused with other myofascial techniques, myofascial pain management is specific. Management, as it has evolved, identifies physical signs and symptoms and treats them according to established parameters.

EVALUATION

Evaluation, regardless of diagnosis, requires adequate knowledge of the underlying cause. For that reason, it is essential to understand what is presently known about trigger points, how MFP presents, and the incorporation of MFP therapy into a total evaluation scheme.

The clinical presentation has been well described by Trav-

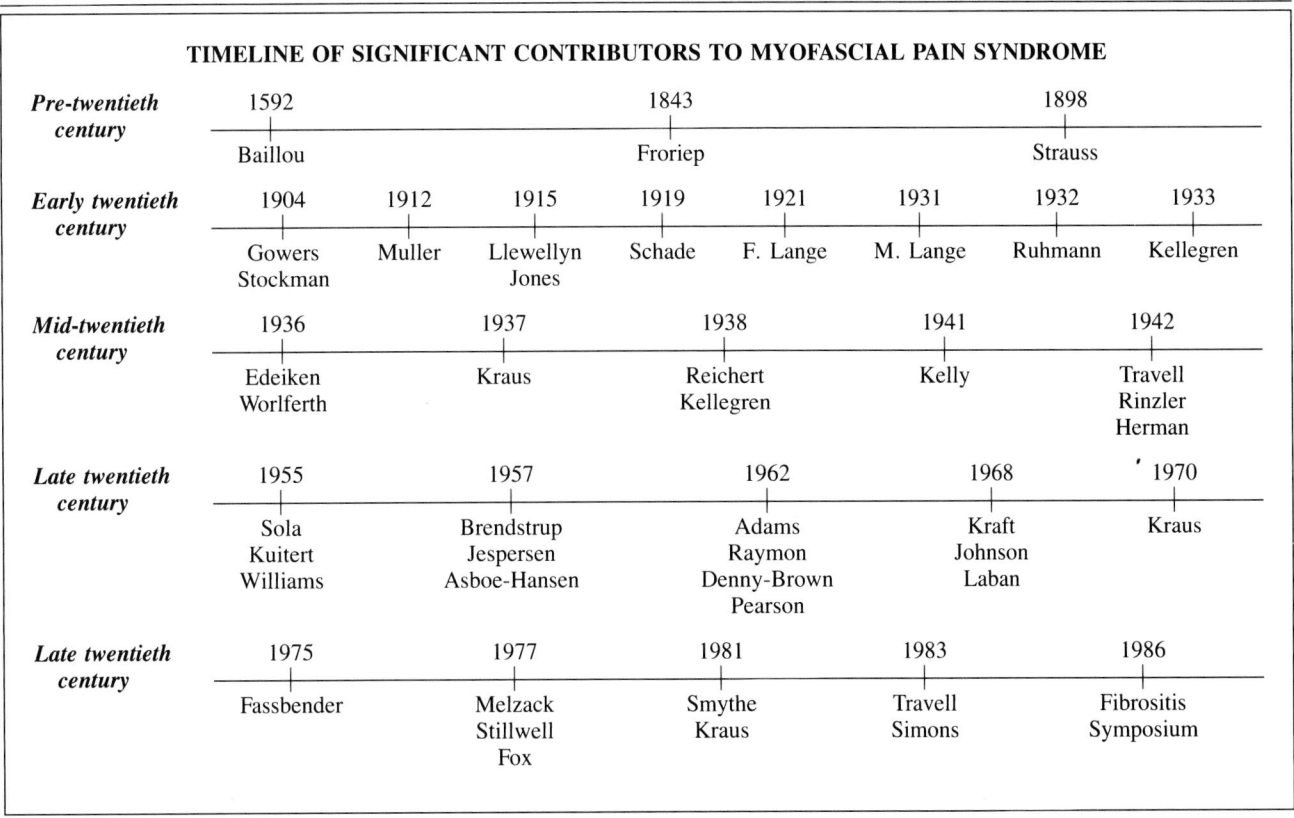

TIMELINE OF SIGNIFICANT CONTRIBUTORS TO MYOFASCIAL PAIN SYNDROME

Pre-twentieth century	1592				1843			1898	
	Baillou				Froriep			Strauss	

Early twentieth century	1904	1912	1915	1919	1921	1931	1932	1933
	Gowers Stockman	Muller	Llewellyn Jones	Schade	F. Lange	M. Lange	Ruhmann	Kellegren

Mid-twentieth century	1936		1937		1938		1941		1942
	Edeiken Worlferth		Kraus		Reichert Kellegren		Kelly		Travell Rinzler Herman

Late twentieth century	1955		1957		1962		1968		1970
	Sola Kuitert Williams		Brendstrup Jespersen Asboe-Hansen		Adams Raymon Denny-Brown Pearson		Kraft Johnson Laban		Kraus

Late twentieth century	1975		1977		1981		1983		1986
	Fassbender		Melzack Stillwell Fox		Smythe Kraus		Travell Simons		Fibrositis Symposium

ell and Simons. Trigger points are small, hypersensitive areas in muscle, ligament, or fascia, which, when stimulated, give rise to referred pain.[83]

Travell and Simons, further define trigger points by classifying them as either latent or active. A latent trigger point is found and can be made to refer pain by palpation. However, when the patient is asked if he has felt this pain at any other time, the answer is "no." If one examined a colleague by palpating a few muscles that commonly contain trigger points, it is quite likely that latent trigger points would be present. Tenderness is perceived over the point palpated, but pain is also perceived at a remote site. An active trigger point is what presents most often clinically, i.e., an irritable area within specific muscle or connective tissue that reproduces the patient's pain. This complaint of pain is termed *referred pain,* which is the presentation of myofascial pain. How pain is referred will be addressed later. The source of the referred pain is the trigger point.

A variety of situations can trigger a muscle to become painful and develop a trigger point: direct trauma, stress, overuse, fatigue, posture, stressful sleeping, and work postures. Often there is a limitation of joint motion produced by adaptive or reflexive shortening of the structure containing the trigger point that crosses that joint.[7,57,82] In a study by Friction and colleagues[17] the clinical characteristics of myofascial pain syndrome were evaluated in 164 patients. Fatigue, stiffness, swelling, and subjective weakness were the chief complaints in 36.9%, 19.5%, 12.2% and 17.7% of the patients, respectively. They also reported the involved muscles were mildly restricted in range of motion and were painful when stretched. For example, if the trigger point is located in the infraspinatus muscle, the limitation of motion will be at the glenohumeral joint in internal rotation and horizontal abduction.

The shoulder musculature frequently contains trigger points, though the diagnosis is usually bursitis, tendonitis, or other pathologic conditions of the shoulder rather than trigger points. Sola and Kuiter examined 100 subjects with shoulder and neck pain.[73] The patients complained of motion loss, pain, and stiffness of the shoulder and neck. Most of these patients had been unsuccessfully treated for diagnosis of bursitis, neuritis, or myositis. Table 57-1 shows the location and the frequency of occurrence of trigger points in 80 of these subjects with the complaint of shoulder pain.

An abundance of articles has been published regarding the effectiveness of treatment of trigger points; unfortunately they fall short of explaining a trigger point. Attempts to explain the existence of trigger points in physiologic, anatomic, or neurophysiologic terms have been frustrating. This excerpt from Sola's 1984 article emphasizes the detail of physiologic explanation:

From an initiation stimulus, such as trauma, fatigue or stress, a physiological response is generated and a particular trigger point begins to send distress signals to the central nervous system. Muscles associated with the trigger point become tense, and soon muscle fatigue is experienced. Local ischemia occurs, leading to change in the extracellular environment of the affected cells, including release of algesic agents. These feed into a cycle of increasing motor and sympathetic activity, which leads to increased pain. Once established as a cycle, a painful event may sustain itself in spite of control of the stimulus which originally initiated the cycle. Thus, proper and adequate treatment of a local injury may not provide alleviation of pain.[72]

Inflammatory etiologic factor

Some authors claim the "distress signals" to which Sola referred might be from inflammation.[1] However, temperature, blood sedimentation rate, and blood cell counts are usually normal, and biopsies have not shown signs of inflammation.[33] In contrast, Frost felt inflammation was an etiologic factor since he found diclofenea, a protaglandin-synthesis inhibitor, to be significantly more effective than lidocine when injected into a trigger point.[18]

Anatomic etiologic factor

In an attempt to uncover the anatomic makeup of trigger points, Kraus described the early work done by Lange, a German orthopedic surgeon.[42] The resistance of muscle to pressure was measured over trigger points and over normal resting skeletal muscles by an instrument called a sclerometer. Lange measured over 250 different muscles in normal subjects and found the resistance (hardness) to be consistent.[46] He then measured resistance over trigger points and found the pressure resistance over trigger points increased up to 50%. Lange also reported that this relative hardness of trigger points persisted even during general anesthesia; therefore, the firmness was not dependent on local muscle contraction.

Connective tissue irritation etiologic factor

Brendstrup and colleagues examined microscopically 11 muscle specimens taken from fibrositis nodules in the sacrospinalis muscles of patients with secondary trigger points.[8] These patients were undergoing surgery for disk herniation. The nodules were located by palpation while the patients were anesthetized. Microscopic investigation of the nodules revealed an interstitial mucinous edema containing acid mucopolysaccharide in the muscle's connective tissue and an accumulation of mast cells. The authors felt this evidence explained the firmness of the trigger points. Chemical analysis revealed a 5% decrease of potassium concentration and a 50% increase in chloride and hexosamine concentration. The increased hexosamine concentration is consistent with findings of connective tissue irritation. Travell and Simons proposed a possible cause for the firmness and the muscle crepitus sometimes felt during palpation. They describe calcium dumping out of the sarcoplastic reticulum as a result of muscle overloading, but this is not confirmed by biopsy.[83]

Ischemia etiologic factor

Ischemia is a commonly reported cause of pain from trigger points.[15,81] Fassbender conducted electron micro-

Table 57-2 Frequency of trigger points in the shoulder region

Muscles	Frequency in 80 cases
Infraspinatus	61
Levator scapula	41
Teres minor	9
Supraspinatus	4
Rhomboid major	3
Trapezius (upper)	2

scopic examination of muscle biopsies taken from trigger points in the medial border of the trapezius muscle in 11 patients.[15]

The following four stages of destruction were seen:

Stage 1: The first stage shows swelling of mitochondria and "moth-eaten" myofilament in the I band region (Fig. 57-1).

Stage 2: Destruction of myofilament is seen in the region of I bands. Z lines are maintained. In large areas, the usual structure of sarcomeres is lost, with remnants of these structures in disarray (Fig. 57-2).

Stage 3: There is isolated condensation of myofilament, and extensive areas show irregular aggregates of contractile substances (Fig. 57-3).

Stage 4: Contractile substance is lost in the proximity of the sarcolemma sheath, leaving fine granules (Fig. 57-4).

Fassbender compared these results to muscle biopsies of normal skeletal muscle. The normal skeletal muscle showed

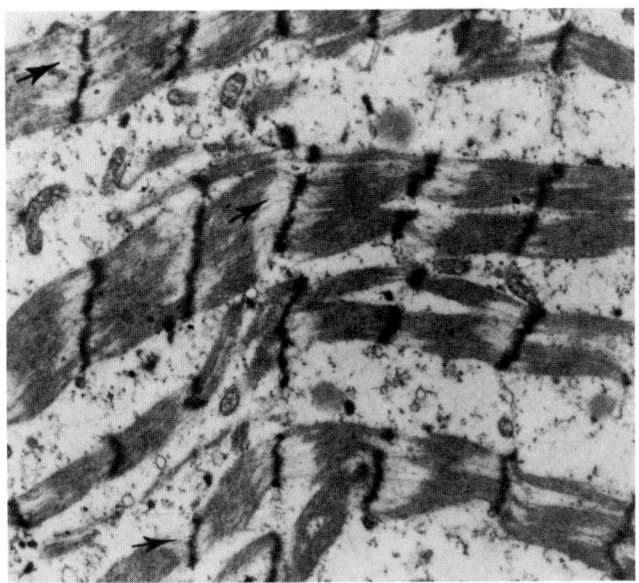

Fig. 57-1 Stage 1, swelling of mitochondria and "moth eaten" myofilament in the I Band region. (From Fassbender HG: Pathology of rheumatic disease, New York, 1975, Springer-Verlag.)

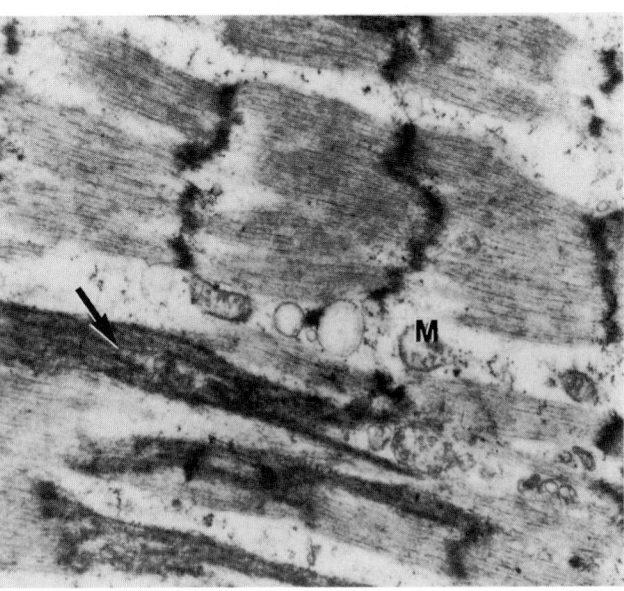

Fig. 57-2 Stage 2, Destruction of myofilaments (arrow), in I Band region with loss of sarcomeres (M). (From Fassbender HG: Pathology of rheumatic disease, New York, 1975, Springer-Verlag.)

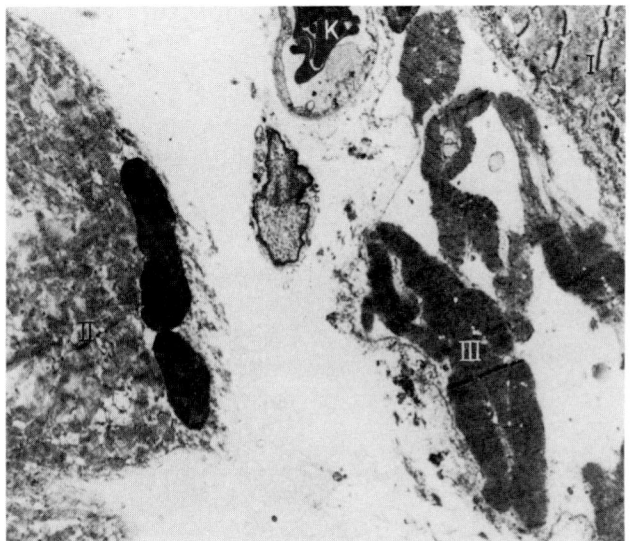

Fig. 57-3 Stage 3, Isolated condensation of myofilament and irregular aggregates of contractile substances (III). (From Fassbender HG: Pathology of rheumatic disease, New York, 1975, Springer-Verlag.)

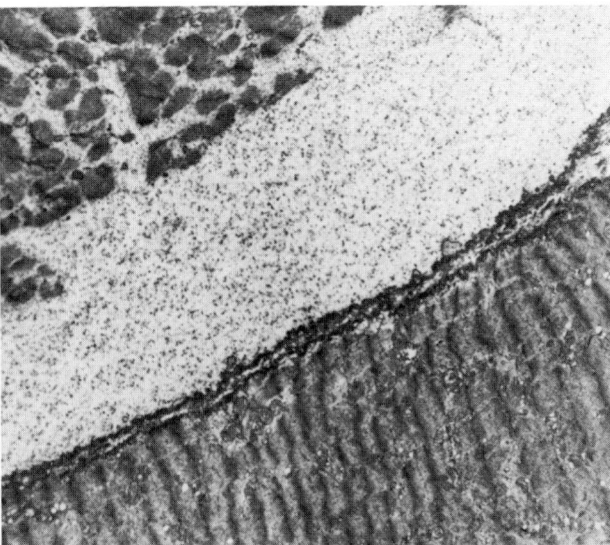

Fig. 57-4 Stage 4, Loss of contractile substance (upper cell). (From Fassbender HG: Pathology of rheumatic disease, New York, 1975, Springer-Verlag.)

a regular arrangement of cross striation, multiple triads, and mitochondria paired on either side of the Z line. He felt the four stages were indicative of a progressive condition of degeneration of contractile muscle elements. The degeneration was caused by prolonged muscle contraction causing damage by reduction of local oxygen tension or hypoxia.[15] Bengtsson, Henriksson, and Larsson's results support Fassbender in that they also found "moth-eaten" and "ragged red" fibers when they examined 77 muscle biopsies in 57 patients with primary fibromyalgia.[4] They felt the chemical and morphologic changes found could be the result of hypoxia because similar findings[29] are found after experimental ischemia; however, overuse could also cause a "moth-eaten" appearance of muscle fibers.

Neurophysiologic etiologic factor

Sola and Williams examined the trigger point from a neurophysiologic perspective.[74] They suggested that an alteration of vasomotor activity existed in the area of a trigger point. They based this on evidence that stimulation of a trigger point with negative galvanic current produced a discrete area of erythema and that skin resistance was decreased over a trigger point.

Altered autonomic nervous system etiologic factor

Travell and Simons described symptoms of dizziness and vertigo especially associated with trigger points in the upper trapezius muscle.[83] They report trigger points in the sternocleidomastoid muscle producing discharge of tears and conjunctiva reddening.

Referred pain

Many authors have demonstrated pain referred from muscle, ligament, and fascia.[31,37,75,83] Travell and Simons have mapped referred pain patterns from almost every muscle in

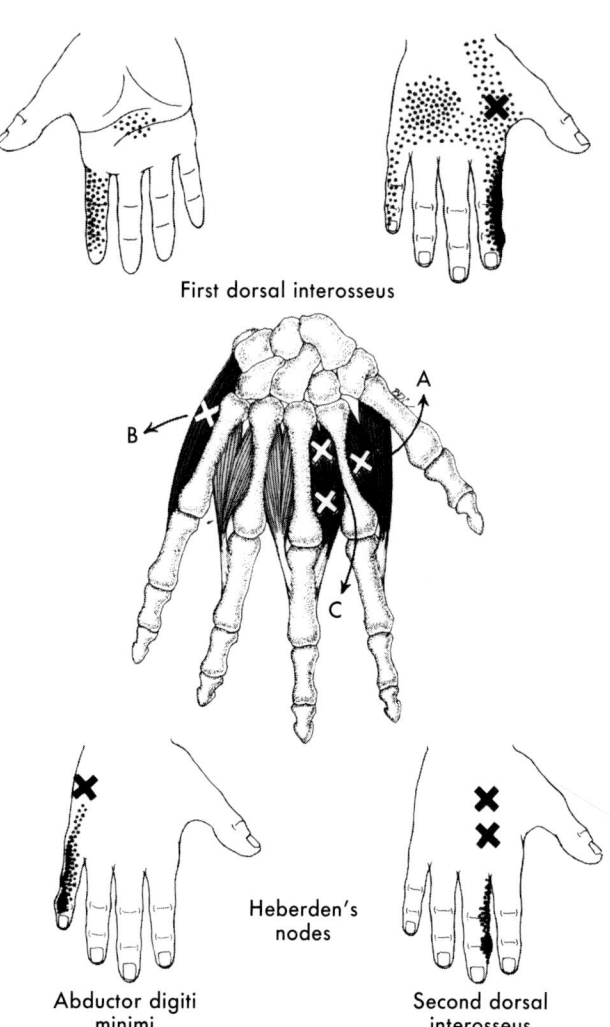

Fig. 57-5 Mapping of referred pain from the interosseous muscles of the hand. *X* denotes the location of the trigger point and *dots* represent the area of referred pain. (From Travell JG and Simons DG: Myofascial pain and dysfunction: the trigger point manual, Baltimore, 1983, Williams and Wilkins.)

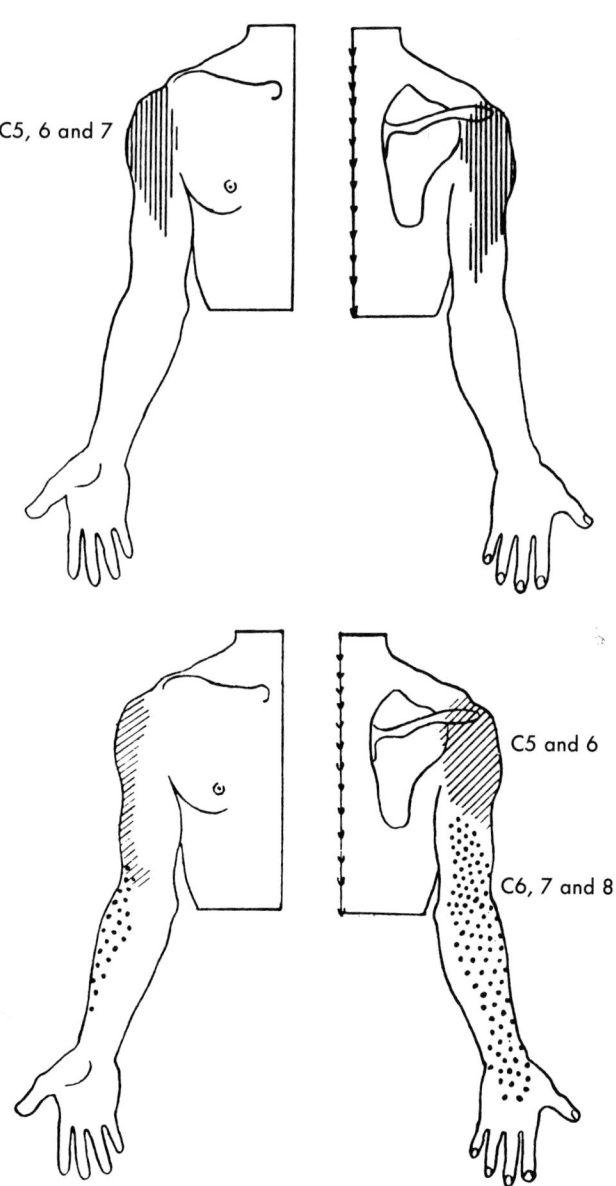

Fig. 57-6 Kellegren's mappings of pain referred from muscles of the upper extremity. (From Kellegren JH: Observation on referred pain arising from muscles, Clin Sci p 175, 1938.)

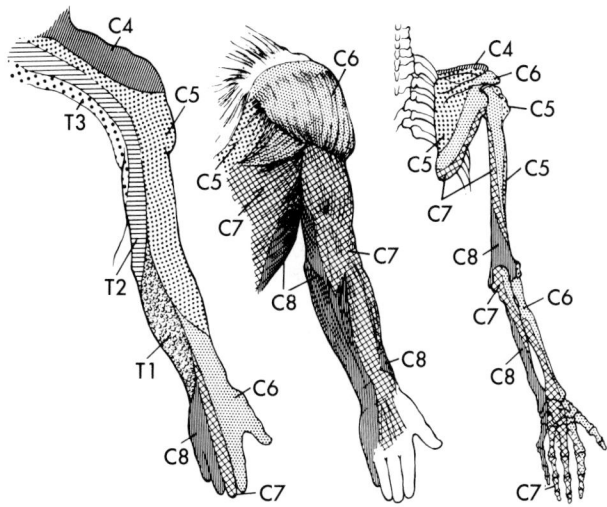

Fig. 57-7 Dermatomes and myotomes of the upper extremity. Note the C6-7 dermatome is the anterolateral shoulder. (From Inman V and Saunders J: Referred pain from skeletal structures, J Nerv Ment Dis 99:660, 1944.)

the upper extremity.[83] They established that pain referred from specific trigger points tends to consistently refer to specific areas. Such an example are the interosseous muscles of the hand (Fig. 57-5).

Travell and colleagues produced their mappings of referred pain areas by dry needling trigger points in over 1000 patients.[82,83] They claim the reference areas are not seg-

mentally related to the trigger point but are referred to as the "fixed anatomical pathways."[80,83]

Rather than mapping the referred pain patterns of existing trigger points, Kellegren mapped out referred pain patterns produced by injecting a 6% solution of sodium chloride into the normal muscle.[37] Fig. 57-6 is a drawing of the referral areas when muscles innervated by that segmental level were injected in his study. Kellegren concluded that pain was not referred to dermatome as classically described by Head and Foester, but he did report a segmental relationship between the irritated tissue and the referred pain site.[16,28] For example, the infraspinatus muscle is innervated by spinal level C5-C6. The dermatome area of C5-C6 is the anterolateral shoulder (Fig. 57-7), which corresponds to the pain mapping.

The comparison of the referred pain patterns of the infraspinatus muscle by Kellegren (Fig. 57-6), the dermatomal mappings (Fig. 57-7), and Travell's mappings (Fig. 57-8) of pain referred from the infraspinatus muscle reveal a marked similarity.

Torejork and colleagues agreed with Kellegren.[75] They electrically stimulated 118 cutaneous and 26 motor nerve fascicles of intact median nerves in normal subjects. When cutaneous fascicles were stimulated, subjects reported pain in the distribution of the median nerve. When the motor fascicles were stimulated, the subjects reported aching, cramplike pain in the forearm and thenar muscles (median nerve innervation), but some reported pain referred to areas clearly outside the median nerve distribution that were segmentally related to the muscle stimulated. For example, pronator teres muscle (C6) pain was referred to the serratus

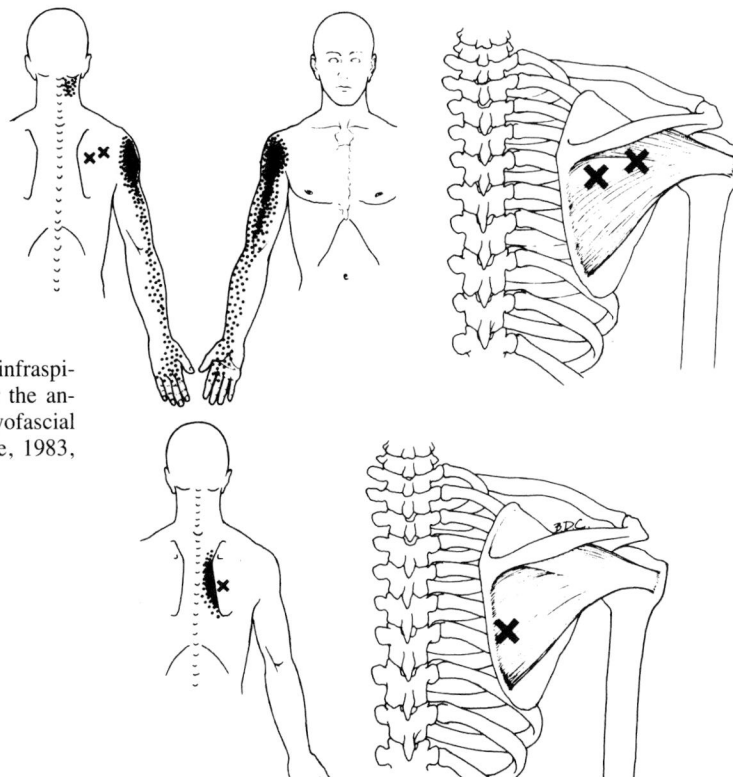

Fig. 57-8 Travell's mapping of pain referred from the infraspinatus muscle. Note the dense area of referred pain over the anterolateral shoulder. (From Travell JG and Simons DG: Myofascial pain and dysfunction: the trigger point manual, Baltimore, 1983, Williams and Wilkins.)

anterior muscle (C6). The pain felt in the referred areas was a deep aching pain with diffuse outlines. The same pain description has been identified by other researchers.[83]

Investigation of a symptom-reproduction examination method (SREM) was reported to determine the local or referred source of low back pain and sciatica symptoms.[59] Ninety-five percent of their subjects with low back pain had their chief complaint reproduced by means of palpation, accessory motion testing, or mechanical tests of position. Of the subjects in whom pain was reproduced, 78.5% of the referred pain sites were located in the dermatome segment related to the irritated tissue. There was an even higher correlation when the dermatome one spinal segment above or below was included. Authors of the most recent literature support this segmental relationship between trigger point and the reference area, but they differ regarding whether the pain is referred to the dermatome or the myotome. Therefore, if one knows the innervation levels of muscle and skin, the possible origins of referred pain can be determined in this manner.

CASE STUDY 1

The following case study will exemplify the aforementioned thought process. This patient was referred to us with the diagnosis of wrist tendonitis. Our traditional evaluation for tendonitis of the flexor carpi ulnaris (FCU) tendon and long finger flexor tendon and possible irritation of the ulnar complex was negative. We continued looking for a myofascial component. Palpation evaluation reproduced her pain from trigger points in the FCU, flexor digitorium profundus (FDP), and extensor pollicis longus (EPL) muscles (Fig. 57-9). After 1 week of treatment, these trigger points were resolved, and she perceived the pain pattern demonstrated in Figs. 57-10, *A* and *B*. Still, evaluation revealed no local source of her pain. All muscles that were innervated by cervical level seven were examined because her description of pain was in the C7 dermatome. The source was the extensor digiti quinti muscle. Palpation reproduced her pain, as did contraction of that muscle. It was also acknowledged that her work as a dental hygienist (Fig. 57-11) exacerbated her symptoms. If an MFP evaluation had not been performed based on examination of all muscles innervated by the same level as the dermatome of the pain presentation, we would not have been able to alleviate her pain.

Neuroanatomic pathways of referred pain

The neuroanatomic pathway that can be traced from the trigger point to the spinal cord level provides a rationale for referred pain. When noxious stimuli from trigger points are

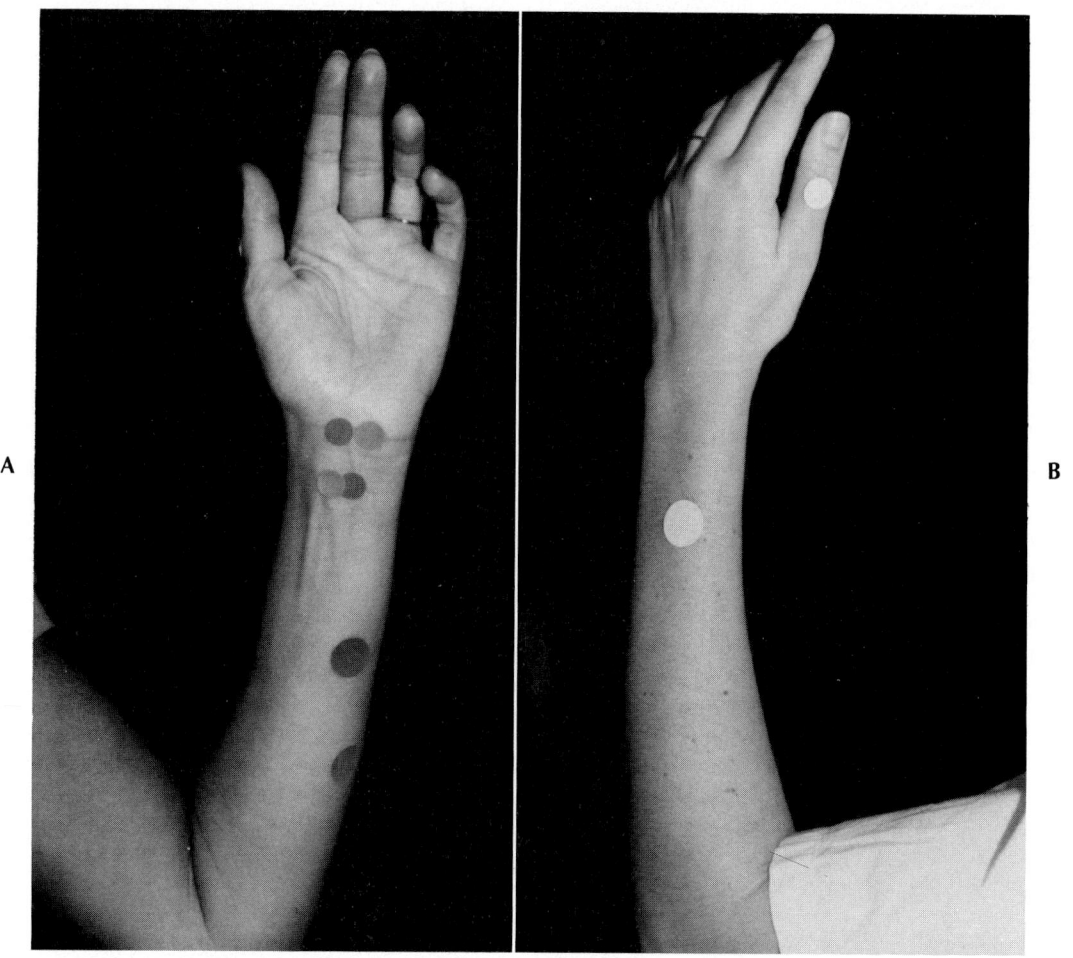

Fig. 57-9　**A** and **B,** Presentation of this patient's pain. The *large dots* denote the trigger points in the flexor carpi ulnaris, flexor digitorium profundus, and extensor pollicis longus mm. The *small dots* show the referred pain distribution.

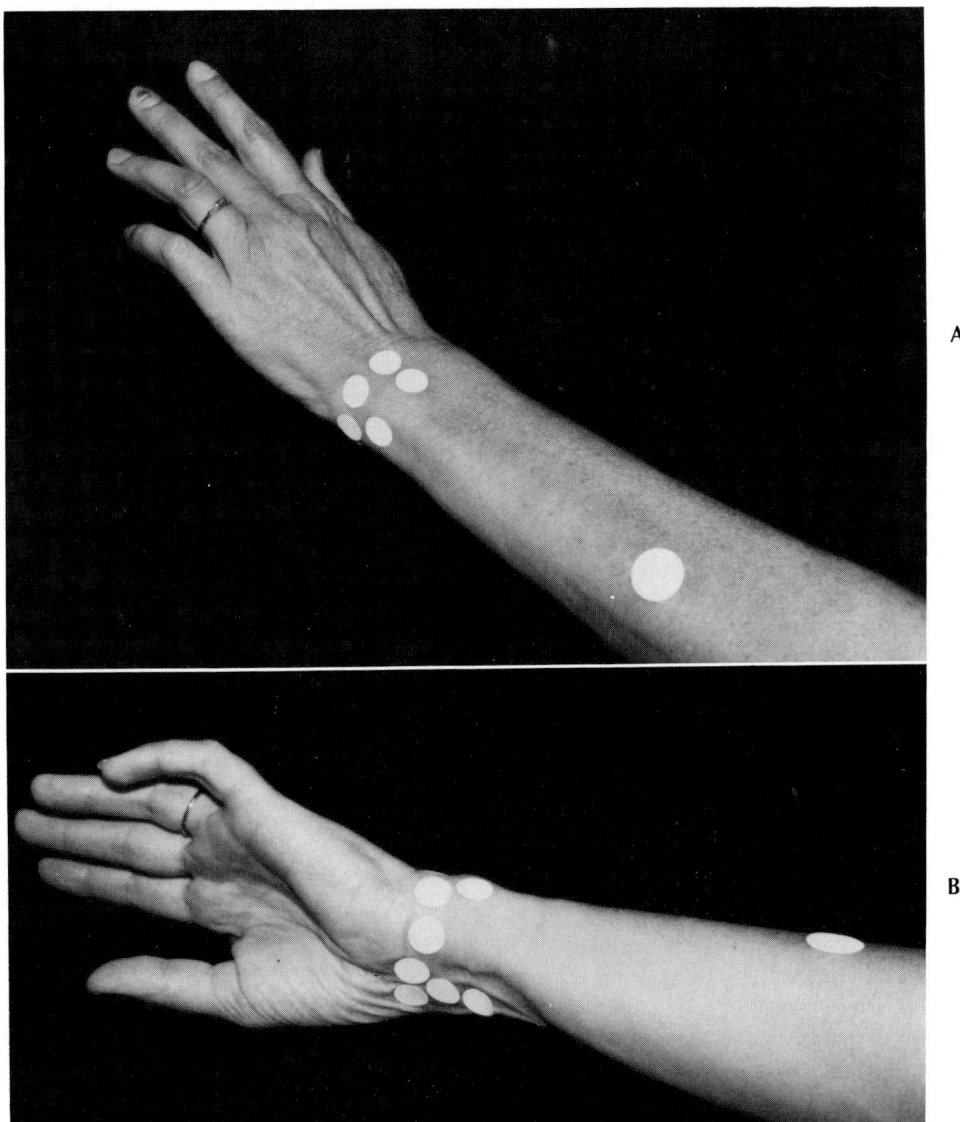

Fig. 57-10   **A** and **B,** Patient's representation of her pain after 1 week of treatment.

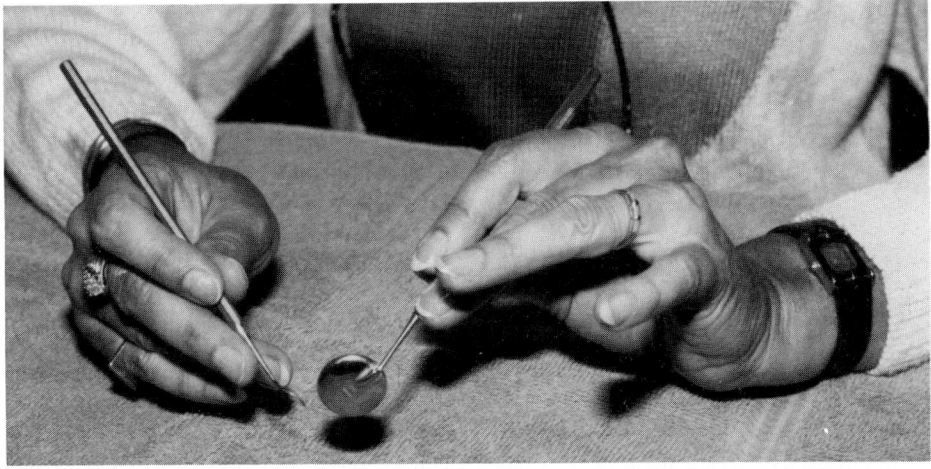

Fig. 57-11   Patient's simulated work posture as a dental hygienist.

strong enough, action potentials are propagated along the axon to synapse in the spinal cord. The fibers bifurcate, most remaining in the same spinal level but some spreading rostrocaudel in the lateral section of the dorsal white matter, including Lissauer's tract. A spread of only two to three segments is believed to occur in man.[45] This anatomic phenomenon can account for the referral of pain one segmental level rostral or caudal, as earlier discussed.

Similar locations of fiber termination at the spinal cord level can also account for the phenomenon of referred pain. The collateral of A delta (Group III) fibers terminate superficially in lamina I, to a small degree in lamina III, and deeper in laminae IV through VI. C-fibers carrying pain terminate almost exclusively superficial in the dorsal horn, but the exact termination is unknown.[19] Unfortunately, most research is oriented toward cutaneous, not muscle, nociception, but researchers have found many muscle nociceptive fiber terminations to be the same as cutaneous nociceptive fiber terminations. Jaeger and Reeves investigated the relationship between pain referral from myofascial trigger points and trigger point sensitivity using a visual analog scale (VAS) and a pressure algometer.[32] The pressure al-

gometer has been proven a valid and reliable measure of trigger point sensitivity in previous studies.[61]

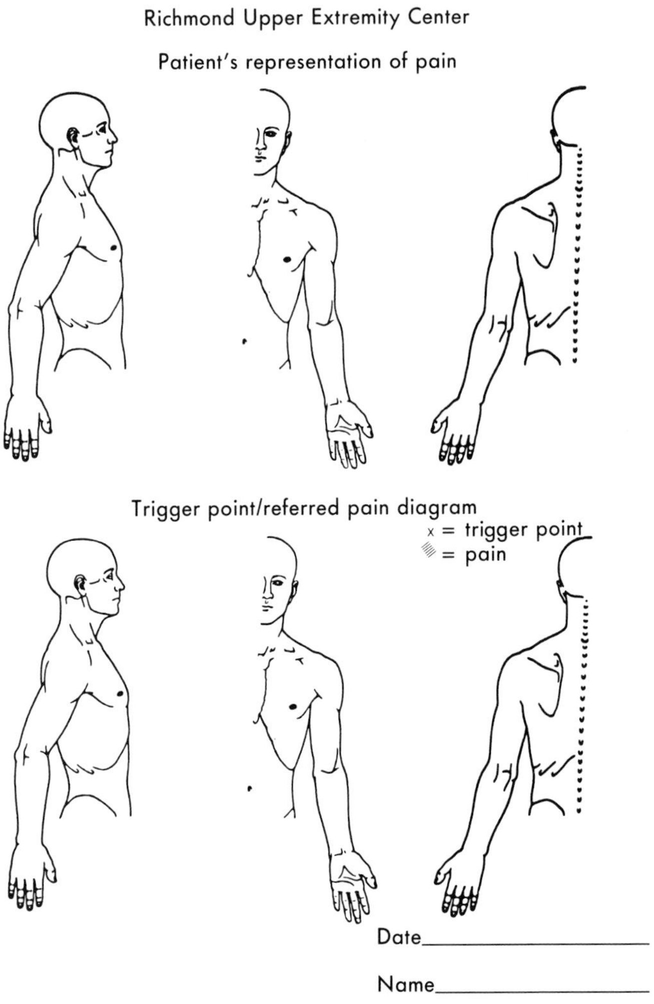

Evaluation process

From this research the characteristics of trigger points and MFP can be understood. First, and most important in evaluation, there are specific patterns of referral that streamline the evaluation. The history may reveal a direct trauma or indirect incident precipitating the pain. The patient may initially have limited range of motion and weakness and there may be autonomic change. The chronicity of the trigger points determines the degree of anatomic change in the muscle and surrounding connective tissue.

Logically, evaluation must begin with an accurate description of the patient's pain. A body chart on which the patient can color in the area of chief pain complaint works well (Fig. 57-12). Letting the patient express his complaints of pain first, and on paper, expedites the evaluation.

The diagram is reviewed with the patient, and a history including the date of onset, nature of the pain (i.e., sharp, dull, deep ache), precipitating factors, and prior treatment and effectiveness is obtained. The intensity of the pain is represented on a pain analog scale (Fig. 57-13).

Traditional evaluation tools are used when appropriate. For example, if the patient complains of numbness, as they often do, Semmes-Weinstein monofilaments and vibrometer testing are used. Most often, complaints of numbness are not substantiated by these tests. Range of motion and strength should also be documented because the patient also frequently complains of stiffness and weakness.

Once a clear picture of the patient's subjective complaints are obtained and objective measurements are recorded, the search for the source of the pain begins. As stated before,

Richmond Upper Extremity Center

Patient's representation of pain

Trigger point/referred pain diagram

x = trigger point

▨ = pain

Date_____

Name_____

Fig. 57-12 A body chart used to represent the patient's pain. The patient colors in the area that represents his/her pain on the top portion. The bottom diagrams are used by the therapist to identify trigger points and the pain referred by each trigger point.

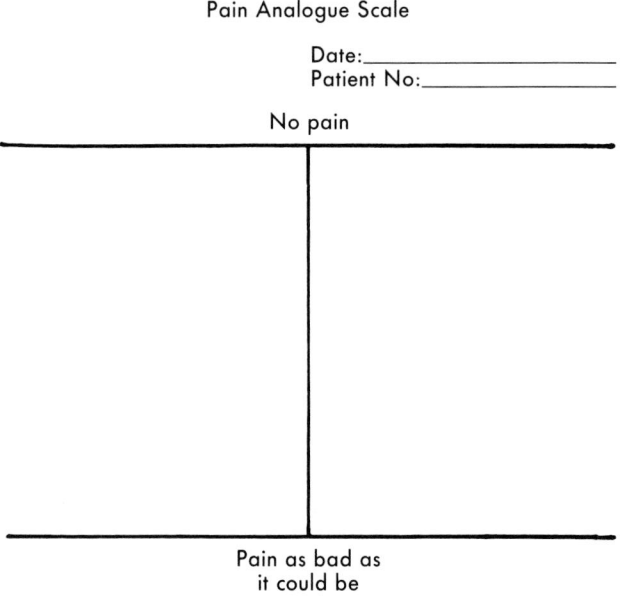

Pain Analogue Scale

Date:_____
Patient No:_____

No pain

Pain as bad as
it could be

*Please mark along this line to indicate

Fig. 57-13 The pain analogue scale is used to objectively measure pain. The line is 15 cm long with one end denoting the most intense pain imaginable and the other end no pain.

the chief complaint can be local, referred, or both local and referred. The traditional evaluation of palpation and accessory motion testing can verify or rule out a local source of pain.

Lastly, information regarding prior treatment helps in determining the initial treatment plan. The information should include not only the effect of prior treatment rendered but, more importantly, where that treatment was administered. If the treatment was applied to the location of the patient's chief complaint of pain, then possible remote origins of referred pain must be considered. If a local source of pain is not found or a secondary source of pain is suspected, the MFP evaluation follows. The area of referred pain is identified for its dermatomal innervation. The muscles of that same spinal level are also identified. Palpation of the entire length of the identified muscle is performed by the therapist. If no source is found, an investigation of the muscles innervated by one spinal segment up or down should be performed. The findings are recorded on another body diagram.

Palpation of muscle for the existence of a trigger point is much the same as palpation for tendonitis. The examiner evaluates for reproduction of pain and tissue turgor. The examiner must transverse the entire muscle, from origin to insertion, applying firm pressure with the pulp of the thumb. First, the patient is asked to inform the examiner if he feels pain, and if he does, is the pain "his pain." Many times the patient will jump and exclaim "that is my pain." That is what Good referred as the "jump sign."[21] The second purpose of palpation, tissue turgor evaluation, can be accomplished by two methods of palpation: skin rolling and lighter palpation using the index finger pulp with the middle finger overlying the index finger nail. Skin rolling is lifting the skin off the underlying muscle, opposing the index finger and thumb, then rolling the skin. We do not use a lubricating lotion and the skin is rolled in all directions. This procedure will be painful over the fascial trigger point. The light palpation is used to sense the depth of the trigger point and to observe for palpable bands, that is, a ropelike structure lying in parallel with the muscle fibers. The findings are recorded on the lower portion of the body diagram (Fig. 57-12). To streamline the investigation, most referred pain is perceived distal to the source of the pain. Travell and Simons identified the following muscles in the upper quadrant that typically refer proximally: sternocleidomastoid, biceps, triceps (long head), supinator, brachioradialis, and adductor pollicis.[83]

Treatment of the source of the pain with resolution of the referred pain is the confirmation of the evaluation. Reevaluation should be performed routinely to assure the source treated is the only source of pain. The following are cases to elucidate the evaluation process described.

CASE STUDY 2

Fig. 57-14 illustrates the trigger points (large dots) and referred pain distribution (small dots) of a 57-year-old male referred with the diagnosis of hand arthritis. The patient had sustained a hyperextension injury from an auto accident 4 months earlier. On the diagram he represented his pain on the dorsum of the ulnar two fingers and the dorsum of the forearm. The pain occurred when he squeezed his hand. Examination revealed irritation of the transverse intermetacarpal ligaments of digits four and five, decreased grip strength, and increased metacarpophalangeal (MCP) flexion

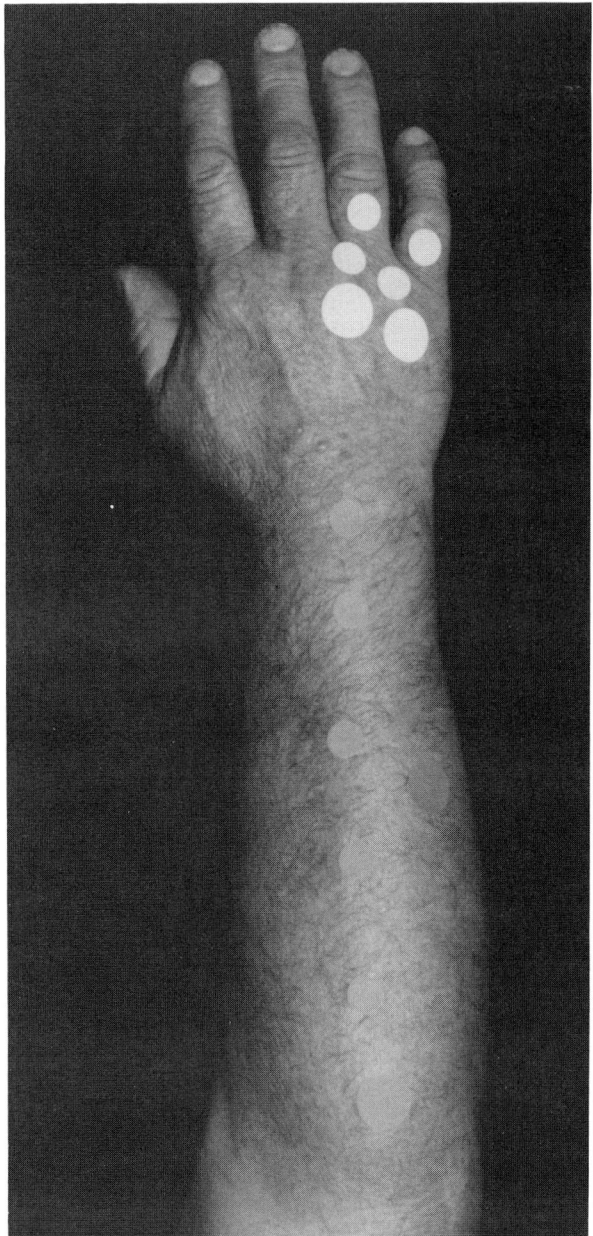

Fig. 57-14 Case study 2, representation of his hand pain.

of digits four and five. MFP evaluation revealed two trigger points: the extensor carpi radialis longus (ECRL) muscle trigger point, in particular, reproduced all of his complaints of pain (Fig. 57-15). Initial treatment produced 48 hours of pain relief.

CASE STUDY 3

This is a 25-year-old male referred with the diagnosis of reflex sypathetic dystrophy (RSD). The patient complained of total upper quadrant pain (Fig. 57-16, *A* and *B*). He carried his right upper extremity in a sling because of stiffness, weakness, and pain. He had limited elbow flexion, elbow extension, shoulder flexion, and external rotation. He rated his pain as 7 on the scale of 0 to 10. His history involved a closed forearm crush involving no fractures 2½

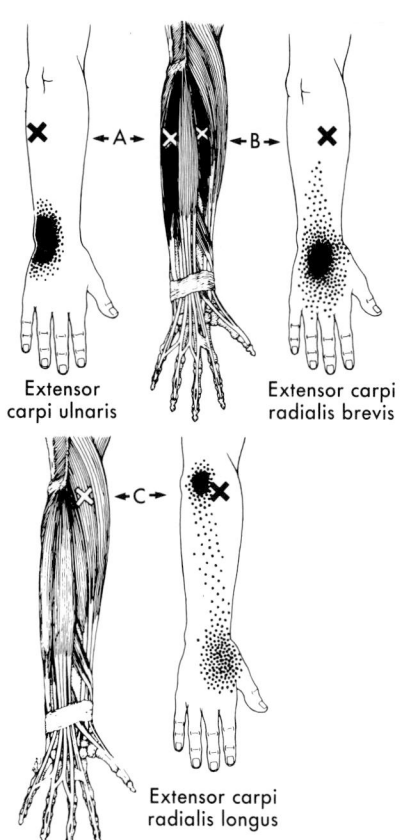

Fig. 57-15 Travell's mapping of referred pain from the extensor carpi radialus longus muscle. (From Travell JG and Simons DG: Myofascial pain and dysfunction: the trigger point manual, Baltimore, 1983, Williams and Wilkins.)

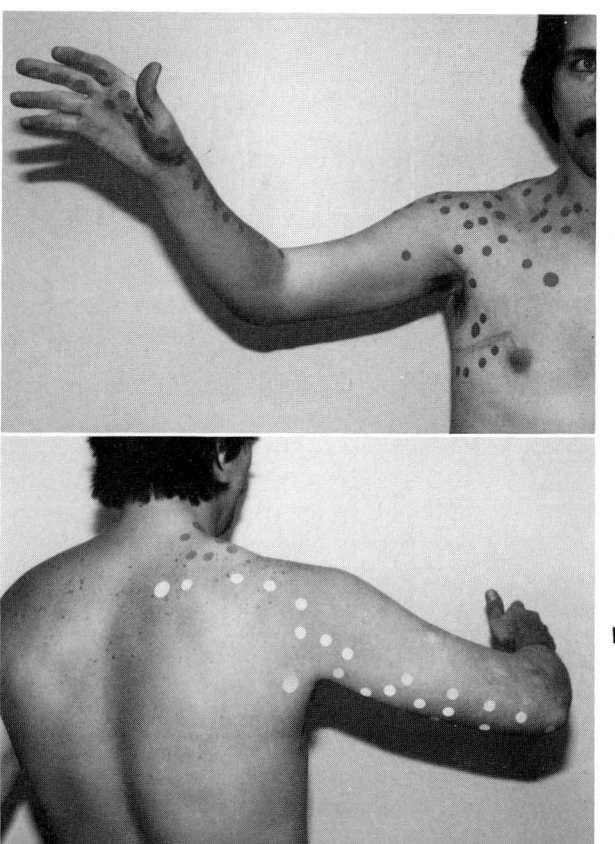

Fig. 57-16 **A** and **B,** Case study 2, representation of his upper extremity pain.

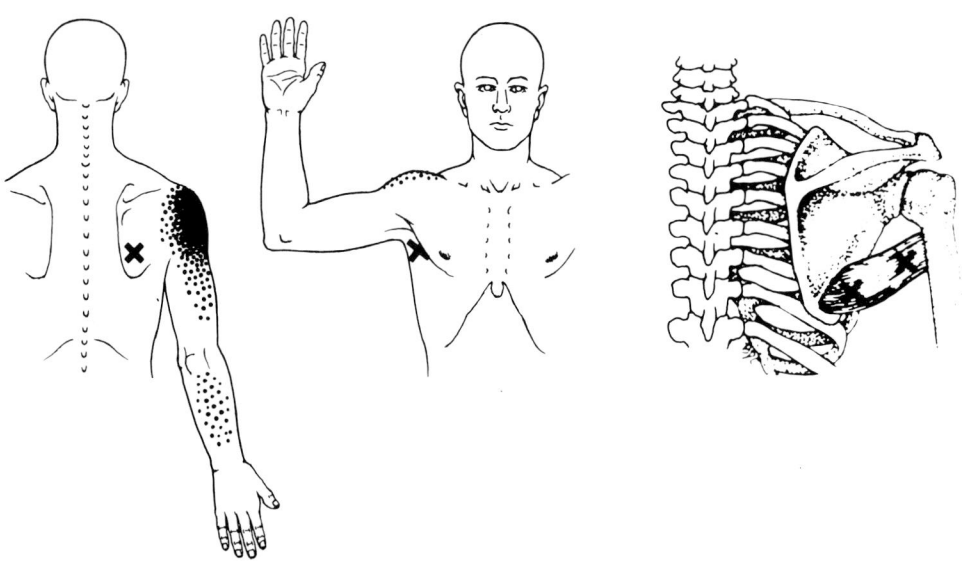

Fig. 57-17 Travell's mapping of pain referred from the teres major muscle to the posterior shoulder and down the arm. (From Travell JG and Simons DG: Myofascial pain and dysfunction: the trigger point manual, Baltimore, 1983, Williams and Wilkins.)

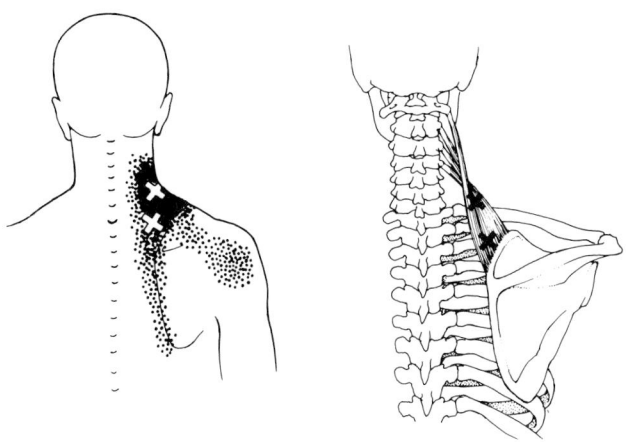

Fig. 57-18   Travell's mapping of pain referred from the levator scapulae muscle to the top of the shoulder. (From Travell J and Simons DG: Myofascial pain and dysfunction of the trigger point manual, Baltimore, 1983, Williams and Wilkins.)

years before being referred to us. His prior medical treatment included casting, hospitalization for intravenous medication, multiple stellate ganglion blocks, and a suggestion by one physician that the arm be amputated. One might wonder where to begin, but when the pain was evaluated muscle by muscle, common referral areas, as described by Travell and Simons, presented themselves. The teres major muscle refers pain to the posterior shoulder and down the arm (Fig. 57-17). The levator scapula muscle is more local, sometimes referring pain over the top of the shoulder (Fig. 57-18). The supraspinatus muscle again refers to the shoulder area (Fig. 57-19). Common referral patterns from the extensor muscles of the forearm refer into the C6-C7 areas of the forearm and hand.

When a patient with upper extremity pain is examined in this manner, the treatment then can be directed toward specific areas. To evaluate such a complex pain, one must take

a step back, refer to the dermatome and myotome charts and to Travell's *Trigger Point Manual*.[83] Then one can solve the puzzle one piece at a time by palpation of muscles that have a potential of referring pain as presented by the patient.

TREATMENT

Treatment of the MFP patient is based on symptoms and body mapping performed in the initial evaluation.[6,9] The therapist must know the locus of the pain to correctly treat and alleviate the discomfort. Simply treating the painful area will not correct the patient's condition. Confirmation of treatment success is made by the patient completing another body mapping and the therapist comparing initial findings to subsequent findings. Other conventional measurements can also be employed such as active and passive range of motion and strength to quantify changes produced by the treatment.

According to the literature, the most popular methods of treatment are injection,* spray and stretch/Fluori-Methane spray,† some form of massage,[7,9,12,13,42] dry needling[24,47] and transcutaneous electrical nerve stimulation (TENS).[13,53,58,60] In this section, all treatments are presented, but those that most easily apply to current clinical practice are discussed. Because the literature rarely presents one treatment alternative but rather a grouping of techniques, multiple treatments are also presented in case study format.

Injection

The most often cited MFP treatment is injection of the trigger point with either procaine, lidocaine, or a corticosteroid (usually a dosage of 0.5% concentration).‡ The medication is injected directly into the trigger point, then the trigger point is rubbed or massaged to dissipate the injected substance. A hot pack is often applied to further disseminate the medication. This treatment choice has proven effective

---

*References 7, 12, 18, 39, 42, 66, 68, 73, 76, 79, 81, 82.
†References 13, 22, 35, 41, 42, 57, 68, 77, 79, 83.
‡References 7, 39, 42, 44, 65, 66, 68, 74, 79, 81-83.

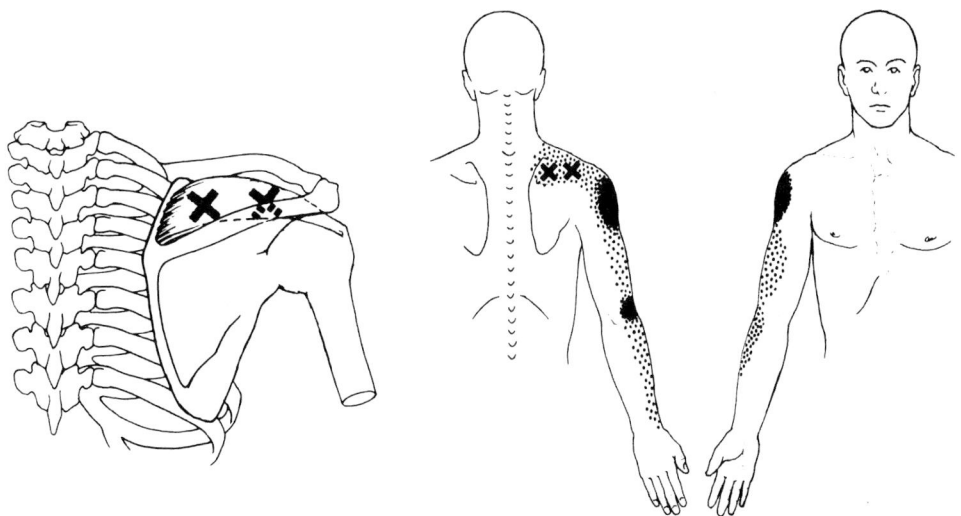

Fig. 57-19   Travell's mapping of pain referred from the supraspinatus muscle to the shoulder area. (From Travell JG and Simons DG: Myofascial pain and dysfunction: the trigger point manual, Baltimore, 1983, Williams and Wilkins.)

in both acute and chronic patient cases, but it is most often effective in acute situations.[42,81,83]

Stretch and spray

The next most popular treatment is stretch and spray, which was originally described by Kraus.* As noted earlier in this chapter, initial treatments were performed with ethyl chloride, but it was found to be too hazardous. Travell introduced the use of Fluori-Methane as the vapor coolant spray for this technique.[83] The vapor coolant provides a mirage of skin impulses over the irritated muscle and the referred zone, which reflexively inhibits the muscle and allows the therapist to stretch the muscle to normal length. The spray is administered at least 18 inches away from the skin surface in a fine spray parallel to muscle fibers of the involved muscle and into that muscle's referred zone (Fig. 57-20). Simultaneously, during the administration of the vapor coolant, the examiner stretches the muscle completely. The therapist performs one to two sweeps of stretch

---

*References 7, 40-42, 57, 65, 68, 76, 79, 82, 83.

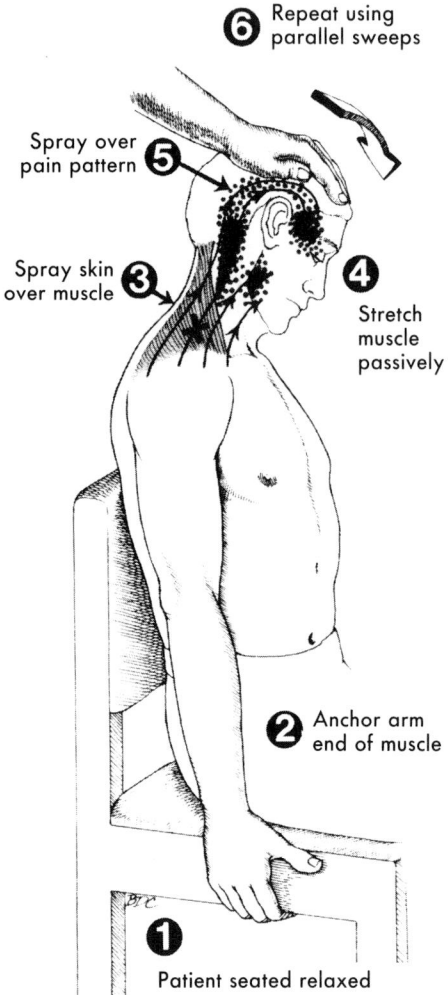

Fig. 57-20 Scheme of application of stretch and spray using vapor coolant spray. (From Travell JG and Simons DG: Myofascial pain and dysfunction: the trigger point manual, Baltimore, 1983, Williams and Wilkins.)

and spray along the width of the muscle's referred zone, followed by hot pack for 5 to 10 minutes, then active exercises afterwards. A gating mechanism that allows the therapist to stretch the muscle completely is thought to inhibit the trigger points.[22,83]

Fluori-Methane spray may be used singularly for trigger point treatment. However, in the experience of the senior authors it is most effective with one other treatment modality such as ultrasound and TENS.

Dry needling

Dry needling is the insertion of a needle and the maneuvering of that needle within the trigger point without removing the needle.[24,42,47,83] It is a very painful technique that theoretically disrupts the pain cycle of the trigger point and physically disrupts the substance of the trigger point. Levit,[47] in 1979, presented his treatment of 244 patients and 312 structures using dry needling as the primary technique. He found that he obtained immediate analgesia in 86.6% of the patients and permanent relief in 92 out of 288 painful structures of these patients. For those patients not receiving immediate relief, Levit recommended other physical therapy treatments to complement the dry needling techniques.

Heat modalities

Heat modalities are infrequently described in the treatment of MFP.[7,49,52] Hot packs are usually mentioned as an adjunct treatment with stretch and spray technique but not used exclusively for treatment.[83] Heat has not been demonstrated clinically effective for MFP treatment. However, McCray and Patton[52] described the use of diathermy and superficial heat. They found diathermy was a significantly more responsive heat modality than hot packs if the trigger points were less sensitive or more acute than chronic. This study is of little help since most hand clinics do not own a diathermy unit. Instead, this study places an interesting perspective on the value of heat in management of this group of patients.

Phonophoresis and iontophoresis

Phonophoresis and iontophoresis are used for delivering corticosteroids and analgesic medications to the trigger point in lieu of injections.[3,27,40] Phonophoresis uses a 10% corticosteroid solution suspended in ultrasonic gel administered to the trigger point with continuous ultrasound. Iontophoresis uses direct current (DC) electricity for medication administration. Both techniques are alternatives to direct injection and are certainly more comfortable for the patient. Treatment frequency is dependent on patient response because resolution of the trigger point is confirmation of treatment process. Most often though, just a few treatments are needed, and typically, phonophoresis treatment interfaces well with ischemic pressure technique and interferential current.

Electrotherapy

A variety of electrotherapy treatments have been cited for the management of MFP. Electrotherapy treatments that are available are hi-volt, electroacupuncture, interferential current, and TENS.[43,53-55,58,60] Historically, electrical management of trigger points is described in a similar fashion as the acupuncture treatment for pain. Melzack noted that many

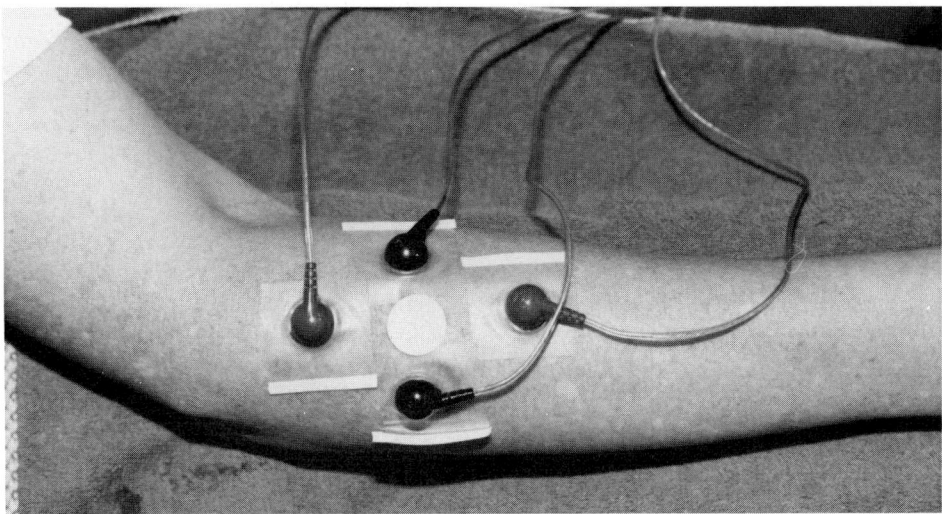

Fig. 57-21 Application of interferential current for treatment of trigger point irritation. Both channels are applied such that crossing of channels occurs at the trigger point.

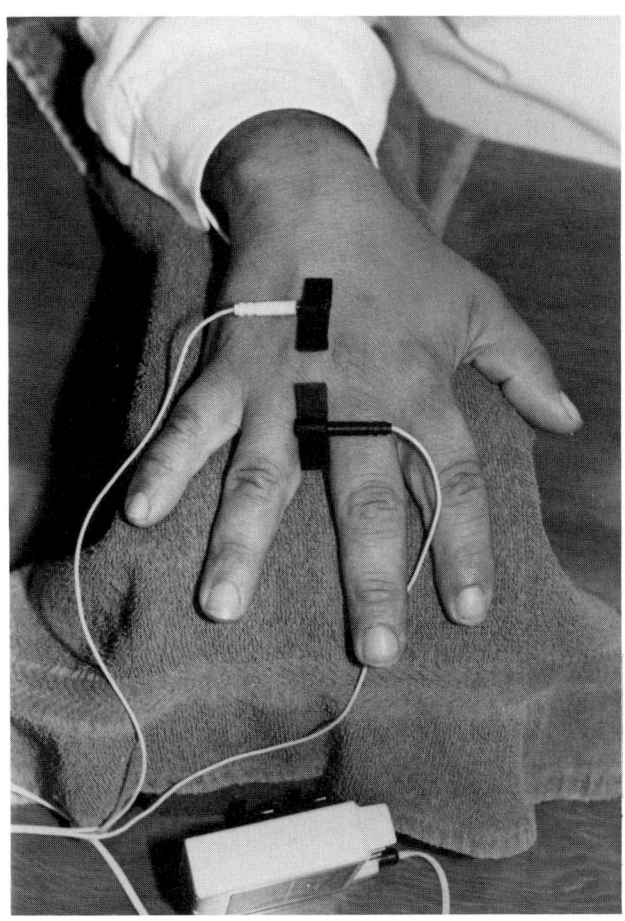

Fig. 57-22 Use of sized electrodes for appropriate treatment of trigger points in small hand muscles.

of the trigger points (78.5%) are located at the same point as acupuncture points.[54,55] He noted in reviewing the available literature, as well as in his clinical experience, that brief, intense TENS stimulation reduced trigger point irritability.[53] Omura described his results using electroacupuncture.[58] Though high frequency electroacupuncture produced quick relief, the carryover of pain relief was short, whereas low frequency electroacupuncture produced a long carryover despite the slowness of the initial relief. He qualified low rate as less than 5 pulses per second.

Procacci and colleagues[60] studied 108 patients with low back pain with a variety of diagnoses to determine what diagnosis responded most effectively to a 15-minute treatment of TENS (50 Hz). TENS provided permanent relief, i.e., relief lasting more than 2 months after discharge, for patients with trigger points and only temporary relief, i.e., return of pain 2 to 3 hours after discontinuation of TENS treatment or within 2 months after discharge, for patients with signs of denervation. They hypothesized that TENS altered the pathologic reflexes that exist in concert with a trigger point.

Also mentioned in the literature is high frequency vibration. Lundberg observed that vibration at 100 to 200 Hz applied over the trigger point provided almost the same effective relief as high and low frequency TENS.[51] Melzack described all of these techniques as hyperstimulation analgesia in offering an explanation of their effectiveness.[53] In our clinical experience, the use of interferential current, TENS, and trigger point vibration have been most effective. The interferential current is applied using both channels, in a fixed or sweep mode, (depending on trigger point irritability) so that the interference wave is formed through the trigger point (Fig. 57-21). The TENS electrodes are sized to treat the trigger points of the small hand muscles (Fig. 57-22), or the probe attachment is used for effective treatment (Fig. 57-23). In certain circumstances, either in cases of trauma-associated trigger points or chronic MFP, the TENS electrodes bracket the trigger point so that stretching exercises can be performed without increasing the irritability of the trigger point (Fig. 57-24).

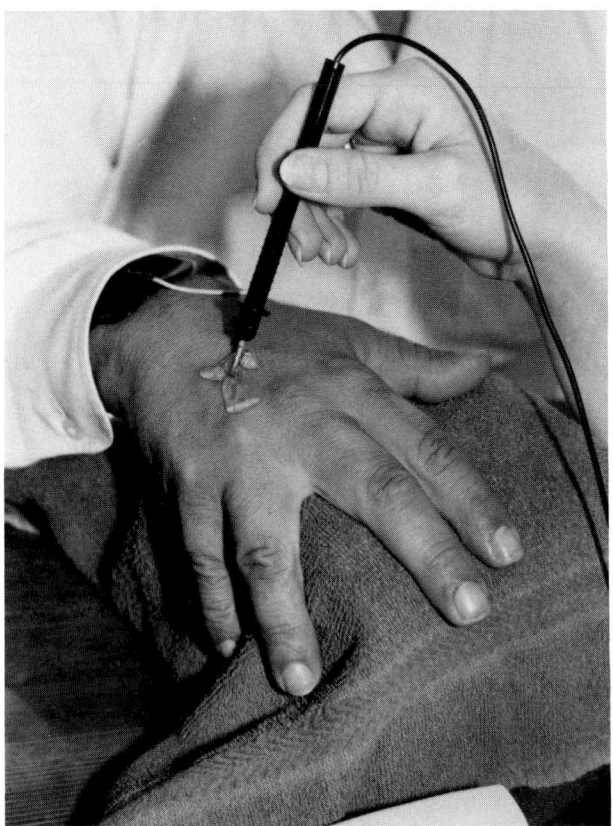

Fig. 57-23 Use of transcutaneous nerve stimulation probe attachment for treatment of trigger points in the small intrinsic muscles.

Connective tissue techniques

The connective tissue technique most often described is the frictioning technique of Cyriax.[7,9,12,65] This is constant application of heavy pressure across the trigger point for the purpose of breaking up adhesions (Fig. 57-25). Skin rolling is another technique that is similar to earlier described massage techniques. This is a very painful technique involving the release of the fascia from the underlying muscle or the skin from the fascia (Fig. 57-26). This technique is used by the therapist for both evaluation and treatment, as mentioned earlier. In chronic cases of myofascial pain, this author frequently uses this technique. Then after 5 to 10 minutes, one can reassess with palpation to observe the trigger point irritability. Those trigger points still irritated can then be treated with ultrasound or interferential current.

Knuckling is another soft tissue technique in which the therapist is performing a stressing technique parallel to muscle fiber (Fig. 57-27). This technique stresses the connective tissue about the muscle fiber, facilitating muscle lengthening during stretching using the therapist's knuckles (proximal interphalangeal, or PIP, joints) as the stress. The flexed knuckles are pulled or pushed along the muscle. While not appropriate in acute patient cases, connective tissue techniques are appropriate in chronic cases where there is adaptive shortening of structures. Capillary breakage is frequently seen in these chronic cases (Fig. 57-28). In these cases, not only is the treatment directed toward trigger point irritability, but also toward lengthening the involved muscles so joint balance and posture can be reestablished. If this aspect of MFP management is not addressed, then trigger point irritation or activation will recur.

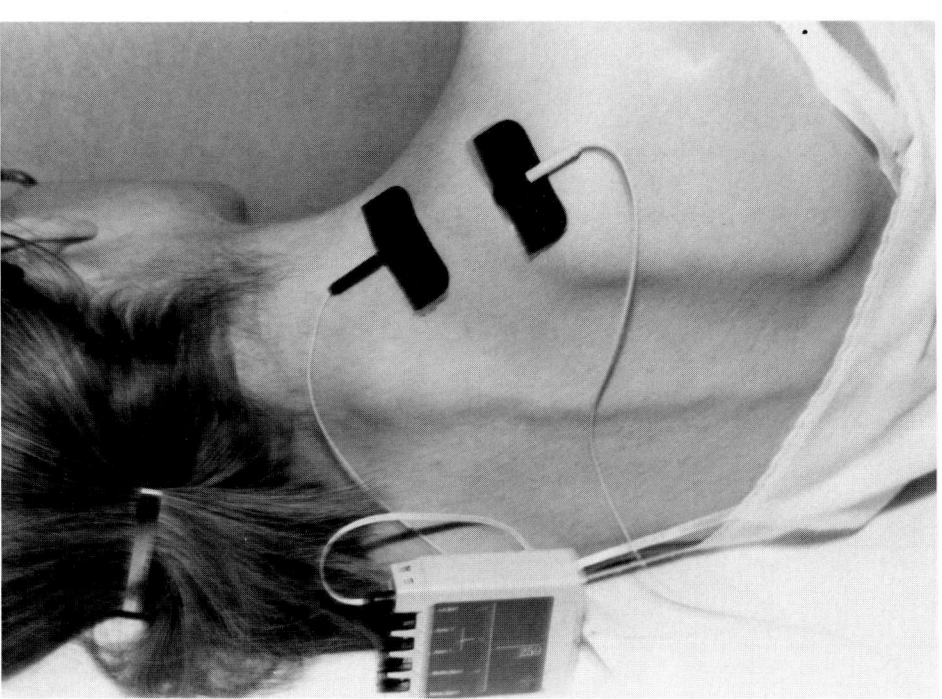

Fig. 57-24 Use of transcutaneous nerve stimulation for treatment of trigger point irritation by bracketing the trigger point with a pair of electrodes.

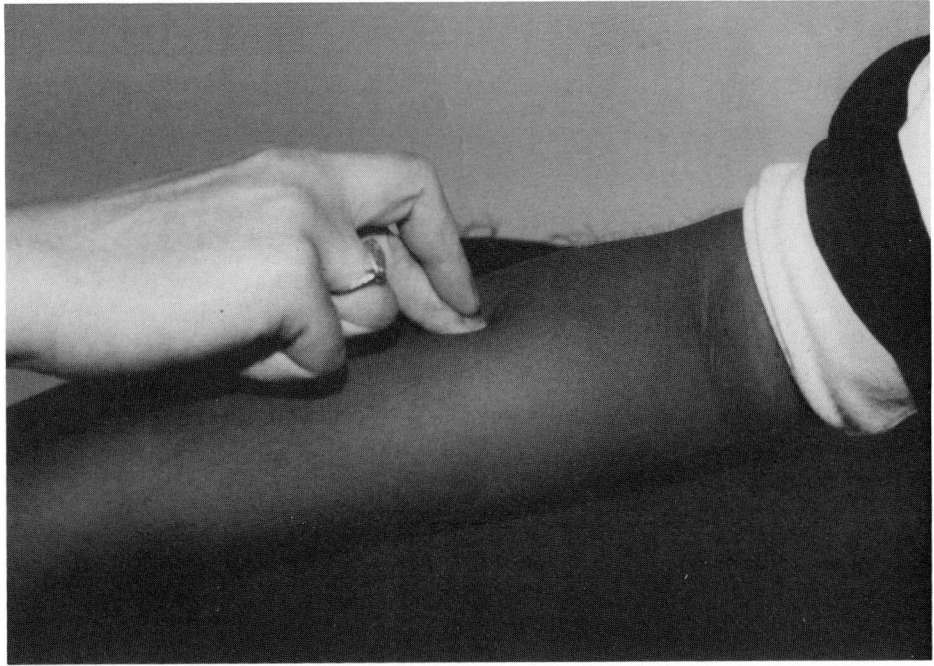

Fig. 57-25   Friction massage techniques as described by Cyriax for disruption of trigger point irritation.

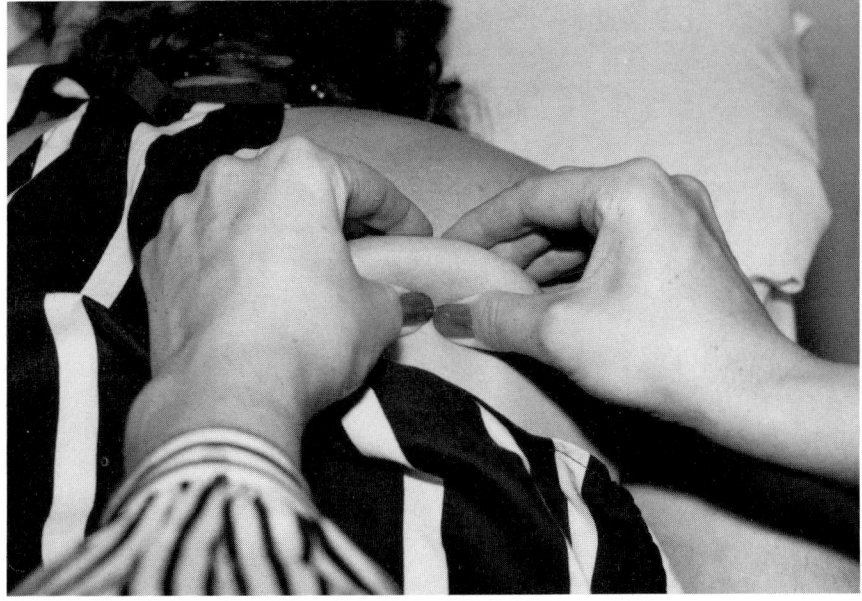

Fig. 57-26   Skin rolling is a connective tissue technique used for evaluation and treatment.

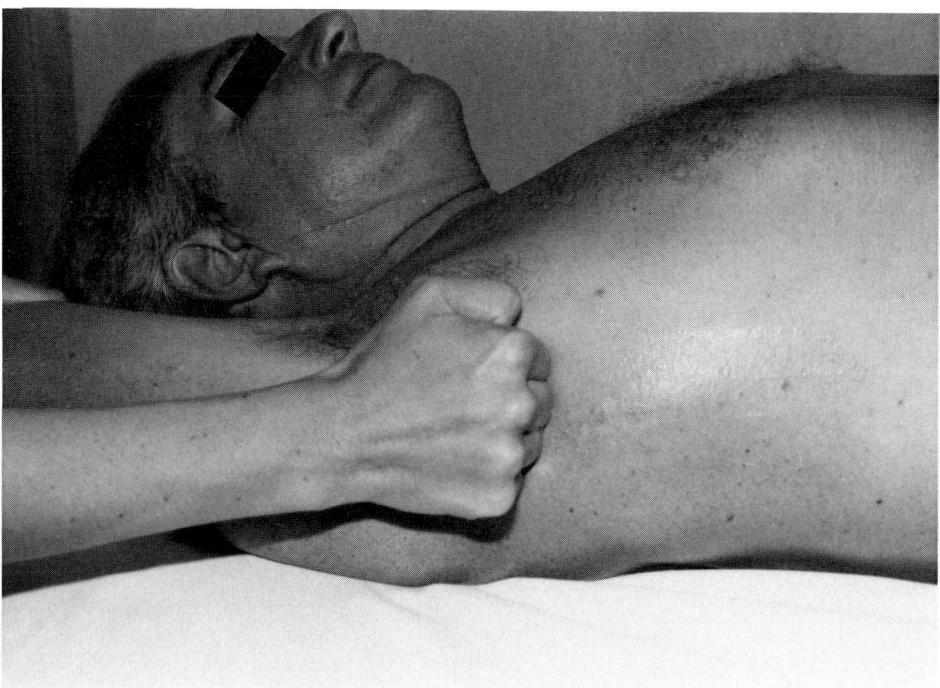

Fig. 57-27   Knuckling is performed parallel to the fibers of the restricted muscle.

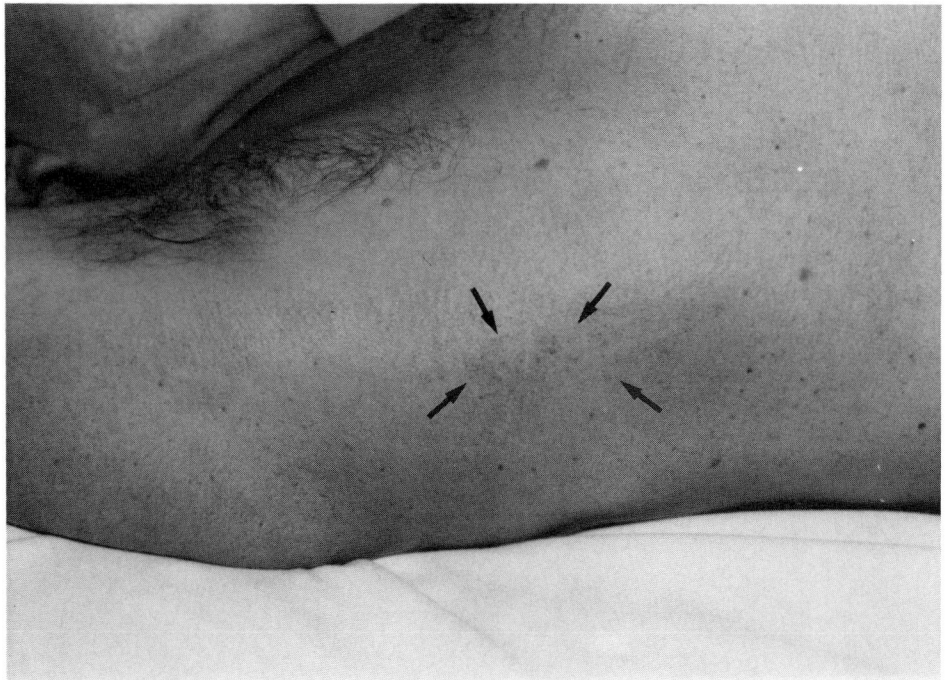

Fig. 57-28   Capillary breakage is a frequent response to skin rolling and knuckling in chronic patient cases.

Ischemic pressure technique

Ischemic pressure technique, as described by Travell, is the use of a graded pressure over the trigger point for up to 60 seconds to provide reflexive inhibition of the trigger point.[83] When the pressure is applied, the patient will report a graded decrease in his pain and resolution of his pain during the 60-second interval (Fig. 57-29). Frequently, the senior authors have used this technique first and, depending on the degree of pain resolution, proceeded to further trigger treatment with TENS or ultrasound. The key to this technique is a *gentle* graded pressure. Increasing pressure is not applied until the patient feels a *decrease* in pain.

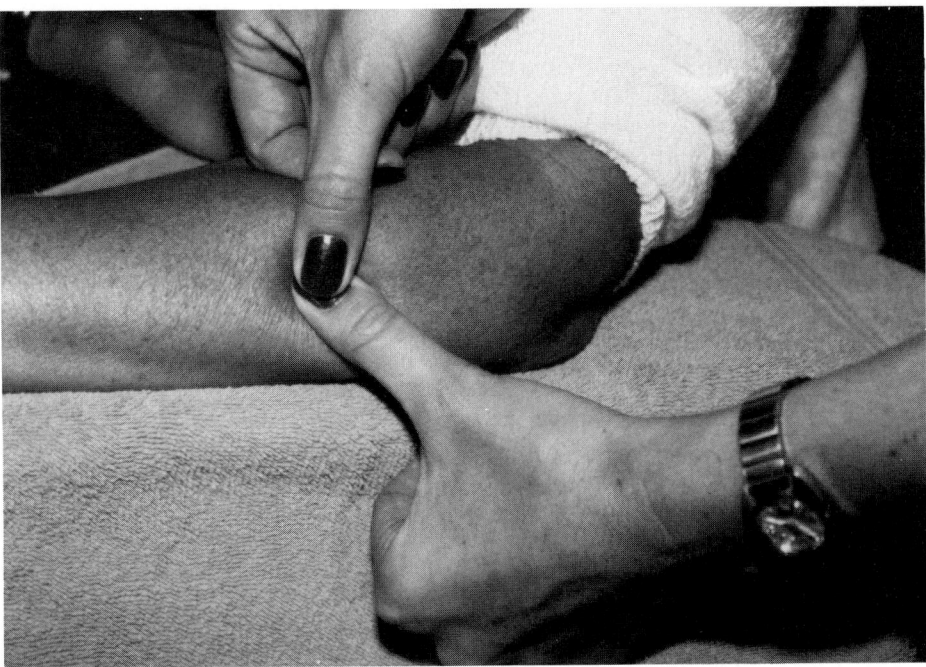

Fig. 57-29 Ischemic pressure techniques as described by Travell involves slow, constant pressure application for disruption of trigger point irritation.

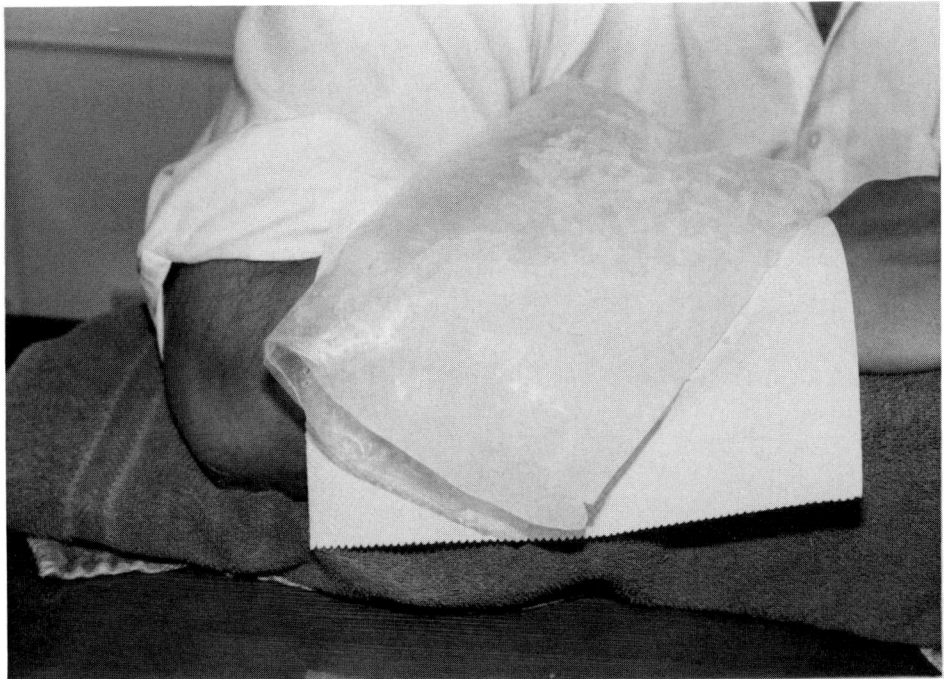

Fig. 57-30 Use of ice slush for quick chill after treatment. Ice bag is positioned over irritated tissue with a paper towel interposed.

Cold modalities

Kraus, Travell, and others have described the use of a vapor coolant spray as an effective cold modality.* Other cold modalities are not recommended because they can ag-

gravate the condition.[83] It is the clinical experience of the senior authors, however, that quick icing is necessary for pain relief and maintaining tissue length in those patients with chronic complaints. These patients require vigorous soft tissue techniques and multiple treatments, which can produce local erythema and swelling. Very often, quick

---

*References 13, 35, 41, 42, 57, 65, 67, 68, 76-83.

icing alleviates the reactivation of a trigger point, but it is strongly recommended that quick icing be used because chilling is a causative factor in MFP. Our clinic uses a particular icing technique combining alcohol and water in a freezer bag. When one part alcohol and three parts water are mixed and frozen, they form a slush. The bag of alcohol slush is applied to the patient's skin with a paper towel interposed for 5 minutes (Fig. 57-30). Longer time or direct skin contact causes frostbite. The skin quickly chills, using this icing technique without the painful sequelae of icing.

Splinting

Static splinting plays an important role in placing the irritated muscle at rest during the early stages of treatment. Splints are used when movement of the involved muscle reactivates the trigger point before regaining full length and strength of the muscle. These movements can be related to normal activity, overuse postures or positions, or trauma-induced postures. Most often, the thumb (adductor pollicis muscle trigger point) and the wrist (wrist flexor muscles trigger points and wrist extensor muscles trigger points) are splinted until the trigger point is completely resolved. Then, as the patient begins strengthening, the splint is gradually weaned. At the Richmond Upper Extremity Center (RUEC), Coban*-wrapping of the distal transverse arch has worked in reducing the irritability of the intrinsic musculature trigger points.

Exercises

Exercises are important for regaining muscle balance about a joint and strengthening in the cases of long-standing MFP. In the literature, descriptions of rhythmic stabilization, specific stretching, strengthening, and work posture

---

*Coban, 3M, Minneapolis.

are reported.* It is most important that the patient learn to move and stretch without creating imbalance again. Often the patient's posture at work or leisure provoked the MFP complaints; therefore, specific stretching is offered and continued after discharge. As soon as the patient demonstrates pain-free range, then active stretching and strengthening begin. In our clinic, the emphasis is on muscular balance about the joint involved. This is particularly true at the glenohumeral joint. Though patients are referred for more distal complaints, the ipsilateral shoulder is often positioned in a protracted posture (Fig. 57-31). Pain-relieving treatments must be accompanied by stretching and strengthening or the trigger points will be reactivated.

These three exercises are usually given as shown in Figs. 57-32 to 34 to the patients to maintain tissue length and balance, provide good posture and joint alignment, and allow for proper stretching. If the myofascial complaint is work related, then stretching exercises to counteract the work posture are provided. The following case study illustrates the effect of work posture on propagating MCP joint complaints.

CASE STUDY 4

(The following case study was outlined in Case Study 1.)

Initially, the patient's pain was identified as arising from the muscle bellies of EPL, FCU, and FDP. These areas were treated with local moist heat and Cyriax friction massage to each trigger point. When the trigger point discomfort decreased after a couple of minutes, stretch and spray was used to provide further pain relief and muscle elongation. The patient was then instructed at the end of this first visit to ice these trigger points at home frequently and not to resume activities.

---

*References 7, 12, 16, 41, 42, 48, 68, 83.

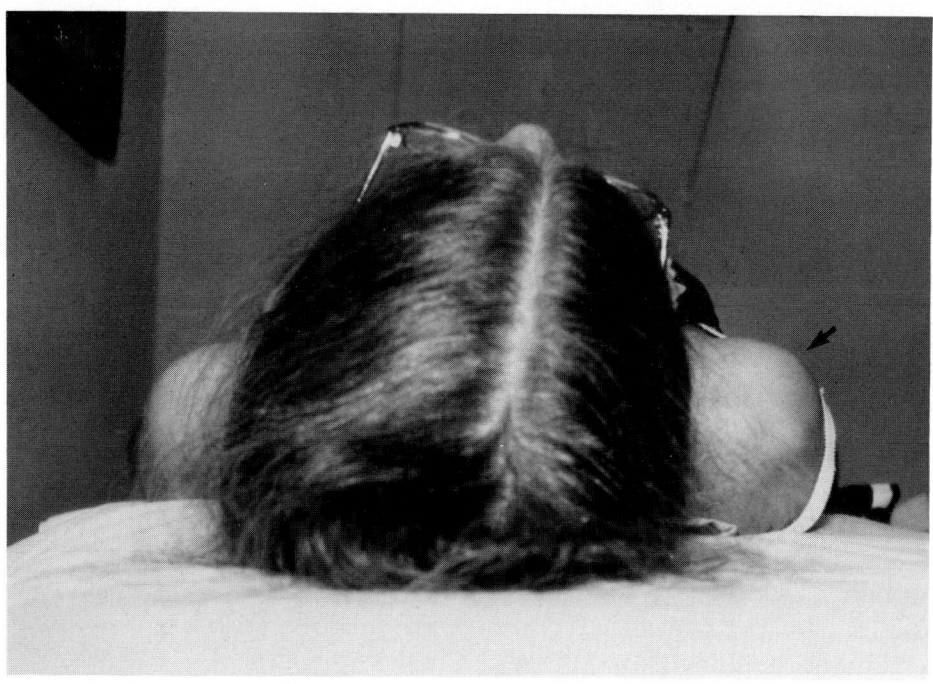

Fig. 57-31 Computer programmer displaying excessive protraction of the glenohumeral joint.

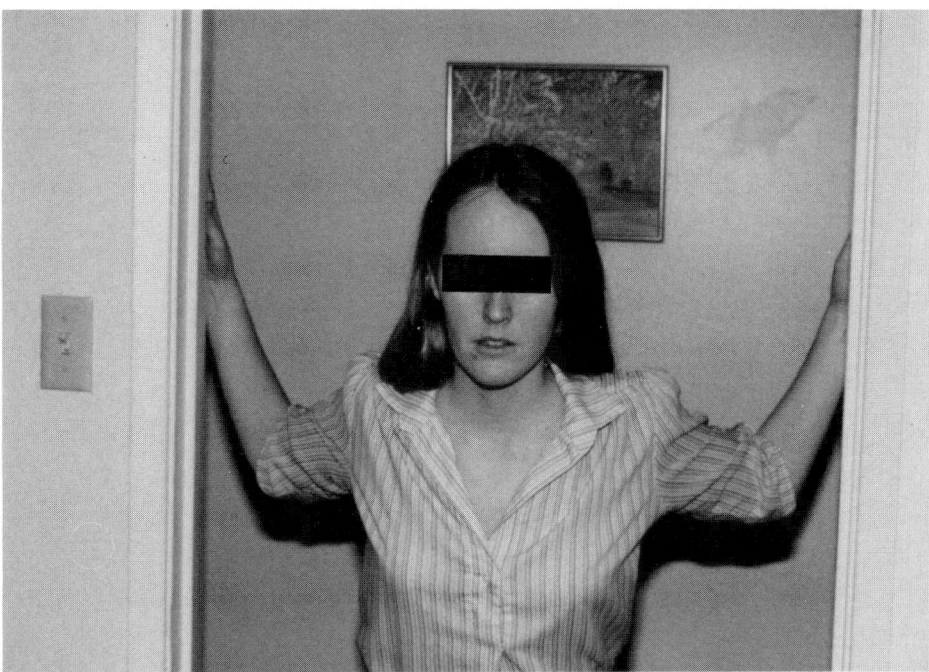

Fig. 57-32 Classical pianist demonstrating the pect stretch that she uses as a warm up exercise and preventative maneuver to avoid recurrence of trigger points in the pectoralis muscle.

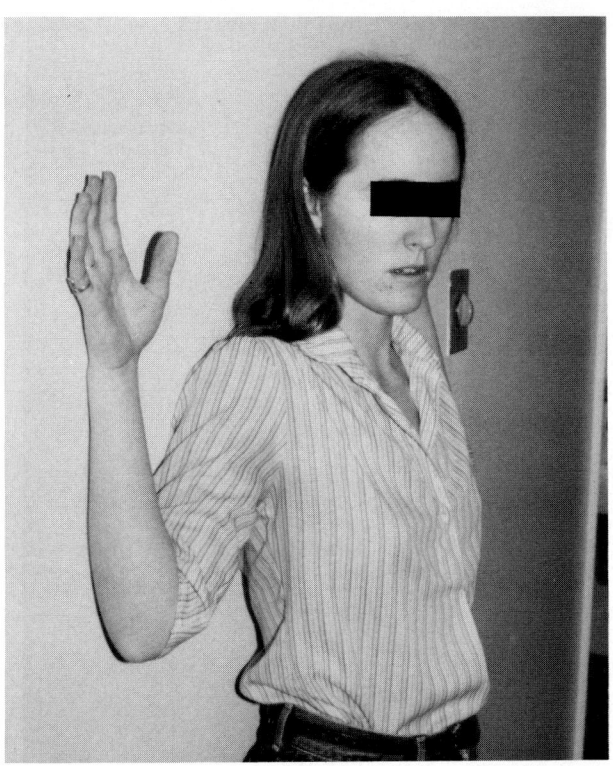

Fig. 57-33 Classical pianist demonstrating the "off the wall" exercise for strengthening the posterior shoulder girdle and stretching the anterior shoulder girdle, which involves maintaining wall contact with her arms as she moves them overhead.

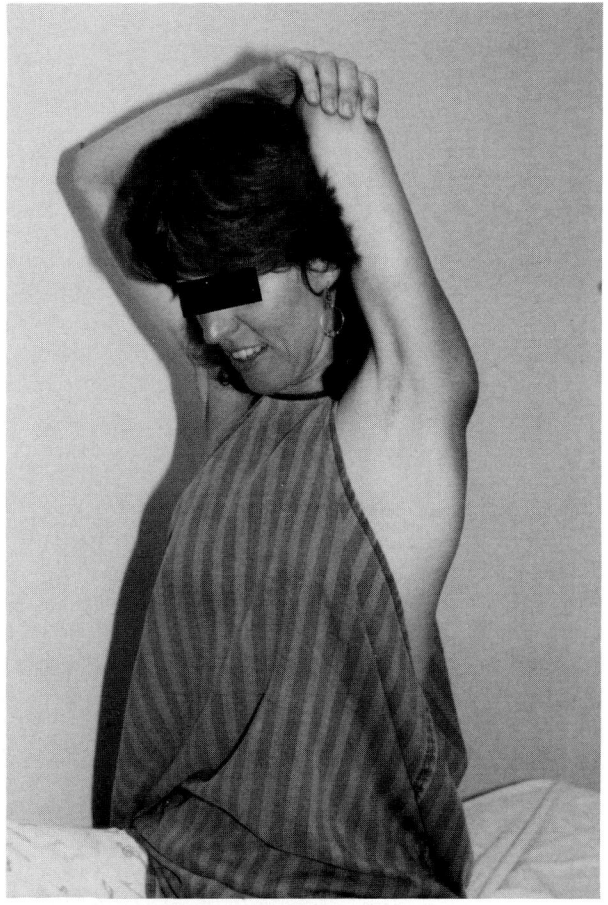

Fig. 57-34 This harpist uses this self stretch exercise to maintain length of the posterior cuff mm and latisimus dorsi muscle.

On the second visit, she reported less pain, but now it was located in a different area. Body mapping and palpation revealed a trigger point located in the ECU muscle referring to the ulnar aspect of her wrist. Treatment then consisted of ischemic pressure technique and stretch and spray to the ECU muscle with resolution of symptoms. By the third visit, the patient reported only mild discomfort between visits. Palpation revealed a trigger point in the extensor digiti quinti

(EDQ) and FCU muscles. The EDQ trigger point referred to the ulnar styloid, which was the area of greatest pain for her from initial evaluation. When asked what postures of work or play provoked a constant strain on the EDQ muscle, the patient observed that she habitually held the fifth MP joint in hyperextension when using her dental tools. Treatment during that visit consisted of ischemic pressure technique, muscle oscillations (which relieved her "thick sen-

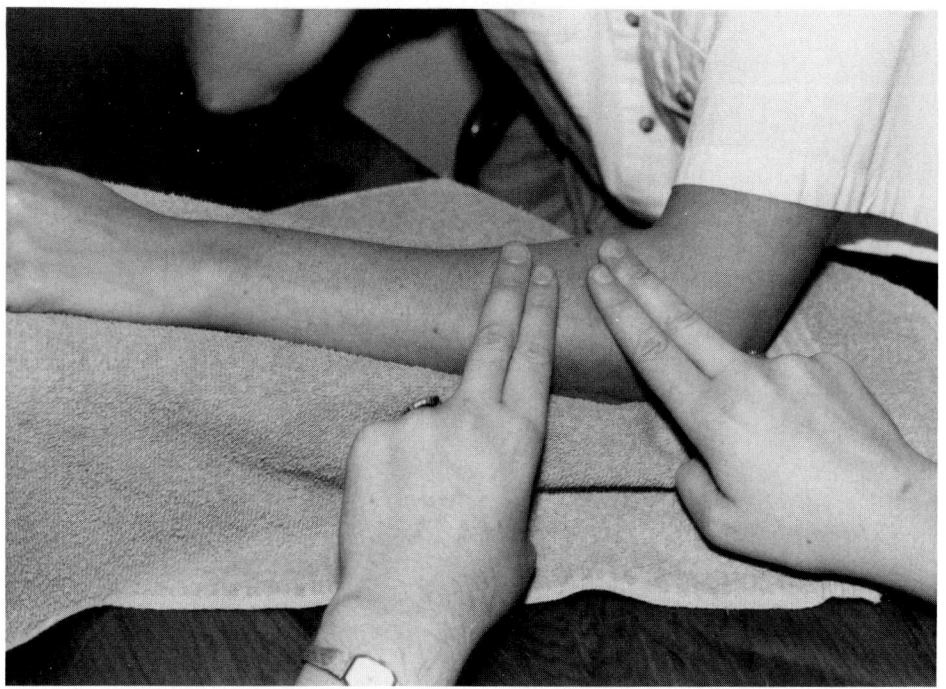

Fig. 57-35   Muscle oscillations are used to decrease "thick" painful sensations.

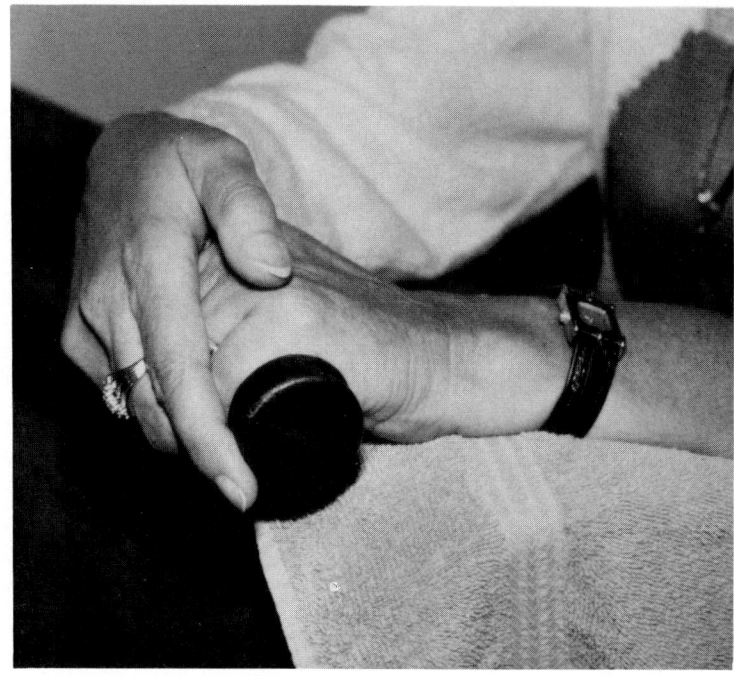

Fig. 57-36   Use of eccentric muscle strengthening for decreasing stress to the previously irritated muscle.

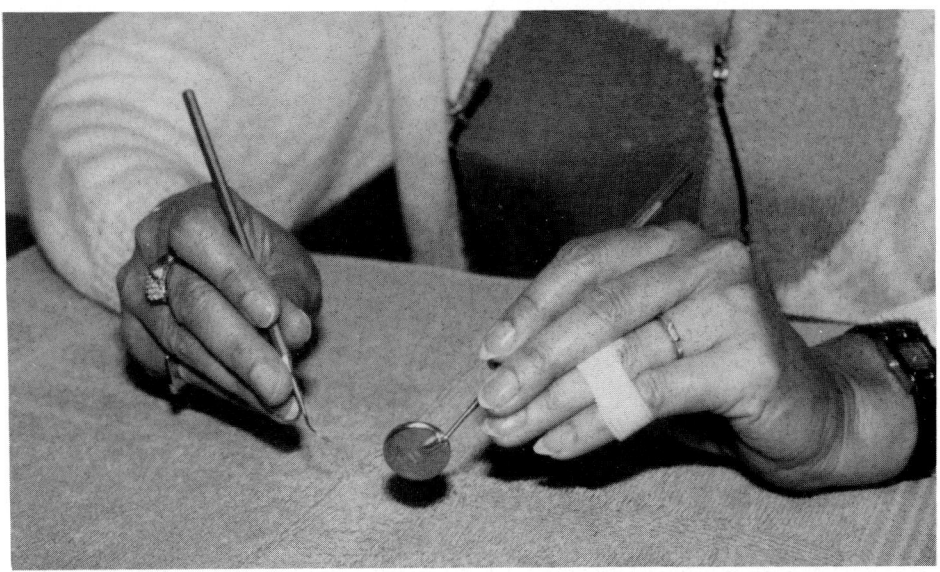

Fig. 57-37 Use of buddy wrap to prevent injurious work posture.

sation") (Fig. 57-35), ice, 1-pound eccentric wrist extension exercises (Fig. 57-36), and work posture modifications. Specifically, at work she used either a Velcro buddy or Coban wrap between digits four and five to prevent MCP joint hyperextension (Fig. 57-37). The FCU trigger point was possibly caused by the habitual position of the fifth MCP joint hyperextension and abduction as described by the patient. This digit posture exerted a constant pull on the FCU insertion.

The patient received three more treatments of ischemic pressure technique, ice, and resistive wrist exercise, and she resumed tennis practice for short periods. She also worked at the dental office during this interval with no discomfort. Throughout, she continued home icing to the EDQ trigger point. Resistive exercises were increased to 5 pounds, and she set up a return appointment in 1 week.

All activities had been resumed during this week without difficulty. She was requested to continue her home program of ice and exercise, plus buddy taping at work. On her return appointment, grip strength was 23.6 kg (right) and 23.3 kg (left) with a couple of flare-ups during the interval. She noted that she could often work without the buddy taping and not place herself in MP hyperextension. She was instructed to continue her home program 1 additional month and then to discontinue formal home care. A visit with the patient 18 months after discharge revealed no recurrence.

CASE STUDY 5

This case study involves the onset of referred pain as the result of trauma. This 36-year-old fireman fell through the floor of a burning structure and sustained a superficial laceration of the left dorsal wrist and left dorsoproximal forearm. Four weeks after injury he was referred because of persistent paraesthesia along the ulnar aspect of the left hand. He had been unable to return to work, despite the lack of evidence of tendon or nerve injury.

On examination, he described stabbing pains at the wrist with deviation and dorsal numbness in left digits four and five. Motion was decreased, as well as strength:

	Right	Left
Wrist flexion	85 degrees	75 degrees
extension	62 degrees	30 degrees
Radial deviation	20 degrees	20 degrees
Ulnar deviation	45 degrees	15 degrees
Grip	31 kg	6 kg
Pinch Lateral	10 kg	8 kg
pulp	6.2 kg	5 kg

Palpation revealed a trigger point at the proximal scar in the left ECU muscle belly referring to an area between the left ulnar head and base of the fifth metacarpal (Fig. 57-38). Local palpation of the left ECU tendon displayed referred pain into dorsal digits four and five.

The first treatment consisted of hand therapy treatments (heat, scar massage, wrist curls) while TENS was bracketed about the scar (Fig. 57-39). Because the scar adherence was provoking the trigger points, scar remodeling was the first priority, not MFP techniques. The TENS served to dampen the trigger points during conventional treatment.

On the second visit, the patient reported a significant decrease in pain and tolerated an increase of weight for wrist curls from 1 pound to 2 pounds. An Otoform* pad was also fabricated for scar remodeling. The third and fourth treatments focused on friction massage and ultrasound to both trigger points, followed by ice.

On the sixth visit, low resistance work simulation was begun with the TENS unit bracketed about the trigger points. For the next eight sessions, this patient continued MFP treatments of friction massage, TENS, and ice, while increasing his work simulation. At the twelfth session, his trigger points had resolved and work hardening commenced for an additional six sessions (Fig. 57-40). He was then discharged and returned to work full time as a fireman.

---

*Alimed, Deedham, Mass.

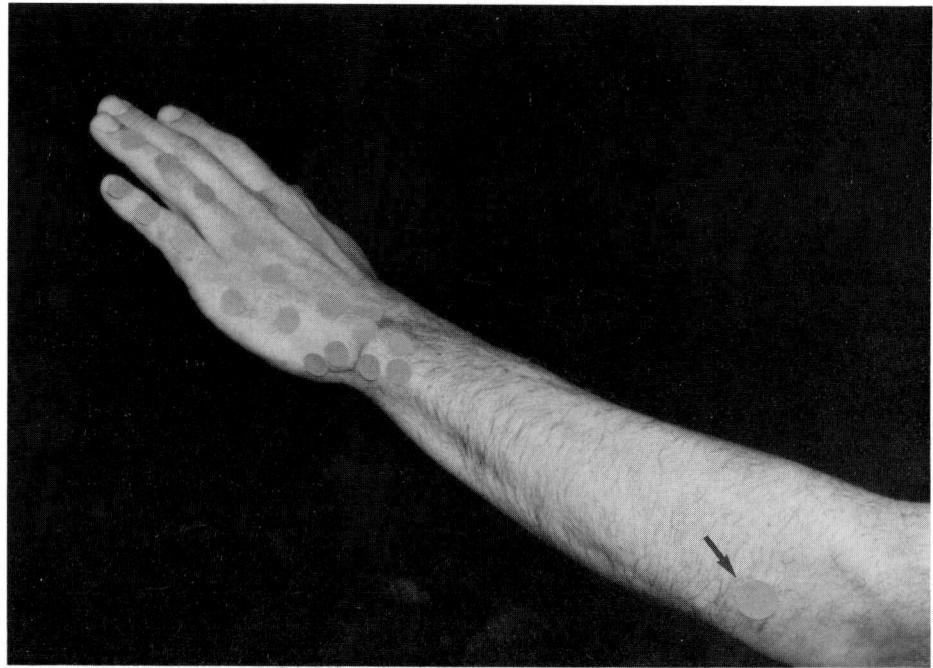

Fig. 57-38   Patient's mapping of pain demonstrating a trigger point in the extensor carpi ulnaris muscle, *arrow,* and its referral pattern to the ulnar head; while distal extensor carpi ulnaris tendon adherence (at ulnar head) refers pain to the base of metacarpal V.

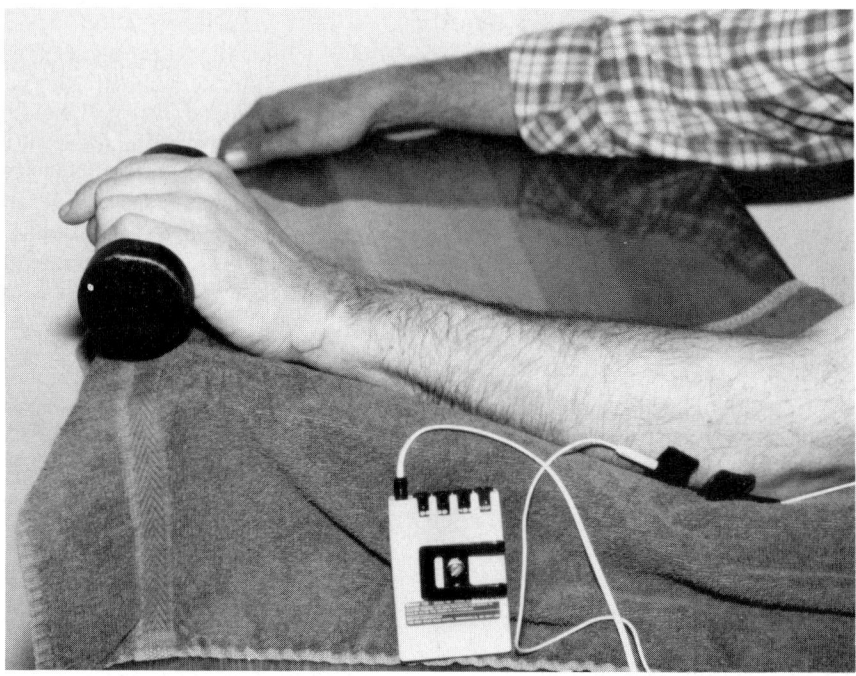

Fig. 57-39   Use of transcutaneous nerve stimulation bracketed about the pain/scar tissue point during performance of wrist curls.

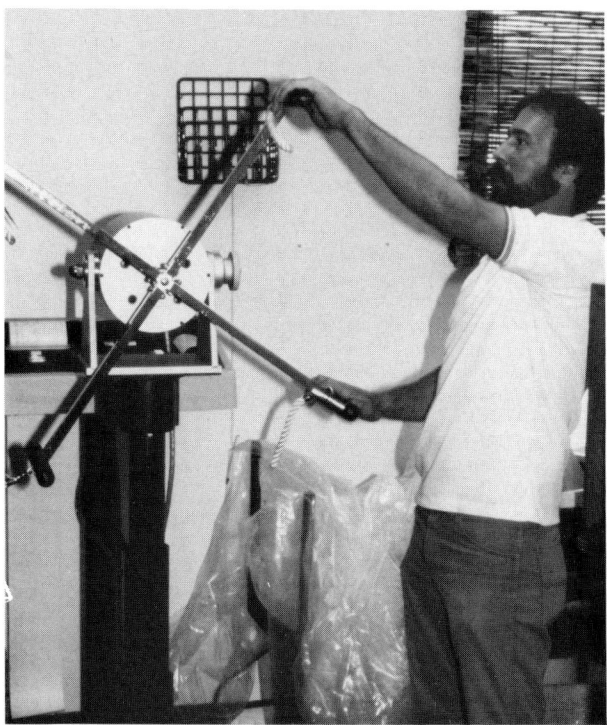

Fig. 57-40   Fireman performing work simulation of climbing a ladder.

Final assessment measurements follow:

Wrist flexion	85 degrees
Extension	60 degrees
Radial deviation	20 degrees
Ulnar deviation	37 degrees
Grip	42 kg
Lateral pinch	7.8 kg
Pulp pinch	6.6 kg

In both case studies, the patient's treatment and selection of specific myofascial techniques depended on their treatment response. Treatment techniques were changed if the patient did not respond to a particular technique. Specifically, techniques are changed after one session if the irritability of the trigger point does not change. This emphasizes the most important feature of treatment for these patients. The "cookbook" method does not apply; instead, treatment techniques are identified during evaluation. Then different sequences are tried and changes in trigger point irritability are noted.

SUMMARY

In summary, this chapter presented a threefold picture of myofascial pain. The historical review provided insight regarding the complexity of the syndrome. A thorough understanding of the potential causes and trigger point structure is necessary to perform a successful evaluation. As outlined, the evaluation follows a sequence of identifying what structures are potentially irritated and what pain patterns are thus displayed. Treatment affirms the evaluation process and manages the pain. A variety of treatment techniques are available; selection is based on tissue response to that treatment. If the treatment does not change the patient's pain,

then reidentification of the pain locus and/or a change in the treatment technique is necessary. Myofascial pain patients offer an exciting challenge for the hand therapist.

REFERENCES

1. Adams RD, Denny-Brown D, and Pearson CM: Disease of the muscle, New York, 1962, Harper and Row.
2. Adler I: Muscular rheumatism, Med Rec 57:532, 1900.
3. Antich T: Phonophoresis: the principles of the ultrasonic driving force and efficacy in treatment of common orthopaedic diagnoses, J Ortho Sports Phys Ther 4:99, 1982.
4. Bengtsson A, Henriksson KG, and Larsson J: Muscle biopsy in primary fibromyalgia. Light microscope and histochemical findings, Scand J Rheumatol 15:1, 1986.
5. Bennett RM: Current issues concerning management of the fibrositis/fibromyalgia syndrome, Am J Med 81:15, 1986.
6. Berges P: Myofascial syndromes, Postgrad Med 53:161, 1973.
7. Bonica J: Management of myofascial pain syndromes in general practice, JAMA 164:732, 1957.
8. Brendstrup P, Jespersen K, and Asboe-Hansen G: Morphological and chemical connective tissue changes in fibrositis muscles, Ann Rheum 16:438, 1957.
9. Chamberlain GJ: Cyriax's friction massage: a review, J Ortho Sports Phys Ther 4:16, 1982.
10. Conference on Therapy, Sternographic Report: Treatment of painful disorders of skeletal muscle, NY St J Med 45:2050, 1945.
11. Correspondence: New treatment for injured joints, Foreign Letters 104:1261, 1935.
12. Cyriax J: Textbook of orthopaedic medicine: Diagnosis of soft tissue lesions, vol 1, ed 6, Baltimore, 1975, Williams and Wilkins Co.
13. Delacerda FG: Comparative study of three methods of treatment for shoulder girdle myofascial syndrome, J Ortho Sports Phys Ther 4:51, 1982.
14. Edeiken J and Wolferth C: Persistent pain in the shoulder region following myocardial infarction, Am J Med Sci 191:201, 1936.
15. Fassbender HG: Pathology of rheumatic disease, New York, 1975, Springer-Verlag.
16. Foester O: The dermatome in man, Brain 1:1, 1933.
17. Friction JR and others: Myofascial pain syndrome of the head and neck: a review of clinical characteristics of 164 patients, Oral Surg 60:615, 1985.
18. Frost A: Diclofenac vs. lidocaine as injection therapy in myofascial pain, Scand J Rheumatol 15:153,1986.
19. Gobel A, Hockfield S, and Ruda MA: Anatomical similarities between medullary and spinal dorsal horns. In Kawamura Y and Dubner R, editors: Facial, sensory and motor functions, Chicago, 1981, Quintessence.
20. Good M: The role of skeletal muscles in the pathogenesis of disease, Acta Med Scand 138:285, 1950.
21. Good M: Objective diagnosis and curability of nonarticular rheumatism, Br J Phys Med 14:1, 1951.
22. Gordon EE and Hass A: A surface analgesic in treatment of musculoskeletal affections, Ind Med Surg 28:217, 1959.
23. Gowers W: Lumbago: its lessons and analogues, Br J Phys Med 1:117, 1904.
24. Gunn C and others: Dry needling of muscle motor points for chronic low back pain, Spine 5:279, 1980.
25. Gutstein M: Diagnosis and treatment of muscular rheumatism, Br J Phys Med 1:302, 1938.
26. Hadler N: A critical reappraisal of the fibrositis concept. Symposium on fibrositis/fibromyalgia, Am J Med 81(suppl 3A):26, 1986.
27. Harris P: Iontophoresis: clinical research in musculoskeletal inflammatory conditions, J Ortho Sports Phys Ther 4:109, 1982.
28. Head H: On disturbances of sensation with special reference to the pain of visceral disease, Brain 16:1, 1893.
29. Heffner R and Barron SA: The early effects of ischemia upon skeletal muscle mitochondria, J Neuro Sci 38:295, 1978.
30. Hench P: Secondary fibrositis. Symposium on Fibrositis/fibromyalgia, Am J Med, 81(suppl 3A):60, 1986.
31. Inman V and Saunders J: Referred pain from skeletal structures, J Nerv Ment Dis 99:660, 1944.
32. Jaeger B and Reeves JL: Quantification of changes in myofascial trigger point sensitivity with the pressure algometer following passive stretch, Pain 27:203, 1986.

33. Jensen K and others: Pressure pain threshold in human temporal region: evaluation of a new pressure algometer, Pain 25:313, 1986.
34. Johnson J: Occupational therapy and the patient with pain. In Chromwells F, editor: Occupation therapy and the patient with pain, New York, 1984, The Haworth Press.
35. Johnson W: Spray 'em, play 'em, Sports Illustrated 6:35, 1981.
36. Jordon HH: Myogeloses: the significance of pathologic conditions of the musculature in disorder of posture and locomotion, Arch Phys Ther 23:36, 1941.
37. Kellegren JH: Observation on referred pain arising from muscles, Clin Sci, p 175, 1938.
38. Kelly M: The nature of fibrositis, Ann Rheum Dis 5:69, 1946.
39. Kelly M: Local injection for rheumatism, Med J Aust 1:45, 1962.
40. Kraft G, Johnson E, and LaBan M: The fibrositis syndrome, Arch Phys Med Rehabil 49:155, 1968.
41. Kraus H: The use of surface anesthesia in the treatment of painful motion, JAMA 16:2582,1941.
42. Kraus H: Clinical treatment of back and neck pain, New York, 1970, McGraw-Hill.
43. Kraus H: Trigger points and acupuncture, Acupunct Electrother Res 2:323, 1977.
44. Kraus H: The causes, prevention and treatment of sports injuries, United States, 1981, Playboy Press.
45. Lamotte C: Distribution of the tract of Lissauer and the dorsal root fibers in the primate spinal cord, J Comp Neuro, 172:529, 1977.
46. Lange M: Die Muskelharten (Myogelosen), Munchen, 1931, JF Lehman, Verlag. Interpreted by Kraus, H: Clinical treatment of back and neck pain, New York, 1970, McGraw-Hill Book Co.
47. Levit K: The needle effect in the relief of myofascial pain, Pain 6:83, 1979.
48. Levit K and Simons D: Myofascial pain: relief by post-isometric relaxation, Arch Phys Med Rehab 65:452, 1984.
49. Lewith G and Machin D: A randomized trial to evaluate the effect of Infra-red stimulation of local trigger points, versus placebo, on the pain caused by cervical osteoarthritis, Acupunct Electro-ther Res 6:277,1981.
50. Llewellyn L and Jones A: Fibrositis, London, 1915, Heinemann. Quoted in Simons D: Muscle pain syndromes, Part I, Am J Phys Med 54:289, 1975.
51. Lundeberg TCM: Vibratory stimulation for the alleviation of chronic pain, Acta Physiol Scand Suppl 523:1, 1983.
52. McCray R and Patton N: Pain relief at trigger points: a comparison of moist heat and software diathermy, J Ortho Sports Phys Ther 5:175, 1984.
53. Melzack R: Prolonged relief of pain by brief, intense transcutaneous somatic stimulation, Pain 1:357, 1975.
54. Melzack R: Myofascial trigger points: relation to acupuncture and mechanisms of pain, Arch Phys Med Rehab 62:114, 1981.
55. Melzack R, Stillwell D, and Fox E: Trigger points and acupuncture points for pain: correlations and implications, Pain 3:3, 1977.
56. Muller A: Der Utersuchungsbefund Am Rheumatisch Erkranten, Muskel Z Klin Med 74:34, 1912. Interpreted by Simons D: Muscle pain syndromes, Part I, Am J Phys Med 55:289, 1976.
57. Nielson AJ: Case study. Myofascial pain of the posterior shoulder relieved by spray and stretch, J Ortho Sports Phys Ther 3:21, 1981.
58. Omura Y: Electro-acupuncture: its electrophysiological basis and criteria of effectiveness and safety. Part I, Acupunct Electrother Res 1:157, 1975.
59. Personius WJ: Low back pain and "sciatica" symptoms—development of a clinical method to identify the sources, unpublished doctoral dissertation, 1984, University of Iowa.
60. Procacci P, Zoppi M, and Maresca M: Transcutaneous electrical stimulation in low back pain: a critical evaluation, Acupunct Electrother Res 7:1, 1982.
61. Reeves JL, Jaeger B, and Graff-Radford SB: Reliability of the pressure algometer as a measure of trigger point sensitivity, Pain 24:313, 1986.
62. Reynolds M: Myofascial trigger point syndromes in the practice of rheumatology, Arch Phys Med Rehab 62:111, 1981.
63. Reynolds M: The development of the concept of fibrositis, J Hist Med Allied Sci 38:5, 1983.
64. Ruhmann W: The earliest book on rheumatism, Br J Rheum 2:140, 1940.
65. Rubin D: Myofascial trigger point syndromes: an approach to management, Arch Phys Med Rehab 62:107, 1981.
66. Schwartz LL: Temporomandibular joint pain—treatment with intramuscular infiltration of tetracaine hydrochloride: a preliminary report. NY St Dent J 20:219, 1954.
67. Simons D: Muscle pain syndromes—Part I, Am J Phys Med 54:289, 1975.
68. Simons D: Muscle pain syndromes—Part II, Am J Phys Med 55:15, 1976.
69. Simons D: FIbrositis/fibromyalgia: a form of myofascial trigger points? Symposium on fibrositis/fibromyalgia, Am J Med 81(suppl 3A):93, 1986.
70. Smith G and Covino B: Acute pain, Stoneham, UK, Butterworths, 1985.
71. Smythe H: Fibrositis and other diffuse musculoskeletal syndromes. In Kelly W and others, editors: Textbook of rheumatology, vol 1, Philadelphia, 1981, WB Saunders.
72. Sola AE: Upper extremity pain. In Wall PD and Melzack R, editors: Textbook of pain, New York, 1984, Churchill Livingstone, Inc.
73. Sola AE and Kuitert JH: Myofascial trigger point pain in the neck and shoulder girdle, NW Med 54:98, 1955.
74. Sola AE and Williams RL: Myofascial pain syndromes, Neurology 6:91, 1955.
75. Torejork HE, Ochoa JL, and Schady W: Referred pain from intraneural stimulation of muscle fascicles in the median nerve, Pain 18:145, 1984.
76. Travell J: Ethyl chloride spray for painful muscle spasm, Arch Phys Med Rehab 33:291, 1952.
77. Travell J: Office hours day and night, New York, 1968, World Publishing Co.
78. Travell J: Myofascial trigger points: a clinical view. In Bonica J and Fessard A, editors: Advances in pain research and therapy, New York, 1976, Raven Press.
79. Travell J: Identification of myofascial trigger point syndrome: a case of atypical facial neuralgia, Arch Phys Med Rehab 62:100, 1981.
80. Travell J and Bigelow NH: Referred somatic pain from skeletal structures, J Nerv Ment Dis 99:660, 1947.
81. Travell J, Rinzler SH, and Herman M: Pain and disability of the shoulder and arm: treatment by intramuscular infiltration with procaine hydrochloride, JAMA 120:417, 1942.
82. Travell J and Rinzler SH: The myofascial genesis of pain, Postgrad Med 11:425, 1952.
83. Travell J and Simons DG: Myofascial pain and dysfunction of the trigger point manual, Baltimore, 1983, Williams & Wilkins.
84. Valentine M: Aetiology of fibrositis: a review, Ann Rheum Dis 6:241, 1947.
85. Wolfe F: Tender points, trigger points and the fibrositis syndrome, Clin Rheum Pract 2:36, 1984.

BIBLIOGRAPHY

Bates T and Grunwaldt E: Myofascial pain in childhood, J Pediatr 53:198, 1958.
Boas NF and Foley JB: Proc Soc Exp Biol Med 86:690, 1954.
Bresler D: Free yourself from pain, New York, 1979, Simon & Schuster.
Caro, XJ: Immunofluorescent studies of skin in primary fibrositis syndrome, Am J Med 81:43, 1986.
Kerr F: Acupuncture and pain. In The Pain Book, New Jersey, 1987, Prentice-Hall, Inc.
McCain A: Role of physical fitness training in the fibrositis/fibromyalgia syndrome, Am J Med 81:73, 1986.
Masi AT and Yunus MB: Concepts of illness in populations as applied to fibromyalgia syndrome, Am J Med 81:19, 1986.
Moldofsky H: Sleep and musculoskeletal pain, Am J Med 81:85, 1986.
Ottoson P: Physiology of the nervous system, New York, 1983, Macmillan Press.
Russell IJ and others: Is there a metabolic basis for the fibrositis syndrome? Am J Med 81:50, 1986.
Simons D: Electrogenic nature of palpable bands and "jump sign" associated with myofascial trigger points. In Bonica J and Fessard A, editors: Advances in pain research and therapy, New York, 1976, Raven Press.
Sinclair D, Weddell G, and Feindel W: Referred pain and associated phenomena, Brain 71:184, 1948.
Smoller B and Schulum G: Pain control: the Bethesda Program, New York, 1982, Doubleday & Co.
Smythe H: Referred pain and tender points, Am J Med 81:90, 1986.
Wolfe F: Development of criteria for the diagnosis of fibrositis, Am J Med 81:99, 1986.
Yunus MB and others: Pathologic changes in muscle in primary fibromyalgia syndrome, Am J Med 81:38, 1986.

58

Management of pain syndromes in the upper extremity

George E. Omer, Jr.

The most common reason for patients seeing a physician is pain.[10] Pain is an unpleasant sensory and emotional experience associated with actual or potential tissue damage or described in terms of such damage.[39] Approximately 75 million Americans are afflicted with pain each year.[6] Over 40 million Americans are either partially or totally disabled by chronic pain. As a result, nearly 700 million work days are lost, which, together with health care costs and compensation, total approximately 50 billion dollars each year.[6]

Chronic pain is defined as pain that persists or recurs at intervals for months or years.[6] Chronic pain is caused not only by pathologic processes in the nervous system, but also by psychopathologic factors and environmental influences. Chronic pain is a wicked force that imposes excessive psychologic, social, and economic stresses on the patient. The treatment of chronic pain problems is most difficult, since pain is such an intensely personal reaction; Aristotle and Plato considered pain to be a "passion of the soul."[14]

PERCEPTUAL PARAMETERS AND PERSONALITY

The pain threshold is the least stimulus at which a patient perceives pain.[39] The pain-tolerance level is the greatest stimulus intensity causing pain that a patient is prepared to tolerate.[39] In the experimental setting, pain threshold and tolerance can be determined by several techniques that show high reliability.[9,63,68,69,77] Age, sex, race, ethnic group, religion, and other factors influence pain tolerance.[55] Personality is the unique blend of intellectual and emotional qualities reflected in individual behavior.[4,71] A number of traits are characteristic facets of personality, such as anxiety, expressiveness, depression, or hypochondriasis.[29] Clinicians may believe that the patient who complains about pain more than the average person does have a low pain threshold, but this is an error. The readiness to communicate the pain is a function of expressiveness, and this in turn is associated with the degree of extraversion.[63] In experimental studies, Lynn and Eysenck[37] found that pain tolerance in college students was negatively correlated with neuroticism and positively correlated with extraversion. Social learning influences expressiveness as well, including that related to pain communication.

Basic personality attributes may be measured by two tests, the Eysenck Personality Inventory (EPI) and the Minnesota Multiphasic Personality Inventory (MMPI). The EPI test measures two dimensions of personality regarded as fundamental because they are related directly to physiologic activity of the central nervous system. These dimensions are stability-neuroticism (N) and introversion-extraversion (E). The higher the patient's N score, the greater the emotional vulnerability shown. The higher the E score, the more the person will be found to be gregarious and cheerful and to have high levels of energy. In general, thresholds for pain are lower for introverts than for extraverts. The EPI can be completed in 10 to 15 minutes.[4] The MMPI is a checklist of physical and emotional symptoms, including both those from the past and those present at the time of examination. High scores indicate the presence of an emotional disturbance. For patients with chronic pain, significantly higher scores are found on those items measuring hypochondriasis, depression, and hysteria. Patients with acute pain show high scores for hypochondriasis and hysteria, but not for depression. One of the attractions of the MMPI is that the personality profiles permit the identification of groups of characteristics, and on this basis patients with pain problems may be categorized.[4] Sternbach and associates[62] found that patients with low back pain of a duration of less than 6 months obtained MMPI profiles within normal limits, while patients with low back pain of longer duration had greatly elevated scores for depression, hypochondriasis, and hysteria. There is a reported clinical correlation of 86.3% between the topographic pain drawing[11] and the MMPI score.

In a practical sense, the attending surgeon or therapist must learn to identify the unstable emotional personality. In such patients the "pain state" becomes a permanent "memory bank," and the total personality may become focused on the pain. These patients will require much more time and explanation to cope with their pain.

TREATMENT

There are only two principles in the treatment of an established pain syndrome involving the upper extremity: (1) relieve the patient's symptoms, and (2) institute active use of the involved extremity.[43-45,49]

Relief of symptoms

One initiates the relief of pain by attempting to divide the source of the patient's symptoms into categories: (1) increased peripheral nociceptive stimulus, which is often a "trigger point" with an associated local disorder, such as a neuroma; (2) reflex sympathetic summation, usually described as "diffuse, burning, sustained" (when symptoms are overwhelming, this should be termed "causalgia"); (3) inflammatory pain of systemic origin, such as peripheral neuritis of diabetes; (4) personality dysfunction pain, which will overlap with all other categories; and (5) cancer pain.[45]

Pain should be evaluated promptly; one should never wait for the full development of an established pain syndrome before initiating aggressive treatment. For example, the osteoporosis of Sudek's atrophy is not evident by roentgenography for 5 to 8 weeks after injury,[52] but the patient has pain from time of injury.

Peripheral nociceptive stimulus. Pain may develop after local trauma for many reasons. The damaged portion of the nerve may develop intraneural fibrosis, or external adhesions may transfix the nerve to its bed. Friction on a nerve will result in inflammatory changes and further fibrosis. The compressed nerve will have venous stasis, capillary leakage, and perineurial edema.[54] Decreased blood flow can be associated with pain, as in any compression syndrome.[15] Any procedure producing vasodilatation may relieve this pain.

A peripheral nerve responds to injury, whether partial or complete, with proliferation of connective tissue and regeneration of damaged axons to form a neuroma. The neuroma becomes symptomatic depending on the quality of regeneration and is influenced by the extent of fibrosis, vascularity, infection, foreign material, and other local factors. Neuromas with inadequate numbers of large myelinated axons or outer fibrous layers develop hyperpathia. Hyperpathia is a painful syndrome characterized by an overreaction or an aftersensation to stimuli.[39] The patient characteristically has extreme sensitivity directly over the neuroma; altered sensibility in at least part of the area supplied by the nerve; and sustained, widely distributed, poorly localized pain.[76]

Percutaneous injection about the painful neuroma should provide local anesthesia. Bupivacaine hydrochloride has a longer duration of anesthesia than lidocaine hydrochloride.[40] Percutaneous injection of triamcinolone acetonide about the neuroma after a cutaneous block with 2% lidocaine hydrochloride has been reported to relieve the pain symptoms in 50% of patients after one injection and in 80% of patients with multiple injections.[59]

Percussion or massage of painful neuromas has been a clinical procedure in amputees since the World War I. Controlled clinical studies have indicated that the technique is useful in selected cases.[21] Rubber mallets, mechanical vibrators, or ultrasonic treatments will provide the repetitious percussion. Anesthesia may be necessary over the trigger area at the onset of treatment, but later the percussion or massage should be done without local anesthesia.

Acupuncture is an ancient technique involving point pressure to relieve pain. Traditional teaching identifies 365 to 400 acupuncture points along the 12 meridian channels that contain the *yin* and *yang* forces that control the energy of life.[72] Modern laboratory studies possibly indicate that acupuncture analgesia is transmitted by the nervous system and requires an intact functional nervous system to be successful.[38,58,70] If an intact dynamic interaction (control gate) among large and small afferent neurons is required, acupuncture should be ineffective in the disrupted nerve, such as a terminal bulb neuroma. An additional neurophysiologic explanation is that some humeral agent may be responsible, and this may explain the generalized alterations in the pain threshold that have been reported in humans.[64] Acupuncture should be more effective in reflex sympathetic summation than in peripheral nociceptive stimulus.

A peripheral chemical sympathetic block may be performed on the ward.[48,49] A 16-gauge needle is inserted near the nerve just proximal to the "trigger point," and a flexible 18-gauge polyethylene intravenous catheter is inserted through the needle. The needle is removed, leaving the catheter in place. A solution of 0.5 ml of 0.5% lidocaine hydrochloride is injected. If the pain is relieved, the catheter is capped and taped in place, allowing exercise activity. Additional periodic injections of lidocaine solution are based on the length of time of pain-free activity. The periodic perineurial infusion has been continued for a few days up to 2 weeks. If there is more than one trigger point, separate catheters should be used. This method has been less effective in those patients in whom the pain has been untreated for 3 or more months.

A neuroma can be classified as a terminal bulb or a neuroma in continuity. A painful partial nerve disruption may benefit from internal neurolysis and graft repair of some fascicular groups.[47,61] If there is no useful distal sensory or motor function, an end-to-end anastomosis should be performed after removal of the neuroma in continuity. Terminal bulb neuromas typically occur in amputation stumps. Although many procedures have been reported, present methods include simple resection of the neuroma, capping of the terminal portion with silicone, or transposition of the entire neuroma to a new site.[24,65,67] The most reliable procedure is transfer of the neuroma, attached to the proximal nerve stump, to a new site where compression is unlikely and traction is minimal. The neuroma should be placed in an area of good circulation with a thick subcutaneous layer that is free of scar.[13,28] Success has been reported in 82% of patients treated by this technique.

Traction injuries to the brachial plexus are often painful initially, but pain should progressively subside.[76] An increase in pain may represent fibrous tissue involvement. The pain from nerve root avulsion is severe, having the characteristics of causalgia, a maximum reflex sympathetic summation.[78]

Reflex sympathetic summation. Many clinical syndromes, including burning pain, abnormal vasomotor response, and trophic dystrophy, have been described. Classic causalgia may have variants that are termed "Leriche's posttraumatic pain syndrome" (minor causalgia), "Sudek's atrophy," or "shoulder-arm-hand syndrome."[29] Phantom pain is identical to reflex sympathetic dystrophy (RSD) but adds postural cramping or squeezing. RSD may not develop immediately but gradually increases to dominate the clinical picture.

The loss of vascular, sudomotor, pilomotor, and muscle tone controls will result in profound nutritional (trophic) changes with atrophy of subcutaneous tissue, skin, muscle, and bone. In the early stages the residual limb is greatly swollen and warm. Hyperesthesia to light touch and sensitivity to cold develop. After 2 to 3 months, fibrotic brawny edema is present. Contractures become fixed because of a lack of active motion. Roentgenograms of the distal bones show patchy osteopenia. A bone scan (technetium 99m–labeled diphosphonate) will be positive before the bone resorption is visible on plane roentgenograms. Six to 9 months after the onset of pain, the extremity becomes pale and cool with either hyperhidrosis or dryness. Pain may dominate or the extremity may be absolutely rejected by the patient.

This syndrome is believed to be a prolongation of the normal sympathetic response to injury.[5] The pain impulses to the cortex are greatly amplified, causing intense discomfort. The hypothesis that a partial injury to a major nerve can result in abnormal cross-stimulation between sympathetic and sensory fibers has clinical support.[12] Others have postulated the liberation of a vasodilator substance (neurokinin) at the periphery as the basis for the pain.[2,7]

In those patients with Raynaud's symptoms associated with pain, it is important to measure digital blood flow.[1] We follow Porter's method[53]: the patient sits quietly for 30 minutes in a warm room with the temperature about 24° C (76° F). The digital pulp temperature is determined with an electronic telethermometer. The patient's hands are then immersed in an ice water mixture for 20 seconds, and the digital pulp temperature measured until the temperature returns to the baseline value for 45 minutes. Normal temperature-recovery time is 10 minutes, with a range from 5 to 20 minutes. The digital temperature test can be supplemented with arteriography to differentiate arterial spasm from organic obstructive disease. Medication to decrease peripheral sympathetic activity should be beneficial for the patient with painful Raynaud's symptoms. A variety of drugs have been proposed for intraarterial injection, including the alpha-receptor blocking drugs tolazoline hydrochloride (Priscoline) and phenoxybenzamine hydrochloride, the beta-adrenergic receptor blocking drug propranolol hydrochloride, and the neuronal norepinephrine depletors reserpine, methyldopa, or guanethidine. Griseofulvin has also been used because it has a direct vasodilator action exclusive of sympathetic innervation. Porter obtained excellent responses in patients with Raynaud's symptoms with repeated brachial artery injections of reserpine (0.25 mg) at approximately 2- to 3-week intervals.[53] Porter also treated 23 patients with oral guanethidine, 10 mg daily, and then increased the level 10 mg each week until there was hypotension or symptomatic improvement. Two patients could not tolerate guanethidine even at the minimal dose of 10 mg daily because of hypotension and were changed to phenoxybenzamine, 10 mg daily. After an average follow-up of 12 months, 19 of the 23 patients had significant reduction in the frequency and severity of the Raynaud's attacks.[53] Similar results have been reported for propranolol hydrochloride in oral dosages of 40 mg every 4 hous.[57]

Chuinard and associates[8] have reported the use of reserpine administered intravenously to relieve pain. The technique is the same as that used for intravenous regional anesthesia. One milligram of reserpine diluted in 50 ml of normal saline solution is injected, and the tourniquet is released after 15 minutes. The authors reported that 21 of 25 patients obtained pain relief.

Hannington-Kiff introduced the regional intravenous sympathetic block technique with guanethidine.[22,23] Wynn Parry[78] records that guanethidine blocks are most valuable and provide instantaneous pain relief. Under tourniquet control, 20 mg of guanethidine in 20 ml of normal saline is injected slowly into a dorsal wrist vein. The tourniquet is deflated in 20 minutes.

Early treatment includes chemical central interruption of the abnormal sympathetic reflex, and a sympathetic block should be performed as a diagnostic test and as a therapeutic procedure. We use solutions of either 1% lidocaine hydrochloride or 1% mepivacaine hydrochloride to produce peripheral warming and loss of sweating, as well as relief of pain. The anterior approach is preferred for the isolated

stellate block, with the technique described by Kleinert[27] being used. A series of four or five blocks should be given on consecutive days; one placebo of normal saline solution given during the series will confirm the value of the sympathetic block. Leffert and colleagues[31] at the Massachusetts General Hospital have developed a technique for continuous sympathetic blockade that uses an indwelling catheter for injection about the stellate ganglion. The initial technique for periodic chemical sympathetic blocks involved the lumbar area.[66]

Transcutaneous electric nerve stimulation (TENS) should be considered for those patients whose pain persists after chemical central sympathetic block. Three sites of electrode placement are used: (1) over a large nerve trunk proximal to the pain site, (2) at the periphery of a painful area if the lesion appears to be primarily cutaneous, or (3) directly over a pain site if proximal nerve trunks are not readily stimulated.[20] The intensity should be varied by the patient because stimuli that are too intense overcome the inhibition mechanism and produce additional pain. Pain relief is complete in less than one third of patients,[19,20,33,34] and the best results are obtained when TENS is initiated within 3 months of the onset of pain.

In 1967 Sweet and Wall[74] implanted electrodes directly on the median and ulnar nerves of a patient with traumatic hyperpathia. Goldner and associates[42] reported 38 peripheral nerves in 35 patients stimulated with electrodes over periods from 4 to 9 years. Successful relief of pain occurred in 53% of patients with upper extremity pain. Direct stimulation to the peripheral nerve is more effective in the upper extremity than in the lower extremity. Current researchers are implanting electrodes to stimulate cells in the periaqueductal periventricular gray matter to release beta-endorphin and obtain analgesia.[25,36]

Surgery should be performed when the burning pain completely responds to central chemical sympathectomy but requires repeated blocks for the long-term relief of pain. The effectiveness of sympathectomy is not related to interruption of a sensory pathway from the extremity, but to elimination of the sympathetic efferent discharge to the peripheral arteries and sweat glands. Surgical sympathectomy will relieve only burning pain; associated painful neuromas or arthritic pain will not be altered. Horner's syndrome often is not present after the transaxillary approach, which permits removal of only the lower half of the stellate ganglion, but it is more often present after the supraclavicular approach and can be most annoying to the patient. Postoperative precise sudomotor function tests should demonstrate complete sympathetic denervation of the involved extremity.

Inflammatory pain. Corticosteroids are useful for the patient with rheumatoid arthritis, diabetes, Reiter's syndrome, or other conditions that are trapped in a massive episode of painful inflammatory stiffness.[17,18] We have used a tourniquet and intravenous regional block with 50 ml of 1% lidocaine hydrochloride and 40 mg of methylprednisolone sodium succinate.[75] During the 20 to 30 minutes of analgesia, one can manipulate stiff joints and stretch contracted web spaces. A different program involves utilization of 250 mg of hydrocortisone sodium succinate intravenously each day for 5 days and then a decrease in the dosage to 100 mg each day for 5 days. These drugs must be monitored and the patients evaluated for adverse reactions. As the pain subsides, the patient is encouraged to employ a gentle lanolin massage and warm water baths. Salicylates should be given to abort ongoing inflammatory metabolic pathways.

Osteoarthritis is managed with aspirin, splinting, physical therapy, and intraarticular steroids as clinically indicated. Compression and massage therapy may be helpful adjuncts, and tissue vibrators at frequencies of 100 to 140 Hz can activate joint mechanoreceptors, which have inhibitory influences in the dorsal horn of the spinal cord. TENS can activate afferent circuits and induce inhibitory influences. Septic complications require appropriate antibiotics.

Personality dysfunction. Optimal management requires a multifaceted and highly individualized program. The patient's general physical condition may have deteriorated because of inadequate sleep, improper diet and exercise, medication abuse, or other complications. Depression may progress to the point that the patient develops an attitude of hopelessness. An occasional tranquilizer for a particular clinical situation may be effective. Narcotics are not indicated.

Medications for emotional instability include phenytoin (Dilantin Sodium), fluphenazine dihydrochloride (Prolixin), carbamazepine (Tegretal), and amitriptyline hydrochloride (Elavil).[75] Phenytoin may be given up to 300 to 500 mg daily in divided or single doses taken with food. This is the safest phenothiazine. Amitriptyline may be given 25 mg at bedtime and at intervals during the day up to 150 mg maximum daily dosage. Phenytoin and amitriptyline may be used together. Benson also advises a phenothiazine such as fluphenazine hydrochloride (Prolixin), which potentiates any narcotic, possesses an analgesic property of its own, and depresses the response to peripheral stimuli.[3] Recommended dosage is 1 mg three times daily; this may be increased to a total of 10 mg per day.[3,76] Carbamazepine (Tegretal) is the most effective drug but is prone to develop toxic symptoms such as nausea, vomiting, or unsteady gait. Because of hematopoietic suppression, it is appropriate to follow up on patients receiving carbamazepine with monthly hemoglobin and white cell count studies.

Electromyographic biofeedback may be used to relieve tension. Pain declined significantly in 12 of 18 patients with tension headaches studied at the University of Washington in Seattle,[51] but significant pain relief was obtained in only one of eight patients with back pain. To be effective, this modality must be given with maximal therapist support.

In the latter part of the eighteenth century, the German physician Franz Anton Mesmer developed modern techniques for hypnosis. Experiments in hypnosis have shown that subjects can distort both perception and motor movements, and through hypnosis one can produce partial to total anesthesia. Successful acupuncture and hypnosis both require the cerebral cortex to activate complex conditioned reflexes that raise pain thresholds, remove anxiety and tension, and relieve depression.[41]

Personality dysfunction may result in the physical presentation of a psychological problem with painful symptoms or clinical state. Examples include the clenched fist syndrome,[56,60] Secretan's disease (or peritendinous fibrosis of the dorsum of the hand[46]) and the S-H-A-F-T syndrome.[73] These patients are far more complex than the malingerer, and require supportive psychotherapy. Attempts to manage the pain symptoms without a multidisciplinary approach are doomed to failure.

Cancer pain. Patients should be considered for an invasive operation when their pain is proved to be intractable to nonsurgical techniques.

Spinal dorsal sensory root rhizotomy through a laminectomy is indicated in patients who have unilateral pain involving the brachial plexus and the involved extremity is functionally useless. Leavens[30] has reported long-standing anesthesia in 50 of 71 patients undergoing this procedure. Other reports of rhizotomy have indicated limited success and disappointing long-term results.[26,32,50] Cordotomy is indicated when the pain is diffuse and involving areas innervated by many roots in a functioning upper extremity. Leavens[30] reported unilateral cervical cordotomy in 37 patients; 15 patients had some pain relief until death from their disease, an average of 3 months after surgery. Twelve of the 37 patients developed pain in the previously nonpainful side, an average of 1½ months after surgery.

Destructive lesions in the thalamus, brainstem, and frontal lobes have been employed for many years. Cingulotomy is the one technique that is still used for patients in whom anxiety and depression are major factors.[35] None of these procedures provides long-lasting pain relief[16]; they are most useful in patients who are expected to live no more than 1 year. The return of pain after surgery is related to increased activity of polysynaptic systems (paleospinothalamic or spinoreticulothalamic) that are widespread in the brainstem and thalamus. These polysynaptic systems are infinitely complex and diffuse and eventually frustrate any surgical ablation procedure.

Institution of functional activity

The second principle in the treatment program of an established pain syndrome is the institution of functional activity. Passive modalities decrease pain and maintain mobility. Passive modalities will improve circulation, decrease edema, and prepare the patient for voluntary participation in active modalities such as athletics. Active modalities build strength and develop dexterity. Active modalities result in an independent patient.

Passive modalities include massage, vibrators, stump wrapping, faradic muscle stimulation, ice packs, hot packs, paraffin packs, microwaves, ultrasound, and inflatable splints with positive and negative pressure. In the apprehensive patient, use of these modalities may have to be preceded by very delicate techniques, such as stroking the skin with a feather. Some passive modalities may be contraindicated, such as the whirlpool bath, because it is dependent on heat and may increase edema. The passive program should maintain joint motion, prevent contracture, and desensitize hyperesthetic areas.[76]

The more important phase is voluntary functional activity. Special care should be directed to warming up key areas of circulation, such as the rotator cuff muscles in the shoulder-arm-hand syndrome. Total body conditioning is important, and the patient should be ambulatory if possible. Function can be developed with diversional games, athletics, assigned work, and activities of daily living. It is important that the health care team be compassionate, yet obtain maximal effort from the patient. The best functional activity occurs when the patient returns to his usual work. With the continued use of functional activity, patients ultimately "cure" themselves.

REFERENCES

1. Balas P and others: Raynaud's phenomenon: primary and secondary causes, Arch Surg 114:1174, 1979.
2. Barnes R: The role of sympathectomy in the treatment of causalgia, J Bone Joint Surg 35B:172, 1953.
3. Benson WF: Treatment of the painful extremity, American Society for Surgery of the Hand Newsletter 50, 1977.
4. Bond MR: Pain: its nature, analysis, and treatment, Edinburgh, 1979, Churchill Livingstone.
5. Bonica JJ: Causalgia and other reflex sympathetic dystrophies, Postgrad Med J 53:143, 1976.
6. Bonica JJ: Current status of pain therapy. In Perry S, chairman: The Interagency Committee on New Therapies for Pain and Discomfort, report to the White House: 111-114, May 1979, US Dept of Health, Education, and Welfare, Public Health Service, National Institutes of Health.
7. Chapman LF and others: Neurohumoral features of afferent fibers in man, Arch Neurol 4:49, 1961.
8. Chuinard RG and others: Intravenous reserpine for treatment of reflex sympathetic dystrophy, J Hand Surg 5:289, 1980.
9. Craig KD, Best H, and Ward LM: Social modelling influences on psychophysical judgments of electrical stimulation, J Abnorm Psychol 84:366, 1975.
10. de Jong RH: Commentary: defining pain terms, JAMA 244:143,1980.
11. Dennis MD, Rocchio PO, and Wiltse LL: The topographical pain representation and its correlation with MMPI scores, Orthopedics 5:432, 1981.
12. Doupe J, Cullen CH, and Chance GQ: Post-traumatic pain and causalgic syndrome, J Neurol Neurosurg Psychiatr 7:33, 1944.
13. Eaton RG: Painful neuromas. In Omer GE Jr and Spinner M, editors: Management of peripheral nerve problems, Philadelphia, 1980, WB Saunders Co.
14. Gelard FA: The human senses, ed 2, New York, 1972, John Wiley & Sons, Inc.
15. Gelberman RH and others: The carpal tunnel syndrome: a study of carpal tunnel pressures, J Bone Joint Surg 63A:380, 1981.
16. Gildenberg PL: Central surgical procedures for pain of peripheral nerve origin. In Omer GE Jr and Spinner M, editors: Management of peripheral nerve problems, Philadelphia, 1980, WB Saunders Co.
17. Glick EN: Reflex dystrophy (algoneurodystrophy): results of treatment by corticosteroids, Rheumatol Rehabil 12:84, 1973.
18. Glick EN and Helal B: Post-traumatic neurodystrophy: treatment by corticosteroids, Hand 8:45, 1976.
19. Goldner JL: Pain: extremities and spine—evaluation and differential diagnosis. In Omer GE Jr and Spinner M, editors: Management of peripheral nerve problems, Philadelphia, 1980, WB Saunders Co.
20. Goldner JL, Nashold BS, and Hendrix PC: Peripheral nerve electrical stimulation, Clin Orthop 163:33, 1982.
21. Grant GH: Methods of treatment of neuromata of the hand, J Bone Joint Surg 33A:841, 1951.
22. Hannington-Kiff JG: Intravenous regional sympathetic block with guanethidine, Lancet 1:1019, 1974.
23. Hannington-Kiff JG: Relief of Sudek's atrophy by regional intravenous guanethidine, Lancet 1:1132, 1977.
24. Herndon JH, Eaton RG, and Littler JW: Management of painful neuromas in the hand, J Bone Joint Surg 58A:369, 1976.
25. Hosobuchi Y and others: Stimulation of human periaqueductal grey matter for pain relief increases immuno-reactive beta-endorphin in ventricular fluid, Science 203:279, 1979.
26. Hosobuchi Y: The majority of unmyelinated afferent axons in human ventral roots probably conduct pain, Pain 8:167, 1980.
27. Kleinert HE, Cole NM, and Wayne L: Post-traumatic sympathetic dystrophy, Orthop Clin North Am 4:917, 1973.
28. Laborde KJ, Kalisman M, and Tsi T-M: Results of surgical treatment of painful neuromas of the hand, J Hand Surg 7:190, 1982.
29. Lankford LL: Reflex sympathetic dystrophy. In Omer GE Jr and Spinner M, editors: Management of peripheral nerve problems, Philadelphia, 1980, WB Saunders Co.
30. Leavens ME: Neurosurgical relief of pain in cancer patients, Cancer Bull 33:98, 1981.
31. Leffert RD, Lenson MA, and Todd DP: The use of continuous sympathetic blockade in the treatment of reflex dystrophy, Personal communication, June 19, 1978.
32. Loeser JD: Dorsal rhizotomy for the relief of chronic pain, J Neurosurg 36:745, 1972.
33. Loeser JD, Black RG, and Christman A: Relief of pain by transcutaneous stimulation, J Neurosurg 43:308, 1975.
34. Long DM: Electrical stimulation for the control of pain, Arch Surg 112:884, 1977.
35. Long DM: Relief of cancer pain by surgical and nerve blocking procedures, JAMA 244:2759, 1980.
36. Long DM: Neuromodulation for the control of chronic pain, Surg Rounds 5:25, 1982.
37. Lynn R and Eysenck HJ: Tolerance for pain, extraversion and neuroticism, Percept Mot Skills 12:161, 1961.
38. Matsumoto T and Levy BA: Acupuncture for patients, Springfield, Ill, 1975, Charles C Thomas, Publisher.
39. Mersky H: Pain terms: a list with definitions and notes on usage (International Association for the Study of Pain [IASP] Subcommittee on Taxonomy), Pain 6:249, 1979.
40. Moore DC and others: Bupivacaine: a review of 2,077 cases, JAMA 214:713, 1970.
41. Murphy TM and Bonica JJ: Acupuncture analgesia and anesthesia, Arch Surg 112:896, 1977.
42. Nashold BS and others: Long-term pain control by direct peripheral-nerve stimulation, J Bone Joint Surg 64A:1, 1982.
43. Omer GE Jr: Management of pain syndromes in the upper extremity. In Hunter JM, Schneider LH, Mackin EJ and others, editors: Rehabilitation of the hand, St Louis, 1978, The CV Mosby Co.
44. Omer GE Jr: Management of the painful extremity. In Ahstrom JP Jr, editor: Current practice in orthopaedic surgery, vol 8, St Louis, 1979, The CV Mosby Co.
45. Omer GE Jr: Nerve, neuroma, and pain problems related to upper limb amputations, Orthop Clin North Am 12:751, 1981.
46. Omer GE Jr and others: Peritendinous fibrosis of the dorsum of the hand in monkeys, Clin Orthop 62:251, 1969.
47. Omer GE Jr and Spinner M: Peripheral nerve testing and suture techniques. In American Academy of Orthopaedic Surgeons: Instructional Course Lectures 24:122, St Louis, 1975, The CV Mosby Co.
48. Omer GE Jr and Thomas SR: Treatment of causalgia: review of cases at Brooke General Hospital, Tex Med 67:93, 1971.
49. Omer GE Jr and Thomas SR: The management of chronic pain syndromes in the upper extremity, Clin Orthop 104:37, 1974.
50. Onofrio BM and Campa HK: Evaluation of rhizotomy: review of 12 years' experience, J Neurosurg 36:751, 1972.
51. Peck CL and Kraft GH: Electromyographic biofeedback for pain related to muscle tension, Arch Surg 112:889, 1977.
52. Plewes LW: Sudek's atrophy in the hand, J Bone Joint Surg 38B:195, 1956.
53. Porter JM and others: The diagnosis and treatment of Raynaud's phenomenon, Surgery 77:11, 1975.
54. Rydevik B, Lundborg G, and Bagge U: Effects of graded compression on intraneural blood flow, J Hand Surg 6:3, 1981.
55. Schachtel HJ: Pain and religion, Cancer Bull 33:84, 1981.
56. Simmons BP and Vasile RG: The clenched fist syndrome, J Hand Surg 5:420, 1980.
57. Simson G: Propranol for causalgia and Sudek atrophy, JAMA 227:327, 1974 (letters section).
58. Sjölund B, Terenius L, and Eriksson M: Increased cerebrospinal fluid levels of endorphins after electro-acupuncture, Acta Physiol Scand 100:382, 1977.
59. Smith JR and Gomez NH: Local injection therapy of neuromata of the hand with triamcinolone acetonide: a preliminary study of twenty-two patients, J Bone Joint Surg 52A:71, 1970.
60. Spiegel D and Chase RA: The treatment of contractures of the hand using self-hypnosis, J Hand Surg 5(5):428, 1980.
61. Spinner M: Injuries to the major branches of peripheral nerves of the forearm, ed 2, Philadelphia, 1978, WB Saunders Co.
62. Sternbach RA and others: Traits of pain patients: the low-back "loser," Psychosomatics 14:226, 1973.
63. Sternbach RA: Modern concepts of pain. In Delessio DJ, editor: Wolff's headache and other head pain, ed 4, New York, 1980, Oxford University Press.
64. Sufian S and others: Acupuncture for chronic pain and anesthesia, Surg Rounds 5:38, 1982.
65. Swanson AB, Boeve NR, and Lumsden RM: The prevention and treatment of amputation neuromata by silicone capping, J Hand Surg 2:70, 1977.
66. Thomason JR and Moritz WH: Continuous lumbar paravertebral sympathetic block maintained by fractional installation of procaine, Surg Gynecol Obstet 89:447, 1949.
67. Tupper JW and Booth DM: Treatment of painful neuromas of sensory nerves in the hand: a comparison of traditional and newer methods, J Hand Surg 1:144, 1976.

68. Tursky B: Physical, physiological, and psychological factors that affect pain reaction to electric shock, Psychophysiology 11:95, 1974.

69. Tursky B and O'Connell D: Reliability and interjudgment predictability of subjective judgments of electrocutaneous stimulation, Psychophysiology 9:290, 1972.

70. Ulett GH: Acupuncture treatments for pain relief, JAMA 245:768, 1981.

71. Vaux KL: Pain: the moral dimensions, Cancer Bull 33:86, 1981.

72. Veith I: Acupuncture in traditional Chinese medicine, Calif Med 118:70, 1973.

73. Wallace PF and Fitzmorris CS Jr: The S-H-A-F-T syndrome in the upper extremity, J Hand Surg 3(5):492, 1978.

74. White JC and Sweet WH: Pain and the neurosurgeon: a forty year experience, Springfield, Ill, 1969, Charles C Thomas, Publisher.

75. Wiley AM, Poplawski ZB, and Murray J: Post-traumatic dystrophy of the hand, Orthop Rev 6:59, 1977.

76. Wilson RL: Management of pain following peripheral nerve injuries, Orthop Clin North Am 12:343, 1981.

77. Wolff BB and Jarvik ME: Variations in cutaneous and deep somatic pain sensitivity, Can J Psychol 17:37, 1963.

78. Wynn Parry CB: Brachial plexus lesions, causalgia, and Sudek's atrophy, American Society for Surgery of The Hand Newsletter 2, 1981.

59

Reflex sympathetic dystrophy

L. Lee Lankford

Homeostasis is defined as a tendency to stability in the normal body states (internal body condition) of the organism and is achieved by a system of control mechanisms activated by negative feedback to return to normalcy any deranged body condition produced by an abnormal stimulus. The body, therefore, has a mechanism designed for the purpose of returning to normalcy (homeostasis) any abnormal state produced by injury or disease. This usually takes place in an orderly fashion, and within the limits of the injury or disease the body will be reinstated in its previous condition. On occasion, however, this orderly mechanism does not function properly and a deranged state persists in the body. Reflex sympathetic dystrophy is an example of such a dysfunction on the part of the body. Instead of an injury or a disease of an extremity healing in the expected fashion, the limb is beset by a condition of increasing pain and dysfunction. Fortunately, this happens infrequently, but because of the devastating effect this has on the extremity and the person as a whole, it behooves us to acquaint ourselves with this condition and its diagnosis and treatment.

WHAT IT IS

Reflex sympathetic dystrophy (RSD) is a diseased state of an extremity that is characterized by very severe pain, swelling, stiffness, and discoloration (Fig. 59-1). It usually

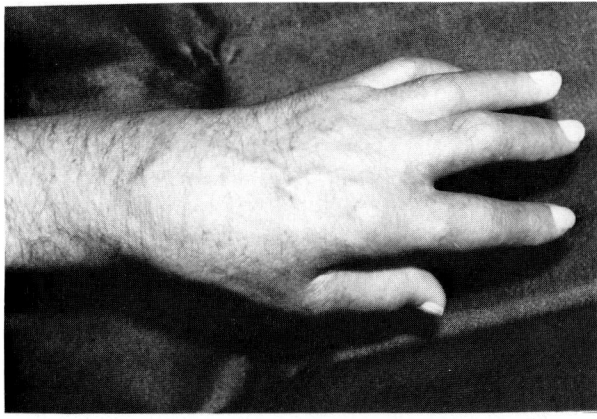

Fig. 59-1 Hand in reflex sympathetic dystrophy is usually swollen and red and has tight, shiny skin. (From Lankford LL and Thompson JE: Reflex sympathetic dystrophy, upper and lower extremity: diagnosis and management. In American Academy of Orthopaedic Surgeons: Instructional course lectures, vol 26, St Louis, 1977, The CV Mosby Co.)

occurs after a trauma or disease of an extremity, is generated by an abnormal sympathetic reflex, and is characteristically treated by the abolition of this increased sympathetic nerve stimulation. RSD is generally considered to be synonymous with "vasomotor and trophic disorders." There are several clinical types of RSD, ranging from a minor involvement of one or more fingers to the severest form, which is major causalgia; therefore RSD presents many different aspects and varying degrees of pain and dysfunction.

WHAT IT IS NOT

It is important to realize that RSD is not the only condition that causes more stiffness, swelling, pain, discoloration, and dysfunction than is normal for a given severity of trauma or disease in the normal individual. Injury (including surgery) or disease in a hand that has a tendency toward excessive fibrosis ("high up on the fibrosis scale") most likely will produce a greater amount of pain, swelling, stiffness, and dysfunction than the same severity of injury or disease in an otherwise normal person. Although one may well think of this as being a "dystrophic" condition, these findings alone do not make it a case of RSD. Conditions that fall in this category are the following: Dupuytren's palmar fasciitis, hypertrophic arthritis, psoriatic arthritis, the primary type of carpal tunnel syndrome (produced by increased fibrosis of the transverse carpal ligament causing thickening and longitudinal contracture of the ligament, thus narrowing the diameter of the carpal tunnel), stenosing tenosynovitis, "knuckle pads" with thickened and inelastic skin over the dorsum of the finger, and long-standing diabetes. One must not be deluded into thinking that all bad results and stiff hands are caused by RSD. It is very important to make this distinction early in the course of the disease so that the appropriate treatment may be given these distinctly different types of dystrophy.

NOMENCLATURE

A Civil War neurologist by the name of Silas Weir Mitchell, working in the Turner's Lane Hospital in Philadelphia, is generally credited with the first accurate description of the condition that we now call "reflex sympathetic dystrophy." Although Mitchell's description[62] remains as the classic, many authors previously had written case reports of patients who may well have had one of the clinical forms of RSD; they are Paré[73] in 1598, Potts[80] in 1736, Denmark[16] in 1813, and Hamilton[31] in 1838. Mitchell, Moorehouse, and Keen[62] published their epochal description in 1864, entitled *Gunshot Wounds and Other Injuries of Nerves*. In the same year, Paget[69] described trophic changes and a glossy appearance of the hand and fingers with severe pain and dysfunction after a nerve injury. Sudeck[87] in 1900 described a condition, which he later called "inflammatory bone atrophy," that produced a reflex sympathetic dystrophy appearance but without specific nerve injury. In 1937 de Takáts[18] described a similar condition, which he called "reflex dystrophy," but in another article[19] in 1945, he used the name "causalgic state." Homans[34] in 1940 coined the term "minor causalgia." In the years after this, many authors who felt the need to recognize the role of trauma and vasomotor dysfunction suggested terms such as "posttraumatic dystrophy," "painful vasodilatation," "posttraumatic osteoporosis," "posttraumatic causalgia," "sympathetic neurovascular dystrophy," "posttraumatic vasomotor disorders," and "reflex nervous dystrophy."

It was not until 1867 that Mitchell[60] in another publication created the term "causalgia" after the Greek words for 'burning pain'—*kausos* plus *algos* plus -ia ("condition").

I[44] believe that all of the above-mentioned vasomotor-trophic conditions are linked together, because all of them owe their existence to an abnormal sympathetic nerve reflex, and therefore all should be classified as RSD. One should also understand, however, that there are several clinical types of RSD. Since Mitchell[60-62] described his condition as a partial injury to a major mixed nerve in the proximal part of the extremity and believed that this condition arose only from a nerve injury, I believe that the term "causalgia" should be reserved for those forms of RSD that involve nerves. The designation of a major causalgia will be given to Mitchell's condition, since not only does it describe the fact that a major nerve is involved but also the symptoms are of the greatest severity. There is, however, a clinical type of RSD that involves the trauma of a peripheral digital nerve and produces, in comparison, minor symptoms and dysfunction, and so in our classification it is called "minor causalgia." More frequently, however, RSD does not involve specific nerve injury but instead involves damage to the soft-tissue, joint, or bone. These non–nerve injury types of RSD are called "minor traumatic dystrophy" or "major traumatic dystrophy," depending on the severity of the inciting trauma or disease and the magnitude of noxious signs and symptoms. The remaining clinical type of RSD is the shoulder-hand syndrome, which is also precipitated by an abnormal sympathetic nerve reflex but is caused either by a trauma of the proximal part of the body or by damage or disease of a viscus.

SYMPTOMS AND SIGNS
Pain

Certainly the paramount symptom of RSD is pain, and it is characteristically described as a burning pain. Most traumas and disease states produce pain, but the distinguishing feature in RSD is that the severity of the pain is all out of proportion to the inciting injury or disease state. In most cases, the first complaint is that of a burning pain, but as times goes on, patients often describe the pain as a pressure, crushing, binding, searing, aching, cutting, or cramping pain. Even though the pain in the patient with well-developed RSD is constant, it certainly is aggravated by either active or passive attempts at motion. Another distinguishing feature is the dysesthesia and paresthesia that is produced by even a light touch of the affected skin. It is difficult to do an examination at times because of the patient's with-

drawal of the hand from the examiner. At first, the pain is more apt to be the expected degree of pain for the involved injury or disease. Later, however, the pain gets worse, and in many cases it does not start until after the cast has been removed. The initial pain, also, is in the expected nerve distribution area of the injury, but it soon spreads to the whole hand, wrist, forearm, and the entire upper extremity. The severity of the tenderness is also quite pronounced, and it is usually worse around the interphalangeal joints of the fingers.

Swelling

Swelling is usually the first physical sign, occurs initially in the involved area, and then slowly spreads to other areas so that eventually it may encompass the hand, wrist, and distal part of the forearm. The swelling in the fingers, which at first produces a fusiform appearance, gradually changes to periarticular thickening at the joints. At first the swelling is that of a soft edema, but in time it becomes a hard, brawny edema and certainly is one of the factors that produces loss of motion.

Stiffness

As in the case of pain, the stiffness in RSD is distinctive because it is profoundly worse than one would expect from the antecedent trauma or disease. A trauma without the presence of RSD would be expected to produce some stiffness, but as times goes on and as the wound heals, the stiffness would normally improve. In the case of RSD, however, one usually finds that the stiffness increases with time. Since any attempt at either active or passive motion is exquisitely painful, it is not hard to understand that the initial lack of motion is attributable to the enforced immobility to escape further aggravation of the pain. Subsequently, the stiffness is attributable to increased fibrosis in the ligamentous structures and adhesion formation around the tendon, which sticks all gliding structures together. All fibrous structures about the joints are thickened and quite hard and inelastic. It is not uncommon to see palmar fasciitis accompanying RSD, and this too, of course, will add to the severity of flexion contractures in the digits.

Discoloration

An ever-present sign is some type of discoloration of the hand. Usually, the discoloration takes the form of redness and initially is most commonly located over the dorsum of the metacarpophalangeal (MP) joints and the interphalangeal joints of the fingers, but it may at times involve the whole hand rather diffusely. At some period of the disease the hand may be pale and at other times grayish to cyanotic. A purplish discoloration may often be seen in the flexor creases of the fingers in the palm; this is particularly true if a palmar fasciitis has developed. The omnipresence of increased coloration of the hand had caused me[42] to call RSD the "red hand disease." Pallor is present, of course, where there is vasoconstriction of both arterial and venous systems, and redness is present when there is dilation of both sides of the vascular tree, but blueness or cyanosis is usually present when there is vasoconstriction of the venous system.

Osteoporosis

The next most common and reliable sign of RSD is osteoporosis, and here again the degree of osteoporosis is distinguished by the fact that it is a great deal more severe than would be expected by the preceding trauma or disease (Fig. 59-2). The initial demineralization in the more severe forms of RSD usually takes place in the carpal bones and produces punched-out areas, which prompted Sudeck[87] to call this condition "inflammatory bone atrophy." There are, however, no distinguishing features of this spotty osteoporosis because with the passage of time the untreated case will progress eventually from the punched-out areas to a diffuse osteoporosis with no particular clinical significance. Also, very early in the disease the demineralization takes place in the polar regions of the long bones of the metacarpals and the phalanges. Although some demineralization would, of course, be present from immobilization alone, the bulk of the washing out of the calcium undoubtedly comes from increased blood flow in the joints. This has recently been shown by Genant.[25]

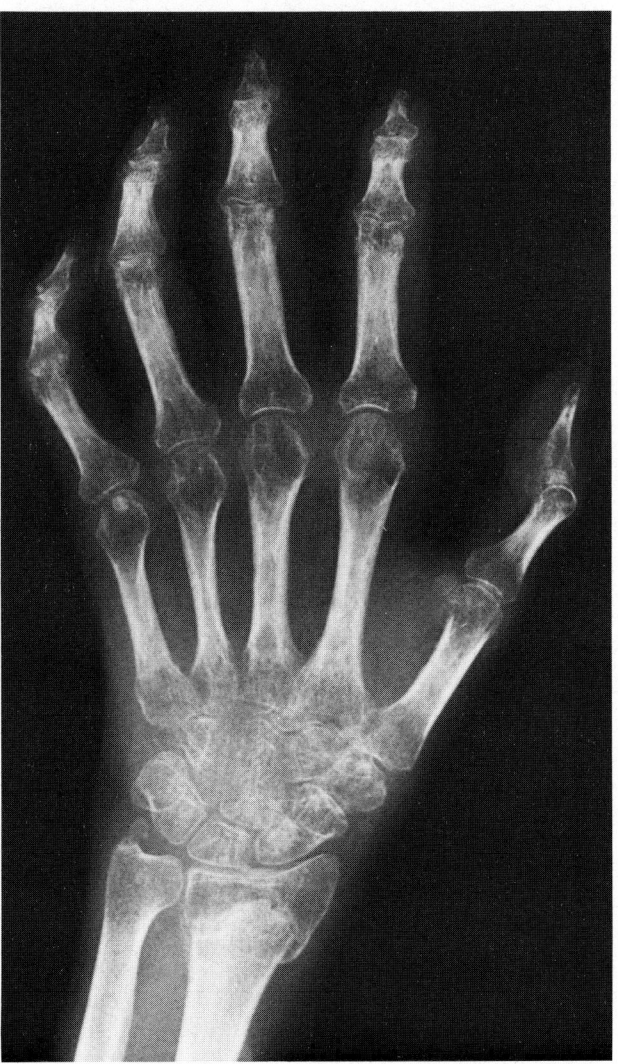

Fig. 59-2 Degree of osteoporosis is distinguished by its being much greater than would be expected in the usual case of trauma with immobilization. (From Lankford LL and Thompson JE: Reflex sympathetic dystrophy, upper and lower extremity: diagnosis and management. In American Academy of Orthopaedic Surgeons: Instructional course lectures, vol 26, St Louis, 1977, The CV Mosby Co.)

Sudomotor changes

Sudomotor changes are usually present but may be variable according to several factors. More often than not the early stages of RSD display hyperhidrosis, though in some severe clinical types dryness may be present initially. In the last stages of the disease, dryness is the rule. At times the diaphoresis is great enough to observe beads of sweat dropping from the hand.

Temperature

The temperature of the extremity involved with RSD also is quite variable. If it is possible to observe the disease at its very earliest onset, one most commonly finds a decrease in the temperature, and this is also usually the case when there is hyperhidrosis. In the early stages when dryness of the hand or redness is present, the temperature is more commonly elevated. When pallor or cyanosis is present, the temperature is nearly always diminished. In some instances, one may find concurrently increased temperature over the reddened joints and diminished temperature in between the joints where there is pallor. Carron and Weller[10] have used thermograms to demonstrate that most patients have increased heat, but they do not state during which stage the thermograms were taken.

Palmar fasciitis

A palmar fasciitis with acute nodules and thickening of the longitudinal bands of palmar fascia in the fingers or in the hand may be seen in several clinical types of RSD. The condition may progress as long as the RSD is not successfully treated. This does, of course, tend to produce flexion contractures of the fingers.

Vasomotor instability

Prolonged capillary refill time is commonly found in RSD, and one may easily demonstrate this by blanching the finger nail with pressure or by pressing on the fat pad areas in the finger. This is generally found with pallor, cyanosis, or excess sweating. A rapid capillary refill may be seen when there is redness in the hand, and this is indicative of vasodilation. In the very early stages of RSD, vasoconstriction is the rule.

Trophic changes

One almost always associates a glossy, shiny appearance of the skin with RSD. In the early stages this appearance is attributable to the swelling and ironing out of the skin wrinkles and is secondary to lack of motion in the joints. Later on, the nutritional (trophic) changes that produce the glossy, shiny surface of the skin are caused by skin and subcutaneous tissue atrophy. This was prominently mentioned by Mitchell[62] and by Paget[69] and many others subsequently. The skin feels quite tight, and one can readily observe a definite decrease in the mobility of the skin over the dorsum of the fingers and particularly the interphalangeal joints. The ends of the fingers may take on a "pencil-pointing" appearance because of the atrophy of the tip of the fat pad and the concomitant downward curving of the fingernail.

STAGES

The difficulty of diagnosis of RSD is attributable in part to the variable signs and symptoms depending on when in the course of the disease the examiner first sees the patient. A particular sign or symptom may be present temporarily but not at a subsequent stage. It is therefore important to be cognizant of the great variations according to the duration of the condition. It is possible to divide the course of RSD into three stages.

Stage I

In the early part of stage I, pain is the most pronounced feature. The pain is usually of a burning nature, and throughout stage I the pain generally increases in severity. Painful paresthesia to light touch may be seen quite early, but aggravation of the constant pain with attempts at motion is seen with greater regularity near the end of stage I. Swelling begins quite early and may cause pitting over the dorsum of the hand if quite prominent (Fig. 59-3). Lack of motion

of the fingers or the wrist is seen early and is progressive throughout this stage. The coloration of the hand is variable but most commonly in the early part of the stage is either pale or cyanotic and near the end of the stage becomes red, especially over the dorsum of the MP joints and the interphalangeal joints. Increased sweating and coolness in the first stage is more frequent than drying or heat, particularly in the early part of stage I. Vasoconstriction or peripheral vasospasm is most commonly noted. Osteoporosis is not present before 3 weeks and often is not seen until the fifth week. The average duration of stage I is 3 months.

Stage II

Pain continues to be one of the most prominent features of stage II, and it continues to get worse during most of this stage unless treated. The swelling changes from a soft

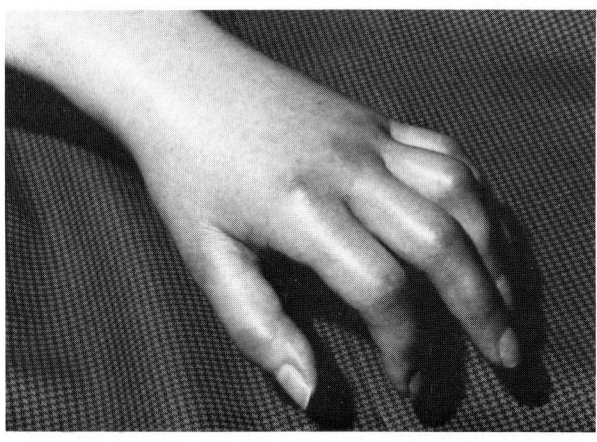

Fig. 59-3 In first stage of reflex sympathetic dystrophy, swelling is usually soft and puffy with redness over joints. (From Lankford LL and Thompson JE: Reflex sympathetic dystrophy, upper and lower extremity: diagnosis and management. In American Academy of Orthopaedic Surgeons: Instructional course lectures, vol 26, St Louis, 1977, The CV Mosby Co.)

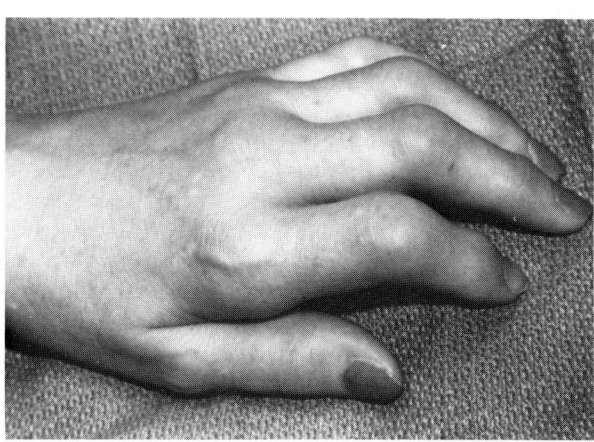

Fig. 59-4 Stage II is characterized by brawny edema with stiffness, as evidenced by flattening out of extensor and flexor wrinkles. (From Lankford LL and Thompson JE: Reflex sympathetic dystrophy, upper and lower extremity: diagnosis and management. In American Academy of Orthopaedic Surgeons: Instructional course lectures, vol 26, St Louis, 1977, The CV Mosby Co.)

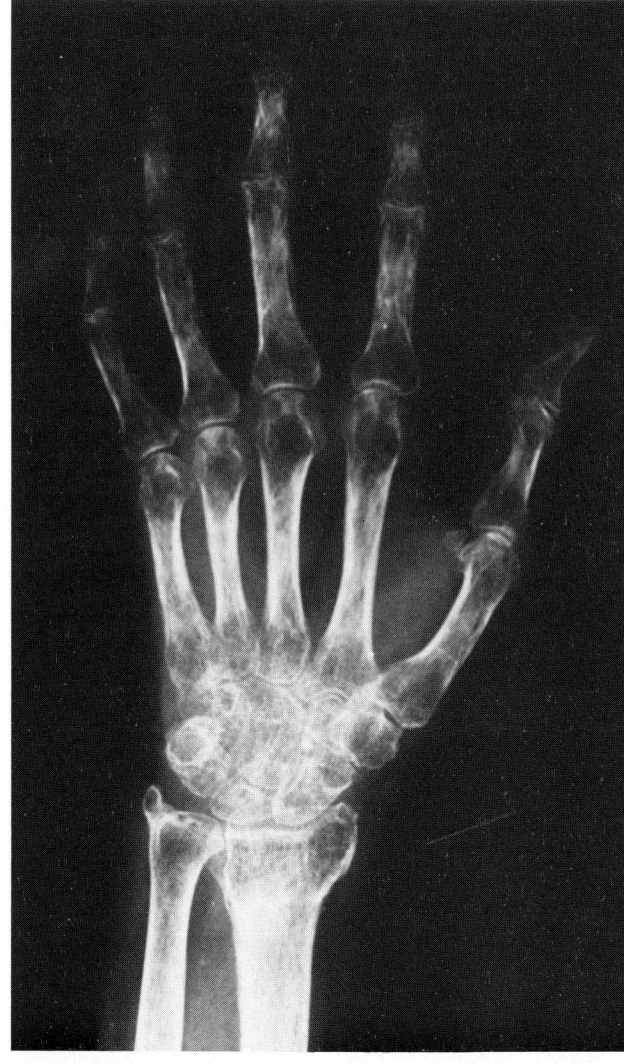

Fig. 59-5 Near end of stage II and early part of stage III, osteoporosis has become uniform and very intense throughout all bones of the hand and wrist. (From Lankford LL and Thompson JE: Reflex sympathetic dystrophy, upper and lower extremity: diagnosis and management. In American Academy of Orthopaedic Surgeons: Instructional course lectures, vol 26, St Louis, 1977, The CV Mosby Co.)

nature to a brawny, hard edema (Fig. 59-4). It is difficult to reduce the swelling by elevation or other standard means during this stage. Stiffness continues to increase throughout most of this stage and again pain is aggravated by attempts at active and passive motion. During stage II redness, increased heat, and decreased sweating are most commonly found. Vasomotor instability is still observed. The demineralization also increases and changes from the spotty demineralization in the carpal bones and the polar demineralization in the long bones of the fingers to a more widespread homogeneous appearance (Fig. 59-5). The glossy or shiny appearance of the skin continues to increase. The duration of stage II is most commonly through the ninth month.

Stage III

The severity of the pain in most instances has peaked in stage III and either remains constant for several months or slowly improves. In many cases, however, the pain continues for at least 2 years and in some cases, indefinitely. John Mitchell, the physician son of Silas Weir Mitchell, continued to follow up on some of his father's cases and reported in 1895[59] that severe pain and dysfunction lasted for more than 20 years. Pain on motion remains fairly severe for several months in stage III even though the constant pain may have subsided somewhat. The fingers and the wrist are usually quite stiff in the untreated case and show very little improvement. The swelling changes from the brawny edema to periarticular thickening of the joints, and such structures as the collateral ligaments are quite obviously thickened. The hand usually becomes pale, dry, and cool. The glossy appearance is usually at its peak in stage III (Fig. 59-6). The skin and subcutaneous tissue atrophy continues with "pencil pointing" of the fingertips at its greatest. Osteoporosis is profound. In most cases the hand is quite dysfunctional. Stage III usually lasts for at least 2 years but in many cases will extend through many years.

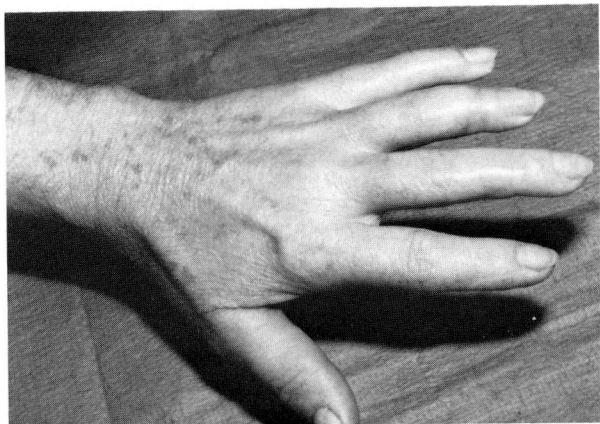

Fig. 59-6   Stage III is characterized by atrophy of skin and subcutaneous tissue, which produces a glossy appearance of skin. (From Lankford LL and Thompson JE: Reflex sympathetic dystrophy, upper and lower extremity: diagnosis and management. In American Academy of Orthopaedic Surgeons: Instructional course lectures, vol 26, St Louis, 1977, The CV Mosby Co.)

CLINICAL TYPES

Evans[23] first suggested that all the many descriptive terms previously used for the various vasomotor conditions be changed to reflex sympathetic dystrophy, since it is apparent that all these conditions are produced by an abnormal sympathetic reflex. I wholeheartedly concur with this name, but at the same time I recognize that there are distinct clinical types and have devised the following classifications[94] of RSD:
1. Minor causalgia
2. Minor traumatic dystrophy
3. Shoulder-hand syndrome
4. Major traumatic dystrophy
5. Major causalgia

Minor causalgia

Since this clinical type of RSD involves a nerve, it is called a "causalgia," and since the nerve involved is a peripheral nerve with the least severe pain and dysfunction, the term "minor causalgia" is used for this condition. A nerve injury in the upper extremity is seen much more commonly in the hand and wrist than in the elbow and upper arm. The symptoms produced are less noxious and involve a smaller part of the hand and may well be limited to only one or two fingers. The degree of pain, swelling, stiffness, discoloration, and osteoporosis is concomitantly less severe. The antecedent trauma is more frequently to the dorsal superficial sensory branch of the radial nerve overlying the radial styloid area of the wrist, and this site is the most vulnerable to injury. If the injury has produced scarring of the nerve or a nerve was severed and repaired, the nerve very commonly binds itself down to the surrounding fixed structures with adhesions and thus produces a "neurodesis" with the fixation of the nerve distal to the wrist. Any flexion of the wrist will produce a stretching of the nerve, and this stretching excites greater fibrous tissue proliferation with the ultimate production of a painful neuroma. In the past I have recommended that severely traumatized radial sensory nerves not be sutured but instead be cut cleanly proximally as far as possible to avoid the formation of the painful neuroma. It was my hope that with the advent of microsurgery the sacrifice of the dorsal superficial branch of the radial sensory nerve might not be necessary, but so far these hopes have not come to fruition.

The palmar branch of the median nerve just proximal to the wrist is quite often injured with lacerations or because of a surgical procedure in this area, and this branch is our next most common nerve injury site in the minor causalgia type of RSD. This nerve is quite often injured inadvertently with the use of a transverse incision in the volar wrist, and for this reason I have avoided the use of this incision.

The next most common site of nerve injury is the dorsal superficial sensory branch of the ulnar nerve and particularly over the dorsal ulnar aspect of the wrist and hand. The common digital and the proper digital branches of the median and ulnar nerves, though less commonly involved in minor causalgia, quite definitely can represent the inciting trauma producing this type of RSD.

Not every painful neuroma, of course, represents minor causalgia. A neuroma of some degree is always produced at the point of an injury of a nerve, and, of course, not all neuromas are painful. If a neuroma is painful only when pressure is applied and not between those times, it should not be considered a minor causalgia. The pain of minor causalgia is constant, and the other features of RSD such as pain on motion, swelling, stiffness, and osteoporosis are much greater than would be expected from a simple painful neuroma. Only when these findings are present can a diagnosis of RSD be properly made.

Minor traumatic dystrophy

Minor traumatic dystrophy is the most common clinical type of RSD because traumas not involving a specific nerve are much more common than nerve injuries and also because minor traumas are more common than major traumas, thereby producing the most frequent painful stimuli. Minor traumatic dystrophy, however, is also the most frequently overlooked type of RSD, since it is not as well known that RSD can involve only a small segment of a hand. The precipitating painful lesion is usually a trauma of minor proportions such as a mashed finger, fracture, dislocation, a sprain, or even a penetrating wound that does not specifically involve a nerve injury. The degree of involvement may encompass only one or a few fingers rather than the whole hand, but the same type of signs and symptoms such as pain, swelling, stiffness, discoloration, and dysfunction are present. The redness is characteristically found over the dorsum of the MP and interphalangeal joints, as well as over the collateral ligaments. A mild degree of palmar fasciitis may also be present. The digits are usually stiffened in flexion.

Shoulder-hand syndrome

The shoulder-hand syndrome usually starts with considerable pain and progresses to stiffness in the shoulder with spreading of the pain into the whole extremity, producing moderate-to-marked swelling of at least the wrist and the hand and sometimes the entire upper arm as well. The causative painful lesion is either a proximal trauma such as a shoulder, neck, or rib-cage injury, or it may well be from visceral sources such as heart attacks, strokes, stomach ulcers, or a Pancoast tumor of the apex of the lung. In most instances in shoulder-hand syndrome, there is a fusiform type of swelling and the fingers are stiffened in extension rather than in flexion (Fig. 59-7). Redness, when present, is more diffuse rather than being solely over the MP and interphalanageal joints, and the hand is usually warmer and dryer than normal. Palmar fasciitis with acute nodules is more likely to be present in this form of RSD than in any other clinical form. The sex distribution of all forms of RSD is heavily weighted toward the female, but the differential is greatest of all in shoulder-hand syndrome. The highest incidence of age distribution is between 45 and 55.

Otto Steinbrocker[85,86] first described this condition in 1947. At that time, apparently he did not fully appreciate the role of the abnormal sympathetic reflex and very likely included in his series several cases of shoulder stiffness that probably should have been diagnosed as adhesive capsulitis or arthritis. It should be emphasized that not all stiff, painful shoulders with swelling in the upper extremities that follow heart attacks or strokes fit into the category of RSD. Statistically, of course, the majority of painful stiff shoulders have their origin in disuse from trauma, rotator cuff tendinitis, or adhesive capsulitis, and if these conditions are

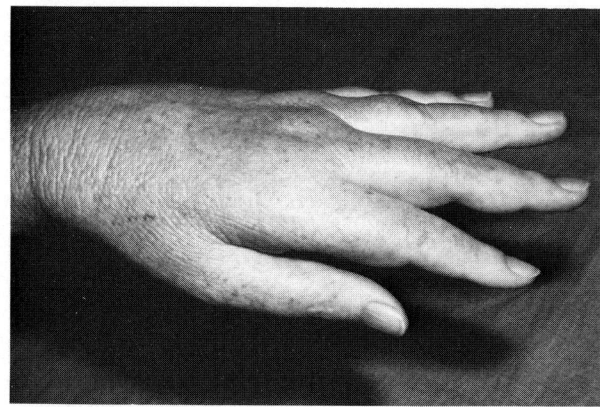

Fig. 59-7 Extension contractures of fingers are usually noted in the shoulder-hand clinical type of reflex sympathetic dystrophy, as contrasted to flexion contractures, which are usually noted in other clinical types. (From Lankford LL and Thompson JE: Reflex sympathetic dystrophy, upper and lower extremity: diagnosis and management. In American Academy of Orthopaedic Surgeons: Instructional course lectures, vol 26, St Louis, 1977, The CV Mosby Co.)

properly diagnosed early, they can usually be successfully treated with physical means. If, however, the degree of pain, swelling, stiffness, dysfunction, and especially osteoporosis is much greater than otherwise expected and the vasomotor component is recognized, they should be considered as possible RSD of the shoulder-hand clinical type and be so treated.

Major traumatic dystrophy

Major traumatic dystrophy is the clinical type that has given RSD such a bad name. The persistent painful lesion that triggers major traumatic dystrophy is usually a major trauma such as a crushed hand, Colles' fracture, or a severe fracture dislocation of the wrist. In a high percentage of cases, this type of trauma produces an acute traumatic carpal tunnel syndrome, which is most likely responsible for the painful lesion that activates RSD.[42] The acute carpal tunnel syndrome, however, need not be from trauma but may well be from an acute flare-up of arthritis. A high percentage of patients with Colles' fracture who have subsequently developed RSD were found to also have carpal tunnel syndromes in our series of cases. Major traumatic dystrophy is the clinical type of RSD that produces the greatest pain, stiffness, swelling, and dysfunction in the non–nerve injury cases. As in all cases of RSD, the degree of pain, swelling, stiffness, dysfunction, and osteoporosis is very much greater than one would expect to find with the same type of antecedent trauma or disease in an otherwise normal person. Flexion contractures of the digits in this type are more frequent than extension contractures. Wrist motion is usually extremely limited, and flexion deformities are present along with a definite limitation of rotary motion of the forearm.

Major causalgia

Major causalgia is the clinical type of RSD that produces the greatest degree of pain and devastation to the patient (Fig. 59-8). This is the clinical type of RSD that was noted

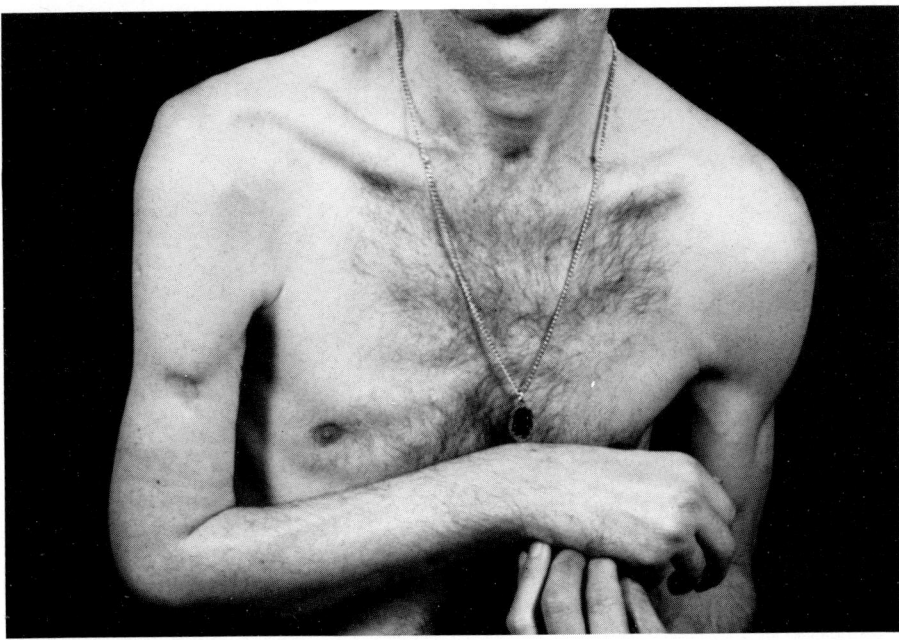

Fig. 59-8   Major causalgia usually produces greatest degree of pain and dysfunction of all types of reflex sympathetic dystrophy. It is usually caused by an injury to a major mixed nerve in proximal portion of extremity. In this case, initiating trauma was a partial injury to median nerve from gunshot wound. (From Lankford LL and Thompson JE: Reflex sympathetic dystrophy, upper and lower extremity: diagnosis and management. In American Academy of Orthopaedic Surgeons: Instructional course lectures, vol 26, St Louis, 1977, The CV Mosby Co.)

by Mitchell,[62] who described the inciting painful lesion as being a partial nerve injury in a mixed major nerve in the proximal part of the extremity. In the case of the upper extremity, the median nerve is usually involved, while in the lower extremity the sciatic nerve is involved more frequently. Sunderland[88] has shown that these two nerves have a much greater sympathetic nerve fiber population than other nerves do, and this is believed to be significant in the production of this clinical type of RSD. Without a doubt, pain is the most prominent symptom of a major causalgia and may, on occasion, begin at the time of injury, but most commonly it makes its appearance within the first week after injury. Characteristically the pain is described as burning. The pain usually progresses through all three stages and becomes extreme. The patient may seek relief by wrapping his hand and upper extremity in wet towels. An exacerbation of the pain may be brought on by light touch of the skin or even by auditory stimuli such as hearing a squeaky noise or by becoming emotionally upset. The vibration of riding in an automobile or even of another person walking across the floor may cause an aggravation of the pain. The pain may, at times, become so severe that the patient will beg for an amputation of the part. There is generally less red coloration in this type of RSD than in other types, and the early stages are almost always pale or cyanotic in color. Sweating and coolness are usually a prominent feature. At first the pain is confined to the distribution of the nerve that was injured but soon begins to spread over the entire hand and eventually the upper extremity. Flexion contractures of the fingers occur, but although the stiffness is extreme, the degree of flexion contracture is often not so great as in major traumatic dystrophy. The pain, stiffness,

and dysfunction, if untreated, may be expected to continue indefinitely.

According to Mitchell[62] his malady developed after the partial injury to a major mixed nerve, but this has subsequently been disproved by Nathan,[65] Kirklin,[37] and Shumacker,[81] who found that it was also caused by complete nerve lacerations. Doupe[20] in 1944 advanced the hypothesis that major causalgia was caused by the loss of the myelin sheath in the afferent sensory fibers in the partially injured nerve and this production an "artificial synapse" that allowed a "short circuiting" of the afferent pain impulses and the efferent sympathetic nerve stimulation. Doupe described a physiologic breakdown of the normal insulating material around the afferent fibers as a "fiber interaction" between the normally nonmyelinated sympathetic efferent fibers and the recently demyelinated pain fibers (Fig. 59-9). With this being the case, the efferent sympathetic fibers could be "short-circuited" in an antidromic direction and would be interpreted by the cerebral cortex as pain. Also, the afferent pain fibers with the loss of their myelin sheath could be "short-circuited" across the "artificial synapse" so that the pain impulses would then be turned distally (antidromic) as sympathetic fiber impulses and cause a greater sympathetic activity. Granit[30] in 1944 has shown in an experimental model that it is possible to produce this cross-stimulation effect from an "artificial synapse."

DIAGNOSTIC CRITERIA

It is of utmost importance to make an early diagnosis in cases of RSD because early treatment is much more effective than treatment at a later stage. This, at times, becomes somewhat difficult because of the varied symptoms in each

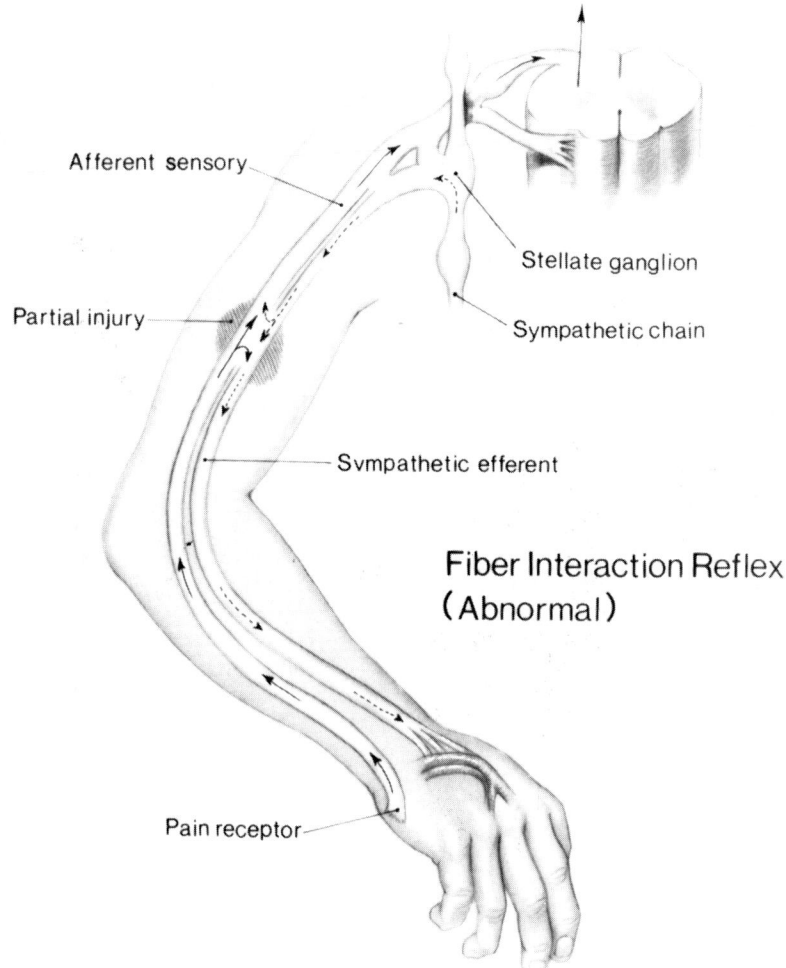

Afferent sensory

Partial injury

Stellate ganglion

Sympathetic chain

Sympathetic efferent

Fiber Interaction Reflex (Abnormal)

Pain receptor

Fig. 59-9 Doupe described a physiologic breakdown of myelin sheath in area of partial nerve injury that produced a "fiber interaction" of efferent and afferent impulses, which results in increased sympathetic nerve activity and increased pain. (From Lankford LL and Thompson JE: Reflex sympathetic dystrophy, upper and lower extremity: diagnosis and management. In American Academy of Orthopaedic Surgeons: Instructional course lectures, vol 26, St Louis, 1977, The CV Mosby Co.)

of the three clinical stages and the variation of the symptoms in the five clinical types of RSD. It is also of utmost importance to rule out other conditions that are characteristically known to produce pain, swelling, stiffness, and dysfunction but do not come under the classification of RSD. As pointed out earlier, traumas or diseases occurring in patients who have a tendency toward increased fibrosis (such as patients with Dupuytren's contracture, arthritis, longstanding diabetes, the primary type of carpal tunnel syndrome, and other collagen disorders) will often produce a stiff-hand syndrome. Although it is not uncommon to see a "flare" reaction in these types of patients after injury or disease, it is very important not to confuse them with RSD.

The dominant characteristic of RSD is that the symptoms and signs are much more intense than ordinarily would be expected from a trauma or disease occurring in an otherwise normal individual. In a normal individual the signs and symptoms will improve with time, but in the patient with RSD they get progressively worse. The four cardinal symptoms and signs are as follows:

1. Pain
2. Swelling
3. Stiffness
4. Discoloration

The secondary symptoms and signs, which are most often present but not necessarily inevitable, are as follows:

1. Osseous demineralization
2. Sudomotor changes
3. Temperature changes
4. Trophic changes
5. Vasomotor instability
6. Palmar fibromatosis

If all four of the cardinal symptoms and signs are present and at least several of the secondary symptoms and signs are found and they exist to a degree much greater than normally expected, a *presumptive* diagnosis of RSD can be made. Actual *confirmation* of this diagnosis, however, comes after interruption of the sympathetic nerve reflex has produced some amelioration of the patient's condition. One cannot, however, rule out RSD upon a single attempt to interrupt the sympathetic reflex arc. At least three or more blocks with completely negative effects should be used so that RSD may be conclusively ruled out. It is also important to make sure that the attempted interruption in the sympathetic reflex arc has been technically successful as evidenced by Horner's sign and by warmth and dryness of the extremity.

DIAGNOSTIC TESTS

Unfortunately there is no single, simple laboratory test that can accurately make the diagnosis of RSD. The lack of a satisfactory animal model has seriously hampered efforts in doing research on RSD. I feel that at some time in the future we will be able to make a definite diagnosis of RSD on the basis of some increase in the ipsilateral blood levels of catecholamines or some of the inflammation-producing substances that are present in RSD—such as bradykinins, serotonin, prostaglandins, or histamines—when compared with the same levels of the contralateral extremity. It is my feeling that most of the inflammatory reaction (and consequently the fibrosis and stiffness) in RSD is caused by prostaglandins. Blumenkrantz[7] in 1972 showed that prostaglandin E_1 causes bone absorption and that prostaglandin F_{1a} causes increased synthesis of collagen fibers. If this indeed is the cause of the severe stiffness and fibrosis in RSD, possibly this fact can be used in the development of a laboratory test.

Radionuclide imaging

In 1975 Genant[25] and later Kozin[39] suggested that the diagnosis of RSD could be made by fine-detail radiography and bone scintigraphy using technetium 99^m-labeled phosphorus complexes injected intravenously. There is increased uptake in the bone and soft tissues of the radionuclide pharmaceutical in the following conditions: (1) increased blood flow, (2) increased inflammatory reaction, (3) increased osteogenic activity, and (4) increased bone metabolism.[36,39,93] Maurer[52] and MacKinnon[50] used a three-phase radionuclide bone scan for the diagnosis of RSD and suggested that the third phase (the delayed image) is consistently positive; this may result from increased vascularity in the region of the focal point of the RSD. While it is true that increased vascularity is one of the reasons for uptake of the radionuclide in the tissues, that in itself is not diagnostic of RSD because of the many other causes of increased blood flow. My experience has been that the three-phase scanning technique has a very high degree of sensitivity but does not do well from the standpoint of specificity. In our experience, it offers very little additional information that cannot be obtained with an ordinary roentgenogram.

Thermography

In recent years attempts have been made to diagnose RSD with the use of thermography using cholesteric liquid crystals, which have the ability to indicate various temperatures because of the specific color changes present. By taking a photograph of the displayed colors, a permanent record can be made that indicates the temperature of the skin of a body part.[74] Uematsu[89] in 1981 reported the use of thermography in the diagnosis of RSD. He contends that a significant decrease in the skin temperature in the affected area would be diagnostic of RSD. I have not found thermography a useful tool in the diagnosis of RSD, because all thermography does is to tell you the temperature of a body part. As pointed out previously, RSD does not always demonstrate decreased temperature and, as a matter of fact, often shows increased temperature. Since many conditions other than RSD show decreased skin temperature, thermography would not be expected to be a reliable test.

ETIOLOGY

Because of the lack of confirmatory laboratory experimentation, the many theories of the etiology and genesis of RSD have yet to be proved. My clinical impression[42] is that the following three factors must occur concurrently before a patient can develop RSD:

1. Persistent painful lesion (trauma or disease)
2. Diathesis (predisposition, susceptibility, or inherent trait)
3. Abnormal sympathetic reflex

If all three of these conditions are present at the same time in the same patient, it is expected that RSD will occur. This explains why RSD develops in only a few persons even though their traumas and treatment may have been identical to those of patients who did not develop RSD.

Persistent painful lesion

A significant characteristic of RSD is that the magnitude of the inciting trauma or disease is not necessarily equivalent to the severity of the patient's symptoms and signs. In general, minor traumas will produce the minor traumatic dystrophy clinical type of RSD and the more severe traumas will produce the major traumatic dystrophy, but almost invariably one is struck by the fact that it is not reasonable to expect the very severe symptoms and signs that are sometimes produced from a very minor trauma. One usually finds himself asking the question, "How could this severe condition result from such a minor injury?"

Most persistent painful lesions that initiate RSD are of traumatic origin, but in some cases pain from a disease will also be sufficient to initiate the process, such as a severe flare-up of arthritis, an acute carpal tunnel syndrome, Pancoast's tumor, tissue ischemia, nerve entrapment, a heart attack, or stroke. Acute traumatic carpal tunnel syndrome has been the initiating persistent painful lesion in a high percentage of my patients with Colles' fracture who developed major traumatic dystrophy. The trauma, however, need not be very severe and may be as inconsequential as a mashed fingertip, a bruised nerve over the radial styloid, or an interphalangeal joint sprain.

Diathesis

I[42,43] have long believed that certain patients are susceptible to the development of RSD and others are not. There appears to be a predisposition, inherent characteristic, natural tendency, a bodily constitutional trait, or diathesis that allows some patients to develop RSD, whereas others receiving the same degree of trauma are not so afflicted. The diathesis in all probability is an inherited trait, which cannot be changed. I have had as patients a mother and daughter who had Colles' fractures (many years apart), both of whom developed RSD after their fractures. Another patient in whom RSD developed in the lower extremity and again several years later in a traumatized upper extremity has been

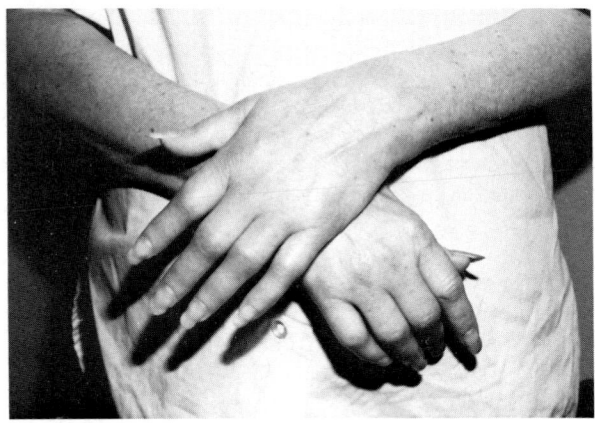

Fig. 59-10 This patient developed bilateral major traumatic type of reflex sympathetic dystrophy from bilateral traumatic carpal tunnel syndromes, which resulted from minimally displaced bilateral Colles' fractures. (From Lankford LL and Thompson JE: Reflex sympathetic dystrophy, upper and lower extremity: diagnosis and management. In American Academy of Orthopaedic Surgeons: Instructional course lectures, vol 26, St Louis, 1977, The CV Mosby Co.)

observed. I have also seen bilateral RSD occurring simultaneously from a bilateral Colles' fracture (Fig. 59-10). Coffman[15] reported in 1975 the occurrence of RSD in the same person on several occasions after different traumas.

Two different types of diathesis are recognized. The first diathesis is the tendency of the patient to be a "hypersympathetic reactor." These patients have increased sympathetic nerve activity.[68] When a history is being taken, the patient is always asked if he has sweaty palms (hyperhidrosis) or other evidence of increased sympathetic nerve activity, such as a history of pallor or excessive coolness of fingers and toes when they are exposed to colder temperatures. On physical examination one often finds evidence of peripheral vasoconstriction and poor capillary refill on the uninvolved extremity. Also, other historical evidence of vasomotor dysfunctions such as fainting, excessive blushing, or even migraine headaches is often obtained in patients with RSD.

The second diathesis has to do with the psychological makeup of the patient. This type of diathesis is more difficult to determine than the hypersympathetic reactor. However, in most patients with RSD it is possible to recognize that they have certain psychological traits that are often described by psychiatrists as "fearful, suspicious, emotionally labile, inadequate personality, chronic complainer, dependent per-

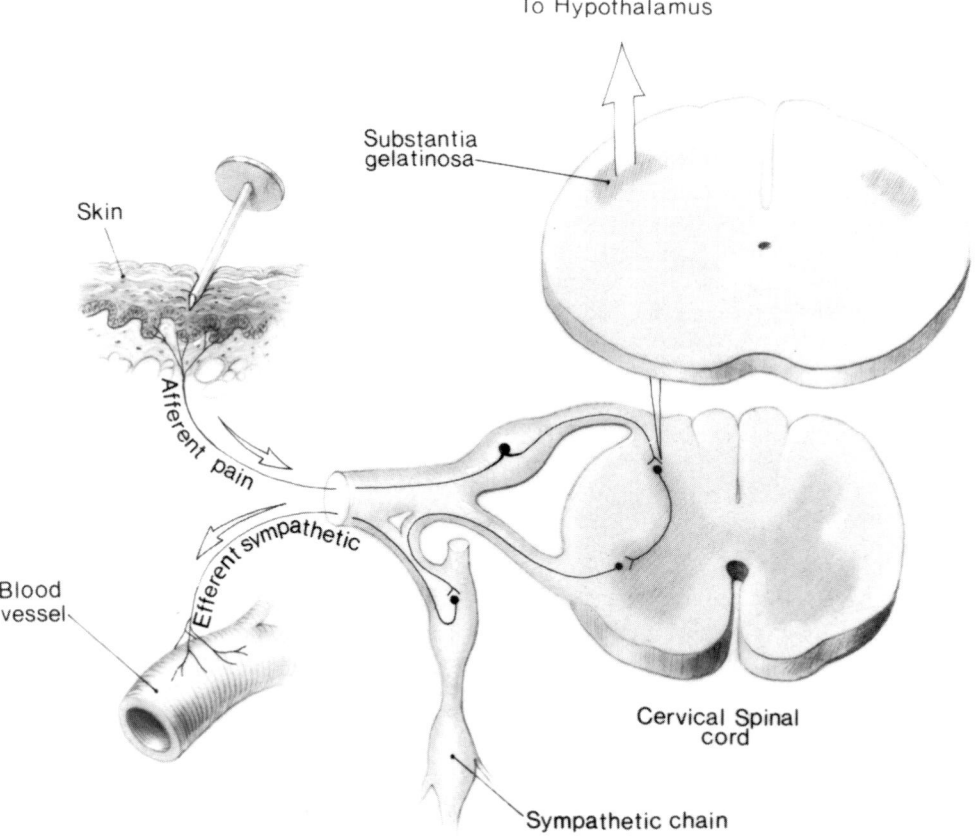

Fig. 59-11 A normal sympathetic nerve reflex arc is set into motion with any painful stimuli; it results in a temporary vasoconstrictive action of the small vessels. However, if this normal sympathetic reflex arc fails to shut down at the appropriate time, an abnormal sympathetic reflex may develop, thus producing one of the etiologic factors of reflex sympathetic dystrophy. (From Lankford LL and Thompson JE: Reflex sympathetic dystrophy, upper and lower extremity: diagnosis and management. In American Academy of Orthopaedic Surgeons: Instructional course lectures, vol 26, St Louis, 1977, The CV Mosby Co.)

sonality, insecure and unstable personality." I almost never discover a psychological trait in a patient with RSD who is described as being stoic or a "Spartan." Patients who develop RSD also have the tendency to have a very low pain threshold. This type of patient will usually not be very cooperative in carrying out the doctor's orders, will think up many excuses for not doing what he is told, and will try to control his own treatment and seek to place the blame for his condition on others.

One therefore would have to be suspicious that a patient has the diathesis for RSD if he has a very low pain threshold and cold, sweaty hands, asks a multitude of irrelevant questions, and tries to manipulate the doctor. This should not be construed to imply that patients with RSD are malingerers. The patient cannot control this diathesis and therefore cannot willfully cause this to happen to himself. However, patient gain or the emotional element can never be fully ruled out of any condition producing pain, stiffness, and dysfunction.

Abnormal sympathetic reflex

Even if a person had a normal tendency toward having increased sympathetic nerve activity, RSD could not take place unless a grossly abnormal situation arose in the sympathetic nerve reflex to perpetuate the extreme increase in sympathetic nerve activity for a prolonged period of time. It would therefore have to be an abnormal sympathetic reflex to cause this to happen.

A normal sympathetic reflex arc comes into play with trauma. When afferent nerves transmit a message of pain from the extremity, these nerve fibers synapse in the posterior root ganglion and then again in the posterior horn and finally in the lateral horn, where the message of pain is transferred to the sympathetic nerve cell bodies. The sympathetic reflex is activated when efferent sympathetic impulses are sent out the anterior horn through the anterior root to the sympathetic chain and then through the white ramus into the sympathetic ganglion, where a synapse occurs; the postganglionic sympathetic fiber then leaves the ganglia through the gray ramus, where it enters the peripheral nerve and goes distally into the extremity to produce vasoconstriction of the small vessels (Fig. 59-11). This is a normal reflex, and it is the body's attempt to begin a process to return the injured tissue to normalcy.

The vasoconstrictive reflex is necessary to prevent excessive bleeding in the injured tissue, but after a few hours it gives way to vasodilation, which is a part of the reparative process in an orderly stepwise progression to healing. If for some reason, however, this normal sympathetic reflex arc does not shut down at the appropriate time but in fact continues on in an accelerated fashion, it will produce ultimately an intense degree of sympathetic nerve activity. The increased vasoconstriction produces ischemia in the tissue, which is painful and causes increased afferent pain impulses to be sent centrally, thus activating the sympathetic reflex arc, and increased sympathetic nerve activity results.[88] This "sympathetic-pain reflex" sets into motion the abnormal sympathetic reflex, which is necessary for the production of RSD. There are many theories about the exact cause of this abnormal sympathetic reflex, but up to now none seems to present a satisfactory explanation.

PATHOGENESIS

The lack of a satisfactory laboratory experimental animal model has hampered the basic research necessary to help answer some of the many questions concerning the pathogenicity of this enigmatic problem.

Livingston,[47] Gerard,[26] and Kennard[35] have further developed a concept first proposed by Lorente de Nó[49] that an abnormal sympathetic reflex was put into play because of an abnormal "feedback mechanism" that occurred in the "internuncial pool" of the posterior and lateral horns of the spinal cord. This increased sympathetic nerve activity that produces tissue ischemia, which in turn generates more pain, turns into a "vicious cycle," which can certainly account for the severe pain and the increased sympathetic nerve activity seen in RSD[44] (Fig. 59-12).

Pool[75] stimulated the proximal end of the distal segment of a severed sensory nerve and produced pain in the sensory distribution of this nerve and found that by blocking adjacent nerves with a local anesthesia he could eliminate the pain produced by stimulation of the cut nerve. This suggests that intensive sympathetic nerve fiber stimulation might well produce a pain-evoking substance. Chapman[13] produced a

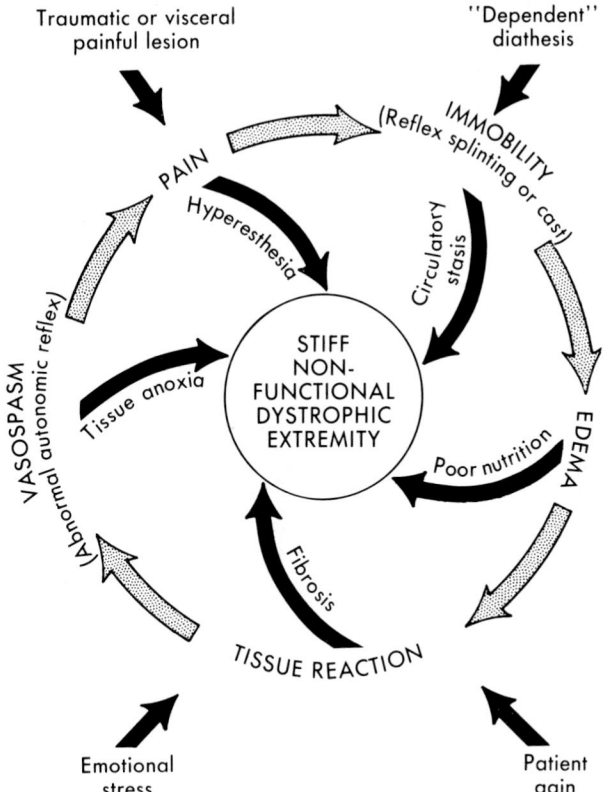

Fig. 59-12 Vicious cycle is produced when tissue ischemia produces greater tissue reaction and pain caused by vasoconstrictive action of increased sympathetic nerve activity, resulting in a painful, stiff, swollen, and dystrophic extremity, as seen in reflex sympathetic dystrophy. (From Lankford LL and Thompson JE: Reflex sympathetic dystrophy, upper and lower extremity: diagnosis and management. In American Academy of Orthopaedic Surgeons: Instructional course lectures, vol 26, St Louis, 1977, The CV Mosby Co.)

substance he called "neurokinin" by electrically stimulating the distal end of a divided nerve. He found that this substance was the mediator of neurogenic vasodilation of skin. This certainly could explain why in RSD we have some areas of vasoconstriction and at the same time in adjacent areas we have vasodilation. When neurokinin was injected subcutaneously, it produced a "flare" reaction, which lowered the pain threshold in the injected area. This might well help to explain the intense dysesthesia noted in patients with RSD when stimulated with light touch. Further evidence of the presence of the abnormal sympathetic reflex is given by Walker[90] and Procacci.[77]

It is generally agreed that afferent pain impulse projection centrally is produced through the small-diameter, slow-conducting, nonmyelinated C fibers and the thinly myelinated A-delta fibers, whereas the heavily myelinated large-diameter A-alpha fibers are responsible for conducting light pressure and proprioceptive sense. Melzack and Wall[57] in 1965 helped to give us some understanding of how some people can perceive a great deal of pain with a minimal stimulus and others feel little or no pain. Their "gate-control" theory of pain proposed that the large-diameter (light touch pressure and proprioceptive sense) afferent fibers have the ability to "close the gate" on the slower conducting nonmyelinated C fibers, which conduct pain. This "modulation" of pain impulses takes place in the substantia gelatinosa of the dorsal horn in the spinal cord. They further propose that there is a central control of the gating mechanism that is activated in the higher centers of the central nervous system that can influence the forward projection of pain (Fig. 59-13). Although not all of the theories of this gating mechanism have been proved in the laboratory, it

goes a long way to help with our understanding of this complex problem. The central control mechanism that alters the forward projection of pain helps to explain how psychological and emotional factors can greatly influence the amount and quality of pain perceived by some patients. It also helps to explain how light touch and gentle exercise tend to eliminate pain in RSD and why painful stimuli will cause a self-sustaining aggravation of pain. Casey[11] in 1973 defined pain as "the private experience of unpleasantness and the interpretation of the stimulation in terms of present and past experience. Moreover, pain is profoundly modified by attention, emotions, and suggestion and by pathologic conditions of a central or peripheral nervous system that can increase or decrease the intensity."

TREATMENT

The old axiom that early diagnosis and early treatment produce the best result has never been more correct than in the case of RSD. Delay in starting the treatment because of the difficulty of diagnosis is certain to produce a greater residual in the form of pain, stiffness, and dysfunction. It is therefore important to rule out other forms of dystrophies that produce similar but not so severe symptoms so that the appropriate treatment for RSD may be given without delay.

It has already been stated that three etiologic factors (persistent painful lesion, diathesis, and abnormal sympathetic reflex) that must be present at the same time before RSD can occur. The treatment is therefore to remove one or more of these factors, and one would hope the vicious cycle can be broken. Although this may stop the forward progress of the disease, it cannot return the patient to normalcy. It would follow therefore that treatment should include attempts to

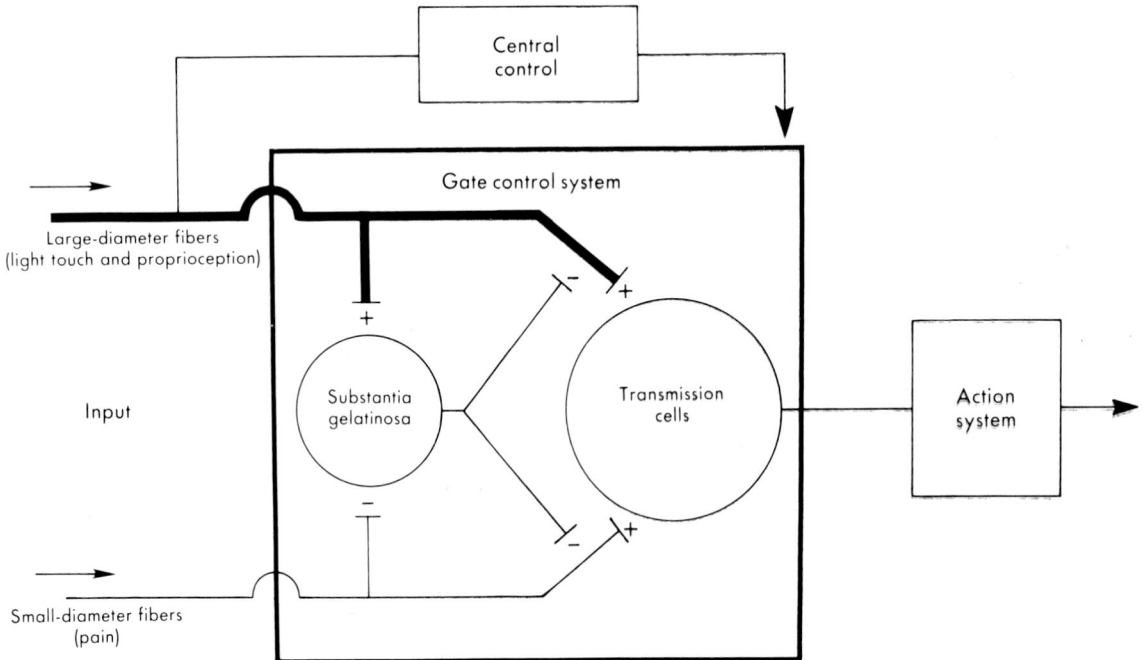

Fig. 59-13 Melzack and Wall's gate-control theory of pain. Melzack and Wall have theorized that large-diameter fibers of light touch and proprioceptive sense impulses can "close the gate" to slower-acting, small-diameter, non-myelinated nerve fibers of pain. On the other hand, absence of large-diameter fiber stimulation will "open the gate" for pain impulses to be projected centrally so that a minimal pain impulse is interpreted as severe pain by the cerebral cortex. (From Melzack R and Wall PD: Science 150:971, 1965.)

eliminate the initiating painful state, modify the patient's diathesis if possible, and interrupt the abnormal sympathetic reflex.

Of these three approaches to the treatment, the elimination of the abnormal sympathetic reflex is usually the easiest to perform and by all odds the most direct and successful approach. Depending on the severity and the duration of RSD, this may be accomplished with the use of one or more of the following regimens: use of sympatholytic drugs, local anesthetic blocks on somatic nerves or trigger points, pharmacologic or chemical blocks of the stellate ganglion and the upper thoracic chain, or use of an upper thoracic sympathectomy.*

Sympatholytic drugs

Sympatholytic medications are alpha-adrenergic blocking agents, which effectively reduce the sympathetic vasoconstrictive action of the peripheral vessels in the involved extremity. This may, at the same time, produce orthostatic hypotension and should therefore be used with caution. Phenoxybenzamine (Dibenzyline)[17,21,24] seems to be the most effective alpha-adrenergic blocking agent, with the only really significant complication being orthostatic hypotension with excessive dosing. A 10-mg capsule is given orally twice a day as a starting dose. If there has been no adverse effect after 5 days, this can be increased to three times a day; and after another 5 days if RSD symptoms are not distinctly improved and no orthostatic hypotension has occurred, the patient may try four times a day. However, with the occurrence of any undesirable side effect, the medication should be either reduced or stopped. As with any medication, one should not operate a machine or drive a car until he has had time to determine whether the medication would disturb him in this activity. When a patient is believed either to have the diathesis for RSD or if he has an obvious vasospastic tendency, phenoxybenzamine may be used prophylactically to help reduce the sympathetic nerve activity and possibly prevent the occurrence of RSD.

Phentolamine (Regitine) and tolazoline (Priscoline) are also alpha-adrenergic blocking agents, but they have definite disadvantages over Dibenzyline. Propranolol (Inderal) has not been found effective in my experience, and it also has some undesirable side effects.

Reserpine is also used for sympathetic blockage because of the catecholamine (norepinephrine)–depleting action at the neurotransmitter junction on the vessel wall. Reserpine may be given by intraarterial injection[76] and regionally by intravenous injection[83] but requires considerable expertise for its use. Oral reserpine (Serpasil) has also been used for the treatment of RSD, but it certainly has limited application because the effective dosage may also bring on undesirable side effects.

Calcium channel blockers

Although the most appropriate treatment for reflex sympathetic dystrophy is the blockade of the sympathetic nervous system, vasodilation of the arterioles by other means also is of some benefit in the treatment of this enigmatic condition. A new class of arteriole vasodilators has been introduced in recent years; these vasodilators are called calcium channel blockers because they inhibit the movement of calcium ions into cells with the resultant inhibition of excitation-contraction coupling and therefore act as a calcium antagonistic agent. One of the more effective calcium blockers is nifedipine (Procardia), which is known as a slow channel blocker. Prough[78] in 1955 reported that he found nifedipine effective in the treatment of RSD in 9 of 13 cases. The FDA has approved the use of nifedipine for treatment of coronary artery vasodilation.

Somatic nerve blocks

A pharmacologic somatic nerve block with a local anesthetic agent does produce an interruption of the abnormal sympathetic reflex inasmuch as the somatic nerves do carry the sympathetic nerve fibers and a blockade at this point would, of course, prevent the increased sympathetic stimulation from reaching the involved area. It is also of benefit because it does, in addition, knock out any afferent nerve impulses of pain that would otherwise help fuel the vicious cycle. Somatic nerve blocks are more commonly used for the minor types of RSD such as minor causalgia and minor traumatic dystrophy. One may accomplish this by giving a median, ulnar, or radial nerve block at the wrist, or even in some cases a metacarpal block in the hand. Ordinarily lidocaine (Xylocaine) or mepivacaine (Carbocaine) is the pharmacologic agent used for the first somatic nerve blocks so that its benefits can be definitely established, and then any future blocks are usually given with bupivacaine (Marcaine). All ordinary precautions are observed, of course, with the use of any local anesthestic agent, and the patients should be made aware that since their digits are anesthetic they must take precautions to avoid injury. Axillary blocks may also be given, as well as median, ulnar, and radial nerve blocks at the wrist. These are less desirable, however, because they leave a greater area anesthetic and temporarily paralyzed. The effective length of time of the sympathetic blockade increases, however, the more proximally the block is performed. The more distal blocks are accepted better by patients than are the more proximal blocks, and they can be given two and three times a week without causing local irritation.

Periodic perineural infusion

Omer and Thomas[66,67] described a method of implanting a small flexible catheter into the site of a trigger point by inserting a large-bore hypodermic needle under local anesthesia into the involved area and periodically infusing it with a small amount of local anesthesia. This method can be quite effective if the trigger point is easily delineated. The same technique can also be used to infuse larger nerves in the forearm, such as the median, ulnar, and radial ones. The exact details of this technique can be found in an anesthesia textbook.

Stellate ganglion blocks

Certainly the most effective treatment for RSD is the interruption of the abnormal sympathetic reflex, and the most effective way to accomplish this is through blockade of all the sympathetic efferent impulses into the extremity by a stellate ganglion block. Although this prevents any sympathetic nerve activity in the extremity, it does not block

---

*References 4, 9, 37, 53, 81, 92.

out any somatic nerve and will therefore not produce a temporary anesthesia or paralysis (unless there is unusual spreading of the anesthetic agent). If a technically satisfactory block has been accomplished, there will be a generalized warming, drying, and return to a more normal coloration of the skin of the entire upper extremity. When the upper two thirds of the stellate ganglion has been adequately perfused with the local anesthetic agent, Horner's sign with drooping of the eyelid, enophthalmos, hyperemia of the conjunctival vessels, constriction of the pupil, and drying and warming of the ipsilateral side of the face will occur. If only the upper thoracic sympathetic ganglia have been blocked, it is possible for the extremity to have been effectively sympathectomized without the presence of Horner's sign, which is usually the hallmark of a successful stellate ganglion block. With the accomplishment of a successful blockade of the sympathetic impulses, the patients are generally amazed at the immediate change in the condition of their hands. There is usually a very prompt and distinct improvement of pain and a generalized feeling of well-being. In our Hand Rehabilitation Unit, for the last several years we have obtained measurements of joint motion, volume, and grip strength of the extremities before and after stellate ganglion blocks, and it has been demonstrated that improvement in all three categories is generally evidenced. Even though there may still be some pain on strenuous joint motion, almost always the burning or constant pain has been relieved after the block. It is only after satisfactory sympathetic blockade that an effective exercise program is beneficial to the patient. Before the block, the pain is usually so great that the patient cannot participate in a vigorous exercise program. It is not wise to subject the patient to strenuous passive exercise before the sympathetic blockade because it is usually very painful and this increased pain simply accelerates the "pain–sympathetic reflex" cycle, and the condition is actually made worse rather than better. The sympathetic block is not only therapeutic but also acts to confirm the diagnosis of RSD. If, on the other hand, the block has been technically unsatisfactory (as evidenced by the absence of drying and warming of the extremity and Horner's sign), or has failed to produce subjective or objective improvement, one cannot on the basis of one block rule out the diagnosis of RSD. In my experience, one patient had four technically successful blocks without any subjective improvement but on the fifth and subsequent blocks showed dramatic improvement.

Generally, not more than one or two blocks are given each week unless the patient is in very severe distress. Only rarely can this condition be completely reversed after only one block. The average number of blocks necessary for the reversal of this abnormal sympathetic reflex is between four and five stellate ganglion blocks. On one occasion it was necessary to use 16 blocks before the forward progress of the disease was reversed. The number of blocks necessary for benefit certainly depends on the duration and the severity of the condition. When blocks alone are used, there is usually a fairly good chance of producing the desired benefit to the patient if sympathetic blockade is started within the first 3 to 4 months. Much later on, however, it is less likely that the sole use of stellate ganglion blocks will be sufficient, and a surgical sympathectomy would need to be considered.

Stellate ganglion block technique. The stellate ganglion block should not be performed by anyone who is not thoroughly familiar with the anatomy and the possible complications of the block. The stellate ganglion lies anterior to the seventh cervical lateral mass and may be located when one first palpates Chassaignac's tubercle, which lies at the level of the sixth cervical vertebral lateral mass. In essence, this is approximately 4 cm lateral to the midcervical line and 4 cm superior to the sternal notch. Before doing the stellate ganglion block, one must be prepared to treat any complication such as an intravascular injection of the anesthetic agent, a "time overdose" (a rapid absorption of an otherwise normal amount of the anesthetic agent), a drug idiosyncrasy reaction, or an anaphylactic shock reaction. Oxygen also should be available in case a pneumothorax has been inadvertently produced. Details of the treatment of a complication of a stellate ganglion block will not be given at this point, but one must understand that a means of giving oxygen and intravenous medication to stabilize the blood pressure should be available.

Moore[43] fully describes the anterior paratracheal approach, which I favor, and for a detailed discussion of this approach I recommend that one use this reference. It is preferred that the first block be done with a short-acting local anesthetic agent with 1:200,000 epinephrine concentration. The short-acting anesthetic agent may be either 1% lidocaine (Xylocaine) or 1% mepivacaine (Carbocaine) for the initial block, and subsequent blocks may be accomplished with 0.5% bupivacaine (Marcaine). The patient should be positioned in a 45-degree semi-Fowler's position with the head not using a pillow and turned 45 degrees to the contralateral side. Chassaignac's tubercle is located by deep palpation while the nondominant index and long fingers are retracting the sternocleidomastoid muscle and the great vessels in the carotid sheath laterally (Fig. 59-14). After sterile preparation and with sterile technique being used throughout, a small wheel of local anesthesia is given with a short 25-gauge needle on a 10 ml Luer-Lok syringe. The point of injection is about 1½ cm inferior to Chassaignac's tubercle, which would make it immediately over the seventh cervical lateral mass. The 25-gauge ¾-inch (2 cm) needle is directed straight posteriorly without angulation and should touch the seventh cervical lateral mass. After this bony landmark has been touched with the needle, one should then withdraw the needle 0.5 to 0.8 cm to clear the prevertebral fascia and muscles and after adequate aspiration (to check for intravascular penetration) inject a test dose of 2 ml (Fig. 59-15). An observation period of 1 minute should be allowed, and if no adverse effects such as ringing in the ear, dizziness, nausea, or cardiac palpitations are detected, 3 ml of the local anesthetic is slowly injected without displacement of the needle. Another period of observation of 1 minute should be allowed, and if no uncomfortable sensations have occurred, the remaining 5 ml of the local anesthetic agent should be injected slowly. A similar technique is employed when bupivacaine is used. In most cases, 10 ml of the anesthetic agent is adequate to get a technically satisfactory block. The first signs of improvement may be apparent within 5 minutes of removal of the needle, but it is not unusual for benefit not to occur for 30 to 45 minutes. Bilateral blocks should not be attempted at the same time for fear of pneumothorax or a bilateral paralysis of the recurrent laryngeal nerve. The patient should remain in the

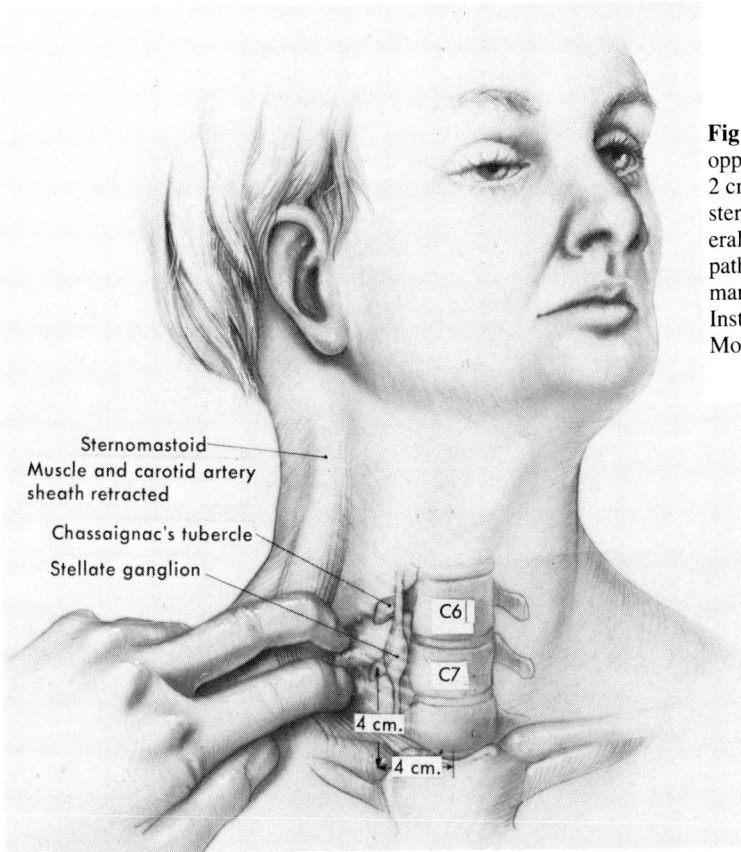

Fig. 59-14   Stellate ganglion of sympathetic chain is located opposite seventh cervical vertebra, which is palpated less than 2 cm inferior to Chassaignac's tubercle and can be found when sternocleidomastoid muscle and great vessels are retracted laterally. (From Lankford LL and Thompson JE: Reflex sympathetic dystrophy, upper and lower extremity: diagnosis and management. In American Academy of Orthopaedic Surgeons: Instructional course lectures, vol 26, St Louis, 1977, The CV Mosby Co.)

Sternomastoid
Muscle and carotid artery
sheath retracted

Chassaignac's tubercle

Stellate ganglion

C6

C7

4 cm.

4 cm.

Fig. 59-15   Anterior paratracheal approach to stellate ganglion is made by inserting needle straight down to seventh cervical lateral mass and then withdrawing it about 0.5 to 0.8 cm to clear prevertebral fascia and muscles. (From Lankford LL: Reflex sympathetic dystrophy. In Evarts C McC, editor: Surgery of the musculoskeletal system, New York, 1983, Churchill Livingstone, Inc.)

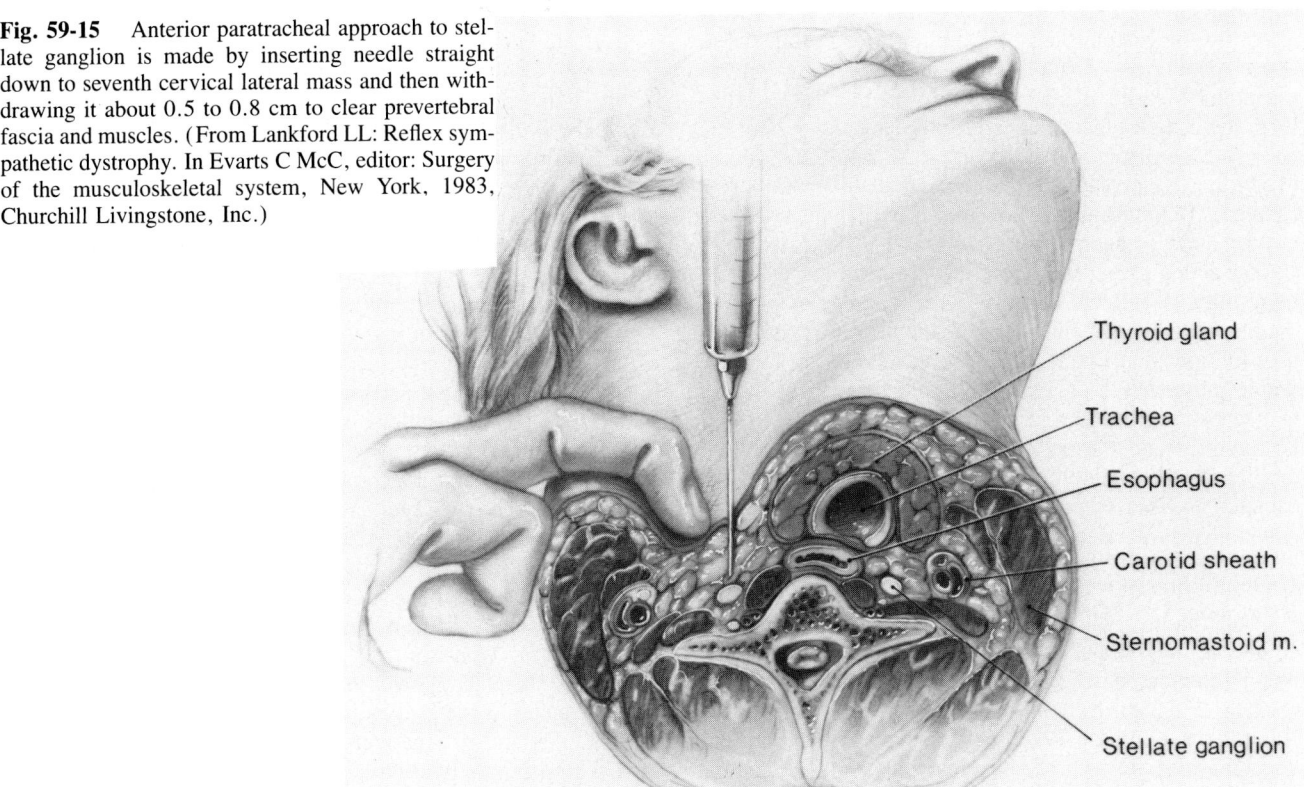

Thyroid gland

Trachea

Esophagus

Carotid sheath

Sternomastoid m.

Stellate ganglion

semi-Fowler's position for at least 30 minutes after completion of the block. Although the normal physiologic interruption of the function of nerve fibers using lidocaine (Xylocaine) and mepivacaine (Carbocaine) is approximately 1½ to 2½ hours and the length of action of bupivacaine (Marcaine) may last from 9 to 18 hours, the benefit as far as the interruption of the abnormal sympathetic reflex is concerned may well last from 1 to 3 days before the sympathetic nerve hyperactivity has regenerated itself to the point that the abnormal sympathetic reflex has again been produced. Because of irritation of the tissues surrounding the stellate ganglion, it is seldom advisable to give more than two blocks per week. If a successful block has been produced, the patient should then be sent to the hand therapy department for physical treatment.

Continuous stellate blockade

Betcher, Bean, and Casten[6] in 1953 described a technique for continuous blocking of the stellate ganglion when it is necessary to produce a longer period of blockade of the sympathetic efferent impulses. Although continuous stellate blockade is not ordinarily advised, it may well be necessary if the patient is having a great deal of pain or is too apprehensive to tolerate interrupted stellate ganglion blocks. A 16-gauge needle is inserted down to the stellate ganglion under local anesthesia and with image intensification roentgenographic control. After the needle has been introduced down to the seventh cervical lateral mass, it is again withdrawn a little over 0.5 cm and a flexible polyvinyl venicatheter is inserted into the 16-gauge needle and the large-bore needle is then withdrawn. The catheter is taped into place and the exact position of the tip of the catheter can be determined by a very small injection of absorbable radiopaque solution. A female Luer-Lok adapter is then attached to the catheter and periodic injections of any of the above-mentioned anesthetic agents are given. In between injections a sterile adapter is used to maintain the sterility. With the catheter taped securely into place the patient may become ambulatory but is requested to minimize motions of the neck and shoulder to prevent dislodgment of the catheter. If bupivacaine (Marcaine) is used, injections need not be more frequent than 18- to 24-hour intervals. The shorter-acting anesthetic agents would need to be injected more often. While the patient is experiencing the benefit of the blockade of the abnormal sympathetic reflex, he should take full advantage of it to perform his exercises and functional activities. If the patient should develop distressing hoarseness or difficulty in swallowing, the catheter should be removed and the patient not allowed to take anything orally until the swallowing function has been regained. The catheter may be left in place for 2 weeks or until there is any evidence of infection around the catheter.

Guanethidine blocks

Guanethidine, which prevents the storage of catecholamines in the sympathetic nerve terminals at the neuroeffector junction, has been used extensively in Europe and Canada as an intravenous regional sympathetic blockade. Hannington-Kiff[32] in 1977 suggested the use of regional guanethidine intravenous sympathetic blockade for the treatment of Sudeck's atrophy. He reported that 17 consecutive cases of Sudeck's atrophy were treated with intravenous

regional guanethidine blocks with "relief" in all patients. He reports that guanethidine displaces noradrenaline stores in the sympathetic nerve endings and its persistent accumulation at these sites prevents the usual re-uptake of noradrenaline, resulting in the depletion of this neuroeffector agent and the production of a very effective sympathetic blockade. A refinement of his technique is described in a subsequent report by Hannington-Kiff[33] in 1984, which is a modification of the Bier block technique. He warns that there is an initial aggravation of the burning pain because of the release of catecholamines by the blocking agent. However, after a short time, there has been an effective sympathetic blockade because of the replacement of catecholamines by guanethidine in the receptor sites. The duration of the block is approximately 5 to 8 days. The effectiveness of the blocks has been essentially comparable to that of a stellate ganglion block as reported by Glynn,[28] Bonelli,[8] and Eriksen.[22]

Reserpine blocks

Regional intravenous sympathetic blockade using reserpine has been reported to be effective in the treatment of Raynaud's phenomenon as reported by Gorsky.[29] The mechanism of action of the sympathetic blockade by replacing the stores of catecholamines in the nerve endings by reserpine is similar in action to guanethidine. Benzon[56] and Chuinard[14] have reported good results in the treatment of RSD with use of intravenous sympathetic blockade using reserpine. McKain[55] found that when comparing regional intravenous blockades of guanethidine and reserpine and using the cold challenge test as the criteria for effectiveness, reserpine was not as effective as guanethidine.

Sympathectomy

If stellate ganglion blocks have not been started early enough in the course of RSD, it may not be possible to break up adequately the abnormal sympathetic reflex with blocks alone. This is especially true in the very severe cases of major traumatic dystrophy and causalgia. If definite benefit has accrued from at least one to three blocks and yet the duration of benefit is not long enough or the relief of pain is less than complete, and especially if the duration of this disease has been at least 4 to 5 months, in all likelihood a surgical sympathectomy will be required to give the patient the desired relief. In many cases, one can reach a decision to do surgery after the second block, but at other times one may need to use four to six blocks before determining whether the intermittent blockade will be sufficient or a surgical sympathectomy will be necessary. If one believes that surgical relief of a carpal tunnel syndrome or some type of reconstructive surgery will be required, I regard that as an indication for sympathectomy. The first four thoracic sympathetic ganglia should be removed for complete ablation of the abnormal sympathetic reflex. If only the upper thoracic ganglia are removed, Horner's syndrome is seldom seen. Some techniques include removal of the lower third of the stellate ganglion with relatively little risk of producing permanent Horner's syndrome. One should expect, however, that the patient with RSD has a diathesis that may make him more likely to complain of pain around the sympathectomy operative site. Fortunately, this post-surgical neuritis seldom lasts more than a few weeks.

After a successful sympathectomy, the greatest benefit to the patient has been the reversal of the process that has given him so much torment. There is usually a dramatic relief of pain, especially of burning or constant pain, though some pain on joint motion may continue, at least for a while. Concomitantly there is a decrease in swelling, improvement in the coloration, and some slow improvement in motion and function. At least after the elimination of the abnormal sympathetic reflex, it is then possible for the patient to do the exercises necessary to improve motion and function (which he was unable to do satisfactorily while he was in the grips of this consuming pain). McGrath[54] in 1974 reported that blood flow in the hands of a sympathectomized patient was increased from sixfold to tenfold over the preoperative state.

On rare occasions when a sympathectomy is needed but the patient for some reason is unable to undergo a surgical operation, a chemical sympathectomy may be indicated wherein the stellate ganglion block is performed with either 50% alcohol or 6% phenol to produce a semipermanent sympathectomy.[9] This, of course, is a somewhat dangerous procedure and should be done only by a person with great expertise in the use of alcohol and phenol for nerve blocks.

Leriche[46] first alluded to the possible connection of an abnormal sympathetic nervous system and Mitchell's causalgia. In 1916 he did a postganglionic sympathectomy of the brachial artery by stripping the adventitia away from the artery. This did provide some relief but only temporarily. Spurling,[84] however, in 1928 did the first successful upper thoracic sympathectomy by removing a portion of the upper thoracic chain. Kwan[41] in 1931 also successfully treated RSD with an upper thoracic chain sympathectomy. The surgical technique for upper thoracic sympathectomy should, of course, be done by someone with special training and will not be discussed in detail in this volume. There are, however, three general types of upper thoracic sympathectomy that are being currently used: (1) the posterior approach, which was first described by Adson[1] and was later modified by Smithwick[82] in 1940; (2) the transthoracic approaches through the axilla suggested by Adkins[3] and Palumbo;[71] and (3) more recently the thoracic endoscopic sympathectomy as described by Kux[40] in 1978. The supraclavicular anterior cervical approach is seldom used at this time unless the posterior or transthoracic approaches are contraindicated by a scar.

Wilkinson[94] in 1984 described a new method of doing upper thoracic sympathectomies using a radiofrequency percutaneous upper thoracic probe from the posterior aspect to interrupt the sympathetic chain and destroy the ganglia.

ADJUNCTIVE TREATMENT

Certainly, the most important treatment for RSD is the interruption of the abnormal sympathetic reflex arc,[92] and this should be done as soon as possible by one of the above-mentioned methods, whether it be a sympathetic nerve block or a surgical sympathectomy. There are, however, other forms of treatment that are helpful and are based on the three etiologic factors. I should emphasize that these methods of treatment should not be used to the exclusion of the blockade of the sympathetic reflex arc.

Treatment of a painful lesion

Since the persistently painful lesion that initiated the RSD continues to fuel this vicious cycle, it may well be of some help to try to eliminate the pain. This is expected to decelerate the vicious cycle. One should do no surgery, however, without making sure that the capability of eliminating the abnormal reflex arc exists. It goes without saying that tight casts or casts with pressure points on bony prominences should be promptly rectified. If there has been painful pressure over a nerve, the cast can be windowed and local injections of an anesthetic agent used on this trigger point. A painful amputation stump may require revision so that there is provision of a loose flap coverage or dissection of a neuroma. I would not, however, advise significant shortening of a ray with the mistaken impression that the neuroma can be eliminated by further amputation. It is especially recommended that a ray amputation not be done for treatment of a painful neuroma. The neuroma should be treated with repeated local blocks of an anesthetic agent. If a "neurodesis" (binding down of a nerve distal to a joint) appears to be causing considerable pain, this may be completely resected proximally in the case of a dorsal superficial sensory branch of the radial or ulnar nerve or of the palmar branch of the median nerve. If the nerve in question is a digital nerve, a nerve graft can be done with no tension on the graft so that this will eliminate excessive fibrosis at the suture site.

Elimination of swelling should be one of our first goals, since it is well known that swelling causes pain and ischemia. Both of these conditions will aggravate the vicious cycle. Patients should be given specific instructions on how to elevate the hand at all times so that the hand is the highest part of the body. If a traumatic carpal tunnel syndrome has occurred secondary to the swelling, this may well need to be treated by elimination of a severely flexed position of the wrist. In many cases, it can be helped by the injection of a long-acting steroid around the flexor tendons going through the carpal tunnel (but not near the ulnar or median nerves). A surgical release of the carpal tunnel may occasionally be necessary but should not be done except under the protection of stellate ganglion blocks.

Transcutaneous nerve stimulation,[91] if used early in the course of the disease, may well help to reduce pain. The electrical stimulation is directed toward the large-diameter myelinated afferent nerve fibers of light touch and proprioceptive sensation. I believe that this constant stimulation of these large-diameter fibers will "close the gate" on the small nonmyelinated slow-conducting C fibers of pain (Fig. 59-13). This is usually accomplished with a small battery-operated stimulator that is connected to the patient with electrodes and can be worn for many hours at a time.[48,58,64] During these periods of reduced pain, it may well be possible for the patient to do his hand exercises or participate in functional activities without aggravating his condition. Unless the transcutaneous electrical stimulator is used very early in the course of RSD, it has little chance of diminishing the pain to a significant degree.

Acupuncture

Acupuncture has been used in the Orient for thousands of years for the relief of pain. Since RSD is an extremely painful condition, it follows that acupuncture would be used for treatment of this enigmatic condition. Chan[12] has reported the use of acupuncture for the treatment of posttraumatic sympathetic dystrophy (Sudeck's atrophy). His findings were reported as showing a 70% marked and permanent improvement in the patient's condition. It is not known exactly how acupuncture works, but Panerai[72] feels that acupuncture stimulates the production of the endogenous opiate beta-endorphin. Lee[45] has shown that acupuncture produces a sympatholytic effect and uses thermography to demonstrate this. This may well be another mechanism of using Melzack and Wall's gate control theory of pain.

Systemic steroids

It is not surprising that steroids would eventually be suggested for use in treating RSD because they are well-known treatments for pain, swelling, stiffness, and dysfunction. Steroids have been suggested by Glick,[27] Rosen,[79] and Steinbrocker[86] for treatment of RSD.

Steroids of a sufficiently high dosage do provide a sense of well-being to the patient and relieve pain to some degree if for no other reason than by reduction of the swelling. Also, it is quite likely that steroids over a long enough period of time may diminish the intense fibrotic reaction that occurs with RSD. It is therefore true that steroids are of some benefit to patients with RSD, but they are not capable of interrupting the abnormal sympathetic reflex, which is the dominant factor in pathogenicity of RSD.

If one uses steroids, he must recognize their limited application, and they should not be used to the exclusion of blockade of the sympathetic nervous system. The use of steroids is certainly not without some risk of producing steroidism, activating gastric ulcers, and producing hypertension and severe osteoporosis. Steroids, however, can be useful for the treatment of the "flare reactions" commonly seen after injury or surgery in patients who have Dupuytren's contracture, hypertrophic or psoriatic arthritis, long-standing diabetes, or other collagen diseases such as primary carpal tunnel syndrome. It is probably because of the benefit to this group (not to be confused with RSD) that some workers[27] have reported good results with the use of steroids for the treatment of RSD. It is much more expedient and effective to produce sympathetic-activity blockade rather than to expose the patient to the complications of high doses of steroids.

We have found that when we wish to treat the increased fibrosis and stiffness seen in RSD and when the use of steroids is contraindicated, we have realized a benefit in the RSD patient by substituting nonsteroidal anti-inflammatory drugs such as indomethacin and naproxen for the inhibition of prostaglandin synthesis and diphenhydramine (Benadryl) as an antihistamine drug.

Calcitonin

In recent years it has been reported that calcitonin, which is a 32-amino acid hormone of the thyroid gland, is beneficial in the treatment of RSD.[2,51] Calcitonin has been used to treat Paget's disease, and because of its ability to produce increased bone formation and reduced osteoclasis, it has been used in the treatment of RSD. It is not felt that calcitonin will reduce the increased sympathetic nerve activity significantly and therefore will not be very useful in the treatment of RSD. McKay[56] found that salmon calcitonin produced reduction in bone absorption, but he did not feel that there would be much symptomatic relief in RSD with the treatment of calcitonin.

Treatment of the diathesis

Since the diathesis for RSD is an inherent trait of the patient, there is little possibility of changing this in any way that will help to break up the vicious cycle present in RSD. Mood-modifying drugs have been suggested for the treatment of RSD[38] such as diazepam (Valium), trifluoperazine (Stelazine), chlorpromazine hydrochloride (Thorazine), chlordiazepoxide hydrochloride (Librium), amitriptyline hydrochloride (Elavil), and fluphenazine dihydrochloride (Prolixin). Although I do not believe that the diathesis can be significantly changed with the use of these drugs, it might well enable a patient to tolerate his condition a little better and make him more receptive to the real treatment of RSD, which is the interruption of the reflex sympathetic arc. Pak[70] has suggested that consultation with a psychiatrist is indicated because he believed that a large number of patients had a psychiatric problem. In general, I have not found that psychiatric consultation offers the patient a great deal more than simply enabling him to understand his condition and become more cooperative in the treatment.

HAND THERAPY

An overzealous therapist who gives passive manipulation of the hand to the point of pain without the patient's abnormal sympathetic reflex having been blockaded or eliminated is very likely to cause a worsening of the patient's condition rather than an improvement of it. The old saying that "pain is gain" is certainly not true in RSD (Fig. 59-16). The patient with RSD is hypersensitive to pain and any painful manipulation will promptly accelerate the vicious cycle and will cause the already painful, swollen, and stiff joint to become even more reactive. It is first necessary to blockade the efferent sympathetic impulses (the "protective umbrella") before it is possible to carry out a vigorous exercise program.

A well-meaning therapist may have the personal opinion that in his hands he can manipulate a joint and obtain increased motion without causing increased pain, swelling, or stiffness by aggravating the reactive process in the joint. Unfortunately, this is not possible in a patient with RSD until his abnormal sympathetic reflex arc has first been eliminated. This does not mean that the patient should not take active exercises, but he should, of course, be warned that in RSD it is possible for active exercises to be done so vigorously that they become painful, thereby worsening the condition.

The basis of any exercise program should be gentle active exercises without coming to the point of pain. It is much better to exercise the hand frequently and for short periods rather than a few longer periods of more strenuous exercises. I believe that more improvement in motion is accomplished by 3 minutes of gentle active exercises every 30 minutes (while awake) than a longer exercise period three or four times a day. It is not until after the sympathetic blockade has decelerated the vicious cycle that it is safe for the patient to be taught gentle passive exercises. The therapist should not do the manipulating himself because he has no way of knowing to what point he can passively manipulate the joint

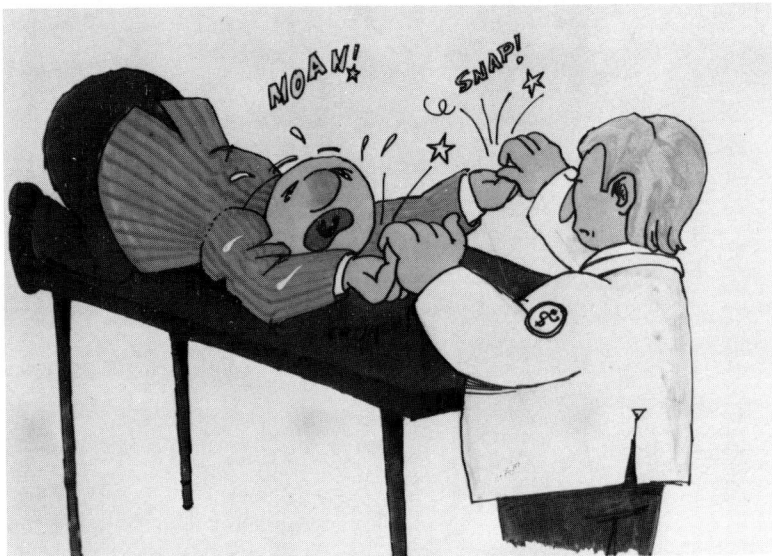

Fig. 59-16   Painful manipulations should be strictly avoided with treatment of reflex sympathetic dystrophy, because these patients are hypersensitive to pain and any painful manipulation will aggravate a "vicious cycle."

just short of pain. The hand therapist should be a teacher and a cheerleader but not a manipulator and should encourage the patient to do the exercises himself without causing pain, so that motion will improve rather than produce greater reaction in the tissues from overzealous stretching.

Exercises

We have learned from the gate-control theory of pain[57] that fast-transmitting, large-diameter, myelinated, afferent nerve fibers that are stimulated by light touch, pressure, and proprioceptive sensation (sensations of joint movement) will "close the gate" to the slower-acting nonmyelinated small-diameter C fibers of pain (see Fig. 59-13). Therefore if we use gentle active exercise and light massage frequently, we should be able to modulate or dampen the slower-acting pain fibers so that the T cells in the substantia gelatinosa will not project the sensation of pain to the higher centers. In other words, we should make the normal-sensation impulses flood the sensorium and "outshout" the pain so that the "good guys" will now become the "vocal majority." If the painful stiff hand of the patient with RSD is not touched or is not moved, the normal sensation will not be heard from, and it will only take a few pain fibers to convey the message of severe pain to the higher centers. It is therefore very important for the patient with RSD to take exercises and massage very frequently (to outshout the pain) but still be careful not to produce pain in so doing, thus preventing these few pain fibers from having a greater and more deleterious effect on the sensorium.

A program called the "three flexion and extension exercises" has been developed by our hand therapy unit, which simply applies the principles of the Bunnell block in the flexion exercises without the use of the block itself by the patient. The first exercise is in flexion; all three joints of all fingers are very gently flexed passively as far as possible without coming to the point of pain, and then an active assist in flexion is provided (while the fingers are still held passively in flexion). This exercise is sustained for 10 seconds, with the use of as much power as possible, just short of pain. Next, the fingers are extended as far as possible without pain, for 10 seconds. In the second exercise, the patient holds each individual finger (or in some cases all four fingers at the same time) with his uninvolved hand so that the MP joint is held in as much extension as possible (without pain). While the MP joint is therefore blocked in extension, the patient makes an active effort to flex the fingers as far as possible just short of pain. This flexion exercise is sustained for 10 seconds, followed by 10 seconds of extension. The third exercise is done the same way, except that this time the patient blocks not only the MP joints but also the proximal interphalangeal (PIP) joints in as much extension as possible without pain and then uses as much active power to flex the distal interphalangeal joint as he can just short of pain (Fig. 59-17). This is also sustained for 10 seconds and again followed by 10 seconds of sustained-effort extension. The "three flexion and extension exercises" are then followed by 10 seconds of light massage of the digits, hand, and wrist. This entire procedure is continued until it has been done for 3 minutes, and the exercise period should be repeated once every 30 minutes. This, of course, requires a great deal of the patient's time, but it must be done frequently to become effective. The patient therefore must become his own primary therapist, because the exercises needed could not be supplied by the hand therapist in the therapy department more often than twice daily. Similar 10-second sustained effort exercises are done for the wrist in all planes of motion (extension, flexion, radial and ulnar deviation, and supination and pronation). If shoulder and elbow joints have also stiffened, they too are exercised.

At first the patient should have a volume measurement of the hand taken before and after the exercise periods, to make sure the exercises are not done too vigorously. Later on, the need for frequent volume measurement is not so

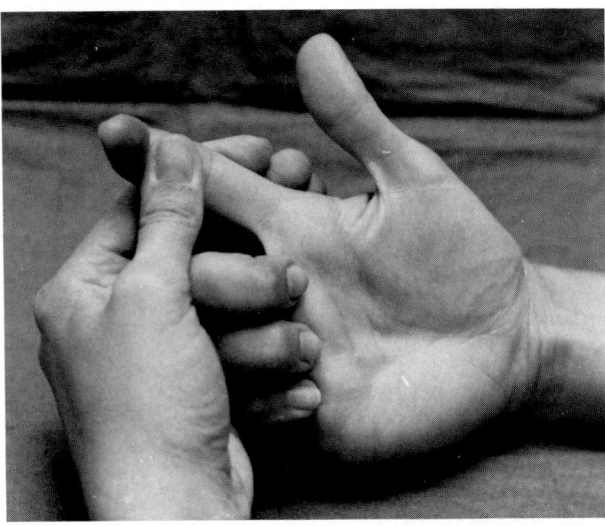

Fig. 59-17 Flexion exercises should be done gently but with 10-second sustained effort and maximum power just short of pain. Note that the proximal two joints are being held in extension so that all of the tendon excursion will be used to flex the distal interphalangeal joint.

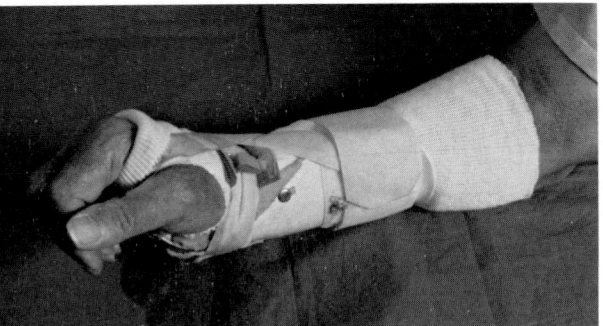

Fig. 59-18 Every effort should be made to obtain wrist extension, because this is the keystone of hand mobilization. Thermoplastic volar wrist splint should be used so that it can be reheated periodically to obtain increased extension of the wrist.

great. With each visit to the therapy department, accurate measurements of active flexion and extension movements of the joints are made and recorded so that the hand therapist can closely monitor the patient's progress or lack of progress. If necessary, the exercise program may then be modified. When the patient is able to show some improvement without any flare-ups in the part involved, his exercise period is then increased to 5 minutes out of each 30 minutes while he is awake.

Heat

In many cases, gentle heat can be used effectively to reduce muscle spasm and to allow the patient to do his exercises with less pain and a greater gain of motion. Heat is helpful, however, only if it is used with elevation. Heat with the extremity in dependence should not be used because this will cause stagnation in the lymphatic and venous system, which will result in greater swelling. This would then eliminate the use of the whirlpool bath in the treatment of RSD for fear of causing increased swelling and reaction. Hot, wet towels, the paraffin bath, and a heating pad all can be used with elevation, however, and can easily be applied at home by the patient after sufficient instructions have been given by the therapist. Swelling can also be reduced with the use of the thermoelastic glove, which will provide warmth and a gentle compression to help control swelling and reduce pain. Patients should be warned that they should avoid cold temperatures because this will increase vasoconstriction; they should always wear warm gloves when going outside in cold weather. Since it has also been shown that smoking of tobacco produces tissue ischemia by increasing vasoconstriction,[15] they should be advised to stop smoking so that at least this factor can be removed from the many causes of tissue ischemia in the patient with RSD.

Transcutaneous nerve stimulation

As already pointed out above, some benefit may well occur from the use of transcutaneous nerve stimulation over the trigger points, and instructions for this are given to the patient by the hand therapist. The patient should wear the stimulation unit while he is doing his exercises and functional activities. It is frequently necessary for the therapist to change the position of the electrodes so that the patient can obtain maximum benefit.[91]

Splinting

The purpose of splinting at first is to rest the hand, to relieve pain on motion, and to relieve muscle spasm. The splints should be light and should be made of a thermoplastic material so that they can be frequently reheated and changed in position. The ultimate goal is to return the position of the hand to the "resting-hand" or "balanced-hand" position, which is approximately 45 degrees of wrist extension, slight ulnar deviation of the wrist, 70 degrees of flexion in the MP joint and 30 degrees of flexion in the PIP joint. The reason we call this the resting-hand or balanced-hand position is that it is the result of all the forces exerted by the extrinsic muscle pull, the intrinsic muscle forces, and the static forces. This position would then be in a balanced state or a resting state. This is the position where fewer deforming forces are being exerted on the joints. Also, fewer pathologic forces are present when the hand is in this position.

The wrist is the "keystone" of the positioning of the hand, and one cannot expect to reduce the extension contractures of the MP joints or the flexion contractures of the PIP joints without first getting the wrist into extension. To accomplish this, a volar thermoplastic splint with Velcro straps is customized for the patient with as much extension of the wrist as the patient can comfortably tolerate (Fig. 59-18).

As time goes on, the splint is periodically reheated and the wrist extension is increased. After reducing the wrist flexion contracture and getting the wrist up into at least mild extension, one can then become more vigorous in reducing extension contractures of the MP joints and flexion contractures of the PIP joints. This reduction is accomplished with a dorsal thermoplastic splint with an outrigger and rubber-band slings to produce a gentle extension force on the interphalangeal joints. It can be achieved, however, only

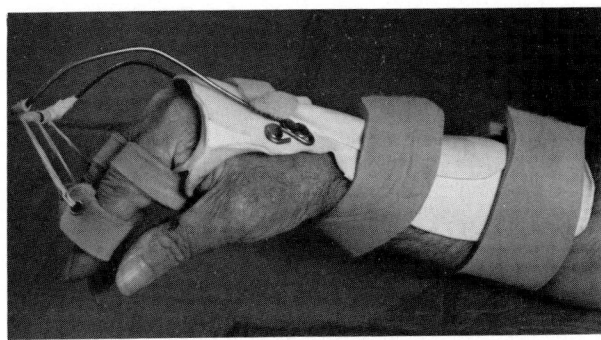

Fig. 59-19 Claw-hand deformities are splinted with a dorsal wrist splint and a dorsal outrigger and slings to produce extension in the proximal interphalangeal joints, but flexion slings must be used on the metacarpophalangeal joints to prevent hyperextension of these joints.

if an equal or greater force is exerted on flexing of the MP joints. This exertion is done by use of a lumbrical bar that presses down on the dorsum of the proximal segments of the fingers (to produce MP joint flexion) with the same or greater force than is used to extend the interphalangeal joints. This can also be accomplished by use of flexion rubber bands and slings affixed to a wristlet band so that a very respectable flexion force can be applied to the MP joints (Fig. 59-19).

These dynamic splints, of course, exert passive motion on the joint, and our rule about never allowing a passive force to become painful certainly applies to splinting. Pain produced by an ill-fitting splint or splint adjusted too tightly can be just as detrimental to the patient's stiff hand as a painful passive manipulation. The splints should be worn most of the time but should be removed every 30 minutes for the prescribed exercise program.

Functional activities

In many cases, the patient with RSD has a very poor self-image and is quite despondent over his wretched condition. Many patients have given up any hope of using their hands again and have, in fact, produced a psychological amputation of the part. It is therefore extremely important to teach the patient how to use his hand again and how to achieve useful function for himself. When the hand is very stiff, certainly there will be only a few types of functional activities in which the patient may participate.

In the beginning, activity may be as simple as placing wooden rings over round pegs or stacking blocks, but as better motion is accomplished and the patient has more confidence, the therapist will be able to teach him to do more sophisticated functional activities (Fig. 59-20). The therapist needs to be very observant so that he can pick up any new degree of motion or power developed by the patient, which can then be put to work doing a different and more advanced type of functional activity. The therapist should be one step ahead of the patient in setting goals for physical accomplishments. Each new accomplishment by the patient is acclaimed with pride and elation, and this spurs him on to even greater heights. The realization by the patient that he has actually made something and performed some useful function provides him with a great psychological boost. Eventually the hand therapist should have the patient doing functional activities that simulate the type of work he will be doing when he returns to his employment.

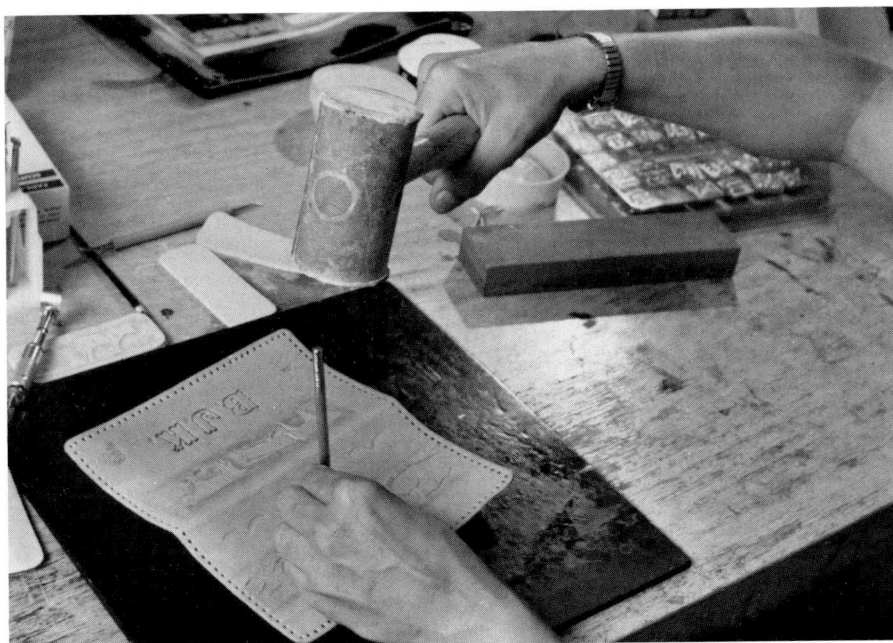

Fig. 59-20 After some motion and power are regained through exercising and splinting, functional activities should be begun to teach the patient how to use his hand again. Initially, functional activities are very simple, but they gradually become more sophisticated, requiring greater motion, power, and dexterity.

REHABILITATIVE SURGERY

It should be the goal of the hand surgeon and the hand therapist to return motion, strength, and function of the hand to as nearly normal a state as possible. In most instances, it is not realistic to expect that this can be completely accomplished with physical methods of exercise, massage, and splinting.

At some point in the recovery of the patient, evaluation must be made according to the needs of the patient about what degree of motion is required and to what extent a contracture can be acceptable for the required degree of function necessary for the patient's well-being. One should have a very limited expectation of regaining a considerable degree of motion after rehabilitative surgery, but at times it may be deemed necessary to gain even a few degrees of motion so that the patient is provided with his required extent of function. There are therefore some very restricted indications for rehabilitative surgery to regain motion in the patient with RSD though this in general should be discouraged.

One should do surgery of any kind only under the protection of either an upper thoracic sympathectomy or stellate ganglion block to eliminate the abnormal sympathetic reflex. Also, the surgery should be delayed until the patient's pain has disappeared or until the reactivity and the excessive fibrosis in the joints have diminished as much as possible and the tissues around the joints have returned to a state of homeostasis to the greatest degree possible. Rehabilitative surgery also should not be done so long as the patient shows progressive improvement with the exercise and splinting and functional activity regimens.

The types of surgical procedures most likely to provide the patient with improved motion are as follows:
1. Capsulotomies of MP joints
2. Capsulotomies of the PIP joint (with or without resection of the volar plate)
3. Capsulotomy of the volar wrist joint to relieve flexion contracture; tenolysis of the flexor tendon with release of the transverse carpal ligament
4. Resection of the tenodesed flexor digitorum superficialis tendon at the level of the PIP joint

If the wrist cannot be passively moved into extension, the transverse carpal ligament should not be simply incised or excised but should be lengthened by the step-cut method so that it will not be binding on the tendons or the nerve but will still function to prevent the tendons from "falling out" of the carpal tunnel. Better results with PIP joint capsulotomies are obtained when the contracture is in extension rather than in flexion.

The exact details of these surgical procedures are found in Chapter 23 and are not repeated here. When the operator starts out to do any of the above-mentioned surgical procedures, he must be prepared to do all of them if necessary. In other words, if he does only a capsulotomy but a tenolysis of the flexor tendons is also indicated, he will not obtain benefit by doing *only* the capsulotomy; instead, he must do everything necessary at that time to regain motion. Postoperatively, very early motion should be started. If the patient's reflex sympathetic dystrophy was eliminated with stellate ganglion blocks only, it is advisable for the patient to have another two to three blocks to help prevent the regeneration of RSD.

SUMMARY

1. "Reflex sympathetic dystrophy" should be the name used for all of the vasomotor-trophic disturbances, which have been given various names in the past.
2. These three etiologic conditions must be present at the same time for RSD to develop:
   a. Persistent painful lesion
   b. Diathesis (patient's susceptibility)
   c. Abnormal sympathetic reflex
3. These are the five clinical types of RSD (listed in ascending order of severity):
   a. Minor causalgia
   b. Minor traumatic dystrophy
   c. Shoulder-hand syndrome
   d. Major traumatic dystrophy
   e. Major causalgia
4. For a presumptive diagnosis of RSD to be made, these four cardinal symptoms and signs should be present:
   a. Pain
   b. Swelling
   c. Stiffness
   d. Discoloration
5. At least several of the following secondary symptoms and signs must also be present before a presumptive diagnosis of RSD can be made:
   a. Osteoporosis
   b. Sudomotor changes
   c. Temperature changes
   d. Trophic changes
   e. Vasomotor instability
   f. Palmar fasciitis
6. The dominant distinguishing feature of RSD is the fact that all the symptoms and signs are very much more severe than would ordinarily be expected for a similar type of inciting painful trauma or disease in an otherwise normal individual.
7. The most important treatment of RSD is some type of interruption of the sympathetic reflex arc so that the abnormal sympathetic reflex is eliminated.
8. The earlier the sympathetic reflex arc is eliminated, the better the result.
9. A confirmed diagnosis of RSD can be made only when the interruption of the sympathetic reflex arc has been shown to produce at least a definite measure of improvement.
10. There is a high incidence of traumatic carpal tunnel syndrome occurring in the major traumatic dystrophy type of RSD; when this condition is found to be present, the compression of the nerve should be relieved surgically.
11. No surgery should be performed on the extremity without having the "protective umbrella" of either a sympathectomy or a stellate ganglion block.
12. The hand therapist should use great care to avoid any painful active or passive exercise on the part of the patient and should be equally as cautious to make sure that no pain is created by the splinting program. The therapist should be only a teacher and not a manipulator.
13. Indications for reconstructive surgery to regain motion should be very restrictive, and the expectations should be limited.

REFERENCES

1. Adson AW and Brown GE: Raynaud's disease of upper extremities: successful treatment by resection of sympathetic cervicothoracic and second thoracic ganglions and intervening trunk, JAMA 92:444, 1929.
2. Ardito S and others: Radioisotope evaluation of the treatment of Sudeck's syndrome with calcitonin, Ital J Orthop Traumatol 4:109, 1978.
3. Atkins HJB: Sympathectomy by axillary approach, Lancet 1:538, 1954.
4. Barnes R: The role of sympathectomy in the treatment of causalgia, J Bone Joint Surg 35B:172, 1953.
5. Benzon HT, Chomka CM, and Brunner EA: The treatment of reflex sympathetic dystrophy with regional intravenous reserpine, Anesth Analg 59:500, 1980.
6. Betcher AM, Bean G, and Casten DF: Continuous procaine block of paravertebral sympathetic ganglions, JAMA 151:288, 1953.
7. Blumenkrantz N and Sondergaard J: Effect of prostaglandins E1 and F1ₐ on biosynthesis of collagen, Nature New Biol 239:246, 1972.
8. Bonelli S and others: Regional intravenous guanethidine vs. stellate ganglion block in reflex sympathetic dystrophy: a randomized trial, Pain 16:297, 1983.
9. Bonica JJ: Causalgia and other reflex sympathetic dystrophies, Postgrad Med 53:143, 1973.
10. Carron H and Weller RM: Treatment of post-traumatic sympathetic dystrophy, Adv Neurol 4:485, 1974.
11. Casey KL: The neurophysiologic basis of pain, Postgrad Med 53:58, 1973.
12. Chan CS and Chow SP: Electroacupuncture in the treatment of post-traumatic sympathetic dystrophy (Sudeck's atrophy), Br J Anaesth 53:899, 1981.
13. Chapman LF and others: Neurohumeral features of afferent fibers in man, Arch Neurol 4:617, 1961.
14. Chuinard RG and others: Intravenous reserpine for the treatment of reflex sympathetic dystrophy, South Med J 74:1481, 1981.
15. Coffman JD and Davies WT: Vasospastic disease: a review, Progr Cardiovasc Dis 18:123, 1975.
16. Denmark A: An example of symptoms resembling tic douleureux produced by a wound in the radial nerve, Royal Med Chir Trans 4:48, 1813.
17. DeSaussure RL: Causalgia, Clin Neurosurg 25:626, 1978.
18. de Takáts G: Reflex dystrophy of extremities, Arch Surg 34:939, 1937.
19. de Takáts G: Causalgic states in peace and war, JAMA 128:699, 1945.
20. Doupe J, Cullen CH, and Chance GQ: Post-traumatic pain and causalgia syndrome, J Neurol Neurosurg Psychiatry 7:33, 1944.
21. Edmundson AS and Calandruccio RA: Drug therapy for causalgia, Mississippi Doctor 34:239, 1957.
22. Eriksen S: Duration of sympathetic blockade: stellate ganglion vs. intravenous regional guanethidine block, Anaesthesia 36:768, 1981.
23. Evans JA: Reflex sympathetic dystrophy: report on 57 cases, Ann Intern Med 26:417, 1947.
24. Fowler FD and Moser M: Use of hexamethonium and Dibenzyline in diagnosis and treatment of causalgia, JAMA 161:1051, 1956.
25. Genant HK and others: The reflex sympathetic dystrophy syndrome, Radiology 117:21, 1975.
26. Gerard RW: The physiology of pain: abnormal neuron states in causalgia and related phenomena, Anesthesiology 12:1, 1951.
27. Glick EM: Reflex dystrophy (algoneurodystrophy): results of treatment by corticosteroids, Rheumatol Rehabil 12:84, 1973.
28. Glynn CJ, Basedow RW, and Walsh JA: Pain relief following post-ganglionic sympathetic blockade with I.V. guanethidine, Br J Anaesth 53:1297, 1981.
29. Gorsky BH: Intravenous perfusion with reserpine for Raynaud's phenomenon, Reg Anesth 2:5, 1977.
30. Granit R, Leskell L, and Skoglund CR: Fiber interaction in injured or compressed region of nerve, Brain 67:125, 1944.
31. Hamilton J: On some effects resulting from wounds of nerves, Dublin J Med Sci 13:38, 1838.
32. Hannington-Kiff JG: Relief of Sudeck's atrophy by regional intravenous guanethidine, Lancet 1:1132, 1977.
33. Hannington-Kiff JG: Pharmacological target blocks in hand surgery and rehabilitation, J Hand Surg 9B:29, 1984.
34. Homans J: Minor causalgia: a hyperesthetic neurovascular syndrome, N Engl J Med 222:870, 1940.
35. Kennard MA: Sensitization of spinal cord of cat to pain-inducing stimuli, J Neurosurg 10:169, 1953.
36. Kirchner PT and Simon MA: Current concepts review: radioisotopic evaluation of skeletal disease, J Bone Joint Surg 63A:673, 1981.
37. Kirklin JW, Chenoweth AI, and Murphey F: Causalgia: a review of its characteristics, diagnosis, and treatment, Surgery 21:321, 1947.
38. Kleinert HE, Cole NM, Wayne L and others: Post-traumatic sympathetic dystrophy, Orthop Clin North Am 4:917, 1973.
39. Kozin F and others: Bone scintigraphy in reflex sympathetic dystrophy syndrome, Radiology 138:437, 1981.
40. Kux M: Thoracic endoscopic sympathectomy in palmar and axillary hyperhidrosis, Arch Surg 113:264, 1978.
41. Kwan ST: The treatment of causalgia by thoracic sympathetic ganglionectomy, Ann Surg 101:222, 1935.
42. Lankford LL: Reflex sympathetic dystrophy. In Omer GE Jr and Spinner M, editors: Management of peripheral nerve problems, Philadelphia, 1980, WB Saunders Co.
43. Lankford LL: Reflex sympathetic dystrophy. In Green DP, editor: Operative hand surgery, ed 2, New York, 1988, Churchill Livingstone.
44. Lankford LL and Thompson JE: Reflex sympathetic dystrophy, upper and lower extremity: diagnosis and management. In American Academy of Orthopaedic Surgeons: Instructional course lectures, vol 26, St Louis, 1977, The CV Mosby Co.
45. Lee MH and Ernst M: The sympatholytic effect of acupuncture as evidenced by thermography: a preliminary report, Orthop Rev 12:67, 1983.
46. Leriche R: The surgery of pain, London, 1939, Baillière, Tindall & Cox (Translated and edited by A. Young).
47. Livingston WK: Pain mechanisms: a physiological interpretation of causalgia and its related states, New York, 1943, The Macmillan Co.
48. Long DM: Electrical stimulation for relief of pain from chronic nerve injury, J Neurosurg 39:718, 1973.
49. Lorente de Nó R: Analysis of the activity of the chains of internuncial neurons, J Neurophysiol 1:207, 1938.
50. Mackinnon SE and Holder LE: The use of three-phase radionuclide bone scanning in the diagnosis of reflex sympathetic dystrophy, J Hand Surg 9A:556, 1984.
51. Martin TJ: The therapeutic uses of calcitonin, Scot Med J 23:161, 1978.
52. Maurer AH, Holder LE, Espinola DA and others: Three-phase radionuclide scintigraphy of the hand, Radiology 146:761, 1983.
53. Mayfield FH and Devine JW: Causalgia, Surg Gynecol Obstet 80:631, 1945.
54. McGrath MA and Penny R: The mechanisms of Raynaud's phenomenon, Part 1, Med J Aust 2:328, 1974.
55. McKain CW, Urban BJ, and Goldner JL: The effects of intravenous regional guanethidine and reserpine, J Bone Joint Surg 65A:808, 1983.
56. McKay NN, Woodhouse NJ, and Clarke AK: Post-traumatic reflex sympathetic dystrophy syndrome (Sudeck's atrophy): effects of regional guanethidine infusion and salmon calcitonin, Br Med J 1:1575, 1977.
57. Melzack R and Wall PD: Pain mechanisms: a new theory, Science 150:971, 1965.
58. Meyer GA and Fields HL: Causalgia treated by selective large fibre stimulation of peripheral nerve, Brain 95:163, 1972.
59. Mitchell JK: Remote consequences of injuries of nerves and their treatment, Philadelphia, 1895, Lea Brothers.
60. Mitchell SW: On the diseases of nerves resulting from injuries in contributions relating to the causation and prevention of disease, and to camp disease. In Flint A, editor: United States Sanitary Commission Memoirs, New York, 1867.
61. Mitchell SW: Injuries of nerves and their consequences, Philadelphia, 1872, JB Lippincott Co.
62. Mitchell SW, Morehouse GR, and Keen WW: Gunshot wounds and other injuries of nerves, Philadelphia, 1864, JB Lippincott Co.
63. Moore DC: Regional block, Springfield, Ill, 1967, Charles C Thomas, Publisher.
64. Nashold BS Jr and Friedman H: Dorsal column stimulation for control of pain, J Neurosurg 36:590, 1972.
65. Nathan PW: On the pathogenesis of causalgia and peripheral nerve injuries, Brain 70:145, 1947.
66. Omer GE Jr and Thomas SR: Treatment of causalgia: review of cases at Brooke General Hospital, Tex Med 67:93, 1971.
67. Omer GE Jr and Thomas SR: The management of chronic pain syndromes in the upper extremity, Clin Orthop Rel Res 104:37, 1974.
68. Owens JC: Causalgia, Am Surg 23:636, 1957.
69. Paget J: Clinical lecture on some cases of local paralysis, Med Times 1:331, 1864.
70. Pak TJ, Martin GM, Magness JL and others: Reflex sympathetic dystrophy, review of 140 cases, Minn Med 53:507, 1970.

71. Palumbo LT: Upper dorsal sympathectomy without Horner's syndrome, Arch Surg 27:743, 1955.

72. Panerai AE and others: Beta-endorphin, metenkephalin, and beta-lipotropin in chronic pain and electroacupuncture. In Bonica and others, editors: Advances in pain research and therapy 5:543, 1983.

73. Paré A: Les œuvres d'Ambroise Paré (histoire de defunct), Roy Charles IX, Tenth Book 41:401, Paris, 1598, Gabriel Buon.

74. Pochaczevsky R and others: Liquid crystal thermography of the spine and extremities, J Neurosurg 56:386, 1982.

75. Pool JL and Brabson JA: Pain on stimulating the distal segment of divided peripheral nerves, J Neurosurg 3:468, 1946.

76. Porter JM and others: Effect of intra-arterial injection of reserpine on vascular wall catecholamine content, Surg Forum 22:183, 1972.

77. Procacci P and others: Skin potentials and EMG changes induced by cutaneous electrical stimulation. II. Subjects with reflex sympathetic dystrophies, Appl Neurophysiol 42:125, 1979.

78. Prough DS and others: Efficacy of oral Nifedipine in the treatment of reflex sympathetic dystrophy, Anesthesiology 62:796, 1985.

79. Rosen PS and Graham W: The shoulder-hand syndrome: historical review with observations on 73 patients, Can Med Assoc J 77:86, 1957.

80. Ross JP: Causalgia, St Barthol Hosp Rep 65:103, 1932.

81. Shumacker HB, Speigel IJ, and Upjohn RH: Causalgia: the role of sympathetic interruption in treatment, Surg Gynecol Obstet 86:76, 1948.

82. Smithwick RH: The rationale and technique of sympathectomy for the relief of vascular spasm of the extremity, N Engl J Med 222:699, 1940.

83. Snider RL and Porter JM: Treatment of experimental frostbite with intra-arterial sympathetic blocking drugs, Surgery 77:557, 1975.

84. Spurling RG: Causalgia of the upper extremity: treatment by dorsal sympathetic ganglionectomy, Arch Neurol Psychiatry 23:784, 1930.

85. Steinbrocker O: The shoulder-hand syndrome: associated painful homolateral disability of the shoulder and hand with swelling and atrophy of the hand, Am J Med 3:402, 1947.

86. Steinbrocker O: The shoulder-hand syndrome: present perspective, Arch Phys Med Rehabil 49:388, 1968.

87. Sudeck PHM: Ueber die acute entzündliche Knockenatrophie, Arch Klin Chir 62:147, 1900.

88. Sunderland S: Pain mechanisms in causalgia, J Neurol Neurosurg Psychiatry 39:471, 1976.

89. Uematsu S and others: Thermography electromyography in the differential diagnosis of chronic pain syndromes and reflex sympathetic dystrophy, Electromyogr Clin Neurophysiol 21:165, 1981.

90. Walker AE and Nulson F: Electrical stimulation of the upper thoracic portion of the sympathetic chain in man, Arch Neurol Psychiatry 59:559, 1948.

91. Wall PD and Sweet WH: Temporary abolition of pain in man, Science 155:108, 1967.

92. White JC: Sympathectomy for relief of pain. In Bonica JJ, editor: Advances in neurology, International Symposium in Pain, vol 4, New York, 1974, Raven Press.

93. Wilkerson RH Jr, Koman LA, Nunley JA II, and others: Radionuclide dynamic imaging of distal upper extremity perfusion, RadioGraphics 2:593, 1982.

94. Wilkinson HA: Radiofrequency percutaneous upper-thoracic sympathectomy, New Engl J Med 311:34, 1984.

60

Therapist's management of reflex sympathetic dystrophy

Janet Waylett-Rendall

BEHAVIORAL PATTERNS IN REFLEX SYMPATHETIC DYSTROPHY

More than 30 terms have been used to describe the symptom complex of reflex sympathetic dystrophy (RSD). Whatever the term, references in the medical literature describe the RSD patient as follows: emotionally labile with low pain threshold, dependent or inadequate personality, introspective, worrying, apprehensive, hysterical, defensive, and hostile.[4-8]

Lanksford[7,8] discussed a predisposition or diathesis for development of RSD that involves (1) abnormal sympathetic reflex, (2) vasoconstrictive reactions resulting in abnormally cold extremities and possible migraine headaches, and (3) predisposing psychologic make-up. The belief that individuals with certain personality traits are most likely to develop RSD is further supported by Ehlers and Zachariae.[5] In their report of a study completed in 1964, 33 male patients with Dupuytren's contracture were seen before surgery by a psychiatrist who assessed each one's character and gave a statement containing a prediction regarding the postoperative course. The surgeon was unaware of the contents of the statement. A few months later the actual course was compared with the predicted postoperative course. "In 30 out of 33 patients there was conformity between preoperative psychiatric statement and the real postoperative course, and the conclusion is that an interested psychiatrist can foretell in a great many cases whether a hand operation will be complicated by postoperative dystrophic symptoms or not.[5]

Because of the frequent frustrations and difficulty in treating this type of individual, Loma Linda University Medical Center Hand Rehabilitation Center and Downey Community Hospital Hand Center became interested in trying to identify some of the more subtle behavioral traits of RSD that might affect such a patient's progress in hand therapy. We noticed that as a group such patients failed to progress as rapidly as other patients and that a few, when seen by the physician after discharge from therapy, had not progressed further on their own.

In 1975 we initiated a survey between our two facilities that involved the standardized Buhler-Coleman Life Goals Inventory[1] and written observations by staff members and students.

BUHLER-COLEMAN LIFE GOALS INVENTORY

The standardized Buhler-Coleman Life Goals Inventory is a self-administered instrument designed to assess personality in terms of an individual's life expectations—what that person wants most and least from life. The four basic tendencies measured by this instrument are as follows:

1. Need satisfaction—need for survival, love, and pleasure
2. Creative expansion—drive toward accomplishment
3. Self-limiting adaptation—limits own needs and satisfaction
4. Upholding the internal order—moral or social values integrated into personality.

We studied three groups of patients. In the *control group* were 17 hand patients—7 women and 10 men—of which 8 had suffered industrial injuries. The *suspected RSD group* consisted of 5 women, 2 of whom had had industrial injuries. In the *diagnosed RSD group* were 12 patients who were known to have the disorder.

In the control group all 17 of the patients evaluated had normal profiles except 1 man. Two of 5 suspected RSD patients had abnormal profiles. Of the 12 diagnosed RSD patients, 5 refused to fill out the inventory and 1 found it too difficult to complete; of the 6 scored inventories, none was in the normal range. In the normally scoring individual, there is a well organized hierarchy of needs. In the diagnosed RSD group, there was a trend toward self-limiting behavior, with conflicting goals. As a group, such patients do not show creative or enterprising tendencies. Because half of this group refused to complete the inventory, one would suspect that these individuals are resistant to the implication that their physical problem is in any way related to their psychologic state.

CLINICAL OBSERVATIONS

It was decided that thorough, written observations, recorded on an observation sheet or an outline, could be the means of identifying the more subtle behavioral traits in RSD patients. Four separate observation sheets were completed for each patient. The observers were a physician, a therapist, a psychologist, a rehabilitation nurse, a secretary, and a student. Three of observers had formed strong opinions about RSD before the observation; the remaining three, for the most part, had not heard of the disorder.

The most obvious observation, of course, is the complaint of the constant, often burning pain that seems to totally preoccupy the patient. Interestingly, our patients did not have acute or severe physiologic problems, such as partial amputations. Another observation made by the staff members was the patient's inability to solve problems, which was seemingly universal among this patient group. This was noted not just in regard to exercises and treatment modalities, which would be unfamiliar to most lay persons, but also in regard to solving very simple tasks. For example, a patient attempted to help in the center by filling a 30-cup coffee maker with water. She did it one cup at a time instead of filling the urn from the faucet. In addition, these patients tended to ignore the most traumatized patients, not displaying any open concern for them.

Behavioral traits based on observations

Control group. The control group demonstrated consistent behavior in at least three of four observations for each question. In addition they displayed the following positive traits:

1. Conversation not dominated by either pain or disability
2. Ability to retain instructions from session to session
3. Ability to perform exercises and use modalities with limited supervision
4. Ability to make decisions about changes needed in splinting (for example, whether rubber-band traction is comfortable, whether straps are becoming worn).

Suspected RSD group. The suspected group was so varied that the results were inconclusive.

Diagnosed RSD group. The traits of the diagnosed group, found in more than 50% of its members, were as follows:

1. Presentation of different picture to each observer, suggesting inconsistent behavior
2. Conversation dominated by either pain or disability
3. Typical initial behavior was to act withdrawn in a room full of people (this gradually changed, but persisted much longer than in control group)
4. Inability to retain instructions from session to session
5. Inability to perform exercises and use modalities without close supervision (for example, did not increase weights when on strengthening program)
6. Inability to make decisions about changes needed in splinting (for example, whether rubber-band traction is comfortable, whether straps are becoming worn)

Conclusions based on observations

The RSD patient requires:

1. Constant supervision initially, which should be reduced only as the patient demonstrates understanding of his condition, which usually takes more time than is necessary for the control group.
2. A highly structured and simplified program, which should include step-by-step teaching by demonstration and written instructions. The use of splints must be explained in a way that is easy to understand, and splints must be easy to apply and wear.
3. Motivation to be an active agent in his own treatment. The idea that he has the *power* to improve must be instilled in him.

A psychologist who reviewed our survey suggested that RSD may represent a form of communication disorder, both receptive and expressive, in which emotional distress is expressed physically. He later tested 12 additional RSD patients with the Minnesota Multiphasic Personality Inventory and found they showed the "conversion hysteria profile." He also expressed the opinion that these patients would probably not benefit greatly from psychologic counseling, since they would resist the implication that anything might be wrong with them emotionally.

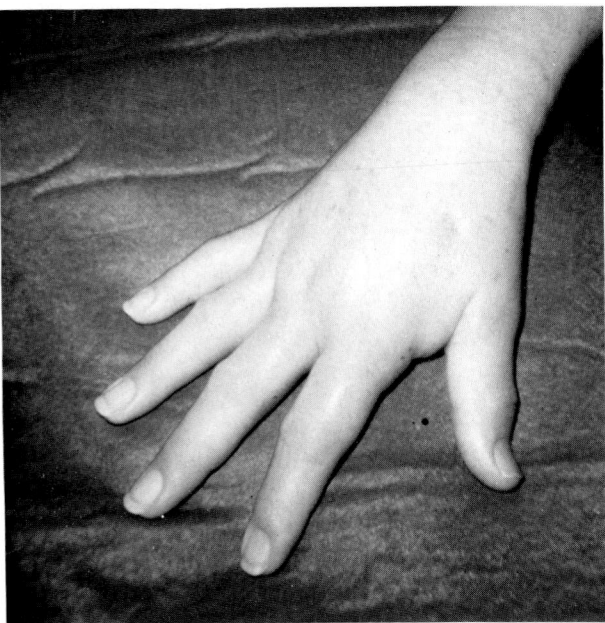

Fig. 60-1 Severe edema as seen in reflex dystrophy.

HAND THERAPY: PHILOSOPHY AND TREATMENT

On the basis of clinical experience and the results of our survey, we believe that treatment should be started very early after injury or operation for individuals whom the physician suspects may be at risk for developing RSD. These patients have pain and swelling out of proportion to the injury.[7,8] For example, there is a high incidence of RSD secondary to wrist fractures,[8-10] and patients should be seen for treatment 1 or 2 days following cast application or external fixator to provide early motion of joints proximal and distal to those immobilized. Early intervention can assist in the prevention of the typical severe edema and trophic changes seen in Fig. 60-1.

EVALUATION

Evaluations that are especially helpful in the assessment of the suspected RSD patient are those for pain, edema, range of motion, and sometimes sensibility. They assist not only the therapist in establishing treatment goals but may also assist the physician in making a definitive diagnosis.

Pain

Before a pain management program is initiated, it is necessary to establish a baseline of perceived pain to better assess the effectiveness of the treatment. There are many scales for assessing pain.[4a,10] We selected the McGill Pain Questionnaire (MPQ), because it was proven to be valid, reliable, consistent, and useful.[4a] It was developed by Melzack and Torgerson from a study that demonstrated high agreement among patients, students, and physicians on the meaning attached to pain adjectives.[8a] The questionnaire is intended to reflect three dimensions of pain: sensory, affective, and evaluative. It also includes line drawings of the body to indicate the spatial distribution of the pain. Pain intensity is recorded as a number on a scale from one to five.

Whichever pain assessment tool is selected, it should determine the intensity, quality, and spatial distribution of the pain.

Edema

The Volumeter is the best evaluation tool, in my opinion, for total hand and wrist edema. Circumference readings are more appropriate when only one or two digits are involved. Evaluations are performed before and after treatment modalities to objectively assess their effect on the edema.

Range of motion

Angular motion is recorded for individual joints, and linear measurements (for example, thumb tip to head of fifth metacarpal) reflect more functional range. The patient can use linear measurements to assess improvement himself.

Sensibility

Sensibility should be evaluated in cases with suspected nerve involvement. Because the median nerve has the greatest number of sympathetic fibers of any nerve in the upper extremity, injury to or compression of this nerve is more likely to result in RSD than injury to any of the other nerves.[8] Evaluation of subtle sensibility changes might include Semmes-Weinstein monofilaments and two-point discrimination. The vibrometer (made by Biothesiometer) might be used to assess hypersensitivity to vibration with comparison made to the contralateral extremity.

TREATMENT
Pain

Treatment of pain may begin with a "stress-loading" program as described by Watson and Carlson.[10] In this approach the weight bearing is begun on the hands and knees with the involved hand scrubbing with a scrub brush a set number of times a day and for a prescribed period of time. Loading the extremity by carrying a weight with the extended arm is another aspect of this program. Watson and Carlson[10] add no other exercises until the pain subsides. In our experience it is often difficult to place the wrist fracture patient in the hands and knees position if the wrist is contracted in flexion. However, limited weight bearing can be accomplished by having the patient sand with a bilaterally adapted handle sander on an inclined plane.

The patient may be given a series of stellate ganglion blocks, each one administered just before therapy so that treatment is comfortable.[8] This treatment regimen may also be used in conjunction with transcutaneous electrical nerve stimulation (TENS)[6] and/or anti-inflammatory drugs.[7,8]

Desensitization as described by Yerxa and associates[11] may also be indicated in cases of nerve involvement.

Heat treatment

Once the swelling has increased the patient can proceed to heat modalities such as hot packs or paraffin bath to relax muscles and soften scar tissue. The paraffin bath is used to obtain finger flexion; the patient's fingers are taped into flexion with paper tape to ensure that maximum passive flexion is maintained throughout the bath. The hand is dipped six times into the bath; the patient then soaks the hand for 10 minutes in paraffin if he can tolerate the heat. After removing the hand from the bath, the paraffin glove is left in place and covered with a plastic bag. With the uninvolved hand the patient passively flexes the involved fingers. Hot packs are used to gain extension range of motion, since their flat, square configuration lends itself well to holding the fingers in extension. Both the paraffin bath and the hot packs are followed by passive or active range-of-motion exercises and strengthening exercises, as indicated by the patient's clinical picture.

Fluidotherapy is a form of heat treatment that can be thermostatically controlled and may be ideal for the patient needing desensitization and softening of scar tissue.

Edema

Jobst treatment. Edema is usually a serious problem in the RSD hand (because of minimal active movement by the patient), and treatment of this problem is begun on initial contact. The Jobst intermittent compression unit (see Chapter 11) is used in combination with elevation and the use of pressure wraps and compression gloves or splints to decrease edema. The Jobst treatment is most effective with patients demonstrating "pitting edema." The treatment lasts 45 minutes to 1 hour in length, with compression being set between 60 to 90 mm Hg. If the Jobst unit is used to increase passive interphalangeal flexion, the compression must be reduced to 30 to 60 mm Hg, and the fingers should be alternately positioned in flexion and extension.

Ice treatment. A 20-minute ice treatment or contrast baths can also be used to decrease edema; however, they are not tolerated by RSD patients as well as the other edema-reducing modalities.

Retrograde massage. Retrograde massage is very helpful with this patient group to decrease edema and at the same time desensitize the fingers and hand and soften any scar tissue present. Retrograde massage is performed for 10 to 15 minutes, with a lanolin-base cream used as a lubricant.

Range of motion

Active range of motion (ROM) is preferred initially because it is less likely to cause pain and anxiety in the patient. In addition, active exercise is excellent for decreasing edema, because the pumping action of the muscles assists in venous return. Tendon gliding can increase active ROM without pain.

The active exercise program must be extremely simple, with a set number of repetitions and predetermined weights. Weight increases must be supervised by either the clinic aide or the therapist.

Skateboard exercises, as shown in Fig. 60-2, are performed on an adjustable-height table and are used to provide gravity-eliminated active exercises to shoulder and elbow in the horizontal plane. These exercises can be made resistive by attaching a weight to the skate through a pulley mechanism. Skateboard exercises are designed to improve shoulder and elbow range of motion, which are often involved in RSD when the patient has a shoulder-hand syndrome.

Reciprocal pulleys are used to provide assistive ROM

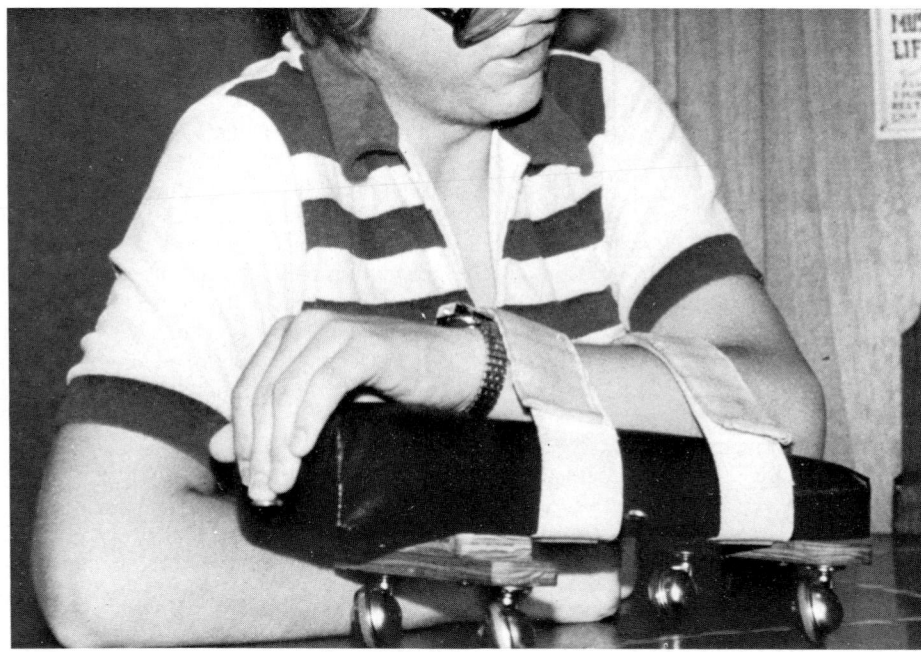

Fig. 60-2 Skateboard exercise for shoulder and elbow.

exercise to shoulder and elbow musculature and are excellent for home use when applied to a doorway.

Dowel or wand exercises, an example of which is shown in Fig. 60-3, are given for home and clinic programs to increase shoulder, elbow, and forearm strength and ROM. A Velcro cuff weight can be added to the dowel to provide resistance.

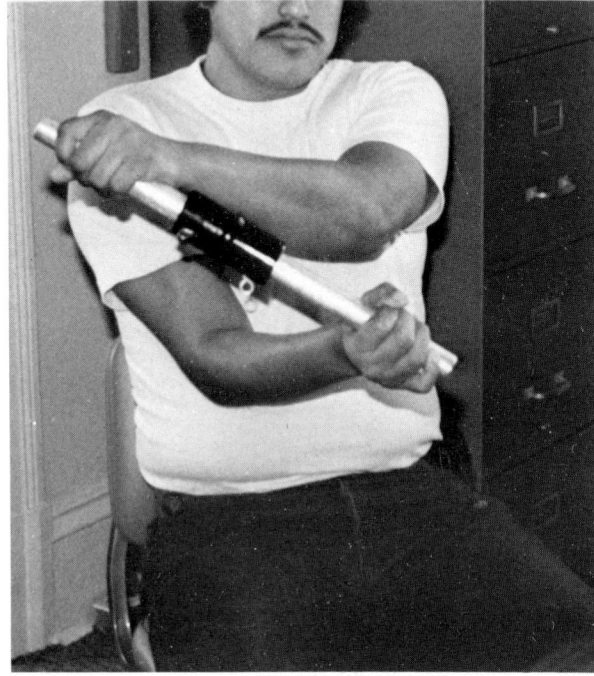

Fig. 60-3 Dowel exercise to increase shoulder, elbow, and forearm strength and range of motions.

RESISTIVE EXERCISE

Progressive resistive exercises (PRE) are the method of choice for increasing the strength of the upper extremity musculature. PRE to finger abductors and adductors is shown in Fig. 60-4. The treppe, or "staircase," method is used to gradually warm up the muscle for maximum exertion without the risk of overstretching the muscle.[2,3] "Treppe" (German for *staircase*) is the term used to describe the phenomenon of increasing muscle contractions against gradually increasing resistance. The system employs a series of 10 contractions against 50% of maximum weight, 10 contractions against 75% of maximum weight and 10 contractions against 100% of maximum weight.[3,4] Isotonic exercises are preferred to isometric exercises, because isotonic

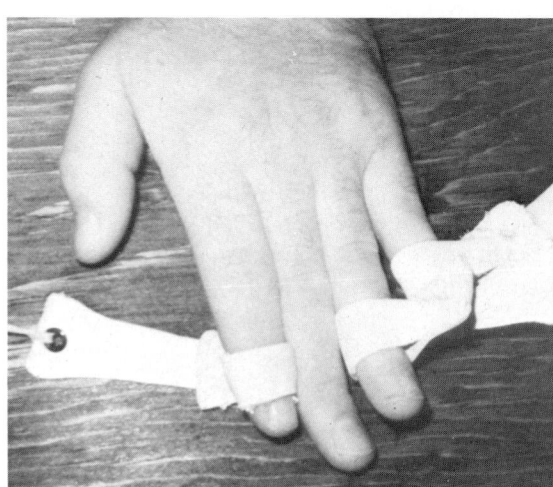

Fig. 60-4 Progressive resistance exercise to finger abductors and adductors.

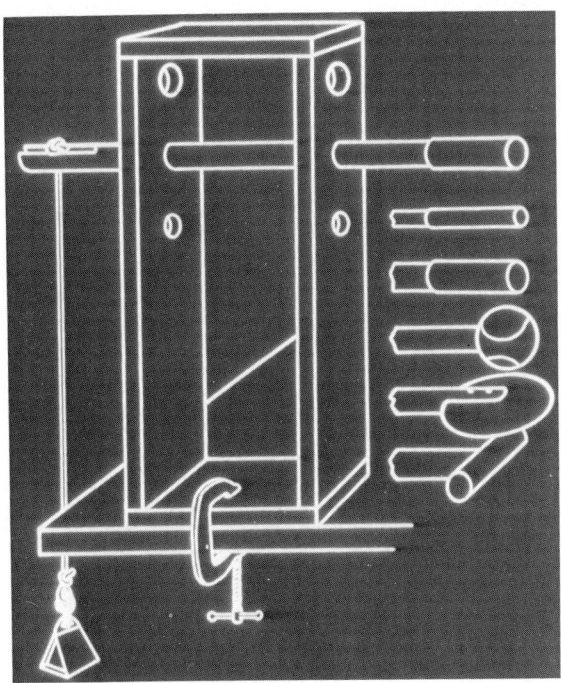

Fig. 60-5   Weight well exercise device with interchangeable handles for wrist and hand exercises.

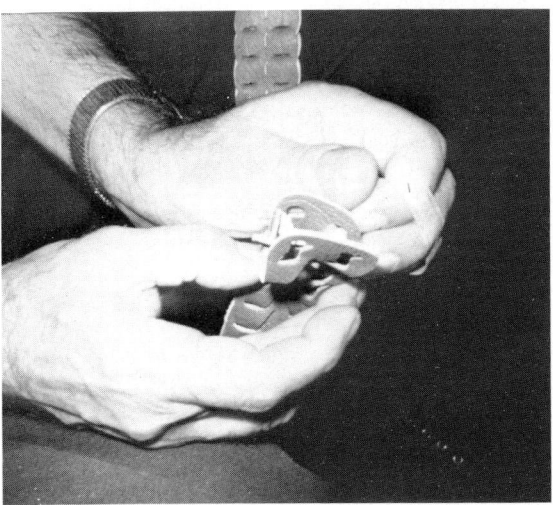

Fig. 60-6   The link belt is a simple rote craft used to rehabilitate the patient with reflex sympathetic dystrophy.

exercises produce joint movement and thereby increase ROM and strength. Patients are seen preferably three times weekly for this strengthening program.

Weight well exercises, as shown in Fig. 60-5, consist of a wide variety of wrist and hand exercises, as demonstrated with the different handles. These exercises also elevate the hand to decrease edema, and they assist venous flow through the pumping action of the forearm and hand musculature. Weight wells can be checked out for home use.

SPLINTING

Splinting follows the basic principles applied to any patient with an injured hand. However, splints must be very comfortable, accomodate for swelling, and be very easy to apply (color-coded straps) with minimal adjustments. Initially, static splints may be tolerated more readily than dynamic splints. Continuous passive motion devices (CPM) could be ideal in theory for the RSD patient in controlling pain and increasing ROM; however, in practice the individual must be very carefully selected for comprehension, mechanical aptitude, and "gadget tolerance."

ACTIVITIES OF DAILY LIVING

Activities of daily living and concurrent craft activities are most important with RSD patients, since these patients characteristically avoid using the involved extremity. They require a highly structured, purposeful activity to reincorporate the spontaneous use of the injured hand into their lives. Simple rote crafts, such as the link belt shown in Fig. 60-6, are excellent because they are bilateral and repetitious and require very little problem solving. Through the initial use of crafts, it is possible to motivate the patient to use the

injured hand in everyday activities, since the rigid RSD patient is often unwilling to accept substandard performances in self-feeding and other activities but has no set expectations about a craft activity that was never before attempted. Through simple accomplishments in craft projects, the patient is made aware that the hand is functional and will begin using it once again. Inquiries should be made frequently about how and when the patient is using the hand at home, so that functional use can be upgraded.

SUMMARY

Understanding the RSD personality, with its dependency, worry, and apprehensive and hysterical behavior, can assist the therapist in directing the patient's treatment program. To alleviate apprehension and worry, the therapist should inform the patient, in simple terms, exactly what is expected of him and when. The therapist should not assume that the patient understands either how to apply a splint or how to perform an exercise until the therapist has observed the patient accomplishing the task properly, because this type of patient does not seem to attend to directions very well (possibly because he is worrying when he should be listening). The RSD patient may not solicit help when he needs it. It is best initially to direct every aspect of the patient's treatment, gradually allowing the patient to assume more responsibility as he demonstrates the ability to do so. This patient group presents a supreme challenge to the therapist's interpersonal skills, because the therapist must relate to the patient socially as an adult peer and in treatment as a dependent or child and at the same time not offend or alienate him.

REFERENCES

1. Buhler C and Coleman WE: Life goals inventory manual, Los Angeles, 1965, University of Southern California School of Medicine.
2. DeLorme TL: Restoration of muscle power by heavy-resistance exercises, J Bone Joint Surg 27:645, 1945.
3. DeLorme TL and Watkins AL: Technics of progressive resistive exercise, Arch Phys Med 29:263, 1948.
4. de Takats G: Causalgic states in peace and war, JAMA 128:699, 1945.
4a. Dubuisson D and Melzack R: Classification of clinical pain descrip-

tion by multiple group discriminant analysis, Exp Neurol 51:480, 1976.

5. Ehlers H and Zachariae L: Mentality and dystrophy, Acta Orthop Scand 1:109, 1964.
6. Headley B: Historical perspective of causalgia management of sympathetically maintained pain, Phys Ther 67:1370, 1987.
7. Kleinert HE and others: Post-traumatic sympathetic dystrophy, Orthop Clin North Am 4:917, 1973.
8. Lankford LL: Reflex sympathetic dystrophy. In Green DP, editor: Operative hand surgery, vol 1, New York, 1982, Churchill Livingstone, Inc.

8a. Melzack R: Neuropsychological basis of pain measurement. In Kruger L and Liebeskind JC, editors: Advances in pain research and therapy, vol 6, New York, 1984, Raven Press.
9. Schutzer SF and Gossling HR: The treatment of reflex sympathetic dystrophy syndrome, J Bone Joint Surg 66(4):623, 1984.
10. Watson HK and Carlson L: Treatment of reflex sympathetic dystrophy of the hand with an active "stress loading program," J Hand Surg 12A(5)(part 1):779, 1987.
11. Yerxa EJ and others: Development of a hand sensitivity test for the hypersensitive hand, Am J Occup Ther 37:176, 1983.

61

Clinical application of transcutaneous electrical nerve stimulator in patients with upper extremity pain

Valerie Holdeman Lee and C. Christopher Reynolds

Transcutaneous electrical nerve stimulation (TENS) has gained universal recognition as a method of producing analgesia in a number of patients with acute or chronic pain. The efficacy of this treatment modality is dependent on a clear understanding of the neuromechanisms for pain modulation. Choosing the proper electrical stimulator and a thorough knowledge of its clinical applicability are equally imperative. The objective of this chapter is to discuss this technique whereby pain management in the upper extremity might be enhanced.

COMPONENTS OF TENS UNITS

The transcutaneous electrical nerve stimulator is an electrical device that emits a pulsed current in the form of a biphasic asymmetric wave form. Pulsed current is neither alternating nor direct but has components of each (Fig. 61-1).

TENS units generally have three controls: (1) output or amplitude, which is expressed in milliamps; (2) pulse rate or frequency, which is expressed in pulses per second, or Hertz (Hz); and (3) pulse width, which is expressed in microseconds.

On some TENS units pulse width is not an option and is set internally. On one commercially available stimulator, the Empi, the pulse width is tied to the amplitude control. As the amplitude increases, the pulse width also increases.

TENS units commonly have either one channel (two electrodes), or two channels (four electrodes). Each channel has the capacity for application of two electrodes. Several models permit additional electrode incorporation on a single channel. This is referred to as a "piggyback arrangement." For patients with upper extremity pain, the two-channel unit is more practical.

Generally, it is not possible to adjust rate and width controls for each channel independently. Characteristically, however, amplitude adjustments maintain their independence on each channel.

Several varieties of electrodes are available. The standard carbon electrode must be covered evenly with conducting gel before it is applied to the patient, to prevent skin irritation or burning. Increasingly popular are the caraya and self-adhesive electrodes. Gel is not necessary and skin reaction is rare. Electrodes are available in various sizes and can be trimmed to meet specific needs. When one is reducing the size of one electrode in a channel, it is important to remember that a 2:1 ratio should not be exceeded, to prevent burning under the small electrode. To assure adequate contact for good electrical conduction, one may need to shave the skin. Commercial skin preparations are also available to enhance conduction.

Precut adhesive patches or hypoallergenic paper tape can be used to secure the electrodes to the patient.

Energy sources for TENS units vary. In most instances rechargeable pencil or transistor batteries with rechargers can be obtained. Other units offer separate rechargeable battery packs.

MODES OF TREATMENT

There are several different treatment modes to choose from when TENS is being used for pain relief. These different forms of stimulation are achieved by adjustment of the characteristics (amplitude, pulse rate, pulse width) of the pulsed wave form and are termed "conventional," "brief intense," and "low-frequency (low-rate) TENS" (Fig. 61-2).

Conventional TENS

The success of conventional TENS is based on the gate-control theory proposed by Melzack and Wall[11] in 1965 and further clarified by more recent studies. Receptors that detect pain (nociceptors) transmit information to the central nervous system via A-delta and unmyelinated (C) fibers. When these nociceptive impulses reach the posterior horn of the spinal cord, a gating or control mechanism determines which signals ascend in the spinothalamic tract to the brain, where pain is perceived. The gate is facilitated or inhibited by peripheral afferents other than those carrying messages and by impulses descending from the brain. The mechanism of this control and its location are unknown, as is the exact function of substantia gelatinosa. The balance between the activity in the A-delta and C fibers may be critical. Increased

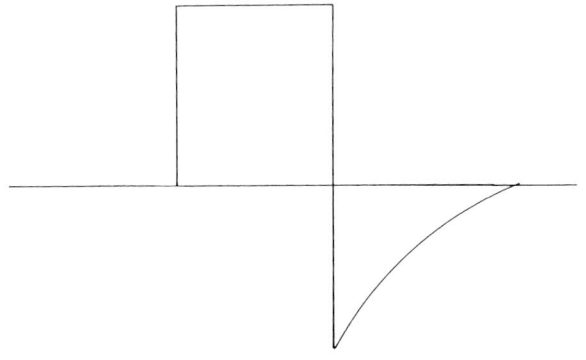

Fig. 61-1 Biphasic asymmetric waveform.

	RATE	PULSE WIDTH	AMPLITUDE
HIGH RATE (conventional)	60 to 120 pps	50 to 100 microseconds	Comfortable No muscle contraction
LOW RATE	1 to 5 pps	150 to 200 microseconds	Slightly uncomfortable Strong muscle contraction
BRIEF INTENSE	60 to 120 pps	200 microseconds	Tolerable Tetanic or sustained muscle contraction

Fig. 61-2   Modes of TENS treatment.

C-fiber action inhibits the gate, allowing passage of impulses, while a relative increase in large myelinated A-fiber activity closes the gate, blocking pain.

The parameters for conventional TENS are as follows: rate, which is high (60 to 120 pulses per second [pps]); width, which is low (50 to 100 microseconds); and amplitude, which is increased until the patient perceives a pleasant, tingling sensation in the area that was previously painful. The onset of pain relief is sudden, and carry-over varies from a few minutes to several hours.

Low-frequency TENS

Pain relief after low-frequency TENS is at present attributed to the release of naturally occurring morphine-like substances called "opioid peptides (endorphins)."[1,5] Elevated endorphin levels have been reported in patients after low-frequency TENS, whereas patients with chronic pain have been reported to have depleted levels of endorphins.[12,13] Naloxone, a specific opiate antagonist, counteracts the pain relief achieved with low-frequency stimulation.[2,4,5] To achieve low-frequency stimulation, the pulse rate must be low (1 to 5 pps), the pulse width high (150 to 200 μsec), and the amplitude increased until a visible muscle contraction occurs. TENS units with a preset width cannot be adjusted adequately for low-rate stimulation. One should keep these factors in mind when acquiring TENS units for clinical

purposes. Low-frequency TENS is perceived by most patients with upper extremity pain to be more comfortable when delivered in a pulsed train or bursting mode. The same low-frequency settings are used, and trains of high-frequency bursts are incorporated in each pulse. Less current intensity is necessary to elicit muscle contraction and stimulation may be more tolerable (Fig. 61-3).[12] Pain relief occurs approximately 15 to 30 minutes after initiation of low-rate TENS or cycle-bursting TENS. Carry-over relief can vary anywhere from 30 minutes to several hours. Because a muscle contraction occurs with this mode of treatment, the patient must be cleared for active exercise before its use.

Brief intense TENS

Brief intense TENS has also been labeled "hyperstimulation analgesia."[9] It is in effect a form of counterstimulation. Melzack suggests that areas in the brainstem act as a "central biasing mechanism" and inhibit formation transmission. He states that intense stimulation would produce a predominantly small fiber input, which would give rise to pain, but would also activate the "central biasing mechanism," which would inhibit pain signals from other areas such as sources of pathologic pain.[8,9] To deliver brief intense TENS, the rate is set high (60 to 120 pps), the pulse width is also set high (200 μsec), and the amplitude is adjusted until a strong muscle contraction occurs. Onset of relief should be sudden, treatment time is short, and carry-over is extremely variable. Brief intense TENS has several useful clinical applications. Procedures such as wound débridement and suture removal may be simplified. In addition to a sustained muscle contraction, sensation is almost completely inhibited within the electrode field. Muscle fatigue occurs rather rapidly, however, and stimulation time must be brief.

Modulation

Accommodation and sensory adaptation may occur during stimulation.[3] To prevent these phenomena from occurring, a number of TENS units provide modulation controls for rate or amplitude or both. These controls may increase effectiveness of treatment and aid in patient comfort.

POSTOPERATIVE TENS

TENS may be used to reduce pain postoperatively. Sterile electrodes are available and may be placed intraoperatively or in the recovery room. Best results with pain relief have been reported when the patient awakes from anesthesia with the TENS functioning. The patient should be seen by the therapist before surgery to experience the stimulation and allay any apprehension. Conventional TENS is usually the

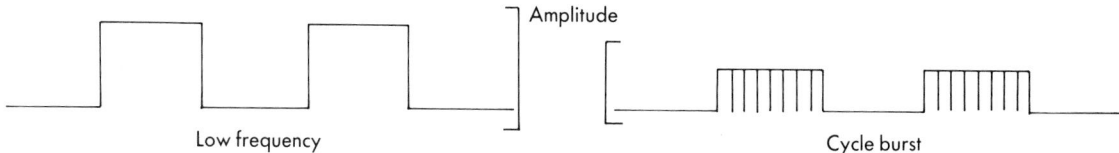

Fig. 61-3   Burst TENS is a variation of low-rate TENS with a more comfortable delivery of "bursts" of low frequency versus "beats" of low frequency.

method of choice. It delivers a pleasant sensation to the patient and provides immediate pain relief, and a muscle contraction is unnecessary.

Postoperative TENS may be extremely beneficial in facilitating early motion in patients with fractures or after such surgical procedures as capsulectomies, neurolysis, and tenolysis and is of particular value with patients who have a history of reflex sympathetic dystrophy (RSD) or a chronic pain problem.

One must, however, remember that pain can be an important feedback mechanism to prevent damage to newly repaired structures. Therefore the therapist must closely monitor the exercise program to prevent the patient from overexercising while experiencing pain relief from the TENS.

USE OF TENS FOR PAIN OTHER THAN POSTOPERATIVE

The use of TENS has been beneficial in a number of upper extremity problems. Particularly, neurostimulators have proved beneficial in reducing pain for persons with a diagnosis of peripheral nerve injury, RSD, or crush injuries. Sensitive scars resulting from fingertip injuries and surgeries about cutaneous branches of peripheral nerves have been desensitized with TENS.

Selection of mode of treatment

Although no set rules have been established, it appears that conventional TENS is best used for initial trial treatment. Onset of pain relief is immediate, and many patients achieve good results with conventional TENS alone. If satisfactory pain relief does not occur after 15 to 30 minutes of conventional TENS, switching to low-frequency TENS may be advantageous. Brief intense TENS should also be used as an alternative. Again, patients must be cleared for active exercise so that either low-frequency or brief intense stimulation may be safely used.

Pre-TENS treatment evaluation includes measurement of grip and pinch (when appropriate), recording of range of motion, and measurement of joint circumference. The therapist must also understand the cause of each patient's pain. The patient is asked to quantitate subjectively his degree of pain on a scale of 0 to 10, with 10 being the highest degree and 0 being pain free. The therapist examines the involved hand and charts color differences, general posturing of the hand and arm, and any changes in sudomotor activity or hair growth.

Before application of the neurostimulator, patients are given a brief explanation of what TENS is and the theory behind its use. TENS must be presented in a positive manner, but it is important not to promise the patient that it will

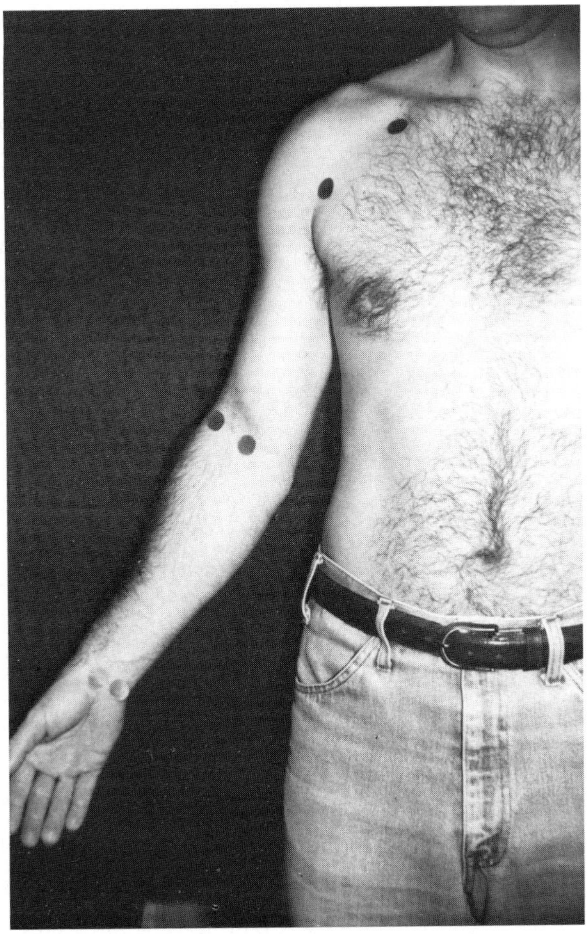

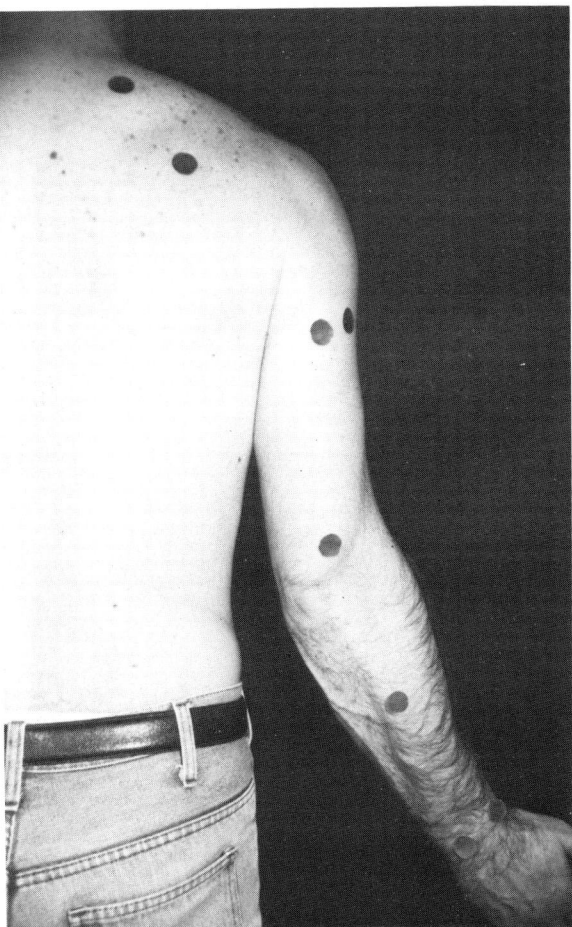

Fig. 61-4   Common sites for TENS, anterior aspect.

Fig. 61-5   Common sites for TENS, posterior aspect.

"cure" his pain. TENS should simply be presented as an adjunct to treatment. For a proper evaluation of TENS, the patient should refrain from taking analgesics 6 to 8 hours before treatment, and the patient should be feeling pain at the time of treatment.

If the patient complains of pain only in the morning, then that is when treatment time is scheduled. Another, more subtle factor that may influence the success of treatment is whether litigation or a compensation settlement is pending. Consciously or subconsciously, the patient may not be ready to let go of his pain if secondary gain is a possibility.

Electrode placement

A critical factor in the success of TENS is electrode placement. In both conventional TENS and brief intense TENS the paresthesias must be perceived in the area that was previously painful. The patient is asked to locate the distribution of pain by outlining on his arm or shading in painful areas on a diagram. The therapist seeks trigger points by palpation and percussion of the extremity, particularly along the course of the superficial peripheral nerves. When one is looking for specific points for stimulation, it is interesting to note that there is a strong correlation between trigger points, motor points, and acupuncture points.[9,10] If they do not occupy the same location, they are often close enough that one electrode may cover both points. One characteristic all three have in common is a lowered resistance

to electrical current.[6] Therefore the therapist should become familiar with the location of motor points, trigger points, and acupuncture points in the upper extremity.

Stimulation sites

Some common sites for stimulation of the upper extremity are shown in Figs. 61-4 and 61-5. Good results may also occur when electrodes are placed in corresponding dermatomes or in segmentally related myotomes.[4] According to the literature, the use of TENS should be avoided over carotid sinuses, across the neck, around the eyes, and in the presence of a cardiac pacemaker. Once location of electrode placement is decided on, the patient is stimulated for 1 hour when conventional or low-rate TENS is being used. Treatment with brief intense TENS should be from 15 to 25 minutes.

Occasionally patients may perceive paresthesias under one electrode of a channel but not the other, a condition that can occur when the area is heavily scarred or there has been damage to the underlying peripheral nerve. In this situation, the electrode may be reduced to one half the size of the remaining electrode. This will increase current density under the smaller electrode.

Patients who complain of diffuse pain over a large area may benefit from having the electrodes placed in an overlapping fashion (Fig. 61-6). In this manner, a greater total area of stimulation is achieved.

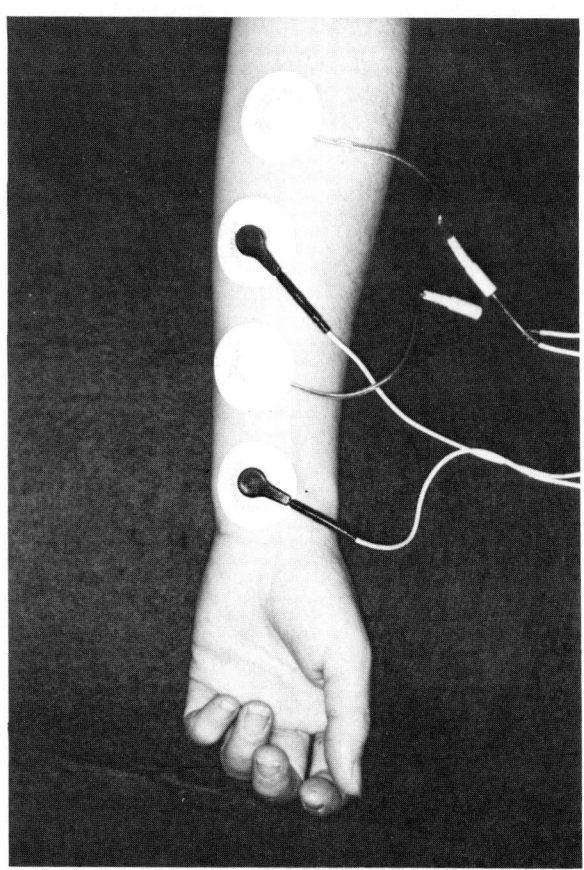

Fig. 61-6 Through overlapping of electrode channels, a large area of stimulation is achieved.

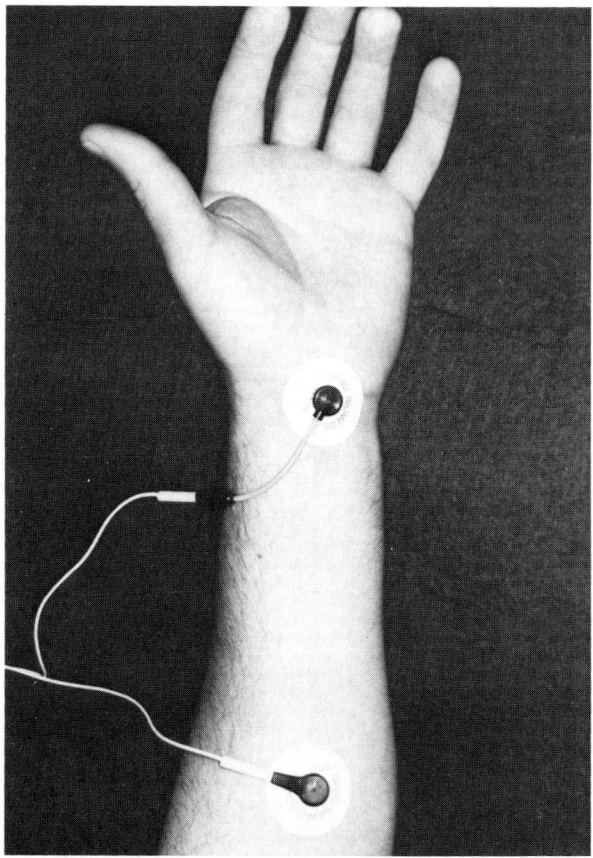

Fig. 61-7 One example of distal electrode placement for patient who has pain resulting from a median nerve injury at the wrist.

Lampe suggests bilateral stimulation if the painful area to be treated has sustained damage to the A fibers, as in a peripheral nerve injury. His suggestion is based on the theory that stimulation of A fibers on the uninjured side would cross over and produce a relative increase in A-fiber activity, which would then trigger the gating mechanism and block C-fiber input.[7] At the end of the first treatment session, patients are asked to record again the level of pain on a 0 to 10 scale. They are also asked to record the duration of carry-over of pain relief. If pain relief is not achieved, electrode placement should be varied. There is no definite formula for electrode placement according to diagnosis, because each patient and condition will vary. The therapist must be willing to spend time with the patient to achieve optimum electrode placement. The following examples demonstrate electrode placement in two different patients. A patient who has suffered an injury to the median nerve at the wrist may complain of pain at the site of the injury and also of pain that radiates proximally into the axilla and anterior chest wall. Distally, one electrode might be placed over the volar wrist crease, with another electrode placed over the proximal third of the volar area of the forearm (Fig. 61-7). Placement of one electrode proximal in the axilla, and the other over the anterior chest wall has proved beneficial (Fig. 61-8).

Prolonged pain after partial or complete amputation of a finger may be referred along the course of the digital nerve. One electrode is placed in the palm just proximal to the metacarpophalangeal (MP) joint of the painful finger. The second electrode is then situated on the dorsum of the hand, also proximal to the MP joint of the injured digit (Fig. 61-9). Paresthesias should be felt over the amputation stump and along the course of the digital nerves involved. If proximal pain is also present, the second-channel electrodes can be placed either in the axillary scalene area as previously mentioned or over the proximal course of the involved nerve. Although experience may enable the therapist to ascertain in just one treatment session whether TENS will be beneficial to a particular patient, a 3-day trial in the clinic

is recommended. This allows enough time for optimal stimulation sites to be located and prevents the patient from experimenting at home on a random basis, which may reduce efficiency. Most insurance companies are now willing to reimburse patients for the cost of TENS with a physician's prescription. At the end of the evaluation period, patients obtaining pain relief receive a rental stimulator unit to be used at home for 1 month. Patients who do not achieve pain relief at the end of the 3-day trial are discontinued from this portion of the program.

If the patient is undecided about whether the stimulator is providing pain relief, treatment with TENS is discontinued. The patient is then reevaluated in 3 days. If without the use of the stimulator the patient has had appreciable increase in pain, consideration is given for further treatment with TENS. When the rental stimulator is delivered, the patient is checked out in his proficiency in attaching the electrodes and adjusting the controls.

The patient is instructed initially to use TENS for 1 hour and then to turn off the stimulator but to leave the electrodes in place. He is then told that if he "senses" that pain is returning, he is to use TENS again for 1 hour. The duration of application depends on the severity of the pain, the duration of carry-over, the patient's pain tolerance, and the functional demands placed upon the patient.

SUMMARY

Treatment with the TENS does not preclude the use of other modalities or procedures. Although some patients present pain as their sole problem, most exhibit edema, decreased joint range of motion, and diffuse hypersensitivity. The purpose of TENS is to decrease pain sufficiently to allow the patient to participate in a complete rehabilitation program and to perform functional activities. TENS should be considered not merely as a modality of last resort but rather as an addition to the treatment regimen of any patient who has pain severe enough to interfere with his rehabilitation program.

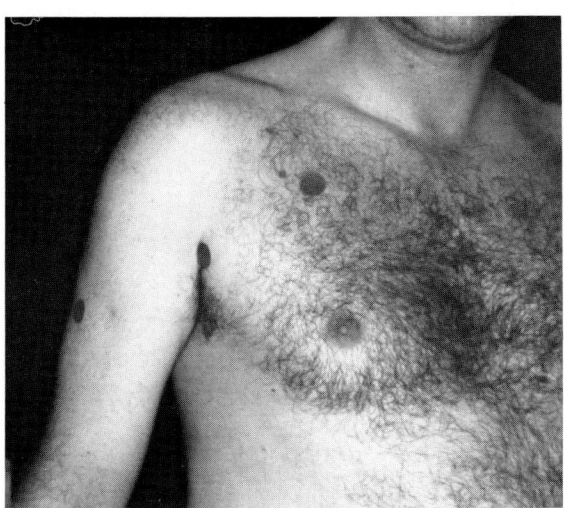

Fig. 61-8   An example of proximal electrode placement.

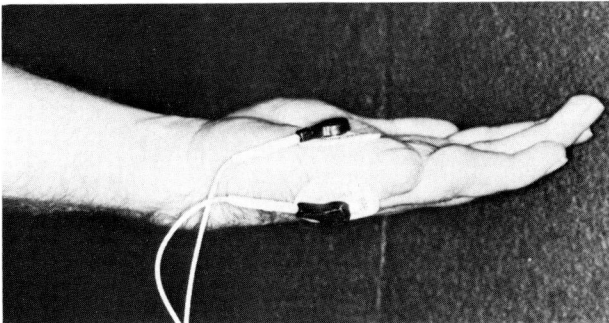

Fig. 61-9   Electrode placement following amputation of little finger. The paresthesias should be felt in the amputation stump and along the course of the digital nerves.

REFERENCES

1. Almay BGL, Johansson F, von Knorring L and others: Endorphins in chronic pain. I. Differences in CSF endorphin levels between organic and psychogenic pain syndromes, Pain 5:153, 1978.
2. Andersson SA: Pain control by sensory stimulation. In Bonica JJ, Liebeskind JC, and Albe-Fessard DG, editors: Advances in pain research and therapy, vol 3, New York, 1979, Raven Press.
3. Empi, Inc: Modulation, 1981, Fridley, Minn.
4. Eriksson M and Sjölund B: Acupuncture-like analgesia in TNS-resistant chronic pain. In Zotterman Y, editor: Sensory functions of the skin, Oxford, 1976, Pergamon Press: Inc.
5. Goldstein A: Opioid peptides (endorphins) in pituitary and brain, Science 193:1081, 1976.
6. Gunn CC and others: Acupuncture loci: a proposal for their classification according to their relationship to known neural structures, Am J Chin Med 4(2):183, 1976.
7. Lampe G: The physical therapists' role in pain management with TENS. In Ersek RA, editor: Pain control with TENS, principles and practice, St. Louis, 1981, Warren H Green, Inc.
8. Melzack R: Phantom limb pain: concept of a central biasing mechanism, Clin Neurol 18:188, 1971.
9. Melzack R: Prolonged relief of pain by brief, intense transcutaneous somatic stimulation, Pain 1:357, 1975.
10. Melzack R, Stillwell DM, and Fox EJ: Trigger points and acupuncture points for pain: correlations and implications, Pain 3:3, 1977.
11. Melzack R and Wall PD: Pain mechanism: a new theory, Science 150(3699):971, 1965.
12. Sjölund B and Eriksson M: Endorphins and analgesia produced by peripheral conditioning stimulation. In Bonica JJ, Liebeskind JC, and Albe-Fessard DG, editors: Advances in pain research and therapy, vol 3, New York, 1979, Raven Press.
13. Sjölund B, Terenius L, and Eriksson M: Increased cerebrospinal fluid levels of endorphins after electro-acupuncture, Acta Physiol Scand 100:382, 1977.

BIBLIOGRAPHY

Lampe GN: Introduction to the use of transcutaneous electrical nerve stimulation devices, Phys Ther 58:1450, 1978.
Melzack R: The puzzle of pain, New York, 1973, Basic Books Inc.
Santiesteban AJ and Sanders BR: Establishing a postsurgical TENS program, Phys Ther 60:789, 1980.
Vander Ark G and McGrath K: Transcutaneous electrical stimulation in treatment of postoperative pain, Am J Surg 130:338, 1975.

VIII

REPLANTATION

62

Surgical aspects of replantation and revascularization

James B. Steichen and Richard S. Idler

One of the greatest technologic advances in surgery made this century has been the ability to revascularize complete and incompletely amputated digits and limbs. Many surgeons dealing with extremity injuries are now well versed in the use of the operating microscope and techniques of microvascular surgery. In major replantation centers throughout the world, survival rates of greater than 80% have been reported in series of digital and major limb replantations.[26,48,64,81,90] These excellent survival rates have come about through better surgical skills developed by experience and through refinements in technique, instrumentation, and suture, as well as the development of stringent criteria for acceptable candidates to undergo replantation. Microvascular techniques that were developed through experience with replantation surgery are now being applied to secondary reconstruction in cases of trauma and congenital deformities. The ability to take free composite-tissue transfers of skin, bone, muscle, nerve, toes, digits, and all combinations of the above and to reestablish a blood and/or nerve supply to these tissues has been made possible through experience gained through replantation surgery.[71]

Although replantation surgery has made the transition from the exotic to the commonplace among surgeons, the lay population and the media still focus on the technical feat rather than the functional outcome of replantation. Although advances in techniques of microvascular surgery have enhanced survival of replanted parts, many problems related to the management of other soft-tissue injuries remain, such as the inability to obtain excellent sensory return or tendon gliding after injury. Many major centers that have been actively involved in replantation surgery are now beginning to report their long-term results. The limitations in functional recovery and the problems of secondary reconstruction in replantation patients are becoming apparent. We hope continued refinement in the selection of candidates for replantation can be made so that the best functional results can be provided. Basic understanding of the response to injury of all tissue types is required to improve the ultimate function of all patients with hand injuries.

HISTORY OF MAJOR LIMB AND DIGITAL REPLANTATION

Successful experimental major limb replantations were achieved as early as the start of this century by investigators such as Hopfner[16] in 1903 and Carrel and Guthrie[6] in 1906. This early experimental work was performed on laboratory dogs; it was supplemented by Reichert[62] in 1931, who reported on 52 replants in dogs. Lapchinsky[31] in 1960 reported on follow-up work performed by Soviet investigators during

the 1950s on experimental major limb replantation. One significant piece of information to be produced from this work was the importance of limb cooling for limb survival. Snyder[70] in 1960 continued experimental major limb replantation and used a pump oxygenator in an attempt to prolong part preservation. In May 1962 the first clinical major limb replantation was performed by Dr. Ronald Malt.[42] Reports of other major limb replantations rapidly followed—from Ch'en[8] in 1963, Horn[17] in 1964, Shorey and others[68] in 1965, and Williams[88] in 1966. Many replantation centers have continued to perform major limb replantation, mainly of the upper extremity, and the Chinese have accumulated fairly large numbers of major limb replantations and are now beginning to report their long-term follow-up.[54,85]

Before digital replantations could be achieved, the development of the operating microscope and microinstrumentation was necessary. The father of the modern operating microscope is considered to be Nylen, who used the scope experimentally for inner ear dissection in rabbits.[11] Clinical introduction of the operating microscope for middle and inner ear surgery was made in the 1920s by Gunnar Holmgren.[15] Experimental work on vessel anastomoses in dogs with vessel diameters from 0.5 to 4 mm was performed by Seidenberg[65] in 1958. Improvements in magnification and instrumentation by Jacobsen and Suarez permitted successful vascular anastomoses in vessels of 2 mm in dogs and rabbits.[22] The first successful clinical application of small vessel surgery took place in November 1962, when Dr. Harold Kleinert anastomosed a digital artery, revascularizing a partially amputated thumb.[23] By applying techniques of microvascular surgery to other clinical examples, Kleinert was able to demonstrate the feasibility and value of revascularization in upper extremity limb salvage.[24,25] In 1965 Buncke and Schulz reported on their experience with replantation of partial hand amputations in rhesus monkeys, achieving one survival out of nine attempts.[4] In July 1965 Komatsu and Tamai reported the first successful replantation of an amputated thumb after several previous failures.[29] Subsequent to this, many attempts at digital replantation were made.

By the early 1970s, large series of digital replantations were reported by O'Brien and Miller,[58] Ch'en,[9] Lendvay,[33] Ikuta,[20] Tsai,[78] and other authors. Continued experimental work was performed during this time to achieve refinements in technique, needles, sutures, and instrumentation. In 1974 O'Brien and Baxter reported on the successful long-term survival of replanted index fingers in stump-tail monkeys, anastomosing vessels of only 0.5 to 0.6 mm.[56] At that same time, Hayhurst and others demonstrated with cooling techniques that successful digital replantation could be performed in monkeys up to 24 hours after amputation.[14] Since the first digital replantation in a human, a wealth of clinical material has been accumulated. This has been supplemented by experimental work in areas such as microscopic changes in vessel anatomy after vessel injury and repair,[1] evaluation of the no-reflow phenomenon,[49] use of intravital stains to identify luminal trauma,[61] and noninvasive techniques of monitoring blood flow.[2] O'Brien in 1977 reported a survival rate of 63% in complete amputations and 80% in incomplete amputations in a series of 103 digits in 74 patients.[55] Recently a number of major replantation centers have reported success rates of greater than 80% after replantation of completely or incompletely amputated digits.[26,48,64,81,90]

REQUIREMENTS FOR REPLANTATION SURGERY

Replantation surgery should be performed only at hospitals with the appropriate equipment and facilities and trained personnel. Although formal replantation centers have not been established in this country, informally several medical centers have established reputations for expertise in replantation surgery. Any center undertaking replantation surgery must have access to emergency transportation systems, particularly if the patient needs transportation over long distances. In digital replantation, because of the absence of muscle tissue, cooling of the part has prolonged the permissible ischemia time. In major limb replantation, however, no more than 6 hours of warm ischemia should elapse, because of the possibility of irreversible muscle death. The primary health care personnel who first manage the potential replantation patient must be educated about evaluation of appropriate candidates for replantation, initial preparation of the amputated part and stump, appropriate means of transporting the amputated part, and management of associated injuries before and during transit. The replantation center must have the capacity to accept a replantation patient at any time and to initiate immediate treatment. Rapid response to this type of an emergency is facilitated by the creation of a replantation team, with each member having an appropriate job and responsibility. Because replantation surgery frequently involves many hours of operative time, the team approach is beneficial in providing fresh personnel who can be alternated during the course of the procedure. Usually a minimum of two fully trained surgeons is required in order to provide an acceptable replantation service. In large centers where several surgeons are available to function on the team, it is advisable that at least one physician, perferably the one who initiates the procedure, remain throughout the course of the entire operation to coordinate the sequence of events. The commitment to replantation surgery requires the availability of a high-quality operating microscope and well-kept microsurgical instruments. Someone should be available to supervise the maintenance of these items at all times. In addition, an animal laboratory is required so that the surgeons are able to maintain their practical skills and to develop new techniques before their application to humans.

Just as important as the operative care is the postoperative management. Immediately after surgery the replantation patient requires close observation, so that any clinical deterioration in the status of his replanted part can be recognized and appropriate treatment instituted. During this period, other support personnel are necessary to manage problems arising from the sociological and psychological disruption produced by a replantation. Finally, a hand therapy center with therapists fully skilled in the rehabilitation of patients with difficult problems of the upper extremity may be the most important factor in achieving the best functional result possible.

DEFINITIONS

If a part has been *completely* traumatically divided from the body and has lost all vascular supply and all tissue connection, the situation is defined as a *complete* amputation. If there is *any* tissue connection, such as skin, tendon, or nerve, even though all or some of the part's vascular supply is lost and the part would die from avascularity without reestablishement of arterial or venous flow or both, then the situation is defined as an *incomplete* amputation, or a devascularization.

The reattachment and repair of the vascular and nonvascular tissues of a completely amputated part are referred to as *replantation*. The repair of the vascular and nonvascular tissues of an incompletely amputated part is termed *revascularization*. Thus the repair and reestablishment of adequate arterial and/or venous flow for both categories is correctly termed *revascularization*, while only the repair and reattachment of parts that are initially completely separate should be defined as *replantation*. This distinction is similar to the distinction between Cognac and brandy; that is, all Cognac is brandy, but not all brandy is Cognac.

INDICATIONS AND CONTRAINDICATIONS IN REPLANTATION SURGERY

In determining whether a patient is a candidate for replantation, one must remember that the goal of treatment is to establish better function in the rest of the injured extremity than would occur if the part were left amputated and the wound closed. This requires return of sensation, adequate skin coverage, a limb free of pain, and the ability to position actively the parts of the limb in a functional manner. Consideration must be given to the type and level of injury, the physiologic age of the patient, his general health, hand dominance, whether the amputation involves single or multiple digits, and the psychological and socioeconomic considerations as well. Many surgeons believe that age is not a major consideration in the evaluation of a patient for replantation.[28,47,80] Systemic disease is not necessarily an absolute contraindication but may influence aftercare and the results.[28] In evaluating the multiply-injured hand one must take care to evaluate the hand in light of other possible concurrent injuries to the same or other extremity. In reconstruction of the hand, attempts should be directed toward achieving at least a thumb, the first web space, and two opposable digits.[26] To accomplish this, one frequently needs to be innovative and to improvise by replanting the best parts in their best sites.

Sophistication in technique has made many amputated parts replantable, but from a functional standpoint, this may not be of benefit to the patient. An effort must be made to discuss with the patient the exact magnitude of his injury, the nature of the surgery, the required period of hospitalization, and the rehabilitative program required after surgery. The alternative methods of treatment must be discussed in detail. Consideration must be given to the needs and motivation of the patient. In the end, however, it is the surgeon who must decide whether to proceed with replantation. The surgeon should not be forced into replanting a part that will not be of functional benefit to the patient.

There is general agreement that any patient with a thumb, multiple-digit, or partial-hand amputation should be considered a candidate for replantation (Fig. 62-1). A child with an amputation of any part, even a single digit, is a reasonable candidate for replantation. Replantation of isolated digits distal to the proximal interphalangeal (PIP) joint is recommended by May,[48] Kleinert,[28] Tamai,[76] and Urbaniak.[81] They base their support for this view on the fact that functional results are generally good, there is reasonable sensory return without neuromas, which might be present after an amputation, and the operating time is usually less than for a more proximal amputation.

Contraindications to digital replantation and revascularization include severe crush or mangle injuries; injuries at multiple levels in the same digit (Fig. 62-2); medical illnesses that make the patient a poor surgical risk; peripheral vascular disease secondary to diabetes, atherosclerotic cardiovascular disease, and so on; mental instability; and injuries in which individual digits are amputated proximally to the flexor digitorum superficialis insertion (except possibly in females and musicians). Other contraindications to replantation surgery include life-threatening associated injuries, warm ischemia time greater than 12 hours, extreme contamination, and previous injury or surgery to the am-

putated part. As mentioned, age is not always considered a contraindication to microvascular surgery; replantations have been attempted in patients from ages 10 weeks[80] to greater than 72 years.[63]

Frequently it is not possible to determine whether a part will be acceptable for replantation until it has been appropriately prepared and examined under the operating microscope in the operating room. Two clinical signs that indicate a poor prognosis for successful replantation are the "red-line" sign[25] and the "ribbon" sign.[83] The red-lign sign, which is visualized on the skin of the amputated part, represents extravasation of blood along a neurovascular bundle, demonstrating a shearing force applied over the length of the neurovascular bundle. The ribbon sign, visualized under the operating microscope, is pronounced tortuosity of the neurovascular bundle secondary to avulsion and represents a relative contraindication to vascular repair requiring resection of the injured length of vessel and vein grafting. Avulsion injuries produce longitudinal trauma to the digital vessels, accounting for the presence of the ribbon and red-line signs. In one series they accounted for 80% of the reoperation rates.[57] Avulsion injuries also carry a poor prognosis because of poor sensory return in avulsed nerves.

Considerations in regard to major limb replantations or revascularizations are similar to those in regard to digital replantation. Although technically major limb replantation may be easier than digital replantation because of the larger size of the vessels, the functional recovery may not be nearly so good, particularly in adults. Pertinent information that is necessary to evaluate in connection with major limb replantation is as follows: age of the patient, occupation, hand

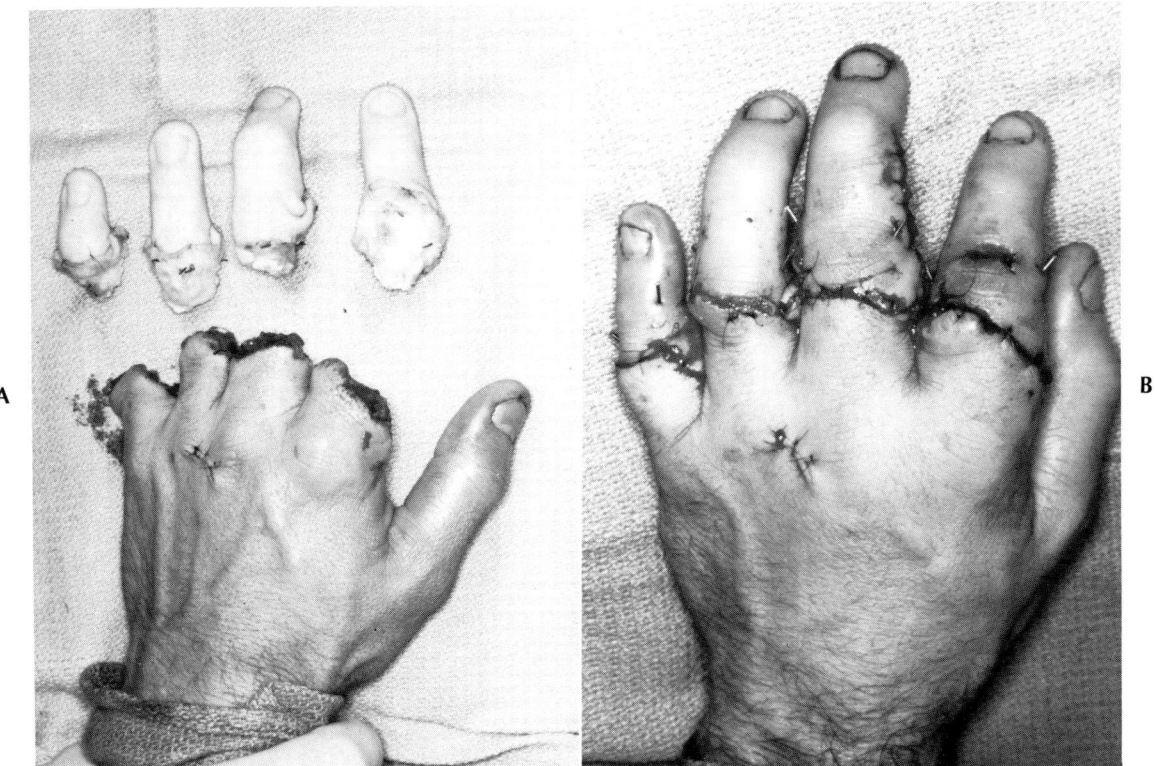

Fig. 62-1   **A,** Complete amputation of four digits of left hand in a belt and pulley in 25-year-old man. **B,** Replantation with primary repair of all structures of all four digits.

Continued.

Fig. 62-1, cont'd **C,** In immediate postoperative period, long finger developed vascular thrombosis but patient would not consent to surgical reexploration. Digit proceeded to develop avascular necrosis, as shown here 3 weeks after surgery. **D,** Roentgenogram 3 weeks postoperatively showing crossed Kirschner-wire fixation of proximal phalangeal fractures of index and ring fingers and fusion of proximal interphalangeal joint of small finger. **E** and **F,** Result 16 months after replantation. Patient refused secondary capsulotomies and tenolyses to improve range of motion and function.

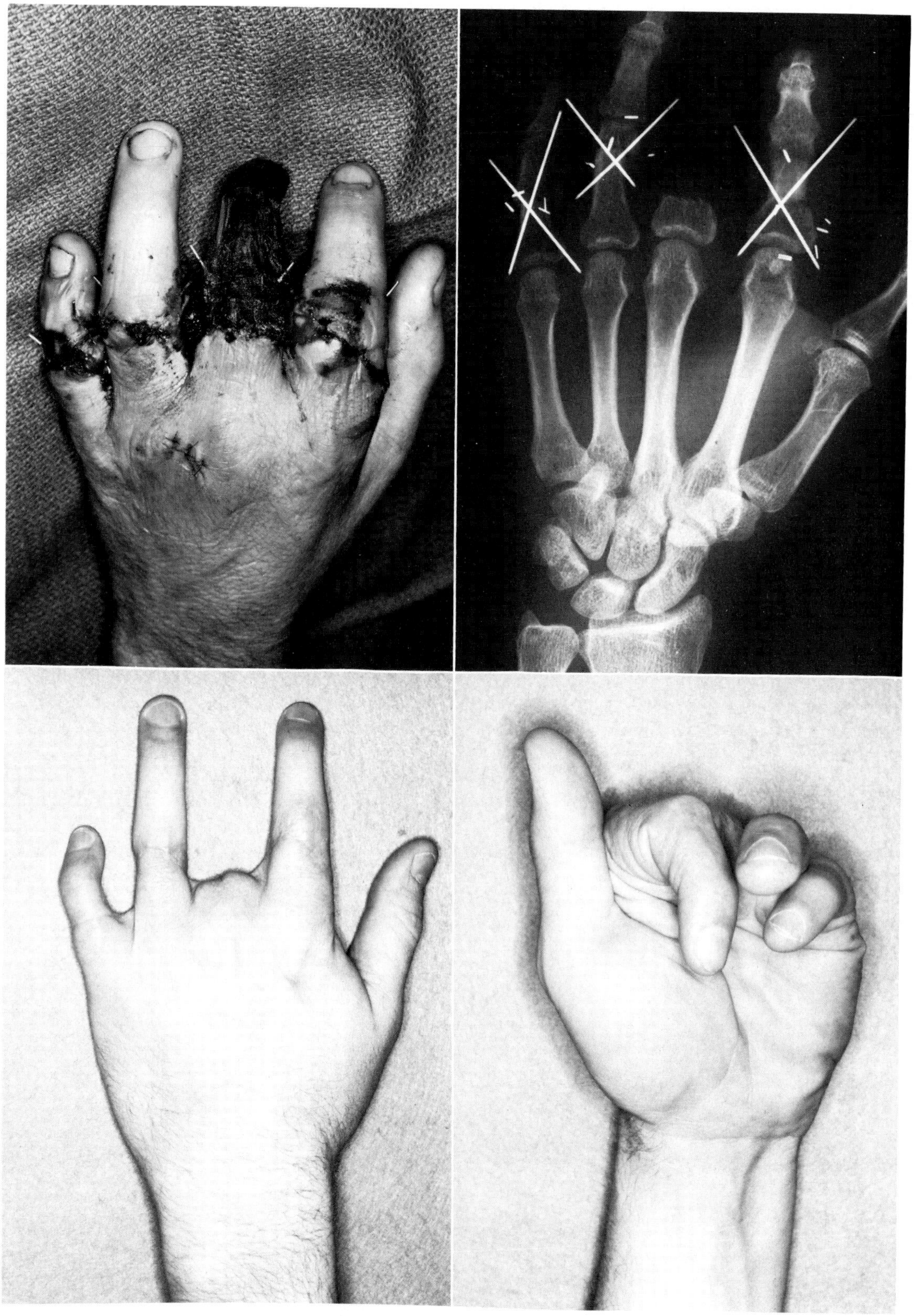

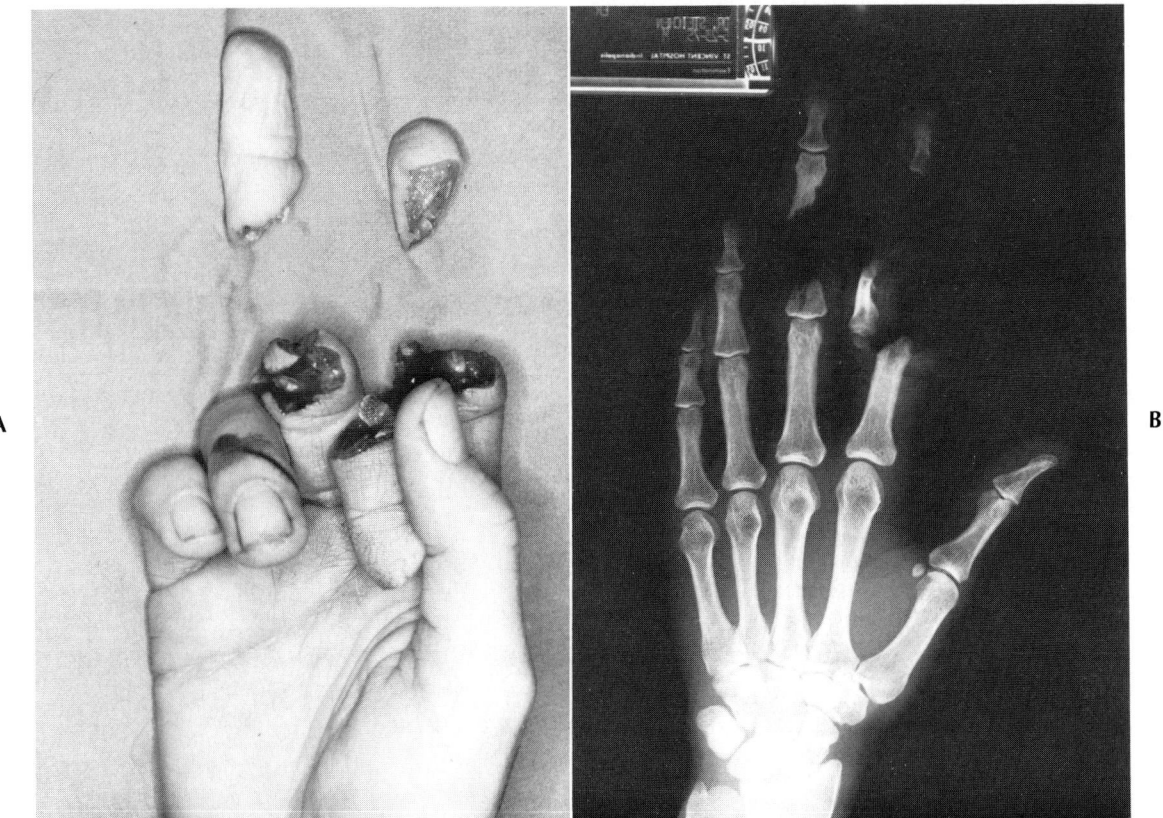

Fig. 62-2 **A,** Woman, 34 years of age, with multilevel amputation of her left index finger and single-level amputation of the long finger caused by a lawnmower injury. **B,** Roentgenogram of injury. Index amputation and devascularization were considered a contraindication to multilevel joint, nerve, and vessel injuries. Long finger was replanted but failed.

dominance, mechanism of injury, associated injury to the other extremities, injuries at other levels of the same extremity, and ischemia time.[46] Children have had the best results in major limb replantation.[43,52] Morrison has suggested an arbitrary upper age limit of 50 years in considering patients for major limb replantation.[52] Sharp amputations occur less frequently in major limb replantations than in digital replantations, but they certainly have a better prognosis than crush or avulsion injuries. Major limb amputations involve higher energy level injuries and subsequently greater soft-tissue injury at the site of amputation. Another factor to consider in major limb replantations is that muscle tissue, which is necessary to make the limb functional, may frequently be traumatically devascularized and crushed. If there has been extensive destruction, devascularization, or contamination of this tissue, then replantation may be contraindicated. Although concomitant injuries in the amputated limb must be taken into consideration, they may be repairable and the limb may be a candidate for replantation. Ch'en has reported on 10 cases involving two-level injury in which limbs were replanted, with six limbs subsequently surviving.[9] Other authors are in agreement that in certain cases two levels of injury of a major limb may not be a contraindication to replantation.[43] However, we believe that in most cases other than those involving children, two-level injury in the same extremity is certainly a contraindication to replantation, because of the poor prognosis for functional return. As with digital replantation, it is not possible to

determine before one enters the operating room whether a major limb replantation is possible or indicated. Certainly if arterial flow is established and most of the muscular compartments of the limb are not perfused, replantation should not proceed.

Indications for revascularization are quite straightforward when there is only a loss of circulation or the injuries to other soft tissues are repairable. With devascularization of the multiply-injured hand, the considerations in regard to proceeding with surgery are the same as they would be in the case of the same injury with complete amputation. If the decision is made to proceed with surgery, an attempt should be made to reestablish the circulation to all parts of the hand, which will be needed for function or which might be useful in later reconstructive efforts.

DIGITAL REPLANTATION: INITIAL MANAGEMENT

The persons caring for the injured patient at the scene of the accident must be trained to recognize potential replantation candidates. In all cases, the amputated part should be retrieved and brought to the hospital for examination by the physician. Initial care of the amputated part involves placing it in a sponge or cloth moistened with water or a physiologic solution and then placing it in as sterile a container as possible, such as a plastic bag or jar. The plastic bag should be placed in iced fluid to reach a chilling temperature somewhere around 4°C. Dry ice should never be used! Care of the amputation site involves topical irrigation with a physiologic solution and attainment of hemostasis with a pressure dressing. It is rare that in digital amputations or amputation of the extremity distal to the wrist that hemostasis cannot be accomplished with the use of a pressure dressing. Appropriate cold preservation of the amputated part is the key to its functional survival; parts appropriately managed have been replanted as long as 37½ hours after the injury. Transportation of the patient and the amputated part from the scene of the accident to a replantation center should be as expedient as possible.

In the emergency room, the patient should be managed with the same care and attention as any other emergency patient. A detailed history should be taken of the accident, so that information is available as to the time of the injury, the mechanism of injury, and whether other injuries were sustained. Other information relevant to making the decision to replant an amputated part consists of the age of the patient, hand dominance, occupation, past medical illnesses, and history of previous injury to the amputated part. A complete physical examination should be performed to establish the patient's ability to withstand lengthy surgery and to determine whether any other injuries that might be life threatening to the patient are present. An x-ray examination should be performed on both the amputated part and the amputation stump. Laboratory procedures of importance include a chest roentgenogram, an electrocardiogram (if the patient is of the appropriate age), hematocrit, urinalysis, prothrombin time, partial thromboplastin time, and type and cross-match for blood. Other laboratory studies may be indicated in specific patients. Before a final commitment is made for replantation, it is important that the patient and his family be informed of the potential surgery, the magnitude of the surgery, the economic considerations involved, the time commitment involved, the potential need for secondary procedures, and a realistic assessment of potential function.

MAJOR LIMB REPLANTATION: INITAL MANAGEMENT

Accidents producing major limb amputations are usually of a greater magnitude than those causing digital amputations and are therefore more likely to result in associated injuries, which might be life threatening. It is important that these injuries be recognized and managed appropriately. Proper preparation of the amputated limb and expedient transportation of the part is of even greater importance in major limb amputations. The reason is that the more proximal the amputation, the greater the amount of muscle tissue contained in the amputated part. Muscle tissue has a poor tolerance for ischemia, incurring irreversible injury after warm ischemia time exceeds 6 hours. With appropriate cooling of the amputated limb, successful major limb replantations have been performed in China more than 30 hours after the original injury.[7,85] The importance of cooling is that it decreases tissue metabolism, the tissue oxygen requirement, and the production of toxic waste products.

Significant blood loss from the stump after a major limb amputation is more likely to be a problem than after a digital amputation. In most cases, because of retraction of the severed artery into the surrounding soft tissue, hemostasis can be achieved with the use of an appropriately applied pressure dressing.

The use of a tourniquet should be avoided. In rare circumstances of uncontrolled blood loss, it may be necessary to achieve hemostasis by cross-clamping of the offending artery or vein. But this technique should be only rarely contemplated; it may cause more harm than good, since a vital nerve or other tissue may be irreversibly damaged.

In the management of incomplete amputations of either digits or major limbs, care must be taken to align the part appropriately to correct or avoid any kinking of the residual intact tissue. The wound needs to be properly topically irrigated, dressed, and immobilized to prevent any additional injury to the part. Measures must be taken to chill the devitalized part just as if it were completely detached, so that the effects of ischemia are minimized. Perhaps the greatest threat of exsanguination exists in cases of incomplete amputation, since partial arterial injuries will continue to bleed because of their inability to retract into the surrounding soft tissue.

Management of the patient with a major limb amputation upon arrival in the hospital is similar to that of a patient with a digital amputation. It is important that the patient's tetanus status be determined and appropriately updated and that the patient be started on antibiotics prophylactically.

DIGITAL REPLANTATION: SURGICAL MANAGEMENT

An axillary block performed with a long-acting anesthetic such as bupivacaine (Marcaine) is the most appropriate anesthesia for digital replantation and most cases of major limb replantation distal to the elbow. An axillary block is easily and reliably performed by competent anesthesia personnel, it is a rapid form of anesthetic that can be given to a patient even if he has eaten a full meal before his injury, it avoids many of the problems associated with a long general anesthetic, and it provides a sympathetic block to the extremity. A general anesthetic will be required for children and uncooperative adults. It has been recommended that in cases in which a general anesthetic is administered, the anesthetic be supplemented with an axillary block because of its ability to provide long-lasting pain relief after the general anesthesia is over and to provide a sympathetic block.[58,87] Because replantation procedures tend to be prolonged, it is important that the patient be positioned on the operating table in a comfortable position, with sufficient protective padding. It may be necessary to provide a heating blanket, particularly for children, so that core temperature can be maintained at an appropriate level. Intravenous lines are necessary for fluid and antibiotic administration. In some instances, transfusions will be required. In all cases, a Foley catheter should be placed in the bladder for fluid management and to avoid the disruption of the patient needing to void during the procedure. It is important that consideration be given to surgical preparation of other parts of the body in case other tissues, such as skin or veins, are required during the procedure. If it is necessary, the patient can be administered a short-acting general anesthetic for the period of time necessary to take whatever graft tissue may be required.

It is important that all instruments and equipment required for the procedure be available and in working order. This is particularly true of the microvascular instruments, which one should check regularly to ascertain if all are functioning and without damaged parts.

The procedure should begin with inspection of the amputated part. Our procedure is to take the amputated part and gently irrigate it and scrub it with an antibiotic soap such as hexachlorophene or povidone-iodine (Betadine). Once the part has been cleansed, it should be returned to its bed of ice so that it is kept chilled. Attention should be directed first to inspection of the part, particularly if one is uncertain about whether the quality of the part is such that it can be salvaged. The part should be inspected under high-power loupe magnification or the operating microscope. It should be possible for the surgeon to work on the amputated part while keeping it on a bed of ice, so that the warm ischemia time is minimized. One prepares the amputated part by first identifying and tagging all structures required for repair. If additional exposure is required for finding the neurovascular bundles, lateral midline incisions are made, allowing a volar flap and a dorsal flap to be mobilized. The flexor and extensor tendons are identified and, if necessary, debrided, and a modified Kessler type of repair or other appropriate intratendinous repair using 4-0 synthetic suture is placed into the end of the tendons. Initial bony débridement is performed only to remove contamination and severely comminuted fragments. Dorsal veins are identified and clipped at their most distal ends for later identification and repair. Sometimes it is necessary to explore for volar veins and venae comitantes if adequate dorsal veins are not present.

A two-team approach is used at this point, with one team working on the amputated part while the other team begins preparation of the amputation stump site. Once it has been determined by the team working on the amputated part that it is replantable, measures are taken by the second team to prepare the amputation stump to receive the part to be replanted. If the amputation stump is on a digit, lateral midaxial incisions are made to achieve exposure of the neurovascular bundles. If the level is more proximal into the palm, zigzag incisions are used to obtain additional proximal exposure. At the amputation stump the neurovascular bundles are identified and tagged at their most distal aspect with a clip, with one clip identifying the artery and two clips identifying the nerve. Dorsal veins are identified and tagged. An attempt is made to retrieve the proximal ends of the flexor tendons with minimal trauma to the flexor tendon system. If necessary, additional proximal incisions are made so that the tendons can be retrieved. Once both the flexor and extensor tendons have been retrieved and identified, sutures similar to those described for the amputated part are placed. Bony débridement is again limited to that necessary to eliminate comminution and contamination.

Because of the frequently complex and lengthy nature of the surgery, it is very important that during the procedure, as the parts are being identified, one make a list of the structures that have been identified, describing their condition and their potential for functional utilization.

When confronted with multiple digital amputations, most surgeons would agree that the most important digits should be replanted first. Certainly the thumb takes precedence as the most important digit when it is involved. When possible, each digit should be revascularized individually. This per-

mits the digits awaiting revascularization to remain cool until needed. Occasionally several replanted digits will be connected by skin bridges. Under these circumstances, if it is believed that important lymphatic and venous channels are present within the skin bridge, the digits need to be replanted as a unit, which means that the warm ischemia time may be significant for the last replanted or revascularized finger.

Regarding the order of tissue repair within each digit, we begin with bony fixation, followed by extensor tendon repair, flexor tendon repair, nerve repair, arterial repair, venous repair, and skin closure. There is some controversy regarding the exact order of tissue repair, particularly the order of venous versus arterial repair. Investigators such as Phelps,[61] Kleinert,[28] and O'Brien[55] believe that venous repair should be performed before arterial repair. It is their belief that this will minimize blood loss and minimize swelling after revascularization, allowing better skin closure. They have not found that thromboses occur at the site of the venous anastomosis while arterial repair is being awaited and have found no difficulty with multiple deflations and inflations of the tourniquet during other vascular repairs. Those who advocate repair of the artery before that of the vein are surgeons such as Urbaniak[81] and Lendvay.[32] It is their philosophy that early arterial repair diminishes the effects of ischemia on the digit and also may facilitate identification of veins for repair.

Bone shortening

Most investigators believe that bone shortening should be performed not only to eliminate contamination and comminution but also to permit easy approximation of the damaged soft tissues, particularly the neurovascular bundles.* In most cases of sharp amputations of the digit or amputations involving limited local crush, 0.5 to 1 cm of shortening is required; however, this is dictated primarily by the amount of associated soft-tissue injury. Urbaniak also believes that shortening the digit makes it less likely to "get in the way" postoperatively and thus facilitates its function.[81] Others, such as Tupper[79] and Phelps,[61] believe that only a minimal amount of bone shortening should be performed for elimination of contamination or comminution, unless there is a complete segmental defect of all soft tissues. Bone shortening only to eliminate a gap between the neurovascular bundles may also be managed by appropriate vein and neural grafts. When bone shortening is to be performed, it should always, whenever possible, be done on the distal amputated part rather than proximally, to preserve proximal length in case of failure of the replantation or revascularization.

Bony fixation

A number of methods are used to achieve bone fixation in replantation sugery. Perhaps the simplest method is use of the single longitudinal intramedullary pin, which is advocated by Urbaniak[80,81] and Lendvay.[32] The advantages of this technique are that it is simple and quick, requires minimal local dissection, provides adequate bone stock for approximation, and allows for rotational adjustment while one is aligning and repairing other soft-tissue structures. Rota-

---

*References 28, 30, 40, 55, 81, 86.

tional control is provided through repair of the adjacent soft tissues, particularly the flexor and extensor tendons, or may also be supplemented by a second longitudinal wire or an oblique Kirschner- (K) wire. Placement of this oblique K-wire should be done before any vascular anastomoses, so as not to jeopardize the vascular repairs in any way. Perhaps the most common method of bone fixation is the use of the crossed K-wire. Other available methods of bone fixation include intraosseous wiring or the combination of K-wires and intraosseous wiring as advocated by Lister,[37] small fragment plates and screws as advocated by Meuli[50] and Tupper,[79] and microscrews as developed by Ikuta and Tsuge.[19] Recently a system of intramedullary screw fixation has been developed independently by Tamai[76] and Irigaray[21] and Yamano.[89] The disadvantage of this system is that it is only applicable to complete amputations and not to incomplete amputations. Leung[36] has recently reported on his experience using autograft or allograft intramedullary bone pegs for fixation. He reported on a series of 25 cases of digital replantation or revascularization and 35 toe-to-hand transfers in which this technique was used. He was able to achieve union in all cases and was able to start motion as early as 3 to 4 weeks postoperatively. Bone union was reported as early as 6 to 10 weeks. No supplemental fixation was required, and the technique was useful with fractures and amputations within 0.5 cm of an adjacent joint. Urbaniak, in his series of more than 200 patients with digital replantations, has had a malunion rate of less that 5% and has performed no secondary procedures for non-union after his method of longitudinal intramedullary K-wire fixation.[81]

For bone fixation of complete or incomplete amputations through the metacarpal level, K-wire fixation is usually chosen. For those familiar with small-fragment plate and/or screw fixation, more stable fixation can frequently be achieved with these techniques, allowing earlier mobilization. For amputations through the level of the carpus, proximal row carpectomy with K-wire fixation may be advised.[44] If substantial damage to either the carpus or the distal radius has occurred, the remaining bony surfaces should be prepared in an attempt to achieve an arthrodesis.

Arthrodesis

When the amputation has taken place near or through the level of the metacarpophalangeal (MP) or interphalangeal joint, one must decide whether an arthrodesis needs to be performed. Most surgeons tend to perform arthrodeses of the joint if it is damaged beyond function. O'Brien recommends arthrodesis of the PIP joint of the index finger in a position of 15 degrees of flexion and arthrodesis of the more ulnar digits in approximately 50 degrees of flexion.[55] Phelps advocates PIP arthrodesis at 25 to 30 degrees regardless of the digit and MP arthrodesis in a position of 30 to 35 degrees of flexion.[61] An alternative to formal arthrodesis, usually performed with crossed K-wires or a tension band technique, is to perform a resectional arthroplasty with the possibility of secondary silicone rubber (Silastic) reconstruction or to perform a primary silicone rubber arthroplasty at the time of replantation.[26] Primary silicone rubber arthroplasty has been performed by investigators such as our group; however, the long-term success of this technique is still not clear. Another innovative technique for

management of amputations near or involving the distal or PIP joint is use of a polypropylene intramedullary peg, as develop by Harrison. Such intramedullary pegs provide rapid stabilization with minimal shortening. A single peg is available for the distal interphalangeal joint and is preangled at 25 degrees. The PIP pins are individualized to the index, middle, ring, and little fingers and are also preangled, progressing from 20 degrees for the index finger through 50 degrees for the little finger. The ultimate goal of these pegs is to provide sufficient stability to permit early motion of the digit while still leading to an arthrodesis. Harrison in his original report had a clinically stable bony arthrodesis achieved in 5 out of 12 digits and reported no infections or extrusions related to use of the pegs.[13]

Tendon repair

Extensor tendon repair is performed using figure-of-eight or horizontal mattress sutures of 4-0 synthetic braided suture to bring about end-to-end approximation of the extensor tendons. Care must be taken that both lateral bands are identified and that these structures are repaired; otherwise one will not achieve adequate extension at the proximal or distal interphalangeal joint.

Flexor tendon repair is performed by reuniting the two ends of the flexor tendon by tying together the ends of the previously placed intratendinous sutures. If the digital amputation is proximal to the insertion of the superficialis tendon, both the profundus and superficialis tendons are repaired. An attempt is made in preparation of the tendons to perform as little débridement as possible—only the amount necessary to rebalance correct tendon length after shortening. The intratendinous suture may be supplemented by a circumferential suture of 6-0 or 7-0 nylon, if necessary, to achieve a smooth repair. The tendons should be handled as gingerly as possible, just as if one were doing an isolated tendon repair. Tendon adhesions and lack of flexor tendon gliding constitute one of the major postoperative problems after replantation surgery, and probably not enough attention to detail is paid while one is performing repair of the flexor tendons (Fig. 62-3). Repair of the flexor tendons may be delayed until after the neurovascular repairs have been performed, because reapproximation of the flexor tendon does tend to put the digit in a position of flexion, which may make subsequent repairs difficult. If the flexor tendon system is not optimal for primary repair, plans should be made for secondary staged tendon reconstruction with silicone rubber rods and tendon grafting.[81] Primary placement of silicone rubber tendon rods has been suggested by Scott,[64] Morrison,[53] and Lendvay.[32,33] Lendvay did report a 20% removal rate after inital placement, but this apparently resulted in no compromise to the digit, and subsequent replacement of the silicone rubber rods without difficulty was possible.

Nerve repair

Many surgeons believe that nerve repair should be performed before arterial repair, because it can be done in a field free of blood. Until now there is no evidence to demonstrate that ischemia time in the appropriately cooled digit affects the quality of sensory return after primary nerve repair in digital replantation.[12,27,57]

In replantations distal to the wrist, nerve repair is per-

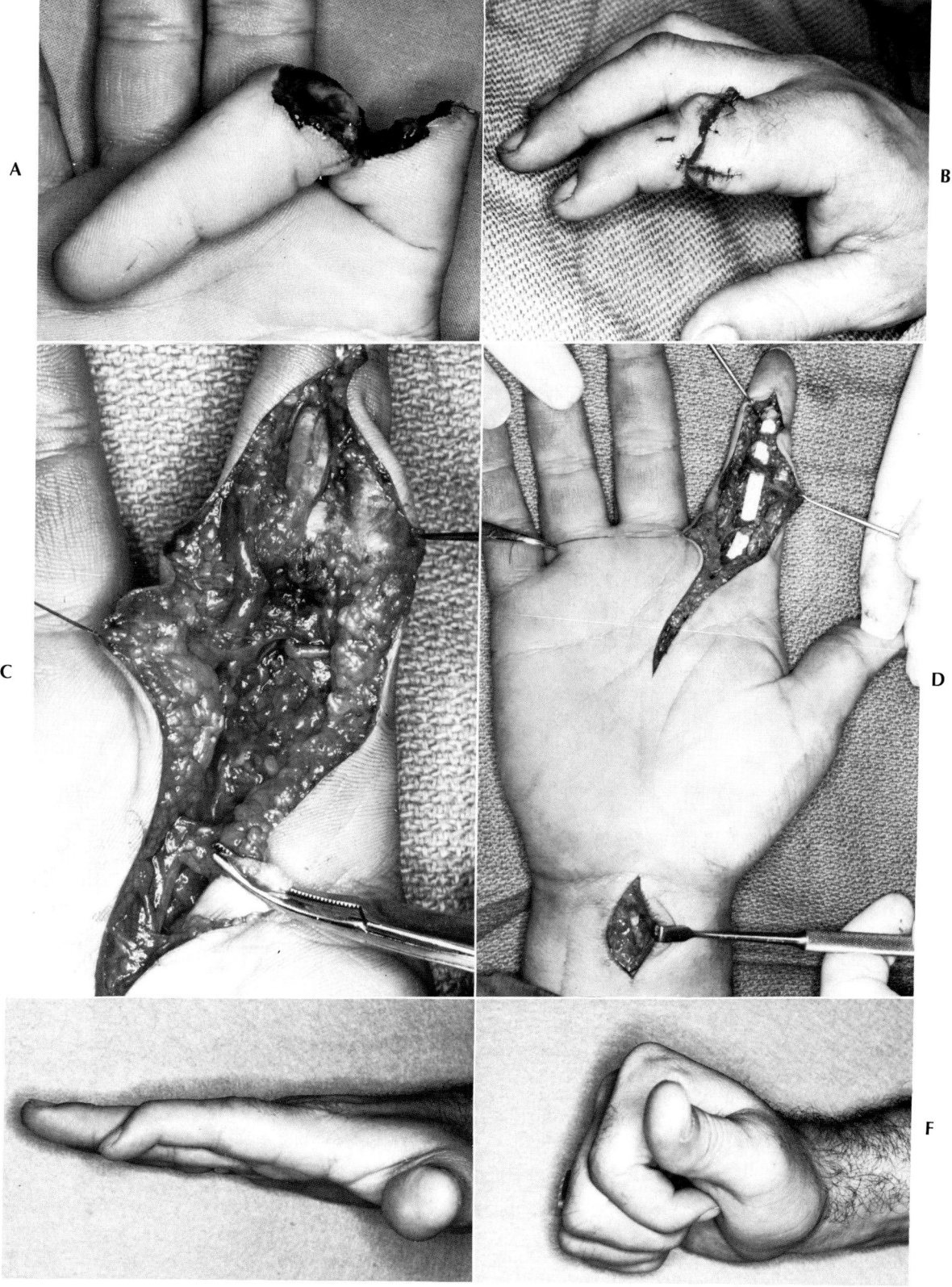

Fig. 62-3   A, Power-saw injury with complete devascularization and incomplete amputation of right index finger in 25-year-old butcher. **B,** Revascularization with primary repair of all structures. **C,** Seven months postoperatively, patient had achieved good passive range of motion but no active flexion, and surgical exploration revealed rupture of repaired flexor tendons. **D,** Two-stage flexor tendon reconstruction was performed with insertion of silicone rubber rod followed by later free-tendon graft. **E** and **F,** Final motion as seen 2 years postoperatively, with some remaining cold sensitivity.

formed with interrupted sutures of 10-0 or 9-0 nylon. The amount of débridement of the nerve required before repair is determined by the nature of the original injury. Using the operating microscope, the surgeon needs to resect the nerve to a level where normal-looking fasciculi with surrounding epineurium are present. It is frequently difficult to identify healthy neural tissue in the acute situation, and especially in avulsion injuries, large defects may be present between two healthy ends of the nerve. For this reason it may be necessary to harvest nerves for interpositional grafting. Available donor sources are the lateral and/or medial antebrachial cutaneous nerves of the forearm, the dorsal sensory branch of the ulnar nerve at the wrist, the sural nerve from either leg, and possibly a digital nerve harvested from a nonreplantable digit. Based on past experience with replantations, primary end-to-end nerve repairs perform much better than secondary repairs.[64,87] It has not yet been determined, however, that primary nerve grafts perform as well. Secondary nerve repairs are complicated by the tremendous amount of scarring that occurs about the unrepaired neuromas and gliomas, which puts the digit at some risk for potential injury to its repaired blood supply.

Arterial repair

The basic principle of arterial repair is to approximate normal intima to normal intima. With avulsion injuries the extent of longitudinal trauma to the artery may be quite significant, and frequently it is very difficult to identify acutely. An attempt has been made to use intravital stains to identify intimal damage, but this has not been consistently accurate.[61] One must closely inspect the vessel under high magnification with the operating microscope to identify any intimal separation from the media or the presence of thrombus formation on the surface of the intima, either of which suggests vessel damage. No arterial repair should be performed under abnormal tension. If the defect created by débridement of the artery is greater than what would permit a primary anastomosis, interpositional grafting must be performed. Ready sources of vein grafts are the volar surface of the forearm and the dorsum of the foot. One should take care to select a vein that is comparable in size to the artery to which it will be interposed. The vein should be reversed from its normal direction of flow so that any valves that may be present in the graft do not obstruct the arterial flow. Care should be taken not to place an interpositional graft that is too long, since it may lead to kinking and subsequent thrombosis. Sometimes it is possible to avoid the use of a vein graft by mobilizing an arterial pedicle from an adjacent normal digit or digit that is not replantable or by crossed arterial repairs within the same digit. In most circumstances, it is the ulnar digital artery that is the largest and most easily repaired in the thumb or the index finger. Most surgeons believe that an effort should be made to repair both digital arteries in the finger so that its vascularity is improved and an insurance policy should one of the arterial repairs become thrombosed. Some surgeons have intimated that repairing two digital arteries as opposed to one results in less cold intolerance and better return of sensation; however, there are no data to support either one of these statements.[12,64]

Arterial repairs distal to the level of the wrist are performed with use of interrupted sutures of 10-0 nylon. In preparation of the vessel, minimal adventitial stripping is performed. Only enough adventitial tissue is mobilized to prevent any loose ends of adventitial tissue from entering the vessel lumen. Approximation of the vessel ends for repair is achieved with an approximator microvascular clamp. Some surgeons, such as Urbaniak, believe that these types of clamps should be used only as necessary and that with appropriate bone shortening or appropriate grafts, vessel anastomoses can be performed without the use of the clamps, with hemostasis being achieved at the time of vascular repair by inflation of the pneumatic tourniquet.[81] Urbaniak,[81] Kleinert,[27] and others[75,77] have reported that intermittent inflation and deflation of the pneumatic tourniquet will not lead to thrombosis at the sites of previous vascular anastomoses, either arterial or venous.

One must determine before vessel repair that there is adequate flow through the proximal limb of the artery. One can do this by release of the pneumatic tourniquet or the microvascular clamp, or both, on the proximal limb of the vessel. In a patient with adequate arterial pressure, a digital artery should have enough pulse pressure to generate a stream of blood that reaches beyond the end of the digit and, one would hope, beyond the operative field. If the arterial stream is sufficiently powerful to reach the end of the hand table, we consider this a positive squirt test and a good prognostic sign for flow. Should good flow not be present, one must determine why this is the case. It may be that there is spasm in the proximal artery, which may be relieved with the use of an appropriate topical vasodilator, such as lidocaine or bupivacaine (Marcaine). Sometimes additional adventitial stripping is beneficial, which produces a local sympathectomy. Occasionally one has to pass a fine dilator into the lumen of the proximal vessel to facilitate the removal of an obstructing clot. It goes without saying that atraumatic technique needs to be used while one performs the arterial anastomoses. Frequent irrigation of the field with a heparinized Ringer's solution is important, to keep the tissues moist and prevent accumulation from developing on the microinstruments, needles, and suture. Once the arterial repair is completed, the pneumatic tourniquet or microvascular clamp is released and good blood flow should return to the digit. Poor flow may exist initially secondary to vascular spasm. This can be relieved by the use of a topical local vasodilator and by topical irrigation with warm physiologic solutions. Restoration of acceptable blood flow to the finger should result in a digit that is pink and that has good capillary refill. The usual number of sutures necessary for a 1-mm vessel ranges from 6 to 10. It is not unusual to have some bleeding at the anastomotic site after release of the clamps, and one can minimize this by gently wrapping adjacent soft tissue about the anastomosis or using a small piece of background material folded over the anastomosis.

Venous repair

Venous repair is performed in a manner similar to arterial repair, although it is technically more difficult because of the thinner, more friable nature of the walls of the veins. It is necessary to perform a venous repair that unites normal venous intima to normal venous intima. Débridement of the vessel ends must be performed before repair. In most digital replantations, the major veins will be found on the dorsum of the finger, although occasionally only a volar vein or vena comitans will be found for repair. Large gaps between vessel ends are best bridged with vein grafts. No venous repair should be performed under tension. Occasionally it is possible to swing over a venous pedicle from an adjacent digit, although one must do this without jeopardizing the venous drainage of the donor digit. An approximating clamp may be used during the venous repair, but great care must be taken to avoid injury to the vessels with the use of this clamp. The recommended ratio of venous to arterial repair is 2:1.[64,81,87] The minimal number of veins repaired per digit should be two.[74] If interpositional venous grafts are necessary to repair the veins without tension, it is important to remember not to reverse the vein graft from its original orientation.

Wound closure

Wound closure at the end of a replantation can be quite difficult because of several factors. Sufficient skin may not be present because of loss from the original injury or removal with débridement. Local swelling after revascularization may prevent closure. No attempt should be made to close skin under tension. Skin should be loosely approximated so that constriction of the vascular repairs is prevented. Circular wounds can be broken up by Z-plasties. If lateral midaxial incisions have been used, no closures of these incisions will be necessary so long as the arterial repairs are appropriately protected by overlying soft tissue. An attempt should be made to provide coverage for any exposed arterial or venous repairs. When this is not possible, split-thickness skin grafts can be applied over vessel repairs.[26,40,64,96] In rare circumstances, there may be indications for performing local flap coverage, such as a dorsal rotation flap or cross-finger pedicle flap, or even for constructing a distant pedicle flap for coverage. The problem with employing such flaps is that should vascular compromise occur during the postoperative period, operative intervention is somewhat hindered by the presence of the flaps.

Thumb replantation

Replantation of a thumb presents several special technical problems. For one thing, preservation of length is the key. Any bone shortening that is being performed to achieve soft-tissue approximation should be done on the amputated part, so that should the replantation fail, the patient will still be left with a stump of maximum bone length.

Reestablishing arterial supply to the thumb can be difficult, because of the anatomy of its blood supply and the difficulty involved in positioning the thumb under the operating microscope at the time of repair. Although in 80% of patients, the princeps pollicis artery will arise from the first palmar metacarpal artery, remember that some patients will have a substantial contribution either from the superficial palmar arch or from the first dorsal metacarpal artery.[60] Usually it is necessary to repair the ulnar digital artery, because frequently the radial digital artery of the thumb is quite small and seemingly clinically insignificant. For amputations or revascularizations distal to the midportion of the proximal phalanx, it is usually possible to achieve a primary end-to-end digital artery repair. For more proximal amputations, however, this is frequently not possible, or if large segmental defects are present because of avulsion injuries, vein grafting should be contemplated. Shafiroff has

recommended that in these circumstances the distal amputated part be prepared as any other amputated digit is prepared for replantation, with appropriate identification of the neurovascular bundles and preplacement of intratendinous sutures. He then sews any required vein grafts into position to the digital arteries and dorsal veins. The amputated thumb is stabilized and its tendons are repaired. It is now possible to take the previously placed arterial vein graft and to anastomose it into either the dorsal branch of the radial artery or into the superficial palmar arch.[67] In Schlenker's series of thumb replantations, 49 patients underwent primary repair of their digital vessels, but 15 patients required vein grafting for arterial reconstruction. He did this by performing an end-to-side proximal anastomosis with the dorsal branch of the radial artery and then taking the vein graft through the first web to the digital arteries, where either an end-to-end or end-to-side anastomosis was performed with the digital arteries, depending on the size discrepancy between the digital arteries and the vein graft. In no cases in which a distal end-to-end vein-graft arterial anastomosis was performed did the cul-de-sac at the end of the vein graft lead to failure of the replant.[63] Another technique that is sometimes used to provide an arterial supply to the thumb is to mobilize an arterial pedicle, such as the radial digital artery from the index finger, with enough length for anastomosis into the distal digital artery of the amputated thumb.[79] Frequently the radial digital artery of the index finger is quite small, and one may need to take the vascular pedicle from another digit, such as the middle finger. This technique has been proposed by Lobay, who transfers the ulnar neurovascular bundle of the middle finger to the ulnar neurovascular bundle of the thumb in cases of thumb avulsion. Using this technique, he has been able to increase his survival rate from 54% to 85%. Use of the ulnar digital nerve from the middle finger to provide innervation to the ulnar aspect of the thumb has not improved sensation in the thumb, and in all cases patients have interpreted stimulation of the ulnar border of the thumb as involving the middle finger.[38]

MAJOR LIMB REPLANTATION: SURGICAL MANAGEMENT

From a surgical standpoint, major limb replantations are quite similar to digital replantations. When possible, an axillary block is used for upper extremity major limb replantations, although with more proximal amputations a general anesthetic is needed. As with digital replantation, when the patient is being prepared and draped it is important to contemplate the possible need for tissue graft donor sites and to prepare these areas. A team approach is valuable in minimizing ischemia time, with one team preparing the amputated part while the other team prepares the recipient stump.

The major difference between a digital replantation and a more proximal major limb replantation is the presence of muscle. This is a tissue that tolerates trauma and ischemia very poorly, yet its presence and survival are crucial for producing a funcitoning extremity. The key to achieving a successful major limb replantation is to perform an adequate débridement and to achieve revascularization of the extremity as quickly as possible. It is extremely important that both the amputated part and the amputation stump be examined quite closely as the structures are being identified and tagged. If substantial muscle damage has occurred beyond the point where function will be possible after replantation, the replantation should not proceed. Another important consideration is the status of the nerves, and the mechanism by which the major limb amputation occurred. Although in the young child one can be quite aggressive about major limb replantation, in the adult the presence of nerve avulsion is an ominous sign and needs to be considered in the decision to proceed further with replantation.

In the past, major limb replantation has proceeded first with bone débridement and stabilization. The amount of bone resection is dictated by that necessary to achieve soft-tissue approximation. Resection of as much as 18 cm of bone has been performed in major upper limb replantations. The techniques of bone stabilization that are the most rapid rather than the most rigid have generally been used, in an effort to minimize warm ischemia time. For that reason, the techniques of fixation have usually been simple screw fixation, crossed K-wire technique, or intramedullary rodding. Recently, Manktelow[45] and Urbaniak[82] have demonstrated that carotid shunts may be placed in both the arterial and venous systems of the replanted major limb, thereby revitalizing the limb and allowing more time to achieve a rigid bony fixation using A-O technique or other methods as preferred by the surgeon. Once bone stabilization has been achieved, attention can then be directed toward removal of the shunts and replacement with a vein graft or primary anastomosis if possible.[45]

The first surgeons having clinical experience with major limb replantations recommended venous repair before arterial repair.[42,45] The reasons for this were to prevent major blood loss and to minimize swelling. Most surgeons performing major limb replantation in the United States now recommend arterial repair before venous repair. This allows the limb to be revascularized and to be purged of toxic waste products that have accumulated during the ischemia time. Deaths have occurred in this country after revascularization of major limb replants in which venous repair was performed before arterial repair.[41] Wang, from China, recently reported a series of 91 major limb replantations in which venous anastomosis was performed before arterial anastomosis and had no episodes of complications arising from toxic metabolites after revascularization of the replanted limb. He attributed this to adequate cold preservation of the part before replantation.[85]

When revascularization of the replanted limb has been achieved, it is paramount that all muscle groups be inspected regarding their viability. It may be possible that some muscle groups are not adequately perfused, and under these circumstances these muscles should be resected to prevent tissue necrosis and possible severe infection.

Achieving a technically good nerve repair is very important in the success of a major limb replantation, because one is trying to provide a limb that is more functional than a prosthesis. One needs a *sensate* limb with actively movable parts, and this can only be accomplished through reinnervation. One may need nerve grafts to achieve an adequate nerve repair without tension. It may or may not be appropriate to perform a nerve graft as a primary procedure at the time of replantation. If a primary nerve repair or graft is undertaken, one must take care to achieve fascicular alignment.

Muscle repair is performed with absorbable sutures to align the muscle groups. Care should be taken to minimize trauma to the remaining muscular tissue. Adequate muscle tissue must remain to make the limb functional. We cannot overemphasize that the key to survival of a major limb replantation is adequate débridement, so that no necrotic muscle or soft tissue is left behind to serve as a potential source of infection. A primary reason for failure of major limb replantations is necrosis and infection.[52,55,85]

In most cases of upper extremity major limb replantation, fasciotomies are indicated in the forearm, carpal tunnel, and intrinsic muscles. In Wang's series of major limb replantations, 65 upper limb replantations were performed and 10 cases of interosseous contracture developed in patients with ischemia times of only 5 to 9 hours.[85]

Skin closure may or may not be possible. Z-plasties and local flaps may sometimes facilitate coverage of vascular and neural repairs. Split-thickness skin grafts may be of great help in achieving wound coverage; in rare circumstances distant pedicle flaps may be used, but they are not normally recommended.

POSTOPERATIVE MANAGEMENT

Postoperative management for both digital and major limb replantations begins in the operating room with the application of an appropriate dressing. The purpose of the dressing is to provide protective, comfortable positioning of the extremity. The dressing must be such that it is able to accept drainage from the wounds but at the same time provide protection from external contamination. Maintaining a warm environment for the extremity is important for prevention of peripheral vasospasm from cold exposure. The dressing must be applied in such a way that it does not inflict injury on the replanted part from pressure or constriction. This is particularly true when the dressing becomes soaked with bloody drainage. Although the dressing should not be applied overly tightly, it should create a gradient of pressure decreasing distally to proximally to control swelling.

The dressing we apply begins with a nonadherent petrolatum-impregnated dressing that is applied over all wounds but does not overlap. This is followed by fluffed sterile gauze pads that are placed between the fingers and over all exposed wounds. Care must be taken in the placement of any dressing material between the digits, particularly in a digital replantation, so as not to create pressure that might compromise the neurovascular bundles. The fluffed gauze dressing is then supplemented with either foam or polyester fiber (Dacron), and the dressing is completed with a plaster splint applied to one side of the extremity. The plaster splint is held in place with a nontensed elastic bandage.

Postoperative orders should include instructions regarding elevation, antibiotics, anticoagulation, frequency of neurovascular checks, and guidelines outlining circumstances under which the physician should be contacted.

Our recommendation for elevation of digital replantations and distal major limb replantations is to use a sling that gently supports the extremity in an elevated position above the heart, with the elbow flexed between 45 and 60 degrees. Phelps recommends avoiding elevation greater than 30 degrees. He believes that at this point, hydrostatic resistance to flow may jeopardize circulation to the extremity.[61] Care must be taken to watch that the elbow is not overly flexed, which might create obstruction to venous drainage.

An antibiotic in the form of a cephalosporin is begun preoperatively and administered for at least 10 days during the postoperative period. Additional oral antibiotics may be indicated in appropriate circumstances.

During the infancy of replantation surgery, great attention was paid to anticoagulation, based primarily on the results of animal experimentation in which survival was improved with the use of anticoagulants.[14] Initial recommendations were the use of aspirin, low-molecular-weight dextran, dipyridamole (Persantin), and continuous systemic heparinization, with the partial thromboplastin time placed at one and a half to two times normal. It was found that heparinization that was begun intraoperatively frequently lead to significant postoperative bleeding. This was somewhat lessened when heparinization was begun 24 hours postoperatively. As surgical techniques in replantation surgery improved, however, it became apparent that the need for extensive anticoagulation was not necessary. Most surgeons now use primarily aspirin or low-molecular-weight dextran, or both, as protection against vascular thrombosis.[38,48,64] Our regimen is to use 600 mg of aspirin, administered orally twice a day, and 500 ml of low-molecular-weight dextran (LMD) in glucose, given intravenously over 4 hours each day, for 5 to 10 days postoperatively. Some surgeons, such as Bright[3] and Kleinert,[26] still recommend systemic heparinization in replantation of severe injuries or in injuries in which technical difficulties are encountered intraoperatively. For major limb replantation, many surgeons recommend no anticoagulation,[55] although the use of aspirin and LMD is prevalent.

During the immediate postoperative period, the patient is restricted to bed rest and his activities are limited. An attempt is made to minimize pain and anxiety, because both of these may be factors in producing peripheral vasoconstriction. It is important that the patient be provided with adequate pain medication around the clock as needed during the initial postoperative period. It is important that the morale of the patient be maintained through supportive contacts with the nursing staff and the surgical staff. If sedation is required, chlorpromazine hydrochloride, 25 mg given orally three times a day, is usually recommended, because of its associated vasodilatory effects.

During the inital 24 to 48 hours the patient is not fed, so that should it be necessary to return the patient to the operating room this can be done without delay. Once the patient is started on a diet, he is restricted from caffeine-containing products, and during the entire postoperative time he is in the hospital, he is prevented from smoking.

The greatest risk to the replant during the postoperative period is vascular occlusion, which occurs most frequently within the first 10 days after surgery. Over 80% of vascular occlusions will occur within the first 24 to 48 hours.[51] Close monitoring of the replanted part is essential to achieve an early diagnosis of this complication and to take appropriate corrective measures. Attempts have been made to improve on constant monitoring of the replant with the use of devices such as ultrasonic Doppler scanners and digital pulse volume flowmeters. The difficulty with these techniques is that they are not capable of identifying venous obstruction until it has progressed to the point that it begins to compromise arterial

function.[3] Constant-temperature probe monitoring has been used effectively by Urbaniak.[82] He uses a three-probe system in which one probe is applied to the replanted digit, one to an adjacent normal digit, and one to the dressing to achieve an ambient temperature. Stirrat[73] reports that normal digital temperature after a replantation is usually 30° to 35° C in the uninjured digit. During the initial postoperative phase, the digital temperature of a replanted digit is frequently greater than that of the normal digit. Thrombosis should be suspected if the temperature of the replanted digit drops more than 2.5° C while the control digit remains unchanged, if the replanted digital temperature drops below 30° C for more than 1 hour, or if the control digit temperature drops below 30° C without an obvious cause. In Stirrat's reported series using temperature monitoring, no replanted digit with a continuous temperature drop below 30° C for more than 12 hours survived.[73]

A healthy replanted digit is warm, it is pinker than a normal digit, and it demonstrates a rapid capillary refill. The pulp of the digit will feel full, with good turgor. Arterial occlusion should be suspected if the digit becomes cool and pale, loses turgor, or demonstrates slow capillary refill. Venous obstruction is usually present if a finger takes on a bluish purple hue, has a drop in temperature, and demonstrates a very brisk capillary refill. Stirrat has been able to correlate these subjective clinical findings with objective temperature changes detected by surface monitoring in replanted digits.[73]

If it is suspected that the digital replant is failing secondary to vascular occlusion, appropriate measures must be taken to correct this. The initial measure is to check the dressing for constriction, usually resulting from hardened blood-stained dressings adjacent to the site of vascular repair. On occasion, adjustment of the position of the arm will improve its circulation. If arterial occlusion is diagnosed, the arm should be lowered below the heart. If venous occlusion is diagnosed, the extremity should be elevated. It is important to rule out diffuse peripheral vascular shutdown as the cause of diminished circulation in the replanted part. At this point temperature monitoring may be helpful, by allowing identification of a drop in temperature of the normal digits. Diffuse peripheral vascular shutdown may result from inadequate hydration, blood loss, pain, anxiety, offending agents such as caffeine and nicotine, or a drop in core temperature. If conservative corrective measures fail to improve the circulation of the replanted part, the patient should be returned immediately to the operating room for exploration of his neurovascular repairs. Frequently, the administration of a stellate ganglion block (in a nonheparinized patient) and a dressing change will result in a return of normal circulation to the replanted part. Under no circumstances should a major dressing change be performed without the benefit of a stellate block, since digits have been lost secondary to vasospasm occurring during dressing change within the first 3 postoperative weeks. Usually the clinical appearance of the digit and its course of demise give some indication about whether the obstruction is arterial or venous. The change in blood flow must be diagnosed early, however, because the pale state of arterial occlusion will soon become cyanotic and will then be difficult to distinguish from venous occlusion.

The hospital stay for a replantation is a minimum of 5 to

10 days. After 3 or 4 days of bed rest, the patient's activities are progressively liberalized. The low-molecular-weight dextran is usually stopped after 5 days, but aspirin is continued for a total of 3 weeks postoperatively. Moderate elevation is usually maintained at all times, and dietary and smoking restrictions continue throughout hospitalization. Phelps has cautioned that the replant must be protected against cold exposure for at least 2 to 4 weeks postoperatively.[61]

A dressing change is not routinely performed until 3 weeks after surgery. At this point, the dressing can be safely removed with minimal concern about vasospasm affecting the viability of the replanted part. At this stage sufficient healing of all involved tissues has taken place to initiate a rehabilitation program. Because open wounds may still be present, continued wound care may be required. Active range-of-motion (ROM) exercises may be started if there is adequate skeletal fixation. Protective static splinting is performed. By 6 weeks postoperatively, passive ROM exercises may be initiated, as well as dynamic flexion and extension splinting, with overnight static splinting. Remember that the replanted part is anesthetic and that passive motion and dynamic splinting should be performed only by persons who are knowledgeable in the use of these techniques and familiar with replantation rehabilitation. Postoperative swelling is common and needs to be managed with appropriate digital and extremity wrapping. Continued elevation remains an important defense against swelling during the rehabilitative phase. Steichen[72] has divided the rehabilitative phase of replantation into three parts. The first 3 weeks represents the immobilization phase. The period 3 to 6 weeks after replantation represents the early mobilization phase. The period 6 weeks to 6 months postoperatively represents the late mobilization phase. Other authors, such as Ikuta[18] and Lendvay,[36] advocate the initiation of therapy on the first postoperative day.

In major limb replantations, the emphasis in therapy will depend on the level of the amputation and the extent of denervation. Distal forearm replantations with functioning proximal muscle bellies will require therapy directed at reestablishment of tendon gliding and active motion of the wrist and more distal joints. In the more proximal major limb replantations, emphasis needs to be placed on maintaining passive motion of the distal joints while reinnervation of the motor units is being awaited.

COMPLICATIONS OF REPLANTATION SURGERY

The most commonly reported complication of replantation surgery and the most common cause of failure in replantation surgery is vascular occlusion.[55,78] Morrison has stated that arterial occlusion is more common than venous occlusion.[51] In the experience of 130 digital replantations in 100 patients reported by Morrison and O'Brien,[51] 49 cases of thrombosis occurred. Thirty-four patients were returned for revision, and at that time, 22 arterial thromboses were documented, 6 were venous, and 6 digits were indeterminate. Other investigators, however, believe that venous obstruction is the more common cause of failure in digital replantation. In Leung's series, 20 digital replantations were reported in 10 patients. Venous congestion was found in 11 of 20 patients versus arterial thrombosis in only 6 of 20 patients.[35] Weiland in 1978 reported on a series of 86 replantations performed in 71 patients. In this series, there

were 54 unsuccessful replantations, with 68.4% being secondary to vascular thrombosis and 31.4% of undetermined cause. The majority of thromboses were found on the venous side.[86]

The recognition of vascular obstruction has already been discussed. The recommended management, in the event of the failure of conservative measures, is to return the patient to the operating room immediately for exploration. Most surgeons advise complete excision of the failed anastomosis with secondary vein grafting or use of a vascular pedicle brought in from an adjacent normal digit.[40] Salvage after vascular obstruction ranges from 34% in Morrison's series[53] to 50% in Schlenker's[63] series of thumb replantations. Eighty percent of vascular occlusions have been reported to occur within the first 24 to 72 hours after surgery. There have been sporadic cases of vascular failure as late as 12 days.[51,55] If the vascular failure occurs early in the postoperative course or is a catastrophic event, there is a strong indication to return the patient to the operating room for exploration. If, however, the deterioration is gradual and the surgeon believes that his original repair was technically competent, the likelihood of salvage on reexploration is greatly diminished.

The rate of infection is surprisingly small in digital replantations. This has been attributed to the débridement performed before replantation, the frequency of irrigation during surgery, the use of antibiotics intraoperatively and postoperatively, and a loose wound closure. In major limb replantation surgery, infection remains the major cause of failure of the replantation, as well as a devastating complication that potentially can cause death as a result of overwhelming sepsis. The key to avoiding this complication in major limb replantations is thorough débridement of all devitalized soft tissues. If this cannot be performed without compromising the potentail function of the limb, replantation should not proceed. Postoperative bleeding was a more significant complication when heparin was used routinely for anticoagulation. Bleeding can be minimized as a potential complication by meticulous attention to hemostasis before wound closure. It is particularly important that any unsatisfied veins be ligated. Loose wound closure will permit drainage and prevent the accumulation of blood beneath skin flaps. It is important that one apply an appropriate dressing; it must be able to accept any postoperative bleeding without compromising the viability of the replanted part. Isolated instances of digital replantation with only arterial repair and open venous drainage have been reported.[10,66,69] Under these circumstances, it is usually necessary to heparinize the patient and blood loss can run into many units, putting the patient at risk for transfusion complications. It is rare that salvage of a digit is worth the risks inherent in this method, and it is mentioned only to be discouraged.

Postoperative swelling is to be anticipated after replantation, and it is not a complication unless it leads to vascular impairment or compartment syndromes. Compartment syndromes are more likely to occur in major limb replantations. It is important that one keep in mind the possibility of compartment syndromes during the operative procedure, and fasciotomies should be performed routinely. Clinical suspicion of postoperative compartment syndromes can be further documented by the use of the various techniques available for measuring compartment pressures.

Perhaps one final complication that deserves mentioning

is an error in judgment that results in replantation of a digit or limb that becomes a liability to the patient. This can be avoided if one adheres to the guidelines developed through previous clinical experience regarding indications and contraindications for replantation surgery. At this time revascularization is technically possible after nearly all amputations, whether complete or incomplete; however, as the Chinese surgeon Ch'en Chung-Wei has stated "Survival without restoration of function is not success."[5]

Late complications that can occur after replantation include nonunions, malunions, joint stiffness, traumatic arthritis, flexor and/or extensor adhesions, tendon ruptures, neuromas, dysesthesias, and scar contracture.

SECONDARY PROCEDURES

The need for secondary procedures is not uncommon after replantation surgery. In Morrison's review of 130 digital replants in 100 patients, a total of 47 secondary procedures were required among the 96 digits that survived replantation.[53] In Scott's series evaluating digital replantation in 100 patients, over 80% of the patients with surviving replants required secondary surgery, with an average number of operations being 2.6 (range 1 to 4).[64]

The incidence of malunion and nonunion in most replantation series is quite small. Morrison's series contained only 1 nonunion and 10 malunions, none of which were of clinical significance.[53] In Leung's series, there were two rotational malalignments and 1 nonunion out of 16 surviving digital replantations.[35] In Urbaniak's series of over 200 digital replantations, his reported malunion rate was less than 5%.[81] If a nonunion or malunion is present and of clinical significance, it must be treated with open-reduction internal fixation and bone grafting. It is important to perform such a procedure, which requires postoperative immobilization, before one proceeds to other soft-tissue reconstruction, which may require movement of the digits for postoperative rehabilitation.

Joints that were partially destroyed in the initial injury and that proceed to deteriorate require either arthrodesis or silicone rubber arthroplasty.

Arthrofibrosis and tendon adhesions can be anticipated in digital replantations through the classic zone 2, or "no-man's-land." Our management of the stiff hand after replantation surgery is to make as many gains as possible through therapy during the first 6 months after replantation. If at that point the patient has plateaued, attention is first directed to the extensor surface of the hand and to the joint capsules. Dorsal capsulectomies and extensor tenolyses of the appropriate digits are performed along with traction tenolyses of the flexor tendons to check the status of the flexores digitorum profundus and superficialis, followed by intensive hand therapy to maintain active and passive motion gained by these procedures. Once an acceptable result is achieved in passive digital flexion after release of the joint capsules and the extensor mechanism, attention is directed to the volar surface of the hand, where flexor tenolyses and volar capsulectomies are performed when indicated. It is our belief, particularly in regard to the replanted digit, that it is quite dangerous to operate on both the volar aspect and the dorsal aspect of the digit simultaneously, because of the severe swelling that follows and the risk of vascular compromise.

Rarely it may not be possible to perform a primary repair of the flexor tendon injuries, and secondary repair must be performed. Surgeons such as Scott,[64] Lendvay,[32,33] and Morrison[53] have suggested or used silicone rubber rods during the primary surgery in reconstruction of the flexor tendon system.

Any injury that results in paralysis of the intrinsic or thenar muscles may require secondary tendon transfers to restore function.

It is recommended that nerve repair be performed primarily whenever possible in replantations or revascularizations. It has been demonstrated in clinical series that the results of primary neurorrhaphy are better than those of secondary repair.[64,87] Attempting to retrieve the nerve endings from the adjacent scar tissue during secondary repair is technically difficult and may place the vascular supply of the extremity in jeopardy. One of the reasons advocated for digital replantation distal to the insertion of the superficialis tendon is that a nerve repair can be performed with less likelihood of painful neuroma formation than an amputation at that same level would produce.[48] Occasionally, disabling paresthesias occurring after replantation will lead to amputation of the digit, as reported by Morrison[53] and Kleinert.[27]

Secondary procedures may be required for revision of scar contractures, particularly when linear scars cross the volar surfaces of flexor creases. With major limb replantations, and subsequent intrinsic contracture, a tight first web that requires release is not uncommon.[52]

FUNCTIONAL RESULTS IN REPLANTATION SURGERY

Several large replantation centers are now beginning to report long-term results of their replantations. Unfortunately, there is no coordinated list of criteria by which these patients are being judged, and so it is difficult to compare the results of these series. Perhaps the most rigorous criteria put forth in the literature up to now have been those of Kleinert, who believes that functional evaluation of replantations should include sensibility rating, grip strength, range of motion, the presence of cold intolerance and information regarding return to work.[26]

One of the primary goals of replantation surgery is to reestablish sensation in the replanted part. In the series reported by Morrison, 90% of the patients demonstrated two-point discrimination between 4 and 15 mm.[53] O'Brien went so far as to state that the result of sensory return in replantation was as good as simple digital nerve repair.[55] In 1979 Urbaniak reported a series of 187 complete or incomplete amputations. Among the surviving 163 digits, protective sensation was present in 90%, two-point discrimination of 15 mm or less was present in 66%, and two-point discrimination of 10 mm or less was present in 50%.[81] In Scott's series of 38 replanted digits, normal two-point discrimination was believed to be present in 40%, two-point discrimination of 6 to 10 mm was present in 8%, two-point discrimination of 11 to 15 mm was present in 18%, and protective sensation or two-point discrimination greater than 15 mm was present in 34%. In the same series, 55 revascularizations were performed and normal sensation was found in 71% as compared with two-point discrimination of 6 to 10 mm in 24%, two-point discrimination of 11 to 15 mm in 3%, and protective sensation in 2%. Scott's conclusion was that the results of nerve repair in replantation were not as good as in simple nerve repair. Based on his series, he drew a correlation between sensory return, vascularity, age, level of amputation, and the type of injury.[64]

In this series, all patients undergoing replantation complained of cold intolerance, whereas 55% of the revascularization patients complained of cold intolerance. Scott found no relationship between the number of digital arteries repaired and cold intolerance.

Gelberman has examined sensory return in detail in a series of 29 patients with 35 replanted digits. These patients were tested not only for two-point discrimination, but also for constant touch, moving touch, 30 and 250 cps tuning fork perception, heat and cold discrimination, sharp and dull discrimination, and number tracing. Gelberman found that patients with two-point discrimination less than 20 mm were able to perceive the other sensory function tests. In his series, he was unable to find any strong correlation between sensory return and the age of the patient, mechanism of injury, digit involved, ischemia time, or the patency of the ipsilateral artery. Sensory return also did not seem to be dependent on whether one or two arteries were repaired, but was dependent on pulse pressure. Poor sensory return and significant cold intolerance were found in patients whose pulse pressure was less than 70% of that of the normal contralateral digit. In his series, two-point discrimination ranging from 0 to 6 mm was found in 9 patients, from 6 to 10 mm in 7 patients, from 11 to 15 mm in 2 patients, and greater than 15 mm in 17 patients. Based on his experience, he also agreed that digital repair in replantation surgery was not as good as simple digital repair.[12] Both Weiland[86] and Scott,[64] in evaluation of sensory return in their series of digital replantations, have stated that the results of primary neurorrhaphy are better than those of secondary nerve repair.

Few studies have given accurate documentation of return of range of motion to replanted digits. Scott in 1981 presented a series of 38 patients with 65 complete digital amputations and 62 patients with 84 incomplete amputations requiring revascularization.[64] Survival rate in his series of complete amputations was 79%, as compared with 97% in the revascularized digits. Average total active motion (TAM) for 21 replantation and revascularization patients was 120 degrees for the digits and 59 degrees for the thumbs. Less than 180 degrees of TAM is considered poor. Eighty-four percent of the fingers were rated as poor, and only 6% were rated as excellent. Total active range of motion was found to be related to the level of injury (being particularly poor in the zone 2 area), nature of the injury (worse with avulsion injuries), age (worse results being obtained in older patients, and concomitant presence of a fracture (in the revascularization group the presence of a fracture decreased the total active range of motion). In Morrison's series of 130 digital replants in 100 patients, joint stiffness was found to be quite common and PIP joint motion averaged 30 to 70 degrees.[53]

It has been stated that the return of function of a replanted part is related to how much it is needed. Scott certainly found this to be true in his series of digital replantations, since isolated digital replants did not achieve significant function.[64] In contrast to this is May's report of digital replantation distal to the insertion of the flexor digitorum superficialis.[48] He reported on 24 digits replanted in 18 patients. The survival rate in this series was 96%, whereas previous survival rates of replant surgery performed at this

level were 24% as reported by Tamai[76] and 35% as reported by Morrison.[53] Although all had some degree of cold intolerance, the mean two-pint discrimination was 11 mm. Active range of motion at the PIP joint averaged 95 degrees and at the (DIP) joint 9 degrees. Nine of the patients treated were workers, who returned to work in an average of 5.1 months. Among the nine students, return to school was accomplished in 1.7 months. It is intimated in the article that even patients with replantations of the index finger used their replanted digits.[48]

The thumb has been considered the most important digit in priority of replantation; however, the literature contains little information on the functional outcome of thumb replantation. Schlenker[63] reported a series of 51 replantations and 13 revascularizations, with a failure rate of 27%. The failure rate in replantation of the thumb was believed to vary with the nature of the injury and the age of the patient. Among the 47 patients with surving thumbs, 12 secondary procedures were required, including tenolysis, tendon grafts, tendon transfers, neurolysis, nerve grafting, first web release, interphalangeal arthrodesis, bone grafting for a proximal phalangeal nonunion, and amputation for disabling hyperesthesias. Twenty-three patients in this series had amputations of digits other than their thumbs, and in 5 of these, 1 of the fingers was transplanted to the thumb position. Only 3 of the 5 succeeded. Twenty-five patients with surviving replanted thumbs were evaluated in follow-up from 6 months to 3 years after replantation. Two-point discrimination was documented as less than 10 mm in 12 patients and greater than 10 mm in 13 patients. Two of the 3 heterotopic thumbs were available for evaluation, and in both cases only protective sensation was present. Joint motion was obtained in 14 patients, and the range of motion at the interphalangeal joint was found to average from 10 to 45 degrees and that the MP joint from 3 to 32 degrees. Seventy-six percent of the patients employed before their accident returned to work at an average of 7 months after surgery. Among 26 patients interviewed about the function of their thumbs, 10 stated that they used their thumbs more than before, 14 less, and 2 not at all. The most common reason for decreased use of the thumb was loss of motion. The 2 patients who claimed that they did not use their thumbs complained of either paresthesias or weakness. Only 4 of the 26 patients did not complain of cold intolerance. Cold intolerance in this series seemed to be most related to age and not to ischemia time, level of injury, mechanism, or number of vascular repairs.[63]

Few series are present in the literature documenting the functional performance of replantation surgery in children (Fig. 62-4). Van Beck presented a series of 8 patients, but presented only case studies and no functional follow-up.[84] O'Brien reported on a series of 31 replantations in children. Four were major replantations, including an incomplete midpalm and forearm amputation and complete leg and foot amputations, and 27 were digital replantations. In this series, all 4 major replanted parts survived and demonstrated continued growth and return of adequate sensation. The survival rate in the digital replantations and revascularizations was 64.5%. The least successful digit regarding survival was the little finger. Only 1 out of 5 replanted little fingers survived. In this series, survival was found to be correlated with age, the level of injury, and the nature of injury. Digital replantation in children less than 2 years of

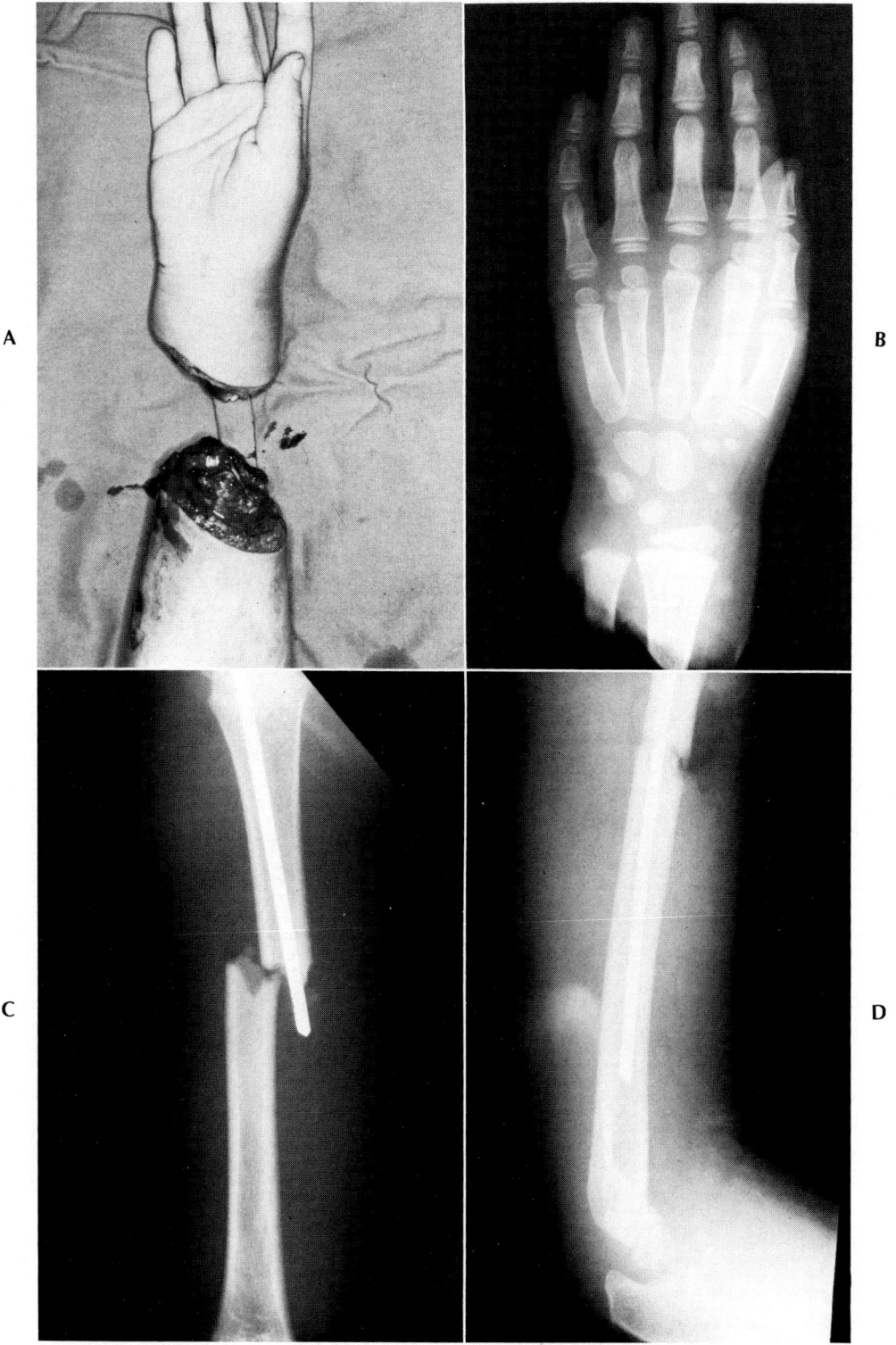

Fig. 62-4   **A,** Boy, 6 years of age, with complete major upper limb amputation caused by a farm-machinery accident. **B,** Roentgenogram showing the level of sharp amputation of the right upper extremity. **C** and **D,** Before replanting of the right wrist and hand, it was necessary to perform an open-reduction internal fixation (ORIF) of an open displaced fracture of the ipsilateral humerus.

Continued.

Fig. 62-4, cont'd **E,** Replantation was performed, with primary repair of all structures, including revision of laceration to prevent a linear scar contracture with circumferential banding. **F** and **G,** Two and a half years postoperatively, replanted hand shows growth and function similar to normal extremity. **H,** Roentgenogram taken 2½ years postoperatively shows normal epiphyseal growth.

age had a survival rate of only 50%, whereas in children greater than 5 years of age the survival rate was 71%. When two-point discrimination could be documented, it was found to be in the range of 2 to 10 mm. Only 4 of 16 had normal motion. Seven patients required secondary procedures, including tenolysis, first-web release, secondary tendon repair, tendon graft, and local flaps.[59]

Wang has recently reported on the results of 91 major limb replantations with a success rate of 77%.[85] The age range in his series was from 2 to 55 years. Ischemia time ranged from 4 to 33 hours, with an average ischemia time of 12 hours. Seventy-two major upper extremity replantations were included in this series, 65 of which were successful. Survival was found to be related to the level of injury and mechanism of injury. Replantations after proximal forearm amputations were found to have the worst survival rate. Causes of failure in this series were seven cases of inability to revascularize the limb, nine postoperative thromboses, and five local complications representing either infection or muscle necrosis. It was reported that venous thromboses were more common than arterial thromboses. Function in these major replanted parts was graded form 1 to 4, or nearly normal to no function. Eighty percent of the surviving replanted limbs were rated as nearly normal or fair in function. Failure to achieve useful function was found to be related to the severity of the initial injury, excessive loss of length, intraarticular fractures, extensive destruction of muscle, irreparable damage to nerves, prolonged ischemia, and inadequate management of soft tissue and bone.[85] Yoshizu presented a series of 99 replantations in 66 patients, which included 20 major upper extremity replantations or revascularizations. The success rate in this series was 92.6%. Evaluation of these major limb replantations demonstrated poor recovery of intrinsic function and only return of protective sensation.[90] Morrison reported on the results of 20 major limb replantations in patients ranging in age from 21 months to 57 years. In this series, there were 16 survivals and 4 failures. All failures occurred in above-elbow amputations associated with avulsion injuries, diffuse crush, ischemia time greater than normal, or subsequent infection. Among the surviving replanted parts in this series were 7 replanted hands and 2 forearms. In the replanted hands, two-point discrimination was documented between 10 and 30 mm, with an average of 17 mm. All patients were found to have light touch and protective sensation. On evaluation of the tendon function in the replanted hands, 2 were found to be nearly normal, 5 required tenolysis, all but 1 had intrinsic paralysis and required opposition transfers, and 5 had first-web contractures. Among the 2 forearm replantations, two-point discrimination was greater than 20 mm. Tendon function was found to be minimal. One pateint was found to have intrinsic contractures.[52]

CONCLUSION

Through technologic advances, surgical experience, and the establishment of reliable criteria for selection of candidates for replantation sugery, most replantation centers are able to achieve success rates of greater than 80% in revascularizing amputated digits and major limbs. As these replantation centers have accumulated their clinical experiences and reported their results, emphasis has evolved from the importance of vascular survival to the establishment of function in the replanted part.

The achievement of the best functional result possible for each patient is dependent on the many factors that have been presented in this review, which has emphasized the nature of the injury to the patient and the surgeon's role in repairing it to the best of his or her ability. The equally important and necessary role of the hand therapist in the patient's rehabilitation is discussed in Chapter 63.

REFERENCES

1. Acland RD and Trachtenberg L: The histopathology of small arteries following experimetnal microvascular anastomosis, Plast Reconstr Surg 60:868, 1977.
2. Bendick PJ and others: A photoplethysmographic technique for detecting vascular compromise: a preliminary report, J Trauma 19:398, 1979.
3. Bright DS and Wright S: Postoperative management in replantation. In American Academy of Orthopaedic Surgeons: Symposium on microsurgery: practical use in orthopaedics, St. Louis, 1979, The CV Mosby Co.
4. Buncke HJ Jr and Schulz WP: Experimental digital amputation and reimplantation, Plast Reconstr Surg 36:62, 1965.
5. Buncke H and others: Replantation surgery in China: report of the American Replantation Mission to China, Plast Reconstr Surg 52:476, 1973.
6. Carrel A and Guthrie CC: Complete amputation of the thigh with replantation, Am J Med Sci 131:297, 1906.
7. Chi Sui-Tan Hospital, Peking, as reported by O'Brien BM: Microvascular reconstructive surgery, Edinburgh, New York, 1977, Churchill Livingstone.
8. Ch'en C-W, Chien Y-C, and Pao Y-S: Salvage of the forearm following complete traumatic amputation: report of a successful case, Chin Med J 82:632, 1963.
9. Ch'en C-W, as reported by O'Brien BM: Microvascular reconstructive surgery, Edinburgh, New York, 1977, Churchill Livingstone.
10. Elsahy NI: Replantation of a completely amputated distal segment of thumb: case report, Plast Reconstr Surg 59:579, 1977.
11. Gelberman RH: A history of microsurgery. In American Academy of Orthopaedic Surgeons: Symposium on microsurgery: practical use in orthopaedics, St. Louis, 1979, The CV Mosby Co.
12. Gelberman RH and others: Digital sensibility following replantation, J Hand Surg 3:313, 1978.
13. Harrison DH and Watson JS: Use of the polypropylene peg for immediate stabilization in digital replantation, J Hand Surg 5:253, 1980.
14. Hayhurst JW and others: Experimental digital replantation after prolonged cooling, Hand 6:134, 1974.
15. Holmgren G: Some experience in surgery of otosclerosis, Acta Otolaryngol 5:460, 1920.
16. Hopfner E: Ueber Gefässnaht: Gefässtransplantationen und replantation von amputirten extremitäten, Arch Klin Chir 70:417, 1903.
17. Horn JS and Lond MB: Successful reattachment of a completely severed forearm, Lancet 1:1152, 1964.
18. Ikuta Y: Microvascular surgery, Hiroshima, 1975, Lens Press.
19. Ikuta Y and Tsuge K: Micro-bolts and micro-screws for fixation of small bones in the hand, Hand 6:261, 1974.
20. Ikuta Y, as reported by O'Brien BM: Microvascular reconstructive surgery, Edinburgh, New York, 1977, Churchill Livingstone.
21. Irigaray A: New fixing screw for completely amputated fingers, J Hand Surg 5:381, 1980.
22. Jacobson JH and Saurez EL: Microsurgery and anastomosis of small vessels, Surg Forum 9:243, 1960.
23. Kleinert HE and Kasdan ML: Anastomosis of digital vessels, J Ky Med Assoc 63:106, 1963.
24. Kleinert HE and Kasdan ML: Salvage of devascularized upper extremities, including studies on small vessel anastomoses, Clin Orthop 29:29, 1963.
25. Kleinert HE, Kasdan ML, and Romero JL: Small blood-vessel anastomosis for salvage of severely injured upper extremity, J Bone Joint Surg 45A:788, 1963.
26. Kleinert HE, Jablon M, and Tsai T-M: An overview of replantation and results of 347 replants in 245 patients, J Trauma 20:390, 1980.
27. Kleinert HE and Tsai T-M; Microvascular repair in replantation, Clin Orthop 133:205, 1978.
28. Kleinert HE and others: Digital replantation: selection, technique and results, Orthop Clin North Am 8:309, 1977.
29. Komatsu S and Tamai S: Successful replantation of a completely cut-off thumb, Plast Reconstr Surg 42:374, 1968.
30. Kutz JE: Preparation for replantation. In Daniller AI and Strauch B, editors: Symposium on microsurgery, St. Louis, 1976, The CV Mosby Co.
31. Lapchinsky AG: Recent results of experimental transplantation of preserved limbs and kidneys and possible use of this technique in clinical practice, Ann NY Acad Sci 87:539, 1960.
32. Lendvay P: Pursuit of function in digital replantation. In Daniel RK and Terzis JK, editors: Reconstructive microsurgery, Boston, 1977, Little, Brown & Co.
33. Lendvay PG: Replacement of the amputated digit, Br J Plast Surg 26:398, 1973.
34. Lendvay PG, as reported by O'Brien BM and MacLeod AM: Digital replantation. In Daniller AI and Strauch B, editors: Symposium on microsurgery, St. Louis, 1976, The CV Mosby Co.
35. Leung PC: An analysis of complications in digital replantations, Hand 12:25, 1980.
36. Leung PC: Use of an intramedullary bone peg in digital replantations, revascularizations, and toe-transfers, J Hand Surg 6:281, 1981.

37. Lister G: Intraosseous wiring of the digital skeleton, J Hand Surg 3:427, 1978.
38. Lobay GW and Moysa GL: Primary neurovascular bundle transfer in the management of avulsed thumbs, J Hand Surg 6:31, 1981.
39. MacLeod AM and O'Brien BM: Replantation surgery in the upper extremity. In Flynn JE, editor: Hand surgery, Baltimore, 1982, The Williams & Wilkins Co.
40. MacLeod AM, O'Brien BM, and Morrison WA: Digital replantation: clinical experiences, Clin Orthop 133:26, 1978.
41. Malt RA and Harris WH: Replantation of limbs, Advancing with Surgery Monograph, Somerville, NJ, 1965, Ethicon, Inc.
42. Malt RA and McKhann CF: Replantation of severed arms, JAMA 189:716, 1964.
43. Malt RA, Remensnyder JP, and Harris WH: Long-term utility of replanted arms, Ann Surg 176:334, 1972.
44. Malt RA, Smith RJ, and May JW Jr: Replantation of the amputated hand. In Daniel RK and Terzis JK, editors: Reconstructive microsurgery, Boston, 1977, Little, Brown & Co.
45. Manktelow RT: American Academy of Orthopaedic Surgeons presentation, Anaheim, Calif, Feb 1982.
46. Matsuda M, Kato N, and Hosoi M: The problems in replantation of limbs amputated through the upper arm region, J Trauma 21:403, 1981.
47. May JW Jr and Gallico GG III: Upper extremity replantation, Curr Probl Surg 17:634, 1980.
48. May JW, Toth BA, and Gardner M: Digital replantation distal to the proximal interphalangeal joint, J Hand Surg 7:161, 1982.
49. May JW Jr: The no-reflow phenomenon in experimental free flaps, Plast Recontr Surg 61:256, 1978.
50 Meuli HC, Meyer V, and Segmuller G: Stabilization of bone in replantation surgery of the upper limb, Clin Orthop 133:179, 1978.
51. Morrison WA, O'Brien BM, and MacLeod AM: Evaluation of digital replantation—a review of 100 cases, Orthop Clin North Am 8:295, 1977.
52. Morrison WA, O'Brien BM, and MacLeod AM: Major limb replantation, Orthop Clin North Am 8:343, 1977.
53. Morrison WA, O'Brien BM, and MacLeod AM: Digital replantation and revascularization: a long term review of one hundred cases, Hand 10:125, 1978.
54. O'Brien BM: Replantation surgery in China, Med J Aust 2:255, 1974.
55. O'Brien BM: Microvascular reconstructive surgery, Edinburgh, New York, 1977, Churchill Livingstone.
56. O'Brien BM and Baxter TJ: Experimental digital replantation, Hand 6:11, 1974.
57. O'Brien BM and MacLeod AM: Digital replantation. In Daniller AI and Strauch B, editors: Symposium on microsurgery, St. Louis, 1976, The CV Mosby Co.
58. O'Brien BM and Miller GDH: Digital reattachment and revascularization, J Bone Joint Surg 55A:714, 1973.
59. O'Brien BM and others: Replantation and revascularisation surgery in children, Hand 12:12, 1980.
60. Parks BJ, Arbelaez J, and Horner RL: Medical and surgical importance of the arterial blood supply of the thumb, J Hand Surg 3:383, 1978.
61. Phelps DB, Lilla JA, and Boswick JA Jr: Common problems in clinical replantation and revascularization in the upper extremity, Clin Orthop 133:11, 1978.
62. Reichert FL: The importance of circulatory balance in the survival of replanted limbs, Bull John Hopkins Hosp 49:86, 1931.
63. Schlenker JD, Kleinert HE, and Tsai T-M: Methods and results of replantation following traumatic amputation of the thumb in sixty-four patients, J Hand Surg 5:63, 1980.
64. Scott FA, Howar JW, and Boswick JA: Recovery of function following replantation and revascularization of amputated hand parts, J Trauma 21:204, 1981.
65. Seidenberg B, Hurwitt ES, and Carton CA: Techniques of anastomosing small arteries, Surg Gynecol Obstet 106:743, 1958.
66. Serafin D, Kutz JE, and Kleinert HE: Replantation of a completely amputated distal thumb without venous anastomoses: case report, Plast Reconstr Surg 52:579, 1973.
67. Shafiroff BB and Palmer AK: Simplified technique for replantation of the thumb, J Hand Surg 6:623, 1981.
68. Shorey WD, Schneewind JH, and Paul HA: Significant factors in the reimplantation of an amputated hand, Bull Soc Int Chir 24:44, 1965.
69. Snyder CC, Stevenson RM, and Browne EZ Jr: Successful replantation of a totally severed thumb, Plast Reconstr Surg 50:553, 1972.
70. Snyder CD and others: Extremity replantation, Plast Reconstr Surg 26:251, 1960.
71. Steichen JB: The microvascular free groin flap. In American Academy of Orthopaedic Surgeons: Symposium on microsurgery: practical use in orthopaedics, St. Louis, 1979, The CV Mosby Co., pp. 279-305.
72. Steichen JB and others: Rehabilitation of the upper extremity replantation patient. In Hunter JM and others, editors: Rehabilitation of the hand, St. Louis, 1978, The CV Mosby Co.
73. Stirrat CR and others: Temperature monitoring in digital replantation, J Hand Surg 3:342, 1978.
74. Strauch B and Terzis JK: Replantation of digits, Clin Orthop 133:35, 1978.
75. Tamai S: Multiple digit replantation. In Daniel RK and Terzis JK, editors: Reconstructive microsurgery, Boston, 1977, Little, Brown & Co.
76. Tamai S: Digit replantation: analysis of 163 replantations in an 11 year period, Clin Plast Surg 5:195, 1978.
77. Tamai S and others: Microvascular anastomosis and its application on the replantation of amputated digits and hands, Clin Orthop 133:106, 1978.
78. Tsai T-M: Experimental and clincal application of microvascular surgery, Ann Surg 181:169, 1975.
79. Tupper JW: Techniques of bone fixation and clinical experience in replanted extremities, Clin Orthop 133:165, 1978.
80. Urbaniak JR: Replantation of amputated hands and digits. In American Academy of Orthopaedic Surgeons: Instructional course lectures, 27:15, St. Louis, 1978, The CV Mosby Co.
81. Urbaniak JR: Replantation of amputated parts: technique, results and indications. In American Academy of Orthopaedic Surgeons: Symposium on microsurgery: practical use in orthopaedics, St. Louis, 1979, The CV Mosby Co.
82. Urbaniak JR: Replantation. In Green DP, editor: Operative hand surgery, Edinburgh, New York, 1982, Churchill Livingstone.
83. Van Beek AL, Kutz JE, and Zook EG: Importance of the ribbon sign indicating unsuitability of the vessel in replanting a finger, Plast Reconstr Surg 61:32, 1978.
84. Van Beek AL, Wavak PW, and Zook EG: Microvascular surgery in young children, Plast Reconstr Surg 63:457, 1979.
85. Wang S-H, Young K-F, and Wei J-N: Replantation of severed limbs: clinical analysis of 91 cases, J Hand Surg 6:311, 1981.
86. Weiland AJ, Villarreal-Rios A, and Kleinert HE: Replantation of digits and hands: analysis of surgical techniques and functional results in 71 patients with 86 replantations, J Hand Surg 2:1, 1977.
87. Weiland AJ and others: Replantation of digits and hands: analysis of surgical techniques and functional results in 71 patients with 86 replantations, Clin Orthop 133:195, 1978.
88. Williams GR and others: Replantation of amputated extremities, Ann Surg 163:788, 1966.
89. Yamano Y and others: Some methods for bone fixation for digital replantation, Hand 14:135, 1982.
90. Yoshizu T, Katsumi M, and Tajima T: Replantation of untidily amputated finger, hand, and arm: experience of 99 replantations in 66 cases, J Trauma 18:194, 1978.

63

Therapist's management of the replanted hand

Paula Breme Kader

In the past two decades, microsurgery, pharmaceutical drugs, and advanced microsurgical training have developed a new type of patient population: those who have successfully survived a complete amputation of a body part and its replantation. The tremendous systemic changes that occur after an amputation and during the subsequent surgery are life threatening and must be carefully managed. This chapter will focus on the therapist's evaluation and management of patients who have undergone hand amputation and replantation.

EVALUATION

When providing therapy for the patient who has undergone replantation, identifying problems, establishing goals, and planning a treatment program is an ongoing process. The multistructural involvement necessitates individual assessment of all the systems, problems, and goals before integrating them into a total treatment program. Compromise may be necessary because a treatment program for one system may be incompatible with another. Continual evaluation allows the introduction of appropriate treatment as soon as possible.

A complete amputation involves five major structures: the vascular system, the skeletal system, tendons, nerves, and skin[1] (Fig. 63-1). Each system has its own rate of healing and protocol for rehabilitation.[5]

Occasionally, surgical repair of a structure may not be possible during the replantation procedure. It is generally more favorable to the final result if everything is repaired during the initial surgery. However, if total replant survival is threatened, secondary surgery is appropriate.

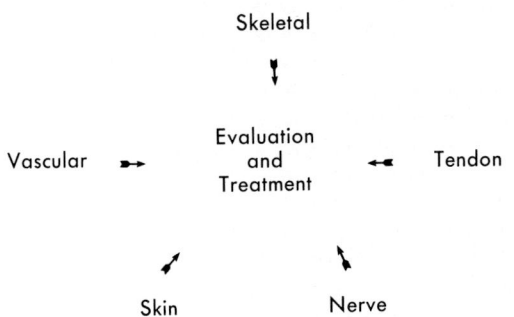

Fig. 63-1 The five systems that are affected by amputation and subsequent replantation must be evaluated separately. Therapy evaluation and the treatment program must take into account the variable healing rates.

Vascular system

Restoration of the blood vessels is the key to a successful replantation. There should be no tension on the vessel's anastomosis.[6,8,9] The optimum ratio for vascularity is two veins for every artery repaired. Because arteries are larger in diameter than veins, this ratio assures an adequate venous return. The surgeon will attempt to repair more veins if possible because the lymphatic system is disrupted and cannot participate in the return of fluid.

Many factors can cause a poor result. As the surgeon prepares the vessels for repair, the edges are trimmed of necrotic tissue until healthy tissue is exposed. It is through this débridement process that the approximated vessel ends may come under tension. In this case, a vein graft may be used to fill in the gap. Grafting creates two anastomosis sites instead of one from which emboli can evolve. The size of the vessel and anastomosis can influence results. The blood vessels in the palm and digits, as well as those in children, are small and difficult to repair.[6,8,9]

Postoperative situations, such as patient compliance and medical management, can affect surgical results. It is difficult to assess a patient's compliance during those frantic hours after amputation and before replantation. For the replanted part to survive, the patient must be willing and able to elevate the hand properly, keep the extremity warm, and avoid caffeine and smoking. This is basic survival for the replanted part. Good medical management is necessary because these patients are susceptible to blood loss, hemostasis, and electrolyte imbalance.[4]

Once repaired, the vascular system heals quickly. During the first few days, indications of vascular compromise may necessitate an emergency trip back to the operating room. As the weeks progress, a collateral circulatory system develops and by 4 weeks is well established.[9]

Skeletal system

Skeletal fixation is the first operative goal and is crucial in the replantation procedure (Fig. 63-2). The shortened length of the bone will decrease tension at the repair site(s) of the adjacent structures. Amputations through a joint may necessitate a fusion or insertion of a silastic spacer. Amputation through the wrist can result in carpectomy of an entire row. Rigid skeletal stabilization allows hand therapy to begin early, before bony union. The method of bony fixation depends on the level of injury. Bone plates are commonly used for amputations through the metacarpals, whereas the wrist and distal joints can be stabilized with percutaneous pins and/or intraosseous wiring.[6,8,9]

Every joint of the involved extremity, both proximal and

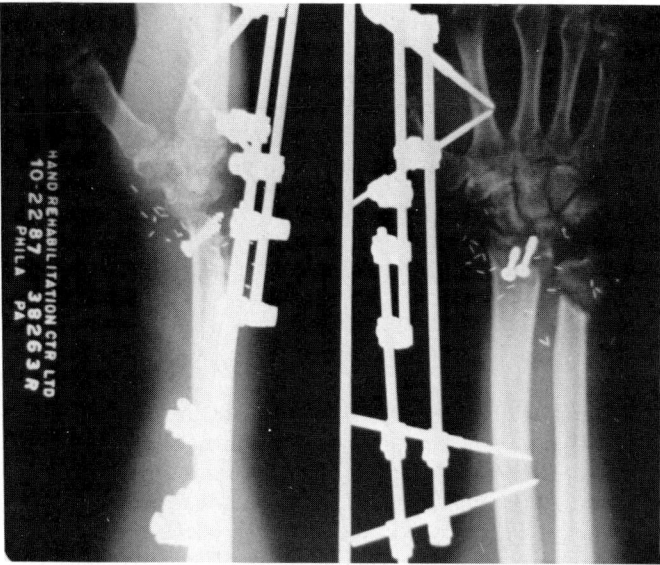

Fig. 63-2 Radiograph of an amputation through the distal ulna and radius of a male factory worker. External skeletal fixation was used to maintain skeletal stabilization.

distal to the amputation, should be evaluated for its potential for early motion. A joint may require total immobilization. Other joints may not need immobilization; however, special positioning is necessary because of soft tissue repair. Joints proximal to the amputation site that do not need immobilization for skeletal or soft tissue repair, such as the elbow and shoulder, should be freely moved to avoid stiffness. Not all amputations occur through a joint. More commonly noted in the digital amputation, bony stabilization may be achieved without immobilization of the proximal or distal joints.

It is important to note that healing of a fracture in the replanted part is slow because of the compromised vascularity of the amputation. Skeletal fixation longer than 8 weeks is not uncommon.

Tendon system

Every attempt is made to repair all the lacerated flexor and extensor tendons at normal tension. Occasionally the superficialis tendon is excised because the profundus muscle will effectively flex the entire digit.[6,8,9] If the tendon pulley system has been disrupted, reconstruction is performed and protection will be necessary. Excessive soft tissue loss on the dorsum of the hand promotes tendon adhesions of the extensor tendons. The insertion of silastic tendon implants and skin grafting allows the formation of pseudosheaths under adequate soft tissue coverage. In a few months, the pseudosheaths area will be ready to accept tendon grafts.[3]

When both flexor and extensor tendons are repaired, the surgeon can visually inspect what joint positions minimize tension on the tendon repairs and the tendency for joint contractures. An intraoperative or early postoperative splint is fabricated to maintain this position of balance between the opposing tendon systems.

Peripheral nerve

The quality of peripheral nerve repair is the indicator of functional recovery; therefore every effort is made to repair lacerated nerves primarily. The surgeon strives to repair the nerve. The nerve repair should be without tension as tension increases scar formation at the anastomosis.[6,8,9] The therapist should inquire as to what joint positions will create stress on the nerve juncture, and then avoid those positions. Fortunately, the length lost through skeletal shortening will generally provide enough slack to permit nerve repair without tension.

Nerve grafts are frequently used if the extent of damage is too great to allow primary end-to-end repair. This procedure may be performed during initial replantation or during subsequent surgery. Regeneration will take longer because there are now two juncture sites for regenerating axon to cross.

Motor and sensory loss can be expected in amputations proximal to the midcarpal level. Sensory loss is noted in amputations distal to this level. Becoming familiar with the innervation sites of the motor units of each nerve will help determine muscular loss in relation to amputation site. Loss of thumb opposition and intrinsic musculature creates significant loss of function in the hand. Regeneration is poor because these muscles are small and atrophy of the motor end plates is quick. Sensibility return can be monitored from the site of amputation to the distal digit.[2]

Wounds

The type of skin closure the physician chooses depends on the amount and condition of the remaining tissue. Tension on the wound should not be strong enough to create ischemia. A primary skin closure is the approximation and suturing together of the skin edges. The wound is relatively clean, skin loss is minimal, and healing is quick. Secondary healing, or healing through secondary intention, occurs when the skin edges are left apart. Tissue granulation occurs from the perimeter and moves toward the center. This technique is often used after fasciectomy or for dirty wounds where drainage is encouraged. Skin grafting is performed over a clean wound when primary closure is not possible (Fig. 63-3). A wound may be left open for a few days to drain, and then a skin graft is performed to speed up closure. Finally, skin flaps are required when there is excessive soft tissue loss. This is commonly performed on the dorsum of the hand where the extrinsic tendons are so superficial that minimal skin loss can lead to exposed tendons.[7]

TREATMENT

Assessment of each system, establishing goals, and developing the treatment plan provide direction in the therapy program. However, treatment indicated for one system may be contraindicated for another during certain specific healing phases. Treatments may need to be withheld until all structures are appropriately healed. Treatment programs are performed in therapy and continued at home if the patient demonstrates ability to follow through accurately.

Postoperatively treatment can be broken down into three stages. The first 8 weeks after replant is the acute phase during which the rate of tissue repair is accelerated. New treatment techniques are added to the therapy program weekly. Care is taken, however, not to overwhelm the vascular system of the replanted part. The subacute phase, from 8 weeks to 4 months, is the period during which healing tissues are still susceptible to change, yet able to withstand progressive demands of function. Therapy must maximize

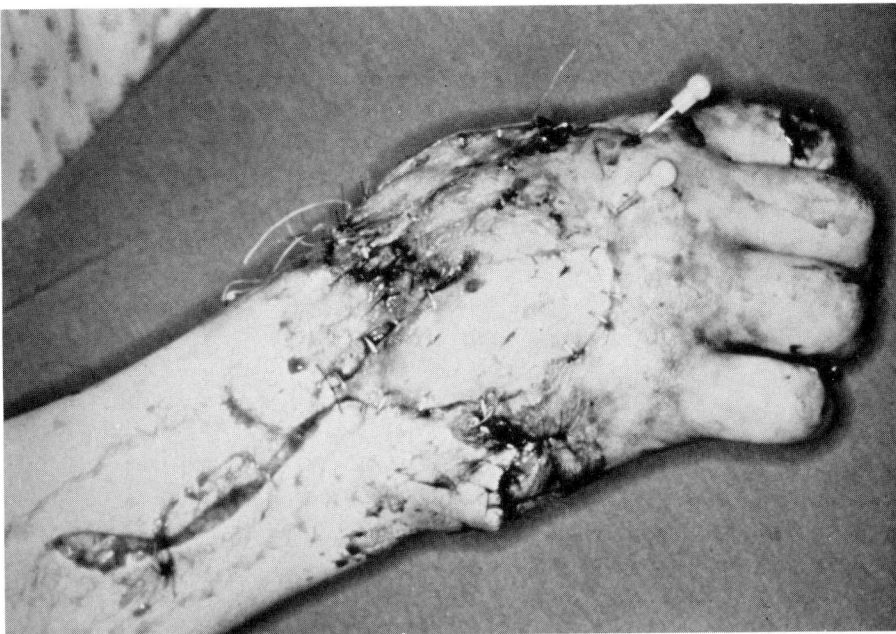

Fig. 63-3   Hand of a young woman who sustained a log splitter injury resulting in amputation at the wrist level. Skin grafting was necessary to close the wound. Because of the proximity of the extrinsic extensor tendons to the skin graft, extensive scarring in this area can lead to limited tendon excursion.

range of motion, strength, and function during this phase. The final chronic phase occurs after 4 months. During this time, decisions are made concerning further surgery. Even after an intensive therapy program, surgery is usually necessary to improve function.

Acute phase

Week 1. During this period the patient remains in the hospital for close observation. Medical personnel make frequent inspection of the replanted part for vascular patency. If necessary, the patient is taken to the operating room for surgical intervention.[6,8,9]

Signs of vascular insufficiency can be monitored in several ways. Visual inspection of a healthy digit finds it pink in color. A bluish, white, or black hue suggests arterial insufficiency. A bright red color along with severe edema indicates venous compromise. Vascular patency can also be observed through capillary refill. Pressure is applied to the end of the digit until it blanches. On release, the color will normally return briskly. With vascular compromise the color returns sluggishly. Finally, use of a digital thermister providing a readout of over 30° C indicates vascular patency.

Hand therapy treatment is generally not instituted during the first postoperative week. The therapist may be introduced to the patient and family to discuss long-term rehabilitation. The therapist can use this time to review the medical chart and prepare an initial treatment plan with the surgeon.

Weeks 2 to 4. Therapy is initiated during this time with priority given to the vascular system and the healing wounds. The greatest amount of healing of these two systems occurs within this first 4-week period.

Vascular system. The therapeutic goal is to maintain optimal condition for vascular repair. Patient education regarding proper care of the replanted part is initiated by the

medical personnel and continued by the therapist. Keeping the extremity warm, especially through the winter months, is crucial. While wearing gloves is impossible, wrapping the hand loosely with a warm scarf and placing it under the coat near the body protects the extremity from cold. The patient must avoid substances that create tissue ischemia. Caffeine, coffee, dark sodas, and chocolate cause vasoconstriction. Nicotine decreases the oxygen in blood, which compromises vascularity in the replanted extremity with limited circulation.

To minimize vascular stress, the extremity must be elevated at all times. However, because of repairs of both vein and artery, elevation must not be excessive. The hand is kept at heart level. As elevation increases, the heart must pump harder, creating more stress on the arterial anastomosis. As elevation falls below heart level, stress to the venous return system is increased.

Good wound care avoids trauma, especially when removing bandages. The proper technique for removing a dressing directly over a wound is to peel the gauze off, keeping it parallel to the skin. This creates less of a force in the tissue than pulling the bandage off in a perpendicular direction.

Temperature biofeedback is indicated when the medical staff is concerned with vascular insufficiency. Thermister readings provide digital temperature. Through techniques of autoimagery, the patient can increase peripheral temperature. (Please refer to Chapter 79 for further information on thermal biofeedback.) The thermister is often used as the treatment progresses to ensure that exercises or splints do not decrease digital temperature (Fig. 63-4).

Wounds. The next therapeutic goal is to promote wound closure. The type of closure and the surgeon's preference will determine wound care. It can be expected that a clean primary skin repair will require minimal bandages and will

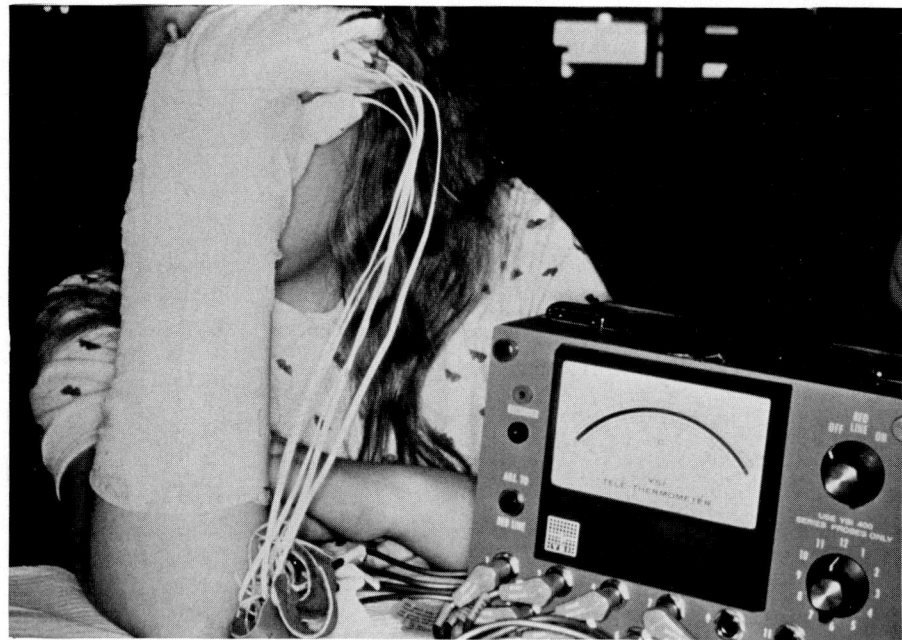

Fig. 63-4 The patient's hand is placed in a splint to maintain an intrinsic-plus position during the acute phase of healing. The thermistor is attached to each digit to monitor the affect of the splint on the patient's vascularity.

heal relatively quickly. A skin graft may require more dressings and complete closure will take longer.

With all wounds, therapy treatments aim to facilitate tissue granulation and prevent infection. This requires a patent vascular system. Keeping the granulating bed free of biologic debris promotes tissue healing. Débridement can be achieved through the use of wet dressings to absorb serous fluids or the surgeon's use of forceps to excise necrotic tissue. The use of sterile technique when handling bandages promotes good hygiene for the patient and health care provider.

Since traumatic amputations do not occur in a sterile environment, chance for infection from the initial injury always exists. Some surgeons prescribe prophylactic antibiotics to reduce the risk of infection. Deep wounds heal from the inside out. A sinus can retain bacteria that can lead to a serious infection. The hallmark signs of infection are redness, increased swelling, odor, localized tenderness, and drainage. The patient must also be alert to these signs.[7]

Additional therapeutic techniques. If vascular and wound healing are stable, the following therapeutic techniques may be instituted. However, if either of the above-mentioned systems are stressed, such as in a massive infection, then further therapy may be contraindicated.

SPLINTS. Protection of healing tissue is the goal of splinting. Several factors may be considered when planning a splint for the replanted part. External stabilization for healing bones and joints may be a necessary adjunct to skeletal fixation. Repaired tendons and nerves must be held in a protected position especially if early motion is to begin. As ligaments heal, the affected joints should be held in a position to maximize ligament length without creating stress on repaired tendons or nerves. Specifically, metacarpophalangeal (MP) joint flexion and interphalangeal (IP) joint

extension of the digits minimize contracture in the opposite direction. Avoidance of shearing force over skin repair is achieved through a well-molded splint. Alternating splints may become necessary if the joints are developing contractures in the position in which they are held. The therapist must keep in mind the repaired tendons when splint changes are made.

PROTECTIVE RANGE OF MOTION. The goal of early range of motion is to maintain full range in all joints that can be safely mobilized. The range is performed passively. As in splinting, consideration is given to the repaired tendon and, to a lesser extent, to the nerve and vessel that cross the joint.

Positions of passive motion should be discussed with the surgeon; however, some guidelines can be given. If the replantation is at the midmetacarpal level or proximal to it, then the hook first (MP extension and IP flexion) (Fig. 63-5) and tabletop (MP flexion and IP extension) positions provide full range of motion to the digital joints while balancing the flexor and extensor tendons. The wrist must be supported in neutral during these exercises. For replantations distal to the midmetacarpal level, the individual joint is flexed with the adjacent joints extended or the individual joint is extended with the adjacent joints flexed. This may be limited if the proximal joint is pinned.

The uninvolved joints of the elbow and shoulder should be placed in full range of motion. Respect to the position of hand elevation must be given. Therefore the patient must perform these exercises in a comfortable supine or side-lying position.

Approximately 3 weeks after replantation, "place and hold" (isometric) exercises may begin. For this, the patient passively places the digit into the hook fist and then attempts to maintain this position through active muscle contraction.

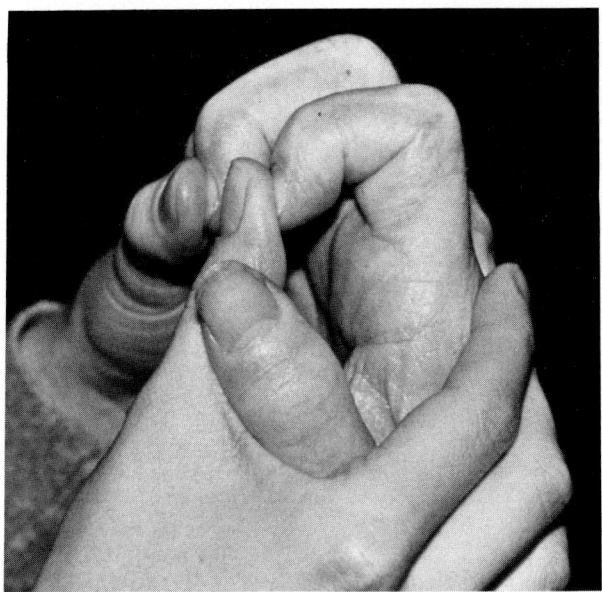

Fig. 63-5 The hook fist allows full extension of the metacarpophalangeal joints and full flexion of the interphalangeal joints, yet does not place the extrinsic extensor or flexor tendons on stretch. After the third postoperative week, the patient attempts to maintain the hook position isometrically after the digits are passively positioned (place and hold).

The tabletop position will be impossible if the intrinsic muscles were denervated.

ONE-HANDED ACTIVITY. Patient independence raises self-esteem and thereby follow-through in therapy. Begin the patient in one-handed activity such as hygiene, dressing, and eating as soon as possible. Use adaptive equipment if necessary, and initiate writing exercises if the dominant side was amputated.

Weeks 4 to 8. During this time period, vascularity is stable as collateral circulation has been established. Wound healing progresses and simple closures may already be healed. Skin grafting any remaining open wounds is performed at this point to expedite healing. Skeletal fixation needs to remain in place because bony healing is not yet complete. Nerve repairs are protected up to the sixth postoperative week. The tendon system will need active exercise and passive range.

WOUND CARE. Wound care continues to be provided as indicated. Whirlpool baths at 92° F to 98° F may be given to loosen the biologic debris in the wound. Cooler temperatures may create vasospasms. Higher temperatures may create excessive edema, especially if the hand is in a dependent position. Whirlpool baths should be followed by copious irrigation with water, at the same temperature, to remove debris from the wound. The bulk of bandages should decrease so the patient is free to use the hand. As wounds heal, scar management should be initiated to influence collagen synthesis in a smooth and organized fashion. This may include massage and pressure appliances, such as Elastomer and Otoform.

EDEMA CONTROL. As the vascular system stabilizes and collateral circulation is strong, edema-reducing techniques become more aggressive. Elevation higher than the heart and retrograde massage are indicated and taught to the patient. If edema is persistent, compression wrapping (leaving the tips exposed), wearing compression gloves, and using an intermittent compression pump may effectively reduce swelling. Because healing nerves and tendons may still require protection, these techniques are carried out with the hand properly positioned.

PASSIVE RANGE OF MOTION. If the joints allowed early mobilization have not obtained full joint motion, passive motion should be continued, keeping the extrinsic tendons on slack as previously described. It is important that all joints have full passive range of motion before addressing muscle-tendon unit tightness.

ACTIVE RANGE OF MOTION. Active motion is added gradually. By 4 weeks, place and hold exercises in full digital flexion and extension are initiated. The patient is asked to use the uninvolved hand to hold the fingers either flexed or extended and then maintain that position as he withdraws the supporting hand (Fig. 63-6, *A* and *B*). Flexor tendon gliding exercises,[10] extensor digitorum communis, and thumb exercises are initiated. Intrinsic function of the hand is lost in wrist level amputations. At 5 weeks after surgery, blocking exercises in both flexion and extension are initiated. By the sixth week, activities to promote range are performed. This includes macramé and light pickups. Providing adaptive equipment with built-up handles will encourage the patient to perform activities of daily living, (ADL) as well as use available hand function. In replants distal to the midmetacarpal level, active motion is usually not initiated until the sixth postoperative week.

SPLINTING. The purpose of splinting is to continue to protect the healing skeletal system. If mobilized joints are beginning to develop contractures, however, splinting is initiated for correction. Because the purpose will be to reduce joint contracture, not muscle-tendon tightness, adjacent joints must be positioned to minimize traction on the tendons and nerves. It is important to monitor digital temperature when using new splints so as not to overstress the vascular system.

SENSIBILITY. Because the patient is now using the hand more, through therapeutic activities and activities of daily living, the therapist must reinforce the need to be visually aware of pressure or friction on the hand. When the patient uses the hand for an extended amount of time, visual inspection is necessary to monitor for red areas indicating pressure or friction. Using the hand around heat, such as when cooking, presents danger because the patient will not feel pain in the replanted part. Burns to an insensate digit can be severe and can provide a quick entry site for bacteria.

Subacute phase

8 Weeks to 4 months. During this period, the vascularity is of minimal concern except when applying splints that may inadvertently compromise circulation. The wounds should be healed or close to it. The tendons and nerves no longer need to be held in protective positioning. At approximately 8 weeks or more, percutaneous fixation is removed as bony union is observed clinically and radiographically.

WOUND CARE AND SCAR MANAGEMENT. The rate of wound healing depends on the extent of injury. As scar tissue matures, the therapeutic goal is to minimize hypertrophic scar-

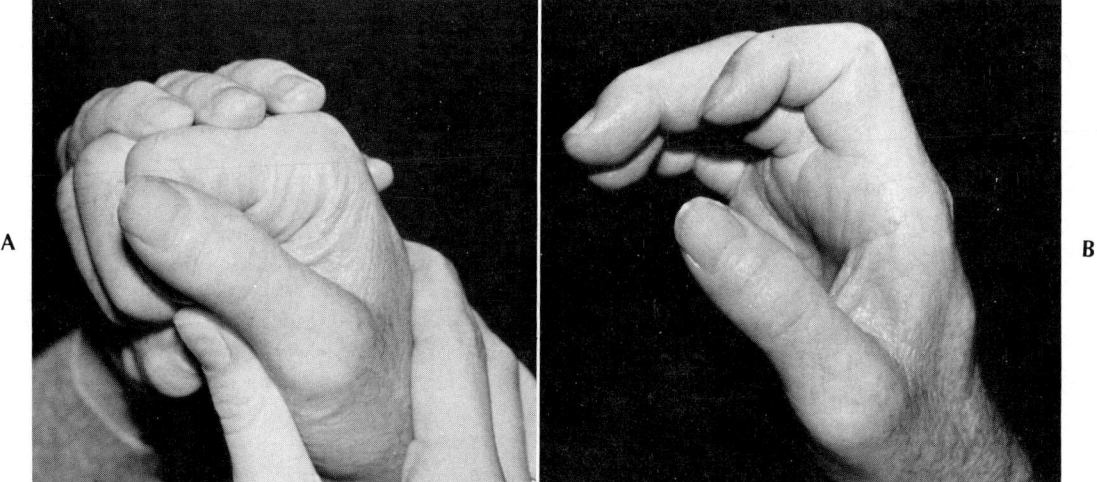

Fig. 63-6 Place and hold exercises. **A,** Patient's hand is placed in a full-fist position. **B,** He attempts actively to maintain the fist as the supporting hand is withdrawn.

ring. The patient is instructed in deep friction massage to loosen skin from the adjacent soft tissue. The use of a soft silastic mold that conforms to the patient's scar will influence the organization of newly synthesized collagen. When the scar responds by becoming flatter, a new mold is needed to conform to the changed scar.

Techniques of scar reduction are applied directly to the skin, and the results can be observed through visual inspection and palpation. The raised, red scar will become flat and pink as scar management succeeds. Skin that was once adherent and immobile over the underlying soft tissue becomes more mobile with therapeutic efforts. A correlation between controlled reorganization of maturing collagen (through signs described above) and the improvement of active range of motion and passive stretch of the adjacent flexor and extensor muscles can be observed. The deep heat of ultrasound applied over scar tissue and the muscle tendon unit will produce a softer scar and increased range of motion. It is important to note that ultrasound produces a quick rise in tissue temperature that lasts a relatively short time. Therefore, if the goal of ultrasound application is to improve active range of motion, the patient must perform active range of motion immediately after its application to take advantage of the thermodynamic effect.

EDEMA. At this stage, edema should be under control through one or more of the previously described techniques. An increase in edema is usually an indication of change in external conditions. For example, aggressive exercise or a tight-fitting splint may produce an increase in hand volume. The external cause should then be modified. As the patient progressively increases activities, the internal pumping system of the hand will reduce swelling and the patient will depend less and less on external edema-reducing techniques. The patient's activities assist in edema reduction during the day; however, wearing a compression glove or using an intermittent compression pump at night may continue as long as edema is unstable.

RANGE OF MOTION. As skeletal fixation devices are re-

moved, previously immobilized joints can begin motion. However, some external protection may be necessary. Amputation and replantation through a joint will create new arthrokinematics and range may never be full and may be painful. Passive range of motion is begun on all joints. Efforts to decrease previously noted joint contractures continue. Passive range of motion may be performed to increase extensibility of the tight musculature (e.g., long flexor muscles). Application of heat before passive stretch increases the patient's comfort and tissue extensibility. If heat is applied to the insensate part, careful monitoring is necessary.

Active range of motion is continued and exercises are added as previously immobilized joints can safely begin to move. Muscle return will be delayed and weak when the amputation occurs proximal to the innervation site. Return of the small muscles of the hand may never occur because atrophy of the muscle is too severe. While the therapist must continue to evaluate for any muscle return, asking the patient to use muscle that has not been reinnervated leads to frustration.

As more joints are available for motion, the patient increases the use of the extremity for functional ADL. Adaptive equipment may still be necessary. Patients measure progress in the amount of time in which they perform ADL. Satisfaction is derived when a patient can discard adaptive equipment and perform tasks independently.

Even though active range of motion may not be full, resistive exercises are gradually introduced. By increasing strength in the available range, further motion is encouraged. Activities such as Velcro checkers and leather work facilitate grasp and can be graded in resistance. Sanding, which increases flexor tendon excursion by increasing flexor muscle strength, can be graded by increasing the time spent sanding or decreasing the width of the handle on the sanding block. Activities assigned to patients take into account the desired hand function, level of strength, and level of endurance. Job simulation tasks are introduced in the therapy program around the twelfth postoperative week. Use of the

BTE Work Simulator* reproduces work tasks at a rate and power similar to the patient's actual job requirements.

SPLINTING. As the bones heal, the need for external splints decreases. When pins are removed, however, a splint may be necessary for additional support for a few extra weeks, especially when the patient performs resistive exercises.

Other splints may be necessary for specific problems, such as joint contractures. It is preferable to allow the joints previously held immobilized to gain motion from active exercise and passive range until a plateau is reached, before splinting is instituted. Excessive motion of these traumatized joints, for which normal arthrokinematics may never return, can create pain and instability.

Splinting may be geared toward increasing extensibility of repaired tendons. Tightness of the extrinsic flexor muscle-tendon unit is commonly noted at this stage of the replantation rehabilitation. Stretch is obtained by placing all the joints over which the tight muscle and tendon cross into extension. Prolonged positioning with a splint that is serially increased over a few days will allow the maturing scar tissue to form in a position of optimal length. The progression can be seen quickly when the patient wears a serial static splint for long periods of time, such as 8 hours while sleeping. Fabricated from plaster, these splints are changed frequently at first—every 5 to 7 days. A new splint is made when passive range of motion improves and the patient can no longer feel a stretch to his muscles when the splint is donned. (Refer to Chapter 90.)

SENSIBILITY. During this phase, sensibility is beginning to progress distally and can be monitored by an advancing Tinel sign. A full sensibility evaluation should be performed when evidence of returning sensory nerve function exists.[2] Such evidence includes a Tinel sign that is significantly distal to the nerve repair, or the patient's report of sensation (paresthesia or hypesthesia) distal to the repair.

Sensory reeducation is initiated when the patient falls into a diminished loss of protective sensation range. The cooperative and motivated patient will have changes in the ability to perceive sensation as he learns how to interpret sensory input. Short yet frequent activities should be changed appropriately to keep up patient interest.

Chronic stage

4 Months and beyond. With respect to the time frame of tissue healing, the first 4 months show a rapid change and therapy has progressed appropriately. At 4 months tissue synthesis reduces, as do the changes in the therapy program. Range of motion and strength will continue to improve. Sensibility continues to be monitored, and sensory reeducation is advanced. The therapist begins to assess the areas

of limitations in respect to the patient's personal, social, and employment needs. With these limitations established, the surgeon can determine if further surgical intervention is necessary. Even in the most ideal situation, further surgery such as tenolysis or tendon transfer is required.

Once secondary procedures are performed, the patient will follow the rehabilitation protocol for that particular surgery.[5] However, keep in mind that the initial problem of vascular insufficiency will always be greater than normal and will slow the healing rate of the affected tissue.

SUMMARY

Therapeutic management of the patient status after replantation is challenging and can be successful if approached in an organized fashion. Assessment includes the five major systems: vascular, skeletal, tendon, nerve, and skin. Evaluation looks at each system separately, yet treatment planning takes into account all systems simultaneously. It is important not to initiate therapy that is appropriate for one system but contraindicated for another. The management after replantation can be broken down into three stages. During the acute phase, which is through 8 weeks, the repaired structures are volatile but react well to a carefully planned therapy program. The subacute stage, from 8 weeks to 4 months, find the structures less fragile and ready to take on the increasing demands of function. The final chronic phase incorporates the time past 4 months when strength and function are maximized and thought is given to further surgical intervention.

REFERENCES

1. American Society for Surgery of the Hand: The hand examination and diagnosis, ed 2, New York, 1983, Churchill Livingstone.
2. Dellon AL: Evaluation of sensibility and reeducation of sensation in the hand, Baltimore, 1981, Williams & Wilkins Co.
3. Hunter JM, Jaeger SH, and Mackin EM: Staged tendon grafting using tendon implants. In Tubiana R, editor: The hand, vol 3, Philadelphia, 1985, WB Saunders Co.
4. Jobsis F, Boyd J, and Barwicki W: Metabolic consequences of ischemia and hypoxia. In Serafin D and Buncke Jr H, editors: Microsurgical composite tissue transplantation, St. Louis, 1979, The CV Mosby Co.
5. Mackin EJ, editor: Hand Clinics, vol 2, no 1, Hand Rehabilitation, Philadelphia, Feb. 1986, WB Saunders Co.
6. Meyer VE: Upper extremity replantation basic principles, surgical technique, and strategy, New York, 1985, Churchill Livingstone.
7. Peacock E: Wound repair, ed 3, Philadelphia, 1984, WB Saunders Co.
8. Urbaniak JR, editor: Hand Clinics symposium on microvascular surgery, vol 1, no 2, Philadelphia, May 1985, WB Saunders Co.
9. Urbaniak JR: Microsurgery for major limb reconstruction, St. Louis, 1987, The CV Mosby Co.
10. Wehbe MA and Hunter JM: Flexor tendon gliding in the hand. Part II. Differential gliding, J Hand Surg 10A:575, 1985.

---

*Baltimore Therapeutic Equipment Co., Baltimore.

IX

BURNS AND COLD INJURIES

64

Acute care and rehabilitation of the burned hand

Roger E. Salisbury, Sandra Utley Reeves, and Phyllis Wright

OCCUPATIONAL THERAPY
Splinting

Philosophies vary regarding the best time to splint an acutely burned hand, and an increasing number of occupational therapists are no longer splinting immediately after injury. Significant edema usually develops during the first 48 to 72 hours, especially in a large-surface-area burn that requires fluid resuscitation. A splint that is applied immediately on admission may not fit several hours later. Splints applied with either straps or dressings may become constrictive as swelling increases and must be closely monitored and modified frequently to accommodate increasing circumferences. Therefore more emphasis should be placed on keeping the hand well elevated and actively exercising to decrease edema and keep joints mobile. The hand should be positioned above the elbow, and the elbow above the shoulder, even if only the hand is burned. This can be accomplished by placing the arm on pillows or suspending it in an overhead sling or positioning device (Fig. 64-1). If the shoulder or elbow is also burned, it should also be carefully positioned. The elbow should be positioned in 5

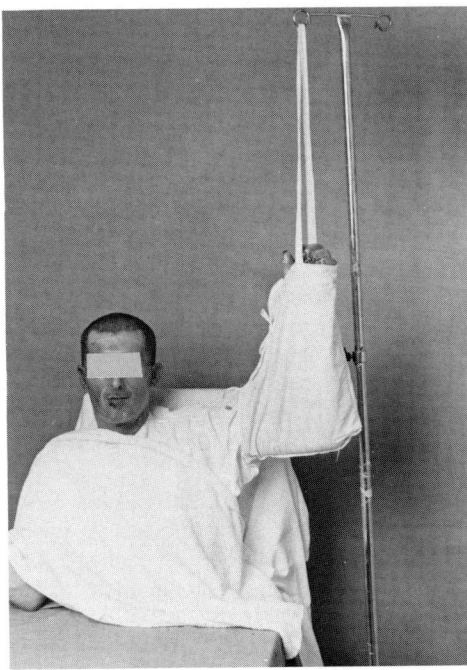

Fig. 64-1 Elevation in a sterile sling is a simple, inexpensive way to reduce edema soon after a burn when elbow is uninvolved.

degrees of flexion to prevent hyperextension stress to the joint. The shoulder should be positioned in 90 to 110 degrees of abduction and externally rotated. The shoulder should not be positioned in greater than 110 degrees abduction for extended periods, which could cause injury to the brachial plexus.

After the edema "peaks," the hand should be splinted at the first signs of decreased mobility or skin tightness. Splints should be worn at night and during periods of rest, with the patient's hands being left free during the day. Patients should be encouraged to use their hands and to actively exercise on their own as much as possible. The splinting program should not interfere with activities of daily living. For instance, splints should be removed at mealtime to encourage self-feeding. Patients who lack motivation, who are unable to actively use their hands, or who are beginning to develop contractures in spite of night splinting may need to wear hand splints during daytime periods of inactivity as well.

The burned hand should be splinted in the "antideformity position" rather than the traditional "position of function." The antideformity position will vary, depending on the location and size of the burn. The goal is to position the hand so that the burned surface area is stretched, thus preventing the skin from "drawing" or contracting as it heals. For instance, in circumferential or volar wrist burns the antideformity position of the wrist is 30 to 40 degrees of extension; neutral (0 degrees) is used for dorsal burns. In dorsal hand burns the metacarpophalangeal (MP) joints should be flexed as much as possible, with the interphalangeal joints in full extension. The thumb should be abducted fully and slightly extended to preserve the first web space. The antideformity position differs from the so-called position of function in that the latter has more MP extension and interphalangeal flexion and less thumb abduction and extension (Fig. 64-2). In the case of hand burns to the palmar surfaces only, the most advantageous position may be that of MP and interphalangeal extension, finger abduction, and thumb extension and abduction, to stretch the palmar skin to its maximum. In a circumferential burn, in which there is a potential for both dorsal and volar contractures, it may be advantageous to alternate between the two splint designs, with the patient wearing the antideformity splint during the day and the palmar stretching splint at night.

Low-temperature thermoplastics such as Polyform and Kay Splint are recommended for hand splint fabrication, since these materials are easily reshaped to accommodate changes in edema or increases in range of motion. A strapping material that is soft, washable, nonabrasive, and non-

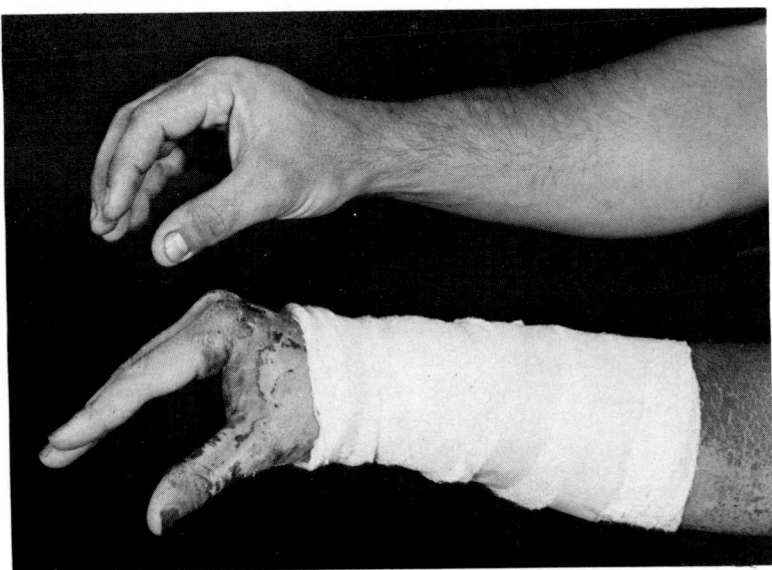

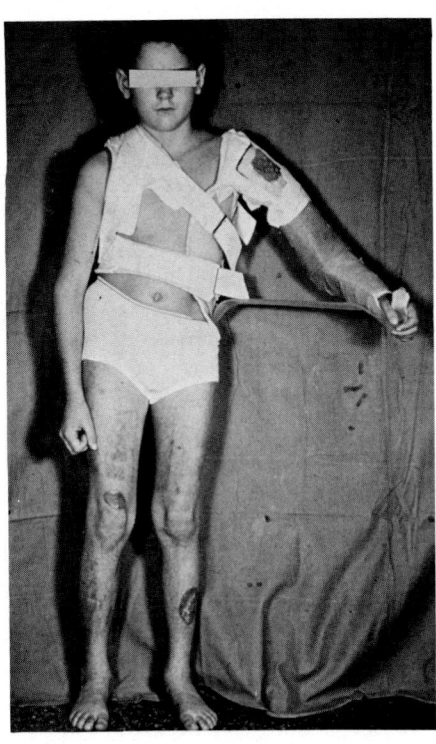

Fig. 64-2 Antideformity position for dorsal burns of hand, *bottom*, has more metacarpophalangeal flexion and interphalangeal extension than position of function, *top*.

Fig. 64-3 Lightweight Polyform splint provides immobilization for humeral fracture after electrical injury but also allows optimum care of burn wound.

constrictive, such as Velfoam or Betapile II is recommended.

When a splint is applied over topical antibiotics, it is especially important that the splint be removed, fresh antibiotics be applied, and the cleaned splint be reapplied, several times per nursing shift. Otherwise the cream will pool under the splint, providing a soupy culture medium in which bacteria may grow. A light gauze dressing over the cream keeps the cream from being rubbed off and helps prevent the splint from sliding distally (which would hold the hand in the position of contracture).

Special splints may have to be designed if peripheral nerve lesions, fractures, or tendon damage were incurred at the time of thermal injury. Early prophylactic splinting can decrease the incidence of secondary deformities and often minimize the number of reconstructive procedures required later in the patient's hospital course. Internal fixation through the burn wound and plaster casting of fractures are not recommended, because of potential wound sepsis. Instead, thermoplastic or aluminum splints are employed, because they are sturdy, light weight, easily cleaned, and cover as little of the burn wound as possible while rendering adequate support (Fig. 64-3).

The success of a grafting procedure is often dependent on the quality of intraoperative and postoperative splinting and follow-up therapy programs. Even wounds covered by thick, split-thickness skin grafts may contract, resulting in joint deformity, if appropriate splinting is not initiated promptly and continued until all evidence of skin tightness is gone. Careful preoperative planning between the surgeon and the occupational therapist is necessary, so that both

understand what is the desired functional result of the surgery. Although preoperative planning makes it possible for most postoperative splints to be made before surgery, often splints must be made in the operating room at the time of surgery, such as in a surgical release of a contracture. In the case of the hand, where no meshed sheet grafts are preferred (for best cosmetic and functional results), immediate and complete immobilization, which allows open treatment of the graft site, is preferred. The size and location of the graft to be treated open will determine the type of postoperative splint to be used. Dorsal hand grafts can be splinted in an antideformity splint, with fingernail traction being used to secure the fingers into the splint (Fig. 64-4).

After the antecubital fossa has been grafted, one of two splint designs can be used to immobilize the surgical site. If the graft is being treated open, a posterior elbow splint (with a hole cut into it to avoid pressure to the humeral condyles, olecranon, and ulnar nerves) can be used. If the graft is being treated closed, an anterior elbow splint can be applied over heavy dressings, a technique that not only provides a more stable splint but also protects the graft site from accidental trauma.

Because the postsurgical position of an axillary graft is difficult to anticipate, the splint in such a case is usually fabricated in the operating room. Whether a three-piece airplane splint (for treating the axilla open) or an axillary conformer over heavy dressings is decided on, caution must be used to avoid splinting the shoulder in more than approximately 110 degrees abduction. As stated earlier, this could cause injury to the brachial plexus as a result of overstretching. It is also recommended that the patient re-

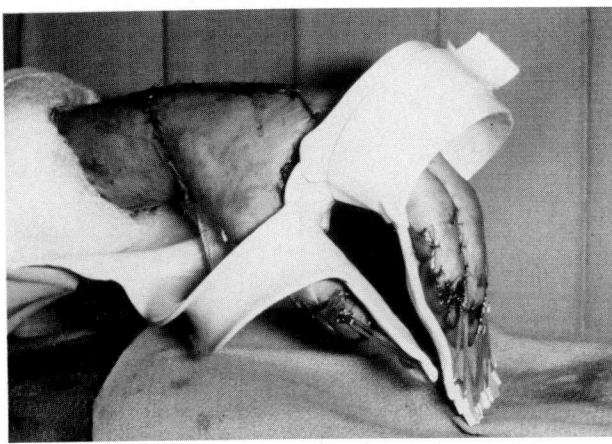

Fig. 64-4 Volar splint with "guard rails" and fingernail traction applied to immobilize the hand and wrist grafts without using dressings.

main supine in bed for at least 3 days after grafting. This is to avoid the downward shifting of the splint during transfers or ambulation.

With any of the previously mentioned postoperative splints, it is best to apply the splint in the operating room while the patient is still under anesthesia. This will lessen the chance of disturbing the graft during transfers or when the patient awakes. This is especially important with children, who tend to move around more as they come out of anesthesia.

Splinting may be necessary on a long-term basis in a hand with more serious, deep second- and third-degree burns. Early contractures of the upper extremity can usually be corrected with serial static and/or dynamic splinting techniques. Serial static splinting works best for correcting shoulder-adduction, elbow-flexion (Fig. 64-5), wrist-flexion, and thumb-adduction contractures. It is used in conjunction with an aggressive exercise program. The joint is splinted at the maximum passive range of motion gained during exercise. The splint is modified each time passive range of motion increases. Serial splinting does not increase range of motion but maintains that which is gained through aggressive therapy.

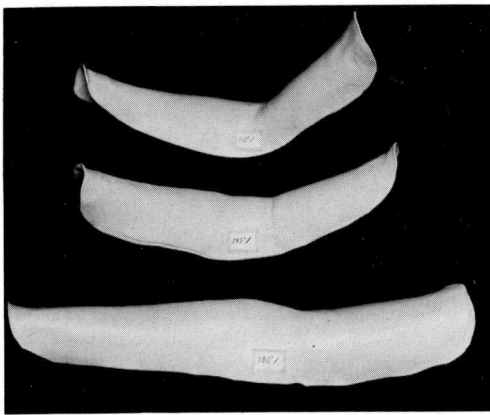

Fig. 64-5 Serial splinting of early elbow-flexion contracture will achieve normal extension with minimal trauma.

Dynamic splinting exerts a steady force to increase range of motion of the involved joint. It is often used to correct finger contractures, such as in increasing MP joint flexion or interphalangeal joint extension. Dynamic splinting often takes the form of rubberband traction, in which soft cuff loops are placed over the fingers or clothing hooks are attached to the fingernails with cyanoacrylate glue. Longitudinal fingernail traction is often used to maintain MP flexion and interphalangeal joint extension in a newly burned or recently grafted hand when straps are not able to adequately maintain proper positioning or cross over newly grafted dorsal burns. Fingernail traction also helps control the longitudinal rotation sometimes encountered in laterally or circumferentially burned phalanges. A burned palm may also be spread open with fingernail traction and a dorsal splint after autografting. Fingernail traction, however, must be done with caution, to ensure that the fingernails are stable and will not pull loose. Also, the fingernail beds may be hypersensitive, making the patient unable to tolerate this technique. Fingernail traction should not be used to correct contractures, because any force that is strong enough to stretch a contracture will cause pain and can damage the nail beds.

Special care must be taken when deep dorsal finger burns are treated, since the integrity of the extensor mechanism is jeopardized. Unlimited flexion could cause disruption of the central slip and result in a boutonnière deformity. The involved joint, therefore, is exercised only with the distal interphalangeal (DIP) and MP joints supported in extension, to prevent stress to the extensor mechanism. The hand is splinted in the traditional antideformity position by means of longitudinal fingernail traction (if possible) when the patient is not receiving wound care or exercise. If the proximal interphalangeal (PIP) joint is open, however, internal fixation with Kirschner wires may be necessary to maintain immobilization. If a boutonnière deformity is present, the joint should be splinted statically in the more functional position of approximately 40 degrees flexion at all times. It is not uncommon for scar to bridge the central slip defect if the joint is completely immobilized, thus preventing a more severe boutonnière deformity or the necessity for joint arthrodesis.

Contractures in the small pediatric hand, once established, can be very difficult to correct nonsurgically. Therefore it is recommended that splinting be initiated the day of injury as a preventive measure. Unlike the adult or an older child's hand, which tends to contract into the "claw" flexing at the MP joint and the IP joints, burns of this type should be splinted in a position of full palmar stretch with the wrist and MP and IP joints extended and the fingers abducted. A wide finger strap padded with T-Stick foam padding is effective in preventing the fingers from flexing while in the splint (Fig. 64-6). Because small finger splints tend to slide off of small hands, it may be necessary to splint the whole hand to correct or prevent contractures in one or two fingers. This is especially true in fifth finger flexion/rotation contractures.

The splints should be worn all night and during naps but should be off during waking hours to allow use of the hands in normal play. If skin tightness develops, time in the splints should be increased.

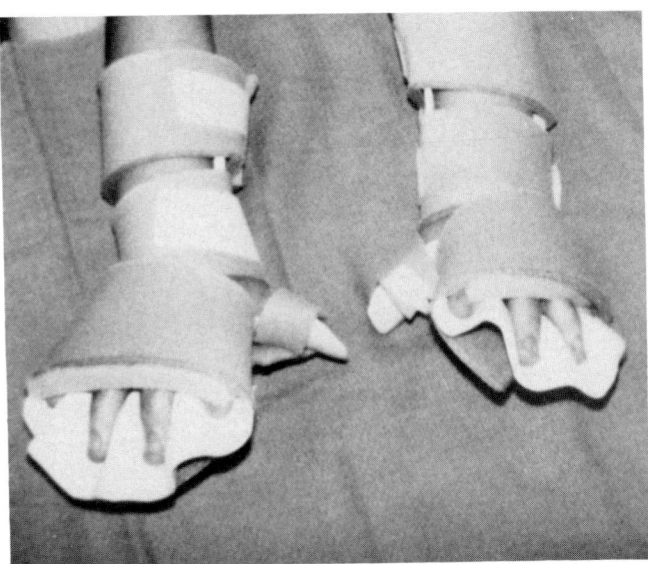

Fig. 64-6 For small pediatric patients with palmar or circumferential hand burns, volar hand splints, which abduct and extend the fingers thereby stretching the palmar skin, are recommended over the adult antideformity position.

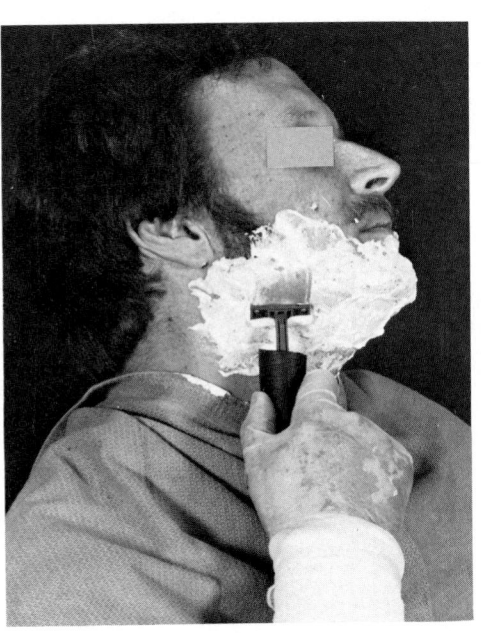

Fig. 64-7 Adaptive devices such as this enlarged razor handle for a patient with limited grasp increases independence in self-care.

Activities of daily living and hand function

As soon as the patient's condition is stable, he is encouraged to become actively involved in self-care and in activities of daily living. These tasks not only exercise the hands but help prevent deterioration of general strength and endurance. An activities of daily living (ADL) evaluation is performed by the occupational therapist at various stages of the patient's recovery to determine what activities the patient is capable of performing, whether special adaptive devices are needed, and, if they are needed, whether they will be required temporarily or permanently. Before offering help, family members and health care personnel alike are encouraged to allow the patient the chance and the time to try to do a task without assistance, to foster an attitude of self-reliance. Adaptive devices are provided only if absolutely necessary, and each device is removed as soon as the patient can perform the particular task without it.

As soon as the patient is allowed nourishment by mouth, he is expected to participate in self-feeding; this is usually the first ADL task attempted by the patient. Initially, simple adaptive devices, such as a large sponge handle for feeding utensils, may be necessary because of decreased hand range of motion and strength secondary to edema and pain.

The next tasks attempted by the patient are basic hygiene care, such as assisting with bathing, dental hygiene, hair care, and shaving. These activities may also require temporary assistive devices provided by the occupational therapist (Fig. 64-7). Wound care, application of Ace wraps, and getting dressed are attempted after general endurance and range of motion improves, since these activities require greater joint mobility and general strength. In many cases, job-related tasks or household activities are simulated prior to discharge, so that any difficulties can be anticipated. Any adaptations to tools or work setting can then be provided

for or planned for, especially in the case of permanent disability (Fig. 64-8).

During the patient's hospitalization graded activities are provided by the occupational therapist to increase hand strength, joint mobility, and fine motor skills. These activities may range from squeezing a sponge during the first few days to help decrease edema, to working on a selected therapeutic craft activity to increase hand mobility and coordination. Throughout the patient's hospitalization and after discharge, hand function is evaluated with both standardized and nonstandardized techniques to monitor changes in joint range of motion, strength, coordination, and sensation (Fig. 64-9).

Scar control

Any deep second- or third-degree burn of the hand has a high potential for hypertrophic scarring, which not only is unappealing cosmetically but also can compromise function. Therefore it is essential that a scar control program be begun as soon as initial healing occurs.

Good basic skin care is taught, including what types of moisturizing lotions and sunblocks to use. Cold cream, petroleum jelly or oil-based lotions serve as moisture barriers and are best used after washing the hand to seal in moisture already absorbed. However, petroleum or oil-based creams and lotions may block pores and cause secondary infections if not thoroughly cleansed from the skin daily. Also, these creams and lotions do not add moisture to skin that is already dry. Nor can they be used when scar compression garments are worn. These substances are absorbed into the material, causing a loss of elasticity as well as grease stains. Water-based lotions (which readily rinse off the skin with water alone) add moisture to the skin, but because they do not

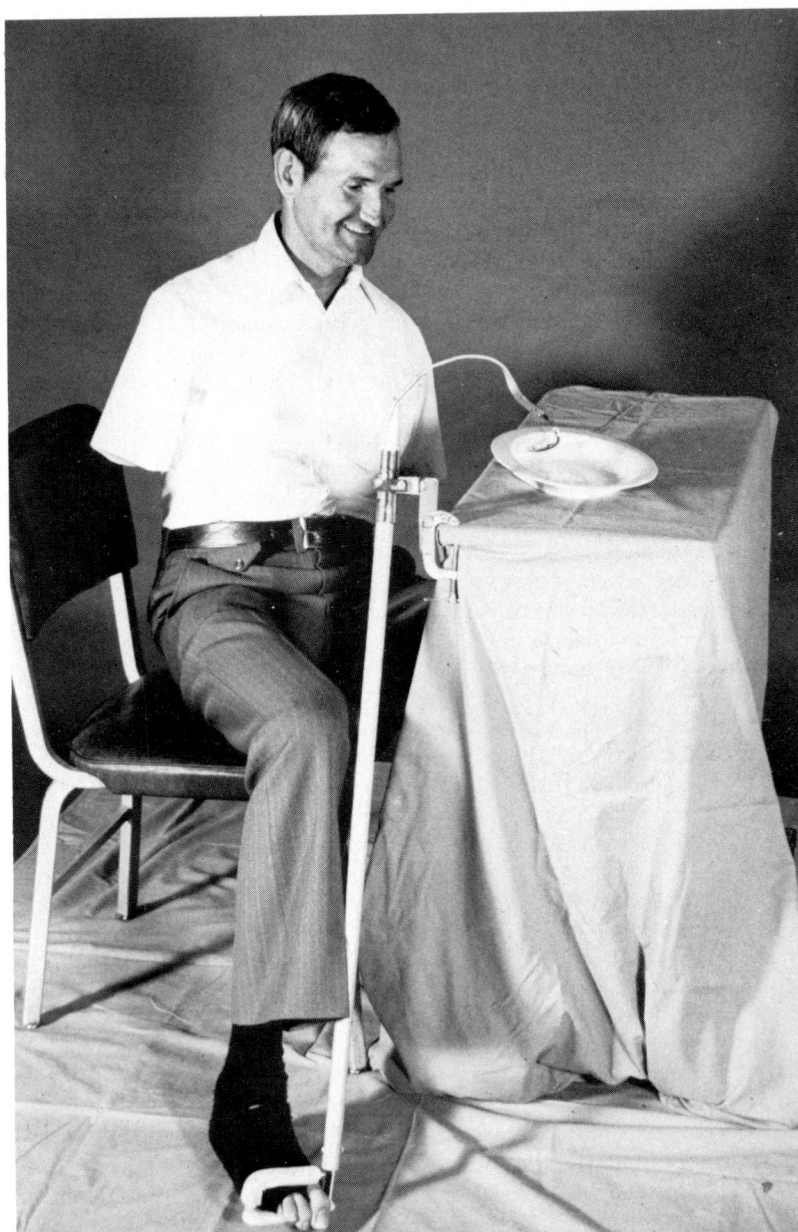

Fig. 64-8 Patient with bilateral shoulder girdle amputations resulting from an electrical injury uses a foot-powered feeding device designed by Larry Smith, Occupational Therapy Adaptive Device Specialist to meet the patient's specific feeding needs.

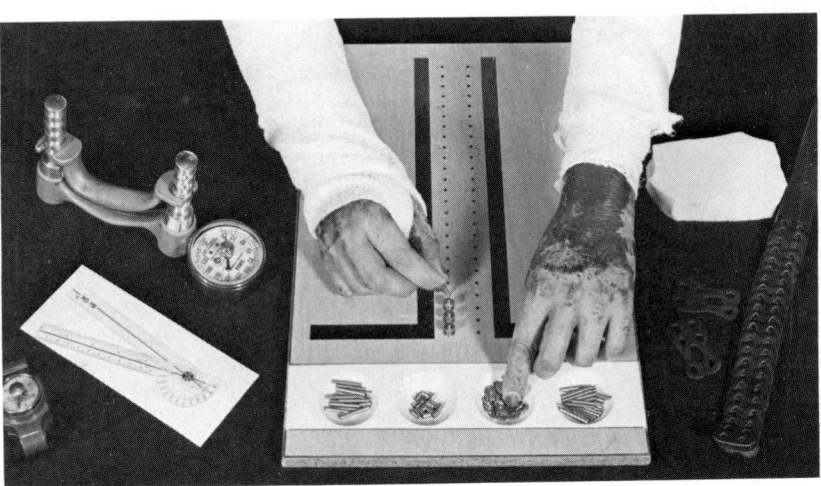

Fig. 64-9 Progress in hand rehabilitation is evaluated by use of standardized tests and completion of functional tasks.

prevent evaporative water loss, they have to be applied more often (two or three times per day). Water-based lotions can be used with scar compression garments without staining them or ruining the elasticity. Moisturizing the skin frequently, especially before exercise, increases the flexibility of the skin and helps minimize itching and breakdown, which occurs to a greater degree if the newly healed burns are allowed to become too dry. Avoidance of direct sunlight on the burn is recommended to prevent sunburn (because a newly healed burn is very sensitive and easily sunburned) and hyperpigmentation. Sunblock lotions of high numerical rating (the higher the number, the stronger the shielding properties) as well as gloves are recommended until the scars have completely matured.

Scar compression is the primary means of preventing the buildup of hypertrophic scarring. Scar compression garments (such as the Jobskin burn compression garments, by Jobst) should be measured for and ordered before discharge, since it may take several weeks for garments to arrive. In the meantime, Isotoner gloves by Aris (with adornments removed and turned inside out so that the seams are outside) along with elastic bandage, serve as the initial compression garments. Tubigrip gloves by Seton come in ready-made sizes and can be used after the skin has stabilized and no longer blistered. Jobst gloves can be ordered with slant inserts to better compress the dorsal web spaces, but they may also require small Betapile or Velfoam pads between the fingers beneath the glove to prevent dorsal hooding scars (Fig. 64-10). Open fingertips can be ordered in the gloves allowing sensory input and visual checking of circulation, but fingertips should be left closed over any finger that has been partially amputated. Zippers may be desirable in the wrists of the initial pair of gloves to increase the ease of application while the newly healed skin is still fragile, so that blistering can be avoided.

It may also be desirable to order the gloves to come 1½ inches above the wrist so that the dorsal hand and wrist receive better compression, since the elastic band at the cuff does not provide adequate compression. An adequate supply of garments will need to be ordered, since the patient will be required to wear the garments at all times, except during

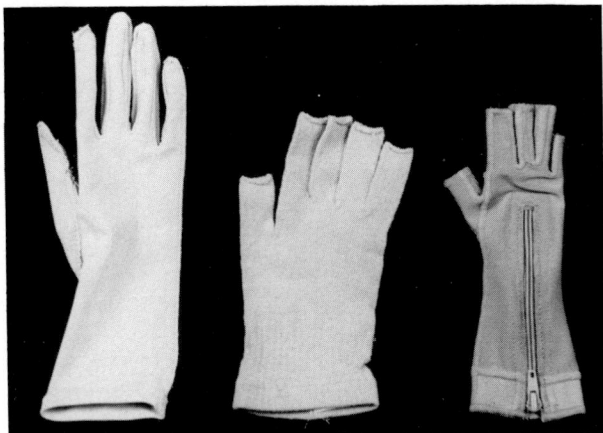

Fig. 64-10 Pictured from left to right are the Aris Isotoner glove, Tubigrip glove (both used with elastic wrap over the palm and wrist), and the Jobst scar compression glove.

meals and baths, until the scars mature. Scar maturation takes an average of 12 to 18 months to occur in hypertrophic scarring and 2 to 3 years in keloid scarring. It is evidenced by a complete fading of the erythema, softening and thinning out of the scars, and an increase in wrinkling and flexibility of the scars.

Certain areas of the hand present special scar problems, which require not only exercise, moisturizing, and compression but also massage to obtain the optimal results in scar control. Scar bands tend to form at the web spaces and palmar surfaces across flexion creases. These areas should be well lubricated with a moisturizing cream before massage or exercise. During massage, firm pressure is applied with the fingers, and the skin is manipulated in a circular motion perpendicular to any existing scar band. At the same time, the skin should be gently, passively stretched to increase the skin surface area.

Discharge

Before discharge the patient is provided with a written home program, including instructions regarding exercises, splinting, activities of daily living to be performed, and scar control techniques. The therapist's phone number is provided in case unforeseen questions arise before the patient's first outpatient visit.

Outpatient follow-up

The patient continues to be seen regularly by the occupational therapist on an outpatient basis for reevaluation in regard to exercise, splinting, activities of daily living, and scar control programs.

Hand function continues to be reevaluated, and adjustments in exercise and splinting programs are made accordingly. When a patient has permanent impairment, the occupational therapist assists the physician in evaluating the patient's current functional level and employment potential and in determining whether he needs to seek a different line of work. A vocational assessment may be performed, with recommendations being made to a vocational rehabilitation or other service agency. The occupational therapist may help the patient to overcome problems that occurred after discharge involving self-care or other activities of daily living, such as cooking, cleaning, and driving. Suggestions for trying new techniques and for arranging the work space more efficiently are made, and, when necessary, self-help devices are provided.

The patient may need to be remeasured for new pressure garments to accommodate changes in weight or, in the case of children, growth spurts. Special conformers, not previously required, may be necessary under the Jobst garments to maximize compression (i.e., Otoform conformer used in the palm).

The occupational therapist will continue to follow the patient as an outpatient (or as an inpatient, if reconstruction procedures are necessary) until the scar control program is discontinued and maximum functional results are obtained. This may take years. The quality of the results is directly related to the motivation and active participation of the patient in the rehabilitation process. Therefore the occupational therapist must emphasize the importance of the patient's involvement in the setting of long-term treatment goals. When rehabilitation of the burned hand is complete, it is the patient who should feel the greatest sense of accomplishment.

Physical therapy

The goals that the physical therapist strives to reach are to maintain the patient's range of motion and stength and to work with the occupational therapist and the surgeon in helping the patient to perform ADL independently. If these goals are reached, numerous surgical procedures for contractures and scar release may be unnecessary. To rehabilitate a patient with upper extremity burns successfully, the physical therapy program must begin in the acute stage of burn care and continue for at least 12 to 18 months. The rehabilitation program includes: (1) proper positioning of the burned joints of the upper extremity when they are not splinted, (2) an aggressive exercise regimen, (3) reinforcing independence in ADL, and (4) comprehensive physical therapy follow-up care.

Positioning

The following positions for upper extremity burns are accepted widely as ideal; however, modifications are often necessary because each patient requires "custom" positioning, with the degree and extent of the burn being taken into account.

Shoulder. If good positioning is not maintained, the shoulder tends to contract in adduction and internal rotation. The ideal position is with a minimum of 90 degrees abduction, shoulder girdle retraction, and neutral rotation, especially after grafting of the axilla, when the shoulder is immobilized for 5 to 7 days.

Elbow. Flexion and pronation contractures occur without adequate physical therapy. The ideal position is in complete extension and neutral with respect to pronation and supination.

Hand. If the hand is not positioned properly, the typical burned-hand deformity can develop. It consists of wrist flexion, MP hyperextension, PIP flexion and DIP flexion or extension, thumb adduction, and interphalangeal extension. Thus the correct positioning for a dorsal hand burn is antideformity, approximately 0 to 30 degrees wrist extension, 90 degrees metacarpophalangeal flexion, 0 degrees proximal interphalangeal and distal interphalangeal flexion (depending on depth of burn), and thumb abduction with slight interphalangeal flexion.

• • •

Correct upper extremity positioning must be maintained (with or without a splint) at all times except during exercise periods. If a patient is motivated, works well on his own, and progresses with his range of motion, splinting need be performed only during long periods of rest. All burned upper extremity joints should be positioned and splinted during sleep.

Communication among surgeon, nurse, occupational therapist, and physical therapist concerning surgical procedures is essential to determine: (1) what area will be debrided and/or grafted, (2) where the donor sites will be, (3) what position the patient will be in postoperatively, (4) if any splints will be needed to maintain the desired position, (5) how and by what means the grafted area is to be supported, and (6) what exercises are permitted. Correct positioning immediately after grafting is critical to the maintenance of range of motion, because all movement of the grafted area is contraindicated for approximately 1 week to allow the graft to adhere to the recipient site. During this period of immobilization, contractures could begin.

Exercise management

In the acute stage of burn care, emphasis is on maintenance of range of motion and muscle tone more than on strength; therefore active and active-assistive exercises are used for the burned joints. In most instances these exercises are done while the patient is in the Hubbard tank, because the warm water tends to increase the pain threshold and tissue extensibility. Thus most patients move more willingly, and greater range of motion is possible. As eschar separates and peripheral nerves regenerate, exercising becomes extremely painful. It is at this stage that contractures can begin to appear. The proprioceptive neuromuscular facilitation techniques of contract-relax and rhythmic stabilization are helpful in maintaining range of motion during this period.

When a patient is taken to surgery for débridement and/or grafting of his upper extremity, the physical therapist accompanies him because this is an opportunity to fully evaluate the patient's "pain-free" range of motion and to exercise an uncooperative patient thoroughly. Joints are not forced at this time, and care must be taken not to tear contracted soft tissue. Physical therapy is not discontinued totally during the week of immobilization after grafting. The patient should be instructed to do isometric exercises to maintain the tone of the muscles that act on the immobilized joints, including uninjured areas. Active and/or resistive exercises should be continued for the joints not grafted. Ambulation should be reinitiated as soon as possible after grafting.

After the period of immobilization for grafting, splints are removed and gentle active exercises are begun. Gradually, the patient's upper extremity therapy program is augmented to include active-assistive, resistive, and stretching exercises. The uninvolved extremities and joints of the burned upper extremity must not be overlooked. Resistive exercises should be applied to these areas during all stages of rehabilitation when the patient's medical status allows. Individual exercises are planned for the shoulder, elbow, wrist, and hand because the patient with only a burned hand will often "splint" the rest of the extremity in an effort to make himself comfortable.

Exercise should be supervised at least twice a day by a physical therapist. A minimum of seven to ten repetitions of each exercise should be done. The ideal goal of physical therapy is to have the patient moving his burned upper extremity at least every 2 hours. To attain this goal, the patient's own motivation and willingness to follow through with instructions are critical. Giving the patient a list of the exercises he is to do and putting it where he can see it or having him commit them to memory have been helpful in encouraging him to exercise more. An exercise list also informs the nurse and other medical personnel of the exercises and number of repetitions the patient should be doing independently. Other medical personnel and the patient's relatives can reinforce the physical therapist's efforts by encouraging the patient to do his exercises when the therapist is not present. Goniometric measurements should be taken at appropriate intervals to document progression or regression objectively.

The following exercises are specific ones that have proven successful in maintaining or gaining range of motion and strength for the burned upper extremity.

Shoulder exercises

1. Simple overhead pulley allows one upper extremity to stretch the other in shoulder flexion and abduction and elbow extension.
2. Reaching for opposite ear across the top of the head helps maintain shoulder abduction.
3. Wall climbing exercises with the patient facing the wall are for shoulder flexion; with the side to the wall they are for shoulder abduction.
4. Shoulder is abducted while the patient is lying on a bench and holding a small weight in each hand; the arms are abducted as much as possible, with the elbows kept locked in a neutral position.
5. Hold a stick or broom handle while in a supine position, bringing the arms back as far as possible over the head while trying to touch the bed. This exercise stretches the shoulder.
6. Hanging from stall bars stretches tight shoulders and elbows. This is reserved for healed and/or grafted wounds in deep second- or third-degree burns; however, it can be used as a maintenance exercise for shoulder and/or elbows of an unburned or superficial second-degree burned upper extremity.
7. Wand exercises are good for shoulder abduction, flexion, and internal rotation (Fig. 64-11).
8. With hands clasped behind the head, pull elbows together and then spread them out to the side and back as far as possible.

Elbow exercise

1. Holding a small weight while walking stretches the elbow into extension.
2. Patient can stretch his own elbow into extension by placing the burned arm on the edge of a table and using the other hand to push down on the forearm.

3. Simple overhead pulley helps in elbow extension (see shoulder exercises).
4. Hanging from stall bars helps in elbow extension (see shoulder exercises).

After grafting, elbow extension can be maintained only through vigorous exercise and splinting. It is easier to maintain complete elbow extension after grafting than to reduce an elbow flexion contracture. One should not be overly concerned, however, if a patient develops decreased elbow flexion from prolonged splinting in extension, because as he gradually resumes his ADL, elbow flexion returns to normal limits. The same is not true for decreased elbow extension. When an elbow flexion contracture begins, it tends to worsen with time because most activities of daily living demand elbow flexion.

Forearm exercises

1. Tuck the flexed elbow against the patient's side and manually assist it into supination.
2. Turning a doorknob improves supination.
3. Working with a screwdriver enhances supination or pronation.

Wrist exercises

1. Prayer exercise—holding palms together in a prayer position and winging elbows out to the side to form a right angle at the wrist helps maintain wrist extension (Fig. 64-12).
2. Rocking wrist—place fingers on a table and gently rock the wrist back and forth, pushing wrist into extension. Wrist flexion is achieved by placing the dorsum of the hand on the table and repeating the exercise.
3. Wall push-ups—with hands flat on wall, feet approximately 2 or 3 feet away from wall, and face close to the wall, push chest away from wall with arms, keeping hands flat. This exercise maintains wrist extension.

Hand exercises. The techniques of exercising an acutely burned hand (before grafting) with deep second- and/or third-degree burns are of utmost importance. One must keep in mind the amount of tension placed on the finger extensor mechanism when administering stretching and active-

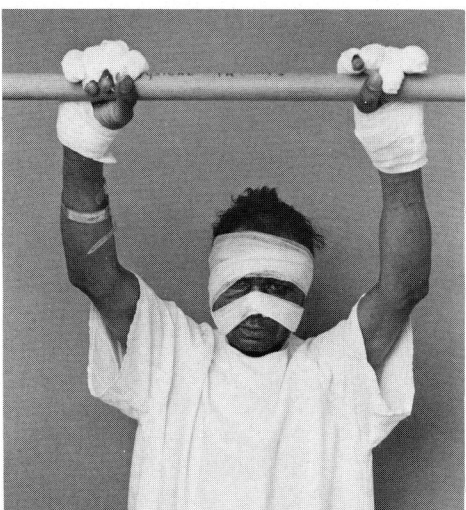

Fig. 64-11 Wand exercises will improve shoulder flexion and increase the strength of weak musculature.

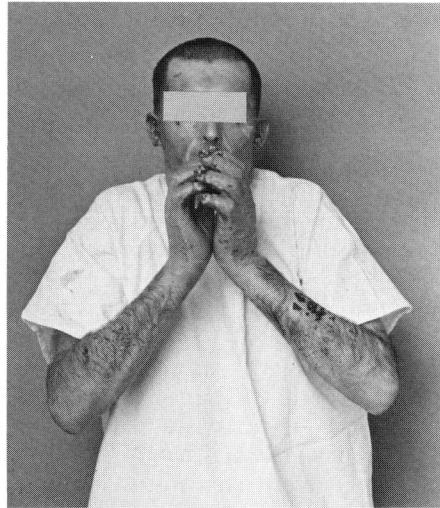

Fig. 64-12 Prayer exercise allows patient to passively stretch his own wrist in extension.

assistive exercises. Pushing fingers into mass flexion to make a fist is dangerous because components of the finger extensor mechanism can slip, split, and be damaged beyond repair. For each individual finger, active-assistive exercises should be performed in the following manner:

1. To accomplish MP flexion and extension, keep the PIP and DIP joints of the same finger blocked in extension.
2. For PIP flexion and extension keep the MP and DIP joints in extension (Fig. 64-13).
3. For DIP flexion and extension keep the MP and PIP joints in extension.
4. Stretch thumb and finger web spaces.
5. For thumb MP flexion and extension keep thumb interphalangeal joint blocked in extension.
6. For thumb interphalangeal flexion and extension keep MP joint of thumb blocked in extension.
7. Thumb opposition—assist patient in touching tip of thumb to base of small finger.
8. Fist making—only active, no assistance.
9. Try to touch the tip of each individual finger to palm—only active, no assistance.
10. Rocking weight on fingertips—place fingertips on table and gently rock body weight against them. This helps to check incipient flexion contractures of the finger.

For less extensive burns of the hand—that is, superficial second-degree burns—more aggressive physical therapy can be done. Active-assistive and passive-stretching exercises, if necessary, should be used to maintain range of motion.

After grafting and/or healing, active-assistive fist making should begin with gentle stretching of each finger joint individually. The patient should be encouraged to exercise his hands on his own at least every hour. Using Theraplast or Be-OK Putty is an excellent way to achieve this goal. Theraplast is a flexible substance patients can use independently for exercising their hands; it helps to increase strength and range of motion in the grafted hand. The patient with arthritis of the hands should squeeze foam rubber instead of

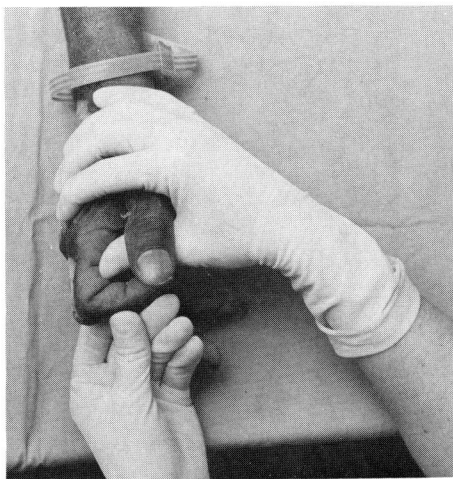

Fig. 64-13 Therapist should support metacarpophalangeal joint in extension while flexing proximal interphalangeal joint to reduce tension on the extensor mechanism.

putty (which is stressful to his joints). By using his burned hands before and after grafting in activities of daily living, the patient is exercising and placing his hands in functional positions.

Follow-up care

Patients with upper extremity burns are discharged with a home exercise program. The period from discharge up to 1½ years after the burn is the most important time. They are scheduled to return at appropriate intervals for evaluation of strength, range of motion, and skin condition. Good physical therapy follow-up care is important because the majority of the healing process takes place at home. Many patients are discharged with normal range of motion, only to return for the first clinic visit with multiple contractures. This problem can be alleviated to a certain extent by intensive follow-up management.

Hypertrophic scars usually make their first appearance after the patient is discharged from the hospital. These scars can be difficult to manage because they can continue to enlarge for 12 to 18 months and if removed surgically they may recur. Antiscar pressure garments have been effective in preventing these unfortunate consequences of burns. Wrapping the burned upper extremity with elastic bandages may help to prevent hypertrophic scars but is not as effective as custom-fitted garments. The patient should be measured for his garments before discharge, since it takes approximately 5 weeks for each custom order to be filled. To produce a beneficial result, the garment must be worn continuously except for laundering or if it inhibits the patient during exercise periods.

Because the nurse spends the most time of any member of the burn team with the patient, he or she may facilitate the patient's recovery and rehabilitation. It is the nurse who must ensure that the doctor's orders are carried out, that the hands continue to be elevated, that the splints are worn as they were intended, that the wounds are covered with topical chemotherapy continuously, that the skin grafts do not get dislodged, and that the patient mobilizes the hands continuously. In smaller hospitals, the nurse assumes many of the duties described previously for other members of the burn team.

Following skin coverage of the burned hand, it is very tempting to begin reconstruction immediately. Because the character of the healing burn wound changes for more than 6 months after injury, it is wise to delay all but the most immediate problems (such as a severe elbow flexion contracture that obviously cannot be splinted into neutral) and for the burn team to plan an outpatient treatment program for the patient. With proper splinting and an exercise program, strength and muscle mass will increase gradually; skin will soften and become more pliable. After several months, the patient's functional problems will be defined more clearly and definitive surgical reconstruction can be planned.

It is imperative that the burn team act in concert with the vocational rehabilitation counselors, representatives of the insurance companies, rehabilitation nurses, and the patient's family and employer, to achieve meaningful rehabilitation. For instance, in North Carolina in 1975, 46,350 days were lost from work because of burn injuries, at a cost of $2,370,000. Early consultation with the vocational rehabilitation counselor ensures that the patient will have a strong ally when he leaves the hospital and, most importantly, a plan for employment. With unemployment a national problem, it is obvious that an employer may be reluctant to rehire an injured person when he can obtain the services of one with normally functioning hands. The surgeon and the burn team must concentrate all their efforts to achieve a functional result that will allow the patient to resume his previous job or compete for a new one.

BIBLIOGRAPHY

Malick MH and Carr JA: Manual on management of the burn patient, Pittsburgh, 1982, Harmarville Rehabilitation Center Educational Resource Division.

Von Prince K and Yeakel M: The splinting of burn patients, Springfield, Ill, 1974, Charles C Thomas, Publisher.

65

Remodeling of scar tissue in the burned hand

Wandra K. Miles and Laurie Grigsby

The objectives of therapy in scar management of the burned hand are to maintain and improve function, prevent deformity, and improve appearance. Because the survival rate of burn patients has increased significantly, we are now faced with the challenge of attempting to control scar formation, the major cause of disability. Early excision and grafting, traction, pressure, ultrasound, and injections are therapies presently being used to manage scar; however, none has proved to be totally effective.[59] This chapter stresses the importance of early management of scar in the burned hand, with special emphasis on the most universal methods being used: exercise, pressure, and externally applied traction through splinting.

Scar formation is a natural sequela in the healing process of burned skin. Although it has been observed that scars do diminish with time,[59] motion must be maintained until scar maturation to prevent or minimize the need for reconstructive surgery. It is important to remember that scarring cannot be prevented; attempting to control it is all that can be done.

CLASSIFICATION OF THERMAL INJURIES

In the burn injury, there are standard classifications to identify depth of injury.[33,34] The superficial partial-thickness burn involves the epidermis and may also involve the upper dermis. These burns are characterized by edema, blister formation, pain, and erythema. The skin will heal spontaneously by re-epithelialization, with good functional ability and appearance. Deep partial-thickness burns, also referred to as deep second-degree burns, involve damage to the epidermis and dermis. Deep partial-thickness burns can heal spontaneously but with decreased function and poor appearance. Full-thickness burns do not heal spontaneously and require grafting for wound closure. Deep partial-thickness burns and full-thickness burns commonly develop contractures and hypertrophic scarring that can result in major deformity and disability. Electrical burns often damage muscle and bone. Because therapy considerations are more complex, electrical burns are not discussed here.

NORMAL WOUND HEALING

There are three sequential stages involved in the process of wound healing: (1) inflammation, (2) migration and proliferation of connective tissue cells and blood vessels, and (3) deposition of a new connective tissue matrix. Each stage appears to be activated by specific molecular signals.[21]

The initial cells entering the injured site produce factors that serve as signals to influence the movement of specialized cells, such as neutrophils and monocytes, to the injured site to repair the tissue[29] (Fig. 65-1, *A*). In the early inflammatory phase, neutrophils infiltrate the site of injury to remove infectious bacteria. Also present are monocytes, which convert to macrophages. This infiltration begins the transition from the inflammatory stage to the second stage of wound healing. In this stage, macrophages function to initiate proliferation and migration of cells that are involved in granulation tissue formation. Granulation tissue is composed of macrophages, fibroblasts, and newly formed blood vessels (Fig. 65-1, *B*).

Some of the proliferating fibroblasts undergo a cell phenotype change and become myofibroblasts. These have characteristics similar to those of smooth muscle cells and have stress fibers rich in actin. The myofibroblasts also have motility and contractile-like properties and are believed to stimulate wound contraction.[37] The postulated mechanism by which this occurs is through the collective force of actin contraction in the myofibroblasts. This contraction then exerts a pull to the linker molecule (fibronexus). However, a recent study by Ehrlich[23] disputes this opinion. He concluded that fibroblasts working as individual units, not myofibroblasts working in unison, are responsible for the forces involved in connective tissue matrix reorganization, wound contraction, and scar contracture. The fibronexus complex plays an essential role in cell-cell and cell-collagen matrix adhesion.[13]

The final stage of wound healing is matrix formation and remodeling. In this stage, fibronexin serves as a template for fibroblasts to synthesize collagen.[13] Collagen is the major protein of the body; it is an important element of skin, tendon, ligament, and bone. During the second week of wound repair, tissue resiliency develops as the glycosamino-chrondroitin-4-sulfate replaces the hyaluronic acid and facilitates the deposition and remodeling of collagen. This leads to a gradual accumulation of fibrillar collagen (types I, II, III), basement membrane collagen (type IV), and type V collagen, which is associated with capillary endothelial cells during granulation tissue development.[13] Initially the collagen that is formed is fragile and resembles a gel-like material with poor tensile strength. Approximately 20% of its final strength is established by the third week. Tensile strength slowly increases over time and mirrors the collagen content of the wound during the remodeling phase. Approximately 70% of its tensile strength is obtained by 2 months.

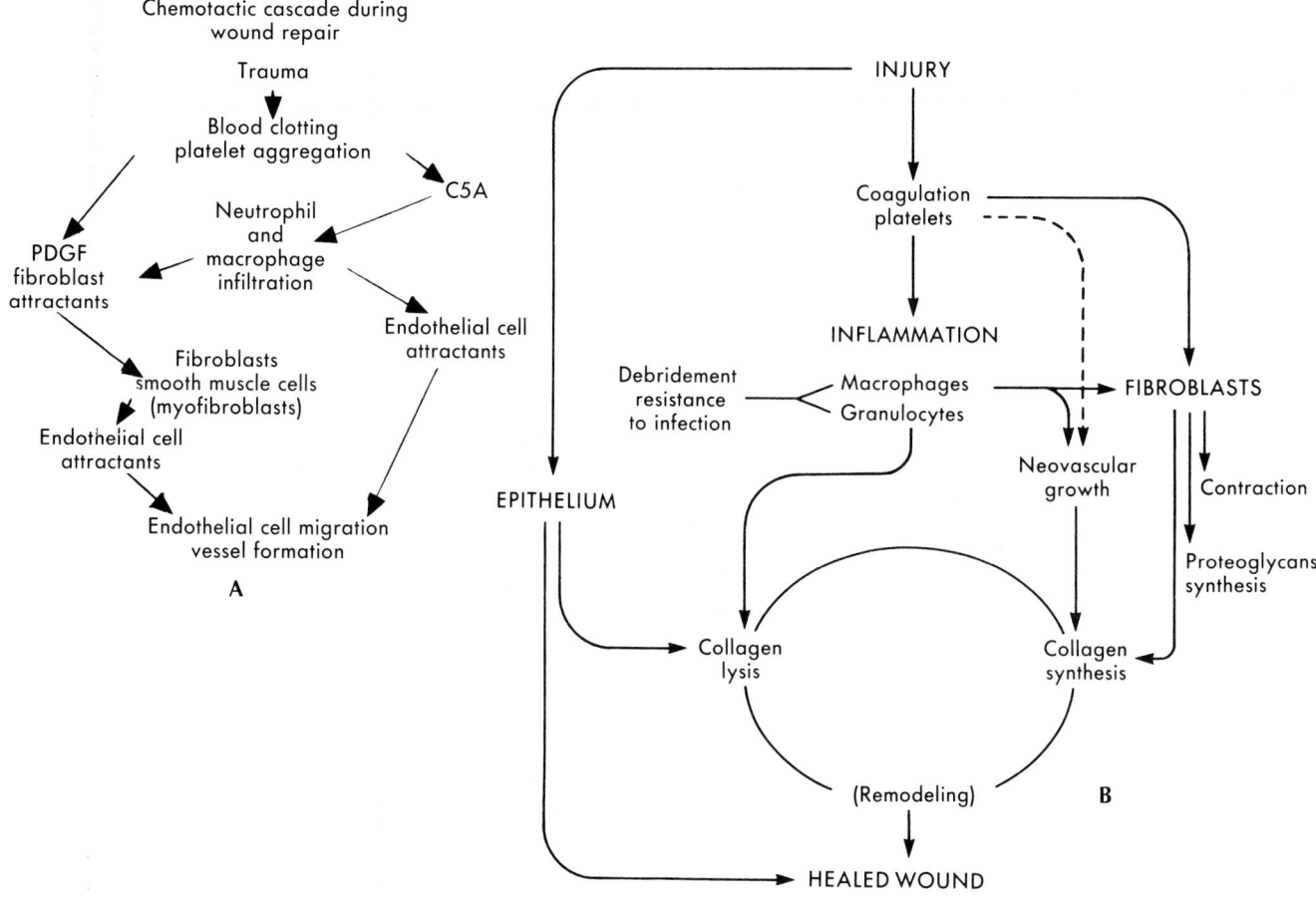

Fig. 65-1 **A,** Chemotactic cascade during wound repair. **B,** Diagram of wound healing. (**A,** Courtesy of Gary Grotendorst, Ph.D., J Trauma 24[suppl 9]:49, 1984. **B,** Courtesy of Dr. Thomas K. Hunt, University of California School of Medicine, San Francisco.)

HYPERTROPHIC SCARS, KELOIDS, AND SCAR CONTRACTURE

Grotendorst[29] has suggested that because the skin fibroblasts typically involved in normal wound healing are destroyed at the site, connective tissue cells from deeper structures are recruited to repair the wound. This process affects the quality of repair, because it leads to a predominance of myofibroblasts. The myofibroblasts synthesize types III and V collagen, which are found in scar tissue.[5] Current evidence suggests that overabundance of myofibroblasts is noted in contracted scars.[65] A contracture has been defined as a shortening of scar, causing limitation of joint or skin movement.

Infection, lack of available donor sites, or poor granulation beds for grafting often can delay wound closure in the thermally injured hand. The excessive collagen deposition then needed to close the wound results in a tight, rigid, nonresilient scar. The overall effect of the excess collagen is the formation of hypertrophic scars and keloids. This can be seen by comparing the organized patterns of normal collagen in Fig. 65-2, *A* with the highly disorganized patterns of hypertrophic scar in Fig. 65-2, *B*.

Hypertrophic scars and keloids result from an imbalance between collagen synthesis and collagen lysis. Hypertrophic scars have been described as excess collagen that stays within the boundary of the wound.[34,59] Keloids demonstrate excessive amounts of collagen that no longer conform to the boundaries of the wound.[34,59] Hypertrophic scars are commonly found in areas of motion such as the joints, because tension along the scar promotes collagen deposits and lessens collagen lysis.[34]

Keloids have been found to occur at a higher incidence in individuals with dark skin. This may because of increased skin pigmentation.[66] Koonin[46] has hypothesized that increased keloid formation in darker skin appears to be attributable to increased reactivity of melanocytes to melanocyte-stimulating hormones rather than to increased tension on the wound. This viewpoint has been supported clinically, because keloids rarely occur on the palms or the soles, where melanocytes are rare.

Keloids often have been described as painful. The hyperalgesia appears to be supported by the presence of numerous nerve terminals found in keloids.[66]

Increased levels of mast cells (which produce histamine and heparin) have been noted in keloids and hypertrophic scars. There is evidence that histamine may accelerate collagen synthesis whereas heparin enhances vascularization of the growing keloids.[68,70] A study by Smith[68] indicated that keloid formers showed a higher incidence of allergic symptoms than did hypertrophic scar formers and normal subjects in the experiment. Studies[15,70] have shown that the

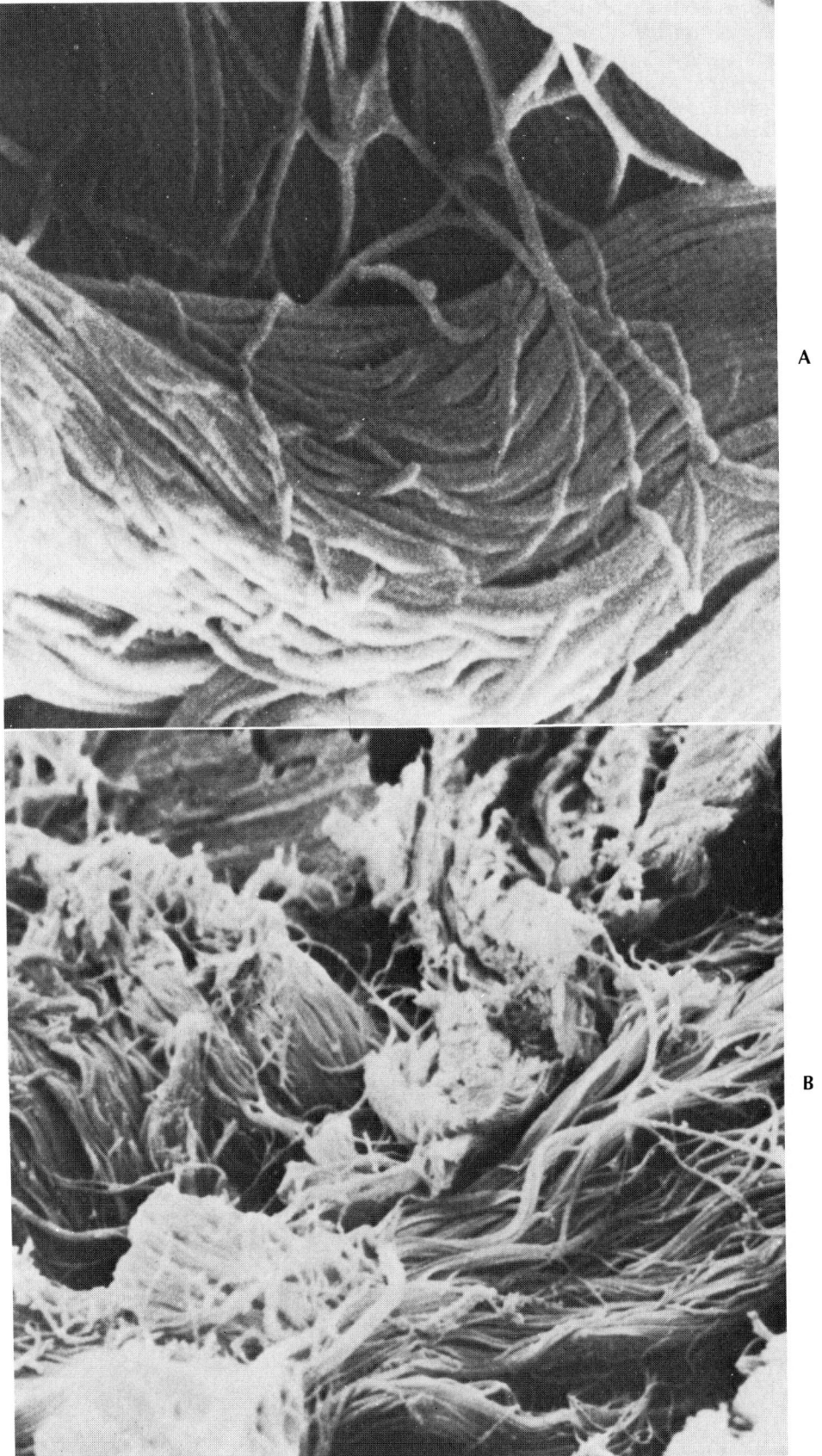

Fig. 65-2   A, Normal skin collagen at 10,000 magnification. Notice uniformity of collagen fibrils. **B,** Scanning electron microscopy of collagen near a rat colon anastomosis. Notice lack of definition and disorganization of new collagen fibrils. (Courtesy Dr. Thomas K. Hunt, University of California School of Medicine, San Francisco.)

commonly reported irritating symptom of itching may be reduced or abolished with the use of pharmacologic antihistamine. Topol[70] has presented the question of whether an antihistamine would be effective in prevention of keloid recurrence if it were administered after excision.

The incidence of hypertrophic scarring has been noted to be greater in children and in adolescents in puberty than in adults, especially the elderly. This may be the result of the accelerated cell growth in the young as well as the decreased tautness and associated lower level of tension in the skin of the elderly.

Overall, the risk of developing hypertrophic scars has been found to be related to burn size and depth, anatomic location of the burn injury, race, and age.[20] The most pre-

dominant factor appears to be the time needed to obtain complete closure of the wound.[20,59]

Scarring in the hand

Several forces throughout the healing of the thermally injured hand can contribute to deformity. Scar hypertrophy and contracture are major ones. Besides the obvious effect scar hypertrophy and contracture can have on the appearance of the hand, without intervention they can have a devastating effect on the structures and function of the hand. In the case of burns of the dorsum of the hand, even where there is not joint or tendon involvement, the force of the contracting scar can pull the metacarpophalangeal (MP) joints into hyperextension with the interphalangeal (IP) joints flexed or

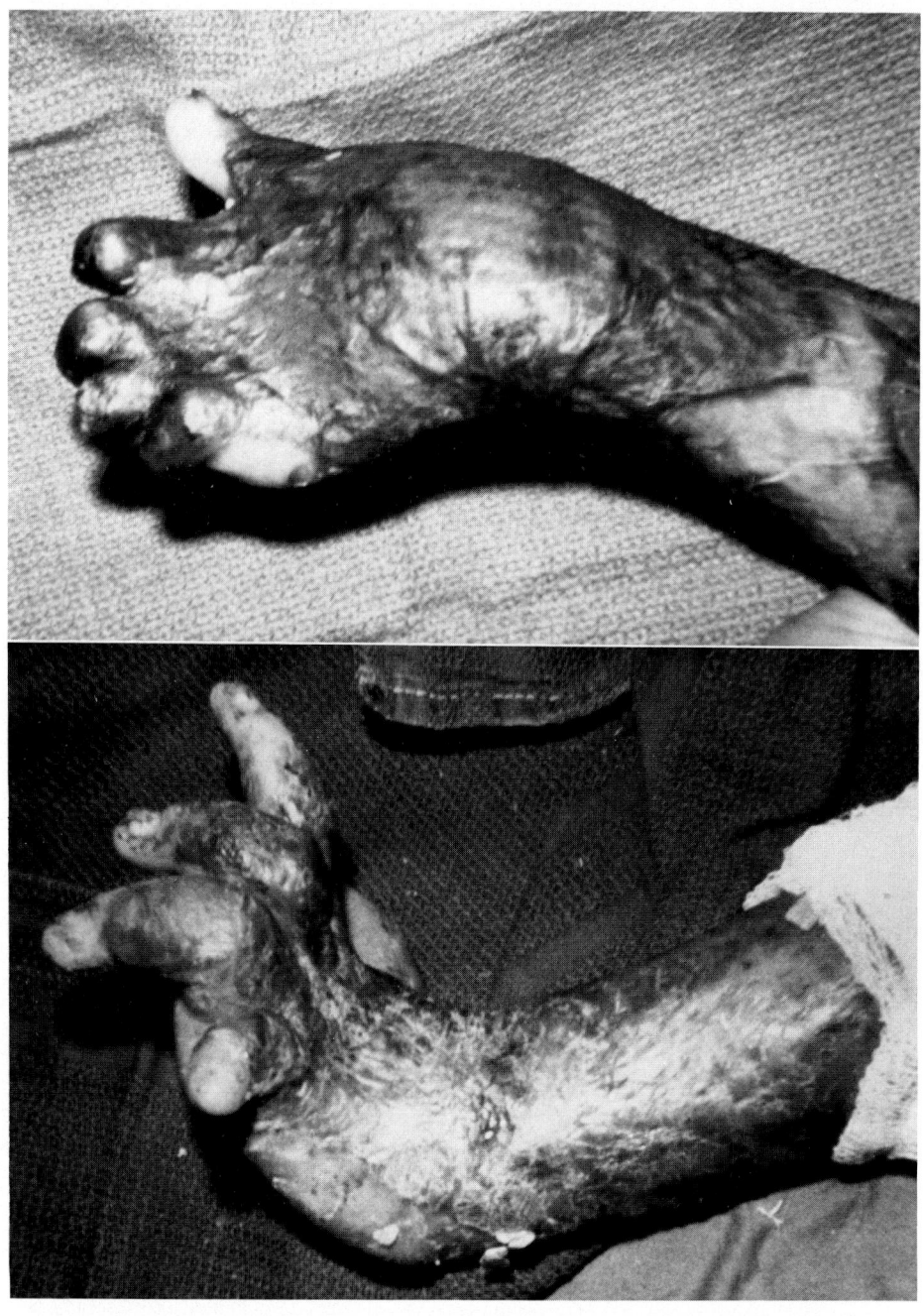

Fig. 65-3 **A** and **B**, Deformities that can result from scarring in the burned hand.

hyperextended. Flattening of the transverse and longitudinal arches occurs, and in more extreme cases, a reverse palmar arch can occur. The fifth digit may be ulnarly rotated. The thumb is pulled into extension and adduction, and the thenar web is contracted. Scarring in the interdigital web spaces pulls the fingers together. Even in the absence of other contractures, this can limit spherical grasp. Essentially, this is a nonfunctional hand: no grasp (except perhaps limited IP flexion or limited thumb adduction), no opposition, and no prehension. What begins as just contracting scar, if unopposed, can lead to shortening of other tissues such as muscles, tendons, and joint capsules, joint subluxation, bone deformities, and muscle imbalance (Fig. 65-3).

Scarring on the palmar surface of the hand can also cause impairment, though usually not to the same magnitude as dorsal scarring. Contracting scar in the palm alone can result in loss of the palmar web, and this can result in loss of thumb and finger extension and abduction.

A 1 cm scar contracture in an adult hand may cause little loss of motion. That same 1 cm contracture in a small child's hand may cause a more significant loss of motion.[30]

PHASES OF BURN RECOVERY

The therapist's role in scar remodeling of the burned hand, particularly concerning exercise, pressure, and splinting, is discussed below in four phases of burn recovery: the emergent phase, the acute phase, the skin-grafting phase, and the rehabilitation phase.

Emergent phase

The emergent phase of burn recovery is generally considered to be the first 48 to 72 hours after injury. The therapist's goals at this time are to control edema and to initiate and maintain active motion.

Edema control. During the first 3 to 5 days after burns to the upper extremity, it is essential to control the hard, immobile edema to prevent fibrosis and ischemic necrosis of the intrinsic muscles of the hand.[9] Madden and Enna[49] have pointed out that evaluation of the radial or ulnar pulses may not be adequate in assessing ischemia. Frequent checks of median and ulnar nerve sensation and of motor power to the intrinsic musculature was believed by Madden and Enna to be more beneficial to determine if there is vascular insufficiency caused by edema. If the therapist notes difficulties, the difficulties should be reported to the surgeon, because an escharotomy may be necessary.

Initially, to help control edema the hand can be elevated at heart level. The arm should be supported in extension with pillows or a foam support from the axilla to the hand. A foam donut can be provided to prevent excessive weight-bearing stress to the olecranon of the elbow, which can result in tingling sensations caused by pressure on the ulnar nerve. Wadsworth and Williams[71] have demonstrated how the prolonged position of the elbow flexed in 90 degrees can cause internal pressure by the arcuate ligament onto the ulnar nerve, and how the prolonged position of forearm pronation can cause external compression on the ulnar nerve. This can result in motor weakness of the intrinsic muscles as well as in impaired sensation in the ulnar nerve distribution in the hand.

Compression dressings should not be initiated during this phase of recovery until vessels begin to regain their normal permeabilities. In approximately 5 days the edema is more mobile and will be responsive to compressive wraps. Where initially the skin felt taut when gently pressed by the therapist's fingertip, there is now more give. One sign of this in a patient who also has facial burns is that the edema will have subsided enough for the patient to open his eyes.

Motion in the control of edema. Active motion, in conjunction with elevation, is also effective in the early control of edema. Simple wiggling of the digits is totally ineffective. The muscle contraction must be forceful enough to serve as a pumping mechanism to help venous blood and lymph return.[6] Exercise sessions should take place during the dressing change, at which time the therapist can evaluate the wound and range of motion. Exercises should be done as quickly as possible because debridement and reapplication of dressings must also be done. The wound must not remain open for long, because extreme heat loss can occur, and increased risk of infection is present when there are extensive body surface area burns.

The goal of therapy is to gain full fist closure, finger extension, and thumb opposition. However, edema may limit full range of motion. Active range of motion exercises can be done by "grouping motions." For example, active fist closure and hooking motions can be done to obtain tendon gliding of the long flexors. The patient should oppose the thumb to each fingertip and make circles clockwise and counterclockwise with the thumb. Emphasis should be placed on MP flexion and IP extension. For older children, modified standard exercise protocols can be followed. Younger children should be encouraged to participate in age-appropriate play activities that facilitate active motion.

Dressing application. The functions of dressings are to (1) protect the wound against infection, (2) maintain contact between the topical agent and the wound, (3) debride the wound, (4) provide pressure for early management of scar, and (5) provide comfort for the patient, particularly during movement. The role of pressure for scar control is discussed in the sections on pressure. The dressings should not be restrictive, because they can inhibit range of motion by discouraging spontaneous movement of the digits and cause isolated pockets of edema.

Different facilities use different dressing techniques, and all are effective. A technique should be chosen that works best for each patient population and setting. One method for dressing the hand is described here. Sterile technique should be observed when applying dressings. A 2 × 2 inch fine-mesh gauze pad is first draped volarly to dorsally around each finger. Two-inch fine-mesh gauze is then wrapped around the hand to cover the dorsal and volar aspects of the palm. The topical agent is applied. As the procedure is repeated, a second layer of bandages is then applied, but Kling* is used in place of fine-mesh gauze. In some facilities the topical agent is applied with a tongue blade directly onto each piece of gauze, which is then applied to the patient. Patients have reported that there is less pain with this method. To complete the dressing, the bandages are secured with Surgifix† (tubular net bandage retainer) to keep them in place and to prevent them from unraveling. When the

---

*Johnson & Johnson, New Brunswick, NJ.
†FRA Surgifix, Inc., Elmsford, NY.

dressing is complete, the therapist instructs the patient to make a fist. If motion appears to be restricted by the dressings, the bandages are loosened or adjusted.

Traction. During the emergent phase, static splinting is used mainly to support the hand and to maintain joint alignment. The majority of burns of the hand involve the dorsal rather than the volar surface. Dorsal edema encourages wrist flexion, MP joint hyperextension, and IP joint flexion. Edema of the intrinsic muscles contributes to proximal interphalangeal joint (PIP) flexion.[49] To counteract the positioning force of edema, it is recommended that the wrist be maintained in 15 to 20 degrees of extension, the MP joints flexed 60 to 70 degrees, the IP joints extended fully, and the thumb positioned in palmar abduction with the IP joint flexed. When younger children are splinted during the emergent phase, the MP joints do not necessarily have to be in as much as 60 to 70 degrees of flexion.

Whether to use a splint acutely is determined by the experienced therapist (in accordance with physician orders) based on the depth of the wound and on the cooperation of the patient. It is not usually necessary to splint the hands of infants and toddlers during this phase unless the wrist needs to be supported. If the child is 3 years or older, splinting should be considered. If a decision is made not to splint the infant or toddler, bulky dressings that support the hand are sufficient. For example, a small roll of gauze that helps maintain the thenar web and the palmar arch can be wrapped in the palm. The therapist should evaluate the patient on a daily basis to determine the need for splinting.

Prefabricated handsplints can be applied initially if a therapist is not immediately available to construct custom splints. They are generally adequate for superficial burns with excessive edema during the first 3 to 5 days after edema formation. For full-thickness burns of the hand where immobile edema is present, customized splints are necessary. If the hand is extremely edematous, it must be forced into the ideal position described above, because this could lead to ischemia caused by loss of capillary integrity. Serial splinting should be initiated as the edema begins to subside. The splint should conform to the person, not the person to the splint.

During the initial 3 to 5 days, the splint should be applied with gauze wraps. Elastic wraps can cause vascular compromise. Straps should not be used because they can cause a tourniquet effect. The splint should be removed on a regular schedule for supervised exercises and for self-care tasks and then reapplied. In the case of children, the splint should be removed for play activities. Adaptive devices such as utensils with built-up handles should be provided as necessary.

Acute phase

The acute phase generally extends from the emergent phase until wound closure. Clark[13] has reported that collagen synthesis can begin as early as 3 days after injury and remain rapid for up to 6 months. After 6 months this process slows and continues for 1 to 2 years after the injury. Therefore, early intervention is imperative for orientation of the collagen fibers that are being deposited in order for deformity caused by scar formation to be minimized or prevented.

Motion. At this time, the therapist should be aware that full active range of motion can be compromised by fibrous

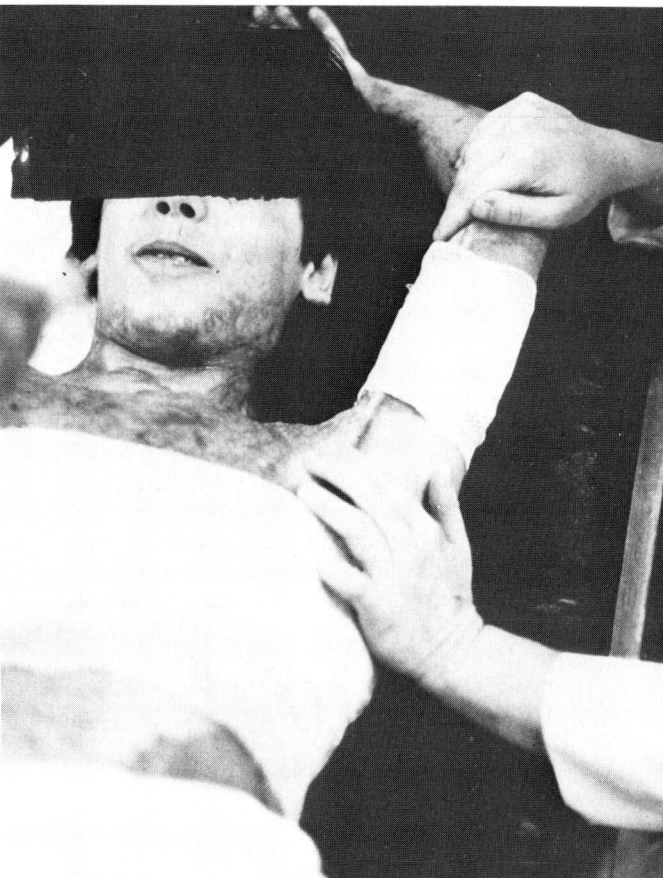

Fig. 65-4 Restriction of forward flexion of shoulder caused by hypertrophic scar banding in axilla.

(not pitting) edema, by inelastic eschar (destroyed nonviable tissue), or by tension from newly deposited collagen. The scar band from newly deposited collagen can appear in the open wound as well as in the closed wound. To help judge if more active motion should be expected from the patient when he appears to be at his maximum range, gently press the scar band to test the tension of the scar (Fig. 65-4). If it is as taut as a stretched rubber band, the patient is indeed at his maximum range. If not, the patient should be encouraged to achieve more motion. Range of motion, particularly in children, may be more accurately assessed while the patient is under anesthesia before surgical procedures.

If a limitation in passive joint range of motion exists, gentle passive or active assistive stretching can be done to increase range of motion. When exercising the burned hand, support the joint proximal to the joint being stretched (Fig. 65-5). To avoid unnecessary pain, provide support where eschar is present rather than on granulation tissue. It is important to stress to the patient that active motion results in less pain than does passive motion. Gentle passive range of motion can be done in the operating room.

Forceful and aggressive passive range-of-motion exercises are totally unnecessary to achieve motion and should never be done. Overly aggressive passive ranging constantly reinjures the fragile new tissue, resulting in an increase of collagen deposition and consequently more scarring.[35]

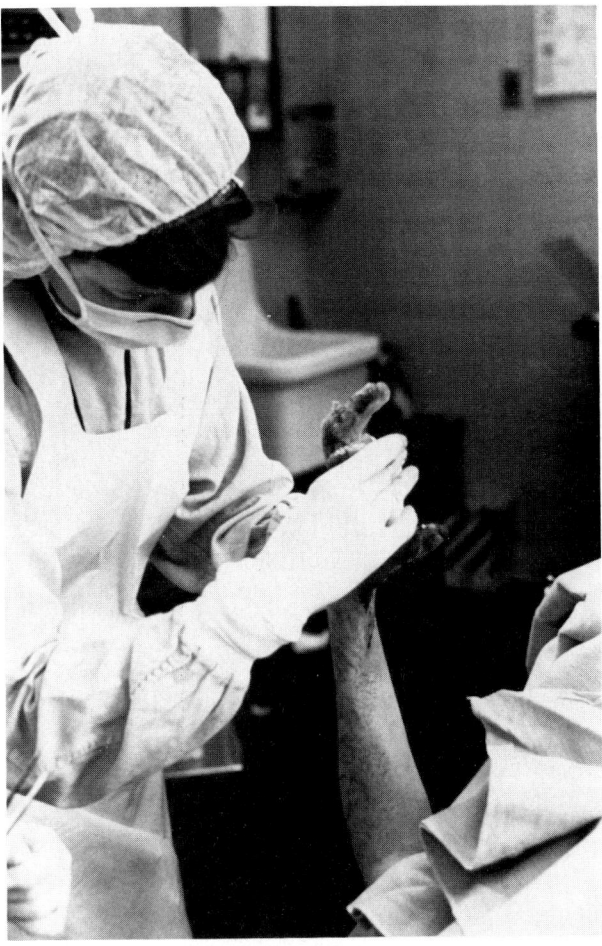

Fig. 65-5   Daily range of motion and evaluation of the burned hand by the therapist are crucial.

The range of motion obtained during dressing changes should be maintained in the patient's independent exercise program at the bedside. Active motion, with emphasis on isometric contraction, should be encouraged during these sessions. The patient should be carefully instructed in his exercise program and then observed to be sure that the exercises are done correctly. At this time spontaneous use of the hand should be strongly encouraged.

Exposed tendons and joints. Evaluation of the wound should continue to be done on a daily basis. As the eschar is debrided, the therapist should look carefully for tendon and joint exposure, since such exposure will make it necessary to adjust the therapy program accordingly. One of the most common sites of an exposed tendon is along the dorsum of the hand where the skin is thinner. The more distal the tendon exposure, the less the functional deficit noted.[36] Unfortunately, the central slip of the extensor tendon and the PIP capsule are often involved, leading to poor recovery.

Once tendon exposure has been noted, the wound must be kept covered with a moist gauze or a hydrophobic dressing to prevent dryness from heat lamps and air. Because of poor autograft take when the autograft is placed directly on the tendon, xenograft or homograft is placed until an adequate granulation bed has been formed. The use of anti-

microbial cream or antibiotic soaks is not recommended, because they can lead to tendon maceration.[36]

The involved tendon and joint should be immobilized to prevent possible rupture, but efforts should be made to ensure motion of the uninvolved joints and to maintain gliding of the involved tendon. For example, when there is exposure of the extensor digitorum communis (EDC) over the MP joint of the index finger, the MP joint and wrist should be extended to put the tendon at maximum slack. Gentle passive extension and active flexion of the PIP and DIP joints can then be done, but no active extension should be allowed. When there is exposure of the extensor slip of the digit, the PIP joint must be maintained in extension during active flexion of the MP joint, but active extension of the PIP joint is prohibited. Gutter splints have been found to be effective for immobilization of exposed tendons of the PIP joint while still allowing MCP joint flexion.[63] All ADL tasks should be monitored to prevent accidental rupture.

If the central slip of the extensor tendon to the PIP joint has ruptured, the involved joint can be immobilized in extension for 6 weeks. This may inhibit the lateral bands from sliding volarly and contributing to the classic burn boutonnière deformity. Beneficially, this also may allow granulation tissue to form over the PIP joint, and a structurally stable scar may extend a finger when there is no discernible anatomically separate tendon.[58]

Traction. Traction provides the opposing forces needed to orient the plastic collagen being deposited during the early stages of wound healing, and it maintains joint alignment as well. Traction can be accomplished through the use of externally applied splints. A thorough knowledge of anatomy is essential for accurate determination of potential deformities. Following a burn injury, the patient often assumes a position of comfort, which is flexion. This can result in the burned hand deformity discussed earlier. Generally, in a superficial burn that is healing without complications, the hand should not be splinted unless there is a limitation in active motion of the MP or IP joints of 20 degrees or greater in extension, or MP or IP joint flexion is less than 70 degrees.

As the patient's wound status changes, so does the splinting program. In cases of burns to both the dorsal and volar aspects of the hand, the therapist should evaluate closely the directions of the deforming forces. For example, if the healing tissue begins to pull the MP and PIP joints into flexion and thereby limits extension, a palmar-based splint that holds the MP and IP joints in extension should be alternated with an MP-flexion/IP-extension splint.

In addition to evaluating the wound, it is important to evaluate the fit of the splint and to check whether it is being applied correctly. If a splint is applied incorrectly and not secured adequately, it can slip forward, contributing to the deforming forces of thumb adduction, MP hyperextension, and IP flexion.

As the patient's range of motion improves, the use of the splint during the day can be decreased. If the patient is unwilling or unable to cooperate, the splint should be worn continuously and removed only for dressing changes, self-care activities, and supervised exercises. The splints should be worn during all hours of sleep. It is not unusual for a patient to lose range significantly because the splint was not applied during the night.

The therapist must be careful not to overimmobilize the patient. This can result in soft tissue adhesions, joint stiffness, and in some cases, calcification of the joint, especially in the elbow. Children can tolerate immobilization for longer than adults because of the elasticity of their joints and soft tissue, but they still need to be monitored. In addition to immobilization caused by splinting, the therapist should note whether the patient is causing the increased joint stiffness by self-immobilization caused by pain.

Pressure. As with traction, pressure should be applied early during the wound débridement phase and not delayed until complete wound coverage has been obtained. For example, burned web spaces should be packed with gauze incorporated into the dressing as soon as the eschar is debrided. Worn over dressings, splints that conform well to both the palmar web and the thenar web can also apply pressure to those areas. Elastic bandages used to secure splints worn over bandages also apply pressure.

Skin graft phase

Early excision of eschar and use of split-thickness skin grafts in deep burns appear to decrease the extent of scar formation.[54] Because the skin graft contains flexible dermis and epithelium, the transfer of vasculature from the wound to the graft is quick, and the scar tends to remain pliable and supple.[35] Rudolph[64] has found that the application of skin grafts, especially full-thickness skin grafts, does not prevent myofibroblast formation. Grafts speed up the life cycle of the myofibroblast and thereby decrease the length of time the active myofibroblasts are present in the wound (Fig. 65-6). The overall result is a decrease in wound contraction. Unfortunately, early grafting must often be delayed because of severe medical complications and infection.

It is crucial to have obtained full range of motion before grafting, because the patient will need to be immobilized for 5 to 7 days after surgery.[27] For most hand burns, a splint maintaining the patient in the burned hand position should

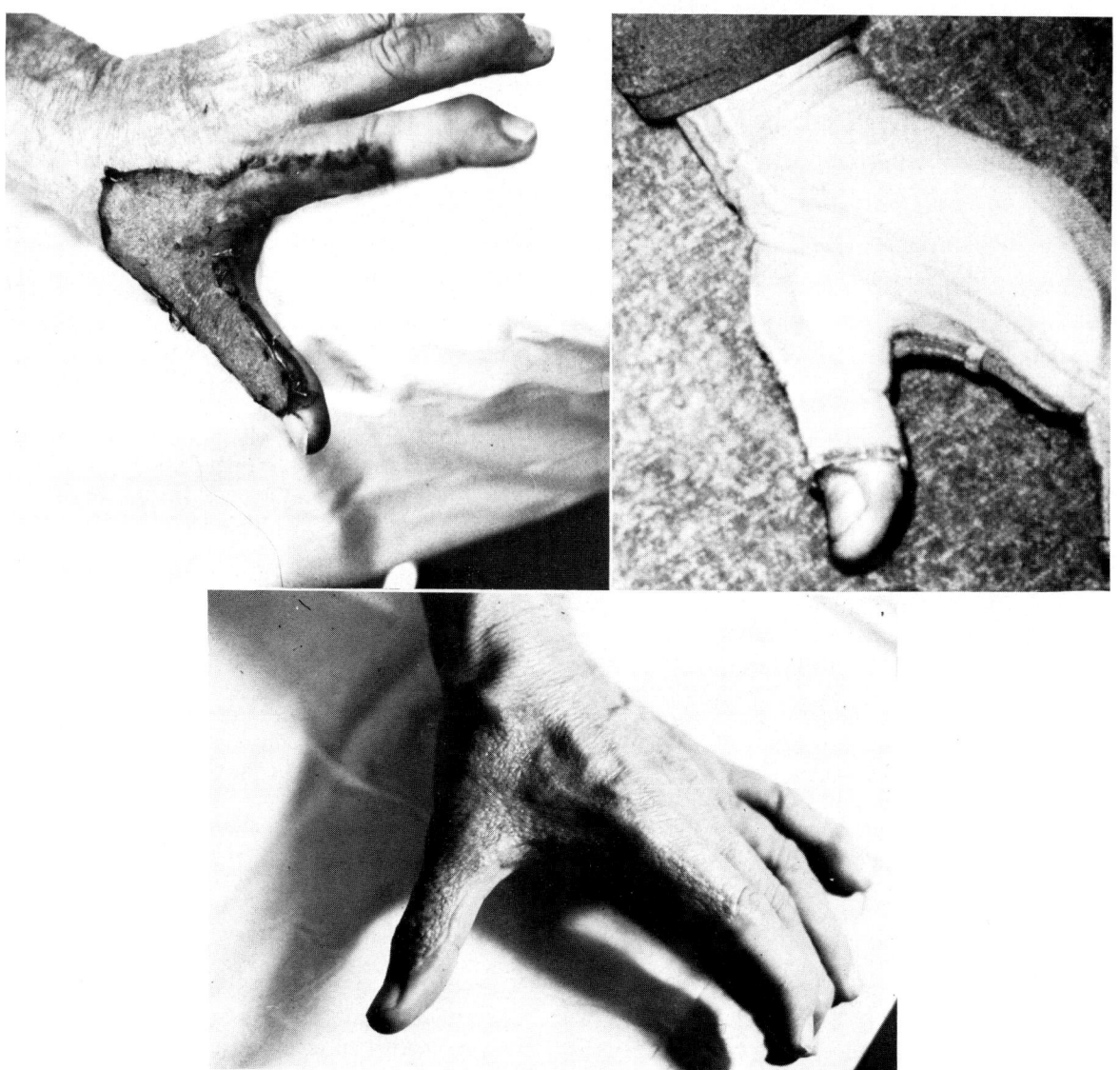

Fig. 65-6 Early grafting and excision, followed by pressure with Aliplast thumb-web stretcher.

be applied in the operating room to prevent loss of graft take caused by mobility while optimally positioning the hand.

Rehabilitation phase

This phase is generally considered to extend from the time of graft adherence or wound closure until scar maturation. The primary goals of therapy at this time are to protect the new spontaneously healed wound or the fragile graft, maintain joint mobility, increase function, increase strength, and inhibit the development of scar contracture and hypertrophy.

Motion. When evaluating range of motion in the recently healed burned hand, the therapist should look at the total range of motion across several joints and evaluate individual joint motion. A patient with a dorsal hand burn may have full passive flexion of the MP and PIP joints individually and still lack a full fist actively. Contracting scar, leading to loss of skin mobility, can also cause loss of active motion in an adjacent, unburned area. For example, the patient with a burn to the dorsum of the hand may be able to actively make a fist with the wrist extended, but, because of scar contracture, may not be able to actively make a full fist with the wrist at neutral or in slight flexion.

The exercise program should consist of isolated tendon gliding exercises for the profundus and superficialis and full EDC extension as well as PIP extension with the MP joint blocked in flexion. Spontaneous use of the hand is strongly encouraged to help the patient overcome fear of potential skin breakdown or pain with use.

Therapists have begun to employ continuous passive motion (CPM) machines in the treatment of hand burns to help maintain or restore range of motion. The machines can be applied over dressings. CPM does not replace the therapist; it is an adjunct to therapy. Also, hand CPMs do not take the patient through the full range of motion.

Covey et al.[18] have reported on the use of CPM with patients with bilateral deep second- or third-degree hand burns that required excision and grafting. Nine hands in a control group underwent conventional hand therapy while nine hands received range of motion through the use of a CPM machine. The results showed that there was no difference between the two groups in length of time to regain total active motion, in reported pain, or in loss of graft attributable to motion.

Resistive exercises and activities that challenge finger dexterity should be increased in pace with the patient's tolerance. The exercises can be done following massage.

Massage. Massage can be effective in maintaining mobility by freeing restrictive fibrous bands and in increasing circulation.[19] It is also helpful in alleviating the commonly reported itching sensation caused by excessively dry and cracked skin resulting from damage to the sweat glands.

Only gentle massage should be done to newly spontaneously healed or recently adherent grafts, because the skin is fragile and friction can result in skin breakdown and blister formation. Fragile skin may appear translucent and wet-looking, be sensitive to touch, or appear as though it will break open with slight pressure. As the skin becomes thicker and stronger, greater pressure can be exerted by massaging in a rotary motion along the scar. Creams that are not water based, such as lanolin and cocoa butter, are recommended because they are good lubricants and are not rapidly absorbed into the skin. One should not massage over small open areas, because this could result in delayed wound healing at that site. The skin should be massaged a minimum of two times a day. After massage, the excess cream should be removed, and approximately 30 minutes should elapse before pressure garments are reapplied. This will help prevent pimple formation and maintain the elastic quality of pressure garments, which can frequently be damaged as a result of overaccumulation of oil in the material.

Vitamin E plays an important role systemically in wound healing. Patients frequently massage with vitamin E cream for scar control. However, a study by Jenkins[38] found no change in scar size or in range of motion following the use of vitamin E topically. Therefore one should ask whether the positive effects reported are really the result of the mechanical aspects of massaging rather than the vitamin E itself.

Pressure

The use of pressure in controlling scars. The flattened, smooth, supple appearance of the scar following application of pressure has been reported clinically, but objective support has been inadequate. Studies[44,47,67] on tissue gases in normal dermis in hypertrophic scars have found that pressure of approximately 25 mm Hg is believed to decrease the blood flow to rapidly metabolizing collagenous tissue. The authors of these studies noted that hypoxia does not appear to result in cell death but does indirectly affect the metabolic pathway (such as collagen formation) of scar growth or maturation. Another viewpoint[39,58] is that pressure only causes dehydration of the scar (by indirectly affecting mast cells) and the temporarily diminished size of the scar noted following application of pressure is caused by the close approximation of collagen cross-linking. Despite lack of objective data, the therapist can take advantage of the positive effects seen clinically of pressure on scar.

A major goal of the therapist at this time is to anticipate which patient population will have the greatest risk of scarring. Therefore the therapist must know the characteristics of scarring and use this information when making a decision on the best way to manage the patient. A preliminary study[32] using a Laser Doppler flowmetry has been done to determine whether monitoring of blood flow would serve as a good predictor of hypertrophic scarring at a graft. The study was on individuals with less than 30% body surface burns. The data showed microcirculatory blood flow to be doubled in both initial and follow-up visits for 6 months in wounds with hypertrophic scars when compared with nonhypertropic wounds. However, this technique is rarely available for use in the clinic.

A quick test to determine whether a patient with superficial burns might develop hypertrophic scars is to lightly rub a finger across the uninjured skin and the healed burned wound with the eyes closed. If no change in tension of the skin can be detected, hypertrophic scarring probably will not develop.

Pressure after graft adherence or wound closure. Once grafts are adherent or wound closure has been achieved, pressure can be applied. The purpose of pressure at this time is not just to inhibit scar contracture and hypertrophy, but also to inhibit vascular and lymphatic pooling and to avert hypersensitive, fragile skin.[10]

Commercially made custom-fitting pressure gloves can be ordered when there are openings no larger than the size of a quarter and any edema appears to be controlled. However, if commercially made custom-fitting gloves are forced on fragile skin too early, the friction caused by the material rubbing against the skin can result in blister formation and skin breakdown.

INTERIM PRESSURE BANDAGES AND GLOVES. Interim pressure bandages or gloves may be used until the patient can tolerate commercially made custom gloves. The type of interim pressure bandage or glove used depends on how much pressure the patient can tolerate, and this should increase over time. There is commonly a progression of interim pressure bandages and gloves that are used until the patient receives commercially made custom gloves. The therapist should postpone application of interim pressure bandages or gloves if the skin appears too fragile.

Elastic bandage wraps, Tubiton,* Tubigrip gloves,* commercially available noncustom gloves (such as Bio-Concepts Redi-Made gloves† or Jobst Pre-Sized gloves,‡ and gloves custom-made by the therapist are among the types of interim pressure bandages and gloves that can be used. The least shearing may be a compression hand wrap. This has been used by therapists for many years but was recently detailed by Rivers.[62] The hand is wrapped with an elastic bandage in a figure-of-eight pattern. Lambswool or a thin equivalent web spacer is used in the healed interdigital web spaces and in the thumb web space. A flexible silicon spacer is used for the thumb when healing is complete. The therapist can construct pressure gloves out of elastic materials. The amount of pressure and the shearing forces depend on the specific material used and technique or pattern employed. Bruster and Pullium[10] described a method for making a temporary pressure glove of Lycra Spandex by tracing the hand.

Using a similar method to that described by Bruster and Pullium, the glove can be fabricated of 3:1 stretch swimsuit Lycra[45] (Fig. 65-7). Apfel et al.[2] have developed a computer program for drafting pressure gloves.

Bio-Concepts also makes custom gloves with a close-knit material that is smoother and stretchier than their so-called regular material, which is otherwise used for their pressure garments. In addition, the therapist can specify to the company how much pressure (mm Hg) the glove should apply in order that the shearing forces of applying and wearing a glove can be reduced.

Any of these pressure bandages or gloves can be worn over small open wounds with light dressings. Even if wounds are not present, a light dressing or protective material may be needed to guard fragile skin against the shearing forces of even interim pressure bandages and gloves.

Commercially made custom-fitting pressure gloves. Commercially made custom-fitting gloves can be ordered from several companies, principally Bio-Concepts and Jobst. Depending on the particular company making the glove, several types of materials, adaptations, and individual custom designs are available. The therapist should select according to the requirements of the individual pa-

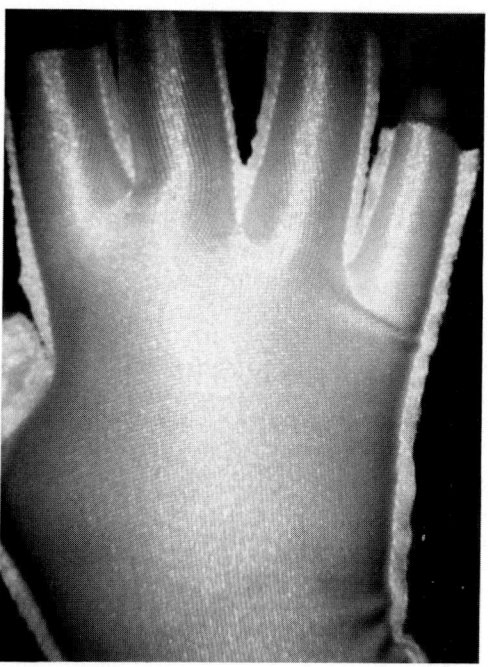

Fig. 65-7 Interim pressure glove constructed by the therapist of 3:1 stretch swimsuit Lycra.

tient, and these may change over time depending on factors such as stage of scar maturation, the need for inserts, the patient's daily activity regimen, and whether the glove is for day or night use.

FINGERTIPS AND CLOSURES. Although closed fingertip gloves may be worn at night (or may be recommended initially also for day use for burns extending to the DIP joints,[50] open fingertip gloves are recommended for day use. This is to allow sensory input to the patient's fingertips and in some patients (children in particular) to monitor circulation. Additionally, when gloves have open fingertips, it seems easier to ensure that the glove web spaces are flush with the web spaces of the hand than when the tips are closed.

Gloves can be ordered with zippers, with Velcro closures, or without either. Zippers (or Velcro closures) can be placed almost anywhere on the dorsal, volar, or ulnar aspect of the glove.

There are pros and cons concerning the use of zippers (or Velcro closures) in gloves. Some therapists may order zippers in the first set of gloves to decrease friction on fragile skin during glove application. Patients and family members may prefer zippers because they make it easier to put on or take off gloves. This is especially so if inserts are used or if the glove needs to be removed and reapplied by the patient at intervals throughout the day and help is not available. Zippers for ease of application also might be ordered for small burns of the hand where most of the scar is covered by an insert or where zippers do not appear to interfere with proper application of pressure.

Other therapists have the opinion that zippers (or Velcro closures) actually decrease or disrupt pressure because they take the place of elastic material, are nonmobile, and ripple, causing disruption of pressure on and around their location.

---

*Seton Products LTD, Tubiton House, Oldham, Lancashire, England.
†Bio-Concepts, Inc., Phoenix.
‡The Jobst Institute, Inc., Toledo.

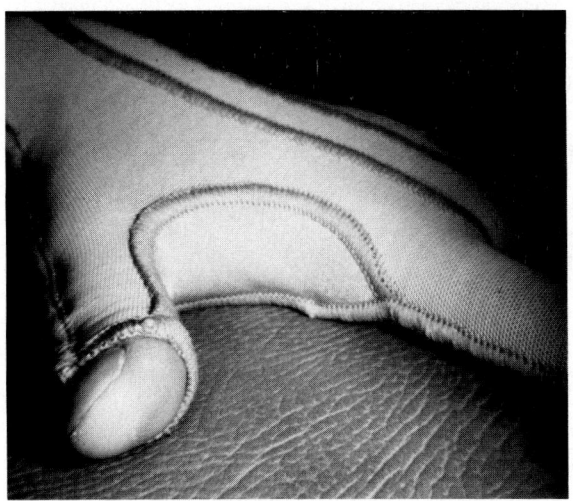

Fig. 65-8 Soft expansion panel in Bio-Concepts glove to reduce abrasion over the thenar web.

This may be particularly true in a pediatric glove where the zipper may make up a proportionally large part of the glove. The situation may also occur where a zipper leaves an indentation on the skin and causes breakdown.

GLOVE MATERIALS AND ADAPTATIONS. As indicated previously, when ordering gloves, a therapist may select from several materials. Bio-Concepts gloves can be constructed from one of three materials (or from a combination of two or more) with each material having its own properties of smoothness and stretch. As also mentioned earlier, gloves can be made from softer material for patients who have more fragile skin or who cannot tolerate regular material. For durability, gloves for children should be made from regular material. Whichever material is used, Bio-Concepts gloves are designed to apply 25 mm Hg unless more or less pressure is requested by the therapist. Bio-Concepts can construct gloves from regular material with "insert material" sewn in substitution of regular material in a specified part of each glove. This insert material is softer and stretchier than the regular material. Expansion panels of insert material sewn into regular gloves can make donning easier. Insert material can be sewn in to reduce abrasion over any particularly fragile area such as over MP joints, over amputation sites, or even over a specified finger surface (Fig. 65-8).

On request, Bio-Concepts or Jobst will sew a dart almost anywhere in a glove to help provide pull in a particular direction. For example, a dart sewn in the area of the thenar eminence may help pull the thumb into opposition.[40]

WEAR AND CARE OF GLOVES. Commercially made custom-fitting pressure gloves are worn 24 hours per day until scar maturation. The glove is removed only for bathing and skin care. Because the glove and any inserts can inhibit full active range of motion when on, it may also need to be removed for exercise. Because of the need for a developing child to use his hand for both sensory and motor experience, a child's glove may need to be removed for specified periods throughout the day. These periods may become progressively longer as scar maturation proceeds.

Since the gloves must be worn continuously, two sets are necessary so that one can be worn while the other is being laundered. With the constant wear and tear that gloves endure, having three sets at a time may be desirable or necessary to ensure that a fresh set of gloves is available.

FIT OF GLOVE. The burn glove should fit snugly but not too tightly. A glove is too loose if the material can be pinched up from the skin. Custom-made pressure garments can lose their elasticity (and, therefore, their pressure) while seeming to fit adequately, so new sets may be necessary about every 2 months to ensure that adequate pressure is being provided. Many factors contribute to the breakdown of elasticity. Some of these factors are normal wear and tear ("normal" can vary widely according to occupation or daily activity), the use of petroleum-based lotions and ointments, ozone (more of a factor in the eastern United States than in the western United States), and laundering. Although daily laundering may be recommended by the manufacturer, it may not always be necessary. Even without wear and tear, gloves may need to be adjusted or new measurements taken to accommodate edema or weight changes or growth in children.

Where contractures or amputations exist or there are problems that make fit difficult, a positive plaster mold of the hand can be sent to the manufacturer.

THE DYNAMICS OF PRESSURE AND THE USE OF INSERTS. Jobst custom-made pressure gloves are designed to provide an average of 30 mm Hg pressure at the fingertips reducing to 10 mm Hg at the wrist.[8] Bio-Concepts gloves are designed to apply an average of 25 mm Hg. Although the gloves are designed to apply a specific amount of pressure over a specific body part, the exact pressure applied by any device may not be able to be determined.[56]

Despite the fact that pressure garments are custom-made and appear to fit well and that pressure may have been applied early to a compliant patient, there still may be problems with hard, thickening, or contracting scar. If this is so, there may be insufficient pressure in those areas. There are many dynamics of applying pressure to the hand. Knowledge of these dynamics can help the therapist anticipate these problems and effectively intervene.

To be effective, pressure must be conforming. The palm of the hand is a concave surface. The best made custom-fitting glove will always bridge across this area, as well as on other concave surfaces, while fitting snugly over convex areas. When a glove is applied to a hand with a burn on the palmar surface, an insert must be used. Many materials can be employed as inserts. Some of these are Elastomer, Otoform,* Soft Sponge,† and Aliplast†. The glove manufacturer can sew a pocket in the palmar, dorsal, or other specified part of the glove to secure an insert. However, a pocket may interfere with the conformity of the insert to the surface of the skin, and therefore care should be taken in this regard.

Interdigital web spaces are concave surfaces that can hypertrophy even when a glove is being worn. These areas are a problem not just because they are concave. In order for pressure to be applied using an elastic glove, there must be an opposing force. For example, pressure applied by a glove to the dorsum of a finger comes in part from the tension of the elastic material being stretched against the

---

*Dreze, Inc., Unna, West Germany.
†Alimed, Inc., Boston.

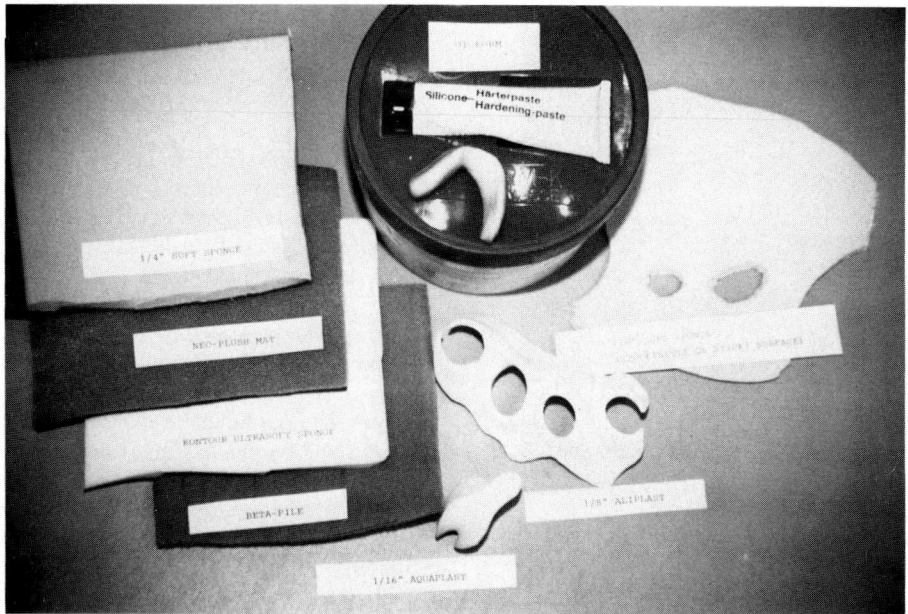

Fig. 65-9   Insert materials that can be used to provide conforming pressure under the glove.

volar surface of the finger. However, when a glove is applied, there is essentially little opposing force for the web spaces. This can be compensated for by using a dynamic web spacer or by adding conforming pressure with the use of inserts. There are many materials from which web spacers can be constructed. Some of these are molded ⅛-inch or ¼-inch Aliplast, Soft Sponge, Neo-Plush Material*, ¹⁄₁₆-inch Aquaplast†, Beta-pile‡, Otoform, and Elastomer (Fig. 65-9). Also, Bio-Concepts can sew web-spacers into the glove.

To maintain the webspace of the thumb, ½-inch molded Aliplast (¼-inch for children) worn under a pressure garment is effective because the thickness of the material holds the thumb in abduction at rest but is flexible enough to allow movement. If thumb abduction is within normal limits, ¼-inch Aliplast is recommended. A more rigid web-spacer for the thumb may be worn at night.

Movement will also change the dynamics of pressure on the glove by either increasing or decreasing it. For example, although a Bio-Concepts custom-made glove is designed to apply 25 mm Hg over the MP joints when the fingers are extended, this pressure can increase to about 60 mm Hg when the fingers are flexed.[61] Movement may also decrease pressure over an area by lifting a portion of the glove away from the skin.

When a custom-made glove is used, pressure is usually greater over harder surfaces of the body than it is over softer ones. Therefore, inserts may be needed over softer surfaces.

Wherever inserts are used, the skin must be checked routinely for maceration or breakdown. Inserts, especially more rigid or bulky ones, can also limit motion or function. For these reasons, even though constant pressure is preferred,

it may be possible to use inserts only part of the day. Softer or less restricting inserts can be used during the day and more rigid inserts used at night.

Other methods of applying pressure to the hand. Although custom-made elastic pressure gloves and inserts are the most common way of applying pressure on scar, other methods may also be employed. Generally, these methods are used when a glove with inserts is not effective in controlling scar. They are often employed to serially correct contractures and decrease scar hypertrophy.

For burns involving only the palmar surface of a child's hand, splints made of Polyform* or Multiform† (sometimes two or three layers for strength and pressure), which are made to conform well to the hand and are attached with an elastic bandage wrap or with Coban‡, can provide excellent conforming pressure as well as provide traction. Splints also can be made of ¹⁄₁₆-inch Aquaplast. Both of these can be easily adjusted regularly as scar or range of motion changes. Because this type of pressure inhibits hand use, it may be desirable for only a brief period of time or may be used solely at night while a glove and an insert are worn during the day.

Other ways of applying pressure to the hand are through the use of a bivalved Silastic Elastomer circumferential mitt and through the use of a prosthetic foam dorsal mitt.[50] The silastic elastomer mitt is constructed by pouring silastic elastomer over the dorsum of a hand that has been placed in a functional position with an empty 35 mm film container in the palm. The film container is removed, and the process is repeated on the palmar surface of the hand. The mitt is bivalved and secured with a Velcro strap or an elastic wrap. The prosthetic foam dorsal mitt has been recommended for

*Dricast Orthopaedics, Inc., Spring Valley, Calif.
†WFR/Aquaplast Corp, Ramsey, NJ.
‡Alimed, Inc., Boston.

*Smith & Nephew Rolyan, Inc., Menomonee Falls, Wis.
†Alimed, Inc., Dedham, Mass.
‡Medical Products/3M, St. Paul, Minn.

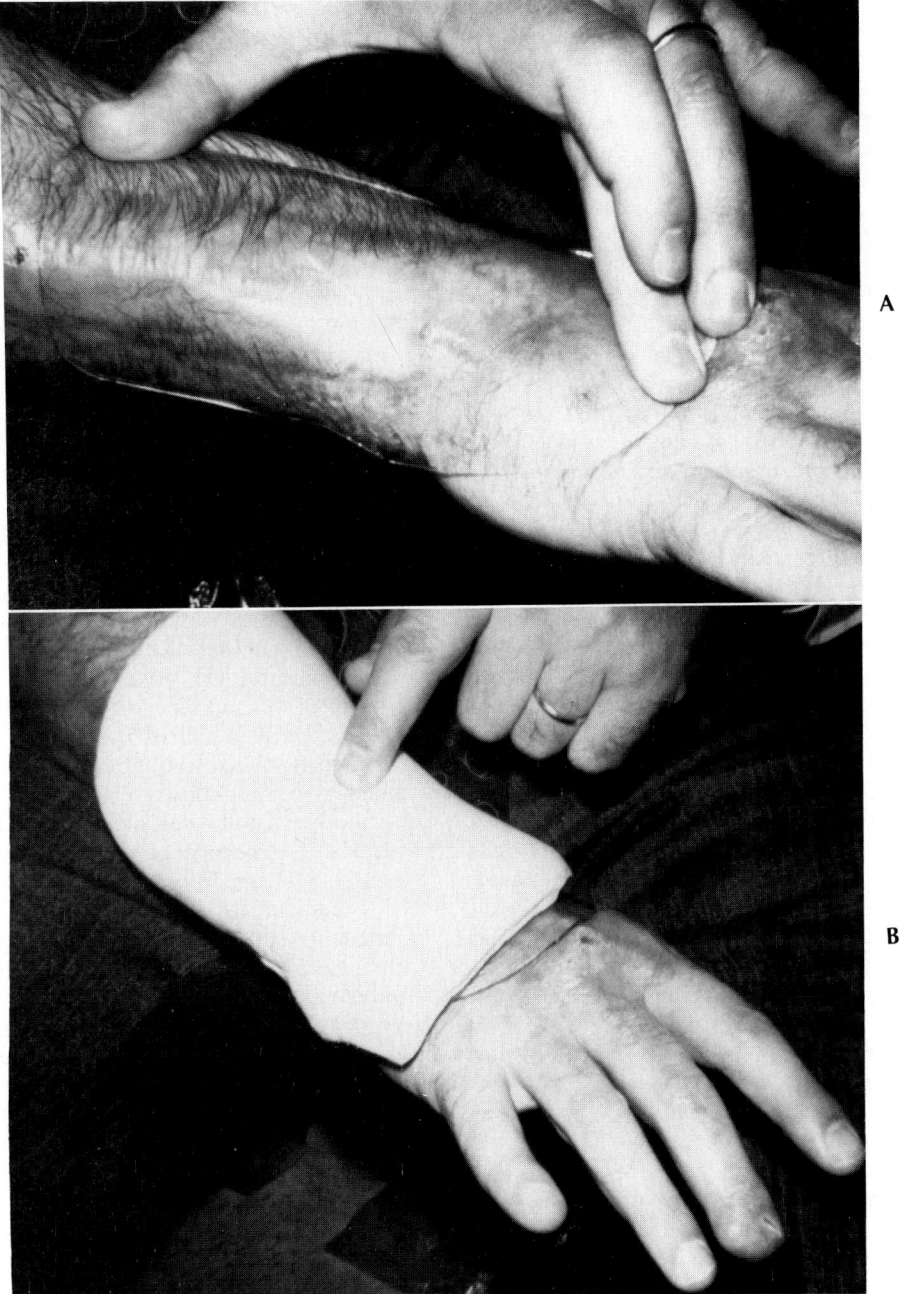

Fig. 65-10 **A,** W-clear insert. **B,** Additional pressure provided by molded Aliplast.

children with severe dorsal burns of the hand. There are several variations of this mitt, but all involve the use of Q7-4290 prosthetic foam applied to the dorsum of the hand and secured with an elastic wrap. Adding elastomer to the prosthetic foam makes a more durable foam.

A similar method to the Silastic mitt and dorsal mitt can be used by substituting Otoform for the elastomer or prosthetic foam. The Otoform is sturdier, heavier, and may be easier to mold. Instead of using a film container, a palmar splint of Polyform or Multiform is molded to the hand with the scar on stretch. With the palmar splint in place and the scar on stretch, the Otoform is then molded onto the dorsum of the hand. The two are secured with Coban or an elastic

bandage wrap. The process is repeated to serially increase motion.

Thick scars of the dorsal wrist can be flattened gradually by using a positive plaster mold made of the patient's hand. A piece of transparent plastic (W-Clear*) is molded over the scar on the positive mold, which has been only partially chiseled and sanded off. This appliance can be worn under a custom-made glove (with sponge or foam for additional pressure) or wrapped securely with an elastic bandage (Fig. 65-10). As the scar flattens, the scar on the positive mold

---

*WFR/Aquaplast Corp., Ramsey, NJ.

can be chiseled and sanded down more, and the W-Clear can be remolded.

Problems with pressure. Although pressure gloves, inserts, splints, and other pressure appliances can be effective in scar management, problems can occur not only from misapplication but also from routine use. Some of these include skin maceration or breakdown, allergic reactions to materials, impedence of circulation, and problems associated with pressure on a nerve. Also reported[48] is narrowing of the palmar arch from use of the glove. Drawbacks or tradeoffs—but not problems—from using pressure can include impedence of sensation and use of the hand. The therapist should carefully monitor the patient's status and pressure program.

Whatever pressure gloves or appliances are used, the therapist should properly educate and train the patient and family in their correct application, use, care and in various precautions. Perhaps as important, the therapist should offer encouragement and support. Application alone can be frustrating to the patient and family. They may need to be assured that skill comes with practice, and that persistance will yield good results.

Skin care. The pressure gloves are worn continuously for scar control, but they also protect the skin from the sun. Because new skin and scar tissue are fragile, they will burn easily. If garments must be removed and the patient is in the sun, a sun block (not a tanning cream) should be used for protection. If the scar is exposed to the sun prematurely, it may also tend to tan darker because of the increased melanin.

Traction. The purpose of traction when used initially during the rehabilitation phase is to maintain range of motion by opposing the force of contracting scar, usually during periods of patient inactivity. Traction is also used to correct scar contractures. Both static and dynamic splints can be used.

Casting. Casting to provide positioning or serial casting to correct contractures can be used at almost any time throughout the acute and rehabilitation phases. Casts can be circular, bivalved, or cover a single surface. They can be applied over dressings.

Casts can be particularly effective in maintaining MP flexion in toddlers while allowing active flexion of the digits,[24] and serial casting can be effective in correcting scar contractures even in small digits of children.

A dynamic plaster casting technique has been described for correcting burn scar contractures in, among other joints, elbows and wrists, that could not be controlled by standard therapy procedures.[42] This technique involves casting, cutting a tranverse wedge in the case at the joint (thus creating a fulcrum) 24 hours later, stretching the contracture, and replastering.

Modalities. Besides the modalities already discussed, there are many modalities that may be beneficial in scar management of the burned hand. More studies and documentation concerning the use and effectiveness of many of these modalities with the burned hand need to be done. Several modalities are discussed below.

Paraffin. The use of paraffin in treating burn scar contractures has been described by Head and Helm,[31] who state that paraffin, when combined with sustained stretch, can increase collagen extensibility, make the skin more pliable,

decrease joint discomfort, and increase joint range of motion. The paraffin is mixed with mineral oil (12 pounds of paraffin to 1 quart of mineral oil), and the temperature is lowered to 115° F.[27] Patients with limited finger flexion make a tight fist around a cone or cylinder before dipping into the paraffin. If the patient cannot tolerate the heat, the paraffin can be painted on.[41] After the paraffin has been applied, the hand is covered with plastic wrap, and the position of finger flexion is maintained with an elastic wrap.

Gross and Stafford[27] describe a modified method for paraffin application. Pieces of coarse mesh gauze are dipped in paraffin and applied on the scar area. A layer of plastic wrap and a towel are then applied. With the wax in place, gentle long stretch and active exercises are performed.

Paraffin should not be used on patients with fragile skin or decreased sensation. Many burn patients appear to have increased sensitivity to heat or may be fearful of hot liquids.

Functional electrical stimulation. A pilot study reported by Apfel et al.[4] investigated the use of functional electrical stimulation (FES) with three patients with three severely burned hands that had not responded to traditional range-of-motion and exercise techniques. The FES was applied to the flexor digitorum superficialis in hands with an intrinsic-plus imbalance. Objective measurement showed late improvement in hand function after the use of FES.

Ultrasound. In 1953, Bierman[7] presented three case studies of scars treated with ultrasound. One patient had a burn injury to the first dorsal web space. The increased range of motion noted following the application of ultrasound suggested that this modality may be able to play a role in scar management. In 1970, Wright[72] conducted a clinical study of six individuals who had developed scar formation from various types of trauma. The scar tissues were treated with ultrasound. The total number of treatments given was 24 and covered an area of approximately 36 cm² for a total of 6 minutes. A rotary method was utilized. The first 12 treatments were of a dosage of 0.5 w/cm², and this was increased to 0.8 w/cm² for the final set. Biopsy specimens and photographs were taken. Wright concluded that ultrasound may have some effect on keloids or hypertrophic scars treated in the fibroblastic stage when there is increased vascularity. Wright also noted that ultrasound was unsuccessful in the treatment of keloids in the later stages when a great deal of hyalinized tissue had developed. He speculated that further experimentation utilizing a larger population with longer treatment might produce better clinical results. According to Dyson's work,[22] ultrasound may effect the rate of wound healing by facilitating fibroblast activity to increase collagen synthesis, thereby altering the collagen fiber pattern. Ultrasound also has been attributed to causing changes in plasma membrane permeability.[22,55]

Additionally, ultrasound has been used in connection with steroids on scar sites. Because no significant changes have been noted with the topical application of steroids alone in reducing scar formation,[38] therapists are experimentally using ultrasound as a means of increasing cell membrane permeability to facilitate introduction of low-dosage steroids into the scar site. Triamcinolone (0.25%) is the agent most frequently used as a coupling medium. The pulse-mode is used on superficial scars, and the length of treatment time varies, because it is based on the size of the scar.[1] Because triamcinolone is used as the coupling medium, application of the ultrasound is given directly on the skin and not under water. Therefore, care must be taken over bony areas. During treatment the scar should be at maximum stretch.

The positive effects seen in the clinic are encouraging and demonstrate that ultrasound may have a role in scar management. Research is still needed, especially on the use of ultrasound coupled with topical agents.

Pharmacologic agents. In 1965, Maquire[52] demonstrated successful regression of a keloid through the use of intralesional treatment with triamcinolone (9 alpha-fluorohydrocortisone acetonide). Positive results[26,43] have been reported through the practice of excising small lesions followed by injection of triamcinolone followed by the reapplication of pressure. Cohen[16] has postulated that triamcinolone encourages keloid regression by removing the inhibitory effects of alpha globulins on callogenase. Eliminating collagenase inhibitors allows degradation of collagen.

Cortisone is generally initiated when the keloid has not responded to conservative management. But if most scars injected with triamcinolone are followed by pressure, it is difficult to determine which factor is actually causing the decrease of scar size.[59] Although controlled studies have been done in which a single scar is injected with triamcinolone on one side with obvious flattening of scar noted, more data are needed to accurately determine the effectiveness of triamcinolone.

Beta-aminoproproinitrile fumarate (BAPN, or D-penicillamine) is a lyslyl oxidase inhibitor that interferes with collagen cross-linkage.[57] Presently, there is a great deal of interest in the low-dosage topical application of BAPN to the early wound healing phase before cross-linkage has been completed.[13,54] This treatment causes a decrease in tensile strength and prevents excessive collagen deposition. The authors of these studies believed the systemmic use of these agents may prove to be too toxic, but topical use may prove to be of some beneift.

The addition of platelet-derived growth factors (PDGF), which act synergistically with other growth factors (such as insulin) on the site of injury, has been suggested to stimulate repair by increasing the rate of proliferation and influx of cells deeper in the wound.[29] Such action will speed up the overall rate of the healing process.

The present viewpoint is to use agents that interfere with the pathway of collagen synthesis rather than to focus on the breakdown of collagen once it has formed. Future studies are necessary to truly assess the role of these agents in the prevention of or decrease in scar formation.

Scar maturation phase

Hypertrophic scars take approximately 6 months to 2 years to reach maturity. Relapse is possible as long as the scar is erythemic.[25] As a scar matures, it should gradually cease to be hyperemic. The purplish or pinkish color should diminish, and the scar should not blanch to the touch. A mature scar should also be less dense to touch and pliable with lessened elevation. A subjective way to assess whether the scar has reached maturity is to have the patient remove the pressure garment for 1 to 2 days and note if any changes occur in the appearance of the scar. Return to normal color should not be expected. The goal is to have obtained a smooth, flat, supple scar.

Reconstructive surgery is usually delayed until the active process of scarring has ceased. However, in the case of MP hyperextension, early surgical intervention may be necessary to restore MCP flexion when therapy has been unable to do so. If surgery is performed, resumption of pressure and traction is necessary. If surgery is performed after scars are mature, a period of therapy is often necessary.

FUNCTIONAL OUTCOMES

Evaluation of the effectiveness of present burn treatment protocols is encouraging. The few assessments of functional return of the thermally injured hand have shown promising results.[3,17] As to be expected, individuals who have sustained the deepest burns requiring grafts appear to demonstrate the greatest dysfunction in range of motion, grip strength, and coordination. For these patients it may take up to 1 year or more for normal function to return. The unburned hand must also be included in the therapy. If not, disuse can often lead to stiffness and muscle weakness.[17]

A great deal of research has been done to assess the extent of diminished sensation of grafted skin.[69] Several variables appear to contribute to this deficit, including depth of injury, type of graft used, time required for healing, and the amount of scar present.[60] In 1980, the results of sensory evaluations done on eight adults (20 years after the burns) who had been burned in early childhood (ages 2 to 5 years) were reported.[53] Normal sensation and tactile gnosis were found with slight hyperesthesia. One conclusion Matev made was that nerve fibers and nerve endings appear to be established before there is even awareness of skin sensitivity. As the child grows, he has the capacity to reproduce these sensations through a process of readaptation of a single nerve ending. This leads to normal sensation in the grafted area by adulthood.

In the adult population, following thermal injuries requiring grafts for wound closure, impaired light-touch sensation appears to return to normal when scar reaches maturity. However, the results for two-point discrimination were varied.[3] It has been suggested that the size of the graft flap and the number of axons available may play a role in the quality of two-point discrimination regained by the patient.[51] Another explanation given for the diminished sensation is that increased scar formation impedes axon regeneration in skin grafts, and it may take 1 or 2 years to achieve final sensory return.[60]

A study by Cadwallader and Helm[11] showed a decrease in the number of functional sweat glands in hypertrophic scar tissue. An increase in activity of functional sweat glands was noted in burned areas as well as in the holes of the meshed split-thickness skin grafts. It was recomended that tests for sweating be done to evaluate potential problems of heat intolerance, especially in patients with large body surface area burns. The presence of dense tissue in the hypertrophic scar appears to affect the water barrier, leading to excessive evaporative water loss. This results in extreme dryness of the skin and is another cause of the patient's common complaint of itching. This was found to be especially true for partial-thickness burns that healed with hypertrophic scars.[12]

PSYCHOLOGY

Many patients believe that once they have been discharged from the hospital, they are completely healed and everything will return to normal. The early introduction of scar management and the extensive time commitment needed for good results are essential. The therapist must explain the scar remodeling process fully to patients and their families to obtain their understanding and cooperation. It must also be stressed to patients that because of the major trauma they sustained, they will never have normal skin, but that deformity and excessive scarring can be prevented. Patients will require a great deal of support and motivation or they are not likely to comply with treatment requirements. Goals regarding function should be set high and in conjunction with the patient. If the therapist expects less, the patient will also expect less.

SUMMARY

Exercise, traction, and pressure can be effective in remodeling of scar tissue in the burned hand. Early intervention is essential. The goals are to maintain and improve function, prevent deformity, and improve appearance.

ACKNOWLEDGMENTS

The authors thank Anne Putnam for her help.

REFERENCES

1. Amier PF, Executive Director, Futuro Medical Inc, Philadelphia: Personal communication, 1988.
2. Apfel L and others: Computer-drafted pressure support gloves (abstract), American Burn Association Meeting, San Francisco, 1984.
3. Apfel L and others: Functional hand assessment after enzymatic débridement and early autografting, J Burn Care Rehabil 5(6):438, 1984.
4. Apfel L and others: Functional electrical stimulation in intrinsic/extrinsic imbalanced hands, J Burn Care Rehabil 8:97, 1987.
5. Barsky SH and others: Increased content of type V collagen in demosplasia in human breast carcinoma, Am J Pathol 108:276, 1982.
6. Beasley RW: Secondary repair of burned hands, Clin Plastic Surg 8:141, 1981.
7. Bierman W: Ultrasound in the treatment of scars, Arch Phys Med Rehabil 35:209, 1954.
8. Blair KL: Prevention and control of hypertrophic scarring and contractures by the application of the custom-made Jobskin Pressure Covers, Toledo, Ohio, 1977, Jobst Institute, Inc.
9. Brown HC: Current concepts of burn pathology and mechanisms of deformity in the burned hand, Orthop Clin North Am 4:987, 999 1973.
10. Bruster J and Pullium G: Gradient Pressure, Amer J Occup Ther 37:485, 1983.
11. Cadwallader C and Helm P: Sweat gland distribution in healed severe burns: quantitative topical distribution and qualitative function, American Burn Association Meeting, San Francisco, 1984.
12. Carnes R, Sollecito W and Salisbury R: Evaporative water loss from healed burn wounds, J Burn Care Rehabil 2(5):239, 1981.
13. Clark R: Cutaneous tissue repair: basic biologic considerations. I. J Amer Acad Dermatol 13(5):701, 1985.
14. Cohen IK: Can collagen metabolism be controlled: theoretical considerations, J Trauma 25(5):410, 1985.
15. Cohen IK and others: Histamine and collagen synthesis in keloid and hypertrophic scar, Surg Forum 23:509, 1972.
16. Cohen IK, Diegelmann RF, and Bryant CP: Alpha-globulin collagenase inhibitors in keloids and hypertrophic scar, Surg Forum 27:61, 1976.
17. Covey MH and others: Return of hand function following major burns, J Burn Care Rehabil 8(3):224, 1987.
18. Covey M and others: Efficacy of continuous passive motion (CPM) devices with hand burns (abstract), American Burn Association Meeting, Washington DC, 1987.
19. Cyriax JH: Clinical application of massage. In Licht S, editor: Massage, manipulation and traction, New Haven, Conn, 1960, Elizabeth Licht Publisher.
20. Deitch and others: Hypertrophic burn scars: analysis of variables, J Trauma 23(10):895, 1983.
21. Diegelmann RF, Cohen IK, and Kaplan AM: The role of macrophage in wound repair: a review, Plast Reconstr Surg 68:107, 1981.
22. Dyson M and Suckling J: Stimulation of tissue repair by ultrasound: a survey of the mechanisms involved (abstract), International Symposium on Therapeutic Ultrasound, London, 1981.
23. Ehrlich HP: Do myofibroblasts produce the contractile forces which organize connective tissue matrices (abstract), ABA, Seattle, 1988.
24. Flesch P: Casting the young and the restless, American Burn Association Meeting, Orlando, Fla, 1985.
25. Fujimori R, Hiramoto M, and Ofugi S: Sponge fixation method for treatment of early scars, Plast Reconstr Surg 42:322, 1968.
26. Griffith BH: Treatment of keloids with triamcinolone acetonide, Plast Reconstr Surg 38:202, 1966.
27. Gross J and Stafford S: Modified method for application of paraffin wax for treatment of burn scar, J Burn Care Rehabil 5(5):394, 1984.
28. Gross, J and Stafford S: Optimal length of immobilization on the postgrafted hand (abstract), American Burn Association Meeting, Chicago, 1986.
29. Grotendorst G: Can collagen metabolism be controlled?, J Trauma Suppl. 24(9):S49, 1984.
30. Deleted in proofs.
31. Head M and Helm P: Paraffin and sustained stretching in the treatment of burn contractures, Burns 4:136, 1977.
32. Hosada G, Holloway G and Heimbach D: Laser doppler flowmetry for early detection of hypertrophic burn scars (abstract), American Burn Association Meeting, 1986.
32a. Hulnick SJ, Burn Center Director and Chief of Plastic Surgery, St. Christopher's Hospital for Children, Philadelphia: Personal communication, 1988.
33. Hunt TK: Mechanisms of repair and spontaneous healing. In Polk H and Stone HH, editors: Contemporary burn management, Boston, 1971, Little, Brown & Co, Inc.
34. Hunt TK: Fundamentals of wound management in surgery—wound healing: disorders of repair, South Plainfield, NJ, 1976, Chirurgecom, Inc.
35. Hunt TK: Spontaneous healing of burns. In Fundamentals of wound management in surgery—selected tissues, South Plainfield, NJ, 1977, Chirurgecom, Inc.
36. Hunt TK and Sato R: Early excision of full-thickness hand and digit burns: factors affecting morbidity, J Trauma 22(5):414, 1982.
37. Hunt TK and Van Winkle W Jr: Fundamentals of wound management in surgery—wound healing: normal repair, South Plainfield, NJ, 1976, Chirurgecom, Inc.
38. Jenkins M and others: Failure of topical steroids and vitamin E to reduce postoperative scar formation following reconstructive surgery, J Burn Care Rehabil 7(4):309, 1986.
39. Jensen LL and Parshley PF: Postburn scar contractures: histology and effects of pressure treatment, J Burn Care Rehabil 5(2):119, 1984.
40. Johnson CL: Bio-Concepts, J Burn Care Rehabil 8:329, 1984.
41. Johnson CL: Physical therapists as scar modifiers, Phys Ther, 64:1383, 1984.
42. Jordan M and others: Dynamic plaster casting for burn scar contracture: an alternative to surgery (abstract), American Burn Association Meeting, San Francisco, 1984.
43. Ketchum L, Robinson D, and Masters F: Follow-up on treatment of hypertrophic scars and keloids with triamcinolone, Plast. Reconstr. Surg 48(3):256, 1971.
44. Kirscher CW and Shetlar CW: Microvasculature in hypertrophic scars and the effects of pressure, J Trauma 19:757, 1979.
45. Knothe B, St. Agnes Medical/Burn Center, Philadelphia: Personal communication, 1988.
46. Koonin AJ: The aetiology of keloids: a review of the literature and a new hypothesis, S Afr Med J 38:913, 1964.
47. Larson D, Abston S, and Evans EB: Splints and traction. In Polk H, and Stone HH, editors: Contemporary burn management, Boston, 1971, Little, Brown & Co, Inc.
48. Leung K, Cheng J, and Ma G: Complications of pressure therapy for postburn hypertrophic scars, Burns 10:434, 1984.
49. Madden JW and Enna CD: The management of acute thermal injuries to the upper extremity, J Hand Surg 8:785, 1983.
50. Malick MH and Carr JA: Manual on management of the burn patient, Pittsburgh, 1982, Harmarville Rehabilitation Center Educational Resource Division.
51. Mannerfelt L: Evaluation of functional sensation of skin grafts in the hand area, Br J Plast Surg 15:136, 1967.
52. Maquire HC: Treatment of keloids with triamcinolone acetonide injected intralesionally, JAMA 192:325, 1965.
53. Matev I: Tactile gnosis in free skin grafts in the hand, Br J Plast Surg 33:434, 1980.

54. Montandon D: Les problèmes de rétraction tissulaire en chirurgie plastique, Médecine et Hygiène 36:817, 1978.
55. Mortimer A: Effects of ultrasound on membrane electrophysiology (abstract). An International Symposium on Therapeutic Ultrasound, Winnepeg, Manitoba, Canada, 1981.
56. Patterson RP and Fisher SV: The accuracy of electrical transducer for the measurement of pressure applied to the skin. IEEE Trans Biomed Eng 26:450, 1979.
57. Peacock EE Jr: Pharmacologic control of surface scarring in human beings, Ann Surg 193:592, 1981.
58. Peacock EE Jr: Wound repair, ed 3, Philadelphia, 1984, WB Saunders Co.
59. Peacock EE Jr, Madden JW, and Triec WC: Biologic basis for the treatment of keloids and hypertrophic scars, South Med J 63:755, 1970.
60. Ponten B: Grafted skin: observation on innervation and other qualities, Acta Chir Scand (Suppl) 257, 1960.
61. Reichenbacher F, President of Bio-Concepts, Phoenix: Personal communication, 1988.
62. Rivers E: A compression hand wrap, J Burn Care Rehabil 5(4):291, 1984.
63. Rivers E and others: The use of individual gutter splints to preserve exposed PIP joints: a case study, American Burn Association Meeting, San Francisco, 1984.
64. Rudolph R: Inhibition of myofibroblasts by skin grafts, Plast Reconstr Surg 63:473, 1979.
65. Rudolph R: Contraction and control of contraction, World J Surg 4:279, 1980.
66. Seghers M: Cutaneous pigmentation and keloids, Transactions of the Fourth International Congress of Plastic Surgeons, Rome, 1967, p. 115.
67. Sloan DF and others: Tissue gases in human hypertrophic burn scars, Plast Reconstr Surg 61:431, 1978.
68. Smith CJ, Smith JC, and Finn MC: The possible role of mast cells (allergy) in the production of keloid and hypertrophic scarring, J Burn Care Rehabil 8(2):126, 1987.
69. Topol BM, Lewis VL Jr, and Benveniste K: The use of antihistamine to retard the growth of fibroblasts derived from human skin, scar, and keloid, Plast Reconstr Surg 68:227, 1981.
70. Wadsworth TG and Williams JR: Cubital tunnel external compression syndrome, Br Med J 1:662, 1973.
71. Wright ET: Keloids and ultrasound, Arch Phys Med 52:208, 1971.

66

Acute care and rehabilitation of the hand after cold injury

Forst E. Brown, Murray P. Hamlet, and Dennis G. Tobin

Optimum management of the frostbitten hand necessitates an understanding of the pathogenesis of cold injury, the nature and extent of the damage, and the expected clinical course.

Cold injuries are common during war and have affected the outcome of numerous campaigns,[60] including Xenophon's Greeks in Armenia (400 BC), the Swedish troops of Charles XII in the Ukraine (1708), Washington's army at Valley Forge (1777-1778), and Napoleon's army fleeing Russia (1812-1813). There were more than 90,000 U.S. casualties from cold injury in World War II, including 12,000 from frostbite. The most dramatic of these were in the waist gunners of bombers who were exposed to high-altitude cold and 200-mph wind chill. There were 9000 casualties from cold in the Korean War; the occurrence in marines at the Chosin Reservoir in the winter of 1950-1951 provided a dramatic example. In these situations, large numbers of individuals were exposed to a significant degree of cold for a sufficient period to overcome the body's homeostatic mechanism for heat maintenance. Unrelieved heat loss at temperatures below 0° C produced tissue freezing or frostbite. In peace, individuals or small groups will experience comparable cold injuries when internal and external factors combine to allow tissue temperatures to drop to critical values.

CHILBLAIN AND IMMERSION INJURY

Cold injuries are usually classified into two major groups: freezing (frostbite) and nonfreezing (chilblain and immersion injury).[55] *Chilblain* is the mildest form of cold injury and occurs in susceptible individuals who are exposed repeatedly to cold without adequate protection. The skin manifests edema, a cyanotic rubor, and a vesicular dermatitis. The acute condition usually subsides within a week but can become chronic. On exposure of the individual to cold, itching and burning recur. The skin becomes erythematous and vesiculated. Ulcers may develop and lead to scarring and local atrophy. Treatment involves primarily protection from cold with maintenance of normal skin temperatures. Biofeedback and conditioning may be helpful.

Immersion injuries are a result of exposure of an extremity to wet cold at a temperature above freezing. The time required to produce injury is inversely related to the temperature. Tissue damage can occur within hours but usually requires days of exposure; the pathophysiology of this injury was described by Ungley and others.[61] Peripheral vasoconstriction is produced by the direct effect of cold on the vessel and by neurally mediated constrictor tone, followed by ischemia, with compromise of endothelial cell function. Loss of intravascular fluid produces peripheral edema and vascular sludging. Thrombosis can occur, particularly in the rewarming or hyperemic phase, and the release of prostaglandins will aggravate the situation. During this phase, neurons show early damage; sympathetic fibers are particularly susceptible. The posthyperemic and chronic phases are characterized by pain, paresthesia, and peripheral neuritis. Raynaud's phenomenon is common, and edema, cold sensitivity, and hyperhidrosis are common sequelae. Treatment involves management of the Raynaud's symptoms and protection from cold. Treatment by a hand therapist may be required to provide preventive or corrective splints and to direct therapy in the management of flexion contractures.

FROSTBITE

Frostbite is the result of crystallization of tissue water and is produced by exposure to temperatures below freezing. Tissue freezes near −6° C. To reduce heat loss and to maintain a core temperature of approximately 37° C, the body responds to cold by peripheral vasoconstriction and heat exchange between cold venous blood and warm arterial blood. Such a reaction would put a cold-stressed extremity at risk of developing frostbite. However, cyclic vasoconstriction and vasodilation have occurred when the hand was exposed to water and air at about 0° C.[33] This is the so-called "hunting reaction" and appears better developed in certain races and in those individuals who live in a cold environment; they are able to maintain the temperatures of their digits at higher levels when cold-stressed.* The primary protection from severe cold in man, however, lies in external insulation or layered clothing. Yet under certain circumstances, these external and internal protective factors can be breached; tissue freezing occurs.

Three physical and health factors contribute to frostbite.[41] They are (1) *those conditions encouraging heat loss* (wet clothing, exposed skin, immobility, fever, injury, hyperventilation, overexercise, and excessive alcohol intake causing vasodilation); (2) *mechanical or physical restriction of the peripheral circulation* (tight boots or gloves, peripheral vascular disease, blood vessel injury, fracture or crush injury, and drug-induced vasoconstriction); and (3) *problems that decrease the ability of the patient to cope with cold* (fatigue or emaciation, dehydration, poor caloric intake, underlying systemic disease, previous frostbite, and mental disorders).

The principal causative factors in producing frostbite are the degree of cold and the duration of exposure.[30] Still air

---

*References 1, 11, 21, 31, 37, 51, 65.

858

allows the development of an air insulation barrier around the body. As wind velocity increases, heat is more rapidly removed from around the body. This was well described by Siple and is the basis of a wind chill chart indicating the danger of freezing.[57] For example, a 10-mph wind at 10° F means a temperature equivalent of − 10° F. Contact with cold metal or moisture will speed heat loss and increase the risk of frostbite. The thermal conductivity (BTU/h/°F/ft) of water is 0.35; steel, 26.0; but still air, only 0.014. This will explain the more rapid temperature drop with exposure to metal or moisture.

Pathophysiology

Clinical frostbite is a slow-freeze process except for rare accidental contact with liquefied natural gas or liquid nitrogen. Slow freezing produces an extracellular ice crystal formation. The growth of this crystal causes an adjacent hypertonic extracellular solution, which draws water out of the cells and thus produces intracellular dehydration. During thawing, the water returns to the cell. There is a possibility that crystal formation may cause mechanical damage to the cell but this cannot be proven. There is a difference in cell susceptibility to this freeze/thaw process that relates more to susceptibility to dehydration than resistance to freezing.[39] Nerves, muscles, and blood vessels are the most susceptible; skin and connective tissue are less susceptible; and bone and tendon are most resistant. The extent and depth of the injury are more pronounced with longer time and colder temperatures. The temperature of the thaw bath is another variable in the formula for cold-induced tissue injury. Hardenburgh and Dawson showed that 42° C provides maximum tissue sparing.[19]

Exposure of tissues to severe cold (< − 22° C) appears to have a direct effect on the cell, which may be distinct from the dehydration associated with ice crystal formation. Muscle fibers show acute cell breakdown with nuclear, mi-

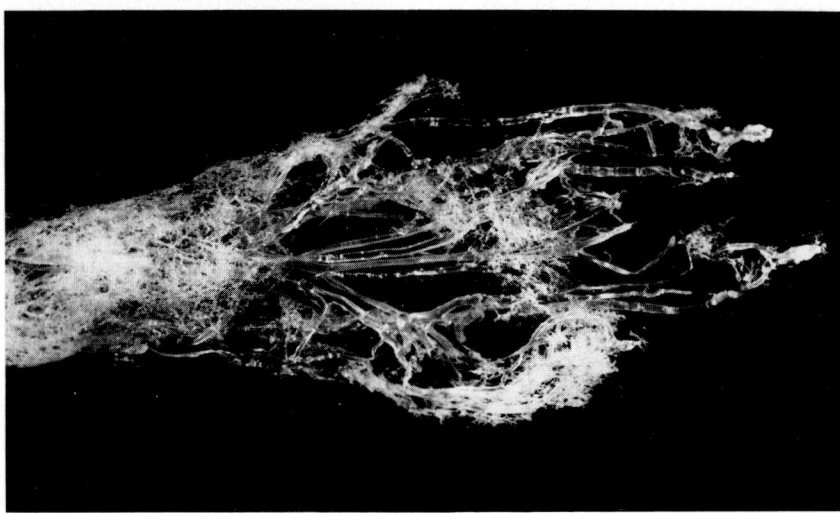

Fig. 66-1 Photograph of entire vascular microcorrosion cast from a frozen hind paw. (From Daum PS and others: Cryobiology 24:65, 1987.)

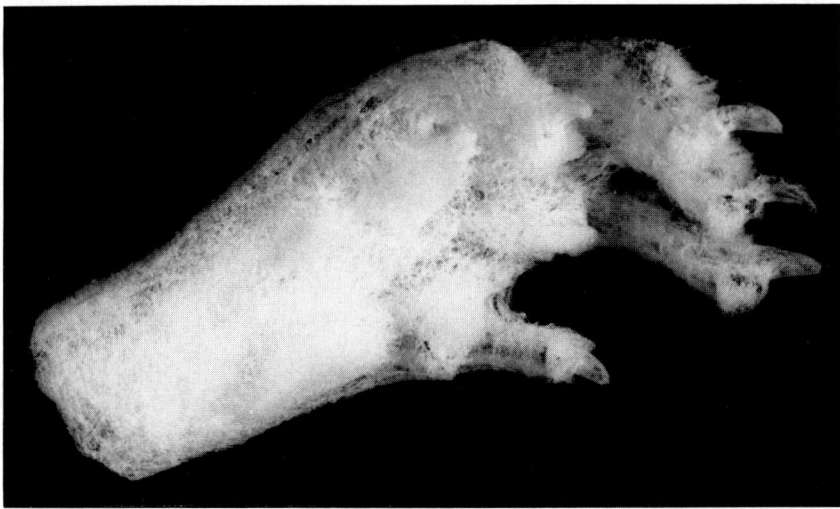

Fig. 66-2 Photograph of entire vascular microcorrosion cast from a control (uninjured) hind paw. (From Daum PS and others: Cryobiology 24:65, 1987.)

tochondrial, and membrane changes, which are evident immediately after freezing.[32] Membrane damage is associated with enzyme leakage. There is lipoprotein denaturation. Active growth centers, such as the epiphyseal plate, are particularly sensitive.

Another major effect of freezing is ischemia caused by both vasospasm and vascular damage. Vasoconstriction is the sum of the three reactions: (1) an intrinsic contractile response of blood vessels to cold exposure, (2) a local vasospastic reflex mediated through the sympathetics, and (3) a systemic response caused by cooled blood passing through the brain's vasomotor center. Endothelial cells are very susceptible to the freeze/thaw cycle. If they are damaged and there is a loss of vessel wall integrity, interstitial edema follows. The resulting intravascular sludging and platelet aggregation can lead to thrombosis. Usually during rewarming there is an initial rapid elevation of blood flow above the preinjury level; this is caused by loss of sympathetic tone in the vessels. Flow subsequently decreases, a result of the rising interstitial pressure, endothelial cell damage, and thrombosis. Injection studies show a marked diminution in the aborization of small vessels in the frostbite wound (Figs. 66-1 and 66-2).[8]

Vasoactive agents, such as thromboxane, may also play a part in the etiology of cold-injury ischemia. Elevated levels of thromboxane and prostaglandin PGF_2 have been demonstrated in frostbite blister fluid, as in the burn wound.[52]

The result of all these factors is ischemia and tissue death. The aim of treatment is the preservation of the maximum amount of tissue that has been subjected to freezing and the sequelae described above.

Classification

The degree of cold injury is usually difficult to determine initially, even after thawing of the frozen extremity. Definitive classification is possible only in retrospect, because deeper tissues may suffer irreparable damage while superficial tissues survive (Fig. 66-3). The standard classification involves four degrees.[63]

First degree. After rewarming, the skin becomes mottled, cyanotic, red, hot, and dry. There may be intense itching or a burning sensation, as well as a deep-seated ache.

Second degree. Hyperemia, edema, and burning pain develop early after rewarming. Light touch and position sense may be absent. Clear blisters appear within 6 to 12 hours, extend nearly to the digit tips, and subsequently dry to form eschars.

Third degree. This injury involves necrosis of skin and subcutaneous tissue. The vesicles that form are smaller, hemorrhagic, and violaceous; they do not extend to the end of the digit. Anesthesia is present early and is followed by sever burning, aching, or throbbing. Eschars separate late, exposing granulation tissue.

Fourth degree. There is necrosis of the entire thickness, including bone. Upon rewarming the skin appears deep red, mottled, or cyanotic. The area is without sensation, and there is no edema and no vesicle formation. There is progression to dry gangrene and mummification.

Most important in the clinical management of the patient with frostbite is a differentiation between superficial and deep injury. This is the basis of a simpler classification of frostbite advocated by Mills and others in 1960.[43] A history

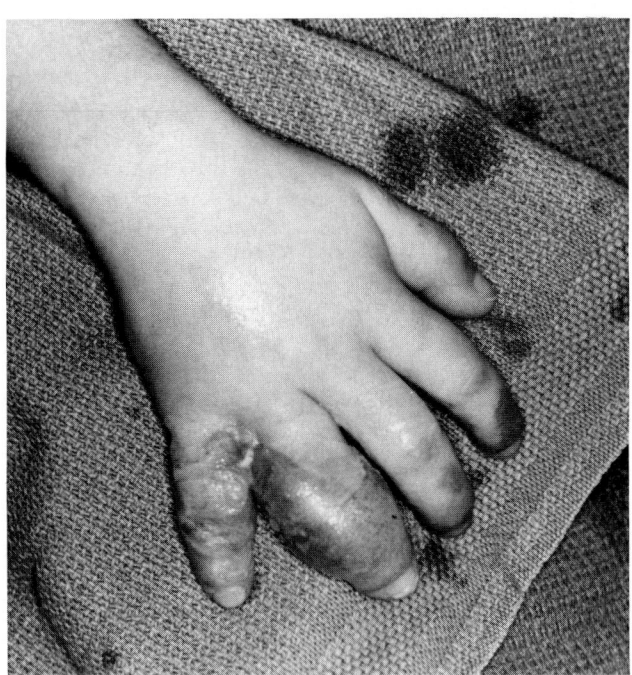

Fig. 66-3 Appearance of right hand of a 3½-year-old boy who 5 days previously had sustained a freezing injury because of exposure to snow at −20° C. Subsequently there was complete skin healing, but epiphyseal damage.

of prolonged exposure, severe temperatures, contact with metal or water, and a freeze/thaw/refreeze cycle suggests deep injury. Further indicators of a poor prognosis include insensitive, cold, white or cyanotic skin after thawing, no blisters, edema, or dark hemorrhagic blebs, early mummification, and constitutional signs of tissue necrosis. Findings suggestive of superficial injury are the following: large, clear blebs developing early; rapid return of sensation and temperature; rapid capillary refill; and mildly erythematous skin.

In an attempt to obtain an earlier prognosis and to better direct treatment, clinicians have tried various diagnostic modalities. *Arteriography* has demonstrated decreased arterial flow with vasospasm, arteriovenous anastomosis, and focal arterial thrombosis after cold injury.[17,58] However, arteriography may not be accurate in the acute phase because of vasospasm. Cold and vasoactive agents will produce vasoconstriction by direct effect on the vessel wall, possibly through an inhibition of the modulating effect of the endothelium on vascular tone.[62] Also, the microcirculation is not portrayed in the angiogram. *Scintigraphy* using technetium-99m has provided a determination of eventual tissue salvage as early as the third day after injury.[22,54]

Treatment

The initial management of the cold-injured patient should be directed toward correction of *systemic hypothermia*. A thermometer that measures <35° C should be inserted 10 cm beyond the anal sphincter. External or surface rewarming using warm water (40 to 45° C) immersion, heating blankets, hot water bottles, or heat cradles is more commonly employed than is internal rewarming (for example peritoneal dialysis, gastric lavage, and extracorporeal circulation). Oral administration of warm liquids aids in the restoration of a normal core temperature and fluid balance. Monitoring of vital signs, electrocardiogram, arterial pH and blood gases, blood chemistries, and urine output is critical. Hypoxia, hypovolemia, acidosis, hyperkalemia, and life-threatening cardiac arrhythmias are usual occurrences in the rewarming phase. Attention must also be given to other injuries and malnutrition.

It is rare for the physician to see a frozen extremity in the hospital emergency department. Advice to those in the field managing the frostbitten limb must emphasize the avoidance of refreezing. The ideal rewarming technique is that popularized by Mills and others.[43] Rapid thawing in a water bath (whirlpool) at a monitored temperature of approximately 42° C provides maximum tissue preservation.[7,15,19] Rewarming is continued until there is a return of a warm flush and sensation to the involved extremity; this usually requires approximately 20 to 30 minutes. The rewarming treatment may be extremely painful, requiring use of intravenous morphine or other analgesics. The intravenous injection of an alpha-blocking drug, such as tolazoline, may also be helpful.[50] During the rewarming cycle, no rubbing or massage should be used. Alcohol is to be avoided, as is exposure to dry heat. After rewarming, the extremity should be gently dried with sterile towels or gauze, then left uncovered. Cotton or other padding can be placed between fingers to prevent maceration. Blisters will appear within several hours after thawing and should be left intact. Surface painting with Betadine is used to decrease surface bacterial count.[20,44] Patients must not smoke. Antibiotics are used only for treatment of infections, and selection is based on culture and sensitivity reports. Tetanus immunization should be current. A high-calorie, high-protein diet with vitamin supplements is provided. Twice-daily whirlpool treatments of the cold-injured hand in a bath with water temperature near 37° C facilitates débridement; a bacteriostatic agent should be added to the bath. This is the ideal time for the hand therapist to work with the patient in a program of active range-of-motion exercises. Active exercises and hand elevation are important to reduce hand edema in the early healing period. Light functional splints of thermoplastic materials may be necessary to prevent contractures. They should be used at night and during rest, but should not interfere with active exercise.

Surgery has no role in the early treatment of the frostbite patient. Premature intervention increases the risk of infection and results in increased tissue loss. The exception is midlateral escharotomy for the release of circumferential eschars that inhibit circulation. Mills also emphasized the occasional need for fasciotomy; persistent cyanosis or pallor after rapid thawing may indicate increased intracompartment pressure.[42] Demarcation of nonviable tissue should be allowed to occur naturally. Full demarcation of nonviable tissue requires 12 to 15 weeks. Partial-thickness injuries usually heal within several weeks.

As in the burn injury, the frostbitten hand has three zones of injury. Distally, there is a zone of tissue destroyed by the freezing process. Proximally, survival will occur without treatment and probably without sequelae. Between these is a zone where optimum tissue survival will depend on interventions designed to improve circulation, reduce edema,

restore acid-base balance, counteract chemical mediators, and improve oxygenation. This is the basis for the use of various modalities in the treatment of the cold-injury extremity. *Ultrasound* was evaluated by Mills and others and found to possibly effect additional tissue damage and increase pain.[44] Experimental studies with *heparinization* early after freezing showed improved tissue survival.[29,45] Clinical studies, as in the Korean War, did not indicate a comparable beneficial effect.[60] However, in that situation heparin use was delayed.

Low molecular weight Dextran (LMWD) was evaluated for its ability to reduce intravascular sludging and increase tissue perfusion. In the experimental rabbit model, LMWD given immediately after freezing and continued for 5 days significantly improved tissue survival,[45] but in the dog model, LMWD caused increased tissue edema and no evidence of improved tissue survival.[47] In addition, Lofstrom demonstrated that hypothermia produced systemic intravascular corpuscular aggregation and defective small vessel perfusion, which was reversed by LMWD.[34] Although there were no controlled clinical evaluations of LMWD's effectiveness, it is an innocuous substance and might well be tried as an adjuvant in the management of the frostbitten extremity.[55]

Antiprostaglandins should be of some help in reducing the vasoconstriction caused by thromboxane and prostaglandin PGF_2.[49,52] McCauley and others reported excellent results with a frostbite treatment protocol that employed aspirin (a cyclooxygenase blocker) and topical aloe vera (thromboxane synthetase blocker).[36]

Regional sympathectomy in the first few days after injury appears to increase circulation, reduce edema, help resolve infection, and provide earlier resolution of pain. Hyperhidrosis is controlled, and sensation appears to return earlier. There is earlier demarcation of tissue necrosis and more prompt healing.[9,16,23,40] Regional sympathectomy may also have a beneficial effect on the late sequelae of frostbite: hyperhidrosis, vasospastic symptoms, and cold intolerance.[16,56] However, Mills is not convinced that sympathectomy preserves tissue and discovered that many of his patients complained after 6 to 12 months that the sympathectomized extremity was "too dry."[40]

Medical manipulation of the vascular supply has been attempted. Intraaterial sympathectomy using reserpine has been reported to be effective in treating acute frostbite,[48] but there are no controlled studies of its effectiveness, and intraarterial use of reserpine is not now available for clinical use. Mills suggested use of Dibenzyline (phenoxybenzamine hydrochloride) for its alpha-adrenergic blocking effects.[42]

SEQUALAE OF FROSTBITE AND THEIR TREATMENT

After the acute and healing phases of frostbite, deep injuries may present management problems. *Mummified tissue* should be allowed to autoamputate, thus preserving maximum functional length of the digit. Secondary closure of the defect is preferred. If there is insufficient skin to close over bone, skin can be grafted to the defect after granulation tissue has developed over the defect. Local flaps may be of value. With the advent of microvascular surgical techniques, distant free flaps may be used to cover large defects and to preserve length.

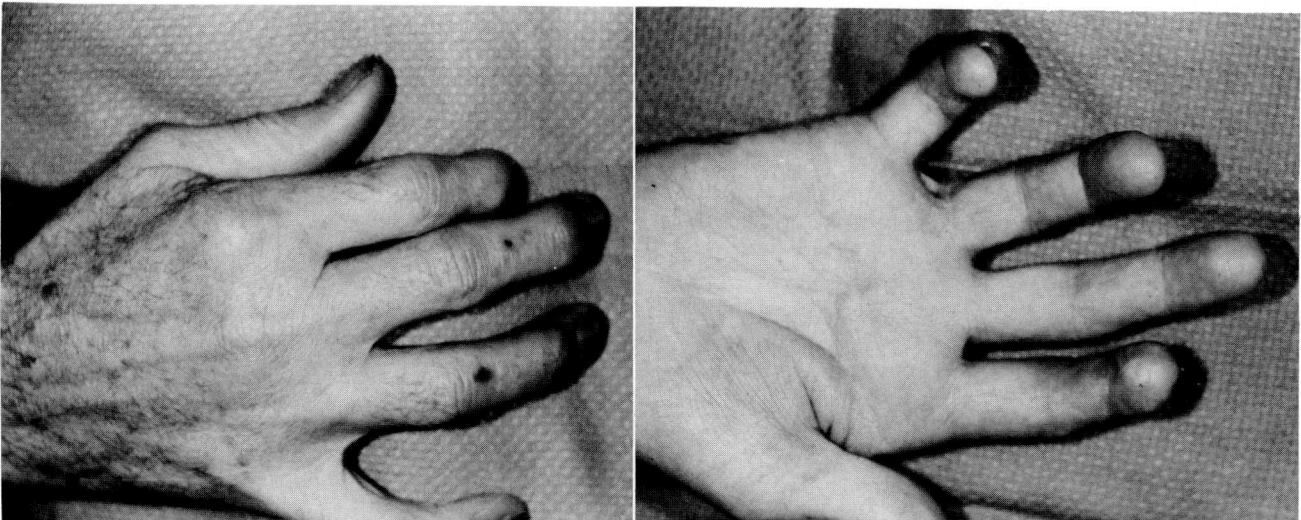

Fig. 66-4   Contracture of interphalangeal joints is noted in the right hand at 1 year after frostbite injury.

Muscle tissue is very sensitive to the effects of freezing and thawing. The intrinsic muscles of the hands are particularly at risk to this injury, as well as to local ischemia. Muscle fibrosis may occur,[12] and *contractures* may require later surgical release (Fig. 66-4). However, maintenance of an active physiotherapy program with early institution of splinting when required will usually prevent joint contractures and preserve motion.

Epiphyseal damage in the juvenile hand has been reported after cold injury.[2,10,18] There appears to be a direct effect of freezing on the sensitive epiphyseal chondrocyte, because there is poor correlation between the extent of soft tissue injury and the subsequent bone change. X-ray examination changes become evident 6 to 12 months after injury and show a distal to proximal progression. There is undermineralization of the phalanges, coarsening of the trabecular pattern, atrophy or absence of the involved epiphyses, and an irregular convolution of the metaphyses. Blunt, short fingers are the result (Fig. 66-5). There may be joint pain, stiffness, and weakness. Rarely is surgical treatment required. In fact, one patient who had epiphyseal damage from frostbite is an accomplished flutist with the New England Conservatory.[6]

Blair and others evaluated 100 servicemen for sequelae 4 years after cold injury in Korea during 1950 and 1951.[3] The most common symptoms were excessive sweating, pain, cold extremities, numbness, abnormal color, and joint problems. Deep injuries produced scars of a punched-out appearance. Nails were thickened and ridged, with an occasionally cyanotic appearance to the nailbed. Stiff joints were present in 20% of those with previous third-degree injury and in 86% with previous fourth-degree injury. X-ray examinations demonstrated early osteoporosis, mutilation of the terminal phalanges, and small cystic or scooped-out defects in the periarticular regions. In such patients, *scar contractures* can be released by skin grafts and/or flaps. *Joint contractures* may be amenable to physiotherapy and splinting, but rarely to surgical release.

The *vasospastic and cold intolerance* problem is usually the most prominent symptom of individuals who have sustained severe cold injury. The symptoms and clinical signs are similar to those of Raynaud's phenomenon. Pain and pallor of intense vasospasm occur after exposure to cold or even cool temperatures. Reactive hyperemia follows rewarming. If the episodes are serious, skin blistering and ulceration may result, with subsequent tissue loss and osteoporosis. The effect of regional sympathectomy has been discussed. In addition, Flatt reported distal sympathectomy at the level of the digital artery to be of value in the management of vasospastic disorders.[13] Medical treatment with phenoxybenzamine, guanethidine,[4] and nifedipine[46,53] can be effective in the management of Raynaud's phenomenon, as can microvascular reconstruction in appropriate situations.[64]

Because previous cold injury is associated with a disturbance of the autonomic nervous system, many researchers have attempted to treat cold intolerance by behavioral methods, such as biofeedback and classical conditioning. The most frequently used method of behaviorally increasing digital blood flow is *operant conditioning*. Digital thermal biofeedback is the usual technique and may be combined with autogenic training and/or frontalis electromyograph feedback. Moderate success in the treatment of Raynaud's syndrome has been reported.[14,24,28,59,64] Kappes and Mills use thermal biofeedback in the management of postfrostbite patients.[27]

Classical conditioning has been demonstrated to increase the skin temperature and reduce the frequency of vasospastic attacks in patients with Raynaud's syndrome.[25,35,38] Jobe and others compared classical conditioning with biofeedback in the treatment of Raynaud's disease.[26] They found that both therapies significantly increased the digital temperature response to cold at the end of the training program, but classical conditioning was more effective at 1-year follow-up. Brown and others also found classical conditioning to be effective in the management of patients with posttraumatic cold intolerance caused by vasospasm.[5] Patients with previous frostbite were included in the study group. This same technique is the one currently used for treating patients with

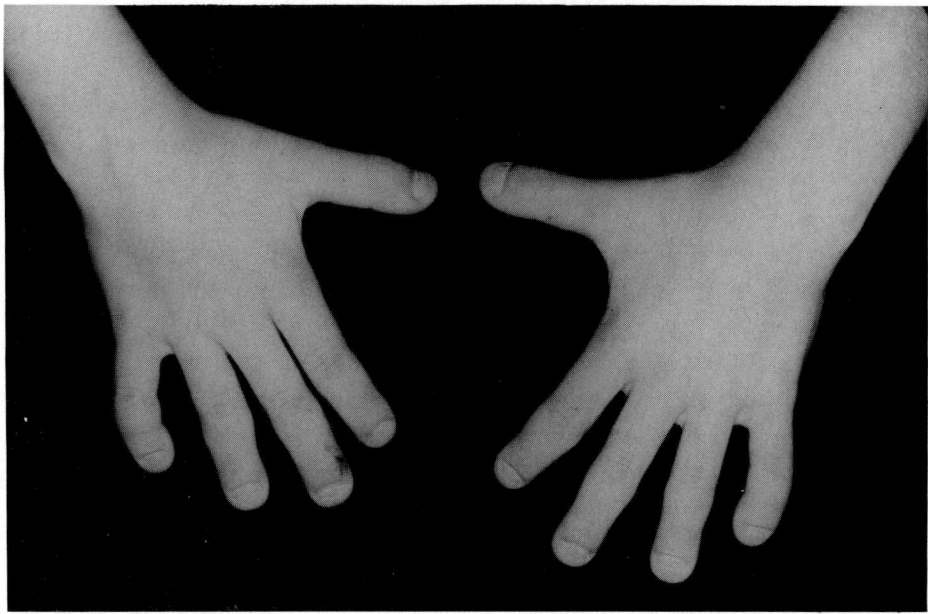

Fig. 66-5   Appearance of juvenile hands 4½ years after frostbite epiphyseal damage.

postfrostbite cold intolerance. Patients immerse their hands in water at 43° C for 10 minutes, 3 times a day, 3 days a week for 6 weeks simultaneously with whole-body exposure in a room of 0° C. Ten-minute rest periods at normal room temperature are interspersed between the treatments.

SUMMARY

The treatment of patients with acute frostbite should follow the program described by Mills and by the U.S. military.[43,60] Physiotherapy and splinting are used to help prevent and to treat contractures. Reconstructive surgery is employed rarely. Classical conditioning is a proven technique for treating postfrostbite cold intolerance/vasospasm.

REFERENCES

1. Adams T and Smith RE: Effect of chronic local cold exposure on finger temperature responses, J Appl Physiol 17:317, 1962.
2. Bigelow DR and Ritchie GW: The effects of frostbite in childhood, J Bone Joint Surg 45B:122, 1963.
3. Blair JR, Schatzski R, and Orr KO: Sequelae to cold injury in one hundred patients, JAMA 163:1203, 1957.
4. Blunt RJ and Porter JM: Raynaud syndrome, Semin Arthritis Rheum 10:282, 1982.
5. Brown FE and others: Induced vasodilation in the treatment of posttraumatic digital cold intolerance, J Hand Surg 11A:382, 1986.
6. Brown FE, Spiegel PK, and Boyle WE Jr: Digital deformity: an effect of frostbite in children, Pediatrics 71:955, 1983.
7. D'Amato HE and Covino BO: Evaluation of various rewarming techniques following general and local hypothermia, U.S. Air Force Arctic Aeromedical Laboratory Technical Note AAL-TN-60 11:1, 1960.
8. Daum PS and others: Vascular casts demonstrate microcirculatory insufficiency in acute frostbite, Cryobiology 24:65, 1987.
9. deJong P and others: The role of regional sympathectomy in the early management of cold injury, Surg Gynecol Obstet 115:45, 1962.
10. Dowdle JA and others: Frostbite effect on the juvenile hand (abstract), Orthop Trans 2:13, 1978.
11. Elsner RW, Nelms JD, and Irving L: Circulation of heat to the hands of Arctic Indians, J Appl Physiol 15:659, 1960.
12. Flatt AE: Frostbite of the extremities: a review of current therapy, J Iowa Med Soc 52:53, 1962.
13. Flatt AE: Digital artery sympathectomy, J Hand Surg 5:550, 1980.
14. Freedman RR, Ianni P, and Wenig P: Behavioral treatment of Raynaud's disease, J Consult Clin Psychol 51:539, 1983.

15. Fuhrman FA and Fuhrman GJ: The treatment of experimental frostbite by rapid thawing: a review and new experimental data, Medicine 36:465, 1957.
16. Golding MR and others: Protection from early and late sequelae of frostbite by regional sympathectomy: mechanism of "cold sensitivity" frostbite, Surgery 53:303, 1963.
17. Gralino BJ, Porter JM, and Rosch J: Angiotherapy in the diagnosis and therapy of frostbite, Radiology 119:301, 1976.
18. Hakstian RW: Cold-induced digital epiphyseal necrosis in childhood, Can J Surg 15:168, 1972.
19. Hardenburgh E and Dawson D: Research Report NM 41-02-00.01.01, Effect of rapid rewarming in time and temperature of exposure on tissue survival in frozen rabbit feet, Naval Medical Research Institute, Bethesda, MD, 1957.
20. House JH and Fidler MO: Frostbite of the hand. In Green DP, editor: Operative hand surgery, ed 2, New York, 1988, Churchill Livingstone, Inc.
21. Hsieh ACL, Nagasaka T, and Carlson LD: Effects of immersion of the hand in cold water on digital blood flow, J Appl Physiol 20:61, 1965.
22. Ikawa G and others: Frostbite and bone scanning: the use of 99m-labeled phosphates in demarcating the line of viability in frostbite victims, Orthopedics 9:1257, 1986.
23. Isaacson NH and Harrell JB: The role of sympathectomy in the treatment of frostbite, Surgery 33:6, 1965.
24. Jacobson AM, Manschreck TC, and Silverberg E: Behavioral treatment for Raynaud's disease: a comparative study with long-term follow-up, Am J Psychiatry 136:844, 1979.
25. Jobe JB and others: Induced vasodilation as treatment for Raynaud's disease, Ann Intern Med 97:706, 1982.
26. Jobe JB and others: Comparison of behavioral treatments for Raynaud's disease, J Behav Med 9:89, 1986.
27. Kappes BM and Mills WJ: Thermal biofeedback training with frostbite patients, Circumpolar Health 84:83, 1985.
28. Keefe FJ, Surwit RS, and Pilon RN: A 1-year follow-up of Raynaud's patients treated with behavioral therapy techniques, J Behav Med 2:385, 1979.
29. Lange K, Boyd LJ, and Loewe L: Functional pathology of frostbite and prevention of gangrene in experimental animals and humans, Science 102:151, 1945.
30. Lapp NL and Juergens JL: Frostbite, Mayo Clin Proc 40:932, 1965.
31. LeBlanc J, Hildes JA, and Heroux O: Tolerance of Gaspe fishermen to cold water, J Appl Physiol 15:1031, 1960.
32. Lewis RB: Pathogenesis of muscle necrosis due to experimental local cold injury, Am J Med Sci 222:300, 1951.

33. Lewis T: Observations upon the reactions of the vessels of the human skin to cold, Heart 15:177, 1930.
34. Lofstrom B: Induced hypothermia and intravascular aggregation, Acta Anesth Scand (Suppl) 3:1, 1959.
35. Marshall HC and Gregory RT: Cold hypersensitivity: a simple method for its reduction, Arch Phys Med Rehabil 55:119, 1974.
36. McCauley RL and others: Frostbite injuries: a rational approach based on the pathophysiology, J Trauma 23:143, 1983.
37. Meehan JP Jr: Individual and racial variations in a vascular response to a cold stimulus, Milit Med 116:330, 1955.
38. Melin B and Fagerstrom KO: Treatment of peripheral vasospasm, Scand J Behav Ther 10:97, 1981.
39. Meryman HT: Mechanics of freezing in living cells and tissues, Science 124:515, 1956.
40. Mills WJ Jr: Frostbite: a discussion of the problem and a review of an Alaskan experience, Alaska Med 15:27, 1973.
41. Mills WJ Jr: Frostbite. In The Encyclopedia Brittanica, ed 15, USA, 1974, HH Benton, Publisher.
42. Mills WJ Jr: Out in the cold. In Cohen IJ, editor: Back to basics: common emergencies in daily practice, New York, 1979, EM Books.
43. Mills WJ Jr, Fish W, and Whaley R: Frostbite: experience with rapid rewarming and ultrasonic therapy, Alaska Med 2:114, 1960.
44. Mills WJ Jr, Whaley R, and Fish W: Frostbite: experience with rapid rewarming and ultrasonic therapy, Alaska Med 3:28, 1961.
45. Mundth ED, Long DM, and Brown RB: Treatment of experimental frostbite with low moleclar weight dextran, J Trauma 4:246, 1964.
46. Nilsson H and others: The effect of the calcium-entry blocker nifedipine on cold-induced digital vasospasm: a double-blind crossover study versus placebo, Acta Med Scand 221:53, 1987.
47. Penn I and Schwartz SI: Evaluation of low molecular weight dextran in the treatment of frostbite, J Trauma 4:784, 1964.
48. Porter JM and others: Intra-arterial sympathetic blockade in the treatment of clinical frostbite, Am J Surg 132:625, 1976.
49. Raine TJ and others: Anti-prostaglandins and anti-thromboxanes for treatment of frostbite, Surg Forum 31:557, 1980.
50. Rasmussen DL and Zook EG: Frostbite: a review of pathology and newest treatments, J Indiana State Med Assoc 65:1237, 1972.
51. Rennie DW and Adams T: Comparative thermoregulatory responses of Negroes and white persons to acute cold stress, J Appl Physiol 11:201, 1957.
52. Robson MC and Heggers JP: Evaluation of hand frostbite fluid as a clue to pathogenesis, J Hand Surg 6:43, 1981.
53. Rodeffer RJ and others: Controlled double-blind trial of nifedipine in the treatment of Raynaud's phenomenon, N Engl J Med 308:880, 1983.
54. Salimi Z: Assessment of tissue viability by scintigraphy, Postgrad Med 77:133, 1985.
55. Shumacker HB Jr: Frostbite. In Flynn JE, editor: Hand surgery, ed 3, Baltimore, 1982, Williams & Wilkins.
56. Shumacker HB Jr and Kilman JW: Sympathectomy in the treatment of frostbite, Arch Surg 89:575, 1964.
57. Siple PA and Passel CF: Measurements of dry atmospheric cooling in sub-freezing temperatures, Proc Amer Phil Soc 89:177, 1945.
58. Smith SP and Walker WF: Arteriography in cold injury, Br J Radiol 37:471, 1964.
59. Surwit RS: Biofeedback: a possible treatment for Raynaud's disease, Semin Psychiatry 5:483, 1973.
60. Technical Bulletin MED 81/NAVMED 9-5052-29/AFP 161-11, 1976.
61. Ungley CC, Channell GD, and Richards RI: Immersion foot syndrome, Br J Surg 33:31, 1945.
62. Vanhoutte PM: The endothelium: modulator of vascular smooth-muscle tone, N Engl J Med 319(8):512, 1988.
63. Whayne TF and DeBakey ME: Cold injury, ground type, Office of the Surgeon General, Dept of the Army, 1958, U.S. Printing Office.
64. Wilgis EF: Evaluation and treatment of chronic digital ischemia, Ann Surg 193:693, 1981.
65. Yoshimura H and Iida T: Studies in the reactivity of skin vessels to extreme cold. II. Factors governing the individual difference of the reactivity on the resistance against frostbite, Jpn J Physiol 2:177, 1952.

X
DUPUYTREN'S DISEASE

67

Dupuytren's disease

Robert M. McFarlane and Ursula Albion

The name of Dupuytren will always be associated with a certain type of flexion deformity of the fingers, because the great French surgeon Baron Guillaume Dupuytren (1777-1835) identified the palmar and digital fascia as the tissue responsible for joint contracture.[2] He demonstrated at autopsy that the flexor tendons were not shortened, as others had suggested. Also, he showed that the skin, although compressed into pits and folds, assumed its normal dimensions when separated from the underlying fascia. Thus he established that the site of disease was the fascia and not the overlying skin or the underlying tendons (Figs. 67-1 and 67-2).

Hueston prefers the term "Dupuytren's disease" to that of "Dupuytren's contracture" because it broadens one's concept of this condition as a disease process.[5] Joint contracture is but the end result of the process. Much is known about Dupuytren's disease because it is so common. It is of genetic origin, behaving as a mendelian dominant, and occurs primarily in people of northern European origin.[9] It is associated with other diseases, such as epilepsy, diabetes, and alcoholism, and with conditions such as carpal tunnel syndrome and trigger finger. A similar pathologic process occurs in the fascia of the penis (Peyronie's disease) and in the plantar fascia (Lederhose's disease). Clinically it is seen more frequently in males than in females, because the disease appears later in women and is less likely to cause a joint contracture that requires treatment. The disease usually appears in the fifth decade in men and somewhat later in women, although it has been noted in teenagers of both sexes. The first sign is a nodule that is usually in the palm, near the distal crease and in line with the ring finger.

Although Dupuytren's disease is progressive, it is not possible to predict how rapidly the disease will progress from the first appearance of a nodule to finger joint contracture. The nodule enlarges and others form, and over a period of months or years tendonlike cords form and are readily palpable in the palm and finger. The metacarpophalangeal (MP) joint is most frequently contracted. The proximal interphalangeal (PIP) joint may be contracted alone or with the MP joint. Occasionally the distal interphalangeal (DIP) joint is contracted (Fig. 67-3).

The initial pathologic changes are not known, but early in the course of the disease there is fibroblast activity.[1,11] This cellular proliferation, accompanied by collagen production, accounts for the appearance of the pathognomonic nodule in the palm or the finger. Later, when joint contracture begins, the myofibroblast appears; presumably this cell is responsible for shortening the fascia and thus contracting the finger joints.[1,3] New collagen is produced, and much of it is of type III, which is the type of collagen found in granulation tissue and scar.[7] This leads us to believe that the pathologic changes of Dupuytren's disease are not unique; rather the changes are those of scar contracture. Why this process begins in the hand and progresses for no apparent reason is unknown. Until the pathogenesis of Dupuytren's disease is understood, our methods of treatment remain empirical.

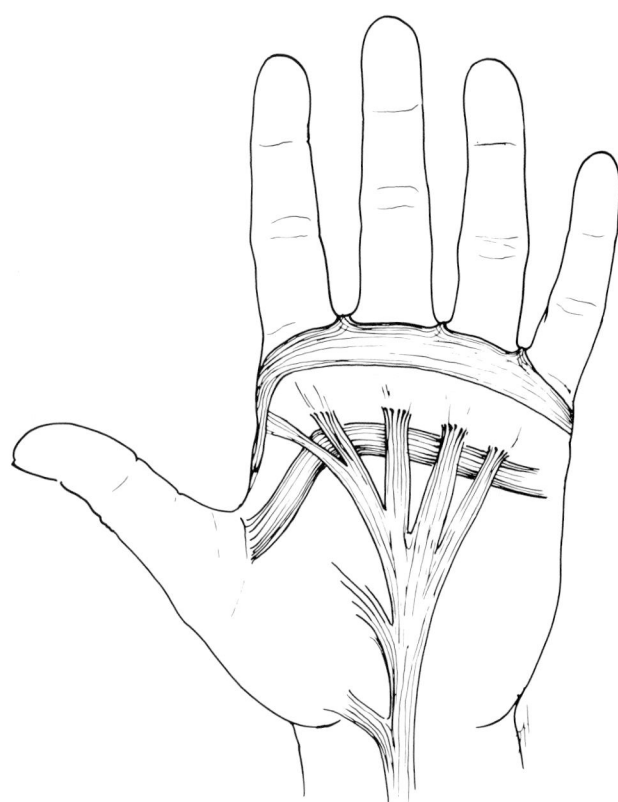

Fig. 67-1 Fascia of palm that becomes diseased consists of palmar aponeurosis and natatory ligament. This ligament extends across distal part of palm, supporting each web space and ending in first web at thumb base. When natatory ligament is diseased, digits cannot be separated. Pretendinous bands of palmar aponeurosis pass toward each digit and end at level of metacarpophalangeal joint by inserting into both skin and tendon sheath. Disease of a pretendinous band results in contracture of metacarpophalangeal joint. Superficial transverse ligament of palm passes across palm, deep to pretendinous bands. Usually this ligament is not diseased, except for the part extending from index finger ray to base of thumb. This part frequently causes an adduction contracture of thumb.

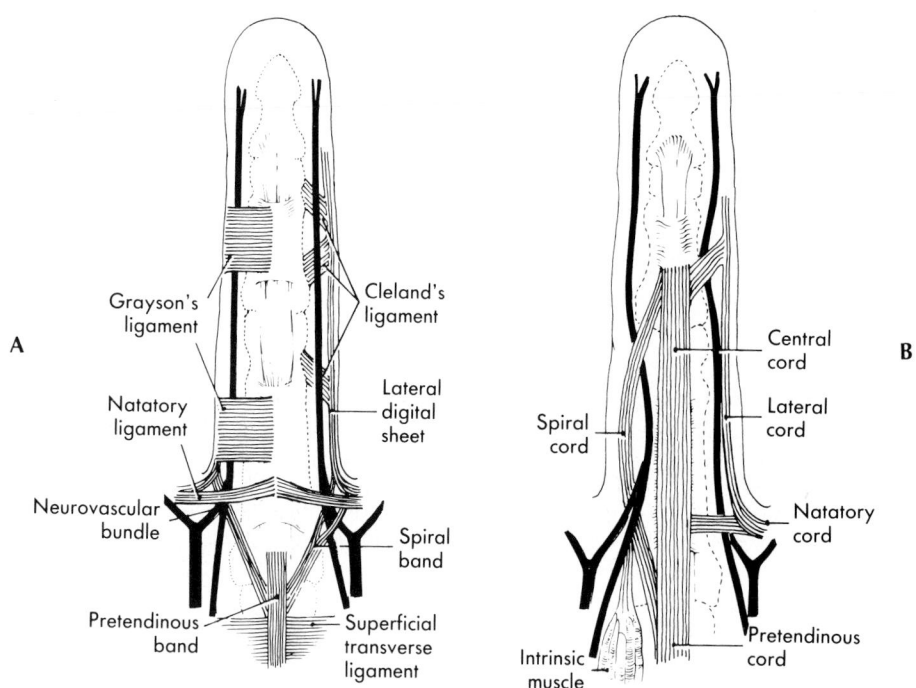

Fig. 67-2 **A,** Components of volar digital fascia that may become diseased. **B,** Diagram of diseased cords that are derived from normal fascia. Central, lateral, and spiral cords may occur alone or in combination, and each one causes contracture at proximal interphalangeal joint.

TREATMENT

There is no proven nonsurgical method of treatment. Vitamin E taken orally and the local injection of steroids may cause some change in a nodule. Attempts at stretching the contracting cord in the early stages of joint contracture are uniformly unsuccessful. Other forms of physical therapy, such as ultrasound, are of no benefit. At this time the only way to alter the course of the disease is to remove the diseased tissue surgically.

The presence of a nodule in the palm or digit is not an indication for operation. Frequently the nodule will be tender when first noted by the patient, but almost invariably the tenderness will disappear when the nature of the "disease" is explained to the patient. Occasionally, a nodule becomes so large that it is troublesome and excision is indicated. Again, on occasion, the skin of the palm may be involved out of proportion to the degree of joint contracture. The skin may be drawn into pits and folds that are difficult to cleanse and become calloused over the large nodules. In such patients early operation is advised so that the skin can be restored to its previous state.

Most patients are candidates for treatment because of finger joint contracture. The indications for operation are somewhat different at the MP joint and the PIP joint. It is always possible to correct MP joint contractures, regardless of their severity, by an appropriate surgical procedure. The collateral ligaments of the MP joints are stretched when the joint is in flexion, and therefore there is no restriction to full extension once the offending fascia has been released. For this reason, there is no urgency to operate when the MP joint only is contracted, because correction is possible at any time. Most patients note some inconvenience or disability with a MP joint contracture of about 30 degrees, and

so this degree of contracture is a reasonable guide to advising a patient when to have an operation.

On the other hand, it is not always possible to correct fully a contracture at the PIP joint.[8] One reason for this is that the collateral ligaments at the PIP joint become shortened in any position of flexion. Release of the diseased fascia may not permit correction of the PIP joint contracture if the contracture has been present for several months. Contracture at the PIP joint of 15 degrees or more is an indication for operation.

Flexion contracture at the DIP joint is not common. It is usually seen in the little finger and may be difficult to correct, for the same reasons that apply to the PIP joint. DIP joint hyperextension is more common and again is most frequently seen in the little finger. It is not attributable to fascial contracture but is compensatory to severe PIP joint flexion.[7] It is difficult to correct even when the extensor tendon is divided.

Disease of the thumb or thumb web is not often of sufficient severity to warrant operation alone. However, contracture in this area should be corrected at the time of operation on other parts of the hand. Tubiana has drawn attention to disease on the radial side of the hand, affecting the thumb, the thumb web, and the index finger, a disease that is aggressive and is often seen in patients with a history of alcoholism.[16] This type of disease, which is uncommon, should be operated on early and aggressively.

Patients under proper medical control of systemic disease are candidates for operation because the type of anesthetic and operation can be modified accordingly. Patients with a strong diathesis, which is not common, are likely to have continuing trouble regardless of the type of treatment. Such patients have a family history of the disease, which begins

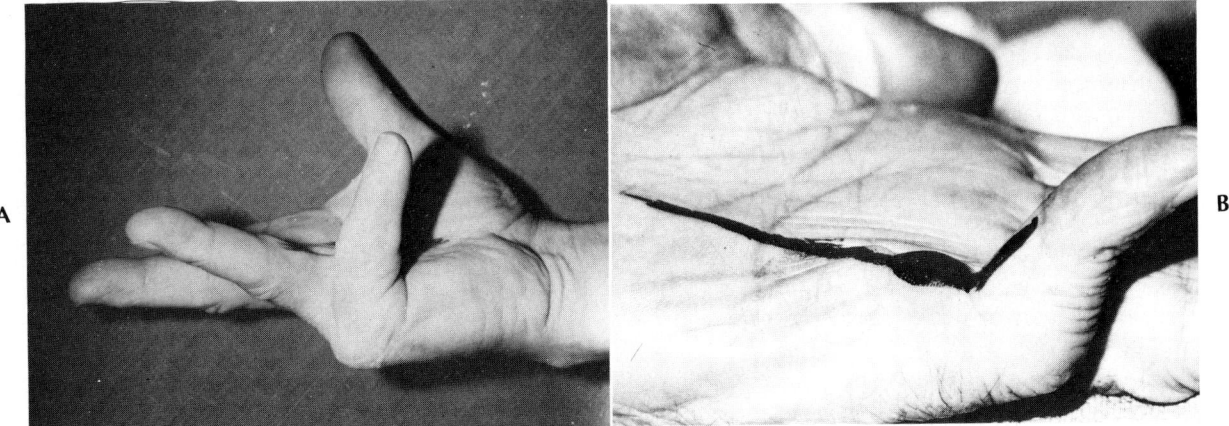

Fig. 67-3   Types of joint contracture. **A,** Contracture at metacarpophalangeal joint only. This patient gained complete hand correction after operation. **B,** Contracture at proximal interphalangeal joint and hyperextension at distal interphalangeal joint. This patient's hand was improved, but not fully corrected, by operation.

at an early age, and show evidence of fibromatoses elsewhere than the volar surface of the hand. Nevertheless, the indications for treatment of these patients are the same as for others. In the same way, patients who are epileptic or alcoholic will not do well with an operation but are still treated according to the state of their disease.

Types of operation

One should distinguish between a type of incision and a type of operation. For example, McCash described a transverse incision in the palm that is left open to heal by second intention.[12] This has nothing to do with what is done to the underlying diseased fascia. King, Exeter, Bass, and Watson described exposure to the fascia by multiple Y-shaped incisions that are converted to V-shaped incisions to make up for the relative shortages of skin.[6] Again this is an adjunct to operation rather than an operation in itself. Incisions should be planned according to the extent of the disease in the palm and the number of digits involved.

Opinions differ about how little or how much fascia need be removed. In the McIndoe operation an attempt is made (through a transverse incision in the palm) to remove all the palmar aponeurosis.[14] This has been called a "radical excision of the palmar fascia." This operation successfully removes the disease in the palm, but hematoma in the palm and morbidity associated with it are common. McCash overcame the problem of hematoma by leaving the wound open, and Skoog did so to some extent by retaining the superficial transverse ligament of the palm.[15]

The antithesis of the McIndoe operation is the subcutaneous fasciotomy of Luck.[10] He believed that because the nodule causes the formation of the contracting cords, only the nodule need be removed. He also believed that in the later stages of disease, when the nodules are not apparent, the contracting cords need not be removed but simply divided. This operation corrects contracture at the MP joint but does not often correct PIP joint contracture. If the cellular process continues, contracture may recur at both the MP and PIP joints.

Gonzales recommends a limited operation, similar to the fasciotomy of Luck, to minimize the postoperative com-

plications of more extensive procedures.[4] He advocates excision of nodules and incision of cords through transverse incisions. On correction of the joint contracture the skin defect is covered with a full-thickness skin graft, thereby holding the ends of the diseased fascia apart.

Radical excision of the palmar fascia is associated with some degree of hematoma formation. If the hematoma is massive, skin loss, infection, edema, and delayed healing will result in prolonged, if not permanent, disability. The patient may not regain either full extension or full flexion of the digits. To overcome this problem, most surgeons have resorted to less extensive dissection in the palm, removing only the diseased fascia (regional fasciectomy). At this stage in our understanding of the disease process this procedure is a good compromise between removal of almost all the palmar aponeurosis, so that recurrence cannot take place, and local incision or excision of a nodule or cord in the palm on the assumption that interruption in the continuity of the contracting tissue will prevent further contracture. With a regional fasciectomy the surgeon removes only the clinically apparent disease, and it should be clear to both the surgeon and the patient that disease elsewhere in the palm may progress.

As Hueston states, "The only difference between a radical and conservative operation is in the extent of the palmar dissection. Digital dissection will be required for interphalangeal joint deformity in any case."[5] This distinction must be emphasized. The surgeon enjoys a considerable choice of methods of treating disease in the palm, and personal preference or bias may well decide the choice. In the finger, however, a direct approach to the disease is essential both to correct interphalangeal joint flexion contracture and to prevent recurrence of contracture. An understanding of the anatomy of the contracting cords and adequate exposure are essential.[13] To correct a contracture at the PIP joint the exposure should be beyond that joint, at least to the distal crease. Because the distal joint may be involved, it is best to include this area in the original dissection.

Therefore the plan of treatment is to perform a regional fasciectomy in the palm to permit full correction at the MP joint and also prevent recurrent contracture. In the affected finger a radical fasciectomy is performed to gain maximum correction at the PIP joint and also to remove potentially diseased tissue that can be a source of recurrent contracture. If only one finger is involved, the operation is performed through a longitudinal incision (Fig. 67-4). If more than one finger is involved, a longitudinal incision is used in the finger, but in the palm a transverse incision is used because it provides better exposure (Fig. 67-5).

Postoperative complications

Hematoma, skin necrosis, and infection are a triad of complications that are intimately related. Extensive opera-

tions in the palm, followed by closure of the wound, very often result in the formation of a hematoma, which then embarrasses the blood supply to the skin that is already compromised. When the edges of the wound become necrotic, infection is inevitable. The result is swelling and stiffness of the hand. These complications are prevented when the palmar wound is left open. Hematoma is less frequent after limited fasciectomy through longitudinal incisions, but skin necrosis and subsequent infection may occur in the small triangular flaps and Z-plasties and prolong recovery.

The digital nerves and vessels may be damaged intra-

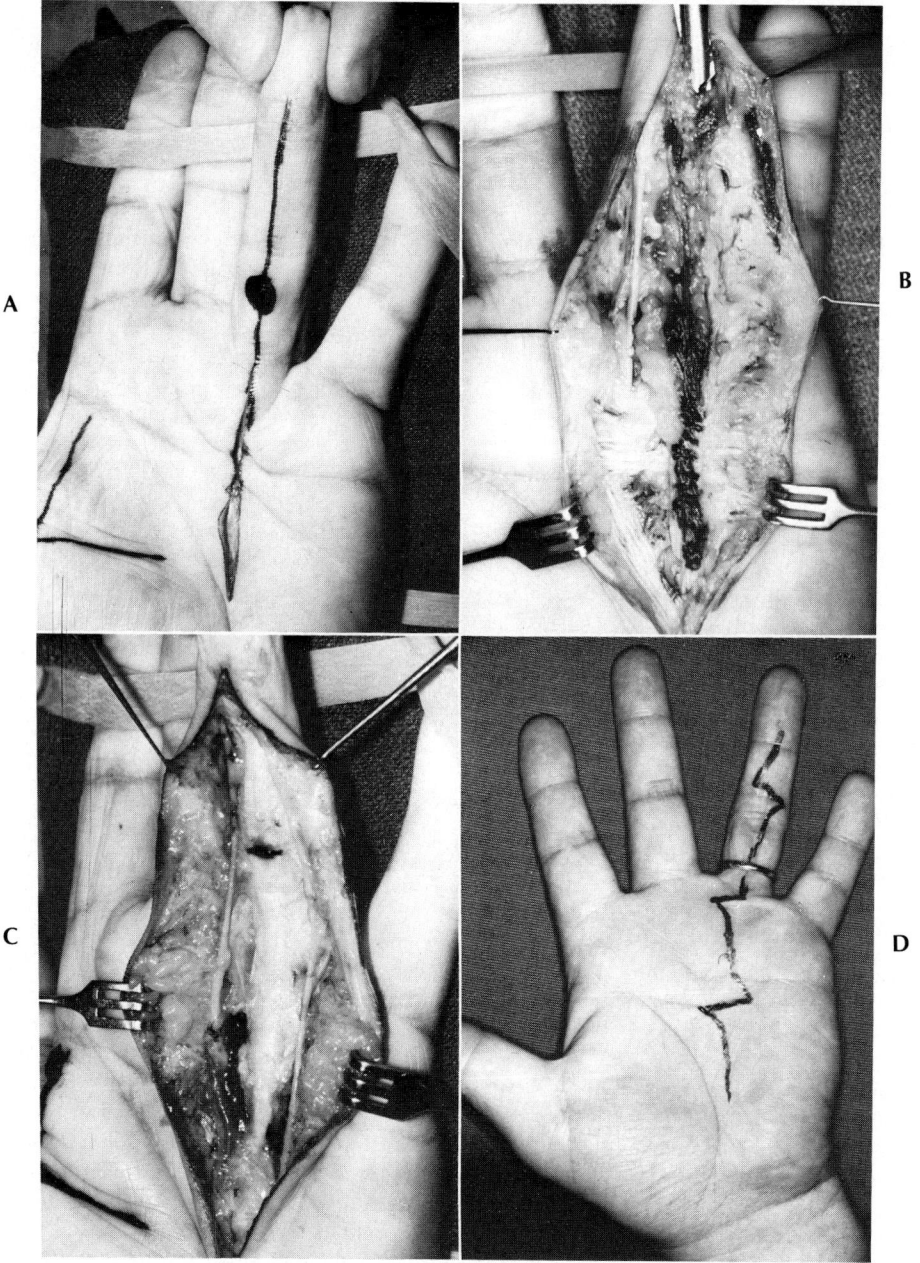

Fig. 67-4 Type of operation performed when only one finger is involved. **A,** Midline longitudinal incision is made from proximal palm to distal crease of finger. **B,** Generous exposure of fascia of palm and finger. **C,** Diseased fascia has been removed. Both neurovascular bundles and the flexor tendon sheath between them have been cleared of fascia. **D,** Appearance of hand 8 years later. Longitudinal incision was broken by three Z-plasties to prevent postoperative scar contracture.

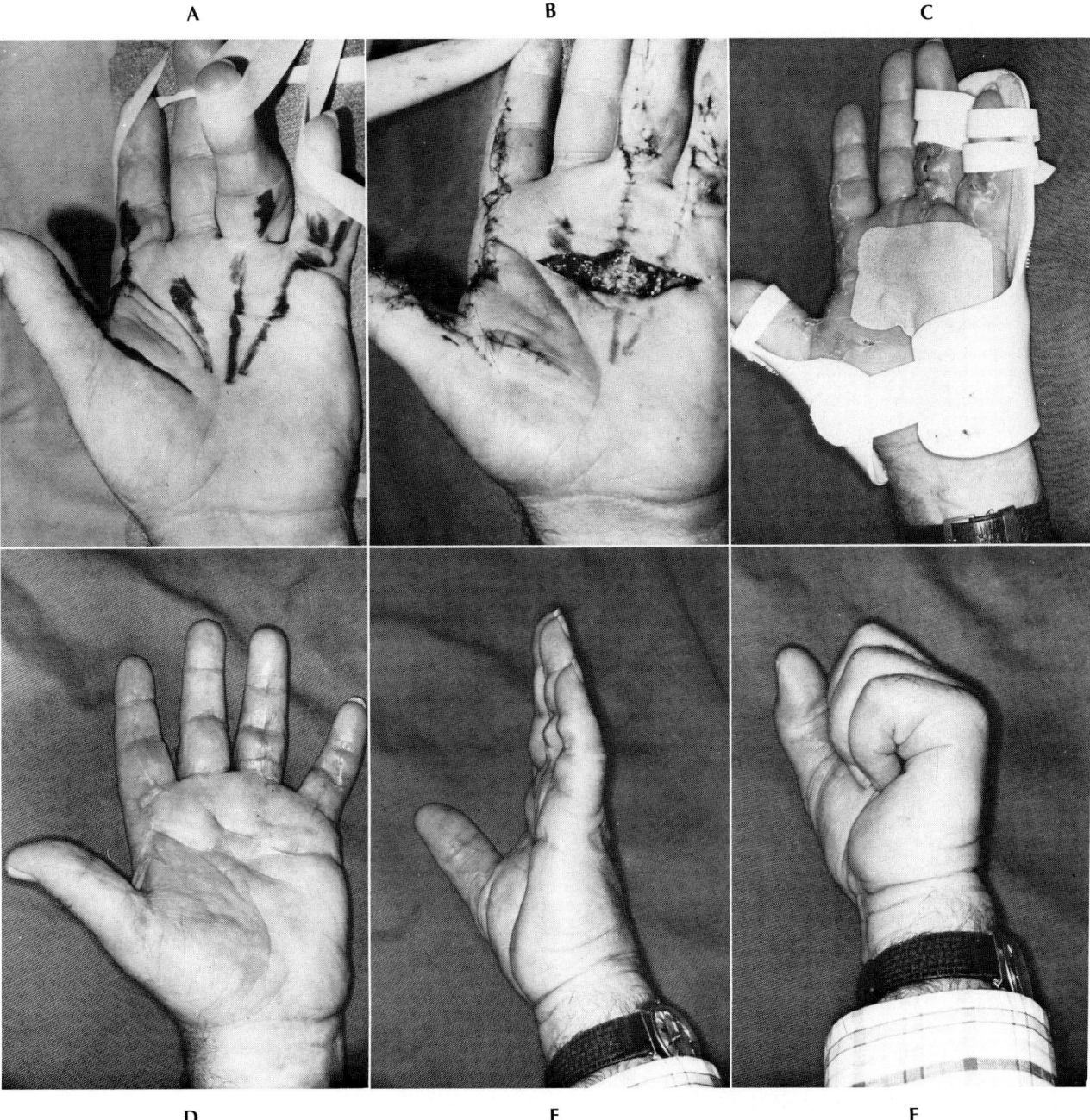

Fig. 67-5   Type of operation performed when more than one digit is involved. **A,** This patient had disease involving pretendinous bands to all five digits, as well as disease causing contracture of proximal interphalangeal joints of little, ring, and index fingers. Natatory ligament in thumb web was also diseased, so patient was unable to fully abduct or extend thumb. **B,** Appearance of hand at end of operation. Longitudinal incisions were made in thumb and index, ring, and little fingers, through which diseased fascia was removed. Incisions were closed by use of multiple Z-plasties. Disease in palm was removed through transverse incision, which was left open. **C,** Three weeks after operation longitudinal incisions were healed. Palmar wound healed in 6 weeks. Patient wore splint most of time for 2 months and at night for another 2 months. **D to F,** Appearance of hand 1 year after operation. Wounds are well healed. Patient lacks full interphalangeal extension but has full flexion.

operatively because they are often surrounded by the diseased fascia. Severance of both arteries will likely result in loss of the digit unless the arteries are repaired. A severed nerve should be repaired. Observation of the patient overnight in a hospital is desirable.

POSTOPERATIVE MANAGEMENT

On the first postoperative day, the dressing is removed and a static dorsal finger-extension splint is molded of a thermal plastic material. Velcro straps are used to fasten the splint to the hand and to hold the fingers in extension (Fig. 67-5, *C*). The purpose of the splint is twofold. The first purpose is to gain the degree of finger extension obtained at operation. One would hope that this will be full extension, but it is unlikely that more extension will be gained by splinting than that obtained by excision of the diseased fascia. It is important to inform the therapist of whether the finger can be expected to extend fully. The second purpose of the splint is to hold the fingers in maximum extension during the period of wound healing.

Usually the splints are well accepted by the patient and finger extension is easily regained. The patient is instructed to tighten gradually the Velcro straps, extending the fingers within pain tolerance, until the fingers have straightened. The patient is given a goal to work toward—for example, achievement of full finger extension in 2 days. In addition, active exercises are essential to prevent joint stiffness and to regain a full range of motion in the fingers. The splint is worn at all times. The patient is instructed to remove the Velcro straps every hour and to actively or with assistance allow the fingers to fully flex and extend. If the patient is to continue these exercises independently at home, it is important that the exercises given are simple and easy to remember. Therefore only complete patterns of motion are stressed—flexion of all fingers to the distal palmar crease and full finger extension. Wrist and thumb exercises may be added if there is any decreased motion. Hand grips and putty can be used to improve grip strength. Progressively resistive exercises to both finger flexors and finger extensors are important in strengthening the hand. Functional activities should be encouraged. When the wounds have healed, hydrotherapy or paraffin wax baths may be used before exercise sessions.

If the fascia has been removed through a longitudinal incision in the palm and digit, the sutures are removed about 10 days after the operation, and the wounds are sufficiently healed in 2 weeks to tolerate most modes of therapy. If more than one digit was involved, the digits are exposed through a longitudinal incision, but a transverse incision is used in the palm. This incision is left open to heal by contraction. The time required for the palmar wound to heal depends on the width of the wound and varies from 3 to 6 weeks after operation. During this time the dressing is changed two or three times each week and the patient wears a splint and is supervised as discussed above. Hydrotherapy is used as described by Fietti and Mackin (see Chapter 68).

The time required to recover from an operation for Dupuytren's disease is variable. Recovery implies a full range of finger motion. Certainly full flexion should be regained, because almost always patients have full finger flexion preoperatively. Full extension is the goal of treatment, but with severe and long-standing PIP contraction, full extension is unlikely, particularly in the little finger.[8] Most patients will be incapacitated for 6 to 8 weeks. The time required to return to work will depend entirely on the job involved, but a laborer will not likely return to work within 2 months of operation.

Having regained full flexion and maximum extension of the fingers, the patient is advised to wear a splint at night for about 3 months. The scar contraction that takes place during this time can cause further joint contracture. Many patients do not wear the splint this long, simply because they are satisfied with the correction obtained. As a result, it is not uncommon to see patients 6 months after operation with 10 to 15 degrees more flexion, especially at the PIP joint, than was present under supervised splinting.

SUMMARY

A successful result after operation for Dupuytren's disease requires the cooperation of the patient, the surgeon, and the therapist. An appropriate operation must be designed for the individual patient. MP joint contracture can always be corrected, but some residual PIP joint contracture may have to be accepted.

REFERENCES

1. Chiu HF and McFarlane RM: Pathogenesis of Dupuytren's contracture: a correlative clinical-pathological study, J Hand Surg 3:1, 1978.
2. Dupuytren G: Permanent retraction of the fingers produced by an affection of the palmar fascia, Lancet, p 222, 1834.
3. Gabbianni G and Majno G: Dupuytren's contracture: fibroblast contraction? Am J Pathol 66:131, 1972.
4. Gonzales RI: Dupuytren's contracture of the fingers: a simplified approach to the surgical treatment, Calif Med 115:25, 1971.
5. Hueston JT: Dupuytren's contracture: the trend to conservatism, Ann R Coll Surg Engl 36:134, 1965.
6. King EW and others: Treatment of Dupuytren's contracture by extensive fasciectomy through multiple Y-V-plasty incision, J Hand Surg 4:234, 1979.
7. Legge JWH, Finlay JB, and McFarlane RM: A study of Dupuytren's tissue with the scanning electron microscope, J Hand Surg 6:482, 1981.
8. Legge JWH and McFarlane RM: Predictions of results of treatment of Dupuytren's disease, J Hand Surg 5:608, 1980.
9. Ling RSM: The genetic factor in Dupuytren's disease, J Bone Joint Surg 45B:709, 1963.
10. Luck JV: Dupuytren's contracture: a new concept of the pathogenesis correlated with surgical management, J Bone Joint Surg 41A:635, 1959.
11. MacCallum P and Hueston JT: The pathology of Dupuytren's contracture, Aust NZ J Surg 31:241, 1962.
12. McCash CR: The open palm technique in Dupuytren's contracture, Br J Plast Surg 17:271, 1964.
13. McFarlane RM: Patterns of the diseased fascia in the fingers in Dupuytren's contracture, Plast Reconstr Surg 54:31, 1974.
14. McIndoe A and Beare RLB: Dupuytren's contracture, Am J Surg 95:2, 1958.
15. Skoog T: The transverse elements of the palmar aponeurosis in Dupuytren's contracture, Scand J Plast Surg 1:51, 1967.
16. Tubiana R and Defrenne H: Les localizations de la maladie de Dupuytren à la partie radiale de la main, Chirurgie 102(12):989, 1976.

68

Open-palm technique in Dupuytren's disease

Vincent G. Fietti, Jr. and Evelyn J. Mackin

In 1831 Baron Guillaume Dupuytren, lecturing at surgical rounds at L'Hotel Dieu in Paris, described a malady that caused contractures of the digits. The following year his lecture appeared in the French literature,[13] and in 1834 his article was published in Lancet.[12] The clinical features of the entity that now bears his name are presented in Chapter 67. Although considerable information has been gathered over the past 150 years, the etiology remains unclear, the prognosis variable, and the treatment debatable.[27] Initially, radical fasciectomy, or removal of the entire palmar fascia and its extensions, as proposed by McIndoe and Beare was popularized,[29] but high postoperative morbidity including hematoma formation, necrosis of wound edges and flaps, infection, swelling, and stiffness soon led to a more limited surgical approach.[37] The subtotal palmar fasciectomy, or removal of only visably involved tissue, is now the mainstay of surgical treatment. The manner in which the palmar and digital skin is managed, however, is still one area where opinions differ. The use of midline longitudinal digital incisions closed by the use of multiple Z-plasties is still favored by many.[17,18] Others excise diseased portions of skin, particularly in recurrent cases, and cover these defects with split-thickness or full-thickness skin grafts.[12,15] Even if skin has not been excised, the release of contractures may result in insufficient skin for closure unless flaps can be widely undermined and sutured under tension. Although the use of grafts is one solution, the hand must be kept immobile during the first postoperative week while the grafts "take," and this immobility predisposes to stiffness of joints.

Although subtotal fasciectomy resulted in lower morbidity than the radical operation, early wound complications in many series were still alarmingly high when incisions were primarily closed or skin grafted. In 1964 C. R. McCash reported his experience with a technique based on Dupuytren's original recommendations in which multiple transverse incisions were made in palm and on digits. These wounds were not sutured but left open to heal "by granulation."[25] The so-called open-palm technique has become popular with many hand surgeons, and as more experience has been gained, its virtues as well as its limitations have become clear.*

TECHNIQUE

Axillary block is our preferred mode of anesthesia, but general or even local anesthesia with sedation has been used. Exsanguination with good tourniquet control of bleeding is a prerequisite. We have used a modification of the McCash technique with a transverse incision across the palm either in the distal crease or just beyond it (Figs. 68-1 and 68-2). The length of this incision is determined by the number of digits involved. A more proximal second incision may be made paralleling the thenar crease if proximal extension of diseased fascia requires further exposure. Instead of transverse "ladder" incisions on the digits, we favor a volar Bruner incision usually connected to the palmar wound (Fig. 68-3). Care must be taken to extend the apices of the volar zigzag to the midaxial line of the digit to prevent subsequent scar contracture. Limited exposure with "blind" dissection beneath intact skin bridges can be extremely dangerous, especially over the proximal phalanx where the neurovascular structures are displaced toward the midline by the spiral cords.[26] The Bruner incision gives excellent exposure in the entire digit. Flaps must be kept as thick as possible. Heavy nodules often have no subcutaneous fat and most be dissected carefully, removing as much nodule as possible. A "button-hole" in the skin in such areas is not uncommon and will not jeopardize healing.

After fasciectomy, the volar digital flaps are sutured in place using a minimal number of nonabsorbable sutures to avoid tension. If additional skin length is needed, the Y-V–plasty incision described by Watson can be used.[20] Gaps in the incision closure are usual and will heal secondarily. With release of the contractures, the transverse palmar incision expands to a diamond-shaped defect (Fig. 68-4). This is left open, and all wounds are covered with nonadherent dressings. Our preference is to apply a full strength povidone-iodine dressing over this with a bulky "fluff" dressing in the palm and between the digits. A light plaster shell is applied, but no attempt is made to forcibly hold digits in full extension (Fig. 68-5). This dressing remains for approximately 3 days. Although informed preoperatively of the nature of the open wound, many patients are surprised at its appearance during the first dressing change. Often formal therapy of whirlpool and supervised exercises is begun at that time. Wound healing occurs both by marginal epithelialization and flattening of contracted skin[32] over 3 to 6 weeks, depending on the size of the defect (Figs. 68-6 to 68-9). The patient is taught to change his dressings daily and perform home soaks. We used a topical antibiotic ointment, Elase,* only in those cases that have suspected superficial infection. This ointment must be used sparingly, because it might promote the formation of hypertrophic granulations (Fig. 68-10). If granulations become exuberant, they respond best to silver nitrate application.

---

*References 1,4,6,7,10,11,19,21-23,31-33,38.

*Parke-Davis, Morris Plains, NJ.

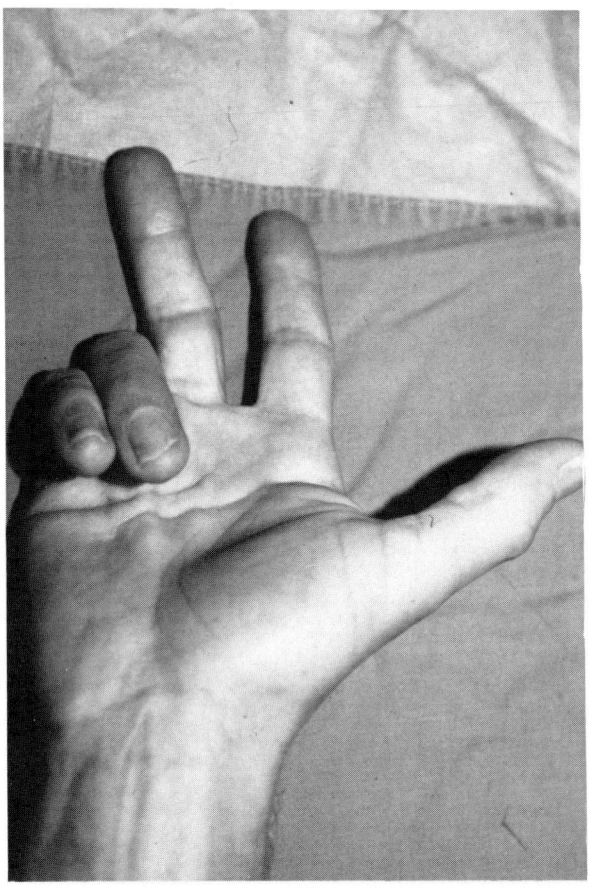

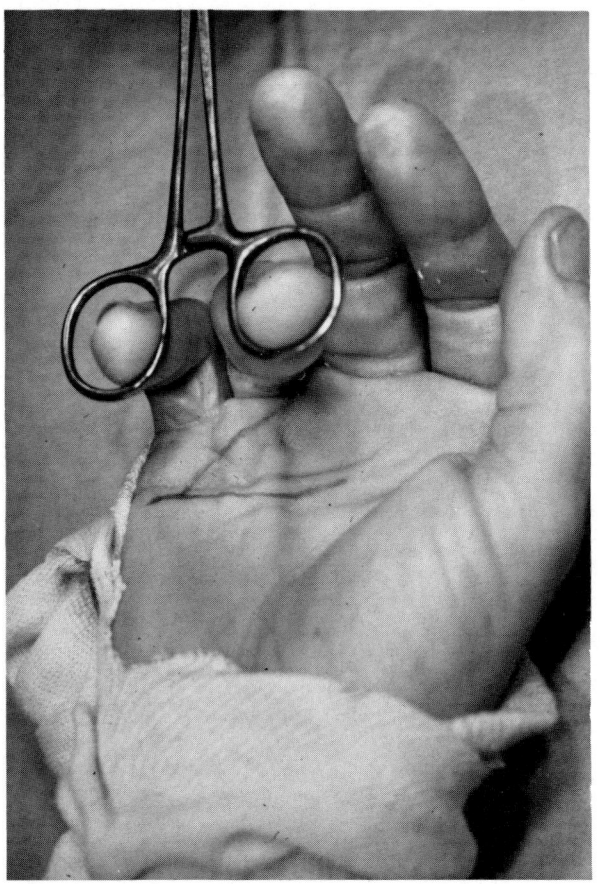

Fig. 68-1 Preoperative status with 60-degree metacarpophalangeal contractures of the ring and little fingers and 90-degree proximal interphalangeal contractures.

Fig. 68-2 Incision is mapped out on the palm and volar zigzag on the fingers.

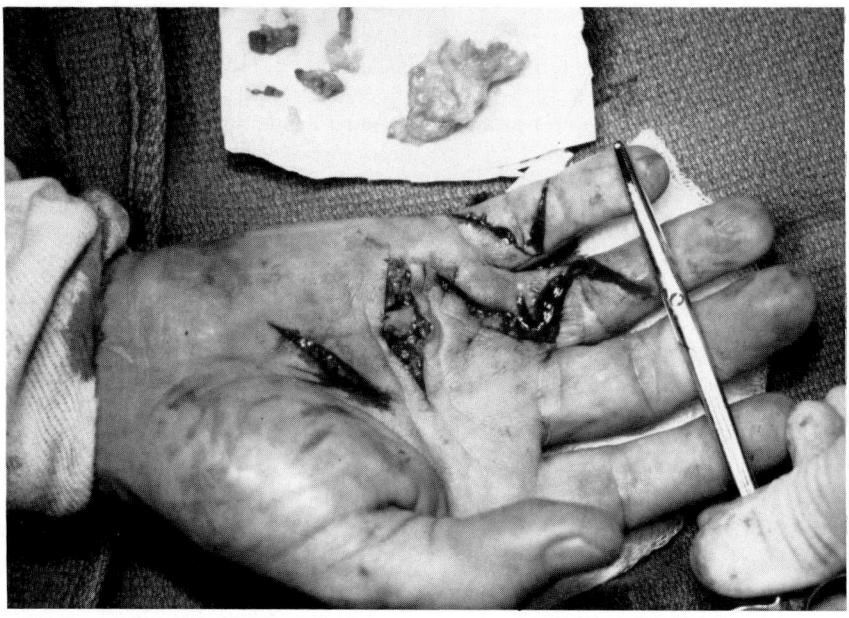

Fig. 68-3 Following fasciectomy volar wounds on digits are sutured. Note the proximal incision paralleling the thenar crease.

There are clear advantages to the use of the open-palm technique. Incision planning is simplified, and there is decrease in operative time. The open wound allows free drainage of blood, which results in no palmar hematomas. No drains are required. Infection of the open wound, theoretically possible, does not occur with proper wound care. Because skin is not sutured under tension, wound sloughs are rare and postoperative pain minimal. With less pain, the patient can mobilize digits better and the incidence of reflex sympathetic dystrophy is reduced. Schneider, reporting on 49 cases, had no infections or wound sloughs.[33] Gelberman compared open with closed treatment in 82 patients in a random prospective study.[14] The patients treated with the open-palm technique had no infections, hematomas, or flap necrosis compared with 18% flap necrosis, 4% infection, and 4% hematomas in the closed group. In another series of 158 patients, Lubahn's open group improved total active motion (TAM) 17%, whereas those with closed wounds improved 10%.

Despite these advantages, the open-palm technique is criticized by some. An earlier objection was the potential danger of the "blind" dissection beneath intact skin bridges. This is eliminated by combining a volar zigzag connected to the transverse palmar wound. Fears of infection have not proven to be justified. Some surgeons seem philosophically opposed to leaving a wound open that might otherwise be closed. It is true that the open-palm technique requires more patient involvement and cooperation than with a closed wound, and full wound healing is about a week longer. These objections do not seem convincing in light of reduced morbidity using the open-palm method.

It is well known that a high percentage of patients will redevelop contractures either because of recurrent disease in a previously operated area or extension of disease into

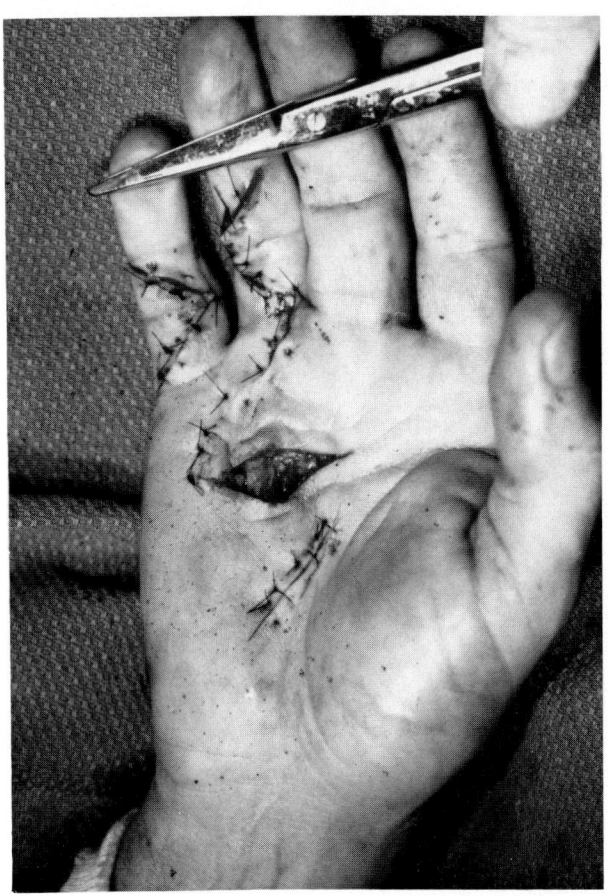

Fig. 68-4 Palmar wound is left open.

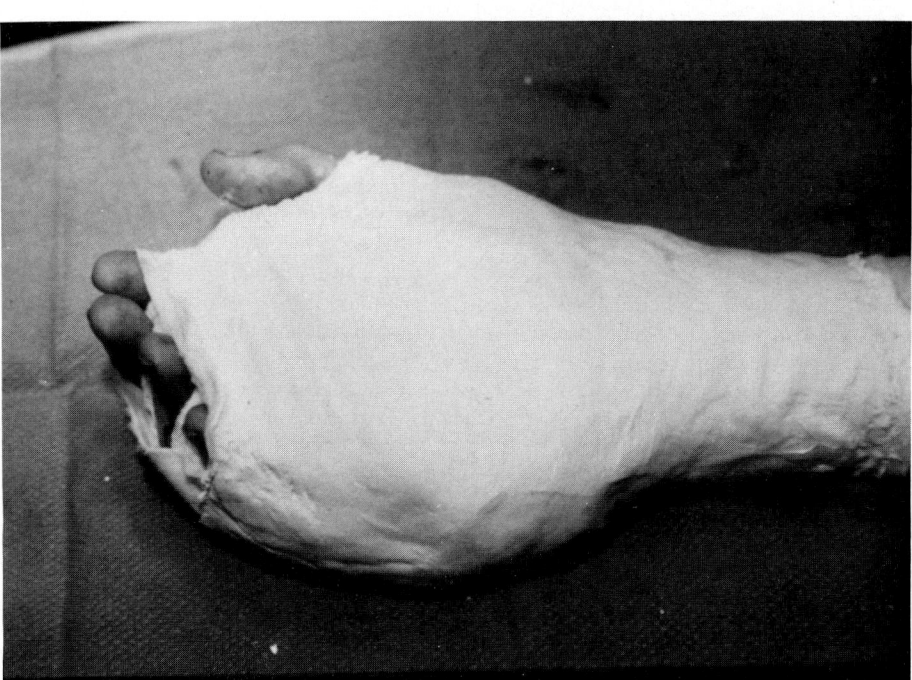

Fig. 68-5 Bulky hand dressing with light plaster shell.

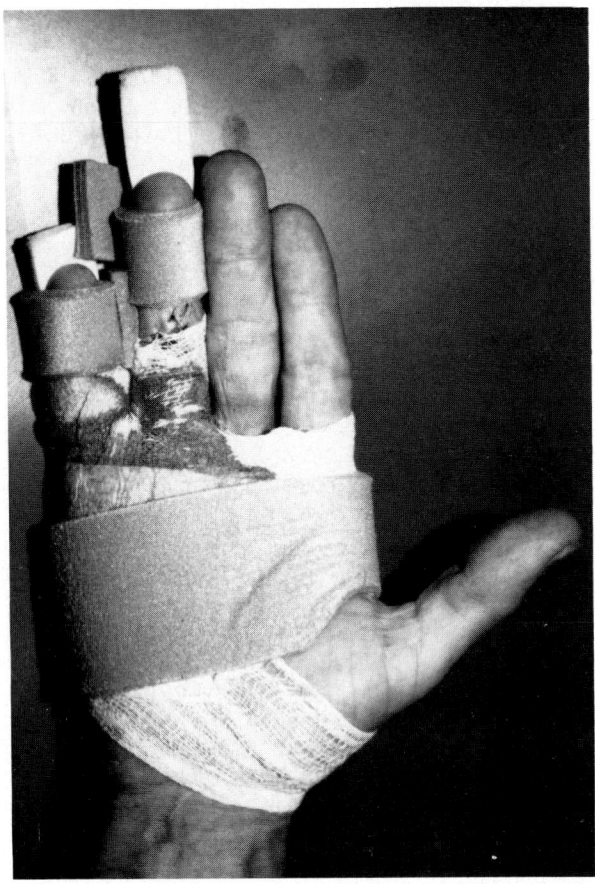

Fig. 68-6 Night extension splinting with dorsal static splints.

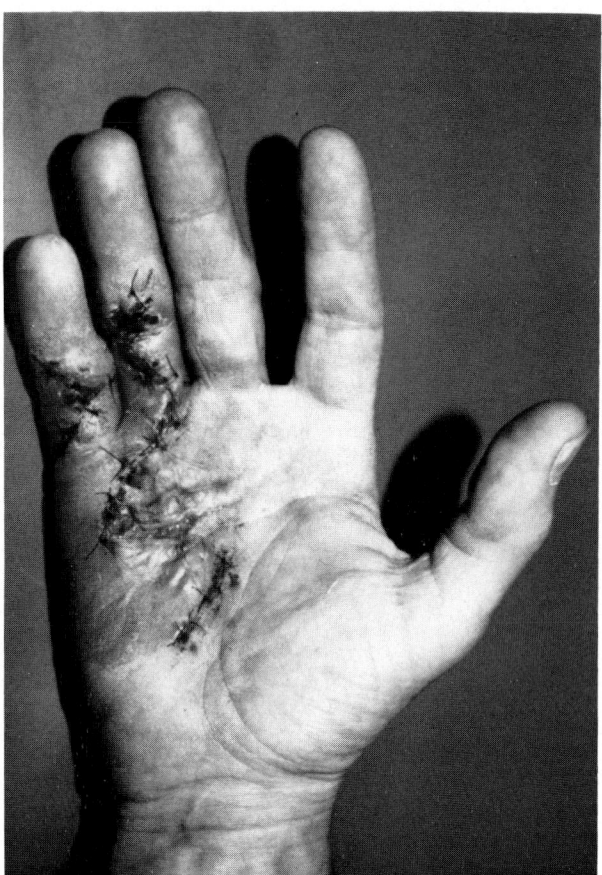

Fig. 68-7 Appearance at 2 weeks when sutures are removed and palmar wound is almost healed.

areas not involved before. The rate of recurrence or extension probably depends more on the aggressiveness of a patient's disease rather than on any other factor. However, published studies have sought to correlate prognosis with the manner of skin closure. Schneider's series followed 5 years revealed 32% recurrence and 48% extension.[33] In a multicenter study coordinated by McFarlane, recurrent contractures of the proximal interphalangeal joint occurred more frequently with open wounds versus Z-plasty closures.[28] It is apparent from the reviewed data and experience that the open-palm technique has a lower incidence of early wound complications but has little or no bearing on long-term prognosis.

POSTOPERATIVE THERAPY

Despite good surgical treatment, some patients recovering from Dupuytren's surgery will develop complications unless a careful postoperative hand therapy program is initiated. Some of these complications are persistent edema, stiffness of the entire hand, hematoma, and early recurrence of flexion contractures. The patient must understand that approximately 1 to 2 months of intensive postoperative therapy and splinting may be required if the good results attained at surgery are to be maintained and that night extension splinting may be necessary for 6 months or longer.[24]

Evaluation

Because the postoperative Dupuytren's hand can change dramatically in as little as a few days because of the dynamics of the healing process, careful evaluation must be performed and documented from the first visit. The evaluation battery should include wound and edema assessment, active range of motion, passive range of motion, and sensibility.

Because patients often are startled at the wound's appearance at the time of the first dressing change, the therapist should reassure the patient that wound healing will progress over the coming weeks. Also at this time the therapist assesses the progress of the wound.

Edema is initially recorded using circumferential measurements taken with a tape measure. These measurements should be taken at specific landmarks to improve reproducibility. When the wounds are healed, volumetric measurements* replace circumferential measures. Volumetrics involve edema measurement through water displacement. If edema persists, measures should be taken before and after treatment.

Active and passive range of motion are measured with a goniometer. Measurement of the distance from the finger

*Volumeters Unlimited, Idyllwild, Calif.

pulp(s) to the distal palmer crease during active flexion is taken, because this measurement relates to the function of grasp.[34] Extension must also be closely monitored. Passive range-of-motion measures at each joint in both flexion and extension are taken.

Sensibility may be affected as a result of Dupuytren's surgery. The diminished sensation often recovers spontaneously but should be monitored, because it may affect functional recovery.

Treatment

Therapy usually begins on the third to fifth postoperative day. It includes wound care, edema control, and active and passive range of motion. As healing progresses, flexion splinting and scar management may also be indicated.

Wound care

The open-palm technique of McCash prevents hematoma and may contribute to the overall reduction of complications.[35] Because the open-palm technique allows free drainage of the wound, whirlpool treatment assists in wound management by cleansing the wound. In this regard the postoperative management after the open-palm technique differs from that after closure with skin grafts or Z-plasties when early hydrotherapy would be inappropriate.

A whirlpool-bath, clear-rinse procedure is used. Betadine* (povidine-iodine complex), an antibacterial agent, is added to the agitating water. Niederhuber and associates[30] stated that "as an adjunctive modality in the treatment of

*Purdue Frederick, Norwalk, Conn.

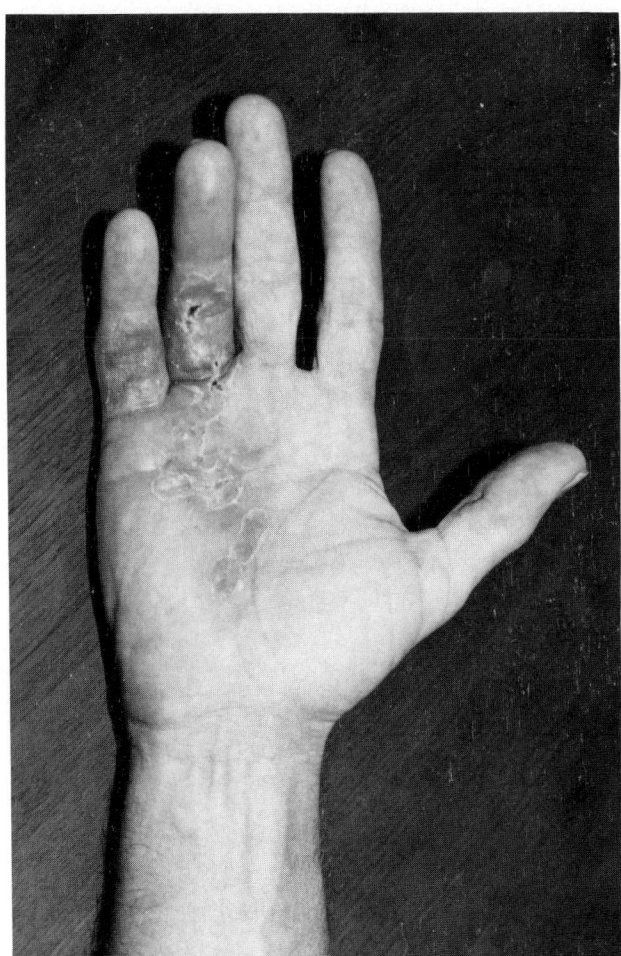

Fig. 68-8 Appearance at 4 weeks with wound completely closed in the palm.

Fig. 68-9 Appearance at 7 weeks.

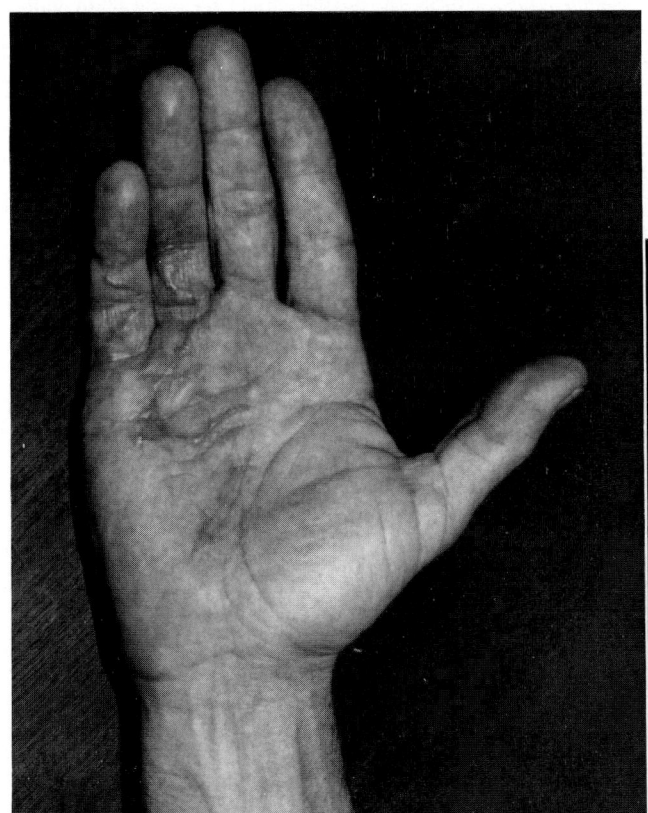

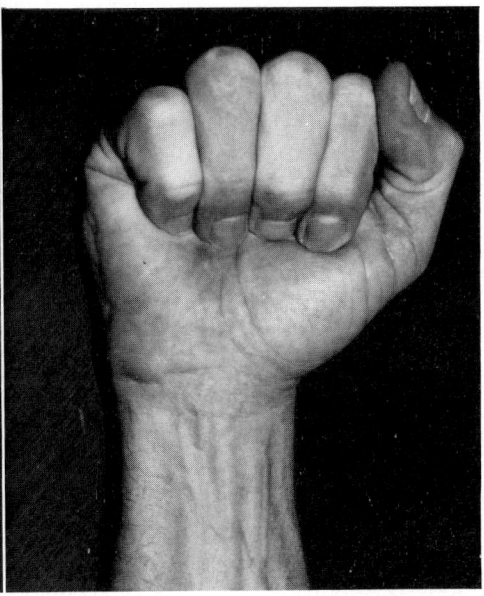

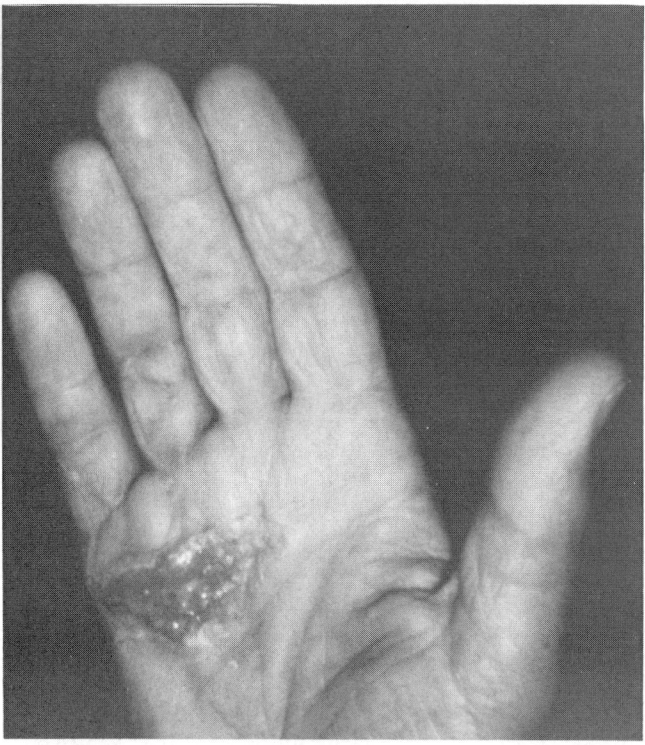

Fig. 68-10 Hypertrophic granulation tissue caused by excessive use of antibiotic ointment.

many types of wounds, the therapeutic whirlpool provides the physiological benefits of heat to promote healing and the atraumatic removal of surface eschar and exudates where bacteria thrive." They found that a combined treatment of whirlpool agitation followed by a clear-water rinse was significantly more effective in removing bacteria than a procedure in which the part was not rinsed after removal from an agitating whirlpool bath. In a later study, Bohannon[5] produced further evidence of the value of rinsing contaminated ulcers, wounds, or burns after removal from a whirlpool bath.

Whirlpool-bath temperature ranges from 98° to 100° F. The patient's extremity is positioned with the elbow in flexion so that the agitating water just covers the hand; thus one can avoid a dependent position. Active flexion/extension exercises are done in the bath. When the whirlpool-bath treatment is completed, the patient's hand is rinsed with clear water. A contraindication to a whirlpool bath is the presence of edema, which may increase with the heat of warm water. The risk of increasing edema is decreased by having the patient remove his hand from the whirlpool and elevate it overhead where he performs active fist-making for 1 minute. This is repeated every 3 to 5 minutes.[8]

Between sessions with the therapist, the patient will do warm saline soaks at home, prepared with one tablespoon of table salt added to a quart of boiling water. The hypertonic solution is bactericidal. The patient lets the boiling water cool to lukewarm temperature and then soaks his hand for 10 to 15 minutes, three times a day. Active motion is done during the soaks. The patient is instructed in redressing the wounds at home in the manner preferred by the surgeon.

Generally, dry sterile dressings are used. They are changed after each whirlpool bath or home saline treatment. The critical factor is to keep the granulating wound clean. A small number of patients will develop superficial infection with increased exudate. As mentioned, this can be treated with a light application of Elase ointment.

If resection into the digit or digits is necessary, the closed digital incision is also bandaged; however, the dressing to the digits must not restrict the patient's exercise program; full active flexion/extension exercises must be possible within the confines of the dressing. A thin piece of gauze cut from a 4 × 4 sterile gauze pad, placed over the incision and covered with a piece of tube-bandage, is effective when the digital incision is bandaged.

If a skin graft was necessary at surgery, it must be closely monitored for vascularity during the early phase of healing. Generally, the volar plaster splint applied at surgery is removed, and a lighter dressing is applied at the first postoperative visit. Care must be taken to apply the dressing so that it does not abrade or cause pressure to the graft during early mobilization. A palmar pan splint is fabricated to maintain extension (see Fig. 68-1).

Control of edema

Edema is the first and most obvious reaction of the hand to injury or surgery. Most wounds have excess fluid content early in the healing process, and this should not cause alarm. It is the continuing edema 2 or 3 weeks postoperatively that is an ongoing complication and has long-term consequences. If edema persists in conjunction with immobilization, which is its advocate, gliding surfaces become adherent and the hand stiffens. Reflex sympathetic dystrophy is a severe complication of Dupuytren surgery and is to be suspected when edema and stiffness are accompanied by significant pain.

Edema is a common reaction in the hand disturbed by the complex surgical dissection required in many Dupuytren procedures. The importance of controlling edema and thereby avoiding complications must be emphasized. Until good muscular activity is restored, we depend on gravity and external measures to assist the return of blood flow through the lymphatic and venous systems.

The patient's hand is elevated after surgery to minimize limb dependency and thus assist in edema control. The elbow should not be acutely flexed, because this will increase venous stasis. During sleep the hand should be elevated on pillows.

In cases of severe pitting edema, an intermittent compression unit is helpful to reduce swelling. The hand is placed in the sleeve with the fingers in extension. The extremity is elevated on a table or pillows to an angle of 30 to 45 degrees to take advantage of the flow of gravity while the intermittent pressure is applied. Use of external compression is not contraindicated in the presence of open wounds as long as sterile dressings are used. Felt pads can be positioned around pins to prevent pressure on them. The amount of pressure is adjusted to the condition. Initial treatment might be as low as 30 to 40 mm Hg for ½ to 1 hour. (To be effective, unit pressure must exceed capillary pressure [25 mm Hg] and be kept below the patient's diastolic pressure.) After mechanical massage by the intermittent compression unit, retrograde massage with lanolin may be applied by the therapist in a further attempt to push the extracellular fluid out of the hand. Care must be taken to avoid contaminating the wound with lanolin.

Coban* wraps applied to the digits and hand also assist in reduction of edema. Coban is applied distally to proximally and must be wrapped without tension. Tightly applied Coban will interfere with circulation of the fingers. An Isotoner† glove, an elasticized glove, may also be helpful in controlling edema while allowing the patient to use his hand with minimal restriction. The tips of the glove may be cut off to allow sensory input.

We have found that an effective exercise that incorporates elevation and active motion is to have the patient elevate both arms over the head and make as firm a fist as possible 10 times each hour. This exercise can also be used to maintain good shoulder and elbow motion.

Macramé and the Valpar* Whole Body Work Sample are examples of activities that may be performed in elevation

*Medical Products Division, 3M, St. Paul.
†Aris Isotoner Inc, New York, NY.

*Valpar Corp, Tucson.

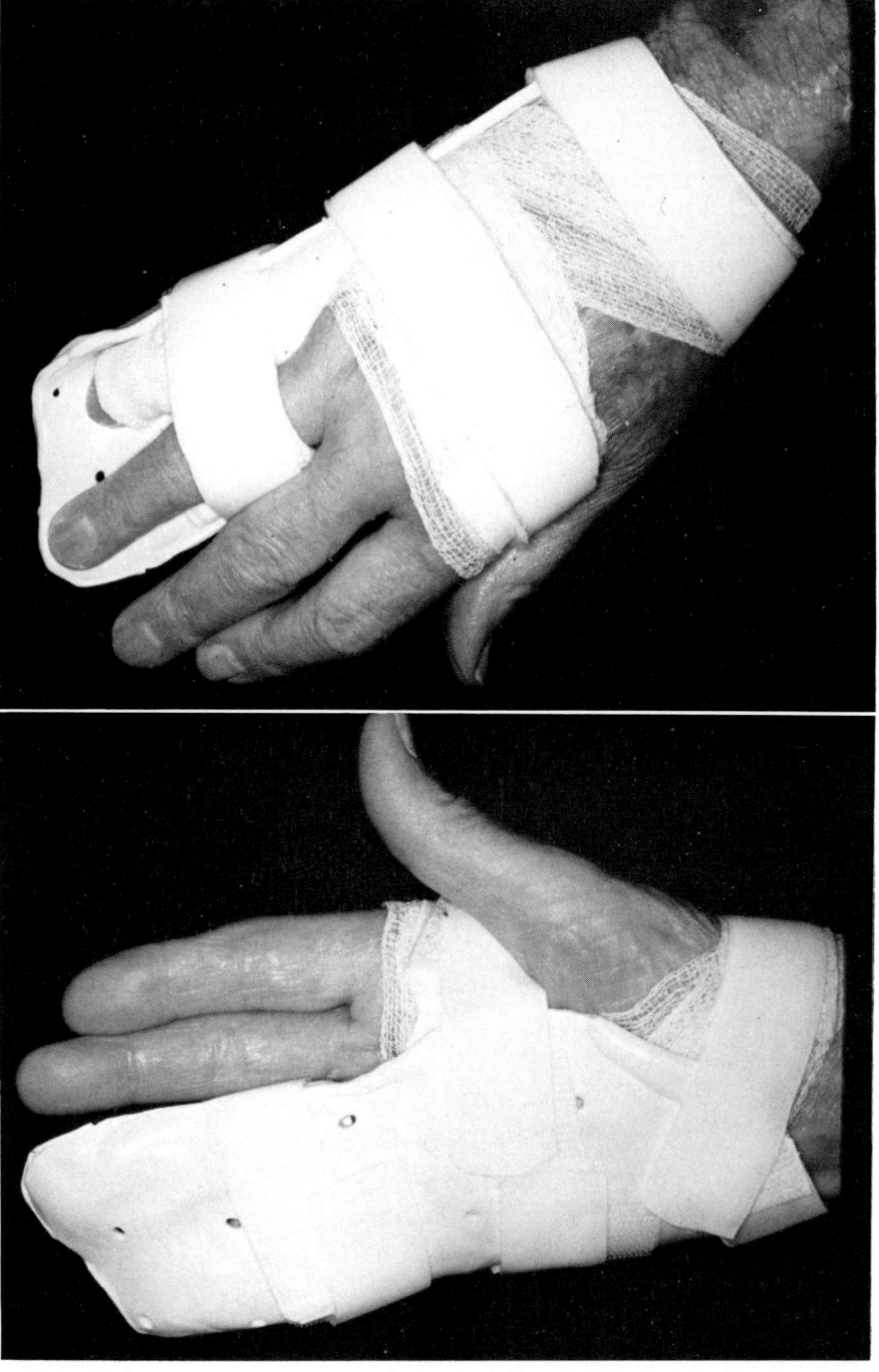

Fig. 68-11   A thermoplastic palmar pan splint.

to decrease edema while increasing active motion and co-ordination.

Splinting

Splinting is an important part of postoperative care. In a few patients with minimal disease and pliable skin and in whom good finger extension has been obtained, postoperative splinting may not be necessary; however, in all other patients a splint to maintain the extension of the digit(s) gained in the operating room is fabricated at the initial therapy session. In some instances the surgeon could not release a proximal interphalangeal (PIP) joint contracture to full extension. It is important to know the intraoperative range of motion and the result the surgeon expects postoperatively so that realistic goals can be set. Awareness of neurovascular status is important in splint application.

Splints must be carefully fitted to gently hold the digit(s) in extension during wound healing. Each time the patient is seen for therapy, the splint should be evaluated so that necessary adjustments can be made. A thermoplastic palmar pan splint (Fig. 68-11) that holds the digit(s) in extension is fabricated. Initially it is removed only for exercise and wound care. As healing progresses, day splinting is gradually reduced but night extension splinting may be necessary for 6 months or longer. The surgeon and therapist may elect to change initial day splinting in specific cases.

In severe cases where a digit shows early signs of recurring contraction (this is most often seen in the little finger PIP joint), a different splint design may be needed. In these cases, a splint designed in our clinic by Callahan[9] specifically addresses this problem. The splint (Fig. 68-12) employs a length of Velcro loop over the outrigger to provide the extension force instead of a finger loop and rubber band. The Velcro provides a static pull. It may be adjusted to provide increased tension as tolerated by the patient between treatments.

Active range of motion

Gentle, basic active finger exercises are begun during the first postoperative visit. The active exercise program includes the following:

1. Thumb opposition to each fingertip, abduction, and extension
2. Finger blocking (DIP joint flexion with the PIP joint and MP joint held in extension with the uninvolved hand, followed by PIP joint flexion with MP joint extension)
3. Flexion of each finger to the thenar eminence
4. Fist-making
5. Finger abduction and adduction
6. Finger extension
7. Full wrist motion and thumb range of motion

Ten repetitions of each exercise are done three to four times daily.

Severe PIP joint flexion contractures of the little finger frequently result in hyperextension of the distal joint, an attitude assumed by the digit to compensate for the PIP joint flexion.[16] When these contractures are released at surgery, the surgeons' approach may be to hold the PIP joint in extension by Kirschner-wire fixation. Early active DIP joint flexion must be emphasized to encourage tendon gliding and restore system alignment.

As motion improves, the exercise program is modified to make the exercises more precise. Usually by the second postoperative week, tendon-gliding exercises can be initiated.[36]

As exercises become "easy," they are discontinued and more difficult exercises and resistance are gradually added. For example, when finger extension is performed easily, the patient may be asked to cross his fingers, such as index over long, long over index, and long over ring. This exercise can be made even more difficult by asking the patient to pass a coin from finger to finger.

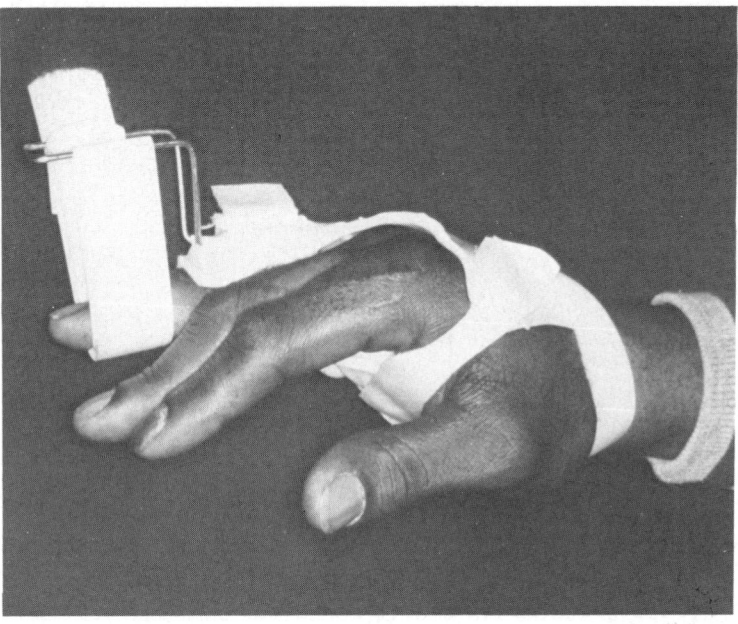

Fig. 68-12 A splint with a Velcro loop over the outrigger to provide extension force.

Putty-squeezing may be instituted at 4 to 6 weeks after surgery. Making a "hot dog" from putty, that is, repetitive squeezing of the putty using only the fingers, strengthens the grip and improves flexion. Exercises should never be overdone. Squeezing the putty 10 times intermittently during the day is a far better regimen than doing it for 10 to 20 minutes continuously, which might result in pain and edema. Patients must be cautioned against this. Putty may also be used for extension exercises.

Active hand use is encouraged in therapy via functional activities. While the palm is still open, light pickups and pinch activities may be initiated. When the wound closes, generally by 6 to 8 weeks, sustained grip activities, such as woodworking and working with leather, help regain full function of the hand. Resistance is increased as tolerated.

Passive range of motion

Patients are instructed in gentle passive range of motion of all joints. If flexion is a problem, flexion splinting may be necessary.

When passive flexion of one or more PIP joints is limited, a web strap provides the necessary passive stretch. The strap is worn over the involved PIP joints and behind the MP joints. The strap is fabricated from a 2.5 cm wide webbing with a 2.5 cm wide buckle. The patient may begin wearing the strap for ½ hour, three times a day. The patient adjusts the tension of the strap until he feels a slight pull on the affected joints. The time the strap is worn may be increased gradually for as long as 2 hours, three times a day (see Chapter 24).

When all the joints of a digit are stiff in extension, a combination web strap is indicated (see Chapter 24). It is comfortable and easily adjusted. The combination web strap, however, is not effective in gaining the final degrees of PIP joint or DIP joint motion. As flexion improves, the combination web strap can be discarded and the web strap or DIP joint elastic is used. The time the combination web strap is worn is the same as for the web strap.

Because of prolonged preoperative positioning in MP joint or combined MP/PIP joint flexion, intrinsic tightness may be a problem. The splinting alternatives mentioned here may not be specific enough to resolve this problem, because addressing it requires MP joint extension with IP joint flexion. An intrinsic stretcher splint may be required in these cases (see Chapter 24).

Specific instructions should be clearly written for the patient, describing the application of the splint and desired time each splint is to be worn. The patient must be instructed to look for changes in color of the fingertips and increase in tingling, numbness, or swelling of the digit or hand as signs to decrease splint tension. Although passive flexion devices may be necessary during the day to increase flexion, night splinting is reserved for extension.

Scar management

When the wound has healed, lanolin massage is helpful to soften scar and maintain tissue mobility. The palm and digits should be massaged before each exercise session for approximately 10 minutes. A small, deep, circular stroke is used for massage over the scar. After massage, the excess lanolin should be removed to prevent skin maceration.

Silastic Elastomer is an effective adjunct in managing digital and palmar scars. A catalyst is added to the material, and it is spread over the scar area. Its advantage is its ability to conform to the entire scar area, thus producing a reusable mold with pressure over all areas of the scar. It can be applied before complete wound closure by placing a piece of nonadhering gauze over the wound and applying the Elastomer over it. Additional pressure is achieved with the palmar pan split. Elastomer is discontinued when the scar is flat and no longer reactive.

Occasionally a patient may experience hypersensitivity over the healed area. This should be addressed through a program of desensitization. Desensitization involves the stimulation of a hypersensitive area with textures that are normally not noxious. The stimulation is applied for about 10 minutes each waking hour and proceeds through a predefined hierarchy, beginning with fur and progressing to vibration.[2,3,24]

SUMMARY

The importance of a carefully supervised postoperative active motion exercise and splinting program cannot be overemphasized. Gosset[16] suggests that 50% of the result of the operation depends on active postoperative movement and that "without this, the best operation will be left with a functional deficit."

REFERENCES

1. Ariyan S: In defense of the open wound, Arch Surg 111:293, 1976.
2. Barber LM: Occupational therapy for the treatment of reflex sympathetic dystrophy and posttraumatic hypersensitivity of the injured hand. In Fredericks S and Brody GS, editors: Symposium on the neurologic aspects of plastic surgery, St. Louis, 1978, The CV Mosby Co.
3. Barber LM: Desensitization of the traumatized hand. In Hunter JM and others, editors: Rehabilitation of the hand, St. Louis, 1984, The CV Mosby Co.
4. Beltran JE, Jimeno-Urban F, and Yunta A: The open palm and digit technique in the treatment of Dupuytren's contracture, Hand 8:73, 1976.
5. Bohannon RW: Whirlpool versus whirlpool and rise for removal of bacteria from a venous stasis ulcer, Phys Ther 62(3):304, 1982.
6. Borden J: The open finger treatment of Dupuytren's contracture, Orthop Rev 3:25, 1974.
7. Breidis J: Dupuytren's contracture: lack of complications with the open palm technique, Br J Plast Surg 27:218, 1974.
8. Byron PM and Muntzer EM: Therapist's management of the mutilated hand, Hand Clin, 2:69, 1986.
9. Callahan AD: Personal communication, 1984.
10. Carroll RE and Conolly WB: Open wound technique for Dupuytren's contracture. In Proceedings of the American Society for Surgery of the Hand, J Bone Joint Surg, 52A:1068, 1970.
11. Conolly WB: The spontaneous healing of hand wounds, Aust NZ J Surg 44:393, 1974.
12. Dupuytren G: Permanent retraction of the fingers produced by an affection of the palmar fascia, Lancet 2:222, 1834.
13. Dupuytren G: Lecons orales de clinque chirugicales faites a l'Hotel Dieu de Paris, vol 1, Paris, Bailliere, p 1.
14. Gelberman RH and others: Wound complications in the surgical treatment of Dupuytren's contracture: a comparison of operative incisions, Hand 14:248, 1982.
15. Gonzolez RI: Open fasciotomy and full thickness skin grafts in the correction of digital flexion deformity. In Hueston JT and Tubiana R, editors: Dupuytren's disease, New York, 1974, Grune & Stratton, Inc.
16. Gosset J: Dupuytren's disease and the anatomy of the palmodigital aponeunoses, In Hueston JT and Tubiana R, editors: Dupuytren's disease, ed 2, New York, 1985, Churchill-Livingstone, Inc.
17. Howard LD Jr: Dupuytren's contracture: a guide for management, Clin Orthop 15:118, 1959.
18. Hueston JY and Tubiana R, editors: Dupuytren's disease, New York, 1974, Grune & Stratton, Inc.

19. Kates J, Burkhalter W, and Mann R: Open palm, open digit technique for Dupuytren's contracture. In proceedings of the American Society for Surgery of the Hand, J Hand Surg 4:287, 1979.

20. King EW, Bass DM, and Watson HK: Treatment of Dupuytren's contracture by extensive fasciectomy through multiple Y-V plasty incisions: short-term evaluation of 170 consecutive operations, J Hand Surg 4:234, 1979.

21. Kleinman WB: Dupuytren's contracture: treatment by the open palm technique. In Strickland JW, and Steichen JB, editors: Difficult problems in hand surgery, St. Louis, 1982, The CV Mosby Co.

22. Jacobson K and Holst-Nielson F: A modified McCash operation for Dupuytren's contracture, Scan J Plast Reconstr Surg 11:231, 1977.

23. Lubahn JD, Lister GD, and Wolfe T: Fasciectomy and Dupuytren's disease: a comparison between the open-palm techinque and wound closure, J Hand Surg 9A:53, 1984.

24. Mackin EJ and Byron PM: Postoperative management. In McFarlane RM, McGrouther DA, and Flint MH, editors: Dupuytren's disease (Hand and upper limb series), New York, Churchhill Livingstone, Inc. (in press).

25. McCash CR: The open palm technique in Dupuytren's contracture, Br J Plast Surg 17:271, 1964.

26. McFarlane R: Patterns of the diseased fascia in the fingers in Dupuytren's contracture, Plast Reconstr Surg 54:31, 1974.

27. McFarlane R: The current status of Dupuytren's disease, J Hand Surg 8:803, 1983.

28. McFarlane R: Personal communication, 1987.

29. McIndoe SA and Beare RLB: The surgical management of Dupuytren's contracture, Am J Surg 95:197, 1958.

30. Niederhuber SS, Stribley RF, and Koepke GH: Reduction of skin bacterial load with use of therapeutic whirlpool, Phys Ther 55:482, 1975.

31. Noble J and Harrison H: Open palm technique for Dupuytren's contract, Hand 8:272, 1976.

32. Salvi V: Personal experience with McCash's "open palm" technique for Dupuytren's contracture, Hand 5:161, 1973.

33. Schneider LH, Hankin FM, and Eisenberg T: Surgery of Dupuytren's disease: a review of the open palm method. J Hand Surg 11A:23, 1986.

34. Tonkin MA, Burke FD, and Varian JPW: Dupuytren's contracture: a comparative study of faciectomy and dermofaciectomy in 100 patients, J Hand Surg 9B, 156, 1984.

35. Tubiana R: Overview on surgical treatment of Dupuytren's disease. In Hueston JT and Tubiana R, editors: Dupuytren's disease, ed 2, New York, 1985, Churchill Livingstone, Inc.

36. Wehbe M and Hunter JM: Tendon gliding, Orthop Rev, 14:416, 1985.

37. Zachariae L: Extensive versus limited fasciectomy for Dupuytren's contracture, Scan J Plast Reconstr Surg 1:150, 1967.

38. Zachariae L: Operation for Dupuytren's contracture by the method of McCash, Acta Orthop Scand 41:443, 1970.

XI
ARTHRITIS

69

*Pathogenesis of arthritic lesions**

Alfred B. Swanson

Arthritis is a ubiquitous disease. Almost 100% of the population is susceptible to some form of arthritis, and if an individual lives long enough, he is almost certain to develop one type or another. It is estimated by the United States Public Health Service's National Center for Health Statistics, in a survey conducted in 1966 and 1967, that there are 16.8 million persons in the United States suffering from some form of arthritis. An estimated 3.4 million arthritis victims are completely disabled at any one time. The annual wage loss and medical care costs combined result in a loss to the national economy of approximately $3.5 billion, whereas the total national investment in research and medical education against arthritis in 1968 was only $15 million. Arthritis is considered the second greatest cause of chronic limitation of major activity; heart diseases rank first in limiting activity only by a slight margin. Although arthritis is a crippling disease that seldom kills the patient, no other group of diseases causes so much suffering to so many people for such long periods. Arthritis therefore has great social and economic repercussions.

Disabling work injuries in the United States totaled 2.2 million in 1970, according to the National Safety Council. Arms were involved in 9% of the cases, hands in 7%, and digits in 17%, for a total of 33% of all injuries incurred. Handling objects and falls were the source of more than half of the temporary total disabilities. Motor vehicle accidents accounted for only 4% and machinery accidents for 6% of total temporary disabilities but gave rise to 19% of the permanent partial disabilities. More than half of the injuries to the hand resulted in permanent partial disability. Many of these patients have joint stiffness or destruction, and their rehabilitation is a significant economic, social, and personal problem.

There are many different forms of joint disease, some caused by known etiologic agents and others resulting from unknown etiologic factors. The numerous terms for certain types of arthritis are also confusing. Many classifications of diseases of joints and related structures have been suggested. All have certain disadvantages and remain a controversial problem. For the sake of simplification, clarity, and unification of terminology, the classification tentatively approved by the American Rheumatism Association has been recommended for general use. Until the etiology of all types of arthritis is known, no grouping can be accurate. The present classifications are based on clinical patterns,

pathologic change in the tissues, and etiology when known. The classification accepted by the American Rheumatism Association is shown in the boxed material.

Rheumatoid arthritis is primarily a generalized disease affecting the synovium as its main target, with secondary changes occurring in the articular cartilage. Osteoarthritis is predominantly a disease of the articular cartilage. The main features of the pathogenesis of the lesions occurring in osteoarthritis and rheumatoid arthritis are briefly presented.

RHEUMATOID ARTHRITIS

It is estimated that 3% of the population is afflicted with rheumatoid arthritis, and although it is responsible for only approximately one fourth of the total number of arthritis patients requiring treatment, it is the greatest crippler from the standpoint of severity and prolonged disability.

Rheumatoid arthritis is one of the unsolved enigmas of medicine. It is a systemic disease whose most characteristic lesion is inflammation of the synovial membranes of joints and tendon sheaths. The swelling, redness, heat, and pain occurring in synovial structures in arthritis are based on this inflammatory reaction, which results in damage to joints, supporting soft-tissue structures, and tendons (Fig. 69-1). The inflammatory stage is usually chronic and persistent in two thirds of the cases.

The most widely accepted theory of the pathogenesis of rheumatoid arthritis is that of an immunologic response taking place in the synovial tissues. There are probably two mechanisms involved in the chronicity of the arthritic inflammation. The first is attributable to the initiating, presumably exogenous, antigen; and the second is attributable to development of an autoimmune response to a new antigen from the host tissues. Normally, when a foreign antigen enters the body, it comes in contact with a defender cell, the lymphocyte. The lymphocyte becomes transformed into a larger plasma cell. The plasma cell manufactures antibodies that have surfaces precisely keyed to fit the surfaces of the antigen so that the two can lock together. As antibodies lock in with antigens and immobilize them, a blood substance called complement is attracted and combines with them. The three-part combinations formed in this way are called complexes. The scavenger phagocytic cells then engulf the complexes. The phagocytic cells have small sacs called lysosomes that contain enzymes. The enzymes destroy the complexes, thus disposing of the intruder. In rheumatoid arthritis the phagocytic cells become incapable of handling the antigen-antibody-complement complex. Some of the lysosomes escape from the cells and attack the sy-

*Text and illustrations taken in part from Swanson AB: Flexible implant resection arthroplasty in the hand and extremities, St Louis, 1973, The CV Mosby Co.

885

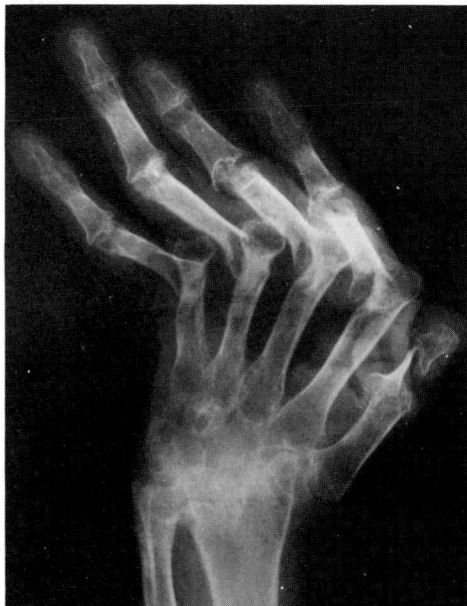

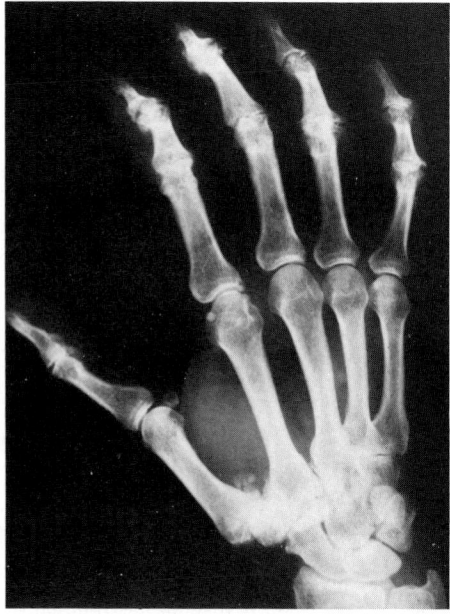

Fig. 69-1 Roentgenogram demonstrating findings in severely involved rheumatoid arthritic hand. There are severe absorptive changes of proximal phalanx of thumb, dislocation of metacarpophalangeal joints, erosive changes in proximal interphalangeal joints, fusions in carpal bones, and subluxation at wrist. Osteoporotic changes are also noted.

Fig. 69-2 Roentgenogram of hand of 50-year-old woman with primary osteoarthritis. There are severe degenerative changes at the first carpometacarpal joint, distal interphalangeal joints, and proximal interphalangeal joints of the fourth and fifth digits. Metacarpophalangeal joints and wrist have been spared. There is no evidence of osteoporosis.

novium and cartilage of the joints. Destruction of cartilage adds to the requirement for more phagocytic activity to clean up the resulting debris. The phagocytes pour out more of their enzymes and further trigger inflammation. Thus, once triggered, arthritic inflammation becomes self-perpetuating.

The inflammatory synovium forms a pannus, a granulomatous mass that grows over the surface of the cartilage, into and around the tendons, and into ligament attachments. If unchecked, this invasion results in loosening of ligaments, destruction of joint surfaces, and disability of tendons to function, all of which are typical of the advanced rheumatoid process. Every derangement or deformity of the musculoskeletal system seen in rheumatoid arthritis is the result either primarily or secondarily of this synovial invasion.

OSTEOARTHRITIS
Incidence

Osteoarthritis is very commonly seen in adults. Roentgenograms of the hands and feet of persons from 18 to 79 years of age show evidence of osteoarthritic changes in 37.4% of the cases. Approximately 8% of all adults are estimated to have moderate to severe clinical symptoms of osteoarthritis of the hands and feet. In a serial survey of 1000 consecutive autopsies, 72% of the patients showed some osteoarthritic changes of the knee joint, with 9% showing severe changes; 38% had changes of the hip, with 5% showing severe changes; and 22% had changes of the shoulder, with 4% showing severe changes. The prevalence of osteoarthritis rises steeply with age. Approximately 4% of the persons between 18 and 24 years of age are estimated to have some degree of arthritis, whereas nearly 85% of all persons 75 to 79 years of age demonstrate roentgenographic

evidence of this condition. In persons less than 45 years old, the prevalence of osteoarthritis is greater in men than in women, suggesting the importance of trauma as an etiologic factor. In the older age groups a larger proportion of women suffer from the disease. The incidence of this condition is not affected by race, geographic location, income, or education. However, the incidence of this disease does appear to be less in certain occupations as compared to others.

Classification

Degenerative arthritis. This more common form is not considered a generalized disease and is usually seen in an increasing percentage of the population as age increases. It most commonly involves the weight-bearing joints and the distal interphalangeal (DIP) joints of the hand.

Primary generalized osteoarthritis. This form of arthritis usually occurs in middle-aged women and is characterized by roentgenographic evidence of osteoarthritic lesions of the interphalangeal joints of the hand, the carpometacarpal (CMC) joint of the thumb, the knee and hip joints, the spine, and the metatarsophalangeal joints of the feet (Fig. 69-2).

Erosive arthritis. This disease is characterized by chronic degenerative changes with intermittent inflammatory episodes. It is usually seen in middle-aged women and involves mainly the hands, feet, and cervical spine (Fig. 69-3). The synovium removed from these inflamed joints resembles that of rheumatoid arthritis. However, the predominance of cartilage destruction, juxtaarticular erosions, and osteophytic formation without the clinical symptoms of rheumatoid arthritis separates it from this group.

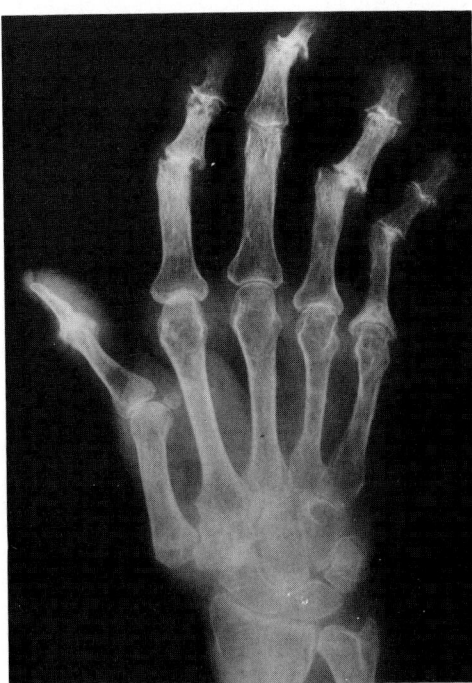

Fig. 69-3 Roentgenogram of 68-year-old woman with erosive osteoarthritis in both hands. Note involvement of first carpometacarpal joint and proximal and distal interphalangeal joints and lack of involvement of wrist joint. There is evidence of erosive changes, moderate osteoporosis, and malalignment of joints.

Pathogenesis

The term "rheumatism," invented about 300 years ago, derived from the Greek word *rheuma* (that which flows as a stream or brook), because an increased flow of mucus was believed to be pathogenetic. Since an increased flow of mucus—that is, an increased synthesis of synovial fluid—and a greater increase in degradation of matrix mucopolysaccharide occur in human osteoarthritis, the term may be an accurate description of the pathogenesis of this disease.

The pathogenesis of osteoarthritis has not been thoroughly established. The precise sequence of histologic changes in this condition cannot be reconstructed. Osteoarthritis may be considered a wear phenomenon in which a breakdown of the normal joint characteristics occurs. Consideration of this problem must be given under several headings. The biology of the cartilage and the changes that occur in its degradation; the lubrication of the joint; the reaction of physical factors; and chemical, genetic, vascular, and bone changes are all interrelated factors in the mechanism of joint destruction.

Biology of cartilage. Articular cartilage is a composite material of cellular and extracellular components. The cellular part is the chondrocyte, and the extracellular portion is a matrix consisting of collagen fibers embedded in a mucopolysaccharide (chondroitin sulfate) ground substance. Cartilage is a living, dynamic, ever-changing tissue responding promptly to alterations in activity, environment, nutrition, and trauma. It takes up and expels water freely from the synovial fluid, thus promptly changing as much as 10% of its volume. It proliferates and grows faster with exercise or work, and it shrinks and atrophies with rest and

disuse. Articular cartilage is composed of three distinct layers:

1. In the surface layer the collagen bundles are predominantly parallel to the surface. There are small ripples on its surface, so that, actually, the microscopic appearance is one of a rough, undulating surface, which is an important factor for the trapped-pool mechanism in lubrication. This layer also shows the presence of old or degenerated cells that are continuously being exfoliated and shed into the joint.

2. In a thicker elastic layer the collagen fibers are angled intermediately to the articular surface. This layer is responsible for much of the elasticity of the normal hyaline cartilage.

3. The basal layer fixes the cartilage to the subchondral bone plate. It is the growth area where cells divide and multiply. Here the fibers are more or less perpendicular to the articular surface and to the subchondral bone.

Cartilage is peculiar in that it is formed mostly by extracellular material surrounding relatively few cells whose main function is to maintain the composition of this extracellular matrix. Articular cartilage is avascular; approximately the outermost two-thirds zone affected by the early events in osteoarthritis receives its nutrition through exchange of substances between the matrix and the synovial fluid. This exchange is increased by the normal use of a joint; compression of cartilage squeezes fluid out like a sponge, and the matrix draws the fluid back in when the compression is released. Increased compression with continued motion causes thickening of the cartilage and cellular proliferation where mitotic failure is observed. In contrast, when all articular motion is experimentally prevented or when there is no surface-to-surface contact of the joint, the cartilage degenerates, apparently because of a lack of nutrition.

The status of the cartilage, whether healthy, active and growing, or sick, inactive, or aged, can be determined by its histologic appearance. When the cartilage is healthy, there are many large nuclei, often showing mitoses in the basal layer. In the elastic layer, the cells show activity by producing mucopolysaccharides, and there is a larger proportion of matrix to nuclei. The earliest pathologic changes in the cartilage have been described differently by various investigators and include focal swelling of the cartilage matrix, loss of chondroitin sulfate from the superficial layers of the cartilage, proliferation of chondrocytes in a disorderly fashion, a diminution of chondrocytes, fatty degeneration in the matrix, and alteration of the collagen fibrils. These changes probably represent a depletion of ground substance and are seen as cartilage surface irregularities in the form of undulations and fissures.

Gross changes in the articular cartilage have been described as localized areas of softening of the cartilage with flaking of the superficial layers and fibrillation, which represents fissures into the deeper layers. Mechanical abrasion of the fibrillated cartilage takes place with progressive loss of cartilage and exposure of the underlying bone. It may be present in areas of shearing stress on weight-bearing surfaces but also may be seen in non–weight-bearing areas of the joint.

The chondrocytes secrete the macromolecular compo-

NOMENCLATURE AND CLASSIFICATION OF ARTHRITIS AND RHEUMATISM
*(tentatively accepted by American Rheumatism Association)**

I. Polyarthritis of unknown etiology
  A. Rheumatoid arthritis
  B. Juvenile rheumatoid arthritis (Still's disease)
  C. Ankylosing spondylitis
  D. Psoriatic arthritis
  E. Reiter's syndrome
  F. Others
II. "Connective tissue" disorders
  A. Systemic lupus erythematosus
  B. Polyarteritis nodosa
  C. Scleroderma (progressive systemic sclerosis)
  D. Polymyositis and dermatomyositis
  E. Others
III. Rheumatic fever
IV. Degenerative joint disease (osteoarthritis, osteoarthrosis)
  A. Primary
  B. Secondary
V. Nonarticular rheumatism
  A. Fibrositis
  B. Intervertebral disc and low back syndromes
  C. Myositis and myalgia
  D. Tendinitis and peritendinitis (bursitis)
  E. Tenosynovitis
  F. Fasciitis
  G. Carpal tunnel syndrome
  H. Others
   (See also shoulder-hand syndrome, VIII E)
VI. Diseases with which arthritis is frequently associated
  A. Sarcoidosis
  B. Relapsing polychondritis
  C. Henoch-Schönlein syndrome
  D. Ulcerative colitis
  E. Regional ileitis
  F. Whipple's disease
  G. Sjögren's syndrome
  H. Familial Mediterranean fever
  I. Others
   (See also psoriatic arthritis, I D)
VII. Associated with known infectious agents
  A. Bacterial
   1. *Brucella*
   2. *Gonococcus*
   3. *Mycobacterium tuberculosis*
   4. Pneumococcus
   5. *Salmonella*
   6. *Staphylococcus*
   7. *Streptobacillus moniliformis* (Haverhill fever)
   8. *Treponema pallidum* (syphilis)
   9. *Treponema pertenue* (yaws)
   10. Others
  B. Rickettsial
  C. Viral
  D. Fungal
  E. Parasitic
   (See also rheumatic fever, III)
VIII. Traumatic and/or neurogenic disorders
  A. Traumatic arthritis (viz., the result of direct trauma)
  B. Lues (tertiary syphilis)
  C. Diabetes
  D. Syringomyelia
  E. Shoulder-hand syndrome
  F. Mechanical derangements of joints
  G. Others
   (See also degenerative joint disease, IV; carpal tunnel syndrome, VG)
IX. Associated with known biochemical or endocrine abnormalities
  A. Gout
  B. Ochronosis
  C. Hemophilia
  D. Hemoglobinopathies (e.g., sickle cell disease)
  E. Agammaglobulinemia
  F. Gaucher's disease
  G. Hyperparathyroidism
  H. Acromegaly
  I. Hypothyroidism
  J. Scurvy (hypovitaminosis C)
  K. Xanthoma tuberosum
  L. Others
   (See also multiple myeloma, XG; Hurler's syndrome, XII C).
X. Tumor and tumorlike conditions
  A. Synovioma
  B. Pigmented villonodular synovitis
  C. Giant cell tumor of tendon sheath
  D. Primary juxta-articular bone tumors
  E. Metastatic
  F. Leukemia
  G. Multiple myeloma
  H. Benign tumors of articular tissue
  I. Others

*From Hollander JL: Arthritis and allied conditions, ed 8, Philadelphia, 1972, Lea & Febiger, p. 4–5.

---

nents. Because the cartilage is avascular, the chondrocytes utilize glucose and other components of the synovial fluid and discharge the waste products of their metabolism into the articular cavity. Cartilage cells must continuously renew the protein-polysaccharide content of the matrix. Irreversible depletion of the matrix and subsequent loss of normal spongelike mechanical properties of the cartilage seriously interfere with the lubrication of the joint.

Lubrication. The diarthrodial joint is a most remarkable mechanical model. There is an extremely low coefficient of friction in this bearing mechanism. Its efficiency in dissi-pating heat, self-lubrication, and ability to continuously repair itself is remarkable. The basic principles of lubrication known to engineers have been studied in human joints, but the general excellent performance of the normal human joint exceeds the expected conditions. It is important, however, to understand basic concepts of lubrication in bearing surfaces to help explain the osteoarthritic joint and also for consideration in prosthetic joint replacement.

The various types of lubrication include the following.
  1. *Fluid-film lubrication* is the development of a film between two opposing surfaces transmitting load.

2. *Hydrodynamic lubrication* occurs when the relative motion of two surfaces draws fluid into the interspace. It is sometimes called the wedge action.

3. *Elastohydrodynamic lubrication* is present when elastic deformation occurs between one or both of the opposing surfaces.

4. *Squeeze-film lubrication* occurs when the opposing surfaces are subjected to a varying load and the lubricating film restores itself before the increased load is again applied.

5. *Boundary lubrication* occurs when the lubrication is governed by the properties of the surface layers of the opposing component.

6. *Hydrostatic lubrication* occurs when the lubricant is supplied under pressure between the surfaces.

7. *Mixed lubrication* is a combination of the various types.

In the human joint the bearing surface is a layer of articular cartilage having an elasticity similar to that of rubber. It is porous, a property that is very important, and the lubricant synovial fluid is contained within a capsule. The surface of the cartilage is undulating, allowing the fluid to be trapped. The fluid-film type of lubrication can also occur because the loading on the joint is intermittent. The elasticity of the cartilage allows elastohydrodynamic lubrication because of the deformation of the substance under contact pressures and the resultant drawing of fluid into the flattened areas. There appears also to be a boundary type of lubrication in which the lipid present in the articular cartilage aids the lubricating mechanism by weeping on the surface of the cartilage. This is a type of self-lubricating mechanism.

The normal synovial fluid gets most of its lubricating properties from hyaluronic acid, which is extremely viscous and elastic. In an abnormal joint the synovial fluid loses much of this quality, which in turn affects the lubricating mechanism.

Physical factors. Local physical factors seem to be important in the pathogenesis of lesions. The chemical and morphologic alterations occur focally in the joint, and it is likely that mechanical phenomena are important. Loading on a joint surface beyond its tolerance can play a significant role in the eventual disorganization of the joint. The energy absorption function of articular cartilage can be overloaded when joints are unstable; when trauma is repeated, as in certain occupations; when the joint alignment is disturbed by fracture, dislocation, or congenital or developmental defects of the skeleton; or when there is aseptic necrosis of the underlying bone. Shear stresses are more destructive than compressive forces.

Chemical changes that may destroy cartilage include repeated bleeding into the joint, inflammation from infection, and deposition of chemicals such as homogentisic acid in the cartilage in cases of ochronosis.

Genetic factors. Genetic factors clearly influence the incidence of osteoarthritis in human beings and may be related in part to congenital structural factors such as posture, joint alignment, or deformity. The levels of various degradative enzymes and the rate of synthesis and breakdown of cartilage cells at rest or in response to stress could be genetically determined.

Vascular factors. The synovial tissue is the least affected portion of the joint in osteoarthritis. However, in the erosive type of osteoarthritis, an inflammatory type of synovitis is frequently seen; it may be a factor in cartilage destruction similar to that seen in rheumatoid arthritis. Fibrosis of the synovial surface and occasional cartilaginous metaplasia may be seen in advanced osteoarthritis. The inadequate synovium cuts down the normal supply of lubricating synovial fluid (synovia). Inflammatory reaction is seen in late osteoarthritis and is probably related to a foreign body reaction to the cartilaginous debris within the joint. In osteoarthritis there is an increased vascular supply at the level of the juxtachondral blood vessels. This is believed to be a secondary reaction to the degeneration of articular cartilage. A subchondral hyperemia of bone occurs, and vessels may enter the cartilage peripherally or through the subchondral plate. This hypervascularity further weakens the structure of the bone beyond the point where it can withstand compression and shearing forces.

Bone changes. Proliferation of bone in the subchondral zone is most noticeable in areas that have been denuded of cartilage. As the force-dampening effect of the cartilage is lost, bone is subjected to increased strain and responds, in part, by hypertrophy. Cystic lesions, however, may also develop immediately beneath the joint surface, and excessive blood vessel formation occurs around them. These cysts may fill with fluid, and their increased tension may cause peripheral rarefaction of bone and gradual enlargement of the cystic space. There also is remodeling of the bone at the level of the joint surface, which is probably related to bone formation from the calcified layer of the basal portion of the articular cartilage. Severe irregularity of the joint surface may be evidenced in the later stages of this process.

The development of marginal osteophytes is typical of the osteoarthritic process. Some of them protrude into the joint space in the intercondylar areas, and others are present at the periphery of the joint and also at the site of capsular and ligamentous attachments. The formation of osteophytes seems to be governed by the lines of the mechanical forces. Osteophytes consist largely of bone and are continuous with the normal bone. They are frequently capped by layers of

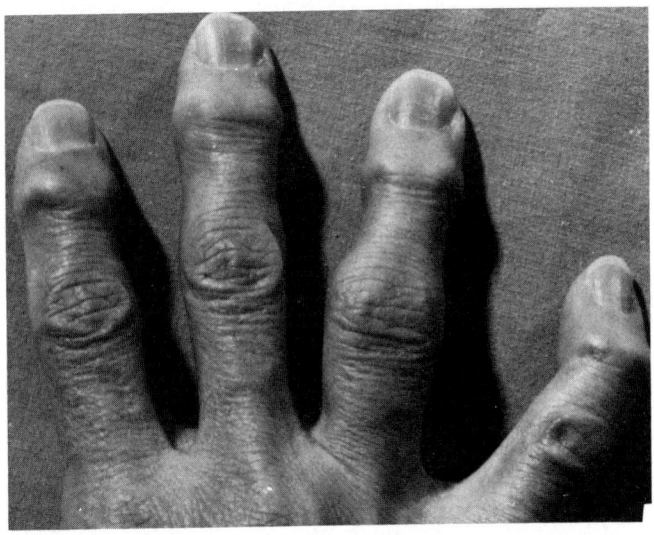

Fig. 69-4   Heberden's nodes are a typical finding in osteoarthritis.

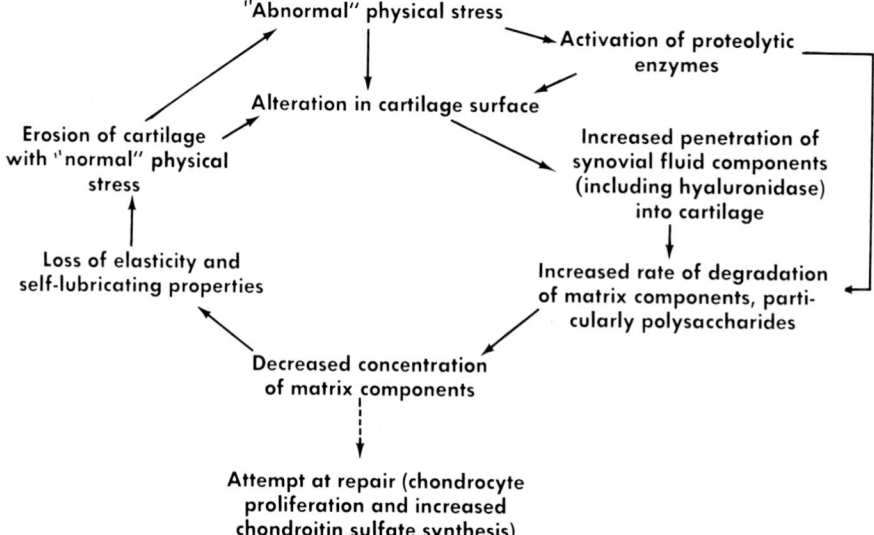

Fig. 69-5 Proposed mechanisms involved in pathogenesis of osteoarthritic cartilage degeneration. (From Bollet AJ: Arthritis Rheum 12:152, 1963.)

hyaline cartilage or fibrocartilage, and some investigators have believed that they are caused by a metaplasia of cartilage debris within the joint.

The nature of the physical stresses on DIP joints deserves comment since these joints are among the most common sites of osteoarthritic changes, and yet they are not weight bearing. The distal phalanx slides along the middle phalanx on the forces applied in pinch and grasp activities, resulting in great shearing stress. Osteoarthritic outgrowths into tendon insertions occur at many sites. The extensor tendon inserts at the extreme proximal end of the bone in the distal phalanx. Extension is produced at a considerable mechanical disadvantage. These stresses associated with the degenerative process of osteoarthritis probably contribute to the severe remodeling of the bone with the presence of so-called Heberden's nodes, which is such a typical finding in this condition (Fig. 69-4).

Mechanism of osteoarthritis. In the destruction of the involved joints, there undoubtedly is an interdependence between the wear-and-tear process and the disturbed biologic state of the articular tissues. Mechanical factors of change in the lubrication power of joint fluid, in conjunction with a loss of the smoothness of the cartilaginous surface, gradual decrease of the dampening property of the cartilage, and chemical degradation of the cartilage and fluid joint, result eventually in collapse of the joint surface, with resultant restriction of motion and angulation of the joint. A vicious cycle of deformity is established.

There may be chondrolytic enzymes from the synovial fluid and also from chondrocytes, which break down articular cartilage. Local physical stress may rupture lysosomes in cartilage cells, thus activating proteolytic enzymes. The movement of lysosomes to the cell surface and discharge of their contents externally could induce digestion of extracellular protein polysaccharide. This relationship between the chemical and morphologic alterations found in joints is noted in Fig. 69-5.

The vicious cycle of destruction and repair efforts in a joint has been stated by Trueta as a process that appears to be an attempt to transform a decaying joint into a youthful one, and for this, as in the miraculous rejuvenation depicted in Goethe's *Faust*, a high price must ultimately be paid.

Gouty arthritis. The joint lesions of gout are related to the deposition of monosodium urate salts. Aside from the destruction of the articular mechanism by tophaceous deposits, the commonest lesion is of the osteoarthritic type. Urate crystals are deposited not only on and in the surface of the articular cartilage but also in the subchondral cysts, where they constitute the so-called punched-out lesions. These deposits of urate crystals in the articular structures of the hand usually become absorbed after medical treatment. Implant resection arthroplasty has rarely been indicated for gouty arthritis in our experience.

70

*Pathomechanics of deformities in hand and wrist**

Alfred B. Swanson

The pathomechanics of deformity in the hand secondary to arthritis relate to the disorganization of the joint and the external forces that are applied to it. Deformities secondary to rheumatoid arthritis are usually more severe than those seen in osteoarthritis. The deformities associated with osteoarthritis are mainly limitation of motion and occasionally angulation. The pathomechanics of deformities associated with rheumatoid arthritis have special significance in treatment.

In the normal hand there is a fine balance between the muscle and tendon system and the architecture of the bones and joints through which they act. If the restraining ligamentous structures of the joints are lengthened by the rheumatoid process, this vulnerable balance is compromised. The normal arch system of the hand is disturbed and the stability and equilibrium necessary for prehension are lost. In the presence of deranged mechanical equilibrium, the use of the hand in daily functional adaptations further compounds the progress of deformity.

An understanding of normal architecture and normal function of the hand is important for the study of pathomechanics and the evaluation of compensatory functional adaptations that become necessary when disability intervenes. A brief outline of the basic architectural considerations is presented for this purpose.

ARCHITECTURAL CONSIDERATIONS

The form of the hand has a certain unique elegance. The skeleton provides the lever arms, the mobile joints, and the stabilizing points around which functional adaptations of the hand take place. A great number of units are compacted

*Text and illustrations taken in part from Swanson AB: Flexible implant resection arthroplasty in the hand and extremities, St Louis, 1973, The CV Mosby Co.

into a small area through which greater power and precision can be applied. The arches of this complex enable the digits to bring objects into the hand and control them. The bony architecture of the hand is arranged in three arches, one longitudinal and two transverse. The proximal transverse arch passes through the carpal area, with its center at the capitate bone. The distal transverse arch is developed across the metacarpal heads, its center being the head of the third metacarpal. The fourth and fifth digital rays offer mobility of the ulnar aspect of the hand around this fixed point. The thumb ray provides mobility around the radial aspect. The digits make up the longitudinal arches, with their apex at the metacarpophalangeal (MP) joints. A break in the longitudinal arch system of the digit may result in a collapse deformity of the multiarticulated structure (Fig. 70-1). Stiffness or deformity of the joints will disturb the normal flexion sequence of the digits and create a loss of integrity of this arch system, with resultant disturbance of functional adaptation patterns.

The ligament system of the finger joints is arranged so that stability is provided as flexion occurs. When the joints are in extension, the collateral ligaments are relatively lax. If the digit is immobilized in extension, these ligaments may contract and flexion will be limited. Therefore, when the injured or diseased part is treated, it is important to place the hand in the functional position with the digital joints in a semiflexed position.

The fingers rotate slightly around the third "metacarpal keystone" to converge toward the scaphoid (Fig. 70-2). Only the middle finger lies in a longitudinal axis of its own. Care must therefore be given to align the reconstructed digits according to this convergence; otherwise the fingers may overlap each other in grasping. The ideal result of treatment of any reconstructive problem in the hand would be to obtain

Fig. 70-1 Bony architecture of the hand is arranged in one longitudinal and two transverse arches. In rheumatoid arthritis palmar subluxation of the metacarpophalangeal joint causes collapse of the longitudinal arch. (Redrawn from Tubiana T: Anatomical and physiopathological features. In Tubiana R, editor: The rheumatoid hand, Group d'Etude de la Main monograph no. 3, Paris, 1969, L'Expansion Scientifique Française.)

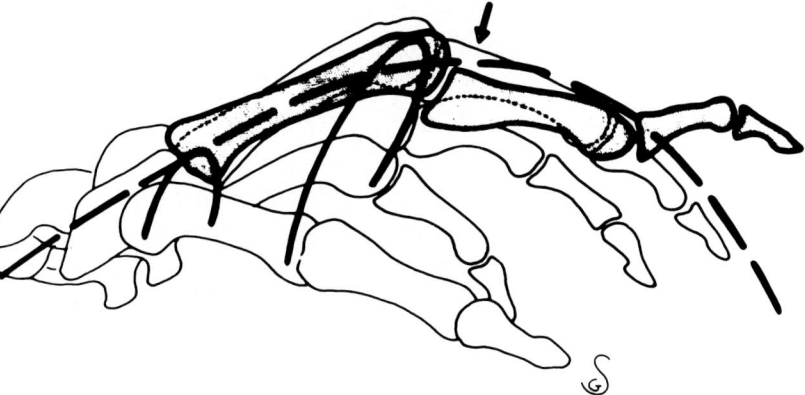

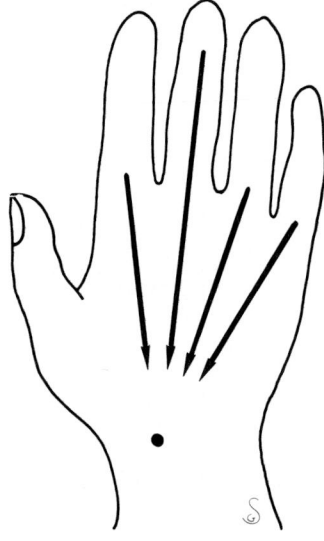

Fig. 70-2   Only the middle finger lies in a longitudinal axis of its own. Other fingers rotate slightly around the third "metacarpal keystone" to converge toward the scaphoid.

mobility, stability, and proper alignment of the lever arm system. This should be the goal of every treatment method.

PATHOMECHANICS OF DEFORMITIES OF HAND AND WRIST IN RHEUMATOID ARTHRITIS

In rheumatoid arthritis the inflammatory synovium forms a pannus. This destructive and invasive granulomatous mass grows over the surface of the cartilage into the ligamentous attachments and into and around the tendons. The result is capsular distension, destruction of cartilage, subchondral erosions, loosening of the ligamentous insertions, impairment of the function of tendons, and, finally, joint disorganization, all of these being typical lesions of the advanced rheumatoid process. Every lesion or deformity of the musculoskeletal system seen in rheumatoid arthritis is the result primarily or secondarily of this synovial invasion, which eventually destroys the normal anatomic relationships. Spe-

cific deformities are related to the location and the intensity of this destructive process.

Distal interphalangeal joint

Synovial invasion of the distal interphalangeal (DIP) joint resulting in specific deformities is uncommon in rheumatoid arthritis. Loosening of the distal attachment of the extensor tendon may cause a typical mallet, or drop, finger (Fig. 70-3). Loosening of the collateral ligament system, erosive changes in the subchondral bone, and cartilage destruction are aggravated by the daily external forces and may result in instability of the distal joint. The severe absorptive changes occurring in arthritis mutilans may totally destroy the joint in rheumatoid arthritis. Most deformities seen at the DIP joint are secondary to the boutonnière or swan-neck collapse deformities.

Proximal interphalangeal joint

The proximal interphalangeal (PIP) collateral ligament system consists of two parts: an oblique and a vertical component. The oblique component connects the middle and proximal phalanges by a ligament from the head of the proximal phalanx to the side of the middle phalanx. The vertical component, frequently called the accessory collateral ligament, is mainly a system for suspension of the palmar plate and the flexor tendon sheath. The flexor tendons are securely contained within this fibrous tunnel. The extensor apparatus consists of the central tendon, which inserts into the dorsal capsule, and the base of the middle phalanx. It is flanked by lateral tendons of the intrinsic muscles. A synovial pouch from the joint extends proximally beneath the extensor tendons. Another synovial pouch extends proximally between the palmar plate and the underlying bone.

Limited movement of the PIP joint may result from (1) articular causes such as disorganization of the joint and fibrinous adhesions, (2) periarticular causes such as adhesions affecting the attachments of the collateral ligaments, and (3) tendinous causes, arising from involvement of the flexor tendons by hyperplastic synovial tissue, which limits the gliding of the tendon and later forms adhesions.

Collapse deformity, or the buckling phenomenon of the

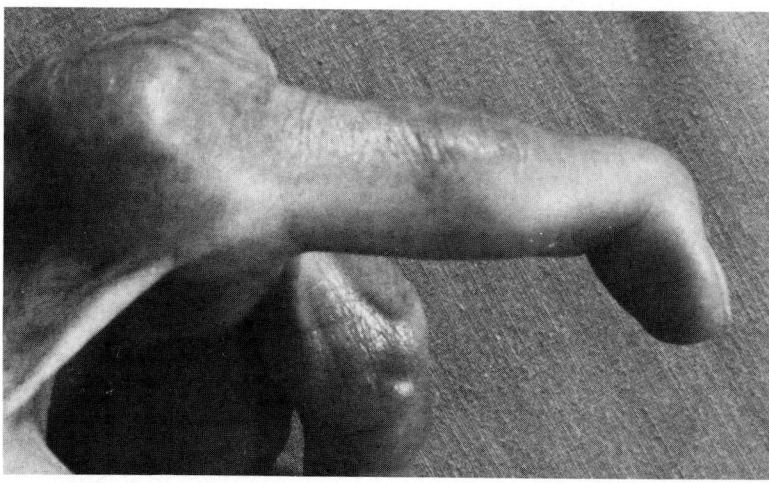

Fig. 70-3   Loosening of the distal attachment of the extensor tendon by synovial invasion of the joint may result in mallet finger deformity. Isolated mallet finger is an uncommon deformity in rheumatoid arthritis.

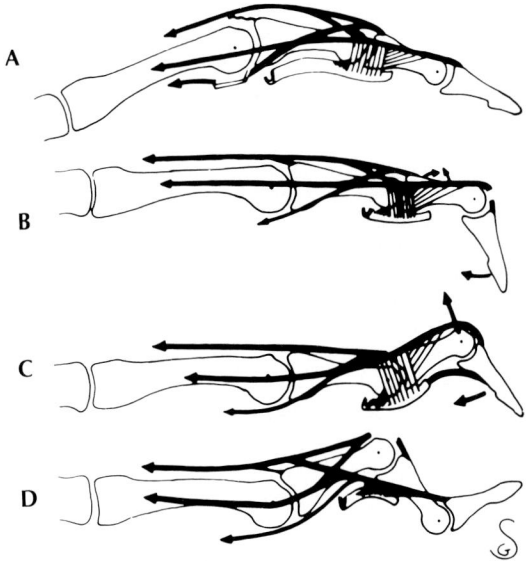

Fig. 70-4 Collapse deformities of the three-joint system are often seen in rheumatoid arthritis and are characterized by hyperextension of one of the joints, with reciprocal flexion of contiguous joints. Balanced tendon mechanisms and ligament restrictions that normally prevent hyperextension are lost. This shows the altered relationship of extensor tendons and bone and joint systems after damage to the extensor apparatus. **A,** Normal finger. **B,** Mallet finger. **C,** Swan-neck deformity. **D,** Boutonnière deformity. (Redrawn from Tubiana R: The mechanisms of deformities of the fingers due to musculotendinous imbalance. In Tubiana R, editor: The rheumatoid hand, Group d'Etude de la Main monograph no. 3, Paris, 1969, L'Expansion Scientifique Française.)

three-joint system of the digit, is seen frequently in rheumatoid arthritis (Fig. 70-4). This disturbance is characterized by hyperextension of one of the joints and reciprocal flexion of the contiguous joints. This zigzag break in the normal flexion-extension pattern of the bony chain is ordinarily prevented by balanced tendon mechanisms and ligament restrictions on hyperextension. The claw, swan-neck, and boutonnière deformities are examples of this dysfunction; the latter two are seen frequently in rheumatoid arthritis. A vicious circle of deforming forces is established. Axially applied forces further aggravate the established deformity.

Boutonnière deformity. The boutonnière, or buttonhole, deformity usually occurs in rheumatoid arthritis through bulging of hyperplastic synovium between the extensor central and lateral tendons. The capsular and bony attachments of the central tendon are weakened, and a relative lengthening of the tendon occurs. The tendon is thus unable to effect normal extension of the middle phalanx. The transverse fibers that connect the lateral tendons to the central tendon are further lengthened by this synovial invasion, allowing the lateral tendons of the extensor apparatus to dislocate in a palmar direction. The lateral tendons are now located below the central axis of the PIP joint and become flexors of the PIP joint. Because the lateral tendons are relatively shortened by their displacement, there is an increased pull on their distal insertion to the distal phalanx, resulting in hyperextension deformity of this joint. Once this collapse deformity is established, it becomes self-perpetuating (Fig. 70-5). The joints may become stiff because of contracture of associated soft-tissue structures, and

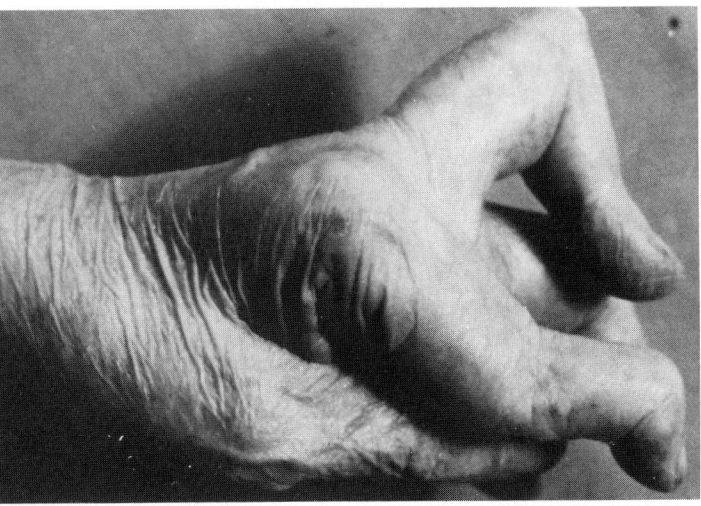

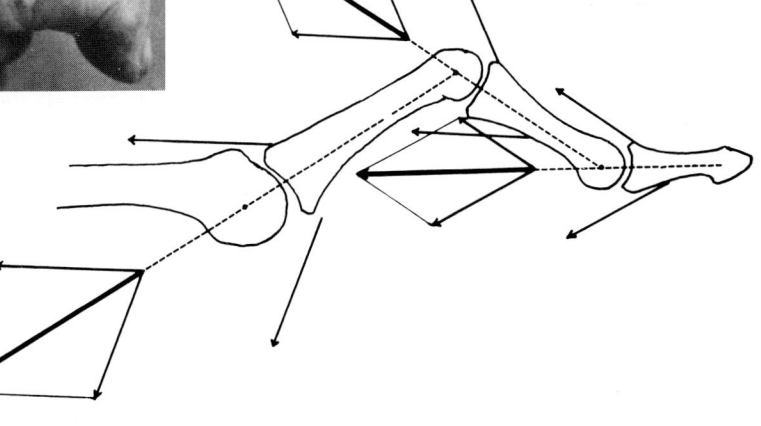

Fig. 70-5 Boutonnière deformity of digits. **A,** In rheumatoid arthritis this deformity usually occurs through weakening of the capsular and bony attachments and relative lengthening of the central tendon by destructive synovial invasion. Lateral tendons are subluxated palmad. **B,** Once collapse deformity is established, resultant axial forces further aggravate the deformity.

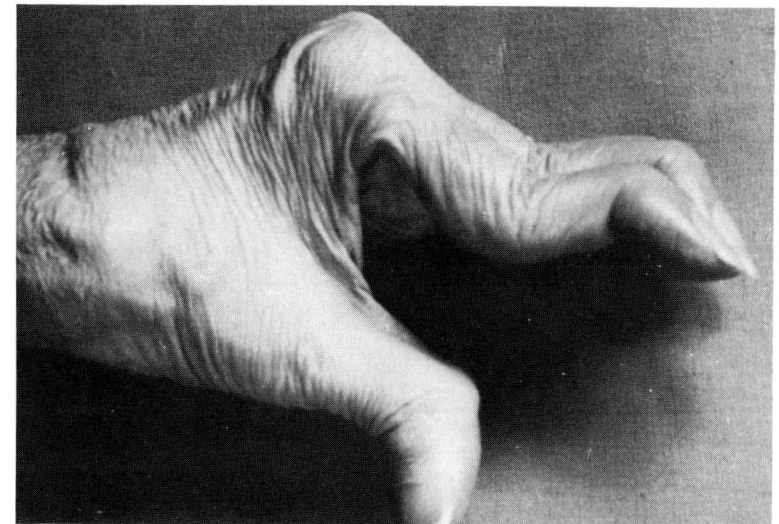

A

Fig. 70-6 Swan-neck deformity. **A,** This deformity is usually caused, in rheumatoid arthritis, by synovitis of the flexor tendon sheaths, which results in restriction of interphalangeal joint flexion. Flexor power becomes concentrated in the metacarpophalangeal joint, and in this position intrinsic muscle pull on the central tendon is facilitated, resulting in unbalancing of forces to the extensor aspect of the joint. Hyperextension of the middle phalanx on the proximal phalanx occurs. **B,** Axially directed forces further aggravate the collapse deformity. Lateral tendons become subluxated dorsally above the axis of rotation of the joint.

B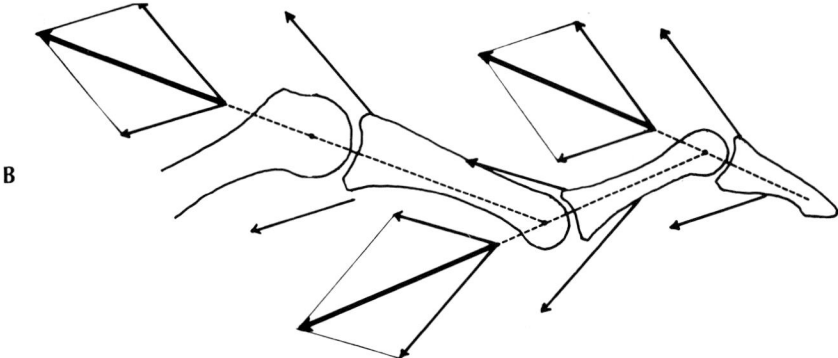

the PIP joint may become further disorganized and subluxated if the disease process continues.

The events taking place in the development of the boutonnière deformity in rheumatoid arthritis can be summarized as follows:

1. Capsular distension of the PIP joint
2. Lengthening of the central tendon
3. Lengthening of the transverse fibers
4. Lateral tendon palmar subluxation
5. Increased extensor tendon pull on the distal phalanx
6. Collapse of the three-level system
7. Joint disorganization

Swan-neck deformity. The swan-neck deformity is characterized by hyperextension of the PIP joint and flexion of the distal joint (Fig. 70-6). It probably is caused primarily by a synovitis of the flexor tendon sheath, with restriction of interphalangeal joint flexion. The main function of the long flexor tendon is to flex the interphalangeal joint, especially during the first part of finger flexion. Patients who have flexor tendon synovitis have difficulty initiating or completing interphalangeal joint flexion, either because of pain or because of mechanical restriction of the flexor tendons. The flexor tendons then concentrate most of their power on the MP tendon joints. This posture of the digit facilitates the pull of the intrinsic muscles to the central tendon across the dorsal aspect of the proximal interphalangeal joint. The failure of PIP flexion therefore gives a greater opportunity for the intrinsic muscles to provide imbalancing forces to the extensor aspect of the joint. The

presence of hyperplastic synovium in the PIP joint and its volar pouch further prevents flexion and causes loosening of the attachments of the palmar plate and the accessory collateral ligaments, thus allowing hyperextension of the joint. Treatment programs for this severely disabling deformity must first be directed at the flexor tendon synovitis. Correction of the hyperextension deformity of the PIP joint through readjustment of the balance of the joint system becomes the main problem.

There is a tendency for perpetuation of the collapse deformity by axially directed forces, resulting in further imbalance of the linked motor system for the chain of joints. As hyperextension deformity is increased, the transverse fibers of the retinacular ligament are stretched out, allowing the lateral tendons to subluxate dorsally, which further magnifies the deforming power through its extensor pull, now located above the center of the axis of rotation of the joint. The oblique retinacular ligaments are stretched, a relative lengthening of the lateral tendons occurs, and the DIP joint becomes flexed by the pull of the flexor profundus tendon. Other deforming forces can increase the mechanical advantage of the extensor pull. Palmar subluxation of the MP joint or the wrist joint, or contracture of the wing-inserted intrinsic muscles secondary to a chronic flexion deformity of the MP joint, will further accentuate the swan-neck deformity. The failure of the long flexor tendons to flex the PIP joint results in permanent joint stiffness. Further destructive changes result in complete joint disorganization and subluxation.

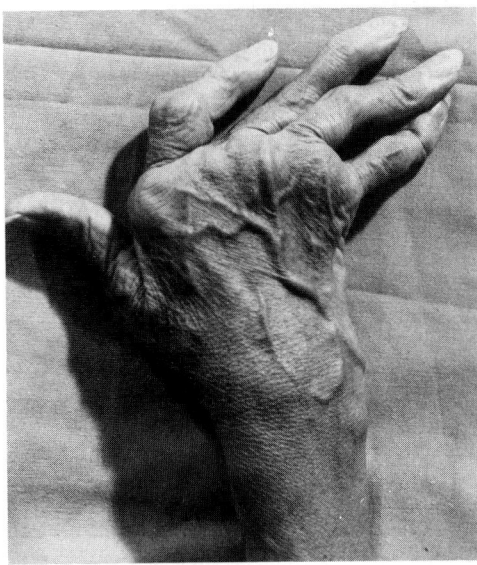

Fig. 70-7 Most common deformities occuring in rheumatoid arthritis are ulnar drift and palmar subluxation at metacarpophalangeal joints. Note swan-neck and boutonnière deformities present in digits.

The events taking place in the development of the swan-neck deformity in rheumatoid arthritis can be summarized as follows:

1. Synovitis of flexor tendon sheath
2. Increased flexion pull on the MP joint
3. Imbalance to the extensor central slip through the long extensor tendons and the intrinsic muscles
4. Stretch of palmar plate of PIP joint
5. Hyperextension of PIP joint
6. Stretching of transverse fibers of retinacular ligament
7. Dorsal subluxation of lateral tendons
8. Reciprocal flexion of DIP joint
9. Joint disorganization

Metacarpophalangeal joint

Deformities of the MP joint in rheumatoid arthritis are usually manifested by increased ulnar drift and palmar subluxation (Fig. 70-7). The MP joint is potentially unstable if normal muscle balance is lost or if the restraining structures of the ligament system are destroyed by rheumatoid disease. The MP joint differs from the interphalangeal joints in that its movements are not simply flexion and extension movements but also involve some degree of rotation, abduction, and adduction. The MP joint, because of its complex movements, which are almost constant during functional adaptations of the hand, is subjected to greater

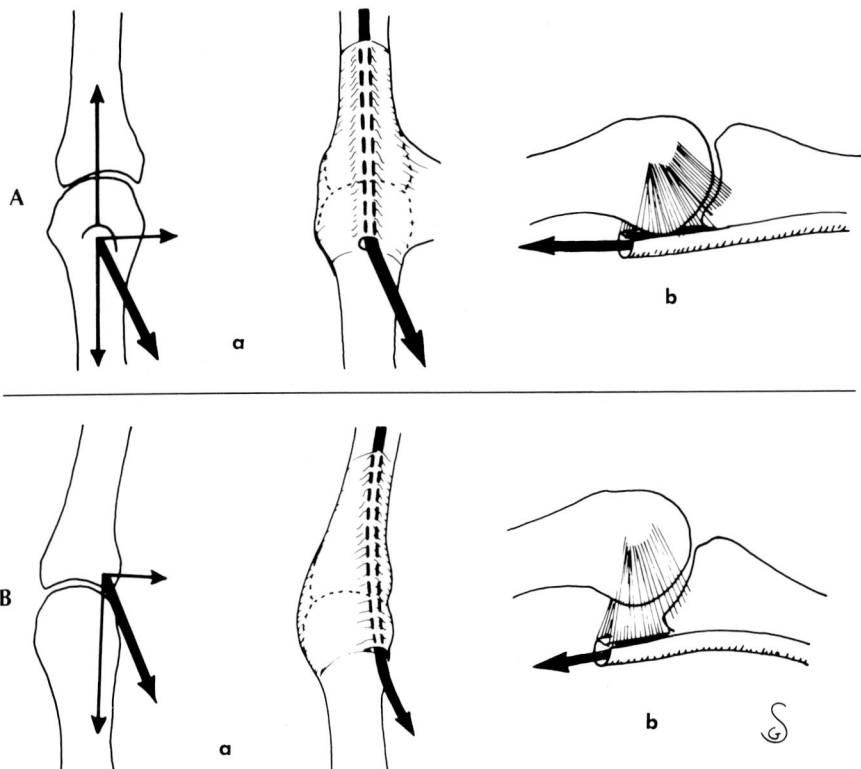

Fig. 70-8 **A,** Common flexor tendons enter fibrous sheath at an angle, and forces produced by their action have ulnar and palmar component. In normal stable metacarpophalangeal joint, ulnar component has little or no displacement effect, *a,* and resistance of capsule and ligaments prevents displacement of sheath inlet, *b.* **B,** When capsule and ligaments of metacarpophalangeal joint are distended and weakened by rheumatoid process, resistance to these deforming forces is lost. Point of reflection of sheath is displaced distally, ulnad and palmad. Base of proximal phalanx is displaced ulnad, *a,* and palmad, *b,* by action of ulnar component of this force. This mechanism is especially deforming at level of index and middle fingers.

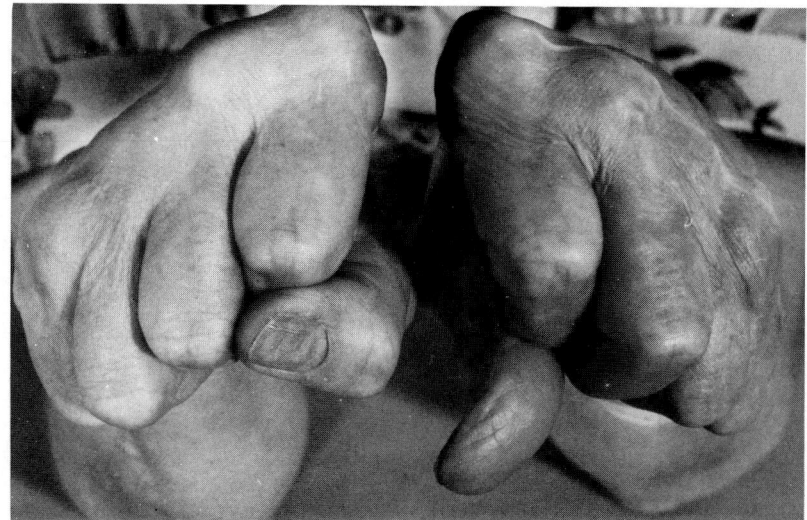

Fig. 70-9   There is increased mobility of fourth and fifth digits in rheumatoid arthritis because of the ligamentous loosening at carpometacarpal joints and dysfunction of extensor carpi ulnaris in the ulnar head syndrome. Resulting increased breadth of the transverse arch can be the cause of ulnar displacement of extensor tendons through the pull on their juncturae tendinum.

stresses. The extensor tendon expansions across the dorsum of the joint are loosely fixed and are vulnerable to disruption. The flexor tendon mechanism and its supporting structures are more complex. The capsule and ligaments of the MP joint are distended and weakened by the rheumatoid process. Forces generated by the long flexor tendons across the fibrous sheath during pinch and grasp activities may act adversely to produce elongation of the supporting accessory collateral ligaments. The palmad and ulnad displaced flexor tendons produce further deforming forces (Fig. 70-8). The intrinsic muscles, which form a bridge between the extensor and flexor systems and, at the same time, provide direct flexor power across the MP joint, can become deforming elements once the restraining structures of the MP joint have been lengthened by the rheumatoid disease. Increased mobility of the fourth and fifth metacarpals is seen frequently in rheumatoid arthritis (Fig. 70-9). It is attributable to ligament loosening at the carpometacarpal (CMC) joints and to the dysfunction of the extensor carpi ulnaris, as seen in the ulnar head syndrome. The increased breadth of the hand in MP joint flexion causes ulnad displacing forces to be applied to the extensor tendons through their juncturae tendinum. When the extrinsic extensor tendon across the MP joint has become displaced ulnad, the balance of the intrinsic extensor tendons is lost. The intrinsic muscles will then further aggravate the tendency toward volar subluxation of the MP joint and toward ulnar drift of the digits. The normal mechanical advantage of the ulnar intrinsic muscles is greatly increased once the deformity is established. Normally the metacarpal heads are symmetric and present an ulnad slope, especially in the index and middle fingers. The collateral ligaments also show an asymmetry that allows ulnar drift to occur. Wrist deformities and ruptured extensor tendons play a secondary role in further aggravating the MP joint disturbances. Once ulnar deviation and palmar subluxation have occurred, muscle pull and forces developed in functional activities and by gravity further accentuate the deformity.

The many anatomic and pathologic entities that play a role in creating deformities in the MP joints are summarized as follows:

1. Normal anatomic asymmetry of second and third metacarpal heads
2. Unequal lengths of ulnar and radial collateral ligaments
3. Wing attachment of ulnar interosseous muscles of the index and middle fingers
4. Forces applied in an ulnar direction on the digits in pinch and grasp activities
5. Postural forces of gravity
6. Hypothenar muscle imbalance to ulnar side of the little finger
7. Attrition of collateral ligaments and bone erosion by the synovitis of the rheumatoid process
8. Stretching of accessory collateral ligaments
9. Synovitis of flexor tendon sheath
10. Subluxation of flexor tendons ulnad
11. Subluxation of extensor tendons ulnad
12. Subluxation of intrinsic tendons volarly
13. Radial deviation and pronation of the wrist
14. Contracture and fixation of intrinsic and extrinsic muscles
15. Associated joint deformities

Thumb ray

The following disabilities are usually seen in the rheumatoid thumb:

1. Postural deformities
   a. Longitudinal collapse deformities
      (1) Boutonnière (primary MP joint disturbance)
      (2) Swan-neck (primary CMC joint disturbance)
      (3) Other
   b. Fixed positional deformities
      (1) Adducted retropositioned thumb
      (2) Other
2. Unstable, stiff, or painful joints

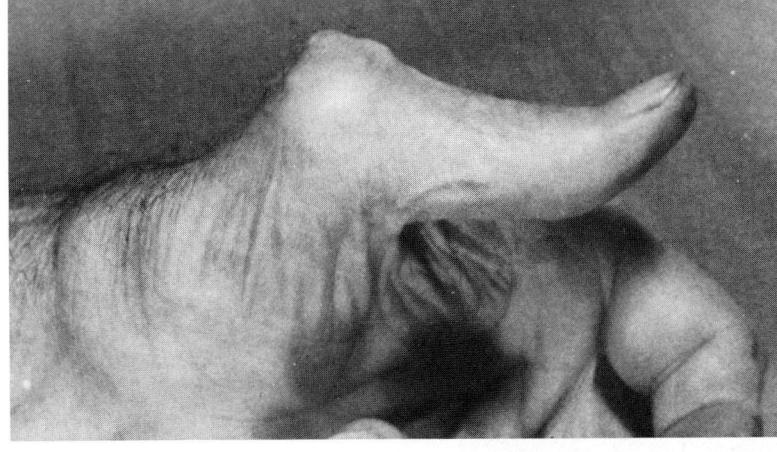

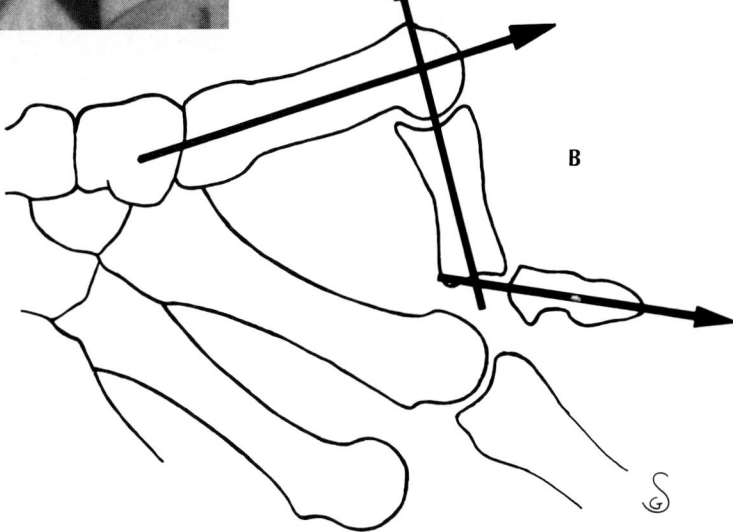

Fig. 70-10 Boutonnière deformity of thumb. **A,** This deformity is a common occurrence in rheumatoid arthritis and starts as synovitis of the metacarpophalangeal joint. **B,** Pinch movements of functional adaptations accentuate the deformity, and a vicious circle of deformity is established.

    a. Interphalangeal joint
    b. MP joint
    c. CMC joint
  3. Tendon disabilities (contracture, displacement, rupture)
    a. Flexor pollicis longus
    b. Extensor pollicis longus
    c. Extensor pollicis brevis
    d. Abductor pollicis longus
    e. Intrinsics

Boutonnière deformity. The most common collapse deformity of the thumb is the boutonnière deformity. Initially, the joint capsule and extensor apparatus around the MP joint are stretched out by a synovitis process. The extensor pollicis longus tendon and adductor expansion are displaced ulnad. The lateral thenar expansions are displaced radially in relation to the MP joint. The attachment of the extensor pollicis brevis tendon to the base of the proximal phalanx is lengthened and becomes ineffective. The ability to extend the MP joint is decreased and results in a flexion deformity of the proximal phalanx. The long extensor tendon and the extensor insertions of the intrinsic muscles apply all their power to the distal joint and produce hyperextension deformity of the distal joint. Pinch movements further accentuate the deformity, and a vicious circle is established: the more the flexion of the MP joint, the greater the tendency for the interphalangeal joint to hyperextend and the thumb

ray to collapse (Fig. 70-10). There is a failure of extension of the MP joint attributable to loss of power of the extrinsic extensor tendon. In time, as contractures occur, the deformity becomes fixed. Destructive articular changes compound the deformity, and disorganization and subluxation of the joint may occur.

Swan-neck deformity. The swan-neck deformity of the thumb is usually initiated by synovitis of the CMC joint, followed by stretching of the joint capsule and radialward subluxation of the base of the metacarpal. Abduction becomes painful and a degree of adductor muscle spasm occurs. This imbalance of forces results in an adduction deformity of the metacarpal with contracture of the adductor pollicis muscle.

As adduction of the thumb becomes more difficult, the distal joints are used to compensate for the lack of movement at the base of the thumb. This may result in hyperextension of the interphalangeal joint, but more frequently of the MP joint and adduction of the first metacarpal. A vicious circle of deformity ensues. Further hyperextension of the MP joint aggravates the adduction tendency of the first metacarpal. This promotes increasing lateral subluxation of the CMC joint and contracture of the adductor muscle. The interphalangeal joint becomes flexed similarly as in a swan-neck deformity of the finger. The deformity is self-perpetuating, and as it increases in one segment, it is aggravated in associated areas (Fig. 70-11). Occasionally severe erosive

A

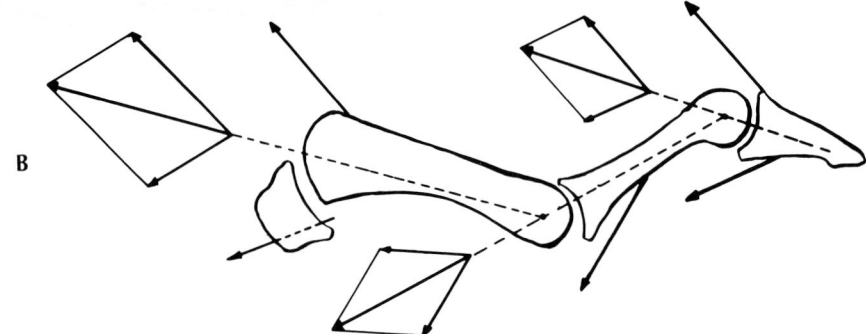

B

Fig. 70-11 Swan-neck deformity of thumb. **A,** This deformity is usually initiated by synovitis of the carpometacarpal joint. It may be accompanied by adduction contracture of first metacarpal joint and subluxation of carpometacarpal joint. **B,** Forces developed in this deformity are self-aggravating. As the deformity increases in one segment, it aggravates deformities in other segments.

changes in the CMC joint and absorption of the trapezium occur. This decompresses the joint, and the severity of the collapse deformity is decreased.

Adducted retropositioned thumb. The adducted retropositioned thumb deformity is seen in less than 5% of the rheumatoid patients and presents difficult treatment problems. Typically the thumb metacarpal is retropositioned, adducted, and externally rotated. It appears that the deformity is initiated by a synovitis at the CMC joint. Awkward positioning of the thumb on a flat board during acute illness can result in a permanent deformity. The ability of the extensor pollicis longus muscle to adduct and externally rotate the metacarpal is predominant. Palmar and radial subluxation of the metacarpal off the trapezium occurs. Consequently, the patient has difficulty abducting the metacarpal and may develop an abduction deformity at the MP joint by stretching the ulnar collateral ligament in grasp activities.

Unstable, stiff, or painful joint. Instability, stiffness, or pain at the interphalangeal, MP, or CMC joint may occur as isolated deformities in rheumatoid arthritis, resulting from synovial invasion and erosive changes of the bone or may be seen in association with other deformities (Fig. 70-12). These deformities are accentuated by the forces applied during pinch activities. Gross destruction of the distal joint may occur also in the late stages of the boutonnière deformity.

Tendon disabilities. Tendon disabilities in the rheumatoid thumb may be related to muscle contracture, tendon displacement, adhesions, or ruptures, similar to that seen in the other digits in the rheumatoid hand.

The extensor pollicis longus tendon is the most commonly ruptured tendon in the rheumatoid thumb; this occurs most often within the third extensor compartment in the area of Lister's tubercle. The rupture of this tendon results in a sudden drop of the thumb MP joint and some loss of extensor power at the distal phalanx. The deformity may be confused with the boutonnière deformity, which is also an extrinsic-minus problem; the hyperextension of the distal joint is, however, not so prominent. The lack of extension of the MP joint is usually associated with less flexion contracture, and, most importantly, the long extensor tendon cannot be prominently palpated on the back of the hand in forced extension and retroposition of the thumb.

Rupture of the flexor pollicis longus is not rare and must be considered in any hyperextended interphalangeal deformity of the thumb. This frequently occurs at the entrance of the digital flexor canal. Careful examination of active flexion will differentiate the hyperextended interphalangeal joint of the thumb from that of the ruptured flexor pollicis longus.

Ruptures of the abductor pollicis longus and extensor pollicis brevis are rare. Disability of the intrinsics usually results from their displacement and secondary contracture caused by synovial invasion and stretching of the dorsal hood of the MP joint of the thumb. The intrinsic attachment to the dorsal hood is consequently displaced palmad, and this results in distortion of its normal function.

The wrist

The wrist is the key joint for proper function of the hand. The wrist joints and surrounding soft tissues are frequently affected by rheumatoid arthritis. Roentgenographic evidence

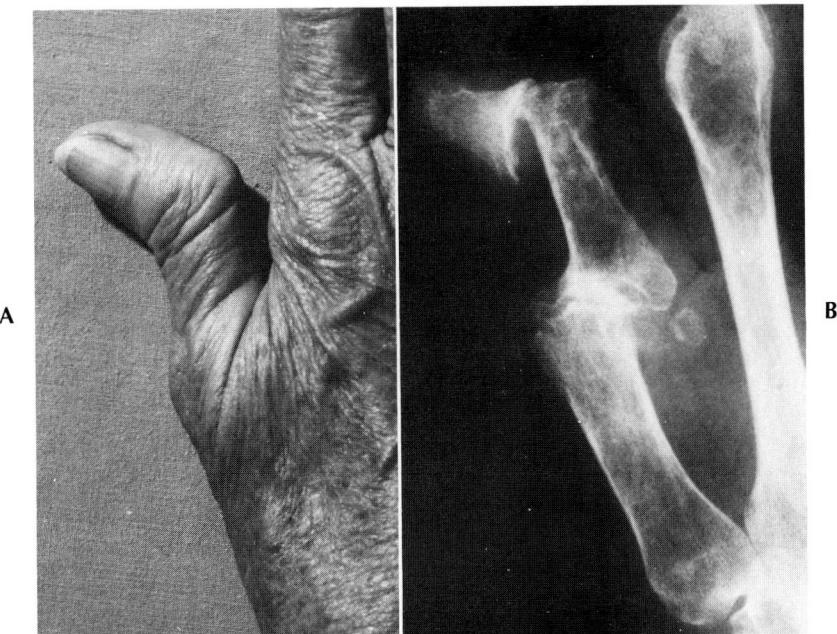

Fig. 70-12 Instability of distal joint of thumb. **A,** Lesions of the distal joint of the thumb may occur as isolated deformities because of synovial invasion and erosive changes and are accentuated by forces applied during pinch movements. **B,** Roentgenogram showing destruction and subluxation of the distal interphalangeal and metacarpophalangeal joints of the thumb.

of arthritic changes was noted in 65% of the rheumatoid wrists studied. Clinically, pain or loss of movement from associated synovitis was present in an even greater percentage of cases. Involvement may be seen early in the course of the disease in the radiocarpal, intercarpal, or radioulnar joints, or in a combination of these joints.

Typical deformities seen in rheumatoid wrists are flexion, pronation, radial or ulnar deviation, palmar subluxation, and associated dorsal subluxation of the ulnar head. Active flexion and rotation movements of the wrist joint are very important for functional adaptations in the normal hand and even more so when digital disabilities are present.

Anatomy. Flexion, extension, and radial and ulnar deviation movements at the wrist occur in both the radiocarpal and midcarpal joints. The proximal carpal row includes the scaphoid, lunate, and triquetrum bones and links the forearm to the distal carpal row and hand. The scaphoid and lunate bones articulate with facets on the radius and also with the triangular fibrocartilage bridging the radius and ulna. These bones are united by means of interosseous ligaments. The distal row of carpal bones includes the trapezium, trapezoid, capitate, and hamate. These bones are also linked by interosseous ligaments. The articulation between the proximal and distal carpal row forms the midcarpal joint. The volar radiocarpal and dorsal radiocarpal ligaments are extremely important to support the carpal area. The fibers of the volar radiocarpal ligament extend distally and obliquely from the radius, the triangular fibrocartilage, and the styloid process of the ulna (Fig. 70-13). A symmetric pattern is formed by its insertions into the scaphoid, lunate, triquetrum, and capitate bones. Short, deep ligamentous bands connect the trapezium and trapezoid to the scaphoid and the hamate to the triquetrum. The ulnar and radial collateral ligaments provide some lateral wrist stability. The dorsal ligamentous struc-

tures are not so dense as the volar ones. The dorsal radiocarpal ligament is connected intimately with the fibrous channels of the digital long extensor tendons located above.

Physiology of movements. Ulnar and radial deviation of the wrist occurs mainly at the radiocarpal joint. However, because a bony crest separates the distal radial surface in two concavities and a strong interosseous ligament unites the scaphoid and lunate bones, about 20% of radial deviation movements also arise at the midcarpal joint, mainly around the head of the capitate.

During wrist extension, the first two thirds of movement are principally located at the radiocarpal joint and the last third at the midcarpal joint. In flexion approximately the first half of excursion occurs at the midcarpal level, and the rest at the radiocarpal level. As noted, the scaphoid bone bridges the midcarpal joint. However, from a functional point of view, the midcarpal joint continues distally between the trapezium, trapezoid bones, and adjacent surfaces of the first and second metacarpals; the thumb, trapezium, and scaphoid act as a unit that plays only a small part in midcarpal movements. Motion around the scaphoid takes place in all three body planes: vertically at its proximal pole, horizontally at the distal pole, and coronally at the scaphoid-capitate articulation.

Integrated movements of the radiocarpal and midcarpal joints are made possible by important displacements of the carpal bones. The shape of the proximal carpal row changes in various hand positions, and the shape of the second carpal row becomes modified accordingly. Link systems are present in the hand as they are in the digits. Proper balance of this link system is dependent on the shape of bones and the integrity and tension of their ligaments. Normal functional adaptations and muscle pull apply external strains across the system. However, when the building blocks or their

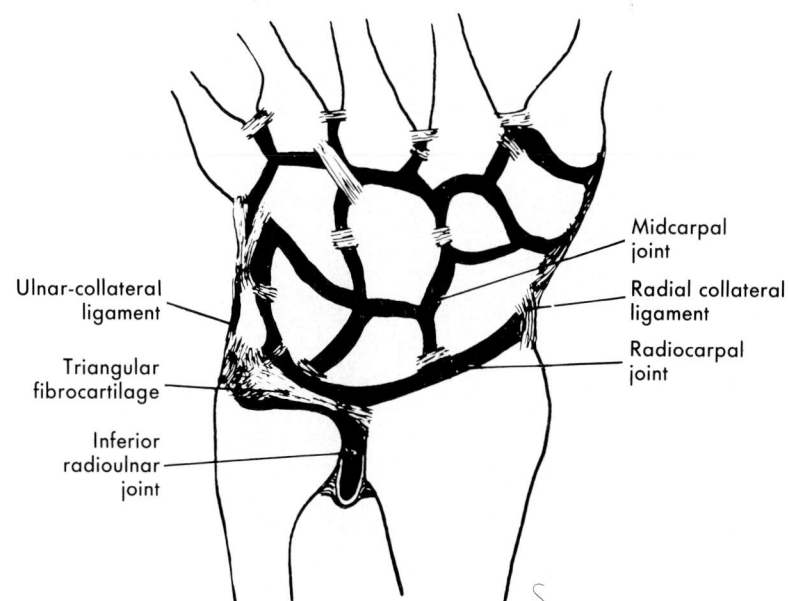

Fig. 70-13 Relationships of wrist ligaments. Triangular fibrocartilage and its important ligamentous attachments between the distal radius and ulna are commonly destroyed in early synovial invasion in rheumatoid arthritis, which allows instability of the distal radioulnar joint.

important ligamentous connections are destroyed, the wrist system can no longer tolerate these external forces and collapses into deformities.

Collapse mechanisms. The proximal carpal row represents a link between the region of the forearm and the distal carpal row and hand. If the midcarpal joint becomes unstable, the lunate rotates dorsally and the capitate becomes hyperflexed. The resultant shortening of the long axis of the carpus causes rotation of the scaphoid, which usually is seen only in normal radial deviation. Instability of the midcarpal joint may follow a hyperextension injury of the wrist in which the volar radiocarpal ligaments are partially ruptured and the joint capsule between the capitate, scaphoid, and lunate bones is damaged. In extreme cases of instability the scaphoid dislocates spontaneously and shifts horizontally, so that its distal articular surface points straight forward. Carpal stability is most vulnerable in dorsiflexion and ulnar deviation. Collapse deformity of the wrist can also occur after dislocations of the lunate or loosening of ligaments of the wrist by an arthritic process.

Radiocarpal joint. The multiple-link system of the wrist is disturbed in rheumatoid arthritis as a result of the loosening of ligamentous structures and deformation of bones by the destructive synovitis. In some cases spontaneous fusion will occur before subluxation, and in severe cases a complete dislocation of the wrist may result (Fig. 70-14). Loosening of the ligaments on the radial aspect of the joint is common and will allow an ulnar displacement of the proximal carpal row, resulting secondarily in a radial deviation of the hand on the forearm. The associated subluxation of the distal radioulnar joint causes a loss of stability on the ulnar aspect of the wrist. In some cases loosening of the volar radiocarpal ligament disrupts the longitudinal axis and is followed by a buckling phenomenon. A palmar subluxation of the proximal row on the radius is more common.

Rheumatoid arthritic changes in the radiocarpal joint are frequent and may be summarized as follows:
1. Erosions in the intercarpal and radiocarpal area, with fusion or fibrosis, or both, and associated stiffness
2. Ulnad shift of the carpus and the radius, which may or may not result in radiad deviation of the hand
3. Palmar subluxation of the carpus on the ulna, with associated absorptive changes in the proximal carpal row
4. Occasional ulnad dislocation of the hand off the radius, which is usually associated with pronounced instability and serious loss of function.

Distal radioulnar joint. Rotation is the most important component for adapting the wrist joint to movements of the hand. The distal radioulnar joint is therefore of great importance. Dysfunction of the distal radioulnar joint in rheumatoid arthritis is a common occurrence. Destructive synovitis at this joint sets off a chain of disabilities that impair the normal function of the wrist and hand. Bäckdahl has described this problem very well in his comprehensive essay *The Caput Ulnae Syndrome in Rheumatoid Arthritis.* Approximately one third of our rheumatoid patients undergoing hand surgery had associated distal radioulnar disability, which is characterized clinically by the dorsal prominence and instability of the ulnar head, with increasing weakness of the wrist, pain and crepitation on movement, especially rotation, and decrease of rotation and dorsiflexion, and there may be an increased flexion of the fifth and fourth metacarpals because of the loss of the normal action of the extensor carpi ulnaris, which is displaced palmad, and ruptures of the extensor tendons of the little, ring, and long fingers, which must be differentiated from the above (Fig. 70-15).

Dysfunction of the extensor carpi ulnaris in this syndrome is an important and frequently ignored problem that can lead to further imbalances in the complex musculoskeletal system

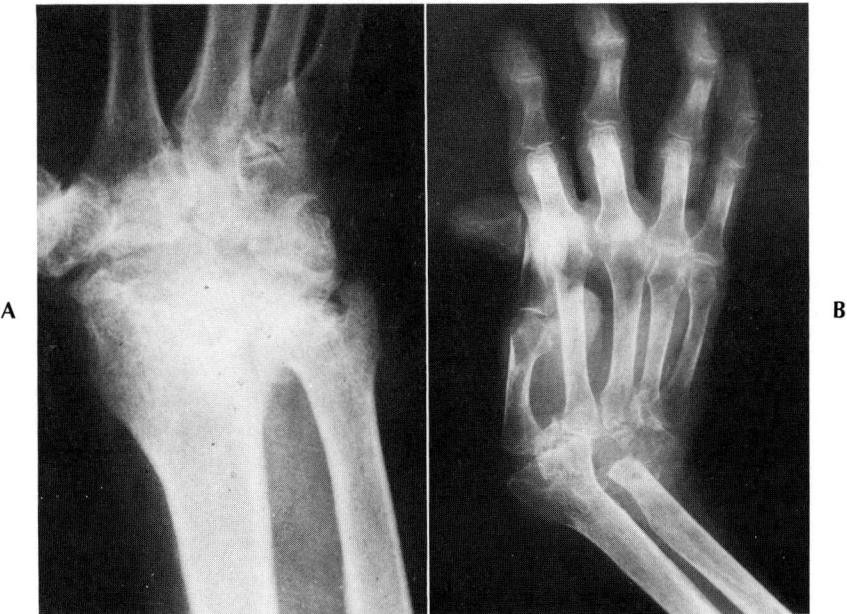

Fig. 70-14 **A,** Disabilities of wrist joints are very common and are seen early in rheumatoid arthritis. Erosive and cystic changes, collapse of bone, fusion, and subluxation—all may occur in the same wrist in either radiocarpal, midcarpal, intercarpal, or distal radioulnar joint. This rheumatoid patient's wrist shows all these roentgenographic findings. **B,** Severe erosive changes occur in the radiocarpal joint, with dysfunction of ligaments, absorption of bone, and wrist subluxation, usually with hand-deviating palmar and ulnad.

disabilities of the rheumatoid hand. Normally the extensor carpi ulnaris acts in dorsiflexion and ulnar abduction of the wrist and helps stabilize the wrist during abduction and extension of the thumb and when the hand is opened for grasp. It also contracts during palmar flexion of the wrist, whereas the other extensors relax. The extensor carpi ulnaris crosses the dorsal surface of the distal ulna to assist in the stabilization of the wrist and to maintain the integrity of the distal radioulnar joint. It helps stabilize the fifth metacarpal through its insertion, and its dysfunction allows greater flexion of the fourth and fifth metacarpals, with secondary deformity and impaired finger function.

As the destructive synovial hypertrophy increases, the ligamentous support of the distal end of the ulna, formed mainly by the triangular fibrocartilage and its ligaments, the ulnar collateral ligament, and the surrounding capsule, undergoes attritional changes; the ulnar head can now dislocate to the line of least resistance dorsally. The sixth dorsal compartment is stretched by the synovial hypertrophy, and the extensor carpi ulnaris is subluxated ulnad and palmad.

Roentgenographic examination may show early dorsal subluxation and erosive changes of the ulnar head and the ulnar notch of the radius. The ulnar head loses its smooth rounded contour and becomes sharp and irregular. The ulnar styloid may become prominent or disappear, or severe absorptive changes of the distal ulna may occur. Extensor

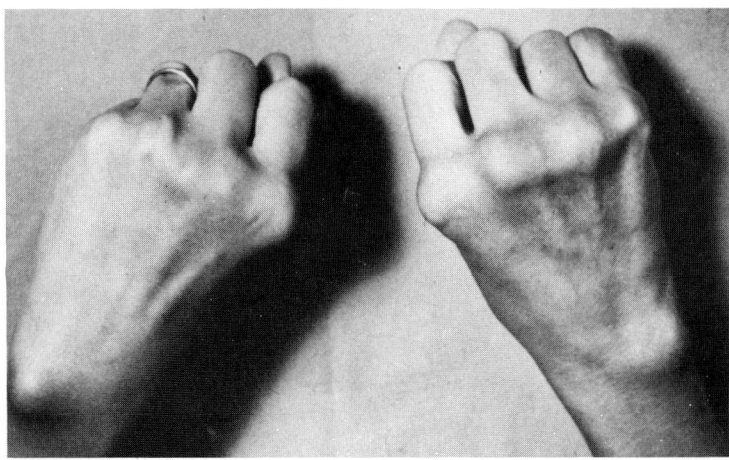

Fig. 70-15 Dorsal subluxation of ulnar head occurs early and commonly in rheumatoid arthritis. This causes painful disability that has many functional implications, such as those described in ulnar head syndrome.

tendons may rupture over the jagged distal ulna or secondary to attritional changes from the invasive synovitis.

Any involvement through arthritic change or trauma that disturbs the integrity of the bones of the wrist or of their ligamentous support can result in severe functional disability. The problem in reconstruction and rehabilitation of the rheumatoid wrist is to regain stability and at the same time maintain the motion that is so important in functional adaptations of the hand.

The discussion of the pathogenesis of digital deformities in rheumatoid arthritis as given is useful for the surgeon who will be called on to do reconstructive surgery for these problems. We have noted that the changes are secondary to invasive characteristics of the pathologic proliferative synovitis, which distends the joint capsule, destroys ligament and tendon attachments, erodes the joint surfaces, and prevents gliding of the tendons. The disturbed balance of the linked tendon system and the collapse of the skeletal structures further aggravate the deformity.

71

The management of patients with rheumatoid arthritis

Cynthia A. Philips

Rheumatoid arthritis is a chronic disease characterized by inflammation of the synovial tissue of the joints and tendon sheaths, and it is frequently combined with other systemic manifestations. The course of the disease is often unpredictable and varies considerably from patient to patient. The clinical course of 20% to 30% of these patients is characterized by episodes of complete or partial remissions.[1,8] The disease in these patients seems to be milder with fewer joints involved, but over time, more joints may be affected. These patients generally do well. In another group of patients, the disease is progressive, leading to severe joint dysfunction and deformity.

Hand involvement from rheumatoid arthritis is common. Characteristically, the wrist, the metacarpal joints, proximal interphalangeal (PIP) joints, and the metacarpophalangeal (MP) joints and carpometacarpal joints of the thumb are most often affected.[7,9,10,13] The distal interphalangeal (DIP) joints are not as frequently involved. Deformities of the distal joints may often be the result of imbalance caused by involvement of the proximal joints. Inflammation of the synovium may lead to weakening of the supporting joint structures, destruction of cartilage, and erosion of bone. This eventually leads to muscle and tendon imbalance, ligamentous laxity, instability, and subluxation or complete dislocation of the joints[7] (see also Chapter 70). In some cases, ankylosis of the joints occurs. Proliferating synovium can also invade the synovial-lined tendon sheaths (tenosynovitis) and can contribute to tendon rupture.[7,10,13] On the dorsum of the hand, the extensor tendons glide in synovial sheaths only at the wrist. The synovial sheaths extend approximately 1 inch above and 1 inch below the extensor retinaculum. This is a common site of tenosynovitis. On the volar aspect of the hand, tenosynovitis can occur at the wrist, palm, or digits, because these are areas where tendons glide in synovial-lined sheaths.[7,10,13] It is no surprise, then, that rheumatoid hand deformities can occur in numerous combinations.

PATIENT EVALUATION

When the therapist first sees a patient with rheumatoid arthritis, it is necessary to do a baseline evaluation to determine appropriate treatment goals. Periodic reassessments will be necessary to monitor the patient's progress and to make any needed modifications in the patient's program. This is particularly important for patients with rheumatoid arthritis, because their course is often variable. The evaluation may be divided into three sections: (1) observation and palpation, (2) subjective assessment, and (3) objective measurement.

Observation and palpation

Observation and palpation give the therapist an indication of the nature of the person's disease. This includes noting abnormal posture of the hand, any observable deformities, the condition of the skin, or any muscle atrophy. If deformities are evident, one should determine how long the deformities have been present and how rapidly they have progressed, because this may determine various treatment options. The therapist should note joint or tendon crepitus, joint stability, and tendon integrity. To test for profundus function, support the finger in extension and ask the patient to flex the DIP joint. To test for superficialis function, hold all the fingers except the one being tested in extension. Then ask the patient to flex the finger. If the superficialis is intact, the patient should be able to flex the PIP joint. The exception may be in the fifth finger where the superficialis may be absent or weak. In patients with severe deformity, it may be difficult to accurately assess tendon integrity. Palpable tendon nodules or evidence of locking should be noted as well. Tenosynovitis proliferating within the proximal portion of the palm may cause snapping and locking as the tendon slides within the tendon sheath. These patients are often able to flex the digit fully, but as the patient attempts to extend the digit, the nodule will catch and cause a snap. Sometimes the digit will become locked in flexion and must be passively extended. Upon examination, one can usually feel a fullness or tendon crepitus as the patient attempts to flex and extend the fingers.[13]

Subjective assessment

The second step of the evaluation is a subjective assessment of pain, fatigue, morning stiffness, and for those patients with deformity, an assessment of cosmesis. Pain is assessed according to how much it interferes with function, as described by Swanson (see Chapter 8). The categories are (1) minimal (is annoying), (2) slight (interferes with activity), (3) moderate (prevents activity), or (4) severe (prevents activity and also causes distress).

Morning stiffness is assessed by how long after rising the stiffness last. Fatigue is evaluated by how much and at what time of day it interferes with daily activities.

Cosmesis is important to evaluate, because it helps the therapist understand how much the patient is affected emotionally by the deformities caused from the disease. Surgery to help correct the deformity for cosmetic reasons may be a valid indication for those patients whose lowered self-esteem prevents them from participating fully in social interactions. Swanson measures both active and passive cosmesis[15] (while the hand is engaged in activity and while the hand is at rest). A point system is then used by both the patient and the examiner to rate the cosmetic effects of the deformity.

Objective measurement

Objective measurement provides a baseline for comparison and helps quantify some of the therapist's impressions. These include evaluation of range of motion, grip and pinch strength, dexterity, information regarding activities of daily living (ADL), and other objective tests as necessary.

Active and passive range of motion should be recorded when possible, because this gives information about the location of the pathologic condition.

Grip strength is recorded with a Jamar dynamometer, because several authors have found it to be a reliable instrument.[5] We have found that a grip strength of at least 20 pounds is necessary for most ADLs. Below this level, patients begin to have difficulty in lifting objects and may require two hands to lift a coffee cup, for example. One should remember that many rheumatoid patients are well below this functional level. Normal grip strength varies with age and sex, but generally the average is between 50 and 60 pounds for a woman and 100 pounds for a man. Some authors recommend the use of a sphygmometer to test grip strength of people with arthritis.[9] However, it is not a reliable instrument for this purpose, because it may be difficult to obtain the exact inflation point at each evaluation. It may also be difficult to stabilize the cuff and obtain the same cuff circumference. This is especially true if a nylon cuff is used. This tool should be used only in situations where it is not possible to use the Jamar dynamometer, as in the presence of severe deformity. Then the therapist should continue the use of the sphygmometer in subsequent reevaluation.

Pulp, three-point, and lateral pinch are tested with a standard pinch meter. We have found that a pinch strength of 5 to 7 pounds, although by no means normal, is adequate for performing most daily tasks. A normal pinch strength is usually between 15 and 20 pounds. Although grip strength is important, pinch strength has particular application when assessing self-care skills, such as holding eating utensils, buttoning clothing, and writing.

Dexterity is tested using a pickup test, consisting of eight items that can be completed by a normal hand in about 5

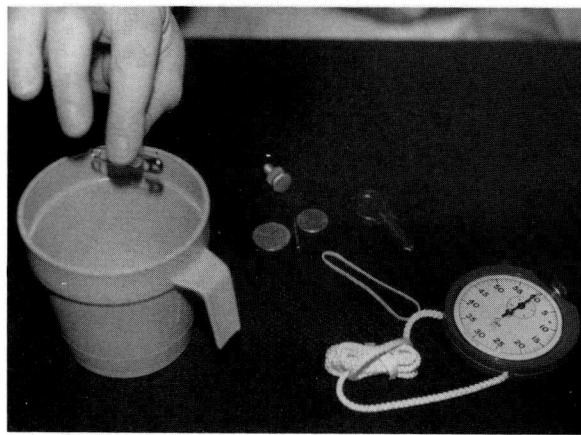

Fig. 71-1 Pickup test for assessing dexterity.

to 7 seconds (Fig. 71-1). Even though this is not a standard test, we use it for several reasons. The test helps note subtle changes in hand function: fine coordination is usually affected early in the course of the disease. Changes in sensibility can also be noted with this test, and further sensibility testing can be done if necessary. Entrapment neuropathies are fairly common in rheumatoid arthritis.[3,12] Because these are often insidious and may be bilateral, the patients themselves may not be aware of the decreased sensibility. A more extensive hand function test, such as the Jebson-Taylor hand function test may be done on those patients with more severe or complex problems.

Activities of daily living

It is important to consider that the severity of the deformity does not necessarily correlate with the patient's level of functioning. Often patients with very severe deformity function well. They have developed compensatory patterns that work well for them. There are a number of ADL evaluations described in the literature and include basic self-care skills, homemaking skills, and communication skills. With a chronic disease, it is important, when possible, to get to know the patient over time to gain a better understanding of the person, the nature of his disease, and what his individual lifestyle and needs are.

TREATMENT

Rheumatoid arthritis, as with other inflammatory diseases, can be divided into three stages: the acute stage, the subacute stage, and the chronic stage. The chronic stage can either be chronic-active or chronic-inactive. Although the goals of treatment are similar in each category, that is, to help the patient maintain a certain functional level, the treatment approaches will vary with the patient's individual situation. Early treatment is essential if many of the severe disabling effects of the disease are to be prevented or minimized. The treatment goals are to decrease pain and swelling, maintain joint mobility, prevent or minimize joint deformity, and maintain a level of general physical fitness. One way these goals can be achieved is through administration of various medications by a rheumatologist in an attempt to control the disease. Often, trials on several medications are necesary to find the appropriate one for the patient. Some of the drugs used may take several weeks or months to become effective. The patient may also receive steroid injections into specific areas to help reduce local synovitis or tenosynovitis. Too many injections into the same area may have negative consequences to the surrounding joint and tendon structures. Therefore they are used judiciously. There can be potential complications with any of the medications used for arthritis. Therefore the therapist should be aware of the drugs the patient is taking and their potential side effects. It is the therapist's role to provide careful and thoughtful splinting, appropriate exercise and activities programs, and instruction in joint protection and energy conservation methods as a part of a comprehensive treatment program. Exercise and activities programs need to be modified according to the stage of the patient's disease and the presence or absence of pain and swelling.

In the acute stage, rest to decrease swelling, pain, and inflammation, proper positioning to prevent contractures, and gentle range-of-motion exercises to maintain joint mobility are used. Gentle exercise is usually done three to four times daily for brief periods. Brief periods of exercise are less likely to cause tissue reaction than one long period. Range of motion can be active, passive, or active-assisted. In cases of acute synovitis associated with pain and muscle spasm, gentle passive range of motion may be less stressful to the joints than active range of motion. Active exercise must be used judiciously during an acute flare-up. Exercises may be done in lukewarm water. The water helps reduce stresses to the joints while making range of motion more comfortable. For those patients who do not have Raynaud's phenomenon or are otherwise cold-sensitive, icing inflamed joints may be helpful in reducing pain and swelling.

In the subacute stage, when pain and swelling begin to subside, exercise and activities are gradually increased as tolerated by the patient. Joint protection principles and energy conservation techniques are introduced at this time. These techniques enable the patient to function more easily and safely.

In the chronic stage, the emphasis is placed on joint protection, activities of daily living, and exercises to increase strength and endurance. Exercises of increasing resistance and isometric exercises may be used. The patient is instructed to monitor his activities and watch for signs of increased inflammation. If this occurs, activity should be appropriately adjusted. For patients in remission, incorporating a program of general physical conditioning may be helpful to minimize the disability during exacerbation periods and to improve overall function. However, as with any exercise program, the patient must be carefully monitored to avoid any harmful effects.[2,4,11,14]

Activities of daily living

Patients may experience functional limitations in any of the stages mentioned. These include dressing, grooming, bathing, toileting, cooking and homemaking activities, writing, and other dexterity skills. This will often vary and may change from day to day in the same patient. These problems may be the result of pain, deformity, loss of range of motion, fatigue, or decreased muscle strength. Some patients may require the use of adaptive equipment to function independently. In some cases, the need for equipment may be only temporary to help the patient through a flare-up and to protect his joints. Any equipment should be suggested prudently after careful assessment. Inappropriate use of equipment could prevent the patient from using his available range of motion and ultimately lead to increased disability.

Joint protection

Joint-protection techniques are methods of performing daily activities with a minimal amount of stress to the joints to reduce pain, preserve joint structures, and conserve physical energy.[9] These techniques consider the implications of the disease process and integrate these with the person's lifestyle. Basic principles of joint protection follow.

Respect for pain. A person's fear of pain can lead to needless inactivity, whereas total disregard for pain can lead to unnecessary joint damage. It is important for the patient to learn to monitor his activities and to stop when discomfort or fatigue begins to develop. If discomfort lasts for more than 1 hour after an activity, that activity should be decreased or in some cases omitted from the patient's schedule.

Maintain muscle strength and range of motion. Exercises are an important part of the overall treatment program. The therapist should help the patient integrate these exercises into his daily routine to help maintain range of motion and enhance muscle strength.

Balance work and rest. A chronic disease, such as rheumatoid arthritis, can put a tremendous strain on both physical and emotional resources. The appropriate use of rest and relaxation during the day's activities can be the most effective weapon against the demands of the disease. The amount of rest necessary must be determined individually. During the active phase of the disease, more rest will be required.

Avoid deforming positions. The patient should be instructed to avoid positions that could ultimately lead to or hasten joint deformities. For example, the patient should be instructed to avoid resting his head on his hands. Proper positioning and proper use of the joints during activities are important parts of this principle.

Use stronger and larger joints when possible. The stresses of the daily activities can, of course, be tolerated more easily on larger joints than on smaller joints. For example, the patient may carry either a shoulder bag or carry a pocketbook on the forearm and thus reduce the stresses on the small joints of the fingers.

Avoid one position for prolonged periods. Muscles can fatigue in an attempt to maintain a static position as well as when engaged in active motion. This can put positional strain on underlying structures and thus lead to joint contractures. Sustained joint compression can lead to damage to articular surfaces. It is therefore recommended that the patient change positions every 20 to 30 minutes. The patient's activities can be alternated to facilitate these positional changes.

Use of necessary adaptive equipment. If it becomes necessary, certain pieces of adaptive equipment can enable the person to maintain his independence while protecting his joints.

Conserve energy. Activities should be assessed, and the most economic way of performing the activity should be determined. Priorities should be set so that those activities that are the most important can be accomplished first. This saves energy for those activities that may have special meaning to the patient.

Most normal functional hand patterns, such as power grip, hook grasp, pulp pinch, and strong lateral pinch, place stress on the joints of the wrist and hand. There are, however, certain techniques that can reduce these stresses and thus improve overall function. For example, the use of a dishcloth when washing dishes encourages a prolonged tight grasp and ulnar deviation of the fingers, both of which should definitely be avoided. The use of a sponge allows the patient to better position the hand and thus avoid the deforming position. Opening jars can also place a strain on the MP joints and wrists. If one uses the palm of the hand and uses the right hand to open the jar and the left hand to close the jar, one minimizes external forces on the hand and wrist and reduces the ulnar deviation forces at the MP joints. The weight of packages should be evenly distributed between the two arms (Fig. 71-2). Using large handled utensils will help reduce the stress on the small joints of the hand by making a tight grip unnecessary (Fig. 71-3).

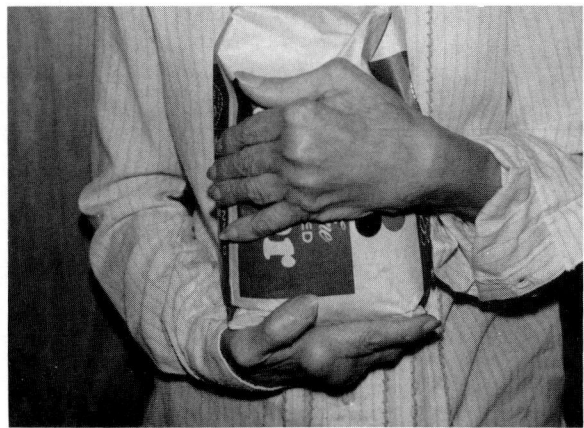

Fig. 71-2 Correct method of balancing the weight of objects between the two arms.

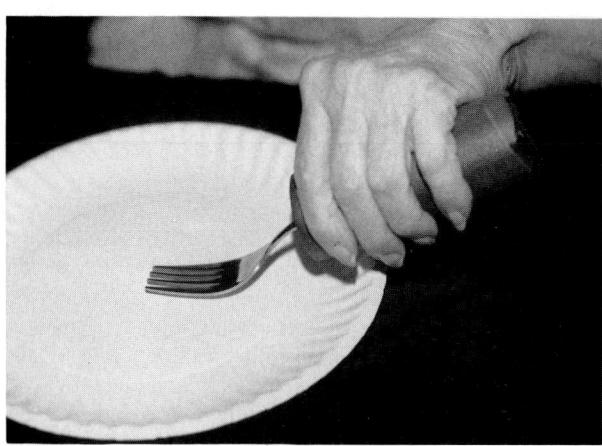

Fig. 71-3 Patient demonstrating the use of a large-handled fork to reduce stress to the small finger joints.

Splinting

As part of the treatment program, the therapist may determine that splinting would be beneficial. The rheumatoid hand may be splinted for the following reasons: (1) to reduce inflammation, (2) to rest and support weakened structures, (3) to properly position joints, (4) to minimize joint deformity, (5) to help in postoperative management, and (6) to improve function. Controversy still surrounds this subject. Most, however, would agree that splinting does have a place in the total management of the person with rheumatoid arthritis, especially in the acute stage when joints are hot and swollen. However, there are few documented or well-established indications for splinting the rheumatoid hand.

Resting-splints, either for the whole hand or wrist, are used when there is swelling and inflammation of the joints. During periods of inflammation, the joints are more vul-

nerable to damage from both internal and external sources. Therefore splinting protects the joints during this time, as well as reduces pain and swelling. A study by Zoeckler and Nicholas showed that 63% of patients who responded to their questionnaire found moderate or great relief from pain and morning stiffness by using splints.[15] It is suggested that splints, when made for this purpose, be worn full-time except for brief periods of gentle range of motion. The splints should, if feasible, be worn at night for several weeks after resolution of acute inflammation.[7] If bilateral splints are necessary, alternating the use of each splint often seems more reasonable to the patient and leads to better acceptance and compliance.

In cases where the MP joints are involved but the PIP joints are not, a resting splint may be fabricated to include the MP joints and leave the IP joints free (Fig. 71-4). This

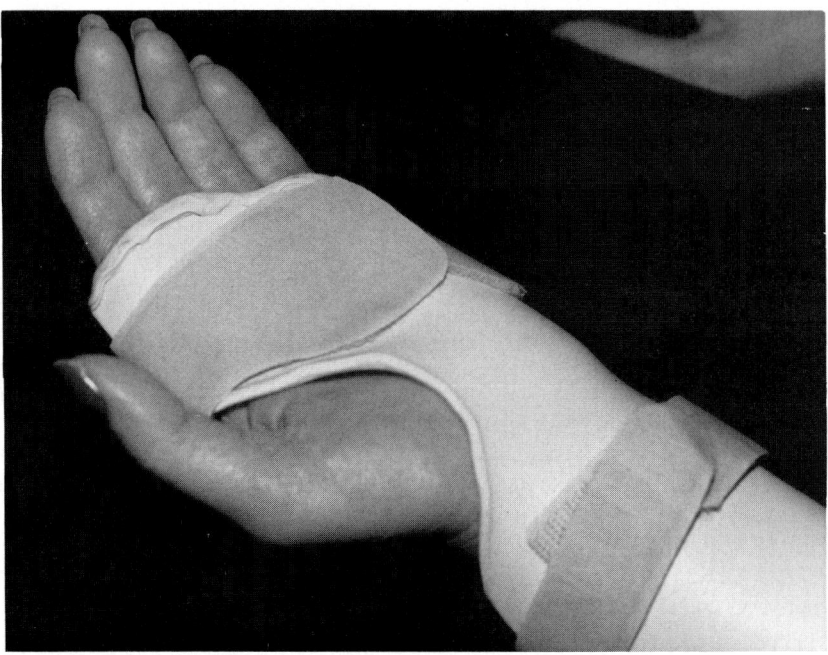

Fig. 71-4 A resting splint to protect the wrist and MP joints while allowing the IP joints freedom to move.

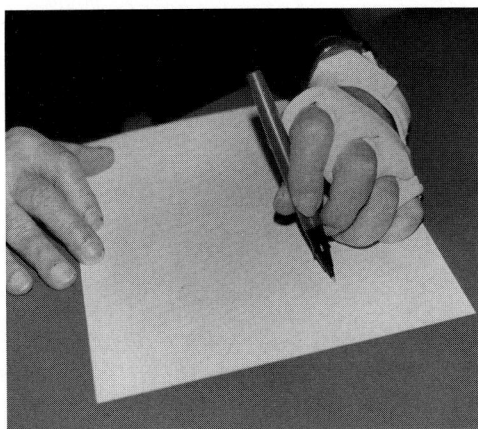

Fig. 71-5   A functional ulnar deviation splint.

may also be used as an exercise splint for the PIP joints when there is evidence of tight intrinsic muscles or PIP joint stiffness.

When positioning an arthritic hand in a resting splint, one should keep in mind the pathomechanics of the disease. The tendency is for the MP joints to sublux volarly. Therefore the MP joints should be held in close to full extension (about 25 degrees of flexion) to provide volar support to the joints and surrounding soft tissues. The PIP joints should be held in slight flexion. The wrist should be positioned in neutral to 10 to 15 degrees of dorsiflexion.[6] Too much dorsiflexion may increase the tendency toward carpal tunnel syndrome.

Splinting also may help improve function. Both static and dynamic splints may be used for this purpose. For example, an ulnar deviation splint may be fabricated to help the patient improve function by realigning the fingers (Fig. 71-5). This splint will, of course, not correct the deformity but will help some patients improve function while wearing the splint. A wrist splint made for a painful wrist may help enhance overall hand function by reducing pain.

Postoperative splinting with either dynamic or static splints may be an integral part of the patient's postoperative management as in MP arthroplasty where proper postoperative splinting is crucial in the development of the new capsuloligamentous system.

VOCATIONAL COUNSELING

Counseling about employment is also important in the overall management of the person with rheumatoid arthritis and is frequently overlooked. Often self-esteem depends on the maintenance of useful and purposeful work, either at home or in the outside workforce. Often it is helpful for the patient to consult with a vocational counselor regarding the outlook for continued employment or vocational training. In these cases, the hand therapist would supply information regarding physical capacities and ADL skills. A creative approach to the person's rehabilitation may prevent the loss of self-esteem and yet help the person accept the realities of his functional limitations.

In summary, treating the patient with rheumatoid arthritis requires a team approach. It is necessary to do a baseline evaluation before treatment, and periodic reassessment to determine treatment goals and treatment plans. Treatment includes various medications prescribed by a rheumatologist, exercise and activities programs, splinting, and joint protection techniques taught by the therapist. This approach helps these patients live and cope more effectively with their disease.

REFERENCES

1. Baker DH and Rabinowitz JL: Current concepts in the treatment of rheumatoid arthritis, J Clin Pharmacol 26:2, 1986.
2. Burchhardt CS, Clark SR, and Nelson DL: Assessing physical fitness of women with rheumatic disease, Arthritis Care and Research 1:38, 1988.
3. Castaldo JE and Ochoa J: Peripheral nerve, structure, function and dysfunction. In Kelley WN and others, editors: Textbook of rheumatology, ed 2, Philadelphia,1985, WB Saunders Co.
4. Ekblom B and others: Physical performance in patients with rheumatoid arthritis, Scand J Rheumatol 3:121, 1974.
5. Fess EE: Documentation: essential elements of an upper extremity assessment battery. In Hunter JM and others, editors: Rehabilitation of the hand, ed 2, St. Louis, 1984, The CV Mosby Co.
6. Fess EE and Philips CA: Hand splinting: principles and methods, ed 2, St. Louis, 1987, The CV Mosby Co.
7. Flatt AE: Care of the rheumatoid hand, ed 4, St. Louis, 1983, The CV Mosby Co.
8. Harris ED Jr: Rheumatoid arthritis: the clinical spectrum. In Kelley WN and others, editors: Textbook of rheumatology, ed 2, Philadelphia, 1985, WB Saunders Co.
9. Melvin JL: Rheumatoid disease, occupational therapy and rehabilitation, ed 2, Philadelphia, 1982, FA Davis Co.
10. Millender LH and Nalebuff EA: Evaluation and treatment of early rheumatoid hand involvement, Orthop Clin North Am 6(3):697, 1975.
11. Minor MA, Hewett JE, and Kay DR: Monitoring for harmful effects of physical conditioning exercise (PGE) with arthritis patients, Arthritis Rheum 29:S144, 1986 (abstract).
12. Nakano KK: The entrapment neuropathies of rheumatoid arthritis, Orthop Clin North Am 6(3):837, 1975.
13. Nalebuff EA and Millender LH: Reconstructive surgery and rehabilitation of the hand. In Kelley WN and others, editors: Textbook of rheumatology, ed 2, Philadelphia, 1985, WB Saunders Co.
14. Youg AG and Minor MA: Physical conditioning exercises (PCE) for arthritis patients: description of method, University of Missouri-Columbia, Arthritis Rheum 29:S144, 1986 (abstract).
15. Zoeckler, AA and Nicholas, JJ: Prenyl hand splints for rheumatoid arthritis, Phys Ther 49:377, 1969.

72

Joint protection for inflammatory disorders

Judy Leonard

Provision of therapy services for the person with rheumatic disease has frequently included use of the educational process for teaching of joint protection principles. The assimilation of new information into one's daily life most frequently requires modification of long-standing habits. Before most people are willing to make changes, it appears that it is helpful for them to understand *why* symptoms exist and *what* external forces of habit, daily activities, or rest positions are contributing to their problems.

Many of these same principles traditionally applicable for those people with rheumatic disease are very appropriate for individuals with other musculoskeletal or musculotendinous diagnoses. Whether offered to the patient with inflammatory or noninflammatory, systemic or nonsystemic diagnoses, the methods have been found clinically to be effective when carried out on a regular basis.

For people with acute phase systemic inflammatory disease the instruction must include direction for general body rest. Adequate nighttime sleep and intentional rest periods during the daytime enable restorative functions to occur within the body. Specific joints involved are at an increased risk from internal pressure with subsequent over-stretching of capsuloligamentous structures and are to be especially protected with resting splints. The joint protection methods of activity, adequate sleep, and intermittent daytime rest are also appropriate for coping with chronic conditions that may not be systemic in nature.

The therapist is usually the major contributor in helping the patient learn protective positions of rest and protective methods for performing work and leisure activities. As the therapist helps the patient understand *why* symptoms exist and understand the influence of his actions, the individual becomes willing to make changes in his life-style. The therapist helps set the stage for this educational process to occur. It is likely that the best results will be derived from direct services over a 4- to 6-week period to enable the patient to begin feeling a difference. Through these direct services it is possible for the therapist to ensure that the patient correctly follows a plan of treatment most appropriate for his condition. Attention at close intervals increases opportunity for future independent carry-over. The voice of a confident therapist reassuring the individual that there is something positive that can be done to help control their symptoms is many times the turning point for an individual who may otherwise be discouraged by facing a chronic problem. Beyond the initial series of educational treatment sessions, the therapist is available as a resource person for assistance with problem solving and monitoring a home routine of appropriate exercise and splinting.

Specific application in postoperative situations requires the therapist to clearly understand the presurgical existing conditions and be thoroughly knowledgeable in the specific reconstructive procedure and the expectations of the surgeon. It would be appropriate for the therapist to review concepts of wound healing and to review the time frames for specific tissue healing. Review of the subject areas of body mechanics, biomechanics of deformity, splinting principles and applications, and the psychological aspects of coping with a chronic problem are well advised.

PRINCIPLES OF JOINT PROTECTION

1. Maintain muscle strength and joint range of motion. Use of lightly resistive putty and Theraband exercises three to four times per week are frequently advised for maintaining strength, and a complete series of mobility patterns are recommended daily for maintaining range of motion. If a flare-up occurs, the strengthening exercises are usually temporarily discontinued while the daily range-of-motion patterns continue, sometimes with fewer repetitions.
2. Avoid positions of deformity.
3. Use strongest joint available for job.
4. Use each joint in most stable anatomic and functional plane.
5. Ensure correct patterns of movement for optimum muscle balance. Use of a mirror for feedback during independent exercises is helpful.
6. Avoid prolonged static positions.
7. Eliminate activities that cannot be stopped immediately if they prove to be beyond one's power to complete.
8. Respect pain. Learn to differentiate between discomfort and pain. Keep in mind that medication may mask pain, requiring extra precautions through visual monitoring. If pain following activity exists longer than 2 hours, modification of the activity is indicated.

APPLICATION OF PRINCIPLES

It is beneficial, particularly in cases of systemic diseases, to allow the entire body (not only the part that hurts) appropriate rest. During acute stages of rheumatic disease 10 to 12 hours of sleep and rest for every 24 hours is frequently recommended. This, along with the appropriate balance between activity and intentional daytime rest, helps to avoid over-fatigue and increase endurance. The concept of stopping activity before over-fatigue helps increase endurance.

The therapist will need to help the individual analytically recognize the activities or postures that increase their symptoms and also help identify those specific postural adjust-

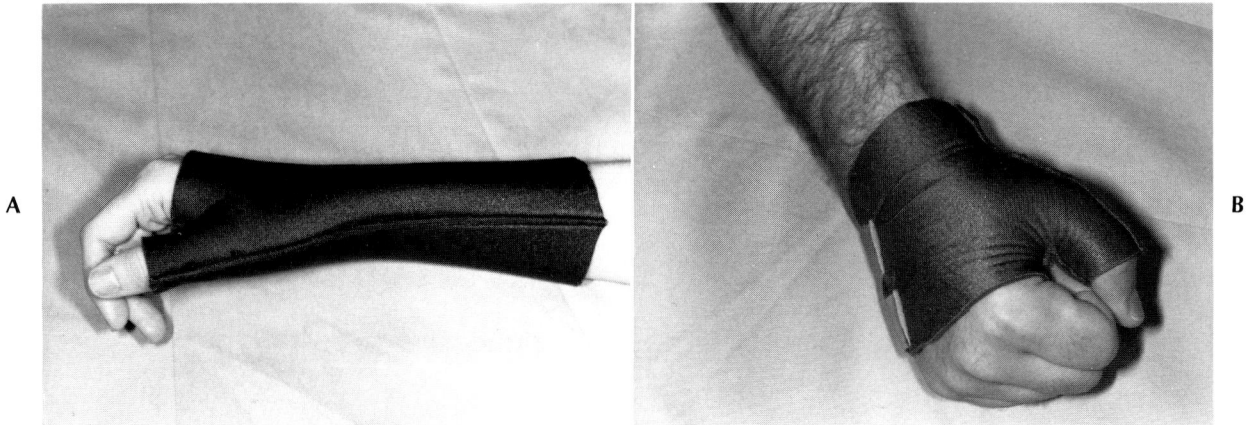

Fig. 72-1   Neoprene soft splints, ⅛ inch. **A,** Support for the first dorsal wrist compartment and abductor pollicis longus (APL) and extensor pollicis brevis (EPB) musculotendinous units of a professional piano player with deQuervain's tenosynovitis. **B,** Support for the right carpometacarpal joint of a police officer after base of thumb reconstructive surgery including excision of right trapezium and trapezoid with ligament arthroplasty using APL tendon and interpositional palmaris longus tendon graft.

ment patterns or rest patterns that provide relief. Learning to recognize the required time, distance, or resistance required in various tasks will help the patient learn pacing techniques. Suggest that the individual organize his responsibilities and delegate those that may be too strenuous.

Encourage the patient to let others help, being certain to communicate his need for help. Teach activity modification, which includes (1) reducing time spent at a given activity, (2) alternating different forms of activity, and (3) considering changes in the method of doing an activity. For example, sit rather than stand, use two hands rather than one, identify the appropriate tool and reduce the degree of force in gripping. The therapist will need to help the individual apply these principles through regular exercise to (1) reach or maintain maximum mobility, (2) practice relaxation, (3) learn specific protective positions of rest, (4) maintain appropriate muscle tone and strength, and (5) maintain appropriate body weight through a balanced diet.

Using work simplification techniques includes planning sequences to minimize energy required and subsequently increase endurance. Time and motion economy is accomplished through appropriate body mechanics, choice of an appropriate tool or equipment, and efficient arrangement of the workplace.

The therapist may need to assist in the patient's understanding that prescription or appropriate levels of over-the-counter medication reduces tissue imflammation and subsequently reduces pain. Use of medication as prescribed or at early onset of recurring symptoms usually controls or resolves the problem in a shorter time.

The educational process used in the series of treatment sessions is modified according to patient need, the patient's individual style of learning, and the individual acceptable level for acquiring new information.

SPLINTING MODALITIES

Resting splints and sometimes working splints are an appropriate means for protecting tendons, joints, capsular and ligamentous structures, and also irritated, surgically

released, or transposed nerves. The resting splint is designed for use when the hands are not involved in performance of activities and therefore are usually rigid or semirigid in design. Splinting principles and methods are well documented. (See Chapter 88.) The critical aspect of the working splint, however, is that adequate fit allow for mobility with the least amount of resistance. If a thermoplastic stay is used in conjunction with a soft splint, the thermoplastic material is chosen to permit flexibility. Soft splints I have found successful (Fig. 72-1) are custom-fabricated ⅛-inch neoprene or sometimes elasticized stockinette, single or double layer. The light tension provided from this external support gives a feeling of protection to the individual during activity. In the practice of this therapist, the neoprene soft splint has most commonly been used for working splints that support the metacarpophalangeal (MP) or carpometacarpal (CMC) joints of the thumb or that support the tendons within the first and third dorsal wrist compartments. Also, custom-fabricated neoprene soft splints have been used suc-

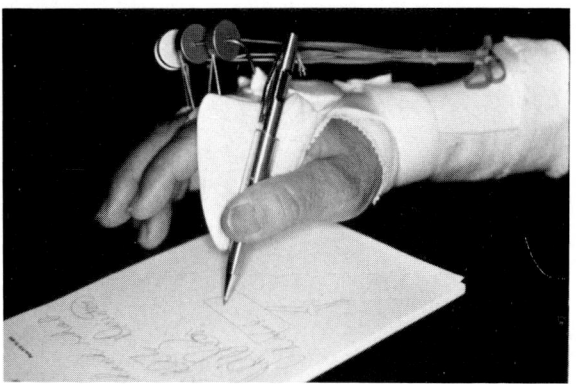

Fig. 72-2   Splint applied after metacarpophalangeal implant arthroplasty to protect reconstructed joints from ulnar-directed forces of early postoperative pinch patterns. (Used with permission from Judy Colditz, OTR/L.)

REGIONAL HAND REHABILITATION SERVICE
Warm Ups - Daily - Preferred in A.M.
BEGIN WITH THREE COMPLETE REPETITIONS

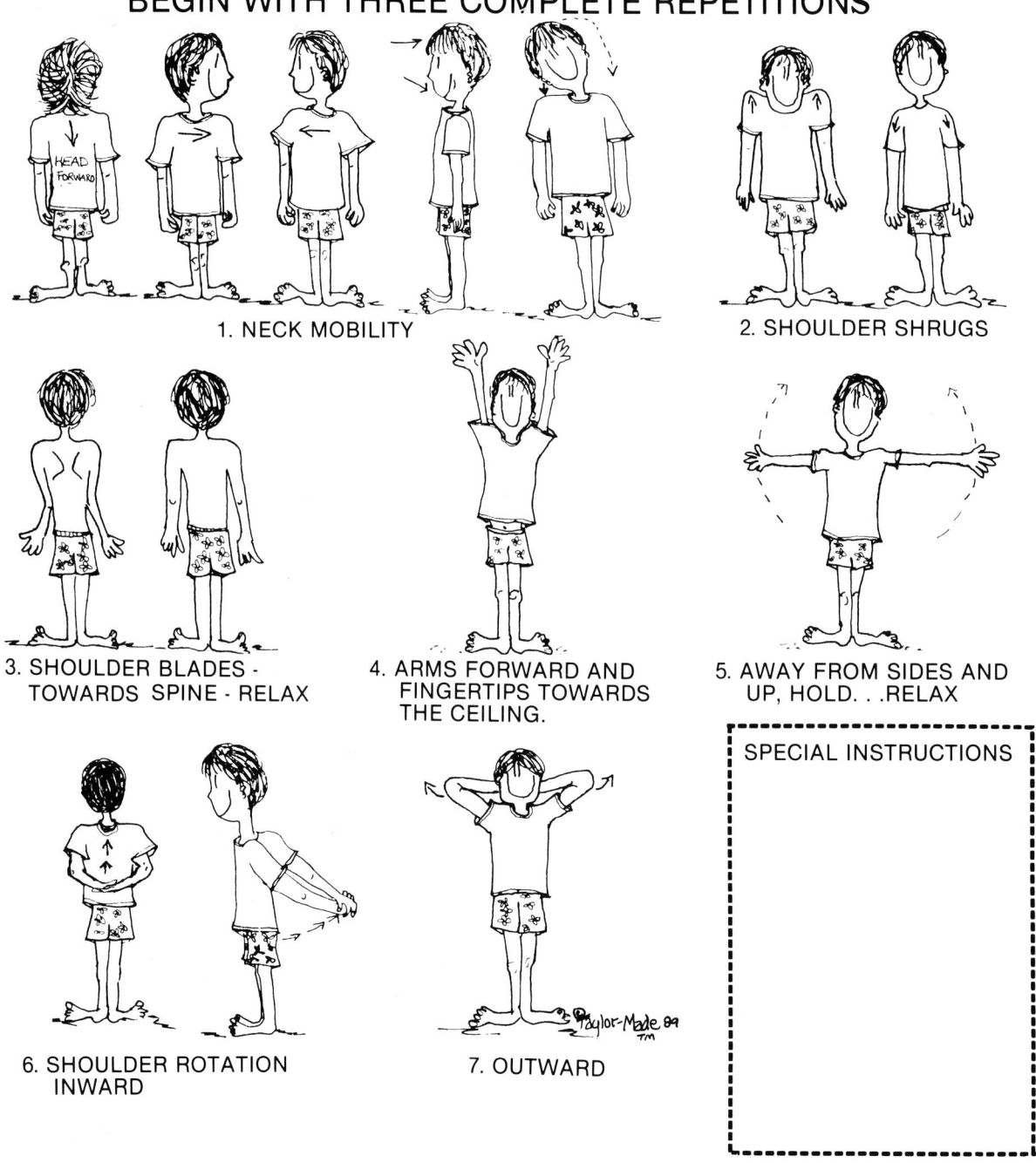

1. NECK MOBILITY

2. SHOULDER SHRUGS

3. SHOULDER BLADES - TOWARDS SPINE - RELAX

4. ARMS FORWARD AND FINGERTIPS TOWARDS THE CEILING.

5. AWAY FROM SIDES AND UP, HOLD. . .RELAX

6. SHOULDER ROTATION INWARD

7. OUTWARD

SPECIAL INSTRUCTIONS

Fig. 72-3   Range-of-motion patterns: (1) Cervical mobility: forward flexion, rotation, lateral flexion, and "chin-tuck" extension, (2) Shoulder girdle elevation and depression, (3) Scapular adduction, (4) Forward humeral flexion-elevation, (5) Humeral 90-degree abduction with external and internal rotation, humeral abduction-elevation, (6) Internal rotation and humeral hyperextension, (7) Outward rotation with elbow flexion and scapular adduction.

cessfully in providing support for the extrinsic flexor tendons at the wrist following median nerve release at the carpal tunnel. Patients have described successful use of soft splints also at the shoulder, elbow, and forearm. The degree of tension within the support must not inhibit venous return or further irritate sensitive tissues. The strap attachments are carefully placed relative to line and direction of pull to accommodate the specific joint or tendon or other irritated areas requiring support.

In selective cases following MP implant arthroplasties, a working splint is fabricated to allow the individual to resume pinch activities at an earlier than usual postoperative date. The protective splint in this type of situation will reduce the risk of recurring ulnar drift following the reconstructive procedure (Fig. 72-2).

MAINTAINING RANGE OF MOTION

This series of exercise patterns (Fig. 72-3) is offered from my experience in working toward the goals of maintaining optimum joint range of motion and musculotendinous length. The approach is to encourage the individual to move slowly and deliberately, holding the maximum arc for 3 to 5 seconds. If in use with an individual in acute stage inflammatory joint disease, the patient is cautioned to use the patterns once daily, aiming toward three full repetitions. Select patterns are particularly helpful as intermittent postural adjustments throughout the day. They have been useful in eliminating or minimizing symptoms for people having musculoskeletal pain and muscle spasm. Successful use by the author of this series in a "warm-up for work" program provided in an automobile parts manufacturing company is also noted. The patterns most frequently used as postural adjustments are lateral cervical flexion and "chin-tuck" extension, scapular adduction with arms at side, and outward rotation with combined elbow flexion and scapular adduction. Whether a worker is involved with desk work, work at a computer terminal, work as a tool maker in a machine shop or an assembly line worker in an automobile plant, these are patterns of motion that contribute to their well-being. Some workers within the company have had pain and muscle spasms occasionally to the degree of incapacitation. Use of the patterns in conjunction with a progressive strengthening exercise series for rebalancing posture has led to reduction in pain and enabled many to more comfortably carry out their work responsibilities.

COMPLIANCE

We increase the likelihood for compliance when we offer periodic reinforcement sessions to ensure accuracy and monitor possible need for regimen changes. The medically trained eye will recognize the often subtle substitute patterns that may mask the lack of accuracy. Living comfortably with a chronic condition requires lifelong commitment to protective measures. The patient's perception of his condition will influence his ability to comply with the treatment program. It is desirable for the patient to play an active role in managing his specific needs.

Recognizing that there will be individual variations in need and learning style, the therapist will individualize the treatment plan and educational process and thereby increase chance for optimum compliance. It is often counterproductive to threaten a patient with potential deformity as a means of teaching joint protection principles.

CONCLUSION

Pacing work and leisure activities and choosing intentional, individualized methods of rest before over-fatigue will reward the patient with increased comfort, less fatigue, less stress, and greater endurance.

The therapist is a resource person who is able to help identify specific individual needs and facilitate problem solving. Listening to the patient and establishing support will lead to productive therapy treatment sessions providing individuals with a greater sense of control over their own symptoms. A receptive patient and appropriate timing of therapy services is a positive step forward to minimizing discomfort, pain, and deformity, while gaining protection and endurance for a more comfortable way of life.

BIBLIOGRAPHY

Brand PW: Clinical mechanics of the hand, St Louis, 1985, The CV Mosby Co.

Carter MS: Joint protection program. In Hunter JM and others, editors: Rehabilitation of the hand, ed 2, St. Louis, 1984, The CV Mosby Co.

Cordery JC: Joint protection—a responsibility of the occupational therapist, Am J Occup Ther 19:285, 1965.

Fess EE and Philips CA: Hand splinting principles and methods, ed 2, St Louis, 1987, The CV Mosby Co.

Madden JW and Peacock EE Jr: Studies on the biology of collagen during wound healing: dynamic metabolism of scar collagen and remodeling of dermal wounds, Ann Surg 174:511, 1971.

Madden JW, DeVore G, and Arem AJ: A rational postoperative management program for metacarpophalangeal joint implant arthroplasty, J Hand Surg 2:358, 1977.

Melvin JL: Rheumatic disease: occupational treatment and rehabilitation, ed 2, Philadelphia, 1982, FA Davis Co.

Swanson AB: Flexible implants section arthroplasty in the hand and extremities, St Louis, 1973, The CV Mosby Co.

Swanson AB, DeGroot Swanson G, and Leonard J: Postoperative rehabilitation program for flexible implant arthroplasty of the fingers. American Academy of Orthopaedic Surgeons: Symposium on total joint replacement of the upper extremity, St Louis, 1982, The CV Mosby Co.

73

Postoperative rehabilitation programs in flexible implant arthroplasty of the digits

Alfred B. Swanson, Genevieve de Groot Swanson, Judy Leonard, and Jeanine Boozer

A successful arthroplasty should be stable, mobile, durable, retrievable, and free from pain. The postoperative care and rehabilitation program are of great significance for the quality of the final result of the arthroplasty. Individual variations presented by patients, especially in the "complex hand" problem, demand the greatest mastery of the many factors involved.

The use of flexible materials as an adjunct to resection arthroplasty provides a new and different approach to joint reconstruction—it allows us to take an easier and safer alternative in helping nature build her own new joint system through the resection arthroplasty concept.

FLEXIBLE IMPLANT ARTHROPLASTY: CONCEPTS

The flexible implant resection arthroplasty concept can simply be expressed by the following:

Bone resection + Implant + Encapsulation = New functional joint

The finger joint silicone elastomer intramedullary stemmed implant is a flexible hinge that acts as an internal mold, around which a new capsuloligamentous system develops (Figs. 73-1 and 73-2). One of the most important functions of a flexible implant is to maintain internal alignment and spacing of the reconstructed joint while early motion is started, with the implant acting as a dynamic spacer. Early guided motion is essential in promoting the development of a new, functionally adapted fibrous capsule. That collagen formation and development can be guided is a basic concept to be understood by the surgeons who would undertake arthroplasty procedures. In the early stages of healing, the orientation and tension of the developing capsule are extremely important. In fact, the immediate postoperative positioning and the control of joint movement during the first 6 to 8 weeks after reconstruction by dynamic splinting and therapy are as important as surgery itself. In the postoperative course, the implant continues to act as a dynamic spacer to support the important fibrous capsule and maintain the integrity of the new joint space. We have named this important phenomenon the "encapsulation process."

The stems of the flexible implant are included in the encapsulation process; the fact that the implant is not fixed to the bone increases the life of the implant because forces developed around the implant on flexion and extension movements are not concentrated in one particular area but, rather, are spread over a broader section. The distribution of forces of stabilization of the implant over a broad area

with a low-modulus material (softer than bone) also decreases interface problems because the bone is less likely to react at the juncture with the implant if the forces are within the strain tolerances of the bone. The implant transmits beneficial loads to the cut end of the bone and cortical shaft. The favorable bone remodeling is seen as new bone formation around the implant stems and thickening of cortical bone. Excessive bone resorption and "pencilling" of the cut bone end as often seen after simple resection arthroplasty does not occur (Fig. 73-3).

In finger joint arthroplasty, the encapsulation phenomenon offers further advantages. Early mobilization can and should be started to ensure a greater eventual range of motion to the joint. The implant can find the best position with respect to the axis of rotation of the joint; a rigid implant would not have this advantage. The capsuloligamentous structures around any flexible implant can be reconstructed to improve the stability, alignment, and durability of the implant; revision procedures to further reinforce or release the capsule and ligaments when necessary are easily performed. Because the implant stems are not firmly attached to the bone, replacement of an implant for either fracture

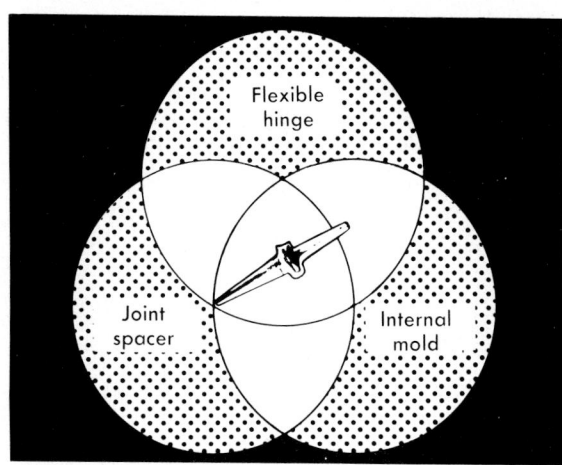

Fig. 73-1 Function of finger joint implant as flexible hinge, internal mold, and joint spacer can be represented in this Venn diagram. Insertion of implant assists nature in development of more predictable and reproducible resection arthroplasty, which has proved to be pain-free, stable, mobile, and durable. (From Swanson AB: Flexible implant resection arthroplasty in the hand and extremities, St Louis, 1973, The CV Mosby Co.)

912

or subluxation is a simple procedure. Furthermore, if a fracture of an implant develops or removal becomes necessary, the joint can continue to function adequately as a simple resection arthroplasty. In case of fracture, the implant continues to function by maintaining the joint and the integrity of the capsular space; in case of implant removal, the implant has fulfilled much of its mission as a spacer to support the development of the capsule-ligament system. If synovitis is present, synovectomy and implant removal or replacement should be considered.

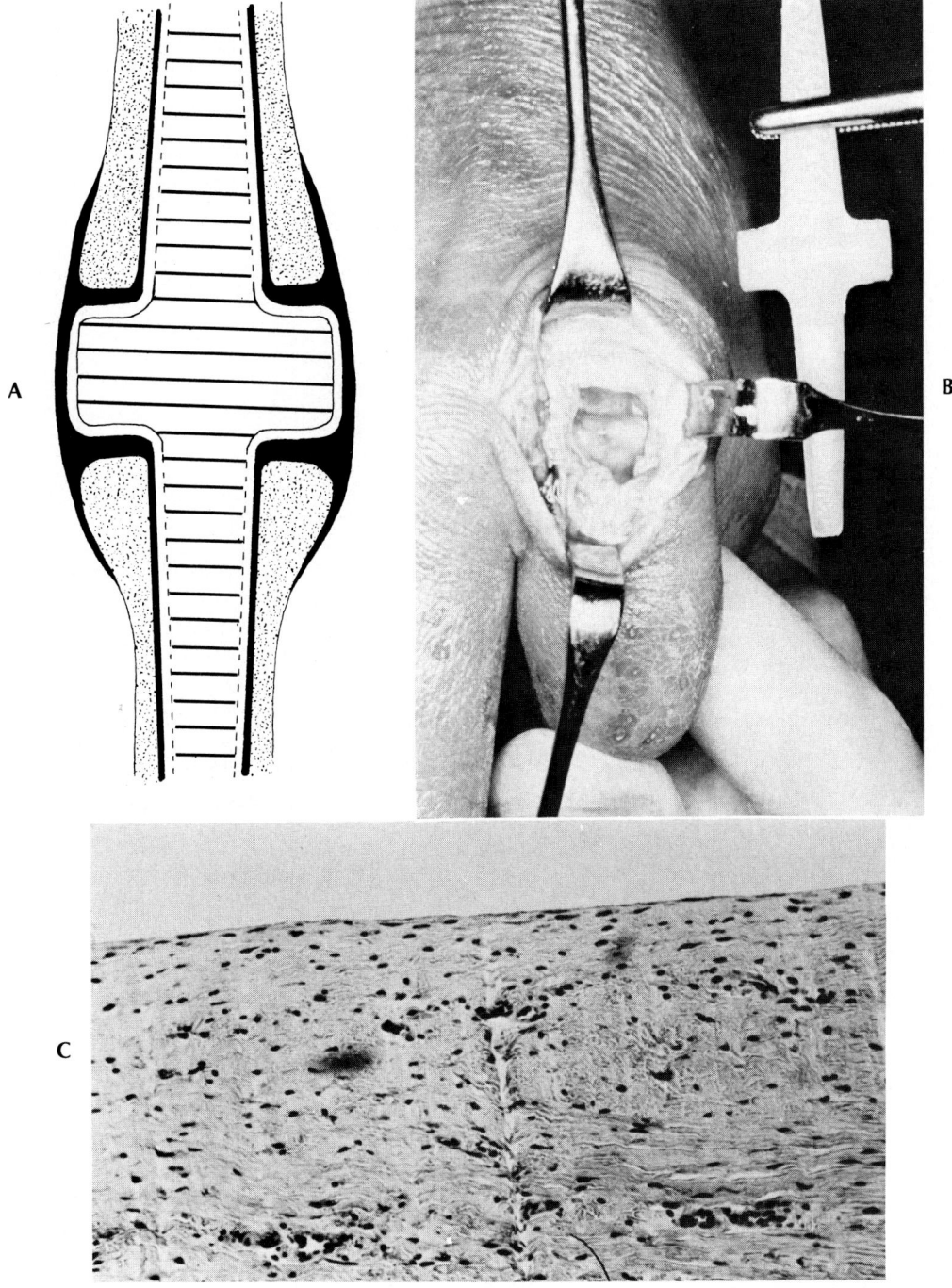

Fig. 73-2 Fixation by encapsulation. **A,** Formation of new capsuloligament system that totally surrounds implant and stabilizes its position. **B,** Implant removed from second metacarpophalangeal joint 1 year postoperatively for purposes of capsulotomy and lipid analysis of implant in prospective research study. Note capsular formation around implant and into intramedullary stems that represents internal mold. **C,** Microscopic sections of capsular specimen in **B** showing organized longitudinal arrangement of collagen fibers, which is not unlike ligament tissue. Single-cell mesothelial lining is noted in upper portion of specimen, which was adjacent to silicone implant. (From Swanson AB: Flexible implant resection arthroplasty in the hand and extremities, St Louis, 1973, The CV Mosby Co.)

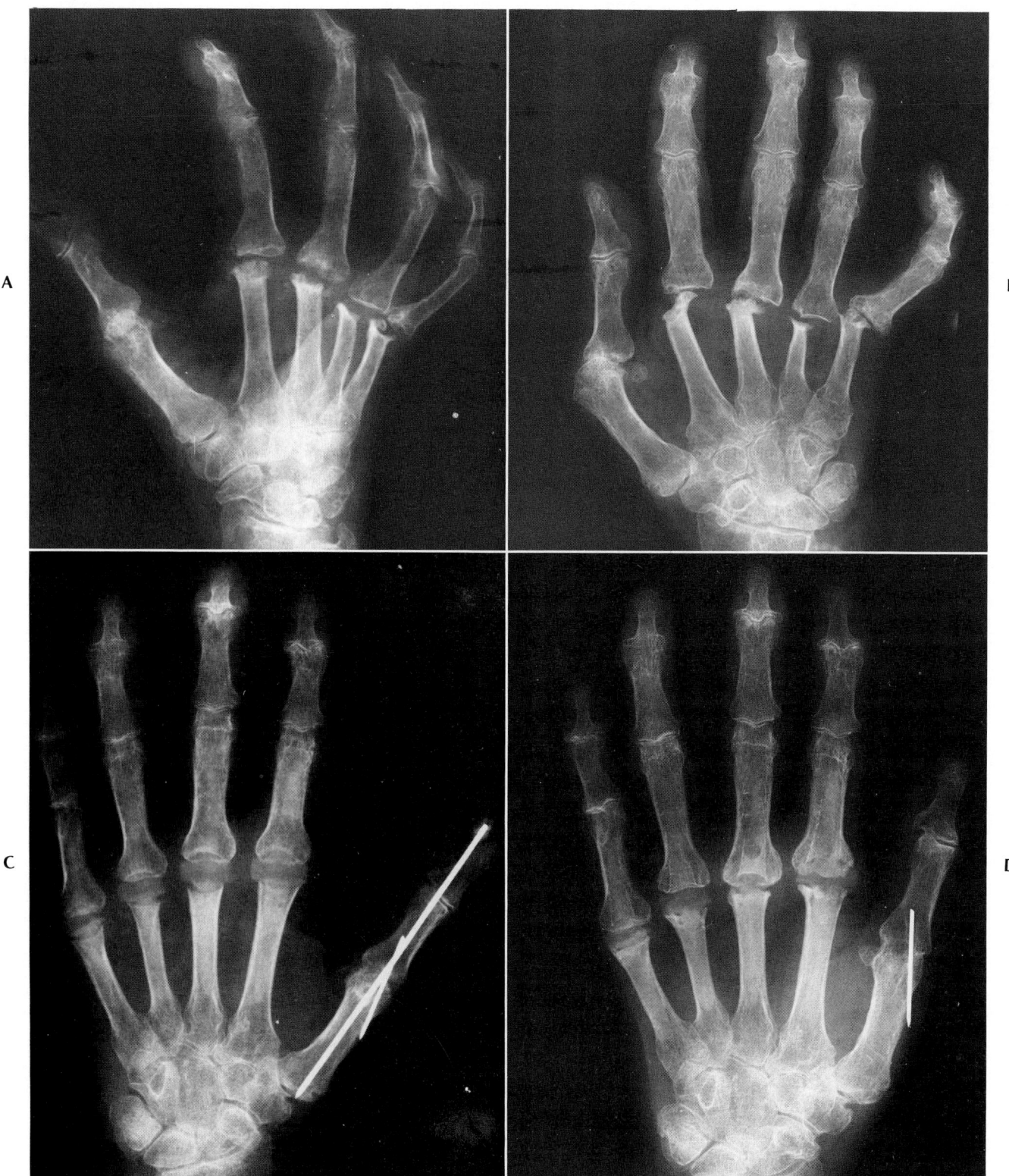

Fig. 73-3 Comparative roentgenograms of right and left hands of rheumatoid arthritic patient soon after surgery and 5 years later. A simple resection arthroplasty was carried out on the right hand. **A,** Roentgenogram of hand taken 6 months after resection arthroplasty of metacarpophalangeal joints of the index, middle, ring, and little fingers. **B,** Roentgenogram showing simple resection arthroplasty 5 years later. Note pronounced remodeling of amputated metacarpal ends. **C,** Early postoperative roentgenogram showing flexible implant arthroplasty of four metacarpophalangeal joints and fusion of thumb metacarpophalangeal joint. **D,** Roentgenogram 5 years after flexible implant resection arthroplasty. Note maintenance of the squared-off appearance of bone ends and the controlled bone remodeling around implant stems. Note fracture of implant of long finger: patient presented no clinical changes. Contour of bone ends has been maintained, as compared with the progressive penciling seen in the opposite hand, because the implant continues to maintain joint space and integrity of capsular structure and bone. (From Swanson AB and Swanson G: Flexible implant resection arthroplasty: A method for reconstruction of small joints in the extremities, the American Academy of Orthopaedic Surgeons Instructional Course Lectures, 27:27, St Louis, 1978, The CV Mosby Co.)

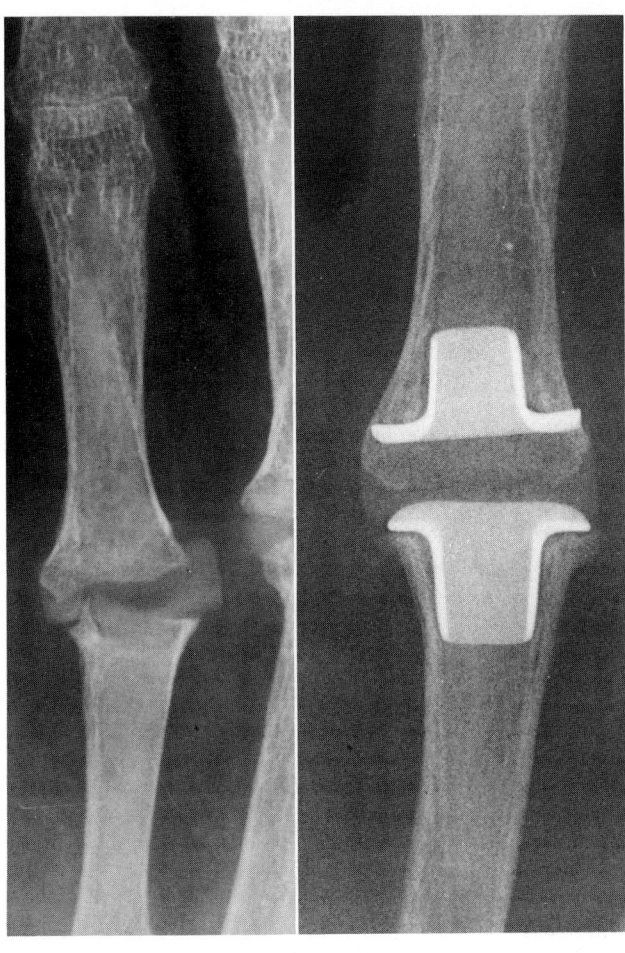

A   B

Fig. 73-4 **A,** Roentgenogram of metacarpophalangeal arthroplasty showing the cutting effect of a sharp metacarpal bone edge into the silicone implant. **B,** Postoperative roentgenogram 24 months after metacarpophalangeal implant arthroplasty using a proximal and distal grommet. Note the increased favorable bone production and remodeling around the grommet.

In 1974 a high performance silicone Elastomer was developed and offered a 400% greater tear propagation resistance over the previous material. However, a 5% incidence of implant breakage of the metacarpophalangeal (MP) and radiocarpal hinges was noted in our clinic. Implant tears are most often initiated by pinching or cutting of the implant by sharp bone edges across a tight subluxating joint or a joint that has become loosened through recurrent synovitis (Fig. 73-4). The tendency for subluxation can be attributed to inadequate surgical correction of the deformity or to increased progression of the synovial disease; this can also be seen when the more proximal joints fall victim to the destructive process resulting in collapse of the longitudinal arch with secondary tendon imbalances distally as seen in the swan-neck deformity. A laboratory, animal, and 3-year human clinical studies for development of bone shielding devices using eight different materials have shown that a titanium metal bone liner (grommet) appears to be most satisfactory. Since 1982 there have been no fractures at 221

distal and 240 proximal hinge sites in 326 MP joints where 461 titanium grommets have been used. Similarly, no fractures occurred at 109 radiocarpal hinge sites protected by a titanium grommet in 58 wrists. Since 1985, 62 grommets have been used in the great toe metatarsophalangeal joint in 30 patients with equally good results. Other recent advances include the development of titanium carpal bone, single stem toe, and radial head implants, and a metal hemiwrist implant.

Because the tissue reaction after surgery alters the physical properties of the host tissues by destroying or replacing their normal structures with scar, an understanding of wound healing reactions and scar formation form the biologic basis for reconstructive surgery of the hand. It seems appropriate in this chapter to review some of the basic concepts of tissue reactions that are so important to achieve a good result.

BIODYNAMICS OF SCAR FORMATION

A general sequence of events occurs after surgery on a joint. Within minutes the wound space is filled with clotted blood, and the components of the acute inflammatory reaction become manifest: white blood cells leave the confines of the vascular walls and accumulate in the wound, fixed tissue macrophages become mobile and active, and a pronounced vasodilatation occurs with accompanying local edema. Injured tissue components and dead cells are removed by phagocytosis. If there has been limited tissue damage, the inflammatory phase is completed quickly.

Within hours of wound closure, the epithelial cells of the basal layer of the skin at the wound edge begin to migrate centrally and completely cover the open surface of the wound within 36 to 48 hours. During the first few days, local cells present within the confines of the wound and identifiable as fibroblasts by their content of large amounts of rough endoplasmic reticulum begin to divide rapidly and migrate into all areas of the wound space. Fibroblasts gradually replace all but a few mononuclear white blood cells.

Although collagen fibers form the bulk of mature scars, fibrils are not apparent microscopically until the fourth or fifth day. Once fibrils begin to form, however, the wound space is rapidly filled with randomly oriented collagen fibers that increase in size and abundance during the first 3 or 4 weeks. Newly synthesized collagen fibers link all portions of the wound within a three-dimensional network of collagen fibers. As the content of scar collagen becomes more abundant, wound cellularity decreases. Fibroblasts, isolated within the collagen network, gradually lose most of their characteristic rough endoplasmic reticulum and become fibrocytes. By the third week, the rate of accumulation of scar collagen is greatly decreased, and the total amount of collagen in the scar becomes stable.

The cohesive forces between the epithelial cells, fibroblasts, and endothelial cells give some strength to the wound during the first few days of healing. These forces, however, are weak, and wounds may be easily disrupted. A rapid gain in tensile strength begins with the appearance of collagen fibrils, and wound strength increases as collagen becomes more abundant. It usually reaches clinical adequacy in 3 weeks.

As noted by Madden and Peacock, early in fibril formation collagen molecules are held together by hydrogen bonds and other weak physical forces. If tension is applied to new aggregates, fibrils are ruptured easily. With time, however, newly formed fibers demonstrate a sharp increase in tensile strength. As fibrils mature, the weak intermolecular forces are supplemented by the formation of covalent bonds, the strongest union between atoms. Ultimately, collagen fibers become giant polymers, each molecule being linked to its neighbor by these strong covalent bonds.

Aggregation and covalent bonding produce a strong flexible fiber that can be woven into many different tissue patterns. The quantity of scar collagen, the anatomic configuration of the fibers, and the density of inter- and intramolecular covalent bonding determine the physical characteristics of the reconstructed joint capsuloligamentous system.

Remodeling of scar tissue

All wounds undergo remarkable changes in color, firmness, and bulk. A well-healed wound 2 months after initial injury bears little resemblance to the same wound 1 year later. The measurable physical properties of incised and sutured wounds regarding strength also change slowly over prolonged periods of time. Collagen gains strength rapidly during the first 3 to 4 weeks but continues to gain strength at a steady rate for 12 months or longer. Alterations in scar architecture are most striking as the scar collagen becomes oriented in parallel bundles. This physical weave of collagen fibrils and the parallel orientation of collagen fibers are the most effective configurations to resist longitudinal stresses.

All the factors that control the morphology of remodeling of scar tissue are not known. Age plays an important role in the remodeling of scars; younger patients tend to remodel scar tissue more rapidly than older ones. The total amount of randomly oriented scar collagen present in a wound also affects remodeling; larger amounts of scar collagen limit effective remodeling. The remodeling changes that occur at a later period may be insufficient to reestablish proper scar morphology if the collagen deposition was too great. For this reason, old previously remodeled scar tissue, present within a new wound, has detrimental effects on the remodeling of the new wound and should be removed during the reconstructive procedure. This is especially important in posttraumatic cases.

Physical forces such as longitudinal stresses and shearing forces acting on the scar-containing area play an important role in the remodeling of collagen tissue. The precise relationship between tension and scar remodeling, however, remains obscure. During the remodeling of bone, electrical field forces generated by deforming tissue play an important role in the organization of collagen fibrils and bony spicules. These same forces may be at work in soft-tissue healing but have not been clearly demonstrated to date. The biologic condition of the tissues at the time of surgery also plays an important role in scar remodeling. There are also significant differences among individuals in their capacity to deposit and remodel collagen.

The deposition and remodeling of collagen around the joint and the implant provide the reconstructed joint with a proper balance of mobility and stability and are of obvious importance to the finger joint reconstruction. The implant acts as an internal mold around which the collagen is deposited and further continues its role in acting as an internal spacer to maintain the integrity of the joint space.

The proper control of scar formation by appropriate rest, protection, and properly applied tension forces during the postoperative period is the basis of the rehabilitation program. It would appear that motion must be started early and continued until the collagen reaction is stabilized. In our experience, early motion must be started within the first week after surgery, and exercises must be continued for at least 3 months in the average patient.

Remodeling of the cut bone end

Bone remodeling occurs from a constant interplay between bone absorption and bone formation. An optimum amount of stress is necessary for production of a satisfactory degree of osteogenesis, which will not occur if the stress is too little or too great. The remodeling of the cut bone ends in an arthroplasty is dependent on both mechanical and biologic considerations. The palmar edge of the sectioned bone end is the most susceptible area. Compression and shear-loading forces, exceeding biologic and mechanical tolerance, will cause bone absorption. The condition of the bone affected by the arthritic process, rough handling and drill burning, fracturing of the bone edges, stripping of the periosteum containing its blood supply, or excessive reaming of its endosteal surface are all important factors that affect the eventual strength of the cut bone end and its resistance to the loads applied to it. Mechanical factors are not solely responsible for bone absorption; biologic factors affected by nutritional and vascular changes are also important in bony response. This especially is true in the active rheumatoid patient.

The following are factors that will help assure a proper remodeling of the bone at the arthroplasty site: (1) correction of subluxating forces to decrease the shear-loading stresses at the interface between the implant and the bone; (2) limiting the amount of flexion at the joint (In our experience, 70 degrees of flexion would appear to be functionally and mechanically ideal. This is especially important if the bone stock is inadequate or too thin.); (3) obtaining more collagen formation around the joint to limit the mechanical stress of increased flexion and also to absorb some of the deforming forces applied to it; (4) appropriate operative technique; (5) the mechanical characteristics of the flexible implant regarding its softness and stress loading; and (6) the proper postoperative care and rehabilitation program. Bone modeling should be carefully evaluated by serial roentgenographic studies in the postoperative period. A long-term study of bone-remodeling phenomena around flexible implants at the MP joint was carried out. This study showed the bone-remodeling process to occur as a newly formed cortical bony shell around the implant stems and thickening of the metacarpal and phalangeal metaphysis. Thickening of the phalangeal midshaft was present. A decrease of the metacarpal midshaft was noted early after surgery and remained permanent; this was related to the surgical reaming. It was concluded that the clinical durability of this procedure was linked in part to the favorable biologic effect of this implant at the bone interface.

Our long-term retrieval studies have shown that the flexible hinge implant arthroplasties have stood up well through the years; the durability of the range of motion, the implant, and the host interface tissue is very good. One of the interesting radiographic observations is the maintenance of

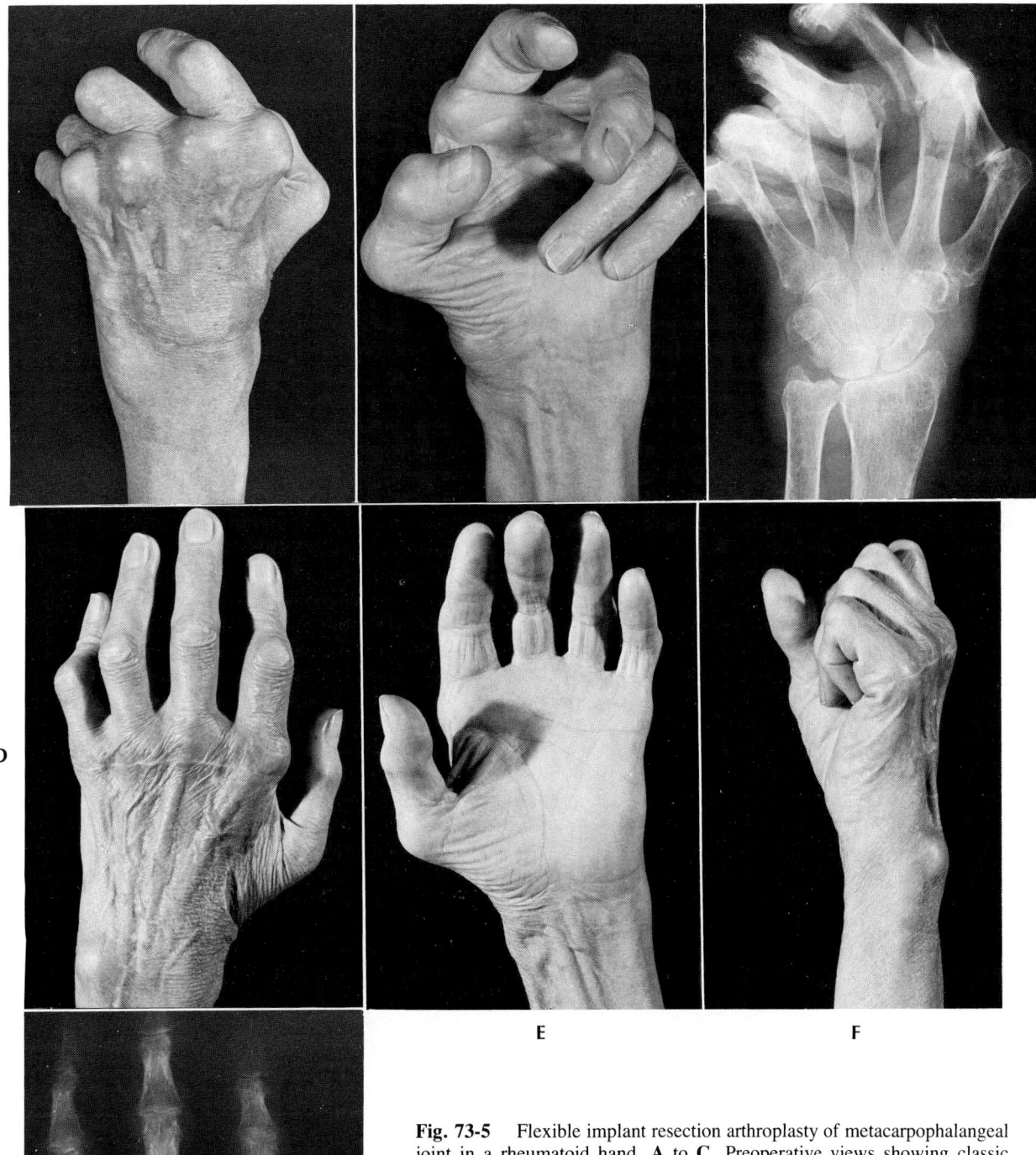

Fig. 73-5 Flexible implant resection arthroplasty of metacarpophalangeal joint in a rheumatoid hand. **A** to **C,** Preoperative views showing classic findings of rheumatoid deformity in hand with severe subluxation of metacarpophalangeal joint, deviation and lack of extension of fingers, ulnar subluxation of extensor tendons, and deformity of thumb. **D** to **G,** Clinical appearance of roentgenogram of same hand 2 years after flexible implant resection arthroplasty of all five metacarpophalangeal joints. Note improved appearance of hand with good correction of deformities. Patient remains pain free and has functional range of flexion and extension.

the shape of the bone where the implant has been used as compared to the simple resection arthroplasty. The implant apparently maintains the anatomic shape of the bone end, and the remodeling process that usually results in shortening and narrowing and spike formation after simple resection arthroplasty does not occur in the presence of the implant.

BASIC OPERATIVE AND EARLY POSTOPERATIVE CONSIDERATIONS

Variations of the arthritic involvement presented by many patients demand special consideration of all factors involved. Reconstructive procedures of weight-bearing joints of the lower extremity that will require walking with crutches should precede upper extremity reconstruction. Ex-

cessive manual labor and awkward hand weight bearing, such as seen in some crutch walkers, should be avoided after surgery. If crutch walking cannot be avoided, a special platform-type of crutches should be used. Multiple reconstructive procedures must be appropriately staged.

In MP joint disabilities associated with severe wrist involvement, the wrist should be treated first. This may involve reconstruction of the distal radioulnar joint, as well as stabilization of the carpal area either by partial fusion, semiconstrained or total wrist implant arthroplasty, or wrist fusion. Tendon repair and synovectomy of tendon sheaths should be done 6 to 8 weeks before joint reconstruction in the rheumatoid hand. However, if the extensor tendons are ruptured and the MP joints are dislocated, arthroplasty of

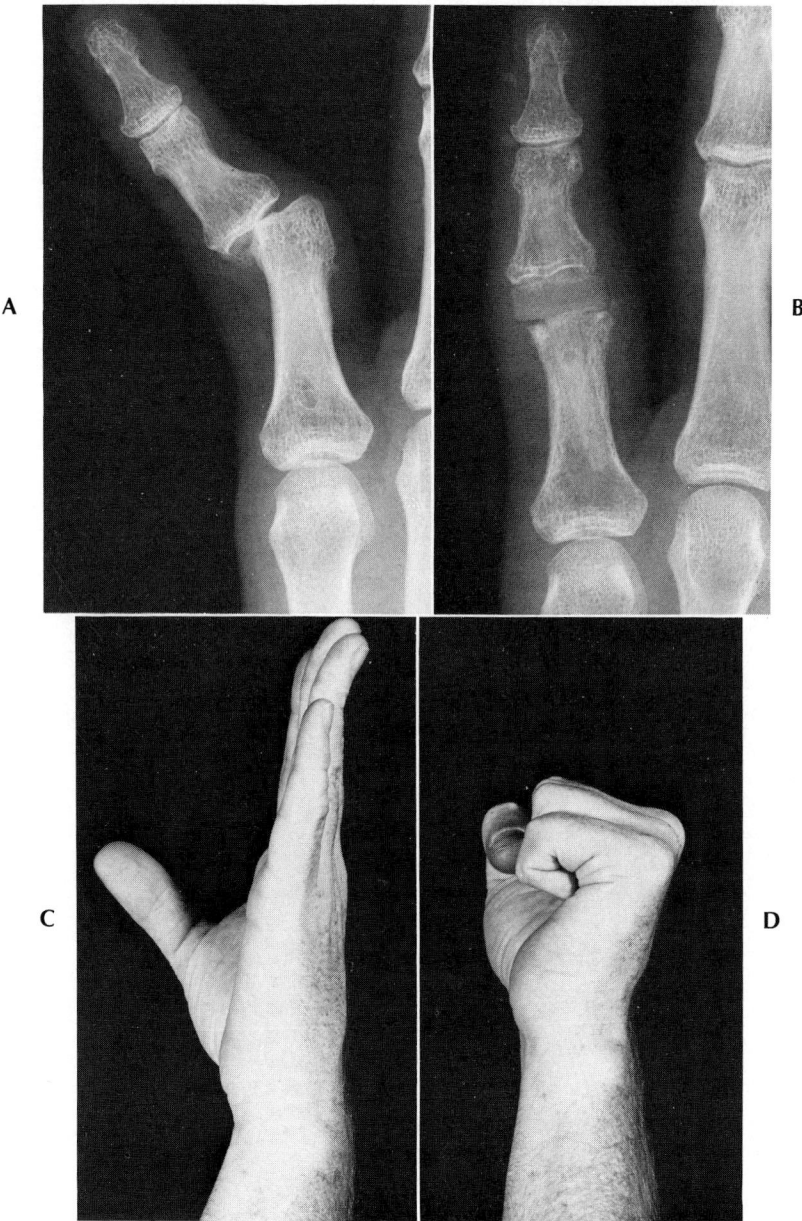

Fig. 73-6 **A,** Long-standing dislocation of proximal interphalangeal joint of little finger in young, athletic male. **B,** Roentgenogram showing excellent position and tolerance of implant 3 years postoperatively. **C** and **D,** Patient recovered full use of his hand with excellent flexion and extension.

the MP joints is done before tendon repair. In swan-neck deformity, arthroplasties of the MP and proximal interphalangeal (PIP) joints are done at the same stage. The use of implants is not recommended for rheumatoid swan-neck deformity. However, in boutonnière deformity, it is preferable to reconstruct the PIP joint before the MP joint. Any tendon imbalance or bone and joint malalignment must be corrected; otherwise, it will affect the long-term result of joint replacement. Precise anatomic dissection, adequate soft-tissue release, respect for gliding surfaces, prevention of edema, and early guided movement in functional planes are essential for good results in arthroplasty procedures (Fig. 73-5).

As noted, wounding of any part of the body results in a vascular reaction and edema. This reaction can result in scar formation, which in turn can cause stiffness. From the early stages of treatment, every measure should be taken to decrease, if not prevent, unnecessary residual stiffness. Stiffness in the hand is in itself a difficult reconstructive problem. Contracture of the elbow and shoulder joints can result in severe loss of function by preventing the hand from being properly positioned in space. Knowledge and strict application of certain basic principles of hand care are therefore essential to avoid these complications. These include proper operative dressing, immobilization in a functional position, postoperative elevation, early motion, and exercises.

Constrictive dressings should be avoided. Proper elevation of the hand and extremity will enhance venous return and decrease the escape of fluids into the interstitial spaces of the injured parts, thus reducing edema. Slings should not be worn when the patient is in the upright position because they may prevent use of the extremity. Early motion is also important to maintain muscle length, reduce edema, prevent ligament contracture, prevent adhesions of tendons and other gliding surfaces, and maintain hand architecture. Motion should be encouraged not only distally but also at the level of the wrist, elbow, and shoulder joints to avoid sympathetic dystrophy and maintain mobility. The rheumatoid patient usually has already some loss of motion and some functional impairment. He should be frequently examined for new loss of mobility of the elbow and shoulder, for even a few degrees of loss of abduction and external rotation may signal an impending shoulder-hand syndrome. Circumduction exercises of the shoulder and active movements of the digits, especially with the hand elevated, if done early and continued throughout the treatment program, will avoid many of the disastrous effects seen in improperly treated patients. Specific exercises for the reconstructed part must follow an organized and supervised regime.

The flexible implant acts as an internal splint that separates the incongruous bone ends; once the released ligaments and scar have healed, they will stabilize the joint in a fashion similar to the function of normal ligaments. As with simple resection arthroplasty, if motion is restricted during the healing phase, there will be poor mobility. The greatest challenge in postoperative rehabilitation of finger joint arthroplasty is to maintain a proper balance between good healing of the surrounding scar tissue and at the same time apply proper amounts of tension across the scar to obtain the desired range of motion. Controlled motion during this period will train the new capsule to have sufficient looseness for flexion and extension and sufficient tightness in the me-

diolateral plane for rotation and angular stability. An adjustable dynamic splint is therefore necessary to guide the motion of the joint in desired planes and to prevent recurrent deformity during the early postoperative course. Scar formation will vary according to the joint involved, the type of surgery performed, and the differences in the collagen reaction in each patient. It is therefore the responsibility of the operating surgeon to control the process by providing a well-organized and preplanned rehabilitation program for his patients. The patients receive specific instructions and are regularly coached through their exercises in the early postoperative period. They are instructed to sit comfortably, to stabilize the proximal joints, including the shoulder, elbow, and wrist, and to concentrate the movement at the reconstructed joints. Using mirrors can be most helpful in assisting the patient's self-evaluation of his degree of movement. Once the sutures are removed, we encourage the patients to precede their exercises with an oil or lanolin massage. The follow-up should be meticulous and include objective measurements of the patient's progress. This is as important to the final result as the surgical procedure. To fail to understand these basic facts is to miss the opportunity of the pleasure of a complete success (Figs. 73-5 and 73-6).

DYNAMIC SPLINT

We have designed a splint (Fig. 73-7) to facilitate early postoperative motion in our patients who have undergone finger joint implant resection arthroplasty. Its use has greatly improved the anatomic and functional results. The splint prevents undue stretching of associated reconstructed tendons and ligaments and also assists the digital extensors and flexors, which are frequently weak because of long-standing deformity, accompanying tenosynovitis, and fibrosis. The dynamic splint has three major functions: (1) to provide complete and adjustable correction of residual deformity; (2) to control motion in the desired plane and range; and (3) to assist flexor and extensor power, ensuring an adequate alternation of complete extension and flexion ranges of movement in the joint.

The basic splint for the finger joint arthroplasty is a dorsal splint that provides a stable base for outriggers and support for the weak or deficient wrist. The splint is available in three basic sizes.* Three transverse straps are attached to the basic dorsal splint and are made of malleable metal to be easily adjusted to the shape and size of the patient's forearm; adjustable Velcro straps are attached to these malleable transverse straps to hold the splint in position. Two Velcro straps are placed around the forearm, and a narrow Velcro strap is placed across the palm; the latter has a palmar pad to help maintain the arches of the hand and prevent rotation of the splint. A transverse bar to which finger slings are attached is fitted onto a dorsal arm. The position of the transverse bar can be adjusted in all three planes. The finger slings are of soft plastic with multiple perforations and are connected to the transverse bar with rubber bands. Short, radially placed outriggers are added for correction of the pronation deformity often present in the index and middle fingers of rheumatoid hands. A longer bar can be used for

---

* Swanson Postoperative Hand Splint, United States Manufacturing Co., Pasadena, Calif.

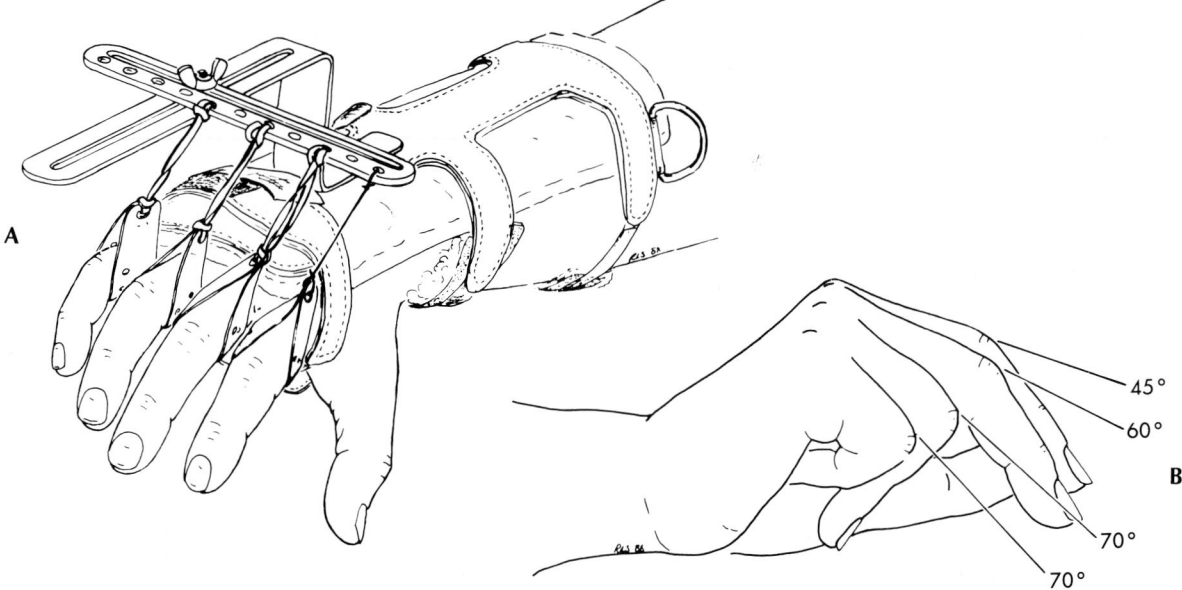

Fig. 73-7   A, Finger slings of dynamic splint are placed on proximal phalanges to assist metacarpophalangeal joint extension and guide alignment of digits. Slings are adjusted to pull from radial side to prevent ulnar deviation. Padding underneath splint with lightweight dressing or a dorsal strip of felt may be necessary. The index finger is supported with a string rather than a rubber band to favor stability over mobility. **B,** Ideal goal of rehabilitation program is to obtain full extension to 70 degrees of flexion at the ring and little fingers, 60 degrees at the middle, and 45 degrees at the index finger. The rubber-band tension may need to be reduced at the little finger to allow 70 degrees of flexion at the metacarpophalangeal joint.

thumb abduction. All of these outriggers are attached with thumb screws.

When weakness of the flexors is present, specific measures must be taken to ensure flexion of the joint through an adequate range of motion. Available devices are discussed later.

METACARPOPHALANGEAL JOINT POSTOPERATIVE PROGRAM
Goals and special considerations

The results of an organized postoperative program for these patients are so much better than those of any other method that all attempts should be made by the surgeon to provide this type of care for his patient. It is extremely useful to have the adjustable dynamic splint available preoperatively for patients undergoing MP joint implant resection arthroplasty to avoid any delay in its application.

The ideal motion to be obtained after implant resection arthroplasty at the MP joints would provide adequate flexion of the ulnar digits, allowing the surface of their pulps to touch the palm at the distal palmar crease for adequate grasp of smaller objects. Full flexion of the index and middle fingers is less critical for grasping because these digits are mainly used for pinch activities. A degree of spreading of the fingers into abduction, especially of the index finger, is important. Full extension at these joints is also important for performance of normal hand activities and maintenance of the balance of the distal joints. Chronic flexion deformity of the MP joints can further aggravate hyperextension tendencies at the PIP joints. Pronation deformity of the index finger and occasionally the middle finger can be a problem

in the rheumatoid hand and can, to some degree, be corrected in the postoperative program.

Patients who have normal PIP joints frequently will not gain the full expected range of motion at the MP joint after arthroplasty because they will rather flex the PIP joint during their exercise program and thus their MP joints will be relatively immobilized. To help localize all flexion forces at the MP joints in these patients, we recommend taping small padded aluminum splints on the dorsum of the PIP joints during exercise periods for the first 3 to 4 weeks after surgery. This seems to improve the range of motion obtained after this surgery. Occasionally, in the presence of associated swan-neck deformity, temporary Kirschner-wire (K-wire) fixation of the PIP joints can also be used for the same functional purpose.

Splint fitting and early postoperative treatment

The voluminous conforming operative hand dressing is left on until the postoperative swelling has decreased, usually in 3 to 5 days. The dynamic splint is applied over a lightly padded dressing after removal of the postoperative dressing. If the splint is not available, one may still obtain guided early motion by applying a lightweight, short arm cast fitted with outriggers and similar rubber band slings.

The dorsal wrist splint with a ¼-inch felt pad placed between the forearm and the splint should be applied loosely enough so that it is not constrictive and yet tightly enough so that it does not rotate on the forearm and hand. If there is a tendency for continued swelling, the splint application is delayed and a bulky conforming dressing is reapplied, taking care to support the wrist in extension with a palmar

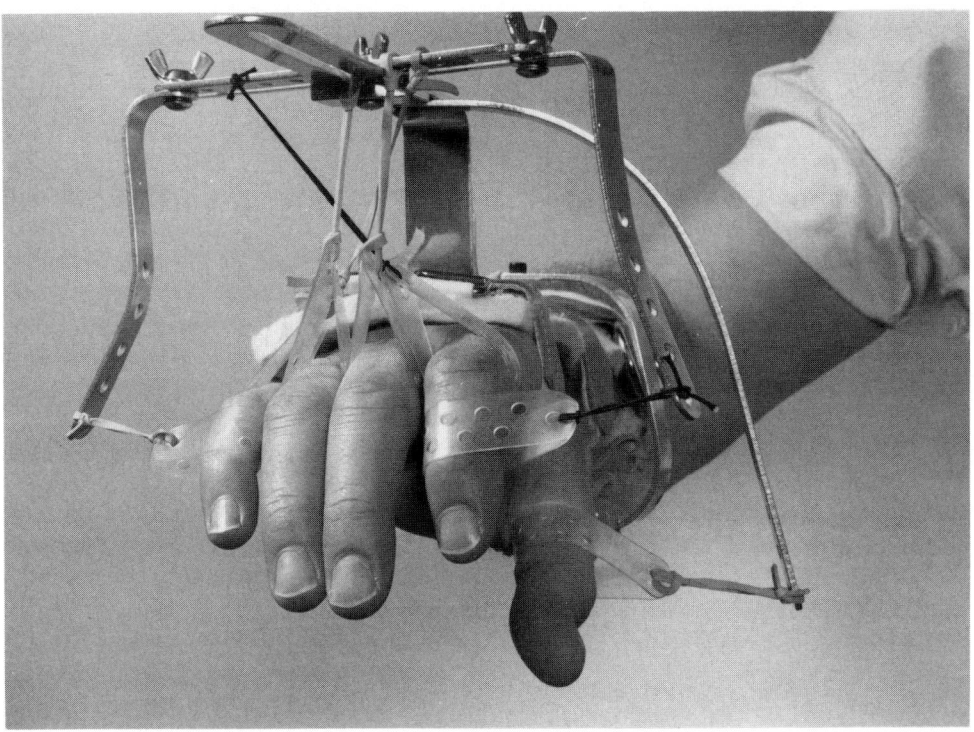

Fig. 73-8   Method of using combined pull of two slings on the index digit to form couple-producing supinatory torque force and limiting range of motion with string during the first 2 to 3 postoperative weeks. This technique can be used to assist in correction of pronation deformity, which is often seen in index and middle fingers in rheumatoid hands. All outriggers are attached for correction of ulnar drift and rotation deformity of index finger, to control abduction of thumb, and to help pronate the little finger.

splint and properly align the digits with gauze strips and tape. The limb is kept elevated and active exercises are carried out in this position.

The slings are placed on the proximal phalanges to guide the alignment of the digits into the desired position. The pull of the slings in the radial direction will require adjustment to prevent recurrent ulnar drift. The tension of the rubber bands should be tight enough to support the digits and yet loose enough to allow 70 degrees of active flexion; this is especially true of the little and ring fingers, which may have weaker flexion power (Fig. 73-7).

Because greater stability than mobility is preferred for the index and middle fingers, a nonelastic material (such as a braided dacron fishing line) is usually substituted for the rubber band at the level of the index finger and occasionally at the middle finger. This static arrangement is often maintained for the first 2 to 3 postoperative weeks. The use of a string for the index and occasionally the middle finger favors stability over mobility of these digits. Rubber bands replace the strings when active range of motion is initiated. The splint may require adjustment once or twice a day in the early postoperative course.

The thumb outrigger may be applied in cases where the patient has a tendency to bring the thumb over to the fingers on flexion. This movement should be avoided because the pressure applied by the thumb to the index finger would be in the ulnar direction, thus aggravating the tendency toward ulnar drift deformity.

If there is a tendency toward medial rotation (pronation)

in the index or middle fingers, additional outrigger bars are applied to provide a rotation force at the MP joint according to the concept of a force couple; a force couple is defined as two equal and opposite forces that act along parallel lines, and it is obtained by applying the loops to the digit that shows a tendency for pronation, as shown in Fig. 73-8. A string is fitted from an additional outrigger to the distal phalanx of the digit showing a pronation tendency. This combined pull of two slings forms a coupling that produces a torque force in the direction of supination on the digit.

The extension portion of the splint is worn continuously day and night for the first 4 to 6 weeks, alternating with specific flexion measures as required and discussed later.

For the middle, ring, and little fingers, the flexion exercises in the splint with the extension slings in position are carried out, starting at 3 days postoperatively, both actively and passively (with no more than 2 pounds of force) on an hourly basis (Fig. 73-9). The ideal goal of 0 degrees of extension to 70 degrees of flexion is constantly stressed at the ring and little fingers. The patient is seen at least three times by the physician or the therapist during the first week, and the splint is carefully readjusted as necessary. Only exceptionally, if there is considerable flexor weakness of the little finger with adequate extensor stability, can the extension sling be removed from this digit during the exercise periods.

During the second and third weeks, the extension portion of the splint is also worn continuously day and night. If there is active flexor weakness and good extension, the

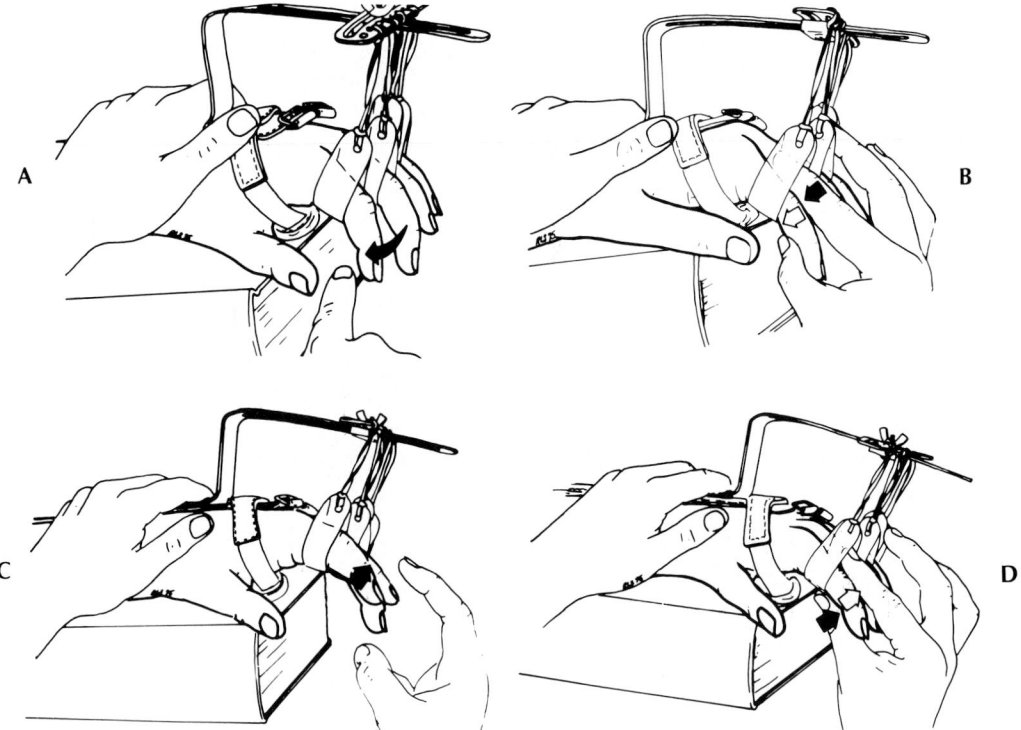

Fig. 73-9 Flexion-extension exercises for metacarpophalangeal joint. **A** and **B,** Active and passive flexion exercises are carried out in the splint starting at 3 days postoperatively. No more than 2 pounds of force should be applied to assist passive flexion. Arm is positioned on a firm surface to help stabilize proximal joints and allow movement of digits. Proper adjustment of the tension of rubber bands is essential to allow full range of motion. Extension portion of splint is worn continuously for the first 3 weeks. **C** and **D,** Active and passive extension exercises are carried out in the splint.

extensor slings can be removed during active range-of-motion (ROM) exercises to achieve greater active flexion of the MP joints of the little and ring fingers. If the patient appears not to be obtaining 70 degrees of flexion, several measures can be taken. Should most of the motion be occurring at the PIP joints, these may be splinted in extension as previously described (p. 920), to help localize the flexion force at the MP joints. The rubber bands may be lengthened to decrease the extension force applied.

At 3 weeks any residual flexor weakness should be energetically treated. The flexion outrigger may be used 3 to 5 times a day for 20 to 30 minutes (Fig. 73-10) to flex

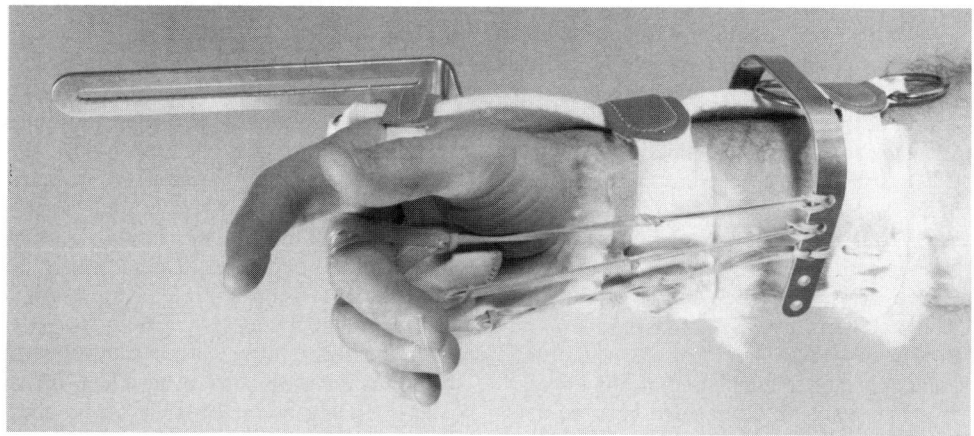

Fig. 73-10 A flexion outrigger is attached as shown to passively flex the metacarpophalangeal joints of the lateral three fingers. The flexion slings can be applied three to five times daily for 20 to 30 minutes and are alternated with the extension portion of the splint.

passively the MP joints in conjunction with active flexion exercises. A figure-of-eight elbow strap may be applied to prevent distal migration of the splint. This method is especially useful and can be started during the early postoperative course in certain cases presenting severe preoperative stiffness or flexor weakness with adequate extensor mechanism. In these difficult cases one can reach a functional compromise by sacrificing a few degrees of extension. Because the index finger requires greater stability than mobility, it is usually not included in this passive flexion arrangement.

The extension portion of the splint is usually worn at night only, starting on the sixth postoperative week for at least another 3 weeks. In a few cases where there is a persistent extensor lag or a tendency for flexion contracture or deviation of the digits, continued part-time day support by use of the splint must be prescribed for several more weeks or even months. The patient should follow a continued exercise program for 3 months postoperatively to maintain the movement obtained in the earlier phase. After this time the final range of motion will have been established.

Collagen maturity and scar contracture vary from patient to patient. The associated tendon deficiencies also vary; therefore the use of the splint in the postoperative period requires tailoring and careful follow-up by the operating surgeon or therapist, or both. The patient's progress is evaluated by measurement of the range of motion with accurate goniometer readings; one observes the movements of the digits without the splint to be sure that the patient is getting the desired result. The reconstructed joints start tightening up during the second postoperative week and will be quite tight by the end of 3 weeks. If the desired range of motion has not been obtained by 3 weeks, it will be difficult to gain further improvement in motion.

THUMB METACARPOPHALANGEAL JOINT

Postoperative care for the thumb MP joint implant arthroplasty differs from that previously described. The goal of this procedure is to obtain adequate stability with limited motion ranging from approximately −10 degrees of extension to 25 degrees of flexion.

At the time of surgery a 0.045-inch K-wire is carefully passed longitudinally through the fingertip into the flexor tendon sheath for temporary internal fixation of the distal and MP joints; this wire is left in place for 2 to 3 days or until the postoperative swelling has sufficiently decreased to allow circumferential bandaging of an external splint. At that time a padded aluminum splint extending distally to the end of the thumb and proximally to the wrist is taped dorsally for 4 to 6 weeks (Fig. 73-11). No special exercises are prescribed after splint removal except normal functional adaptations. Forceful activities should be avoided for 6 to 8 weeks postoperatively.

PROXIMAL INTERPHALANGEAL JOINT POSTOPERATIVE PROGRAM

The type of postoperative care for the PIP joint varies with the preoperative deformity and the surgical reconstruction. There are four basic situations: (1) reconstruction of a stiff PIP joint, (2) reconstruction of a PIP joint with lateral deviation, (3) reconstruction of a swan-neck deformity, and (4) reconstruction of a boutonnière deformity.

When the implant arthroplasty has been performed for a *stiff PIP joint*, active movements of flexion and extension may be started within 3 to 5 days after surgery in posttraumatic cases having good soft tissue structures. The ideal range of motion after this surgery is 0 degrees of extension to 70 degrees of flexion at the ring and little fingers, 60 degrees of flexion at the middle finger, and 45 degrees of flexion at the index finger. Small, padded aluminum splints, or splints made of a low-temperature plastic, are used to hold the finger in extension between the hourly exercise sessions. These splints are worn for at least 6 weeks postoperatively depending on the degree of extension lag present and are often worn at night for at least 3 months after surgery (Fig. 73-12, *A*). Active flexion and extension exercises can be performed with a variety of exercise devices such as those described later in this chapter. Resistive flexion exercises using the Grip-X (a "finger-gripper" exercise device) to support proper alignment of the digits are started 6 weeks after surgery. If one needs to do so, the DIP joint may be temporarily pinned with a K-wire to concentrate the action of the flexor profundus at the PIP joint. There are almost always a few degrees of extension lag in these types of cases.

Implant arthroplasty of a laterally deviated PIP joint requires reconstruction of the central slip and collateral ligament(s). The soft tissue reconstruction is protected with an extension splint for at least 2 to 3 weeks. The splint can be applied slightly laterally to correct any residual deformity (Fig. 73-12, *B*). When active ROM exercises are started, they are carried out while wearing a protective device such as a buddy-system strap or a radial outrigger (Fig. 73-12, *C* and *D*). Active exercises are carried out 3 to 5 times a day, and the static splint is worn between the exercise sessions for at least 6 to 8 weeks. Night splinting is continued for at least 3 to 6 months.

Implant arthroplasty of the PIP joint is rarely indicated for rheumatoid arthritic swan-neck deformities.

If the implant resection arthroplasty has been done for a *swan-neck deformity* in association with a tendon recon-

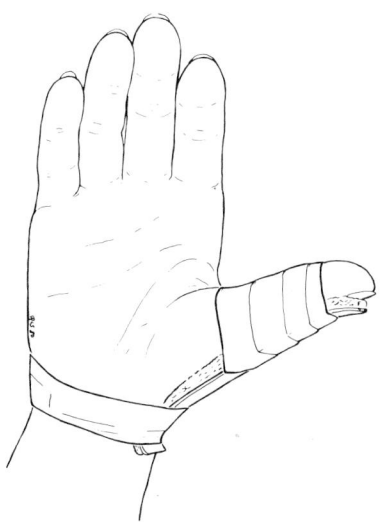

Fig. 73-11 Dorsal thumb-extension splint extending distally to end of thumb and proximally to wrist.

struction procedure, a padded, taped-on aluminum splint is usually placed on the digit after the postoperative edema has subsided. The joint is immobilized in 30 to 40 degrees of flexion, and the splint is left on for 2 to 3 weeks until the exercises are begun. When the active exercises are started, they are carried out while wearing a blocking splint to prevent hyperextension of the joint for 6 weeks after surgery (Fig. 73-12, *E*). It is important to obtain at least 20 degrees of flexion contracture of these joints to prevent recurrent hyperextension tendencies. Unless the central slip has been released, there may be an imbalance of the joint in favor of extension. To obtain adequate correction of the swan-neck deformity, one must not let the distal interphalangeal (DIP) joint remain in too great a flexion, and this

may require pinning in 0 degrees of extension. Resistive exercises using the Grip-X to maintain proper finger alignment during flexion are started at 6 weeks. Night splinting is continued for 4 to 6 months as necessary.

If implant resection arthroplasty has been done to correct a *boutonnière deformity,* it is important to maintain the extension of the PIP joint and to allow flexion of the DIP joint (Fig. 73-12, *F*). The reconstruction of the extensor mechanism should be protected with an extension splint applied after the postoperative swelling has decreased. The splint, in this situation, should immobilize only the PIP joint in extension; the distal joint should be allowed to flex freely. Active flexion and extension exercises are usually started 2 to 3 weeks after surgery. The extension splint is worn be-

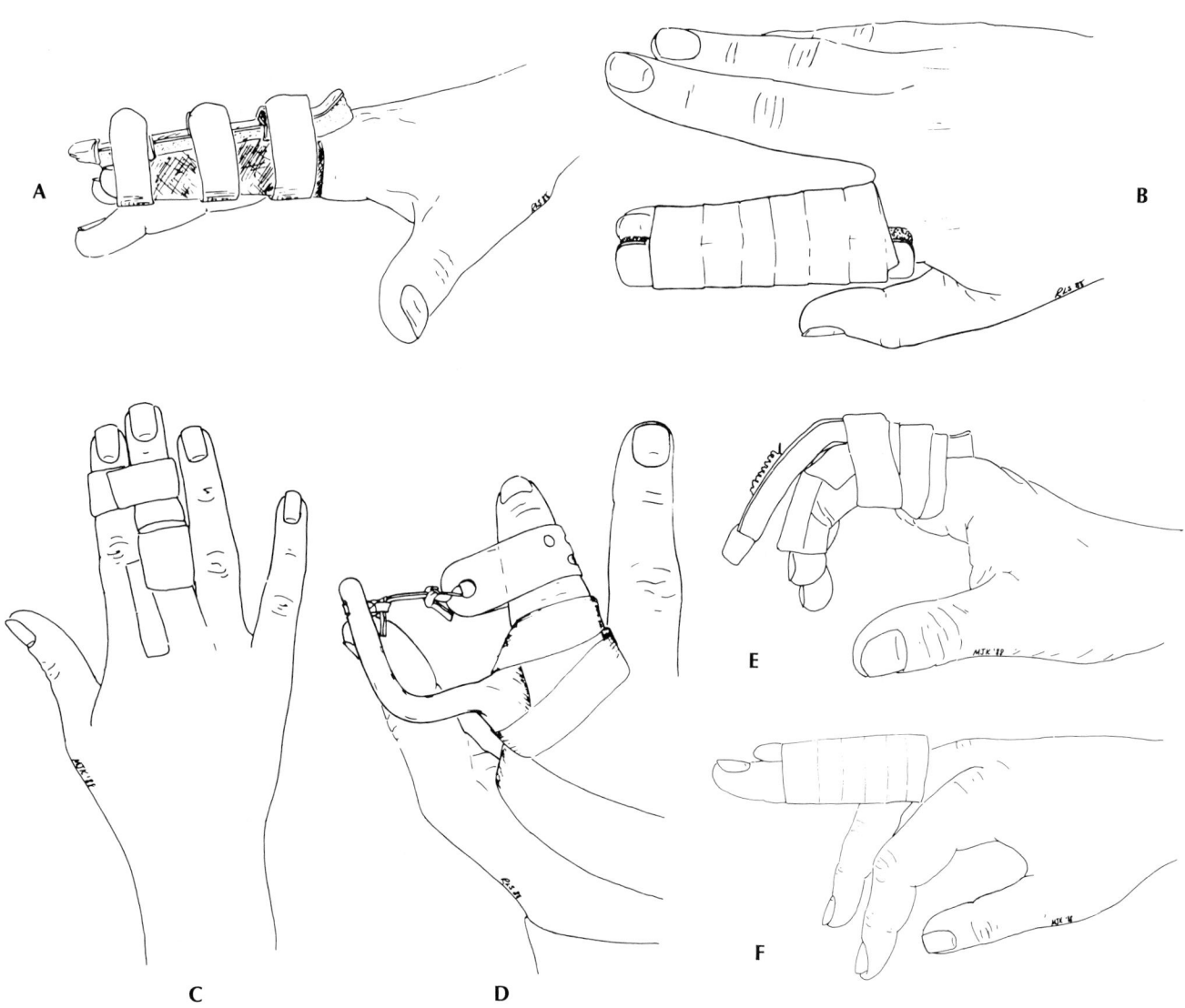

Fig. 73-12   **A,** Small padded aluminum splints or splints fabricated from low-temperature plastics hold the digit in extension between exercise sessions. The splints are secured with Velcro straps. **B,** The splint is applied laterally in digits that demonstrate any associated deviation. **C,** The buddy system protects digit alignment and provides a slight extension assist during active range-of-motion exercises. **D,** A radial outrigger for protecting the index digit alignment and providing a slight extension assist during active range-of-motion exercises. **E,** A blocking splint to prevent full extension yet allow flexion following reconstruction of the swan-neck deformity. **F,** If the implant resection arthroplasty has been done to correct a boutonnière deformity, the splint should allow active flexion of the distal interphalangeal joint.

tween exercise sessions and at night for at least 6 to 8 weeks after surgery to hold the PIP joint in extension until its position is stable. Resistive exercises are started at 6 weeks. Night splinting is continued for at least 3 to 6 months. There is almost always a few degrees of extension lag in these cases.

A K-wire passed into the flexor sheath through the fingertip can be used as a temporary internal splint for immobilization of either the DIP or PIP joints. A 0.035-inch wire is very carefully passed into the flexor sheath through the fingertip distally to proximally; the wire should touch the palmar aspect of the proximal end of the proximal phalanx and is left in place for several days or until the postoperative swelling has decreased sufficiently so that splints with circumferential bandaging can be used.

Exercises for the PIP joint can be carried out actively and passively, with care always being taken to support the MP joint in extension. This can be done with the opposite hand,

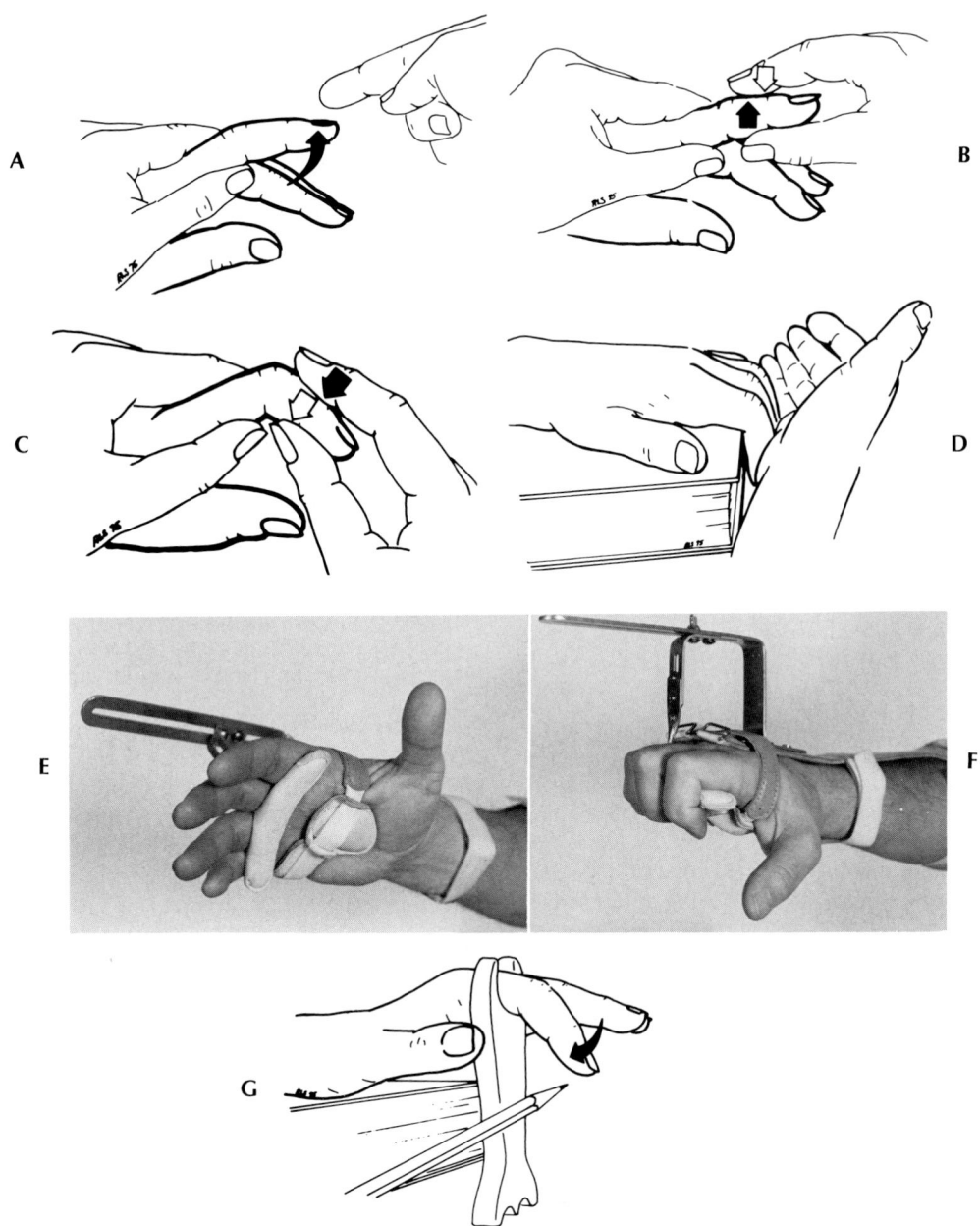

Fig. 73-13   Flexion and extension exercises for proximal interphalangeal joint. **A** and **B,** Active and passive extension exercises are carried out while stabilizing the proximal phalanx. **C** and **D,** Passive flexion exercises can be carried out with the opposite hand while the proximal phalanx is stabilized either over the edge of a book or by an assistant. **E,** A reverse lumbrical bar can be used to support proximal phalanges and eliminate motion of metacarpophalangeal joints during flexion exercises. Note palmar pad used to maintain transverse arches of hand and help prevent rotation of brace. **F,** Flexion of proximal interphalangeal joints over reverse lumbrical bar. Flexion slings attached to the flexion outrigger can be applied to gently encourage flexion if it appears to be necessary. **G,** We designed "finger crutch" to help support the proximal phalanx in extension during flexion exercises.

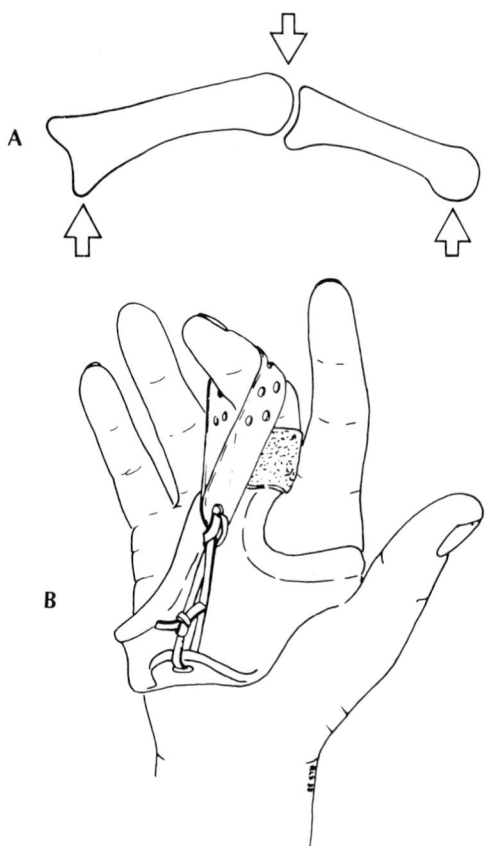

Fig. 73-14 **A,** Passive stretching of joint requires use of three-point principle of pressure application. **B,** A method of obtaining passive flexion of proximal interphalangeal joints after arthroplasty. Splint provides support to proximal phalanx and limits motions of metacarpophalangeal joint.

over the edge of a book, or with a variety of orthotic devices (Fig. 73-13). Extension of the MP joints can be supported with the reverse lumbrical bar attached to the dynamic splint or to a special hand splint. Passive flexion at the PIP joints can be obtained with gentle rubber band traction from a PIP flexion splint (Fig. 73-14, *A* and *B*). One can carry out passive stretching of flexion contractures of the PIP joint by blocking hyperextension of the MP joint with the lumbrical bar and applying extension force to the middle phalanx with the extension rubber band slings of the dynamic splint. We have developed a small finger crutch that we have used in a similar fashion to the Bunnell wood block to support the proximal phalanx during exercises; this is made of ¼-inch plywood or hard rubber material (Fig. 73-13, *G*).

DISTAL INTERPHALANGEAL JOINT POSTOPERATIVE PROGRAM

Treatment of the DIP joint must be considered in reconstructive procedures of the PIP joint, especially if it is deformed. In reconstruction of a stiff PIP joint, the DIP joint may be temporarily pinned with a K-wire to concentrate the action of the flexor profundus at the PIP joint. These pins can be removed after approximately 3 weeks.

In reconstruction of a swan-neck deformity, the DIP joint

may also be temporarily pinned in a neutral position if a severe flexion deformity of the joint is present. This will localize the flexion forces at the PIP joint and help the recovery of movement.

In the reconstruction of a boutonnière deformity, one should release the DIP joint, if in severe hyperextension, by sectioning the lateral tendons over the middle phalanx or by relatively lengthening the lateral tendons. Flexion exercises specifically located at this joint are important to recover movement of this joint and also to help correct the imbalance of the PIP joint.

POSTOPERATIVE PROGRAM FOR COMBINED PROCEDURES

Patients who present a "complex hand" show involvement at multiple joint levels. Knowledge of hand function and of surgical principles is essential for selection of the proper timing of surgical procedures. As a rule, the proximal joints are given priority in the surgical and rehabilitation program. In combined involvement of the MP and PIP joints of the same digit, the MP joint should receive priority. However, the goals and principles of each reconstructive method at each specific level are always respected so that a balance of functional motion is obtained.

If two different involvement levels are presented in separate digits of the same hand, the above principles apply as described in the following example: MP joint reconstruction of the index and long fingers and PIP joint reconstruction of the ring and small fingers for boutonnière deformities. The described protocol for MP joint arthroplasty is followed for the index and long fingers; the described postoperative protocol for a boutonnière deformity is followed for the ring and small fingers. In this case, however, we would favor including the ring and small fingers in the slings of the dynamic splint to provide a balanced tension within the hand.

If reconstruction of the MP and PIP joints of the same digit is carried out at the same seating, the described postoperative program for each level and specific deformity is followed, giving priority to the MP joint.

In all cases and even more so in these complex cases, it is critical that oral and written instructions be given clearly and that the patient understands his responsibility.

OTHER MODALITIES OF POSTOPERATIVE TREATMENT

General physical and occupational therapy modalities should be considered in most patients; however, if such modalities are not available, most patients can be managed by the surgeon.

Some simple heat applications may be of benefit in the postoperative course after complete wound healing. We occasionally will use paraffin or contrast baths for their heating and analgesic benefits. The methods for these baths are described in the following.

Paraffin bath for the hands

This bath requires four cartons of paraffin and one 10-ounce bottle of baby oil.
1. Put these materials in a large can or double boiler. Heat slowly to melting point, approximately 100 to 110° F.

2. Dip hand in quickly to 2 inches beyond the wrist, keeping hand over can; repeat 12 times or until ¼ inch of wax remains on hand.
3. Wrap the paraffin-covered hand for 15 minutes in plastic and a large bath towel. Exercise fingers with wax on. Keep the hand elevated.
4. Remove paraffin by stripping it off while holding the hand over the can.
5. Massage and exercise warm fingers with the hand elevated.

This bath may be repeated two or three times a day. There should be no open wounds or unusual swelling of tissue or skin reaction.

Contrast bath for the hands

1. Sit at the side of a sink that has a mixing faucet to regulate hot and cold water.
2. Fill one basin with water at 55 to 65° F and a second basin with water at 100 to 110° F.
3. Active flexion and extension exercises of the fingers are carried out with the hands under the water.
4. The hot water should be used first for 10 minutes; switch to cold water for 1 minute, hot water for 4 minutes, cold water for 1 minute, hot water for 4 minutes.
5. The hands are then dried and hand lotion is rubbed into the skin.

Active exercises

The patient may increase the range of motion and the strength of the reconstructed joints through a variety of exercises over devices such as the Bunnel block or modifications thereof, cylinders of progressive sizes, or a variety of special hand-exercise devices that are commercially available. These devices should maintain the architecture of the hand and should not force the digits into deforming positions (Fig. 73-15). To be efficient, they must support the bone proximal to the reconstructed joint to obtain the best mechanical advantage; with these goals in mind, we devised a "finger-gripper" exercise device (Grip-X). Isotonic movements in which joint movement accompanies the exercise effort are important for the gliding mechanism of the joint. Isometric exercises, as in grasping around a solid object or the Grip-X, are especially good for muscle strengthening. Resistive exercises using the Grip-X are usually started 6 weeks after surgery. However, close communication be-

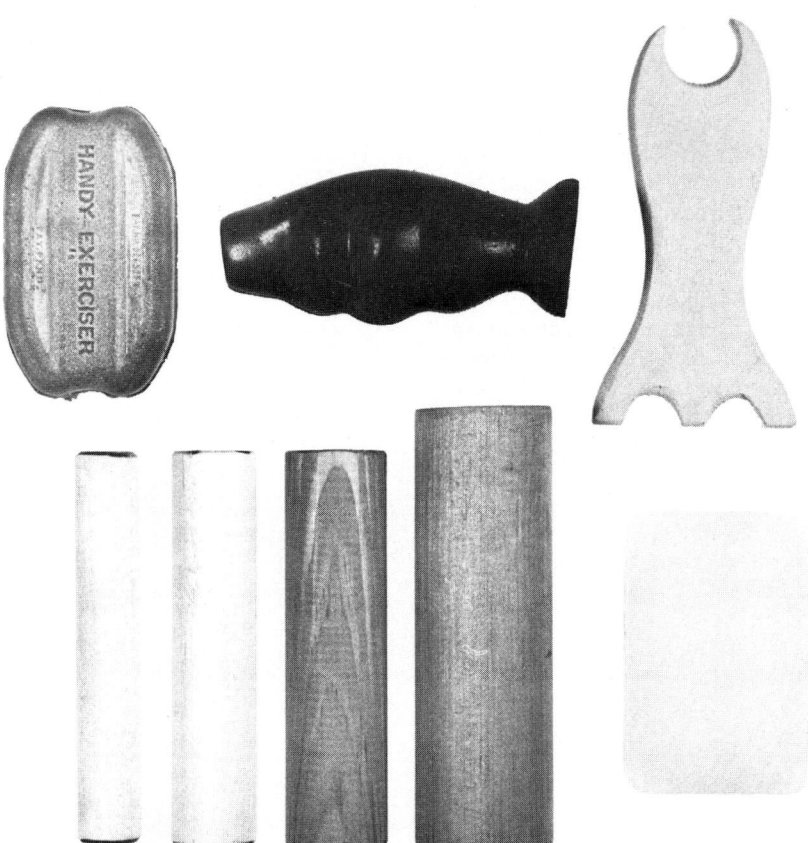

Fig. 73-15   Variety of exercise devices used to increase joint range of motion and strength. *Top (left to right),* Rubber modified Bunnel block; "finger gripper" shaped to maintain proper anatomic position of digits and arches of hand; "finger crutch" designed to help support proximal phalanx during flexion exercises of proximal interphalangeal joint. *Bottom (left to right),* Progressively sized wooden dowels; plastic modified Bunnel block.

tween the therapist and surgeon is required to properly evaluate individual needs and progress for each patient. The use of progressively smaller objects to grasp, such as various sizes of wood dowels, is also a good way of obtaining an improved range of motion.

It is advisable for the patient to use his hand protectively during the early postoperative phase. The postoperative rehabilitation program must be continued for at least 3 months after surgery because of the tendency of these previously stiffened joints to tighten up. It is best to discontinue the exercises gradually, rather than abruptly, and it is wise to follow a weekly self-evaluation of the range of motion. After this, the patient can safely use his hand for activities of daily living and vocational skills. However, the patient should continue to exercise and splint as necessary for at least 1 year after surgery.

A very cooperative patient following a good rehabilitation program can obtain an excellent range of motion using the implant resection arthroplasty method.

Stretching of contractures

Most contractures around joints can be progressively stretched by application of splints or plaster casts, which slowly elongate the tissues without causing the secondary reactions after overzealous movements that tear the collagen. If bone adhesions are not involved in the contracture, diligent stretching by repeated applications of splints can be of benefit.

Manipulation

Manipulation of joints to correct contracture deformities is usually not indicated. Gentle progressive stretching is preferred. Occasionally, if the contracture has not been long established, gentle manipulation of the joint with or without anesthesia may achieve better positioning of the joint. We have used this technique very infrequently in our practice. If a manipulation is done, temporary fixation in the corrected position is usually indicated.

Rehabilitation techniques are highly individualized with each reconstructive surgeon. A physical, occupational, or hand therapist and other trained personnel, when available, can be of valuable assistance in carrying out postoperative therapy programs. However, close communication between the therapist and surgeon is required to properly evaluate individual needs and progress for each patient. An understanding of the basic concepts of the flexible implant resection arthroplasty and the development of good rapport with the patient can allow the operating surgeon to obtain ideal results from this method.

BIBLIOGRAPHY

Madden JW and Peacock EE Jr: Studies on the biology of collagen during wound healing: dynamic metabolism of scar collagen and remodeling of dermal wounds, Ann Surg 174:511, 1971.

Madden JW, Arem A, and DeVore G: A rational postoperative management program for metacarpophalangeal implant arthroplasty, J Hand Surg 2(5):358, 1977.

Swanson AB: A flexible implant for replacement of arthritic or destroyed joints in the hand, NYU Interclin Inform Bull 6:16, 1966.

Swanson AB: Flexible implant resection arthroplasty in the hand and extremities, St Louis, 1973, The CV Mosby Co.

Swanson AB: Flexible implant arthroplasty in the hand, Clin Plast Surg 3:141, 1976.

Swanson AB: A grommet bone liner for flexible implant arthroplasty, Bull Prosthet Res Rehabil Eng Res Devel BPR10-35 1:108, 1981.

Swanson AB: Bone remodeling phenomena in flexible (silicone) implant arthroplasty in the metacarpophalangeal joints—long-term study, Orthop 205:254, 1986.

Swanson AB and de Groot Swanson G: Bone remodeling phenomena in flexible (silicone) implant arthroplasty in the hand: long-term study, Kappa Delta Award Lecture, forty-ninth annual meeting of Orthopaedic Surgeons, New Orleans, Jan 21-26, 1982, Orthop Rev 11(7):129, 1982.

Swanson AB and de Groot Swanson G: Joint replacement in the rheumatoid metacarpophalangeal joint. In Inglis A, editor: Symposium on total joint replacement of the upper extremity, American Academy of Orthopaedic Surgeons, St Louis, 1982, The CV Mosby Co.

Swanson AB, de Groot Swanson G, and Leonard J: Postoperative rehabilitation program for flexible implant arthroplasty of the fingers. In Inglis A, editor: Symposium on total joint replacement of the upper extremity, American Academy of Orthopaedic Surgeons, St Louis, 1982, The CV Mosby Co.

Swanson AB and de Groot Swanson G: Osteoarthritis in the hand, J Hand Surg 8(Part 2):669, 1983.

Swanson AB and de Groot Swanson G: Flexible implant arthroplasty in the rheumatoid metacarpophalangeal joint, Clin Rheum Dis 10:609, 1984.

Swanson AB and de Groot Swanson G: The complex hand—treatment considerations and priorities of finger deformities, Rheumatology 11:6, 1987.

Swanson AB and others: Long-term review of flexible implant arthroplasty in the proximal interphalangeal joint of the hand, J Hand Surg 10A:796, 1985.

Swanson AB and Netter FH: Reconstructive surgery in the arthritic hand and foot, Ciba Clin Symp 31(6), 1979.

Swanson AB, de Groot Swanson G, and Winfield DL: The pronated index finger deformity in the rheumatoid hand, Bull Hosp Joint Dis 44:498, 1984.

74

The rheumatoid thumb

Edward A. Nalebuff and Cynthia A. Philips

The bad news is that rheumatoid arthritis frequently involves the all-important thumb, resulting in significant deformity and functional loss. The good news is that it is possible to understand the various deformities and to carry out both nonsurgical and surgical treatment to prevent and correct them, with restoration of function. Disruption of the normal thumb biomechanics often leads to significant loss of the patient's ability to carry out activities of daily living. Such activities as buttoning of clothing or the manipulation of small objects is greatly diminished if the patient lacks either control or stability of the thumb joints. Before embarking on a discussion of our current treatment program, we will review the most common thumb deformities and determine the factors that lead to their development.

DEFORMITIES OF THE RHEUMATOID THUMB

The deformities encountered in the rheumatoid patient are varied and are the result of changes taking place both intrinsically and extrinsically to the thumb. Synovial hypertrophy within the individual thumb joints not only can lead to destruction of articular cartilage, but also can stretch out the supporting collateral ligaments and joint capsules. As a result of this, each joint can become unstable and react to the stresses applied to it both in function against the other digits or as a result of the deforming forces of the extensor or flexor tendons acting upon it. A number of years ago one of us (E.N.)[5] proposed a classification in which the deformities were divided into three types. The type I deformity was believed to be the most common and was characterized

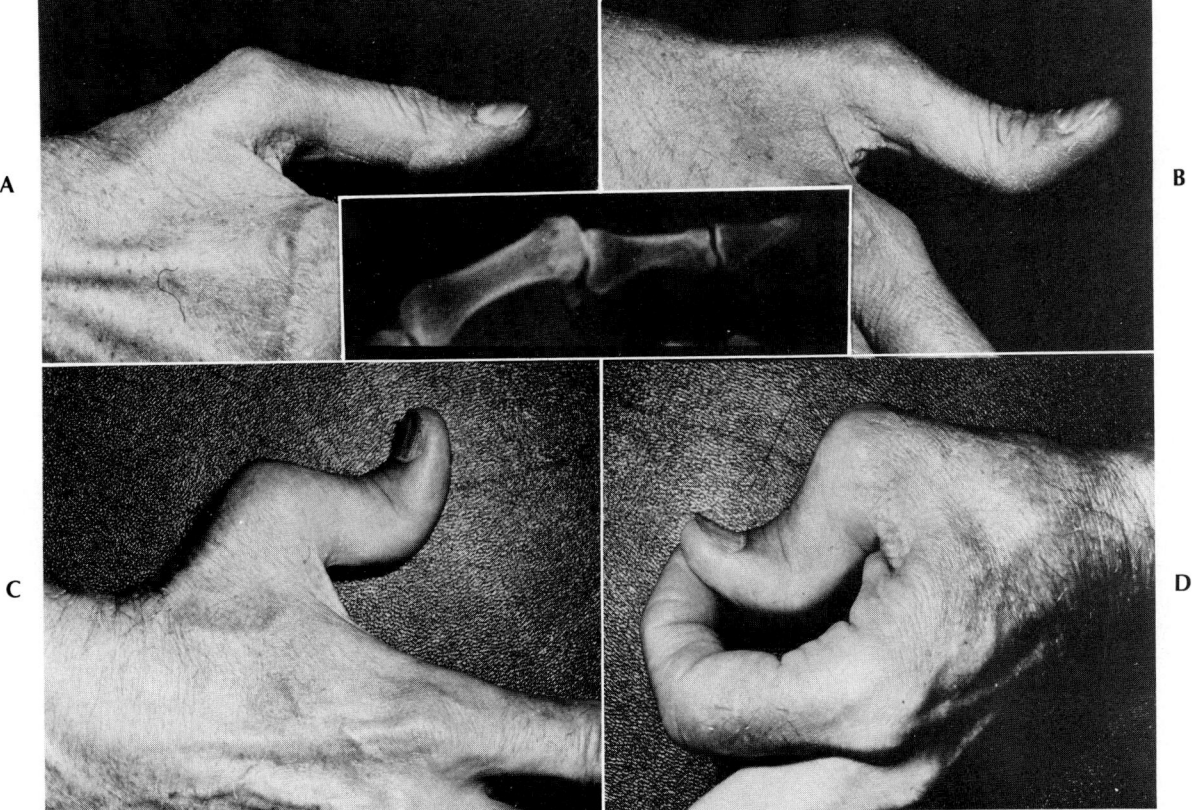

Fig. 74-1 **A** and **B,** Development of the common type I thumb deformity with early metacarpophalangeal joint flexion. Roentgenogram shows associated volar subluxation of the joint. **C,** Metacarpal abduction and distal joint hyperextension, as patient tries to straighten the thumb. **D,** Deformity is accentuated with pinch.

by metacarpophalangeal (MP) joint flexion, distal joint hyperextension, and metacarpal abduction. Others have called this the "Boutonnière deformity" of the thumb,[12] which is confusing because the flexion deformity in this thumb deformity is at the MP joint rather than at the proximal interphalangeal (PIP) joint as in a digit. The usual sequence of events leading to this particular deformity is as follows: Synovitis of the MP joint stretches out the extensor mechanism made up of the extensor pollicis brevis and extensor pollicis longus tendon. After this, the proximal phalanx tends to subluxate volarly or assumes a flexed position. Although the patient may maintain passive extension, there is an inability to extend the joint actively. As a compensating mechanism, the patient will abduct the first metacarpal and hyperextend the distal joint. This hyperextension of the distal joint and the flexion of the MP joint as well is accentuated when pinch forces are applied to the thumb. This particular deformity is best described as an "extrinsic-minus" deformity (Fig. 74-1). As stated above, the most common site for the initial change is at the MP, and it is the lack of extrinsic extensor power that starts the sequence of events. Not only can this be the result of changes occurring at the joint level itself, but also a rupture of the extensor pollicis longus at the wrist level can lead to the same deformity (Fig. 74-2). Although this particular deformity of the thumb

most commonly originates at the MP level with the distal joint hyperextension being a secondary factor, the reverse can also occur. As a result of stretching of the volar plate of the distal joint or rupture of the flexor pollicis longus tendon, the distal joint hyperextension can be primary, with MP joint flexion being secondary (Fig. 74-3). In these patients the metacarpal abduction is usually not a significant factor. Therefore, when faced with a patient having a type I deformity, one should evaluate not only the extensor tendons controlling the MP joint but also the flexor tendon controlling the distal joint to determine the primary site of imbalance.

In the original classification of thumb deformities, deformities of type II and type III were described.[5] In both of these instances the original alteration was at the carpometacarpal (CMC) joint level with subluxation of the first metacarpal, which then assumed an adducted position. In some of these patients the MP joint and interphalangeal joint assumed positions identical with the type I deformity in that the MP joint was flexed and the distal joint was hyperextended. This particular combination of metacarpal adduction with MP joint flexion and distal joint hyperextension (type II) (Fig. 74-4) is not common and assumes importance only in that it should be recognized as different from the type I deformity because of the metacarpal adduction. A much more common sequence of events after CMC joint subluxation and metacarpal adduction is MP joint hyperextension and distal joint flexion (type III) (Fig. 74-5). This deformity is the opposite of the common type I deformity in all respects. It has been called a "swan-neck deformity" of the thumb, but since the hyperextension is at the MP joint rather than the PIP joint, it is a confusing term and we believe should be avoided in classifying thumb deformities. At first, the MP joint hyperextension is passively correctable. In fact, with time the range of MP joint flexion diminishes and ultimately the joint is fixed in either a straight or hyperextended position. Any attempt to correct the type III deformity requires the first metacarpal to be abducted. If the CMC joint is subluxated, abduction can often only be accomplished by surgery. With restoration of metacarpal abduction the MP joint hyperextension deformity may correct itself, but if fixed hyperextension persists, this joint must also be treated, either by arthrodesis, tenodesis, or capsulodesis in a flexed position.

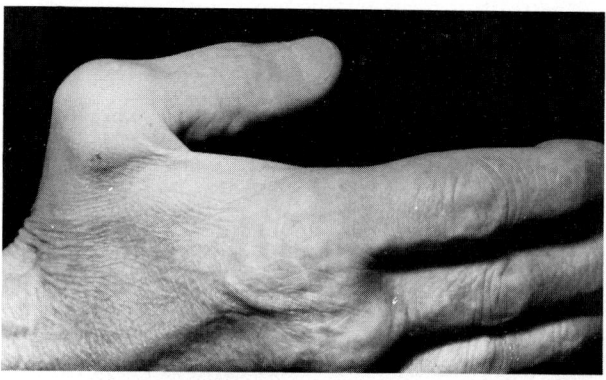

Fig. 74-2 Metacarpophalangeal joint flexion deformity of the thumb caused by rupture of the extensor pollicis longus tendon at the wrist.

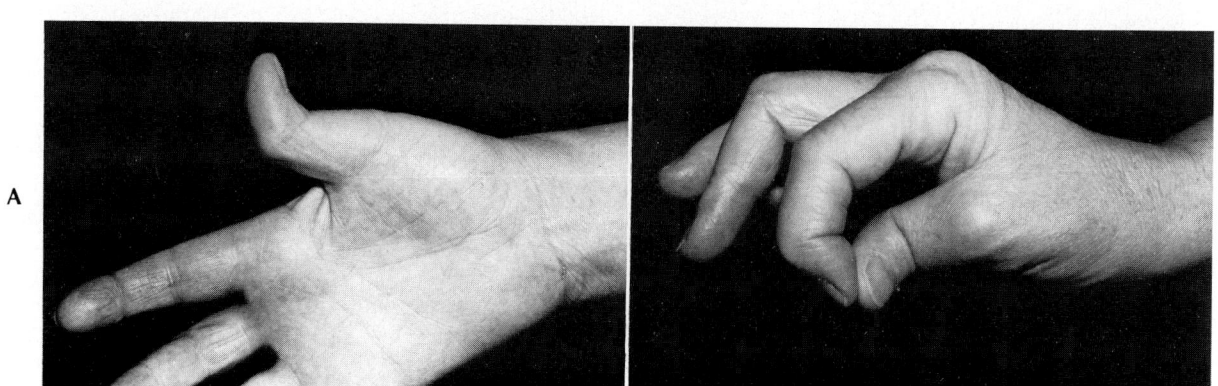

Fig. 74-3 Type I thumb deformity caused by distal joint hyperextension. **A,** Hyperextension of the distal joint, as a result of stretching out or rupture of the volar plate. **B,** Accentuation of the deformity with pinch.

THE RHEUMATOID THUMB **931**

Since our original description of these three thumb deformities, we have encountered a number of patients with deformities that at first glance appear similar to the type III deformity but originate at the MP joint level. The most common of these, which we call type IV (Fig. 74-6), is the result of stretching out of the ulnar collateral ligament of the MP joint as a result of synovitis. As the proximal phalanx deviates laterally at the MP joint level, the first metacarpal secondarily assumes an adducted position. After this, the first dorsal interosseous and adductor muscles are shortened and the web space between the thumb and index finger becomes contracted. Although the first metacarpal is adducted in these patients, there is no subluxation at the CMC joint. The key to treatment with this deformity is to restore stability to the MP in a corrected position and to release the first web space contracture. A Z-plasty of the skin in the first web space may be needed. Surgery is ordinarily not necessary at the CMC joint level. Another thumb deformity, type V, should also be recognized. There are patients in whom the major deforming factor is instability or stretching

out of the volar plate of the MP joint of the thumb. As a result of this, the MP joint hyperextends and the distal joint assumes a flexed position (Fig. 74-7). In these patients, however, the first metacarpal bone need not assume an adducted position and the CMC joint is usually not involved. This particular deformity is best treated by stabilization of the MP joint either by a fusion or a capsulodesis in a flexed position. These five thumb deformity patterns are the result of imbalances occurring between the various joints of the thumb. One can see that in each of these cases the alteration of posture at one level has an affect upon the adjacent joint. However, there is another type of thumb deformity, type VI (Fig. 74-8), which should be mentioned in which the major element is a collapse or loss of bone substance.[7] Patients with arthritis mutilans develop thumbs that become quite short and are characteristically unstable with what appears to be abundant skin in relationship to the underlying skeleton. Although this condition can be isolated at the thumb level, it is ordinarily associated with similar difficulties in the other digits.

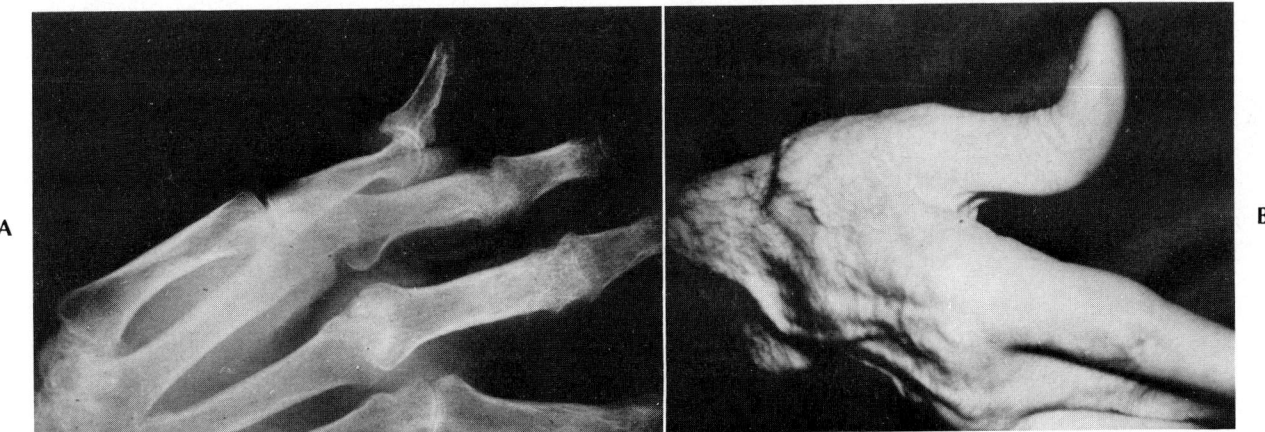

Fig. 74-4 Uncommon type II thumb deformity with metacarpal adduction and metacarpophalangeal joint flexion and distal joint extension. **A,** Metacarpal adduction at the carpometacarpal joint. **B,** Clinical appearance of the thumb.

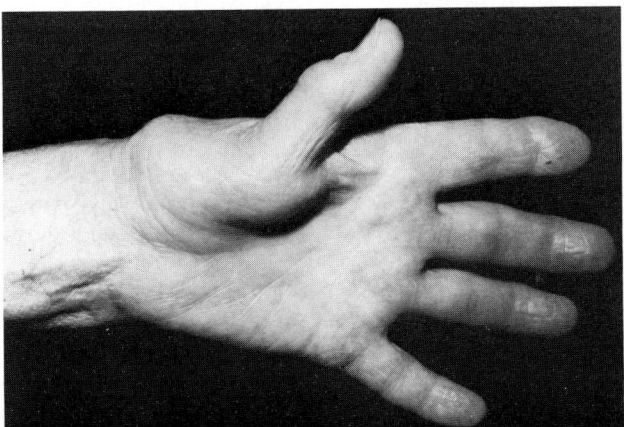

Fig. 74-5 Type III thumb deformity—metacarpal adduction with metacarpophalangeal joint hyperextension and distal joint flexion. Initial stage of this deformity is subluxation of the carpometacarpal joint.

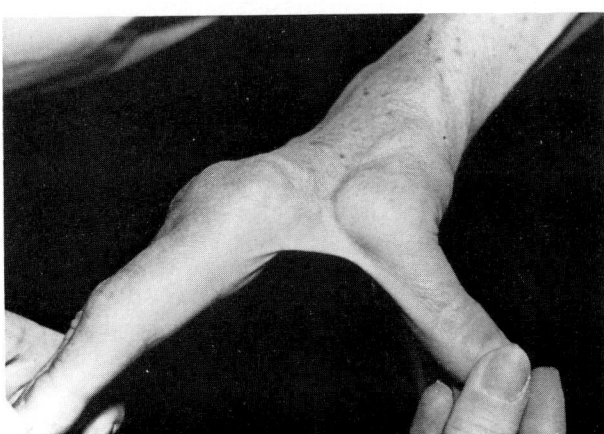

Fig. 74-6 Type IV thumb deformity demonstrates adducted metacarpal with abduction of metacarpophalangeal joint. Initial stage of this deformity is stretching of the ulnar collateral ligament. Metacarpal adduction and tight web space are secondary.

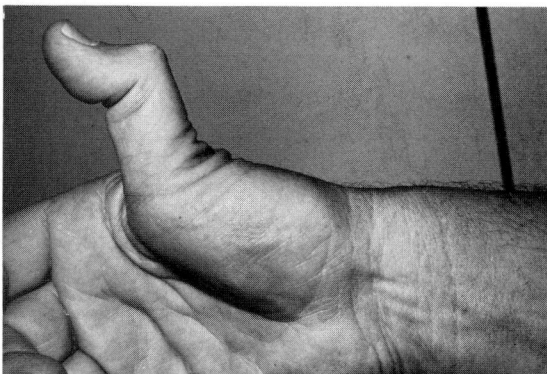

Fig. 74-7 Type I thumb deformity with hyperextension of the metacarpophalangeal joint caused by stretching of the volar plate. In this case metacarpal adduction was caused by the metacarpophalangeal hyperextension. The carpometacarpal joint was preserved.

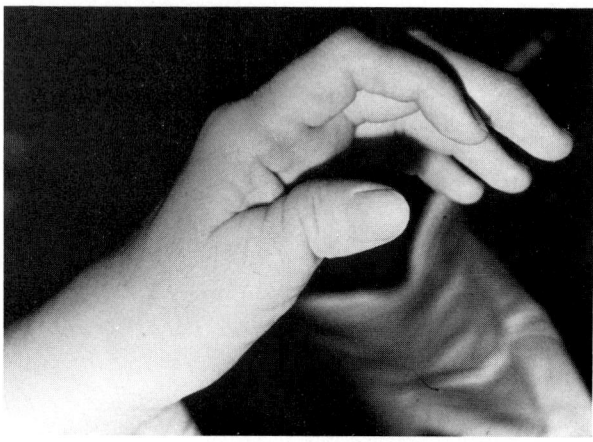

Fig. 74-8 Type VI thumb deformity showing collapse with loss of bone substance. In this case major bone loss involves the area adjacent to interphalangeal joint.

The six patterns of thumb postures described above unfortunately do not exhaust the deformities one encounters in rheumatoid arthritis. It is possible, for example, for the patient to stretch the supporting structures of a joint causing either a flexion, extension, or lateral deformity. However, instead of the adjacent joint assuming the opposite posture, it may assume an abnormal position secondary to a tendon rupture. Thus a patient might have hyperextension of both the MP and PIP joints or in fact flexion at both levels. When patients are encountered with adjacent joints deformed in the same direction, it usually implies that a combination of factors have brought this about. The examiner should check each individual joint for instability and also the controlling tendons for their integrity.

EVALUATION OF THE THUMB

Although it is of value to recognize the various thumb deformities and gain an understanding of their development, it is still necessary in each case to evaluate the individual joints of the thumb to determine appropriate therapy. One should, of course, not limit the evaluation to the thumb but instead assess the whole hand and upper extremity, since the thumb does not act in isolation in hand function. Our evaluation ordinarily includes a recording of the active and passive ranges of motion, pinch strength, and grip strength, as well as a functional status of the hand. Ranges of motion are recorded with a goniometer. Grip strength is recorded with a Jamar Dynamometer, and pinch strength is recorded with a standard pinch meter. Normal grip strength varies with age and sex. However, a normal grip strength for a man is around 100 pounds.[2] We have found that a grip strength of at least 20 pounds is necessary to perform most daily activities. One must keep in mind that many people with rheumatoid arthritis have grip strengths far below this functional level. Pulp, lateral, and three-jaw chuck pinch are also tested. Although grip strength is, of course, important, pinch strength has a particular application when one is assessing self-care skills. These include holding eating utensils, buttoning clothing, writing, and manipulating small objects for precision grip. Normal pinch strength ranges between 15 and 20 pounds.[2] We have found that a pinch strength of 5 to 7 pounds is necessary to accomplish most daily activities. Many rheumatoid patients have less than this. Therefore they encounter considerable difficulty in accomplishing even simple activities.

Functional assessment is also done as part of our examination. We use the Moberg pickup test to evaluate dexterity[4] (Fig. 74-9). We may also use other objective tests such as the Purdue Peg Board Test if the situation merits additional testing. In more complex cases we may also use the Jebsen Hand Function Test.[1]

The types of deformities encountered and the mechanism of these deformities have been previously discussed. Initially they are passively correctable. At this stage, the goal of hand therapy is to help maintain joint mobility and to help protect the joint through splinting and joint protection procedures. When the CMC joint becomes involved, the synovitis stretches out the joint capsule. As stated previously, this stretching can lead to joint subluxation or dislocation, with the metacarpal assuming an adducted position. The goal of therapy at this joint is to help prevent the adduction contracture and to maintain a functional range of motion. To accomplish this goal, we fabricate a CMC joint splint to maintain the thumb web space and to stabilize and protect the CMC joint. The splint extends distally to the interphalangeal joint level and proximally past the CMC joint to a level reaching the middle or proximal area of the forearm (Fig. 74-10). In this way, the CMC joint has good stabilization and the MP joint can be maintained in a corrected position. We advise patients to wear this splint at night. They are also encouraged to wear the splint during the day as much as possible while performing functional activities. Patients are instructed to remove the splint at least three times a day to take the thumb through a gentle range of motion. In our experience, a short opponens splint is not effective in stabilizing and positioning the CMC joint of the thumb.

In cases where the MP joint is involved, the goals are to prevent the deformity from becoming fixed and to help protect the joint from external forces that can produce further joint damage and deformity. One way this can be accomplished is through the use of a small splint for the MP joint.

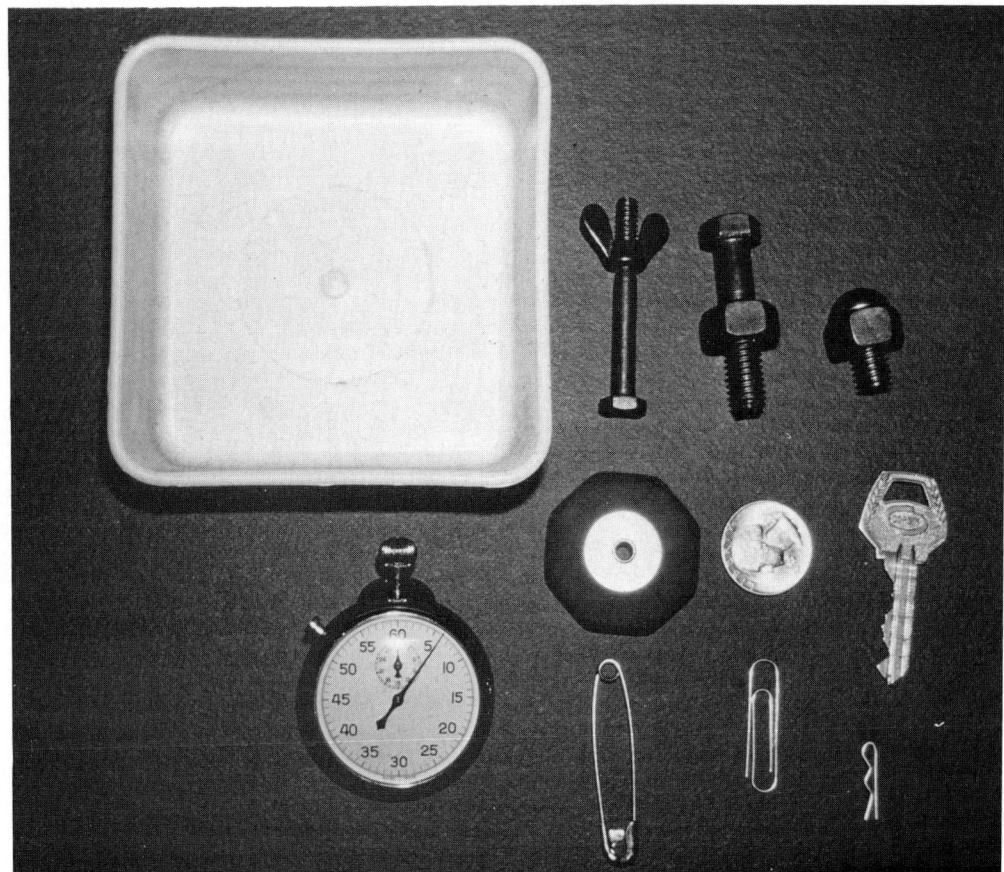

Fig. 74-9 Materials used to perform Moberg pick-up test. Nine objects of varying shapes and sizes are used. Patient picks these objects up and places them in a basket, first with eyes open and then with eyes closed. A stopwatch is used to record speed.

One can do this by taping an aluminum foam splint to the MP joint or by fabricating a MP splint from a thermoplastic material (Fig. 74-11). Since immobilizing one joint can cause added stress to adjacent joints, the therapist must watch for signs of increased synovitis or pain in these areas. The splint is worn during the functional activities and removed several times a day for range-of-motion exercises.

The interphalangeal joint can also be protected by the use

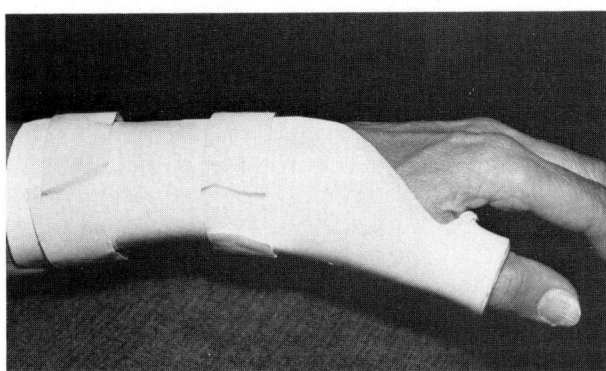

Fig. 74-10 Splint used for stabilizing the carpometacarpal joint. This is used both for relief of pain and as a protective device for patients with carpometacarpal involvement.

of an aluminum and foam splint taped to the joint (Fig. 74-12). This provides both stability and protection to the interphalangeal joint. If this joint becomes unstable, splinting helps to improve pinch while the person is awaiting corrective surgery. These small splints should be changed frequently to prevent any skin maceration.

One of the most important aspects of treatment is to teach the patient techniques of joint protection. The joints of the thumb are subject to great external stresses during activities of daily living (ADL). When the joints are swollen with synovitis, they are even more vulnerable to these outside forces. Therefore we instruct patients in general joint protection principles and specifically those that will minimize stress to the joints and soft-tissue structures of the thumb. Special devices are recommended for use during certain activities. One of the most stressful activities for the thumb is the opening of a car door. A piece of dowel that can be kept in the patient's pocket or purse can be used for car doors with a push button. The patient uses the dowel to push the button rather than placing the strain on the thumb (Fig. 74-13). There are also commercially available car-door openers. Turning a key can also be both stressful and difficult for patients with severe thumb involvement. A commercially available key holder can be used or a device can be created using thermoplast materials (Fig. 74-14). One tries to provide a greater surface area for grip. This will

Fig. 74-11 Use of metacarpopha-langeal splint for the thumb to facilitate functional use of the hand.

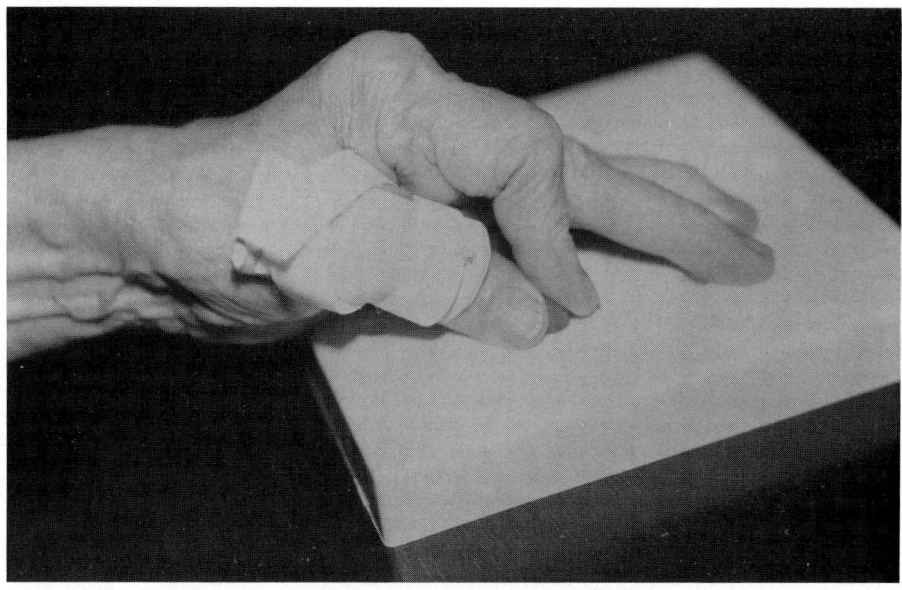

Fig. 74-12 Interphalangeal joint protected with aluminum foam splint during activities. This is used when a patient shows involvement at that joint.

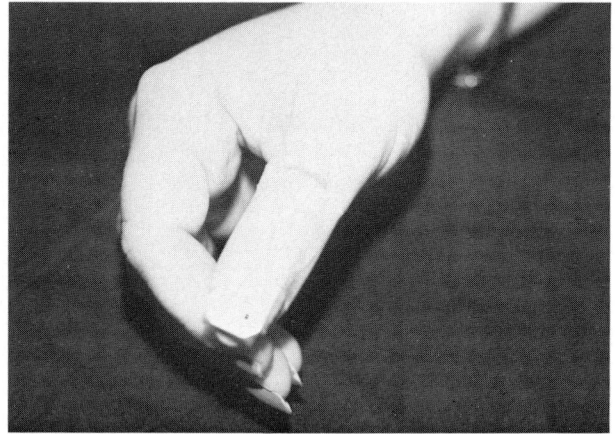

Fig. 74-13 Patient using dowel to open car door to minimize the force to joints of the thumb.

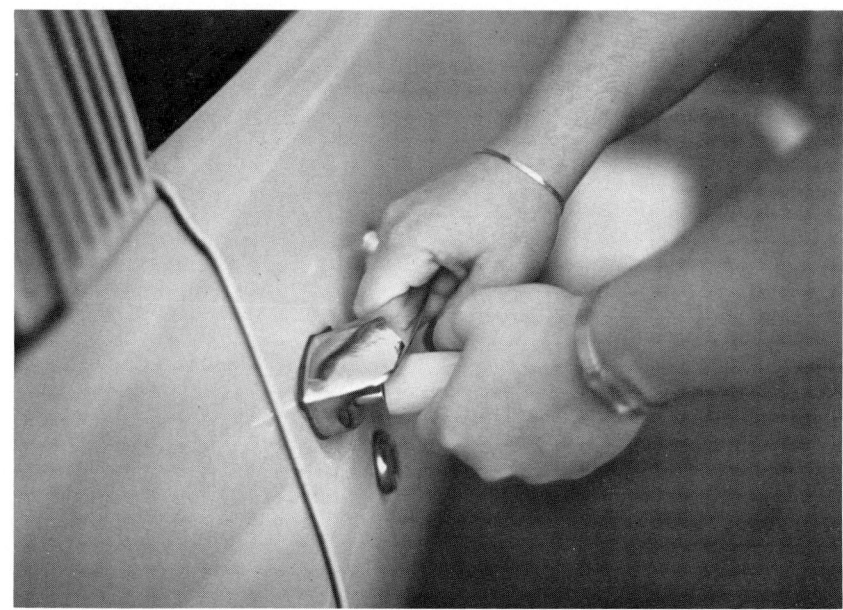

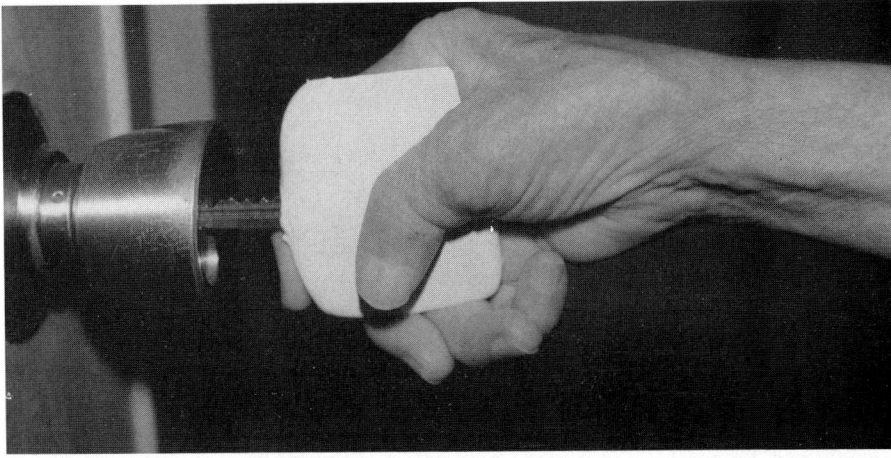

Fig. 74-14   Use of an adaptive key holder to distribute the force on the thumb when turning the key.

reduce the stress to the thumb and the index finger as well. We also advise patients to use built-up pens or large-diameter pens, which are available in stationery stores, to help minimize the stress to the thumb when writing. It takes less strength for the patient to stabilize the large-diameter object. Patients may find felt-tip pens easier to use because of reduced friction on the paper. Eating and other utensils can also be built up to reduce the external forces not only on the thumb but on the whole hand. We encourage patients to use as many lightweight utensils as possible. Activities such as wringing out clothes or a washcloth can put a great deal of strain on the wrist and thumb, particularly the CMC joint. This stress can be reduced by wrapping the cloth around the water faucet rather than twisting it with the hands. The cloth is wrapped around the water faucet and then is squeezed rather than twisted (Fig. 74-15). Certain repetitive activities such as the use of scissors are particularly stressful to the CMC joint and should be avoided as much as possible. We also advise patients to limit knitting and crocheting. These activities often lead to increased pain in the thumb and to symptoms of carpal tunnel syndrome.

These activities also keep the hand and wrist in very poor positions, actually the position of deformity.

These suggestions for alteration of ADL and the use of splints can afford these patients considerable relief. They may also slow the progression of deformity. However, surgical therapy is often the final treatment to correct the deformity, provide stability, and relieve pain.

SURGICAL TREATMENT

Despite the fact that there are various deformities affecting the thumb leading to bizarre alterations in posture at multiple levels, the surgical procedures that are applicable are more determined by the joint involved than by the specific type of deformity encountered. For this reason, we discuss the surgical procedures commonly performed at each joint level rather than discussing the individual deformities and their specific treatment.

INTERPHALANGEAL JOINT

The terminal joints of the thumb can, as a result of stretching of supporting structures, assume either a flexed, ex-

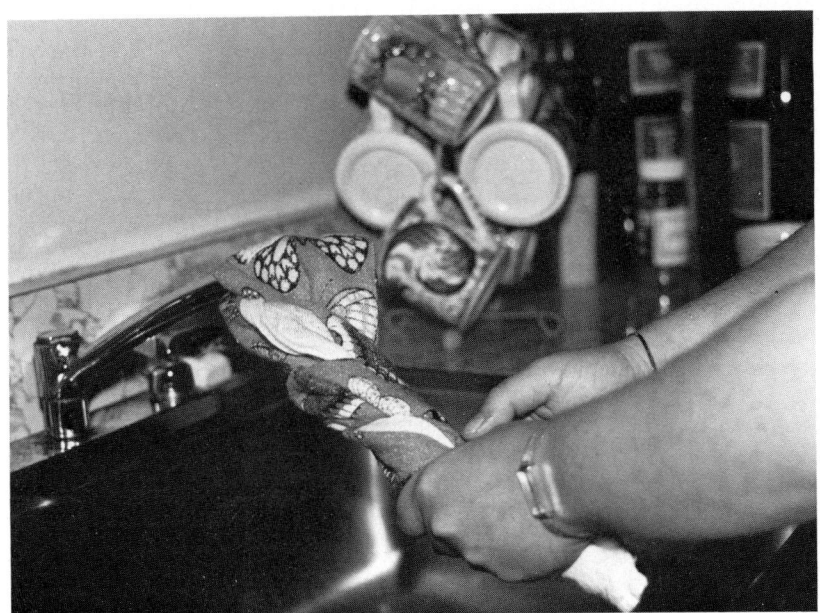

Fig. 74-15   Patient wringing out a dishcloth in a way that decreases stress to the thumb, wrist, and other digits.

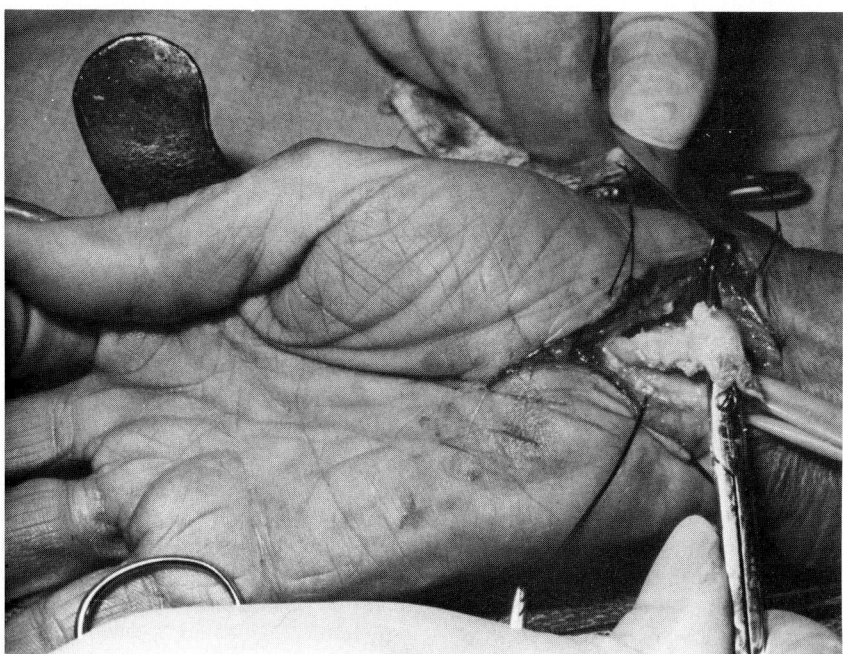

Fig. 74-16   Volar view of wrist, demonstrating rupture of the flexor pollicis longus tendon at the wrist. This is an attrition rupture on the bony spicule of the scaphoid.

tended, or laterally deviated position. Flexion and extension deformities at this level can result from ruptures of the extensor or flexor pollicis longus tendons. In these particular instances restoration of tendon function is attempted if the articular surface and supporting structures of the joint are intact. In the case of loss of extensor power, the tendon usually ruptures at the wrist level. With retraction of the muscle it is ordinarily not possible to carry out end-to-end tendon repairs, and restoration of extensor pollicis longus function is ordinarily achieved by transfer of the extensor indicis proprius to the extensor mechanism over the MP joint of the thumb.[6] In evaluating extensor tendon ruptures of the thumb affecting the distal joint one must check the extensor apparatus both at the wrist level and at the MP level where local ruptures can also be encountered. Because of the strong flexor power that is present with the intact flexor pollicis longus tendon, any extensor repair should be splinted for at least 5 weeks before one encourages active motion with force. The ruptures of the flexor pollicis longus tendon are quite common in the rheumatoid patient. The most frequent site of rupture is at the volar aspect of the wrist in the region of the carpal scaphoid[8] (Fig. 74-16). A portion of the scaphoid bone ordinarily erodes through the volar joint capsule and acts as a sharp edge against which the flexor tendon ruptures. When faced with a patient who has lost active flexion of the distal joint of the thumb, which is usually in a hyperextended position, one should assume that the tendon rupture is at the wrist level. In those instances in which the distal joint of the thumb is irregular or unstable so that restoration of active motion does not seem worthwhile, one might consider stabilizing the joint by bony fusion. However, if the diagnosis of flexor pollicis longus rupture has been made, it is suggested that the volar aspect of the wrist also be explored with removal of any bone

spicule in the carpal region. If this is not performed, the adjacent flexor tendons of the index finger are in jeopardy and, if left untreated, would sustain the same fate of spontaneous rupture. When one attempts to restore flexor pollicis longus function, it is also unusual to be able to carry out an end-to-end repair. Short "bridge" tendon grafts have been found useful, and in other patients tendon transfers using the superficial flexor of the ring finger can be carried out. In those patients in whom the joint is grossly unstable with or without intact extrinsic tendons, one should seriously consider an arthrodesis. Fusion of the terminal joints of the thumb does not cause significant functional loss and in fact improves the patient's ability to pinch objects with force. Fusion at this level often makes it possible for one to correct rotation deformities of the thumb by putting the terminal joint in a slightly flexed and pronated position. In patients with the collapse type of deformities, the use of supplemental bone grafts is required not only to achieve fusion but also to restore length (Fig. 74-17). The most common fixation technique for interphalangeal joint fusion in the rheumatoid thumb is the use of a longitudinal Kirschner (K) wire that is kept in place for at least 8 weeks (Fig. 74-18). An external aluminum splint can be used to protect the joint allowing mobility at the MP level. In patients in whom volar instability is present but the joint surface is intact one could consider a flexor tenodesis using one half of the flexor pollicis longus attached distally to the proximal phalanx.[8,12] Arthroplasties for interphalangeal joint involvement in the rheumatoid thumb are rarely indicated, because they do not provide good lateral stability.

METACARPOPHALANGEAL JOINT

The surgical procedures found useful about the MP joint in the rheumatoid patient include synovectomy, extensor

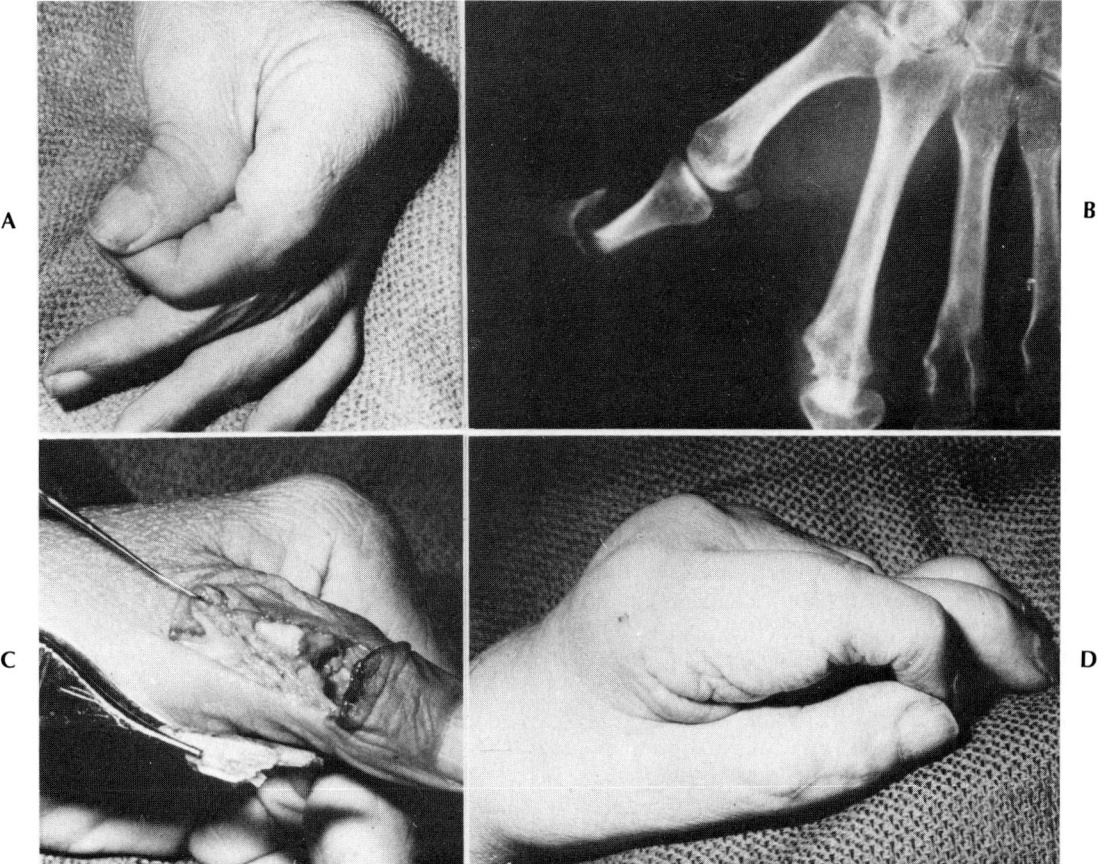

Fig. 74-17   Surgical treatment for unstable thumb with collapse deformity. A bone graft was used to restore length. **A,** Preoperative pinch with collapse. **B,** Roentgenogram showing loss of bone substance. **C,** During surgery bone graft was prepared for insertion. **D,** Postoperative pinch stability was restored.

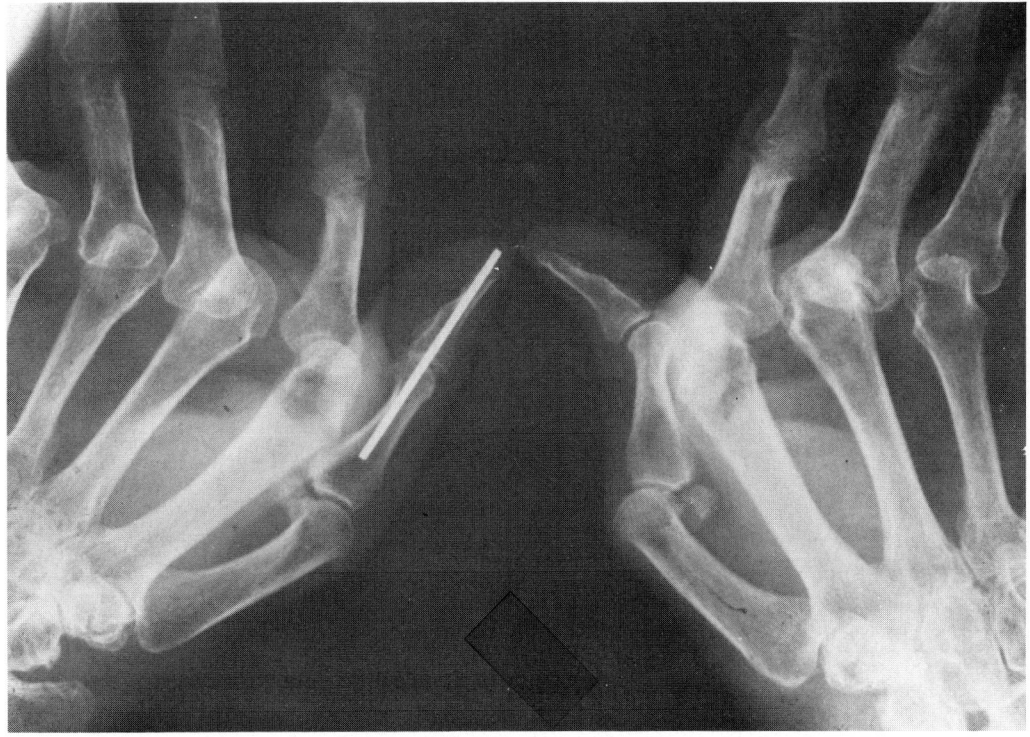

Fig. 74-18   Roentgenogram showing correction of type I thumb deformity with distal joint fusion, using longitudinal Kirschner wire. Thumb on the opposite hand demonstrates untreated type I thumb deformity.

pollicis longus rerouting, arthrodesis, arthroplasty, and capsulodesis. Synovectomy is advisable in those patients in
whom the joint is chronically swollen and whom x-ray evaluation reveals that the joint surfaces are still well maintained.
When synovectomy is performed for the rheumatoid thumb,
one often encounters a stretching out or elongation of the
extensor mechanism. In these cases, it is advisable to carry
out some shortening of the extensor mechanism followed
by splinting so that the rapid onset of a flexion deformity
is prevented. In patients in whom a flexion deformity has
occurred but passive extension is still possible, a reinforcement of the extensor forces to the MP joint can be performed. A number of techniques have been advised, but
one of us (E.N.)[5] has been pleased with the use of an extensor pollicis longus rerouting procedure, in which the long
extensor tendon is rerouted through the dorsal capsule of
the joint to provide additional extensor force at this level.
When this procedure is done, the intrinsic muscles of the
thumb, the flexor pollicis brevis and abductor pollicis brevis,
act as extensor forces for the distal joint (Fig. 74-19).

For the MP joint that is grossly unstable or in which the
articular cartilage has been destroyed one must choose between arthrodesis or arthroplasty. For those patients with
flexion deformities it is possible to correct the deformity by
resection of a portion of the adjacent joint surfaces and
insertion of a Swanson flexible implant.[9-11] This procedure
is ordinarily supplemented by a reinforcement or shortening
of the extensor mechanism (Fig. 74-20). Patients undergoing arthroplasties at this level ordinarily are not started
on early motion. It is important to splint these thumbs in
almost full extension for 4 to 5 weeks before allowing unrestricted motion. We tend to limit the use of the implant

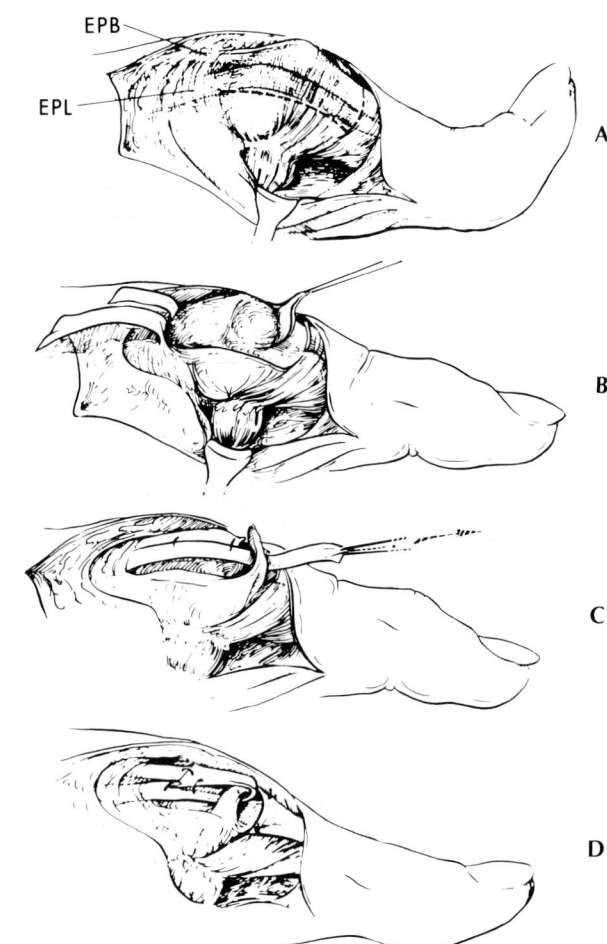

Fig. 74-19 Technique of extensor pollicis longus rerouting to
restore active extension to the metacarpophalangeal joint.

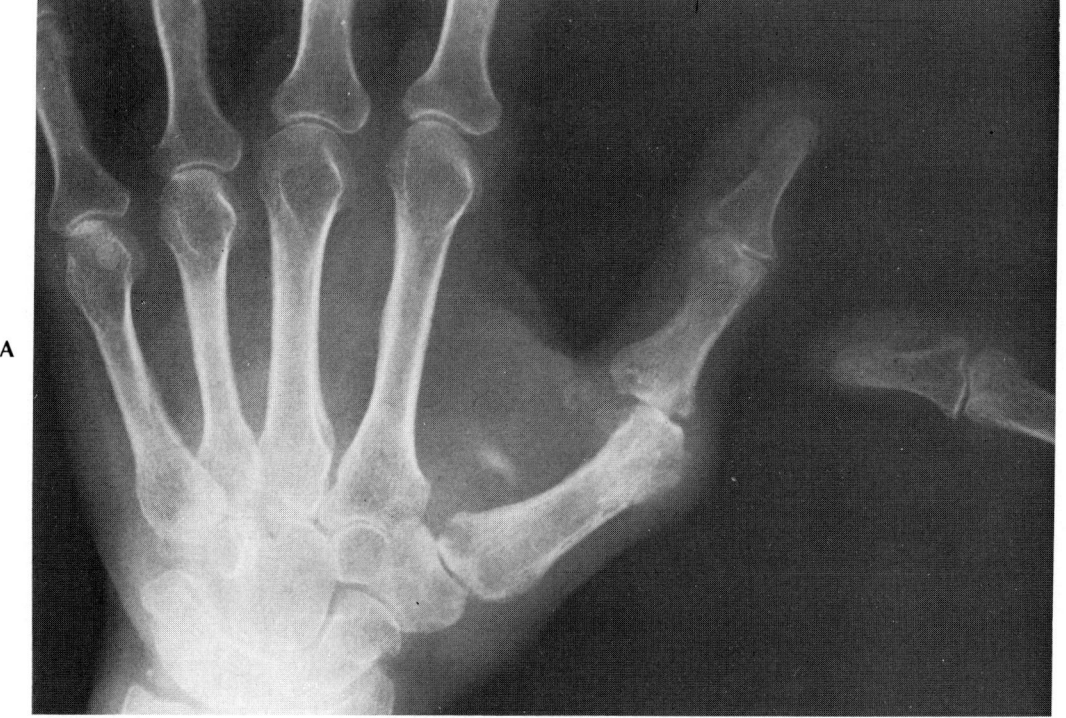

Fig. 74-20 Type I thumb deformity treated with arthroplasty of the metacarpophalangeal joint and the extensor
pollicis longus rerouting procedure. **A,** Roentgenogram of subluxation of the metacarpophalangeal joint showing much
irregularity and loss of bone substance.

arthroplasty at the MP level to those patients having flexion deformities. In patients with hyperextension deformities arthrodesis of the MP joint in a slightly flexed position is advisable. We are reluctant to insert a flexible implant in these patients because of the lack of volar stability. When one is performing an arthrodesis of the MP joint of the thumb, the position to strive for is 15 degrees of flexion, 5 degrees of abduction, and 20 degrees of pronation (Fig. 74-21). For fixation we usually use two crossed K-wires. Supplementary bone grafts are advisable if there has been some previous bone collapse or loss. It is important in these patients to start early postoperative interphalangeal joint motion, because there is a possible risk of the extensor mechanism becoming adherent at the fusion site. Fusions of the MP joint in slight flexion to correct the hyperextension deformity are particularly important. By fusing the MP joint in slight flexion one takes considerable strain off of the CMC joint. This is particularly important in those patients who have undergone or will require an arthroplasty at that level. In patients with full flexibility of the MP joint but a tendency

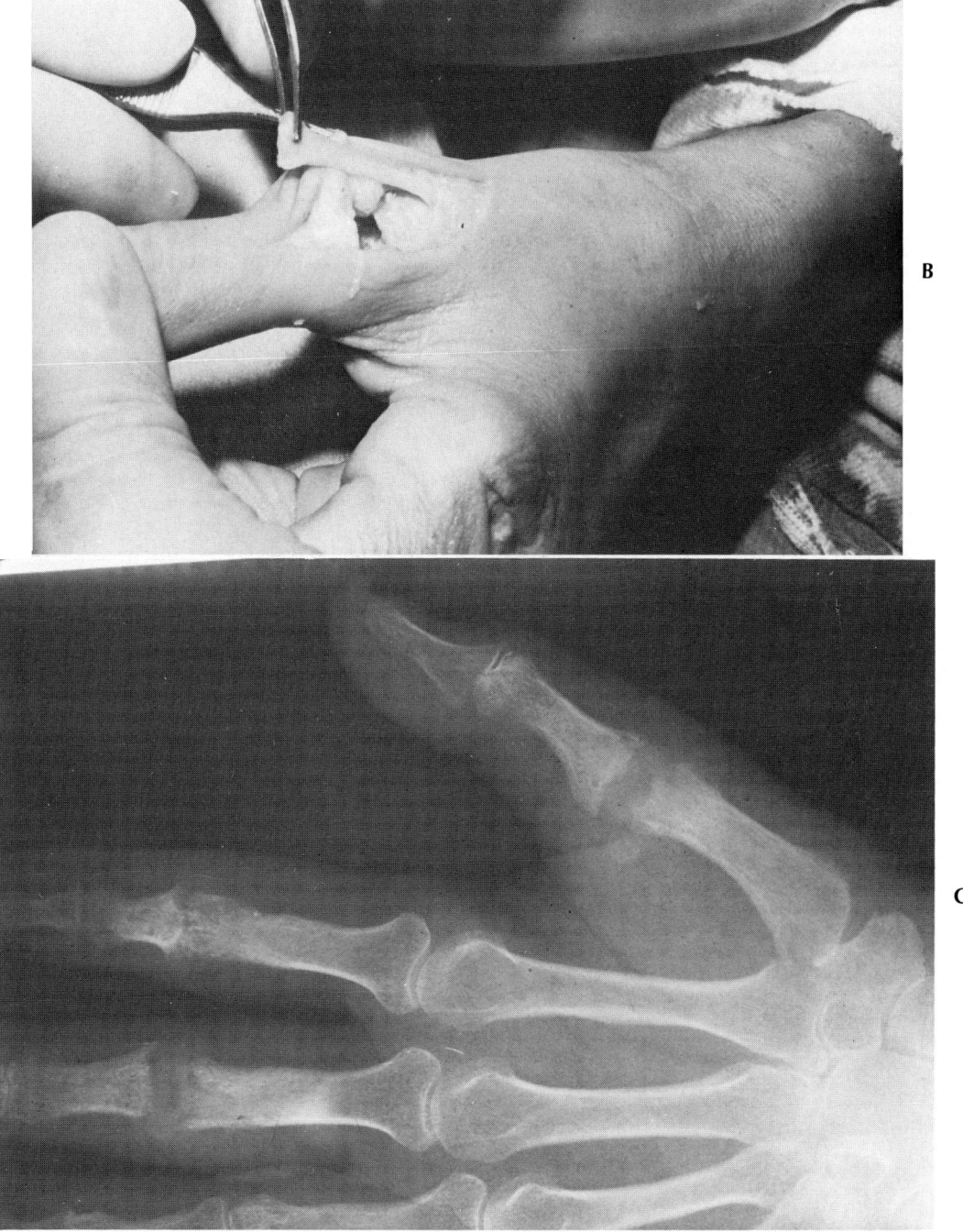

Fig. 74-20, cont'd   **B,** Appearance during surgery with resection of the joint before insertion of the prosthesis and reattachment of the extensor pollicis longus. **C,** Postoperative correction of a deformity with Swanson flexible implant arthroplasty in place.

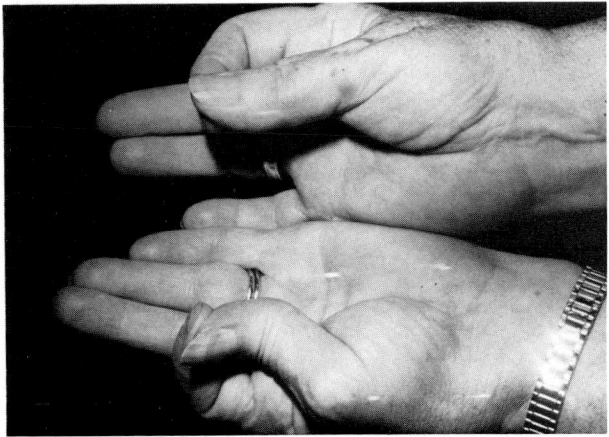

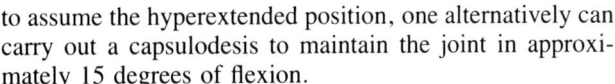

Fig. 74-21 *Right hand,* Correction of type I thumb deformity with arthrodesis of the metacarpophalangeal joint. *Left hand,* Preoperative appearance with collapse of the thumb on pinch.

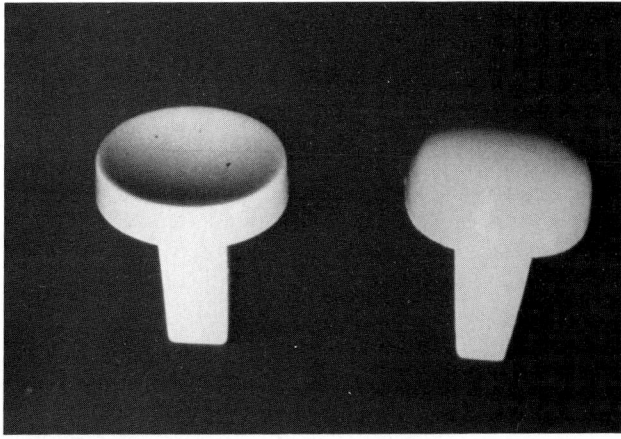

Fig. 74-22 Two types of prostheses used for hemiarthroplasty at the base of the thumb. *Left,* Concave prosthesis. *Right,* Convex condylar prosthesis.

to assume the hyperextended position, one alternatively can carry out a capsulodesis to maintain the joint in approximately 15 degrees of flexion.

At the CMC joint the surgical procedures performed include various types of arthroplasties and in specific instances arthrodesis. Because rheumatoid arthritis commonly affects multiple joints, it is ordinarily not advisable to fuse the CMC joint. Subsequent involvement at the MP joint level requiring fusion would leave the patient with very little mobility. An exception to this rationale is the patient with lupus erythematosus.[9] In this condition, articular cartilage seems to be spared, and the major problem is an instability with subluxation of the joints. Therefore arthrodesis of the CMC joint can provide a solid foundation for the thumb. However, in most cases surgical treatment of the CMC joint implies some form of arthroplasty. Because carpal involvement is common in rheumatoid patients, the trapezium implant commonly used in degenerative arthritis is not used in these patients. The type of arthroplasty we commonly carry out at the CMC joint level in the rheumatoid arthritic patient is a resection arthroplasty in which bone is removed to allow the first metacarpal to assume an abducted position. Soft-tissue interposition using a piece of tendon is often helpful.[3] In other patients a hemiarthroplasty using either a concave or convex hemiprosthesis (Swanson) with a single stem inserted into the first metacarpal has been found to be worthwhile[12] (Fig. 74-22). It is important after any CMC joint arthroplasty in the rheumatoid patient to maintain the thumb in a position of abduction for approximately 5 to 6 weeks before starting motion. As stated in the discussion of MP joint surgery, it is imperative that one not leave a hyperextended MP joint when performing an arthroplasty at the CMC joint level. If the MP joint is allowed to collapse into hyperextension, the forces are quite strong to adduct the first metacarpal, leading to subluxation of any implant.

POSTOPERATIVE HAND THERAPY

Hand therapy is instituted very early in the postoperative management and is important in rehabilitating these patients. The therapy after thumb reconstruction is geared toward the functional use of the thumb. Periodic postop-

erative assessments are done to monitor the patient's progress. Postoperatively the thumb is immobilized for approximately 6 weeks. During this immobilization we encourage the patient to perform ROM exercise of the other digits to prevent stiffness.

When the splint is removed, active and active-assistive ROM exercises are started. These include circumduction, abduction, and opposition exercises. Initially, warm-water soaks may be helpful when one is initiating motion. Dexterity activities are then introduced into the program. The functional use of the thumb is gradually increased as tolerated by the patient. Increasing the program too rapidly can cause pain and increased swelling and should be avoided. However, if this should occur, the thumb must be rested before the therapy program is resumed.

After MP arthroplasty of the thumb, immobilization is maintained for 5 weeks to ensure capsular healing. The goal is to provide a stable, pain-free joint for pinch. After the immobilization period, active and active-assistive exercises are started. Dexterity activities are introduced gradually over the next few weeks. Our goal is not to achieve a large range of motion, but enough to be functional. One does not need a great deal of MP motion to have good hand dexterity and pinch strength. In fact, this joint has a wide variation in range of motion in the normal population.

In many cases other hand-reconstructive procedures may be done at the time thumb reconstruction is undertaken. Naturally one must keep that in mind when planning the patient's treatment program.

SUMMARY

Although the thumb is frequently involved in rheumatoid arthritis, causing significant function loss, as well as pain and deformity, much can be done both nonsurgically and surgically to alleviate the condition and restore function to the patient.

REFERENCES

1. Jebsen RH, Taylor N, Trieschmann RB and others: An objective and standardized test of hand function, Arch Phys Med 50:311, 1969.
2. Melvin JL: Rheumatic disease: occupational therapy and rehabilitation, ed 2, Philadelphia, 1982, TA Davis Co.

3. Millender LH and others: Interpositional arthroplasty for rheumatoid carpometacarpal joint disease, J Hand Surg 3(6):533, 1978.

4. Moberg E: Objective methods of determining functional value of sensibility in the hand, J Bone Joint Surg 40:454, 1958.

5. Nalebuff EA: Diagnosis, classification and management of rheumatoid thumb deformities, Bull Hosp Joint Dis 29:199, 1968.

6. Nalebuff EA: The recognition and treatment of tendon ruptures in the rheumatoid hand. In American Academy of Orthopedic Surgeons: Symposium on Tendon Surgery in the Hand, St. Louis, 1975, The CV Mosby Co.

7. Nalebuff EA and Garrett J: Opera-glass hand in rheumatoid arthritis, J Hand Surg 1(3):210, 1976.

8. Nalebuff EA and Millender LH: Reconstructive surgery and rehabilitation of the hand. In Kelley WN and others: Textbook of rheumatology, Philadelphia, 1981, WB Saunders Co.

9. Nalebuff EA and others: The surgical treatment of hand deformities in systemic lupus erythematosis, J Hand Surg 6(4):339, 1981.

10. Swanson AB: Silicone rubber implants for replacement of arthritic or destroyed joints in the hand, Surg Clin North Am 48:1113, 1968.

11. Swanson AB: Flexible implant arthroplasty for arthritic finger joint, J Bone Joint Surg 54A:435, 1972.

12. Swanson AB: Flexible implant resection arthroplasty in the hand and extremities, St. Louis, 1973, The CV Mosby Co.

75

Preoperative assessment and postoperative therapy and splinting in rheumatoid arthritis

Gloria L. DeVore

In this chapter I discuss the method of patient selection for implant arthroplasty and the postoperative splinting and therapy employed at Hand Therapy Associates, Inc., in Tucson, Arizona. This protocol has evolved over 10 years in the evaluation and diagnosis of hundreds of patients. We believe it contributes greatly to our excellent results and satisfied patients.

In the development of the following evaluation techniques, we know that some portion of each aspect of the process must be used to some degree but the exact amounts are controlled and adjusted by the patient, the surgeon, and the therapist—the team. We seldom see rheumatoid arthritic patients in the beginning stages of their diseases; instead, most of them are referred to us when they are in the last stages of deformity.

PHILOSOPHY

So that you understand our approach to upper extremity reconstruction for the rheumatoid hand, I will present the manner in which we approach the patient: The surgeon might ask, "How can I help you, Ms. Jones?" The answer almost invariably is, "I have arthritis and I would like you to fix my hands." Surgeon: "What is the problem with your hands, Ms. Jones? Where would one start to fix your hands?"

In looking at the hands (Fig. 75-1, *right hand*), you can appreciate the problem that confronts the surgeon. Before

him are 24 finger joints, six thumb joints, and two wrists, all badly needing reconstructive surgery.

The question then becomes, "Where would one start?" From the viewpoints of the surgeon and therapist, many possibilities for surgical reconstruction exist. But would our viewpoints answer for the patients the questions of what and where their primary problems are located?

We start to help the patients define their problems by having them participate in a complex evaluation, which includes the following questions: In which joints are the problems located? Am I having difficulty because of pain, power, or position?

The following printed diary instructions and examples are reviewed and given to the patients. They are asked to keep a diary for at least 1 week.

Diary instructions

The purposes of this diary are:
1. To increase your awareness of yourself
2. To increase awareness regarding your particular disability
3. To aid us in accurate diagnosis and management of your disability
4. To make *you* an active participant in diagnosis and management of your disability

Before we get into the specifics of your diary, please begin by listing:
1. Current and past medications. Give frequency and doses of

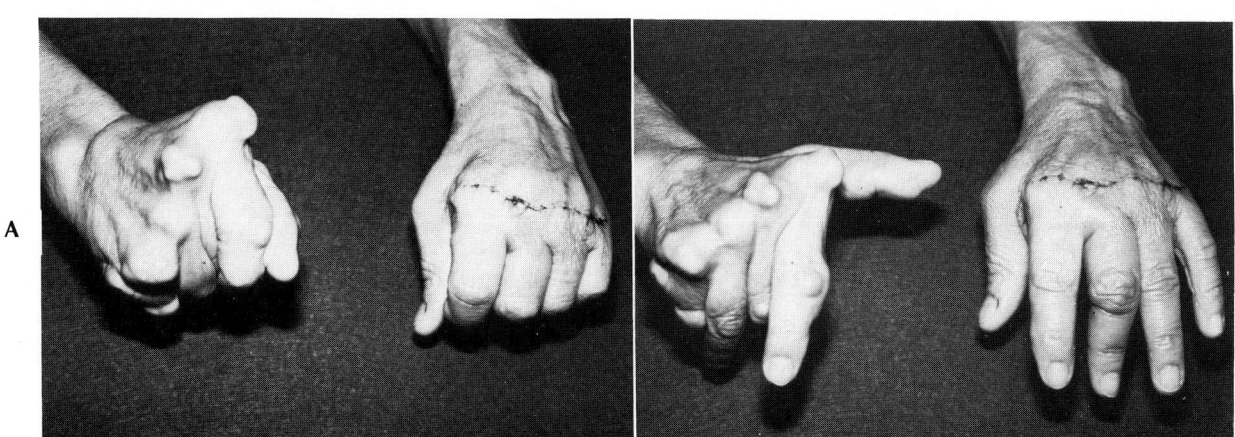

Fig. 75-1 **A,** Patient making a fist, 3 weeks after metacarpophalangeal implant arthroplasty on left hand. **B,** Patient extending fingers. Notice the improved appearance of left hand. Surgery was performed on the right hand 3 months later.

current medications only (example: Clinoril, 100 mg 4×
daily).
2. Surgeries. List surgeon, operative date, and the procedure.
3. Wish list. Pretend your doctor and your therapist have a
magic wand and are able to grant you three wishes as we
begin to discuss your problems.

We hope this diary will raise your level of consciousness about
yourself. As you complete your diary, you will discover many
things about your hand that you have not been aware of previously.
By doing this, your awareness and understanding will increase.
All of this will be of great help to you, your doctor, and your
therapist.

As you go through your daily routines and you come across
activities that you used to do but are now unable to accomplish,
or have difficulty accomplishing, write them in your diary under
"Activity." Break the activity column into three components:
1. Pain
2. Position
3. Power

If you experience *pain*, list it in the pain column. A check (√)
is not enough. We need *location* of the pain and a description of
what the pain feels like—the more adjectives used the better. If
you become confused about a particular joint, just place your hand
on the attached diagram and then identify the joint.

Next, think about the activity and decide if you are unable to
accomplish the task successfully because you cannot *position* your
hand correctly *on* or *around* the object. List the joint and the
position that you are having difficulty achieving. Again, if you get
confused about the name of the joint, place your hand on the
diagram.

And last, ask yourself if your inability or difficulty in accomplishing the task is a result of lack of *power* or of *strength*, or
both. In this column, you may simply place a check (√). However,
if you would like to make a comment, please do so.

You may construct your chart like the one below. The results
of your diary may vary with each activity. There is no need to list
activities twice. Please identify the hand in which you are experiencing the problem.

Read the examples carefully.

Bring your diary with you when you come to us for your functional evaluation. Your therapist will review your activities with
you.

If you should have any questions, please feel free to call us.

The patients return to the clinic with their completed
notes, and the functional evaluation is performed in one and
sometimes two periods. It should be noted that functional
evaluations are not limited to the upper limbs; the diaries
can be used for various problems involving the entire body.

FUNCTIONAL EVALUATION
History

Extensive histories of the patients are first taken so that
a data base and the patients' attitudes toward their chronic
disease can be established. Included are medications, past
and present progress of the disease, other medical problems,
and present home setting. It is of great importance that
patients become aware of their position on the team. Patients
must come to understand that all future decisions made
regarding their care must be made with their understanding
and commitment and that they hold the ultimate responsibility for their own care.

As we continue to gather our data base, range-of-motion
(ROM) and ulnar drift measurements are taken for all joints
in both upper extremities. This is done for objective documentation of their status on that date.

Joint protection

To continue the evaluation, we use questions clustered
around broad topics. Inevitably, joint protection becomes a
topic of conversation. A patient facing the therapist across
the table will eventually rest his head on his hand, with the
fingers being pushed off into ulnar deviation. This provides
a perfect opening to discuss the best physiologic and mechanical way to rest the head on the hand without causing
further damage.

Activity	Pain	Position	Power
Holding a coffee mug	MP joints of fingers and CMC joint of thumb	Can't grab cup with MP joints—extend ulnar deviation	Because of ulnar drift and position
Opening or unscrew- ing pill bottle or lids	Right wrist—ache MP joints MP joint of thumb	Can't grasp because of ulnar drift and inability to tightly flex MPs and PIPs	No power because of inability to position
Combing hair	Shoulder—ache and tight Elbow—same Wrist—same	Unable to lift shoulder, flex elbow, and extend wrist, hold brush simulta- neously	Yes, because of position and pain
Lifting pan off stove	Wrist and CMC joint of thumb—burning, pulling, dull ache	No problem	Yes, because of pain and weakness
Using keys for door or car—turning or twisting motion	MP joint (index, long) CMC and MP joints of thumb and wrist	Can't pinch hard enough with thumb, index, and long	Yes, limited by posi- tion and power
Writing	MP joint of all fingers, carpal area, and ulnar burning, pulling	———————	Maintaining position is difficult

We then ask for demonstrations of how patients get up from their chairs. Many patients are no longer at a stage where even the most widely accepted standards can be used in getting up from a chair. A trial-and-error session must take place to provide a way of getting them to their feet without causing undue forces in the wrong direction, especially if any type of joint replacement is to be considered. This is always a difficult task, because these established habit patterns are very difficult to change, and it is sometimes too traumatic to try.

Muscle testing

Muscle testing and evaluation of tendon continuity are performed carefully. We believe there must be evidence of muscle contraction in all muscle groups surrounding a joint being considered for possible replacement. Tendon rupture always changes the complexity of reconstruction and serves as an indicator of the extent of the disease process on the tendons. We have observed clinically that when one tendon has ruptured, patients are in great danger of further ruptures. A discussion now takes place regarding the synovial linings around the tendon sheaths. We explain that early in the disease a synovectomy with removal of the diseased tissue acts as a deterrent to tendon rupture.

Further discussions about the anatomy of the dorsal surface of the wrist, the volar surface of the wrist, the metacarpophalangeal (MP) joints, and the proximal interphalangeal (PIP) joints are carried out. We point out the differences between dorsal and volar compartments. Many times patients believe their problems are isolated only on the dorsum of their hands, because of the obvious deformities. We explain to them that significant hidden volar problems often exist.

We find it easier for patients to understand the involved anatomy when we use a plastic skeleton of the wrist. We demonstrate how the tendons on the volar surface are trapped, along with the median nerve, in the carpal tunnel by the transverse carpal ligament. Dorsally the tendons are all held in place by a wide band, the extensor retinaculum (retinaculum extensorum). Under this band, the tendons are surrounded by sheaths so that they glide back and forth.

Sensation

Sensation is tested by light-touch sensory testing, with the right and left hands being compared. We ask about being awakened at night by the hands going to sleep. We go into further detail regarding the volar compartment and discussion of the median nerve, which often gets compressed by the hypertrophic synovium, which cannot be seen as readily on the volar surface as on the dorsal surface. On many occasions, we find that the sensory problems are not at the wrist at all but are much more proximal, often in the neck. This is tested by having the patient assume the position that causes the paresthesia.

By this point in the evaluation, patients are beginning to have more understanding of their complex problems and can speak with us regarding the progression of their disease in terms other than a decrease in their sedimentation rate.

Exercises

Only very specific exercises are given in our clinic. Some patients who have had arthritis for over 20 years are still trying to do the same exercise program they were given when the disease was first diagnosed. As a consequence of this experience, we are unwilling to give patients three pages of by-the-number exercises. We believe we can do this only when we are assured of being able to observe the patients and only if we can design a program when the exercises are active and under direct control of the patients.

Flatt has stated that joint range without sufficient muscle control is of no value and leads to joint instability. Our clinical observation bears this out. Can you visualize patients continuing to do finger exercises of thumb-to-fingertips opposition when every MP joint is subluxated and intrinsic tightness is already severe? Many patients continue to try to do radial exercises when structurally it is no longer possible.

There are two mobility plans we are willing to give patients that, if they should continue for 20 years, would keep them much more functional and make for a better life-style. One is the overhead-pulley exercise for shoulders, with a piece of adaptive equipment that we make in our clinic. The other is hip abduction. Hip abduction mobility over the years becomes crucial; many patients in the process of their evaluation talk to us about the loss of this motion.

Sometimes at the end of the assessment, patients come to the realization that their problems are not in their hands as they suspected, but that the lack of power and position are caused by shoulder pain and immobility.

We have all experienced the often-repeated story of inability to get the hands where they need to be to carry out the tasks required (such as dressing or taking care of toilet needs). This is a shoulder problem and not a hand problem.

Diary assessment

Now we come to the special part of the evaluation, the diary, examples of which follow.

Wish list—J.M., early forties, pipe salesman in construction industry

Would like to wear gloves
Would like to put baseball glove on left hand
Would like to pass baseball or football with sons
Would like to be able to use a hammer, screwdriver, or any tool in the proper manner
Would like to hold a gun to hunt and a fishing rod to fish
Would like to be able to shake hands; when I try now the other man's grip hurts my knuckles

Diary excerpt—B.M., 59-year-old woman, retired teacher

In a public restroom, unable to open door after it was unlocked. Had to knock to get out.

Turning on T.V., had to use both hands to hold remote control unit in proper position to punch on program.

In looking at recent photographs, I notice I always try to hide my hands; however, they usually show anyway and their deformity. A more "normal" appearance would be pleasing to me.

Writing this is bad for me psychologically. I was never aware of so many dreads and difficulties. I didn't know I was having such a hard time as I was busy and happy. Now, I look for trouble. Habitually, I have always just gone along doing the best I could and ignoring most difficulties. I really don't like being made so acutely aware.

Diary excerpt—B.Q., 44-year-old woman, not employed

When applying hair spray, I am unable to use any type or size of bottle except a 4 oz nonaerosol. Anything larger I am unable

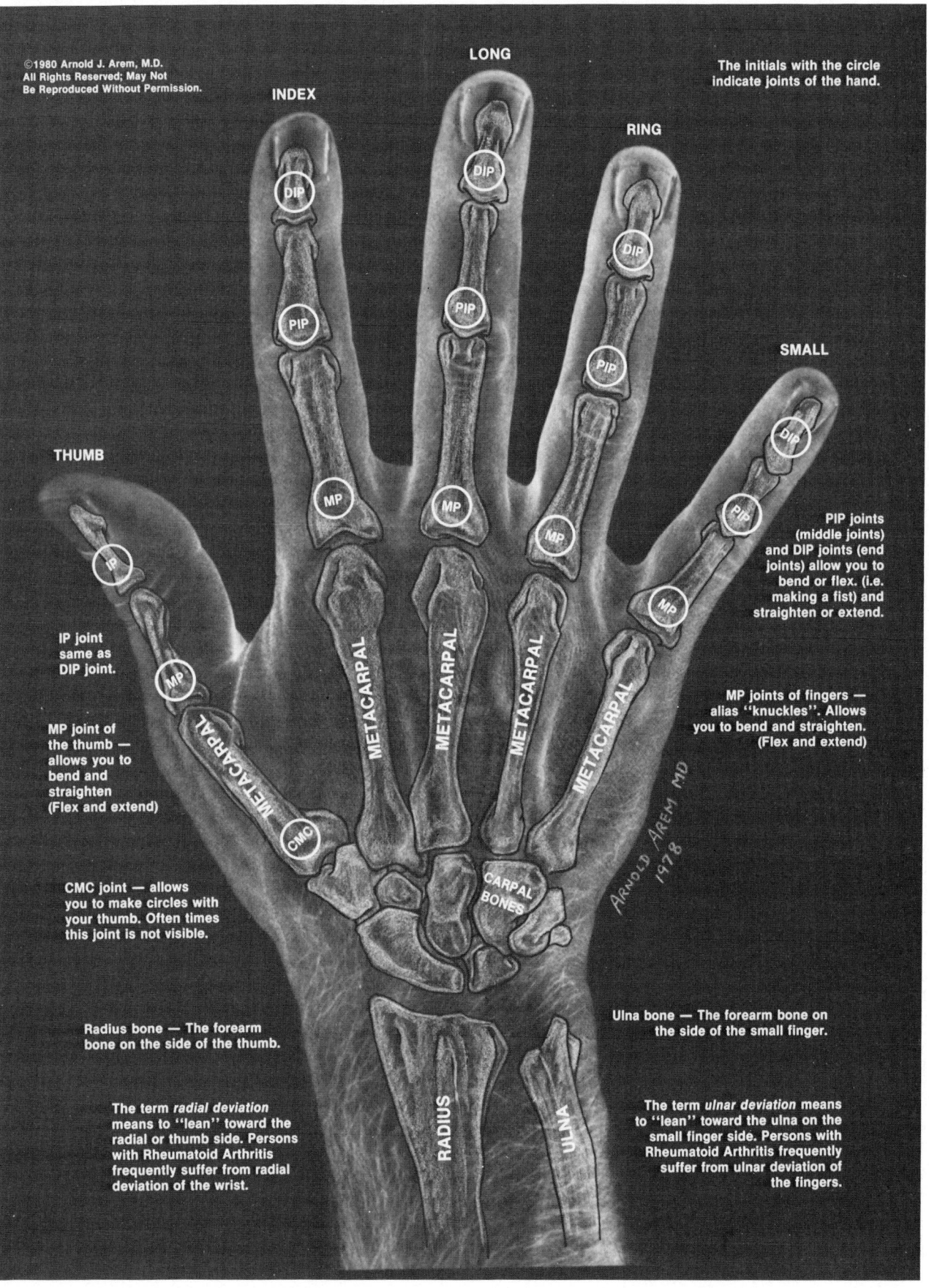

to reach the back of my head. The sides and front of my hair I can manage with the spray quite easily, but in spraying the back, I am holding a mirror in one hand to see the back of my head. Not only do my fingers and wrists not work normally or in the way I wish them to, but pain and stiffness in my shoulders also limit my ability in that area.

While shopping I need to use both hands to pick up items. Any item I am unable to reach because it might be too high or in an otherwise difficult position, I am not at all bashful about asking a stranger for help in reaching it for me.

I always keep ice cubes in a milk carton in the freezer; that makes it easier and saves time. When drinking a glass of ice tea, I must lift the glass with both hands. It is impossible to lift with only one hand.

Actually, I believe I have more strength in my hands than people would ever believe from looking at them, that is, a lot of power for certain jobs. On the other hand, for another type of job, no strength at all. No strength to remove a lid from a jar but enough strength to put one on tightly. My husband wonders how I am able to get the lid on his thermos so tight.

Diaries come to us in many different forms; sometimes they read like novels. Initially, many patients complain bitterly at having to enter into this process actively. They do not like to concentrate on their problems and have spent many years trying not to notice their disabilities. What they are really telling us is, "I do not want to be bothered; you make the decision." The diary exercise forces them to define the problems as presented in Fig. 75-1. The diary helps them focus on many insidious problems that they have stopped thinking about and that they no longer consider problems. Now, the norm is any way that they can get the job done. They will tell us they can do everything they ever did. They have forgotten the long-ago episodes of painful synovitis and entrapment of the flexor tendons, leading to early development of swan-neck deformities and the inability to grasp objects firmly.

It does not matter whether the result will be a surgical procedure or whether patients come to the realization that the more significant problems are in their feet, knees, hips, shoulders, elbows, wrists, neck, or hands, because they can now start to make choices. Patients then begin to become active participants in their programs. Unfortunately, sometimes the choice is not to be bothered any further with the details of the arthritis.

As part of their diaries, the patients make "wish lists," in which they record in order of importance their wishes regarding their hands and upper extremity function. In evaluating these wishes, I invariably notice that never first on the list but second or third is that patients would like their hands to look better. Number one usually has to do with the area in which patients feel most frustrated in hand function—that is, the ulnar drift, which reduces all hand-position functions and contributes to deformity of other joints and reduces their power as well. As diary items are reviewed, a continuous teaching situation occurs. Patients are shown an easier way of performing the functions, and we go over the adaptive devices that are available and might help with their particular problems. We never suggest adaptive devices unless the patients have brought them to our attention. The clinic offers to obtain the appropriate devices if the patients can see that the devices might help their problems. After many years in rehabilitation, it is obvious to us that patients accept suggestions for devices much better

if they believe the ideas are their own. Therefore we acquaint patients with the devices and leave the choices up to them.

Diary descriptions are converted into medical terms. For example, an observation might be that a patient has difficulty putting on pajamas because of an inability of one of the shoulders to get into the sleeve. This is defined in relation to pain or position and is listed by the therapist under shoulder problems. The next item might be a problem in switching on lamps. This is translated into a key-pinch problem, which has to do with position and which is caused by ulnar drift, volar subluxation, and Z-deformity of the thumb. This is listed under hand problems.

After we have gone through a patient's diary, converting the problems into medical terms and listing them under the classifications feet, knees, hips, shoulders, elbows, wrists, hands, and neck, we see which classification contains the largest number of problems. Some patients eliminate themselves from the program in this way. Many times a patient realizes it is not his hands that need to be fixed and that are causing all his problems. Perhaps, it is an edematous knee, a painful hip, or even a shoulder without proper range of motion that prevents him from being able to carry out most functions. However, having gone through the laborious task of maintaining a diary, a fair number of patients are able to reach the conclusion that they need more stability either in their MP joints or in their wrist to rid themselves of pain and perhaps gain more power.

The surgeon or therapist could have outlined the program quite nicely without involving patients to this degree. However, our team finds it difficult to make the above-described decisions for the patients. We prefer to use this procedure as an effective way to involve them actively in their care. Since they are the most important members of the team, the patients must assume their part of the responsibility. They must understand that although the surgeon can give the potential for good hand function and the therapist can supervise, teach, and splint, the patients are the ones responsible for all the hard work.

POSTOPERATIVE GOALS AFTER IMPLANT ARTHROPLASTY

Let us consider the rationale for implant arthroplasties and the use of silicone rubber implants. There are two goals regarding postoperative care to consider: (1) development of scar for stability and (2) development of scar for allowing motion. The patients must understand that the implants are not joints but only spacers that prevent the two raw ends of bone from rubbing together. We hope the patients are beginning to understand that the remnants of their joints will be gone and that *all* stability will then be gone as well. Until the areas develop scars around the implants, they will continue to be unstable and may fall off into ulnar deviation when the patient tries to move the joints.

How are we to accomplish our two goals? We demonstrate to the patients how they will be given the potential for stable motion in the proper plane and that it is up to them and the therapist to develop flexion and extension while not allowing any lateral motion.

Splinting

Our first goal, stability, will be assured by splints that are made especially for the patients on the fifth postoperative

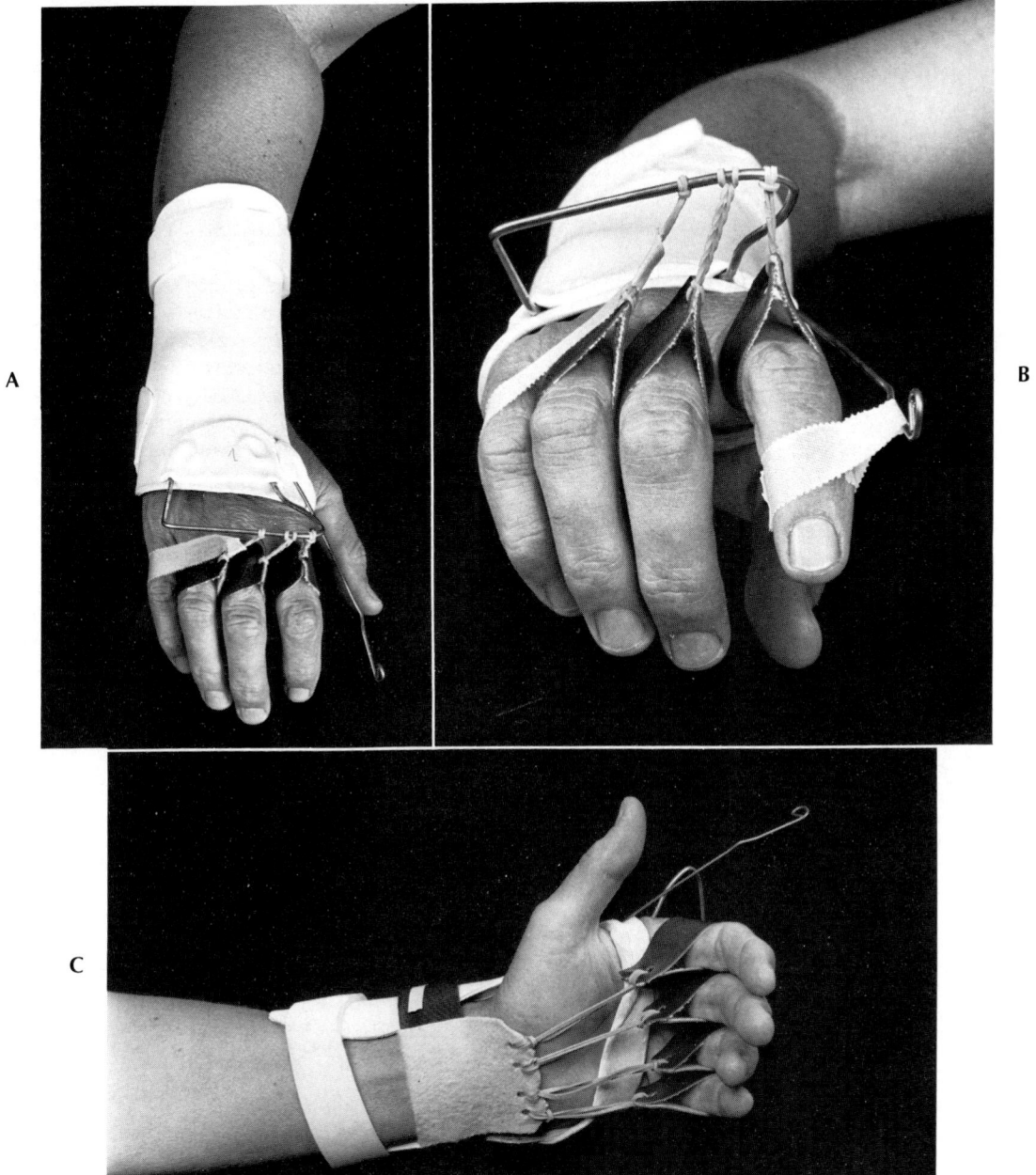

Fig. 75-2 **A,** Dynamic splint with extension outrigger. Notice that there is no padding and small finger is taped to ring finger. **B,** Dynamic splint with small finger taped using Dermicel tape to ring finger and outrigger for pronation or supination problems. Microfoam tape, which stretches, controls pronation or supination of index and long fingers but allows flexion and extension. **C,** Splint with flexion bands.

day, when they come out of their bulky hand dressings. Some centers use commercially available splints for this aspect of the program, but we believe universal splints do not suffice in many cases because they do not accommodate the residual deformities in rheumatoid patients and are cumbersome. Our splints (Fig. 75-2) are molded from one of the many thermoplastic materials on the market. The splints are cut from this material with patterns that usually look like that in Fig. 75-3. The three areas that usually deviate from this basic pattern and need to be modified on any splint depend on the patient's thumb (Fig. 75-3, *1*), the location of the suture line (Fig. 75-3, *2*), and the length of the

forearm (Fig. 75-3, *3*). To the dorsal surface of this splint (Fig. 75-3, *2*) a welding rod (³⁄₃₂ inch diameter) outrigger is added. This wire should be bent in such a way as to be low profile and yet hold the fingers in the proper position, that is, 10 degrees of radial deviation and just holding, not pulling, into extension to compensate for ulnar motion when the patient flexes hard. If patients have pronation or supination problems, a smaller piece of welding rod (¹⁄₁₆ inch diameter) can be attached to the radial side of the splint to help control this (Figs. 75-2, *B,* and 75-3, *4*).

The height of the outrigger should be such that a number 10 rubber band through the finger loop is just the right

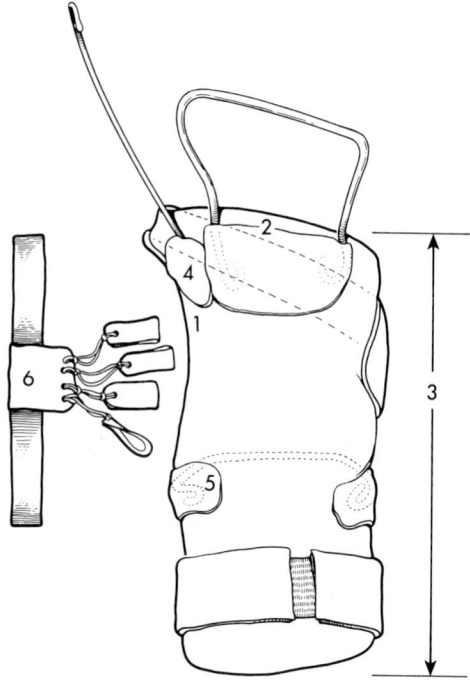

Fig. 75-3 Dynamic splint with low-profile extension outrigger and flexion band. *1,* Thumb area—splint accommodates thumb deformities. *2,* Attachment area of extension welding rod (³⁄₃₂ inch diameter) outrigger distal edge of splint should not hit on suture line. *3,* Length of forearm—splint should cover two thirds of forearm. *4,* Outrigger—use ¹⁄₁₆-inch–diameter welding rod for pronation and supination problems. *5,* Flexion rod outrigger for patients with "stiff" arthritis. *6,* Flexion band, made from Velcro and moleskin.

tension to hold the finger in proper alignment. The small finger does not get a finger loop or rubber band because it obliterates the distal palmar arch and becomes stiff much faster than the other digits do. It is simply taped to the ring finger (Fig. 75-2, *A*). Padding should not be used as a substitute for a proper splint fit. I believe that clinically this splint, as described, will provide stability with no lateral motion for the 6 weeks the patient is required to wear the splint. At the end of 6 weeks, we start to wean the patient from the splint during the day and have him continue to wear it at night in either flexion or extension, depending on the particular requirement, for a full 3 months. We make this determination based on the total active motion (TAM) recorded on the measurement sheets.

The second goal to be accomplished during this 6-week period is to mold or stress the scar in a flexion and extension plane to remodel the scar dynamically to allow motion in flexion and extension. Weekly measurements are taken, with the therapist's goal being to develop at least a 90-degree total passive motion (TPM) at the MP level and a 70-degree TAM. If the patients do well with the program and our two goals are met during their first 2 weeks of daily therapy, the visits to the clinic over the next 4 weeks are greatly reduced.

The dynamic-flexion part of the splinting program is started anywhere from 10 to 21 days postoperatively. This judgment is based on the TPM and TAM measurements.

Also of primary consideration is whether patients have "stiff" or "floppy" arthritis. Those having stiff arthritis start the flexion bands earlier, and those with floppy arthritis sometimes never need flexion bands. This band is worn initially 1 to 2 hours each day, and the time is increased until the patients can stay in the band during sleep. They then wear extension bands during the day to allow for activities of daily living and flexion bands at night. The flexion band can be attached in two ways: (1) by a volar welding-rod outrigger (Fig. 75-3, *5*) for attachment of the loops and bands to provide the proper angle of pull for those with stiff arthritis, or (2) when bridging is not necessary, by Velcro strap and moleskin (Fig. 75-3, *6*). If patients have enough TPM to use the Velcro straps, it is much more comfortable for them and can be adjusted proximally or distally by attachment of a Velcro holder (Fig. 75-3, *5*) to the splint. One begins resistive extension exercises when the flexion band is initiated, by having the patient extend the fingers against the rubber band.

Rehabilitation and management

Therapy requires a time commitment from the patient *because the procedure takes about 2 hours daily* to complete. In therapy we use moist heat in the form of hydrocollator packs (hot packs) so that the positions of the fingers are always under control. This takes about 15 to 30 minutes. After this, massage and passive range-of-motion exercise are carried out simultaneously. *No lateral motions are allowed.* We strive to obtain at least a 90-degree TPM during these sessions so that the patients will end up with a 70-degree TAM.

If the patients have difficulty of any sort, such as edema, excessive stiffness, or more pain than expected, they are treated in short sessions several times during the 2-hour period.

After the splint is back in place, we work on active long extensor gliding through the dorsal scar.

The home exercise program is of the utmost importance during the period of joint capsule formation. Active flexion and extension exercises within the dynamic splint, with the finger loops in place, are carried out on an hourly basis. Flexion exercises are performed in an intrinsic-plus position, maintaining interphalangeal extension and MP flexion so that the flexion force is concentrated at the MP joints. Should most of the force be occurring at the PIP joints, the joints may be immobilized with removable small dorsal aluminum splints or plaster casts. Immobilization of the PIP joints localizes the force at the MP joints, thereby increasing active MP flexion.

Patients are shown how to activate their extensor tendons in an intrinsic-minus position, extending the MP joints while maintaining the interphalangeal joints in flexion.

In addition to the active flexion and extension exercises in the dynamic splint, patients perform passive flexion and extension exercises demonstrated by the therapist.

At 6 weeks, when daytime splinting is discontinued, the patient may begin resistive flexion exercise using putty.

CONCLUSION

The procedures described in this chapter have proved to be clinically successful in the accomplishment of the goals as originally outlined: (1) the surgeon gives the patient the potential for good motion, (2) the therapist provides instruction and splinting, and (3) the patient provides the hard work.

This treatment protocol was outlined in our study described in the November 1977 issue of the *Journal of Hand Surgery* in which we made an effort to simulate 70 to 80 degrees of motion in the implanted MP joints. However, during the past 10 years, we have come to realize it is not possible to make man-made materials function like "normal" joints. Our goals for range of motion have been altered somewhat now and each patient's goals are set individually. The factors that must be weighed for setting postoperative goals for range of motion after an MP joint arthroplasty include (1) the amount of range of motion present in the interphalangeal joints, (2) the overall soft tissue and extensor tendon integrity at the MP joints, and (3) the surgical procedures performed. Thus the deserved range of motion can vary for each joint within the hand and from patient to patient. Function and joint stability are our primary criteria as we guide our patients through the rehabilitation process.

With this understanding, the therapist and the patient return to the surgeon's office, and the results of the functional evaluation are discussed with the surgeon. Included are the decisions reached by the patient regarding what he believes needs to be "fixed." The unwritten contract and time commitment to the program are complete.

BIBLIOGRAPHY

Arem A and Madden JW: Effects of stress on healing wounds. I. Intermittent non-cyclical tension, J Surg Res 20:93, 1976.

Flatt AE: Care of the rheumatoid hand, ed 3, St Louis, 1974, The CV Mosby Co.

Madden JW, Arem A, and DeVore G: A rational postoperative management program for metacarpophalangeal implant arthroplasty, J Hand Surg 2(5):358, 1977.

Swanson AB: Flexible implant arthroplasty in the hand, Clin Plast Surg 3:141, 1976.

XII
HEMIPLEGIA AND TETRAPLEGIA

76

Rehabilitation of the upper extremity after stroke

Robert L. Waters, Dorothy J. Wilson, and Charlotte Gowland

Rehabilitation of the upper extremity after a stroke involves a careful evaluation of the patient's motivation, cognition, motor control, peripheral sensation, and sensory integration. The goals of both surgical and nonsurgical therapy are to maximize functional use of the upper extremity and to prevent contractures or pain caused by spasticity. Treatment always includes therapy to prevent contractures whether the potential for use of the arm or hand is present or not.

The largest portion of spontaneous neurologic recovery in the stroke patient occurs within the first 2 months. Because the majority of the function of the upper extremity will be present at 2 months, therapy is directed toward integration of the involved side of the body into normal movement patterns using neurodevelopmental principles.[3] Symmetric alignment of the trunk and weight bearing are critical to allow the upper extremity to be used to its greatest potential.[17] Function of the involved upper extremity may range from being used as a minimal stabilizing assist to incorporation in all bilateral tasks.[19]

EVALUATION

The patient's cooperation with the assessment of function is dependent on the therapist's ability to guide the patient through activities giving needed physical or verbal direction that produces the patient's maximum response.[3] To determine the difference between a communication impairment and a physical or cognitive impairment, all tests are first performed on the normal side. Communication with the patient should be conducted at a level that produces the most accurate responses. For example, some patients cannot understand spoken communication but will respond to written communication or gestures. Other patients will respond to simple phrases but not to complex sentences. The speech therapist can determine the optimum method of communication.

Cognition and communication

Cognition is one of the most important factors in determining upper extremity function. It determines the ability of the patient to profit from a rehabilitation program. The patient must be capable of following simple verbal or pantomimed instructions and have sufficient memory ability to retain what is taught. If problem-solving ability, memory, organization, and attention span are severely impaired, the patient may not function well enough to learn modified activities of daily living (ADL). Most patients without bilateral cortical involvement have sufficient cognition to learn routine independent self-care activities. The ability to learn

and retain new skills must be assessed over several sessions with the patient. Only then can one determine whether the patient is educable and therefore a rehabilitation candidate.

Sensation and sensory perception

The final steps in sensory perception occur in the cerebral cortex where basic sensory data are integrated into more complex sensory phenomena. If the cerebral infarct involves the entire sensory cortex, the patient will respond to touch and pain. However, the more complex aspects of sensation (shape, texture, point localization, proprioception, and so on) will not be present. If such a patient has intact motor function, observation and questioning his family will reveal that he may use the hand on request, using the eyes for visual sensory feedback, but he will not spontaneously use the affected extremity unless he has a task that can be performed only with two hands.

Sensory evaluation should measure proprioception and two-point discrimination.[22] These are accurate tests of the patient's ability to receive and interpret sensory information for function (Fig. 76-1). Object identification is often difficult to use as a test in stroke patients because of their motor inability to handle objects and determine texture and shape.

Hemiplegic patients will not use their affected hand unless proprioception is intact and they can discriminate between two points applied simultaneously to the fingertips less than 1 cm apart.[1] The exception is the extremely motivated patient with an important task to perform that can be performed only with two hands. These patients use the eyes for sensory feedback and have intact visual perception.

Even slight sensory deficits limit the use of the affected extremity to assist in performing functional tasks because the patient will have persistent problems performing fine manipulative tasks.

Stroke patients may also have other sensory-integration problems: distorted perception of sensory input, interpretation of that input, and integration of the input with the available motor control to perform purposeful tasks. These deficits are manifested by lack of kinesthetic awareness of body parts, the relation of these parts to each other, and their position in space. Inability to organize and sequence motor acts and denial or neglect of the affected extremities are other higher sensory deficits.[30]

Kinesthetic awareness may be checked by positioning the involved arm in space while the subject looks toward his intact extremity. The patient is then instructed to duplicate the same posture on the uninvolved side. Patients who spontaneously use their involved hand as an assist without visual feedback can duplicate the posture of the involved extremity

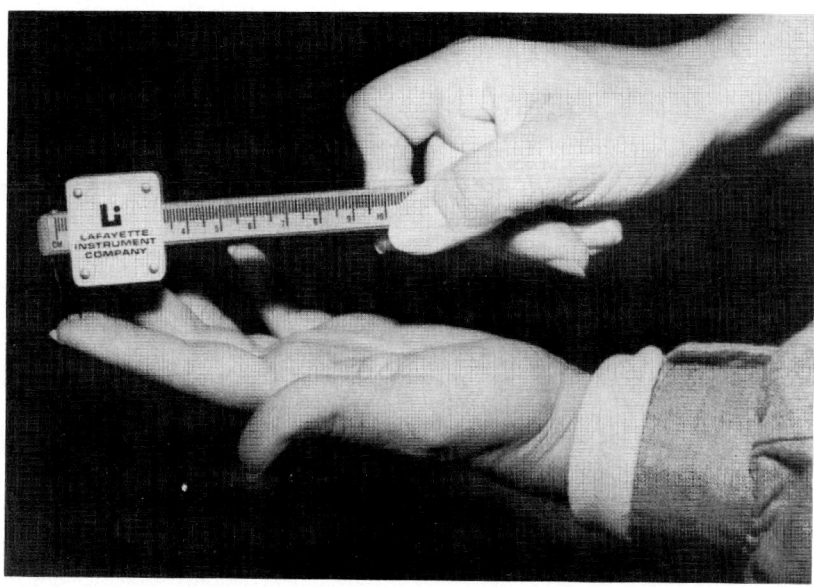

Fig. 76-1 Two-point discrimination is one of the sensory tests used to determine a patient's ability to interpret sensory input.

within a few degrees at the shoulder, elbow, forearm, wrist, and metacarpophalangeal (MP) joints.

Observing the patient's attempts to perform functional tasks or purposeful movements is an excellent method to evaluate visual perceptual deficits. Some screening tests of visual perception, such as foreground-background discrimination, rotation of forms in space, and eye-hand coordi-

nation, are useful paper-and-pencil tools to identify likely areas of functional problems to observe. Observation of motor tasks that require sequential planning and execution of individual motions should be included in the sensory-integration evaluation[26] (Figs. 76-2 and 76-3).

Ataxia is often present when severe sensory loss is present, even when the eyes are used for visual feedback. As-

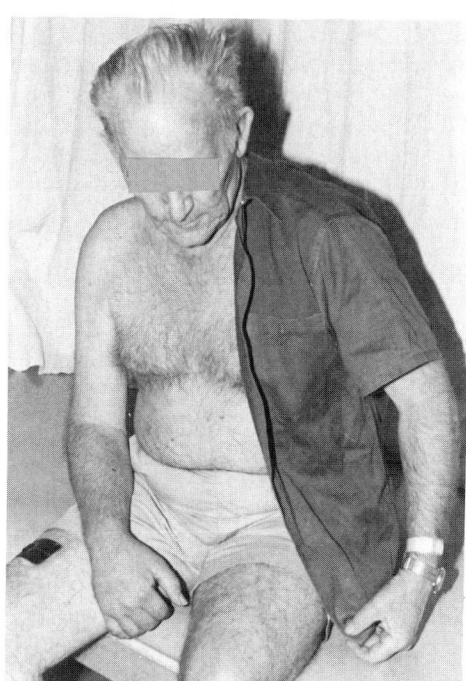

Fig. 76-2 Patient with right hemiplegia attempting to put on shirt, unsuccessfully because of an inability to organize and sequence activities.

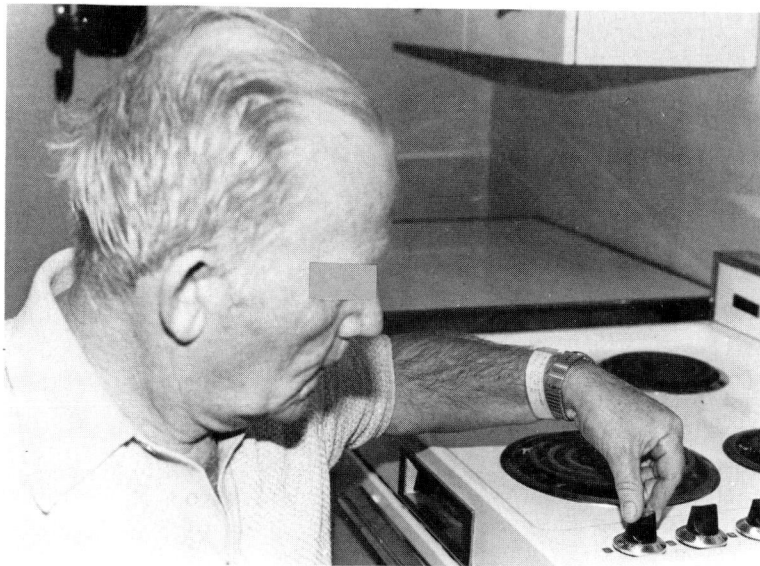

Fig. 76-3 Observation of patient's behavior during kitchen evaluation allows therapist to determine if the patient is safe and able to use good judgment while operating a stove.

sessment of speed and precision during motor acts and the patient's ability to cross midline or change direction should also be included in the sensory and perceptual evaluation. Sensory integrative deficits greatly influence the patient's rehabilitation because they interfere with the motor performance of the normal limb as well.

Vision

Evaluation of visual acuity and visual perception identifies problems of visual perception and the effects of these aberrations on the patient's functional ability.[5]

Homonymous hemianopsia often occurs after a stroke; the patient is unable to see objects placed on his affected side. This impedes function because the patient is unable to see one half of what is in front of him (Fig. 76-4). Most patients learn to compensate by turning the head. Even when homonymous hemianopsia is not present, the patient may have distortions of verticality or visual neglect in the contralateral visual field.

Balance and body handling

Use of the upper extremities depends on trunk stability, balance, and body-handling skills. Trunk stability is important for upper extremity use and is a prerequisite for sitting and bed activities[12] (Fig. 76-5). Most hemiplegic patients with unilateral involvement recover sufficient balance and body-handling skills for independent sitting activities within 6 weeks of the onset of the stroke if placed on a rehabilitation program.

Motor control

The patterned synergistic movements and abnormal reflexes in the stroke patient represent the failure of cortical regulation of normal subcortical responses. John Hughlings Jackson first recognized the hierarchic organization of the nervous system. The spinal reflexes comprise the basic or-

ganizational unit. Supraspinal reflexes involving the midbrain and medulla modify the excitability of the spinal reflexes. The cerebral cortex provides the versatility and precision of willed movement and can act directly on the anterior motor neurons through the corticospinal pathways or indirectly through the extrapyramidal system. Several recent reviews detail the role of these mechanisms in the central nervous system–damaged patient.[14,20,23,25]

The degree of functional return of the hand and arm depends on the type of volitional movement present. Normal use of the upper extremity requires versatile and precise motion. The accomplishment of routine tasks requires a wide variety of normal upper extremity movements at all joints. The functional test for the hemiparetic upper extremity developed by Wilson gives an accurate and immediate assessment of the use of the upper extremity in functional activities.[33] This allows the therapist to plan an effective treatment program for improving function and for measuring the improvement in meeting those functional goals.

An understanding of the flexion and extension synergy patterns is necessary for assessment of the hemiplegic patient's motor control. Impairment of motor control in stroke patients can be manifested in minimal loss of fine motor control, motion of the extremity only in pattern movements, or complete paralysis of the extremity.[27] The most common flexion synergy in the arm is abduction, extension and external rotation of the shoulder, elbow flexion, forearm supination, and flexion of the wrist and fingers. The most common extension pattern is forward flexion, adduction and internal rotation of the shoulder, extension of the elbow, forearm pronation, and extension of the fingers and thumb.

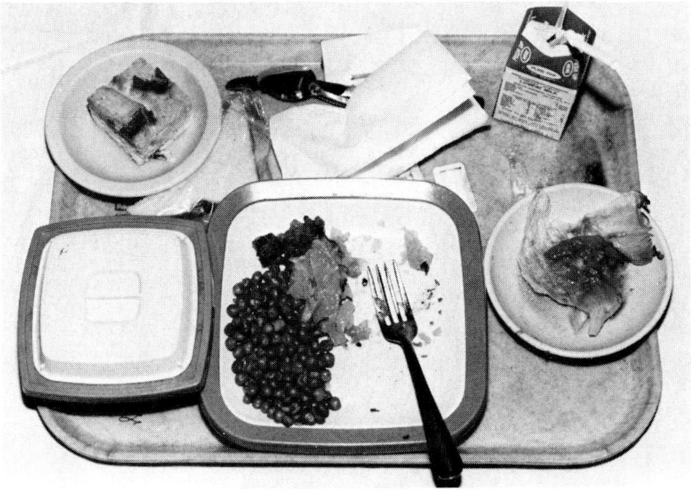

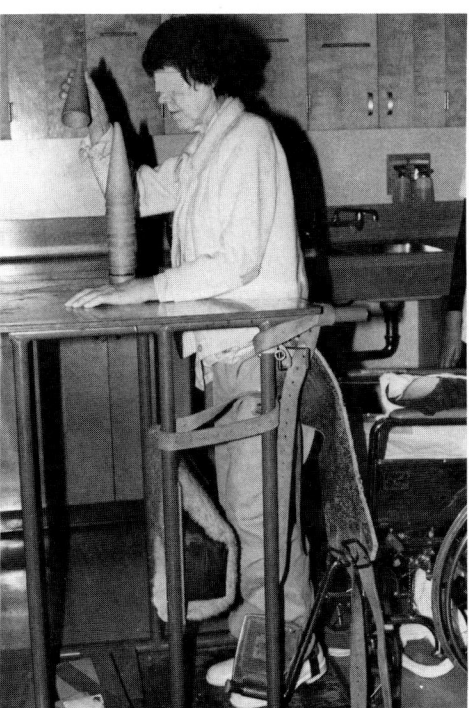

Fig. 76-4 Patients with homonymous hemianopsia, or visual neglect, frequently ignore food on half of the tray, unless they are trained to compensate for this problem.

Fig. 76-5 Development of standing balance and body-handling skills is an important prerequisite for obtaining functional use of the upper extremities.

The actual posture of the limb and exact movements vary considerably among patients, since these movements themselves produce secondary stretch-reflex responses.[31]

Return of voluntary motion in the completely paralyzed limb first occurs as flexion of the shoulder, followed by flexion of the elbow, wrist, fingers, and, last, supination of the forearm.[27] At that time, any movement of the affected extremity causes simultaneous flexion at all joints. Flexor spasticity is greatest at this period. If recovery stops at this stage, the patient will develop contractures if the joints are not passively extended and positioned daily to counteract flexion forces.

By the time the flexor synergy includes the wrist and fingers, extensor motion at the shoulder and elbow has usually occurred. At this point there is a wait of several seconds between the order to execute muscle movement and the time contraction or relaxation occurs. The ability to flex all joints of the upper extremity selectively without invoking a total flexor synergy response usually returns first at the shoulder and elbow. Once selective extension has been reestablished, there is a notable reduction in flexor spasticity, as well as improvement in speed and precision of flexor motor control.

Simultaneous flexion and extension of all fingers occur before the ability to selectively flex and extend one finger only. The index and middle fingers are usually the first to acquire this ability. Thumb opposition, when first performed, is done with the thumb opposed to the side of the index finger (key pinch). Last, the thumb can be opposed to the tips of each finger. Complete selective motion may return, as well as normal speed and control and normal reflexes.

The preceding events can be summarized as follows: In the flaccid limb joint, flexor spasticity develops before voluntary flexion. Voluntary motion in the mass flexor synergy pattern occurs before the development of extension in the mass extensor synergy. Selective flexion precedes selective extension, and the amount of flexor spasticity varies with the quality of extensor control. Usually both pattern and selective motion begin at proximal joints and are later acquired at distal joints.

Most hemiplegics will not use their affected hand as an assist unless recovery has reached the stage where selective finger or thumb extension is present without simultaneous extension of the elbow in a mass extensor synergy. When recovery is arrested at a level where pattern movements meet upper extremity demand and some selective extension in the fingers or thumb is present, but incomplete because of mild flexor spasticity or myostatic contracture, the surgeon can improve function by lengthening the flexors to increase active extension.[24,29]

Posture and tone

Reaction of the muscles of the hemiparetic upper extremity to quick (phasic) stretch by the therapist is used to determine the extent of spasticity. The response may be graded as no abnormal response (none); a palpable response that does not block continued passive motion (minimal); a response that blocks passive motion but can be overcome by slow, steady tension (moderate); or a response that produces block to further passive motion that cannot be overcome (severe). The exaggerated flexor response to stretch represents a failure of normal cortical inhibition. When that re-

sponse is present, there is also a failure of the normal relaxation action of the flexors during extensor movements (reciprocal inhibition) directly and indirectly interfering with the strength, speed, and range of extension. Clinically, the amount of flexor spasticity is inversely proportional to the amount of extensor control. Repetitive voluntary flexion and extension increases the amount of spasticity.

The precision and speed of normal hand function makes the least degree of spasticity conspicuous. Even minimal spasticity is associated with loss of fine motor control. If spasticity is moderate or severe, contractures of the elbow, wrist, and fingers will occur if the patient is not placed on a preventive therapy program. Also, functional use of the hand is limited to gross grasp when moderate spasticity is present in the fingers or thumb. Some patients with moderate flexor spasticity may manually open the hand with their intact extremity and then grasp objects to perform activities that can only be performed two-handed.

The influence of body position on the posture and tone of the hemiplegic upper extremity should be determined.[12,17] The tonic labyrinthine reflex arises from end organs in the inner ear and is activated when the head is in the upright position. This reflex activates the fusimotor fibers in the muscle spindle, increasing the excitability of the stretch reflex. Thus flexor spasticity is greater when the subject is sitting or standing than when supine. Proprioceptive righting reflexes involving the position of the neck, trunk, and limbs also influence spasticity and the voluntary response. For example, patients with limited wrist and finger extensor strength may have greater electromyographic activity during a voluntary contraction if the shoulder and elbow are extended rather than if they are restricted in flexion.

Range of motion

Range of motion (ROM) is evaluated by the muscle response to slow stretch. The joint is slowly extended over a period of several minutes. This is to avoid the velocity-sensitive components of the muscle spindle that are responsible for causing the monosynaptic phasic stretch reflex. Even when the extremity is extended slowly, some tonic activity may persist. Differentiation between what is presumed to be myostatic contracture and persistent muscle activity can be determined only after anesthetic block of the peripheral nerves or examination of the patient under anesthesia.

Most patients require minimum active ranges of joint motion to perform tasks. Minimum functional shoulder range should be flexion to 100 degrees, abduction to 90 degrees, external rotation to 30 degrees, and internal rotation to 70 degrees. The elbow range of motion should be flexion to 120 degrees and extension to 30 degrees. The forearm should have full pronation and 60 degrees of supination. The wrist should extend to −30 degrees, and the fingers should have at least −30 degrees of MP and proximal interphalangeal (PIP) flexion. The thumb should abduct to 30 degrees and have full interphalangeal extension.

NONOPERATIVE TREATMENT

Once evaluation has been completed, a treatment program is planned. The first objective in treating the spastic upper extremity is to prevent contracture. Proper extremity positioning, exercises, and electrical stimulation (of the extensor muscles) may be used. Now that most patients receive early therapy aimed at preventing contractures, severe deformities at the shoulder, elbow, and wrist are seen only in the neglected patient.

Most hemiplegic patients can be taught to do exercises using their unaffected arm and hand to passively move the joints of the affected extremity. The exercises can integrate the principles of neurodevelopmental treatment, which include trunk symmetry, weight bearing, mobilizing the scapula, and positioning of the body to decrease the abnormal tone, which allows for good upper extremity range of motion (Fig. 76-6). If the exercises are done properly, an adequate amount of joint range can be maintained. Range-of-motion exercises should be performed slowly to prevent triggering the stretch reflex and aggravating spasticity. They should be performed only within the patient's pain-free arc of motion, since pain also increases spasticity. If the patient is unable to perform these important exercises independently, the family or nursing personnel must assist or perform these for the patient.

Positioning the upper extremity is important, particularly if the patient has neglect or the resting position of the upper extremity interferes with trunk symmetry and alignment and increases abnormal tone. Some equipment used to position the upper extremity in the wheelchair include the half-lapboard and commercially available arm troughs.[28] The equipment should accomplish good body alignment, positioning the upper extremity within the visual field and protecting the upper extremity if neglect or decreased sensation is present. In addition, inhibiting spasticity throughout the extremity allows for increased motor control and use.

Serial casts are often helpful in the neglected patient with flexion contractures of the elbow, wrist, or fingers. Correction of flexion contractures of the elbow is obtained by a dropout cast applied to the extremity in maximum extension.

The posterior half is removed above the elbow to allow for further extension (Fig. 76-7). For severe problems, the serial casting may be done in conjunction with anesthetic blocks. For example, an anesthetic block of the musculocutaneous nerve temporarily decreases the abnormal spasticity in the biceps and gains elbow extension. Until maximum range of motion has been achieved, the cast is changed weekly.

Electric stimulation may be used to correct or prevent flexion contractures of the wrist and hand.[8] Electrodes are applied cutaneously over the extensor muscles of the wrist and fingers, and these muscles are cyclically contracted. Follow-up of patients receiving stimulation shows that not only can contractures be prevented and extensor muscles strengthened, but also mild flexion contractures can be corrected.

The shoulder deserves special attention. A variety of different factors may contribute to shoulder pain, glenohumeral subluxation, shoulder-hand syndrome, spasticity, central pain, degenerative changes about the shoulder, and referred pain resulting from cervical spondylosis. If early range-of-motion exercises within the pain-free arc are performed and the extremity is properly positioned to reduce subluxation, severe or chronic pain at the shoulder is rarely seen. When pain is present, patients should be examined to determine if the shoulder pain is related to degenerative changes and can be treated by methods such as aspirin and localized steroid injections. Methods to increase control of musculature that help hold the head of the humerus are also indicated when subluxation is present. Each of these techniques is successful with some patients; however, none is reliable for all patients. The exception is the patient with pain of central origin; no specific treatment is available for this cause of pain. These patients require positive psychologic reinforcement, and the use of narcotics should be avoided.

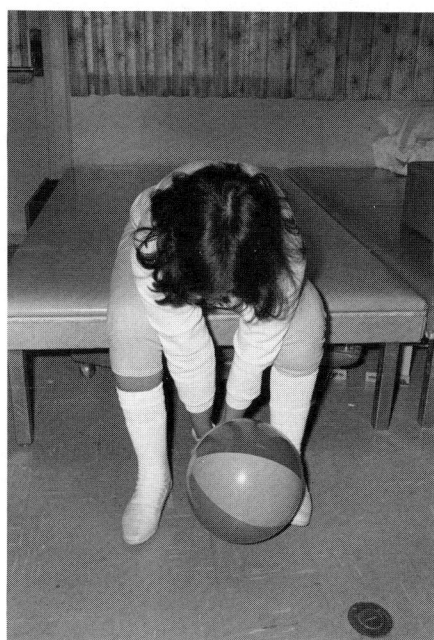

Fig. 76-6 Self–range of motion using neurodevelopmental treatment principles.

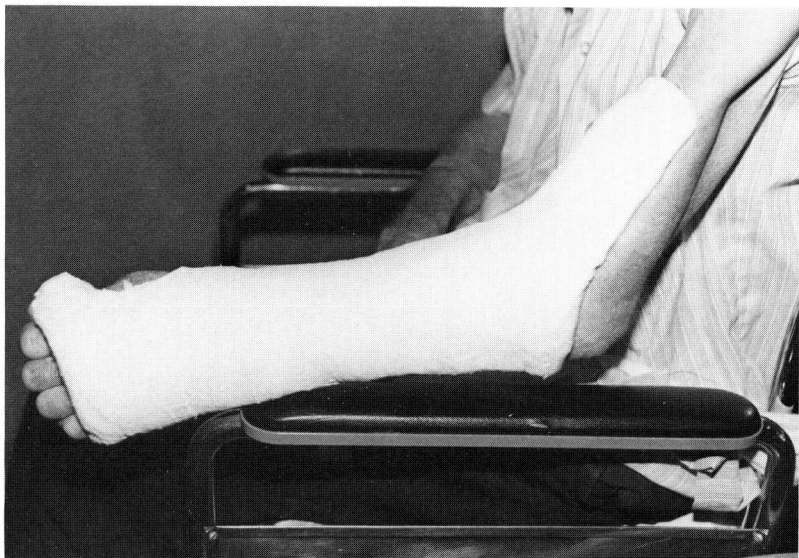

Fig. 76-7 Drop-out cast with posterior half of humeral cylinder removed to allow future elbow extension range.

Edema

Edema contributes to joint contracture in the nonfunctional, flaccid upper extremity. The shoulder-hand syndrome is a common cause of pain and swelling in stroke patients. Elevation is the most important method of preventing and controlling edema. The extremity should be supported by a sling while the patient is ambulating and elevated in a good position while he is in a wheelchair. Intermittent or continuous positive pressure can be externally applied by pressure machines such as the Jobst. Although not as effective, an edema mitt that is applied directly to the edematous hand has the advantage of giving positive pressure to the hand while one is walking.

Motor-sensory reeducation

Facilitatory techniques to increase motor control depend on the amount and type of control present and the length of time since the stroke. What is perceived as a rapid performance of a complex motor act only occurs after practice and the development of motor engrams. Although the normal person can easily learn to activate and control the discharge frequency of individual motor units, the time interval for perception and motor response is sufficiently prolonged (300 m per second) so that even during slow movements a person can consciously control only two or three motions at a time. This is readily apparent when a person attempts to perform a new, unpracticed movement; he becomes aware that he cannot regulate multiple motions. Just as a normal person learns new motor tasks, it is possible for stroke patients to increase the strength and precision of the motor response impaired by stroke and learn new patterns of motor behavior.[18]

Hemiplegic patients who have made some spontaneous neurologic recovery and who are seen within the first 6 weeks after a stroke may benefit from therapy directed to elicit motion.[9] Motion may be elicited by strong muscular contractions of the uninvolved extremity. Rapid tapping, vibration, or electrical stimulation of the muscle belly may also activate the voluntary response. These techniques are usually not indicated for patients who are more than 6 weeks after a stroke and who still have no voluntary motion.[3,4,8,13,21]

Patients with some limited motion may profit from techniques that strengthen or improve existing motor control. Weak selective motion can be strengthened by treatment and equipment that assist active motion once it has been initiated by the patient. As the patient progresses, increased extremity strength and precision are gained through the use of exercise or recreational activities.

Patients with primitive synergistic motion who begin to develop some selective movement are often restricted by moderate spasticity. Upper extremity function may be improved by treatment that inhibits spasticity. These depend on body and limb positioning, equilibrium and balance reactions, and proximal joint stability designed to inhibit the influence of spasticity and allow for use of available motor control.

Improved motor performance has been reported after biofeedback training.[2] During this training, electromyography is usually used to detect muscle contraction. In this instance the signal is amplified and displayed by means of audio and visual signals, and the patient is instructed to maximize this response.

Functional electric stimulation (FES) facilitates motor recovery in the stroke patient. Electric stimulation of the extensors increases muscular strength and inhibits spasticity in the antagonistic flexor musculature. After stimulation of the wrist and finger extensor muscles, voluntary extension is temporarily improved in some patients.[1,16] By electrically contracting the muscle, the patient becomes more aware of the actual sensation of muscle contraction and is better able to initiate a motor command. Also, afferent pathways from peripheral sensory receptors in skin, muscles, tendons, and joints are stimulated, and such stimulation may increase excitability of the anterior motor neurons.

Biofeedback and functional electric stimulation have been combined in an experimental program at Rancho Los Ami-

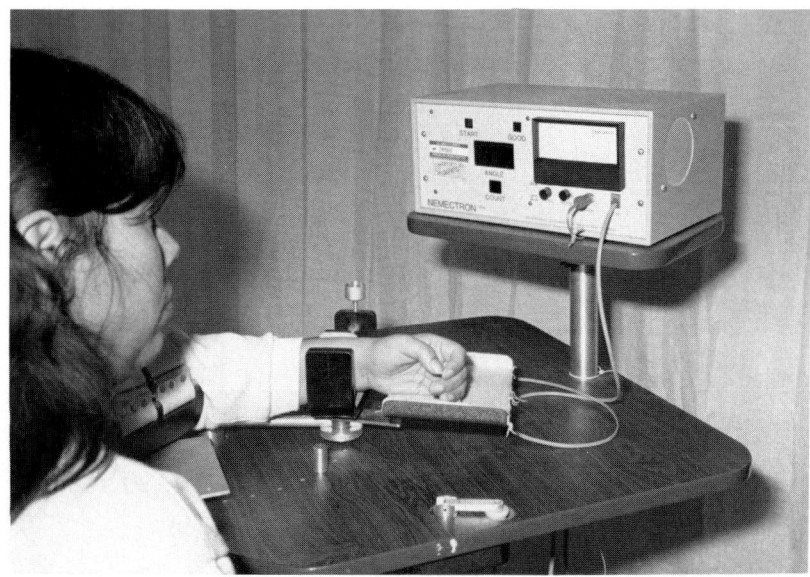

Fig. 76-8 Combination of electrical stimulation and biofeedback is used to increase motor control and strength of the wrist extension of the hemiparetic upper extremity.

gos Medical Center to maximize elbow, wrist, and finger extension in hemiplegic patients. A goniometer attached to the affected wrist provides audio and visual biofeedback in proportion to the amount of extension. Electric stimulation is then used to complete extension once the patient's maximum has been attained (Fig. 76-8).

Once a patient has recovered sufficient motion, an activity program incorporating functional gains is begun. The essence of the therapy program becomes practice and repetition to develop motor engrams enabling functional use of the extremity. The methods for retraining the upper extremity can be functional activity, craft activity, recreation, or exercise.[11,18] The appropriate approach is based on the muscles or muscle groups involved and whether the patient's control is localized at a specific joint or if the lack of control is caused by an absence of strength in the total extremity.

Simple tasks need to be broken down into several steps. These steps are taught separately and then gradually combined into the single task (Fig. 76-9).

Training in daily-living activities

Routine self-care activities such as dressing and feeding are basic skills for every person. Home and community skills such as cooking, cleaning, marketing, and driving are considered to be higher level tasks that are evaluated and training implemented when appropriate (see Fig. 76-3). The goal of rehabilitation is to achieve the highest possible level of self-care, home, and community skills.[10,15,32]

SURGICAL TREATMENT OF THE FUNCTIONAL UPPER EXTREMITY

Surgery to improve extension of the wrist, thumb, or fingers is performed when there is a restriction of extension caused by mild spasticity or myostatic contracture. The following general rules will help the surgeon select hemiplegic patients who will reliably benefit from surgery.

1. Nine months have elapsed after the stroke, and the patient has intact cognition and is well motivated.

2. Selective extension is present at the fingers or thumb.
3. The patient already spontaneously uses the hand for some functional activities, even if only as a passive paperweight.
4. Proprioception is intact and two-point discrimination is less than 10 mm at the palm or fingertips.
5. The patient has no fixed joint contractures.

Local anesthestic block of the median or ulnar nerves is used to differentiate spasticity from contracture. It is also used as a preoperative demonstration of whether the patient will benefit from surgery. If restriction of extension is attributable to spasticity, improved extension will occur after the block.

Extensor strength is often temporarily greater after local anesthetic block of the median nerve. Extensor strength commonly improves for several months after flexor tendon lengthening. This leads to the conclusion that spastic flexors not only act directly to mechanically restrict extension, but also act indirectly through neurologic pathways to inhibit the extensor anterior motor neurons. Clinically the surgeon can generally count on increased extensor strength and increased active range of motion after flexor tendon lengthening in the spastic patient.

Fingers

Active finger extension, restricted by mild spasticity or contracture, may be improved by flexor tendon lengthening. Surgical release of the flexor pronator origin has been advocated in the past as a method of treating spastic wrist and finger flexion deformities.[6] This procedure requires extensive dissection; in our experience, supination deformity has often resulted, and lengthening of the individual flexor tendons has proved to be a more reliable procedure.

Myostatic contracture shortens the active range of muscle (AROM) excursion. Lengthening of spastic flexor tendons results in partial loss of voluntary flexor strength and contractile range. Because of these factors, overlengthening of the flexor tendons resulting in a loss of flexion range and

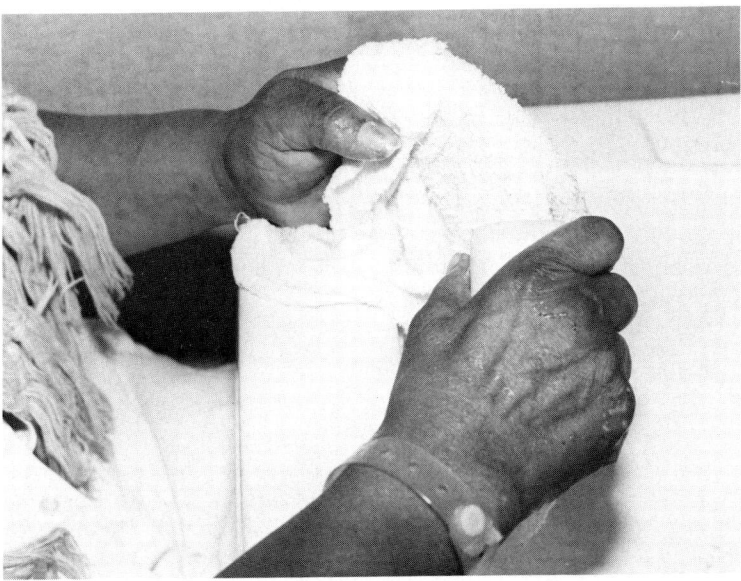

Fig. 76-9 Use of any improved control in hemiparetic hand should be incorporated immediately into the performance of basic self-care tasks.

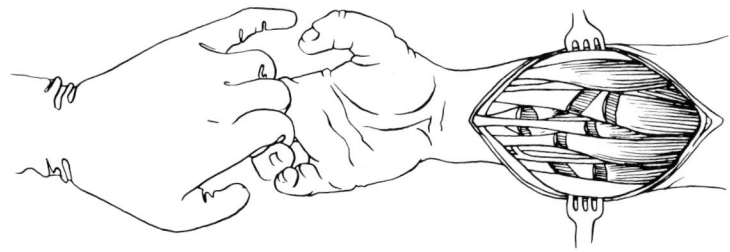

Fig. 76-10 Fractional lengthening is performed by making one or two transverse cuts in the flexor tendon proximal to the most distal insertion of muscle fibers on the same tendon. Surgeon extends fingers to obtain desired amount of lengthening. Underlying muscle fibers preserve continuity. (From Waters RL: Upper extremity surgery in stroke patients, Clin Orthop 131:30, 1978.)

strength is the most common surgical error. The amount of tendon lengthening performed is determined preoperatively. The tendon is lengthened only one half of the length necessary (usually 1 to 1.5 cm) to extend the finger from the point of restriction of the voluntary extension to full extension.[24,29] The surgeon should resist the temptation to perform further lengthening.

Passive extension of the fingers often reveals that only the sublimi appear to restrict motion. However, lengthening of the sublimi alone often uncovers restrictive spasticity in the profundi. Accordingly, both tendons are lengthened an equal amount.

Either fractional lengthening or multiple Z-plasties of the individual tendons are performed (if only one or two fingers are involved) (Fig. 76-10).[29] The hand is splinted for 3 weeks after surgery. A vigorous hand rehabilitation program after removal of the splint is essential to a successful result. Therapy is scheduled for 1 to 2 hours a day, 5 days a week for a minimum of 2 weeks. The program includes FES of the wrist and finger extensors and gentle passive range of motion to the wrist and finger flexors. Treatment is progressed to include active exercises and activities that maximize wrist and finger-extension response and full grasp of the hand.

Fixed contracture of the PIP joints may be present in long-standing deformities. If so, surgical release is performed at the time of flexor tendon lengthening. After a dorsal longitudinal incision is made, the skin is retracted laterally on either side of the PIP joints to expose the collateral ligaments, volar plate, and flexor sheath, which are contracted. The proximal attachments of the collateral ligaments and volar plate are released and the flexor sheath is excised. If the skin on the volar surface now restricts extension, Z-plasty is performed. The PIP joint is transfixed with a Kirschner (K) wire at 25 degrees of flexion for 3 weeks to prevent subluxation.

Thumb

Patients with voluntary key pinch between the thumb and side of the index finger commonly have restricted extension because of spasticity in the adductor pollicis or flexor pollicis longus muscles. The contribution of the adductor pollicis is assessed by anesthetic block of the ulnar nerve. If improved extension occurs after the block, the patient will benefit

from adductor release. The adductor pollicis tendon is released distally. Significant loss of lateral pinch strength or late MP instability has not been seen after this procedure.

When the interphalangeal joint of the thumb flexes during thumb extension, the flexor pollicis longus is restricting terminal extension. The flexor pollicis longus is lengthened in the forearm one half the amount necessary to extend the thumb from the position of restriction of voluntary extension to full extension (usually 1 cm). Stability is ensured by fusing the interphalangeal joint. Commonly, adductor release, flexor pollicis longus tendon lengthening, and interphalangeal joint fusion are performed at the same time.

Fusion of this joint is indicated also in patients with paresis of the flexor pollicis longus and hyperextension at the interphalangeal joint hindering pinch.

Wrist

Patients with shortening of the wrist flexors, because of spasticity or myostatic contracture, may also have shortening of the finger flexors. Before a decision is made to lengthen the wrist flexor tendons, it is important to determine whether the patient will still be able to extend the fingers if only the wrist flexor tendons are lengthened and be unable to extend the fingers if wrist flexion deformity is corrected. To do this, the wrist is manually held in the corrected position. If satisfactory finger extension is still present, wrist flexor tendon lengthening can be performed safely.

It is important to determine which wrist flexor tendons to lengthen. Manual palpation usually reveals the flexor carpi ulnaris (FCU) is active during attempted hand opening. Anesthetic block of the ulnar nerve, which innervates the FCU, determines to what extent this muscle hinders wrist extension. If satisfactory wrist extension occurs after the block, only this tendon is lengthened. If wrist extension is still inadequate after the nerve block and the palmaris longus and the flexor carpi radialis (FCR) are taut on palpation, these should be lengthened as well.

When excessive flexor spasticity is present at both the wrist and fingers preventing functional use, lengthening of both sets of tendons is performed. Once again, it is important to lengthen the tendons only one half the amount necessary to correct the wrist and fingers to a neutral position.

We have not found it advisable to transfer the flexor tendons to the wrist extensors in stroke patients. Electromyograms of the wrist flexors reveal different patterns of abnormal phasic activity. There are no guidelines to determine how to secure the transferred tendon under the proper amount of tension. If secured too tightly, wrist hyperextension will occur or wrist flexion may be restricted, preventing release. Fortunately, stroke patients with selective finger extension have sufficient strength to extend the wrist if the wrist flexors are lengthened.

Postoperative treatment

After lengthening of the spastic flexor tendons, the patient is placed in a short arm cast with hand included for 3 weeks after surgery. The case and sutures are then removed, and an anteroposterior splint is made at that time. If the patient has active finger flexion, one can cut away the volar portion of the cast over the fingers to allow active flexion while protecting against overstretching.

The therapy program at this time consists of cyclic FES

to finger and wrist extensors for 30 minutes twice a day, with the patient attempting to extend the wrist and fingers actively through as much range as possible with stimulation. It may be necessary to stimulate the wrist and fingers separately so that a good extensor response is obtained. In addition to extensor stimulation, passive range of motion is performed to maintain the range of wrist and finger flexion.

As active finger and wrist extension are gained, FES is used in conjunction with grasp and release activities. The stimulation is used to assist in extension and releasing objects. Various sizes of blocks and pegboards of graded sizes are used. When the patient is able to complete the full available extension range actively, stimulation is discontinued and active finger and wrist extension exercises are initiated. The patient is progressed to theraplast exercises when muscle power is F+ and can take some resistance, usually within 6 weeks after surgery. At this time also, passive range of motion into extension can be initiated, if needed, without damage to the surgical site being imposed.

Once strength and range are regained, the patient is instructed and encouraged to incorporate his new release abilities into all upper extremity functional tasks.

SURGERY IN THE NONFUNCTIONAL UPPER EXTREMITY

Surgery in the nonfunctional upper extremity is indicated to correct flexion deformities of the hand, elbow, or shoulder that cause pain or prevent adequate hygiene.

Hand

The temptation to release all finger and wrist flexors should be resisted; the wrist may become hyperextended and dislocated dorsally if extensor tone was unmasked after surgery.

When severe wrist and finger flexion deformities are present, the sublimis to profundus transfer is an excellent method of achieving the flexor tendon lengthening necessary to obtain correction.[7] Through an incision on the volar aspect of the forearm, all the sublimis tendons are divided distally and all the profundus tendons are divided proximally. The proximal end of the sublimis is sutured en masse to the distal end of the profundus. Sufficient lengthening is allowed so that the wrist and fingers can be extended to neutral position without tension. Unless finger flexion deformities are long-standing and the skin is contracted on the volar surface, fixed contracture of the finger joints can be corrected by gentle passive manipulation. Passive manipulation should not be performed in the functional hand, since it results in greater postoperative edema and stiffness than what occurs after surgical release. The wrist flexors and flexor pollicis longus may be lengthened through the same incision.

When excessive finger flexion is present without wrist flexion, a sufficient flexor tendon lengthening can be obtained by fractional tendon lengthening. As in the case of the functional hand, usually only the sublimis tendons appear tight on passive stretch of the fingers; however, the profundus tendons should be lengthened as well. Lengthening of the sublimis alone will unmask spasticity in the profundus tendons, preventing satisfactory correction.

When finger flexion deformity is present, the intrinsic muscles are commonly spastic. If surgical attention is di-

rected only to the flexor tendons, the fingers will assume an intrinsic-plus posture after surgery. Evidence of intrinsic spasticity is sought preoperatively by examination of the thumb. If the adductor pollicis is spastic, the intrinsic muscles of the fingers also may be presumed spastic. Neurectomy of the motor branch of the ulnar nerve performed at the time of flexor tendon lengthening will improve the cosmetic appearance of the fingers and relieve adductor spasticity of the thumb as well. Conspicuous intrinsic atrophy is not a problem and is obscured by slight edema and subcutaneous fat, which is present in most nonfunctional hands if the patient is well nourished.

Because some patients lack extensor tone, the wrist may remain in a flexed position because of gravity after flexor tendon lengthening if the forearm postures in a pronated position. A wrist splint may be prescribed or extensor tenodesis performed at a second operation. The three wrist extensors (extensor carpi radialis brevis, extensor carpi radialis longus, extensor carpi ulnaris) are divided longitudinally and one half of each tendon inserted through two holes in the dorsum of the radius (Fig. 76-11). The wrist is protectetd in a splint in 20 degrees of dorsiflexion for 8 weeks after surgery.

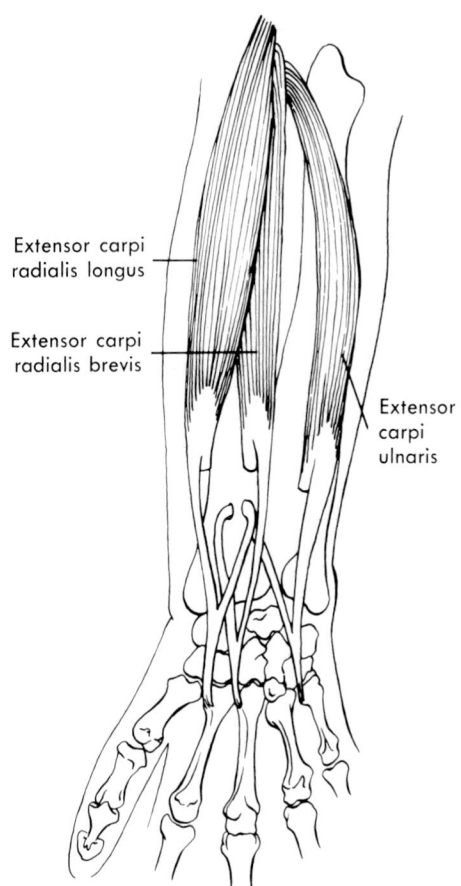

Fig. 76-11 Wrist extensor tenodesis is performed by securing one half of the extensor carpi radialis longus, extensor carpi radialis brevis, and extensor carpi ulnaris to the radius. Remaining portions of the wrist extensor tendons are left intact. (From Waters RL: Upper extremity surgery in stroke patients, Clin Orthop 131:30, 1978.)

Elbow

Most stroke patients receive early range of motion therapy after a stroke, and elbow flexion contractures are not common. It is common for the elbow to assume a flexed posture while the patient is walking, and it may bounce up and down because of clonus. Patients will purposefully slow their walking speed to decrease clonus. Musculocutaneous neurectomy will improve cosmesis and eliminate clonus. The loss of elbow flexion strength is not important, since nearly all stroke patients with excessive elbow flexion have nonfunctional hands. Since the brachioradialis is innervated by the radial nerve, which is left intact, some elbow flexion will persist after surgery. To ensure the brachioradialis is functioning, an anesthetic block can temporarily weaken the biceps. The loss of musculocutaneous sensation is not bothersome to the hemiplegic patient.

When elbow flexion contracture is present, lengthening of the biceps tendon alone will not significantly improve elbow flexion deformity and attention must be directed to the brachialis muscle as well. X-ray examination is performed to ensure that heterotropic bone is not present. Myostatic contracture is differentiated from spasticity by anesthetic block of the musculocutaneous nerve (axillary nerve block) or by examination of the patient at surgery. If there is less than 75 degrees of fixed deformity, musculocutaneous neurectomy is performed. Residual deformity is corrected after surgery by dropout or serial casts.

Musculocutaneous neurectomy is performed through a longitudinal incision extending distally from the tendon of the pectoralis major in the interval between the short head of the biceps and coracobrachialis muscles. This incision can be extended proximally or distally if further exploration to locate the nerve is required. A 1 cm segment of nerve is excised.

In the long-standing elbow flexion deformities, if the amount of fixed deformity is more than 75 degrees, release of the elbow flexor muscles is performed instead of musculocutaneous neurectomy. Surgery is performed through a lateral incision over the origin of the brachioradialis. After release of the origin of the brachioradialis, the biceps tendon and brachial muscle are divided. About 45 degrees of correction is obtained before excessive tension is placed on the brachial artery or median nerve, which are usually also shortened. However, further correction is obtained postoperatively by serial casting.

Shoulder

As at the elbow, passive range-of-motion exercises begun immediately after a stroke prevent severe contractures, which usually only occur in the neglected patient. Once a common deformity, it is now rare.

Surgical release is indicated when spastic contractures cause severe pain or prevent axillary hygiene.

Four muscles are responsible for adduction and internal rotation contractures of the shoulder. These are the pectoralis major, subscapularis, latissimus dorsi, and teres minor.[34] To determine which muscles contribute to the deformity, one abducts the arm and rotates it externally. All but the subscapularis are clinically palpable. If, with the arm at the side, the humerus resists external rotation, the subscapularis may be presumed to be spastic as well.

Surgery is performed through an incision over the inser-tion of the pectoralis major tendon. The pectoralis major and subscapularis are released and also the teres major and latissimus dorsi if the latter muscles were tight preoperatively.

The range-of-motion program initiated immediately after surgery by the therapist and continued after hospital discharge by the patient or his family is essential to the success of the surgery.

REFERENCES

1. Baker L and others: Electrical stimulation for hemiplegic patients, J Am Phys Ther Assoc 59(12):1495, 1979.
2. Basmajian JV and others: Biofeedback treatment of foot-drop after stroke compared with standard rehabilitation techniques: effects on voluntary control and strength, Arch Phys Med Rehabil 56:231, 1975.
3. Bobath B: Adult hemiplegia: evaluation and treatment, London, 1978, William Heinemann.
4. Bobath B and Cotton E: A patient with residual hemiplegia and his response to treatment, J Am Phys Ther Assoc 45:9, 1965.
5. Bouska MJ and Kwatny E: Manual for application of the motor free visual perceptual test to the adult population, Philadelphia, 1980.
6. Braun RM, Mooney V, and Nickel VL: Flexor-origin release for the pronation-flexion deformity of the forearm and hand in the stroke patient, J Bone Joint Surg 52A:907, 1970.
7. Braun RM, Vise GT, and Roper B: Preliminary experience with superficialis to profundus tendon transfer in the hemiplegic upper extremity, J Bone Joint Surg 56A:466, 1974.
8. Brunstrom S: Movement therapy in hemiplegia: a neurophysiological approach, New York, 1970, Harper & Row, Publishers, Inc.
9. Caldwell C, Wilson DJ, and Braun R: Evaluation and treatment of the upper extremity in the hemiplegic stroke patient, Clin Orthop 63:69, 1969.
10. Davies P: Steps to follow, Berlin, 1985, Springer Verlag.
11. Eggers O: Occupational therapy in the treatment of adult hemiplegia, Rockville, Md, 1984, Aspen Systems Corporation.
12. Fisher B: Effect of trunk control and alignment on limb function, J Head Trauma Rehabil 2:72, 1987.
13. Flanagan EM: Methods for facilitation and inhibition of motor activity, Am J Phys Med 46(1):1006, 1967.
14. Fugl-Meyer AR: Assessment of motor function in hemiplegic patients. In Buerger AA and Tobis JS, editors: Neurophysiologic aspects of rehabilitation medicine, Springfield, Ill, 1974, Charles C Thomas, Publisher.
15. Gee ZL and Passarella PM: Nursing care of the stroke patient, Pittsburgh, 1985, Aren Publications.
16. Gracinin F and Dimitrijevic MR: Application of functional electrical stimulation in rehabilitation: the use of reflex mechanisms in reeducation of mobility, Praha, 1969, Blanea.
17. Horak FB and others: The effects of movement velocity, mass displaced, and task certainty on associated postural adjustments made by normal and hemiplegic individuals, J Neurol Neurosurg Psychiatry 47:1020, 1984.
18. Johnstone M: Restoration of motor function in the stroke patient, New York, 1978, Churchill Livingstone, Inc.
19. Jordan C, Hrynczak C, and Wilson D: Rehabilitation potential: is it predictable from initial findings? In Contemporary concepts of stroke rehabilitation: physical management, Downey, Calif, 1980, Professional Staff Association of Rancho Los Amigos Medical Center.
20. Kottke FJ: Facilitation and inhibition as fundamental characteristics of neuromuscular organization. In Buerger AA and Tobis JS, editors: Neurophysiologic aspects of rehabilitation medicine, Springfield, Ill, 1974, Charles C Thomas, Publisher.
21. Knott M and Voss DE: Proprioceptive neuromuscular facilitation: patterns and techniques, New York, 1956, Harper & Row, Publisher, Inc.
22. Moberg E: Criticism and study of methods for examining sensibility in the hand, Neurology 12:8, 1962.
23. Mooney V: A rationale for rehabilitation procedures based on the peripheral motor system, Clin Orthop 63:7, 1969.
24. Perry J and Waters RL: Surgery. American Academy of Orthopaedic Surgeons: Instructional course lectures 24:40, St Louis, 1975, The CV Mosby Co.
25. Perry J and others: The determinants of muscle action in the hemi-

paretic lower extremity (and their effect on the examination procedure), Clin Orthop 131:71, 1978.

26. Siev E, Freishtat B, and Zoltan B: Perceptual and cognitive dysfunction in the adult stroke patient: a manual for evaluation and treatment, Thorofare, NJ, 1986, Slack, Inc.

27. Twitchell TE: The restoration of motor function following hemiplegia in man, Brain 74:443, 1951.

28. Walsh M: Half-lapboard for hemiplegic patients, Am J Occup Ther 41:8:533, 1987.

29. Waters RL: Upper extremity surgery in stroke patients, Clin Orthop 131:30, 1978.

30. Weinstein EA and Friedland RD, editors: Hemi-inattention and hemispheric specialization. In Advances in Neurology, Vol 18, New York, 1977, Raven Press, Publisher.

31. Wilemon WK and others: Hemiplegic upper extremity posture and tone analysis. Paper presented at American Academy of Orthopaedic Surgeons meeting, San Francisco, March 1971.

32. Wilson D: Adult hemiplegia: a treatment guide for occupational therapist, unpublished guide, Downey, Calif, 1968, Rancho Los Amigos Medical Center.

33. Wilson DJ, Baker LL, and Craddock JA: Functional test for the hemiparetic upper extremity, Am J Occup Ther 38:159, 1984.

34. Zarins B: Evaluation of the painful shoulder in hemiplegia using EMG. In Orthopedic Seminars, Downey, Calif, Rancho Los Amigos Hospital 5:459, 1972.

77

Helpful upper limb surgery in tetraplegia*

Erik Moberg

A NEW APPROACH

More can now be accomplished by using reconstructive surgery to help the victims of cervical spinal cord lesions increase function of their upper limbs than is generally believed. My opinion is derived from my experience with approximately 300 handgrip reconstructions and elbow extensor transfers and additional knowledge of about half as many similar operations performed by surgeons I have instructed.

Very important earlier work in this field should not be forgotten.[9,20,23,35,38] Only the following names are mentioned here: Freehafer, Lamb, Lipscomb, McDowell, Nickel, Perry, and Zancolli.

The results of this reconstructive surgery are limited, and it is of paramount importance not to give rise to unrealistic expectations. On the other hand, one should remember what Sterling Bunnell said: "If you have nothing, a little is a lot." It is no wonder that in most centers for tetraplegia reconstructive surgery has been almost a forbidden field, because trials have sometimes resulted in loss instead of gain. But today, when suitable facilities are available, it is hardly fair to let these patients, so severely handicapped, go without the help surgery can afford.

The results of the Third International Conference on the Surgical Rehabilitation of the Upper Limb in Tetraplegia, held May 14 to 16, 1983, in Göteborg, Sweden, are incorporated here.

First of all, to get positive results, a new basic approach is required, including:

1. A new concept of physiology for gripping function.[29,32]
2. A useful way to examine sensibility, because this factor is so important for evaluation.[32]
3. A new classification.[28,30]
4. A new goal for gripping function.[28,29]
5. A new functional follow-up treatment method.

Of course, adequate hand surgical skill and resources are also required just as is other basic training.

Poor results can be expected if:

1. The patient is, for one reason or another, bedridden when examined or treated.
2. The patient does not want surgery or is mentally too inactive.

3. The patient does not yet fully understand his prognosis and has not accepted the fact that dependence on a wheelchair will continue for a lifetime.
4. The patient's remaining motor activity is of abnormal *quality*. However, spasticity in some of the muscles is not always a contraindication.
5. Adequate nursing facilities for tetraplegics are lacking.
6. The surgeon in charge cannot direct all details himself, beginning with the examination and ending with the follow-up treatment.

It is my opinion, based on experience, that if conditions are adequate, some help can now be offered to at least 80% of all tetraplegia cases. This number can probably be increased. Already it is time to make surgery a *routine* part of tetraplegia treatment. This, however, will require a surgeon at each center with enough time and sufficient interest to oversee all this work. It is clearly inadequate to perform this surgery without specially trained staff for the follow-up treatment. One should start with the simpler cases, with arms here classified as good (OCu:2) or a bit better, and then gain experience and advance slowly. Even with increased experience, one has to remember that the patients left with very little mobility will need help more than those with more functional capabilities to start with.

New concept of physiology for gripping function

The motor area has always been regarded as the predominant part of grip function. If sensibility has been mentioned at all, it has been in regard to so-called feedback function. This mistake has dominated the literature on the tetraplegic hand, just as it is still dominating prosthetic work. Now the problem must be put into proper perspective. Every useful motor grip is just a response to *afferent* impulses, coming from cutaneous sensibility, vision, or the auditory system. People have to learn their gripping functions the hard way, by training. During the act of learning, a person has to build up a new program on his computer system, which enables him to perform ordered activities and even very complicated activities with *skill and speed* and leaves his conscious mind free for other purposes. Afferent impulses from muscles, tendons, and perhaps joints *do not* signal the conscious mind and are therefore useless for learning motor skills. These impulses are "private to the muscles"[6] but very important to the trained system's computer functioning. Tetraplegic extremities that are operated on have to learn new functions, so afferent impulses to the *conscious* mind are required. The majority of these come from tactile gnosis through the skin if this function has been preserved (in about 50%).

*This work was supported by a grant from Greta and Einar Askers Stiftelse, Göteborg, and made possible through the cooperation of University Departments of Surgery and Rehabilitation in Göteborg, Copenhagen, Helsingfors, and Stockholm. It was followed up by me during a stay as visiting professor at the University of California (Irvine), at Rancho Los Amigos Hospital, Downey, and Veterans Administration Hospital, Long Beach, California.

Vision is almost the only source of afferent impulses if tactile gnosis is lost but also helps very much in cases where it is preserved. Very few impulses come from other sources.

Another most important factor here is proprioception. The control of position, motion, and power load depends, to a great extent, on cutaneous stimulation. What part the joints play must be regarded as unknown. Proprioception must be understood and checked in tetraplegia surgery. Sometimes it is lost up to and including the elbow level.

Useful way to examine hand sensibility

Because tactile gnosis is the only quality of sensory function that can "put an eye" on the fingers to let them know what they are doing and where they are, the majority of current tests for sensibility are useless here. For example, pinprick, cotton wool test, figure writing, tests for temperature, and tests for distinguishing the difference between sharp and blunt must be totally abandoned. The Weber two-point discrimination test, performed in the modern version with an instrument made of a 0.9 mm paper clip wire and applied with not more than 10 g of pressure is the only one I have found of value. Because the skin provides proprioception, the same method is useful for determining the absence or the presence of this function. This factor can be evaluated segment for segment in a digit, and the result can be given numerically. Worse than 10 mm means that neither tactile gnosis nor proprioception is present in adequate quality. But even if present on only one of two gripping surfaces, a useful grip, though less precise, can result.

Classification

Without an adequate classification no comparison between results and no scientific discussion are possible. Therefore my classification does not consider the injury level in the cord or whether the lesion is complete or incomplete; it simply records what function is present. Because 50% of all tetraplegics have important differences between their two upper extremities, every patient is given one classification for the right and one for the left upper extremity. The afferent impulses that are most important head the grouping: hands that must rely on only *ocular* afferents belong to group "O." If they also have *cutaneous* afferents of enough quality, their group is "OCu."

Each of these groups are divided according to the number of muscle groups of grade 4 or better, including and distal to the brachioradialis. Thus a hand with tactile gnosis at least on the thumb pulp and having the brachioradialis and the radial wrist extensors in function with grade 4 power would be classed as OCu:2, whereas an arm with insufficient sensibility for tactile gnosis and only brachioradialis in function with grade 4 would be classed as 0:1.

Of 321 arms classified according to this system, 12% belonged to 0:0, 24% to 0:1, 16% to OCu:1, 27% to OCu:2, and only 8% belonged to the OCu:3 group. Only 6.5% were better than this. Other groups existed but were very small. First, from the OCu:3 group a majority of the extremities had useful triceps function. The figures given are from my own experience in Scandinavia and in the United States. In some countries considerably fewer high-level cases are available for reconstructive work, which means that on the average more complicated hand reconstructions with better results can be performed and fewer elbow extensor transfers

are needed. The higher-level cases, however, are the ones for whom surgical reconstruction is most needed.

A difference of two or three neurologic levels between the two arms, or between sensory and motor level in the same arm, is not uncommon.

New concept for restoration of gripping function

Previously the aim here was to provide two- or three-point pulp pinch against the thumb as well as opposition and finger flexion. This requires a lot of motor function, and therefore only a few tetraplegics could be offered surgery. Only a minimum of motors is required for key grip, and therefore I try to restore this capability. If only a grade 3 wrist extensor is available or can be obtained through the transfer of the brachioradialis, a useful grip is achievable. The tetraplegic does not have to pick up needles or small objects but needs to handle his utensils for eating or to perform other simple activities.

Follow-up treatment

Follow-up treatment requires more brain work than hand work. It is easy, unfortunately, to undo the surgical work with "routine" physiotherapy. This is especially the case with the elbow extensor procedure.

The surgeon should train an interested hand therapist and create an atmosphere of cooperation.[1,29] All exercise must be *active*. No passive tension produced by the human hand is permitted. A variety of splints is used.

IMPROVEMENT OF ELBOW EXTENSION*

One of the results of the recent meeting was the consensus that the reconstruction of the elbow extension for the 70% of patients who have lost this function is here to stay. Often this improvement is evaluated higher by the patients than what can be done for the hands. This reconstruction is even useful when, for example, because of paresthesia, no help can be given to the hands. From Edinburgh it was reported that of the patients who had undergone one elbow extensor operation, all came back to have the same operation performed on the other arm.

It was also clear that modifications of the first published method of the deltoid transfer to the triceps tendon could considerably shorten the time required for postoperative treatment. This finding was very valuable because a long recuperative period was found to be difficult for most patients because of the necessity for help and their diminished independence. Whether this shortening should be achieved by use of a reflexed extensor carpi ulnaris tendon,[22] use of artificial tendon plus fascia lata,[2] or in other ways is still under discussion.

Following are some technical details of the original method, which, in contrast to the hand operations, can be standardized.[28] The posterior part of the deltoid, separately innervated, was transferred.

Surgical procedure

Using a long, curved incision over the posterior part of the deltoid, one exposes the posterior margin of this muscle, and from there the rest of the distal two thirds of the muscle can be mobilized. It is possible to palpate a line of separation

*References 2, 7, 8, 10-15, 19, 21, 24-31, 33, 34, 35, 38, 39.

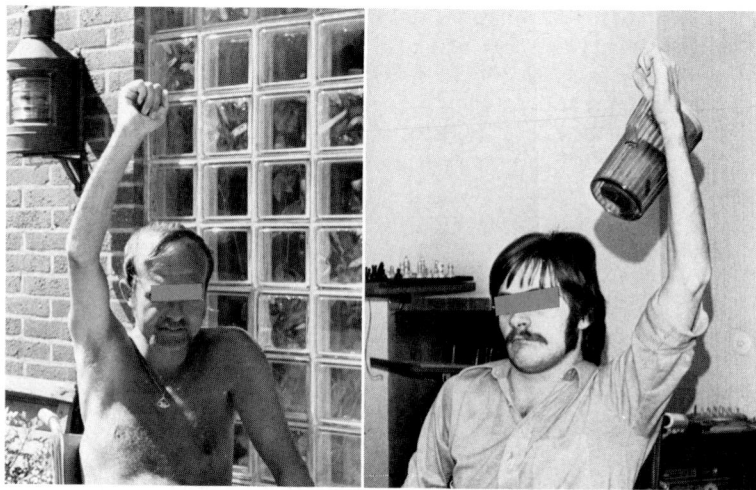

Fig. 77-1   Results of elbow extensor procedures.

between the anterior and posterior portions, through which one can proceed to the humerus. From under the posterior margin of the deltoid a curved pair of scissors can be brought in close to the humerus under the muscle and out through the separation line. From this location it is easy to free the muscle, first distally with its fibrous insertion and later bluntly in the proximal direction. Great care must be taken not to harm the innervation. The muscle must be freed sufficiently to allow about 3 cm of distal elongation when the muscle is gently pulled. Careful hemostasis is necessary during this procedure because many circumferential vessels cross the field (Fig. 77-1).

The original method used three toe extensor tendons as free grafts to bridge the distance to the triceps tendons. Some are now advocating the use of the tibialis anterior tendon as graft, using the fascia later in different ways, and so forth. Some anchor the grafts in the triceps tendon; others prefer the olecranon. To give a more solid anchoring of tendons in the distal end of the deltoid, which previously has no tendon, we created, in a single case so far, some weeks before the transfer a "tendon" to this muscle by interlacing fascia lata strips there. It produced the expected result.

An elbow extensor created by transfer of the biceps to triceps, earlier often used by Zancolli,[38] was tested and reported in new series. No doubt this method can give useful results, and it is clear that the 30% loss of power in elbow flexion was not found by the patients to be a minus. The method can, of course, be used only when a supinator is present, but this muscle is only rarely paralyzed. More experience is needed before it can be said whether or even when a biceps instead of the deltoid should be used. It is difficult to train a biceps to extend the elbow. The deltoid can perform this function without training.

To be useful to a patient, the new elbow extensor does not need much power. Control of the arm is the main requirement. Very few patients will transfer in another way after surgery. This surgery can help patients gain the independence when bedridden to, for example, feed themselves or smoke. It can help a patient achieve better driving skills, write without the aid of the other arm, increase the range of motion, sit up from a lying position, swim, and so forth.

THE HAND

With the increasing number of surgeons now active in the field, some having more patients with more sensibility and muscle left, others with patients worse off, opinions often differ about problem details. There is, however, a general agreement that when both hands can be operated on, it is wise to make them different to be used for different purposes.

Should surgery be performed on one or both hands? With which hand should one start? In my experience there is no doubt about the answers to these important questions. If only ocular afferents can be relied on, only *one* hand can be given an independent grip. The first hand operated on should always, even in cases with enough afferents for surgery to both hands, be the hand that is presently the leading one. Should surgery begin with the elbow or with the hand? If surgery to both is planned, I always try to start with the elbow extension operation. If, as was done earlier, we began with the hand and it started to become useful after surgery, immobilization after the elbow procedure took away this already appreciable gain for several months. This was a most tiresome period for the patient.

But there is another point of view that makes starting with the elbow important.[5,20,24-26,33,37] The brachioradialis muscle, for example, when used to reinforce the wrist extensors or to act as a finger flexor, needs an antagonist to act properly. When no triceps is present, this means that surgery must start with the elbow extensor.

One important principle is that no surgery should impair function that is already present, especially not the ability to transfer or to handle wheelchairs. Nor should the hand be less useful for human contact. Therefore, if at all possible, every surgical procedure should be reversible. If the patient wants to return to his preoperative condition, it should be possible to do so. This means that rarely should an arthodesis be performed in a finger without a previous test with a temporary Kirschner-wire tenodesis.

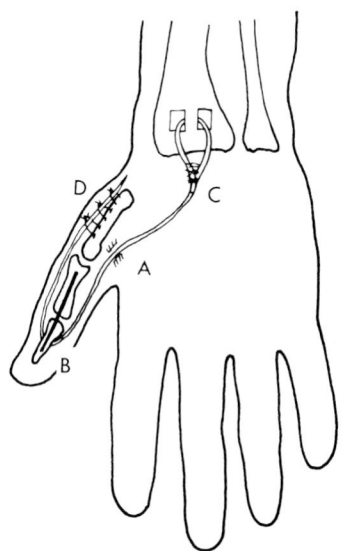

Fig. 77-2 Basic old procedures for key grip.

BASIC SURGICAL PROCEDURE

My basic surgical procedure, recommended for the majority of tetraplegic hands, uses the preserved wrist extensor system as the basis for a flexor-hinge key grip, with the thumb gripping against the radial side of the flexed index finger. If the wrist extensors are paralyzed, it is necessary to transfer the brachioradialis to the extensor carpi radialis brevis. The next steps (Fig. 77-2) are (A) release of the flexor pollicis longus tendon from the annular ligament over the metacarpophalangeal joint so that bowstringing and increased power are created, (B) stabilization of the distal thumb joint with a longitudinally inserted 2 mm Steinmann pin, (C) tenodesis of the flexor pollicis longus tendon to the distal end of the radius with loop fixation through bone windows, and (D), if necessary, tenodesis of the long thumb extensors over the metacarpal shaft to reduce joint flexion if the metacarpophalangeal joint has passive flexion beyond 40 degrees.

After completion of these procedures, the thumb flexor tenodesis will bring the thumb pulp in a broad pinch against the radial side of the index finger when the wrist is dorsiflexed. When the wrist, by gravity, moves into flexion, the thumb releases.

For the majority of cases this method is now modified to the *transpalmar* one, shown in Fig. 77-3. This way makes step (A) in Fig. 77-2 unnecessary and often also step (D). The last mentioned tenodesis was difficult to make resistant enough, gave way often, and less grip power resulted.

The Zancolli thumb method, which starts with an arthrodesis of the thumb carpometacarpal joint, is now a valuable variation, especially if more motor power is present.[38]

OTHER SURGICAL PROCEDURES

In addition to the basic procedures just mentioned, a number of other procedures and variations can be indicated. These include resection of the extensor retinaculum at the wrist to permit bowstringing and thereby increase wrist extensor power, transfer of the brachioradialis to the abductor pollicis longus to get active thumb abduction, transfer of

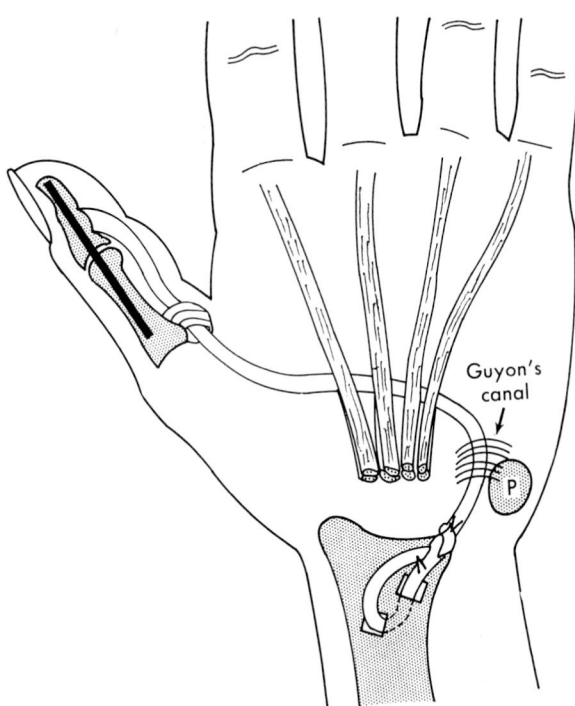

Fig. 77-3 Brand-Moberg transpalmar new technique for key grip. (From Hunter JM, Schneider LH, and Mackin EJ, editors: Tendon surgery of the hand, St Louis, 1987, The CV Mosby Co.)

the same muscle to the extensor pollicis brevis or a rerouted extensor pollicis longus to get similar function, and sling procedures to get a brachioradialis to act not only as a wrist extensor but also as a weak pronator when this function is lost.[*]

When good active wrist extension exists in tetraplegic patients, good finger flexion can be restored in more cases than was previously believed.[†] Such flexion is usually achieved through the transfer of the extensor carpi radialis longus. But this can be done only if the brevis is strong enough to act alone as a good wrist extensor. This power must be evaluated through open exposure under local anesthesia. If the brevis can lift 5 kg, it is good enough.

Several cases have been seen where this examination was not performed before a transfer and the patient lost wrist function. The risk of a late contracture when finger flexors without extensors are constructed must always be remembered. In better cases the thumb can often be given an active flexor by transfer of the brachioradialis, pronator teres, or flexor carpi radialis.

The extensor part of this surgery for the hand is much less important than is the flexor side. If necessary extension is not handled by the natural tenodesis or by trick movements, tenodesis of the extensor tendons to radius is usually enough. A transfer of brachioradialis is sometimes useful.[38]

Different forms of surgery to solve the occasional occurrence of clawing or other intrinsic problems are often discussed but still pending and therefore not discussed in detail here.[39]

---

*References 3, 4, 6, 16-17, 28, 38.
†References 3, 8, 10-12, 13-18, 22, 25-26, 33-34.

HAND SURGERY EVALUATION (TETRAPLEGIA)*

Hospital: _____

_____

_____

Date of examination: _____

Examiner's signature: _____

Patient's name: _____

Born: _____ Sex: _____

Home address: _____ Telephone number: _____

Ward: _____ Doctor: _____

Occupation before accident: _____

Occupation now, if any: _____

Date of injury: _____ Type of accident

Level of skeletal injury:

Driving _____

Diving _____

_____

Leading arm/hand before:

Gunshot _____

Other _____

_____

Leading arm/hand now:

_____

Use of wheelchair

Handdriven _____

Electric _____

Other _____

Can raise seat in wheelchair?

Can turn over in bed without help?

Can transfer without help from bed to wheelchair:

Can transfer without help from wheelchair to car and back again?

Eating with: _____ Grip: _____ Tools: _____

Method of grooming: (shaving, makeup) _____

Method of writing: _____

Stabilization in wheelchair: _____

Right   Left

Spasticity: _____

Contractures: _____

Missing parts: _____

Unusual lack of joint stability: _____

Group: Right   Left

| O | Cu | : ☐ | O | Cu | : ☐

Tr ☐   Tr ☐

Motor examination:

Spasticity (significant):

Muscles available:

Grade

Right   Left

Trapezius
Latissimus
Deltoid
Serratus
Rotators out
Rotators in
Pectorals
  Sternoclavicular
  Costal
Triceps
Biceps brachii
Brachioradialis
Extensor carpi
  radialis longus and brevis (together)
Supinator
Pronator

Name: _____

Shoulder: _____ Wrist: _____

Elbow: _____ Hand: _____

Sensibility (only two-point discrimination test with paper clip of value; includes proprioception):

Results in millimeters

Right   Left

Thumb pulp
Index
Middle
Ring
Little

Dorsal radial area
Dorsal ulnar area
Unusual features and remarks:

*Courtesy Rancho Los Amigos Hospital, Downey, Calif., and Veterans Administration Hospital, Long Beach, Calif.

HAND SURGERY EVALUATION (TETRAPLEGIA)—cont'd

Right   *Left*

Finger extensors
Thumb abduction
Thumb extension
Flexor carpi radialis
Flexor pollicis longus
Extensor carpi ulnaris
Finger flexors
Intrinsics
Passive range of flexion:
Thumb metacarpophalangeal
    joint in degrees:

Right   *Left*

Patient's main hand and arm problems:

Suggestions for improvement by splinting or surgery:

Patient's understanding:

Cooperation expected:

In patients with lower cord–level lesions where more muscles are available, tactile gnosis and proprioception are often normal. In these patients the approved reconstruction of the hand will be similar to that after a trauma. But even in cases with higher-level lesions the Zancolli "lasso" operation can help counteract hyperextension in the metacarpophalangeal joints.[38]

Resection of nerves to spastic muscles to let functional muscles overcome resistance is sometimes useful. In a very few cases wrist fusion is of value in reducing a difficult flexion contracture, but never to get more muscles for transfer.

All procedures must be modified and combined with respect to the results of a careful individual examination. Useful evaluation sheets are shown on pp. 968-969. Of course, often many more details must be examined and recorded. The aim must be, except for the small group (6% to 8%) with lower-level lesions, to concentrate all available resources in one or two strong actions. To list all that is lost and attempt to substitute for too many functions is unrealistic and can lead to disappointment. One must not forget that functional loss in tetraplegia is far beyond that which a superficial examination will reveal. This is especially true in the sensory area.

Plaster fixation is an important part of the surgical procedure. Pressure sores must be avoided, and the correct position for different parts must be found, along with the right moment for removal of the plaster splint. Usually after 3 weeks the plaster splint can be removed and active training started. The surgeon must direct the aftercare with all the attention to detail it requires. Of course, the training necessary to do this comes with experience. As I have found, the surgeon will gain knowledge with each cared-for patient. Tenodeses are apt to slacken in the postoperative period, and so they should be put in a bit on the tight side. If at

surgery the flexor pollicis longus tenodesis produces a steady grip with the thumb pulp against the side of the index finger when the wrist is brought to 5 degrees of extension, tension is adequate.

Separation or elongation where tendons are joined can occur and might need early resuture. To secure diagnosis of them in time, Ejeskar[8] is using stainless steel wire indicators in the donor as well as in the recipient tendon, followed by early and regular X-ray controls, a recommended procedure.

RESULTS

The complications of this reconstructive surgery have not been significant and are discussed elsewhere. It is difficult to evaluate the results because they depend on patient variation and on the patient's mental condition. Of 46 hands operated on in the early Scandinavian series, only four did not gain improved function. None lost any function. Of all the operations performed to date, only one has resulted in a serious loss of function. During anesthesia the neurologic level dropped down half a level. Another patient who gained much improvement in the better arm lost some deltoid power in the other arm. All the rest achieved some important improvement (Fig. 77-4). One elbow extensor reconstruction failed totally but resulted in no loss. A few obtained only weak elbow extension but enough to allow the patients to eat lying on their backs.

This tetraplegia surgery is now firmly established in Argentina, Australia, Denmark, Finland, France, Japan, Norway, Scotland, Spain, Sweden, Switzerland, and the United States.

SUMMARY

By the establishment of realistic goals, important functional improvement can be offered through surgery to a large

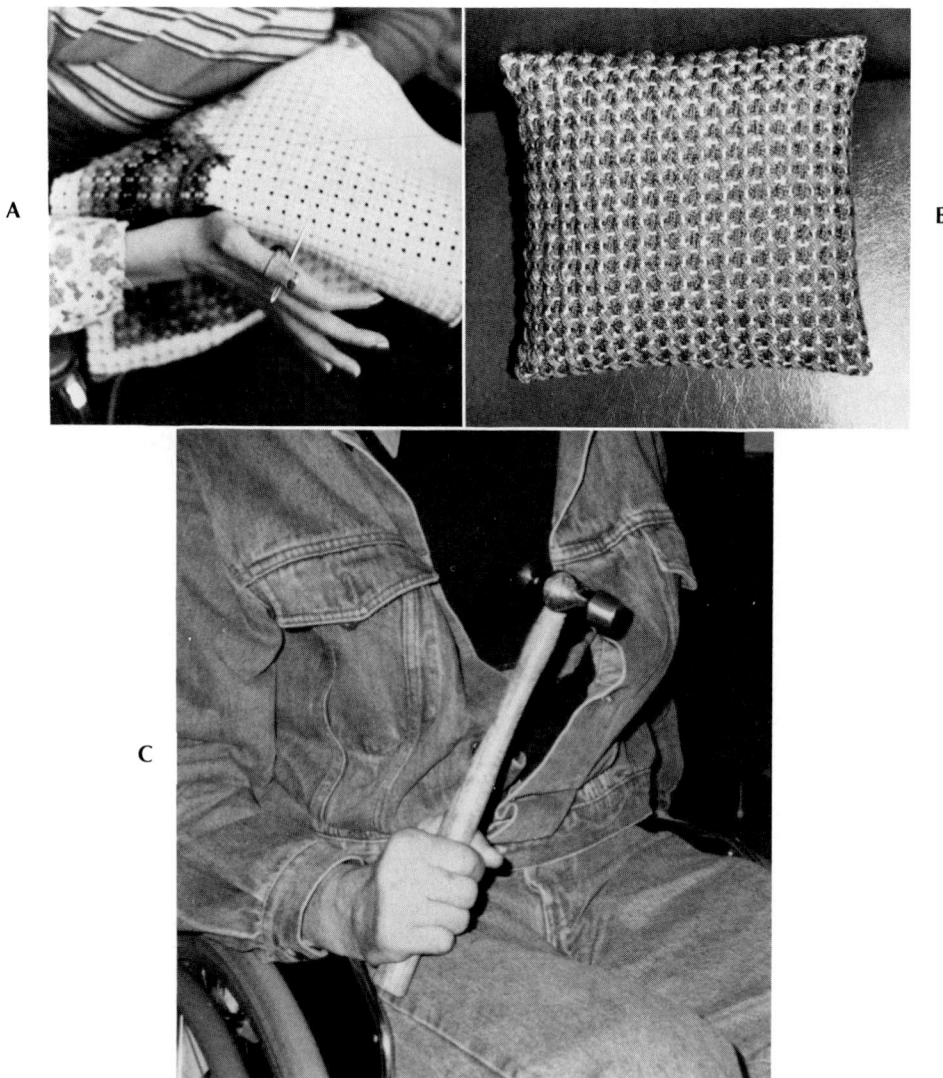

Fig. 77-4 **A,** Key grip with needle. **B,** Result of needlework performed with key-grip hand. **C,** Strong hammer grip obtained by transfer of the extensor carpi radialis longus to the flexor profundi tendons II to V.

number of tetraplegic patients. The procedures described, being reversible, can be offered without fear of reducing these patient's already limited function. Careful attention to all the details of evaluation, selection, surgery, and aftercare is essential to success.

REFERENCES

1. Ainsley J, Voorhees C, and Drake E: Reconstructive hand surgery for quadriplegic persons, Am J Occ Surg 39(11):715, 1985.
2. Allieu Y and others: Reanimation du l'éxtenseur du coude: 21 Cas, Revue Chir Orth 71(3):195, 1985.
3. Beasley RW: Surgical treatment of hands for C5-C6 Tetraplegia, Orth Clin North Am 14:893, 1983.
4. Brummer H: The winsch operation, which can be used even where no forearm muscles are left. In Moberg E: Current treatment program using tendon surgery in tetraplegia. In Hunter JM, Schneider LH, and Mackin EJ, editors: Tendon surgery in the hand, St Louis, 1987, The CV Mosby Co.
5. Brys D and Waters L: Effect of triceps function on the brachioradialis transfer in quadriplegia, J Hand Surg 12A:237, 1987.
6. Colyer RA and Kappelman B: Flexor pollicis longus tenodesis in tetraplegia at the sixth cervical level, J Bone Joint Surg 63A:376, 1981.
7. DeBenedetti M: Restoration of elbow extension power in the tetraplegic patient using the Moberg technique, J Hand Surg 4:86, 1979.
8. Ejeskär A and Dahllöf A-G: Results of reconstructive surgery in the upper limb of tetraplegic patients, Paraplegia 26:204, 1988.
9. Freehafer AA, Vonhaam E, and Allen V: Tendon transfers to improve grasp after injuries of the cervical spinal cord, J Bone Joint Surg 56A:951, 1974.
10. Freehafer AA, Kelly CM, and Peckham PH: Tendon transfer surgery for restoration of upper limb function following cervical spinal cord injury, J Hand Surg 9A:887, 1984.
11. Freehafer AA, Kelly MP, and Peckham PH: Tendon transfer surgery for restoration of upper limb function following cervical spinal cord injury, J Hand Surg 9A:887, 1984.
12. Freehafer AA, Kelly PM, and Peckham PH: Planning tendon transfer in tetraplegia: "Cleveland technique." In Hunter JM, Schneider LH, and Mackin EJ, editors: Tendon surgery in the hand, St Louis, 1987, The CV Mosby Co.
13. Hentz VR and Keoshian LA: Changing perspectives in surgical hand rehabilitation in quadriplegic patients, Plast Reconstr Surg 64:509, 1979.
14. Hentz VR, Brown M, and Keoshian LA: Upper limb reconstruction in quadriplegia: functional assessment and proposed treatment modifications, J Hand Surg 8:119, 1983.
15. House JH, Gwathmey FW, and Lundsgaard DK: Restoration of strong

grasp and lateral pinch in tetraplegia due to spinal cord injury, J Hand Surg 1:152, 1976.

16. House JH and Shannon MA: Restoration of strong grasp and lateral pinch in tetraplegia: a comparison of two methods of thumb control in each patient, J Hand Surg 9A:22, 1985.

17. House JH: Reconstruction of the thumb in tetraplegia following spinal cord injury, Clin Orthop 195:117, 1985.

18. Johnstone BR and others: Surgical rehabilitation of the upper limb in quadriplegia, Aust NZ J Surg 57:917, 1987.

19. Lacey SH and others: The posterior deltoid to triceps transfer: a clinical and biomechanical assessment, 11A:542, 1986.

20. Lamb DW: The management of upper limb in cervical cord injuries. In Proceedings of a Symposium held in the Royal College of Surgeons of Edinburgh, June 7 and 8, 1963, London, 1963, Morrison & Gibbs, Ltd.

21. Lamb DW: Current situation in the management of the upper limb in tetraplegia, Int Rehabil Med 1:135, 1979.

22. Lamb DW and Chan KM: Surgical reconstruction of the upper limb in traumatic tetraplegia: A review of 41 patients, J Bone Joint Surg 65:291, 1983.

23. Lipscomb PR, Elkins EC, and Henderson ED: Tendon transfers to restore function of hands in tetraplegia, especially after fracture-dislocation of the sixth cervical vertebra on the seventh, J Bone Joint Surg 40A:1071, 1958.

24. McDowell CL, Moberg E, and Smith AG: International conference on surgical rehabilitation of the upper limb in tetraplegia, J Hand Surg 4:387, 1979.

25. McDowell CL: Tetraplegia. In Green DP: Operative hand surgery, vol 2, New York, 1983, Churchill Livingstone, Inc.

26. McDowell CL: Tetraplegia. In Green DP, editor: Operative hand surgery, vol 2 in ed 2, New York, 1988, Churchill Livingstone, Inc.

27. McDowell CL: Tetraplegia: early stage of treatment of the upper ex-tremity. In Hunter JM, Schneider LH, and Mackin EJ, editors: Tendon surgery in the hand, St Louis, 1987, The CV Mosby Co.

28. Moberg E: Surgical treatment for absent single-hand grip and elbow extension in quadriplegia, J Bone Joint Surg 57A:196, 1975.

29. Moberg E: Reconstructive hand surgery in tetraplegia, stroke and cerebral palsy: some basic concepts in physiology and neurology, J Hand Surg 1:29, 1976.

30. Moberg E: The upper limb in tetraplegia: a new approach to surgical rehabilitation, Stuttgart, 1978, George Thieme Verlag.

31. Moberg E: Upper limb surgical rehabilitation in tetraplegia. In McCollister-Evarts C: Surgery of the musculoskeletal system, 18:471, New York, 1983, Churchill Livingstone Inc.

32. Moberg E: The role of cutaneous afferents in position sense, kinaesthesia, and motor function of the hand, Brain 106:1, 1983.

33. Moberg E: Current treatment program using tendon surgery in tetraplegia. In Hunter JM, Schneider LH, and Mackin EJ, editors: Hand tendon surgery, St Louis, 1987, The CV Mosby Co.

34. Moberg E: The present state of surgical rehabilitation of the upper limb in tetraplegia, Paraplegia 25:351, 1987.

35. Nickel VL, Perry J, and Garrett AL: Development of useful function in the severely paralyzed hand, J Bone Joint Surg 45A:933, 1963.

36. Raczka R, Braun R, and Waters RL: Posterior deltoid-to-triceps transfer in quadriplegia, Clin Orthop 187:163, 1984.

37. Waters R and others: Brachioradialis to flexor pollicis longus tendon transfer for active lateral pinch in the tetraplegic, J Hand Surg 10A:385, 1985.

38. Zancolli EA: Functional restoration of the upper limbs in traumatic quadriplegia. In Structural and dynamic bases of hand surgery, Philadelphia, 1968, JB Lippincott Co.

39. Zancolli EA: Surgery for the quadriplegic hand with active, strong wrist extension preserved: a study of 97 cases, Clin Orthop 112:101, 1975.

XIII
BIOFEEDBACK

78

Myoelectric feedback in treatment of upper motor neuron conditions

John V. Basmajian

In hand rehabilitation, myoelectric biofeedback has its greatest usefulness in the treatment or training of stroke patients and other patients with upper motor neuron conditions caused by intracranial lesions. With lower motor neuron conditions and with spinal-cord lesions, the limitations are much greater in the application of feedback-retraining methods.[3] Scattered episodes of great success do occur, but they are not the rule.

One cannot view the stroke patient's hand in isolation, for it is part of the upper limb complex. Thus our efforts to restore hand function are wrapped up with training of the whole limb. In the United States, 120 to 170 people per 100,000 population suffer a stroke annually. Of these, 75% survive beyond the early mortality period.[7,10,11,14] Vast sums of money are spent on rehabilitation of the hemiplegic arm, producing limited results. Little has been reported on the percentage of patients that attain functional activity. Joshi and co-workers[9] and Adams[1] have found it to be 4% and 5%, respectively. Findings in a study of 229 patients from the Chedoke Rehabilitation Centre in Hamilton, Ontario, indicated that only 5% of the patients showed recovery in which progress through more than one of the six Brunnstrom recovery stages ended in at least stage 4.[8] Bard and Herschberg[2] found that about 40% of their subjects recovered full voluntary motion; however, they pointed out that voluntary motion was not synonymous with upper limb function. Although the results of the therapy reported up to now are very discouraging, much in the literature suggests that significant improvement in the function of the upper limb is possible. Substantial recovery of neurologic function occurs after a stroke.

Taub[12,13] promotes the theory that lack of functional recovery is attributable to "learned disuse." He demonstrates that monkeys who were subjected to deafferentation of one limb can relearn functional activities, that is, useful hand skills, after immobilization of the unaffected limb and retraining of the affected limb with operant conditioning methods. If such a monkey were not carefully retrained, his upper limb would remain useless. Although our patients have more involved central nervous system deficits than Taub's monkeys, we believe from our clinical experience and our pilot study that his theory is applicable to stroke patients. Because of the trauma of the initial insult to the brain, the person learns that the involved arm is useless and proceeds to train and use only the uninvolved arm. Over time, even though the initial neurologic trauma has been minimized, only the uninvolved arm is used.

Physiatrists and physical therapists have developed elaborate, expensive, neurophysiologically based conventional rehabilitation programs that use techniques based on the work of Kottke, Knott and Voss, Rood, Bobath and Brunnstrom (described in Basmajian[4]). Currently they are being criticized for failing to have validated, in proper, randomized, clinical trials, that these programs do, in fact, lead to greater improvement in functional outcomes than would occur with less expensive treatment regimens.

In two randomized clinical-outcome studies,[5,6] our group showed that an integrated behavioral and physical therapy approach (experimental) has the potential of being significantly more efficacious than the conventional therapeutic method (control). Our hypothesis is that the integrated behavioral and physical therapy approach is superior to the currently advocated exercise physical therapy methods. Positive results of this ongoing research will have a profound significance for future physical therapeutic approaches to the treatment of stroke arms. The financial implications for both patients and society are obviously enormous with either of the two possible outcomes. If the new therapy is practical and useful, the improved therapy will reduce the costs of chronic disability in many ways. If the approach is found to have no clinically worthwhile benefits, its further spread can be limited on scientific grounds.

STRATEGIES

By a system of trial and error, various teams have worked out differing strategies. For example, our former team at Emory University[3] approached the upper limb and hand somewhat differently from the way our present team at McMaster University[6] does. The following is for guidance, not dogma.

Shoulder region

We have been able to decrease and often eliminate subluxation by remobilizing the shoulder girdle and shoulder joint, using the knowledge of normal shoulder function. We did this by giving the patient feedback from the upper part of the trapezius for elevation, middle part of the deltoid for abduction, and its anterior part for flexion. These muscles are easily monitored and give the patient an accurate picture of the movement desired. Feedback from the scapular muscles (which seems ideal) can be confusing to the patient because it is difficult to imagine contracting an obscure muscle, such as the serratus anterior. By gaining control and strength, the patient also gains the scapular movements necessary to allow smooth movement.

Initiating activity in the upper part of the trapezius can

be first learned by various easy procedures. After applying the electrodes over the muscle belly, the therapist may ask the patient to shrug both shoulders while looking in the mirror. Resistance given in the uninvolved shoulder often elicits activity in the involved muscle, which is made obvious by the feedback equipment. Although movement may not be apparent, the feedback should be emphasized and used as a guide until enough strength is gained to produce overt movement of the shoulders.

The middle of the deltoid is easily monitored for training of abduction. The therapist's taking the arm through abduction several times will give the patient a good idea of the movement to be learned. If either the patient is unable to understand the movement or the extension synergy dominates attempts at abduction, the goal-oriented approach may be helpful, such as having the patient put his elbow on the arm of the chair.

To monitor the anterior part of the deltoid, the electrode placement must minimize pickup of activity from either the middle deltoid or the pectoralis major nearby. Flexion seems to be the most difficult for patients. Placing and holding the patient's other hand on the affected shoulder allows the patient to concentrate on moving the elbow. The arm can be passively brought into shoulder flexion and the patient asked to hold that position. By monitoring the anterior deltoid the therapist encourages the patient to assist with the affected arm and can reinforce the early appearance of new activity.

The pectoralis major muscle is a strong component of the extension synergy. It often becomes hyperactive and restricts the passive range of motion. Its frequent recruitment when the patient flexes or abducts at the shoulder interferes with the gaining or greater range of motion. With electrodes placed over this muscle, the patient is instructed to maintain electrical silence in it because both passive and active movements are carried out at the shoulder.

If the only way the patient can initiate activity in the target muscle is by bringing in the synergy, then initially the synergy is tolerated until the target muscle is strengthened. The patient must then learn to separate the voluntary contraction of the specific muscle from the synergy by increasing the sensitivity of the biofeedback apparatus. This permits feedback before the synergistic movements occur.

Elbow region

Electrodes placed over the triceps brachii will usually pick up activity from the flexors and vice versa, unless the electrodes are placed very close together. Control of spasticity of the flexors of the elbow can usually be taught to the seated patient with electrodes over the biceps. The elbow is positioned so that the flexors are quiet, and then the elbow can be passively moved into extension while the patient tries to maintain electrical silence in the flexors. Initially the electromyograph sensitivity should be set so low that there is very little feedback for the patient to reduce. The speed of the passive movements can be gradually increased as the patient gains control of the spasticity. For complete control, the patient must be able to relax both the biceps and brachioradialis.

With a satisfactory electrode placement, one can elicit flexor activity by resisting flexion of the uninvolved elbow or by placing the hand close to the patient's mouth (that is,

elbow flexion) and having him attempt to hold it there while the therapist gently extends the elbow. Holding the patient's hand so that the forearm is supinated seems to inhibit the tendency toward elbow extension. If he tends to go into the extension synergy, active elbow flexion can be enhanced by the therapist's holding the forearm in supination.

Wrist and fingers

Flexor spasticity of the wrist and fingers often interferes with effective extension. Collectively the wrist and finger flexors are easily monitored, and a wide electrode placement during initial training through passive stretch is wise. To reduce forearm flexor spasticity, one follows the same course as for the elbow. First the limb should be positioned so as to quiet the flexors. The patient then tries to maintain relaxation during passive extension of the wrist and fingers. Once this skill is acquired, he is taught to perform the passive movement using his uninvolved hand, with emphasis on feeling the difference in resistance because the feedback indicates different amounts of spasticity. As he performs the passive extension, not only is he learning an effective method of practicing the targeted relaxation at home (without any feedback apparatus), but he is also learning to isolate the activity of one arm from the other.

After the patient has mastered control of the spastic flexors, the next task is to maintain relaxation during active extension. A standard vibrator may be used here to facilitate the extensors without causing interference to the biofeedback electrodes over the flexors. The patient also should be instructed to help raise the wrist and fingers, because vibration is not usually enough stimulation to effect movement of the joints. Initiating extension can be attempted in one of two ways. The most direct is to place electrodes over the extensors and have the patient attempt extension or try to hold the extended position. The feedback generated as a result of the extensor muscle group activity can be used as encouragement until visible movement occurs. With thin patients care must be taken with electrode placement because "cross talk" of muscle potentials from the flexors can be picked up and display a "false" feedback; this reinforces the wrong response from the patient. Very close electrode placement over the extensors can help to prevent or reduce this problem.

The flexors can be monitored to help the patient learn extension. Often as the patient attempts extension, the first muscle response is flexion. After the patient has mastered control of the flexors through stretch, he is asked to attempt active extension or to hold the extended position without bringing in the flexors. In this case the feedback is used as negative reinforcement.

Initiating finger extension is often difficult for the patient, partly because of the dominance of the flexors. One way to work on finger extension is to combine it with wrist extension, to take advantage of any mass extension response that may take place. Electrode placement over the extensor digitorum will usually pick up some wrist extensor activity because of the proximity of the muscles. Interference from the wrist extensors can be minimized by careful placement and use of the stretch reflex to ensure that the extensor digitorum is being monitored.

A useful strategy to elicit mass extension is to have the hand flat on a firm pillow. With the forearm stabilized at the wrist to prevent elbow flexion, cutaneous stimulation in the form of brushing is given to the dorsum of the hand and finger, and the patient is instructed to raise his hand and fingers straight up off the pillow. This strategy requires the patient to extend the wrist past neutral; the intense effort on the part of the patient coupled with the cutaneous stimulation may be helpful in bringing in the finger extensors.

The above strategy requires that the flexors be well relaxed and not dominant during attempts at extension. For those patients who do not demonstrate a great deal of control, the following strategy might be more useful. The forearm is placed in the neutral position between supination and pronation. The patient's wrist and fingers are flexed completely, and the therapist's hand covers the patient's hand. The patient is instructed to attempt to open up his hand—to push his fingers into the therapist's overlying fingers. The therapist will need to stabilize the wrist to prevent extension at that joint. This position reduces the tendency to go into flexion because the flexors are as slack as possible; the extensors are put on maximum stretch to facilitate their activation.

The thumb

Electrode placement over the muscles of the thumb must be very close together. Optimal electrode placement can be confirmed by use of the stretch reflex of specific muscles. One can usually minimize extraneous activity by positioning the hand, such as maintaining the neutral position to minimize activity from the pronator quadratus. With surface electrodes it is very difficult to isolate the extensor pollicis brevis from the abductor pollicis longus. When one is first teaching the patient to initiate activity from these thumb muscles, either movement is acceptable. Once the patient has control of one movement, it is usually easier to attempt the other. The proper position of the hand helps the patient gain the proper movement; the neutral position tends to assist thumb extension, while the supinated position tends to assist abduction. Good control of the thumb flexors is essential to prevent attempts at extension or abduction from being diverted to the flexors.

To assist in abduction, one places the electrodes over the area of the abductor pollicis longus and "scratches" the thenar eminence area over the abductor pollicis brevis. This helps stimulate the brevis and give the patient an idea of which direction to try to move the thumb. Spasms can be put to good use when one is working with the thumb, since appropriately placed electrodes will pick up activity of a muscle spasm. The muscle can often be set off into a spasm by repeated quick stretches. One should have the patient relax the spasm and then quickly reactivate the muscle before he forgets which muscle it was he controlled by relaxation. This has worked well with thumb extension and abduction. Another strategy along the same line is to bring in the muscle through a reflex response, such as quick supination and pronation of the forearm several times, ending in supination to recruit the thumb extensors. The patient can be instructed to first relax the muscle and then quickly reactivate it, or he can be asked to assist the reflex at the appropriate time.

Movement artifact (electrical interference caused by gross movements of electrodes and wires) may interfere with the training session because of the amount of movement in-volved. This problem can be minimized if the electrodes are placed in such a manner as to allow the wires to be secured to a part of the arm that is fairly stable. The therapist can best judge where to secure the wires after working with this strategy a few times.

The thenar eminence can be monitored with widely spaced electrodes when one is teaching a patient to isolate thumb and finger movements. The patient is instructed to maintain silence in the thumb muscles while attempting finger movements. Visual reinforcement can be used while the patient moves the thumb and tries to keep the fingers relaxed.

CONCLUSION

As noted earlier, the combined behavioral–physical therapy approach is more comprehensive than current standard physical therapy approaches, and it appears to be superior in retraining hand function in the brain-damaged person. The integrated behavioral and physical therapy methodology is still semi-experimental and being developed. The method is designed to take full advantage of the concepts of motor skill acquisition, cognitive behavioral therapy, and electromyographic feedback. Great importance is placed on the patient recognizing that it is he who possesses the ability to make the arm and hand functionally active.

The therapist initially teaches the patient the elements of motor skill acquisition. Cognitive strategies and electromyographic feedback allow the patient and the therapist to identify how best to initiate the definite motor program. Feedback shows the patient that self-generated repetitive movements and conscious control result in improved performance. The repetition of goal-oriented performance is constantly stressed. Because repetition is essential, the repetitive performance of selected activities outside of the clinic is structured and monitored.

This approach allows the patient to master the appropriate cognitive strategies and thus gain the necessary elements of motor skill acquisition. Once having applied the process of regaining a functional skill, the patient is then able to generalize the elements of skill acquisition and the cognitive behavior model to acquire additional functional activities.

REFERENCES

1. Adams GF and McComb SG: Assessment and prognosis in hemiplegia, Lancet 2:266, 1953.
2. Bard G and Hirschberg GG: Recovery of voluntary motion in upper extremity following hemiplegia, Arch Phys Med Rehabil 46:567, 1965.
3. Basmajian JV, editor: Biofeedback: principles and practice for clinicians, ed 3, Baltimore, 1989, Williams & Wilkins Co.
4. Basmajian JV, editor: Therapeutic exercise, ed 4, Baltimore, 1984, Williams & Wilkins Co.
5. Basmajian JV and others: EMG feedback treatment of upper limb in hemiplegic patients: a pilot study, Arch Phys Med Rehabil 63:613, 1982.
6. Basmajian JV and others: Stroke treatment: comparison of integrated behavioral-physical therapy vs traditional physical therapy programs, Arch Phys Med Rehabil 68:267, 1987.
7. Feigenson JS and others: Factors influencing outcome and length of stay in a stroke rehabilitation unit, Stroke 8:651, 1977.
8. Gowland C: Recovery of motor function following stroke: profile and predictors, Physiotherapy Canada 34:77, 1982.
9. Joshi J, Singh N, and Varma SK: Residual motor deficits in adult hemiplegic patients. Proceedings of World Conference for Physical Therapy, seventh international congress, Montreal, Canada, June 1974.

10. Moskowitz E, Lightbody FEH, and Freitag N: Long-term follow-up of the post-stroke patient, Arch Phys Med Rehabil 53:167, 1972.

11. Steinberg FV: The stroke registry: a prospective method of studying stroke, Arch Phys Med Rehabil 54:31, 1973.

12. Taub E: Clinical Biofeedback Course, 1979, Chedoke Rehabilitation Centre, Hamilton, Ontario, Canada, Unpublished presentation.

13. Taub E and Berman AJ: Movement and learning in the absence of sensory feedback. In Freedman SJ, editor: The neuropsychology of spatially oriented behavior, Homewood, Ill, 1968, The Dorsey Press, Inc.

14. Waylonis GW, Keith MW, and Aseff JN: Stroke rehabilitation in a midwestern county, Arch Phys Med Rehabil 54:151, 1973.

79

The use of biofeedback in hand rehabilitation

Susan M. Blackmore and Diana A. Williams

Within the past few decades, the health care industry has seen an increasing application of biofeedback to the treatment of many disorders. Basmajian has defined biofeedback as a

technique of using equipment (usually electronic) to reveal to human beings some of their internal physiological events, normal and abnormal, in the form of visual and auditory signals in order to teach them to manipulate these otherwise involuntary or unfelt events by manipulating the displayed signals. Unlike conditioned responses, a human being must want to voluntarily change the signals because he/she desires to meet some goal.[7]

A mix of technologically advanced equipment and an individual's ability to influence the state of his own health renders biofeedback a valuable tool in the treatment of individuals with hand injuries. Not only does biofeedback provide new avenues to enhance patient motivation and performance, but it also yields objective data to evaluate treatment effectiveness and efficiency.

The purpose of this chapter is to familiarize the therapist with three types of biofeedback used for the hand-injured individual: electromyographic, thermal, and electrokinesiologic biofeedback. Each has special indications and techniques. When used appropriately, biofeedback can assist in the rehabilitation of upper extremity function.

EMG BIOFEEDBACK
Historical background

Biofeedback emerged in the 1920s from the fields of psychophysiology and electronics.[1] Jacobson[24] suggested that deep relaxation exercises were an essential component of his intervention with psychoneurotic patients. To evaluate the effectiveness of muscular relaxation, Jacobson used unsophisticated electrical equipment. He monitored muscle tension as the patient was practicing progressive relaxation techniques.

As psychological relaxation techniques, such as those used by Jacobson, became refined, practitioners in the neuromotor field began using electronic equipment in their clinical arena. Initially, electromyography (EMG) was used as a diagnostic test to determine neuromotor function. Only later would EMG activity be applied to patient treatment techniques as biofeedback.

In the development of EMG as a diagnostic test, Adrian and Bronk[2] in 1929 demonstrated that the electrical functions in muscles are an accurate reflection of the functional activity of muscles. Smith[33] further clarified the diagnostic accuracy of EMG signal as a true measure of muscle function. Based on evidence that little to no inherent EMG signal exists in muscle/motor units, Smith concluded that EMG recorded activity is a valid measure of motor unit activity in the muscle.

As scientists became assured of the accuracy of EMG measurements when using indwelling needle electrodes, treatment applications of the measurement of motor unit activity emerged.[5,20,26] Over a 20-year span, beginning in the 1950s, Basmajian developed significant treatment application principles. Much recognition needs to be given to Basmajian, who has been called the father of biofeedback. His works have provided the foundation that has given the field of medicine a valuable adjunct in the restoration and reeducation of neuromotor and musculoskeletal function.

Numerous studies have been conducted on the use of biofeedback for treatment of an injured population. Information theory, learning theory, constructs from physiology, and borrowed concepts from psychology can all be seen in the development of the literature on biofeedback.[40] The behaviorist model served as the initial theoretical underpinning for biofeedback. It was believed that patients who were immediately rewarded for a type of response would then demonstrate that the response could be shaped and controlled. As the application of biofeedback grew, other theories were used to explain the process of learning through biofeedback. Cognitive learning was particularly dominant.[1] As the patient gained an awareness of a response, he could gain control over that response.

Many studies support[28,29,30] and outline the limitations[3] of biofeedback. Middaugh[28] demonstrated that there was a significant difference in the amount of voluntary muscle contraction obtained when subjects with both central and peripheral nervous system injuries used biofeedback reinforcement versus a nonfeedback condition. He repeated the study with a normal population and obtained the same results.[29] Morasky[30] demonstrated that EMG biofeedback has been shown to be effective with training relaxation of a single muscle. Morasky[30] studied eight musicians and found that muscles used during the playing of instruments maintained a lower activity level without affecting musical performance following biofeedback training, for both short and extended time periods. Biofeedback intervention ultimately served to control unnecessary muscle tension during musical performance.

The treatment and research applications of biofeedback continued to grow within many separate fields.[8] In 1969 the Biofeedback Research Society (now known as the Biofeedback Society of America*) was formed as a source for communication and certification in biofeedback principles.

EMG biofeedback has become popular in training for

---

*Biofeedback Certification Institute of America, Wheat Ridge, Colo.

sports performance and strengthening.[41] Lucca and Recchiuti[27] compared three different strengthening programs for the quadriceps in 30 female subjects. They found that the use of EMG biofeedback provided the subjects with a higher peak torque output than the other two methods of exercise. Croce[17] described essentially the same findings as Lucca. He suggested that strength gains result from the muscle tissue changes brought about by muscle tension and learning coordinated patterns resulting in maximal muscle contraction. He attributed the effectiveness of biofeedback to the learning of neuromuscular patterns and to its service as a motivational factor. From the theoretical perspective, learning theories continue to be explored as a basis for the success of biofeedback.

The historical development and research on EMG biofeedback have created a solid foundation upon which the strategies for the use of biofeedback are anchored.

Purpose and strategy

EMG biofeedback monitors activity in skeletal musculature. The activities actually monitored are the impulses sent from the brain through the peripheral nerves to the motor end plate in the muscle. These impulses cause muscle fibers to contract by eliciting a motor unit potential. The ionic membrane activity is detected through surface electrodes and relayed to the EMG amplifier. The activity of the muscle is translated into visual and auditory signals and is displayed by the amplifier to give the patient increased awareness of skeletal muscle function.[9]

Based on Basmajian's[6] research demonstrating that a subject could gain control over a single motor unit, contemporary use of EMG biofeedback with hand-injured individuals focuses on gaining control of as many motor units as possible, either to restore functional coordinated movement or to facilitate muscular relaxation.

The theory supporting motor unit training is based on the notion that voluntary effort must be reinforced by some type of sensory feedback mechanism. "The quality of a motor response is governed by the quality of perception of sensations."[32] According to Abildness, "EMG biofeedback signals can substitute for inadequate proprioceptive signals by shaping responses more sensitive than the signals generated by a therapist's observation."[1]

For the hand-injured patient specifically, EMG biofeedback is used for muscle facilitation, relaxation, or a combination of the two, such as in situations when muscular cocontraction occurs. The diagnostic or postsurgical categories that can benefit from EMG biofeedback intervention include amputation, arthritis, crush injury, fracture, peripheral nerve injury, pollicization, reflex sympathetic dystrophy (RSD), replantation, tendon laceration with subsequent repair, tenolysis, tendon transfer, and toe-to-thumb transfer. Individuals with central nervous system disorders can also benefit from EMG biofeedback (see Chapter 78).

Turning to strategies and guidelines for the use of EMG biofeedback, clinicians and researchers have noted that initially a patient relies on the visual and auditory cues to condition the random attempts at muscle control. This process then progresses to controlled initiation of a movement or motor response. Brundy notes that with biofeedback "retention persists even after withdrawal of sensory feedback, suggesting that new sensorimotor integration is taking place as a result of such therapy."[16]

To learn to control a muscle, a patient must have at least a few functioning motor units in the muscle monitored. It is helpful to have initial and routine electromyographic and nerve conduction studies to assist treatment planning for muscle reeducation.

The patient must also be able to understand the link between the biofeedback signals and his own muscle activity. This understanding is not very difficult. Even small children can learn the connection quickly. To facilitate the understanding, electrodes may be placed first on the uninjured extremity to demonstrate the connection between muscle activity and the display signals. Further, drawing an analogy between the electrodes and a microphone aids the patient in understanding that the electrodes are placed on the muscle to pick up or amplify any muscle activity.

A final guideline for the use of EMG biofeedback was noted by Ince,[23] who found that continuous feedback was more effective than intermittent feedback. In addition, the least amount of delay between patient output and machine display of visual or auditory signals is desired. Thus the purposes of EMG biofeedback span a spectrum of uses and disorders. Specific strategies to enhance the likelihood of success involve assessing the patient for his or her potential to benefit from biofeedback and then presenting the tool in a manner that can be easily understood and independently used.

EMG biofeedback equipment

To obtain maximum benefit from biofeedback, the clinician must be aware of the variety of equipment that is currently marketed and must then make a choice based on the purpose of the intervention.

Available equipment ranges from portable single channel units to computerized component systems with multiple physiologic sign monitoring. Computerized clinic model biofeedback units having an electrical stimulation component are available. With this type of equipment, when the patient achieves an identified goal level of muscular activity, the electrical stimulation is automatically activated to complete the patient's muscle contraction. Regardless of the type of machinery, it is essential for the equipment to be accurate and provide proportional feedback consistent with the patient's physiologic response.

The choice of equipment will vary according to the setting and type of patient population treated. The Biofeedback Society of America and Biofeedback Strategies[1] are sources that give complete descriptions of the components and terms associated with biofeedback equipment.

There are three basic component parts in most types of EMG biofeedback equipment[1]:
1. Transducer or sensing elements: The electrodes.
2. Amplifier: The signal modifier or processor, which is an electric circuit used for increasing strength of an electrical signal; the main housing of the biofeedback unit.
3. Output displays: These audiovisual elements can be light series, graphic displays, or tones or can be attached to other electrical equipment.

Electrodes. Surface electrodes are used for clinical EMG biofeedback. The electrode functions as a transducer. The electrode converts the ionic membrane activity of muscle fibers into an electrical potential which is carried through

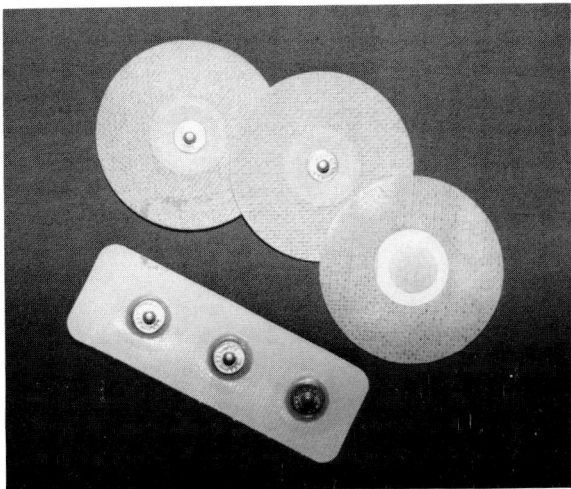

Fig. 79-1 Two varieties of 5-mm biofeedback surface electrodes useful in the treatment of individuals with hand injuries. The three electrodes pictured on top are pregelled with electrolyte gel.

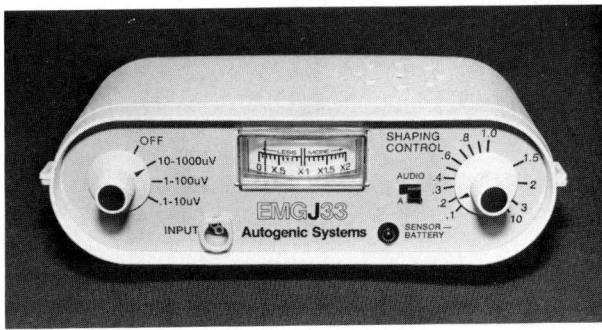

Fig. 79-2 The range on this portable EMG biofeedback unit can be set by the control on the left. This allows patients whose muscle strengths are different to use the same biofeedback unit.

the biofeedback unit. The electrodes range in diameter from 5 to 15 m[42] (Fig. 79-1).

Amplifier. The amplifier is the main housing of the biofeedback unit. Here the range of microvolt activity can be set. The range is the upper and lower levels of voltage recorded and often is broken into various levels. This arrangement enables the patient who is reactivating only a few motor units to work on a range from 1 to 10 mV, whereas a patient with greater muscle activity can work on range from 10 to 100 mV. The range levels will vary among biofeedback equipment[1] (Fig. 79-2).

The goal toward which the patient works is also determined by controls on the amplifier. The type of feedback (audio and visual modes) is chosen by adjusting controls on the amplifier.

Output displays. Output displays vary with the type of machinery chosen. The visual displays can be line graphs on a video display terminal, meter deflection, oscilloscope, pen recordings, and light series (Fig. 79-3, *A* and *B*). Audio feedback can be tones or clicks. Some biofeedback units can be used as bioconvertors so that electrical appliances can be run once the patient achieves the goal set. This functional output can be especially motivating for children.[14]

Clinical application

Once the proper equipment is selected, the following steps are taken:
1. Skin preparation and electrode placement
2. Positioning the patient
3. Establishing a baseline
4. Training techniques for facilitation and relaxation
5. Re-evaluating the training

Skin preparation and electrode placement. Clinical application of EMG biofeedback uses surface electrodes even though research applications may use indwelling needle electrodes. When using surface electrodes, the skin must be prepared to remove the superficial layer of dead skin and oils, which causes impedance to good electrical monitoring. The skin is scrubbed with an alcohol pad until slightly red-

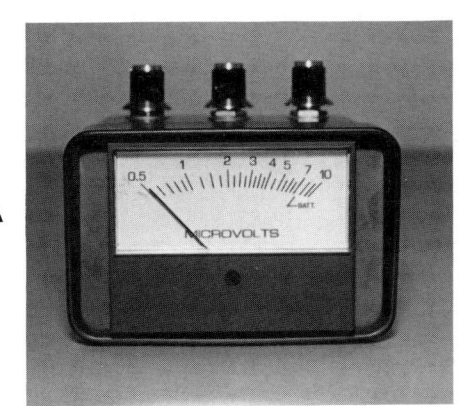
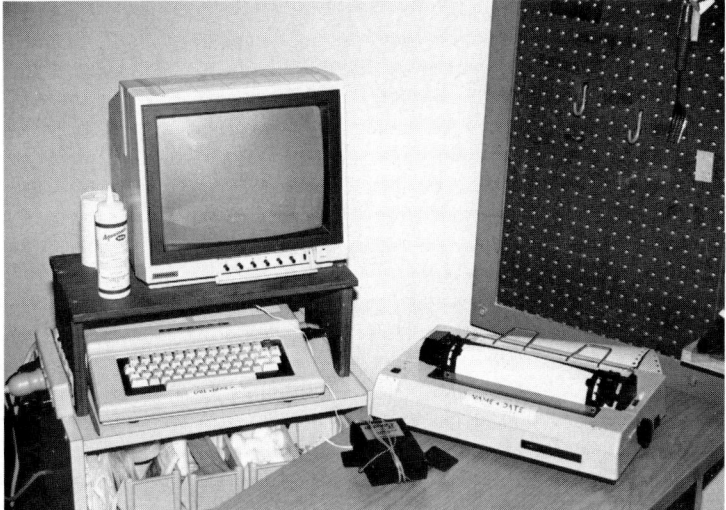

Fig. 79-3 **A,** Output displays can be a simple meter deflection or **B,** A video display with equipment.

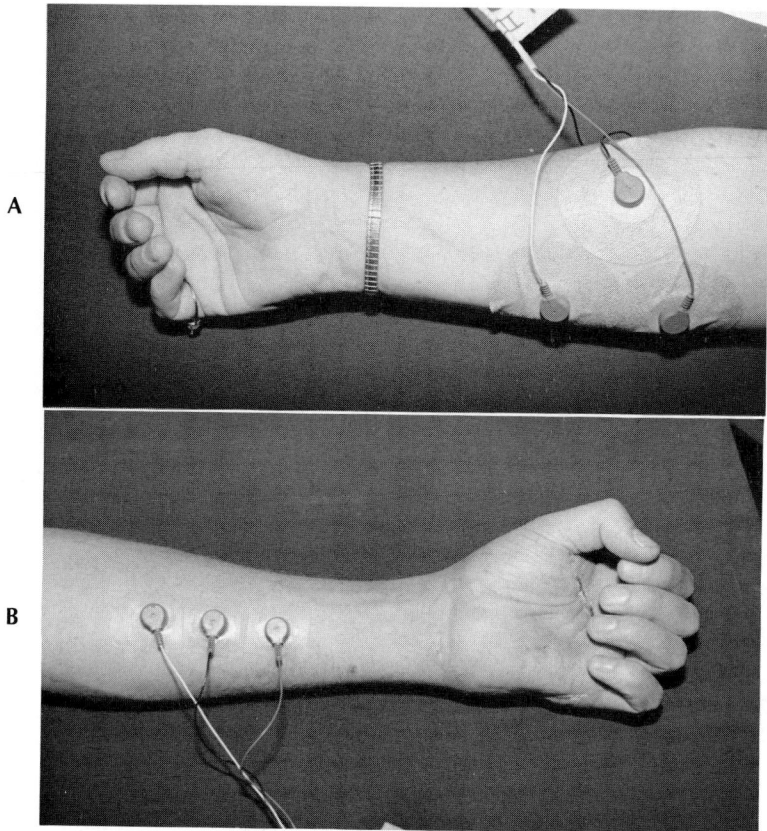

Fig. 79-4   **A,** The ground electrode can be placed either equidistant from the two active electrodes or **B,** Directly between the two active electrodes.

dened. The skin must be dry before the electrodes are applied. If high impedance is evident, then reapplication of the electrodes may be indicated. If hair is present on the skin surface of the area monitored, shaving the hair will improve the electrical contact. Also, rubbing a small amount of conductive gel onto the skin at the electrode site will improve the contact. Placement of electrodes on bony prominences, scarred areas, and fatty areas should be avoided if possible.[9,42]

There are two active and one inactive (ground) electrodes with EMG biofeedback. Conductive gel must be applied to the electrode's surface or sponge covering before attaching it to the patient's skin. The two active electrodes are placed parallel to the muscle fibers. When there is a large distance between the active electrodes, more muscle activity will be recorded. Placing the two electrodes at opposite ends of the muscle belly may be necessary to monitor trace muscle contractions. However, the possibility of inaccurate readings is increased with the electrodes widely spaced. A shorter distance between the active electrodes provides more accurate muscle activity readings and may limit the possibility of unintentionally monitoring neighboring muscles. The electrodes may be placed adjacent to each other, but then the patient must recruit a very strong muscle contraction to obtain feedback. In our clinical experience, placement of active electrodes on the forearm muscles 2 inches apart is effective for most cases.

The ground electrode is used to decrease electrical arti-

fact. Sources differ regarding the best placement of the ground electrode. There may be some advantage to placing the ground electrode between or equidistant from the two active electrodes (Fig. 79-4, *A* and *B*).

Once used, if the electrode is not disposable, it must be cleaned completely to prevent conductive gel buildup.[9,42] The larger the size of the electrode, the less impedance it produces. However, in hand rehabilitation often the small-sized electrode is needed for accuracy with electrode placement so that adjacent muscles will not be monitored. In this case, skin preparation must be thorough to compensate for the higher impedance with the use of small electrodes.[9] Refer to Basmajian and Blumenstein[9] for more detailed information on electrode placements.

The lumbricals and interossei (with the exception of the first dorsal interosseous) cannot be accurately monitored with surface electrodes. The electrodes cannot exclusively isolate these small muscles of the hand. In this case, goniometric feedback is considered a superior treatment intervention.

Positioning the patient.   The treatment environment should be quiet and free of distractions. This is especially true when the patient is working on muscle relaxation. Patients are given a thorough explanation of the process and rationale of biofeedback before initiating treatment. Biofeedback can be used when active range of motion is allowed. The patient's upper extremity is placed in a position where the monitored muscle can function optimally. For a zero-to-poor graded muscle, the patient is placed in a position where gravity is eliminated for that muscle. Muscle function is usually optimal when the muscle is elongated and the patient is asked to attempt a contraction of the muscle through its full range of motion.

If substitution occurs, then placing the extremity in the desired position and asking the patient to hold the position may facilitate use of the appropriate muscle.[9]

Establishing a baseline. After initial trial and error efforts have been made and the patient is more consistently activating or relaxing a muscle, a baseline record of muscle activity should be obtained.

Abildness suggests motor behavior can be assessed by attending to four variables:

1. Frequency: the number of times a response is performed
2. Duration: the length of time a response is maintained (i.e., endurance)
3. Intensity: the magnitude or strength of the response
4. Latency: the amount of time until a response is performed[1]

The component of motor activity that a therapist chooses to monitor is dependent on the patient's presentation. For example, if the patient displays disuse atrophy and is recruiting only a few motor units, intensity and frequency are the most important elements to monitor. When a patient is learning to activate a tendon transfer, the duration and latency are most important initial foci. These variables can be documented manually, or data can be analyzed from computer printouts when computerized equipment is used.

Once baseline measurements are documented, the patient and therapist have a basis for determining the effectiveness of selected treatment techniques.

Training techniques for muscular facilitation. Muscular facilitation or reeducation is indicated when patients display minimal active contraction with an identified muscle or muscle group. Causes of these muscle disorders may be nerve impairment, disuse atrophy, immobilization, pain, or a patient's inability to isolate a specific movement because of cocontraction of the antagonist muscle. The goal of reeducation is for patients to reactivate voluntary control of the muscle. Brown states, "EMG biofeedback is not a muscle strengthener as much as it is an aid in reeducation. By gaining more appropriate feedback the patient can then work on strengthening his muscles."[7]

When the patient is working with a weak muscle, initially the intensity of the motor unit activity and the frequency of the muscle contraction are emphasized. The active electrodes may be placed further apart to obtain more microvolt activity monitoring. Treatment sessions should be short and end when fatigue is noted by a decreasing ability of the patient to achieve the set goal level. Rest periods lasting 15 to 30 seconds between muscle contractions are recommended. The patient should be working within a microvolt range challenging enough such that the recorded muscle activity does not consistently exceed 75% of the total range.

As the patient gains muscle strength, he or she is encouraged to sustain the muscle contraction for a longer period of time to work on endurance. Functional activities then can be used with the biofeedback in place to facilitate carry-over into daily life tasks (Fig. 79-5).

If the patient has difficulty recruiting the muscle activity

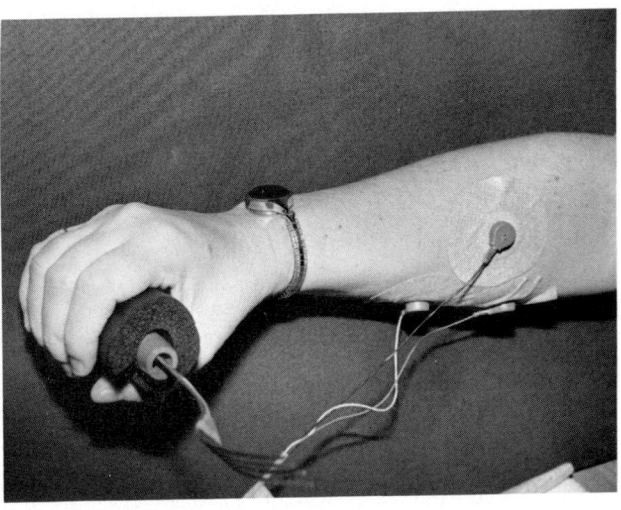

Fig. 79-5 Patient attempting to use finger flexor musculature while attempting to use a fork in a functional task.

initially, there are several conjunctive treatment techniques to facilitate muscle function. For example, he may be able to hold the shortened position of the muscle action after the therapist places the extremity in the desired position (i.e., place and hold exercises). The therapist can slowly carry the patient's extremity through desired motion as the patient attempts to perform the muscle action. Muscle facilitation techniques as described by Brunnstrome[38] and Rood[38] can also be used, including tapping over the muscle belly or resisting the opposite extremity in the desired motion.

Muscular cocontraction is often seen in the hand-injured population. The patient develops a motor pattern of contracting the muscle or muscle group antagonistic to the desired action. This maladaptive motor pattern is often seen after a tendon repair or with RSD. A biofeedback machine with two input channels can be an effective treatment intervention when attempting to decrease abnormal muscle cocontraction. The patient can then observe the level of activity in the opposing muscle group as he attempts to activate the desired muscle. Following a flexor tendon repair, the patient attempts to increase long finger flexor function while keeping the finger extensors relaxed (Fig. 79-6). Electrode placement must be very well defined for the finger extensors to avoid monitoring wrist extensors, which will be activated with strong fisting efforts. The patient is instructed to increase the intensity of flexor muscle activity only if finger extensor activity remains at a minimum. Control is learned before strength is emphasized.

Training techniques for muscular relaxation. Muscular relaxation techniques should be used in the presence of abnormally increased muscle activity. This increase in muscle activity is seen as guarding an extremity because of pain or extensor habitus and is discussed below. (For a discussion of treatment of increased muscle tone caused by central nervous system dysfunction refer to Chapter 78).

Even before the EMG monitoring is used, frequently patients are asked to listen to a relaxation tape to facilitate a decrease in overall muscle tension. The training strategies initially involve patients actively contracting and then relaxing the muscle with increased activity. As patients un-

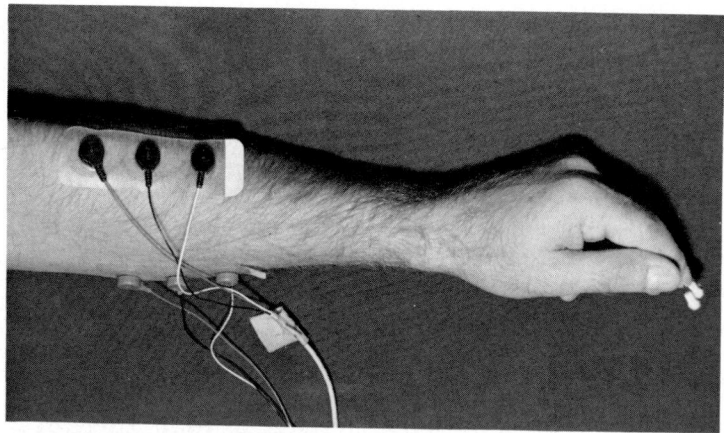

Fig. 79-6   Finger extensors and flexors of this patient are both monitored with EMG biofeedback to enable the patient to decrease cocontraction of his finger extensors as he attempts to make a fist after undergoing a flexor tenolysis procedure.

derstand the process, specific relaxation training begins. If one set of electrodes is used, they are placed on the muscle the patient needs to relax. In some cases, two sets of electrodes may be used to monitor both the muscle that needs to be relaxed and its antagonist. Patients attempt to maintain a low level of microvolt activity with the limb at rest. As this level of rest is accomplished, the patient attempts to move the opposing muscle group while maintaining a low level of microvolt activity in the muscle with increased tension.

The therapist should be aware that eccentric muscle activity will also be monitored through EMG biofeedback. What may appear as increased muscle concentric contraction may in reality be the monitoring of an eccentric contraction. The eccentric contraction tends to be displayed by the biofeedback unit as a low and constant level of microvolt activity, whereas the concentric contraction displayed by the unit tends to have a quality of spikes of motor unit activity.

As the patient learns how to use biofeedback and benefits from it, reevaluation of progress and subsequent modification of the biofeedback program should be undertaken.

Reevaluation. The measurements of frequency, duration, and latency can be compared between sessions. Thus EMG biofeedback provides measurable data to assess the effectiveness of the treatment intervention. It is also very important to use clinical tests such as range of motion, manual muscle testing, dynamometer testing, and coordination testing to provide a view of biofeedback's impact on the patient's functional abilities.[1]

The intensity levels of microvolt activity may be compared at the beginning and end of each biofeedback session. In our clinical experience, a 10% improvement in microvolt activity seen with one session justifies continued use of this treatment modality. A comparison of intensity levels between sessions should be avoided. Different electrode placements and skin preparation between sessions may result in differing baseline microvolt activity. The maximum microvolt activity may appear to be higher in one session if the baseline resting microvolt activity was high during that session.

If EMG biofeedback has been effective in clinic treatment, then it is appropriate to use biofeedback on a home program basis. Rental units or teaching the patient the area to palpate where muscle activity can be felt are techniques to facilitate carryover outside clinical treatment time.

In response to reevaluation findings, EMG biofeedback programs can be modified to more effectively and efficiently enhance patient function.

THERMAL BIOFEEDBACK
Historical background

Another area of application of biofeedback for the hand-injured individual is thermal monitoring. Studies on thermal biofeedback emerged from concepts of operant conditioning of autonomic responses. In 1967 Miller demonstrated the ability of curarized rats to change heart rate, blood flow, and vasodilation using operant conditioning principles.[1] In 1978 a study was performed in which the control of the magnitude of finger pulse volume was reinforced with biofeedback when the pulse volume changed direction. Thus vasoconstriction of digital vessels was trained independently of heart rate or respiration.[36]

As the treatment application of thermal biofeedback grew, further control over vasomotor events was demonstrated by using adjunctive treatments along with biofeedback. These include hypnosis, meditation, or relaxation techniques. Today's literature supports the simultaneous use of thermal biofeedback and an adjunct treatment to achieve control over vasomotor activity.[21]

Applications of the above findings to humans have moved beyond the behaviorist's conclusions. "It has been demonstrated that the human visceral system can respond to a variety of behavioral demands in a manner which represents an adaptive functional CNS reaction designed to maintain body homeostasis."[1]

Based on conclusions about the potential of humans to influence their autonomic processes, temperature training was developed and continues to be used for a variety of purposes in the treatment of hand injuries.

Purpose and strategy

Temperature training focuses on increasing peripheral temperature, which denotes relaxation of the sympathetic system.[1] Peripheral vasoconstriction signals sympathetic arousal and results in lower skin temperature. Conversely, vasodilation indicates sympathetic relaxation and results in higher skin temperatures. In 1977 Taub[35] presented one of the first pieces of evidence demonstrating that voluntary hand warming was capable of overriding thermoregulatory homeostasis mechanisms. The use of thermography equipment for feedback with relaxation and warming techniques has been effective for learning self-regulation of tissue temperature.[21] Today there is much support for the use of thermal biofeedback as a treatment intervention for Raynaud's disease or phenomenon.[34,35,36] Patients with Raynaud's phenomenon display vasoconstriction of digital, palmar, and plantar arteries. Decreased blood flow causes pain, skin discoloration, and possible ulceration. The decrease in blood flow can be initiated by a cold environment or from emotional upset. At the present time, there is no adequate pharmacologic treatment for Raynaud's phenomenon.

Yocum supports the use of thermal biofeedback as a treatment for Raynaud's phenomenon. In his retrospective study, 23 patients with Raynaud's phenomenon who used thermal biofeedback demonstrated elevated baseline temperatures, described subjective improvements, and experienced a decrease in skin ulcers. These improvements persisted 1 year after treatment.[44]

Thermography equipment is used to increase internal sensitivity, which in turn provides the patient with the knowledge of internal events (in this case, blood flow to the hands). Through relaxation and visualization, blood flow can be increased to the hands. Again, once voluntary internal control is established, the thermography equipment is not needed, with the exception of occasional monitoring and reinforcement.

As is the case with EMG biofeedback, the purposes and strategies of treatment can be accomplished only if the practitioner selects the proper equipment.

Thermal biofeedback equipment

Thermal biofeedback units have transducers called thermisters or temperature probes. The temperature probe detects peripheral skin temperature through arteriole blood flow. The skin's surface temperature varies directly with the amount of blood flow to the area. The use of several temperature probes (i.e., one on each finger) is suggested so that training will not be isolated to only one finger. There is usually a 1- to 3-second delay in the equipment's ability to translate temperature information to a visual display signal in the amplifier (Fig. 79-7).

Equipment for absolute temperature training allows the patient to modify the temperature in one region of his body. Equipment for differential training allows two sites to be selected for monitoring whereby the patient can attempt to move blood from one region to another.[1] For example, differential training would translate warmth (blood flow) from the head to the hands. Once the proper equipment is selected, treatment can then begin.

Clinical application

No singular training strategy has proven to be the most effective. However, the following suggestions by Green[5] are a useful training paradigm:
1. Discuss and identify the patient's own goals.
2. Present methods of controlling symptoms and precipitating causes.

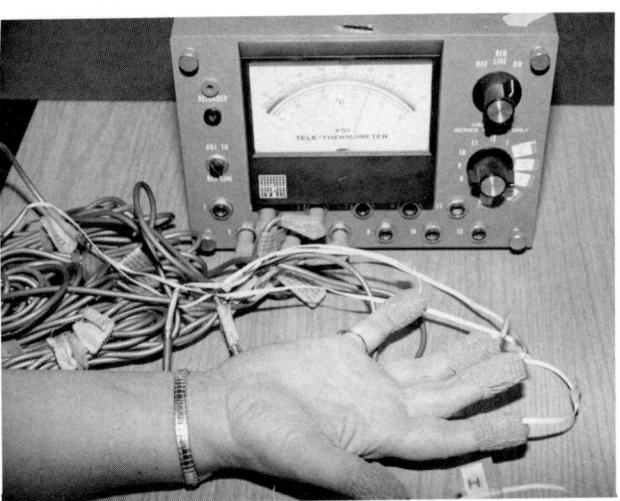

Fig. 79-7   This thermal biofeedback unit is capable of monitoring 10 separate areas for skin temperature. The patient is attempting hand-warming techniques while monitoring the distal digit temperature.

3. Explain the thermography equipment.
4. Establish a baseline resting temperature in any of the following manners:
    a. The patient may monitor his temperature daily with the thermography equipment for 1 week before treatment.
    b. At the initial treatment session a baseline resting temperature can be obtained after a 2 minute adjustment period. A baseline cold temperature can also be obtained after a cold application for 3 minutes. (The patient is instructed to place his hands around a container of ice water.)
5. Treat in a draft-free room where the temperature is from 75° F to 89° F. The patient is seated or reclined in a supportive chair.
6. Instruct the patient in autogenic relaxation and hand-warming techniques. The thermography equipment then is used as feedback while the patient tries these techniques. Sessions usually last for 30 minutes.
7. Repeat procedures in the clinic and on a home program basis. Finger tape temperature monitors are available for home use (Fig. 79-8). In other instances, the patient can be instructed in hand temperature assessment by placing their fingertips on their forehead.
8. Perform reassessment evaluation.
9. Carry-over continues.

Some patients may find it more effective to explore their physiologic response to various stimuli through watching the feedback display as they try different warming techniques. However, a few patients may initially produce a paradoxical stress reaction when in an attempt to warm their hands, they actually decrease the temperature. Simply by trying too hard to increase the temperature in their hands, the patients may actually stress themselves. It is also possible for patients to practice hand warming in only one specific location. To prevent a localized response, temperature readings can be taken from all five digit tips. In all cases, the therapist should be aware that there is a possibility

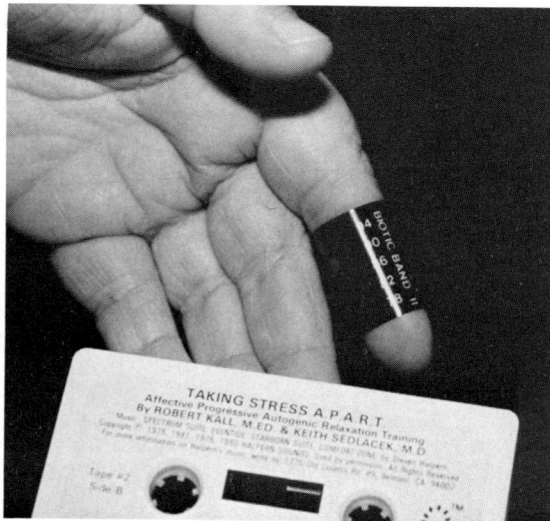

Fig. 79-8 Finger tape temperature strips, used to monitor digital temperature, are useful for the patient's home program, ensuring carryover of relaxation and subsequent hand warming.

of causing too great an increase in blood flow to be directed to the hand.

The best form of adjunctive relaxation technique used with thermal biofeedback has yet to be determined and is most likely dependent on individual needs. Abildness[1] recommends instituting another type of treatment intervention if no treatment improvement is noted after seven sessions with biofeedback.

If thermal biofeedback is effective within the first 10 sessions, Sedlacek[7] recommends an additional 10 to 30 treatments to ensure carryover of thermal regulation to a nontreatment environment. Even though the patients may be able to regulate their vasospasms within 2 to 3 months, they will still need to practice stress reduction techniques over the following 8 months.[7] Ongoing performance of autogenic techniques such as relaxation and hand warming may be necessary for some patients to control hand temperature on a long-term basis.

Thermal biofeedback provides an opportunity for the patient and the therapist to evaluate the physiologic outcome of relaxation and hand-warming techniques. Carry-over of maintained hand warming to functional improvements has been demonstrated by Sedlacek.[7]

GONIOMETRIC FEEDBACK
Historical background

As previously stated, earlier literature and devices were based on single motor unit EMG and kinesiologic studies performed by Basmajian.[6] In the 1950s and 1960s the need for a more specific tracking device for joint motion prompted the development of electrokinesiologic feedback. The feedback goniometer was originated in the late 1950s by an exercise physiologist, Peter Karpovich.[25] He developed a basic linkage system that would drive a potentiometer, which in turn would operate recording equipment. This linkage system was based on a parallelogram configuration and was constructed to study various joint motions.

Through their work on feedback goniometers, Thomas and Long[37] found that they were able to obtain accurate kinesiologic observations through the parallelogram linkage and use of potentiometers that maintained a linear relationship between joint angular displacement and the recorded voltage.

The area of feedback goniometers was also addressed by DeBacher and Brown.[18] They developed a comprehensive set of plans and directions that allowed individuals the opportunity to construct a single joint finger goniometer that tracks active joint motion. Through the work done by Brown, DeBacher, and Hudson, it was determined that feedback goniometers could maximize motivation through a shaping process to attain a specific motor response.[15] These publications led to an increased awareness and interest in feedback goniometers in hand and upper extremity rehabilitation.

Other researchers[4,13,15,22,31] examined treatment applications for patients with central nervous system disorders. From their work, training programs have been developed to enhance functional limb use. A variety of devices[11,12,15,19] have been designed to give positional feedback not only for limb use, but also for sitting balance. Any device must be easily applied by the patient to facilitate use in the clinic and at home.

The equipment and techniques for electrogoniometric feedback continue to be developed. The following discussion addresses the application of feedback goniometers for hand injuries.

Purpose and strategy

The purpose of goniometric feedback is to simply and efficiently monitor joint angles without interfering with motion. Using a goniometer and a simple open-closed circuit system, the patient is able to obtain visual and/or auditory responses from joint movement. Once the movement is under conscious control, this creates an awareness of proper motion, which frequently can be altered as a result of injury or disease processes. By setting parameters in small increments along the arc of the goniometer, patients easily learn to use the devices. They are able to obtain a high level of success in a short period of time, which maximizes motivation to increase range of motion in limited joints.

Patients from all ages easily learn to don and doff the devices and to set appropriate ranges. They can be captivated by these gamelike instruments and become absorbed in meeting goals, which can quickly and easily be changed. The preoccupation with meeting goals frequently overrides any fears and difficulties they may initially have. Patients quickly begin to take an active role in goal-setting, which challenges them to increase their range of motion.

Through specific active motions as monitored by feedback goniometry, tissue structures can be stressed. This stress can assist in altering scar tissue, which leads to permanent improvement in active range of motion. Once motion is achieved, patients are instructed to hold the end range for 5 to 7 seconds. This not only ensures active pull-through within a specific arc of motion, but also encourages patients to perform a sustained holding contraction, which maximizes tissue extensibility.

The onset of muscle fatigue can occur rapidly with these devices, so a brief 10- to 15-minute session can effectively promote many biomechanical factors that alter the restoration of connective tissue structures. The use of feedback goniometers for short durations of time proves most helpful during the early controlled motion phase when patients need to actively move within a designated pain-free range.

Feedback goniometers can do the following:

1. Stimulate active range-of-motion (AROM) exercises, which, at times, can be difficult for patients because they are frightened of disrupting repaired osseous or soft tissue structures.

2. Encourage active motion work within a "set" range, thus stimulating the natural muscle contraction necessary to assist in reducing edema.

3. Allow patients a negotiable amount of control while providing a motivational factor. This is especially important when pain thresholds are low and patients are reluctant to allow the therapist to assist motion. Patients can relax when they feel they have some amount of control over their environment, particularly where pain is concerned.

4. Allow active movement within a protected range. This is useful for patients who have unstable articular and/or periarticular structures that must be moved within a restricted arc of motion.

Goniometric feedback equipment

Finger feedback goniometers (Fig. 79-9, *A* and *B*), both single and dual joint, have appeared to be the most popular among practitioners. Clinically, they have been beneficial for isolated proximal interphalangeal and metacarpophalangeal flexion-extension problems where the primary diagnosis involves fibroosseous structures. Categories such as digital crush injuries, intraarticular fractures, phalanx fractures, volar plate injuries and repairs, digital replantations with gross sensory return, and burns and arthroplasties are all disorders in which goniometric feedback has been useful in restoring motion. These devices can be easily adjusted to attach over dressings for clinic or bedside treatment. Tendon repairs and tendon transfers appear to benefit from feedback goniometers when coupled with sustained positioning with purposeful activity.

The Intrinsic Stretching Device (Fig. 79-10) was designed

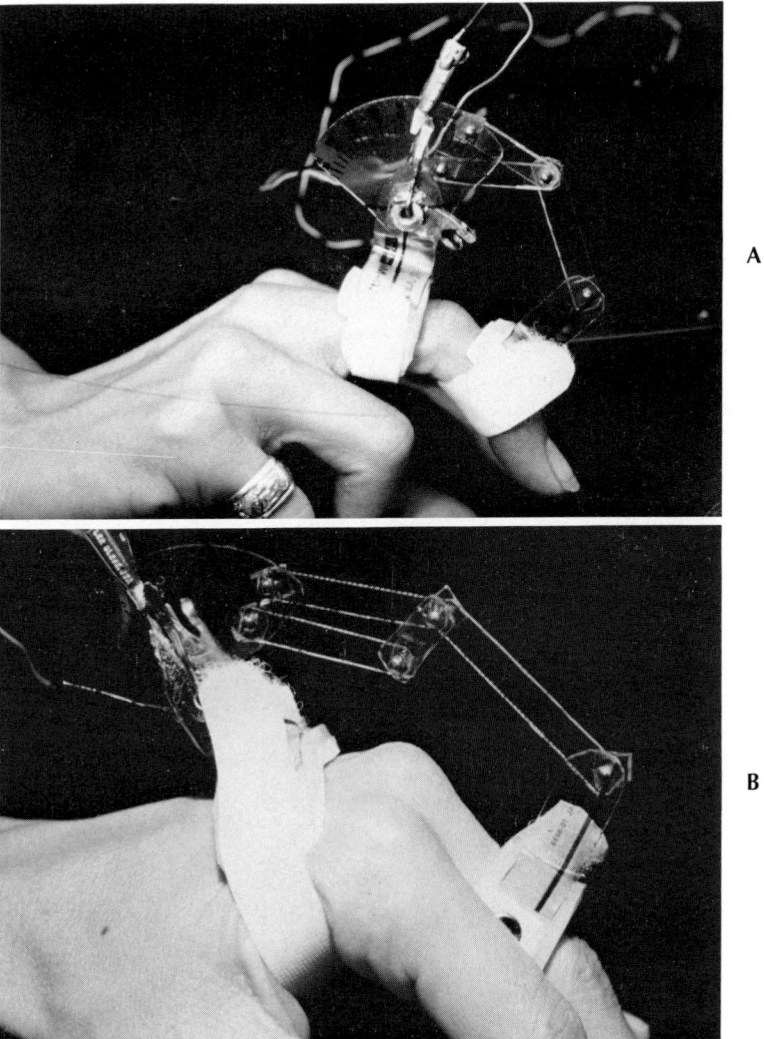

A

B

Fig. 79-9 **A,** Single-joint finger goniometer with open/closed circuit system. Based on designs from Emory University. **B,** Single-joint device for metacarpophalangeal function.

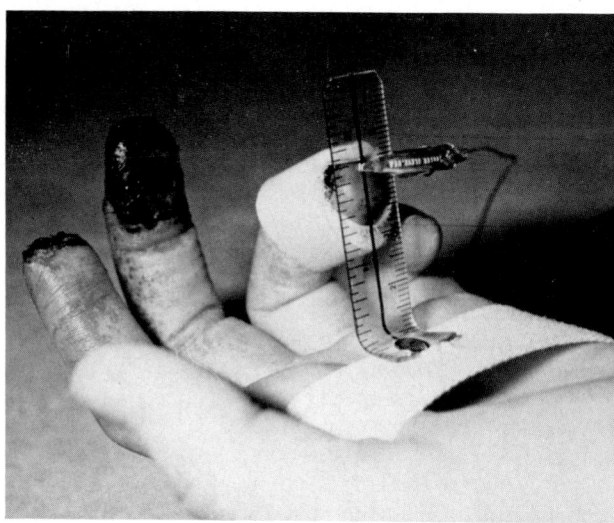

Fig. 79-10   Intrinsic-stretching feedback device designed by D. Williams. Basic principal is to encourage active intrinsic minus position through visual and auditory feedback.

to overcome extensor habitus, i.e., the habit of holding a digit "out of the way" in extension so as to protect the digit. When the finger is healed, the patient is unable to activate the flexors because of the sustained position of extension. Often patients who have undergone Dupuytren's release or have sustained a fingertip injury develop this abnormal pattern. When attempting to perform composite flexion of the digit, the patient uses the extensor and intrinsic muscles rather than the flexors. This can result in marked intrinsic and extrinsic tightness with secondary joint stiffness.

The intrinsic device consists of an 8-cm segment of ruler attached to a palmar strap with a small electrode attachment for the digit and a clip electrode for the upright section. The patient's goal is to make contact with the two electrodes without applying touch pressure to the flexible upright seg-

ment, thus discouraging intrinsic plus position. As contact is properly achieved, the clip electrode is gradually placed closer to the bottom of the ruler, the base of which rests over the distal palmar crease, thus encouraging active intrinsic excursion and decreasing extensor habitus.

The wrist goniometer (Fig. 79-11) has proven highly successful with patients who have sustained fractures, burns, and crush injuries. Many of these individuals attempt to use the secondary motors of the wrist, i.e., the finger and thumb extensors, to straighten the wrist. This patterning adds to disuse and a deconditioned state of an already weakened wrist. Through combined active gentle fisting, which is performed by grasping the palmar strap of the feedback device and active extension, the wrist moves to meet the parameters set along the goniometer. This produces a natural tenodesis type of response as the patient learns to use the wrist extensors without recruiting the finger extensors. This device can also be used to train patients to actively flex and extend, which proves valuable in repetitive grasp, carry, and release activities.

Frequently (Fig. 79-12, *A*) patients in the early phases of recovery feel unsure of how far they can move. They tend to use accessory motions to accomplish movements in an effort to protect the injured structure.[15] During this early recovery phase, it is sometimes difficult for patients to discern pain from soreness, which contributes to their overall reluctance to move. With feedback goniometers, patients can actively control their motion within a given range set by the therapist. By introducing early controlled active motion, patients appear to gain a better understanding of proper movements, which can eliminate unnecessary accessory motions.

A thumb goniometer has proven successful in eliminating substitute patterns (Fig. 79-12, *B*). This device can be used to increase thumb extension or abduction and is useful with patients who have sustained crush or degloving injuries or have undergone replantation.

Supination and pronation can be difficult for the patient to achieve, especially after sustaining a Colles fracture or a

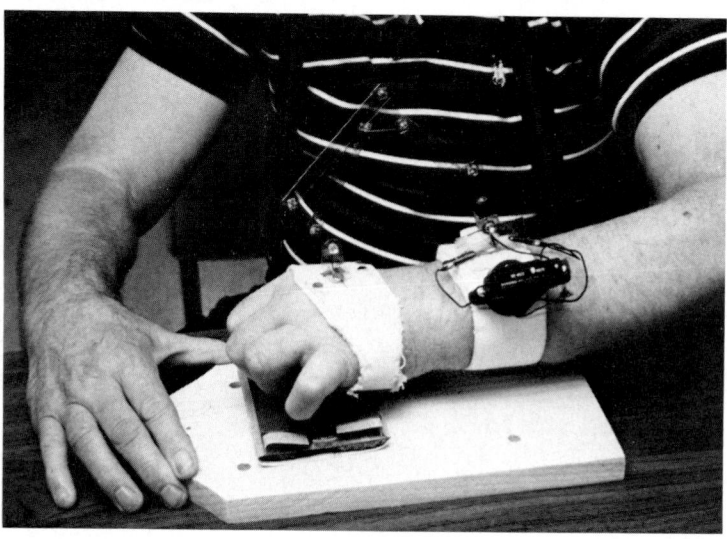

Fig. 79-11   Wrist goniometer based on designs from Emory University. The patient uses the device to increase flexion/extension while performing goal-directed activity.

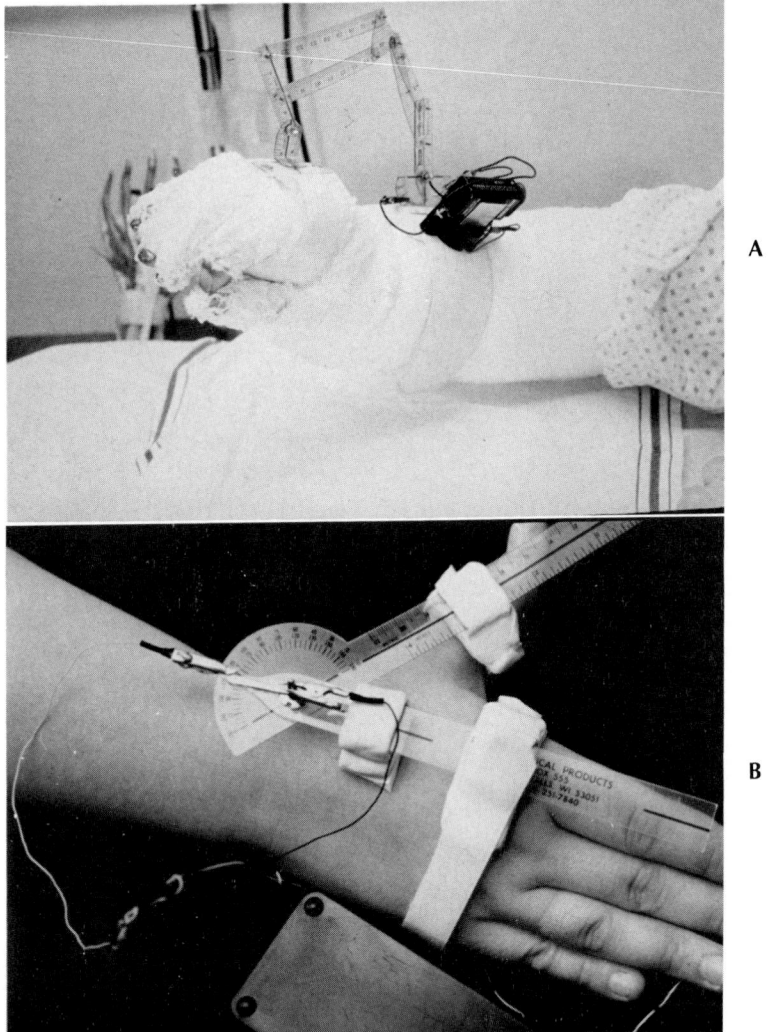

Fig. 79-12 **A,** A wrist goniometer used by a burn patient during the acute phase of rehabilitation. **B,** A thumb goniometer developed to increase extension at the first webspace.

comminuted shaft fracture where exotosis could possibly occur. With the use of two feedback goniometers (Figs. 79-13, *A* and *B,* which are based on designs from Emory University), patients can isolate forearm supination and pronation motions. Initially, a long arm device is used, which runs the length of the forearm and across the wrist joint and is anchored around the distal transverse palmar arch. The patient is encouraged to gently grasp the palmar strap. The long arm eliminates attempts to use the long thumb extensor or flexor, as well as wrist extensors or flexors, to supinate or pronate the forearm. Substitute motion is a common problem that often occurs when patients are concentrating on goal-directed activities, and efforts to accomplish the activity mask proper movement patterns. The strategic placement of the goniometer at the proximal aspect of the forearm also rules out any attempts of substitute motion by the shoulder rotators.

Once the patient can activate the forearm supinator and pronator muscles properly, a short version of the goniometer can be introduced. This is used to liberate the hand during functional activities and strengthening exercises and further enhances the shaping process.

Elbow injuries can also prove difficult to mobilize (Fig. 79-14). Again, substitute patterns of motion involving the shoulder occur commonly. Patients can work extremely hard to extend the elbow only to find they are protracting their shoulder girdle. The use of an elbow goniometer requires isolated joint motion through facilitation of specific muscle contraction. This, in turn, creates a more efficient means of active exercise. Patients with total elbow replacements or fracture-dislocations have found it helpful to use the feedback goniometers when required to move within a restricted range. Through the use of the elbow goniometer, they can safely move without risk of dislocation. This same device has also been converted for knee-injured patients.[12,43]

Clinical application

In measuring joint motion, many of the problems encountered when using EMG biofeedback for specific patient populations appear to be resolved. Because of the light-

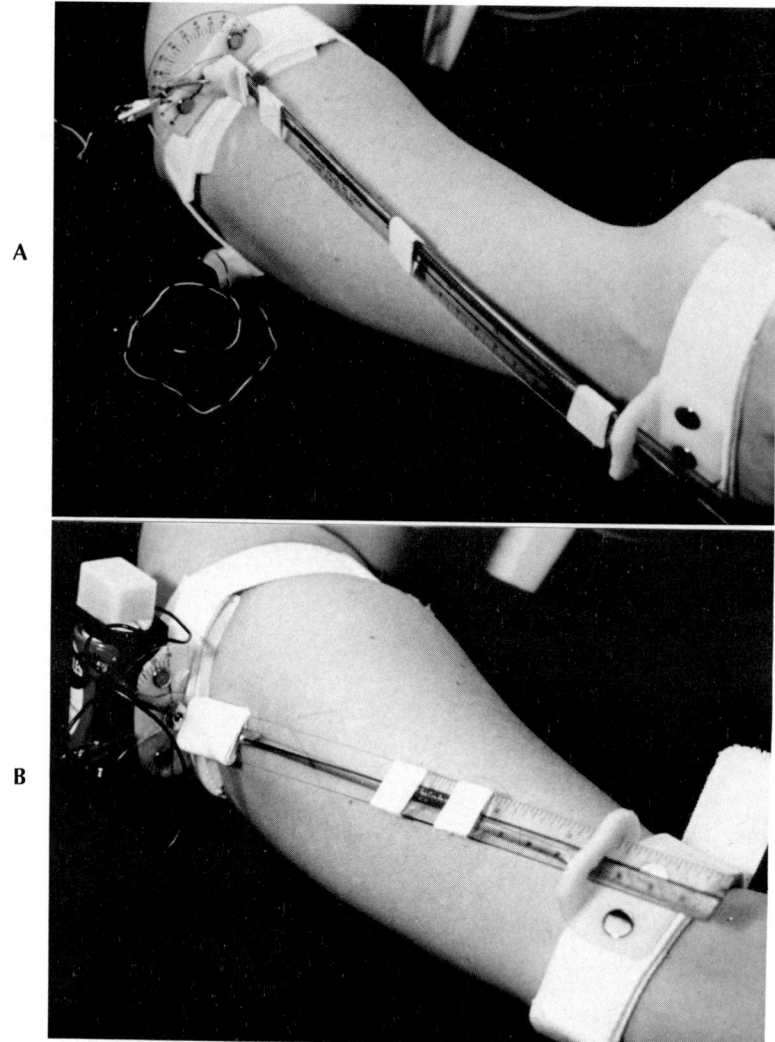

Fig. 79-13 **A,** A long forearm supination/pronation device based on designs from Emory University, used initially to prevent substitution of the wrist and thumb motors for supination/pronation muscles. **B,** The goniometer can be shortened to allow freedom for wrist range of motion.

weight design[18] of the goniometric feedback devices and a simple Velcro cuff system, they can be donned and doffed easily. The devices measure joint motion rather than an ionic membrane changes, so interference is not an issue.

In measuring active block motion rather than muscle response, feedback goniometers are not greatly altered by "spillover," which can be created by mass muscle contractions or accessory motions. Frequently, patients will demonstrate "spillover" in an effort to accomplish a specific task. Since feedback goniometers measure only an arc of motion, they tend to filter out the opportunity to cheat using mass muscle contractions. Altering a specific joint motion is difficult, and patients cannot easily substitute movements or initiate inappropriate responses. Through the isolated and concentrated response, which ultimately requires a specific muscle contraction, patients often fatigue quickly, thus tolerating only a 10 to 15 minute training session. Clinically, patients have found the devices challenging, as well as self-motivating. This has been quite apparent when dealing with adolescent and burn populations. Goniometric feedback ap-

pears to enhance functional mobility in a relatively pain-free range without frustrating the patient. Used throughout a repetitive movement program, feedback goniometers provide an immediate and positive reinforcement.

Patients initially work to meet goals set by the therapist. Once the initial parameters are determined and it is established that there are no restrictions in the arc of motion, patients can and often do set their own goals with little encouragement needed from the therapist. From the acute management phase to the final rehabilitation stage, patients appear to benefit from feedback goniometers.

Feedback goniometer reinforcement with purposeful activity

Active movement is an essential modality of hand therapy.[10] One can also see in the treatment sequence that active goal directed activity is one of the final steps performed in the clinic and the home program. Additionally, active movement coupled with goniometric feedback can increase motion almost 3 to 1.[39] Following initial modalities and hands-

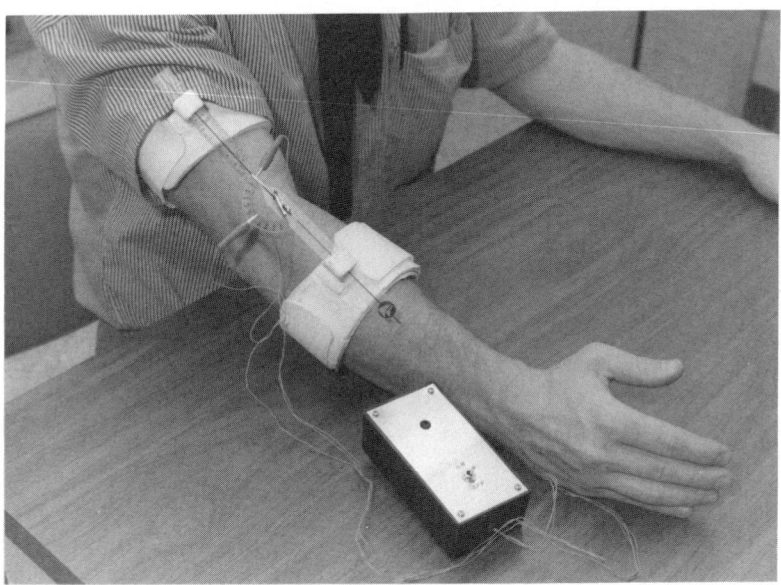

Fig. 79-14   Elbow/knee goniometer designed by D. Williams. This can be used for both elbow and knee disorders to increase isolated joint motion.

on treatment, goniometric feedback can assist in maintaining lengthened periarticular and musculotendinous structures by encouraging active stress loading through sustained holding patterns in a predetermined arc (Fig. 79-15). Isolated motion exercise with a feedback goniometer facilitates edema reduction and decreased joint stiffness and provides for proprioceptive input.

As a component in the rehabilitation process, goniometric feedback has many benefits. Feedback goniometers promote high levels of motivation, which can lead to a more expedient shaping process. Although they are not advocated as a substitute for direct therapist's hands-on care, they can prove highly important as an instant and relatively accurate reinforcer. Although sensitive to the need to succeed through positive reinforcement, the therapist cannot supply the in-

stant feedback on a continuous basis that these devices offer. Even though active exercise and EMG feedback are vital in remodeling tissue structures that restrict motion, feedback goniometers can also be valuable in overcoming these limitations. The devices are simple, cost-effective, and portable so they can be used during performance of functional activities and exercises.

Patients have found feedback goniometers enjoyable and challenging because they do not allow substitute movements. After one session with proper instruction and supervision, the patient can take charge of his or her feedback program and set personal goals with little outside encouragement from the therapist. The major problem with using these devices is keeping the patients from overusing them. Although quickly fatigued, patients have a tendency to want

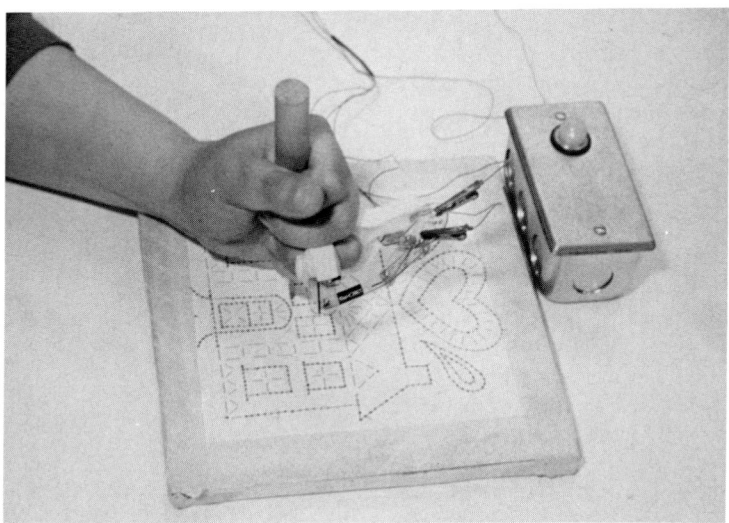

Fig. 79-15   This patient is working on stippling while using a proximal interphalangeal feedback goniometer to enhance flexion pattern.

to keep working to increase their range of motion. It's a bit like playing a video game; once you have the technique, it's hard to stop playing the game.

More clinical research is needed not only to prove the worth of feedback goniometers, but also to maximize the appropriate use in the rehabilitation process.[6]

Choosing an appropriate feedback application: EMG biofeedback versus goniometric feedback

Brown and his associates[15] at Emory University completed a 4-year study to determine the value of feedback goniometers in hand trauma, both before and after surgery. Their conclusion was that these devices proved to be significant for increasing range through properly controlled motion. It must, however, be understood that EMG feedback can, in certain circumstances, be more effective than goniometric feedback. When comparing the two, one must realize that they are quite different and each has their own advantages and disadvantages. Each can be valuable in the realm of rehabilitation but with its own succinct purpose. When considering EMG versus goniometric feedback, it is important to look at the motor function you wish to alter, the neurologic status of the body part you are attempting to condition, the wound status, the pain level, and the patient's attitude. All are important factors when deciding which type of feedback you want to use.

Literature review and clinical observation, nevertheless, have indicated common problems that clinicians have had with the application of EMG feedback for hand and upper extremity injuries. Although valuable, as has been stated, EMG devices frequently take extended periods of time to put on because of skin preparation and electrode placement. There can be interference from the surrounding environment (such as static electricity), which results in lost treatment time while corrections are made.

When using EMG feedback to isolate specific responses from small or deep compartment muscles, electrical overflow or "spillover" has also proven to be a significant problem. This, too, has led to increased training time and frustration for both the patient and the therapist. Also, with the close compartmentalization of both anterior and posterior forearm components, mass muscle responses have been easily elicited, which has afforded the patient an opportunity to "cheat." Isolating specific deep compartment or intrinsic muscle responses without recruiting surrounding motor components is difficult and placement of the surface electrodes can be nebulous when attempting to locate the motor points for these same muscle groups. Another problem with EMG feedback is its inability to be used when open wounds are present over the muscle belly being monitored. When any of these factors are present, the therapist has an alternative available—goniometric feedback.

Limitations in the use of goniometric feedback occur in such instances where motor activity is too weak to cause any joint movement. The application of a feedback goniometer in the above-mentioned case would be an inappropriate therapeutic choice. In some cases of muscular co-contraction, the patient may only be able to break the maladaptive motor pattern by observing two levels of muscle activity. Dual channel EMG biofeedback can provide the patient with this opportunity. Once muscle activity is altered, then joint motion can be changed. At this point in time, feedback goniometers are fabricated by the therapist using them and can be quite fragile. On the other hand, EMG biofeedback equipment is commercially available and rarely needs maintenance.

SUMMARY

Because biofeedback is an effective method by which patients with hand injuries can influence their recovery and function, therapists should be aware of the broad scope of available biofeedback interventions. Patients receive immediate feedback from equipment, which in turn provides empirical evidence to the patient of his or her progress toward therapeutic goals.

Biofeedback can be effectively used to influence the following physiologic processes for the hand-injured individual: muscle activity, digital skin temperature, and joint motion.

Clinical biofeedback is used to provide patients with increased self-control of physiologic functioning, ultimately producing a positive effect on health and wellness. The self-control promotes an increase in the responsibility that patients take in both their preventative and corrective health needs.[40] The therapist acts as a coach to clarify goals and to provide activities and exercises to enhance a patient's performance. It is essential to remember that "the real efficacy of biofeedback lies in the patient's ability to transfer the skills training to practical daily life application."[1]

ACKNOWLEDGEMENTS

The authors wish to acknowledge D. Michael Brown, OTR/L, for his significant contribution to the field of occupational therapy through his work in biofeedback and Elizabeth De Poy, Ph.D., OTR/L.

REFERENCES

1. Abildness AH: Biofeedback strategies, Rockville, Md, 1982, American Occupational Therapy Association, Inc.
2. Adrian ED and Bronk DW: The discharge of impulses in motor nerve fibers, the frequency of discharge in reflex and voluntary contractions, J Physiol 67:119, 1929.
3. Alexander AB, White PD, and Wallace HM: Training and transfer of training effects in EMG biofeedback assisted muscular relaxation, Psychophysiology 14(6):551, 1977.
4. Annual Report of Progress, no 6, Downey, Calif, Rancho Los Amigos Rehabilitation Engineering Center.
5. Basmajian JV: Conscious control of individual motor units, Science 141:440, 1963.
6. Basmajian JV: Muscles alive: their function revealed by electromyography, ed 3, Baltimore, 1974, Williams & Wilkins.
7. Basmajian JV, editor: Biofeedback principles and practice for clinicians, ed 2, Baltimore, 1983, Williams & Wilkins.
8. Basmajian JV, editor: Therapeutic exercise, ed 4, Baltimore, 1984, Williams & Wilkins.
9. Basmajian JV and Blumenstein R: Electrode placement in EMG biofeedback, Baltimore, 1980, Williams & Wilkins.
10. Beasley RW: The mutilated hand. In Hunter J and others, editors: Rehabilitation of the hand, vol 1, St Louis, 1978, The CV Mosby Co.
11. Bjork L and Wetzel A: A positional biofeedback device for sitting balance: suggestions from the field, Phys Ther 1692, 1984.
12. Bohannon R and Short D: Compact device for positional biofeedback—suggestions from the field, Phys Ther 1692, 1984.
13. Bowman BR, Baker LL, and Waters RL: Positional feedback and electrical stimulation: an automated treatment for the hemiplegic wrist, Arch Phys Med Rehab 60(11):497, 1979.
14. Brown DM: Current concepts and capabilities of electromyographic and electrokinesiologic feedback in the total management of traumatic hand injuries. In Hunter J and others, editors: Rehabilitation of the hand, ed 2, St Louis, 1984, The CV Mosby Co.

15. Brown DM, DeBacher G, and Basmajian JV: Feedback goniometers for hand rehabilitation, Am J Occup Ther 33:458, 1979.

16. Brudny and others: EMG feedback: a review of treatment of 114 patients, Arch Phys Med Rehab 57:55, 1976.

17. Croce R: The effects of EMG biofeedback on strength acquisition, Biofeedback Self Regul 11(4):299, 1986.

18. DeBacher G and Brown DM: A simple feedback finger goniometer, Atlanta, 1979, Emory University Regional Rehabilitation Research and Training Center, Center of Rehabilitation Medicine.

19. Harris F, Spelman F, and Hymer J: Electronic sensing aids in treatment for cerebral palsied children, Phys Ther 54:354, 1974.

20. Harrison VF: Voluntary control of threshold motor unit potentials in the neuromuscularly skilled individual, Anat Rec 145:237, 1963.

21. Hayduck A: Increasing hand efficiency at cold temperatures by training hand vasodilation with classical conditioning—biofeedback overlap design, Biofeedback Self Regul 5(3):307, 1980.

22. Herman R: A program of assessment and remediation of neurosensory disabilities, Philadelphia, Pa, 1971, Krusen Center for Research Engineering, Moss Rehabilitation Hospital.

23. Ince LP, Leon MS, and Christidis D: Experimental findings of EMG biofeedback with upper extremity: a review of the literature, Biofeedback Self Regul 9:3, 303, 1984.

24. Jacobson E: Electrical measurements concerning muscular contraction and the cultivation of relaxation in man: studies of arm flexors, Am J Physiol 107:230, 1933.

25. Karpovich PV: The electrogoniometer: a new device for the study of joints in action. Presented at the Research Section of the American Alliance of Health, Physical Education, and Recreation national convention, Portland, Ore, March 31, 1959.

26. Lindsley DB: Electrical activity of human motor units during voluntary contraction, Am J Physiol 114:90, 1935.

27. Lucca J and Recchiuti J: Effect of EMG biofeedback on an isometric strengthening program, Phys Ther 63(2):200, 1983.

28. Middaugh SJ and Miller MC: Electromyographic feedback: effect on voluntary muscle contraction in paretic subjects, Arch Phys Med Rehab 61:24, 1980.

29. Middaugh S and others: EMG feedback: effects on voluntary muscle contracting in normal subjects, Arch Phys Med Rehab 63:254, 1982.

30. Morasky R, Reynolds C, and Stowell L: Generalization of lowered EMG levels during musical performance following biofeedback training, Biofeedback Self Regul 8(2):207, 1983.

31. Progress Report No 4, Philadelphia, Pa, 1975, Krusen Center for Research and Engineering, Moss Rehabilitation Center.

32. Simard T and Basmajian JV: Methods of training the conscious control of motor units, Arch Phys Med Rehab, Jan:12, 1967.

33. Smith OC: Action potentials from single motor units in voluntary contraction, Am J Physiol 108:629, 1934.

34. Surwit RS, Pilon RH, and Fenton CH: Behavioral treatment of Raynaud's disease. Paper presented at annual meeting of Biofeedback Society of America, Albuquerque, NM, 1977.

35. Taub E: Self-regulation of human tissue temperature. In Schwarts GE and Blatty J, editors: Biofeedback theory and research, New York, 1977, Academic Press.

36. Taub E and Stroebel CF: Biofeedback in the treatment of vasoconstrictive syndromes, Biofeedback Self Regul 3(4):363, 1978.

37. Thomas D and Long C: Electrogoniometer for the finger: kinesiologic tracking device, Am J Med Electronics 3:96, 1964.

38. Tromby CA and Scott A: Occupational therapy for physical dysfunction, Baltimore, 1977, Williams & Wilkins.

39. Williams D: Electrokinesiologic feedback: an adjunct in therapeutic restoration of hand rehabilitation. Presented at the Scientific Papers Section of American Society of Hand Therapists, Las Vegas, 1985.

40. Winer LR: Biofeedback: a guide to clinical literature, Am J Orthopsychiatry 47(4):626, 1977.

41. Wolf S: EMG biofeedback in exercise programs, Phys Sports Med 8(11):61, 1980.

42. Wolf S: Essential considerations in the use of EMG biofeedback, Phys Ther 58(1):25, 1978.

43. Wooldridge C, Leiper C, and Oston D: Biofeedback training of knee joint position of the cerebral palsied child, Physiotherapy Can 28:138, 1976.

44. Yocum DE and others: Use of biofeedback training in the treatment of Raynaud's disease and phenomenon, J Rheumatol 12(1):90, 1985.

XIV
AMPUTATION AND PROSTHETICS

80

The management of the nonfunctional hand: reconstruction versus prosthesis*

Sterling Bunnell

In tribute to Sterling Bunnell

GEORGE E. OMER, JR.

Twenty years following his death, the creative genius and organizational contributions of Sterling Bunnell continue to dominate reconstructive surgery of the hand. He published concise, innovative papers on tendon repair, tendon transfers, atraumatic technique, the pull-out suture, reconstruction of the thumb, nerve grafts, intrinsic muscle contracture, dynamic splinting, and many more.

During World War II, Sterling Bunnell gave up his private practice and devoted himself to instruction in hand surgery in the nine centers established in army general hospitals. This salubrious effort resulted in great interest in the discipline of hand surgery and culminated in the organization of the American Society for Surgery of the Hand. Sterling Bunnell was instrumental in encouraging the formation of hand surgery clubs or societies in Scandinavia, England, South America, and Japan.

The first edition of his monumental book, Surgery of the Hand, *was published in 1944 and achieved worldwide distribution; it was the standard text in all military hospitals. His exposure to a great number of crippled hands during World War II stimulated Sterling Bunnell to emphasize the physical rehabilitation of hand injuries. The volume on hand surgery in the medical history series of the U.S. Army Medical Department on World War II was edited by Sterling Bunnell and includes a long chapter written by himself. This chapter stresses rehabilitation and contains illustrations and instructions for constructing and fitting static and dynamic splints; the danger of tight casting and prolonged immobilization are discussed; and the equipment and methods for occupational therapy and reconditioning are detailed. Sterling Bunnell continued to emphasize the physical rehabilitation of hand injuries and to study the prosthetic fitting of the partial or totally amputated hand. His publication in* Artificial Limbs, *"The Management of the Nonfunctional Hand—Reconstruction vs. Prosthesis," was in press at the time of his death in 1957. The principles presented in this comprehensive paper remain valid today.*

In the course of routine practice, the orthopedic surgeon is frequently confronted with the task of dealing with hands that are damaged by trauma or disease or that are otherwise nonfunctional owing to any of a variety of causes. In all such cases, he is called upon to decide whether or not to undertake amputation of parts of the hand or amputation through the wrist, with the expectation of later applying a suitable prosthesis, or whether, with the prospect of long-continued treatment and the possibility of ultimate failure, to attempt surgical construction of a functional hand from such anatomical elements as can be saved. The considerations involved are many and varied, and rarely do two cases resemble each other in more than a remote way. Each individual case must therefore be evaluated on the basis of its own merits.

There has been in the past dozen years a great advancement in the development of hand prostheses, so that in the case of major hand problems one might be inclined to choose wrist disarticulation over attempts at surgical reconstruction. But during the same period surgical reconstruction also has advanced remarkably, so that in judging any individual case there should be a careful analysis as to which procedure is the better to follow. Doing so usually results in a sort of compromise reconstruction, if reasonably possible, being chosen first, a prosthesis being applied when proven necessary, major amputation being considered only as a last resort. It is the purpose here to attempt to extract from many years of clinical experience with hand surgery certain general principles that may offer guidance in making the choice. Generally, the current rule of "save all length possible," now applicable at most other levels of amputation, is applicable in the case of damaged hands also.

The fundamental difference between a reconstructed hand and any present-day hand prosthesis lies in the absence of direct sensation in the latter. Although the wearer of a modern hook or artificial hand may receive indirect sensory impulses through shoulder harness or cineplastic muscle pin, the conventional arrangement constitutes only a crude and inefficient signal system which must be supplemented and directed by sight. A hand prosthesis is of little use in the dark. In contrast, there is the exquisite appreciation we receive from the normal hand by feeling. By light touch, coarse touch, response to heat or cold, and compass-point discrimination, we appreciate texture, and by muscle, joint, and tendon sense we appreciate size and shape. By combining these sense impressions in our cerebral cortex in the opposite parietal lobe, we can identify from memory an object held in the hand. This is stereognosis, a phenomenon replaced by no artificial hand now available. To quote Kirk,[6] "No hand is so badly crippled that, if it is painless, has

*Reprinted from *Artificial Limbs*, 4:76-102, 1957, with permission from Krieger Publishing Co., Inc., Huntington, New York.

sensation, and strong prehension, it is [not] far better than any prosthesis." This being the case, it is generally desirable to preserve any and all hand structures that can reasonably be counted on to have adequate nerve and blood supply. Eventual application of a prosthesis may or may not be indicated, depending upon individual circumstances and the particular demands of occupation.

Before considering any hand amputation, then, one should weigh well the possibility of surgical reconstruction, especially with the idea of restoring natural sensation and strong prehension. Whenever reasonably feasible, surgical reconstruction of a damaged hand or arm should be attempted first. Often the result will be such that a prosthesis will not be necessary. In any case, a reconstructed hand stump is apt to be much better adapted to application of a prosthesis. As a matter of fact, reconstruction and use of a prosthesis are so interrelated that they should be considered together in each individual case. Every useful part of a limb, and every bit of skin that has sensation, should be preserved, thus giving more useful material for reconstruction and, finally, for the fitting, if necessary, of a prosthesis.

Reconstruction may often be done in one operation; in other cases multiple operations are required over a period of a month to a year. But considering that the goal is to provide a useful hand for the remainder of an individual's life, it seems worthwhile. Nevertheless, it should not be undertaken unless there is reasonable assurance that a good practical result can be obtained.

METHODS OF SURGICAL RECONSTRUCTION

Although the hand does the work, the arm places and innervates the hand. Accordingly, if any particular hand is to be truly useful, it is necessary to have good shoulder, elbow, and wrist function and also good pronation and supination half furnished by the shoulder and half below the elbow. Because they supply the hand, the nerves of the arm are particularly important. In the hand itself there should be a good quality of sensation as well as mobile units that can

work against each other with at least a pinch grasp or hook action to simulate normal prehension.

Hands coming in for repair usually evidence partial amputations, stiffening in the position of nonfunction, flexion contracture from scar formation, malalignment of bones, loss of motion from injury to tendons and nerves, loss of sensation from injury to nerves, ischemic contracture, or painful states from vasomotor causes or from tender neuromata. Usually the surgeon's problem is composite, dealing with cover, joints, bones, nerves, and tendons.

For each of these conditions there is much that can be done surgically.[2] For partial amputation, clefts between digits may be deepened, and digits can be built out and made to appose each other. Tender stumps may be corrected. For stiffening in the position of nonfunction, the joints may gradually be drawn around to the position of function by spring or elastic splinting and can be mobilized surgically. Scar tissue of flexion contracture can be replaced by good pliable skin giving good cover and improving nutrition. Malalignment of bones may be corrected so that the mechanics of tendon action are correct. Substitute thumbs may be formed. Tendons and nerves may be repaired or transferred, or new ones may be furnished. A hand thus affected can regain some function. Painful states may be corrected by sympathectomy, and tender neuromata may be removed.

Partial amputation

Arm stumps resulting from amputation through the wrist or through the carpometacarpal joint, or those without the thumb and with amputation through the metacarpals or proximal phalanges, require a prosthesis (Fig. 80-1). Hands retaining a good thumb working against one or more fingers (as in Fig. 80-2), or even against a surgically constructed post (as in Fig. 80-3), do not. Sometimes the usefulness of a sound thumb may be much enhanced by surgical procedures conducted on other remaining hand parts (as for example in Fig. 80-4). Other partial hands (like those shown in Figs. 80-5 and 80-6 for example) when reconstructed

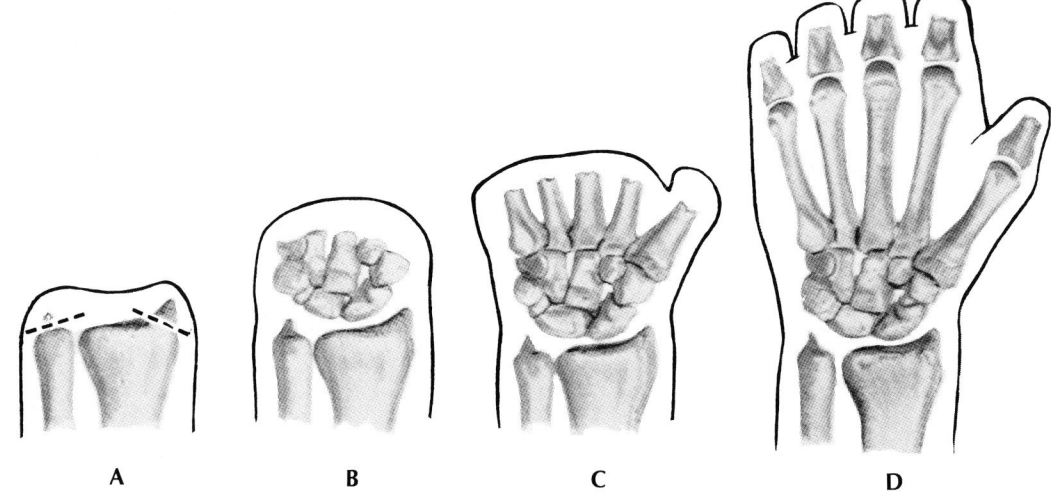

Fig. 80-1 Levels of hand amputation requiring prosthesis. **A,** Wrist disarticulation, including removal of the distal prominences of radius and ulna. **B,** Amputation through the carpometacarpal joint. **C,** Transmetacarpal amputation. **D,** Amputation through all proximal phalanges. In **B** some useful wrist motion may be retained. In **C** hand remnant may be used as a wrist motor to power a prosthesis or simply to point one. In **D** hand stump may be made to work against some prosthetic device, residual sensation offering a substantial advantage over **A, B,** or **C.**

usually are more functional than a prosthesis. Some with a partial hand amputation use remnants of the hand for fine work and a prosthesis for heavy work.

In partial amputations it is best, if possible, to retain the metacarpal heads and hence the full width of the palm for firm grasp of tools, but the metacarpal head of an index or of a little finger that has been amputated through the metacarpophalangeal joint is best beveled off so that it will not snag on entering a pocket. The metacarpal of an index or little finger off through the shaft is best removed obliquely at its base (Fig. 80-7). The interosseous muscle is then transferred to the adjoining digit to give abduction.

A hand amputated through all metacarpophalangeal joints or proximal phalanges may be improved by mobilizing the fifth metacarpal, cutting the transverse metacarpal ligament, and perhaps removing the metacarpal of the ring finger and covering the cleft by a plastic maneuver (Fig. 80-4). The ulnar side of the hand thus becomes a movable part. Motion may be increased as much as 2 in. If the second and fourth metacarpals are deleted, there will remain three digits, consisting of the metacarpals of the thumb and of the long and little fingers, and the thumb cleft will be wide and deep.

Phalangizing the metacarpals gives considerable useful mobility so that one can dress oneself, use knife and fork, and so forth. The metacarpals of the thumb and little finger are cut across at the base and bent toward each other for better grasp (Fig. 80-8). A similar osteotomy may be performed on a hand having only two remaining digits, as for example thumb and little finger (Fig. 80-9), or even when only one complete digit remains, as in Fig. 80-10.

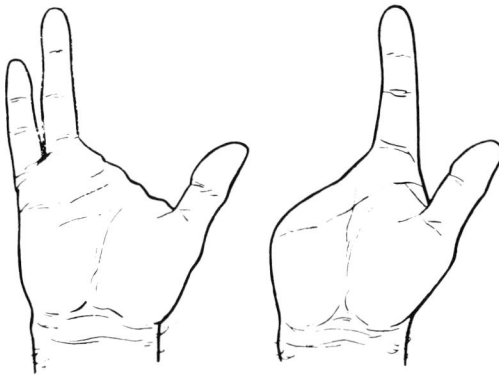

Fig. 80-2 Examples of partial hands requiring no prosthesis. When the thumb can work against one or more fingers, function usually is better than that obtained with a hand substitute.

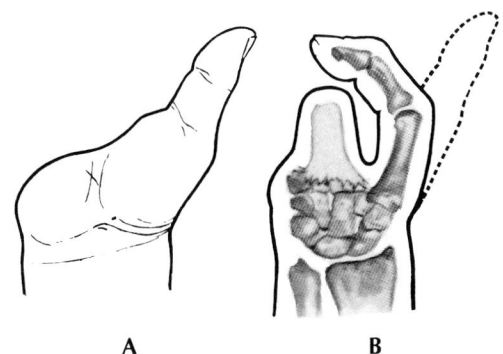

Fig. 80-3 **A,** Partial hand. **B,** Result of reconstruction, no prosthesis needed. When, in the absence of all the fingers and much of the palm, a good thumb remains, it is possible, by means of pedicle and bone graft, to build up a post for the thumb to appose. Function thus obtained is likely to be better than that to be had from a hand substitute.

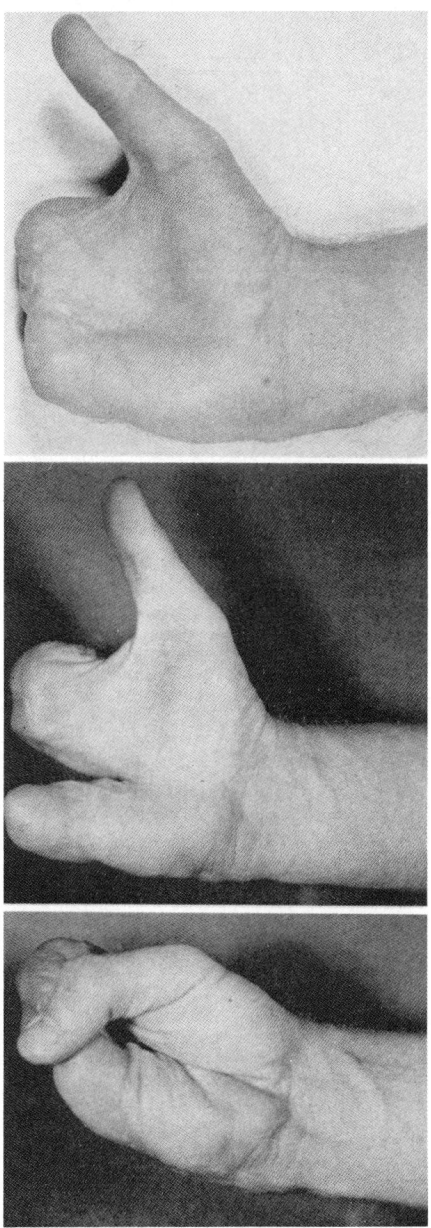

Fig. 80-4 Case M.S. Fingers lost between a sprocket and chain. Excised the tender neuromata of the stumps. Undermined and drew skin down for better coverage. Excised metacarpal of ring finger, covering sides of new digit by plastic maneuvers, to give more mobility (2 in.) to the metacarpal of the little finger. Deepened thumb cleft by Z plasty (see Fig. 80-21). The patient obtained a strong and useful grasp between the thumb, the phalangized index and long "fingers," and the little "finger." (From Bunnell: Surgery of the hand, ed 3, Philadelphia, 1956, Lippincott.)

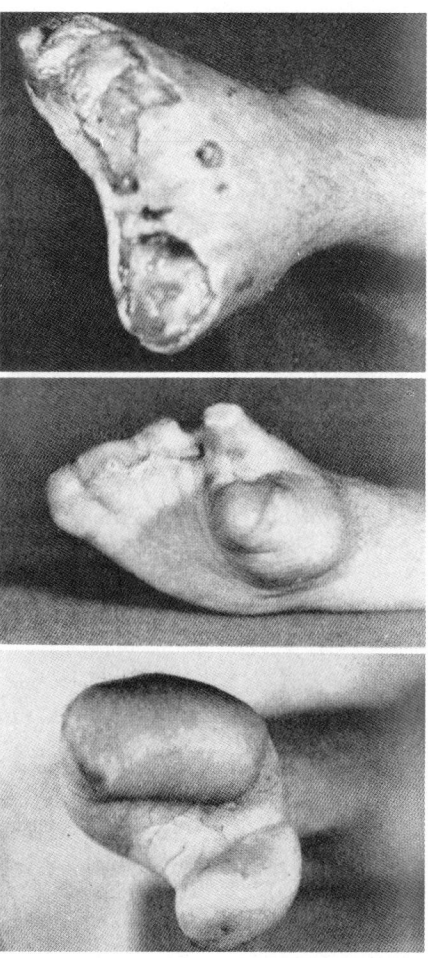

Fig. 80-6 Case B.P. Partial amputation by power saw. Split-grafted next day. Pedicle graft applied and thumb cleft deepened. Index metacarpal removed for wider cleft. Rotary osteotomy was performed on all metacarpals for better apposition. Pinning with Kirschner wires. A good "hand," with good prehension, was obtained. (From Bunnell: Surgery of the hand, ed 3, Philadelphia, 1956, Lippincott.)

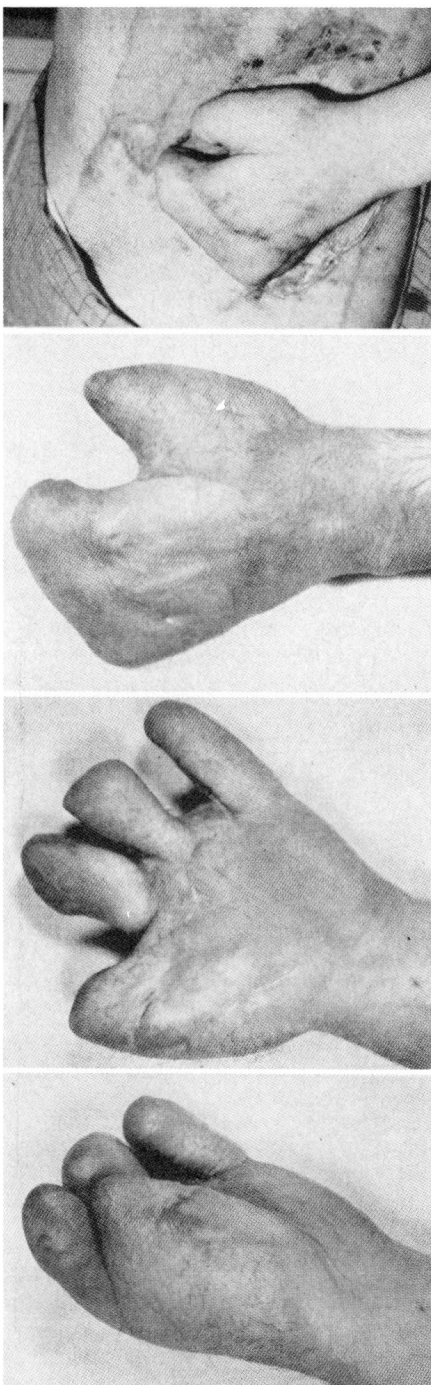

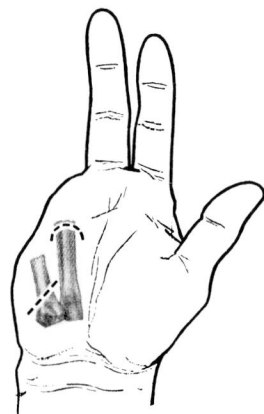

Fig. 80-5 Case P.L. Hand caught between two rollers. Debrided and skin grafted. Later, pedicle flap applied, then interdigitation. Sensation gradually returned throughout. A useful hand was obtained. (From Bunnell: Surgery of the hand, ed 3, Philadelphia, 1956, Lippincott.)

Fig. 80-7 Typical example of loss of the fourth and fifth rays through the shafts of the metacarpals. In such a case, it is best to delete the stub of the fifth metacarpal and round the stub of the fourth. A corresponding procedure is advisable in the event of loss of the second digit, or of the second and third digits, by transmetacarpal amputation.

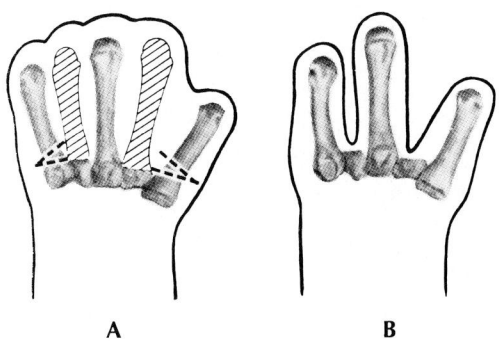

Fig. 80-8 Reconstruction procedure for loss of all digits through the metacarpophalangeal joints. **A,** Second and fourth metacarpals are deleted, clefts are covered by plastic maneuver, first and fifth metacarpals are osteotomized. **B,** Functional three-finger "hand" results.

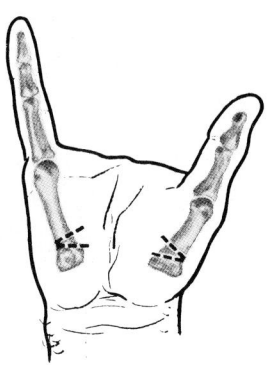

Fig. 80-9 Angulatory osteotomy of first and fifth metacarpals to aid apposition of thumb and little finger. Sometimes it is necessary to effect a tendon T transfer also (see Fig. 80-31).

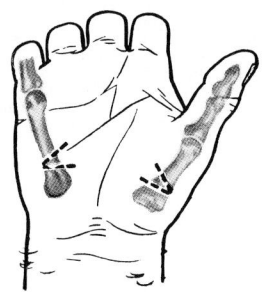

Fig. 80-10 Angulatory osteotomy of first and fifth metacarpals to bring thumb and ulnar side of the palm into easy apposition. Tendon T transfer may be needed here also (see Fig. 80-31).

Frequently a finger or hand stump is so hypersensitive from poor terminal padding and sensitive neuromata that it prevents all of the remaining parts of the hand from functioning. Crushing injuries to fingers present the most difficulty because, in such cases, the fingers usually have been damaged well proximal to the site of amputation. In revising such stumps, the digits must often be shortened enough to give good, well-padded cover, but it is possible to swing a visor flap from the dorsum over the end of the stump and then to skin-graft the dorsum. Still another possibility of furnishing good tactile cover over the end involves use of a cross-finger flap and then skin-grafting the back of the donor finger. Nerves in hands and fingers have a special tendency to proliferate. If they terminate in scar tissue or close under the skin, the neuromata formed may be extremely sensitive and give, on slight tapping, the sensation of an electric shock. These are corrected by uncovering the nerve, dissecting it well back, and cutting it off in good tissue free from scar. Neither alcohol injection nor ligation is used.

Stiffening in the position of nonfunction

Following injury, infection, or paralysis, a hand frequently stiffens in the position of nonfunction so that the digits can no longer touch each other and the hand is therefore useless. In the position of function (Fig. 80-11), the wrist is extended 35 deg., the joints of the fingers are moderately flexed, and the thumb is in moderate apposition, as in holding a baseball. In the position of nonfunction (Fig. 80-12), the wrist is flexed, the metacarpophalangeal joints are hyperextended, the remaining finger joints are flexed, and the thumb is at the side of the hand or even back of it. Although such a hand is totally useless, in general it should not be amputated. For if the joints can be pushed around into the position of function, the available motion will be useful for picking up and holding objects, and the hand will be used more and more from then on.

The first approach to hands stiffened in the position of nonfunction involves use of a system of elastic or spring splinting by which joints can gradually be drawn around into positions of function. Usually the joints are kept active and are not damaged, and the muscles and all tissues are activated, a matter which greatly improves their condition. If, however, the response to such treatment is unsatisfactory, surgical means are resorted to, starting with capsulectomies (Fig. 80-13) and, where there is damage to bone structure, resorting to arthroplasties.

Capsulectomies are usually performed on the metacarpophalangeal joints but sometimes also on the proximal interphalangeal joints. Usually the trouble is found to lie in the fact that the two collateral ligaments are too short and thick to permit the joint to flex. Excision of these structures

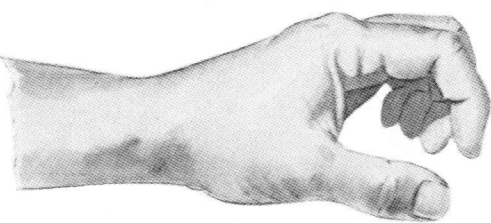

Fig. 80-11 The position of function.

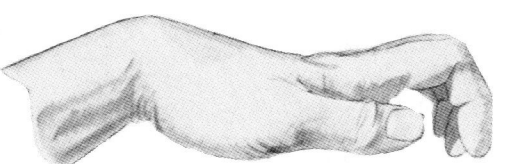

Fig. 80-12 The position of nonfunction.

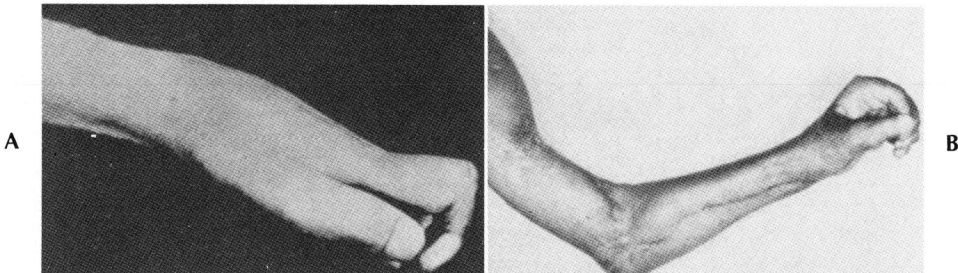

Fig. 80-13   Case E.T. **A,** preoperative position of nonfunction from shark bite on upper arm, severing nerves and vessels. **B,** Correction to a position of function by fusion of the wrist, capsulectomies and opening of the cleft of the thumb, and transfer of the extensors of the wrist to the flexors of the fingers. A tendon transfer through a pulley constructed at the pisiform was used to give apposition to the thumb. No prosthesis needed. (From Bunnell: Surgery of the hand, ed 3, Philadelphia, 1956, Lippincott.)

Fig. 80-14   Case J.D. **A,** Old dislocation of metacarpals on the carpus, upsetting muscle balance, thus resulting in the useless position of nonfunction. **B** and **C,** Dislocation reduced, restoring muscle balance in the position of function. A pedicle graft was applied to the dorsum of the hand and to the open thumb cleft. Freeing of the extensor tendons, together with capsulectomies, allowed the proximal finger joints to flex. No prosthesis needed. (From Bunnell: Surgery of the hand, ed 3, Philadelphia, 1956, Lippincott.)

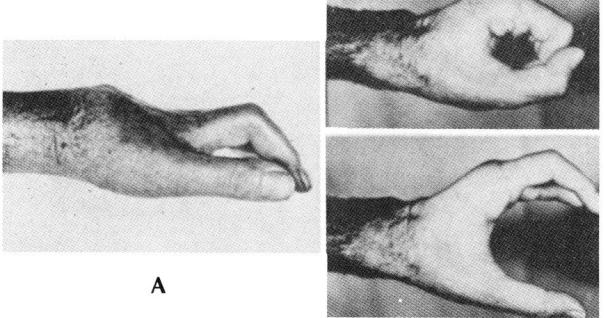

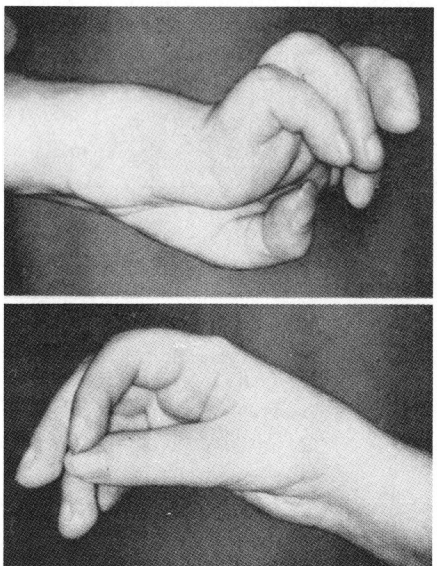

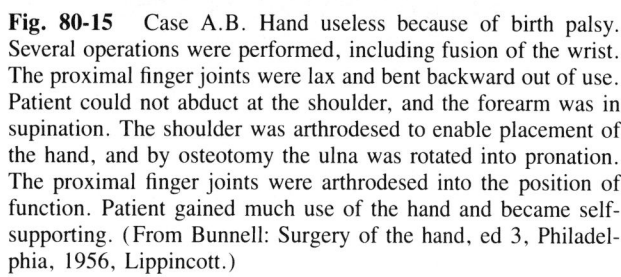

Fig. 80-15   Case A.B. Hand useless because of birth palsy. Several operations were performed, including fusion of the wrist. The proximal finger joints were lax and bent backward out of use. Patient could not abduct at the shoulder, and the forearm was in supination. The shoulder was arthrodesed to enable placement of the hand, and by osteotomy the ulna was rotated into pronation. The proximal finger joints were arthrodesed into the position of function. Patient gained much use of the hand and became self-supporting. (From Bunnell: Surgery of the hand, ed 3, Philadelphia, 1956, Lippincott.)

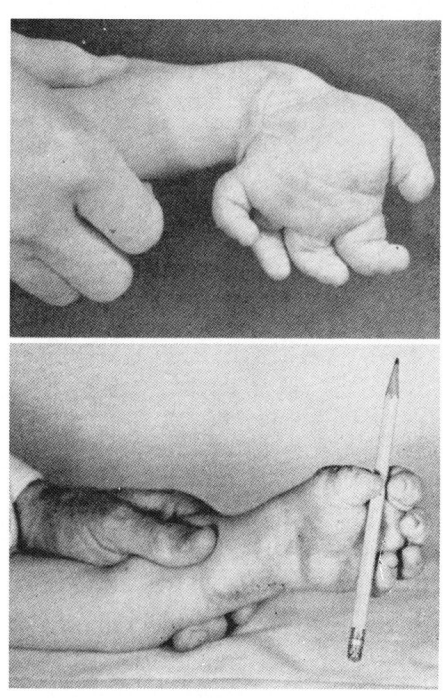

Fig. 80-16   Case J.M. From birth the cicatrix from a tear at the ulnar side of the wrist so distorted the growth of the hand that there was no function. The scar was excised, the ulna elongated, and a pedicle applied. Two years later osteotomies were performed on all metacarpals, the thumb cleft was deepened, and a pulley operation was performed to improve apposition. Three years later the hand was reported to be quite useful. (From Bunnell: Surgery of the hand, ed 3, Philadelphia, 1956, Lippincott.)

makes flexion possible. Often it is necessary also to free the long extensor tendons (Fig. 80-14) and to clean out the volar pouch of the joint. In performing an arthroplasty, the metacarpal head is shortened and reshaped, and a hood of fascia is fastened over it.

Arthroplasty is not often done on the wrist joint; arthrodesis is used instead. In many cases, however, removal of a mass of scar tissue from the volar aspect of the wrist allows the wrist to extend. When pronation and supination are retained, arthrodesis of the wrist or of the proximal finger joints into the position of function gives very little disability (Fig. 80-15).

Flexion contractures and furnishing new cover

Most reconstruction commences with excision of a big plaque of scar tissue that is drawing the hand into flexion contracture and strangling the rest of the tissue (Figs. 80-16 and 80-17). The skin is then undermined and allowed to retract, thus freeing the hand for better nutrition. New cover is then provided, sometimes by a free graft but usually by a pedicle graft from the abdomen (Fig. 80-18), thus giving good, pliable skin with a layer of soft fat beneath. Doing so releases the whole hand and makes it possible to reconstruct the deeper parts, joints, bones, tendons, and nerves. Although the refinements of stereognosis never return to such skin, eventually sensation to light touch and pin prick develops.

Skeletal malalignment

The bones of the hand constitute the framework along which the muscles and tendons function in their proper planes. The joints allow the digits to flex and extend in their proper positions for adequate grasp. After fracture, bones often unite at such odd angles that the whole mechanics are thrown out of true. If, after healing, there is an angle of the bones along the length of the limb, the tendons over the convexity will be tight, over the concavity loose. Such a circumstance upsets the whole nicely adjusted muscle balance so that the joints are pulled into deformity all the way from the site of angulation to the end of the limb. To make the hand function properly again, realignment is necessary. The bones are chiseled or sawed across, a wedge being removed when necessary to place them in proper contact and alignment. They are then pinned so by Kirschner wires, the latter being withdrawn in two months when union is solid and the framework of the hand is restored.

When the thumb does not entirely contact the ring finger

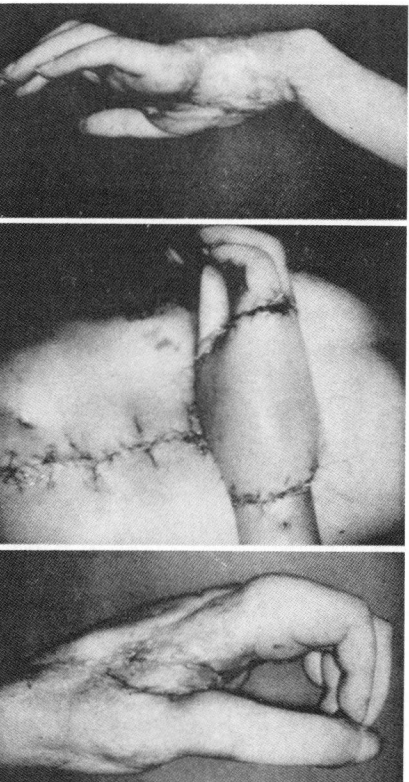

Fig. 80-18   Case A.C. Hand badly crushed between rollers. Poor skin surface, nonfunction position, entire hand and joints stiff, extensor tendons adherent, thumb at side, amputation contemplated. First operation: excised all skin from both dorsal and volar surfaces, covered with one large pedicle graft, and spread thumb from hand; brought joints around by elastic splints. Second operation: freed extensor tendons and placed fat beneath; did capsulectomies on proximal joints; used sublimis of long finger for apposition; freed flexor tendons, placing fat beneath; and defatted pedicle. The hand made a remarkable recovery in nourishment, function, and position. There was good grasping power and a complete change in the morale of the patient. No prosthesis needed. (From Bunnell: Surgery of the hand, ed 3, Philadelphia, 1956, Lippincott.)

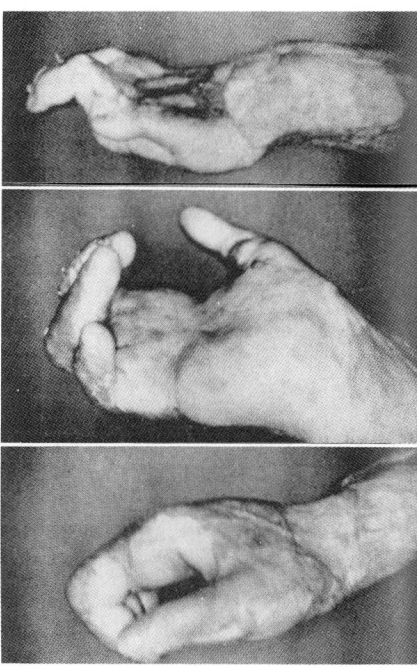

Fig. 80-17   Case D.C.M. Hand severely burned in oil fire so that all digits pointed backward out of use. Fingers were webbed, and middle joints were exposed. There was no thumb cleft, the thumb being at the rear of the hand with the metacarpal arch reversed. In this position of nonfunction, the hand was entirely useless. Excised all dorsal skin, including nails. Sawed away exposed bone. Corrected webs. Established thumb cleft and positioned thumb. Positioned fingers by capsulectomies. Covered all with free skin graft. Patient returned to his job as locomotive engineer. No prosthesis needed. (From Bunnell: Surgery of the hand, ed 3, Philadelphia, 1956, Lippincott.)

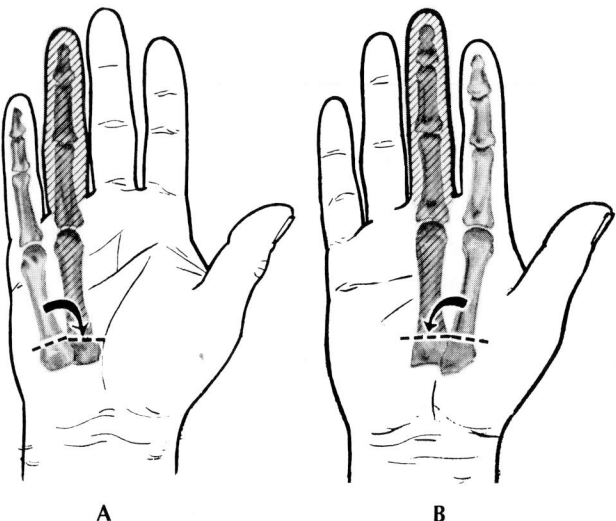

Fig. 80-19 Reconstruction procedure recommended in the event of serious damage to, **A,** the fourth digit or to **B,** the third digit. In **A,** delete the much-injured fourth ray and jog the fifth ray over to its place. In **B,** delete the much-injured third ray and jog the second ray over to its place. The result in either case is a functional four-digit hand.

or the little finger, the metacarpal of either or both may be severed at the base and the digits angulated toward each other in such a way as to provide for easy contact. Similarly, in the absence of a thumb, two or more fingers may be angulated and rotated to give them the ability to work against each other.

When a metacarpal, including the soft tissues about it (tendons, nerves, interosseous muscles, and skin) is badly damaged, it may be excised. If it is one of the central rays, the metacarpal of the adjoining ray, either index or little, as the case may be, is cut across at its base, jogged over to the base of the excised metacarpal, and pinned near and parallel to the next ray (Fig. 80-19).

When a metacarpal head is missing, the lack of support causes the adjoining metacarpals to rotate so that the fingers cross on flexion. In such a case, the metacarpal can be excised and one of the adjacent ones jogged over. Or the proximal phalanx of the ray in question can be recessed, or set back, so that its head will take the place of the missing metacarpal head.

Often it is advisable to arthrodese a joint to place it rigidly in the position of function. This procedure can be carried out on either of the two distal joints of the fingers but rarely on the proximal joints. It is done on the wrist and can be done on the elbow. In the latter case, the choice must be made between arthrodesis, a block operation, muscle transfers, or the wearing of a prosthesis to activate a flail elbow. When the arm cannot be abducted at the shoulder but when muscles around the scapula are good, arthrodesis of the shoulder will allow the arm to position the hand for useful function (Fig. 80-20).

Thumb problems

So essential to prehension is the thumb that every possible bit of an injured one should be saved. Amputation of the thumb through the metacarpophalangeal joint results in a

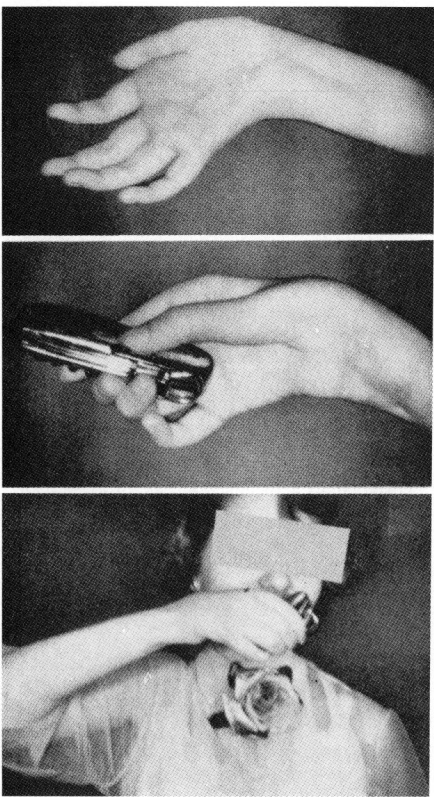

Fig. 80-20 Case L.M.W. As a result of polio, arm was flail at the shoulder, and there were no flexors in the hand. Arthrodesed shoulder and wrist simultaneously so the patient could place the hand. Transferred extensor carpi radialis to flex fingers, palmaris longus to abduct thumb, and the long extensor of the ring finger for apposition. Slit the proximal pulleys so long flexors could flex the proximal joints. Patient gained much use of hand, was able to grasp a piece of paper or a tumbler, could place the hand well, and gained a position in a bank. No prosthesis needed. (From Bunnell: Surgery of the hand, ed 3, Philadelphia, 1956, Lippincott.)

partial digit almost too short to be useful, but a new thumb cleft can easily be made by a Z-plasty operation (Fig. 80-21), meanwhile scraping the adductor origin down from the third metacarpal. The thumb is thus made relatively longer. If the shaft of the index metacarpal projects into the web so as to interfere with grasping, it should be excised at its base to widen and deepen the cleft (Figs. 80-22 and 80-23). Whenever possible, the tip of the third metacarpal should be preserved to provide a concave palm for the remnant of the thumb to work against (Fig. 80-22). Preservation of the broad tip of the third metacarpal is particularly desirable when a complete thumb remains (Fig. 80-24).

The range of motion of a normal thumb extends from a position at the side and slightly back of the hand, with the nail at right angles to the palm, through a wide ellipse toward the volar aspect until it is opposite the fingers, the nail being then parallel to the palm. In the latter position, the thumb is available to participate with the fingers in grasping large objects. The motion is effected by the ten muscles, long and short, that control the thumb. In paralysis of the median

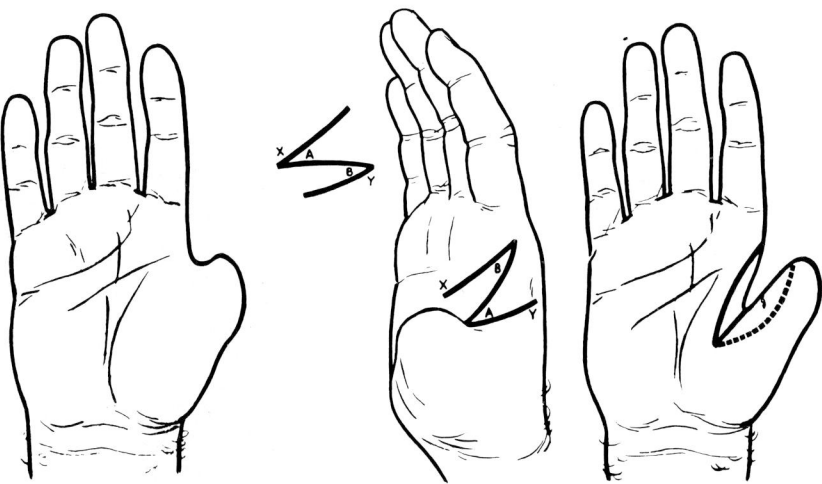

Fig. 80-21   Phalangization of the thumb cleft by Z plasty. *Left,* Hand with short and more or less useless thumb stump. *Middle,* Location of Z-shaped incision. Flap *A* is carried to fixed point *X* and flap *B* to fixed point *Y,* so dorsal flap just covers defect on volar side whereas volar flap just covers defect on dorsal side. Resulting suture line is as shown in inset. *Right,* Result, showing deepened thumb cleft.

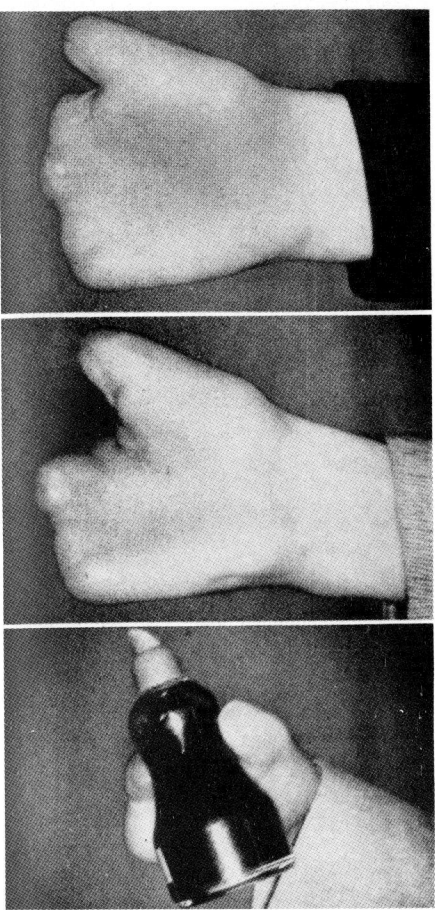

Fig. 80-22   Case C.H. Amputation by meat grinder. Thumb cleft deepened by Z plasty. Index metacarpal removed to give good grasp. (From Bunnell: Surgery of the hand, ed 3, Philadelphia, 1956, Lippincott.)

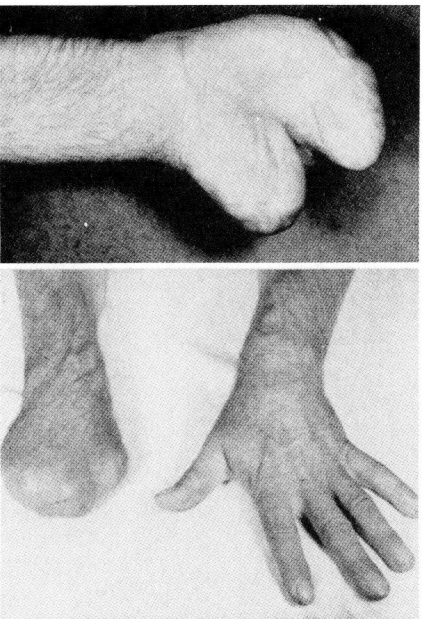

Fig. 80-23   Case H.G. Amputation, by power saw, of all digits through the proximal phalanges, leaving a mitten hand but no thumb cleft. By a plastic maneuver and removal of the index metacarpal, a thumb cleft ¾ in. deep was constructed. It opened ¾ in. and closed against the hand. Patient could write and hold objects. Limited facility can be combined with the use of a prosthesis. (From Bunnell: Surgery of the hand, ed 3, Philadelphia, 1956, Lippincott.)

nerve, in injury to the thenal muscles, in stiffness of the carpometacarpal joint of the thumb, or in flexion contracture on the dorsum of the web, normal range of motion of the thumb is lost. If the other parts of the hand are mobile, the ability to appose the thumb can readily be provided by a simple tendon transfer that draws the thumb toward the pisiform bone and pronates it. When this is not possible, the thumb may be held permanently in a useful position by a bone graft at the base of the first metacarpal.

When a thumb is closely bound to the rest of the hand by scar, it can be spread away by excising the scar tissue and cutting across the cleft from a point opposite the hinge of the first two metacarpals on the dorsal side to the corresponding point on the volar side. The thumb is spread to

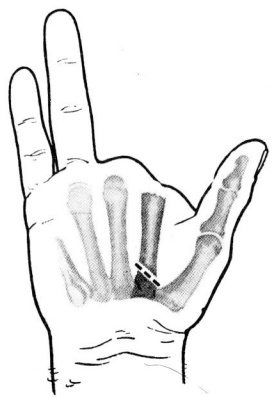

Fig. 80-24 Operative procedure for loss of the second and third digits. Excision of the second metacarpal, but with retention of the third, furnishes easy apposition for the sound thumb.

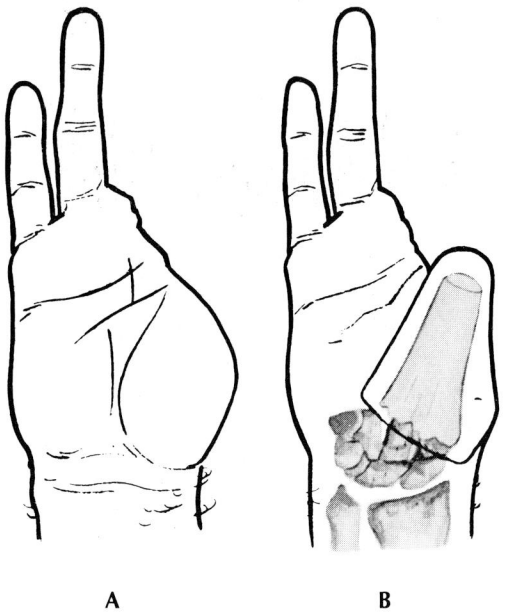

A   B

Fig. 80-25 Surgical construction of a new "thumb." **A,** Poorly functioning partial hand retaining digits four and five only. **B,** Serviceable partial hand made by constructing new "thumb" with pedicle and bone graft. Function is apt to be better than if a prosthesis were applied.

the side and front of the hand, and the large denudation of skin is covered either by a large diamond-shaped free skin graft or, better, by a pedicle graft from the abdomen. In three weeks, pedicle grafts are detached from the abdomen and laid smoothly on the hand.

Although the thumb stump remaining after amputation through the metacarpophalangeal joint usually is not very

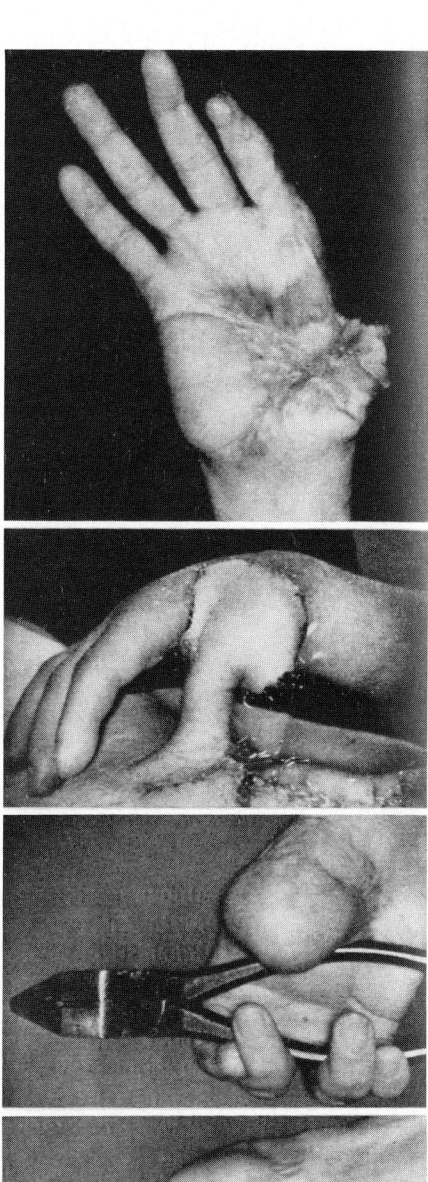

Fig. 80-26 Case C.B. Injury from hand grenade. Pedicle graft covered the thumb, and arthrodesis was performed on the trapezium by a graft from the ilium. Abduction was furnished to the index finger by a proprius tendon graft. A very useful hand resulted. No prosthesis needed. (From Bunnell: Surgery of the hand, ed 3, Philadelphia, 1956, Lippincott.)

serviceable, it may be built out by pedicle and bone graft. If a thumb is amputated proximal to the metacarpophalangeal joint, it should in any case be built out longer. If the thenar muscles and the stub of the metacarpal remain intact, the thumb will be quite movable. A short thumb is a good thumb. Various motions, such as apposition, extension, and flexion, may be furnished it by tendon grafts.

In the case of total loss of the thumb, a new one can be supplied in various ways. The simplest approach is to raise a tube pedicle from the abdomen, attach the pedicle to the hand, and place in it a bone graft from the iliac crest (Figs. 80-25 and 80-26). Although this expedient gives sensation, it does not provide much stereognosis. Nevertheless, a reconstructed thumb is apt to be very serviceable and considerably better than a prosthesis. The graft should be grounded on some other bone rather than connected by a joint. It may be placed on the carpus to make a pad in the base of the palm, or it may be placed on the trapezium or on the stub of the metacarpal.

The requirements of a new thumb are three in number: motion, sensation, and proper placement. The best new thumbs are made by pollicization of a finger, preferably the index finger but sometimes the long finger. Often, as part of the injury, the index finger is already somewhat shortened. In such a case, the finger, or a portion of suitable length, is transferred together with a bridge of skin and with its nerves, blood vessels, and tendons intact (Figs. 80-27 and 80-28). It may even be transferred on a neurovascular pedicle circumscribing the skin all around (Fig. 80-29). When this procedure is possible, it makes for easy and exact placement. The tendons are brought over with the new "thumb" and joined up so as to give motion. The fingers should work directly against the new "thumb" and also, by their side motion, should pass to the side of it and close against the palm. Stereognosis and vascularization are provided by the neurovascular pedicle.

Should a newly constructed thumb not have sensation in its tactile area, a flap of skin may be exchanged for the nontactile skin by a Z-plasty. Or tactile skin can be furnished by using a neurovascular pedicle passed beneath the skin at the base of the thumb. A living thumb, with motion, sensation, and proper positioning, is, of course, far superior to any prosthetic thumb.

Tendon repair

Tendons are frequently lacerated, thus losing their function of transmitting muscle power to provide motion in joints. They can, however, readily be repaired (Fig. 80-30), the most difficult cases being the flexor tendons in the digits and in the distal part of the palm, where the resulting juncture tends to adhere to the surrounding parts. Frequently a tendon graft must be used to bridge the tendon over areas where adhesions are likely to form. Adherent tendons may be freed, and slippery material, such as paratenon and fascia, may be grafted between them and the bones so as to allow the tendons to glide again. Defects in tendons are readily bridged by free tendon grafts from spare tendons in other parts.

The upper limb interdigitates at the ends of the metacarpals, and the tendons normally have individual motion. If either an extensor or a flexor tendon is sutured over a finger stump, it will hold back all of the tendons pulled from the

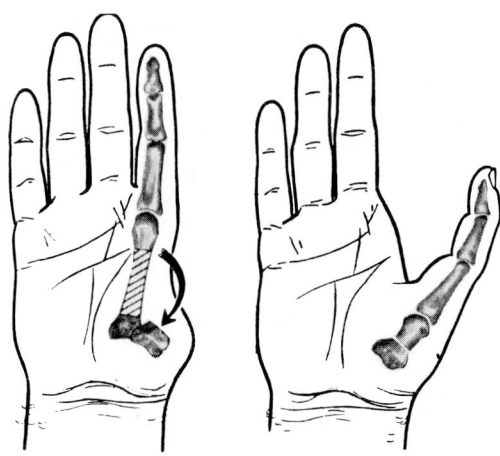

Fig. 80-27   Pollicization of the index finger.

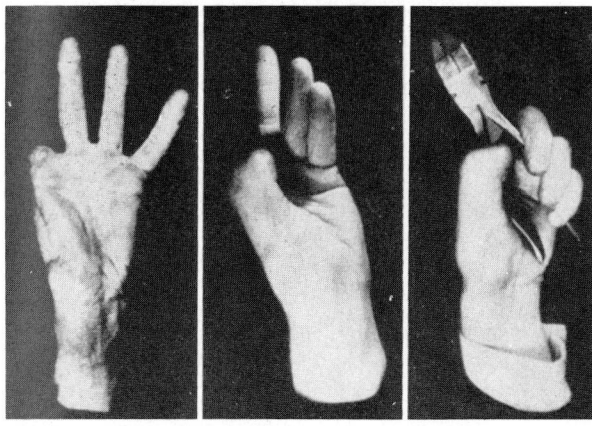

Fig. 80-28   Case H.W.W. First (1929) physiological reconstruction of the thumb by pollicizing the remains of the index finger. Metacarpal lashed to trapezium, nerves and vessels carried over, and all tendons and muscles connected up. "Thumb" had strong motion and normal sensation and was well positioned. Patient worked well as a carpenter for 20 years. Superior to prosthesis. (From Surgery, gynecology, and obstetrics.)

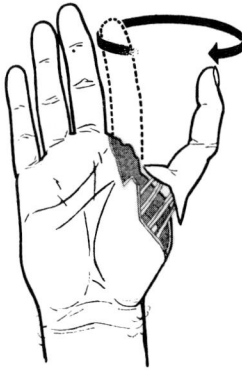

Fig. 80-29   Pollicization of index finger by neurovascular pedicle. Skin is circumscribed, and the index finger is pinned on to the stub of the metacarpal of the thumb in proper position. Tendons furnish motion, vessels furnish nutrition, and nerves furnish sensation.

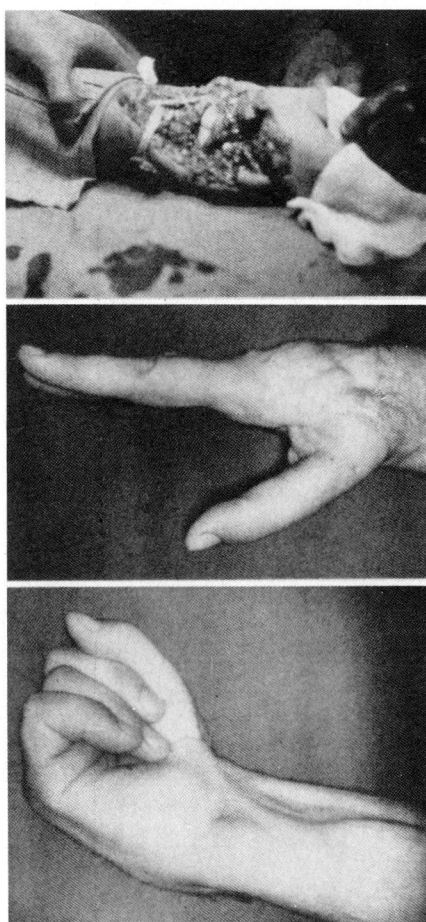

Fig. 80-30 Case F.E. Charge from a shotgun entered palm and emerged dorsally, shattering the carpus and the lower radius and severing many tendons, extensors of the wrist, thumb, and fingers, and the median nerve. Dèbrided, filetted the index finger, and skin-grafted. Considerable infection followed. First operation: excised scar and placed a pedicle. Second operation: furnished tendon grafts plus paratenon to extent thumb and fingers; freed the flexor tendon of the thumb; did a pulley operation for apposition; sutured median nerve to its four branches. The wrist became fused. But sensation, motion, and apposition returned, so a very useful hand requiring no prosthesis resulted. (From Bunnell: Surgery of the hand, ed 3, Philadelphia, 1956, Lippincott.)

same muscle. But when all of the tendons are cut at the end of a carpal or metacarpal stump, they should all be sutured together over the end to provide for movement of the stump.

Isolated digits may be made to provide prehension if they are furnished with new flexor and extensor tendons. To make the fingers appose each other, the tendons can be placed diagonally across the hand, or a tendon T transfer, which consists of one cross-bar tendon from digit to digit and a longitudinal one looped about the first, can be made (Fig. 80-31). When the muscle concerned is contracted, the "T" assumes the shape of a "Y" and the two digits are drawn toward each other. This procedure is particularly useful in median and ulnar paralysis, where it will provide adduction of the thumb and little finger while curving the metacarpal arch of the palm. When some digits have been amputated, great strength can be given to the remaining fingers by

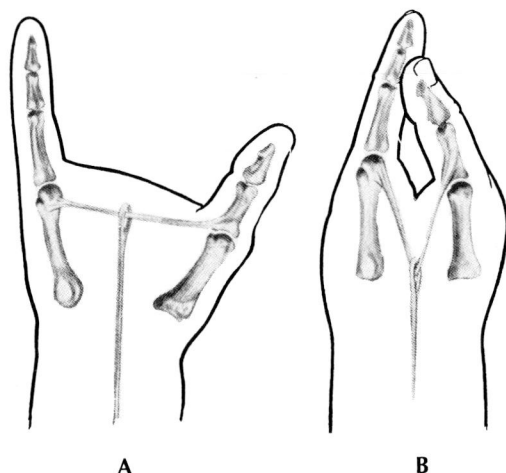

Fig. 80-31 Lobster hand formed by tendon T transfer. **A,** Arrangement of tendons to form the "T." **B,** Contraction of the longitudinal tendon converts the "T" to a "Y" and thus effects apposition of the thumb and little finger.

transferring in the forearm the tendons of the amputated ones to those of the remaining ones.

Especially in paralysis are tendon transfers useful. Good, strong muscle and tendon are transferred to the tendons of the paralyzed muscles. This operation may be performed, without fusing the wrist, to give very good return of function so that splints are discarded. In the case of any two nerves paralyzed high in the arm, the wrist can first be arthrodesed in the position of function, an expedient which results in very little disability. Thereupon the five tendons previously wrist movers become available as digit movers, and the resulting motion is more natural than that obtained using a prosthesis. The patient soon learns to adapt so that the motion becomes natural. A rule is to decide what movements are needed and then to consider the number of muscles available for transfer. For paralysis within the hand—that is, from the median and ulnar nerves—many transfers are available to restore muscle balance, thus correcting the position of the claw hand by substituting for the paralyzed intrinsic muscles.

Another principle is tenodesis, a procedure in which the tendons that move the digits are fastened to the forearm bones. Then, when the wrist is flexed, the extensor tendons tighten and extend the digits; when it is extended, the flexor tendons tighten and cause the digits to flex so that thumb and fingers appose each other. These automatic movements are useful when only one or two strong muscles are available. When no muscles are available, the hand can be converted to a useful hook by tenodesis of the flexor tendons to the forearm bones.

Nerves

Movement and sensation in the hand, which are its two most important functions and which are of equal value, depend entirely upon the nerves. The three large nerves that course down the arm (the ulnar nerve, the median nerve, and the radial nerve) control the hand, and any injury to them is as damaging to the hand as is an injury to the hand itself. When a nerve is severed, it should be rejoined at once. Otherwise fibrous degeneration in both the lower portion of the nerve and in the muscles supplied by it will be so progressive that, after two years, muscle action will not return and, after five years, neither will sensation. A gap of several inches can be overcome and the nerve sutured directly. Even the little nerves in the hand itself can be repaired.

After nerve suture, there is about 80 percent of functional recovery. Nerves can be sutured directly, transferred, or even free-grafted. All of these procedures are successful, but nerve grafts must be used from the same person; if grafted from another person, they will melt away. From loss of nerve supply, the hand if neglected goes into the position of nonfunction, stiffens, and atrophies. Splinting should be by spring or elastic splints sufficient just to substitute for the paralyzed muscles and to hold the hand in the position of function so it can work. When the nerves are irreparable, as for example when too great an interval has elapsed since the time of injury, muscle function in the hand can be provided by tendon transfers. Paralysis in the hand and forearm from ischemic contracture can be overcome to a considerable degree, although never completely cured. In vasomotor disorders, surgery seldom need be weighed against prostheses.

PROSTHESES FOR PARTIAL HANDS

The literature on prostheses for the partial hand is meager, and therefore when a hand is damaged there is a distinct preference on the part of prosthetists to have a wrist disarticulation or a long-below-elbow amputation. In the event they are confronted with a partial hand amputation, many limbfitters prefer to enclose the wrist immobile (as in Fig. 80-32) rather than to construct a partial hand prosthesis. Even those who furnish cosmetic-glove prostheses (as in Fig. 80-33) prefer to enclose the whole hand in the glove and to substitute, for the missing parts, foam filler reinforced with pliable wire. Although a long-below-elbow amputation offers the advantage that many more or less standard terminal devices may be applied (a split hook, a mechanical hand, perhaps some special tools), a partial hand, whatever can be saved, can often be fitted with considerably more success. If the thumb alone is spared, a casing over the palm and wrist can support a pad or other suitable device against which the remaining digit can work (Fig. 80-34). If only the palm, perhaps with a few remnants of phalanges, remains, a casing over the forearm can support a similar pad against which the palm can be pressed by wrist flexion (Fig. 80-35).

By the combined talents of engineers, physicists, prosthetists, orthopedists, and others, there have been in the last ten years many advances in hand and arm prostheses. Accordingly, there has been developed the policy of saving as much of any limb as is likely to be functional and, particularly, as much of the hand as possible. Any portion of skin with sensation should be preserved because of the possibility of placing it in a functional part. Digits with sensation can do light work and, if necessary, a prosthesis can be applied to do heavy work (as in Figs. 80-36 and 80-37).

For the wrist-disarticulation, below-elbow, above-elbow,

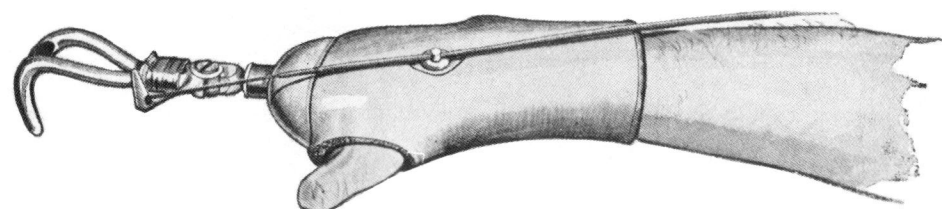

Fig. 80-32   One form of prosthesis for partial hand amputation, with thumb free, wrist encased, and split hook activated by shoulder harness, as in the case of wrist disarticulation. The disadvantages are numerous including the excessive length of the device as a whole, the elimination by the long cuff of possible wrist motion, and obviated residual tactile sense, except in the thumb remnant.

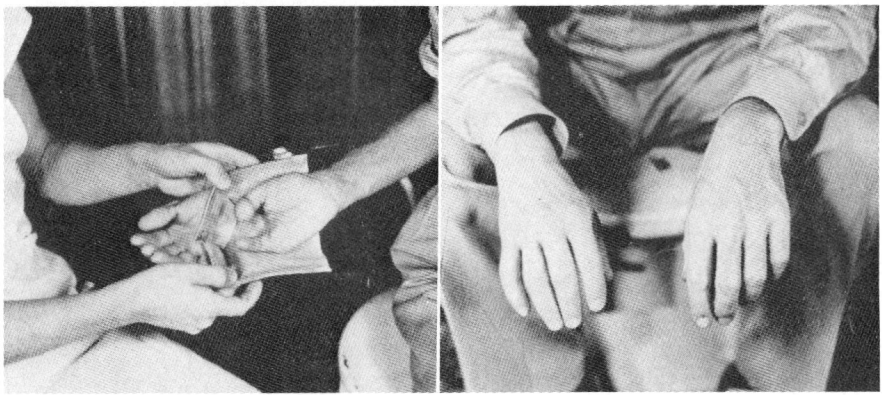

Fig. 80-33   Cosmetic hand for partial amputation—glovelike and zippered at the wrist. Fingers are filled out by foam filler and stiffened by armature flexible enough to hold any shape. (Courtesy Prosthetic Services of San Francisco.)

and shoulder-disarticulation prostheses, many new devices have been developed. They include the alternator elbow lock for the above-elbow case,[3,5] the outside-locking elbow hinge for elbow disarticulation,[1,3,5] the polycentric elbow joint for below-elbow cases,[1] the variable-ratio step-up hinge for the very short below-elbow case,[1] the flexible cable units to allow pronation and supination for the very long below-elbow and wrist-disarticulation cases,[8] and the elbow-coupled shoulder joint for shoulder-disarticulation amputees.[7] For the arm amputee, these devices help to carry the terminal device (hook of artificial hand) to a place of usefulness. The *Manual of Upper Extremity Prosthetics*[11] gives a full account of these and other devices that comprise a full armamentarium for upper-extremity amputees. But the case of the partial hand amputation is not included.

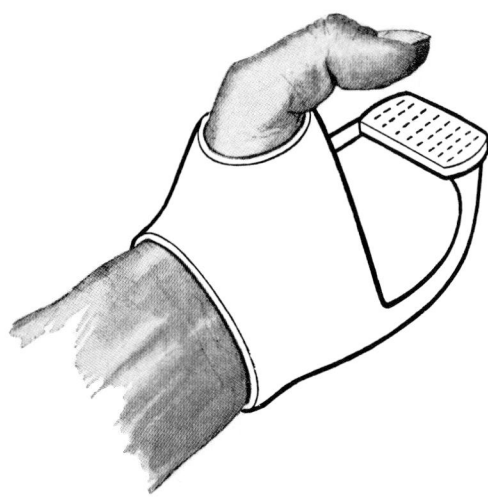

Fig. 80-34 Simple prosthesis for loss of all digits except the thumb.

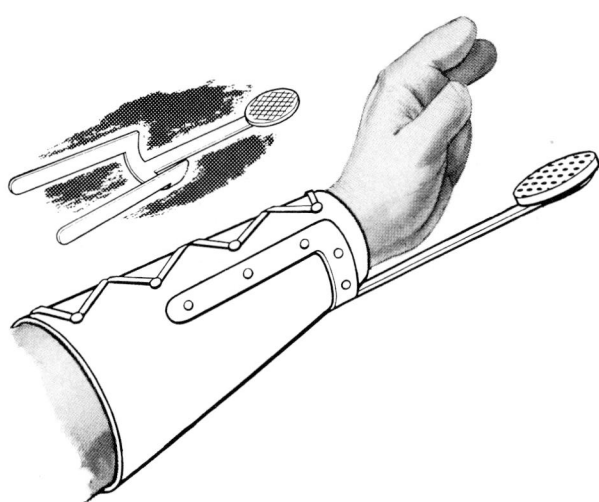

Fig. 80-35 Simple prosthesis for major losses of most of the digits. Wrist serves as motor, hand working against prosthesis. Residual tactile sensation is used.

Prosthesis for one-digit hands

For most practical purposes, loss of one or more distal phalanges does not require application of a prosthesis. Nevertheless, there are exceptions. An accomplished violinist, losing the distal phalanx of even one string finger, for example, is incapable of managing the strings properly. This could mean an occupational change for such a person. A good prosthetic replacement may enable him to continue his occupation. The same occasionally occurs with an organist, a pianist, a typist, or other person in any occupation where finger dexterity means the difference between success and failure. A suitable prosthesis for such a case can be made using thin stainless steel for the socket and extension framework and then dipping the device in flexible vinyl plastic to form the tip cushion and finger build-up. The socket portion may be split along one side to allow it to expand and contract, thus ensuring snugness of fit.

For amputation of all of the fingers at the metacarpophalangeal joint, or approximately half an inch distal thereto such that the volar crease of the metacarpophalangeal joint remains, a ⅛-in. rod framework of stainless steel can simulate the socket while leaving a maximum amount of ex-

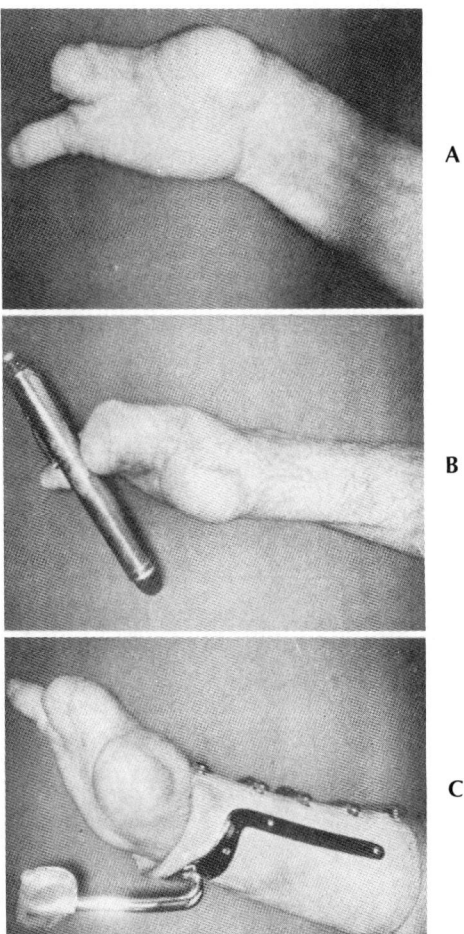

Fig. 80-36 Partial hand capable of prehension. **A** and **B,** Digital motion for light work. **C,** Wrist motor for heavy work. (From Bunnell: Surgery of the hand, ed 3, Philadelphia, 1956, Lippincott.)

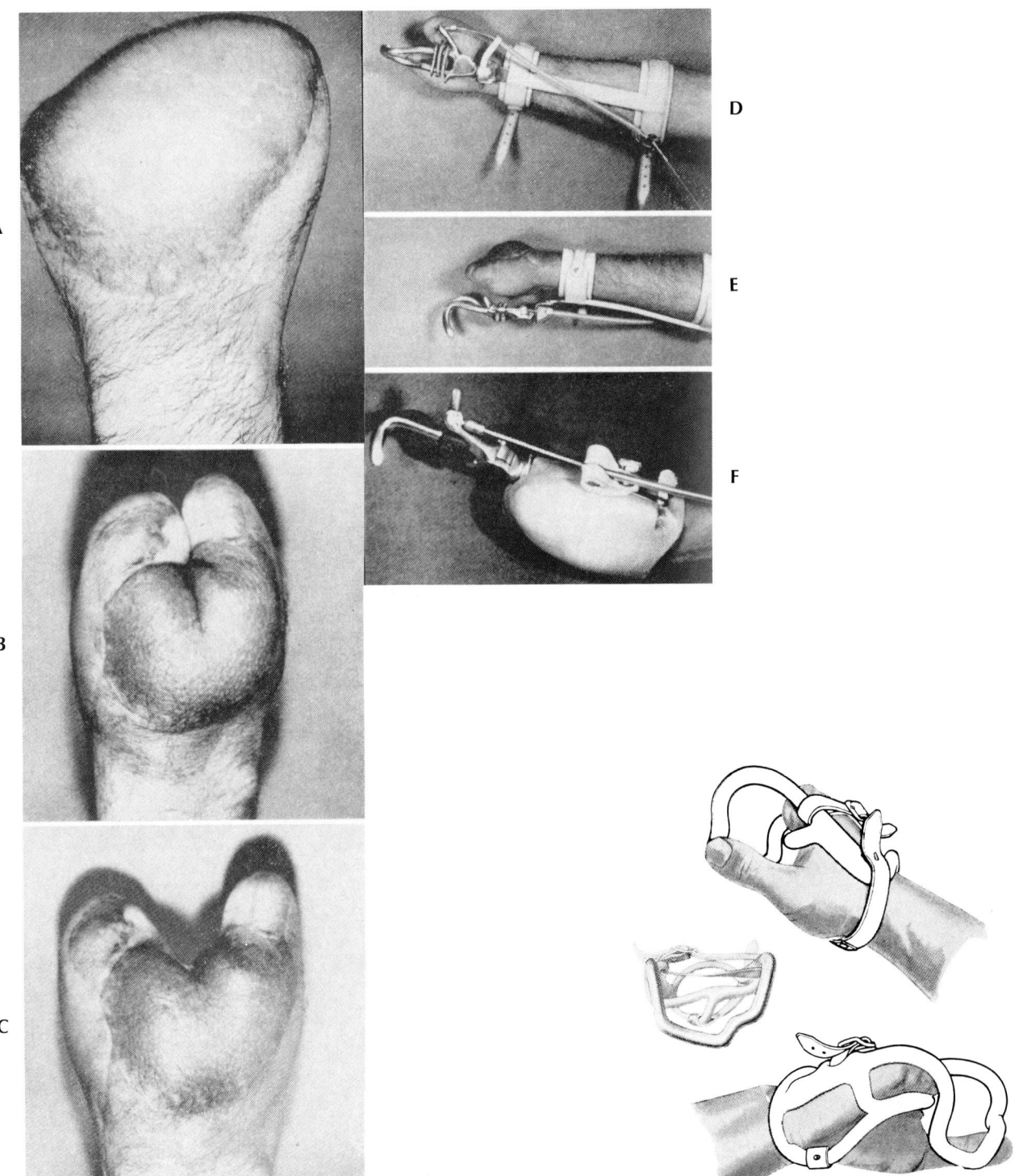

Fig. 80-37   Case E.E. **A, B,** and **C,** Right hand pulled into hay chopper. Dèbridement and abdominal pedicle. Later a two-digit hand was made with a tendon T operation for prehension and a spread of 1½ in. **D** and **E,** A prosthesis that enabled the hand to work against a hook, later discarded because it was too unstable. **F,** A prosthesis made by Robin-Aids Manufacturing Company, Vallejo, Calif., that was very satisfactory. It preserved residual wrist motion and could be removed when fine digital motions were required.

Fig. 80-38   Prosthesis for loss of all the fingers at, or slightly distal to, the metacarpophalangeal joint line. Metal ring, covered with vinyl plastic, is so shaped as to furnish one large hook, representing the index finger, and one small hook, representing the little finger. Thumb works against ring throughout the range of the carpometacarpal articulation. (Courtesy Robin-Aids Manufacturing Company, Vallejo, Calif.)

posed palm for traction and sensation (Fig. 80-38). The distal portion of the framework is bent to simulate the finger tips, the little-finger side being curved to form a hook for pulling or lifting and the index side shaped to appose the thumb as would the first two fingers in three-jaw-chuck prehension.[4] This arrangement provides for prehension between the simulated index finger and the remaining thumb. A similar appliance can be made for an amputation proximal to the metacarpophalangeal joint, but in such a case the remainder of the hand must be fitted with a plastic, metal, or leather socket for attachment to the formed rod (Fig. 80-39). The notable disadvantage is the coverage of surfaces otherwise capable of sensation. In both instances, the rod framework is dipped in flexible vinyl plastic to provide a surface with adequate traction.

Fig. 80-40 shows a single stainless rod curved in hook fashion and mounted to a stainless-steel plate, which in turn is attached to a molded hand and wrist socket. The hook is so positioned as to give apposition to the thumb, and the thumb is exposed to utilize its capability for sensation. This

single hook, being small and smooth, allows easy entry into pockets and other tight places.

Since the thumb is the most important single digit of the hand, it would seem a sound principle not to involve it as a motor for powering other mechanisms. A collar around the thumb would appear to diminish tactile surface, and any mechanical linkage would seem to lessen mobility and dexterity. In general, wrist flexion-extension provides a far more desirable motor with less hindrance to function. But these principles have only general applicability and are not specific. For certain special needs, a thumb-powered mechanism may be desirable. In any individual case, the selection of equipment must be left to the mutual judgment of the patient, the doctor, and the prosthetist. Figs. 80-41 and

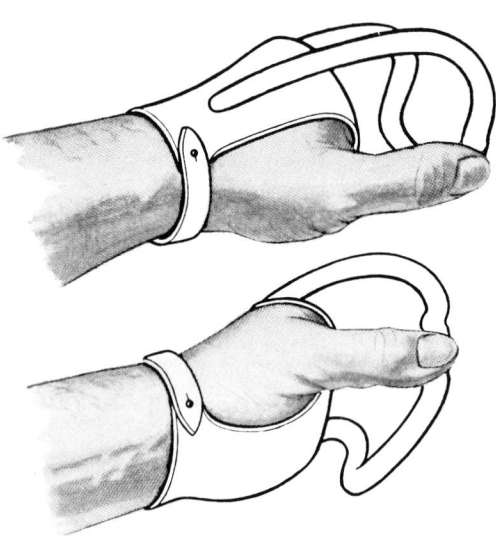

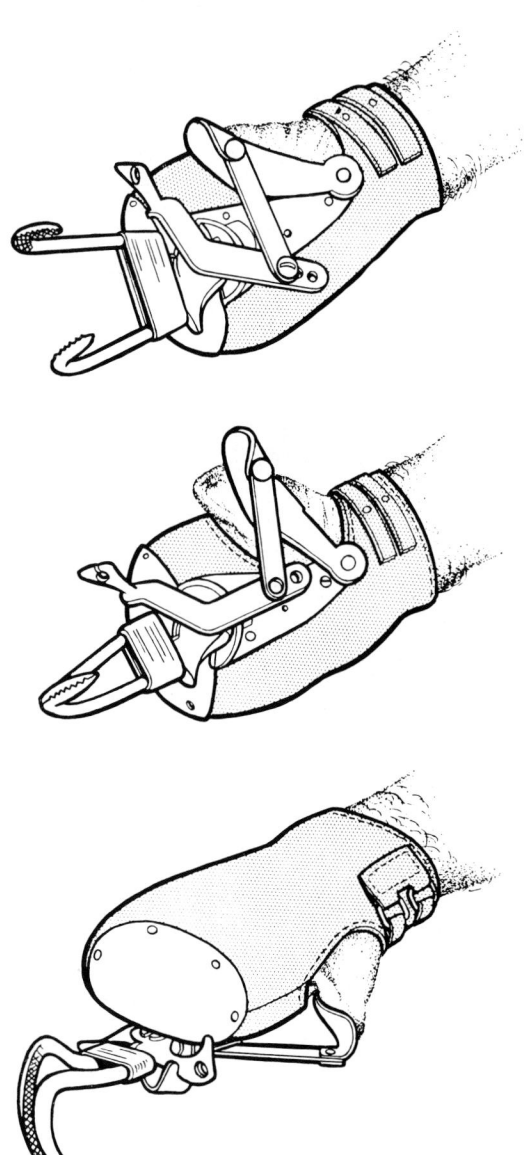

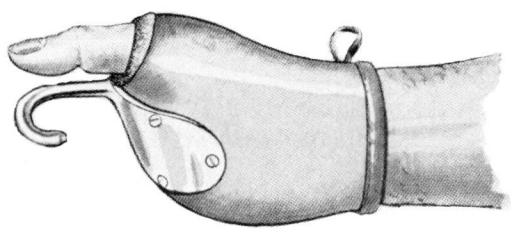

Fig. 80-39 Prosthesis for transmetacarpal amputation. Socket may be of leather, molded plastic, or hammered stainless steel. Metal ring, covered with vinyl plastic, is shaped to simulate fingers, as in Fig. 80-38. (Courtesy Robin-Aids Manufacturing Company, Vallejo, Calif.)

Fig. 80-40 Simple prosthesis for loss of most of the palm but with retention of the thumb. Wrist and hand stump are encased in a socket to which is attached a single stainless-steel hook. The hook may be used by itself or as a member for apposing the thumb.

Fig. 80-41 Prosthesis for amputation of all fingers at the metacarpophalangeal joint line with retention of the thumb. Socket about wrist and hand stump supports split hook, which is powered by the thumb. (Courtesy Navy Prosthetics Research Laboratory, U.S. Naval Hospital, Oakland, Calif.)

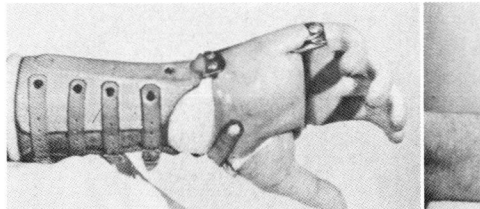
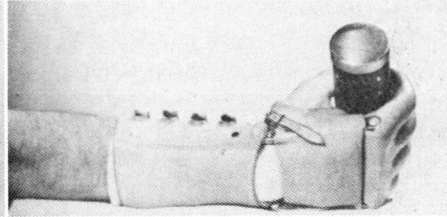

Fig. 80-42 Prosthesis for loss of all digits but the thumb. Hinged at and powered by the wrist, this device provides for prehension by virtue of a thrust rod. (Courtesy Robin-Aids Manufacturing Company, Vallejo, Calif.)

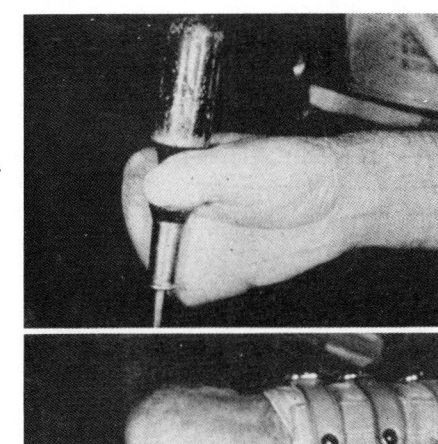

A

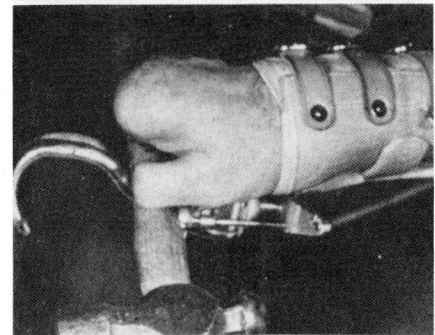

B

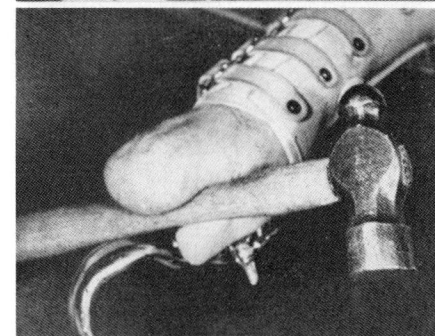

C

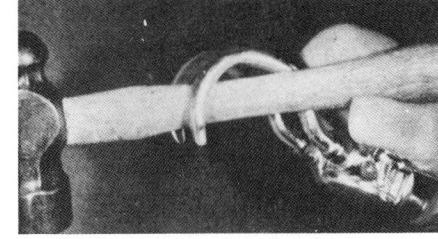

D

Fig. 80-43 Amputation of the fingers at the metacarpophalangeal joint line and of the thumb at the interphalangeal joint; thumb phalangized for deeper cleft. **A,** Holding with thumb unassisted. **B,** Use of hook (powered in this case by shoulder harness) as a device to appose palm. **C,** Holding with thumb, hook available for auxiliary function if needed. **D,** Holding with hook, thumb as stabilizer.

80-42 illustrate the principles involved but show the distinct differences to be found in individual cases.

In the arrangement shown in Fig. 80-43, the hand, wrist, and forearm socket give versatility for the accomplishment of either light tasks or heavy-duty work. For light tasks, the thumb stump is free to appose the remainder of the hand or to contact a small metal post or spoon attached to the hook. The forearm socket allows freedom of wrist motion but provides hook stability for heavy-duty work. Since the thumb stump is also free to appose the hook-activating lever, no shoulder harness is required.

For a hand retaining only the thumb, without fingers or even without their metacarpals, a special prosthesis designed by the United States Navy gives reciprocal motion and active prehension powered by the thumb (Fig. 80-44). To a simple hand cuff and wrist strap is attached a metal plate, which, on the radial side, supports a lever for the thumb to appose and, on the ulnar side, bears a metal finger pivoted on an axis near the base. Apposition of thumb and metal finger is effected by a linkage between the two lever systems.

Prosthetic thumbs

Figs. 80-45 and 80-46 illustrate fixed prostheses for partial or complete loss of the thumb. Two features are essential. First, the prosthetic thumb must furnish proper apposition to the fingers, and its tip should be of such material as to provide adequate traction. Second, the thumb must provide a shaft and a crotch so as to make it possible to hold objects too large for the fingers themselves to encircle. A two-position thumb, such as the thumb from an APRL hand,[3,4] can be used on a prosthesis for disarticulation of the thumb at the carpometacarpal joint. The result is that a larger selection of objects can be held in the hand.

Fig. 80-47 depicts the application of a mobile artificial thumb, powered by the wrist, to a partial hand possessing only the little finger. Attached to a hand cuff, which in turn is hinged to a forearm cuff, the thumb pivots about an axis near its base. Linkage between thumb and wrist hinge is such that wrist flexion causes the thumb to approach the little finger. In the example shown, the small finger has been rotated surgically toward the radial side of the arm to give better placement for apposition.

Prosthesis for loss of all digits

In the case of a hand too crippled or too paralyzed to be of much use in the direct operation of a prosthesis, a split hook may be attached to a forearm cuff and positioned in the palm. This arrangement (Fig. 80-48) allows the palm to work against the hook for some types of prehension and still provides for the hook to be operated by shoulder harness in the usual way. The stainless-steel hand plate shown in Fig. 80-49 provides a simple, light, and cool means of mounting a split hook to a hand stump that is too short to grasp objects without a prosthesis.

Still another way of accommodating for loss of all digits is to enclose the base of the hand in a leather cuff linked to a forearm cuff, a split hook being attached to the hand cuff (Fig. 80-50). The cuff and forearm members are connected by a rod working levers in such a way that, when

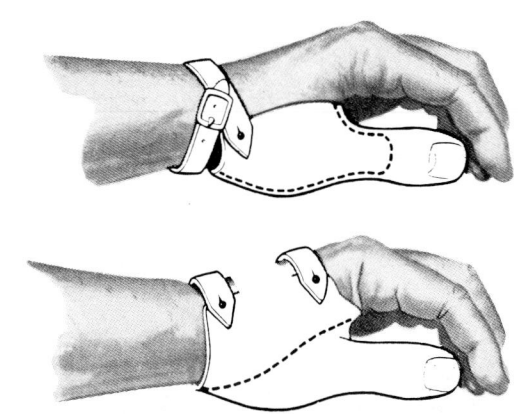

Fig. 80-45 Prosthesis for partial or complete loss of the thumb. Fingers work in apposition to fixed member. *Above,* Prosthesis for amputation of the thumb at the metacarpophalangeal joint, thumb web deepened surgically to provide cylindrical stump proximal to the site of amputation. *Below,* Variation suitable for amputation of the thumb at the carpometacarpal joint.

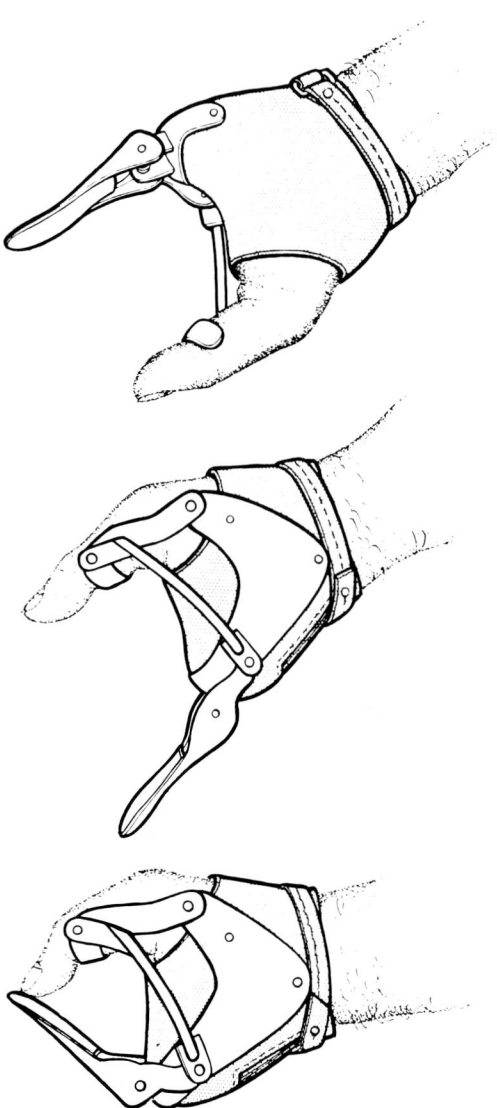

Fig. 80-44 Prosthesis for transmetacarpal amputation with retention of the thumb. Power supplied by the thumb activates metal finger, which is otherwise held in extension by a spring at its base. (Courtesy Navy Prosthetics Research Laboratory, U.S. Naval Hospital, Oakland, Calif.)

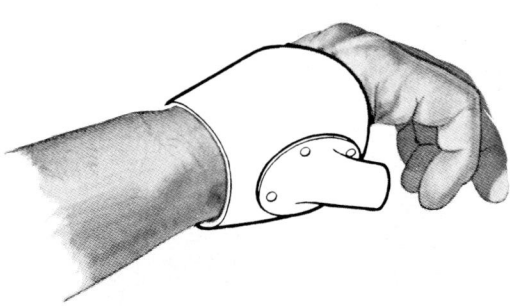

Fig. 80-46 One form of fixed prosthesis for total loss of the thumb.

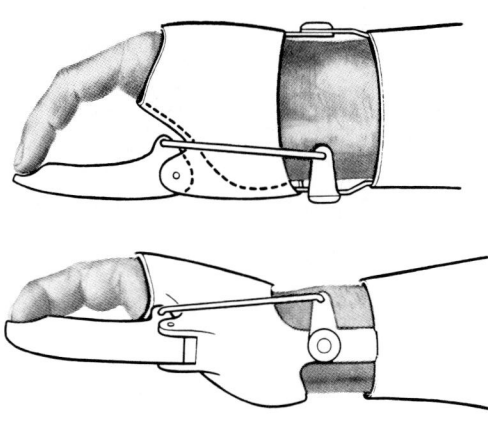

Fig. 80-47 Prosthesis for loss of all digits except the little finger. Laminated plastic socket, hinged to leather or plastic forearm cuff, supports plastic covered metal thumb, which is so linked to forearm piece as to be driven by the wrist motion. Little finger has been rotated surgically to provide better apposition with respect to the prosthetic thumb. (Courtesy Robin-Aids Manufacturing Company, Vallejo, Calif.)

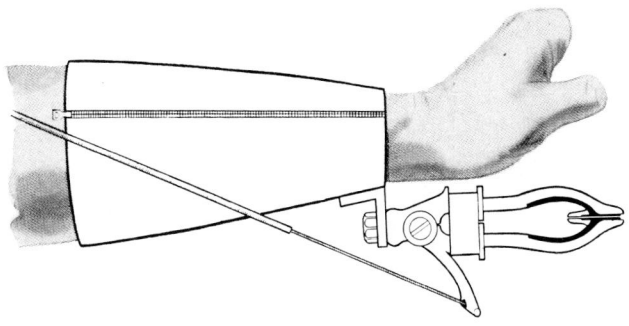

Fig. 80-48 Prosthesis for loss of virtually all digits. Palm can work against hook, or hook can be operated in conventional way by virtue of the cable attached to the shoulder harness.

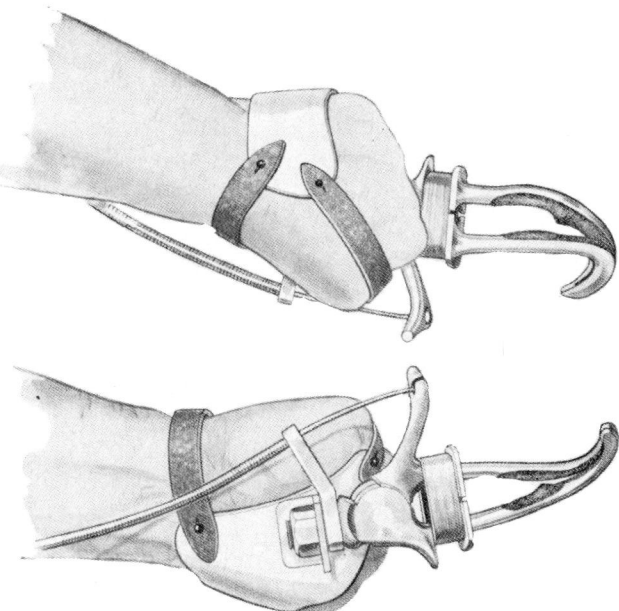

Fig. 80-49 Method of attaching a split hook to a short hand stump. Mobility of the wrist is maintained.

Fig. 80-50 Prosthesis for loss of all digits. Wrist supplies power and excursion for operation of split hook. No shoulder harness needed.

the wrist is flexed, the split hook opens; extension of the wrist closes the hook.

NEW DEVICES FOR PARALYZED ARMS

For the paralyzed arm, many new devices have come forth in the past five years. They all have the same essential purpose—that of carrying the useful, or partially useful, hand to a place where it can operate to advantage. But in these cases there is an additional hurdle to be jumped. Whereas an arm prosthesis can be built to almost any desired weight, in the case of a paralyzed arm the weight of that arm must be overcome before motion can be reacquired. Equipment such as the shoulder suspension hoop, the locking-lever arm brace, the alternator elbow-lock arm brace, suspension slings, and single, double, or triple rocker feeders or arm balancers can do this job.[10]

Once a paralyzed arm can be positioned in a place of usefulness, hand function must be restored, either by surgical or by prosthetic means. Some of the terminal devices intended for arm amputees can be utilized for patients with paralyzed or badly disabled hands. A good example of the management of the paralyzed hand is to be found in the application of the "Handy Hook."[9] It constitutes a simple but effective means of positioning a split hook in the palm of the hand and fastening it there to a metal or plastic palmar plate, which is held in place by straps around the dorsum of the hand (Fig. 80-51). In the event the wrist also is flail, a simple brace on the forearm constitutes a suitable modification (Fig. 80-52).

For a hand that is lacking in one or more features of normal motor power but which retains valuable sensation, there is still another assistive device, the "Handy Hand."[9] Figs. 80-53 and 80-54 show two variations out of numerous possibilities, each designed to accommodate specific motor losses (flexion or extension of fingers, flexion or extension of wrist, and so on). In Fig. 80-53, finger opening may be brought about voluntarily (or, if necessary, by rubber bands), closure being effected by shoulder harness. In Fig. 80-54, active wrist extension effects finger closure.

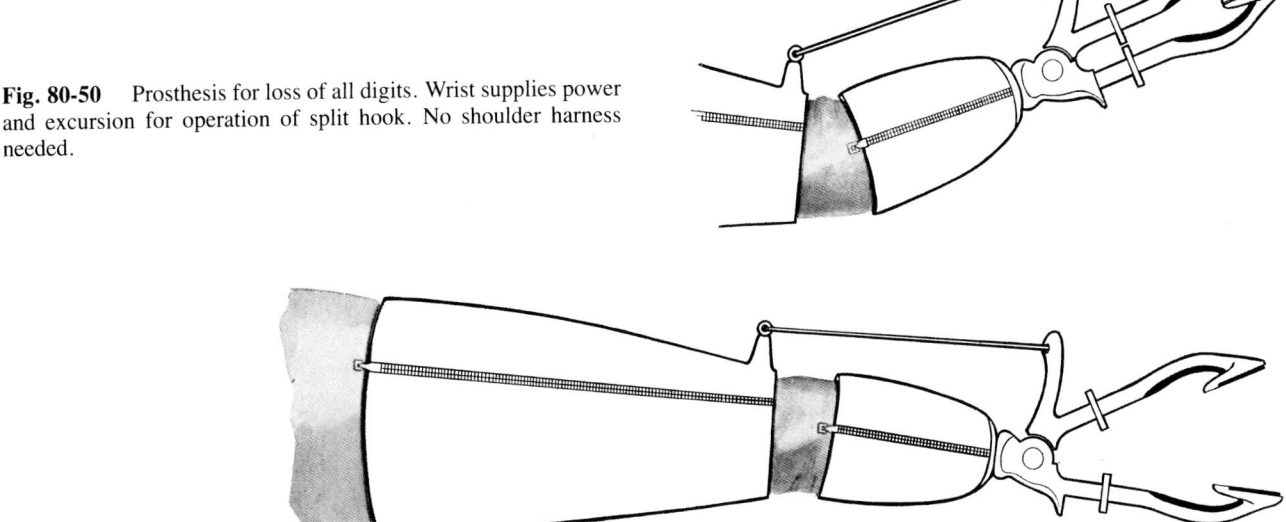

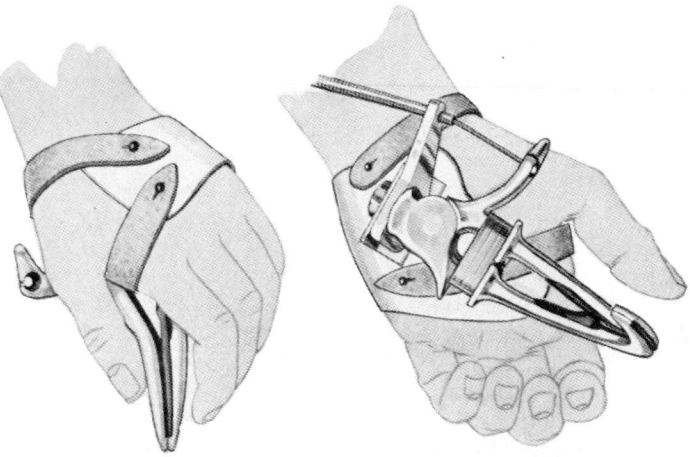

Fig. 80-51 The "Handy Hook" as applied to a flail hand. Positioned in the palm by means of a plate passing over the dorsum, it is powered by a shoulder harness. Hand sensation is preserved. (Courtesy Robin-Aids Manufacturing Company, Vallejo, Calif.)

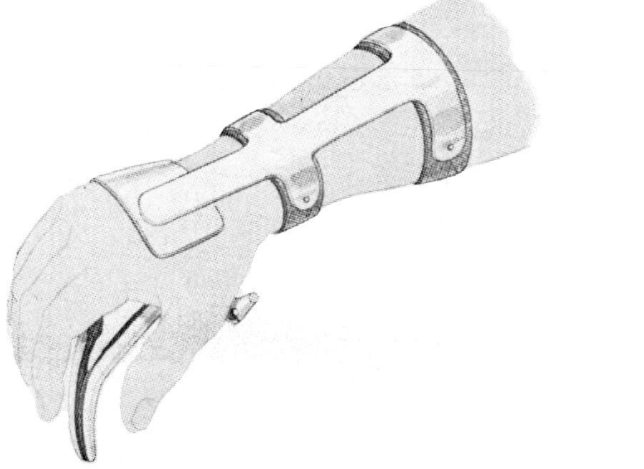

Fig. 80-52 The "Handy Hook" as applied to a flail hand when the wrist also is flail. (Courtesy Robin-Aids Manufacturing Company, Vallejo, Calif.)

CONCLUSION

So vast and so laden with potentialities is the subject of surgical reconstruction of the hand, and so also is that of partial hand prostheses, that a single article such as this can constitute only a very brief introduction to either. But even a brief review of some of the recent advances, both in reconstructive surgery and in prostheses for partial hands, may offer valuable guidance in selecting the best procedure for any given case. In the absence of a well-developed literature, the whole field of work with partial hands is long apt to remain highly empirical and largely dependent upon the experience, judgment, and skill of individual surgeon and prosthetist. Since, unlike the more conventional amputation stump, the partial hand is invariably a special problem, the approach to its solution, whether surgical or prosthetic or both, also invariably calls for special departures. The most that can be said is that from long practice and much trial and error it is possible to extract certain principles generally applicable to the more common types of hand losses.

In any event, it is apparent that the surgeon who would undertake reconstructive hand surgery ought first to be intimately familiar with the best that can be done with prostheses for partial hands. Similarly, the specialist in partial hand prostheses needs to be acquainted with what can be accomplished through surgery. Both, separately and together, must consider each case individually not only from the standpoint of the patient's life and work but also with a view toward his ability to afford the financial outlay incident to surgery and recuperation. Fortunately, insurance has in recent years played a large part in eliminating the economic considerations otherwise involved.

The strongest argument that can be advanced for reconstructive hand surgery is that it preserves the highly desirable facility of tactile sensation. Among the disadvantages are the fact that the result does not always present the best cosmetic effect and the additional one that the reconstructed hand may not be able to perform heavy work as well as could a full prosthesis. The particular requirements of the

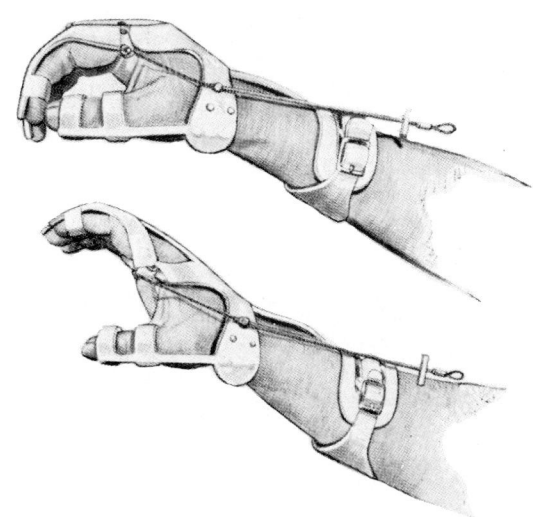

Fig. 80-53 The "Handy Hand" as applied to a flail hand when the wrist also is flail. Extension of the fingers may be effected voluntarily or, if necessary, by rubber bands. Flexion of the fingers is brought about by means of a shoulder harness. (Courtesy Robin-Aids Manufacturing Company, Vallejo, Calif.)

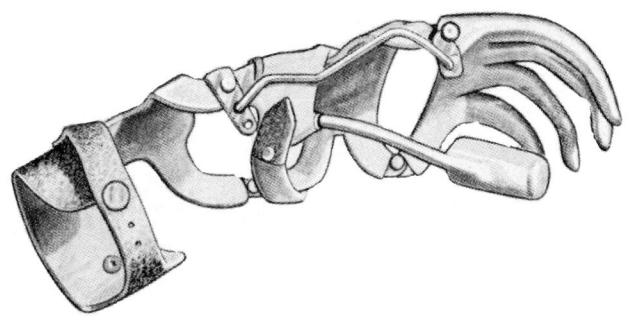

Fig. 80-54 The "Handy Hand" as applied when extensors of wrist and fingers are active, finger flexors inactive. Extension of the wrist effects flexion of the fingers. (Courtesy Robin-Aids Manufacturing Company, Vallejo, Calif.)

individual therefore exercise a strong influence upon the choice between the partial hand and the wrist disarticulation. As has been seen, the most practical result is often best obtained through some combination of surgery and prosthetics, the two complementing each other in such a way as to provide a wide range of functional regain.

Of course there will always be hands with too much wrong with them to justify attempts at reconstruction. Where such appears to be the case, amputation at the lowest possible level, followed by application of a good, functional prosthesis, obviously offers the best solution. But in the face of a rapidly growing technique in hand surgery including special manipulations with muscles, tendons, nerves, and vessels it would appear wise always to choose the most conservative course possible. That would mean reconstruction whenever the anticipated result is likely to serve satisfactorily the needs of the individual concerned. The possibilities outlined here are representative of what might reasonably be expected under a given set of circumstances.

ACKNOWLEDGMENT

For much valuable information on partial hand prostheses that have proved successful, the author is indebted to George B. Robinson, of the Robin-Aids Manufacturing Company, Vallejo, Calif. The drawings accompanying this article are the work of George Rybczynski, free-lance artist of Washington, D.C.

REFERENCES

1. Alldredge RH and Murphy EF: Prosthetics research and the amputation surgeon, Artificial Limbs, Sept 1954.
2. Bunnell S: Surgery of the hand, ed 3, Philadelphia, 1956, JB Lippincott Co.
3. Fletcher MJ: The upper extremity prosthetics armamentarium, Artificial Limbs, Jan 1954.
4. Fletcher MJ and Leonard F: The principles of artificial hand design, Artificial Limbs, May 1955.
5. Fletcher MJ and Wilson AB Jr: New developments in artificial arms. Chapter 10 in Klopsteg and Wilson's Human limbs and their substitutes, New York, 1954, McGraw-Hill, Inc.
6. Kirk NT: Amputations, a monograph from vol III of Lewis' Practice of surgery, Hagerstown, Md, 1944, WF Prior Co.
7. Navy Prosthetic Research Laboratory, U.S. Naval Hospital, Oakland, Calif., Cineplastic above elbow prosthesis (congenital bilateral arm amputation), Interim Progress Report [on] Research Project NM 007 084.26, 1 Nov 1954.
8. Pursley RJ: Harness patterns for upper-extremity prostheses, Artificial Limbs, Sept 1955.
9. Robin-Aids Manufacturing Co, Vallejo, Calif, Functional arm bracing and artificial arms, 1956.
10. Schottstaedt ER and Robinson GB: Functional bracing of the arm, J Bone Joint Surg 38A(3):477; 38A(4):841, 1956.
11. University of California (Los Angeles), Department of Engineering. In Aylesworth RD, editor: Manual of upper-extremity prosthetics, 1952.

81

Restoration of thumb function after partial or total amputation

James W. Strickland

Perhaps no problem has challenged the armamentarium of the hand surgeon more than restoration of function after partial or total amputation of the thumb. Numerous technical advances in reconstructive surgery of the upper extremity have resulted from ingenious efforts to design procedures that would return function to this important part. This chapter is an attempt to sort out and identify the most effective of these procedures and to indicate their application based on the experience of the author. Although most of the important contributions are referenced, specific historical documentation and detailed considerations are beyond the scope of this discussion.

RECONSTRUCTIVE CONSIDERATIONS

The functional requirements of the thumb include adequate sensation, enough length and mobility to oppose the other digits, joint stability to allow strong function without collapse, and freedom from pain.[104] Careful consideration of each of these factors is important to the surgeon when one is planning a reconstructive procedure after thumb injury.

With regard to thumb length, there is some controversy about the amount of thumb shortening that may be permitted before a significant impairment of function occurs.[30] It would appear that at least 2 cm of proximal phalanx is the minimum effective length of the thumb[146] and that amputations occurring through the distal one third of that phalanx will function quite well with no need for surgical lengthening or web space–deepening procedures.[47,138,141,169] Thumb loss at the base of the proximal phalanx or through the metacarpophalangeal (MP) joint results in a residual stump that is inadequate for many pinching and grasping functions.[143]

A restored or reconstructed thumb with minimal sensory perception is of little functional value, and every effort must be made to provide satisfactory tactile sensation and stereognosis at the time of primary thumb repair or reconstruction.* Before a patient will consistently use the thumb after an injury, the thumb must have painless skin that is resistant to normal usage and sensation that is at least protective and preferably of near-normal quality.[169] The use of magnification and better instrumentation for nerve repair has increased the quality of sensory regeneration after nerve interruption, and the use of neurovascular island pedicle techniques and other methods of transferring innervated skin has greatly improved the hand surgeon's ability to restore sensation in thumb salvage or reconstruction.

The position and mobility of the thumb are also of considerable importance. If it is not in the correct anatomic area where it can be brought into position to oppose the adjacent fingers or to grasp objects, it will not carry out any useful function.[24,119,146,165] Although motion is not necessarily required at the MP or interphalangeal joints, thumb function is dependent on carpometacarpal (CMC) joint motion for rotation away from or toward the palm.[24,67,119,146] If an immobile post must be created, it is important that it be positioned in near–full abduction-opposition so that the other mobile digits can be flexed to meet it. It is also important that the three thumb joints are sufficiently stable to provide strong resistance without collapse.

Numerous procedures for salvage and reconstruction of the badly injured thumb have been described, and an excellent historical review of many of these techniques is provided by Littler.[103,104] Unfortunately, very little attempt has been made to define the specific indication for these techniques or to consider which procedures are most applicable in certain circumstances. Factors that must be taken into consideration when one is planning a restorative effort include age, sex, occupation, hand dominance, and the specific desires of the patient. One must acknowledge that not all patients require or desire elaborate reconstructive procedures and that many will adjust to the loss of thumb length, particularly when good contralateral hand function is present. When reconstruction is desirable, however, the exact level of thumb loss is probably the most important single factor in determining the proper procedure to be selected.[6,115,143,167,169] In this chapter I discuss injury and amputation of the thumb at various levels with indications as to the procedures that would appear to best provide restoration of the functional requirements at each level.

PARTIAL AMPUTATION OF THE DISTAL PHALANX

As with distal phalangeal injuries of other digits, a wide assortment of avulsion and amputation injuries may occur in the thumb. Reparative considerations in this area include the need for good, painless skin and subcutaneous tissue with satisfactory sensory perception. Procedures for accomplishing these goals vary depending on the amount and depth of tissue loss.

Guillotine amputation of thumb tip

Small transverse loss of skin and subcutaneous tissue from the terminal aspect of the distal phalanx may be managed by free skin grafts, lateral triangular advancement flaps,[49,93] or the V-Y advancement technique.[4] The advantages of small split-thickness skin graft on this type of lesion lie in its high

---

*References 23, 24, 67, 119, 146, 165, 169.

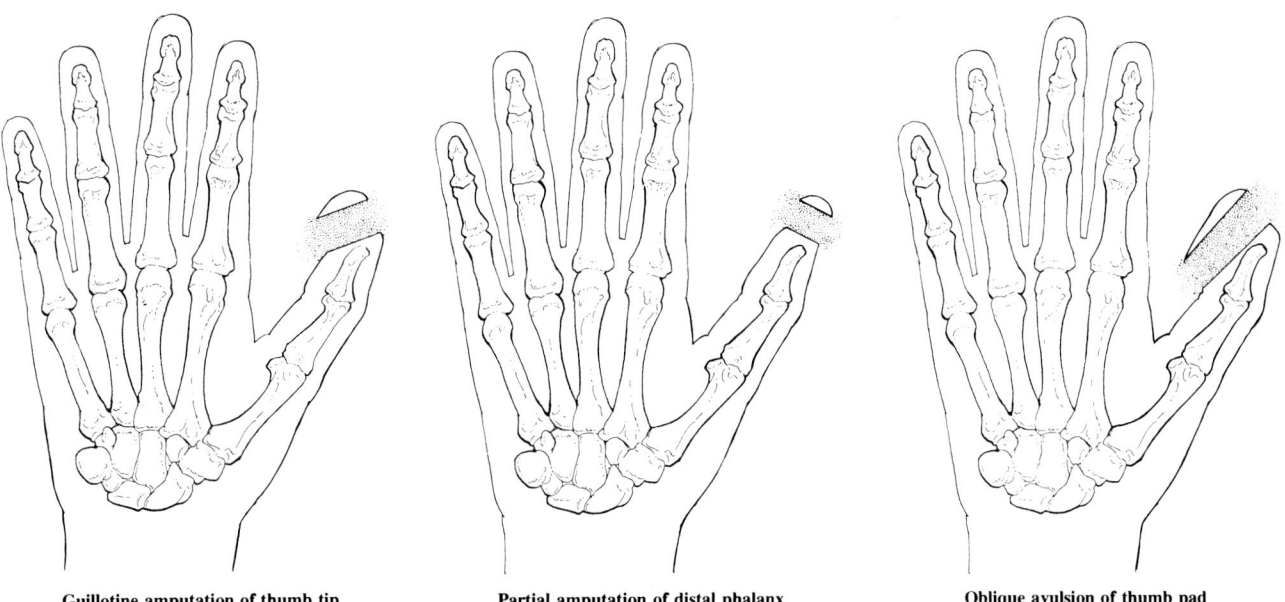

Guillotine amputation of thumb tip   Partial amputation of distal phalanx   Oblique avulsion of thumb pad

percentage of successful "take" and the ultimate contractility of the graft, which results in a minimal defect with near-normal sensation.[29,159]

Oblique avulsion of thumb pad

Larger avulsions of the thumb pad involving approximately 50% of the volar portion of the distal phalanx are well managed by the advancement of a large volar flap containing the neurovascular structures, with or without proximal skin release and grafting.[88,113,137] This technique

has the advantage of bringing well-innervated volar thumb skin distally to resurface the pad lesion and restoring near-normal sensory perception with durable skin and subcutaneous tissue.

Avulsion of entire volar pad of thumb

When the entire volar surface of the distal phalanx of the thumb has been avulsed, free grafting will provide inadequate long-term coverage, and the volar advancement technique becomes technically difficult. A cross-finger flap de-

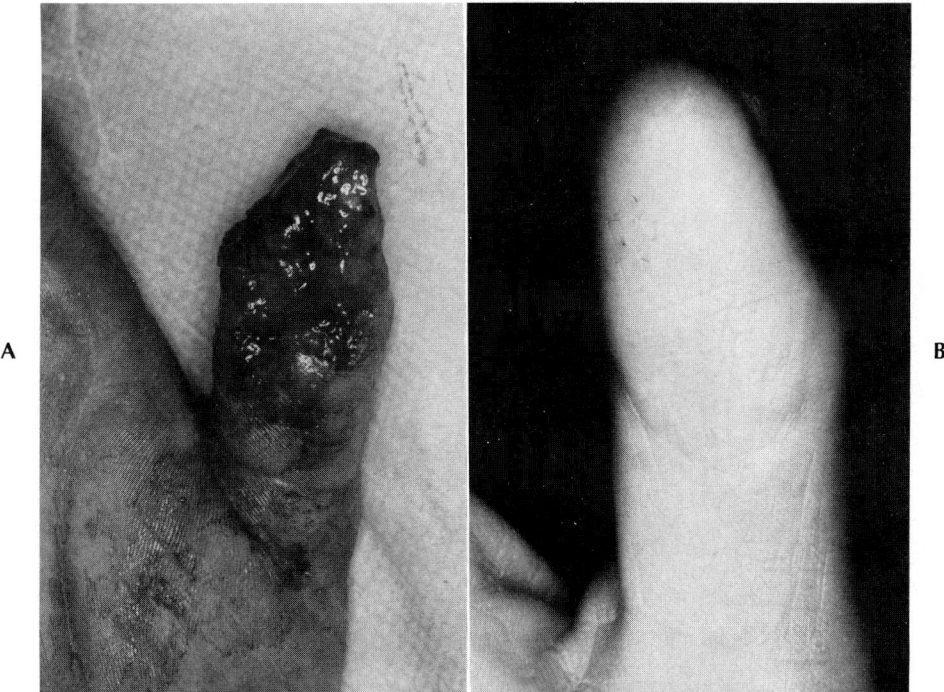

Fig. 81-1   **A,** Avulsion of entire volar pad of thumb. **B,** Thumb appearance 6 months after resurfacing with cross-finger flap from dorsum of proximal phalanx of index finger. Sensory perception is adequate.

signed from the proximal phalanx of the index finger will often provide the best coverage of this type of injury with satisfactory skin and subcutaneous tissue and the expectation of a satisfactory sensory recovery* (Fig. 81-1). The primary use of a neurovascular island pedicle flap may occasionally be indicated[161] and other more elaborate procedures, including the use of the tip of the fifth finger,[172] a one-stage advancement rotational flap combination,[84] or the use of a flag flap,[80] increase the degree of difficulty with little improvement on the reliable performance of a cross-finger pedicle flap.

---

*References 5, 37, 72, 109, 125, 136, 138, 142, 160.

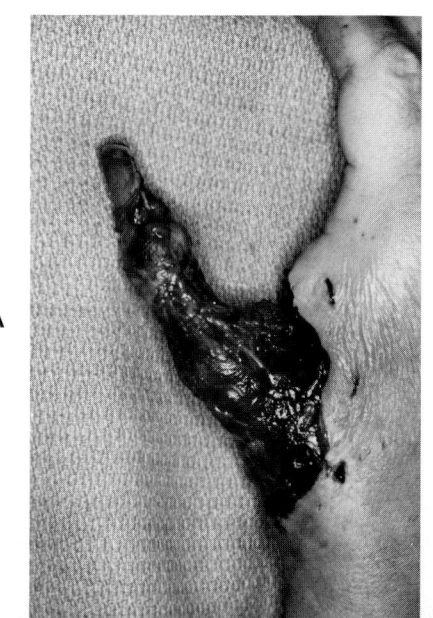

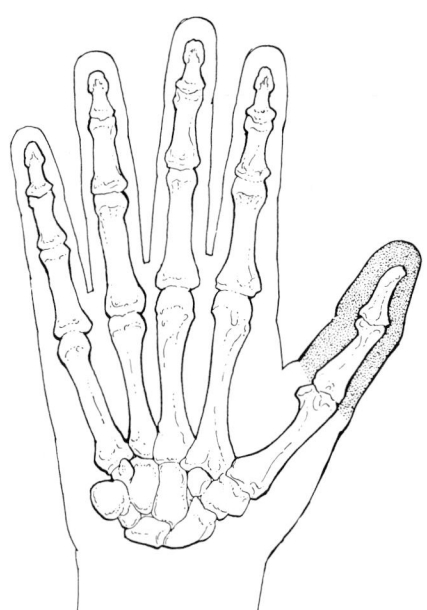

Degloving injury of thumb

DEGLOVING INJURIES OF THE THUMB

The occasional degloving injury to the thumb with loss of all skin and subcutaneous tissue is a major reconstructive challenge. The importance of thumb function would preclude amputation in this type of injury, and because revascularization of the denuded skin is only occasionally successful using microvascular techniques, it is necessary to resurface all or part of the thumb and in most instances to provide sensory input. The use of a tubed abdominal pedicle

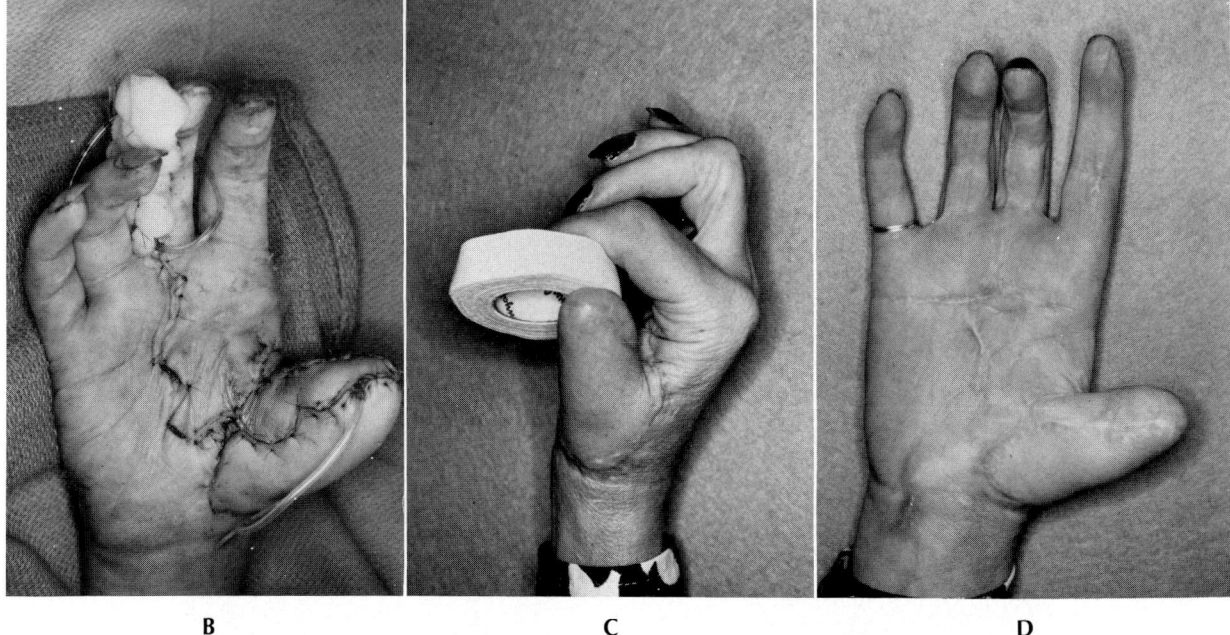

Fig. 81-2   **A,** Total deglovement of skin, subcutaneous tissue, and neurovascular bundles from thumb. **B,** Resurfacing of thumb after amputation of distal phalanx with tubed groin flap and neurovascular island pedicle taken from ulnar side of long finger. **C** and **D,** Appearance of thumb at 1 year after defatting procedure. Function and sensation were good. (Courtesy Dr. James B. Steichen.)

flap followed by the addition of a neurovascular island pedicle flap taken from the long and ring fingers appears to be the best method of restoration after deglovement.[143,146] It is usually necessary to remove the distal phalanx to achieve the correct length, and it should be emphasized that the ability to provide sensory perception to the resurfaced thumb is the critical factor in returning it to a satisfactory functional state. The neurovascular island pedicle transfer, as described by Moberg and Littler[99,100] and extended by others,[75,121,144,158,166] has become an extremely important technique in the armamentarium of the hand surgeon, particularly as an adjunct in reconstructive procedures in which no other method of sensory restoration is possible. In the

degloved thumb that has been resurfaced by an abdominal pedicle flap, the island pedicle technique has proved to be of great value (Fig. 81-2).

Avulsing thumb injuries may result in the loss of large amounts of skin and soft subcutaneous tissue without total deglovement. Resurfacing in these situations may be accomplished by the use of free grafts or, when the transfer of sensory innervated skin is necessitated, local tissue flaps based on the first web space,[109] neurovascular island pedicles, or the transfer of sensory innervated cross-finger flaps.[1,11,55] Particularly in those cases in which there has been longitudinal loss of the entire volar thumb with its neurovascular structures, the use of a large cross-finger ped-

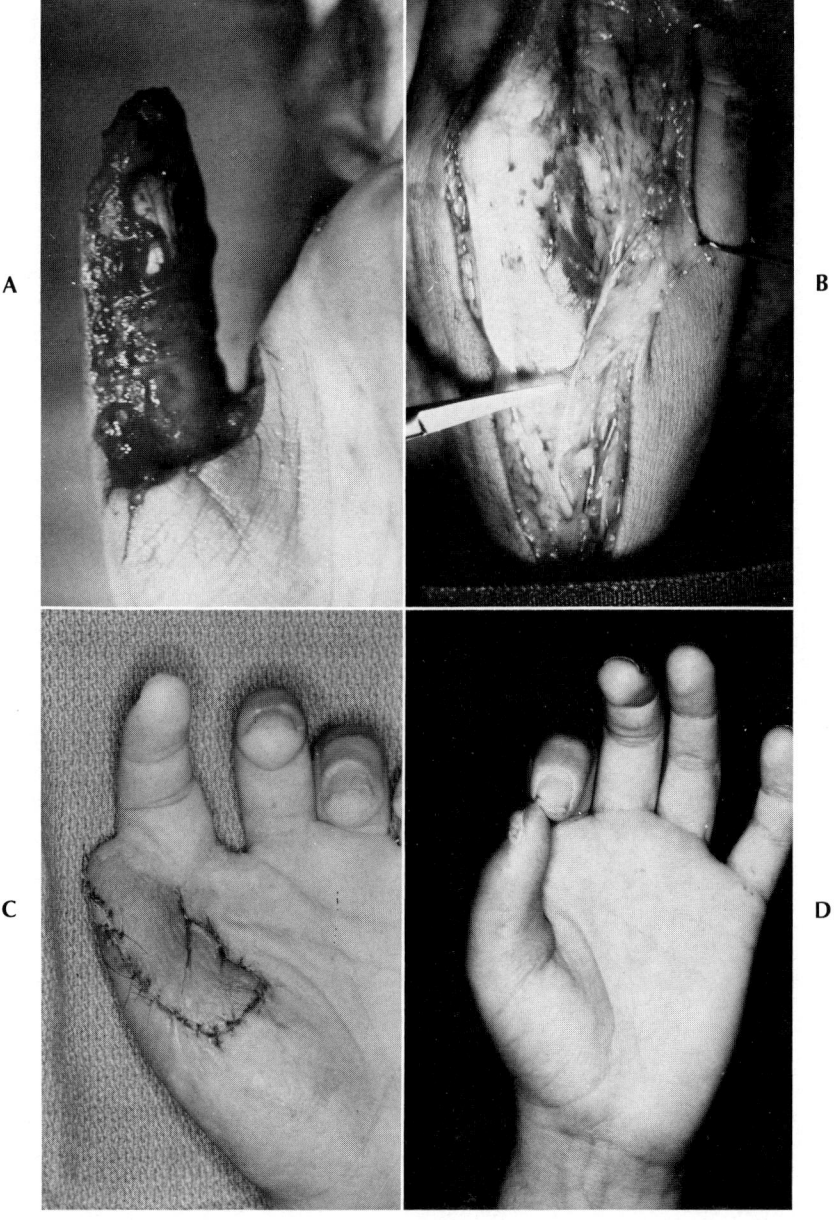

Fig. 81-3 Longitudinal avulsion of entire volar thumb. **A,** Avulsion of entire volar thumb caused by removal of circumferential pipe. **B,** Use of sensory innervated cross-finger flap from second metacarpal and index finger. Scissors point at nerve branch within the flap. **C,** Appearance of transferred sensory innervated cross-finger flap at the time of detachment (3 weeks). **D,** Satisfactory resurfacing with excellent motion and sensation at 9 months.

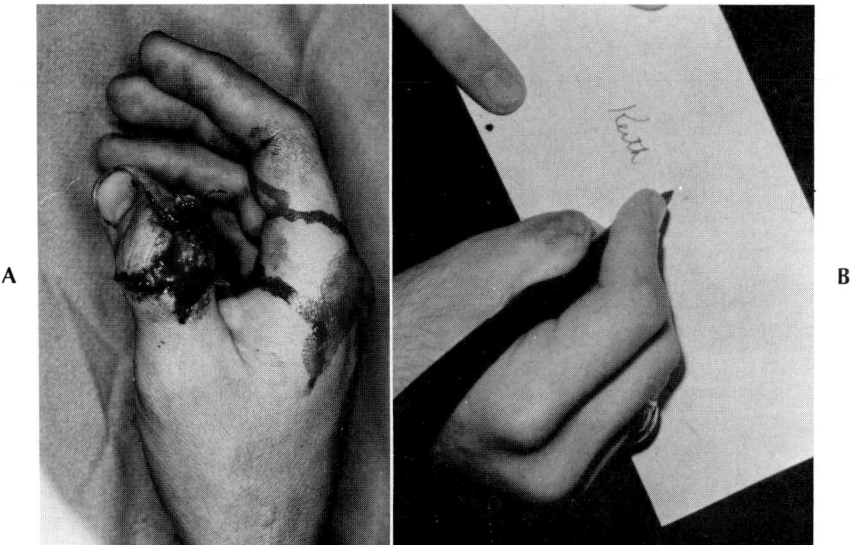

Fig. 81-4   Amputation at interphalangeal joint. **A,** Near-complete amputation through interphalangeal joint of the thumb with loss of significant dorsal skin. **B,** Appearance of thumb 4 months after dorsal resurfacing with split-thickness skin graft to prevent the necessity of further shortening.

icle flap that carries a sensory branch of the radial nerve has proved effective (Fig. 81-3). An alternative technique should be the use of a remote pedicle flap (chest, abdomen, or arm) with the addition of a neurovascular island pedicle flap.

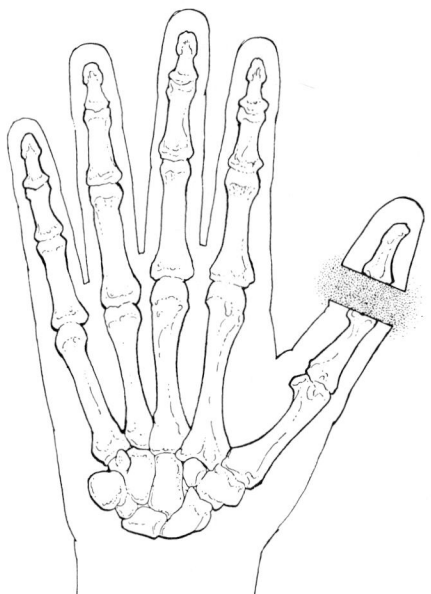

Amputation near interphalangeal joint

AMPUTATION NEAR THE INTERPHALANGEAL JOINT

It has already been shown that amputation distal to, through, or just proximal to the interphalangeal joint is consistent with satisfactory length for nearly all thumb functions. The requirements after amputation at this level are that the resulting stump be left pain free with good sensation.

The best procedure to achieve that goal is primary amputation closure with minimal additional shortening. It is important that that closure be carried out with good amputation principles, including the careful identification and proximal resection of the digital nerves.[35,46,74,111] On occasion, the use of a small dorsal skin graft will be necessary when the obliquity of the amputation has resulted in sufficient dorsal skin loss that bone shortening would be necessary for amputation closure using local skin (Fig. 81-4).

REPLANTATION OF THE AMPUTATED THUMB

The rationale for attempting replantation after thumb amputation is undeniable. A successful replant with the re-

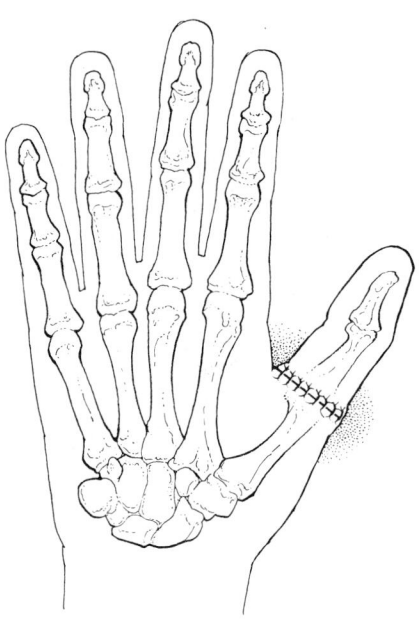

Replantation of amputated thumb

covery of at least protective sensation will prove more functionally satisfactory than any other type of thumb-reconstructive technique, even with some shortening and the loss of motion at both the MP and interphalangeal joints. It is therefore important that the possibility of thumb replantation be recognized in emergency care facilities so that transfer of patient and part to a microvascular replantation center can be facilitated as quickly as possible.

The requirements for replantation of an amputated thumb include sharp severance with minimal avulsion or crushing in a patient in the proper age group. It is important that the part be cooled and that transfer to a microvascular center be carried out within a few hours. The replantation team will proceed with the sequential repair of the phalangeal bone, flexor pollicis longus, extensor pollicis longus, digital nerves, at least one digital artery, several digital veins, and the skin. Extended hospitalization with careful observation of the replanted thumb and anticoagulation are often necessary, but the long-term functional result after successful replantation will justify this additional effort (Fig. 81-5). Numerous reports of successful thumb replantations have

appeared,* and there can be no doubt that it is the procedure of choice for amputations proximal to the interphalangeal joint when the proper requirements are met.

AMPUTATION THROUGH THE MIDPROXIMAL PHALANX

When unsalvageable amputations occur at the midproximal phalangeal level, satisfactory thumb function can usually be achieved by procedures designed to deepen the first web space and create an adequate thumb index cleft. These procedures have been called "phalangization" and use methods that deepen the interdigital cleft so that the first metacarpal and remaining proximal phalanx are relatively lengthened. This may be achieved by a simple Z-plasty,[23,50] by a four-flap Z-plasty technique,[177] by free skin grafts, by dorsal rotational flap techniques,[14,100,131,152,155] or by the use of remote pedicle flaps. The indications for these techniques vary according to the amount of thumb web contracture, the

---

*References 16, 79, 91, 92, 154, 174.

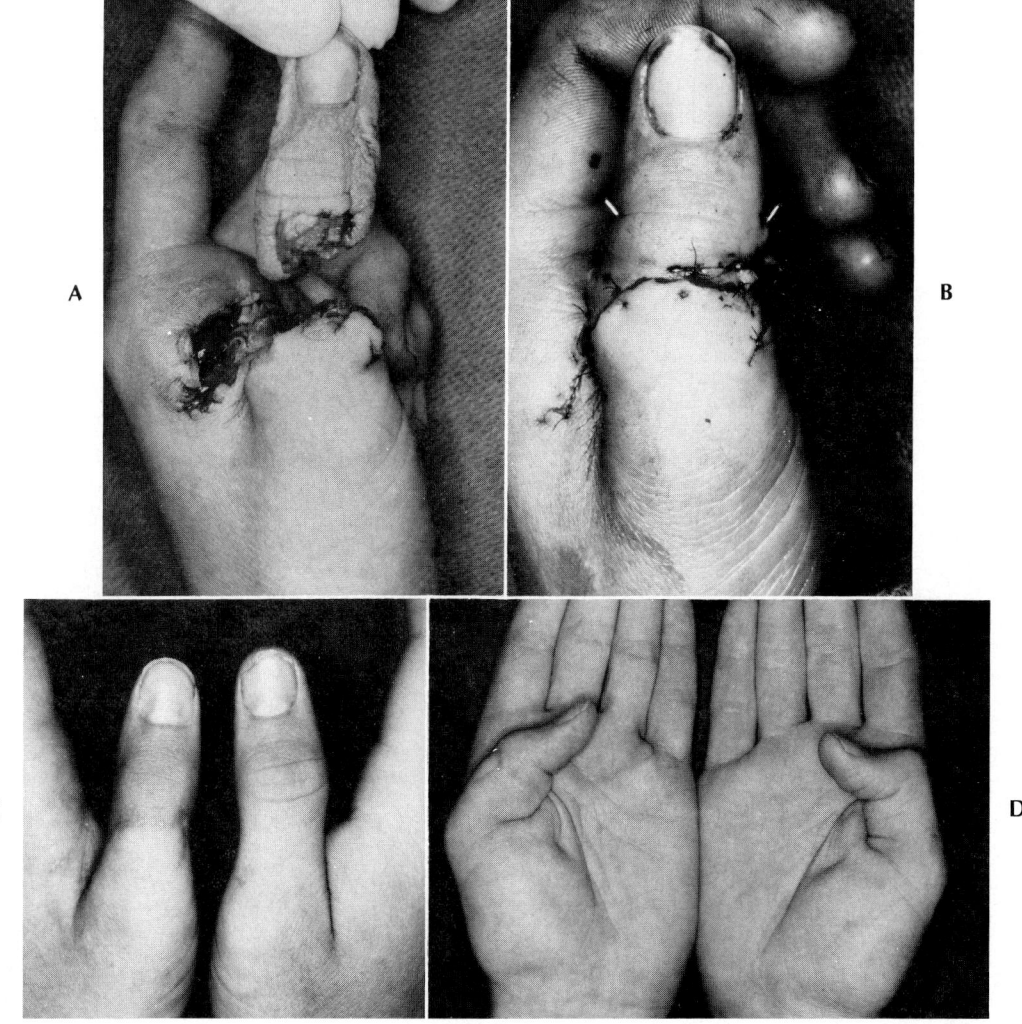

Fig. 81-5   Replantation of amputated thumb. **A,** Complete amputation through proximal phalanx. **B,** After replantation. **C,** Appearance of thumb, *left,* at 6 months. **D,** Thumb at 6 months demonstrating satisfactory flexion. Sensation and strength were good.

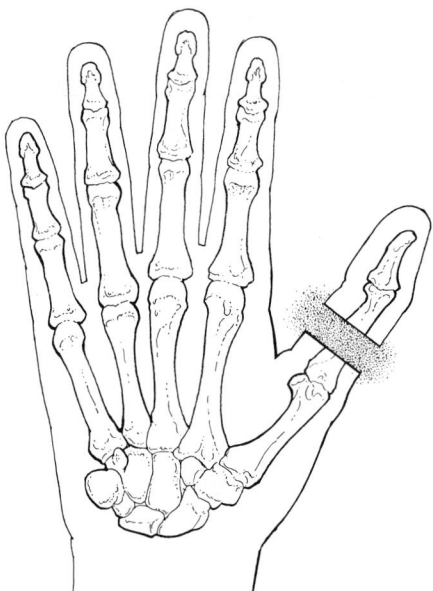

Amputation through midproximal phalanx

loss through the proximal phalanx will also result in considerable adjacent tissue injury with a poorly surfaced thumb remnant and a tight contracture of the first web space. In these instances a rotational flap technique has been effective in providing deepening, mobilization, and partial resurfacing of the metacarpal-phalanx unit. This phalangization technique employs sequential division of all restraining skin, muscles, scar, and capsular adhesions and can result in a very satisfactorily functioning thumb unit[14,100,131,155] (Fig. 81-7).

mobility of the first metacarpal, and the condition of the web-space skin and muscle.*

The simple or four-flap Z-plasty techniques are adequate to achieve web-space deepening when the first metacarpal is mobile and there is no muscle contracture[23,50,177] (Fig. 81-6). Occasionally the injury that has resulted in thumb

*References 3, 13, 14, 50, 60, 73, 77, 97, 98, 105, 114, 123, 152.

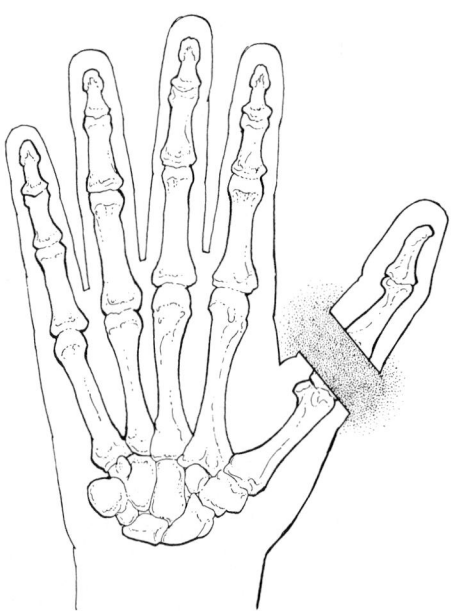

Amputation near metacarpophalangeal joint

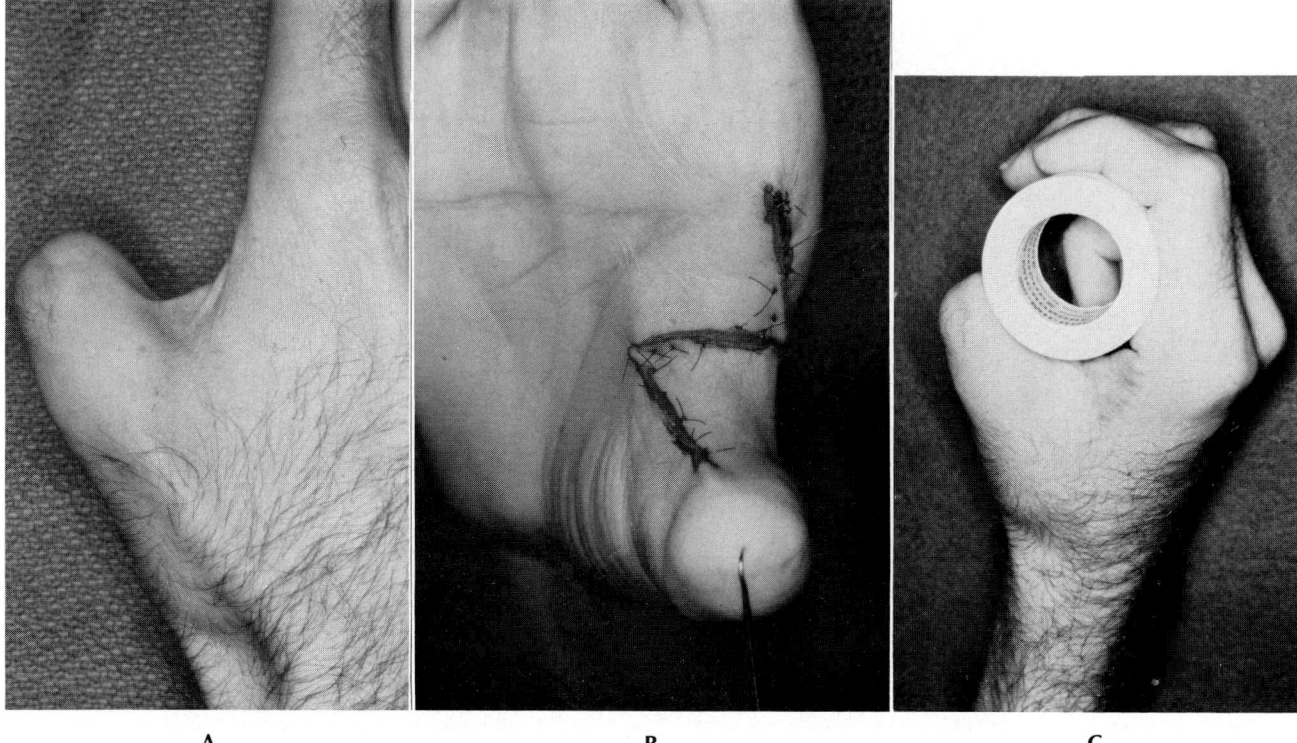

| A | B | C |

Fig. 81-6 Z-plasty deepening of first web space. **A,** Limited thumb-index cleft after amputation through the distal proximal phalanx. **B,** Thumb web deepening using simple Z-plasty. **C,** Improved grasping function at 6 months.

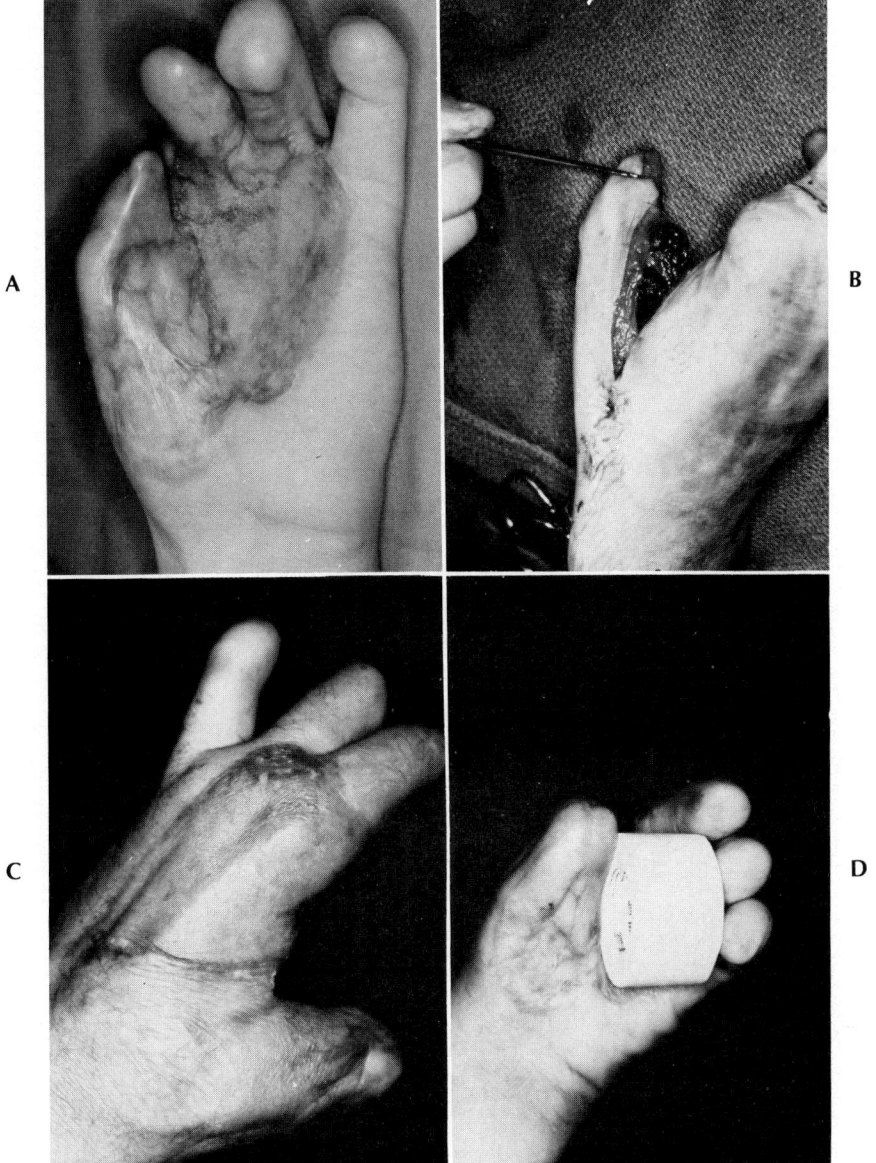

Fig. 81-7   Phalangization of badly damaged metacarpophalangeal unit. **A,** Tightly contracted metacarpal and proximal phalanx with poor skin coverage after crush burn. **B,** Mobilization of metacarpal and division of contracted web, excision of poor skin and scar, and recession of first dorsal interosseous and adductor pollicis muscles. **C,** Proved abduction of phalangized thumb at 4 months. **D,** Improved grasp and pinch at 4 months.

AMPUTATION NEAR THE METACARPOPHALANGEAL JOINT

When unsalvageable thumb amputation occurs near the MP joint, the resulting stump is inadequate to carry out many of the important functions of the thumb.[143,149] In these instances added length of 1 to 2 cm is required with the transference of satisfactory perception.

In the acute injury, autograft techniques may be used with skin and subcutaneous tissue removed from the amputated part. The remaining thumb, consisting of bone and tendon, is either replaced primarily or preserved in an abdominal pocket and reattached after several weeks or months. Reconstruction is then carried out in a manner similar to that described for the degloved thumb. Although this procedure

is not widely used, several authors have considered it worthwhile and have emphasized that when the thumb is cleanly amputated but cannot be replaced, the autograft technique can provide a very satisfactory return of thumb function.*

When the deformity created by the loss of the thumb at the MP joint level is already in existence, reconstruction may be carried out by pollicization of an adjacent injured or partially amputated digit or by the use of a "cocked-hat flap." Other alternatives include the use of osteoplastic reconstruction techniques involving the use of a bone graft covered by a tubed pedicle flap and the addition of an island

---

*References 56, 59, 70, 124, 139, 143, 144, 146, 148, 176.

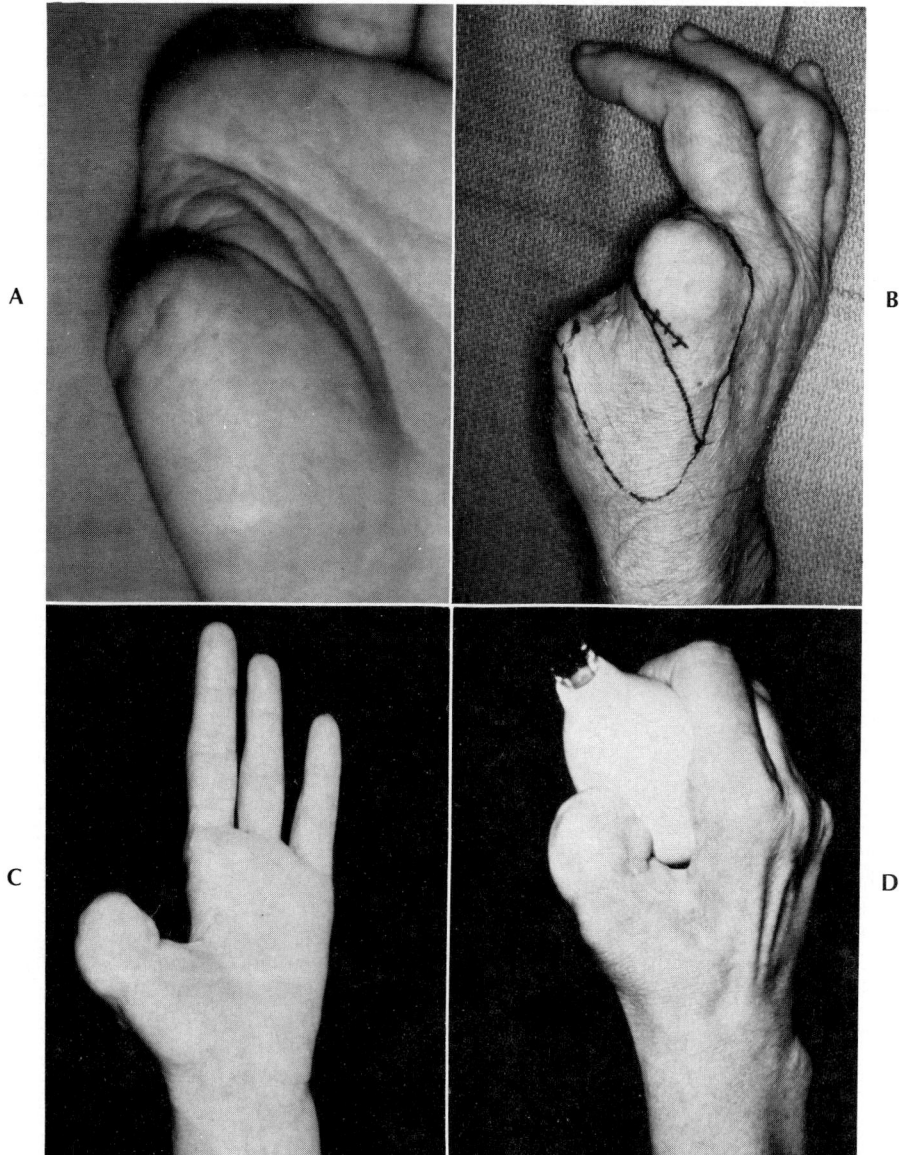

Fig. 81-8 Pollicization of second metacarpal stump. **A,** Old amputation of the thumb and index finger through the metacarpophalangeal joints. **B,** Incisions outlined for pollicization of index stump to first metacarpal. **C,** Appearance of transferred index metacarpal at 6 months. **D,** Excellent restoration of pinch and grasp after this transfer.

pedicle flap or pollicization of the middle and distal phalanges of the normal ring finger.[61,70,95,104]

Because injuries that result in the loss of the thumb quite often involve destruction of adjacent digits, it is occasionally possible to transfer part of the injured digit or metacarpal to the base of the proximal phalanx or the first metacarpal to add length and sensory perception.* Careful planning before making this composite tissue transfer is necessary so that sensation can be preserved and the vascular status of the transferred digit ensured. When the second or third metacarpal stump is transferred, the cosmetic appearance of the reconstructed thumb may be somewhat bulbous, but the functional improvement resulting from this lengthening procedure can be substantial, and the patient is usually satisfied[28,30,32,33] (Figs. 81-8 and 81-9).

The use of the "cocked-hat flap" as originally suggested by Gillies[59] is also a reconstructive possibility when the thumb amputation is at the MP joint level, and an adjacent injured digit is not available. This procedure, which involves local mobilization of skin and subcutaneous tissue from the dorsum and lateral aspects of the first metacarpal to cover a length of iliac bone graft up to 2½ cm, provides a useful increase in thumb length with at least protective sensibility.* Although some authors have found the procedure disappointing, it has proved beneficial provided that close attention to the details of the technique are carried out (Fig. 81-10).

The technique of first metacarpal lengthening that has been described by Matev[107,108] would also have application for thumb loss at the MP joint level. Continued investigation

---

*References 20, 38, 57, 62, 63, 87, 97, 98, 119, 131, 143, 149, 165.

*References 58, 79, 143, 146, 150, 167.

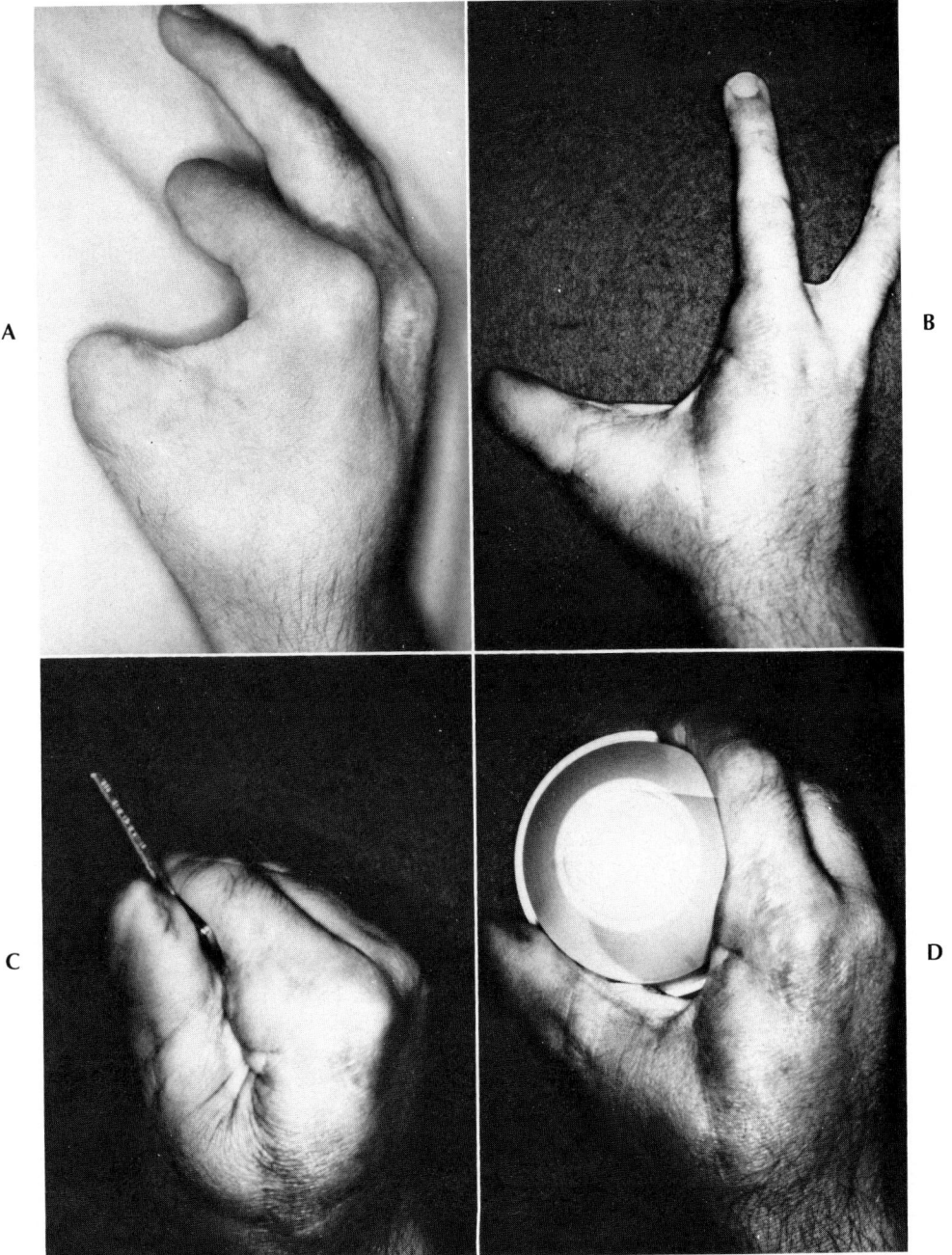

Fig. 81-9 Pollicization of middle finger remnant. **A,** Old amputation of the distal thumb, index ray, and distal two thirds of the long finger. **B,** Nine months after transfer of the proximal phalanx of the long finger. **C,** Satisfactory pinch. **D,** Satisfactory grasp.

of these lengthening techniques may prove them to be safer, more reliable, and more esthetically pleasing than either the transfer of an injured adjacent digit or the "cocked-hat" technique.

AMPUTATION THROUGH THE DISTAL ONE THIRD OF THE METACARPAL

When the thumb amputation has occurred through the distal one third of the first metacarpal, an additional 2 to 4 cm of length are necessary in order to achieve satisfactory thumb function. Again, the need for restoration of adequate sensory perception is important and pollicization of an ad-

jacent injured digit is the best procedure. In the absence of such a digit for transfer, osteoplastic thumb reconstruction using a bone graft, tubed abdominal pedicle flap, and an island pedicle flap would become the best method of restorative surgery.

As with thumb loss at a more distal level, the use of an injured digit, whether it be intact or partially amputated, to add length with sensation is an excellent procedure after amputation through the distal first metacarpal. Despite the fact that the joints or tendons of the transferred digit may not be functional, the added length and sensory perception will result in a substantial improvement in function. Joint

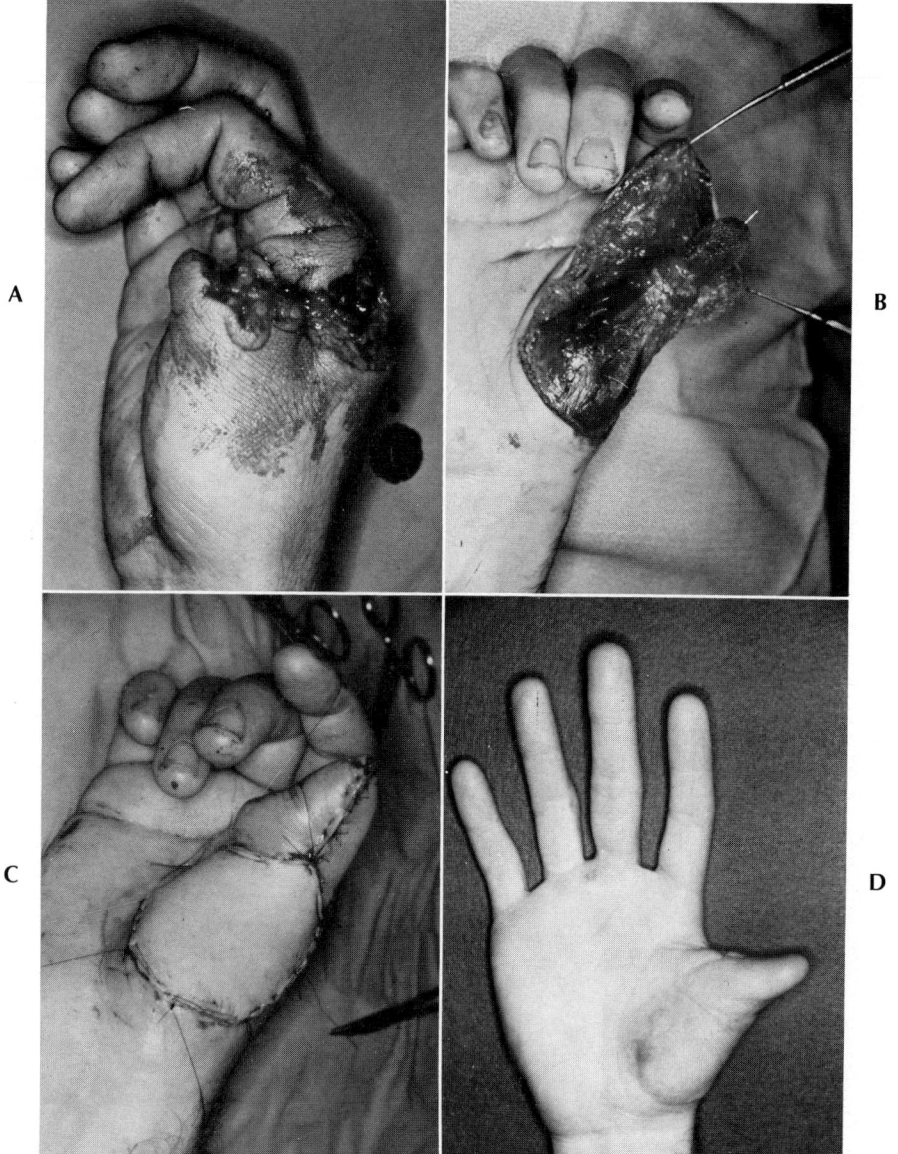

Fig. 81-10 **A,** Power-saw amputation of thumb at metacarpophalangeal joint with concomitant injury to the index finger. **B,** First metacarpal lengthening using 2 cm of iliac bone graft and local flap from the dorsal radial aspect of the first metacarpal. **C,** Appearance of lengthened metacarpal unit at conclusion of surgery with full-thickness skin graft resurfacing of the donor area. **D,** Satisfactory functional improvement at 6 months.

stabilization procedures may be indicated, and great care should be taken to ensure near-normal thenar muscle function and first metacarpal rotation. The techniques of transfer are similar to those of pollicization of a normal digit, and the same attention to preservation of the neurovascular structures is mandatory (Fig. 81-11).

With the advent of refined and predictable microneurovascular techniques, other methods of transfer of digits or metacarpals from an otherwise irreparably damaged hand to the opposite hand may occasionally be indicated. Although the clinical circumstances favoring this type of reconstruction are admittedly rare, the result may be quite satisfactory.[15,157]

Osteoplastic thumb reconstruction has been carried out

by use of various techniques since it was first attempted (but apparently aborted) by Nicoladoni[126] in 1897. Although there were many reports of successful thumb reconstruction before 1955 using bone graft and tubed pedicle flap techniques,* the results of these techniques were generally considered to be unsatisfactory because they failed to provide adequate sensory perception to the reconstructed thumb and because there was usually significant resorption of the bone graft inside the pedicle. After the suggestions of Moberg[116,118] and Littler[99,100] that neurovascular island pedicle transfer be incorporated in osteoplastic reconstruction

---

*References 2, 6, 7, 9, 40, 45, 63, 64, 106, 126, 127, 132, 133, 135, 140, 150, 162, 173.

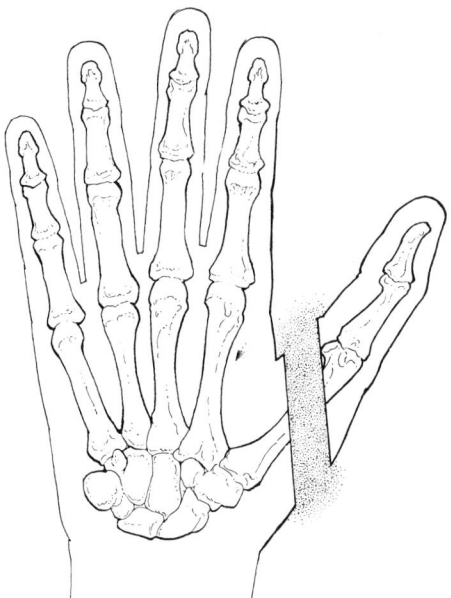

Amputation through distal one third of metacarpal

of the thumb, many surgeons have developed techniques that have proved to be considerably more successful.* Some authors continue to believe that this multiple-staged technique has questionable merit,[118,131,151] and the problem of resorption of the bone graft that compromises the long-term result of this procedure still exists (Fig. 81-12). Nevertheless, osteoplastic techniques have regained popularity as a method of thumb reconstruction at this level when the other

fingers are normal or too badly damaged to be transferred and the first metacarpal has satisfactory rotation.[103] It is interesting to note that there have been several reports of osteoplastic procedures since 1955 using neurovascular sensory transfer.[12,90]

As osteoplastic reconstruction has been modified over the years, the number of stages and the time interval required to complete the thumb reconstruction have been reduced, with most techniques now requiring two stages.[39,110,120,144] Although the tibia[7,106] or the clavicle[2,40,110] have been used as the source of bone graft, iliac bone is believed to be the best type of graft for this reconstruction. Unfortunately, no graft source seems to be free of the tendency toward gradual resorption. The tubed pedicle flap has in most instances been raised from the abdomen or groin, with some surgeons preferring a deltopectoral flap[120] or an inframammary flap.[7,40] Flaps taken concomitantly with the removal of iliac crest[12,48] or clavicle bone[110] may speed union and decrease resorption.[48] The use of a sensory innervated cross-finger flap in this type of reconstruction[1,96] has also been advocated rather than the use of a neurovascular island flap,[115] and various other ingenious procedures often using local flaps have been described.[130,148,168]

An excellent technique of osteoplastic repair consists in a reconstruction as described by Reid[1,44] and emphasized by DeOlveira.[39] It consists in adding an iliac bone graft 2 to 4 cm in length to the distal metacarpal stump, followed by the application of a thin, tubed pedicle flap usually from the upper abdomen. On occasion it may be possible to salvage intact phalangeal bone from the amputated part of sufficient length to use as a bone graft with the hope that there may be less tendency for resorption. The length of the grafted bone should not exceed the level of the normal thumb interphalangeal joint or it will be too long to function ef-

---

*References 1, 23, 29, 31, 39, 48, 72, 75, 96, 104, 110, 120, 130, 131, 144, 148, 156, 158, 166, 167, 170.

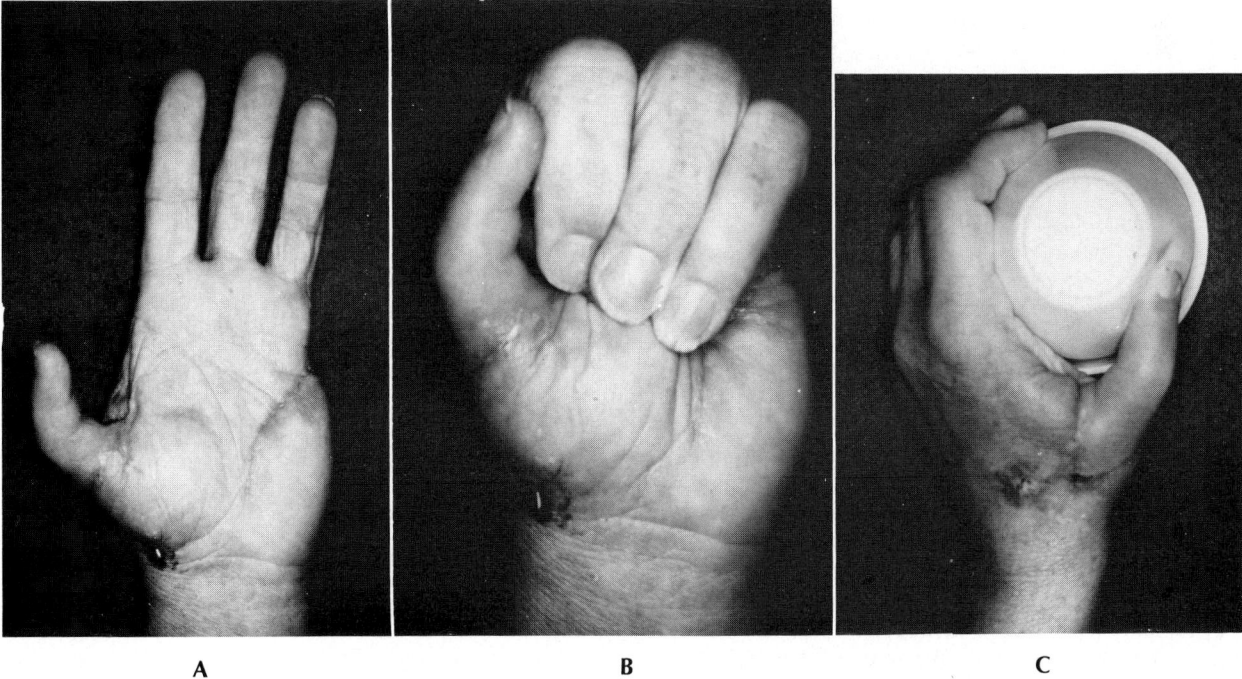

A   B   C

Fig. 81-11   Pollicization of small finger. **A,** Forty-seven-year-old woman 2 months after pollicization of poorly functional finger to the first metacarpal stump. **B,** Satisfactory pinch. **C,** Satisfactory grasp.

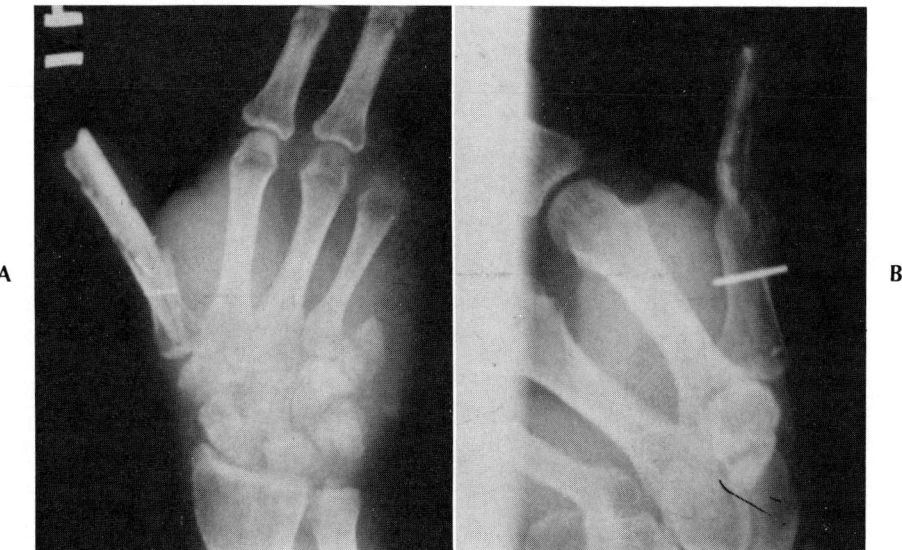

Fig. 81-12   Resorption of bone graft and remote pedicle flap. **A,** Appearance of fibular bone graft 2 months after osteoplastic reconstruction using upper-abdominal, tubed pedicle flap. **B,** Appearance of same graft at 18 months.

fectively. At 3 weeks the tubed pedicle is detached and a neurovascular island pedicle flap, usually from the ulnar side of the long finger, is immediately implanted in the desired tactile area of the bone tube extension. The extended neurovascular flap technique[75,158] is used and provides an adequate area of sensory perception for both pinch and grasp functions. In this manner there has been a rapid and effective restoration of thumb length and sensation, with the patient able to resume functional activity within 6 to 8 weeks in most instances (Fig. 81-13).

The sacrificing of a normal digit to achieve thumb function may occasionally be indicated after amputation at the distal first metacarpal level, although, when a mobile first metacarpal with satisfactory thenar muscle and basilar joint function is present, osteoplastic reconstruction would seem a more logical alternative.

AMPUTATION THROUGH THE PROXIMAL TWO THIRDS OF THE METACARPAL

When amputation of the thumb involves loss of the entire thumb and the majority of the first metacarpal, a procedure designed to provide total thumb reconstruction is required. Because the required length of the reconstructed thumb will usually be in excess of 5 cm and the mobility achieved in a short first metacarpal stump may be limited, osteoplastic reconstructive procedures are probably not indicated. Pollicization of an injured or partially amputated digit would remain as the procedure of choice, with pollicization of a normal digit, usually the index finger, as an alternative. Transfer of the great toe may be occasionally considered in those patients who are poor candidates for pollicization procedures.

The use of adjacent injured digital structures for thumb reconstruction remains applicable for amputations with a shorter first metacarpal stump. Because of the frequent loss of basilar joint rotatory motion, it is desirable for the transferred digit to have at least some motion, preferably at the MP joint, that can provide some power flexion in the thumb

position (Fig. 81-14). Even if little or no motion is present in the injured digit, careful attention to positioning can allow it to function as a satisfactory post against the remaining digits.

The pollicization of a normal finger into the thumb position before the advent of neurovascular transfer techniques was an extremely difficult and hazardous operation, requiring the mobilization of large tissue segments, with the ultimate performance of the transferred digit often being marginal by present standards.* In some instances abdominal flaps were used to fill the cleft left by the digital transfer,[41] whereas in other techniques tendons and nerves

---

*References 6, 38, 41, 81, 83, 119, 171.

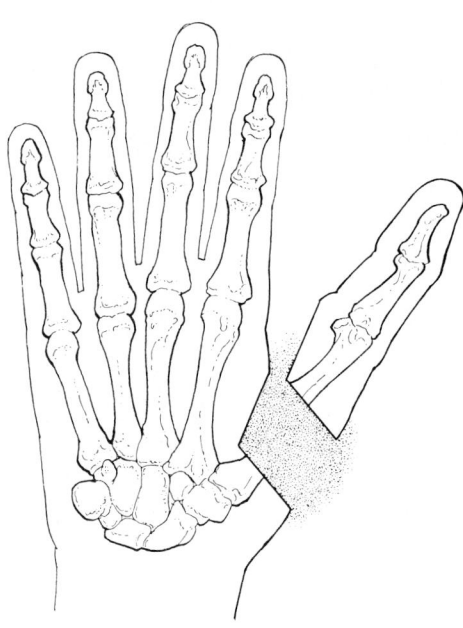

Amputation through proximal two thirds of metacarpal

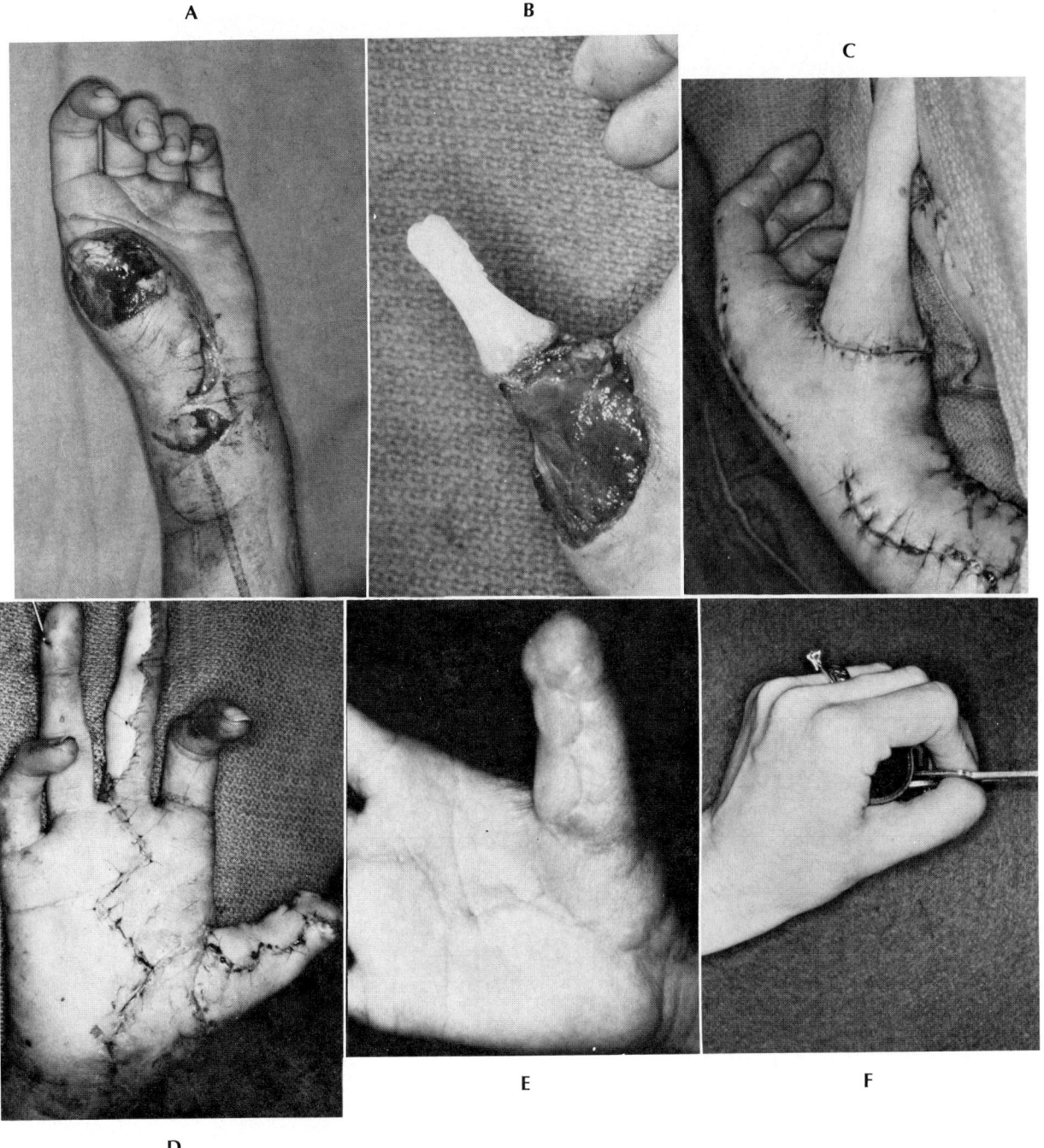

Fig. 81-13   Osteoplastic reconstruction of thumb. **A,** Traumatic amputation of thumb through the distal first meta-carpal. **B,** Bone graft using preserved proximal phalanx and amputated thumb. **C,** Application of upper-abdominal, thin, tubed pedicle flap. **D,** Transfer of neurovascular island pedicle flap from ulnar aspect of long finger at the time of the pedicle flap detachment (3 weeks). **E,** Appearance of thumb unit at 6 months. **F,** Satisfactory pinch and grasping function at 6 months.

were not joined.[171] The first true pollicization of an index finger, using neurovascular dissection and transfer techniques, was carried out in 1949 by Gossett,[61] with similar pollicization of the long finger being carried out shortly thereafter by Hilgenfeldt.[70] Since that time the procedure has been modified with technical considerations emphasized by Littler,[97-99] Harrison,[68,69] and others.* Although most authors have tended to favor the index finger as the digit to be transferred, the use of the long finger,[70,83] ring finger,[25,54,95,151,167] and even the small finger[89] have been ad-

---

*References 10, 18, 22, 25, 54, 89, 95, 111, 134, 151, 167.

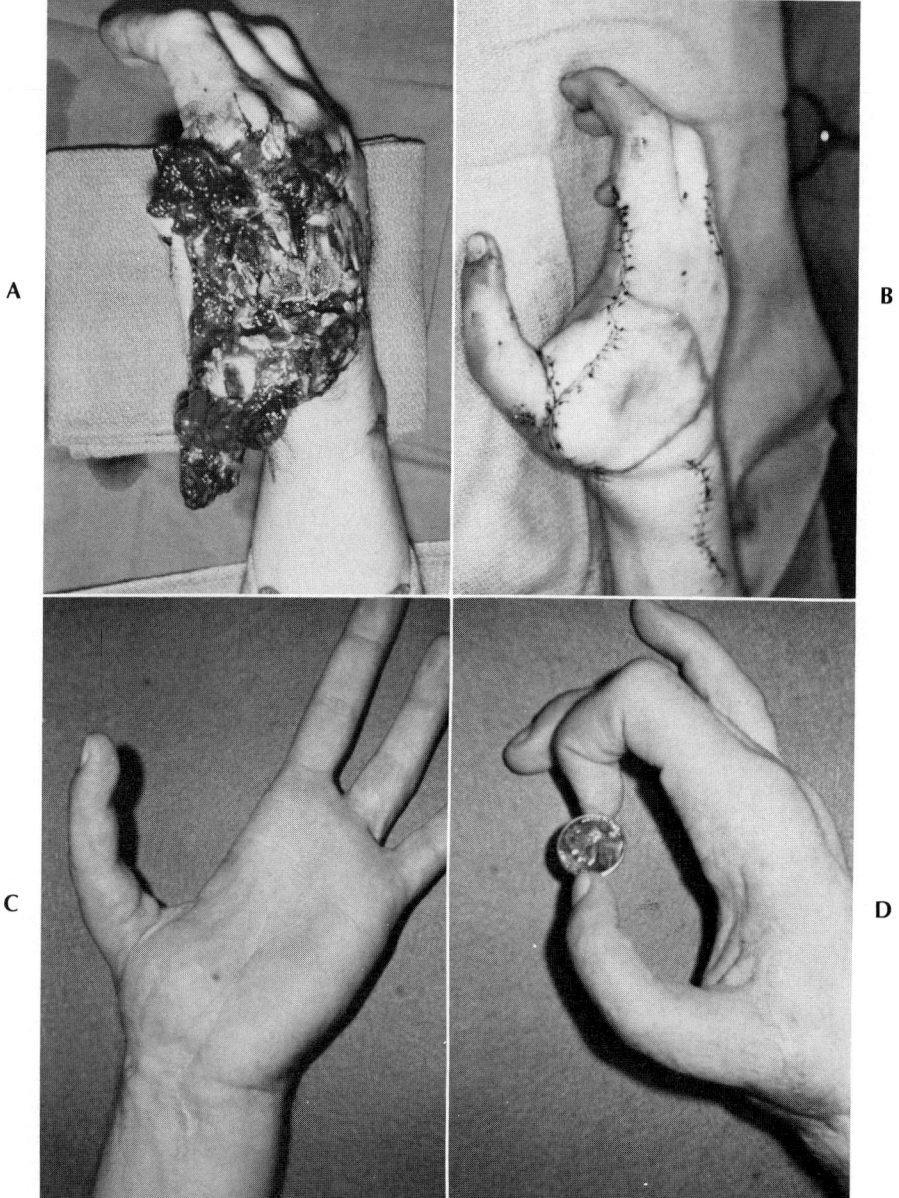

Fig. 81-14   Pollicization of injured index finger. **A,** Mutilating injury resulting in thumb amputation and destruction of the second metacarpal and extensor tendons. **B,** Appearance of hand at 2 months after abdominal pedicle resurfacing and pollicization of the damaged second metacarpal-index finger ray. **C,** Appearance of hand at 3 years. **D,** Ability to carry out fine pinch and strong grasp.

vocated by some surgeons. In recent years careful consideration of the fundamental priorities and technical considerations to restore muscle balance, proper length, and the correct rotation have been emphasized.[68,69,102-104,111] In addition, the contribution of surgeons carrying out pollicization in congenital absence of the thumb has added further modifications of the technique for use after traumatic thumb loss.[17,43,67,94,179]

The pollicization of a normal finger on the stump of the first metacarpal has the advantages of being a one-stage procedure that maintains at least some functional joint motion and has near-normal sensation and vascularization.[170]

I have been satisfied with the use of the index finger for pollicization employing the technique described by Littler[102] (Fig. 81-15).

Surgical efforts to transfer a finger from the opposite hand[85,86] or toes to replace a thumb have been occasionally carried out since Nicoladoni's first toe-to-hand transfer in 1900.[127] Before the advent of predictably successful microvascular anastomoses, the staged transfer of a toe (usually the big toe) to the hand was extremely difficult and fraught with complications. Although hand function may have been improved by this transfer, the technical difficulty, cosmetic appearance, poor sensation, and marginal performance of

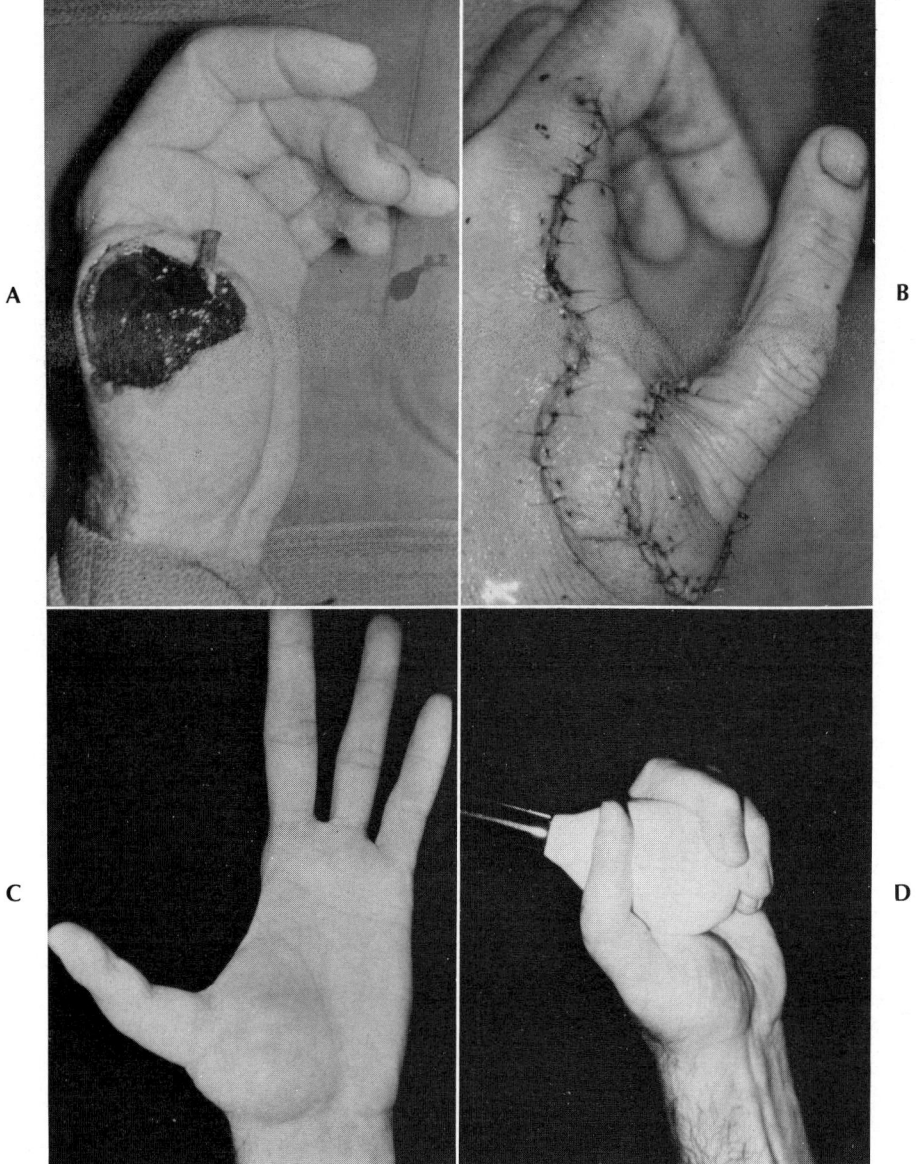

Fig. 81-15 Pollicization of normal index finger. **A,** Complete amputation of thumb through midfirst metacarpal. **B,** Pollicization of the index finger. **C,** Appearance of the pollicized index finger at 1 year. **D,** Satisfactory functioning of the pollicized index finger.

the transferred part served to prevent this method of reconstruction from becoming popular.* After the experimental work of Buncke,[18] Cobbett,[36] Buncke,[19] O'Brien,[129] and Tamai[164] have successfully described and refined procedures for the free transfer of the great toe to the thumb position with vessel, nerve, and tendon repairs.

At the present time toe-to-thumb transfer should be reserved for patients who are poor candidates for other reconstructive techniques and are of the proper mental and physical status for the prolonged procedure and subsequent rehabilitation. The procedure should only be carried out by trained microvascular teams, and the patient should be aware of and in agreement with the possibility of failure that would

compound the thumb amputation by loss of the great toe. The technique of O'Brien[129] simplifies the procedure by allowing for transfer of the great toe on the dorsalis pedis artery and dorsal veins, obviating the necessity for the difficult plantar dissection of vascular structures (Fig. 81-16). Perhaps as microvascular skills improve and more centers are established, and the repugnance for this procedure on the part of reconstructive hand surgeons diminishes, toe-to-thumb transfer will increase in popularity and take its place as an important reconstructive possibility after thumb loss.

LOSS OF THUMB AND ALL DIGITS

The occasional amputation of the thumb and all digits results in a catastrophic functional loss to the hand. The reconstructive surgeon faced with this deformity must assess

---

*References 8, 27, 31, 32, 34, 52, 59, 178.

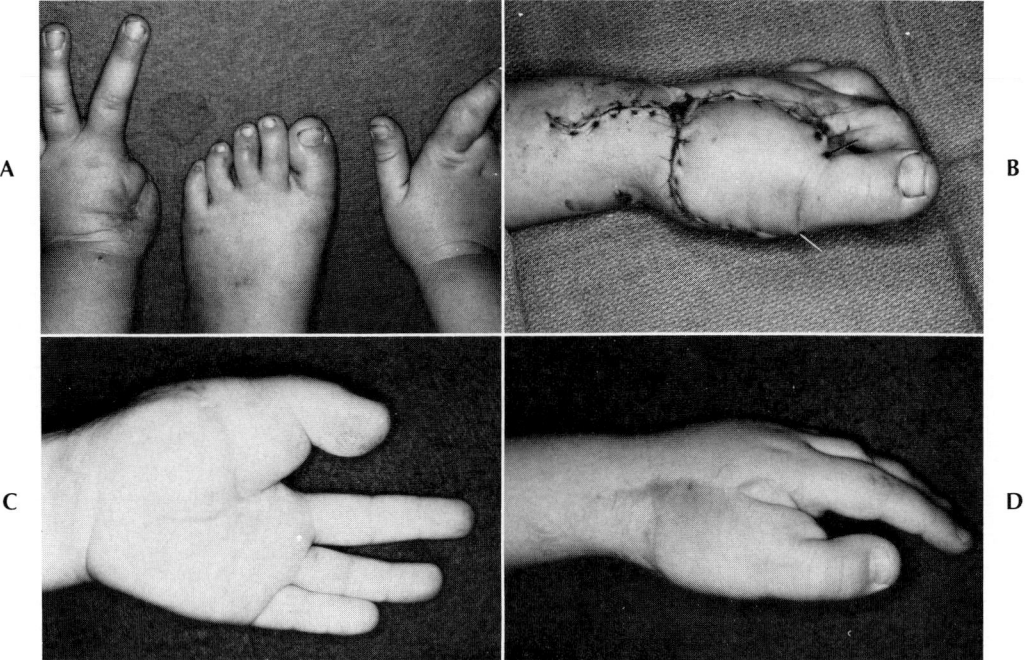

Fig. 81-16   Toe-to-thumb transfer. **A,** Loss of thumb and index finger in left hand of child, with appearance of child's left foot and badly injured right hand also shown. **B,** Immediately after transfer of left great toe to thumb position. **C,** Appearance of transferred toe at 8 months. **D,** Appearance of toe at 8 months with satisfactory pinch, grasp, strength, and sensation. (Courtesy Dr. James B. Steichen.)

the possibility of restoring two opposable rays with strong motion in at least one. Techniques that provide length by the addition of bone grafts and insensitive abdominal flaps usually provide little long-term functional improvement and should be generally condemned. When there are phalangeal remnants present, it may be possible to phalangize mobile

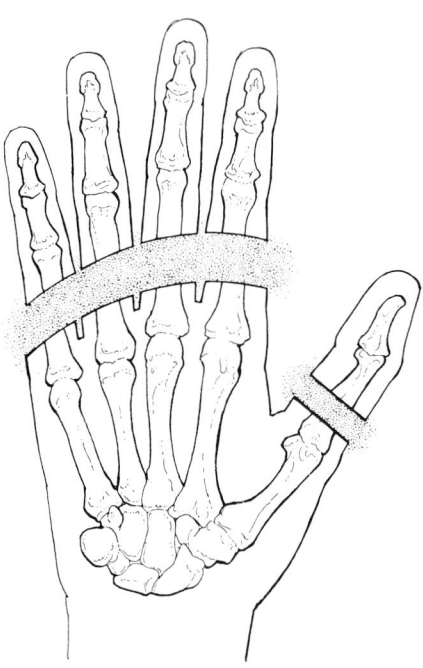

Loss of thumb and all digits

metacarpal segments with satisfactory strength and sensation to accomplish crude pinch and grasp functions.[115] These procedures have varied from phalangization of the first metacarpal,[13] to "reverse pollicization" of the second metacarpal to the first metacarpal,[44] to clefting operations between the first and third metacarpals with removal of the second or second and third metacarpals.[63] By using these or similar techniques,[23,66,112,131] one can hope to achieve a wide enough cleft for an opening and closing pincer function (Fig. 81-17).

Technical considerations for phalangization procedures include removing enough metacarpal and often distal carpal row to provide a satisfactory cleft and at the same time attempting to preserve as much adductor and abductor pollicis function as possible to ensure the mobility of the first metacarpal ray. In those patients with no phalangeal remnants or short metacarpal segments, the procedure may often prove technically impossible. Although small increments of length may occasionally be gained by interpositional or add-on grafting, usually with use of portions of the metacarpals excised to create a cleft, the results may prove disappointing if one cannot ensure a satisfactory midray space, opposable strength and motion of at least one ray, and satisfactory sensory perception on the opposing sides of the pincer.

DISCUSSION

One may note from this chapter that there are many esoteric and technically difficult procedures available for the reconstruction of thumb function after partial or total loss. Emphasis has been placed on a careful evaluation of the functional requirements necessitated at each level of thumb

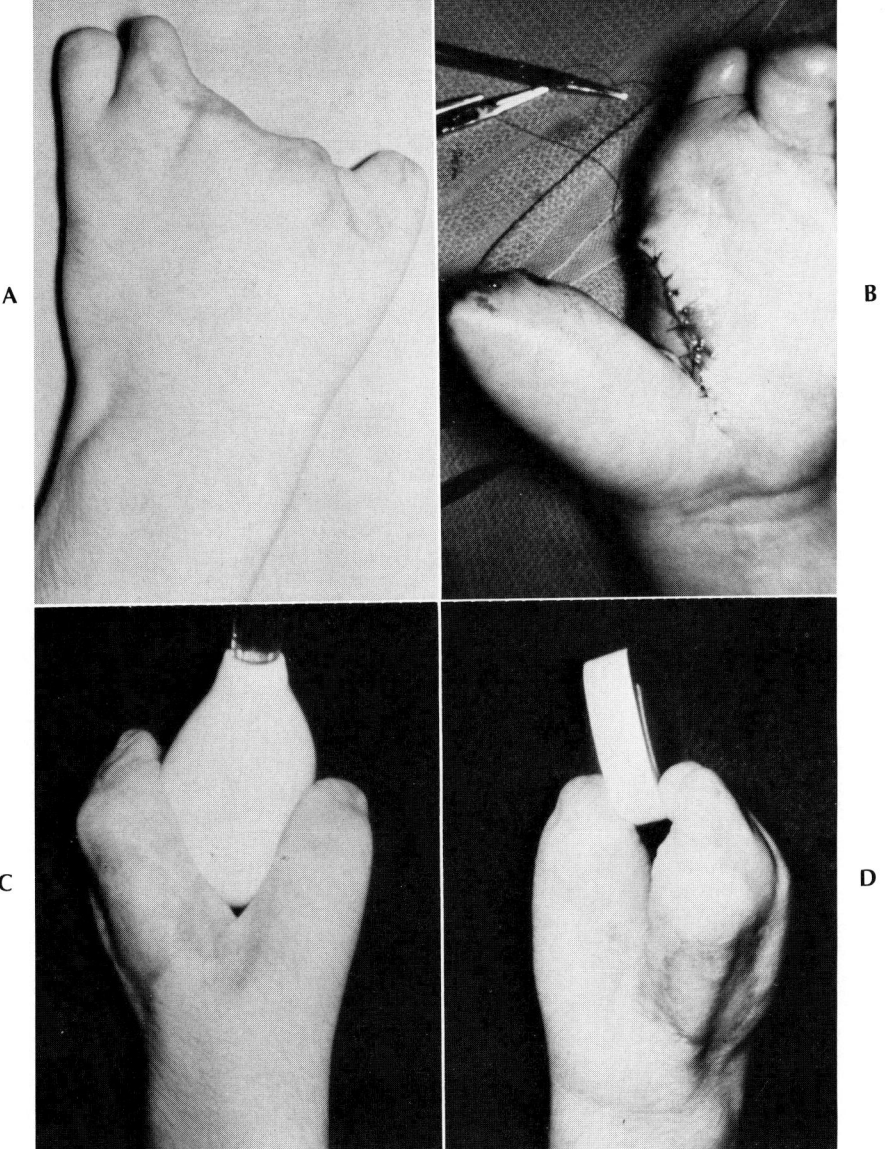

Fig. 81-17   **A,** Appearance of hand after amputation of all digits and thumb, with only short phalangeal remnants present over the first, second, and fifth metacarpals. **B,** Immediately after phalangization of the first metacarpal with midhand clefting permitted by excision of the second and majority of the third metacarpals and trapezoid. **C,** Appearance of hand at 6 months with satisfactory grasping function. **D,** Appearance of hand at 6 months demonstrating pinch.

amputation, and procedures that best meet those requirements are suggested (Fig. 81-18). A genuine consideration of the specific desires of each patient is mandatory, and it is the obligation of the reconstructive surgeon to explain in detail the realistic goals of each restorative procedure and the possible complications. A sufficient time interval after thumb amputation should elapse before any secondary reconstructive procedure is undertaken in order for the patient to adjust to the hand function necessitated by thumb loss so that he may knowledgeably participate in decisions relating to reconstruction. Finally, it should be emphasized that these procedures require not only a cooperative patient but a highly skilled hand surgeon familiar with intricate reconstructive procedures of this nature and, one would hope,

the availability of hand rehabilitation unit to aid in the restoration of thumb function after surgery. Any compromise in these basic considerations will almost inevitably lead to disappointing results.

SUMMARY

The surgeon dealing with the patient whose hand performance is severely impaired by partial or complete loss of the thumb, and in whom a reconstructive effort is indicated, must decide from a wide variety of surgical possibilities. Careful consideration must be given to the level of amputation with an understanding of the specific requirements for satisfactory rconstruction that are necessitated at each level. Proper length, position, mobility, stability, and,

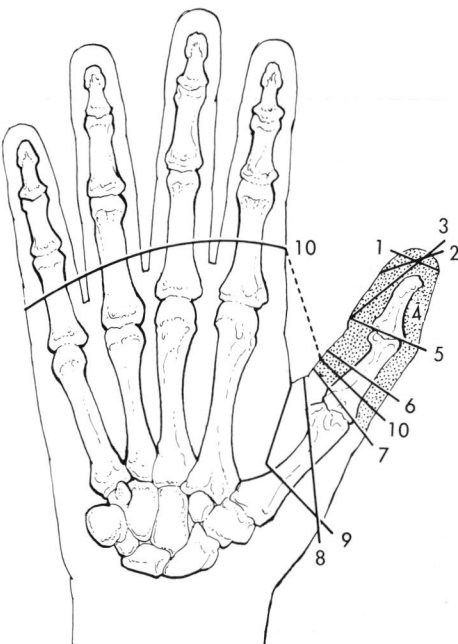

Fig. 81-18 Diagrammatic summary of best procedures for thumb loss at various levels. *Level of thumb loss: 1,* Guillotine tip; *2,* oblique avulsion; *3,* entire volar pad; *4,* deglovement; *5,* interphalangeal joint; *6,* midproximal phalanx; *7,* near metacarpophalangeal joint; *8,* distal one-third of first metacarpal; *9,* proximal two-thirds of first metacarpal; *10,* thumb and digits. *Best reconstruction procedures: 1,* Split-thickness graft; *2,* volar advancement flap; *3,* cross-finger flap; *4,* tubed flap and neurovascular island pedicle flap; *5,* primary closure; *6,* web deepening; *7* (a), pollicize adjacent injured digit, (b) "cocked-hat" flap, (c) first metacarpal lengthening; *8* (a) pollicize injured digit, (b) osteoplastic reconstruction; *9* (a) pollicize injured digit, (b) pollicize normal digit, (c) toe transfer; *10,* phalangization of first metacarpal.

above all, sensory perception must be achieved without sacrificing significant function from other areas of the hand or body. An attempt has been made to describe the best procedures for each level of thumb amputation, with the recognition that a number of other factors may play an important part in the ultimate restorative decision.

REFERENCES

1. Adamson JE: Sensory rehabilitation of the injured thumb, Plast Reconstr Surg 40:53, 1967.
2. Albee F: Synthetic transplantation of tissue to form a new finger with restoration of function of the hand, Ann Surg 69:379, 1919.
3. Arana GB: Phalangization of the first metacarpal, Surg Gynecol Obstet 40:859, 1925.
4. Atasoy E and others: Reconstruction of the amputated finger with a triangular volar flap, J Bone Joint Surg 52A:921, 1970.
5. Barclay TL: The late results of finger tip injuries, Br J Plast Surg 8:38, 1955.
6. Barsky AJ: Restoration of the thumb by transplantation, plastic repair and prosthesis, Surgery 23:227, 1948.
7. Beardsley JM and Zecchino U: Reconstruction of thumb, Am J Surg 71:825, 1946.
8. Blair VP and Byars LT: Toe to finger transplant, Ann Surg 112:287, 1940.
9. Blake HE: Notes on the reconstruction of the thumb, Br J Plast Surg 1:119, 1948-1949.
10. Bowe JJ: Thumb construction by index transposition, Plast Reconstr Surg 32:414, 1963.
11. Bralliar F and Horner RL: Sensory cross-finger pedicle graft, J Bone Joint Surg 51A:1264, 1969.
12. Broadbent TR and Woolf RM: Thumb reconstruction with contiguous skin-bone pedicle graft, Plast Reconstr Surg 26:494, 1960.
13. Brown H and others: Phalangizing the first metacarpal, Plast Reconstr Surg 45:294, 1970.
14. Brown PW: Adduction-flexion contracture of the thumb—correction with dorsal rotation flap and release of contracture, Clin Orthop 88:161, 1972.
15. Brownstein ML: Thumb reconstruction by free transplantation of a damaged index ray from the other hand—a case report, Plast Reconstr Surg 60(2):280, 1977.
16. Bruner JM: Salvage of the "all-but-amputated" thumb, Plast Reconstr Surg 14:244, 1954.
17. Buck-Gramcko D: Pollicization of the index finger: method and results in aplasia and hypoplasia of the thumb, J Bone Joint Surg 53A:1605, 1971.
18. Buncke HJ, Buncke CM, and Schulz WP: Hallux-to-hand transplantation, utilizing micro-vascular anastomoses, Br J Plast Surg 19:332, 1966.
19. Buncke HJ and others: Thumb replacement: great toe transplantation by miocrovascular anastomosis, Br J Plast Surg 26:194, 1973.
20. Bunnell S: Physiological reconstruction of a thumb after total loss, Surg Gynecol Obstet 52:248, 1931.
21. Bunnell S: Opposition of the thumb. J Bone Joint Surg 20:269, 1938.
22. Bunnell S: Digit transfer by neurovascular pedicle, J Bone Joint Surg 34A:772, 1952.
23. Bunnell S: The management of the nonfunctional hand—reconstruction vs. prosthesis, Artif Limbs 4:76, 1957. (See Chapter 80 of the present book for reprint.)
24. Bunnell S: Reconstruction of the thumb, Am J Surg 95:168, 1958.
25. Butler MB: Ring-finger pollicization (with transplantation of nail bed and matrix on a volar flap), J Bone Joint Surg 46A:1069, 1964.
26. Byane MB and Clarkson P: Traumatic amputations of the fingertips. In Flynn JE, editor: Hand surgery, Baltimore, 1966, Williams & Wilkins Co.
27. Chandler R and Clarkson P: A toe-to-thumb transplant with nerve graft, Am J Surg 95:315, 1958.
28. Chase RA: An alternative to pollicization in subtotal thumb reconstruction, Plast Reconstr Surg 44:421, 1969.
29. Chase RA and Laub DR: The hand, therapeutic strategy for acute problems, Curr Probl Surg 27:64, 1966.
30. Chase RA and others: In thumb repair, is length most crucial? Mod Med, p 75, Aug 20, 1973.
31. Clarkson P: On making thumbs, Plast Reconstr Surg 29:325, 1962.
32. Clarkson P and Furlong R: Thumb reconstruction by transfer of big toe, Br Med J 2:1332, 1949.
33. Clarkson PW: Reconstruction of hand digits by toe transfers, J Bone Joint Surg 37A:270, 1955.
34. Clarkson PW and Chandler R: On making thumbs, Plast Reconstr Surg 17:393, 1956.
35. Clifford RH: Evaluation of three methods of finger tip injuries, Arch Surg 65:464, 1956.
36. Cobbett JR: Free digital transfer (report of a case of transfer of a great toe to replace an amputated thumb), J Bone Joint Surg 51B:677, 1969.
37. Curtis RM: Cross finger pedicle flap in hand surgery, Ann Surg 145:650, 1957.
38. Cuthbert JB: Pollicization of the index finger, Br J Plast Surg 1:56, 1948.
39. DeOlveira JC: Some aspects of thumb reconstruction, Br J Plast Surg 57:85, 1970.
40. Dial DE: Reconstruction of thumb after traumatic amputation. J Bone Joint Surg 21:98, 1939.
41. Dunlap J: The use of index finger for the thumb: some interesting points in hand surgery, J Bone Joint Surg 5:99, 1923.
42. Dykes ER: Reconstruction of the thumb, Hawaii Med J 26-27:33, 1966-1968.
43. Edgerton MT, Snyder GB, and Webb WL: Surgical treatment of congenital thumb deformities (including psychological impact of correction), J Bone Joint Surg 47A:1453, 1965.
44. Elsahy NI: Reverse pollicization of thumb reconstruction, Hand 63:233, 1974.
45. Esser JFS: Island flaps, NY J Med 106:264, 1974.

46. Flatt AE: The care of minor hand injuries, St. Louis, 1963, The CV Mosby Co.
47. Flatt AE: An indication for shortening of the thumb (description of technique and brief report of five cases), J Bone Joint Surg 46A:1534-1539, 1964.
48. Finseth F, May JW, and Smith RJ: Composite groin flap with iliac-bone flap for primary thumb reconstruction, J Bone Joint Surg 58A:130, 1976.
49. Fisher RH: The Kutler method of repair of finger tip amputations, J Bone Joint Surg 49A:317, 1967.
50. Flynn JE: Adduction contracture of the thumb, N Engl J Med 254:677, 1962.
51. Flynn JE and Burden CN: Reconstruction of the thumb, Arch Surg 85:56, 1962.
52. Freeman BS: Reconstruction of thumb by toe transfer, Plast Reconstr Surg 17:393, 1956.
53. Freiberg A and Manktelow R: The Kutler repair for fingertip amputations, Plast Reconstr Surg 50:371, 1972.
54. Garcia-Velasco J: Thumb reconstruction using the ring finger, Br J Plast Surg 26:406, 1973.
55. Gaul JS: Radial-innervated cross-finger flap from index to provide sensory pulp to injured thumb, J Bone Joint Surg 51A:1257, 1969.
56. Gillies Sir H: Autograft on an amputated digit, a suggested operation, Lancet 1:1002, 1940.
57. Gillies Sir H and Cuthbert JB: Operation for pollicization of an index finger, Medical Annual, 202, Bristol, 1943, John Wright & Sons Ltd.
58. Gillies Sir H and Millard DR: The principles and art of plastic surgery, Boston, 1957, Little, Brown & Co.
59. Gillies Sir H and Reid DAC: Autograft of the amputated digit, Br J Plast Surg 7:388, 1955.
60. Gordon S: Autograft of amputated thumb, Lancet 2:823, 1944.
61. Gosset J: La pollicisation de l'index, J Chir (Paris) 65:403, 1949.
62. Graham WC: Reconstruction of the thumb, NY J Med 49:49, 1949.
63. Graham WC and others: Transposition of fingers in severe injuries of the hand, J Bone Joint Surg 29:998, 1947.
64. Greeley CPW: Reconstruction of the thumb, Ann Surg 124:60, 1946.
65. Guermonprez F: Notes sur quelques résections et restaurations due pouce, Paris, 1887, Paselin.
66. Haas SL: Operation for the loss of all fingers of both hands, Am J Surg 36:720, 1936.
67. Harrison SH: Restoration of muscle balance in pollicisation, Plast Reconstr Surg 34:236, 1964.
68. Harrison SH: Pollicisation in cases of radial club hand, Br J Plast Surg 23:192, 1970.
69. Harrison SH: Reconstruction of the thumb. Proceedings of the Second Hand Club, 1956-1957, Brentwood Essex, 1975, Westbury Press.
70. Hilgenfeldt O: Operativer Daumenersatz, Stuttgart, 1950, Ferdinand Enke Verlag.
71. Holevich J: A new method of restoring sensibility to the thumb, J Bone Joint Surg 45B:496, 1963.
72. Hoskins H and Curtis RM: Versatility of cross-finger pedicle flap, J Bone Joint Surg 41A:778, 1959.
73. Howard LD: Contracture of the thumb web, J Bone Joint Surg 32A:267, 1950.
74. Howard LD Jr: Plastic procedures in hand surgery, 1963, Manual Distributed at American Academy of Orthopaedic Surgeons, Instructional Courses Lectures.
75. Hueston J: The extended neurovascular island flap, J Bone Joint Surg 18:304, 1965.
76. Hughes NC and Moores FT: A preliminary report on the use of a local flap and peg bone graft for lengthening a short thumb, Br J Plast Surg 3:34, 1950-1951.
77. Huguier PC: Replacement due pouce par son métacarpian, par l'agrandissement du premier espace interosseux, Arch Gen Med 1:78, 1874.
78. Hydroop GL: Transfer of a metacarpal with or without its digit for improving the function of a crippled hand, J Plast Reconstr Surg 3:533, 1948.
79. Ikuta Y and others: The reattachment of severed fingers, Hiroshima J Med Sci 22:131, 1973.
80. Iselin F: The flag flap, Plast Reconstr Surg 52:374, 1973.
81. Iselin M: Reconstruction of the thumb, Surgery 2:619, 1937.
82. Jeffrey CC: A case of pollicisation of the index finger, J Bone Joint Surg 39B:129, 1957.
83. Jepson PN: Transformation of the middle finger into a thumb, Minnesota Med 8:552, 1925.
84. Joshi BB: One-stage repair for distal amputation of the thumb, Plast Reconstr Surg 45:613, 1970.
85. Joyce JL: A new operation for the substitution of a thumb, Br J Surg 5:499-504, 1917-1918.
86. Joyce JL: The results of a new operation for the substitution of a thumb, Br J Surg 16:362, 1928-1929.
87. Kaplan I: Primary pollicization of injured index finger following crush injury, Plast Reconstr Surg 37:531, 1966.
88. Keim HA and Grantham SA: Volar-flap advancement for thumb and finger-tip injuries, Clin Orthop 66:109, 1969.
89. Kelleher JC and Sullivan JG: Thumb reconstruction by fifth digit transposition, Plast Reconstr Surg 21:470, 1958.
90. Kelly AP: Subtotal reconstruction of the thumb, Arch Surg 78:582, 1959.
91. Kleinert HE, Kasdan M:, and Romero JL: Small blood vessel anastomosis for salvage of severely injured upper extremity, J Bone Joint Surg 45A:788, 1963.
92. Komatsu S and Tomai S: Successful reimplantation of a completely cut-off thumb, Plast Reconstr Surg 42:374, 1968.
93. Kutler W: A new method for finger-tip amputations, JAMA 133:29, 1947.
94. Laico J: Total reconstruction of thumb in a thumbless hand, J Phillipine Med Assoc 30:381, 1954.
95. Letac R: Pollicization of the ring finger, J Int Coll Surg 22:649, 1954.
96. Lewin ML: Sensory island flap in osteoplastic reconstruction of the thumb, Am J Surg 109:226, 1965.
97. Littler JW: Subtotal reconstruction of the thumb, Plast Reconstr Surg 10:215, 1952.
98. Littler JW: The neurovascular pedicle method of digital transposition for reconstruction of the thumb, Plast Reconstr Surg 12:303, 1953.
99. Littler JW: Neurovascular pedicle transfer of tissue in reconstructive surgery of the hand, J Bone Joint Surg 38A:917, 1956.
100. Littler JW: The prevention and correction of adduction contracture of the thumb, Clin Orthop 13:182, 1959.
101. Littler JW: Neurovascular skin island transfer in reconstructive hand surgery, Edinburgh, 1960, E & S Livingstone, Ltd.
102. Littler JW: Digital transposition. In Adams JP, editor: Current practice in orthopaedic surgery, vol 3, St. Louis, 1966, The CV Mosby Co.
103. Littler JW: On making a thumb: one hundred years of surgical effort, J Hand Surg 1:135, 1976.
104. Littler JW: Reconstruction of the thumb in traumatic loss. In Converse JM, editor: Reconstructive plastic surgery, vol 6, ed 2, Philadelphia, 1977, WB Saunders Co.
105. Lyle HM: Deformity of the hand—formation of a new thumb from the stump of the first metacarpal, Ann Surg 76:121, 1922.
106. Maltz M: Reconstruction of thumb, Am J Surg 58:429, 1942.
107. Matev IB: First metacarpal lengthening for thumb reconstruction, Ortop Travmatol Protez 6:11, 1969.
108. Matev IB: Thumb reconstruction after amputation at the metacarpophalangeal joint by bone lengthening, J Bone Joint Surg 52A:957, 1970.
109. McFarlane RM and Stromberg WB: Resurfacing of the thumb following major skin loss, J Bone Joint Surg 44A:1365, 1962.
110. McGregor I and Simonetta C: Reconstruction of the thumb by composite bone-skin flap, Br J Plast Surg 17:37, 1964.
111. Metcalf W and Whalen WP: Salvage of the injured distal phalanx—plan of care and analysis of 369 cases, Clin Orthop 13:119, 1959.
112. Michon J and Dolich BH: The metacarpal hand, Hand 6:285, 1974.
113. Millender LH, Albin RE, and Nalebuff EA: Delayed volar advancement flap for thumb tip injuries, Plast Reconstr Surg 52:635, 1973.
114. Minkow FV and Stein F: Phalangization of the thumb, J Trauma 13:648, 1973.
115. Miura T, Yoshitake K, and Nakamura R: Reconstruction of the mutilated hand, Hand 8:78, 1976.
116. Moberg E: Discussion of paper. In Brooks D, editor: Nerve grafting in orthopaedic surgery, J Bone Joint Surg 37A:305, 1955.
117. Moberg E: Aspects of sensation in reconstructive surgery of the upper limb, J Bone Joint Surg 46A:117, 1964.
118. Moberg E: Discussion. In Reid DAC: Policization—an appraisal, Hand 1:31, 1969.
119. Moores FT: The technique of pollicisation of the index finger, Br J Plast Surg 1:60, 1948-1949.

120. Morgan LR and Stein R: Method for a rapid and good thumb reconstruction, Plast Reconstr Surg 50:131, 1972.
121. Murray JF and Gavelin GE: The neuro-vascular island flap, J Bone Joint Surg 49A:1285, 1967.
122. Murray RA: The injured or abnormal thumb: recommendations for treatment, South Med J 52:845, 1959.
123. Mutz SB: Thumb web contracture, Hand 4:236:1972.
124. Nemethi CE: Reconstruction of the distal part of the thumb after traumatic amputation, J Bone Joint Surg 42A:375, 1960.
125. Nichols HM: Manual of hand injuries, ed 2, Chicago, 1960, Year Book Medical Publishers, Inc.
126. Nicoladoni C: Daumenplastik, Wien, Klin Wochenschr 10:663, 1897.
127. Nicoladoni C: Daumenplastic und organischer Ersatz der Fingerspitze (Anticheiroplastik und Daktyloplastik), Arch Klin Chir 61:606, 1900.
128. Nicoladoni C: Weitere Erfahrungen über Daumenplastik, Arch Klin Chir 69:697, 1903.
129. O'Brien B and others: Hallux-to-hand transfer, Hand 7:128, 1975.
130. Orticochea M: Reconstruction of the thumb using two flaps from the same hand, Br J Plast Surg 24:345, 1971.
131. Peacock EE Jr: Reconstruction of the thumb. In Flynn JE, editor: Hand surgery, Baltimore, 1966, The Williams & Wilkins Co.
132. Petersen N: Plastic reconstruction of the thumb, S Afr Med J 17:137, 1943.
133. Pierce GW: Reconstruction of thumb after total loss, Surg Gynecol Obstet 45:825, 1927.
134. Pohl AL, Larson DL, and Lewis SR: Thumb reconstruction in the severely burned hand, Plast Reconstr Surg 57:320, 1976.
135. Polonsky B: Reconstruction of a missing thumb, S Afr Med J 23:812, 1949.
136. Porter RW: Functional assessment of transplanted skin in volar defects of the digits, J Bone Joint Surg 50A:955, 1968.
137. Posner MA and Smith RJ: The advancement pedicle flap for thumb injuries, J Bone Joint Surg 53A:1618, 1971.
138. Pringle RG: Loss of distal thumb need not be severe disability, Injury 3:211, 1972.
139. Prpić I: Reconstruction of the thumb immediately after injury, Br J Plast Surg 17:49, 1964.
140. Rank BK: Reconstruction of opposition digits for mutilated hands, Aust NZ J Surg 17:172, 1947-1948.
141. Ratliff AHC: Amputations of the distal part of the thumb, Hand 4:190, 1972.
142. Reid DAC: Experience of a hand surgery service, Br J Plast Surg 9:11, 1956.
143. Reid DAC: Reconstruction of the thumb, J Bone Joint Surg 42B:444, 1960.
144. Reid DAC: The neurovascular island flap in thumb reconstruction, Br J Plast Surg 19:234, 1966.
145. Reid DAC: Pollicisation—an appraisal, Hand 1:27, 1969.
146. Reid DAC: Thumb injuries, Hand 2:126, 1970.
147. Riordan DC: In Milford L, editor: The hand, St. Louis, 1971, The CV Mosby Co.
148. Robinson OG Jr: Primary reconstruction of the thumb using amputated part and tube pedicle flap, South Med J 66:1025, 1973.
149. Sallis JG: Primary pollicisation of an injured middle finger, J Bone Joint Surg 45A:503, 1963.
150. Sanders GB: Reconstruction of the thumb, Am J Surg 83:347, 1952.
151. Sels M: Present methods of reconstruction of the amputated thumb, Plast Reconstr Surg 32:672, 1963.
152. Sharpe C: Tissue cover for the thumb web, Arch Surg 104:21, 1972.
153. Shaw MH and Wilson ISP: An early pollicisation, Br J Plast Surg 3:214, 1950-1951.
154. Snyder CC, Stevenson RM, and Browne EZ: Successful replantation of a totally severed thumb, Plast Reconstr Surg 50:553, 1972.
155. Spinner M: Fashioned transpositional flap for soft tissue adduction contracture of the thumb, Plast Reconstr Surg 44:345, 1969.
156. Stefani AD and Kelly AP: Reconstruction of the thumb: a one-stage procedure, Br J Plast Surg 15-16:289, 1962-1963.
157. Steichen JB and Strickland JW: Successful pollicization of thumb from irreparably damaged hand to opposite hand, Unpublished manuscript, 1977.
158. Storvik HM: The extended neurovascular island flap in thumb reconstruction, Scand J Plast Reconstr Surg 7:147, 1973.
159. Strickland JW and Dingman DL: Avulsions of the tactile finger pad: an evaluation of treatment, Am Surg 35:756, 1969.
160. Sturman MJ and Duran RJ: Late results of finger-tips injuries, J Bone Joint Surg 45A:289, 1963.
161. Sullivan JB and others: The primary application of an island pedicle-flap in thumb and index finger injuries, Plast Reconstr Surg 39:488, 1967.
162. Szlazak J: Total reconstruction of the thumb, Plast Reconstr Surg 8:67, 1951.
163. Tajima T: Treatment of open crushing type of industrial injuries of the hand and forearm: degloving, open circumferential, heat-press, and nail-bed injuries, J Trauma 14:955, 1974.
164. Tamai S and others: Hallux-to-thumb transfer with microsurgical technique: a case report in a 45 year old woman, J Hand Surg 2:152, 1977.
165. Tanzer RC and Littler JW: Reconstruction of the thumb (by transposition of an adjacent digit), Plast Reconstr Surg 3:533, 1948.
166. Tubiana R and Duparc J: Restoration of sensibility in the hand by neurovascular skin island transfer, J Bone Joint Surg 43B:474, 1961.
167. Tubiana R, Stack HG, and Hakstian RW: Restoration of prehension after severe mutilations of the hand, J Bone Joint Surg 48A:455, 1966.
168. Uzelac O: Reconstruction of the thumb: another possibility, Br J Plast Surg 23:85, 1970.
169. Verdan C: The reconstruction of the thumb, Surg Clin North Am 48:1033, 1968.
170. Verdan C and others: Transactions of the Third International Congress of Plastic Surgery, Washington, DC, 1963, p 25.
171. Verrall PJ: Three cases of reconstruction of the thumb, Br Med J 2:775, 1919.
172. Watman RN and Denkewalter FR: A repair for loss of the tactile pad of the thumb, Am J Surg 97:238, 1959.
173. Weckesser EC: Reconstruction of the distal portion of the thumb, Ohio State Med J 44:602, 1948.
174. Weiland AJ and others: Replantation of digits and hands: analysis of surgical techniques and results in 71 patients with 86 replantations, J Hand Surg 2:1, 1977.
175. White WF: Fundamanetal priorities of pollicisation, Br J Bone Joint Surg 52B:438, 1970.
176. Wilson JB: The autografting of an amputated thumb, Transactions of the Third International Congress of Plastic Surgery, Washington, DC, p 1012.
177. Woolf RM and Broadbent TR: The four-flap Z-plasty, Plast Reconstr Surg 49:48, 1972.
178. Young F: Transplantation of toes for fingers, Surgery 20:117, 1946.
179. Zancolli E: Transplantation of the index finger in congenital absence of the thumb, J Bone Joint Surg 42A:658, 1960.

82

Aesthetic hand prosthesis: its psychologic and functional potential

Jean Pillet and Evelyn J. Mackin

To lack beauty
Is not to be ugly:
Ugliness is displeasing
To the eye.

(PATIENT REFERRING TO HIS STUMP)

When the first aesthetic hand prostheses were made in the 1950s, everyone—surgeons, physicians, and therapists—viewed them as being a beautiful accomplishment but, at the same time, an extravagance that an amputee could permit himself so long as he did not actually use it. Their attitude was that, because the prosthesis was inert, insensitive, and nonfunctional, it could only be likened to a mere gadget.

Thirty five years have gone by, and more than 6000 amputees have been fitted. In the reviews of these patients, it has become clear that this prosthesis not only provides an aesthetic advantage, but in many cases increases function of the involved extremity. To more accurately reflect its dual benefits of aesthetics and function, it is now called the Pillet Passive Functional Prosthesis.

It is always difficult for surgeons and therapists to realize that certain patients need an aesthetic aid, because these professionals come into contact mainly with the recent amputee, a severely handicapped person to whom they wish to give functional help. However, the futures of such persons are hard to predict. In addition, surgeons and therapists often have no experience with agenetic patients, because such patients never have been physically injured and have not required their assistance.

ATTITUDE OF THE UNILATERAL DISTAL AMPUTEE

After amputation, the amputee experiences a major functional handicap. He believes in the miracles of surgery and the possibilities of a prosthesis. It is a period of illusions, but progressively the amputee adjusts to reality during the period of fitting, reeducation, and vocational rehabilitation. It is a period mixed with hope and frustration, during which doctors, therapists, and psychologists all have important roles to play.

Some amputees become invalids, never able to accept their amputations. They hide their stumps and refuse to use them. They wear their functional prostheses but do not make use of them, as if the mere presence of the prostheses justified their behavior. Others accept their amputations only too well—they are delighted to be helped and to be treated as children, and their attitude reflects a psychologic need.

Contrary to this small group, the majority of amputees get down to the business of leading a normal life. They reintegrate with their families and society and are able to do so because they have succeeded in making a realistic assessment of their disabilities. In conjunction with the stump the remaining hand becomes increasingly skillful, to the amazement of not only immediate family members but also the amputee himself.

Thus one may say that for certain amputees it is the unaesthetic aspect of the stump rather than the functional handicap that is the inhibiting factor and causes the amputee to blame his amputation for his failures. Such transfer of blame clearly exists, and most amputees suffer from it. No functional prosthesis is going to eliminate it. Most patients finally grow accustomed to their physical impairments, learning to disregard them and even to forget about the function that has been lost. However, even this group may feel for a long time, and perhaps forever, aesthetic frustration like that experienced by the congenital amputee.

THE UNILATERAL DISTAL CONGENITAL AMPUTEE AND HIS PROSTHETIC REQUIREMENTS
Functional needs

In the senior author's experience unilateral distal congenital amputees almost never ask spontaneously for a functional prosthesis. In the very rare exceptions encountered, it has been relatively easy to discern the influence of parents or family practitioners, both equally misinformed.

When one is treating a congenital amputee, it is common to commit a dual error by considering him as a disabled person and by wishing to fit a functional prosthesis.

That thinking is wrong concerning such a person. He is not a true amputee but rather has an imperfect development because of a congenital deformity. He has established his own perception of his body, which differs from our perception of it. He sees himself as being complete and normal. This mistaken reasoning whereby we imagine ourselves to have undergone an amputation as we try to "put ourselves in his shoes" is not exclusive to normal people. Congenitally deformed persons themselves are astonished when people with more pronounced deformities than theirs are able to carry out the same tasks as they, and even just as quickly and just as well.

To suggest fitting a functional prosthesis for a patient with unilateral agenesis, however perfect the prosthesis may be, is tantamount to encumbering a normal person with a third hand. In fact, that was the reaction of such a patient when I asked why he did not have a functional prosthesis. "Doctor," he said, "What would you want with a third hand?"

Congenital unilateral amputees are therefore disabled, but essentially in our eyes only. Whatever their ages, they manage all activities of daily living without any prostheses. For each need they use a technique that differs from ours. Naturally they have some frustration from not being able to do certain things, and this varies from one person to another. As among normal people, there are lazy and also clumsy agenetic persons, and giving them insensitive functional prostheses will not make them any more dexterous.

In the sixteenth century, Ambroise Paré reported seeing "an armless man do almost all the things any one else could do with his hands."

Aesthetic needs

Unlike the amputee, an agenetic person is not submitted to the initial emotional shock of losing a hand. Only gradually does he come to realize that he is not like other people. This discovery comes rather late, between the ages of 6 and 8 years. The realization is not spontaneous, but rather the work of those around him. As long as the child is confined to the family circle, he usually is unaware of his anomaly. This protective phase is, however, critical. Those who use their stumps very little or awkwardly are invariably found to have had abnormal upbringings, cut off from others by ill-advised parents who hid them and helped them do everything. This misapprehension condemns those unfortunate children to suffer from a dual psychologic and physical handicap.

Generally speaking, awareness of their anomaly begins when children start school and their school friends show their curiosity. They begin to fear medical checkups and gym.

Finally, the hurdle of adolescence is most important. A young person often tends to blame his malformation for all his teen-age troubles.

The congenital amputee considers himself from the outset as being normal from a functional point of view, but he suffers from being different. These patients have the same aesthetic need felt by the amputee who has had a traumatic or surgical loss.

AESTHETIC IMPORTANCE OF THE HAND

The aesthetic prosthesis fulfills a deep-rooted need of both the agenetic person and the amputee: the wish to go unnoticed and have two hands like everybody else. That is the

Table 82-1 Level of amputation of patients fitted with prostheses

Level of amputation	Percentage of patients
Arm	5
Forearm	30
Total hand	15
Metacarpal bone	20
Fingers	30

Table 82-2 Cause of amputation in patients fitted with prostheses

Level of amputation	Agenesis (%)	Trauma (%)
Arm/forearm	50	50
Total hand	45	55
Metacarpal bone	10	90
Fingers	3	97

whole problem. It demonstrates the importance of the beauty of the hand.

One must understand that for some patients the hand not only is a functional tool but also possesses expressive beauty: the appearance of the stump may seriously inhibit adaptation. For such patients the hand is the bearer of trophies; it emphasizes the beauty of gesture, the gracefulness of a movement.

The manner in which aesthetics is perceived varies from one person to another and from one ethnic group to another. In Europe, our patients, for example, are mostly of Latin origin. Very few come from Britain or Germany, and even fewer are Scandinavian. We have tried to determine whether the same pattern is encountered in the United States. The Latin and Anglo-Saxon people differ in their perceptions of the aesthetic importance of the hand. With the intermingling of ethnic groups over many generations, attitudes have become attenuated, but they have never quite disappeared. The problem is quite different in the case of amputees in the Middle East. There it seems that some request an aesthetic prosthesis to become whole once more.

The distribution of our patients fitted with prostheses according to the level of amputation is shown in Table 82-1.

The distribution of our prosthesis patients between agenesis and traumatically acquired amputations is also interesting, with the percentages being more or less equal for the arm and forearm but with a decisive preponderance of traumatic cause in the hand proper (Table 82-2).

ESSENTIAL CHARACTERISTICS OF AESTHETIC PROSTHESIS

To be of real and lasting benefit, aesthetic hand prostheses must be technically of high quality, matching well in details to the individual patient (Fig. 82-1). This is especially true for fingers, because they are viewed alongside normal fingers and thus generally require preparation of expensive molds for each person. Fingernail details are especially important; the nails must be fabricated of hard, translucent

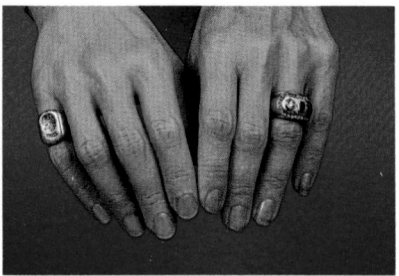

Fig. 82-1 Well-worn but fine esthetic, custom-fabricated prosthesis is compared with normal hand. Prosthesis must be of high quality to be of much benefit. (From Pillet J: Orthop Clin North Am 12:961, 1981.)

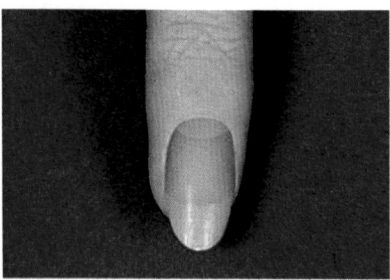

Fig. 82-2 This fingernail was carefully fashioned to match those of the corresponding normal hand and inlaid for perfection. Such fingernails can be polished, if desired, like normal fingernails. (From Pillet J: Orthop Clin North Am 12:961, 1981.)

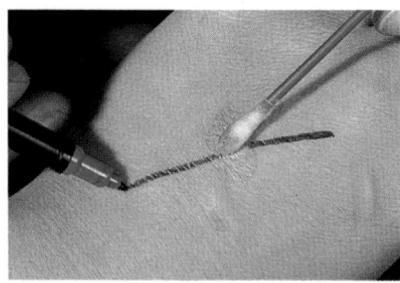

Fig. 82-3 Ink does not stain the silicone prosthesis and is readily removed with a moist applicator. (From Pillet J: Orthop Clin North Am 12:961, 1981.)

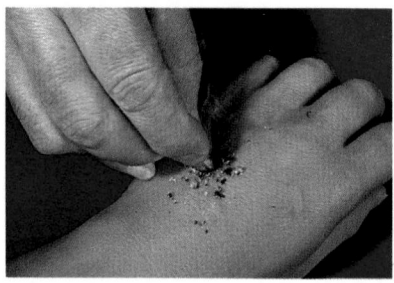

Fig. 82-4 Silicone prostheses are not subject to ordinary thermal damage. (From Pillet J: Orthop Clin North Am 12:961, 1981.)

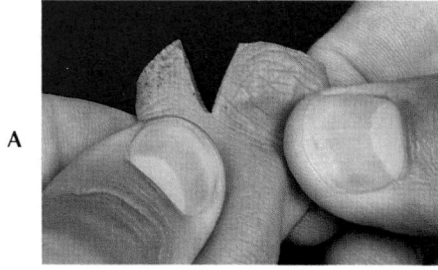
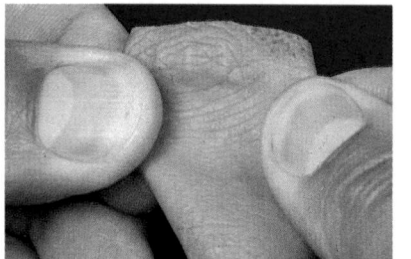

Fig. 82-5 **A,** Tear in the thin proximal end of a fine silicone finger prosthesis. **B,** Repair of the tear cannot be detected. Small tears in a silicone prosthesis can be perfectly repaired, but mutilation requires replacement. (From Pillet J: Orthop Clin North Am 12:961, 1981.)

materials, be inlaid in the prosthesis, and be able to accept lacquer without problems (Fig. 82-2). The material must accept permanent pigmentation to correspond to normal skin color but not be stained by ordinary materials such as newsprint (Fig. 82-3). It must be strong and flexible and resistant to hardening and burning (Fig. 82-4). A lack of all of these qualities has been the reason for the failure of the commonly used polyvinyl chloride prosthesis. Satisfactory material should be translucent like skin and approximate the texture and fine details of skin. The material must not be irritating or incite dermatologic reactions. It must be able to be readily repaired if damaged (Fig. 82-5).

Fixation of the prosthesis must be secure, comfortable, and simple. If the materials are supple, like reinforced silicones, and the fitting is perfect, attempts at removal create a negative pressure that must be broken, or removal is impossible even with very short sockets.

In areas of wide variations in climate, each patient should have two prostheses, one with its color adjusted to the average winter pigmentation and the other to the summer. This does not increase the total cost, because two prostheses will wear twice as long as one. Also, this plan provides a prosthesis to be worn if the other needs repairs.

FUNCTIONAL POTENTIAL OF AESTHETIC PROSTHESES

The first objective of the aesthetic prosthesis is purely psychologic. It is to restore the appearance sufficiently close to normal to eliminate to a high degree the stigma associated with the disfigurement. Often the severity of disfigurement is more in the mind of the patient than real, but this is not important, for it is in fact on the basis of the patient's interpretation that behavior will be predicated. There is little relation between the degree of actual physical loss and the psychologic weight each individual patient will give to it and the degree to which it will influence performance. The man who finds himself unable to take his hand from his pocket, even though it is very "functional," may be as handicapped as if it were lost. Thus, in a global sense of function, the aesthetic prosthesis may be beneficial even if it at times introduces some restriction of the prehensile capability of remaining parts. In allowing use of a stump that the amputee considers too repulsive to expose and use, the prosthesis may well improve overall function.

Sometimes the prosthesis may be indicated in conjunction with surgical efforts by which the part remains too grotesque for public presentation. The patient continues to amputate it mentally and keeps it constantly bandaged to preclude use. Covering the reconstructed part with a thin, flexible, high-quality prosthesis may provide the essential element to realizing the most from the reconstruction, by giving it a socially acceptable presentation.

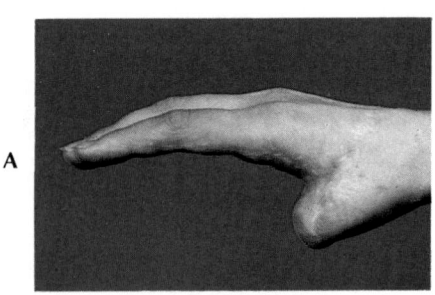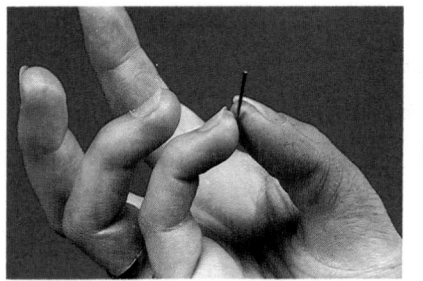

Fig. 82-6 **A,** Patient had a thumb amputation through the base of the proximal phalanx. **B,** Esthetic and functional improvement with a prosthesis. Thinness of the silicone prosthesis permits reasonably good sensibility through it. (From Pillet J: Orthop Clin North Am 12:961, 1981.)

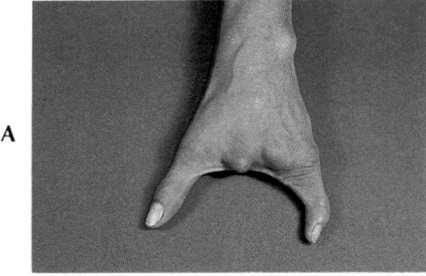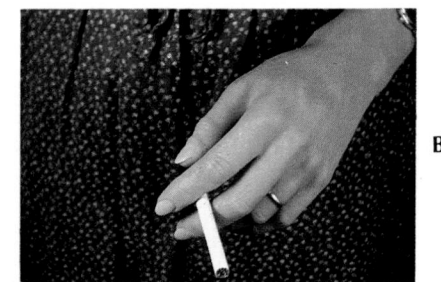

Fig. 82-7 **A,** Patient suffered from unesthetic appearance. **B,** Silicone prosthesis that is nearly identical to the normal contralateral hand resolved the problem of self-consciousness and improved function. Prosthesis is very thin over thumb to preserve both sensibility and mobility. Single finger is placed in the ring-finger position in the prosthesis for best relation to the thumb for prehension. Satisfactory prosthetics for subtotally amputated hand present the most difficult problem and challenge in prosthetic fabrication. (From Pillet J: Orthop Clin North Am 12:961, 1981.)

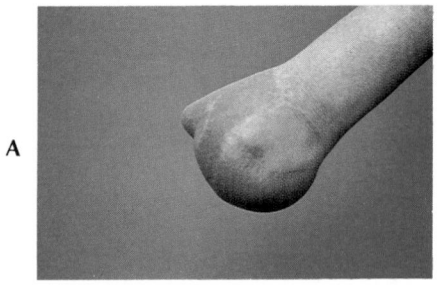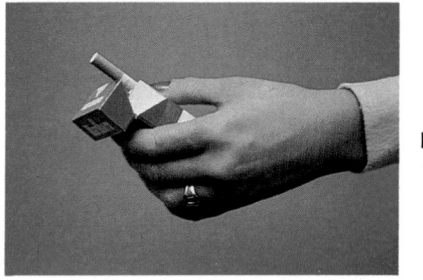

Fig. 82-8 **A,** From prosthetic point of view, transcarpal amputation is same as amputation through the wrist or lower forearm. **B,** Passive total hand prosthesis can be "loaded" to offer some useful assistance in addition to removing the social stigma of loss. (From Pillet J: Orthop Clin North Am 12:961, 1981.)

In the incompletely amputated hand the passive aesthetic prosthesis can often provide an essential physical part against which remaining parts can oppose. This part may lengthen a short thumb (Fig. 82-6), or it may be a stable thumb post against which remaining mobile digits can work. Since potential combinations are innumerable, fitting such a hand with the optimal prosthesis is most difficult and demands the greatest ingenuity but often is also the most rewarding (Fig. 82-7). Fabrication of these prostheses is made possible by the availability of tough, thin, strong, flexible new materials with which good mobility and useful skin sensibility can be preserved. Occasionally, function will be improved just by the protective effect of covering a tender stump to free the injured person from fear of using it. Often the prosthesis can be useful for holding light objects that are placed in it, even though it is totally passive (Fig. 82-8).

Obviously, both psychologic improvements and improvements in physical capacity contribute to a better rehabilitation potential for the amputee. When a professional activity involving frequent contacts with the public has been interrupted, the prosthesis often is the key to returning to the employment for which the patient is already prepared. When retraining is required, the prosthesis broadens greatly the number of vocational possibilities that one can realistically consider.

AESTHETIC PROSTHESES FOR CHILDREN

If the stump does not have a pinch mechanism, fitting of a prosthesis may be carried out at a very early age—usually between 6 and 18 months. However, there are often skin-related problems before 18 months.

If the stump has a useful pinch mechanism, the prosthesis will be functionally more bothersome than useful. In these circumstances it is preferable to postpone fitting until the child has attained adolescence, at which time he will be more motivated.

Sometimes, however, it is necessary to fit a child with a prosthesis if the parents are suffering from psychologic trauma. In such cases, it is the parents we are treating through the child. This is not a conventional approach.

AESTHETIC PROSTHESIS FOR BILATERAL AMPUTEES

Physical impairment is so great for the bilateral amputee that it overshadows the aesthetic concern, but such a concern is in fact not diminished in these patients. Benefits may be derived in the bilateral amputee by fitting one side with an aesthetic prosthesis, but the need for sensibility of a part on at least one side precludes useful bilateral fitting.

PROSTHETIC CONSIDERATIONS ACCORDING TO LEVEL OF AMPUTATION
Loss of fingernail only

The appearance of a finger cannot be good if the fingernail has been lost. Fabrication of a fingernail of good likeness is not a problem, but secure fixation to the digit remains difficult. If there is partial nail loss with a trouble-free remnant remaining, cementing to this can be satisfactory, but cementing to skin is a consistent failure. When a nail fragment exists, the prosthetic nail needs to be made to conform to it.

Commercially available nails are tedious to apply, fit imperfectly, are easily broken, and rarely have a natural appearance. Surgical fixation of fingernails, as with formation of a skin-lined pouch, is unsatisfactory, having a poor appearance with frequent cellulitis and skin complications. The only method yet available for secure fixation of a normal-looking fingernail involves covering the entire distal phalanx with a very thin prosthesis like a thimble, but the disadvantages are obvious. Secure fixation remains a problem without a good solution.

Phalangeal amputations

Satisfactory prosthetic fitting of the finger requires a minimum stump length of 1.5 cm. It should be tapered with pain-free healthy skin coverage. A smaller size than that of the corresponding normal part is desirable. Skin should not be loose and redundant. Sometimes in borderline situations sufficient length for secure fixation can be gained by surgical recession of the interdigital webs.

The proximal end of the prosthesis is feathered to a thin edge without pigmentation, making the break in skin relatively inconspicuous. When the juncture lies over the proximal phalanx, use of an ordinary ornamental ring perfectly disguises the juncture, except in the case of the thumb. In the latter case, if a better disguise of the juncture is desired, it is best achieved if one wears a small skin-colored Band-Aid or medical tape, as if covering an ordinary minor scratch.

Prosthetic fitting of the middle or ring finger when the stump is too short for secure fixation can sometimes be achieved by suspension, with ornamental rings worn on the adjacent digit, but the arrangement is complicated and fixation is less than secure.

The firmness and flexibility of the prosthesis depend on the functional needs. If the proximal interphalangeal joints of the fingers are present, the prosthesis is made flexible at this level to allow motion. If amputation is through the proximal phalanx, the prosthesis is stiff and semicurved in opposition to the thumb, for prehension. Individual fitting of all four fingers is feasible if the stump is of adequate length for secure individual fixation; otherwise a glove is required, usually with the thumb exposed if it is in good condition, so that one of the opposing parts has good sensibility. Obviously, the number of possible physical combinations is almost as great as the needs of individual patients, all of which must be given careful consideration if the best solution is to be offered (Figs. 82-9 and 82-10).

Metacarpal amputations

Metacarpal amputations can be transverse, central, or oblique (in a direction such that the thumb, or alternatively the small finger, is preserved). In the case of transverse amputations, the prosthesis is essentially a total hand.

When only a portion of the thumb remains, it is generally covered with a total hand prosthesis that extends the length of the thumb to normal and provides it with a natural-looking fingernail. In such a case the prosthesis is made very thin in appropriate areas to allow free motion of the thumb remnant and sensibility through the cover. The fingers are made firm in a semiflexed position to serve as opposition parts for the mobile thumb.

When a normal thumb has been preserved, one has the

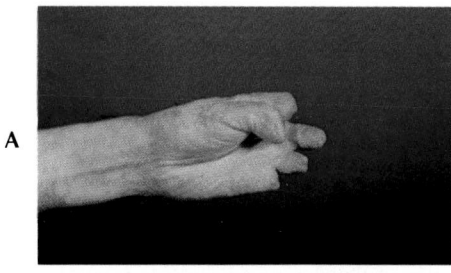 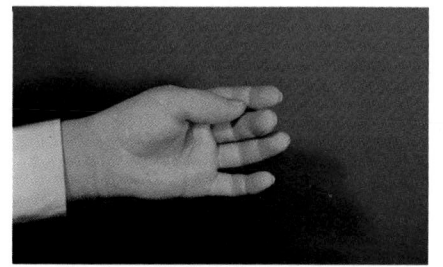

Fig. 82-9 **A,** Hand of chemical engineer severely burned in an industrial accident. **B,** Total hand prosthesis is both esthetic and functional. Prosthesis replaces missing fingers and covers hand scars. It permits opposition of the thumb to the other fingers, whereas this was difficult without prosthesis. Patient has been wearing his prosthesis daily for the past 6 years, from morning until night, both at work and at home.

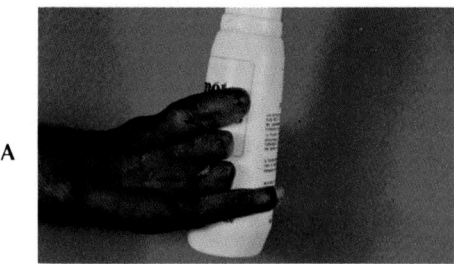 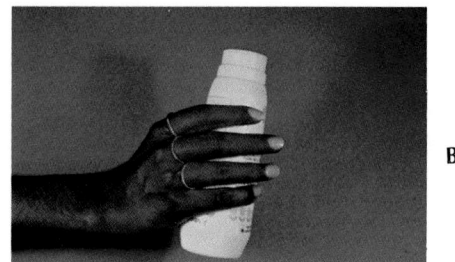

Fig. 82-10 **A,** Several digit amputations. **B,** Prostheses lengthen fingers and facilitate prehension.

option of using a complete glove prosthesis made very thin on the part covering the good thumb or allowing the thumb to protrude freely through the glove. The latter method presents the problem of disguising the opening in the glove, but for most activities it is so functionally superior that it generally is recommended.

When a useful small finger remains after an oblique metacarpal amputation in which all or most of the thumb is lost, it is best that the second metacarpal be surgically resected and the small finger fitted into the ring finger of the prosthesis. This not only is more functional, with the single finger having a better working relation to the thumb post, but also allows the prosthesis to be fabricated to the exact size of the other hand.

A prosthesis with a small finger long enough to slip over the remaining small finger must be conspicuously larger than the other hand; thus a good aesthetic result is precluded. Placing the small finger in the ring finger of the prosthesis solves this problem with no disadvantage.

When a metacarpal amputation is central, involving index, middle, and ring fingers, such as that often resulting from a punch press, both thumb and small finger are preserved. Functionally, it is best to leave both thumb and small finger protruding from the prosthesis if they are normal. This presents little problem for the small-finger juncture, since it can be naturally disguised with an ordinary ring. Also, leaving the thumb and small finger exposed avoids the problem of having to make the prosthesis appropriately thin over these parts (see Fig. 82-7).

Prosthetic fitting of partially amputated hands is a most difficult problem. The variety of physical problems encountered is enormous, and potential solutions must be care-

fully weighed against the needs of the patient, which are almost as variable. The absence of any perfect solution gives rise to a great variety of possibilities that one must carefully consider.

Amputations through the wrist or more proximal levels

Patients with amputations through the wrist or more proximal levels have strong indications for total hand prostheses, and the prosthetic problems chiefly involve the best socket arrangement. When amputation is through the carpus, the prosthesis is made thin over the palm area, so that useful sensibility can be readily transmitted.

With wrist disarticulation it is desirable that the patient be able to take advantage of the sensibility of the long stump. Only in rare instances will this degree of shortening be obvious or visually disturbing.

New materials and techniques, in contrast to the traditional fiberglass, have made possible fabrication of prosthetic sockets that are light, soft, flexible, and secure, even for shoulder disarticulations. Those for amputation distal to the shoulder usually require no straps for completely reliable fixation. These improvements in sockets represent a major step advancement in prosthetics (Fig. 82-11).

ACCEPTANCE AND UTILIZATION OF AESTHETIC PROSTHESES

A review of our patients revealed a high percentage of continued use of their aesthetic prostheses in general. This may in part reflect considerable selectivity in patients fitted, those without strong motivation usually being detected and rejected at the outset. All were unilateral amputees. Most

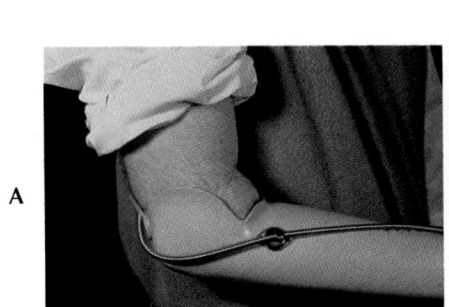
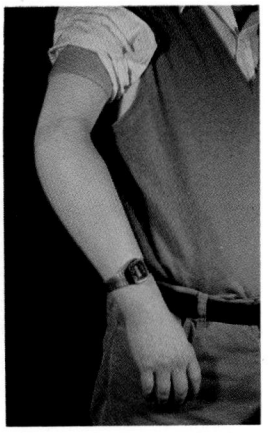

Fig. 82-11 **A,** Traditional fiberglass. **B,** New materials and techniques have made possible fabrication of prosthetic sockets, even for shoulder disarticulations, that are light, soft, flexible, and secure. These improvements in sockets represent a major step in progress with prosthetics.

of the patients were found to fall into a well-adjusted group, which in turn could be subdivided into two subgroups. Some put on their prostheses each morning and removed them only for sleep, making the devices much a part of themselves. Others treated their prostheses much as clothing, wearing them regularly when out of the home but being frequently without them within the confines of the family circle.

A small number were found to have established peculiar attitudes toward their prostheses, but all still had a need for them. A few wore their prostheses day and night, removing them only for skin care. Others kept them available but in fact wore them only rarely—for special occasions such as holiday celebrations or family events. A very small group never wore their prostheses but refused to give them up, keeping them in readiness "in case of emergency."

There seems to be little difference in use between patients with amputations and patients with agenesis. The highest satisfaction was in the age group of 15 to 40 years. The quality of the prosthesis was a major factor as one would expect, because its purpose is primarily aesthetic.

Finally, if the prosthesis is set aside, that may not imply failure of the prosthesis, but rather the excellent effects of psychologic treatment. The patient gives up his prosthesis because he has returned to a normal life. He has been cured; he no longer requires taking his medicine, and so he just stops. The prosthesis has simply helped him come through a difficult period of his life.

CONTRAINDICATIONS TO AESTHETIC PROSTHESES

An absolute contraindication to the provision of an aesthetic prosthesis is a patient without motivation or one with unrealistic expectations as to what the device is expected to accomplish.

There are also patients in whom borderline indications for fitting exist. These patients will seek an aesthetic prosthesis despite the fact that such a device may be uncomfortable, result in significant functional loss, or even achieve a poor aesthetic result. For example, with disarticulation of several digits, the prosthesis must cover the hand completely

for adequate fixation. Attempts at fixation in short stumps can result in trophic skin changes that will make the prosthesis unbearable. Even with stumps long enough for good fixation, several digital prostheses on the same hand reduce its sensibility as well as its gripping functions. When there are bulky or badly aligned stumps, aesthetically pleasing prostheses may not be constructable without prior surgical revision. It should also be noted that in bilateral amputations an aesthetic prosthesis should be provided on only one side.

THERAPISTS' ROLE IN THE PROSTHESIS PROGRAM[1]

Hand therapists often must deal with the task of dealing with the psychologic and aesthetic concerns of patients whose hands have been damaged by disease or trauma. In such cases the treating therapist can assist by telling the patient that at the appropriate time in his recovery the Pillet Passive Functional Prosthesis can help address his emotional and physical needs. The prosthesis provides an aesthetic advantage and often a functional advantage. For example, by extending a short thumb to its normal length, it can provide the patient with the ability to oppose. By extending short digits to their normal length, it will increase the working surface of the hand. Aesthetically perfect, the prosthesis may not even be detected by friends or acquaintances.

Patients are evaluated and fitted for prostheses at various geographic locations in the United States and abroad. In those areas where patients are seen at a hand rehabilitation center, a hand therapist may coordinate the program. This often involves scheduling patients, evaluating patients as to their candidacy for a prosthesis, and assisting during the stages of fabrication. This can be an interesting and gratifying experience.

PATIENT REFERRAL

Patients may be referred from a wide area and multiple sources, including physicians, therapists, rehabilitation nurses, employers, attorneys, insurance carriers, patient referral, and self-referral. The referral source should provide the necessary information about the patient's medical, surgical, or accident history. This must also include photographs (dorsal and volar views) of both the involved and uninvolved hand.

The therapist in return explains to the referral source what the prosthesis is, what function can be anticipated, the cost, and how the insurance carrier or patient should proceed in order to obtain it. A brochure is helpful in showing what the prosthesis looks like. It is important to convey the disadvantages (for example, the absence of direct sensation) as well as the advantages of the prosthesis.

FABRICATION OF PROSTHESIS

Fabrication of the prosthesis can be divided into three stages: the initial stage, the intermediate stage, and the follow-up stage. Stages may be modified to meet the requirements of individual patients.

Initial stage

Patient interview. During this stage the therapist acts as a screener by evaluating the patient to determine the patient's candidacy for a prosthesis. In addition to the examination of his hand, his psychologic, social, vocational, and avocational needs can be determined. A history based on the information obtained from the referral source, and interviewing of the patient should include the patient's age, hand dominance, occupation, and avocations.

Age. Although patients of all ages can be fitted with a prosthesis, a child's growth rate may defer the fitting of a prosthesis until adolescence, and an adolescent may not fully appreciate the care of a prosthesis. A question such as, "What do you do with your clothes at night when you go to bed?" may help ascertain whether a 14-year-old is ready for a prosthesis. If, instead of hanging her clothes on a hanger, she throws them on the floor, she is not ready. She will be told to return in 6 months to 1 year when the same question will be asked again. A prosthesis is costly to parents. It is like a special dress and requires special care.

Hand dominance. When the amputation is the result of injury or disease, the interviewer inquires as to his previous and current hand dominance. What is the patient not able to do now that he could do before the injury?

Occupation. Many patients who sustain amputations are industrial workers whose jobs require the use of two hands to operate various tools and machinery. What does the patient expect from the prosthesis? This last question is important. It is necessary to know his thinking with regard to return-to-work plans and the use of the prosthesis. Is he planning to return to the same job or to a modified job, undergo vocational rehabilitation, return to school, or seek a new occupation? A welder who has sustained amputations of the index, long, ring, and little fingers will be well aware that he will be unable to wear his prosthesis while at work. An occupational change may be necessary. However, a secretary, typist, pianist or any other person who requires finger dexterity who has lost the distal phalanx of a digit may find his functional ability enhanced with a prosthesis. Young adults unable to perform their former job tasks often explore alternative occupations. Many patients from this age group choose to return to college, and in these instances the importance of an aesthetic prosthesis cannot be overestimated!

Avocations. The patient's avocational interests need to be appreciated in the planning of a prosthesis. A prosthesis may enable the patient to participate in his hobby. In the fingertip amputee, a thimblelike prosthesis may provide the needed length to enable a violinist to play the violin again.

The interview will help determine the patient's motivation for obtaining a prosthesis and whether he has a realistic understanding of the advantages and disadvantages. It is necessary to convey that the prosthesis may impede function and reduce sensation in an area. Unrealistic expectations can never be fulfilled. They result in an unhappy patient. Successful results with the prosthesis require a well-motivated, realistic, and compliant patient. The patient who arrives for the interview with his hand concealed in his pocket many months after his injury has not accepted the appearance of his hand. This patient is sure why he wants a prosthesis. He is willing to lose a little sensation and function for improved appearance.

Assessment. Once it has been determined that the patient is realistic in his expectations of the prosthesis and appreciates its capabilities and functional limitations, his hand is examined for edema, length and shape of the stump, and hypersensitivity.

Edema. Although patients are anxious to obtain their prosthesis as soon as possible, it is necessary that edema measurements have stabilized. Circumferential measurements by means of a flexible tape measure are taken at various anatomic locations. When these measurements have stabilized, the patient is ready for fabrication of the prosthesis. Generally, this occurs 2 months or longer after amputation.

It is important that early postoperative care address edema control through elevation, retrograde massage, compression wrapping, and active and gentle assisted range-of-motion exercise, modalities, and therapeutic activities. Coban wrapping helps reduce edema and promote stump shrinkage and contour of the stump for the prosthesis. Coban is applied in a distal-to-proximal, figure-of-eight fashion without tension.

Length of stump. Satisfactory prosthetic fitting of the digit requires a minimum stump length of 1.5 cm. When the length is barely 1.5 cm, the Coban is wrapped circumferentially around the proximal and mid portions of the stump, leaving the distal end free. The distal end then becomes relatively bulbous. The result is that the short stump is better able to anchor the prosthesis.

Shape of the stump. The ideal digit stump should be cylindrical in shape. The skin should be well healed with minimal fleshiness.

Hypersensitivity. Hypersensitivity is a condition of extreme discomfort or irritability in response to normally painless tactile stimulation. Patients commonly complain of shooting pain, "electric shocks," and the extreme irritability to the touch. A painful stump cannot tolerate a prosthesis. Desensitization techniques reduce these paresthesias and help prepare the stump for the prosthesis. The use of constant pressure such as Elastomer caps secured with Coban wrapped in a figure-of-eight distal-to-proximal manner can also help diminish hypersensitivity. When no progress is made with the desensitization techniques, the surgeon might consider surgical resection of the neuroma.

Intermediate phase

The intermediate phase is the period of prosthetic fabrication. Using the patient interview and assessment information and his own consultation with the patient, Dr. Pillet makes the final determination as to whether the patient is a candidate for a prosthesis. If the patient is a candidate, he is told what type of prosthesis he will need.

Digital amputee. The fabrication process begins the same day as the consultation. For the digital amputee, measurements and imprints of the involved digits are completed. The patient will return at a later date for coloring and fitting of the prosthesis. Two visits are generally necessary.

Partial and total hand amputee. For the partial and total hand amputee the consultation with Dr. Pillet includes the selection of the appropriate-size glove. Coloring is also completed. Fitting and adjustments are completed on later visits. Three visits are generally necessary for the partial hand amputee and two for the total hand amputee.

Follow-up phase

The complete prosthesis is assessed for fit. The patient is instructed in the donning and doffing of the prosthesis, and his performance of these procedures is examined. Clear and careful instructions must be provided so that the patient does not damage or tear the prosthesis.

Written instructions explaining the importance of skin care and proper care of the prosthesis are given to the patient. Information regarding a backup prosthesis is provided; however, it is generally recommended that the patient wear the initial prosthesis for 6 months before beginning fabrication of a backup prosthesis. This allows the time for any necessary adjustments and to determine whether the patient proves to be a good prosthetic wearer.

SUMMARY

A high-quality aesthetic prosthesis with passive function can be equally helpful to an amputee and to a patient whose loss is attributable to agenesis. Restoring near-normal appearance improves a patient's function in a global sense, enabling him to better use what he has in the complex socioeconomic environment of today's mobile society. The prosthesis often also gives some prehensile assistance, providing an opposition part for remaining digits or thumb.

The needs of each patient must be carefully considered, and the prosthesis must conform to the high standards of quality outlined. Its use is primarily for the unilateral amputee who is making a good adjustment to the loss, with realistic expectations.

REFERENCE

1. Koehler M: The passive functional prosthesis: therapist's role. Presented at the Surgery and Rehabilitation of the Hand Symposium, Philadelphia, 1987.

83

Fabrication of an early-fit prosthesis

Loretta M. Maiorano and Patricia M. Byron

A useful tool in the management of upper extremity amputees is the immediate or early-fit prosthesis. An immediate fit is fabricated in the operating room or very shortly thereafter. An early-fit prosthesis is fabricated within the first 2 weeks after amputation.

Application of a prosthesis in the early postinjury period offers numerous advantages. It improves the amputee's acceptance of a prosthesis and encourages maintenance of bilateral activity patterns. When a lag is permitted between the time of injury and the application of a prosthesis, as when fit is delayed until the patient is ready for a definitive fitting, the amputee will usually learn to compensate for the loss by development of unilateral use patterns. By this point the amputee has little use for a functional prosthesis. The early-fit prosthesis also helps in the reduction of edema, pain, and phantom-limb sensation because of early contact of the stump with the rigid socket.[1,2]

Materials used in fabrication of an early-fit prosthesis for the below-elbow amputee are the following:

Tubular cotton stockinette
Polyester fluff
4-inch elastic plaster bandage
3-inch standard plaster bandage
Figure-eight harness
Triceps pad
Flexible elbow hinges
Standard cable
Cable housing
Housing cross-bar assembly

Retainer
Base plate
Hanger
Triple swivel terminal
Friction wrist with anchor straps
Terminal device
Equipment needed to fabricate an early-fit prosthesis includes the following:
End nipper (Fig. 83-1)
Crimper (Fig. 83-1)
Rivet setter

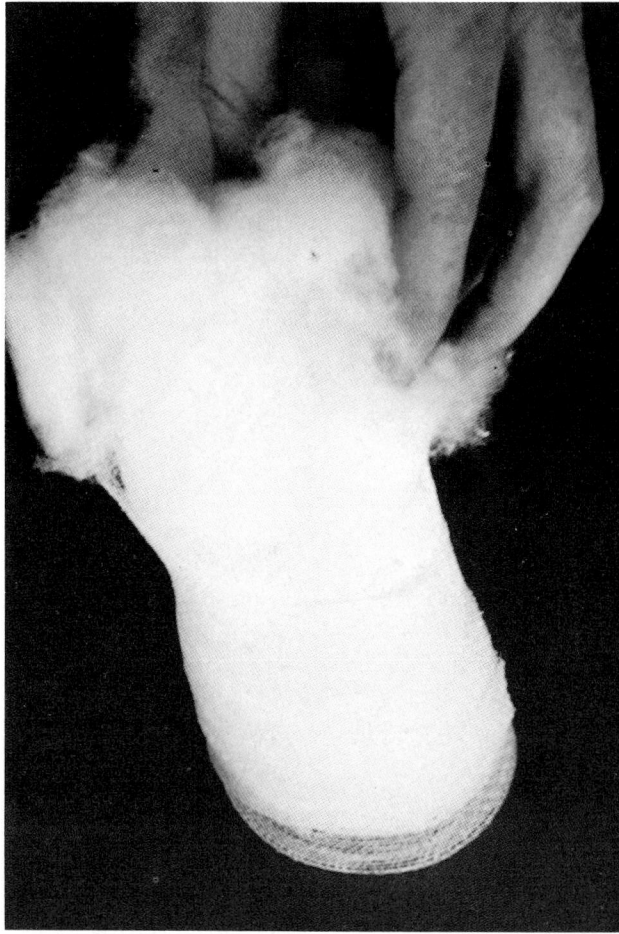

Fig. 83-2 Dacron fluff is applied over the dressing and secured with a sewn stockinette.

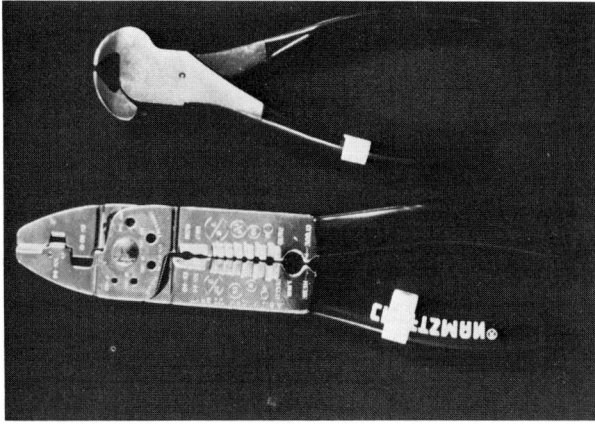

Fig. 83-1 End nipper and crimper.

SOCKET FABRICATION

1. At surgery, a sterile nonadherent gauze is placed over the amputation site, followed by a light sterile dressing. If socket application is done later and the wound is healed, a light dressing is applied as a buffer for the end of the stump.
2. Place polyester (Dacron) fluff over the distal end of the stump as a buffer between the stump and the rigid plaster socket (Fig. 83-2).
3. Measure and cut a single stockinette 2 inches longer than the length of the amputated forearm. Stitch one end of the single stockinet. Place this over the stump and Dacron with the seam side out.
4. To form the rigid plaster socket to the stump, wrap one roll of 4-inch elastic plaster in a figure-eight manner distally to proximally. For a snug fit, elastic plaster is preferred over nonelastic plaster because it can be stretched when wet and it contracts as it dries. Shape the socket by applying pressure to the anterior and posterior surfaces of the forearm. The trim lines of the socket should allow full elbow flexion anteriorly and come up to the elbow posteriorly (Fig. 83-3).

5. When the plaster is dry, place a wrist unit with anchor straps over the socket (Fig. 83-4). If the amputation is at midforearm or shorter, an extention piece must be added to the socket. Do this by adding a paper cup over the plaster socket and wrapping plaster to incorporate this cup into the forearm. The wrist unit is then added to this extension piece as above (Figs. 83-5; 83-6, *A, B,* and *C;* 83-7).
6. The base plate serves as an anchor for the housing. It should be secured to the lateral proximal forearm section of the socket by nonelastic plaster (Fig. 83-8).
7. Wrap a roll of 3-inch nonelastic plaster onto the socket proximally to distally to secure the elbow hinges, base plate, and the wrist unit.

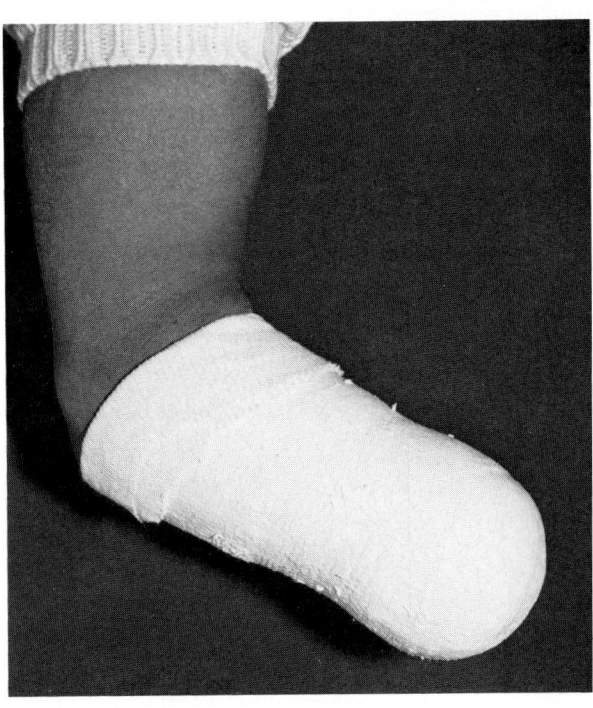

Fig. 83-3 The plaster is wrapped posteriorly up to the elbow to allow full elbow flexion. The stockinette is folded over the distal edge of the socket to produce a smooth edge close to the patient.

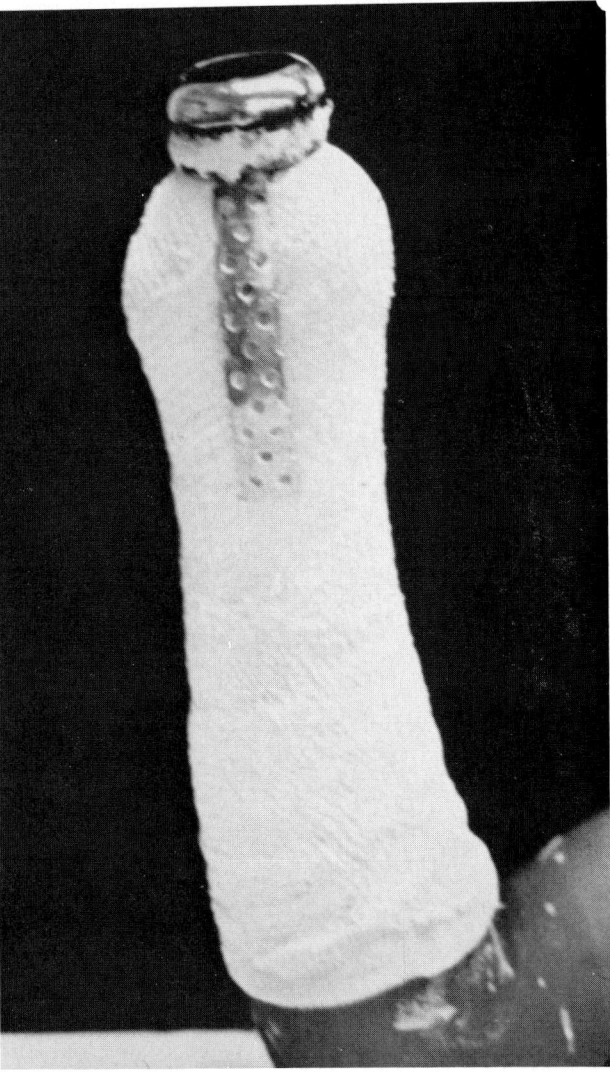

Fig. 83-4 A wrist unit with anchor straps. The anchor straps are placed midlaterally with the extremity in "thumbs up" position.

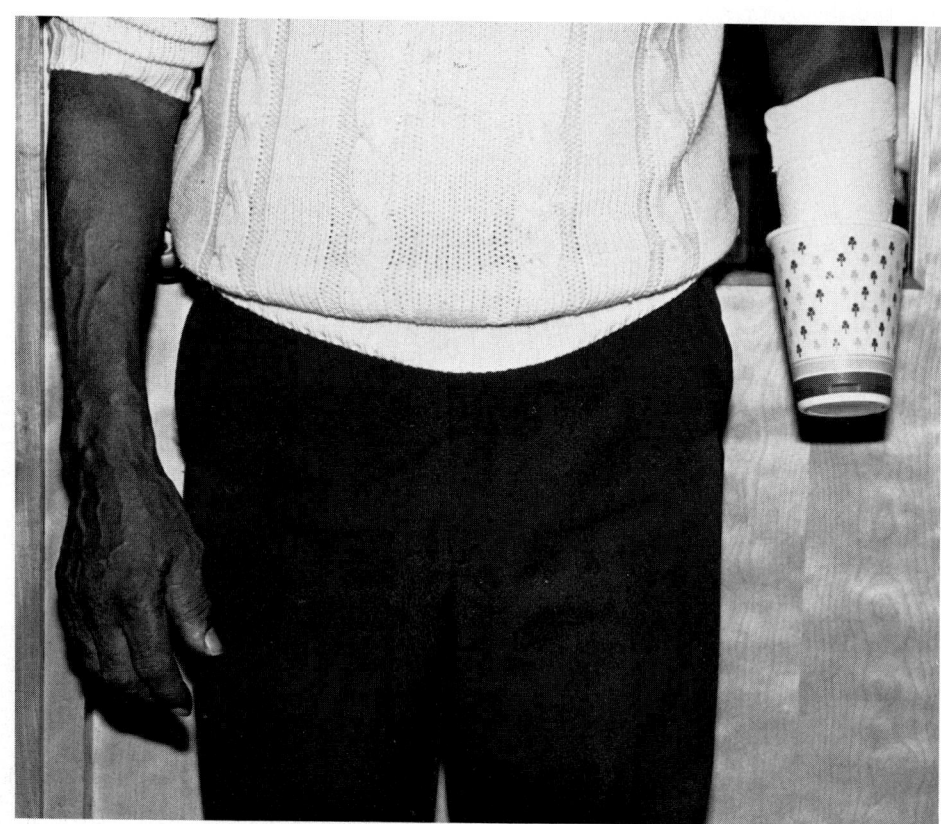

Fig. 83-5   A paper cup is applied at the distal end of the socket to replace lost length.

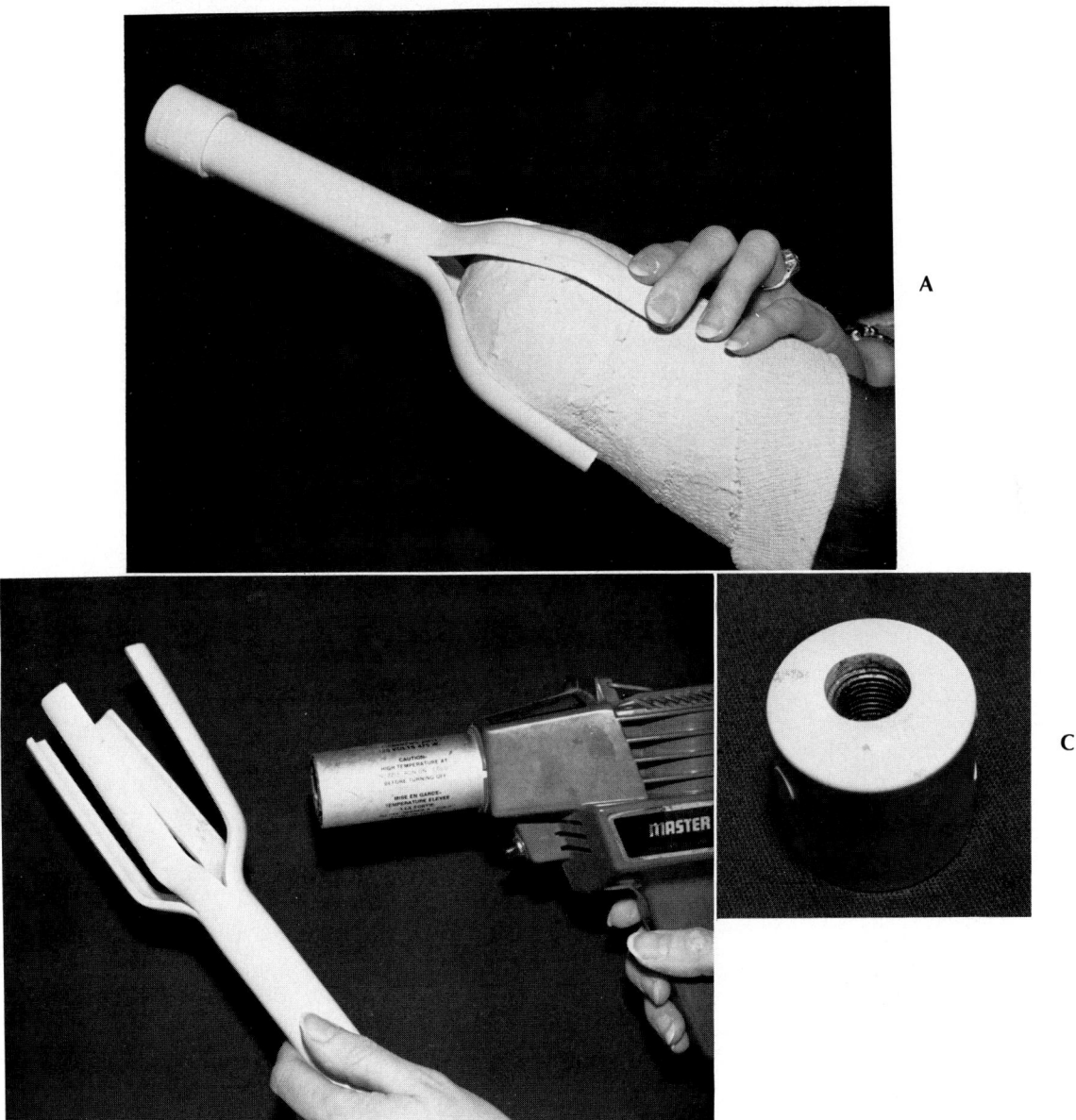

Fig. 83-6   **A,** PVC pipe, with the proximal end split in four sections, can also be used to add length. **B,** The pipe is heated to a moldable consistency with a standard heat gun. It is then wrapped with an Ace wrap or Coban to obtain conformity with the socket. The pipe will be hot and must not be touched by either patient or therapist while it is being molded. The pipe can be cut with a saw to the desired length. **C,** A pipe cap is drilled and threaded to match the terminal device. The cap is glued to the pipe after the pipe has been sized. With the addition of a heavy rubber washer, the cap becomes a friction wrist unit.

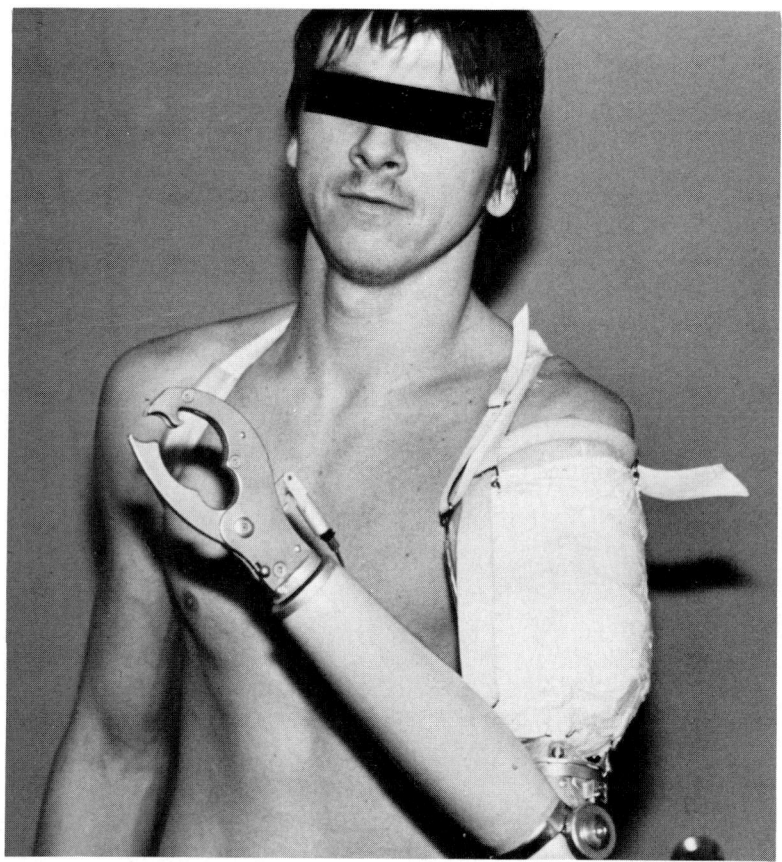

Fig. 83-7   Amputees with above-elbow limb deficiencies can be fitted with a prosthesis by using a method similar to that described for patients with deficiencies below the elbow. Anchor straps are applied to the elbow unit of a prosthesis and then secured to the socket.

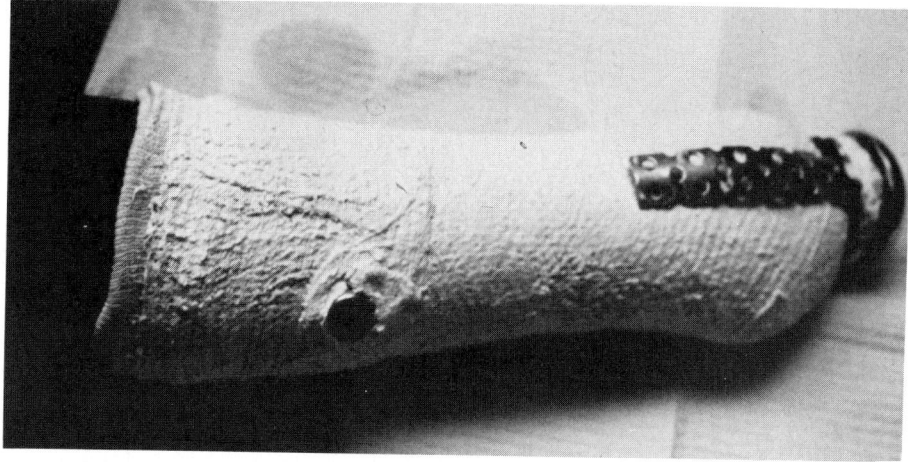

Fig. 83-8   Base plate, which serves as the distal cable reaction point, is secured to the socket.

FABRICATION AND APPLICATION OF THE HARNESS

The harness can be fabricated in advance to accommodate either the right or left side. Use of the Northwestern ring allows for easy adjustment of the harness at the time of application.

Triceps pad assembly

1. Rivet the cross-bar leather to the center of the triceps pad (Fig. 83-9).
2. Rivet the flexible elbow hinges to the distal end of the triceps pad (Fig. 83-10).
3. Rivet two small buckles to either end of the proximal end of the triceps pad.
4. Burn three holes in each end of the inverted-Y strap so that it can be placed through the buckle at the proximal end of the triceps pad (Fig. 83-11).

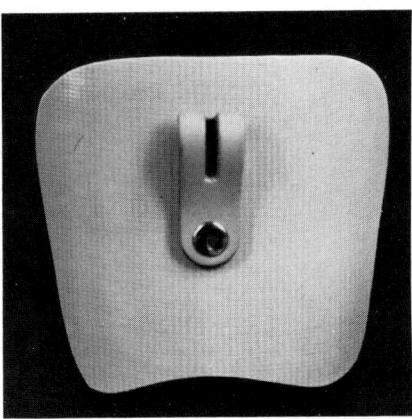

Fig. 83-9 The crossbar serves as the proximal reaction point for the cable. Here the crossbar is shown riveted to the triceps pad.

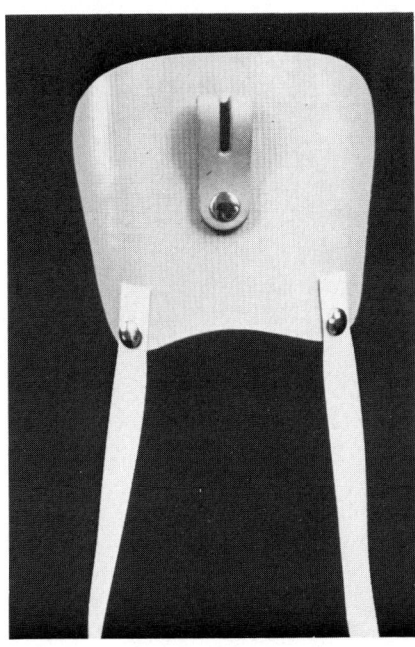

Fig. 83-10 Flexible hinges help with socket suspension. Here they are riveted to the triceps pad. They may also be attached, as is the inverted "Y" (step 3), by small buckles attached to the triceps pad. This increases adjustability of the harness.

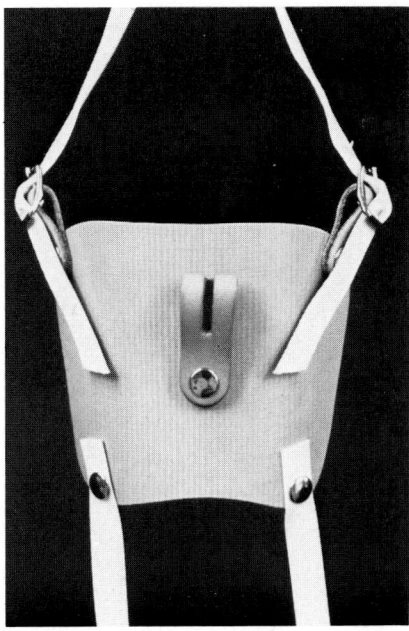

Fig. 83-11 Distal ends of the inverted "Y" strap buckled to the triceps pad.

Harness assembly

The figure-eight harness consists of an axilla strap, suspensor strap and a cable or control strap (Fig. 83-12).

1. The axilla strap encircles the uninvolved side. It is adjusted so that the O-ring sits toward the unamputated side just below the C7 vertebra.
2. The suspensor strap or inverted Y is attached to the ring by means of a four-bar buckle. It attaches distally to the triceps pad.
3. The control strap attaches to the hanger of the control cable assembly.

APPLICATION OF CABLE AND TERMINAL DEVICE

1. Screw the retainer to the distal end of the housing and the cross bar to the proximal end of the housing (Fig. 83-13).
2. Thread the control cable through the metal housing.
3. Crimp the ball terminal to the distal end of the cable (Fig. 83-14).
4. Attach the cable and the housing to the socket by fitting the retainer into the base plate.
5. Attach the cable in the housing to the triceps pad using the cross-bar assembly (Fig. 83-15).

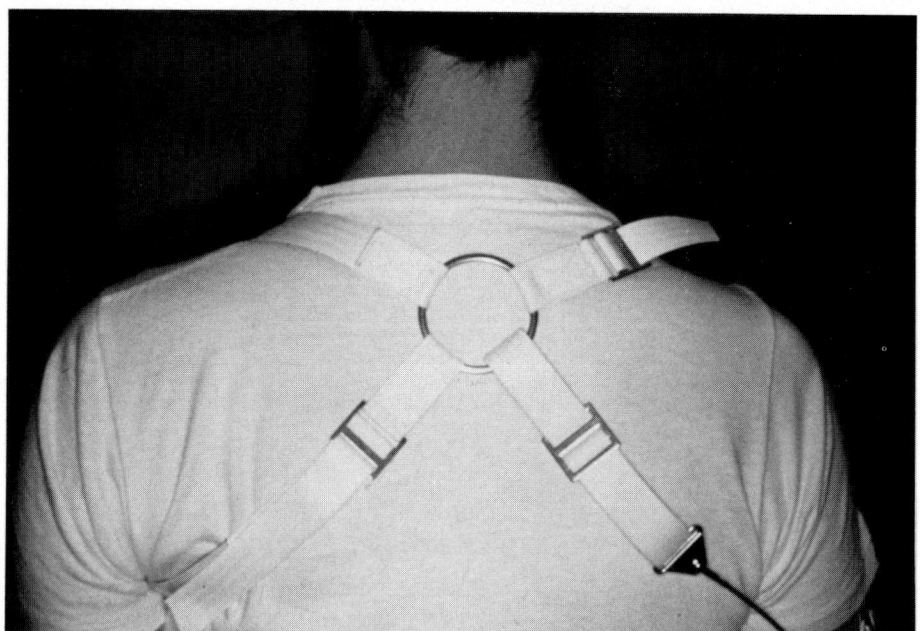

Fig. 83-12 The figure-eight harness with axilla loop, suspensor strap, and control strap.

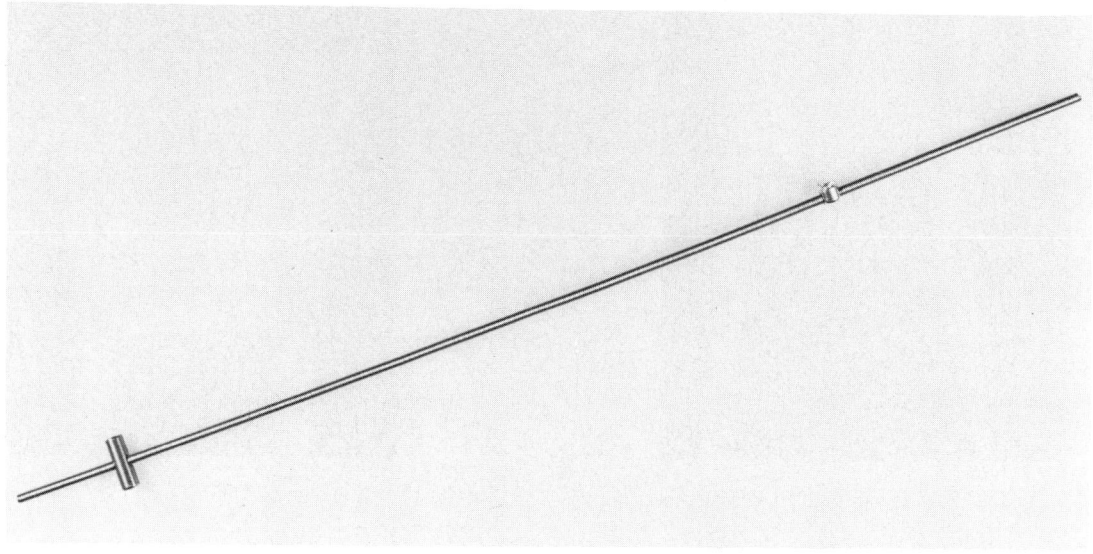

Fig. 83-13 Retainer and crossbar screwed to cable housing.

6. Crimp the hanger to the proximal end of the cable (Fig. 83-16).
7. Attach the hanger to the control strap of the figure-eight harness.
8. Screw the terminal device into the wrist unit and attach it to the cable by the triple swivel terminal.

9. To ensure proper functioning of the terminal device, the patient is observed as he performs ipsilateral forward flexion of the shoulder (Fig. 83-17). If the terminal device does not open or close fully, adjustments must be made in the length of cable, relation of cable housing to retainers, or the harness (Fig. 83-18).

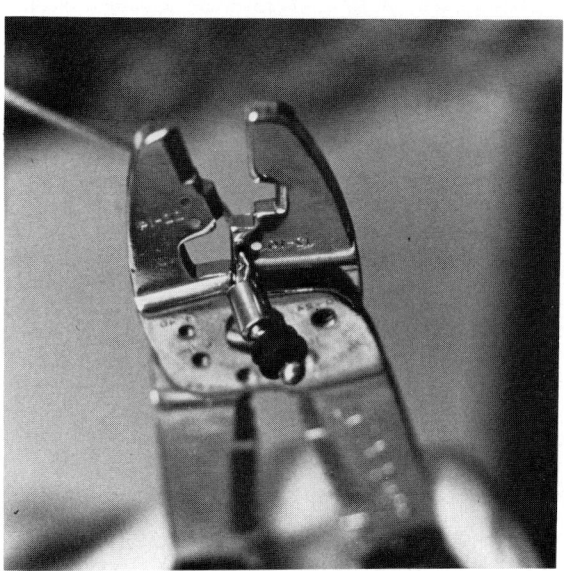

Fig. 83-14 Ball terminal crimped to cable.

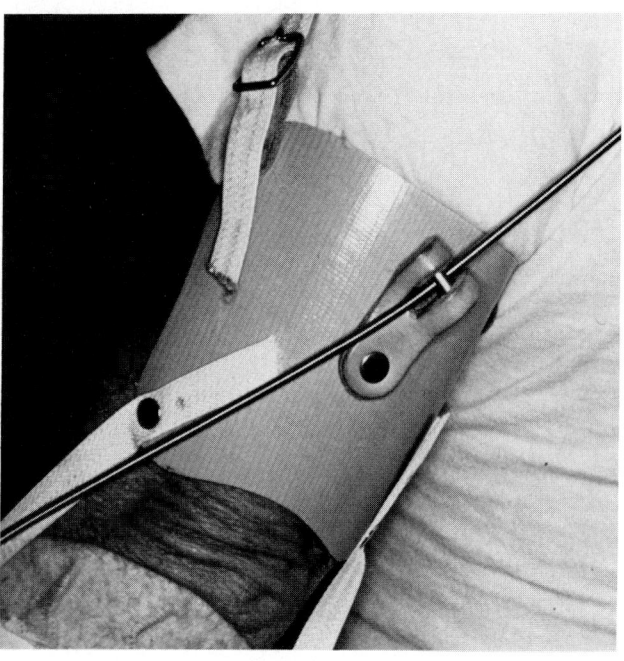

Fig. 83-15 Completed crossbar assembly.

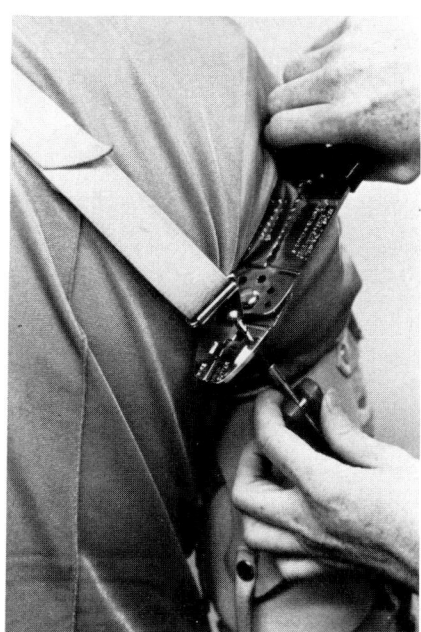

Fig. 83-16 Hanger crimped to control cable.

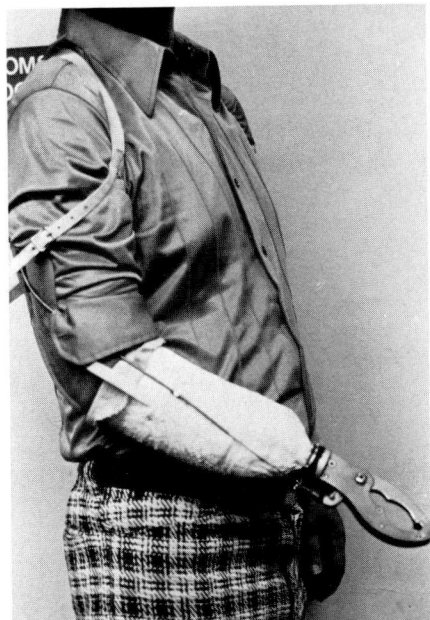

Fig. 83-17 The terminal device is activated by ipsilateral forward flexion of the shoulder.

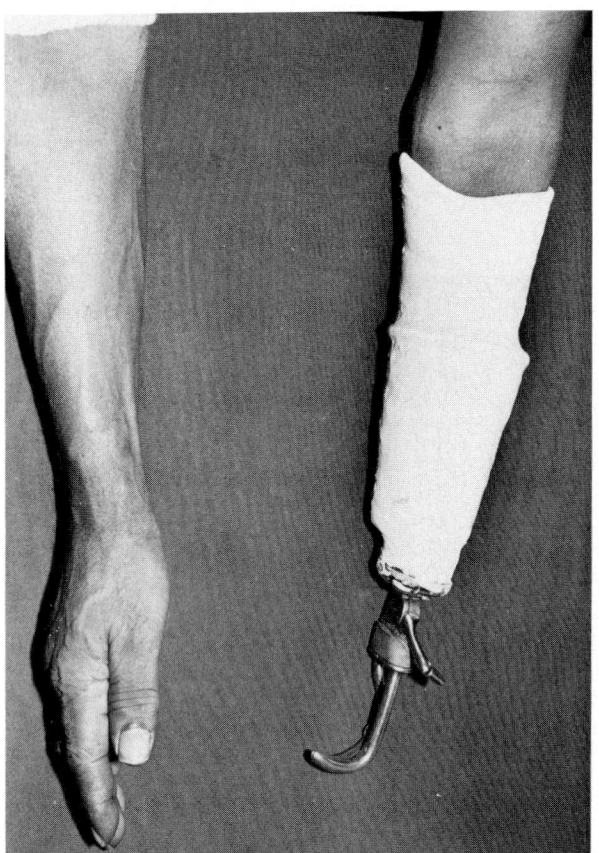

Fig. 83-18 The completed below-elbow prosthesis, including wrist unit and terminal device, should be 1/4 to 1/2 inch shorter than the uninvolved side. When the prosthesis is worn, its weight will cause it to slip approximately 1/4 to 1/2 inch distally. The final visual effect will be that the prosthesis is equal in length to the uninvolved side. (The above-elbow prosthesis should be 1/2 to 3/4 inch shorter than the uninvolved side.)

EARLY PROSTHETIC TRAINING

Ipsilateral-shoulder forward flexion activates the terminal device. The patient performs various control drills to develop a good feel for the amount of muscle activity necessary to operate the terminal device. Drills include the following:

1. Opening and closing the hook in different body positions, such as at the mouth or waist, above the head, and at floor level
2. Picking up objects of different sizes by opening the hook just wide enough to accommodate the object; opening it too wide wastes energy
3. Picking up objects of different densities and making sure he maintains the object's shape by maintaining appropriate tension on the cable.

SUMMARY

Use of an early-fit prosthesis has been shown to improve the amputee's use of the prosthesis and to encourage bilateral use of the extremities (Fig. 83-19). It can also help reduce edema and phantom pain.

REFERENCES

1. Burkhalter WE, Mayfield G, and Carmona LS: The upper-extremity amputee: early and immediate post-surgical prosthetic fitting, J Bone Joint Surg 48A(1):46, 1976.
2. Jacobs RR and Brady WM: Early post surgical fitting in upper extremity amputation, J Trauma 15(11):966, 1975.

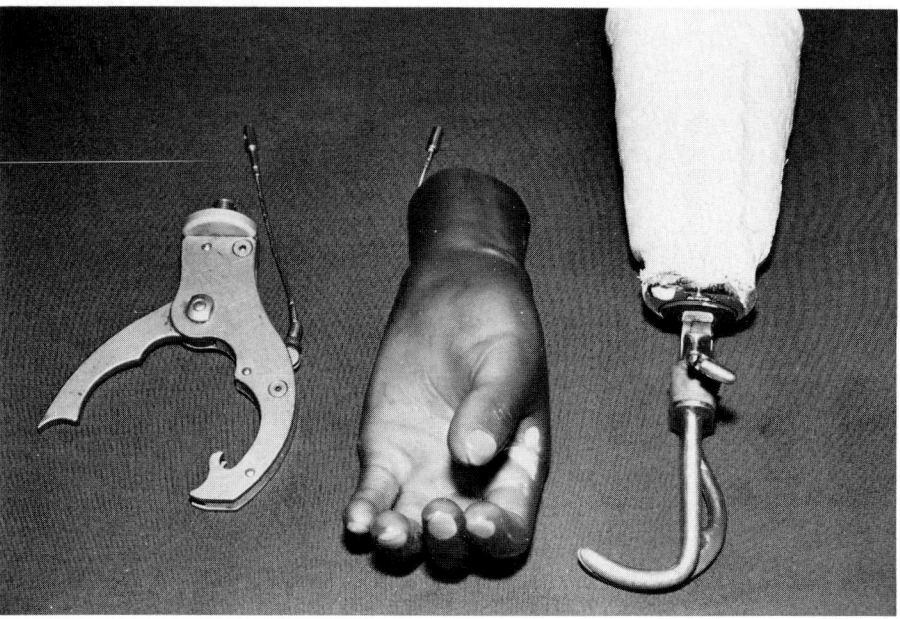

Fig. 83-19 Use of an early-fit device can allow the amputee the opportunity to experiment with various terminal devices before definitive fitting to determine which terminal device best meets the patient's needs.

84

Adult amputee management and conventional prosthetic training

Bonnie L. Olivett

Throughout history there have been reports of humans designing replacements for amputated hands. Certainly the loss of a hand has been and will continue to be a great catastrophe to the individual person in society, since the functional and aesthetic losses are potentially devastating. The rehabilitative problem today is that these two concepts—that is, function and aesthetics—may be incompatible, a situation that probably accounts for the fact that there is no simple answer regarding the "best prosthesis" to satisfy all needs.

The purpose of this chapter is to discuss the functional value and use of the conventional prosthesis with the adult acquired amputee. The importance of an early fit and prosthetic training will be stressed, because this will enhance the amputee's use of the prosthesis functionally.

HISTORY OF UPPER LIMB PROSTHETICS

In 1958 the Smithsonian Institution reported the discovery of a skull dating back about 45,000 years. It was deduced that the skull belonged to a person who must have been an upper extremity amputee, because of the appearance of the teeth, which seemed to have been used functionally to compensate for the loss of a hand.[24]

From the Middle Ages come written accounts along with paintings and museum pieces showing soldiers being fitted with artificial limbs to be worn in battle. The first recorded use of an artificial hand involved the Roman general Marcus Serquis. He reportedly lost his hand during the Second Punic War (218-201 B.C.), and subsequently instructed his armorer to fit him with an iron hand to be clamped onto his shield during battle. Possibly of similar design was the Alt-Ruppin hand, made of iron (Fig. 84-1), which was recovered along the Rhine River in 1863. This hand, along with other artificial limbs of the fifteenth century are on display at the Stibert Museum in Florence, Italy.[24]

Ambrose Paré, who lived during the sixteenth century, can be credited with the most significant contributions to amputation surgery and prosthetics.[20] Paré designed and manufactured ingenious devices that expressed his interest in rehabilitating the amputee. His drawings of the hand and upper extremity prostheses were technically described in his *Dix Livres de la Chirurgie* in 1564. No volitional control was used in his protheses, which used the principles of articulated joints (Fig. 84-2).

Peter Baliff, a Berlin dentist, designed in 1818 the first below-elbow prosthesis, which was operated by harness-controlled pull cords. Also reported during the nineteenth century were various assistive devices for upper extremity amputees, such as a sponge clamped onto a tray and a nail brush fastened upside down. These devices were described by Captain George Derenzy in 1822, after he lost his right arm near the elbow.

The first split-hook terminal device was developed in 1912 by D.W. Dorrance. He designed this hook in an attempt to replace the function of his own amputated hand. Although this hook has been refined, the original version is still used in prosthetics today because of its simplicity and durability.

It was not until after World War II, which produced great numbers of amputees, that an organized attempt was undertaken to produce functional, lightweight, yet inexpensive, prostheses. This impetus, along with the commercial development of plastics, created major advancements in prosthetic fitting for the upper extremity amputee.

INCIDENCE OF AMPUTATION

Approximately 43,000 major amputations occur yearly in the United States.[18] Of the 311,000 amputees reported in

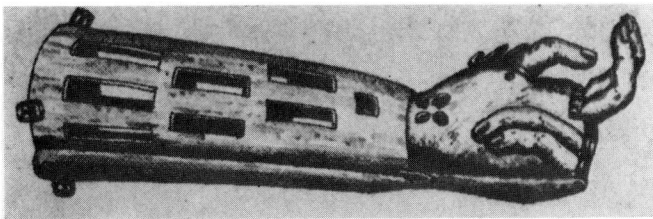

Fig. 84-1 Alt-Ruppin hand, recovered along the Rhine River in 1863.

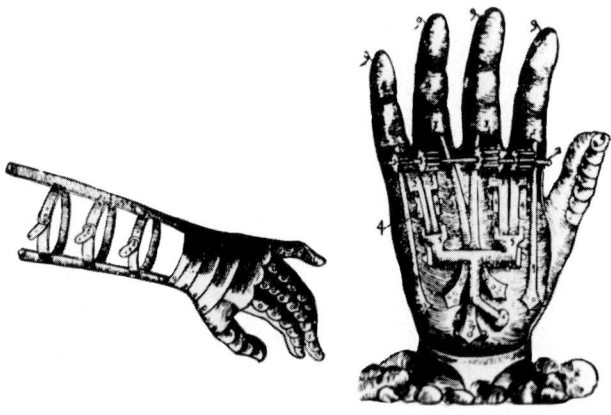

Fig. 84-2 Engraving of a prosthetic hand with articulated joints designed by Ambrose Paré. Published in 1573.

the United States in 1970 by the National Center for Health Statistics, 32% involve the upper extremity. There is a peak between 20 and 40 years of age, with nearly 90% of all the upper extremity amputations resulting from trauma.[1-3] The injuries are equally divided between the right and left sides; however, males outnumber females 4 to 1.[1-3] Possibly, the higher incidence of injuries in males is attributable to the hazards of physical vocational and avocational work in which men engage. According to the *Newsletter of the Amputee Clinics,* October 1972, only 50% of the amputees fitted continued to wear their prosthetic limbs.[5]

PROSTHETIC ADVANCEMENTS

Unfortunately, we all are subject to some rather unrealistic expectations about current prostheses because of the sensationalism of the media. Certainly the field of prosthetics is making greater strides than ever before with the use of external power, myoelectric controls, and sensory feedback systems. These components and designs tend to be expensive, making availability limited to only a few.

Many powered components and designs developed between 1955 and 1970 did not satisfy needs sufficiently to even warrant commercial production.[19] Prosthetic systems using external power and supplementary sensory feedback systems are primarily available in the United States today through major prosthetic research centers, such as Northwestern University, U.C.L.A., Rancho Los Amigos Hospital in Downey, California, Southwestern Research Institute in San Antonio, Texas, and the Veterans Administration Prosthetics Center in New York.

The consensus of several researchers is that myoelectrically controlled prostheses have no significant functional advantage over the standard cable-controlled system, and even with sensory feedback the performance is no better and may only reach a level equal to the conventional cable-operated prostheses.[12] Although new materials and techniques have made available passive cosmetic devices that are meeting very high standards, these devices fall short of the ideal goals of motion and sensibility.[18] As Beasley states, "It is important to dispel the concept of the artificial hand, for such will probably never exist."[4]

CONVENTIONAL METHODS

The conventional prosthesis continues to play an important role in the field of prosthetics because of availability and ease of maintenance and upkeep. According to Burk-

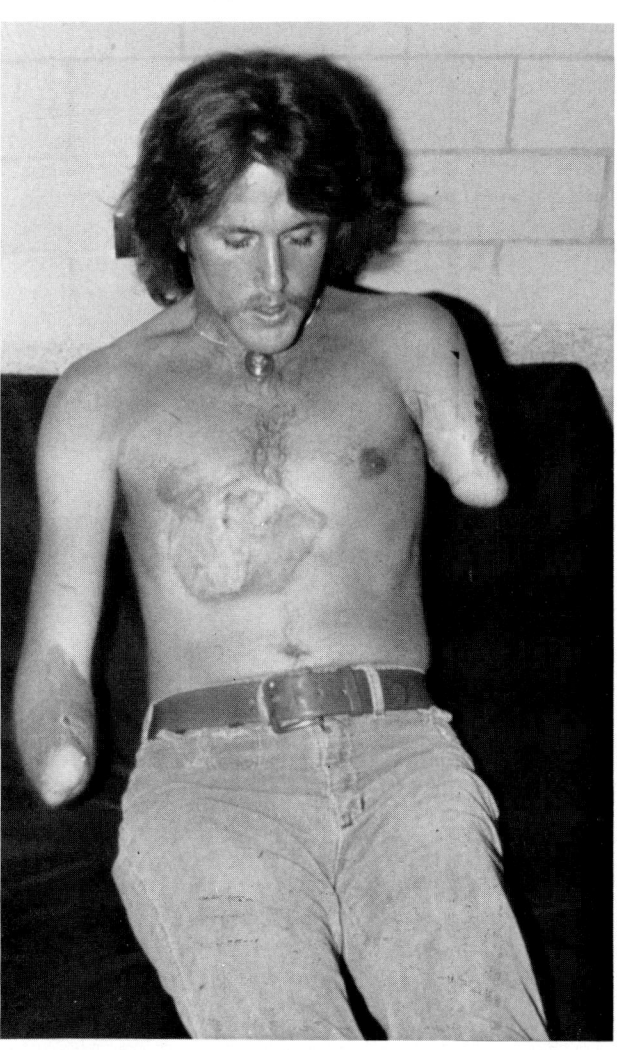

Fig. 84-3   Sit-ups for generalized conditioning.

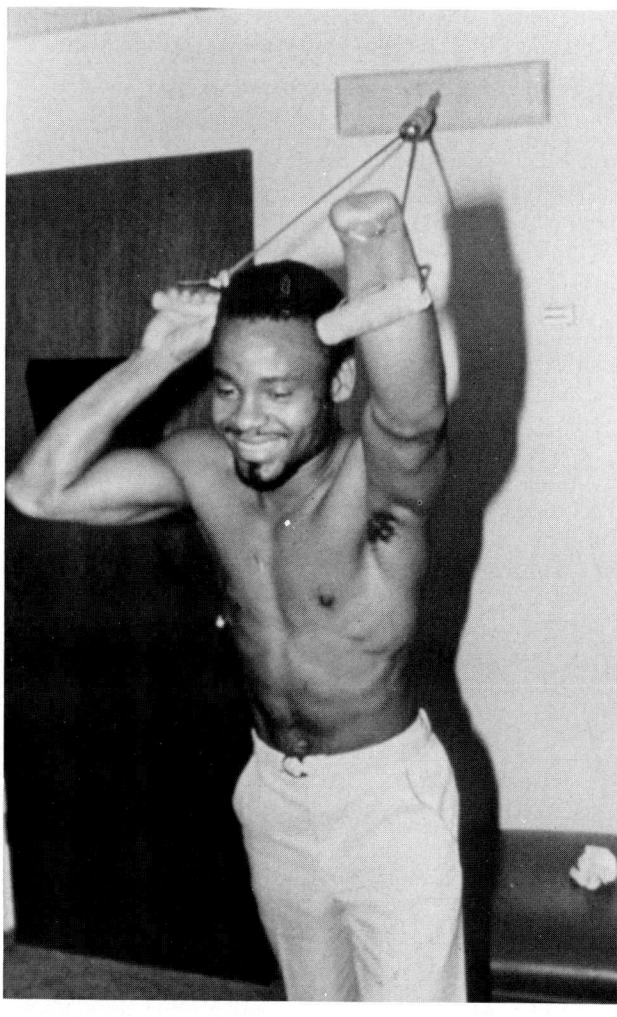

Fig. 84-4   Pulleys used for range of motion and strengthening.

halter,[8] "The vast majority of upper limb amputees still use standard and conventional components that are activated by body powered control."[8]

PREOPERATIVE CARE

Although preparation of the patient before the amputation is not always possible, there are cases when the patient knows in advance that an amputation is inevitable. It is helpful to show the patient what an artificial limb looks like and to begin making him aware of what function can be anticipated. It is also important to convey, if possible, the functional limitations of the prosthesis.

Range of motion and strength of the upper extremity should be assessed bilaterally, if the patient's condition is stable. The general condition of the patient should be noted and his intellectual, psychological, social, vocational, and avocational needs appreciated so that one may begin planning the patient's prosthesis.

POSTOPERATIVE CARE

The period of early postoperative care is one of the most crucial phases. During this time the attitudes of the patient are in flux and his reactions can be dealt with most effectively. The early postoperative goals are to maintain range of motion and strength while preventing the development of contractures and assisting in the conditioning of the stump. Elevation of the stump should be encouraged to prevent edema, thereby decreasing pain.

Frequent active exercises may generally begin 24 hours after surgery, along with gentle assisted stump range-of-motion (ROM) exercise within the patient's tolerance. The use of exercises will help to improve circulation, while increasing strength, which according to Friedman[10] helps prevent "alienation" of the muscles of the stump after the

trauma of amputation. Resistive exercises of the stump are contraindicated until the muscles are well healed.

As the general condition of the patient improves, strengthening exercises include exercises for the trunk and upper extremities, such as sit-ups, one-arm push-ups, and pivot-prone exercises (Fig. 84-3). Cuff weights, Theraband and pulleys are effective treatment techniques for strengthening (Fig. 84-4). Equipment may also be adapted to incorporate the involved upper extremity to promote range of motion, strength and endurance before prosthetic fitting (Fig. 84-5 and 84-6).

The patient is encouraged to care for himself and to assist with the dressings and bandaging if soft compressive dressings are used (Fig. 84-7). Postural awareness must be emphasized, because all amputees have the tendency to carry the stump side higher or lower than the other shoulder until they have regained the sense of balance. Certain pieces of adaptive equipment may be useful, including a suction-cup brush (Fig. 84-8) and a one-handed knife (Fig. 84-9), along with instructions for tying shoelaces with one hand.

DOMINANCE CHANGE

If the dominant hand is amputated, a change in hand dominance is recommended. The normal limb with sensation will be more useful for fine manipulation. One-handed activities that help develop coordination and dexterity during dominance change are copper tooling, painting, or writing.

PREPROSTHETIC MANAGEMENT

An immediate or early fitting can be beneficial to the trauma-induced amputee.[10] If an immediate fit is used, the below-elbow amputee should have a cast applied in the shape of the Münster below-elbow socket (Fig. 84-10) but constructed higher than the Münster socket to utilize the

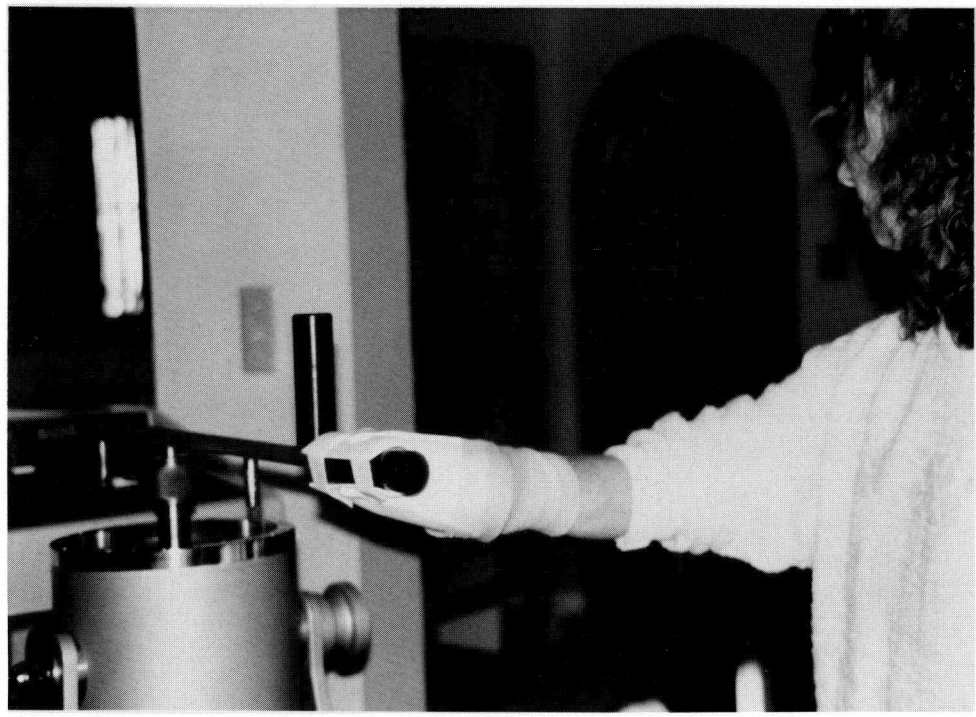

Fig. 84-5   The BTE Work Simulator can easily be adapted for amputee training.

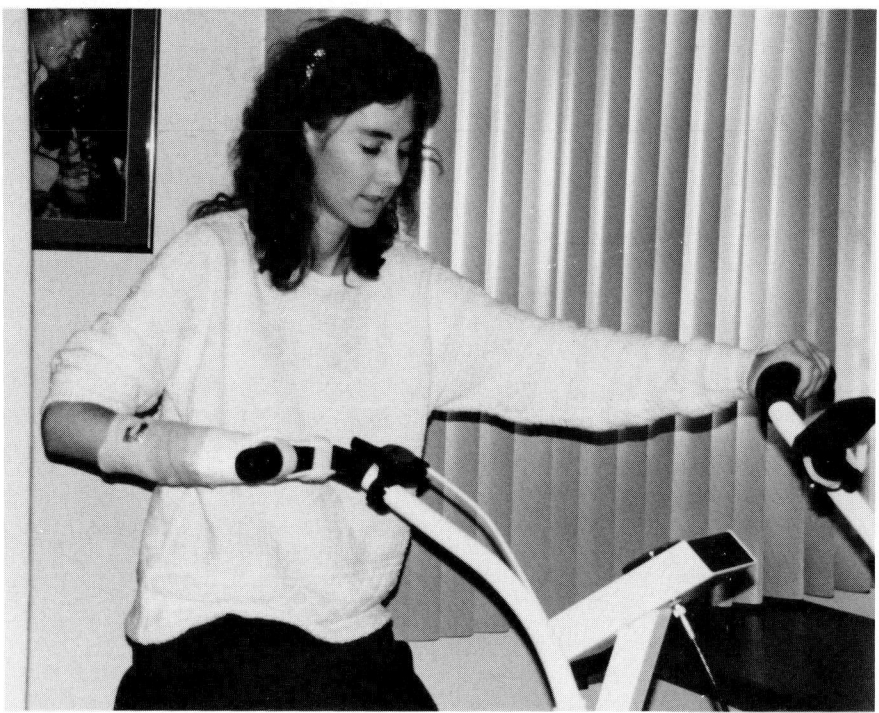

Fig. 84-6 The Pana Plus Panasonic Bicycle is useful for encouraging range of motion and endurance.

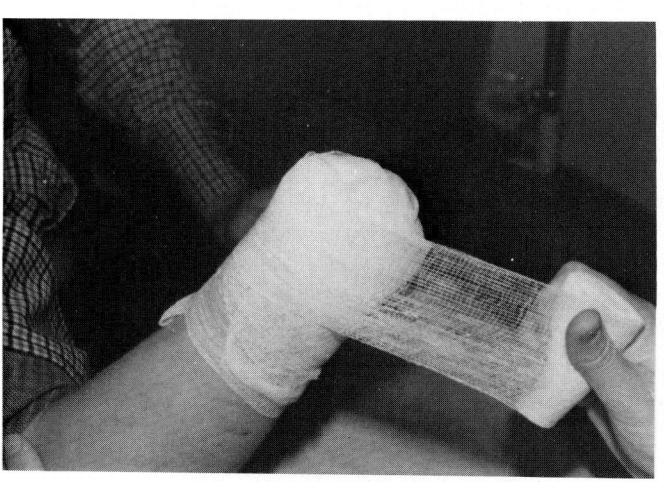

Fig. 84-7 Patient applying dressing, using oblique, distal-to-proximal figure-eight configuration.

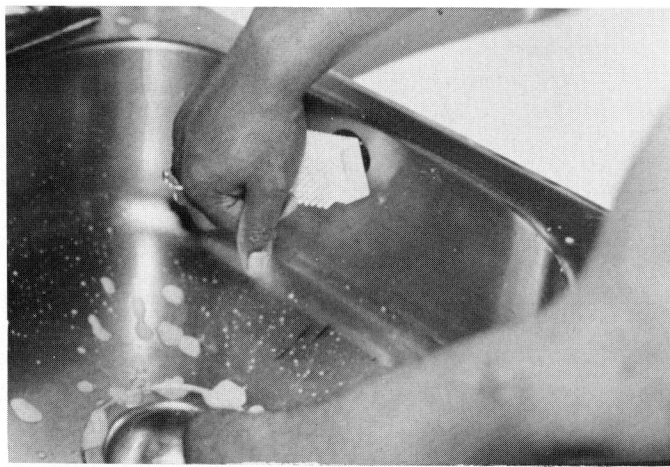

Fig. 84-8 Suction-cup brush for cleansing hand and fingernails.

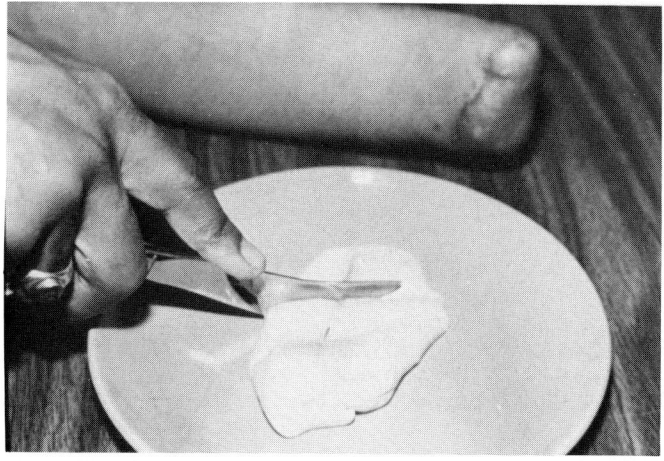

Fig. 84-9 Rocking knife used for one-handed cutting while patient awaits prosthetic fitting.

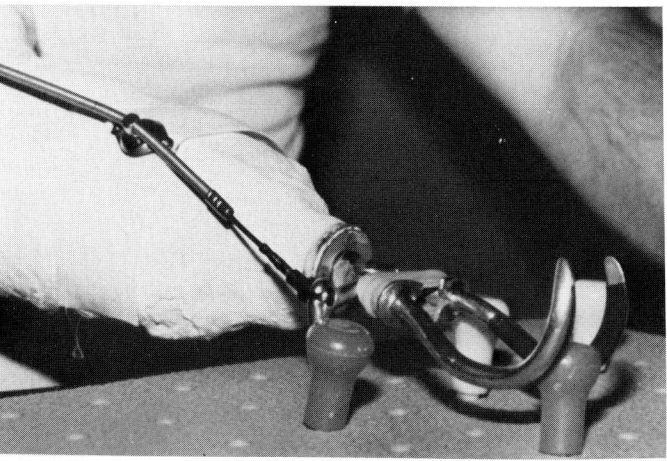

Fig. 84-10 Immediate fit with a cast applied in the shape of a Münster below-elbow socket.

humeral condyles to assist with suspension. The above-elbow amputee should have a socket constructed in the shape of a shoulder spica.

For the bilateral amputee, I recommend fitting one side with a functional prosthesis and placing a rigid total contact plaster cast on the other side to reduce pain and edema.[13]

A temporary or mock-up prosthesis fabricated from thermoplastic materials may be useful when there are postsurg-ical complications or if fitting may be delayed while one is awaiting scar maturation. A prosthesis of this type is used for early training and to provide early function (Figs. 84-11 and 84-12).

Another benefit of the immediate postsurgical fit is that surgeons have become more aware of early functional restoration of the amputee, thus directing the emphasis away from the surgery itself and toward a return of function.[6]

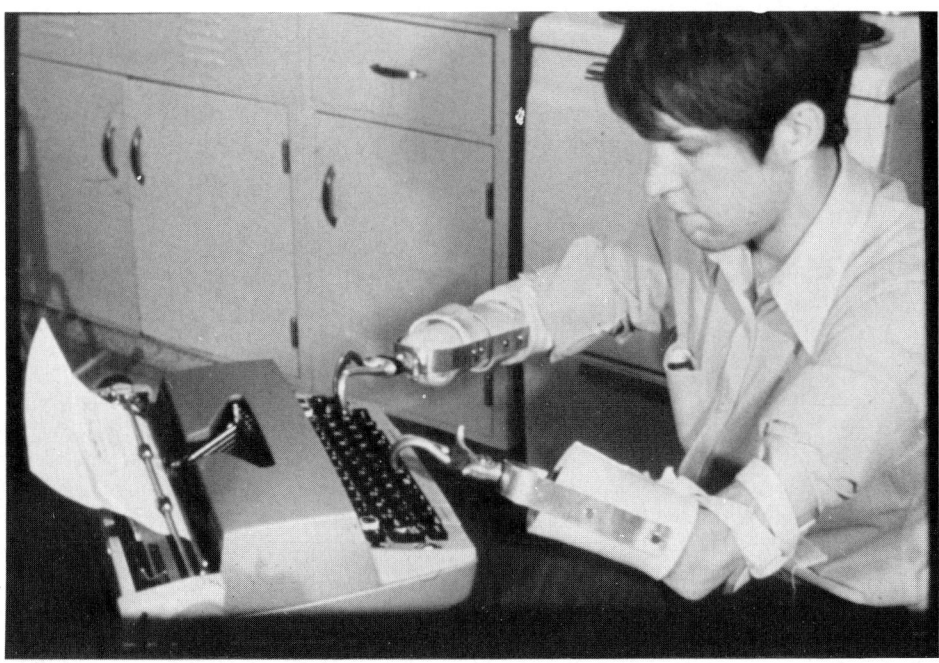

Fig. 84-11 Temporary thermoplastic prosthesis may be useful for early training and function.

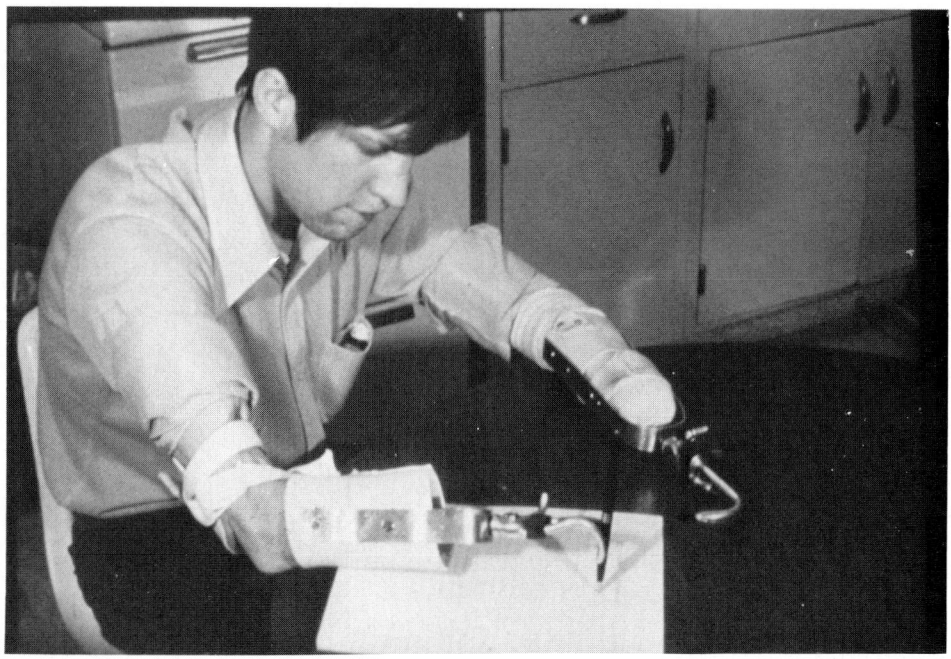

Fig. 84-12 Mock-up prosthesis may be used for early function and training.

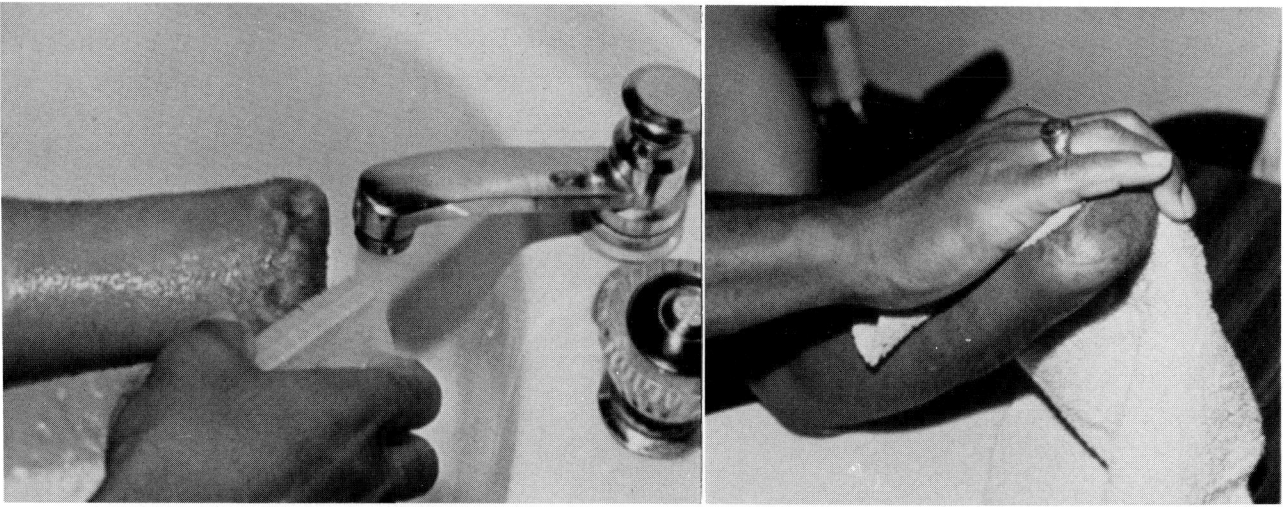

Fig. 84-13   Early desensitization techniques being used to reduce paresthesias.

CONTRACTURES

A joint contracture is a complication that is occasionally inevitable because of the posture of the stump during healing. A slow, steady stretch might be useful while one is attempting to correct a contracture. However, stretching, using the technique of inhibition of antagonist muscles through proprioceptive neuromuscular facilitation, is generally more effective. The use of thermoplastic night splints, such as a three-point splint at the elbow, may help avoid or reduce a contracture. Serial casting might also be utilized to help reduce a contracture.

PREPARATION AND CONDITIONING OF THE STUMP

The adult traumatic or acquired amputee will have phantom sensations, described as the ability to perceive cortical images of the lost limb. Some of these sensations may be disagreeable,[9] such as "pins and needles," "cramping," "twisting," or "burning" sensations. Although the upper

limb phantoms are stronger and longer lasting than those of the lower limb, they tend to be more annoying than painful.[17]

My experience has been that early desensitization techniques greatly reduce these paresthesias and help prepare the limb for the prosthetic socket. Patients generally respond first to deeper pressure such as brushing and massage (Fig. 84-13) to help soften and stretch adherent scarring. As the stump becomes desensitized, lighter touch such as tapping, vibration, and working with textures are all helpful modalities (Fig. 84-14). The use of physical agents, such as heat or cold, electrical muscle stimulation, and transcutaneous nerve stimulation (TENS), can also help diminish phantom sensations.

Tensor bandages may be prescribed to help reduce edema and promote stump shrinkage to prepare the contour of the

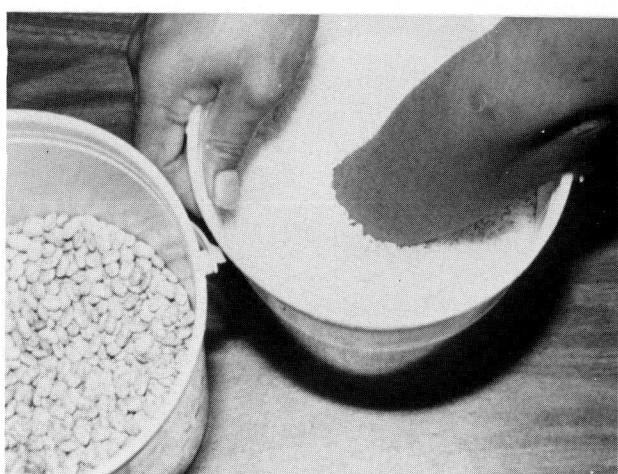

Fig. 84-14   Modalities used for desensitization.

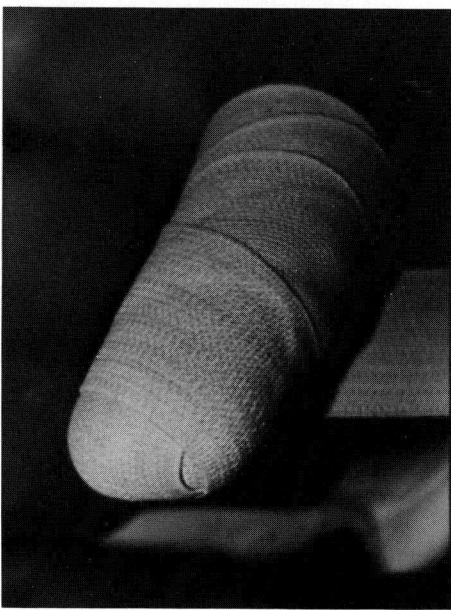

Fig. 84-15   Tensor bandages provide constant compression to promote shrinkage.

stump for prosthetic fit. A constant distal-to-proximal, oblique, figure-eight compression is used. Because it is difficult to establish and maintain proper pressure, frequent reapplication of the bandages is recommended (Fig. 84-15).

For most people, cosmetic function is of primary importance. At this preprosthetic stage, attention should be directed to teaching the amputee to move in a natural manner. Once the prosthesis is received, continued attention should be directed towards good posture and natural movement.[23]

PROSTHETIC COMPONENTS
Terminal devices

Terminal devices are designed for prehension. There is a wide variety available. Some are designed and shaped to look like a hand with one or more movable fingers, and some are designed as two-fingered devices with a hook type of configuration. The terminal device must be suited to the person according to his psychological, vocational, and avocational needs. A hook is recommended if bilateral skills requiring manual dexterity are desired.

Cosmetically, prosthetic hands are superior to hooks (Fig. 84-16) and may be preferred by the individual in a socially oriented vocation. The hands may be active or passive terminal devices. Functionally they are a poor comparison to the hook. The functional and cosmetic hands are commonly covered with a polyvinyl chloride glove, which tends to be sensitive to sunlight, temperature, dyes, and chemicals. Recent use of polymers of dimethyl siloxanes has shown better results, because they are not altered by temperature appreciably and are more resistant to soiling.[14]

Voluntary-opening hooks are prescribed more frequently than any other terminal device, because of their mechanical simplicity and ease of operation.[11] The Hosmer/Dorrance name is associated with a wide range of voluntary-opening hooks. These terminal devices may be prescribed with canted fingers to permit better visualization and manipulation of small objects, or they may be lyre or contour shaped, making it easier to grasp or hold rounded objects (Figs. 84-17 and 84-18). The contour hook is the most recent design by Hosmer/Dorrance. Because of the contoured shape and design, this terminal device is better for office work or for holding objects such as glasses. The force of prehension is determined by rubber bands placed at the base of the hook fingers. As a general rule, each band produces approximately 1 pound of prehensile force.

Voluntary-closing hooks allow the prehension force to be increased progressively by increasing tension, enabling the amputee to adopt a force suited to the object being handled. A clutch or locking mechanism is generally used if grasp is required for a long period of time. The Grip I and Grip

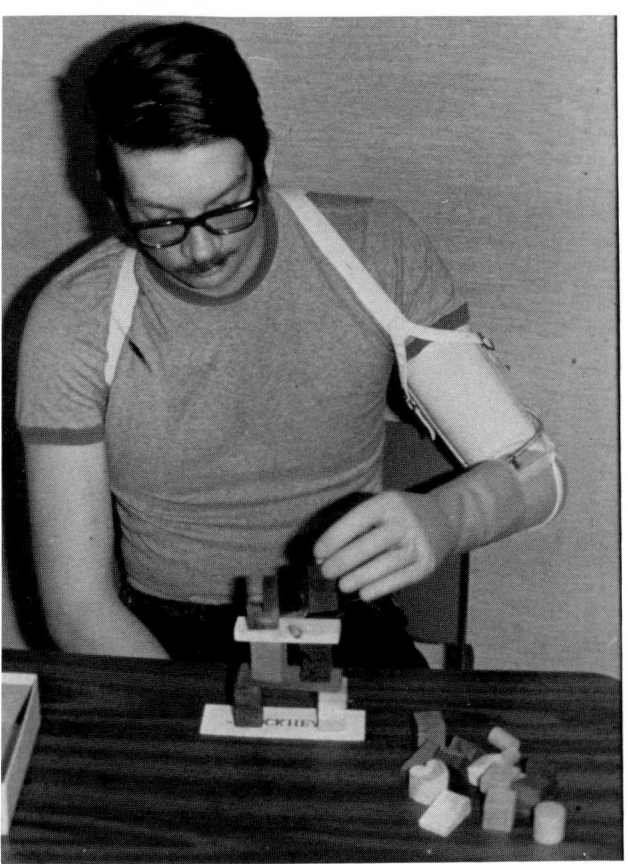

Fig. 84-16 Prosthetic training with a Dorrance functional hand.

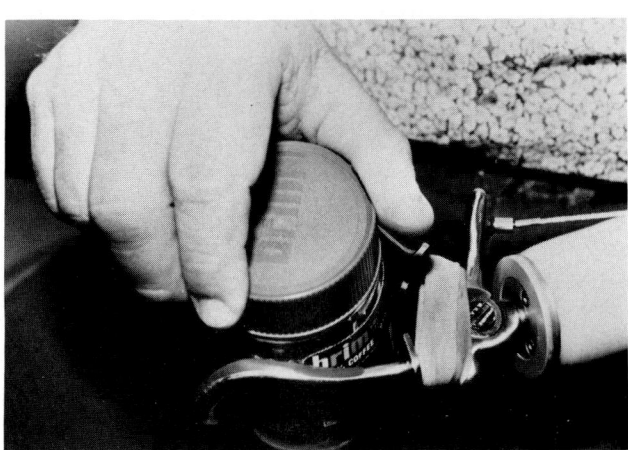

Fig. 84-17 Lyre-shaped fingers help grasp and hold rounded objects.

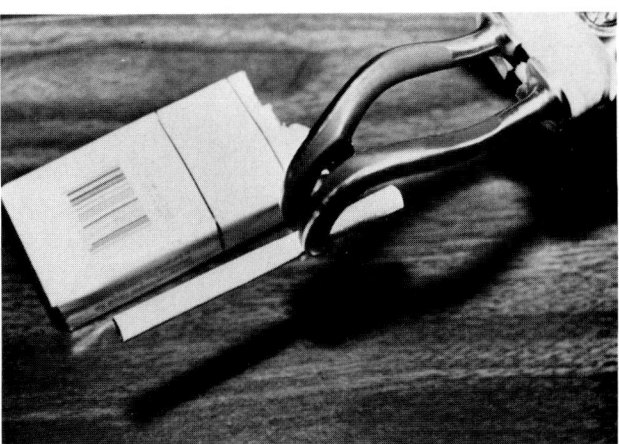

Fig. 84-18 Voluntary-opening hooks permit easy visualization for manipulation of small objects.

II* have been designed as voluntary-closing devices. Prehension is obtained by using the muscle power of the user. The advantages of the terminal device are similar to those of the voluntary opening heavy-duty terminal devices designed for holding, grasping, chiseling, or using carpentry tools and manipulating long-handled implements, such as shovels and rakes. (Fig. 84-19)

Wrist units

A wrist unit connects the terminal device to the prosthetic forearm and provides pronation and supination to the user. The most common unit is the wrist friction unit, which consists of a nylon washer that provides a friction hold

---

*T.R.S., Inc., Boulder, Colo.

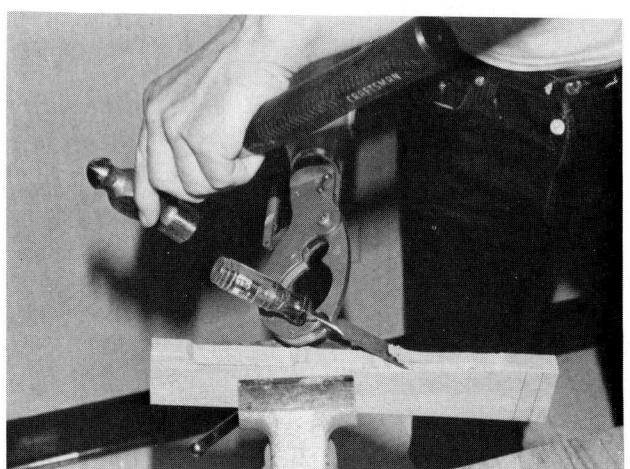

Fig. 84-19 Training using Grip I.

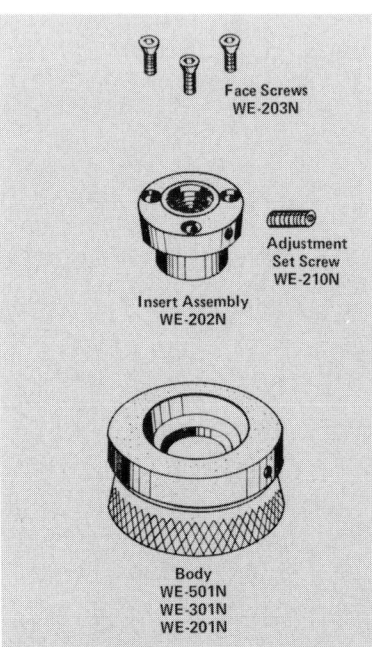

Fig. 84-20 Constant-friction wrist unit. (Courtesy Hosmer/Dorrance Corp, Campbell, Calif.)

during prepositioning (Fig. 84-20). A minimum space of 6 cm is required for placement.

The wrist flexion unit has the same friction feature as the wrist friction unit; however, it allows three positions of flexion: neutral, 25 degrees of flexion, and 50 degrees of flexion. This unit is essential for the bilateral amputee to enable him to work the terminal device close to his body (Fig. 84-21).

The quick-change wrist unit allows a quick change of the terminal device. This unit is not commonly recommended because it wears poorly.

Hinges

The use of flexible or rigid elbow hinges is a form of suspension and part of the transmission of power for the wrist disarticulation or below-elbow amputee. Rigid hinges provide torsional stability at the elbow against the rotational stress of the prosthesis.

Elbow units

The standard elbow unit is an internal multiple-locking unit that is manufactured by Hosmer/Dorrance Corporation. This unit allows 5 to 135 degrees of flexion with 11 locking positions of the forearm (Fig. 84-22). The locking mechanism is controlled through the suspension system. A minimum space of 8 cm is required for the use of this unit.

The external unit, which is an outside-locking elbow, is designed for the long above-elbow or elbow disarticulation amputee (Fig. 84-23). The disadvantage of this unit is its bulkiness, which often damages clothing.

Harness and control systems

The figure-eight harness is most commonly used to suspend the conventional body-powered prosthesis and control the terminal device, since it is the least bulky and provides good control (Fig. 84-24). The disadvantage of this type of harness is the pressure exerted on the axilla of the opposite extremity. If the amputee must lift heavy loads or perform strenuous activities, a shoulder-saddle type of harness or chest strap may be better tolerated (Fig. 84-25).

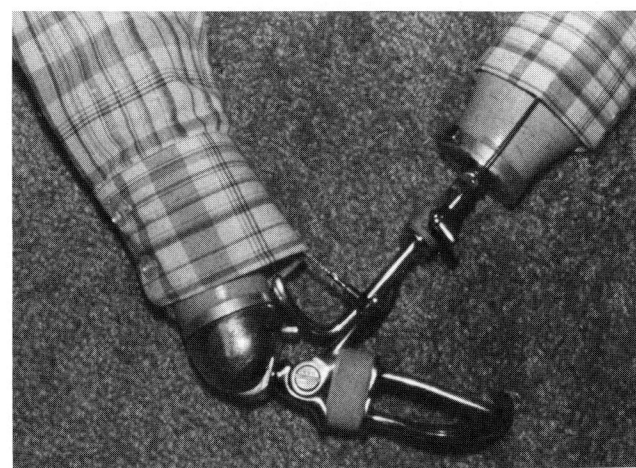

Fig. 84-21 Wrist flexion unit being activated by a bilateral amputee.

The cable is used to provide the force necessary to operate the terminal device. The Bowden cable is used for the below-elbow amputee. It consists of an inner tension cable and an outer housing. The housing maintains a constant length regardless of the motion involved. A dual-control cable is a split-housing cable that activates the forearm lift or the terminal device, or both, depending on whether the elbow lock is in the locked or unlocked position. If the elbow is unlocked, the forearm will lift when tension is placed on the cable. When the elbow is locked, the terminal device will open as tension is applied to the cable. This control system is used for the above-elbow and elbow disarticulation amputee.

Socket

The socket is the most important component of the prosthesis. It must provide support, stability, and comfort. Al-

most all upper extremity sockets are total contact and double-walled to provide better control and proprioception. The internal wall is contoured to fit the stump, following the principle of total contact. The external wall is contoured to match the normal limb. For a detailed review of the upper limb prosthetic systems, the suggested reading is Chapter 9 of *Atlas of Limb Prosthetics*.[7]

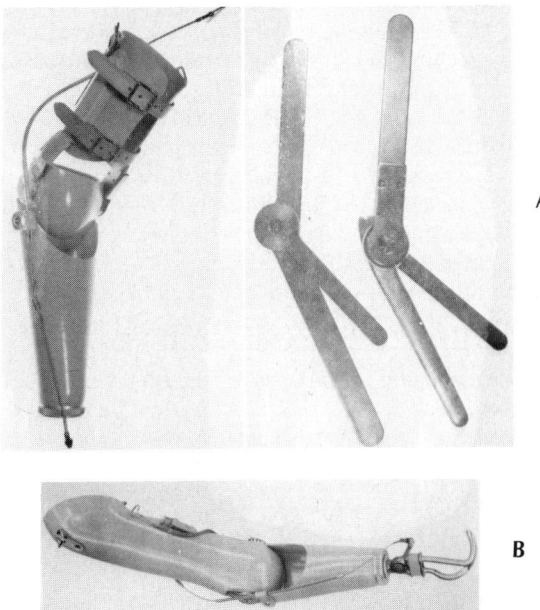

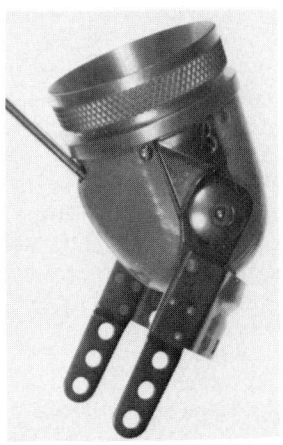

Fig. 84-22 Internal multiple-locking unit.

Fig. 84-23 **A,** Rigid, stump-activated locking hinge for very short below-elbow amputation. **B,** Outside-locking hinges used in elbow unit designed for elbow disarticulation and transconylar levels of amputation. (Courtesy Hosmer/Dorrance Corp, Campbell, Calif.)

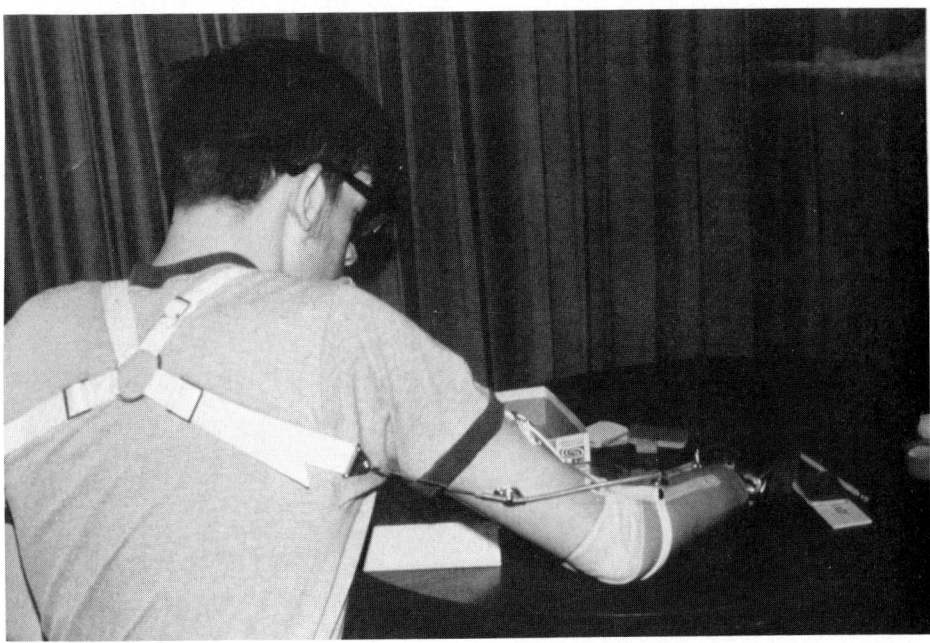

Fig. 84-24 Figure-eight harness worn by a below-elbow amputee.

Flexible sockets are also being designed for upper extremity amputees. Although the flexible socket is not as durable as the standard socket, it is lighter in weight and tends to be more comfortable because it allows for some expansion.

AMPUTEE REHABILITATION

As far back as 1918, Mayer stated that the "greatest educator of the stump is the artificial limb itself."[15] The point he was stressing so long ago was that early fitting is highly recommended whenever possible. Emphasized by Slocom[21] is the placing of the amputee "back into the normal life of his community." This goal can only be realized when the patient has a satisfactory and durable stump, a well-fitted and properly constructed prosthesis, and very diligent training in the use of his prosthesis. All these factors are interdependent and require a healthy attitude on the part of the amputee toward his disability. The "psychological" health of the patient is of utmost importance.[10]

PROSTHETIC CARE AND HYGIENE

When prosthetic training commences, the use of a T-shirt is recommended to avoid irritation from the harness. Later the use of a T-shirt is optional. Women might prefer using Kleinerts Short Sleeve Garment Shields, number 1206.*

Athletic tube socks or stump socks are generally preferred by the upper extremity amputee because they help absorb perspiration and give a sense of warmth and padding. A clean sock should be applied daily. The importance of daily stump hygiene must be stressed to avoid skin infections and irritations. The prosthetic socket should also be wiped clean daily, and the harness washed when soiled. Two harnesses should be supplied so that one can be laundered while the other is being worn.

EVALUATION AND CHECKOUT

The appearance, comfort, and function are evaluated when the prosthesis is received. The socket should closely match the color and contour of the normal limb and must be smooth with the edges slightly rolled away from the patient's skin. The length of the prosthesis is correct if the tip of the terminal device ends at the tip of the thumb on the remaining limb while the prosthesis is hanging at the patient's side.

All movable parts must function smoothly permitting maximal range of motion. The patient's ability to open the terminal device is examined at different levels of the body. There should be no sharp bends in the cable, and it should slide in and out of the casing smoothly. The control-system efficiency is a measurement to determine the amount of force lost between the terminal device and the harness. Although minimum standards are set by the prosthetic and orthotic

*Kleinerts, Inc., Kutztown, Pa.

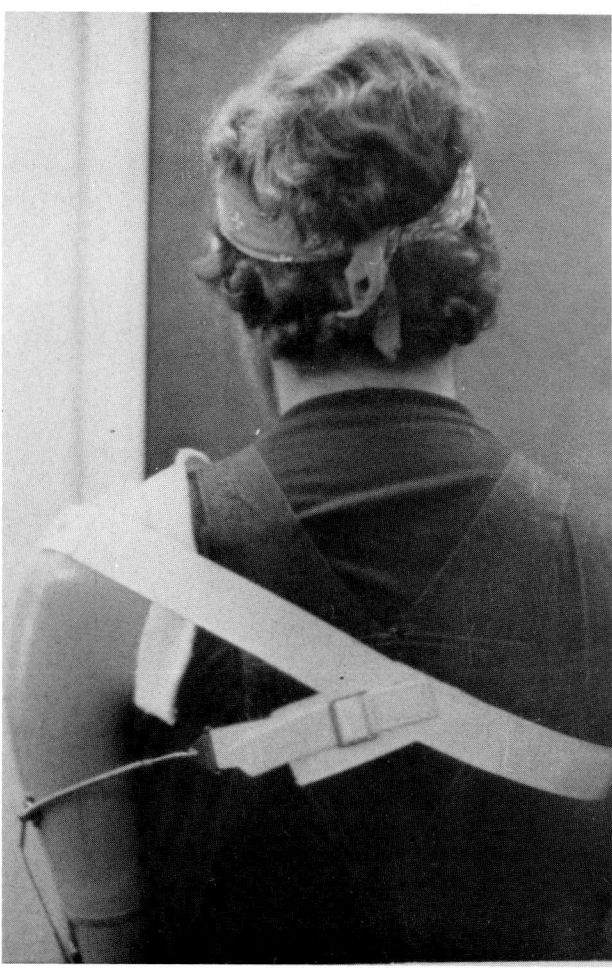

Fig. 84-25 A very short above-elbow amputee using a chest strap harness.

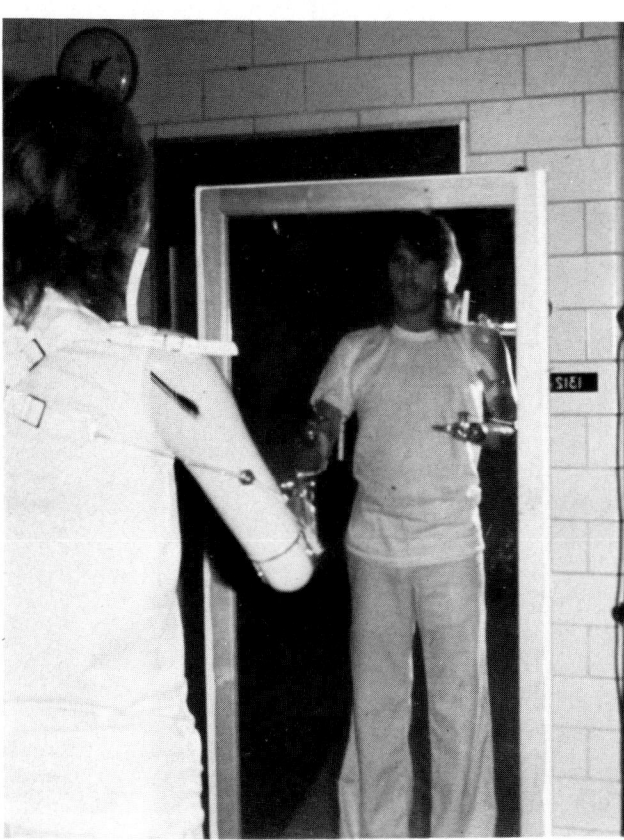

Fig. 84-26 Controls training and postural awareness.

schools, I have found that this efficiency can be increased more than 80% with the use of a Teflon-lined cable.

The points that have been mentioned here are the major areas of importance when a new prosthesis is evaluated. For complete and detailed evaluations on prosthetic efficiency and mechanical checkout, various forms are recommended and may be obtained through Northwestern University, through New York University (Prosthetic-Orthotic Center), or in Santschi's *Manual of Upper Extremity Prosthetics.*[22]

CONTROLS TRAINING

Controls training teaches the patient to be aware of the body motions necessary to operate the prosthesis. The person being trained needs to appreciate the difference between muscular contraction, holding, and relaxation, both for mo-

tion and stabilization. Training should take place in front of a mirror (Fig. 84-26) because this helps the patient develop correct posture and also a proprioceptive awareness of the limb without looking directly at the prosthesis.

With the below-elbow amputee the power is transmitted for one purpose only, prehension. A single-control system using humeral flexion is the major power source used to operate the terminal device, with the opposite shoulder acting as a stabilizer.

For the above-elbow amputee, power is transmitted to substitute for prehension, forearm motion, and elbow function. A dual-control system using humeral flexion is the major power used to operate the terminal device and forearm. The major source of body power used to operate the elbow lock is humeral extension and scapular abduction.

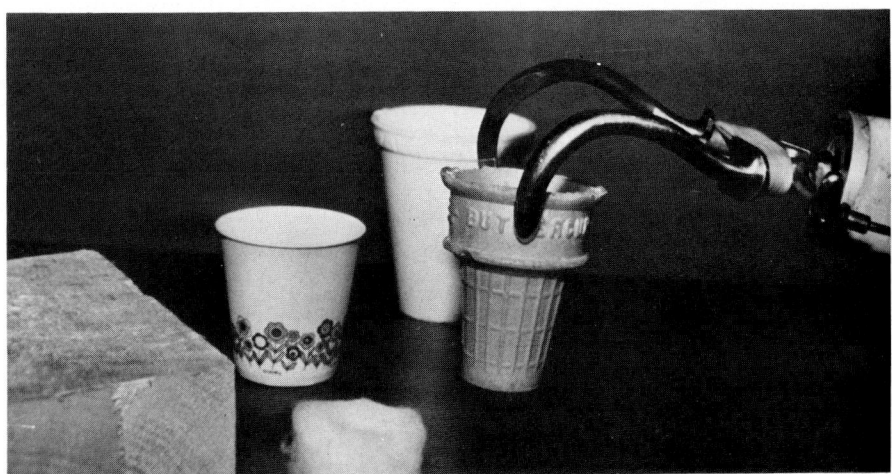

Fig. 84-27 Various weights and textures are employed for grasp and release training.

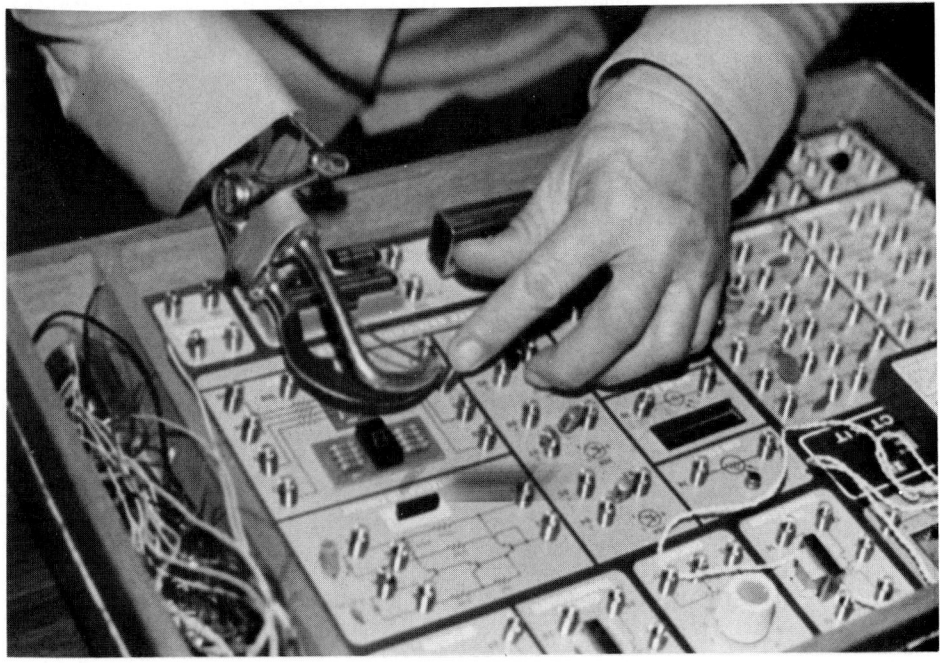

Fig. 84-28 Use training to improve speed, coordination, and dexterity.

FUNCTIONAL TRAINING
Use

Once the controls become smooth and natural and the body-controlled motions become barely perceptible, functional application commences. Activities requiring grasp and release of objects are employed, and the objects used are of various sizes, weights, and textures (Fig. 84-27). During this time close attention is given to the correct prepositioning of the terminal device to minimize unnecessary and awkward positions. As the ability to grasp and release objects improves, repetitive drills and activities are used to achieve speed, coordination, and dexterity (Fig. 84-28).

Activities of daily living

The concept of functional training is geared toward a problem-solving approach in which the patient is guided through an activity with different methods being used to determine which method is easiest and most comfortable.

The amputee will learn to develop sensory feedback through the harness, because a part of the training is learning how much tension should be exerted to hold onto varied objects (Fig. 84-29). The bilateral amputee is trained to use the longer limb with better motion as the dominant extremity.

The aim of treatment is for the patient to become as self-sufficient as possible in all aspects of daily living, including personal hygiene, eating, dressing, and household tasks (Fig. 84-30). This area of training is pursued until the patient feels confident in his abilities. The more he is able to do for himself, the more successful will be his emotional and physical rehabilitation.

Modifications in clothing may be required, as well as prosthetic adaptations and special devices for activities such as driving (Fig. 84-31). Amputees may further benefit from adaptive hand tools (Fig. 84-32).

Avocational and vocational skills are also important aspects of prosthetic training. Recreational activities with or without the use of the prosthesis are encouraged (Fig. 84-33), and the use of adaptive equipment may help the patient continue to pursue a special interest (Fig. 84-34).

Prosthetic use can help an amputee achieve a higher level of function, subsequently broadening occupational opportunities. Vocational skills are an integral aspect of training (Fig. 84-35). A study of more than 1000 industrial amputees at the Ontario Workers Compensation Bureau revealed that 89% returned to work after amputation. Amputees who reported wearing their prosthesis frequently were more likely to be employed. One might speculate that the same positive attitude and motivation required for successful prosthetic use results in a successful return to work.[16] After initial prosthetic training is successfully completed, periodic follow-up should be arranged. Follow-up evaluations are

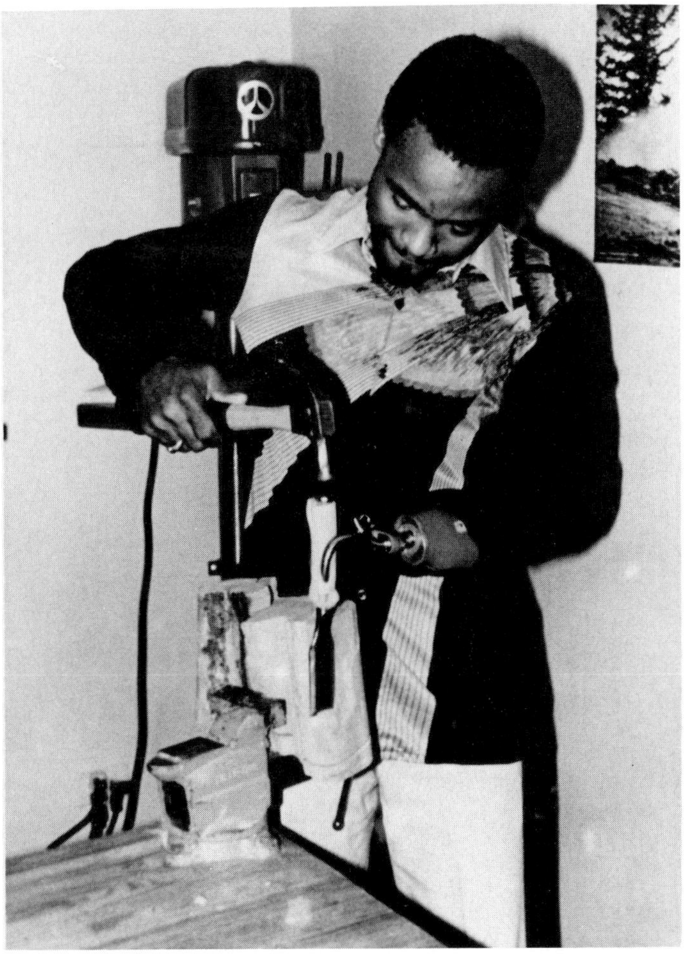

Fig. 84-29   Training should include holding a variety of objects.

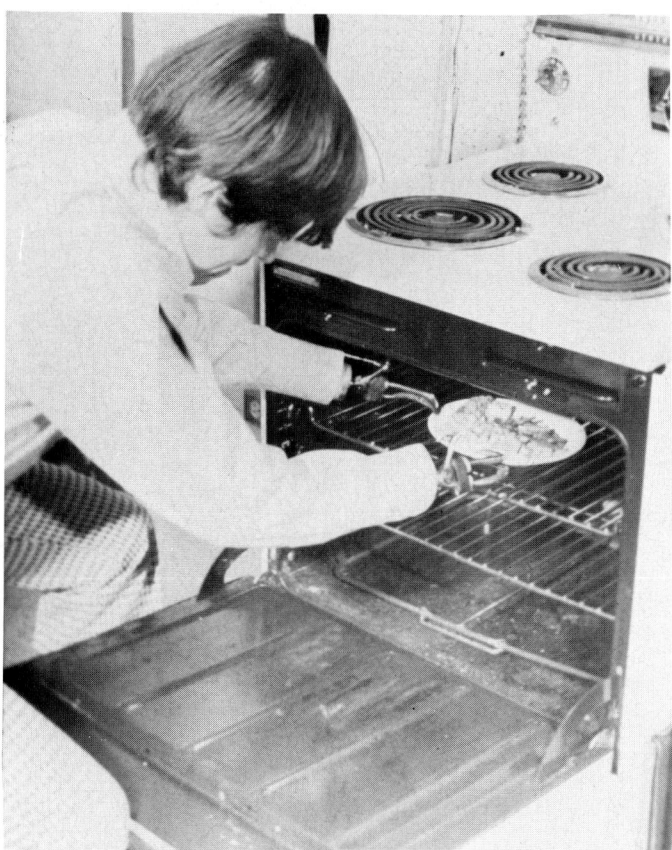

Fig. 84-30   Functional training to improve household skills and independence.

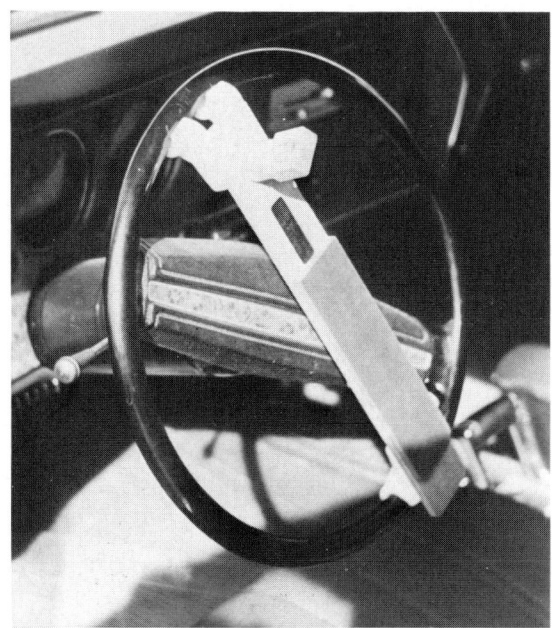

Fig. 84-31 Adaptive driving aid. (Mobility Products & Design, Inc, 709 Kentucky St, Vallejo, CA 94590.)

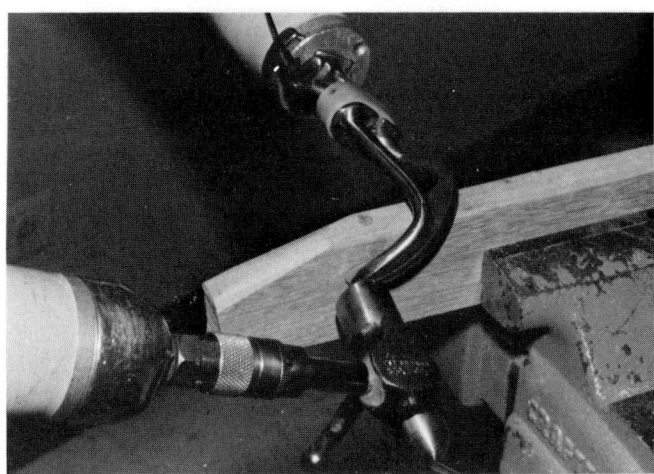

Fig. 84-32 Adaptive Ampu-Tool set. (Wright & Filippis Inc, 19326 Woodward Ave, Detroit, MI 48203.)

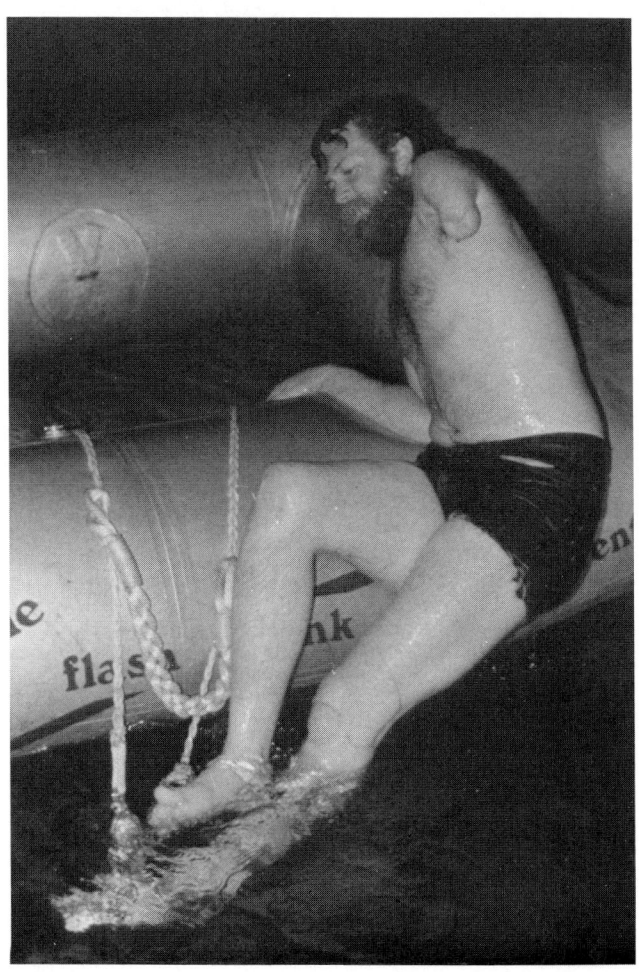

Fig. 84-33 Pursuit of certain sports without using the prosthesis is encouraged.

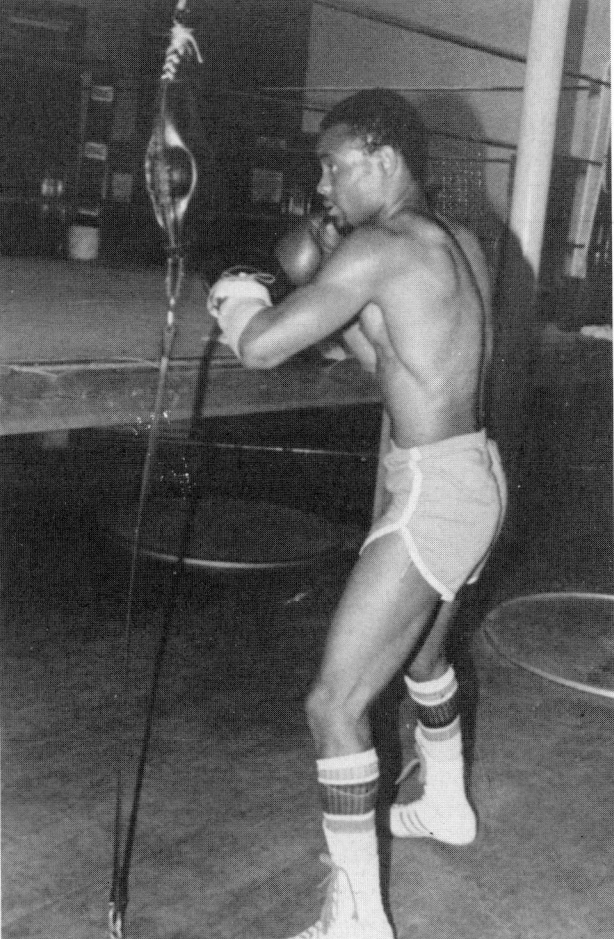

Fig. 84-34 Adaptive equipment may help a patient pursue a special interest.

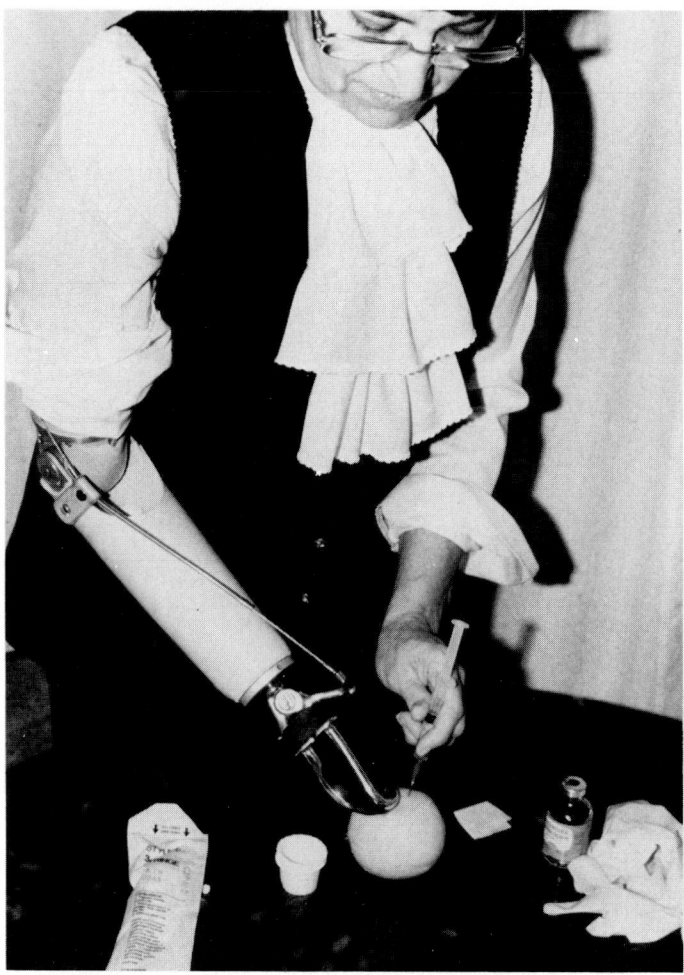

Fig. 84-35 Vocational skills are important aspects of prosthetic training.

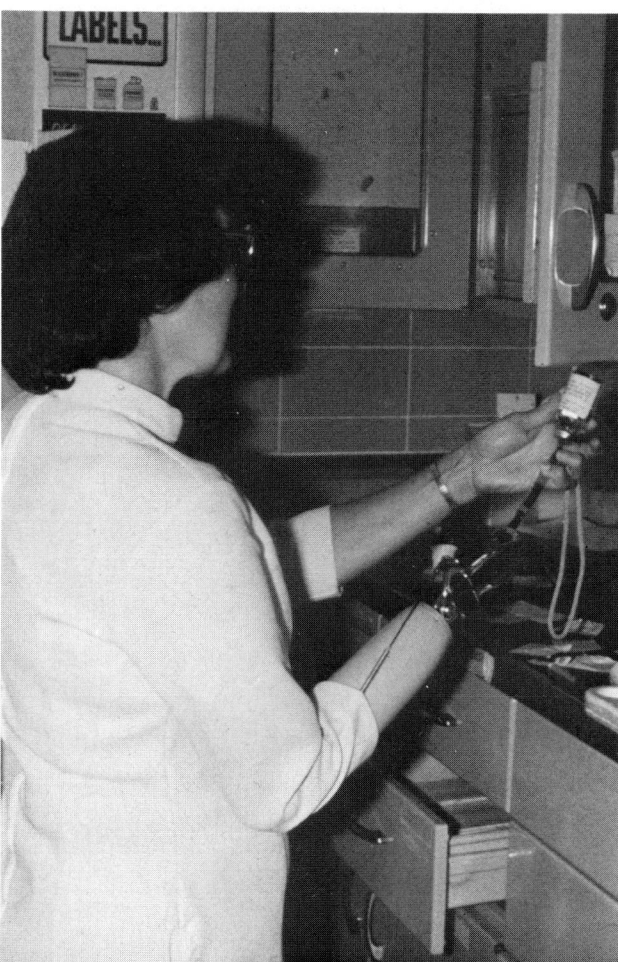

Fig. 84-36 Motivation and training result in a successful return to work.

important to assess prosthetic fit, in addition to ascertaining if functional capacity is being maintained, particularly during the first year.

CONCLUSION

Historical accounts suggest that when an artificial device is designed to replace a lost limb, the primary goal of both the designer and the amputee is to restore the function of that limb. Although there have been many recent advancements in the field of upper extremity prosthetics, there still is no prosthesis that is capable of simultaneously duplicating the function, sensibility, and cosmesis of the human hand.

According to Beasley,[4] "90% of the activities of daily living can be accomplished with one normal hand." This fact may account in part for the high percentage of upper extremity amputees who discard their prostheses. No doubt, the prognosis is influenced by the level of amputation, the quality of the stump, the quality of the prosthetic fit, and the quality of training. Certainly, the prognosis is also influenced by the social needs and the psychological adjustment of the patient. Success is more likely achieved if the patient is given a full appreciation of the limitations of the prosthesis both functionally and cosmetically. Once the limb

is fitted, training should include the establishment of the desire within the patient to make the effort required to accept the prosthesis as a functional part of himself. The skill with which the patient is trained may well be the difference between acceptance and rejection of the limb.

REFERENCES

1. Baumgartner RF: Active and carrier-tool prosthesis for upper limb amputation, Orthop Clin North Am 12:961, 1981.
2. Baumgartner RF: Management of bilateral upper limb amputees, Orthop Clin North Am 12:971, 1981.
3. Baumgartner RF: The surgery of arm and forearm amputations, Orthop Clin North Am 12:805, 1981.
4. Beasley RW: General considerations in managing upper limb amputations, Orthop Clin North Am 12:743, 1981.
5. Burgess EM: Current status of immediate post-surgical prosthetics, Newsletter of the Amputee Clinics 4:11, 1972.
6. Burgess EM: General principles of amputation surgery and postoperative management. In American Academy of Orthopaedic Surgeons: Atlas of limb prosthetics, St Louis, 1981. The CV Mosby Co.
7. Burgess EM: Principles of amputation surgery in upper limb. In American Academy of Orthopaedic Surgeons: Atlas of limb prosthetics, St Louis 1981, The CV Mosby Co.
8. Burkhalter W, Hampton F, and Smeltzer J: Wrist disarticulation and below-elbow and shoulder disarticulation and forequarter amputation. In American Academy of Orthopaedic Surgeons: Atlas of limb prosthetics, St Louis, 1981, The CV Mosby Co.

9. Frazier SH and Kolb CC: Psychiatric aspects of pain and the phantom limb, Orthop Clin North Am 1:481, 1970.
10. Friedman LW: The surgical rehabilitation of the amputee, Springfield, Ill, 1978, Charles C Thomas, Publisher.
11. Fryer C: Upper limb prosthetic components. In American Academy of Orthopaedic Surgeons: Atlas of limb prosthetics, St Louis, 1981, The CV Mosby Co.
12. Körner L: Afferent electrical nerve stimulation for sensory feedback in hand prostheses: clinical and physiological aspects, Orthop Scand Suppl 178:52, 1979.
13. Kritter AE: The bilateral upper extremity amputee. Orthop Clin North Am 3:397, 1972.
14. Law HT: Engineering of upper limb prostheses. Orthop Clin North Am 12:929, 1981.
15. Mayer L: The orthopedic treatment of gunshot injuries. Philadelphia, 1918, WB Saunders Co.
16. Millstein S, Bain D, and Hunter GA: A review of employment patterns of industrial amputees: factors influencing rehabilitation, Prosthet Orthot Int 9:67, 1985.
17. Omer G: Nerve, neuroma and pain problems related to upper limb amputations, Orthop Clin North Am 12:751, 1981.
18. Pillet J: The aesthetic hand prosthesis, Orthop Clin North Am 12:961, 1981.
19. Peizer E: Research trends in upper limb prosthetics. In American Academy of Orthopaedic Surgeons: Atlas of limb prosthetics, St Louis, 1981, The CV Mosby Co.
20. Rang M and Thompson G: History of amputations and prostheses. In Kostuik J, editor: Amputation surgery and rehabilitation: the Toronto experience, New York, 1981, Churchill Livingstone, Inc.
21. Slocum DB: An atlas of amputations, St Louis, 1949, The CV Mosby Co.
22. Santschi WR: Manual of upper extremity prosthetics, ed 2. Berkeley, 1958, University of California Press.
23. VanLunteren A and others: A field evaluation of arm prostheses for unilateral amputees, Prosthet Orthot Int 7:150, 1983.
24. Wilson AB: The modern history of amputation surgery and artificial limbs, Orthop Clin North Am 3:276, 1972.

BIBLIOGRAPHY

Barcome DF and Eickman L: Prosthetic management of high bilateral upper limb amputees, Orthop Prosthes 34:22, 1981.

Beasley R and de Bese G: Upper limb amputations and prostheses, Orthop Clin North Am 17:3, 1986.

Bender LF: Prostheses and rehabilitation after arm amputation, Springfield, Ill, 1974, Charles C Thomas, Publisher.

Burgess EM: Immediate postsurgical prosthetic fitting: a system of amputee management, Phys Ther 51:139, 1971.

Charles D, James K, and Stein R: Rehabilitation of musicians with upper limb amputations, J Rehabil 25:3, 1988.

Clippinger FW, Avery R, and Titus B: A sensory feedback system for an upper-limb amputation prosthesis, Bull Prosthet Res 10:247, 1974.

Derenzy GW: Enchiridion: or a hand for the one-handed, London, 1822, Underwood, Publisher.

Edwards JW: Orthopaedic appliance atlas, vol 2, Ann Arbor, Mich, 1960, American Academy of Orthopaedic Surgeons.

Ficarra BI: Amputations and prostheses through the centuries, Med Rec 156:94, 1943.

Graupe D and others: A multifunctional prosthesis control system based on time series identification of EMG signals using microprocessors, Bull Prosthet Res 10:4, 1977.

Harris R: Common stump problems. In Kostuik J, editor: Amputation surgery and rehabilitation: the Toronto experience, New York, 1981, Churchill Livingstone, Inc.

Harris R: Principles of amputation surgery. In Kostuik J, editor: Amputation surgery and rehabilitation: the Toronto experience, New York, 1981, Churchill Livingstone, Inc.

Hunter G and others: The upper limb amputee: experience of the Workman's Compensation Board of Ontario Amputee Team. In Kostuik J, editor: Amputation surgery and rehabilitation: the Toronto experience, New York, 1981, Churchill Livingstone, Inc.

Kato I: Trends in powered upper limb prostheses, Prosthet Orthot Int 2:64, 1978.

LaBlanc KP and Mason CP: The VAPC functional elbow orthosis, Orthop Prosthet 34:13, 1980.

Lamb D: Prosthetics in the upper extremity, J Hand Surg 8:5, 1983.

Marshall M: 1981. The upper extremity in children. In Kostuik J, editor: Amputation surgery and rehabilitation: the Toronto experience, New York, 1981, Churchill Livingstone, Inc.

MacDonald J: History of artificial limbs, Am J Surg 19:76, 1905.

Mason CP: Practical problems in myoelectric control of prosthesis, Bull Prosthet Res 10:39, 1970.

Mital M and Pierce D: Amputees and their prostheses, Boston, 1971, Little, Brown & Co.

Northmore-Ball M, Heger H, and Hunter G: The below-elbow myoelectric prosthesis, J Bone Joint Surg 62:3, 1980.

Prior R and Lyman J: Electrocutaneous feedback for artificial limbs: summary progress report (Feb 1, 1974-July 31, 1975), Bull Prosthet Res 10:3, 1975.

Prior R and Lyman J: Supplemental sensory feedback for the VA/NU myoelectric hand: background and preliminary designs. Bull Prosthet Res 10:170, 1976.

Sherman and others: Phantom pain: a lesson in the necessity for careful clinical research on chronic pain problems, J Rehabil 25:2, 1988.

Stein R and Walley M: Functional comparison of upper extremity amputees using myoelectric and conventional prostheses, Arch Phys Med Rehab 64:29, 1983.

85

Prosthetic management of complete hand and arm deficiencies

John N. Billock

Advancements in the development of prosthetic control systems and components over the past 25 to 30 years have led to a considerable transition in the clinical management and rehabilitation of individuals with acquired and/or congenital complete hand and arm deficiencies. The introduction of electric-powered control systems and components, along with the previously existing variety of bowden cable control systems and mechanical components, has greatly increased the complexity of determining the most appropriate design for a functional upper limb prosthesis. The variety of myoelectric and electric switch control systems for actuating an electric-powered elbow, wrist, and hand or hook component has also led to advancements in the clinical assessment procedures and prosthetic interfacing techniques traditionally used in the design and development of upper limb prostheses. The use of diagnostic interfaces and diagnostic prostheses, as well as temporary prostheses, has become essential in the proper assessment of an individual's particular needs and functional capabilities. These diagnostic and clinical assessment procedures have become key factors in appropriately determining the specific design of an individual's definitive prosthesis and the successful management of his rehabilitation.

INITIAL REHABILITATION CONSIDERATIONS

Planning prosthetic rehabilitation management and care first requires a thorough understanding of the individual's physiologic, social-psychological, vocational, and avocational needs. The social-psychological aspects of the individual's disability will initially become the most significant problem to deal with and must be appropriately understood if successful prosthetic rehabilitation and functional use of a prosthesis is to be achieved. The congenital or acquired absence of any portion of the hand and arm results in a significantly visible and functional disability. If an individual does not accept the loss or absence of a limb, it is unlikely successful prosthetic rehabilitation and functional use of a prosthesis will be achieved. In the case of a child with a congenital limb deficiency or a traumatic limb loss, the parents' acceptance must become the primary focus. Dembo, Leviton, and Wright[10] clearly identified the social-psychological problems that individuals, as well as those around them, have to deal with in accepting a limb loss and the importance those problems play in the total rehabilitation process.

Dr. Howard A. Rusk, recognized by many as the "father of physical medicine and rehabilitation," identified motivation and timely rehabilitation services as being key elements to achieving successful rehabilitation of an individ-

ual's disability.[17,18] An individual can receive the best rehabilitation services available and be provided with the best prosthesis today's technology has to offer; however, if he is not motivated toward accepting the disability and adjusting to it, acceptable rehabilitation is unlikely. Likewise, the child born with a congenital limb deficiency will not be encouraged to adapt to or functionally use a prosthesis if the parents have not accepted their child's disability or the prosthesis.

The hand and arm represent the most complex and challenging structure of the body to replace and restore with a functional external prosthesis. The human hand itself is an extremely complex terminal device, which moves with a precision and dexterity that has long challenged the minds of researchers in medicine and engineering. Beyond its kinematic capabilities, the hand is also one of the most complex sensory mechanisms of the human body with proprioceptive and sensory feedback capabilities that are unequaled. With this in mind, it is not difficult to understand why hand and hook prosthetic terminal devices of today offer very little in the way of true functional restoration to individuals with upper limb or complete hand deficiencies. This is not meant to be critical of past developments but to put into proper perspective the complexities and challenges of duplicating the human hand. Further emphasis of this is identified by Murphy,[16] who stated, "Though engineers and prosthetists have made substantial contributions, they need perspective and humility to inspire and guide the very long, sustained efforts required to replace even a few of the roles of the hand." This challenge will no doubt continue to keep researchers in prosthetics, and now those involved in robotics, busy with the task of trying to duplicate the kinematic and sensory capabilities of the human hand for years to come.

TRAUMATIC UPPER LIMB AMPUTATIONS

In cases involving traumatic upper limb amputations, it is important to appropriately and knowledgeably address the individual's prosthetic rehabilitation needs because of the combined medical, physiologic, and psychological aspects of his disability. Because of the complexities involved in designing and developing an appropriate upper limb prosthesis, a thorough understanding of an individual's needs and expected capabilities is essential before a rehabilitation plan and development of a prosthesis can be pursued. A thorough review of the individual's admission history and physical and operative reports relative to the amputation can provide valuable information for planning meaningful prosthetic rehabilitation goals and objectives. Close interaction

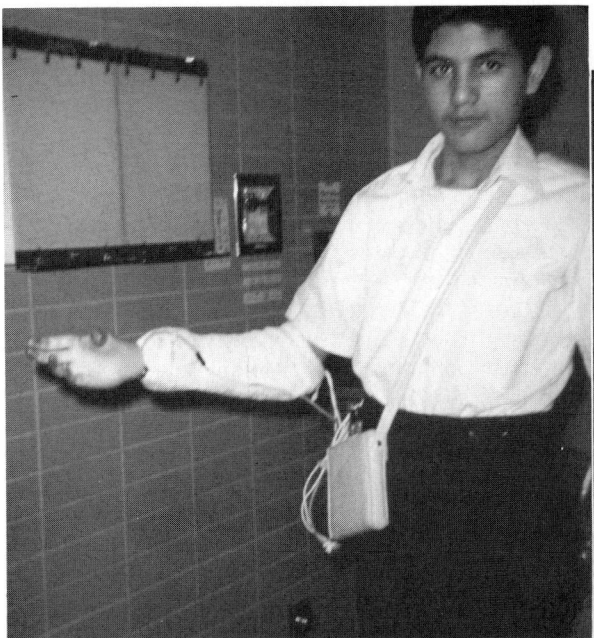
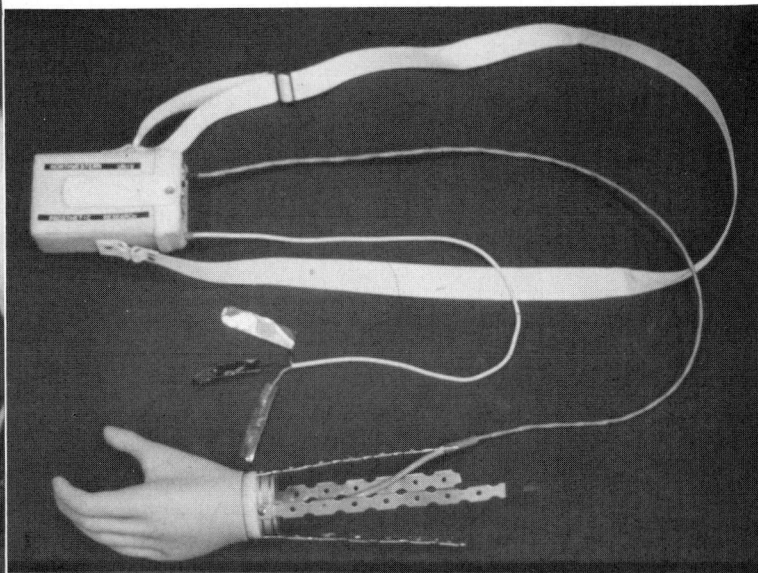

A
B

Fig. 85-1   **A,** Patient provided with an immediate postsurgical below-elbow myoelectrically controlled hand prosthesis. Surface EMG electrode wires extend from the plaster prosthetic interface to a shoulder-sling–supported container, which houses the electronic components and batteries of the system. **B,** The basic components of the immediate postsurgical system include an electric-powered hand, stainless steel foil EMG electrode set, and the myoelectric control system.

between the attending physician, prosthetist, and therapist becomes essential in establishing realistic rehabilitation goals and objectives that will be consistent with an individual's prognosis and overall medical condition. This close interactioin is particularly important when an immediate or early fitting prosthesis is being considered, and it should begin to involve other appropriate members of the rehabilitation team, such as a psychologist, rehabilitation counselor, rehabilitation nurse, and social worker. The early introduction of an immediate or early postsurgical prosthesis, illustrated in Fig. 85-1, can be extremely beneficial, as indicated by Childress and associates[8] and Malone and others[15]; however, if the individual's condition is not appropriately managed, the results can be meaningless and even detrimental. Additionally, a thorough understanding of the factors affecting an individual's social-psychological status relative to his limb loss becomes essential in planning meaningful goals and objectives. Again, it is important to understand that the social-psychological aspects of an upper-limb amputation can present the greatest barriers an individual must overcome if successful prosthetic management and rehabilitation are to be achieved. Personal acceptance of the disability and motivation to return to society is essential to successful rehabilitation.

CONGENITAL LIMB DEFICIENCIES

The complexities of designing and developing an appropriate prosthesis for a child with a congenital limb deficiency are similar to that of the adult; however, the social-psychological aspects of the parents' acceptance of their child's disability also must become the primary focus of the re-

habilitation process. In the case of a child, the early introduction of a passive hand prosthesis by at least the age of 3 months, provided there are no medical contraindications, can be extremely helpful to the parents' adjustment to their child's disability. Further, the early introduction of the prosthesis enhances the child's acceptance during the key developmental stages of early childhood. Along with this, it is equally important for parents to understand the future course of their child's prosthetic management. A passive hand prosthesis will address initial concern regarding aesthetics and begin to develop the child's tolerance to a prosthesis. The passive hand will also provide gross opposition during the early developmental stages of eye-hand coordination. Consideration for introduction of a functional hand prosthesis should occur at or before 6 months of age, depending on the child's status of normal childhood and gross motor development. Typically, a child develops gross palmar prehension and hand dominance at approximately 8 months of age as indicated by Erhardt;[11] therefore the prosthetic rehabilitation plan should be consistent with this.

The role of the child's prosthesis and the parents' acceptance of it cannot be overemphasized. If the parents do not accept the prosthesis, their adjustment to their child's disability will be more difficult and they will not encourage the child's use of and normal development with the prosthesis. The acceptance of the child's disability and prosthesis by immediate family members and friends also plays an important role in the parents' and child's acceptance. Many chidren, as well as adults, have rejected a prosthesis, not because of their own feelings, but because of the reactions of others.

TERMINAL DEVICE CONSIDERATIONS

There exists today a significant number of upper limb prosthetic terminal devices for treating both adult and juvenile complete hand deficiencies. These terminal devices are designed as either mechanical or electromechanical systems and are either biomechanically or electrically powered. Biomechanically powered terminal devices function by using forces generated through body movement or motion as described by Taylor.[23,24] An electric-powered terminal device functions by using the electrical energy stored within a battery to generate force. Further, these sources of power can be used in different ways to activate or control a terminal device. The three most commonly used control systems are bowden cable control, myoelectric control, and switch control. To fully understand the functional potential of a particular terminal device, one must understand the control approach or system being used to actuate the device.

Although controversy continues regarding the appropriateness and functionality of a hand or hook terminal device, it is important to realistically assess and understand an individual's social-psychological, vocational, and avocational needs. The terminal device is the most important component of the prosthesis, just as the hand is the most important part of the normal upper limb. The prosthetic terminal device should be thought of as an assistive device to the sound hand, just as the nondominant normal hand is to the dominant normal hand. Many have felt that the ability to perform fine motor prehension activities with a prosthetic terminal device is important, and this has been a major argument in favor of hook terminal devices. The majority of individuals with upper limb deficiencies are, however, unilaterally involved and do not use their prosthesis for fine motor prehension activities, just as one does not typically use his nondominant hand for such activities. The prosthetic terminal device is most important for gross grasp and release prehension activities, such as holding and stabilizing objects while the sound hand performs the fine motor prehension activities. An electric-powered hand terminal device, with adequately controlled functional prehension, will best serve this need for the majority of tasks performed during activities of daily living.

Billock[2,3] and Sauter[19] have indicated that an electric-powered hand should be considered first over a hook terminal device because of the forceful prehension it provides and its obvious aesthetic value in consideration of the individual's social-psychological needs. Their clinical experiences have indicated that an electrically powered prosthetic hand terminal device, which is controlled using myoelectric electromyographic (EMG) potentials from opposing muscle groups within the residual limb, provides one of the most acceptable and functional upper limb prostheses. Their philosophy is largely based on the fact that almost everything we encounter in our activities of daily living is designed to be held in a hand and most individuals, for aesthetic reasons, would prefer to have a hand over a hook terminal device.

These criteria are obviously not the case for everyone with an upper limb deficiency. However, it is felt to be true for the majority and especially those with unilateral upper limb involvement. If the individual's vocational and avocational needs clearly indicate the need for a hook terminal device, this must be clinically tested and proven or the individual must personally desire the hook terminal device.

Again, it must be remembered that the individual's social-psychological needs should be of primary concern initially and should be taken into consideration before vocational and avocational needs can be effectively addressed.

PROSTHETIC EVALUATION AND ASSESSMENT

With adequate information gathered in the initial prosthetic evaluation, further clinical assessment and evaluation procedures should be carried out to determine the most appropriate residual limb interface, control source, and components for use in the development of the prosthesis. This should initially involve the development of a diagnostic interface for evaluating the desired fitting and suspension technique to be used in the design of the prosthesis. A variety of interface designs and suspension techniques exist for both adults and juveniles at all levels of upper limb deficiencies that require the development of an appropriate diagnostic interface. The development of a diagnostic interface, illustrated in Fig. 85-2, is also necessary for use in determining definitive EMG potential sites when myoelectric control is being considered. If EMG potentials are not adequate and the patient requires further EMG testing and biofeedback controls training, the diagnostic interface becomes essential for maintaining consistent muscle potential sites. The diagnostic interface further allows the practitioner to specifically evaluate optional control sources and components by developing a diagnostic prosthesis (Fig. 85-3). This further allows training before the actual prosthesis is put on and evaluation of the total prosthesis before the development of a definitive prosthesis is carried out. The diagnostic prosthesis is also essential in evaluating hybrid and system design approaches for the definitive prosthesis.

PROSTHETIC CONTROL SYSTEMS

Professional opinions vary considerably regarding the most appropriate control system to use in the design and development of a functional upper limb prosthesis. Bowden cable control systems harness the biomechanical motions and forces generated by gross body movements to actuate

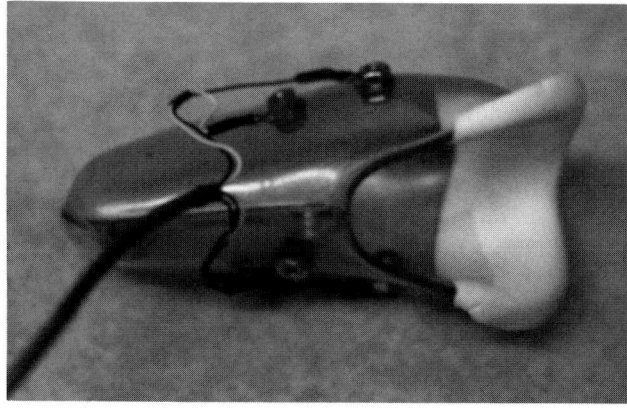

Fig. 85-2 A transparent diagnostic-type residual limb interface allows visual analysis of possible localized tissue and skeletal pressure points. Also, soft tissue changes that occur during muscle contractions or as external forces are applied to the interface can be more appropriately assessed. The interface shown includes surface-type EMG electrodes for assessment of myoelectric control and a supracondylar interface liner.

Fig. 85-3 **A,** A diagnostic prosthesis consists of the diagnostic residual limb interface attached to a temporary forearm segment and terminal device. This allows assessment of the functional control, acceptance of the prosthesis, and the length and angular alignment of the terminal device. **B,** This diagnostic prosthesis on a 22-month-old child is being assessed for the development of a self-contained and self-suspended hybrid-type, two-site/two-function myoelectrically controlled electric-powered hand prosthesis. The interface also includes a supracondylar interface liner for growth adjustability and comfort.

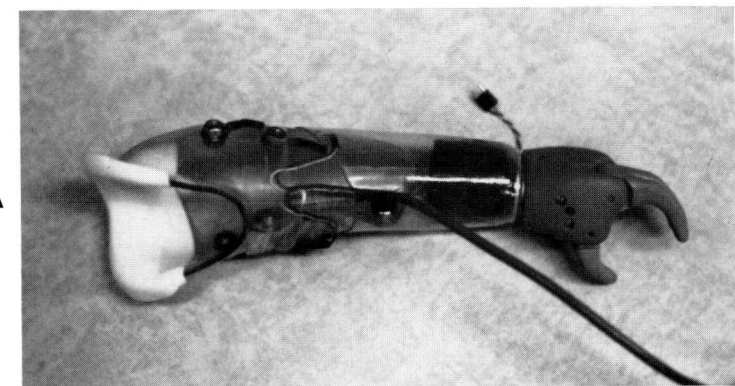

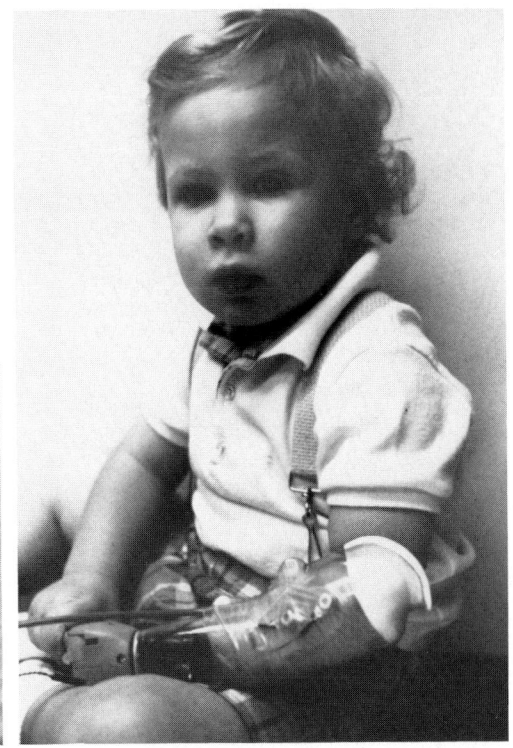

and control a mechanical elbow and/or hook or hand terminal device. These devices require an adequate degree of force and excursion to achieve actuation and functional control of a mechanical upper limb prosthesis as described by Gwynne[12] and Taylor.[23,24] The most common example of this would be the bowden cable control system of a totally mechanical below-elbow prosthesis (Fig. 85-4).

This type of bowden cable control system harnesses the biomechanical motion and forces generated primarily by shoulder flexion-abduction movements for acutation and control of the terminal device. Biscapular abduction and

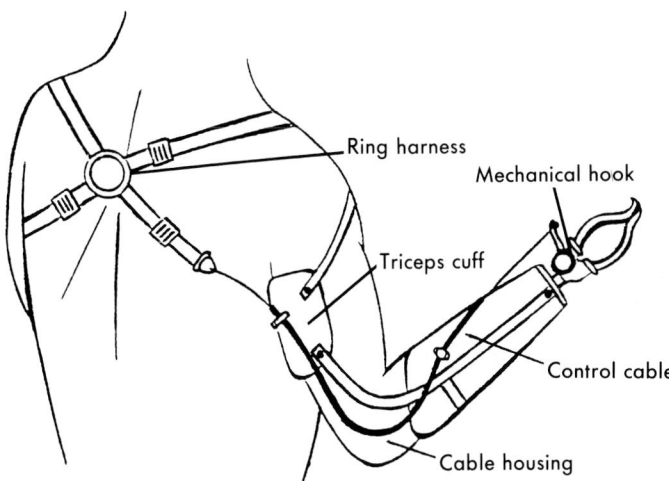

Fig. 85-4 A typical, conventional-type, body-powered Bowden cable-controlled below-elbow prosthesis with a mechanical hook terminal device actuated by "gross" body movements. (From Billock JN: Upper limb prosthetic terminal devices: hands versus hooks, Clin Prosthet Orthot 10(2):59, 1986. Published by the American Orthotic and Prosthetic Assoc., Alexandria, Va.)

elbow flexion movements can also be used to further augment actuation and control of the terminal device. Additionally, the forces and excursion generated in this manner can be used for actuation of either a voluntary opening or voluntary closing mechanical hook or hand terminal device. It is important to note this form of control does produce a certain degree of sensory feedback, related to force and position, through the control system harness because of its contact with the body.

Myoelectric control systems use EMG potentials generated from the residual neuromuscular system for actuation and control of an electromechanical terminal device. A typical myoelectrically controlled below-elbow prosthesis is illustrated in Fig. 85-5. EMG potentials are monitored with skin suface electrodes placed over appropriate agonist-antagonist muscles and/or muscle groups within the residual limb and are used for either digital or proportional control of an electric-powered terminal device. In the below-elbow prosthesis, as illustrated in Fig. 85-5, EMG potentials from the forearm flexors would be used to close the hand and the forearm extensors to open the hand. This type of control is considered to be quite natural, since it uses the existing residual neuromuscular system and provides voluntary control of both opening and closing of the terminal device, which is not achievable in a bowden cable control system control.[2-4] This is especially true when synergistic muscle contractions, particularly those related to natural hand functions, can be selected for actuation and control of the terminal device. The use of myoelectric control enhances the feasibility of designing a totally self-contained and self-suspended prosthesis, which has proven to be an acceptable and reliable design approach.[1-3,5,6,8,9]

Myoelectric control systems can vary considerably depending on the desired function and availability of adequate EMG potential sites to actuate various electric powered com-

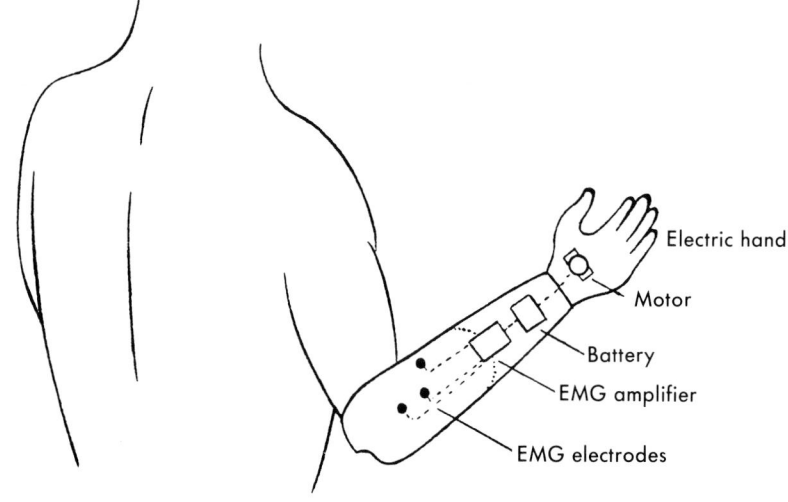

Fig. 85-5 A typical, electric-powered, myoelectrically controlled below-elbow prosthesis with an electromechanical hand terminal device actuated by EMG potentials. (From Billock JN: Upper limb prosthetic terminal devices: hands versus hooks, Clin Prosthet Orthot 10(2):59, 1986, Published by the American Orthotic and Prosthetic Assoc., Alexandria, Va.)

Electric hand

Motor

Battery

EMG amplifier

EMG electrodes

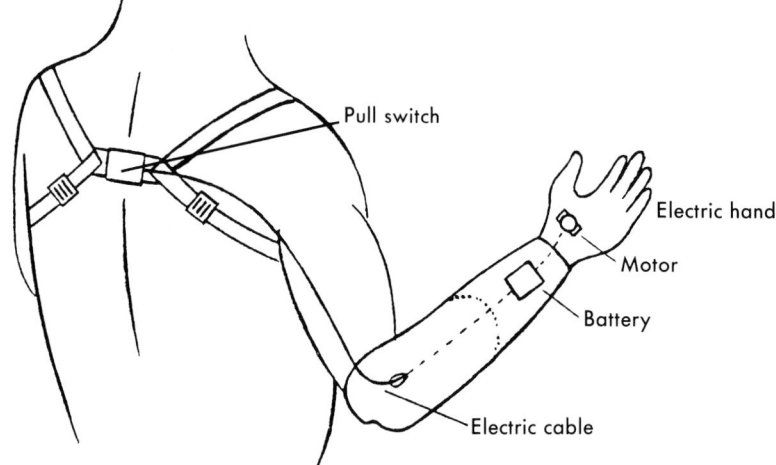

Fig. 85-6 A typical, electric-powered, switch-controlled below-elbow prosthesis with electromechanical hand terminal device actuated by "fine" body movements. (From Billock JN: Upper limb prosthetic terminal devices: hands versus hooks, Clin Prosthet Orthot 10(2):59, 1986, Published by the American Orthotic and Prosthetic Assoc., Alexandria, Va.)

Pull switch

Electric hand

Motor

Battery

Electric cable

ponents of a prosthesis. In some cases, it is necessary to use more than one type of myoelectric control system to achieve the desired functions in a total prosthesis. This is referred to as a *hybrid* control approach. Some myoelectric systems use a single EMG potential from a single site to control a single function.

The Otto Bock* and Veterans Administration–Northwestern University (VA-NU) myoelectric control systems use two EMG potential sites to control two functions, hand opening and hand closing. This type of control is referred to as two site–two function myoelectric control. The University of New Brunswick (UNB) system, described by Scott,[21,22] uses a single EMG potential from a single site to control two functions. This system uses one EMG potential site to control two functions. This is achieved by a light or low level contraction to produce one function and a strong or high level contraction to produce another function. This type of control is referred to as one site–two function myoelectric control. Another common system is the *Utah arm* myoelectric control system, as described by Jacobson and associates,[13] which requires two EMG potential sites to con-

trol actuation of an electric-powered terminal device and elbow. In this system, each EMG potential site controls opposing functions of either the terminal device or elbow, equaling four independent functions. A fifth function requires a cocontraction of the opposing muscle sites to unlock the elbow. The system is either in the terminal device mode or elbow mode. The elbow automatically locks when stopped for a specified period of time and switches to the terminal device mode. This myoelectric control technique is referred to as two site–five function myoelectric control.

Switch control systems are those that use the motions and forces generated by fine body movements to actuate and control an electromechanical component. They require considerably less force and excursion than a bowden cable control system to actuate and control the component. A typical switch-controlled below-elbow prosthesis is illustrated in Fig. 85-6. Switch control systems can incorporate a variety of different types of switches, such as, pull, rocker, push-button, or toggle switch for activation of the terminal device. A basic example of these types of switches is illustrated in Fig. 85-7. This type of control is typically indicated in situations where limited biomechanical movement and force are available for bowden cable control and/or EMG potentials are inadequate or inappropriate for myo-

---

*Otto Bock Orthopaedic Industry, Inc., Duterstat, West Germany, and Minneapolis.

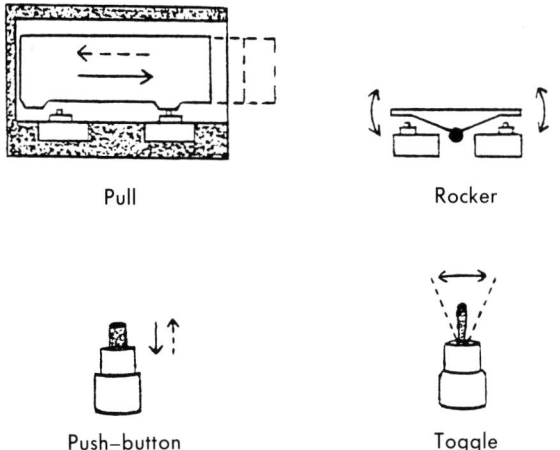

Fig. 85-7 The actuation characteristics of typical pull-type, rocker-type, push-button, and toggle-type switches are illustrated. Switches are generally designed to produce one or more functions with considerably less force and excursion than a Bowden cable-controlled prosthesis. (From Billock, JN: Upper limb prosthetic terminal devices: hands versus hooks, Clin Prosthet Orthot 10(2):59, 1986, Published by the American Orthotic and Prosthetic Assoc., Alexandria, Va.)

electric control of an electric-powered component.

Switch control systems also vary considerably depending on the desired function and availability of biomechanical force and excursion to actuate them. In many cases, to achieve the desired functions in a switch-controlled prosthesis, various types of switch control systems must be incorporated by using a hybrid design approach. The most commonly used switch control system has a pull switch actuated by a single body motion to actuate two functions, such as hand opening and hand closing. This switch control technique is referred to as one motion–two function pull switch control. Another type of system has a push-button switch actuated also by one body motion to acutate one function of the prosthesis and, in most cases, another push-button switch to operate the opposing function. It is suggested that this switch control technique be referred to as one motion–one function push-button switch control. Another common control system has a rocker switch actuated by two body motions to actuate two functions in the prosthesis, which in most cases oppose each other. This control technique is referred to as two motion–two function rocker switch control. In all multifunction switch control systems, the first active position should close the terminal device to avoid inadvertent release of an object or extension of the elbow to keep the terminal device from flexing into the individual.

MECHANICAL TERMINAL DEVICES

After World War II and especially since the development of the APRL Voluntary Closing Hand and Hook in 1945, considerable controversy has existed regarding the functional aspects of hands versus hooks as prosthetic terminal devices. Before the introduction and clinical use of electric hands in the early 1960s, this controversy related only to mechanical hands and hooks. Mechanical hands, although certainly more aesthetic, were felt by many professionals

to be too heavy and awkward for fine prehension activities. A mechanical hook, on the other hand, weighs approximately one third as much as a mechanical hand and provides the dexterity of a pair of tweezers. Mechanical hooks were also considered to be more durable because of their simplistic mechanical design and the lack of need for an external cover to protect internal mechanisms or provide aesthetics. Because of the functional advanatages of the mechanical hook versus the hand, very little regard was given to the social-psychological advantage and need of a prosthetic hand. In fact, it became common practice within prosthetic clinics and teaching institutions to encourage the use of a hook terminal device first before providing the individual with a hand terminal device. The primary purpose of this practice, which continues to some degree today, was to develop the individual's appreciation for the functional advantage of the mechanical hook over the mechanical hand. Further, it was the opinion and experience of many physicians and prosthetists that many individuals, if provided a hand and hook terminal device simultaneously, tended to reject the hook for aesthetic reasons and not develop an appreciation for its functional advantages. As Le Blanc[14] reports, conservative estimates indicate that approximately only 50% of those individuals provided with the conventional type of mechanical prostheses are wearing them; however, this does not relate to actual functional use versus simply wearing the prosthesis. Billock[3] has reported that the introduction of a hook terminal device in the early stages of the prosthetic rehabilitation process may, in fact, be the primary cause of the high incidence of total prosthetic rejection because this philosophy does not address social-psychological aspects of the individual's disability.

The most commonly used mechanical terminal devices today are classified as either voluntary opening or voluntary closing. The Hosmer-Dorrance* hook terminal devices, illustrated in Fig. 85-8, have been the most widely used in the United States since World War II.

Another mechanical terminal device widely used is a

---

*Hosmer-Dorrance Corp., Campbell, Calif.

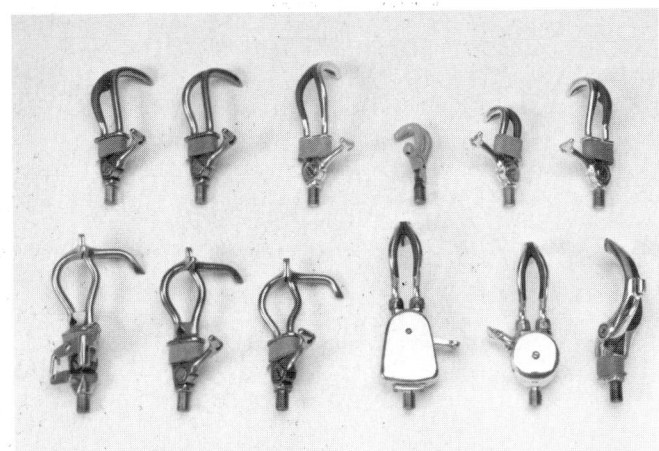

Fig. 85-8 The Hosmer/Dorrance hook terminal devices are available in a variety of materials, shapes, and sizes that can be matched to the particular functional needs of a child or adult. (Courtesy of Hosmer-Dorrance Corp.)

grasping device referred to as the GRIP.* The GRIP device provides voluntary prehension control to achieve a variety of specific functional activities as illustrated in Fig. 85-9. This device uses a shoulder harness and bowden cable control system for actuation. The advantage of this device is felt to be the provision of a greater degree of proprioceptive feedback for the individual through the harness and cable system because of the voluntary prehension control. Additionally, this device has proven to be highly functional for physically active individuals who require a rugged terminal device.

Mechanical hands, although not widely accepted as previously indicated, continue to be used by certain individuals for very specific reasons. For example, most individuals

---

*GRIP Therapeutic Recreation Systems, Inc., Boulder, Colo.

who prefer and require a mechanical hook terminal device will use a mechanical hand for social occasions when the aesthetics of the prosthesis is essential. Totally passive non-functional hand terminal devices also exist; these have limited application for infants and adults where low weight and aesthetics are a primary concern.

ELECTRIC-POWERED TERMINAL DEVICES

The introductioin of electric-powered hands into clinical practice in the early 1960s brought about a new era in prosthetic terminal devices. Early acceptance of these "electric hands" by the prosthetics profession was much slower in the United States than in the European countries where they were initially developed. They are, however, still considered by many not to be as functional as the mechanical hook terminal devices. It is felt much of this belief is because

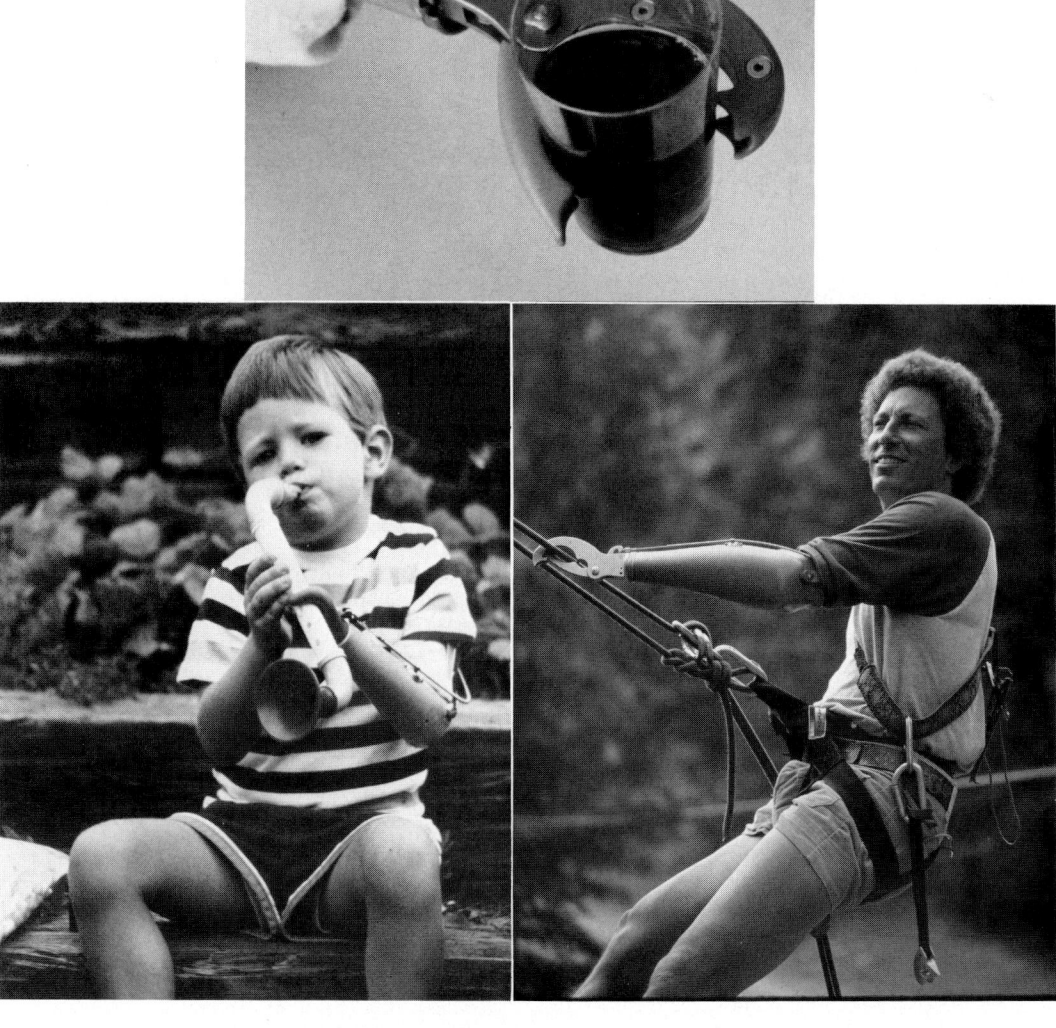

Fig. 85-9 The "GRIP" voluntary-closing terminal device is available in both adult and child versions. It allows an individual to achieve a variety of forceful and delicate prehension activities.

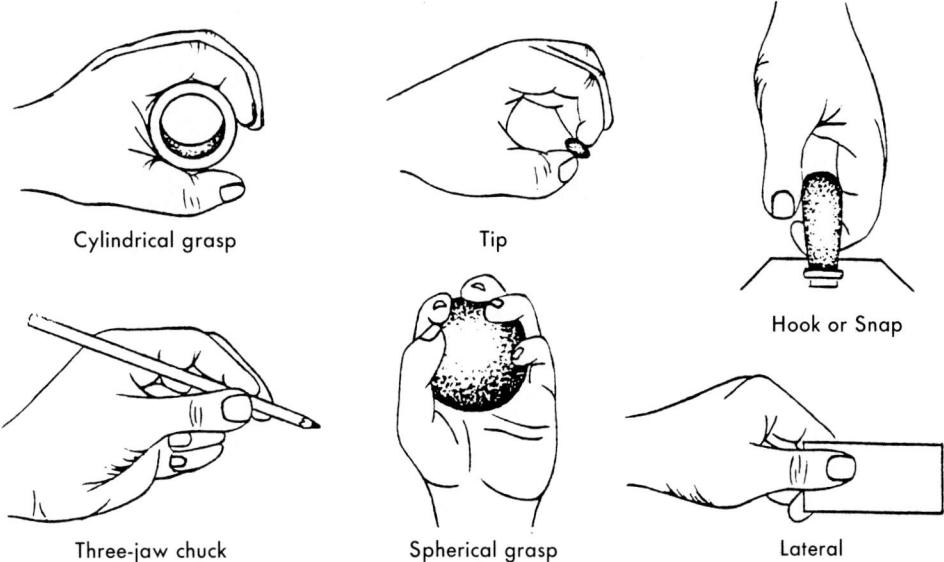

Cylindrical grasp   Tip   Hook or Snap

Three-jaw chuck   Spherical grasp   Lateral

Fig. 85-10   The six most commonly used hand-finger prehension patterns. "Three-jaw chuck" palmar type, tip-type and lateral-type prehension are considered to be used the most often during activities of daily living. (Modified from Schlesinger G: Ersatzglieder and Argeitshilfen, vol 3, Berlin, 1919).

of the attitudes toward mechanical hands being less functional than mechanical hooks. Electric-powered hands, however, have one primary major functional advantage over mechanical hooks and hands. Electric hands can produce finger prehension force equal to, and in some cases greater than, that of the adult or juvenile human hand. The average adult male, for instance, can produce an average of 20 to 24 pounds of finger prehension. The average tolerable amount of prehension for an adult male with a bowden cable controlled prosthesis and the more commonly used voluntary opening mechanical hook terminal device is approximately 8 to 10 pounds. Voluntary closing mechanical hands and hooks obviously are able to provide greater finger prehension than voluntary opening hooks or hands; however, they have not been widely accepted or used. Another key advantage of an electric-powered hand is its forceful "3 jaw chuck" palmar prehension. This type of prehension was identified by Schlesinger[20] as early as 1919 as the most commonly used hand-finger prehension pattern for picking up and especially holding objects in our activities of daily living. The most commonly used prehension patterns identified by Schlesinger[20] are illustrated in Fig. 85-10. Table 85-1 shows their percentage of use to pick up and hold objects. The predominance of "3 jaw chuck" palmar prehension in our activities of daily living accounts for the

reason all mechanical and electric-powered hands of today are designed with the thumb in opposition to the second and third fingers. The forceful palmar prehension of the electric-powered hand, therefore, enhances its overall functional value as a prosthetic terminal device.

The only electric-powered hook available for clinical use at this time is the Otto Bock "Griefer," which was introduced in the United States in the late 1970s. As an electric-powered terminal device, it also has the unique quality of providing forceful prehension. Along with this, it is uniquely designed with multiaxis fingers to keep the grasping sufaces parallel during the entire range of opening and closing (Fig. 85-11). This design feature allows for even pressure throughout its range of opening and closing, which enhances its grasping ability over mechanical hooks. The grasping surfaces of a mechanical hook angle away from one another as the active finger moves in relationship to the stationary finger, as is illustrated in Fig. 85-12. Therefore the larger the object to be held in the mechanical hook terminal device, the less contact with the object and, consequently, the more force required to stabilize the object, depending on its shape. The "Greifer," on the other hand, is heavier and bulkier than the largest stainless steel mechanical hook and is not as durable primarily, because its design is more complex than the single-axis mechanical hooks.

Very soon to become clinically available is the VA-NU Hosmer-Dorrance Synergistic Prehension Hook, as shown in Figs. 85-13 and 14. This electric-powered hook prehension device uses a unique two-motor drive system to achieve both high speed and torque. Childress[4,7] describes the functional advantages of providing high speed and high torque as being essential characteristics of a prosthetic terminal device because it better simulates the functional characteristics of the human hand. This is achieved with a high speed motor-drive system to provide quick response and when the prehension surfaces contact an object, the device automat-

Table 85-1   Frequency of prehension patterns

Function	Prehension type		
	Palmar (%)	Tip (%)	Lateral (%)
Pick up	50	71	33
Hold for use	88	2	10

From Schlesinger G: Ersatzglieder and Argeitshilfen, vol 3, Berlin, 1919.

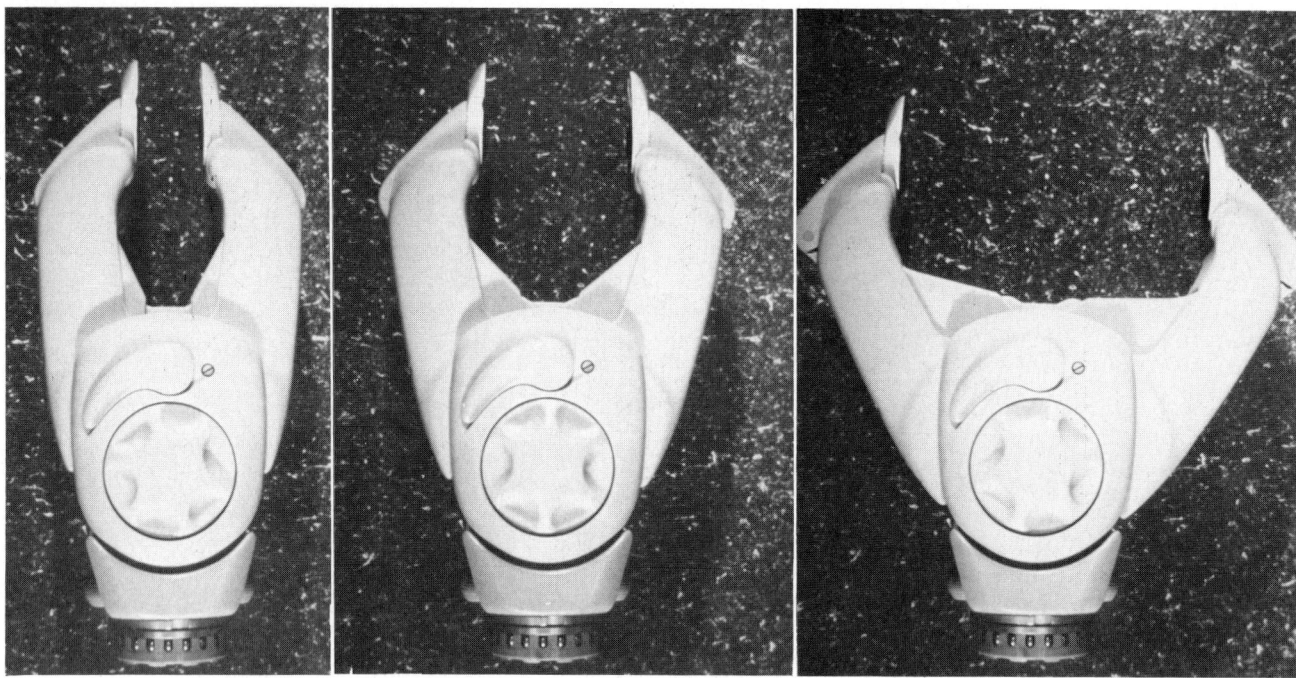

Fig. 85-11   The Otto Bock "Greifer," as shown through its range of opening and closing, maintains parallel grasping surfaces as a result of its "multi-axis" design. (Courtesy of Otto Bock Orthopaedic Industries.)

ically shifts to the high torque motor-drive system to provide forceful prehension up to approximately 30 pounds.

MECHANICAL AND ELECTRIC WRIST DEVICES

Mechanical wrists, which provide passive friction or positive locking positioning of the terminal device are still the most commonly used in the design of either an electric-powered or mechanical prosthesis. The Otto Bock electric powered wrist is the only device of its kind available, and it provides 360 degrees of continuous supination or pronation. It does not provide forceful rotation and therefore is primarily a positioning device for the terminal device. The use of a powered wrist rotator becomes more essential for individuals with bilateral amputations above the elbow and higher. When used in the design of a bilateral upper limb prosthesis, some consideration must be given to in-

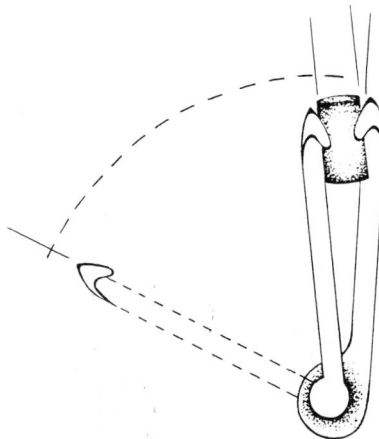

Fig. 85-12   This illustration shows the angular relationship of the grasping prehension surfaces of a "single-axis" prehension device with one stationary finger and the object being held, such as in the Hosmer/Dorrance mechanical hook series. (From Billock JN: Upper limb prosthetic terminal devices: hands versus hooks, Clin Prosthet Orthot 10(2):59, 1986, Published by the American Orthotic and Prosthetic Assoc., Alexandria, Va.)

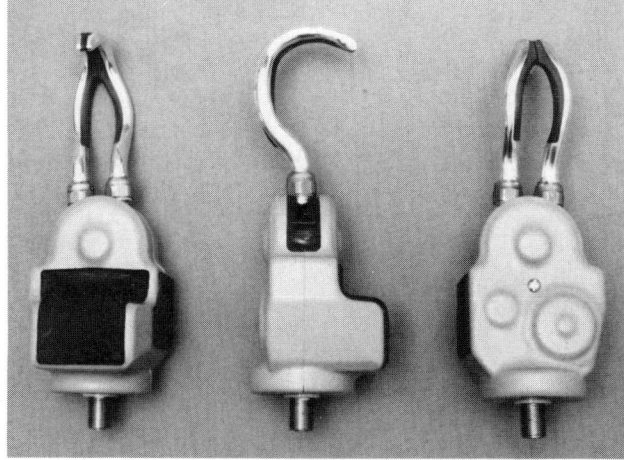

Fig. 85-13   The Synergistic Prehensor, as shown, uses the Hosmer/Dorrance No. 555 hook-finger style with neoprene-lined finger surfaces. (Courtesy of the Northwestern University Prosthetic Research Laboratory, Chicago, Ill.)

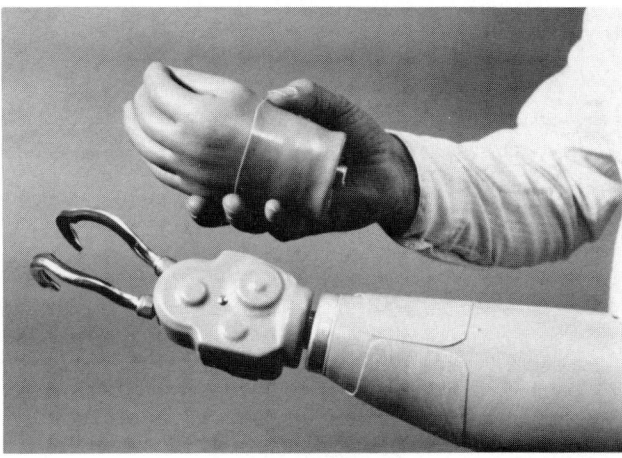

Fig. 85-14 The Synergistic Prehensor has been designed to be interchangeable with an adult electric-powered hand when appropriate. (Courtesy of the Northwestern University Prosthetic Research Laboratory, Chicago, Ill.)

corporating wrist flexion devices proximal to the electric-powered wrist to better achieve midline functional activities (Fig. 85-15).

SHOULDER DEVICES

The only shoulder joint devices available are mechanical in design and allow for passive friction positioning or "free swing" of the prosthesis. One of the most commonly used mechanical shoulder joints is illustrated in Fig. 85-16. Providing electric-powered control at the shoulder joint presents a significant problem because of the forces involved and the availability of control sources to actuate desired movements of a total arm prosthesis. Research aimed at addressing this complex problem has been under way for several years.

MODULARLY DESIGNED PROSTHESES

Because of the complexities involved in designing an appropriate upper limb prosthesis, some researchers and developers have worked toward developing total system prostheses for the various levels of upper limb deficiencies. These systems generally are designed around a modular component concept, where the batteries, electronics, microswitches, and electrodes, are packaged within individual modules for easier handling and assembly. They are also designed with a common electrical connection system, which may or may not be compatible with other available components and control systems. The modular systems approach reduces the overall complexity of designing a total prosthesis; however, it does not always provide the individual with the most appropriate prosthesis when his individual physiologic and psychological needs are considered. In these situations consideration must be given to the possibilities of developing a hybrid prosthesis to achieve a design that best meets the individual's needs.

HYBRIDLY DESIGNED PROTHESES

Hybridly designed prostheses using various components and control methods from various systems can, in many cases, result in a prosthesis that is better functionally de-

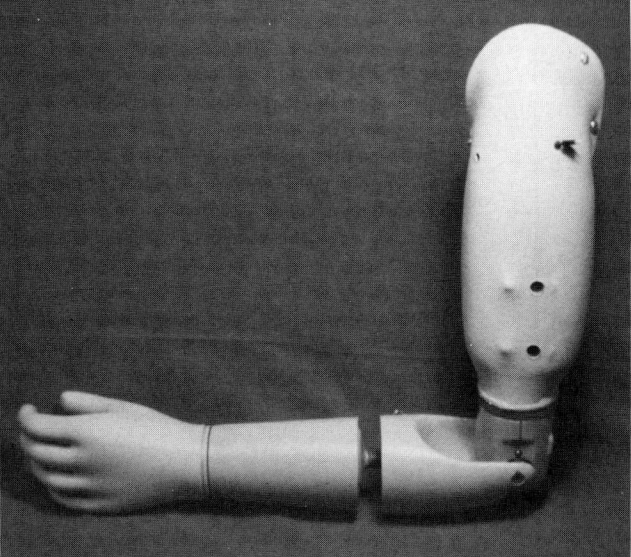

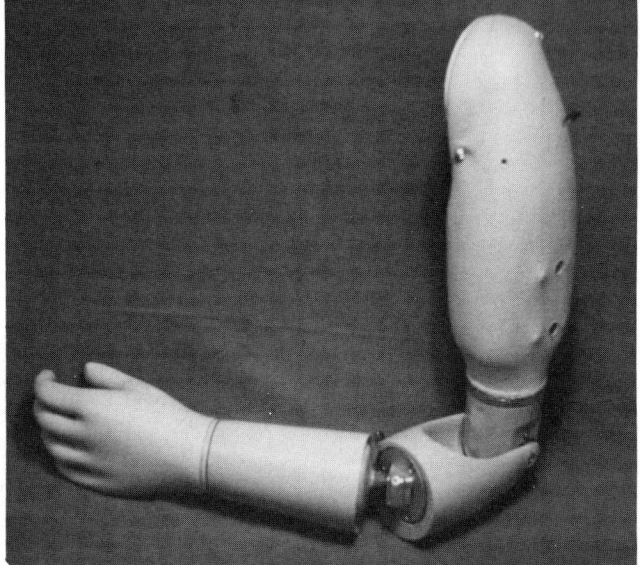

Fig. 85-15 This hybridly designed prosthesis illustrates the use of a forearm flexion device in conjunction with the Otto Bock electrically "Powered Wrist Rotator," **A,** with the forearm in neutral and **B,** full flexion of 45 degrees. One additional position of 25 degrees is also achievable.

signed and more acceptable to the individual. Hybrid design approaches become even more apparent when working with individuals with upper limb deficiencies above the elbow and higher. In many cases, a combination of electric-powered switch and/or myoelectrically controlled components and mechanical body-powered bowden cable controlled components are required to design and develop an appropriate prosthesis. A classic example of this situation would be in designing an above-elbow prosthesis for an individual with a distal humeral level of amputation. A limb deficiency at this level generally does not require the use of an electrically powered elbow because the individual should have sufficient range of motion at the shoulder joint and adequate muscle strength to control a mechanical elbow. A

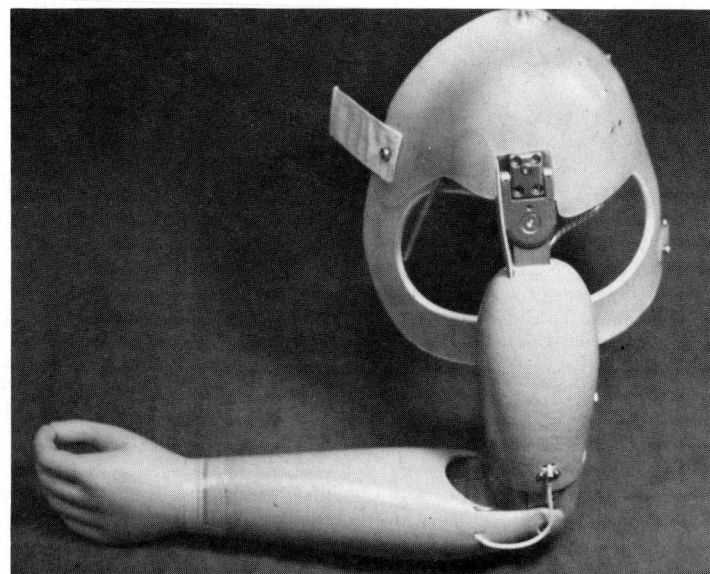

Fig. 85-16 The Hosmer/Dorrance "Flexion/Abduction Shoulder Joint," shown attached to a shoulder disarticulation–type prosthesis, provides passive mechanical range of motion in flexion to 90 degrees and abduction to 135 degrees. An extension stop is provided to restrict extension.

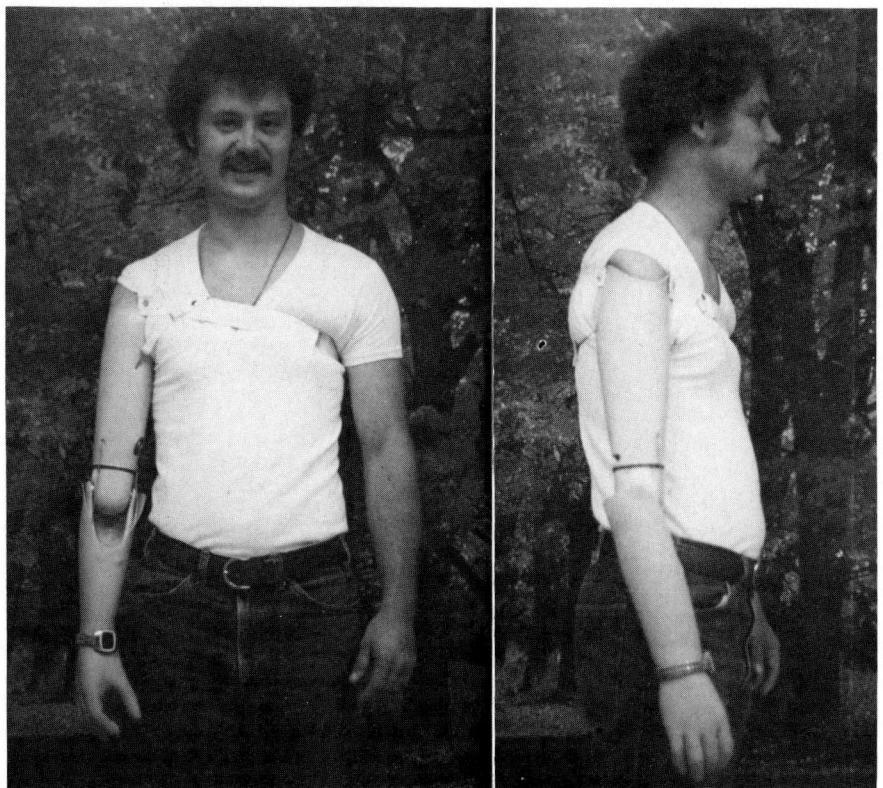

Fig. 85-17 This "hybrid" above-elbow prosthesis uses a thoracic suspension and control harness for total suspension of the prosthesis and actuation of the Bowden cable-controlled mechanical elbow and locking mechanism. The batteries and electronic components for myoelectric control of the hand are self-contained within the upper arm of the prosthesis.

myoelectrically controlled hand introduced into the design of the prosthesis, in this case, can significantly improve its functional capabilities and aesthetics. This particular hybrid design approach allows the individual to independently control the elbow and hand simultaneously. An example of this hybrid type of prosthesis is illustrated in Fig. 85-17. Individuals with this particular hybrid design infrequently use the mechanical elbow lock mechanism to maintain the hand and forearm in a fixed position for functional use. The overall control of the prosthesis is more natural because the elbow lock is not necessary for the majority of functional activities.

Unfortunately, many of the electric-powered components and control systems are not designed for hybrid use at all levels of upper limb deficiencies, even though they may have application. In many cases, they are not electrically or mechanically compatible and require electronic and/or mechanical engineering changes to ahieve an appropriately designed prosthesis that best meets an individual's needs. Prosthetic practitioners of today must be able to appropriately modify these components and systems when necessary. The application of hybrid design concepts requires a sound knowledge of the components and control systems available. Myoelectric and switch control systems can be used in conjunction with each other, depending on their functional and electrical compatibility. The application and ability to use myoelectric, switch, and/or body motion controls for actuation of the primary components of a prosthesis are essential in properly evaluating and developing an appropriate prosthesis.

When body motion is being used in a hybrid manner, along with switch and/or myoelectric control to actuate a bowden cable control system, one should always remember to use the primary body motion for actuation of the mechanical component. The theory behind this approach is that a bowden cable–controlled system requires significant muscle activity and body motion to produce the force and excursion necessary to actuate a mechanical component. Myoelectric and switch control systems require significantly less muscle activity to produce the force and excursion necessary for actuation of a component.

CONCLUSIONS

In summary, the design and development of an upper limb prosthesis should involve a careful evaluation and assessment of an individual's particular needs. Because the terminal device is the most important component of the prosthesis, it is necessary to choose the control technique that will provide the most appropriate actuation of that device. It is felt that myoelectric control provides the most physiologically natural source of control, and whenever possible, it should be given consideration. It is further felt the majority of individuals with upper limb deficiencies generally prefer a hand as a terminal device. In many cases, this desire may be purely psychological, and as professionals, we should respond to that need. The majority of individuals with upper limb deficiencies are unilateral, with the prosthesis obviously becoming the nondominant side. Therefore it is important the prosthesis first meet the individual's physiologic and psychological needs, and secondly, that it be easily controlled and provide adequate prehension for stabilizing objects, which is the primary function of the

nondominant side during bilateral hand activities. This would obviously seem to indicate that myoelectric control, which best uses the residual neuromuscular system, and an electric-powered hand, which provides forceful prehension, should be the first choice in developing a functional prosthesis.

Electric-powered components have been felt by many not to be sufficiently reliable and durable for use in the design of an upper limb prosthesis. This, however, has not proven to be the case when they are appropriately incorporated into the design of a prosthesis and the patient is properly oriented in their care and use. There are those individuals and situations that are abusive to an electric-powered prosthesis, as well as to a mechanical prosthesis. They, however, are not the majority and require appropriate consideration before design and development of an appropriate prosthesis. Hybrid design concepts can also be used to enhance the reliability and durability of a prosthesis by self-containing components within the prosthesis that would otherwise be external.

Hybridly designed prostheses can significantly improve the functional restoration and rehabilitation of an individual with an upper limb deficiency. They are an important consideration in the prosthetic management of individuals with upper limb deficiencies and can be the difference between total rejection or functional use of a prosthesis. Unfortunately, upper limb prostheses of this type will most likely continue to be provided in specialized centers and not find their place in common practice unless developers and manufacturers work toward making their components more compatible and interchangeable with other systems.

REFERENCES

1. Billock JN: The Northwestern University supracondylar suspension technique for below elbow amputations, Orthot Prosthet 26(4):16, 1972.
2. Billock JN: Upper limb prosthetic management—hybrid design approaches, Clin Orthot Prosthet 9(1):23, 1985.
3. Billock JN: Upper limb prosthetic terminal devices: hands versus hooks. Clin Orthot Prosthet 10(2):57, 1986.
4. Childress DS: An approach to power grasp. In Gavrilovic MM and Wilson AB, editors: Advances in external control of extremities, Belgrade, Yugoslavia, 1972.
5. Childress DS: Powered limb prostheses: their clinical significance, IEER Trans Biomed Eng BME-20(3):200, 1973.
6. Childress DS and Billock JN: Self-containment and self-suspension of externally powered prostheses for the forearm, Bull Prosthet Res 10-14:4, 1970.
7. Childress DS and Grahn EC: Development of a powered prehensor, Proceedings of the thirty-eighth annual conference on Engineering in Medicine and Biology, 1985.
8. Childress DS, Holmes DW, and Billock JN: Ideas on myoelectric prosthetic systems for upper-extremity amputees. In Herberts P and others, eds: The control of upper-extremity prostheses and orthoses, Springfield, Ill, 1974, Charles C Thomas, Publisher.
9. Childress DS and others: Myoelectric immediate postsurgical procedure: a concept for fitting the upper extremity amputee, Artif Limbs 13 (2):55, 1969.
10. Dembo T, Leviton GL, and Wright BA: Adjustment to misfortune: a problem of social-psychological rehabilitation. In Selected articles from Artif Limbs, Huntington, NY, 1970, RE Krieger Publishing Co Inc.
11. Erhardt RP: Sequential levels on development of prehension, Am J Occup Ther 28:592, 1975.
12. Gwynne G: Mechanical components. In Santschi WR, ed: Manual of upper extremity prosthetics, ed 2, Los Angeles, 1958, Department of Engineering, University of Southern California.
13. Jacobsen SC and others: Development of the Utah arm, IEEE Trans Biomed Eng BME-29 (4):249, 1982.

14. Le Blanc MA: Patient population and other estimates of prosthetics and orthotics in the USA, Ortho Prosthet 27(3):38, 1973.
15. Malone JM and others: Immediate early and late post-surgical management of upper-limb amputations, J Rehabil R and D 21(1):33, 1984.
16. Murphy EF: Commentary. In Selected articles from Artif Limbs, Huntington, NY, 1970, RE Krieger Publishing Co Inc.
17. Rusk HA: Rehabilitation, JAMA 140:286, 1949.
18. Rusk HA: Advances in rehabilitation, Practitioner 183:505, 1959.
19. Sauter WF: Myoelectric and switch controlled upper extremities prostheses, Amputation surgery and rehabilitation. The Toronto experience, New York, 1981, Churchill Livingstone.
20. Schlesinger G: Der mechanishe aufbau der kunstlochen glieder, Ersatzglieder und Arbeitshilfen, vol 3, 1919.
21. Scott RN: Myo-electric control of prostheses, Arch Phys Med Rehabil 47(3):174, 1967.
22. Scott RN: An introduction to myoelectric prostheses, Fredricton, NB, Canada, 1984, and Bio-Engineering Institute, University of New Brunswick.
23. Taylor CL and Schwarz RJ: The anatomy and mechanics of the human hand. In Selected articles from Artif Limbs, Huntington, NY, 1970, RE Krieger Publishing Co Inc.
24. Taylor CL: Biomechanics of control. In Selected articles from Artif Limbs, Huntington, NY, 1970, RE Krieger Publishing Co Inc.

86

Prosthetic management of the upper limb–deficient child

Steven M. Wenner

The prosthetic management of the upper limb–deficient child requires consideration of multiple variables: level of limb deficiency; functional and cosmetic loss; possibility of successful surgical reconstruction; advantages of prosthetic restoration; and specifics of prosthesis selection, including socket, suspension, harness, power source, and terminal device. It is the purpose of this chapter to review these considerations as they apply to each type of upper limb deficiency. Special concerns in the care of the child amputee and his family will be addressed, and the setting in which such care is proffered—the children's limb deficiency clinic—will be described.

Approximately 80% of children who attend an upper limb deficiency clinic have a congenital cause for their loss. The other 20% is composed of posttraumatic and posttumor resection amputees.[3]

GENERAL CONSIDERATIONS

Sensky[17] and others[10] have stated that an infant with a congenital limb deficiency does not see himself as "abnormal" as an adult might. Rather, a child who grows up without an arm incorporates this defect into his image of himself. Early prosthetic fitting allows the artificial limb to become incorporated into his body image. Conversely, an individual who suffers an amputation (traumatic or surgical) sustains a disintegration of body image.

The congenital upper limb amputee should be fitted with his initial prosthesis in the first year of life. This will ensure better acceptance of the prosthesis by both the child and his parents.[13,14] Such acceptance usually results in an improved functional outcome and more nearly normal patterns of bilateral upper limb function. In addition to being an assistive device in tasks of self-care and mobility, the prosthesis will be an effective tool for learning.[4]

In our clinic we prescribe the initial prosthesis at 6 months of age. Most children are beginning to sit up at this time; a prosthesis helps to maintain sitting balance. Additionally, the restoration of length to the upper limb permits more normal performance of those bimanual activities that are performed at arm's length from the body. The initial prosthesis is a passive device. With appropriate neuromuscular maturation, an activated terminal device is applied; suitable harnessing and suspension are added.

The best candidates for prosthetic restoration are those children whose deficiency is terminal transverse, such as below-elbow or above-elbow. Patients with longitudinal deficiencies, such as those with absence of the thumb or ulnar dysmelia, are less frequently in need of a prosthesis. These

deformities are often amenable to improvement by surgical reconstruction.[9]

ABSENCE THROUGH THE CARPUS

Children with a congenital limb deficiency through the carpus are not very well managed by either surgical reconstruction or prosthetic restoration. The surgical treatment that can be considered is transcarpal distraction lengthening, followed by syndactyly division to separate the distal osseous mass into separate "digits." This is not a commonly pursued treatment program, and we have no personal experience with it.

Prosthetic restoration can take two different forms. The more commonly employed method is to offer the patient a plastic orthosis, which is placed along the volar surface of the wrist and stump and is strapped to the distal forearm with Velcro straps. The child then holds objects between it and the carpal remnant (Fig. 86-1). Such a device can be used effectively only if the patient has an arc of wrist motion of at least 45 degrees. This permits him to effect a "grasp-and-release" pattern against the device.[16] Such a device allows a child to benefit from the sensibility of the stump when handling objects. It is easily removed and reapplied with the normal hand and it does not require suspension or harnessing other than the Velcro straps. Accordingly, the youngster can don the device for those activities requiring an object to be held independently on the limb deficient side. He can remove it for those bimanual activities that are made easier by unimpeded access to the sensible volar surface of the stump and for which the full power of the upper limb is beneficial. An alternative orthoprosthesis that can be tried is the CAPP multiposition post. This device is fitted to the distal forearm and wrist and has a hinge-attached plate against which objects can be held.

The second method of nonoperative management is conventional prosthetic fitting. The use of a standard body-powered or myoelectric terminal device eliminates the natural benefit of a sensible stump. Additionally, harnessing and suspension are an unpleasant encumberance. Scotland and Galway[18] reported a 59% incidence of prosthetic rejection in this group; our experience has been similar to theirs. If prosthetic fitting is attempted, a double wall socket with a volar cutaway to permit voluntary protrusion of the stump for sensory feedback and a voluntary opening hook are the recommendation of Lamb and Scott.[16] We use the same technique. The harness is in a figure eight. The elbow has flexible hinges. The wrist can be either constant friction or quick disconnect, depending on whether the patient ex-

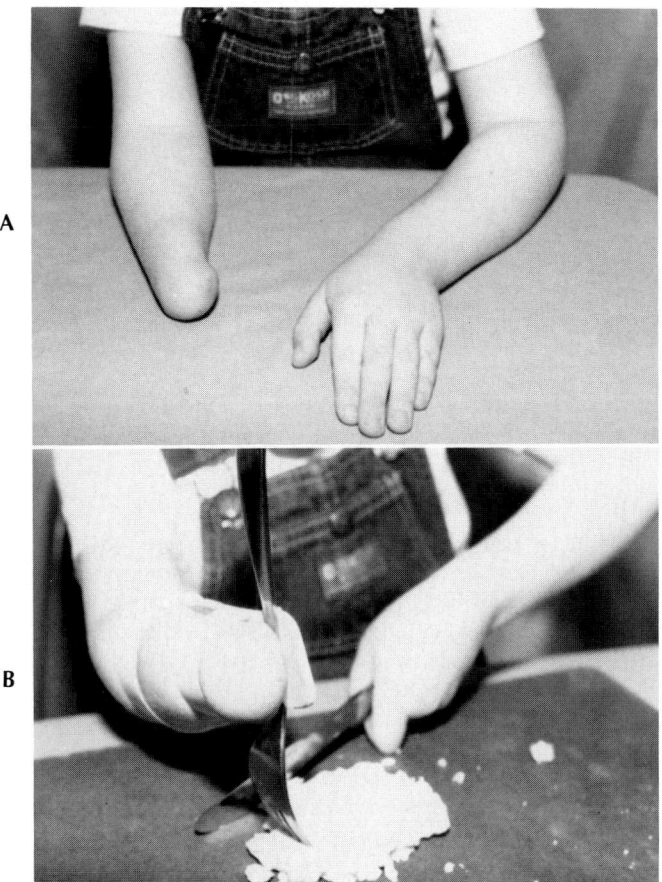

Fig. 86-1 **A,** Six-year-old boy with transverse deficiency through the carpus. **B,** Same child using volar plate orthosis. Patient is infrequent user of orthoprosthesis.

changes the hook for another terminal device (TD) such as a body-powered hand. A single cable operates the TD.

A myoelectric prosthesis can be used instead of a body-powered hook or hand. The advantages of it are self-suspension, elimination of the harness, activation of the TD by isometric forearm muscle contraction rather than by shoulder girdle movement, and its high-tech appeal. The disadvantages of it are partial loss of elbow motion and significant loss of forearm rotation because of Münster socket fitting and the excessive length of the limb when a myoelectric prosthesis is fitted to a patient who has full forearm plus partial carpal length.

Despite the functional advantages of the volar plate orthosis, the body-powered hook, and the myoelectric prosthesis, the rate of patient rejection of these devices is high. This is so because of the excellent overall function these children enjoy despite their limb deficiency. These youngsters, however, often do choose to wear a cosmetic glove while they are at social events.

ABSENT THUMB

The importance of the thumb in hand function is well recognized. The thumb is estimated to represent 40% to 50% of normal hand function; to the patient who loses his

thumb, surely the disability seems greater than this. The requirements for satisfactory thumb function include adequate sensibility, size, strength (pollex), and mobility. Loss or compromise of any of these factors causes impairment of function. For instance, partial thumb amputation will shorten the thumb and impair fine sensibility; the consequence of this is decreased function.

Surgical reconstruction of the missing or inadequate thumb is frequently feasible. A child who has a hypoplastic but articulated thumb may benefit from operations to improve joint stability (capsulodesis and arthrodesis), increase length (distraction lengthening), and improve active movement (tendon transfer). A child whose thumb is either entirely absent or hypoplastic and not articulated (pouce flotant) will benefit from either pollicization of an adjacent digit or free tissue transfer (toe to hand).[22]

The alternative to surgical management of the missing or inadequate thumb is orthoprosthetic fitting. This orthoprosthesis, an opposition post, is strapped onto the hand and presents a stable post against which the palmar digits can work. The drawbacks to it are its lack of sensibility, except for the pressure felt when an object is held firmly against it, and its lack of mobility. Because of these limitations, such prostheses are often rejected by the patient. Therefore we recommend appropriate surgery for these children if they are suitable candidates.

ABSENT FINGERS

The functional deficit that results from inadequate fingers, be they too few in number, too small in size, insufficiently mobile or not strong enough because of joint instability or tendon inadequacy, can frequently be improved by staged surgical reconstruction. Distraction lengthening of existing short digits, arthrodesis/capsulodesis of unstable joints, tendon transfer to move digits more effectively, osteotomy to correct deformity or to create a more functional position for an immobile finger, digital transposition, and free tissue transfer (toe to hand) can be used to improve function of the hand.[22]

Orthoprosthetic restoration with the use of an opposition post will provide a stable, large enough opposite part against which the thumb can press when holding objects. The disadvantages of this method of management include the lack of sensibility of the post, the immobility of it, and its failure to provide cosmetic improvement. For these reasons, patients frequently use such devices in a very limited manner and only for selected activities that require bilateral prehension. Such children are often pleased to have the option of wearing a cosmetic glove, especially at social events.

BELOW-ELBOW LIMB DEFICIENCY

The child with a below-elbow deficiency, whether it is of congenital, posttraumatic or posttumor resection cause, has an ideal level for prosthetic management. In the congenital case with a short or very short stump, surgery is not performed except for minor stump modifications. Occasionally, the skin at the end of the stump will be invaginated and adherent to the bone ends. Such an area can be difficult to keep clean and stump revision is advisable. In the posttraumatic case, skin and soft tissue coverage of the stump may not be stable or sturdy enough to permit prosthetic fitting; this necessitates revision. In no instance of short below-elbow amputation can independent grasp and release be provided without prosthetic fitting.

In the instance of a long below-elbow amputation or a wrist disarticulation, the Krukenberg operation can be considered. This procedure divides the radius from the ulna and provides individual muscle control to each bone. This creates pincer function between the forearm bones and preserves a sensible end organ. The operation is only used in the case of bilateral below-elbow amputation, and then it is generally reserved for the blind patient. The forearm must be at least two thirds of normal length for the procedure to be effective.

The typical congenital below-elbow amputee has a level of deficiency in the proximal one third of the forearm. Elbow motion is usually normal or nearly so. The radial head is frequently dislocated posterolaterally. The discussion of the prosthetic management of the below-elbow amputee will center on this typical very short level. Where appropriate, the differences in technique that apply to the long below-elbow and wrist disarticulation level will be described. The advantages of prosthetic treatment for these children are improved independence in and performance of bimanual activities (in part because of equalization of limb lengths), provision of independent grasp and release on the limb deficient side, and better cosmesis of the limb if a body-powered hand or myoelectric hand is used.

In our upper limb deficiency clinic we fit the child with his first prosthesis at 6 months of age. Early fitting enables the child to incorporate the prosthesis into his body image, which increases the likelihood of long-term prosthetic acceptance. At 6 months of age most youngsters begin to sit. The prosthesis enables the child to touch down on the limb-deficient side and thereby improves his sitting balance. The prosthesis also helps the child to do bimanual activities at arm's length. The parents more readily accept the appearance of the prosthesis when it is fitted at an early age. We employ a figure eight harness, double-wall socket with a triceps cuff, a preflexed forearm, and a passive hand, which is an inactive terminal device. The lower tabs of the triceps cuff are centered at the elbow joint and permit flexion and extension to occur. At 18 months of age we activate a terminal device. Our patients are fitted with a figure eight Dacron harness with either a metal ring or a sewn cloth junction, a double-wall socket with a surlyn liner, triceps pad or cuff, flexible elbow hinges, a constant friction wrist unit with a neoprene-covered voluntary opening hook TD (Fig. 86-2, A-C). A single cable operates the terminal device. Protraction of the shoulders results in opening of the hook; relaxation of the shoulders allows the rubber bands that connect the two limbs of the hook to close it. The number of rubber bands determines the tension in the terminal device; more rubber bands result in stronger grasp.

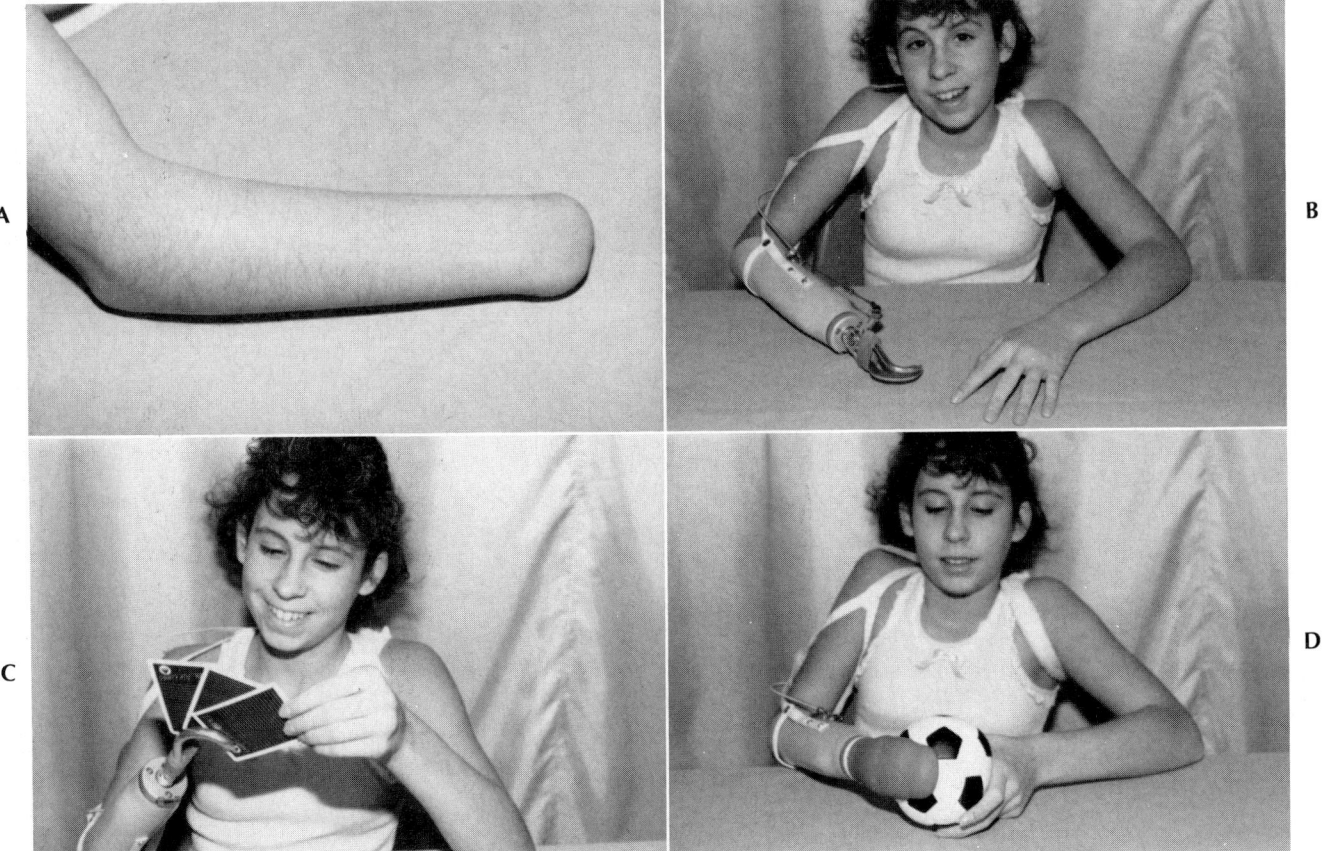

Fig. 86-2   A, Thirteen-year-old girl with wrist disarticulation. **B** and **C,** Same patient using conventional prosthesis with figure-eight harness, triceps pad, double wall socket, quick disconnect wrist, and voluntary-opening split hook operated by single cable. Child is full-time prosthesis user. **D,** Same patient with sports mitt instead of split hook.

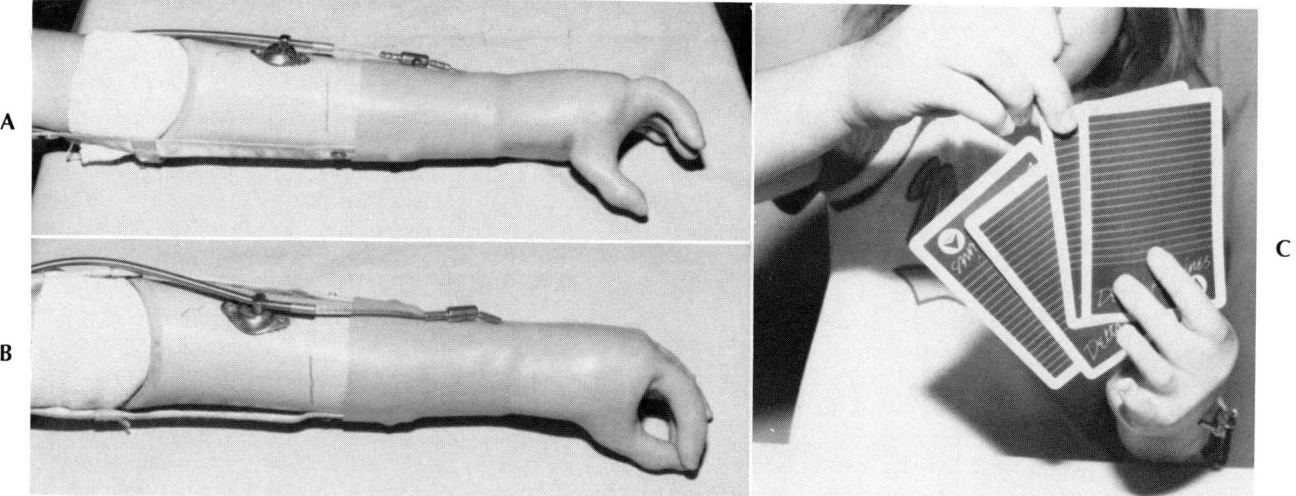

Fig. 86-3 **A** and **B,** Short below-elbow limb deficiency in a patient who has been fitted with a body-powered hand, operated by a single cable. Child is a full-time prosthesis user. **C,** Child using the prosthesis while at play.

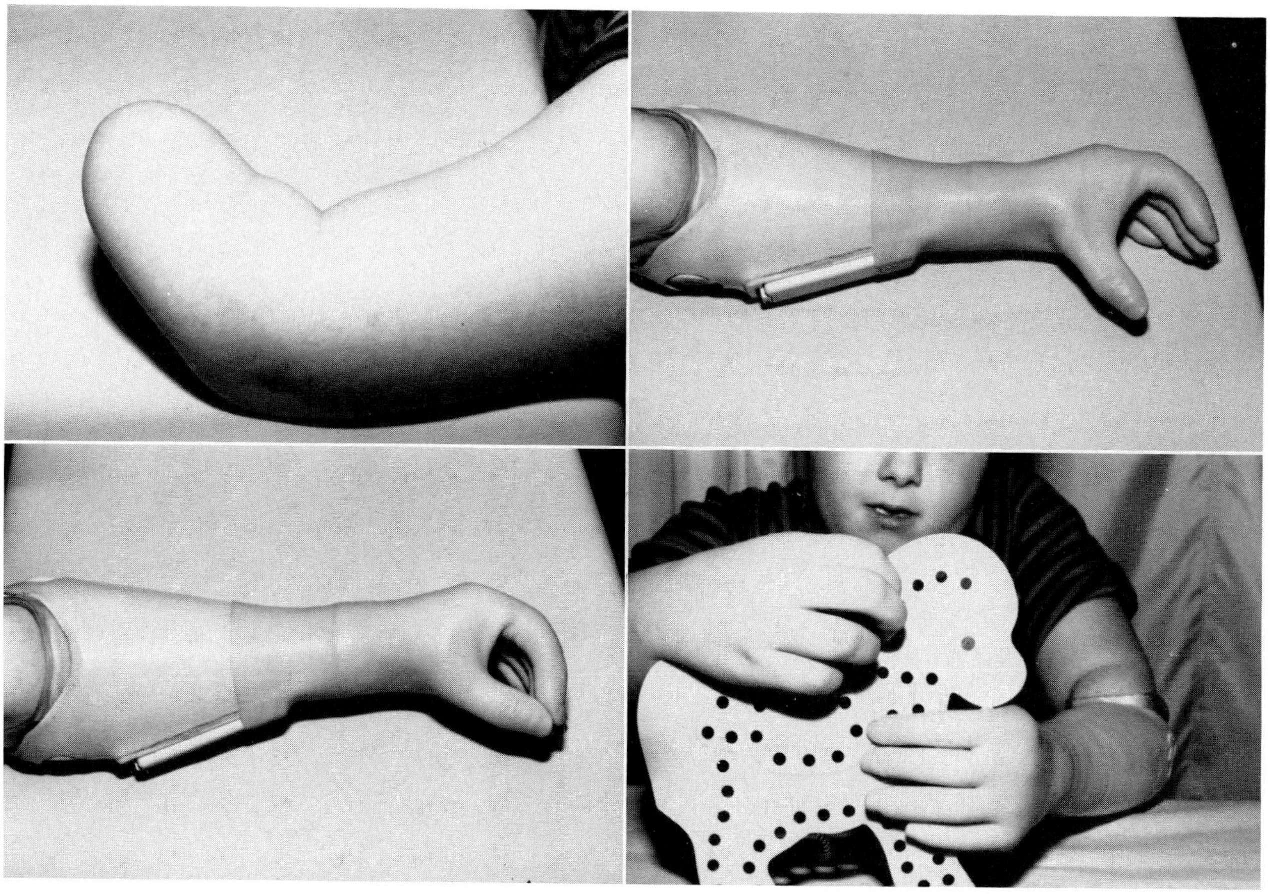

Fig. 86-4 **A,** Six-year-old child with short below-elbow limb deficiency. **B** and **C,** Same child demonstrating opening and closing of myoelectric prosthesis; Münster socket and position socket and position of battery pack can be seen. Patient is full-time prosthesis user. **D,** Same patient using myoelectric prosthesis while at play.

Once the terminal device has been activated, a period of training with an occupational or physical therapist helps the child to master the use of the prosthesis and teaches the parents as they assist the youngster in this learning process. Wendt and Shaperman[22] have recommended that formal training begin when the child uses the normal hand to open the hook. We institute such a training-therapy program as soon as we activate the terminal device. Acceptance of a body-powered prosthesis in the patients with a below-elbow amputation is approximately 85% to 90% if a protocol such as ours is followed. Delay in initial fitting beyond 2 years of age may result in a significant increase in the rate of prosthetic rejection.[18]

As the child matures, other terminal devices may be considered for use. A sports mitt can be interchanged with a split hook; it is useful in athletic activities (Fig. 86-2, *D*). Such a prosthesis should have a quick-disconnect wrist to permit easy terminal device interchange. Also, a body-powered hand can be used instead of the hook; this is useful for the patient who prefers a body-powdered prosthesis but desires the improved cosmesis of the hand (Fig. 86-3). Finally, instead of a voluntary opening hook, the child can be fitted with a voluntary closing hook. This enables the prosthetic user to exert finer control over the force of grasp when he closes the jaws of the terminal device.

Myoelectric prostheses were originally reserved for teenagers and adults (Fig. 86-4). Sorbye[19] introduced their use in young children in Sweden in 1971. Since then a number of other investigators have advised their use in preschool children.[7,12] The advantages of such prostheses are well recognized: self-suspension and the elimination of the harness, improved pinch strength, superior cosmesis, and elimination of the need to move the entire upper limb (including shoulder girdle) to activate the terminal device. The disadvantages include increased weight, potential difficulties with maintenance (now an infrequent problem), and the restriction of elbow and forearm motion because of münster socket, which is necessary for self-suspension.[21] Additionally, sensory feedback (proprioception) is not so good with a myoelectric as with a body-powered prosthesis; that is, it is difficult to tell how much force is being exerted on an object. In the child with a very long below-elbow level, a myoelectric prosthesis may make the length of the upper limb unacceptably long. Nonetheless, overall patient and family acceptance of and enthusiasm for this prosthesis is excellent and we frequently prescribe it for our patients. The accomplished myoelectric user can interchange the customary terminal device with a griffer, an electrically operated pincer that can generate substantial pinch force (40 kg); it is very useful in heavy mechanical work.

In our clinic, we do not encourage fitting with a myoelectric prosthesis before 5 years of age. We prefer to have the youngster master the use of a body-powered voluntary opening hook first. If at 5 years the patient or the family requests fitting with a myoelectric prosthesis, we gladly accommodate them in this regard (Fig. 86-4). Although there are centers in North America where myoelectric prostheses are prescribed at age 2 years, we have not followed this approach.

Training for use of a myoelectric prosthesis is mandatory. The first step entails identification of muscles suitable for control of the prosthesis. Next, a one- or two-channel control system must be chosen. Finally, the muscle(s) must be trained to operate the terminal device.

In our clinic, we make every effort to work with the below-elbow amputee and his family in an effort to keep the child in a prosthesis of his liking as long as it is a sensible solution for the particular situation. It is our philosophy that most every unilateral (and bilateral) below-elbow amputee will have significant functional benefit from using a prosthesis with an activated terminal device. Therefore we exercise patience and offer encouragement as the limb-deficient child and his family work through the occasional (temporary, we hope) problem of prosthetic rejection. We keep such patients supplied with a useable prosthesis, even if it is rarely used, with the hope that as he matures he will try using it once again. Overall, the majority of these children treated in our upper limb deficiency clinic remain full-time users, 8 hours or more each day. A small number of youngsters use their prostheses only for a selected group of activities (part-time users), and an even smaller number reject the prostheses entirely.

ABOVE-ELBOW AND SHOULDER DISARTICULATION

The above-elbow limb-deficient child may appreciate great gains with the use of a prosthesis. Our first goal in prescribing prostheses for these children is to improve function and our second objective is to enhance cosmesis. Specifically, the prosthesis should restore limb length and provide motion and control at the elbow and grasp and release with the terminal device. Occasionally, surgical intervention is necessary in these children. Stump revision may be needed if the skin is invaginated at the distal end. Vestigial digits at the end of the stump should be left alone, especially if the child can move them voluntarily; they may be usable for activation of switch controls in a electrically-powered prosthesis. Spiking of the humeral bone end may require a stump capping operation (Marquardt). Finally, the patient with a very short humeral segment that is difficult to fit may be helped by distraction lengthening of the humerus.

At our clinic, children with this deformity have their initial prosthetic fitting at 6 months of age, for the same reasons as those given for the below-elbow amputee. Youngsters whose deficiency is posttraumatic or follows tumor resection should be fitted as soon as wound healing and skin conditions permit.

The initial prosthetic prescription is for a figure eight Dacron harness, a double-wall socket, a preflexed elbow and a passive hand. At 18 months, the passive hand is exchanged for a single cable activated voluntary opening split hook. This is attached to the socket by a constant friction wrist. The remainder of the prosthetic prescription remains the same (Fig. 86-5). In particular, a working elbow joint is not yet applied. Once the patient is able to use the terminal device purposefully, a conventional body-powered cable operated elbow can be prescribed. Other terminal device attachments can be interchanged as noted in the section on below-elbow amputees. Later, a myoelectric or switch-controlled prosthesis can be considered. The elbow alone or both active units can be so powered. The studies of Glynn and associates[5] and Heger and associates[6] indicate that unilateral above-elbow amputees prefer the myoelectric prosthesis to the body-powered one and that they are more likely

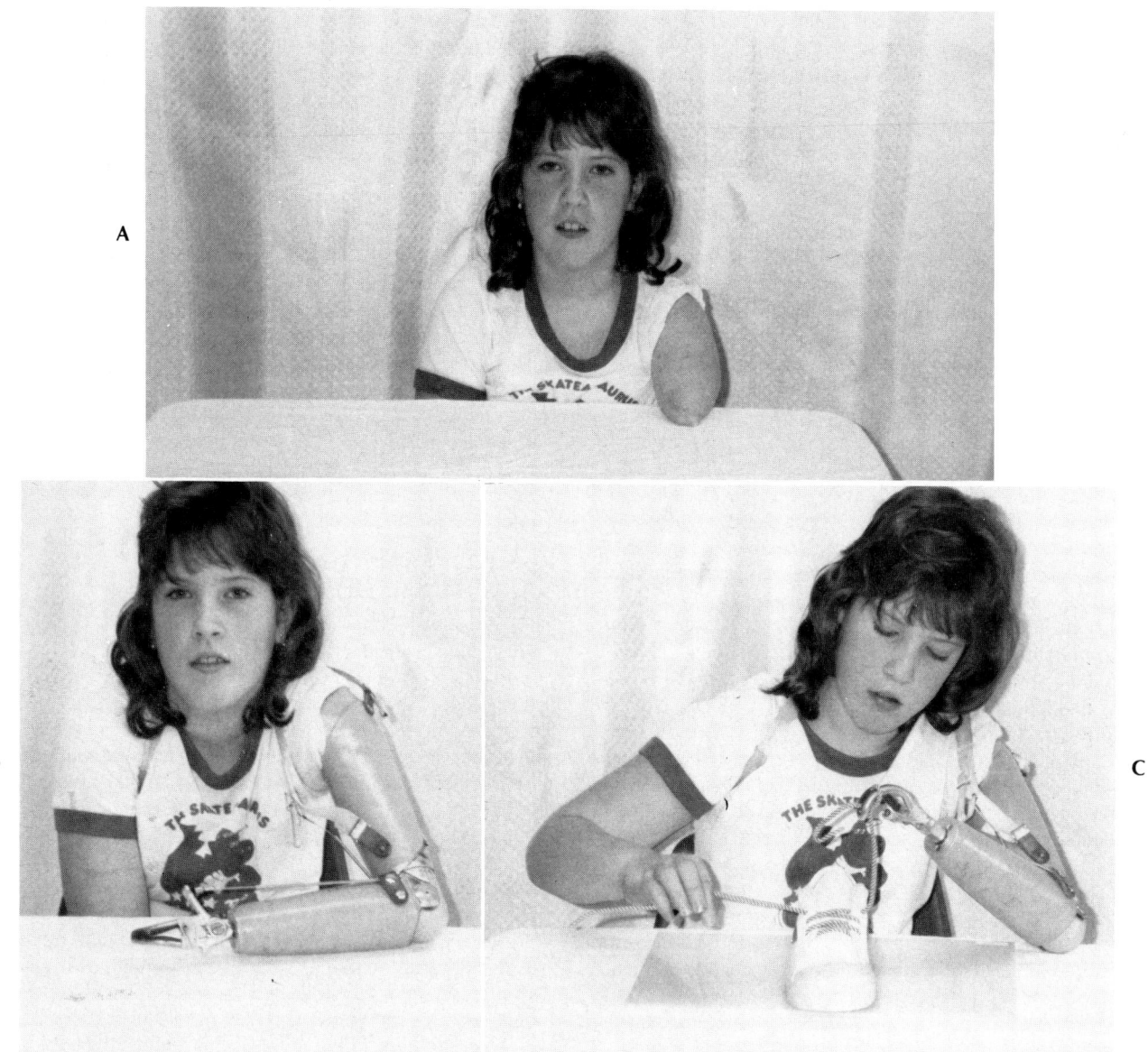

Fig. 86-5 **A,** Eleven-year-old child with above-elbow limb deficiency. **B** and **C,** Same patient fitted with figure-eight harness, double wall socket, and dual cable–operated above-elbow prosthesis with constant friction wrist and split hook. Child is a full-time prosthesis user.

to be full-time users if fitted with a myoelectric prosthesis. Our experience is that about equal numbers of children select myoelectric and body-powered above-elbow prostheses. In the bilateral above-elbow limb-deficient child, only one myoelectric unit should be prescribed. The excessive weight is a drawback to bilateral myoelectric fitting.

BILATERAL PHOCOMELIA AND AMELIA

A large body of literature discusses the problems of and solutions for this unfortunate group of children. The bilateral amelic child has no possibility of independent upper limb function without prostheses. The bilateral phocomelic child will sometimes be capable of handling objects with his hands. Frequently, however, the articulation between hand and trunk is unstable or the motivating musculotendinous units are weak. Either situation will make it difficult for the

hands to manipulate heavier objects. Another difficulty is that the total upper limb length is so short that these youngsters cannot reach the perineum for hygiene. However, they will often be able to handle utensils for self-feeding. As a consequence of these restrictions, they become remarkably adept in the use of their feet. They will often times independently perform nearly all activities of daily living with foot prehension.* Every effort should be made to keep their lower limb joints flexible and their shoes should be easily removed. Prosthetic fitting of these children is met with an incredibly high rate of complete rejection — almost 100%.[11] Their function by foot prehension is excellent; strength, flexibility, and sensibility all contribute to this. The prostheses are heavy and bulky, and donning them is dif-

---

*References 1, 2, 8, 9, 14, 20.

ficult. If the child and family desires a prosthesis, it should be as lightweight and trim as possible. Electrical power should be used for the elbow and the terminal device. The amelic child will need myoelectric controls, whereas the phocomelic patient can often operate switches with the vestigial digits. Frequently, these youngsters will request passive prostheses that they can wear for cosmetic benefit. We accommodate them in this regard.

THE CHILDREN'S LIMB DEFICIENCY CLINIC

The children's limb deficiency clinic is a unique place. It brings together a diverse group of specialists, all of whom share an interest in these youngsters. The children and their parents benefit from the experience of and interaction among the team members—surgeon, prosthetist, and therapist. Nurses and case workers provide emotional and social support for the patients and families. Additionally, the youngsters and their families are afforded the chance to talk with others who share a similar problem. None of these opportunities would exist in the office of a private surgeon.

The opposite side of the coin is that the clinical staff—surgeon, prosthetist and therapist in particular—have the opportunity to become expert in the field of prosthetics for the juvenile amputee. Such expertise comes only with a critical level of experience. Regional limb deficiency clinics provide the necessary volume of patients to educate us well, whereas private office practice does not afford us the same chance. Clearly, then, both patient and professional are well served by this arrangement.

ACKNOWLEDGMENT

The author gratefully acknowledges the advice and assistance of Leon M. Kruger, M.D., Surgeon-in-Chief, Shriners Hospital for Crippled Children, Springfield, Mass. Under his supervision, the author has learned a sensible and sensitive program of management for the upper limb-deficient child. His professional encouragement and warm personal friendship have been invaluable.

REFERENCES

1. Aitken GT: Management of severe bilateral upper limb deficiencies, Clin Orthop Rel Res, 37:53, 1964.
2. Aitken GT: The child amputee, Orthop Clin North Am 3(2):447, 1972.
3. Angliss VE: Habilitation of upper limb deficient children, Am J Occup Ther 28(7):407, 1974.
4. Downie GR: Limb deficiencies and prosthetic devices, Orthop Clin North Am 7(2):465, 1976.
5. Glynn MK and others: Management of the upper-limb–deficient child with powered prosthetic device, Clin Orthop Rel Res, Aug (209):202, 1986.
6. Heger H, Millstein S and Hunter GA: Electronically powered prostheses for the adult with an upper limb amputation, J Bone Joint Surg 67B (2):278, 1985.
7. Hubbard S, Galway HR, and Milner M: The myoelectric training methods for the preschool child with congenital below-elbow amputation, J Bone Joint Surg 67B (2):273, 1985.
8. Kritter AE: The bilateral upper extremity amputee, Orthop Clin North Am 3(2):419, 1972.
9. Lamb DW and others: Congenital absence of the upper limb and hand, Hand 3(2):193, 1971.
10. Lamb DW and Scott H: Management of congenital and acquired amputation in children, Orthop Clin North Am 12(4):977, 1981.
11. Marquardt E: The multiple limb-deficient child. In American Academy of Orthopaedic Surgeons: Atlas of limb prosthetics, St Louis, 1981, The CV Mosby Co.
12. Mendez MA: Evaluation of a myoelectric hand prosthesis for children with a below elbow absence, Prosthet Orthot Int 9:137, 1985.
13. O'Shea BJ and Dunfield VA: Myoelectric training for preschool children, Arch Phys Med Rehabil 64:451, 1983.
14. Sauter WF: Prostheses for the child amputee, Orthop Clin North Am 3(2):483, 1972.
15. Schmidl H: The I.N.A.I.L. experience fitting upper limb dysmelia patients with myoelectric controls, Bull Prosthet Res 10:17, 1977.
16. Scotland TR and Galway HR: A long term review of children with congenital and acquired upper limb deficiency, J Bone Joint Surg 65B(3):346, 1983.
17. Sensky T: A consumer's guide to "bionic arms," Br Med J July, 1980.
18. Smith RJ and Lipke RW: Treatment of congenital deformities of the hand and forearm, New Eng J Med 300(7):344, 1979.
19. Sorbye R: Myoelectric controlled hand prosthesis in children, Int J Rehabil Res 1:15, 1977.
20. Swanson AB: Severe congenital malformations of the upper limb considerations for classification and treatment, Ann Chir 29(5):433, 1975.
21. Weaver SA, Lange LR, and Vogts VM: Comparison of myoelectric and conventional prostheses for adolescent amputees, Am J Occup Ther 42(2):87, 1988.
22. Wendt JD and Shaperman J: The infant with a cable-controlled hook, Am J Occup Ther 24(6):393, 1970.

XV
SPLINTING

87

The forces of dynamic splinting: ten questions before applying a dynamic splint to the hand

Paul W. Brand

A dynamic splint is one that achieves its effect by movement and force. It is a form of manipulation. It may use forces generated by the patient's own muscles or externally imposed forces using rubber bands or springs.

Whenever passive movement and manipulation of the hand are used, there is a danger that too much force will be used by a surgeon or therapist who is anxious to get results in the limited time available at the clinic. The result is often that the patient has pain; the hand gets swollen, and the short-term gain in mobility is followed by long-term stiffness. We prefer to encourage active exercise and work-related movements because these are controlled by the patient who keeps within the limits of pain. Brain-hand reflexes and coordination, which are essential to real hand health are restored.

However, in many cases, it is not possible to achieve a full range of motion by active exercises alone. They may need to be replaced or supplemented by a dynamic splint. Sometimes active movements are used during the day, and then a splint is worn at night. However, even in such cases the splint may have the same bad results as manipulation of the hand unless the surgeons and the therapists exercise stern discipline to ensure that the forces they impose are well controlled. Too little force will do no good. Too much will do harm. *How much is just right?*

To obtain consistently good results from dynamic splinting, I believe that we have to develop a whole new approach. We have to measure, and we have to calculate. It is not enough to say "rubber-band traction" or "not too much force" or "be gentle." We have to be quantitative. Pharmacology would still be in the dark ages if we continued to prescribe a handful of this medicine or a mouthful of that. We now use milligrams and milliliters. So in terms of force on the hand, we must use units. Then we can begin to compare results, and we shall begin to develop a science. Most books and articles about splints are concerned with design. I want to deal only with measurements and objectives here.

We first must realize that a splint by its very presence on the hand is doing harm. It is inhibiting the free movement and use of the hand. It is only justified if the specific good that it will do compensates for the general harm and restriction.

Thus the first step is to define the object of the dynamic splint for the specific hand we are dealing with and for the specific joint or joints that we want to mobilize or modify. Then we need to ask ten questions in relation to the forces we propose to use: (1) How much force? (2) Through what surface? (3) For how long? (4) To what structure? (5) By what leverage? (6) Against what reaction? (7) For what purpose? (8) Measured by what scale? (9) Avoiding what harm? (10) Warned by what signs?

HOW MUCH FORCE?

In most dynamic hand splints the force is provided by rubber bands or steel springs. At the present time these are not marketed for our profession with information about force or tension. Orthodontists use graded rubber bands, but these are too small for our purpose. Thus each therapist or splint-maker has to purchase rubber bands and springs in batches that appear uniform and then test them for tension. A simple stress-strain diagram should be prepared for each batch to be a guide for future use. I use five points on a curve from 100 to 500 gm and measure the length of the band as it hangs with each of those five weights hooked one by one into its end. Fig. 87-1 shows the curve for one of our rubber bands. If a dynamic splint requires a pull of 200 gm from an outrigger 6 cm from the finger, a quick glance across our graphs will show which band we should use and how far we should stretch it. At the time it is applied we can check the tension with a spring scale (Fig. 87-2).

In most dynamic splints there will be a range of movement that will result in lengthening and shortening the rubber band or spring. Thus the tension will change. This too should be noted. For example, when Dr. Harold Kleinert has done a primary suture on a severed flexor tendon, he likes to use a rubber band from the fingernail to a wrist band. The purpose of this is to hold the finger flexed when it is at rest and to allow the patient to extend his finger against the tension of the rubber band by using the extensor muscles. The rubber band should be strong enough to pull the finger back into flexion without the use of the flexor muscle-tendon unit. For such a purpose, I would use a rubber band that was 5 cm long at rest (no tension) that would have a tension of 200 to 300 gm at 15 cm length.

If one is using a spring-steel wire that exerts force at right angles to its length, this may be calibrated ahead of time with a similar stress-strain curve or may be checked after it is in position by pulling it with a spring scale through the same range that it will act on the finger.

Thus in many cases the question "How much force?" is answered by two figures—for example, 250 gm when the finger is extended and 50 gm when the finger is flexed.

To many surgeons and therapists such figures will be

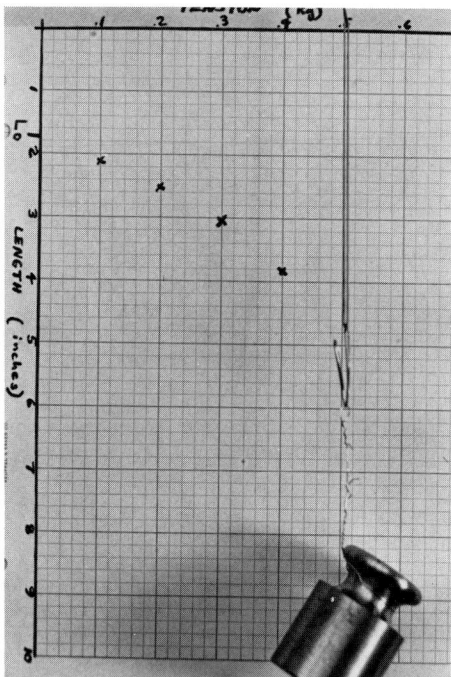

Fig. 87-1 Rubber band being tested by hanging a succession of weights from its end and marking its length on the force-elongation curve.

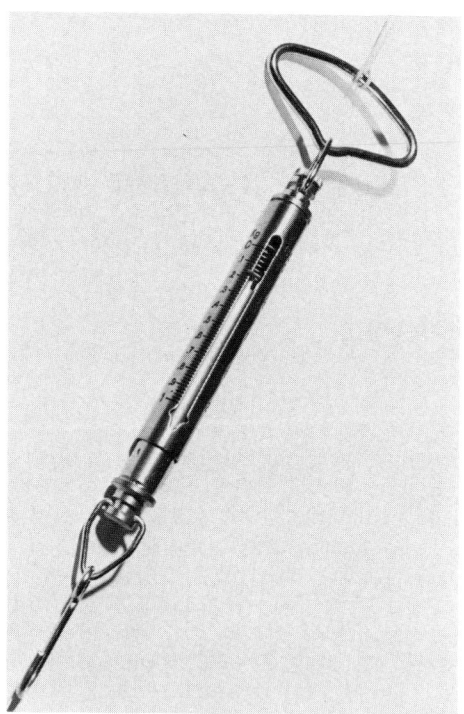

Fig. 87-2 Spring scale.

meaningless because they have not used them before and do not know what 100 gm feels like. If so, it is time to start to learn. Check a tension that "feels right" on the hand and then measure how much tension there is by using a spring scale.

THROUGH WHAT SURFACE?

Every applied force may be presumed to act on the bones or on the musculoskeletal system. However, it has to act *through* the surface of the body. Often the limits on the amount of force we can use are set more by what the skin can stand than by what the joint can accept. Most forces in a hand splint are applied through a sling around a finger and most are quite comfortable at the time they are applied. However, as times passes, they become uncomfortable and finally painful because of ischemia from pressure. This is probably the commonest cause of patients discarding a splint or becoming "uncooperative." If they were more cooperative, they would keep the splint on all night (taking pain-killing medication) and come to the doctor the next day with gangrene under the sling.

Both the ischemia and the pain are caused by *pressure* not just by force. Pressure is force divided by area. Thus a given force may be safe if the sling is wide, and unsafe if it is narrow.

A good general rule is that if a force is to be applied continuously, it should not result in a pressure of more than 50 gm/cm². This is about the same as 35 mm Hg, which is within the margin of safety for long-term pressure on soft tissues. Note that 35 mm Hg is higher than actual capillary pressure, but capillaries in normal tissue can withstand higher pressures.[1] Thus a 200 gm pull needs a 4 cm² area

of sling. All 4 cm² should take equal pressure. If the sling includes curved areas that take oblique stress, it would be better to have 6 cm². This, in old terminology, means that 8 ounces of pull need a full square inch of sling.

A special danger from pressure occurs when a sling becomes tilted. Perhaps the finger changes its angle because the whole splint is loose. Now the same force acts only on the *edge* of the sling. The actual effective surface of the sling may now be less than a quarter of what it was, and so the pressure is multiplied by four. Result—the patient becomes "uncooperative" or else endures pain.

Pressure is relatively unimportant if it is intermittent. It is the sustained pressure that keeps the blood supply from the skin. This is what hurts and then kills the skin.

FOR HOW LONG?

Time is important in two respects—the total time the splint is on the hand and the time that the actual force is pressing on the tissues. If the force acts only in certain positions or when certain muscles pull against it, it is intermittent and the question of ischemia may not airse. If there is any risk from continuous pressure, it is better to use the splint for only 4 or 5 hours at a time and then remove it and look at the skin to see if a flush of reactive hyperemia, or a "hot spot," indicates that the skin has been short of blood. If all is normal, the splint may be worn for gradually longer periods of time.

If the object of the splint is to lengthen a scar or to stimulate the development of free loose skin where previously tight skin has limited joint motion, then time has another kind of importance.

We sometimes speak of "stretching" skin or scar. Stretch

is a passive action that results in the elongation of elastic elements in skin, scar, or ligament. Every bit of elongation of tissue that is accomplished by *stretch* will shorten again when the force is relaxed. When a rubber band is pulled, it becomes longer. It is "stretched." When the pull is relaxed, it returns to its old length. If it is pulled harder, it may break. It is the same with living tissue. The immediate lengthening of tight skin that is produced by pulling will be lost when it is relaxed. If it is pulled too hard, microscopic ruptures in the tissue result in inflammation and later scar formation. The last state may then be worse than the first.

The real true lengthening of any living tissue results from the activity of living cells as they constantly take up and absorb old tissues and lay down new tissues. Old collagen is absorbed; new collagen is laid down in new patterns responsive to new needs. Cells in the skin multiply and proliferate in response to need. Our responsibility is not to try shortcuts by "stretching" or breaking the old tissues but to *stimulate* the living cells to do the work. We do this by keeping the tissues in a physical state that demonstrates the need. The cells will then sense the need and will make changes to meet that need.

The best way to lengthen tissues is to keep them constantly in a state of mild tension. This requires less tension than most of us use, but it needs to be maintained longer than most of us do. A good test is blanching of the skin. If we pull so hard that the skin is blanched, that may be too much. However the tension should be maintained for many hours every day, or even for all day. I often prefer to use cylindric plaster casts reapplied every day to hold the joint in its daily fresh optimal position. However, a good dynamic splint that exercises fairly constant tension is nearly as good and involves fewer visits to the therapist. However, it is of no use unless it is kept in position almost 24 hours a day.

TO WHAT STRUCTURE?

In dealing with stiff joints we have to determine what the limiting structures or tissues are. If we decide that the tissues all around the joint are tight and inflexible, the patient probably should not be in a splint except for pain or inflammation. He should be exercising freely and using his hand. However, if the tissues are free on one side and tight on the other, a corrective splint may be of value. Even so, it is good to know which is the target tissue.

On the flexor side of a proximal interphalangeal (PIP) joint, for example, tight skin or connective tissue will probably remodel with constant tension. An adherent tendon or volar plate, however, may not respond. A good general test is to pull the finger gently toward extension. If it comes to a slow stop and if the skin blanches a little on further attempted movement, this suggests the skin may be short; the prognosis for improvement with a splint is good. If the joint moves freely to a certain point and then stops dead, the prognosis for conservative treatment is poor, and splinting may be a waste of time.

BY WHAT LEVERAGE?

When it is determined which structure or layer around the joint is in need of lengthening, it is possible to visualize the problem in terms of levers around the axis of the joint. The axis of movement of most joints of the hand is at about the midpoint of the head of the proximal bone. Thus, if the palmar skin of the PIP joint is tight, it may be about 1 cm from the axis of the joint in an adult male. Thus, if a sling is placed 3 cm down the finger and hooked up to a force of 250 g to pull the finger straight, the leverage will be 3 to 1, and the skin will experience a tension of 750 g (Fig. 87-3, *A*). If the skin is bowstringing across the joint, it will be farther from the joint axis and will have a longer lever arm. It will be more difficult to get an effective tension to it without producing pressure effects under the sling.

We use the term *mechanical advantage* to express the ratio between the length of the lever through which force is applied and the length of the lever arm through which the force is delivered. In the case of hand splinting this is commonly a number between 2:1 and 5:1. We use the *length* of the finger or hand to *apply* the force, and half the *thickness* of the finger or hand to *deliver* the force. When muscles are moving the fingers from inside the hand, they have very small mechanical advantages because they use levers related to finger thickness to apply their force and have to move levers related to finger length to deliver the force. Thus their ratios are inverted and are commonly 1:5. This is why active exercises are safer than passive movements. They use small leverages and are less likely to do violence to the tissues.

I do not seriously suggest that the mathematic ratios of leverages must be worked out on paper every time a dynamic splint is applied. I do suggest that it is good to work it out sometimes as an educational exercise, and that it should be *thought about* every time. Once a therapist starts to think in terms of leverages and mechanical advantages, he or she is much less likely to make the mistake of overstressing or understressing the key tissues we are trying to modify.

AGAINST WHAT REACTION?

"To every action there is an equal and opposite reaction." Newton knew about this 300 years ago, but we forget it every day. We make a sling to spread the pressure on a finger where we pull, but we forget that the *pull* on the finger results in a *push* on the hand. In the reaction, as well as in the primary action, the damage is done most often by pressure rather than by force. Pressure is force divided by area. Our areas are too small, and so our pressures are big. Consider a simple and common example. A finger has a PIP joint that is stiff in flexion and a metacarpophalangeal (MP) joint that is freely mobile. A splint is applied to provide traction in a dorsal direction to result in tension on the palmar side of the PIP joint. Using our previous figures, the dorsal pull is 250 g at 3 cm from the axis of the PIP joint, resulting in a 750 g tension on the volar skin.

How much force will be needed as a *reaction* or stabilizing force to hold the proximal phalanx steady so that the distal force can act on the PIP joint? If no other force is applied, the finger would *hyperextend* at the MP joint where it is not stiff and the PIP joint would not benefit.

So, *how much?* I find that most therapists and orthotists assume that the *reaction* force should be the same as the *action* force, that is, in this example it would be 250 g. If you pull north with 250 g, you can balance it by pushing south with 250 g. Right? Wrong! Think about leverages and moments. The PIP joint is stiff and will not move much. The movable joint is the MP joint. The 250 g force is applied 3 cm distal to the PIP joint, which means it is about 8 cm

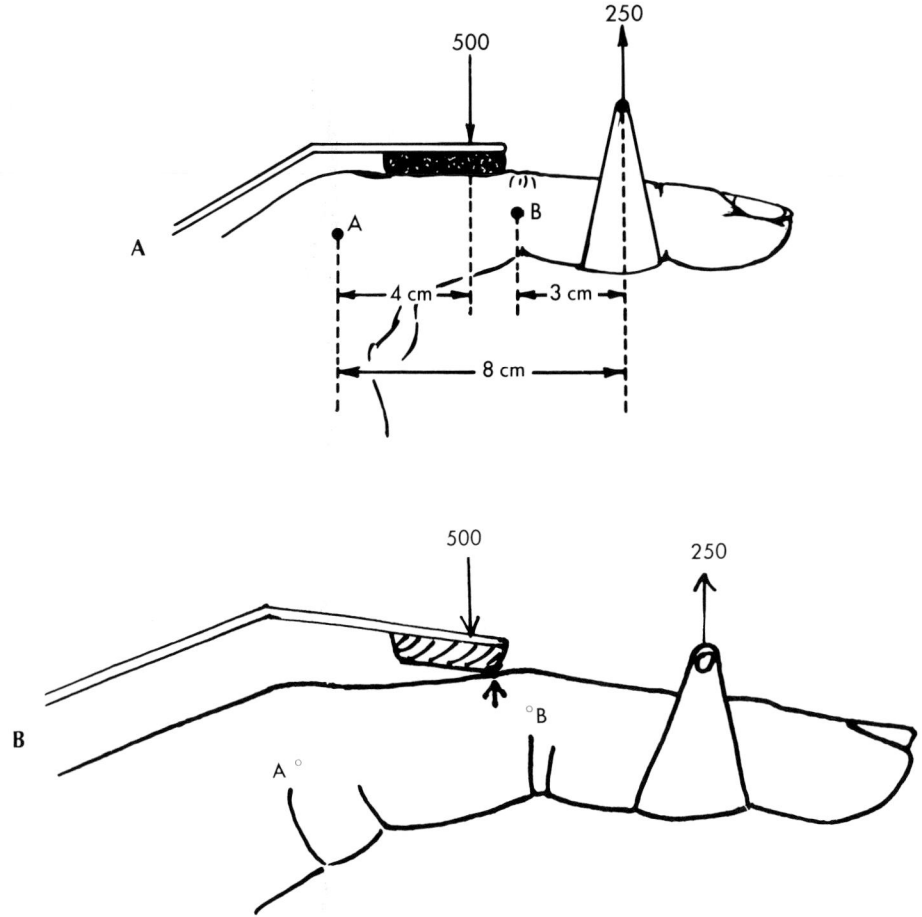

Fig. 87-3 **A,** Diagram of finger subjected to force of 250 g through sling 3 cm from axis, *B,* of the interphalangeal joint. Proximal segment of the finger is held in flexion by a felt pad, which is 4 cm from axis, *A,* of metacarpophalangeal joint. This pad receives thrust of 500 g to balance force on the sling; 500 g × 4 cm = 250 g × 8 cm. **B,** Same finger as in **A,** but because proximal part of hand was not supported, the whole finger has tilted. Now only the edge of the felt pad presses on the finger, creating high pressure.

distal to the MP joint. Thus its moment for extending the PIP joint is 750 gram-centimeters, but for the MP joint it is 250 × 8 g-cm = 2000 g-cm. Now to oppose that moment at the MP joint, 2000 g-cm is needed in the opposite direction. If the restraint on the dorsal surface is placed 4 cm distal to the MP joint, 500 g of force will be exerted on the restraining pad to balance the moment of 2000 g-cm: 500 × 4 = 250 × 8. So it takes double the force on the proximal phalanx to balance the force farther down the finger (Fig. 87-3, *A*).

Splintmakers commonly use a flat bar across the proximal phalanges to balance a sling around the finger. A sling spreads the force around the fingers; a flat bar presses only on the dorsum.

Furthermore, the volar side of the finger is soft and compliant, while the dorsal side is bone and skin. This is why both the pain of a splint and the damage from the splint are more common from the dorsal reaction bar than from the pull on the volar side.

Recognizing how common dorsal problems are, most orthotists and therapists take care to use a broad plate and have it padded. However, the breadth of the plate is of no significance if the finger does not remain in total contact with it. The elastic pull on the finger, failing to straighten

the PIP joint, may use the reaction bar as a fulcrum and tilt the finger upward and the MP joint downward, resulting in the finger pressing only on the edge of the plate. *Result?* The force becomes concentrated on a narrow edge: small area = high pressure = pain or gangrene, or both (Fig. 87-3, *B*).

The way to prevent all this is to think ahead and think in numbers, leverages, moments, and axes. Also, use snug total contact fitting for the proximal support of the hand so that the proximal phalanx cannot move in relation to the hand or the splint (Fig. 87-4).

FOR WHAT PURPOSE?

It has already been stated that before a splint is prescribed, there must be a definition of its specific object. In such a definition it is necessary to bear in mind the harm that comes to the whole hand and perhaps to the patient's own will to recover by keeping him tied up for a long time in a splint. Thus a typical statement of objective might read "to overcome the flexion contracture of the PIP joints of the index and middle fingers and to restore full passive range of motion. The splint may be judged useful as long as 10 degrees of improvement are being recorded per week."

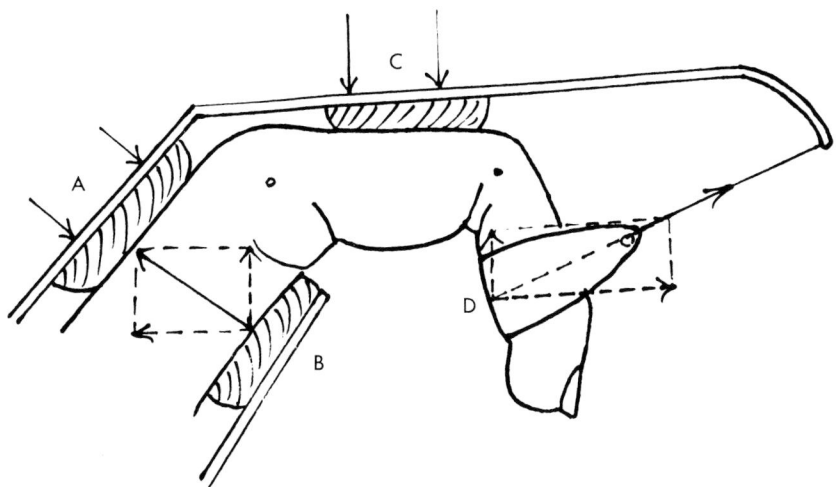

Fig. 87-4 Vector diagram to show how both horizontal and vertical forces need to be balanced. Whereas in Fig. 87-3, *A*, the sling was pulling dorsally, here it pulls obliquely because the interphalangeal joint is flexed. Vector diagram of force of sling, *D*, shows that the horizontal vector is double the dorsal vector. Thus felt pad *C*, which balances dorsal force, will not take much force. However, felt pad in palm, *B*, must be capable of considerable horizontal restraint. It also has dorsal vector, which keeps hand snug against pad *C* and prevents the tilting shown in Fig. 87-3, *B*. Pad *A* has no force to exert or absorb. It is there to stabilize against pad *B* and prevent unexpected shifts of position of hand as a whole.

MEASURED BY WHAT SCALE?

The introduction of specific objective criteria that are time related should ensure that splints are discontinued as soon as their job is done or as soon as they have stopped contributing to total improvement.

In other cases the criteria may be related to muscular strength, reeducation, or some other factor. However, some way should be found to link it to a scale of numbers that may be periodically checked and graphically recorded. Both the therapist and the patient should use the graph and share in the evaluation of the progress and of the value to the patient of the objective that has been chosen.

AVOIDING WHAT HARM?

In addition to the general frustration and harm that comes from confinement in an obtrusive splint, there are sometimes specific problems that arise. These are different for different patients and for different diseases and splints. This is why it is good to pause at the beginning and ask oneself what possible harm could come to *this* hand from *this splint*. One example is when too much force is used to mobilize a stiff joint. The result is inflammation of the periarticular tissues followed by swelling and subsequent increased stiffness. Another example is in rheumatoid arthritis (Fig. 87-5) when a dynamic splint applies force distally on the fingers to extend stiff MP joints. Frequently, there is already some degree of volar subluxation of these joints and a tight volar plate. Distal force will then angulate the finger backwards at the MP joint without true gliding of the joint. This results in intense pressure on the dorsal lip of the proximal articular surface of the phalanx, which presses into the head of the metacarpal because this is now the fulcrum of this abnormal movement. Finally, the lip wears away and complete subluxation ensues. This common problem can only be prevented if the therapist and the patient understand how the

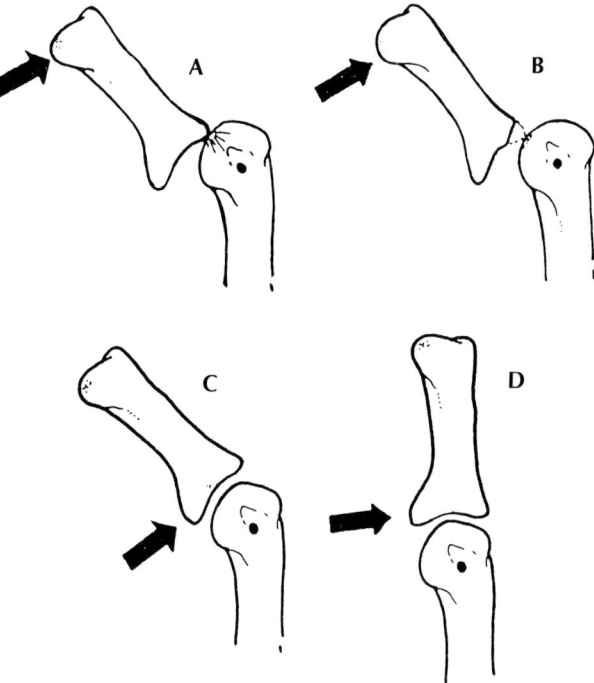

Fig. 87-5 In rheumatoid arthritis if a phalanx begins to subluxate into flexion on the metacarpal head and lies in chronic flexion, it is tempting to use passive external force to extend the joint. If the force is applied distally, **A,** it results in *tilting,* and that results in high stress on the dorsal lip, which becomes absorbed, **B.** If the external force is applied at the *base* of the phalanx, **C,** it tends to restore joint congruence and correct the subluxation, **D.** (Modified from Brand PW: Clinical mechanics of the hand, St Louis, 1985, The CV Mosby Co.)

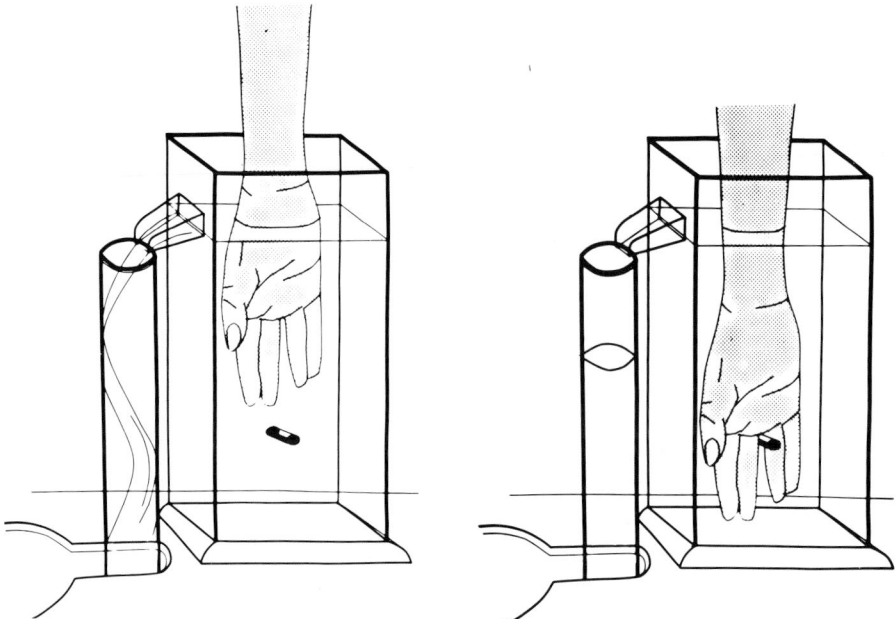

Fig. 87-6 Water displacement volumeter. (Details of this may be obtained from the Rehabilitation Branch, PHS Hospital, Carville, Louisiana 70721.) (From Brand PW: Surgical treatment of primary deformities of the hand. In McDowell F and Enna CD, editors: Surgical rehabilitation in leprosy, Baltimore, 1974, The Williams & Wilkins Co.)

joint works and are warned never to try to extend a subluxating joint by external force unless the force is applied *close to the joint* at the base of the finger, where it will stimulate gliding at the joint not just angulation.

A third problem is that the presence of a big splint sometimes results in the disuse of other, previously normal, joints. These may then become stiff. This is especially true in elderly, arthritic, and apprehensive patients.

Prevention consists in being forewarned and in the institution of regular range-of-motion exercises to all joints that might be affected.

WARNED BY WHAT SIGNS?

When potential dangers are identified, all members of the team need to be alerted to the signs that might indicate the beginning of actual harm.

I like to have a graphic record of hand volume and joint temperatures for problem hands. A water-displacement, hand volumometer gives a quick record of changes in hand volume (Fig. 87-6). Volume goes up when patients keep their hands hanging down or when the hand gets inflamed from excessive use of force. A simple skin thermometer or thermistor probe may be used to keep a record of temperature differentials between a given joint and a contralateral normal joint. Rising temperatures suggest inflammation. Low temperatures may sometimes be associated with sympathetic dystrophy. A careful inspection of the surface of the hand and the feel of the hand by the sensitive palm of the therapist will often pick up redness or swelling or hot spots. A very important modality is the changing reaction of the patient who has been educated and alerted to the potential benefits and problems of any treatment method. The patient experiences a constant feedback that is more significant than some artificially contrived biofeedback apparatus. His or her brain adds up and analyzes a stream of information from skin, joint, and muscle and integrates it with an awareness of personal priorities. The subconscious mind, more flexible and better programmed than any computer, comes up with an evaluation of a splint that should be taken seriously by any physician or splintmaker. We may be specialists treating a single limb with a scientific instrument, but we must be guided by the whole individual—body, mind, and spirit—who has to decide the extent to which he is prepared to place his whole person at the service of one of his digits and restrict his whole freedom and activity to improve a single joint.

The art of a therapist is to remain poised and flexible, responsive to the input of science and technology on the one side and to the human values of a patient on the other. This is a challenge that is constantly different and keeps us constantly alert. You are a hand therapist and spend your time adjusting rubber bands? Look higher! You are in the business of rebuilding human lives.

REFERENCE

1. Daly CH and others: The effect of pressure loading on the blood flow rate in human skin. In Kenedi RM and Cowden JM, editors: Bed sore biomechanics, Strathclyde Bioengineering Seminars, London, 1976, The Macmillan Press Ltd.

88

Principles and methods of splinting for mobilization of joints

Elaine Ewing Fess

Although significant advances have been made in materials and techniques during recent decades, application of external devices to alter upper extremity deformity is not a contemporary concept. Early descriptions of hand splints emanate from the mid-1600s (Fig. 88-1), and surprisingly the primitive appearance of many of these appliances belies a relative sophistication of design. Obvious predecessors to current splints, these inventions often provided serial adjustment in tension through mobilizing forces applied with leather strings, chained loops, or metal screws.

Today's thermoplastic materials facilitate the construction and fitting phases of splint preparation, but these technologic advancements have not automatically led to better understanding of splint design and use. Far too often a splint is exactingly reproduced from a picture without an understanding of the underlying pathologic conditions of the hand and the realistic goals expected of the splint and without utilization of the principles of mechanics, design, fit, construc-

tion and use of dynamic assists that must be correctly applied to achieve effective results. Unfortunately, this "cookbook" approach to splinting often ends in frustration, failure, and undue expense for the patient. Of paramount importance is the understanding that there are no rote splinting solutions to combatting pathologic conditions of the hand. Splints must be individually created to meet the unique needs of each patient, as evidenced by designs that incorporate the variable factors of anatomy, physiology, kinesiology, pathology, rehabilitation goals, occupation, and psychological status.

PURPOSES AND CLASSIFICATION OF MOBILIZING SPLINTS

Mobilizing splints may be used to correct existing deformity through application of gentle forces that gradually cause collagen realignment, tissue growth, and concomitant increased passive range of motion; or they may substitute

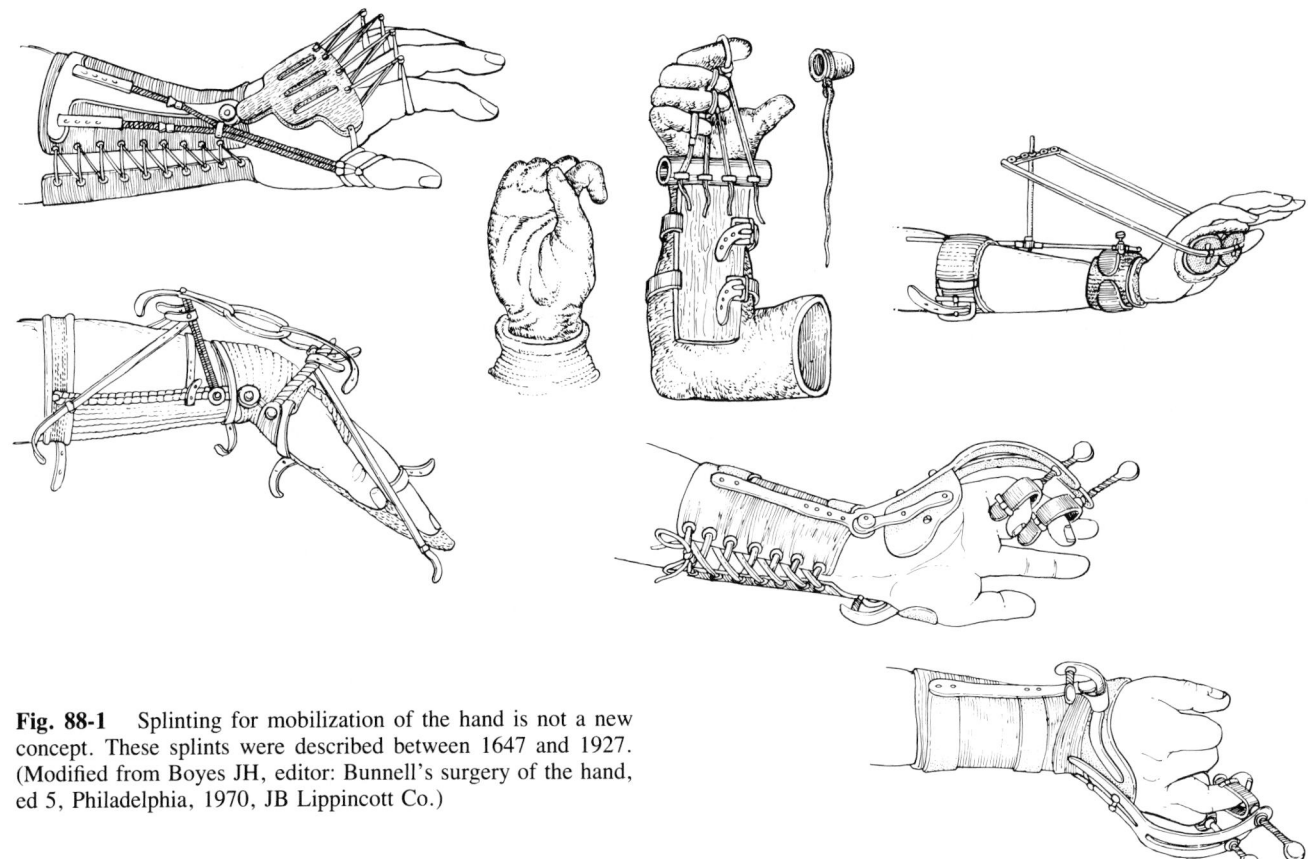

Fig. 88-1 Splinting for mobilization of the hand is not a new concept. These splints were described between 1647 and 1927. (Modified from Boyes JH, editor: Bunnell's surgery of the hand, ed 5, Philadelphia, 1970, JB Lippincott Co.)

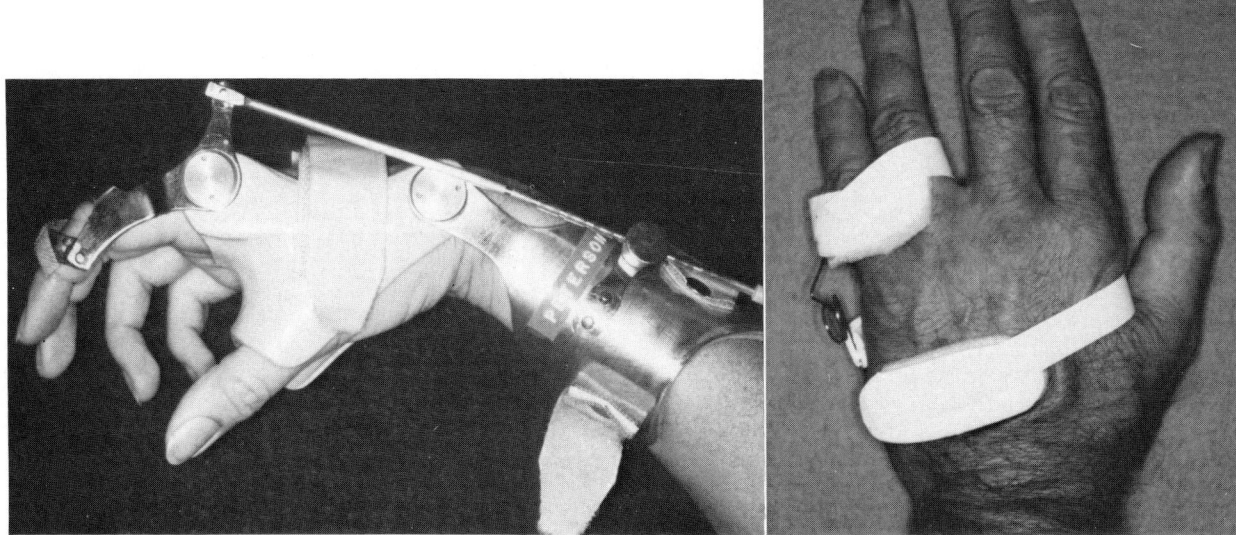

Fig. 88-2 Requiring passive mobility of joints, these substitution splints enhance functional use. (From Fess EE and Philips CA: Hand splinting: principles and methods, ed 2, St. Louis, 1987, The CV Mosby Co.)

for lost active motion, thereby enhancing functional use of the hand. Requiring full passive joint motion, control or substitution splints are often fabricated of more-durable, less-adjustable materials because of their expected length of use (Fig. 88-2). If full joint excursion is not present, a different type of splint is necessary to first decrease existing deformity. Splints designed to improve passive joint motion are usually temporary and should be constructed of materials that are easily altered, because of recurring configuration changes that must be made as range of motion improves. By selecting an inappropriate design option, one may create a splint that is ineffective or that actually contributes to the existing pathologic condition. Control splints frequently do not incorporate the type of forces necessary to alter fixed

deformity; conversely, correctional splint designs may temporarily impede functional use of the hand (Fig. 88-3). It is therefore imperative that a splint design accurately reflect the purpose for which the splint is intended.

Historically, splints have been classified according to purpose of application, configuration, power source, material, or anatomic site. One of the most commonly used classification systems was that of grouping splints according to inherent mechanical characteristics, resulting in two major subdivisions. Static splints had no moving components and were used to provide support and immobilization, whereas dynamic splints employed traction devices such as rubber bands, springs, or cords to apply corrective forces to stiffened joints. However, with the advancement of splinting

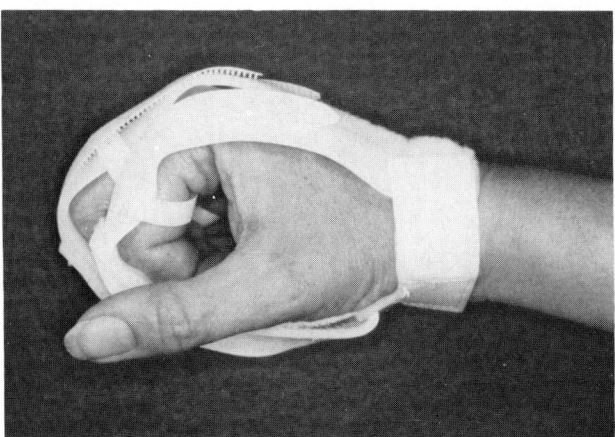

Fig. 88-3 Designed to improve joint motion, this simple finger flexion splint does not allow functional use of the hand during wearing periods. (From Fess EE and Philips CA: Hand splinting: principles and methods, ed 2, St. Louis, 1987, The CV Mosby Co.)

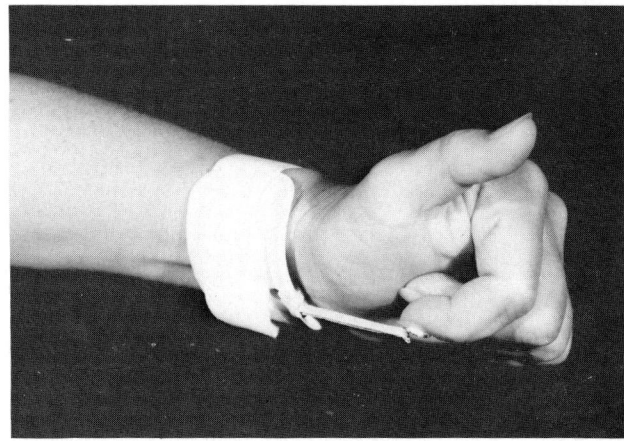

Fig. 88-4 Classified as a simple finger flexion splint, the traction device exerts a similar mobilizing force on the three successive digital joints. (From Fess EE and Philips CA: Hand splinting: principles and methods, ed 2, St. Louis, 1987, The CV Mosby Co.)

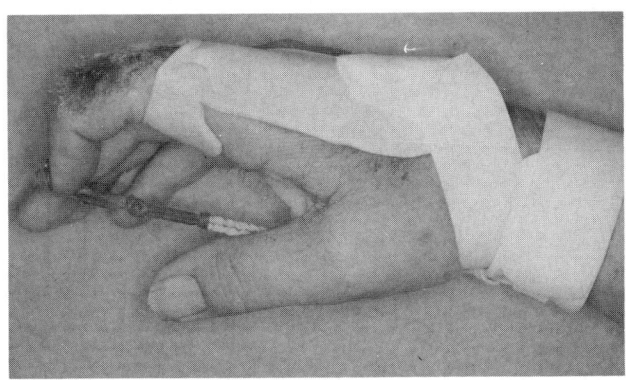

Fig. 88-5 The normal metacarpophalangeal joint is immobilized in this compound proximal interphalangeal joint flexion splint, allowing the flexion force to be directed to the proximal interphalangeal joint. (From Fess EE and Philips CA: Hand splinting: principles and methods, ed 2, St. Louis, 1987, The CV Mosby Co.)

experience and knowledge, the value of using "static" splints to improve range of motion through consecutive configuration changes was recognized and the limitations of this classification method became increasingly apparent.

Based on three independent variables—(1) splint forces and the planes in which they occur, (2) the anatomic site of emphasis, and (3) the primary kinematic goal of the splint—a descriptive classification system provides a more definitive means of grouping splints. Splints are described in terms of these three variables, which in essence consist of the "how," "where," and "why" of splint design and application. The first of the three variables describes the complexity of the forces used within a given splint; in this regard splints can be divided into simple, compound, and long categories. The second variable is the anatomic site to which the mobilizing forces are directed—thumb, index proximal interphalangeal (PIP) joint, ring metacarpophalangeal (MP) joint, and so on. The third variable is the intent or kinematic direction of the splint—in other words, flexion, extension, rotation, or abduction. A simple finger flexion splint applies a similar mobilizing flexion force to all joints incorporated in the splint (Fig. 88-4), whereas a

compound PIP flexion splint uses a series of differing forces to simultaneously control and mobilize the sequential joints of the digit, with the primary mobilizing force of the splint directed toward flexion of the PIP joint (Fig. 88-5). Simple and compound splints are designed to improve articular and capsular motion, but because they do not control the wrist, they do little to effect extrinsic tendon excursion. Providing an additional level of control to the open upper extremity kinetic chain, long splints control wrist motion and therefore may be used to increase passive glide of extrinsic tendons in addition to digital joint motion (Fig. 88-6).

A descriptive splint classification based on well-defined categories that accurately and reliably groups and defines the seemingly endless array of splints is fundamental to the continued development of splinting knowledge and professional communication. This method of classification also allows the splint designer considerable latitude for creating splints that meet the unique needs of patients. Types of forces, materials, surface of application, and splint configurations are options that are left to the discretion and creativity of the person designing and fitting the splint. Latitude is important if splinting is to advance beyond the "cookbook" stage and be used to its full potential as a viable and integral aspect of hand rehabilitation.

ASSESSMENT

Assessment provides a foundation for splinting programs by delineating baseline pathologic factors from which splints may be individually created and progress may be monitored. The evaluation process involves gathering and integrating information derived from many sources. A finished splint should not only reflect anatomic and physiologic requirements, but also should meet the patient's psychologic and socioeconomic needs. Astute observation, detailed interrogation, careful inspection, and concise measurement guide the hand specialist in creating splint designs that are uniquely adapted to meet specific requirements.

Using instruments proven to be reliable and valid, measurements of extremity mass, temperature, range of motion, strength, sensibility, and dexterity provide concrete numerical data about given components of hand function. These measurements are essential to establishing and monitoring splinting and exercise programs. Often exhibiting rapid change, a healing hand must be constantly and carefully

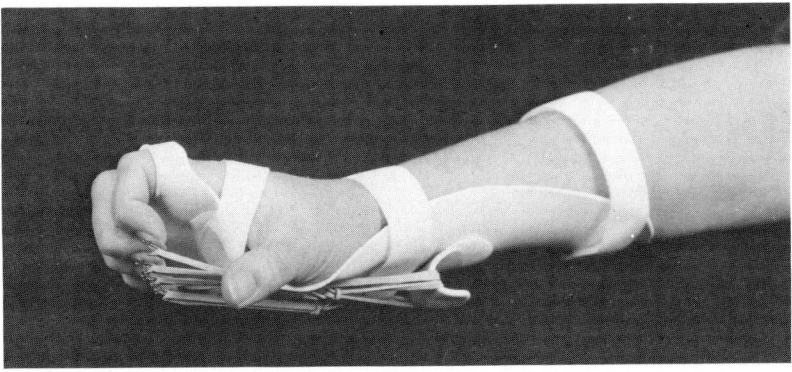

Fig. 88-6 This complex interphalangeal joint flexion splint controls the positions of the wrist and metacarpophalangeal joints in addition to providing mobilizing forces to the interphalangeal joints. (From Fess EE and Philips CA: Hand splinting: principles and methods, ed 2, St. Louis, 1987, The CV Mosby Co.)

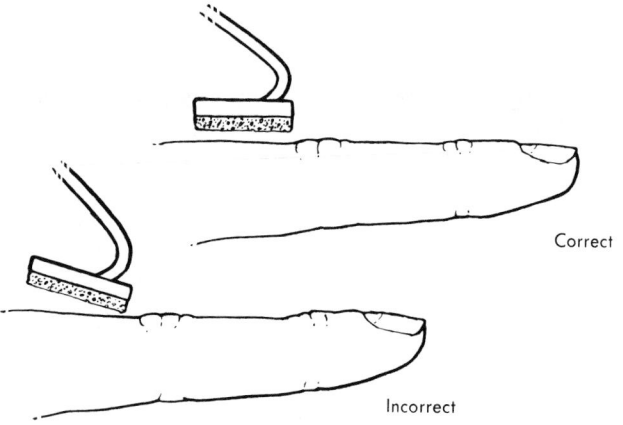

Correct

Incorrect

Fig. 88-7 To reduce pressure, narrow splint components should be carefully fitted to achieve contiguous contact between splint part and hand. (From Fess EE and Philips CA: Hand splinting: principles and methods, ed 2, St. Louis, 1987, The CV Mosby Co.)

monitored for the therapist to direct appropriate and efficient adaptation of splints and exercises.

PHYSIOLOGIC FACTORS

Splinting is one of the most effective means of improving passive mobility of stiffened joints. When used appropriately, it produces a gradual rearrangement or lengthening of the pericapsular structures and an elongation of adhesions through directed gentle traction. It is important, therefore, to thoroughly understand the stages of wound healing and how they apply to specific tissues. The careful integration of these concepts into splinting and exercise programs provides the foundation on which efficacious therapeutic intervention is based. Dictated by the rate and method of the reparative processes of healing tissues following injury, splinting programs must be designed to judiciously use and manipulate the physiologic process of collagen formation.

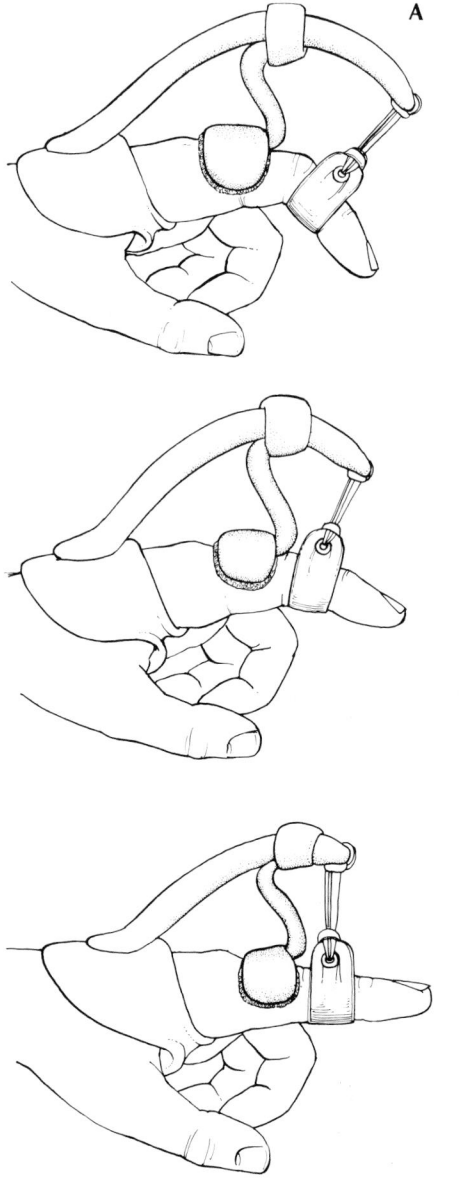

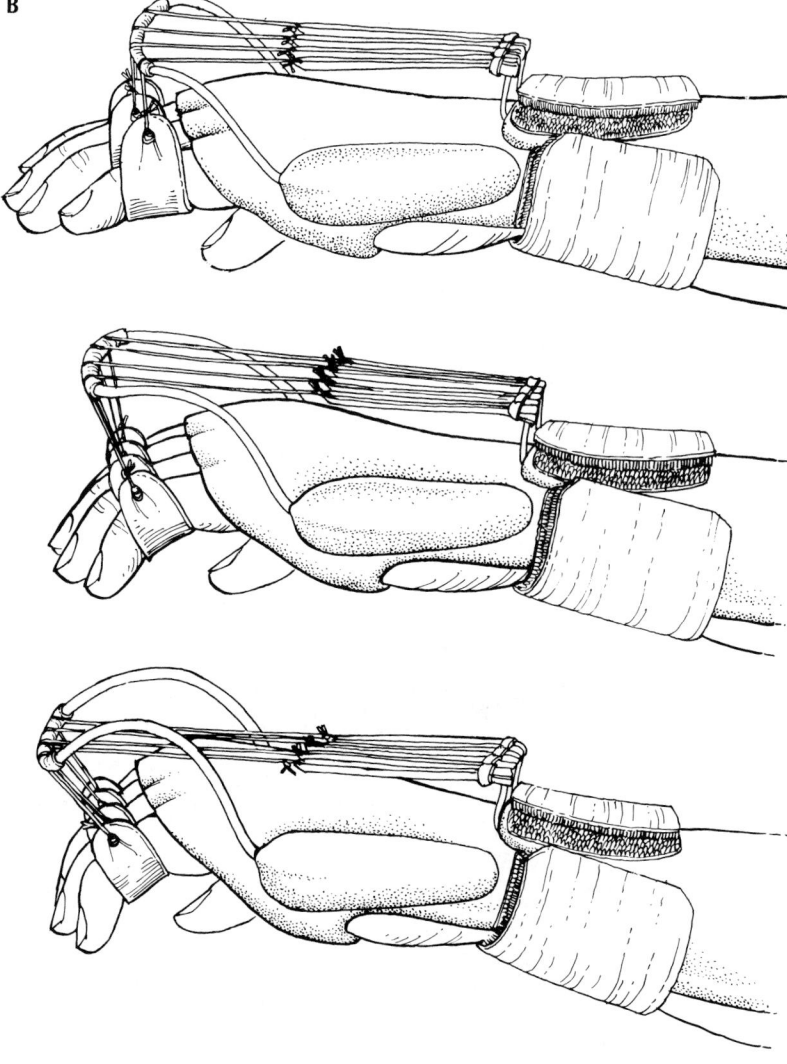

Fig. 88-8 A 90-degree angle of the dynamic assist to the mobilized segment must be maintained as passive joint motion changes. **A,** High profile. **B,** Low profile. (From Fess EE and Philips CA: Hand splinting: principles and methods, ed 2, St. Louis, 1987, The CV Mosby Co.)

PRINCIPLES OF MOBILIZATION SPLINTING

Basic rules apply to all phases of splint preparation regardless of the purpose of application and ultimate splint configuration. These principles define fundamental elements that contribute to the creation of an effectively working splint that is comfortable, durable, and cosmetically acceptable and that successfully meets individual patient requirements. Failure to incorporate these principles may result in splints that are eventually discarded because they are uncomfortable and ineffective or, worse, splints that, if worn, cause additional damage to the hand through pressure sores, attenuation of ligaments, compression or distraction of joint surfaces, or inappropriate application of force direction or magnitude to healing structures. The decision to apply mobilizing forces to an injured or diseased hand is a serious consideration; it should involve close communication between the physician, the therapist, and the patient. It is important that the goals of fitting a splint be realistic and that all those involved thoroughly understand and accept the responsibilities of such an endeavor.

Mechanical principles

Because splinting consists of external application of forces to the extremity, an understanding of basic mechanical engineering concepts is an essential prerequisite to the design, construction, and fitting of all hand splints. One may control or diminish pressure from the splint on the extremity by widening the area of force application and by increasing the mechanical advantage of lever systems. Clinically, this means that splints that are longer and wider are more comfortable, and a contiguous fit of narrow components and over bony prominences is of paramount importance (Fig. 88-7). Elimination of the translational component of an applied force by maintenance of a 90-degree angle of approach to the segment being mobilized (Fig. 88-8) is also of utmost importance when one is designing and fitting splints. This allows the full magnitude of the rotational force to be directed toward correcting the joint deformity and excludes force components that cause compression or distraction of the articular surfaces. Additionally, understanding of torque and the integrated effects of reciprocal parallel forces allows identification and control of the magnitude of corrective and stabilizing forces as they relate to the placement of specialized splint parts. The relative degree of passive mobility of successive joints also plays an important role in splint design. If mobilizing forces are dissipated at normal or less involved joints, the potential for increasing passive motion of stiff joints within the same longitudinal segment is diminished considerably. Splints therefore must be designed to apply corrective forces to only those joints that lack passive motion (Fig. 88-9).

Because excessive shear stress leads to tissue breakdown and ulceration, understanding the effects of shear on soft tissue is also imperative in designing, constructing, and fitting splints. High shear effects may be avoided by rounding splint edges, by keeping pressures low, and by eliminating unwarranted motion and friction. Finally, for a more effective method of increasing splint durability than the retrospective trussing of layers of plastic, one may increase material strength by designing contour into the splint. Mechanical principles determine splint effectiveness, comfort, and durability and should be carefully incorporated into the design, construction, and fitting phases of splint preparation.

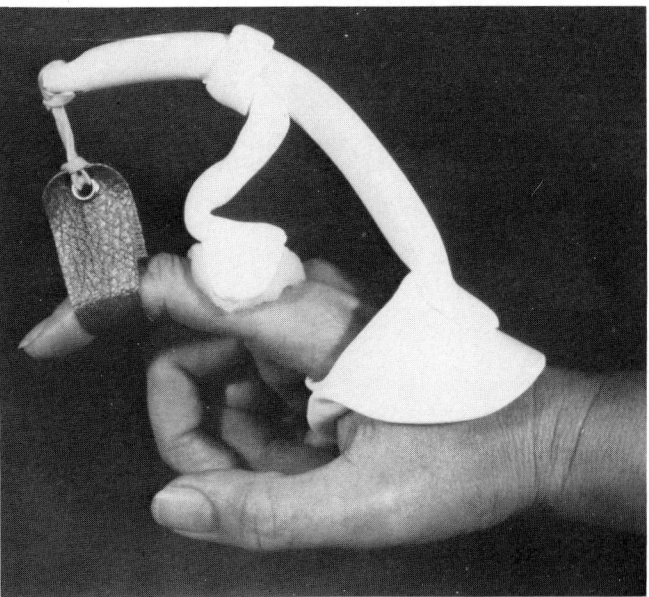

Fig. 88-9 A compound splint allows the mobilizing force to be directed to a single joint when relative joint motion is dissimilar along the digital ray. (From Fess EE and Philips CA: Hand splinting: principles and methods, ed 2, St. Louis, 1987, The CV Mosby Co.)

Principles of using dynamic assists

Regardless of their external configuration, splints that are designed either to improve motion of stiff joints or to substitute for loss of active motion must have a means of generating forces. Depending on the purpose of splint application, these forces either apply prolonged gentle pull to influence collagen alignment of stiffened joints or they move passively supple joints to enhance hand function.

The two key words associated with application of force to mobilize stiffened joints are (1) *prolonged* and (2) *gentle*. Splints designed to improve passive range of motion must be worn for a long enough period of time to allow collagen realignment to occur. Wearing a splint for 1 or 2 hours a day is not sufficient time for tissue growth to take place. For example, it would not be unusual for a patient to be instructed to remove his splint only for periods of exercise every 2 or 3 hours throughout the day. Wearing schedules must, of course, be modified to meet the specific requirements of each situation, but the concept of the application of traction over a long period of time is fundamental. The second word, *gentle*, is of equal importance. Forces that are too great cause further injury to soft tissue structures, resulting in pain, increased inflammatory response, and additional scar formation (Fig. 88-10). The devastating and debilitating cyclic pattern of forceful traction (through splinting or manipulation), tissue injury, pain, inflammation, and production of additional scar must be avoided at all costs.

When using dynamic assists to provide traction to stiff joints, identification, control, and maintenance of force magnitude is critical. Generally speaking, forces between 100 and 300 g are felt to be acceptable. It has been shown that experienced hand therapists adapt the amount of pull within this range to accomodate variations in diagnosis and physiologic timing.

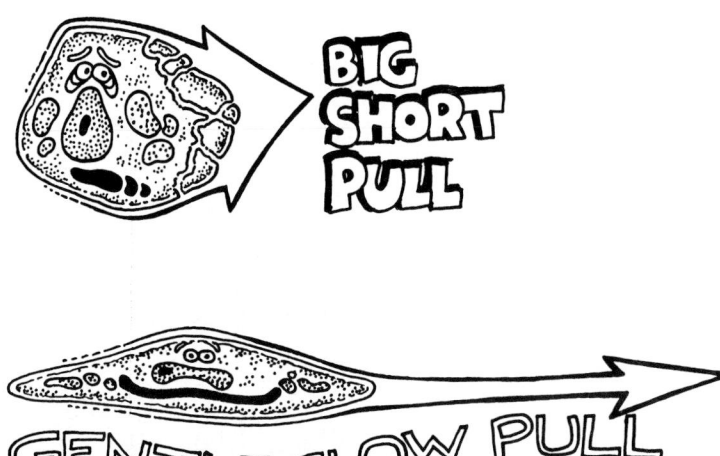

Fig. 88-10   Too much force over too little time creates tearing of soft tissues, resulting in increased inflammatory response and additional scar formation. (From Fess EE and Philips CA: Hand splinting: principles and methods, ed 2, St. Louis, 1987, The CV Mosby Co.)

Actual measurement of force magnitude for substitution or control splints is not necessary since the joint(s) being moved is supple and the required force is that which is sufficient to move the segment(s) into a desired posture.

The range of forces generated by a dynamic assist depends on inherent physical properties of its base material and on the specific design of the assist. Forces created by rubber bands depend on thickness, length, and quality of rubber; springs rely on gauge, tensile strength, and diameter and length of coils. Shelf life also influences some dynamic assist materials. The physical properties of the dynamic assist should be correlated with patient requirements and with splint design. For example, an assist that requires frequent adjustment would not be an appropriate choice for a patient who has difficulty returning to the clinic, and an assist that depends on considerable length to provide consistent tension would be inappropriate for a hand-based splint design.

Mechanical and fit principles must also be taken into consideration. A dynamic assist should apply force in a direction that is 90° to the segment being mobilized and perpendicular to the axis of joint rotation. Pressure on attachment devices such as finger cuffs and nail hooks should be carefully monitored and maintained at minimum levels, and friction and shear should be avoided.

Design principles

The principles of design may be divided into basic groups—general considerations and specific considerations. General principles incorporate broad concepts that result in a splint that is practical for both the patient and the therapist, while the more specific guidelines are concerned with the unique pathologic conditions exhibited by individual patients. Factors such as age, ability to accept responsibility, independence, and occupational demands contribute to the overall design of a splint, as do anticipated use time and prescribed exercise regimens. Splints should allow maximum function and sensation and should be as

simple in design and appearance as possible. Construction time should also be within reason. Specific principles of design encompass concepts that individualize splints to the existing requirements of pathology, anatomy, physiology, and kinesiology. Is the splint intended to substitute for absent active motion, or is it designed to correct existing deformity? Will elastic or inelastic forces be more effective? What splint components are required to control which joints, and what type of mobilizing forces will provide the greatest potential for increasing passive motion of stiff joints? Which mechanical principles should be used to increase effectiveness, comfort, and durability? These and many other questions must be anticipated and answered before design concepts reach the finality of pattern construction.

Component designing lends an organized and rational approach to creating splints that meet individual patient needs. Problems are identified and splint parts are mentally assembled to control or diminish the projected pathologic situation. This approach requires that the designer be fully cognizant of the uses and ramifications of each splint component. For example, low-profile outriggers have been shown to lose adjustment more quickly than do high-profile outriggers (Fig. 88-11). This however, is a viable concept only if one is dealing with correctional forces. If the purpose of a splint is to substitute for active motion, full passive joint motion is a prerequisite and the need for sequential adjustments to accomodate motion improvements is nonexistent. Low-profile outriggers are appropriate design options for control or substitution splints because sequential adjustments are not needed. Conversely, high-profile outriggers provide longer increments of near 90-degree angle of pull than do the low-profile designs, indicating that for correctional splints the higher design option will require fewer adjustments as improvements in motion are gained. Whether this is an important concept in the designing of a correctional splint is entirely dependent on the patient's capacity to return to the clinic for adjustments and the time demands of the therapist's case load.

Splint designing should never be approached in a rote or

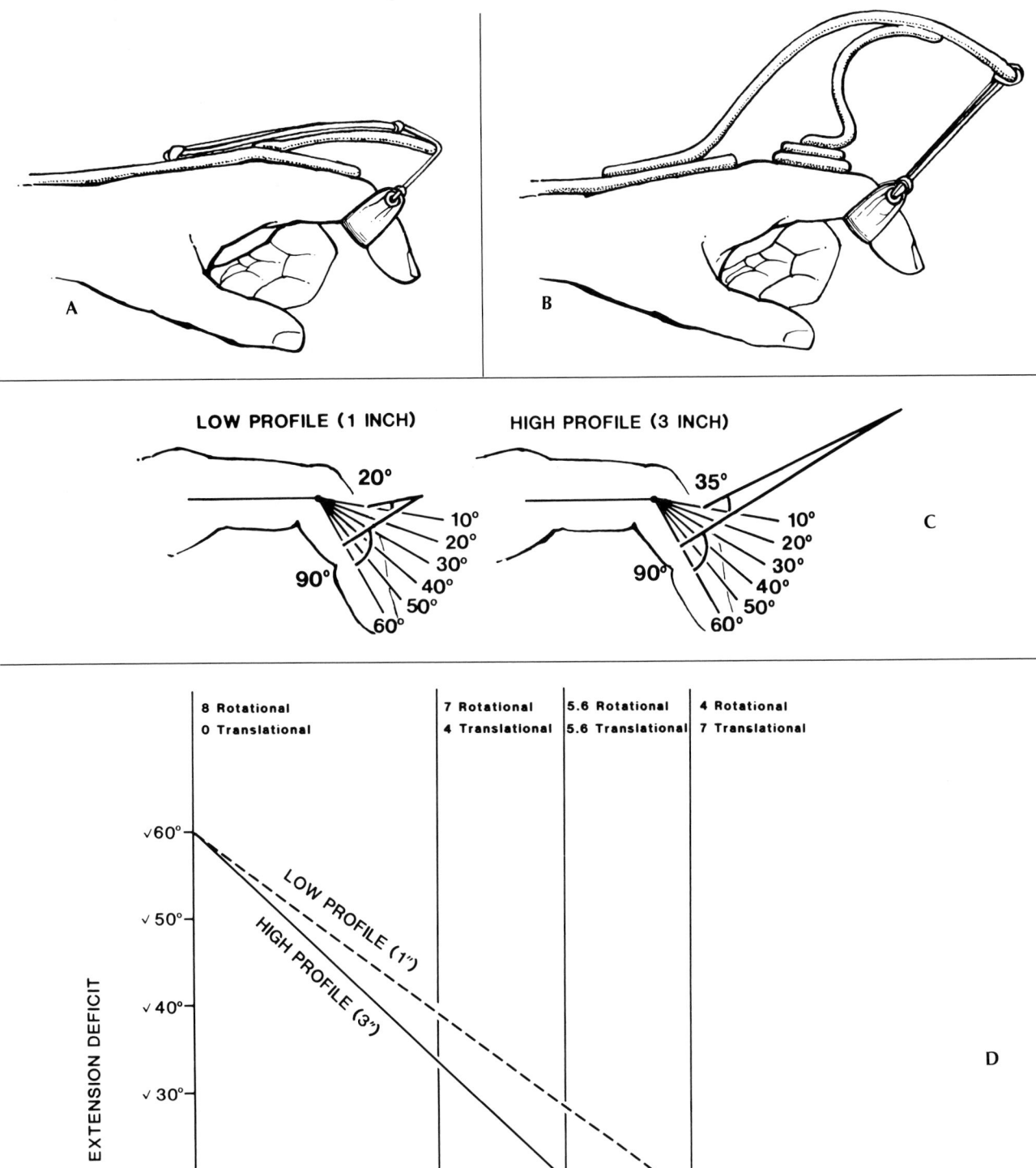

LOW PROFILE (1 INCH)

20°

90°

10°
20°
30°
40°
50°
60°

HIGH PROFILE (3 INCH)

35°

90°

10°
20°
30°
40°
50°
60°

C

8 Rotational
0 Translational

7 Rotational
4 Translational

5.6 Rotational
5.6 Translational

4 Rotational
7 Translational

PIP EXTENSION DEFICIT

√60°
√50°
√40°
√30°
√20°
√10°

LOW PROFILE (1")

HIGH PROFILE (3")

90° 80° 70° 60° 50° 40° 30° 20° 10° 0°

ANGLE OF APPLIED FORCE

D

Fig. 88-11   Schematic representations of low-profile outrigger, **A,** and high-profile outrigger, **B.** Comparison of low-
and high-profile outriggers indicates that as passive motion improves, the high-profile design maintains a better angle
of pull without adjustment than does the low-profile design, **C** and **D.**

Fig. 88-12 To avoid attenuation of a collateral ligament because of unequal force application, **C,** a mobilizing force should be applied in a direction that is perpendicular to the rotational axis of the joint, **B. A,** Correct alignment. (From Fess EE and Philips CA: Hand splinting: principles and methods, ed 2, St. Louis, 1987, The CV Mosby Co.)

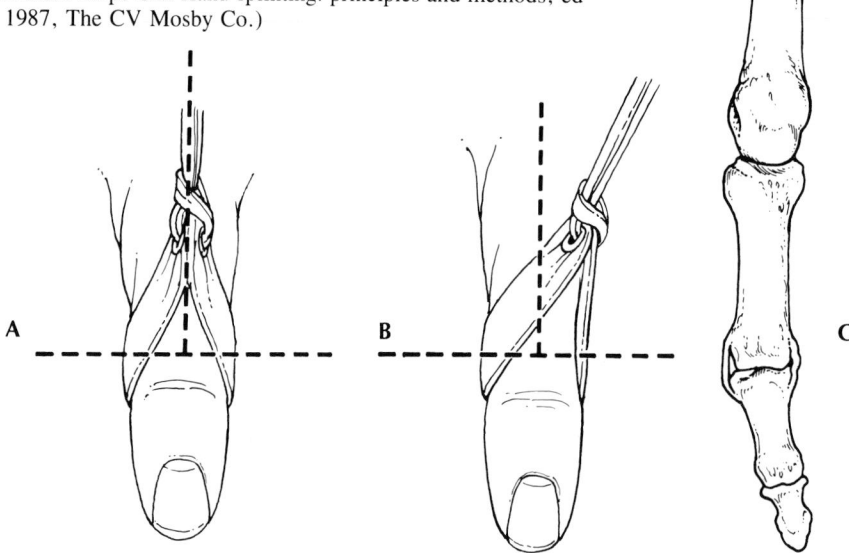

routine manner. Although patients may have similar diagnoses, the pathologic conditions presented are unique, as are the patient's intellectual and emotional capacities to deal with injury and dysfunction. One must approach each case anew to attain maximum rehabilitation potential, using splints designed efficaciously, realistically, and practically for all those involved.

Construction principles

Observing proper construction principles and selecting equipment and methods appropriate to the materials used will help to ensure the durability, cosmesis, comfort, and usefulness of the finished splint. Splint corners should be uniformly rounded, edges smoothed, joined surfaces stabilized, rivets finished, and straps and padding secured. Mechanical principles should be analyzed and incorporated to enhance durability and comfort, and careful adherence to safety precautions when one is working with splinting equipment is important. The equipment and the type and temperature of heat should be selected to meet the demands of the splinting material used. Failure to adhere to construction guidelines may result in splint disuse because of patient discomfort, lack of acceptance, or splint breakage from mechanical failures, all of which represent loss of time and needless expense for both the patient and the members of the rehabilitation team.

Principles of fit

Fitting principles may be divided into four groups—mechanical, anatomic, kinesiologic, and technical. Mechanical factors include use of forces that are perpendicular both to the bone being mobilized and to the axis of joint rotation (Fig. 88-12). When traction is applied simultaneously to several joints within a digit, care must be taken to ensure that the pull is perpendicular to the rotational axis of each joint. Additionally, pressure reduction through contiguous fit and application of lever systems in fitting splint

components is important. Anatomic factors encompass the use of skin creases as guidelines for splint boundaries, identification and adaptation to bony prominences, support of longitudinal and transverse arches, understanding of ligamentous stress, and proper alignment of splint and anatomic joint axes. A hand in motion presents a multiplicity of differing external configurations and internal muscle dynamics as it moves through various planes. Kinesiologic considerations, which include kinematic and kinetic principles, are very important to splint design and fitting phases. Splint parts must be fitted to allow motion, and they must be placed appropriately to control or augment motion, depending on individual requirements. Technical considerations emphasize efficiency and include developing patient rapport, developing work skills, and adapting methods to the materials used. A splint must be continually reevaluated to ensure a proper fit. As the hand heals and motion improves, one must recognize changes that occur and for which appropriate adaptations must be incorporated into the splint. Failure to do so will invariably render the splint less effective, impeding the advancement of the rehabilitation process.

CONCLUSION

Mobilizing splints play an important role in the rehabilitation process of the diseased or injured hand. These splints may provide correctional or substitutional forces and are designed and fitted according to specific requirements unique to each patient. It should also be emphasized that splinting programs should be augmented with appropriate exercise routines and activities that encourage functional use of the extremity. Splints alone do not produce the active motion necessary for hand use. It is the astute combination of passive motion, provided through splinting endeavors, and active exercise programs that forms the foundation for hand rehabilitation techniques and that allows the patient to return to a productive life-style.

89

Spring-wire splinting of the proximal interphalangeal joint

Judy C. Colditz

HISTORY

The proximal interphalangeal (PIP) joint is vulnerable to injury, since it lies midway between the long lever arms of the proximal and middle phalanges. Its tight anatomic construction and intricate anatomy are unforgiving of forces crossing it in any plane but the normal flexion or extension. Residual flexion contracture of the PIP joint is a frequent complication after phalangeal fractures, PIP joint dislocation, volar plate injury, flexor tendon repairs, chronic boutonnière deformity, partial or complete tear of a collateral ligament, or major hand trauma resulting in edema and immobilization.[2,3,12,15] The powerful flexor tendon system with its efficient pulley system is far more effective in gaining flexion of the PIP joint than the primarily intrinsically

powered dorsal hood mechanism is in gaining extension. The last range of full PIP joint extension can be gained most effectively by a gentle prolonged stretch to the tissues toward full extension to reestablish the balance of motion.

Splint design

PIP joint splinting is effectively achieved by a low-profile spring-wire splint incorporating only the finger, as first described by Capener.[8,9] This is a splint of a three-point design with spring coils lying at the axis of the PIP joint laterally (Fig. 89-1). This design is frequently referred to as the Capener splint,[13,16-19] and many commercially available splints using the lateral coil are sold as "Capener" splints.

Bunnell illustrates the use of both clock-spring splints and

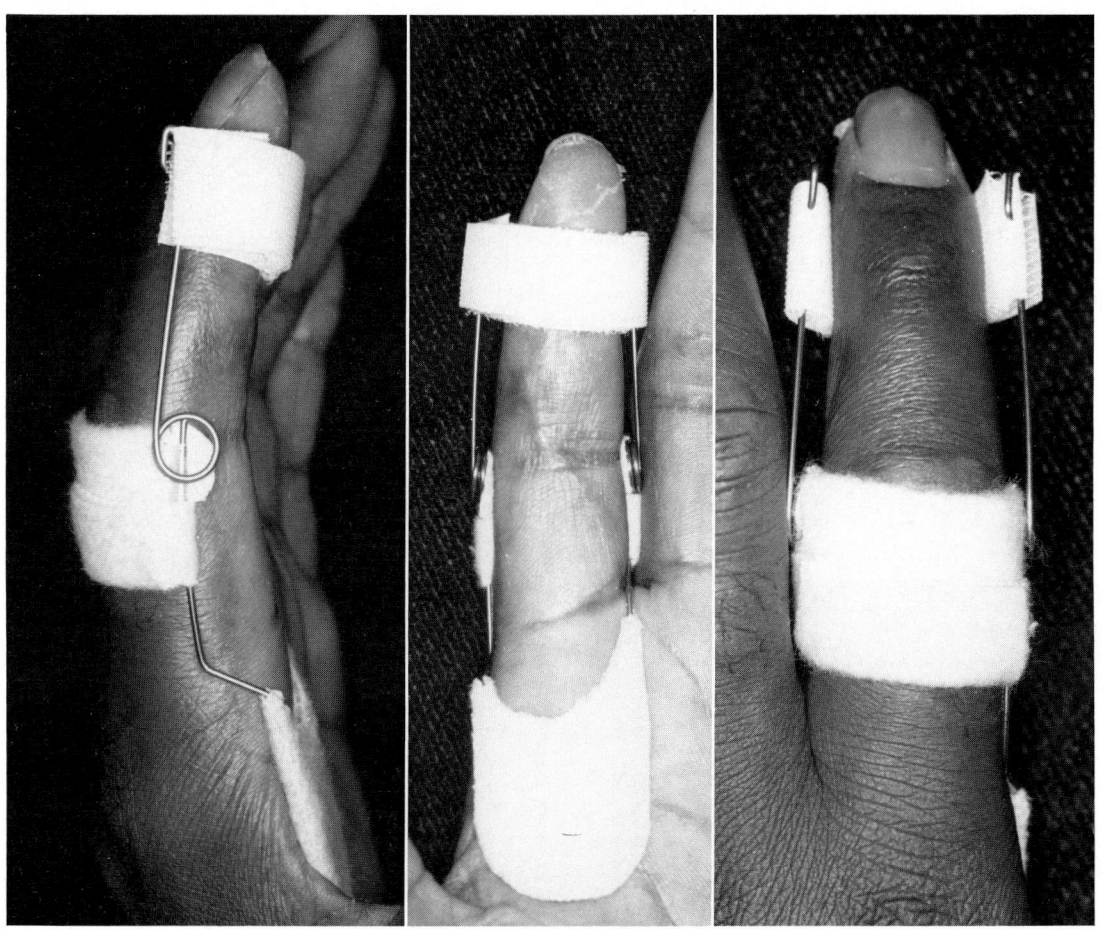

Fig. 89-1 Multiple views of low-profile spring wire splint for PIP joint extension.

spring-wire splints to extend PIP joint flexion contractures.[6] Wynn Parry illustrates in detail the construction of spring-wire finger splints after Capener but describes the spring as being used primarily for resistance for finger flexion after flexor tendon repair or for full-time wear for immobilization in extension, as with a boutonnière deformity.[18] The gauge of wire, the increasing diameter of the coils, and the number of coils described by Wynn Parry provide a lower tension than the technique described below.

Commercially available Capener splints follow Capener's original design of increasing diameters of the coils. Fess has studied the forces generated by these splints and found the forces to be variable within the same design and, as one would expect, variable based on the degree of the flexion contracture of the finger, because the splint is constructed to rest with the extension arms at 0 degrees.[10] Some forces were alarmingly high. Callahan and McEntee also observe that commercial splints provide varying amounts of tension. They express concern about the difficulty of commercial splints fitting accurately and about the force being distributed over a smaller surface area than that of a custom splint.[7]

The design described in this chapter has two coils of identical diameter and is routinely constructed from the same grade of spring steel piano wire. Force generated by this splint can be altered in many ways: the addition of more coils decreases the force applied, the extension arms can be bent to partially accommodate the flexion contracture (thus decreasing force and increasing long-wear tolerance), a lighter gauge wire could be used to alter tension, and the design of the Velcro loop allows the patient some adjustability in force applied. Although many clinicians have empirically suggested force levels for splinting, no clinical study validates these force recommendations.[4,5,10,11,14] Patient comfort and objective measurements demonstrating joint improvement in the absence of any complications have proven the splint design in this chapter to be an effective tool for correction of the mild PIP flexion contracture based on our 16 years of clinical experience with it.

Callahan and McEntee offer a modification of the spring coil splint, which they recommend for PIP joint contractures that have a "hard end feel"[7] (Fig. 89-2). They feel this combines the advantages of ease of application of the Capener splint with the constant force offered by serial casting. They suggest the use of brass welding rod as a superstructure, which gives a static force to the joint, with

the force being altered by the tightness of the Velcro strap. Spring steel piano wire may also be used; the memory in the wire provides a dynamic force without the coils.

Whatever the splint design choice, it must be based on a clear rationale of prolonged gentle stress to the joint with the force being applied using sound mechanical principles.

The technique described below is of greater ease and speed of construction than the soldering of tin as described by Wynn Parry. The splint described is designed with the goal of correcting only the mild flexion deformities (less than 45 degrees) of the PIP joint.

CUSTOM SPLINTING

The advantage of the custom-made splint over the commercially available splint is obvious in that the length of the splint can be made to exactly match the length of the available lever arms and the coils can be located at the exact axis of the joint. Additionally, the dorsal piece lying over the proximal phalanx can be of maximum size, and it ends exactly at the axis of the PIP joint (Fig. 89-1), thus distributing pressure well on the dorsum of the finger, where there is little natural padding. The Velcro strap on the volar aspect of the distal end of the middle phalanx offers the patient adjustability of the tension so as to keep it within comfortable tolerance. Since the resting position of the splint force arms is at 0 degrees of extension, this design does not have the danger of hyperextending the PIP joint, as the reverse knuckle bender can. The use of spring wire elimi-

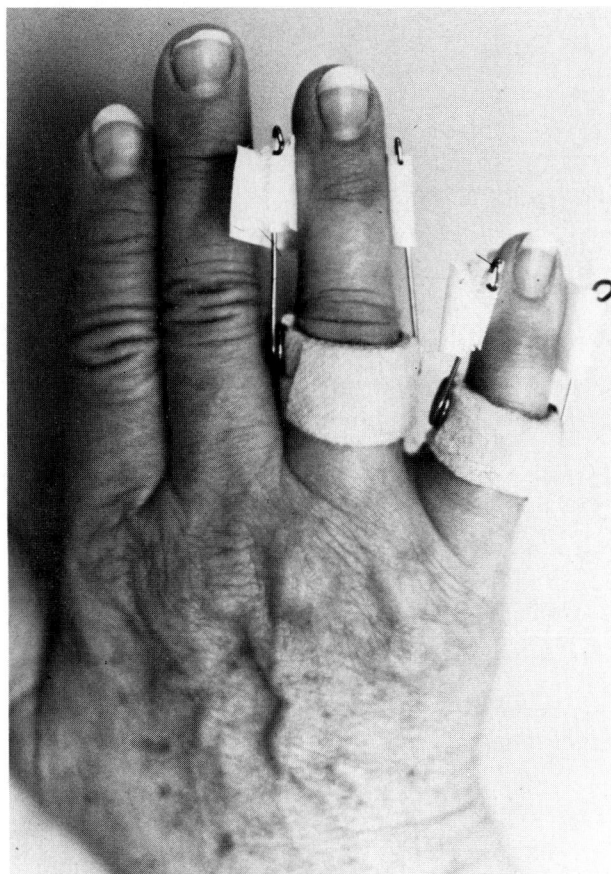

Fig. 89-3   Two spring-wire splints can easily be tolerated on adjacent fingers.

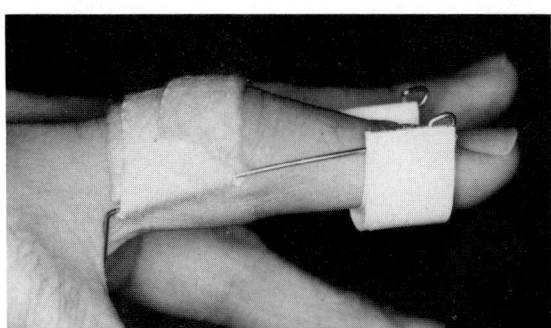

Fig. 89-2   Three-point extension splint without coils.

nates the fatigue factor one encounters with the rubber band outrigger systems; therefore the splint is effective for long-term use without adjustments.

The lateral coil system is effective only for flexion contractures of approximately 45 degrees or less, since a severely contracted finger will provide a counterforce that is at a right angle to the dorsal splint piece and thus the splint itself slips distally, being ineffective in gaining PIP joint extension. If clinical examination of a flexion contracture slightly greater than 45 degrees reveals a springy joint that responds to passive stretch, one can perhaps begin with the spring-wire design with realistic anticipation of early gains. The spring can be fitted initially so that the force arms of the splint rest in a somewhat flexed position, decreasing the tension being applied on the joint. At the next therapy visit it is often possible to bend the wire up to the 0-degree resting position, because the tolerance to the force has increased. In cases of severe (more than 45 degrees) long-standing flexion contractures of the PIP joints, one needs to devise a molded splint base with outrigger arms to provide effective extension force. Serial casting is often most effective with these severe deformities.

Not only does this three-point design provide an efficient extension force, but also by its low profile design it is easily tolerated by the patient. It allows movement of the metacarpophalangeal joint of the splinted finger and does not impede motion of the other fingers. The size of the splint allows it to be carried in the pocket for easy and frequent application. Two splints may be worn on adjacent fingers (Fig. 89-3), but if three fingers are involved, a hand-based splint with outrigger system is recommended for ease of application, removal, and diminished bulk between the fingers.

Patients frequently state that the wearing of the splint offers a distinct relief to the tight feeling within the joint, and they demonstrate an eagerness to wear the splint. For these reasons this splint is considered to have a high rate of patient compliance. For the experienced therapist it requires no longer than 10 minutes to construct.

INSTRUCTIONS FOR WEAR

As with any dynamic splinting program the forces applied must be tolerable over an extended period of time to effect change in the collagen formation. It is important to instruct the patient that after use of the splint the flexion deformity will temporarily recur. Explain to the patient that this is a normal phenomenon and that a period of stretch may gain full extension but that it will not yet have permanently relieved the tightness of the tissues. Patients who have full flexion of the PIP joint are frequently instructed to wear the extension splint at night and are advised to observe how long after removal of the splint the deformity recurs. If it recurs during the waking hours, the patient is then instructed in additional periods of wear during the day, with the splint being removed for flexion exercises. Instruct the patient that the goal is to be able to maintain full extension for longer and longer periods when the hand is out of the splint. When only a slight lag develops after a full day out of the splint, it is appropriate to go to a routine of night splinting only. These instructions vary depending on the nature and extent of the injury and whether flexion range is also limited and flexion splinting and/or exercises need to balance off the extension force. Only an experienced hand therapist can evaluate the balance of motion and the amount of tightness and devise an appropriate splinting schedule.

CONSTRUCTION OF SPLINT
Materials

The materials used for the construction of the spring-wire splint are readily available (Fig. 89-4).

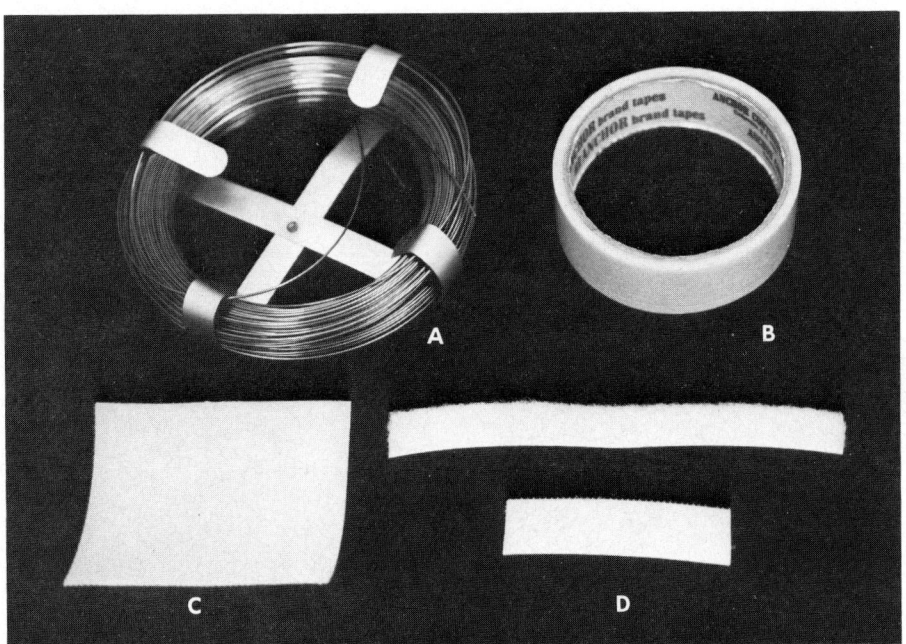

Fig. 89-4   Materials for spring-wire splint include: *A*, spring-steel piano wire; *B*, 1-inch filament tape; *C*, adhesive moleskin; and *D*, Velcro loop and pile.

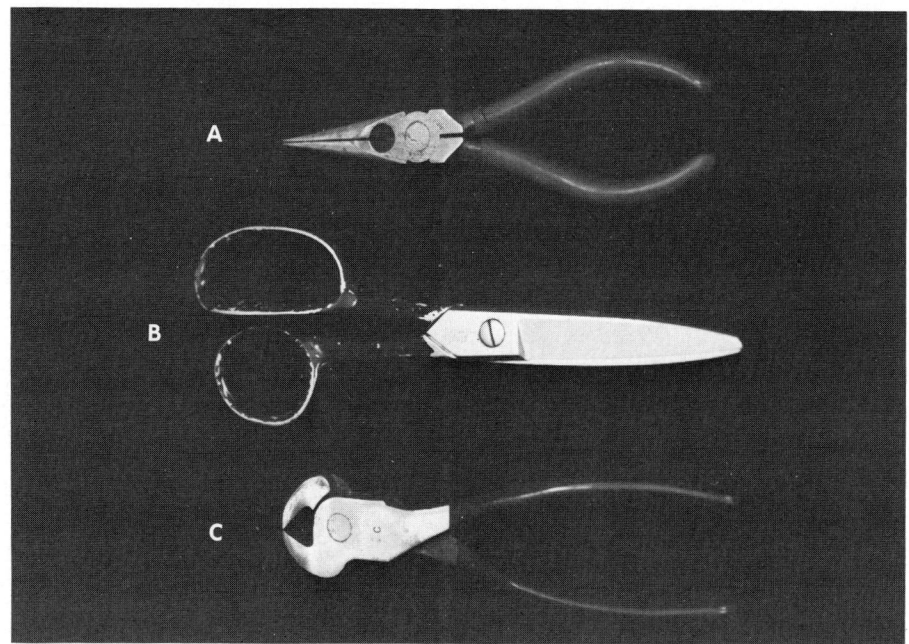

Fig. 89-5 Tools required for making spring-wire splint include: *A,* flat-jawed needle-nose pliers; *B,* leather scissors; and *C,* end-cutting nippers.

Spring-steel wire of 17.0 gauge (0.039 inch in diameter) is recommended and may be obtained from a local piano tuner or a piano supply company. One-pound coils (approximately 248 feet) are available and allow easy procurement of an appropriate length of wire. Spring steel has an inherent resistance to deforming forces and therefore must be overbent to obtain the desired shape. Avoidance of sharp bends will prevent the wire from snapping.

Filament tape used for packaging is used to cover the wire superstructure and may be obtained from any office supply company. A 1-inch width is most workable for this technique, and it is important that no substitutions be made, because the filaments provide the necessary strength for long-term durability.

Adhesive-backed moleskin, available from splinting or surgical suppliers, is used to cover the filament tape for both its padding and cosmetic effect.

One-half inch Velcro fasteners are used for the distal strap, with the adhesive-backed hook providing easy attachment of the strap to the wire and the Velcro loop providing the strap itself.

Tools

As with any technique, it is the correct tool that creates ease and efficiency in the construction (Fig. 89-5).

Firmly constructed flat-jawed needlenosed pliers are necessary to bend the resistant spring steel. Smooth or round jaws allow rotation of the wire. Six- or 8-inch flat-jawed needlenosed pliers with teeth are recommended. Wire-cutting pliers called "end-cutting nippers," which have a broad cutting area, are helpful, since the last step of construction requires cutting of the wire where it is inaccessible to the cutting jaws on the needlenosed pliers.

Sharp scissors with short blades so as to be effective in cutting at the tip of the scissors are necessary for easy trimming and cutting in the small tight areas. Leather shears are excellent for this purpose.

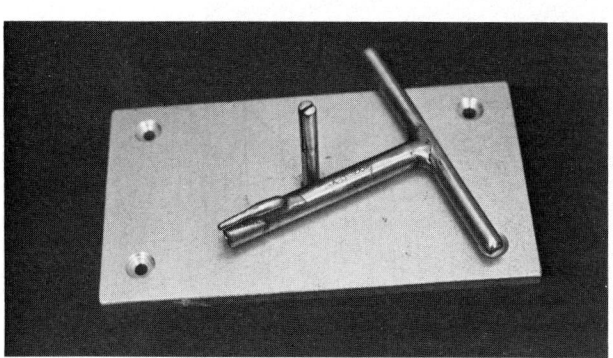

Fig. 89-6 Special jig for turning coils for spring-wire splint.

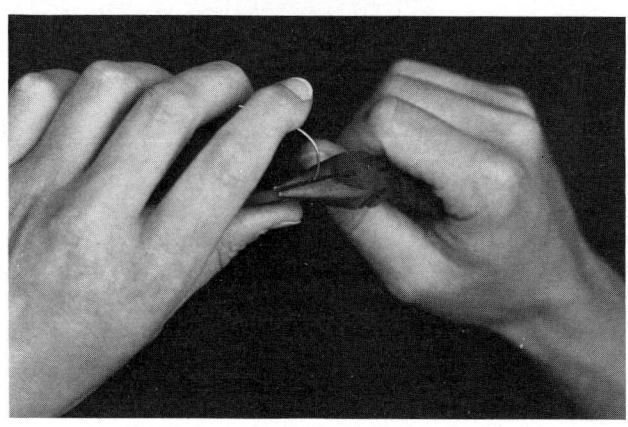

Fig. 89-7 Step 2. Bending initial curve.

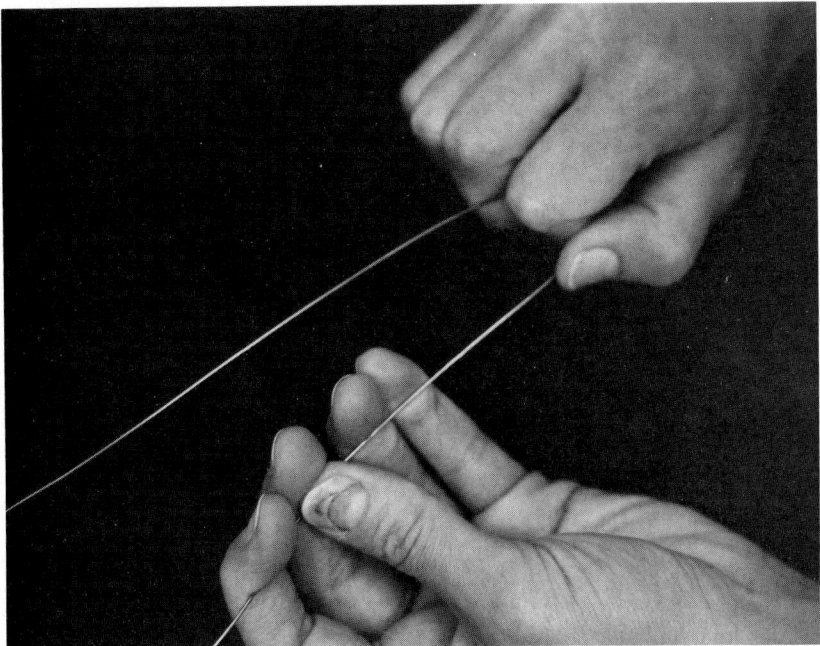

Fig. 89-8   Step 3. Straightening wire ends, making ∪ shape of wire.

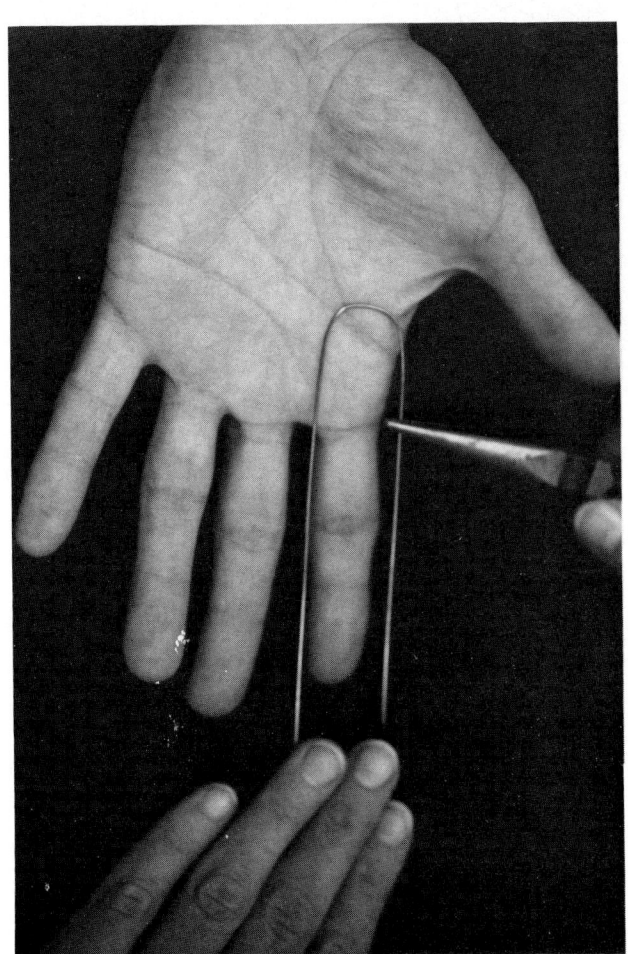

Fig. 89-9   Step 4, measuring width of splint superstructure, and step 5, marking location of the bend to carry wire to the lateral aspect of finger.

The spring wire coil is effectively turned by the use of a special jig fashioned after the design illustrated by Wynn Parry.[18] Use of the commercially available jig illustrated (Fig. 89-6) or an alternate design, the Rescap Bending Jig,* allows one to turn a tight and compact coil, which is difficult when attempted manually with pliers. The dimensions of the jig are specifically for the 17-gauge wire used for the PIP joint splint, although the jig may be used for other splint designs.

Procedure
1. Cut a length of 17-gauge piano wire approximately 14 inches in length.
2. Form a U-shape in the wire by holding the wire with the pliers and bending the wire gently with the fingers. Keep the wire and the pliers moving back and forth to create a smooth-curved shape (Fig. 89-7).
3. After the initial curve is made in the wire, it will retain the curved shape. With the fingertips apply a force to bend the wire in the direction opposite the resting curve. Slide the fingertips down the wire while applying force to straighten the wire (Fig. 89-8).
4. Working on the palmar aspect of the finger, adjust the wire shape so that it is slightly wider than the width of the finger (Fig. 89-9). It is important at this stage and throughout the splintmaking that the wire be parallel in all planes. At this stage it should lie flat on a smooth surface.
5. With the wire U-shape positioned on the palmar aspect of the finger and the curve resting at the distal palmar crease, mark the point of the wire just distal to the finger-web space (Fig. 89-9).

---

*Available from WFR/AQUAPLAST, Ramsey, NJ.

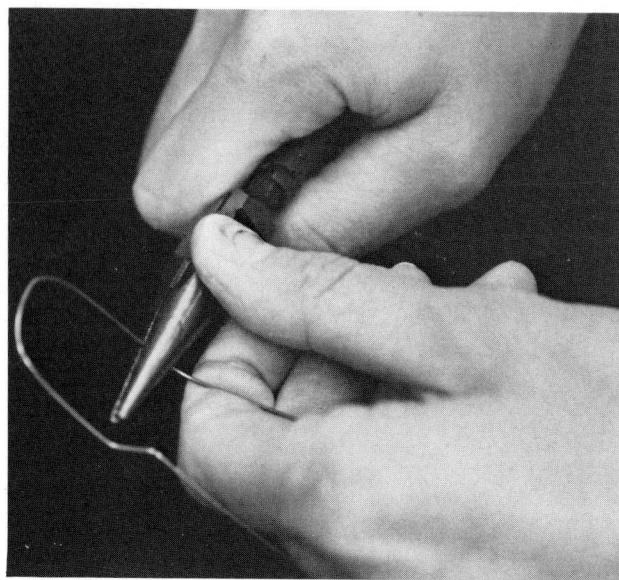

Fig. 89-10 Steps 6 and 7. Bending wire at 60-degree angles.

6. Bend the wire at a 60-degree angle so that it is between the fingers. Pay special attention to the finger webs, measuring carefully on both the radial and ulnar aspects, since they differ on each finger. Hold the wire with the wide part of the jaws of the pliers, and bend the wire sharply at the edge of the pliers by applying force with the fingers (Fig. 89-10).
7. Bend the wire again at a 60-degree angle so that it now lies in a position midlaterally on the finger. Again check to be sure the wire is parallel (Fig. 89-11).
8. Replace the splint on the palmar aspect of the finger, and mark the location of the axis of the PIP joint. One easily determines the axis by locating the apex of the middle palmar finger crease.
9. Place this point of the wire in the middle of the slot in the jig base (Fig. 89-12). Place the jig handle over the jig base, and while maintaining a downward pressure on the wire, turn two complete revolutions (Fig. 89-13). It is important during this procedure to hold the splint superstructure with a bit of torque so that the coil is turned at exactly a 90-degree angle to the

Fig. 89-11 Steps 6 and 7. Lateral view of parallel wire superstructure.

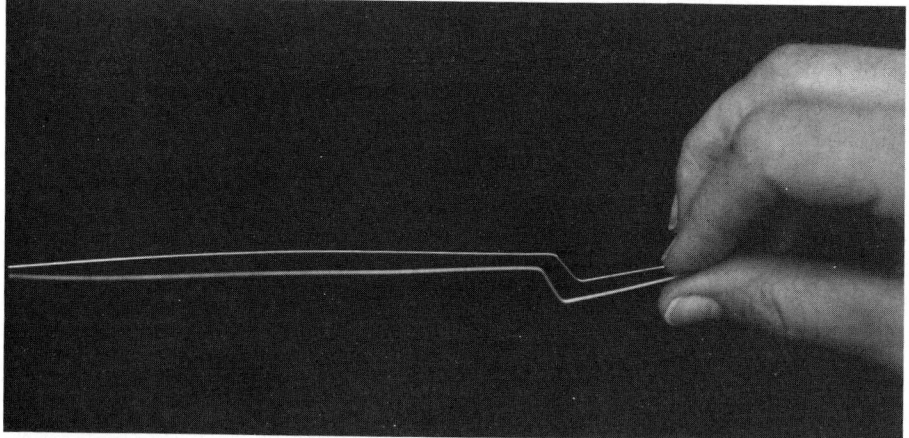

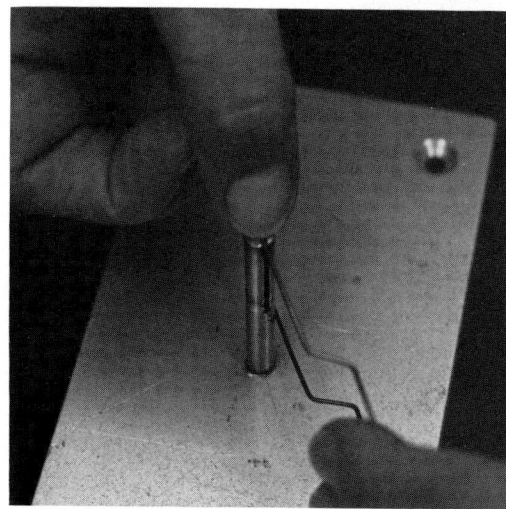

Fig. 89-12 Step 9. Placement of joint axis location in center of the jig slot.

axis of the parallel wires. Since the wire superstructure cannot rest directly under the coil being turned, the coil will not be parallel unless this torque is applied (Fig. 89-13). It is important to remember that for extension splinting of the PIP joint the coil is always turned toward the palmar aspect of the finger.

10. Replace the splint with one coil turned on the volar aspect of the finger, and mark the remaining axis location (Fig. 89-14).
11. Repeat step 9 to turn the second coil (Fig. 89-15).
12. Pad the base of the splint by wrapping six to eight layers of filament tape around the curved area. Trim it with scissors to fit the shape of the wire curve, and cut out a curved shape at the bend of the wire that goes into the finger-web space (Fig. 89-16).
13. Slide a piece of filament tape under the coil, with the sticky side of the tape toward the splint (Fig. 89-17). Wrap tape around the opposite side, and once again ease it under the coil. The nonsticky side of

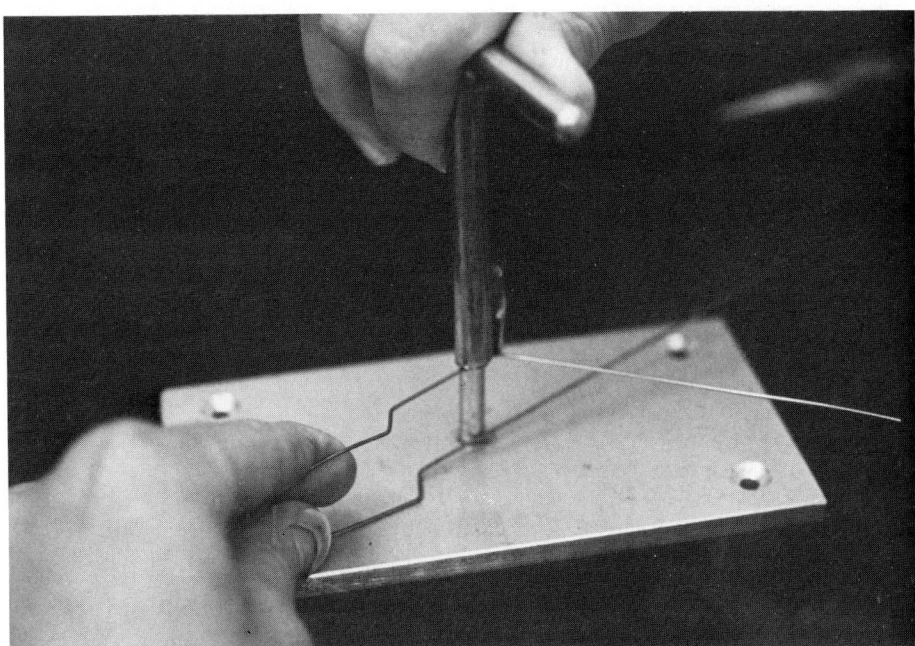

Fig. 89-13 Step 9. Turning initial coil.

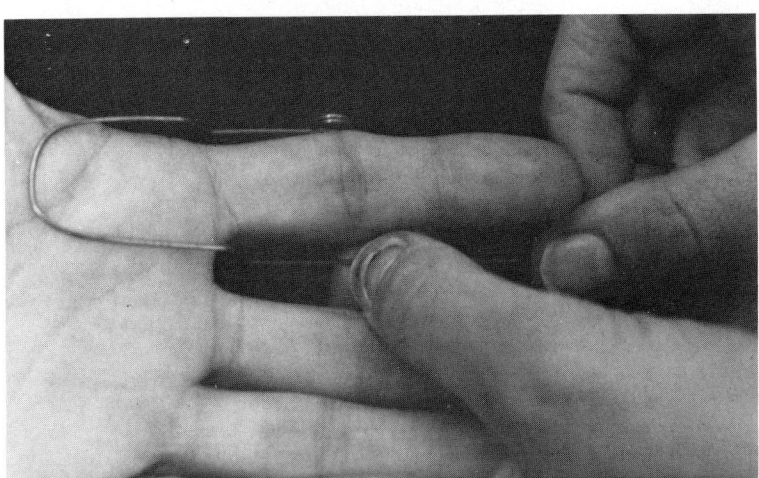

Fig. 89-14 Step 10. Marking second-joint axis location.

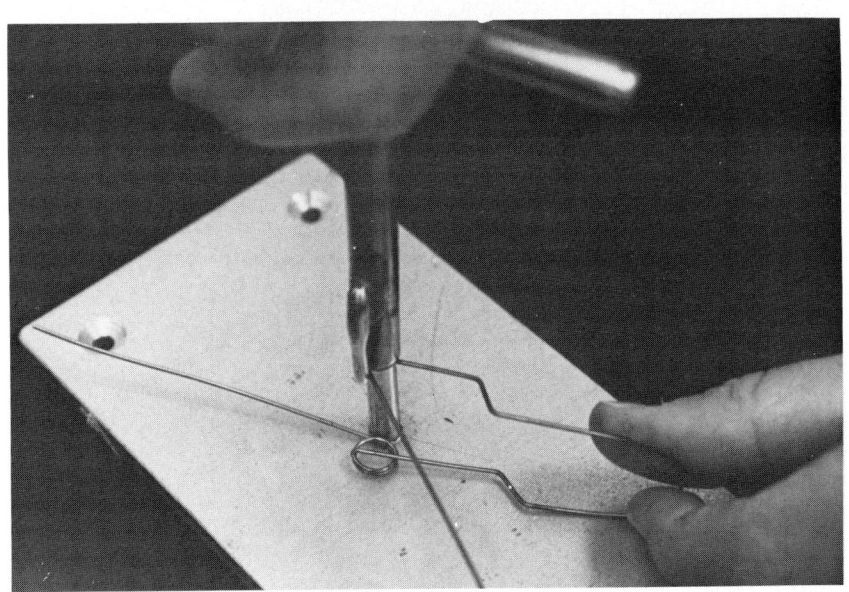

Fig. 89-15 Step 11. Turning second coil.

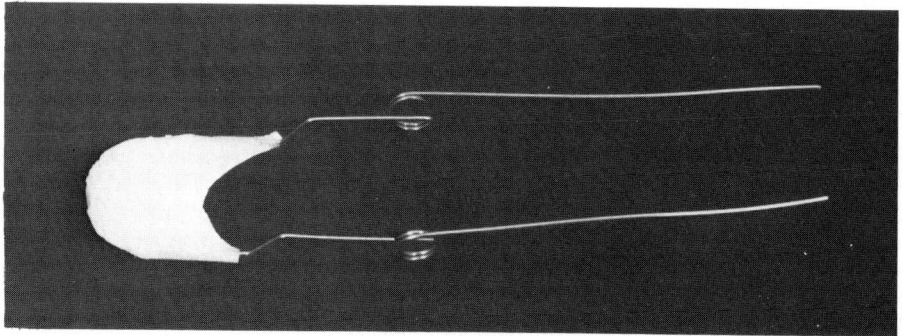

Fig. 89-16   Step 12. Covering proximal area with tape padding.

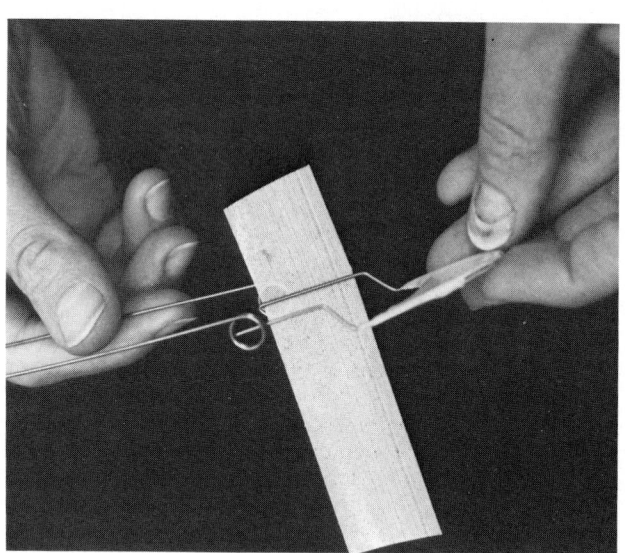

Fig. 89-17   Step 13. Applying dorsal hood piece.

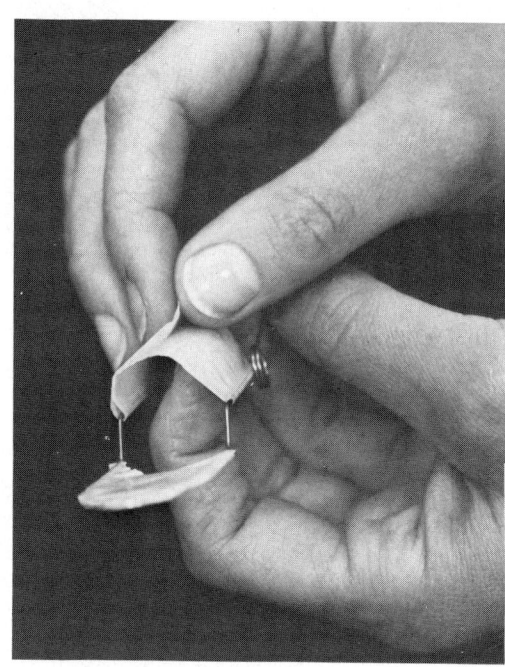

Fig. 89-18   Step 13. Applying dorsal hood piece.

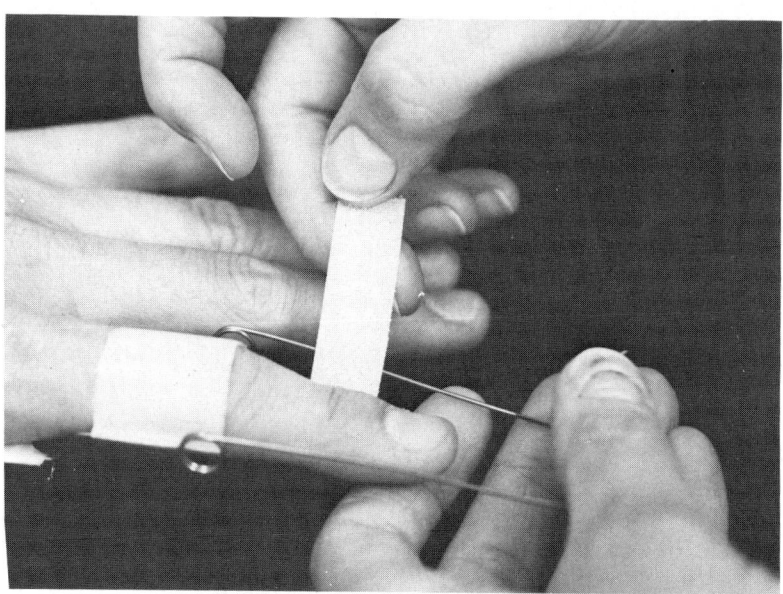

Fig. 89-19   Step 14. Applying Velcro hook.

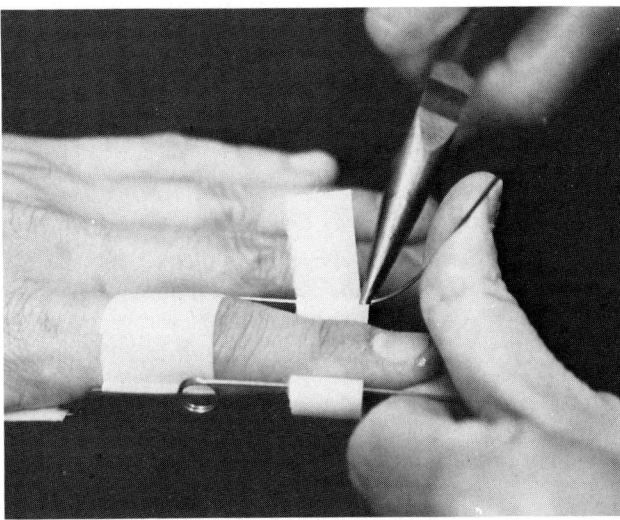

Fig. 89-20   Step 15, Applying Velcro loop to complete strap, and step 16, marking end of splint.

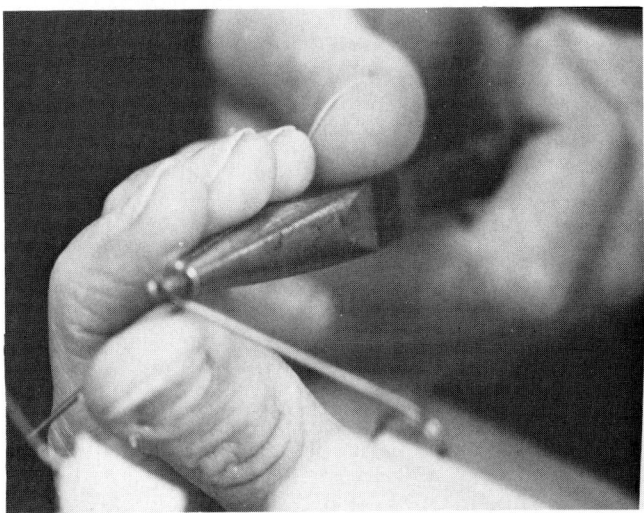

Fig. 89-21   Step 17. Making end coil.

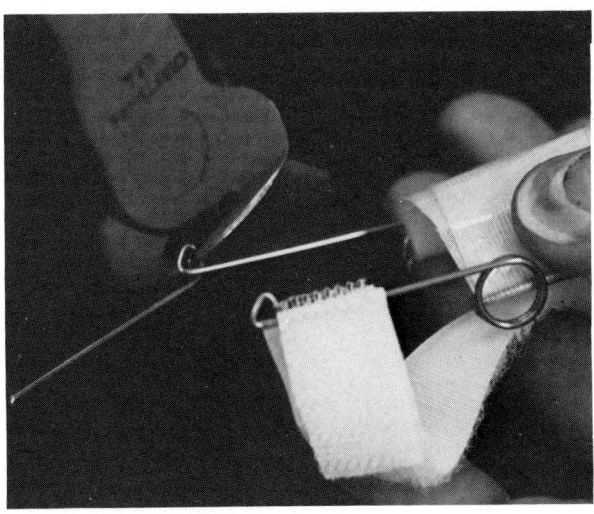

Fig. 89-22   Step 17. Cutting end coil.

the tape should lie against the skin of the finger. Fit the splint on the patient's finger, and adjust the length of tape so that the coils lie exactly in the midlateral position of the finger, at the PIP joint axis. After adjusting the length of the tape, attach it to itself securely (Fig. 89-18).

14. Place the splint on the finger, locating coils at the axis of the joint. Slide a piece of adhesive-backed Velcro hook (½ by 1½ inches) between one side of the finger and the lateral wire, with the sticky side toward the wire (Fig. 89-19). Fold the Velcro over the wire at the level of the distal interphalangeal (DIP) joint crease. Adhere the Velcro to itself, making sure that the unit is pointing palmarly.

15. Apply a ½ inch by 4- to 5-inch piece of Velcro loop to the Velcro hook on the side touching the palmar aspect of the finger. Take this piece of Velcro up dorsally between the finger and the wire, and loop the Velcro over the wire, carrying it palmarly again to adhere to the Velcro hook (Fig. 89-20). The Velcro thus forms a sling under the finger and allows adjustability, since the sling length can be determined by the amount of pull exerted on the Velcro loop.

16. With the splint still on the finger, mark the wire at the point where the splint should end (Fig. 89-20). The point should be just distal to the DIP joint crease, since the strap should lie directly under the DIP joint.

17. Remove the splint and turn a tight coil around the end of the needlenosed pliers at the point marked for the end of the splint (Fig. 89-21). Make sure to have a few inches of wire to work with, because it will make the turning much easier. Cut off the wire with the end-cutting nippers after the coil is turned (Fig. 89-22).

18. Cover the taped areas with adhesive-backed moleskin, trimming it close and making sure no seams are on the inside of the splint (Fig. 89-23).

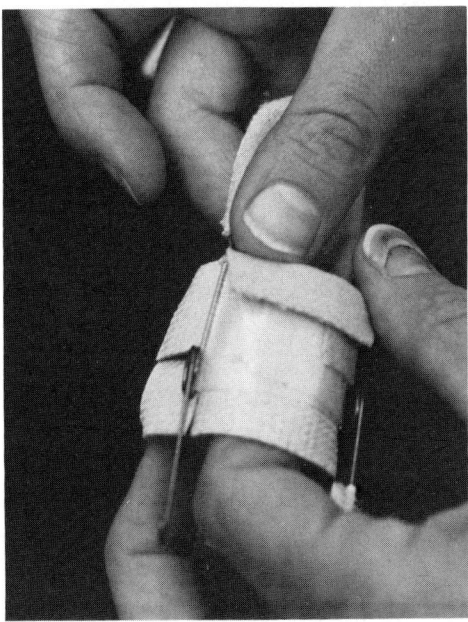

Fig. 89-23   Step 18. Covering taped areas with moleskin.

19. Apply the splint to the patient's finger, and check for proper fit, adequate circulation, and adequate distribution of pressure (Fig. 89-24).
20. Require the patient to apply and remove the splint independently. It is mandatory that the patient be able to demonstrate correct application of the splint.

Splint adjustments and modifications

As with any custom-made splint, minor adjustments and attention to detail ensure the long-term comfort of the splint on the patient. One of the most common problems is the bulbous, enlarged state of the PIP joint after injury. Because the finger is normally cone shaped, the enlarged PIP joint will receive pressure when the distal strap is tightened, since the tip of the finger is narrower than the joint. This situation can be particularly bothersome, since the collateral ligaments of the joint frequently have been injured and direct pressure over the area elicits exquisite tenderness. This problem can be alleviated by incorporating a piece of thin plastic or cardboard material over the dorsal hood area, reinforcing it so that it becomes like an arch and does not easily compress. A small piece of splinting material molded under the distal strap so that it holds the ends of the splint apart can also alleviate this problem. It has the additional advantage of better distributing pressure at the tip. Frequently the leading edge of the Velcro strap will be constricting to the distal pulp, and this molded pad greatly increases comfort (Fig. 89-25). An enlarged PIP joint may also be a problem when a spring-wire splint is fitted after a proximal phalanx fracture, since frequently the shape of the bone is deformed and one must adjust the dorsal hood piece so that it conforms to the bulbous shape of the proximal phalanx.

Although by far the most common use of a spring-wire splint is to correct a PIP joint flexion contracture, it can be

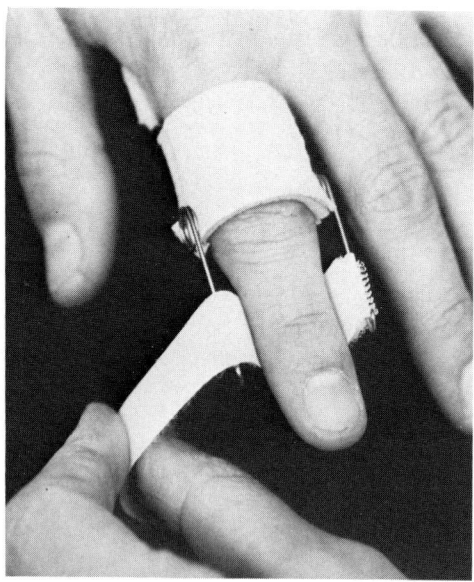

Fig. 89-24 Step 19. Applying splint to check for fit, circulation, and pressure.

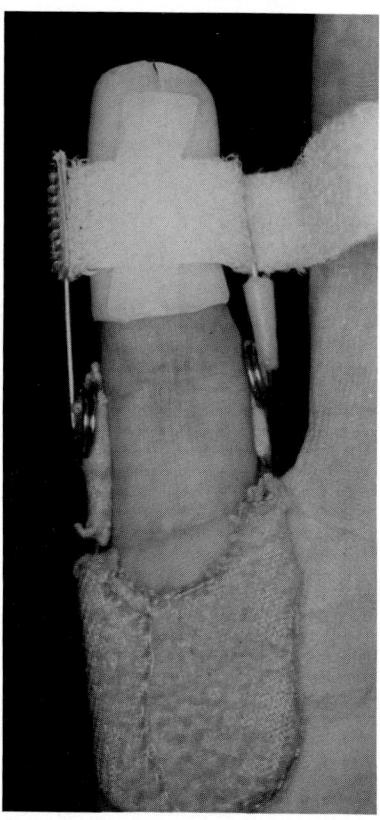

Fig. 89-25 Use of a piece of thermoplastic splinting material to maintain width of splint and better distribute pressure over distal part of pulp.

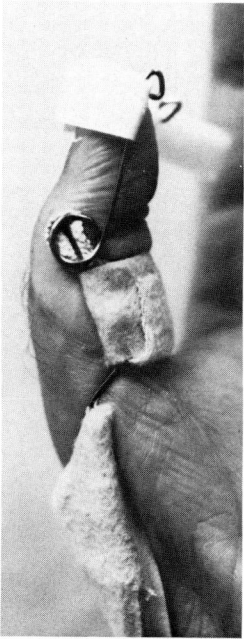

Fig. 89-26 Use of spring wire in reverse direction to achieve the first ranges of flexion of the interphalangeal joint of thumb.

modified to achieve other interphalangeal joint motions. It can easily be adapted to fit the interphalangeal joint of the thumb (Fig. 89-26). The direction of pull may be reversed for either thumb or finger interphalangeal joint flexion. It is important to note, however, that this design is effective to gain only the first ranges of flexion, since the line of pull will force the splint to slide off the finger in the latter ranges of flexion. Numerous other splint designs using spring wire are applicable to hand splinting, for which one should refer to other authors.[1,8]

SUMMARY

The low-profile spring-wire splint first described by Capener is of significant clinical value because of its easy tolerance by the patient. A custom-made splint that exactly fits the length of the finger and applies force at the axis of the joint frequently offers advantages over a commercially available splint. The steps for construction are offered with the hope that this splint can become part of the armamentarium of the skilled hand therapist.

REFERENCES

1. Barr N: The hand: principles and techniques of simple splintmaking in rehabilitation, Boston, 1978, Butterworth Publishers.
2. Bowers WH: Sprains and joint injuries in the hand. In Mackin E, editor: Hand rehabilitation, hand clinics, vol 2, no 1, Philadelphia, 1986, WB Saunders Co.
3. Bowers WH and others: The proximal interphalangeal joint volar plate. I. Anatomical and biomechanical study, J Hand Surg 5:79, 1980.
4. Brand P: External stress: forces that effect joint action. In Brand P: Clinical mechanics of the hand, St Louis, 1985, The CV Mosby Co.
5. Brand P: The forces of dynamic splinting: ten questions before applying a dynamic splint to the hand. In Hunter JM and others, editors: Rehabilitation of the hand, ed 2, St Louis, 1984, The CV Mosby Co.
6. Bunnell S: Active splinting of the hand, J Bone Joint Surg 28:732, 1946.
7. Callahan A and McEntee P: Splinting proximal interphalangeal joint flexion contractures: a new design, Am J Occup Ther 40(6):408, 1986.
8. Capener N: Lively splints, Physiotherapy 53:371, 1967.
9. Capener N: Physiological rest, Br Med J 2:761, 1946.
10. Fess EE: Force magnitude of commercial spring-coil and spring-wire splints designed to extend the proximal interphalangeal joint, J Hand Ther 1(2):86, 1988.
11. Fess EE and Phillips CA: Hand splinting: principles and methods, ed 2, St Louis, 1987, The CV Mosby Co.
12. Kuczynski K: The proximal interphalangeal joint: anatomy and causes of stiffness in the fingers, J Bone Joint Surg 50B:656, 1968.
13. Mackin EJ and Maiorano L: Postoperative therapy following staged flexor tendon reconstruction. In Hunter JM and others, editors: Rehabilitation of the hand, ed 2, St Louis, 1984, The CV Mosby Co.
14. Malick M: Manual on dynamic hand splinting with thermoplastic materials, ed 2, Pittsburgh, 1978, Harmarville Rehabilitation Center.
15. McCue FC and others: Athletic injuries of the proximal interphalangeal joint requiring surgical treatment, J Bone Joint Surg 52A:937, 1970.
16. Wilson RE and Carter MS: Joint injuries in the hand: preservation of proximal interphalangeal joint function. In Hunter JM and others, editors: Rehabilitation of the hand, ed 2, St Louis, 1984, The CV Mosby Co.
17. Wilson RE and Carter MS: Management of hand fractures. In Hunter JM and others, editors: Rehabilitation of the hand, ed 2, St Louis, 1984, The CV Mosby Co.
18. Wynn Parry CB: Rehabilitation of the hand, ed 3, Boston, 1978, Butterworth Publishers.
19. Wynn Parry CB and others: New types of lively splints for peripheral nerve lesions affecting the hand, Hand 2:31, 1970.

90

Serial plaster splinting

Susan M. Tribuzi

Plaster of paris is the oldest, most versatile, and most widely accepted splint material used in the medical community. While the development of low temperature thermoplastics revolutionized hand splinting, plaster of paris can still be a benefit to the hand therapist. Plaster of paris is very effective in the fabrication of serial-static splints, including volar/dorsal stretchers, circumferential metacarpophalangeal (MP) stretchers, and digital cylinder casts. Serial-static plaster splints provide the therapist with an alternative splinting technique for use in the management of complex hand injuries. By gaining an appreciation of its history, advantages and disadvantages, and principles of application, therapists can become as proficient in the use of plaster of paris as with thermoplastic materials.

HISTORY OF PLASTER OF PARIS

Plaster of paris is a fine white powder composed of amorphous anhydride calcium sulfate. It is prepared by heating stone gypsum at temperatures of 100° to 200° C until 93% of the water crystallization is lost. When water is added to the plaster the following exothermic chemical reaction occurs:

$$(CaSO_4)_2 \cdot H_2O + 3H_2O \rightarrow 2(CaSO_4 \cdot 2H_2O) + HEAT$$
$$\text{plaster of paris} \qquad\qquad \text{gypsum}$$

During this reaction long crystals rapidly form, which contributes to the strength of plaster. This process of recrystallization is commonly referred to as "setting."[1,24,29]

The Arabs were credited with being the first to use plaster for medical purposes. Rhazes in the ninth century A.D. used an early form of plaster by mixing lime (calcium oxide) and egg white to fabricate a cast for immobilization of fractures. The material was strong and water resistant. The lime, however, caused irritation to the skin and was gradually replaced with calcium sulfate, the substance used in modern plaster of paris.*

European physicians were gradually introduced to the use of plaster in the 1700s. Lavoisier,[20,29] a French chemist, in 1768 described the chemistry involved in converting gypsum to plaster of paris. It was believed that the term "plaster of paris" was derived from the fact that gypsum was mined in Paris.[4,24] The use of plaster was promoted through the publication "A Survey of the Turkish Empire," published by Eton,[4,6,21,23] a British consul in Basora in 1798. In his writings he described the methods used in the eastern parts of the empire to enclose broken bones in plaster of paris. He commented on the strength of the material and its prop-

erty to conform to the shape of the limb and solidify in minutes. In 1816 Hubenthal[1,4,12,21,23] reported on his use of a combination of plaster of paris and ground blotting paper to form an anterior and posterior shell-type cast. German physicians Koyl and Kluge[4,21,23] in 1828 reported on their technique of pouring liquid plaster of paris in a wooden box mold placed around the injured extremity. The wooden box was then removed after the plaster had set. This method using a box mold was cumbersome and not well received by their colleagues. A similar technique using a box mold was described in the United States in Biglow's *Manual of Orthopaedic Surgery* in 1845.[1]

A significant advancement in the use of plaster occurred in 1852. Anthoius Mathysen,* a Dutch army surgeon published a pamphlet on his technique using bandages of plaster of paris. Mathysen took finely powdered plaster, rubbed it into strips of coarse, meshed cotton, and then rolled the strips into bandages. Mathysen developed this technique of impregnated plaster bandages for the treatment of the wounded on the battlefield. These plaster bandages were used extensively during the Crimean War (1845-1856), even though the bandages frequently needed to be soaked in urine because of the shortage of water.

Just after the Civil War in the United States, Samuel St. John[21,23] advocated the use of a single layer of cotton wadding or soft blanket between the skin and plaster. He also promoted the use of a shoemaker's knife to cut down the front of the plaster to help preserve circulation. St. John was a strong believer in the use of plaster of paris and taught "that the splint should be fitted to the limb, and not the limb to the splint."[21,23] German physicians during the Franco-Prussian War advocated the use of wooden ribbons between the layers of plaster for cast reinforcement.[21,24]

During World War I, World War II, and the Spanish Civil War, further advancements were made in the use, preparation, and storage of plaster bandages. The large scale use of radiology during World War I prompted the standardized use of plaster of paris in the treatment of fractures.[23] During World War II, plaster that turned blue when immersed in water was used, so that the casts were camouflaged at night.[24]

The first commercial company to market a ready-made plaster bandage was Johnson & Johnson, an American company that originated in 1900. The company marketed a loose, coated type of bandage known as "Orthoplast."[4,13] The bandage was similar to Mathysen's original design; however, the plaster easily became dislodged from the band-

---

*References 1, 4, 9, 21, 23, 24.

*References 4, 9, 19, 21, 23, 28.

age during transportation and use and was discontinued in 1952. In 1927 Johnson & Johnson devised a process to prepare a hard-coated plaster bandage. This bandage became known as "Specialist."[4] During this process, the plaster was bound to the cloth by a starch, gum, or resin binder. The bandages were then packaged in waterproof envelopes. This process eliminated the problem of the plaster becoming dislodged from the bandage. In Europe the first production of ready-made plaster was in Germany in 1931. A "Cellona" bandage was developed using an open-meshed cloth with a special leno weave. This cloth was found to be easier to mold than the previously used crinoline cloths. The name changed from "Cellona" to "Gypsona" in 1947.[4]

In 1944 Edwin Geckeller,[8] an orthopedic surgeon, published his text on plaster of paris technic. Geckeller described his techniques of fabrication and application of plaster bandages and commented that "commercially made plaster bandages are not as satisfactory for general use as those made by hand."[8] During this time salt, warm water, and hard water were often used to accelerate the setting process, whereas sugar, borax, cold water and soft water were used to retard the process. However, the overuse of accelerating and retarding agents was found to cause the plaster to become brittle.

Since the 1940s continued advances in the research, marketing, and use of plaster of paris have occurred. A large number of commercial companies now manufacture plaster of paris, including Johnson & Johnson, Smith & Nephew Rolyan, Carpace and Lohmann, to mention only a few. Plaster of paris is currently processed using either a batch process or a continuous mix process developed by Johnson & Johnson. In batch processing the ingredients are added in a sequence, whereas in continuous mix the ingredients are synchronized. Batch processing is less expensive; however, uniformity and consistency in the product is often lost. Johnson & Johson contends that continuous mix assures a more consistent quality in the final plaster product.[14] Today the three most commonly used types of plaster of paris include fast setting, extra fast setting, and elastic impregnated plaster. The setting time is 2 to 4 minutes for extra fast setting plaster and 5 to 8 minutes for fast setting and elastic plaster. Elastic plaster bandages are manufactured similar to the fast and extra fast plaster bandages with the exception of the addition of elastic fibers to the gauze during processing. These elastic fibers enhance the conformability of the plaster; however, the strength of the plaster is compromised and cannot withstand weight bearing. Elastic plaster bandages are most commonly used in the fitting of a prosthesis after amputation or as the initial layers in cast fabrication.

ADVANTAGES AND DISADVANTAGES OF PLASTER OF PARIS

The advantages of using plaster of paris in splinting seem to far outweigh the disadvantages. Plaster is an easy material to apply and requires minimal supplies and setup. The material sets with water in a short period of time to form a rigid casing. One of the greatest advantages in using plaster over other materials is that it conforms nicely to the shape of the body part to which it is applied. Pressure points are less likely to develop because of the nature of plaster's conforming properties and its tendency to distribute forces throughout the length of the cast. Plaster also allows for adequate air circulation, which decreases the chance of skin maceration. Furthermore, plaster is readily available and relatively inexpensive when compared to thermoplastic materials. Plaster's shelf life under normal dry storage conditions is 5 years or more.

Though the disadvantages of plaster are few, they cannot go without mention. The main disadvantage is that it is not water resistant. When plaster becomes wet, it will soften and lose its strength and its integrity. Plaster is also heavier in weight than thermoplastics; however, the weight of a cast can be greatly reduced by controlling cast thickness. Finally, though plaster is messier in application than thermoplastic materials, in time a minimal mess and cleanup can be achieved by the experienced plaster user.

PRECAUTIONS AND PRINCIPLES IN PLASTER USE

When working with plaster one needs to be aware of the thermal effect (exothermic crystallization) and possible allergic reactions from the plaster, stockinette, or cast padding used during casting. Becker,[2] Grazer,[10] Haasch,[11] Schultz,[25] and Kaplan[16] have all reported cases of thermal burns following the application of plaster bandages. Test results from plaster manufactured by one company indicated that heat given off during recrystallization may range from 32.2° C to 82.2° C, with the tendency on the lower end of the scale.[16] Other manufacturing companies contend that the quantitative amount of heat produced by a given amount of plaster is a constant figure. Research by Diack, Schultz, and Nohlgren[5] demonstrated that full-thickness skin burns can result from temperatures of 50° C sustained for a period of 5 to 10 minutes. Most casts will reach maximum temperature in 5 to 15 minutes after application. Several variables have been identified that could contribute to increasing the temperature given off during application of plaster. These include higher room temperature, higher humidity, cast thickness of more than eight plies, undersaturation or oversaturation of the plaster when immersing it in water, use of plaster with faster setting time, dipping temperatures, and inadequate ventilation during the drying period. Inadequate ventilation can occur from overwrapping of freshly applied plaster with cotton or elastic bandages, covering with blankets, or placing the cast or splint near a pillow or mattress.[14,16,17]

The water-dipping temperature used when working with plaster has been shown to be of critical importance and a possible key factor to the cause of thermal burns. Kaplan[16] recommends dipping temperatures to be less than 40° C, and Wehbe[30] identified a safe dipping margin from 30° C to 40° C, with the temperature feeling "comfortably warm to the user's hand." The manufacturing instructions from one company recommend use of dipping temperatures between 21° and 24° C, with the water feeling cool to touch. Lavalette and others[17] found in their study that dipping temperatures of 32° C could be high enough to cause burns; they recommend using temperatures below 24° C. Clean water should always be used because the plaster residue left in the dipping container from previous casts will act as an accelerator and increase the exothermic reaction.

Plaster casts should not be applied directly to the skin. Stockinette or cast padding should be used as a barrier between the plaster and the skin. Contact sensitivity to plaster and plaster bandages, though rare, has been reported.[18,26] When applying plaster, stockinette, or cast padding, the skin should be routinely monitored for possible irritation.

To facilitate a positive experience when working with plaster of paris, review the instruction pamphlet accompanying the product before its initial use. When molding plaster, care should be taken to smooth the plaster, filling the meshes in the gauze. This aids in increasing the strength of the material. Little or no motion should occur during the molding and initial setting phase (3 to 8 minutes depending on material, water temperature, and other factors). Casts will often appear dry on the surface; however, moisture is often contained in the deeper layers. Thin casts may dry completely in several hours, whereas casts with ¼ inch thickness may require up to 72 hours to dry completely.

As with any splint, basic hand splinting principles should be applied when splinting with plaster. Several key principles include providing contour to increase strength, increasing force area to decrease pressure, applying uniform pressure over bony prominences, and attending to finishing touches to assure comfort and cosmesis.[7] For more detailed information regarding basic splinting principles and precautions please refer to Chapter 88.

INDICATIONS FOR THE USE OF SERIAL PLASTER STRETCHERS

Serial plaster stretchers can be successfully used in overcoming muscle-tendon unit tightness, as well as increasing or maintaining joint range of motion (ROM) at the metacarpophalangeal (MP) or wrist joints. However, the use of plaster stretchers often takes a back seat to the use of thermoplastic splints. Plaster casting for interphalangeal joint contractures is presented in detail in Chapter 91 and therefore will not be addressed in this chapter.

Muscle-tendon unit tightness often needs to be addressed in the patient's rehabilitation program. Extrinsic tendon tightness may develop in association with protective positioning, adhesion formation following fractures, extensive soft tissue injury to the hand or wrist, crush injuries, replantations, and tendon and nerve lacerations. Successful reduction of muscle tendon tightness can be obtained

through the appropriate application of serial plaster stretchers. Although plaster stretchers are more commonly advocated in the use of flexor tendon tightness, a dorsal plaster stretcher (Fig. 90-1) can be effectively used in reducing extrinsic extensor tendon tightness before the use of thermoplastic static and dynamic splints.

In addition to muscle-tendon unit tightness, limitations in ROM at the MP and wrist joints are frequently encountered in the variety of "stiff hands" from acute to chronic. Splinting to increase or maintain motion at these joints may also be necessary following surgical procedures. Circumferential plaster stretchers are very effective in maintaining the flexion gained in surgery following a capsulectomy. The use of plaster allows the therapist to achieve a nice conforming mold to the MP joints, thus eliminating the problem of the MP joints slipping into extension, a problem that commonly occurs when using thermoplastic materials.

The theory in application of serial plaster stretchers is based on Brand's work of using plaster in the remodeling of soft tissue. Through serial application of plaster stretchers, a gradual elongation of tissues and collagen realignment can occur.[3,27] This procedure is continued until maximum correction is obtained or when an increase or plateau in joint ROM is observed. Plaster stretchers provide a small continuous force in the desired direction of correction. Dorsal or circumferential stretchers are most effective in gaining flexion, whereas volar stretchers are used to increase extension.

When applying plaster stretchers following surgical procedures, a light force may need to be used initially during the inflammatory phase to avoid disturbance of the healing wound. As healing progresses through fibroplasia and scar maturation, the wound will be able to tolerate an increase in stress and force.

TECHNIQUE IN APPLICATION OF PLASTER STRETCHERS
Volar and dorsal stretchers

Materials needed for fabrication of volar and dorsal plaster stretchers include 4 × 12-inch strips or bandages of extra fast setting plaster, cast padding, stockinette, bowl of dipping water between 20° and 30° C, plaster scissors, band-

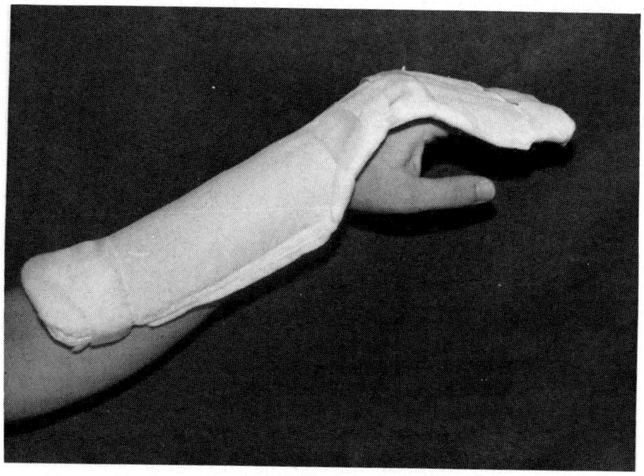

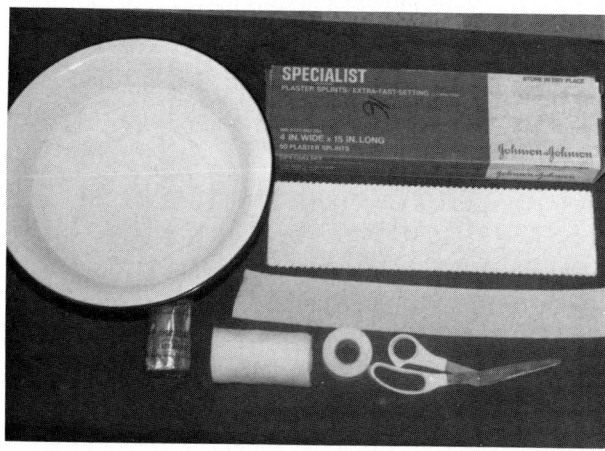

Fig. 90-1 Dorsal plaster stretcher.

Fig. 90-2 Materials needed for fabrication of serial plaster splints.

ing metal or thermoplastic scraps for reinforcement, and tape for finishing. An arm support or positioning device is helpful (Fig. 90-2).

Before application of the plaster, the patient's forearm, wrist, and digits should be prepositioned. When fabricating stretchers for muscle-tendon unit tightness, the wrist should initially be kept in neutral, with the force directed toward the metacarpal and interphalangeal joints. The direction of the force is in extension for flexor tendon tightness and in flexion for extensor tendon tightness. When full extension or flexion of the digits is obtained, the force is then redirected to the wrist. When applying plaster stretchers to gain motion at the MP or wrist joints, the force is directed at the respective joint and in the desired direction of correction. For example, when fabricating a stretcher to increase MP flexion, the force is directed at the MP joints in the direction of flexion.

Stockinette can be applied to the arm before molding; however, this is not necessary, and extra care must be taken to prevent wrinkles from occurring when applying the plaster. Six to eight strips of plaster are then measured to include

the patient's hand and two thirds of the forearm (Fig. 90-3). The medial and lateral borders should extend half the width of the forearm. When a width greater than 4 inches is required, overlap two sets of plaster strips for desired width. The corners can be rounded and a semicircular area cut away for clearance of the thenar eminence. Three layers of cast padding are used between the patient's skin and the plaster and should extend beyond the plaster at both the proximal and distal ends (Fig. 90-4). Layers of stockinette can be used in the absence of cast padding. The six layers of plaster are then immersed as a group into the dipping water for 5 to 10 seconds, taking care not to undersaturate the material. The plaster is then removed and lightly squeezed to remove the excess water. The wet plaster can then be positioned on the cast padding on a flat surface and smoothed before placing it on the patient, or be placed directly on the patient's arm that has cast padding already applied (Figs. 90-5, A and B).

When smoothing the plaster before and during molding, one should attempt to mold all six layers of plaster-filled gauze strips into one single strong unit. The therapist then molds the plaster to the arm while contouring the forearm, the arches, the spaces between digits and over bony prominences. Begin to apply a stretch first at the wrist, then

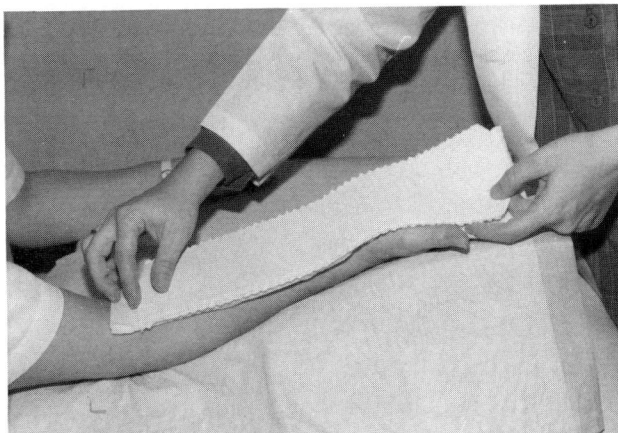

Fig. 90-3 Measure plaster strips to include the patient's hand and two thirds of the forearm.

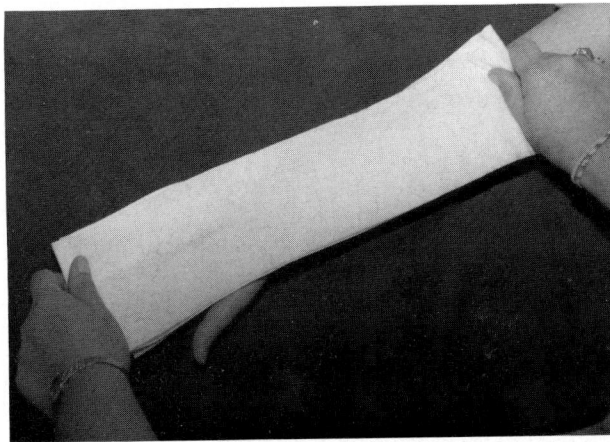

Fig. 90-4 Application of cast padding for volar forearm stretcher.

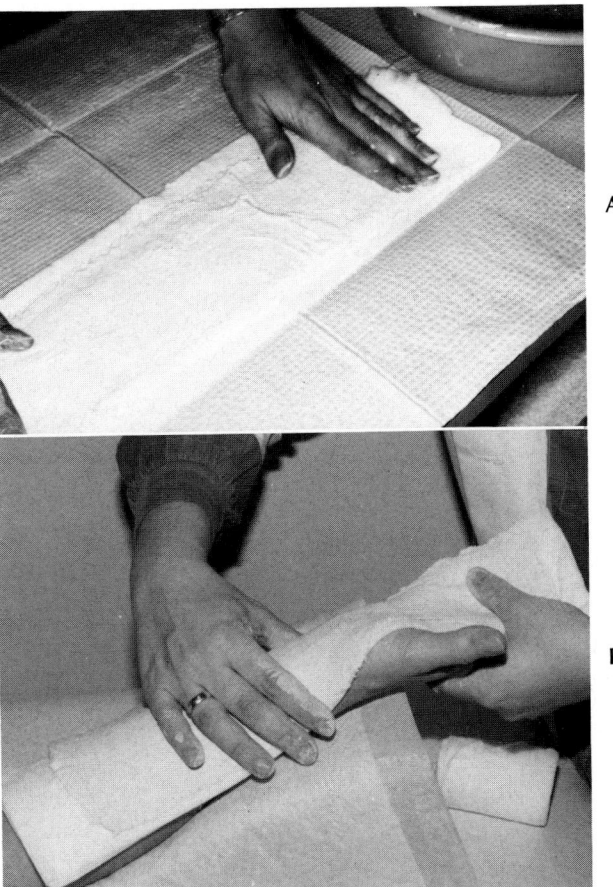

A

B

Fig. 90-5 **A,** Placing wet plaster on cast padding and smoothing on a flat surface. **B,** Placing plaster directly on arm, which has had cast padding preapplied.

proceed to stretch the digits. It is important that uniform pressure be applied and the position of the wrist be maintained during the molding phase. Care should be taken to avoid direct pressure at the distal phalanges to avoid the development of pressure points. A gentle stretch is applied until the plaster is set, approximately 2 to 4 minutes (Fig. 90-6). The plaster stretcher can then be removed for application of the reinforcement bar and for finishing touches.

A contoured reinforcement bar is recommended to provide additional strength to the plaster stretcher. Either banding metal or a strip of thermoplastic material can be used as a reinforcer (Figs. 90-7, *A* and *B*). The reinforcement bar should extend almost the entire length of the stretcher and be covered with two to three layers of plaster to secure it in place (Fig. 90-8).

Finishing touches include cutting away rough edges and overlapping the edges with cast padding or stockinette to prevent the skin from becoming irritated. Velcro and tape will not stick directly to the plaster and, if used, needs to be applied back to itself (i.e., tape to tape). Stockinette can be worn under the stretcher for comfort and to aid in absorption of perspiration, but again it is not necessary and should be left up to the patient's preference (Fig. 90-9).

The plaster stretcher is then secured into place with an elastic bandage or bias-cut stockinette, wrapping in a figure eight or spiral direction from distal to proximal (Fig. 90-10). The tips of the digits can be left visible for the patient

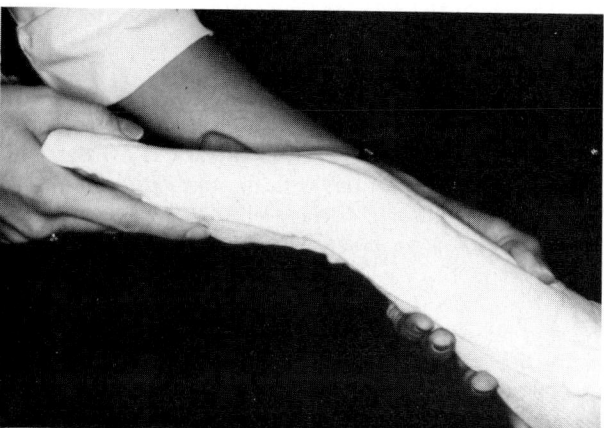

Fig. 90-6 A gentle stretch is applied and held until the plaster has set.

to check color and temperature when diminished sensation is present.

Fabrication of new volar or dorsal stretchers varies with each patient and depends on the patient's tolerance for stretch and the response of the tissues to splinting. Several guidelines helpful in determining the need for a new stretcher include improvements in passive range of motion (PROM), when the digits can be actively or passively extended from the volar stretcher or flexed from the dorsal stretcher, or when the patient no longer perceives a stretching sensation. Generally, a new stretcher will need to be fabricated at least every 7 to 10 days. However, in fact, rapid progress can be achieved by changes daily or every 2 to 3 days.

Circumferential stretchers

Circumferential stretchers used to increase or maintain MP flexion require a slightly different fabrication process. The materials required are essentially the same as for the volar or dorsal forearm stretchers with the exception of using one half to two thirds of a 3-inch roll of extra fast setting plaster instead of plaster strips. The patient's hand is pre-

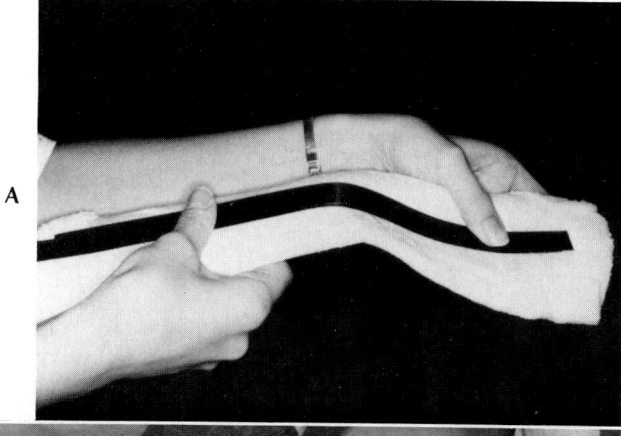

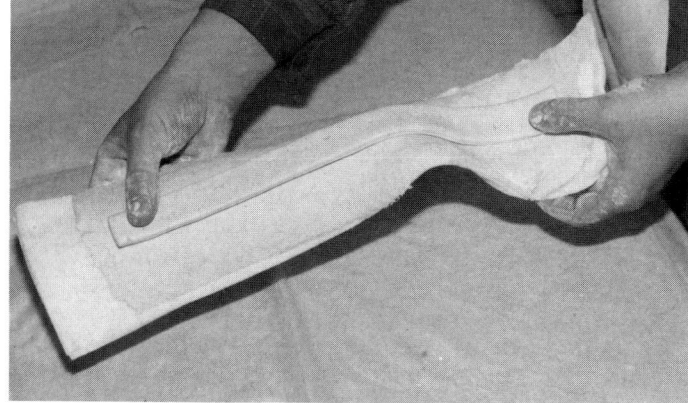

Fig. 90-7 **A,** Reinforcement of plaster stretcher using banding metal. **B,** Reinforcement of plaster stretcher using thermoplastic strip.

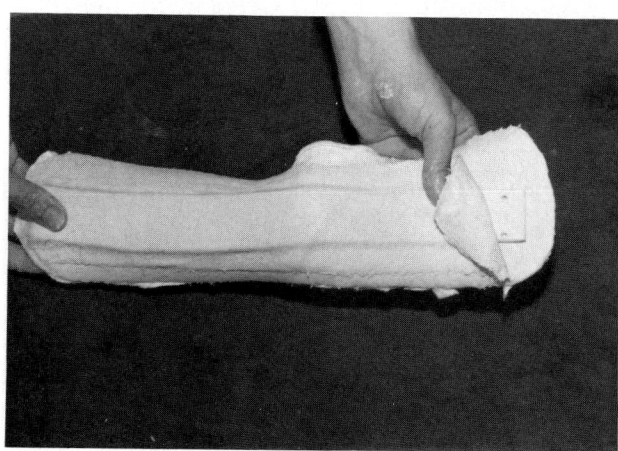

Fig. 90-8 Reinforcement bar is covered with two to three layers of plaster to secure the reinforcement bar in place.

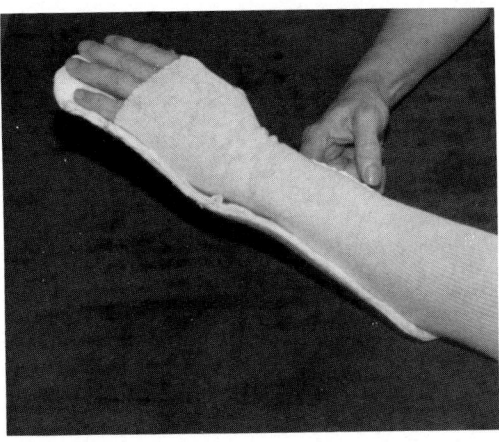

Fig. 90-9   Stockinette can be worn under the plaster stretcher.

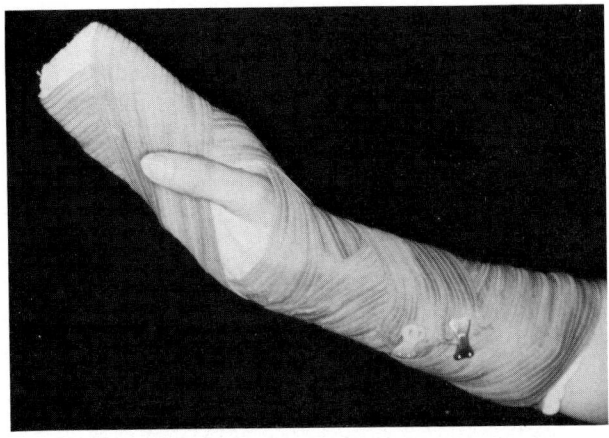

Fig. 90-10   Securing plaster stretcher in place with ace wrap.

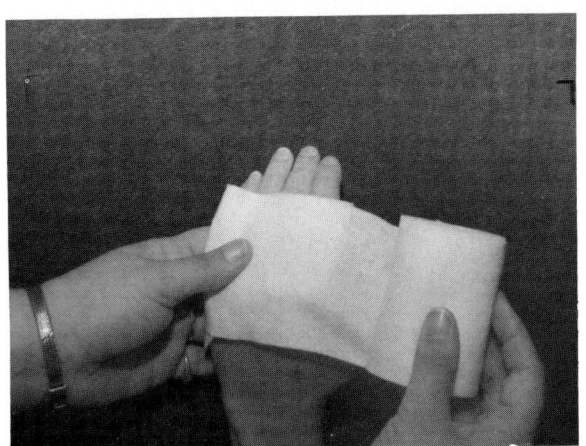

Fig. 90-11   Application of cast padding for circumferential metacarpophalangeal stretcher.

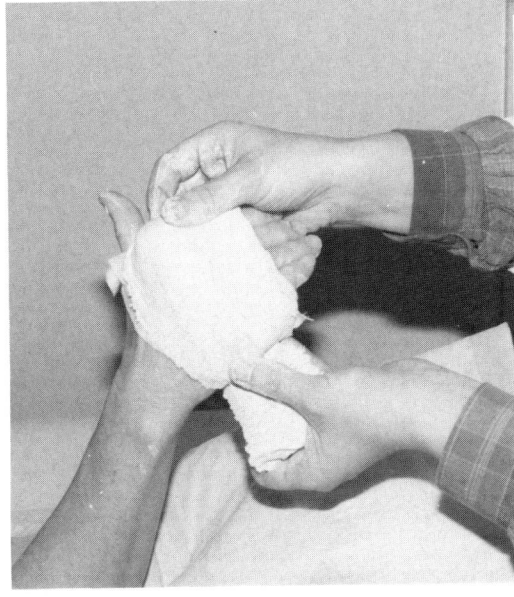

Fig. 90-12   Application of plaster for circumferential plaster stretcher.

positioned with the MP joints in flexion and the wrist in neutral. Three layers of cast padding are preapplied circumferentially before the plaster is molded. The cast padding should extend beyond the interphalangeal joints and into the thumb web space, so that padding can be rolled back during molding to provide a smooth edge when the patient flexes and extends the interphalangeal joints or opposes the thumb (Fig. 90-11). The same technique for immersing and removing excess water from the plaster is used as described on p. 1123. The plaster is then applied circumferentially around the MP joints (Fig. 90-12). Begin wrapping at the proximal phalanges, working in a distal-to-proximal direction. Three layers of plaster are applied, and then the cast padding is rolled back and two to three additional layers of plaster are applied. The plaster should extend approximately two thirds down the dorsal and volar surfaces of the hand, leaving the wrist, thumb, and interphalangeal joints free. A

gentle stretch is then applied to the MP joints in the direction of flexion while contouring the plaster to the arches and over the metacarpal joints (Fig. 90-13).

Special care during the molding phase is crucial to obtain a proper mold. Dorsally mold over the metacarpal heads, into the metacarpal valleys, and mold contouring over each proximal phalanx. Volarly mold into the distal palmar crease, contouring to the transverse metacarpal arch. A well-molded circumferential stretcher is the key to preventing the MP joints from migrating into extension during interphalangeal motion. However, excessive local pressure should be avoided when applying any circumferential cast, because pressure can result in skin breakdown, nerve palsies, or vascular compromise.[9]

Following application of circumferential stretchers, skin color and temperature should be evaluated to assure that circulation has not been compromised by the plaster.

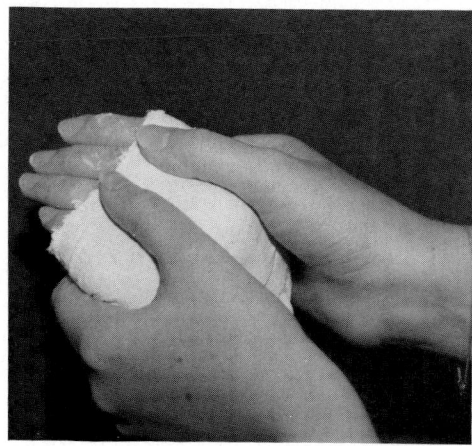

Fig. 90-13 Applying stretch during molding phase.

WEARING SCHEDULE

Plaster stretchers are most beneficial when worn for prolonged periods. However, as with any new splint it may be necessary to initially have the patient wear the stretcher for short periods and gradually increase the wearing time. Kader[15] recommends applying the stretcher in the evening following the patient's last exercise session, then sleeping with the stretcher in place. Kader further advises using the stretcher intermittently throughout the day. Parry[22] advises using a full correction stretcher for 1½-hour periods during the day and sleeping in a stretcher that has less than maximum correction. Stretchers that position the wrist in flexion are not recommended for nighttime wear, since wrist flexion for prolonged periods can compromise lymphatic flow and circulation.

Circumferential stretchers are worn at all times between therapy sessions. The patient should be instructed in how to remove the cast in case of severe discomfort, numbness, or compromised circulation. Removal of circumferential stretchers can be accomplished in several ways. If available

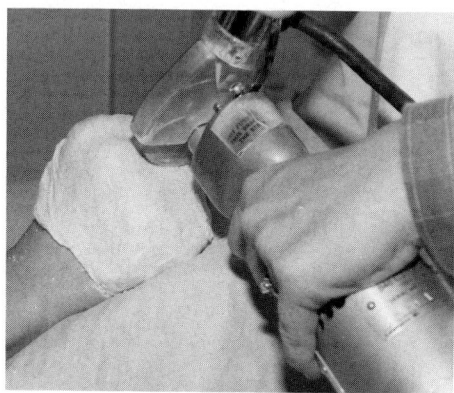

Fig. 90-14 Cutting cast using oscillating cast cutter.

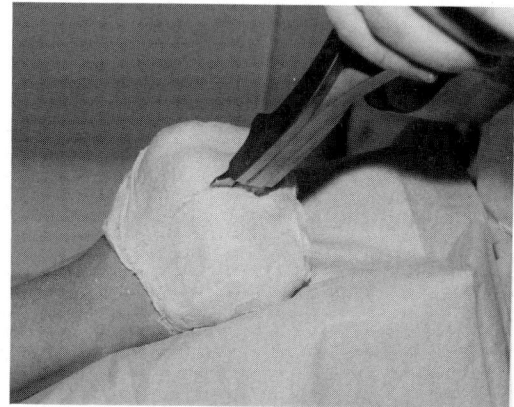

Fig. 90-15 Spreading cast with cast spreaders.

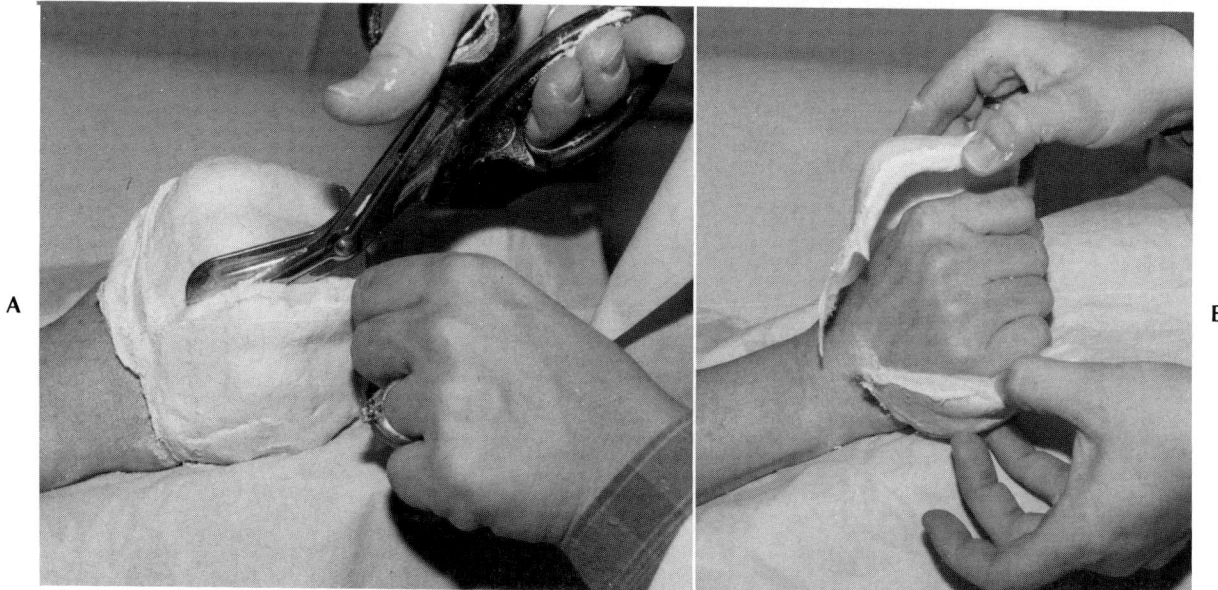

Fig. 90-16 **A,** Cutting cast padding with bandage scissors. **B,** Removing cast.

for the therapist's use, an oscillating cast cutter and cast spreader provide the quickest means for cast removal. When using an oscillating cast cutter, reassure your patient because their first experience can often be frightening. When cutting the cast, use repeated successive short cuts until you feel a lack of resistance or give in the plaster, then move down the cast until you have completed the desired cut (Fig. 90-14). A cast spreader can then be used to separate the two pieces (Fig. 90-15). Then proceed to cut the cast padding with bandage scissors and remove the cast (Fig. 90-16).

When the above cast removal equipment is not available, removal can be accomplished by having the patient soak his or her hand in warm water to soften the cast. The cast can then be removed by cutting with bandage scissors or having the patient wiggle free from the cast. This soak-soften technique for removal should be the technique patients are instructed in for self-removal, if needed. The soak-soften method is also recommended when removing children's casts.

SUMMARY

Splinting with plaster of paris is an art that can be mastered with practice and patience. Its diversity in clinical applications should not be underestimated in hand splinting. Serial plaster stretchers—either volar, dorsal, or circumferential designs—are only a few examples of the possible uses of plaster of paris in hand splinting. A sound knowledge of plaster of paris as a splinting material facilitates its use and proper application in the management of hand injuries.

REFERENCES

1. Atkinson E: Plaster casts, their preparation in the hospital, Walpole, 1937, Lewis Manufacturing Co.
2. Becker D: Danger of burns from fresh plaster splints surrounded by too much cotton, Plast Reconstr Surg 62:436, 1978.
3. Bell J: Plaster casting for the remodeling of soft tissue. In Fess E and Philips C, editors: Hand splinting principles and methods, ed 2, St Louis, 1987, The CV Mosby Co.
4. Cameron D: Plaster of paris—a history, Am J Orthop 3:8, 1961.
5. Diack A, Schultz R, and Nohlgren J: Technique for quantifying low temperature burns, J Surg Res 4:270, 1964.
6. Eton W: A survey of the Turkish Empire, London, 1798. As quoted by Monro J: The history of plaster of paris in the treatment of fractures, Br J Surg 23:257, 1935.
7. Fess E and Philips C: Hand splinting, principles and methods, ed 2, St Louis, 1987, The CV Mosby Co.
8. Geckeller E: Plaster of paris technic, Baltimore, 1944, The Williams & Wilkins Co.
9. Gibson D and Lindsey R: Plaster of paris—its history, functional properties and potential complications, Conn Med 49:525, 1985.
10. Grazer F: Danger of burns from fresh plaster splints surrounded by too much cotton, Plast Reconstr Surg 63(4):560, 1979.
11. Haasch K: Verbrennungen unter dem Gisverband, Hefte Unfallheilkd 78:264, 1964.
12. Hubenthal: Nouvelle Maniere de Traiter les Fractures, Nouv J Med 5:210, 1819. (Interpreted by Atkinson E: Plaster casts, their preparation in the hospital, Walpole, 1937, Lewis Manufacturing Company.)
13. Johnson & Johnson: Plaster of paris bandages, their composition, manufacture and modes of application, New Brunswick, NJ, 1927, Johnson & Johnson.
14. Johnson & Johnson Orthopaedic Division: Fracture Management Orthopaedic Learning System Reference, New Brunswick, NJ, 1985, Johnson & Johnson.
15. Kader P: Serial static plaster splinting and its use on muscle tendon tightness, The International Network, Publication of the American Society of Hand Therapists 4:8, 1986.
16. Kaplan S: Burns following application of plaster dressings, J Bone Joint Surg 63A:670, 1981.
17. Lavalette R, Pope M, and Dickerstein H: Setting temperatures of plaster casts: the influence of technical variables, J Bone Joint Surg 64A:907, 1982.
18. Lovell C and Staniforth P: Contact allergy to benzalkonium chloride in plaster of paris, Contact Dermatitis 7:343, 1981.
19. Mathysen A: Du Bandage Platre et de son Application dans le Traitement des Fractures, ed 2, Liege. (Interpreted by Monro J: The history of plaster of paris in the treatment of fractures, Br J Surg 23:257, 1935.)
20. Mckie D: Antoine Lavoisier, Philadelphia, 1936, JB Lippincott Co.
21. Monro J: The history of plaster of paris in the teatment of fractures, Br J Surg 23:257, 1935.
22. Parry W: Rehabilitation of the hand, ed 4, London, 1981, Butterworth and Co.
23. Rang M: Anthology of orthopaedics, London, 1966, E & S Livingstone Ltd.
24. Salib P: Plaster casting, New York, 1975, Appleton-Century-Crofts.
25. Schultze R: Verbrennungsschaden im Gipsverband, Hefte Unfallheilkd 9:236, 1967.
26. Staniforth P: Allergy to benzalkonium chloride in plaster of paris after sensitization to centrimede, J Bone Joint Surg 62B:500, 1980.
27. Stolov W: Musculoskeletal problems, mobility problems of the muscle-joint unit. In Basmajian J and Kirby L, editors: Medical rehabilitation, Baltimore, 1984, Williams & Wilkins.
28. VanAssen J and Meyerding H: Anthonius Mathijsen, the discoverer of the plaster bandage, J Bone Joint Surg 30A:1018, 1948.
29. Weeks P: Acute bone and joint injuries to the hand and wrist: a clinical guide to management, St Louis, 1981, The CV Mosby Co.
30. Wehbe M: Plaster uses and misuses, Clin Orthop 167:242, 1982.

91

Plaster cylinder casting for contractures of the interphalangeal joints

Judith A. Bell-Krotoski

Plaster cylinder serial casting of the interphalangeal joints of the fingers began as an idea in The Hand Rehabilitation Center established in the 1950s in Vellore, India, by Paul Brand, M.D.[2] It began in the concept of the "inevitability of gradualness" that was to be the hallmark of the center and of Dr. Brand's work. Familiar with the traditional use of force and then of "wedge casting" of clubfeet in children, Dr. Brand began to understand that the early benefits of force were often undone by later contraction of the deep tissue scarring. He felt sure that there must be a way of correcting a deformity without such force on the tissues and on the child. Under his direction, the infant was not fed before having treatment but was put to nursing while Gypsona* plaster of paris was placed in single layers directly on the foot to be corrected. While the plaster was setting, the foot was gradually moved into a corrective position until the child turned his eyes and "looked" without stopping its feeding. Correction of the foot would always stop before the point at which the child would begin to cry. The foot would be held in this position gently but firmly, and the plaster allowed to set. Successive and frequent recastings would be by the same procedure. The method was so successful that the idea was applied to the interphalangeal joints of severely clawed hands found in patients with leprosy. (Patients with leprosy often develop a neuritis of the peripheral nerves resulting in an anesthetic clawed hand with essentially normal extrinsic musculature.) The technique

*Acme Cotton Products Co., Inc., Valley Stream, NY.

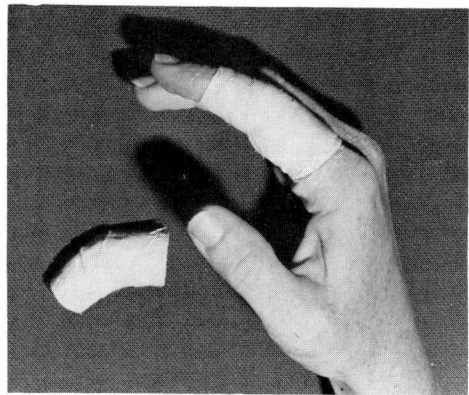

Fig. 91-1 Progressive casting of index interphalangeal joint into extension.

met with equal success and has continued as a successful treatment technique for interphalangeal joint stiffness in India up to now (Fig. 91-1).

As explained by Brand, the technique is not one of progressive "stretching" but of "growth."[2] The cells of the contracted tissue are stimulated to grow and become internally rearranged or modified by being held in the maximum possible extension. This is why the process takes time and the position must be held for a period of time—there is no chance for the remodeling to take place in an hour or two. Each day or every other day the joint can be recasted, having gained a few more degrees, taking advantage of the vital living cell modification.

Steve Kolumban,[5,6] a therapist working with Brand at the Christian Medical College and Hospital in Vellore, India, conducted two studies with leprosy patients supportive of the cylinder casting of contracted proximal interphalangeal (PIP) joints of the hand in 1967. In a study of 50 samples from 24 outpatients with contractures of the interphalangeal joints, Kolumban compared splinting with regular physiotherapy technique. Regular physiotherapy given to 25 of the patients consisted of wax baths, oil massage, and exercise (passive and active-assistive). At the end of the study the group with the splinting was significantly superior. The percentage of degrees straightened from the total possible number was 45.7% with splinting and 0.9% without splinting. Out of the 25 fingers in the group without splinting, 12 joints ended with a greater contracture than that with which they began.

In a study of 26 patients with 52 samples of contracted interphalangeal joints, Kolumban compared cylinder serial casting with dynamic splinting.[4] An attempt was made in the study to match fingers from both groups into pairs of six variables: age, contracture angle, joint resiliency, length of the finger, length of splinting, and applied straightening force. A straightening force of 250 gm was applied in both methods of splinting. At the end of the study, the results showed a strong indication that the casting was superior to dynamic splinting. The percentage of degrees straightened from the total possible with serial cylinder casting was 47.8% and with dynamic splinting, 34.9%. Injuries from splinting (many of the patients had anesthetic hands) were none for the cylinder splinting and 7 for the dynamic splinting.

Brand brought the technique for cylinder serial casting of the joints to the United States in the treatment of leprosy patients at the United States Public Health Service Hospital in Carville, Louisiana. The adaptation of this technique of treatment for joint stiffness from causes other than leprosy was always advocated by Brand, and under his influence the technique began to be used for patients with a wide variety of conditions resulting in joint contractures of the hand. I used the technique at the New Orleans United States Public Health Service Hospital in 1973, and later at the Hand Rehabilitation Center, Ltd., in Philadelphia, Pennsylvania, for joint contractures other than those caused by leprosy. Conditions in which the casting has been used successfully to reduce finger contractures include arthritis, reflex sympathetic dystrophy (RSD), Dupuytren's contracture, congenital contractures, joint dislocations, burns, boutonnière deformities, swan-neck deformities, and contractures after fractures and tendon repairs.

INDICATIONS FOR CASTING

As in the use of any type of splinting, the casting is not used for patients responding well to simple positioning, range of motion, and physiotherapy techniques. For patients with mild contractures, often a simple augmentation to therapy using night gutter splints or traction splints will be all that is necessary to achieve desired results. For moderate-to-severe contractures, in most cases I prefer cylinder casting. I have used dynamic splinting methods since 1968 and cylinder casting since 1973. Experience with the casting teaches the following:

1. The supplies needed are simple and readily available, making the method of treatment available and adaptable to a variety of circumstances—hospital wards, intensive care units, and so on.
2. Once the plaster is applied, the joint has no choice except to stay at the position casted, whereas dynamic splinting comes out of adjustment easily either by itself or by the patient. Dynamic splinting has to be continually checked to assure that traction is at the angle desired and the specific gram traction desired. The one certain thing about rubber bands used for traction is that they do get old quickly and must be changed frequently. Even after slow traction with splinting, the tissues often will not tolerate enough traction to prevent an annoying recurrence of joint stiffness that can compromise an otherwise expected progressive improvement in range.
3. Swelling is never increased by the plaster cast and is often decreased because the cast keeps the joint quiet for periods of rest. Dynamic splinting can cause an increase in swelling—if not by the amount of traction, then by decreased circulation resulting from the restriction of the finger cuff.
4. Since casting is not a stretching or a wedging, pain is not increased by cylinder casting and is often decreased. This is particularly important in patients with RSD, where even a slight increase in pain is a step in the wrong direction. Traction by dynamic splinting can cause soreness, particularly with hypersensitive fingers.
5. Cylinder casting can be used over lacerations and ulcers. The technique is used in leprosy patients to protect insensitive fingers so that they can heal without further trauma.
6. Cylinder casting can be used in the treatment of old fixed deformities and, in fact, is indicated where the use of dynamic traction often fails.

PADDING

The most damaging force to skin is not from direct pressure but from shear force. Plaster that is not padded will conform precisely to the skin and adhere slightly to the skin, preventing sheer force under the cast when the fingers are moved. For this reason, no padding or only padding that is absolutely necessary is used. Wounds are covered very lightly. If irritation has developed over the interphalangeal joint, casting technique should be rechecked; a small, thin fluff of cotton may be placed over the dorsum of the joint before it is recasted. Occasionally, the dorsal skin over the interphalangeal joint is so fragile that this small amount of padding is required for successful casting. For patients with fragile skin, small, thin fluffs of cotton may also be added, if necessary, at the distal and proximal volar edges of the cast when the finger is casted. Plaster allows the skin underneath to breath somewhat and does not macerate the skin if applied directly, as happens with some other splinting materials.

TECHNIQUE

Supplies needed
1. Twelve- to 15-inch strip of plaster bandage, 1 inch wide
2. Scissors—suture or small bandage
3. Water—small paper cup
4. Paper towel
5. Tube of lanolin or other oil

Instructions
1. Prepare finger to be casted (with lanolin if to be removable, light bandage if wound).
2. Dip the plaster strip in water and drain excess water on paper towel.
3. Fold ⅛-inch edge on plaster strip for 2 inches to make a smooth edge (Fig. 91-2).
4. Begin wrapping the finger with the folded edge of the plaster strip just distal to the metacarpophalangeal joint (MP). Over-

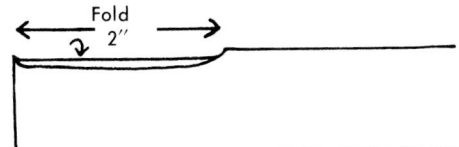

Fig. 91-2 Plaster strip 1 inch wide (cut from 2-inch wide plaster).

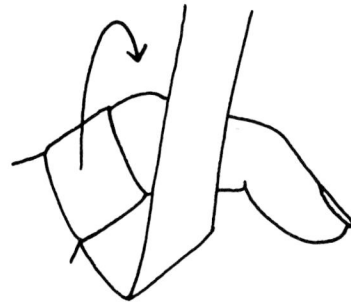

Fig. 91-3 Wrapping of plaster. Finger may be wrapped distal to the proximal finger if believed necessary, but it is usually not necessary because plaster is for positioning of the joint only and wrapping should not compress tissue.

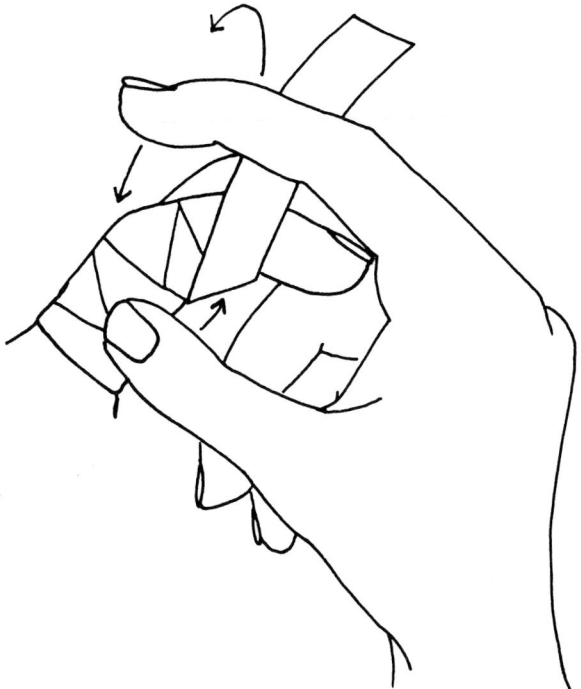

Fig. 91-4   Wrapping of finger while it is being supported in position.

lap the plaster strip as you wrap distally to the fingertip. Two overlapping wraps of plaster is enough to make a firm cast (Fig. 91-3).

5. Support the finger in extension while wrapping if trying for interphalangeal extension; support the finger in flexion while wrapping if trying for interphalangeal flexion.

6. Use a constant motion of your fingers and thumb in a clock-wise direction to maintain the position of the finger and to smooth the cast (Fig. 91-4).

7. Wrap to the distal interphalangeal (DIP) crease if later DIP movement with use of the cast is desired. Wrap past the DIP crease if
   a. The profundus tendon is tight when casting for extension.
   b. The extensor mechanism is tight when casting for flexion.
   c. The improvement in range of movement is also desired at the distal interphalangeal joint.

8. To finish the cast at the distal tip, fold the edge of plaster strip under to make a smooth edge.

9. After wrapping is completed, continue to support the finger in the desired position of correction by continued clockwise movement of the fingers, avoiding any point pressure until the cast is firm.

OR

Apply *slight* traction to the finger by placing the MP joint in flexion, supporting the palm with the thumb of one hand while holding the distal tip of the casted finger (uncasted portion) in corrected position with your index finger and thumb until the cast is firm (Fig. 91-5).

I should emphasize that the method described is not intended to wedge cast the finger or to apply force other than a slight traction to the joint. Too much force applied during casting will shortly be apparent in an angry-looking interphalangeal joint with red, shiny skin. Used correctly, casting is a nontraumatic way of gaining additional flexion or extension range. Circulation of the finger is always checked after cast application to make sure the vascular supply is not compromised. The patient is always instructed to remove the cast later if it appears too tight, but this is not usually necessary.

Brand[2] recommends, when possible, that the cast be left on and removed only for exercise in therapy. The casting is most effective if it is left on continually and changed

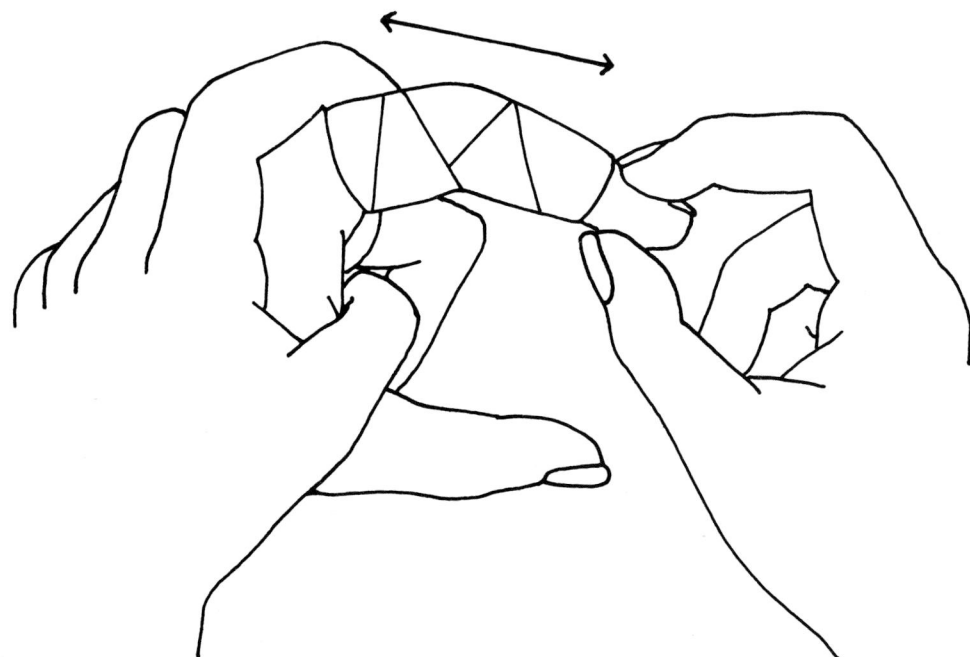

Fig. 91-5   Positioning of finger for traction. Care should be taken to avoid any point pressure on the plaster.

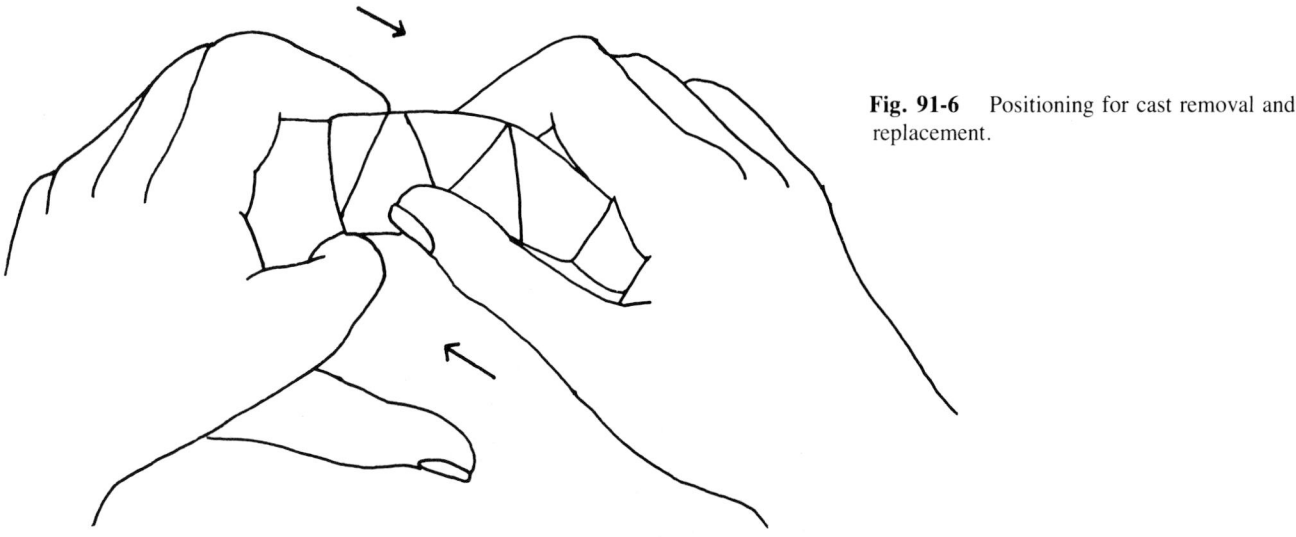

Fig. 91-6 Positioning for cast removal and replacement.

every day or every other day. It can be changed every day if possible, but it must be changed at least twice a week and the jonts exercised to maintain their full mobility. After exercise, a new cast can be applied in what will probably be a few degrees more extension or flexion depending on the direction casted.

Although the cast is a total-contact plaster, one can easily remove it at the time of therapy by immersing the hand in water and unwrapping it or by squeezing the cast from side to side, which cracks the eggshell thickness and makes the whole splint quite pulpy and soft. At this stage it is easy to find the end of the plaster bandage and it is unwrapped. Some therapists mark the end of the bandage or even fold the end back at the time the cast is applied, so that the end will be easy to find.

The casting may be continued so long as improvement is made. Wax baths and oil rubbed into the fingers at exercise times are considered of value.

REMOVABLE CYLINDER CASTS

Occasions arise in which it is necessary to make the cylinder casts removable. The most obvious cases are those in which it is most important to move tendons frequently to prevent adhesions, as in the weeks after a tendon repair or in casts in which the patient can attend therapy only infrequently. Experience has taught me that casting is often not used because of a fear on the part of the surgeon or therapist that flexion of the finger in question will be lost. Flexion is not usually lost with casting, and careful measurements will assure that this is not a problem.[3] However, by making the cylinder casts removable, one can often increase flexion range of motion during casting the finger into extension by exercise of the joint at the time of cast change.

The application technique is the same as has already been described, except that the cast is removed.

Instructions
1. After the cast is firm, grasp along the length of the cast and gently loosen and remove it from the finger. IMPORTANT: The cast must be removed at this point if it is going to be removable for exercise of the joint (Fig. 91-6).
2. Check the finger and cast for point pressure. If need be, trim the edge of the cast for clearance of MP or DIP flexion.
3. Clean the excess plaster off the finger, apply another light coat of lanolin to the finger, and replace the cast.

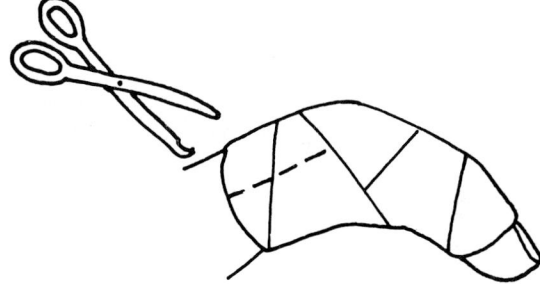

Fig. 91-7 Cast removal for swollen interphalangeal joint.

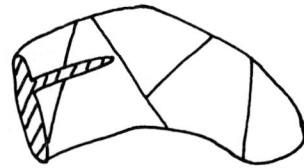

Fig. 91-8 Trimming of cast for replacement.

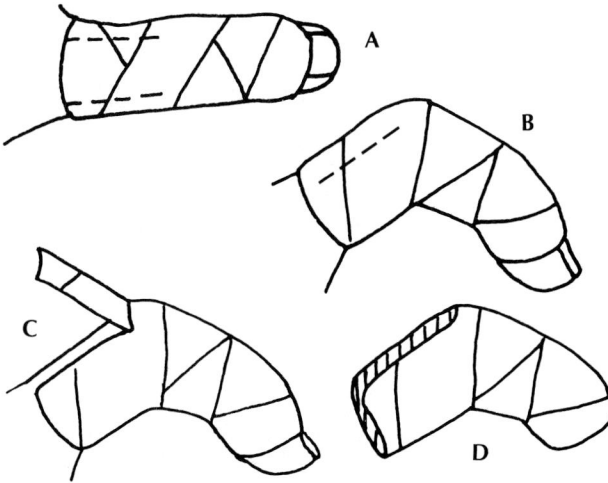

Fig. 91-9 Cast removal for severely flexed interphalangeal joint. **A,** Dorsal view. **B,** Lateral view. **C,** Flap. **D,** Cast.

4. If the interphalangeal joint is too swollen to allow easy removal of the cast, a slight cut can be made in the dorsal radial portion of the cast at the proximal phalanx. This cut is extended toward the interphalangeal joint until the cast can be removed (Fig. 91-7).

5. Once the cast is removed, the cut edges can be trimmed slightly and the cast replaced without losing its correction (Fig. 91-8).

6. If the finger is in a position of too much flexion to allow removal of the cast, one can make a window in the cast with scissors by first making cuts in the dorsoradial and dorsoulnar sides of the cast at the proximal phalanx. The flap is lifted, and the cast is removed. The flap is trimmed with scissors, and the cast can then be replaced and secured at the proximal phalanx with a small strip of adhesive tape (Fig. 91-9).

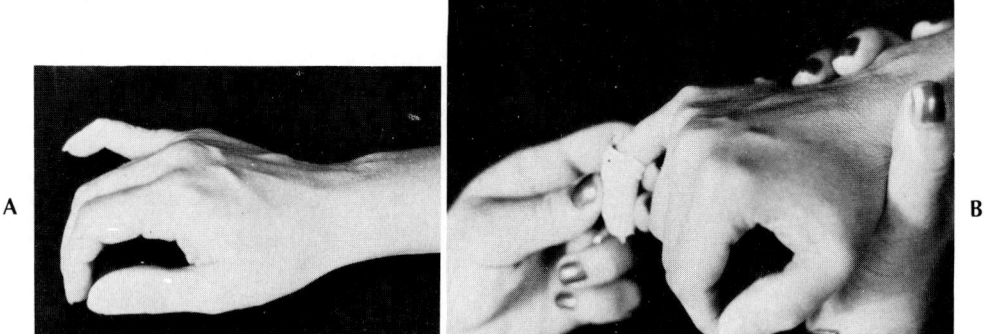

Fig. 91-10 **A,** Swan-neck deformity of left fifth digit with fixed hyperextension of the interphalangeal joint. **B,** Technique of casting for correction in two planes. Once the distal interphalangeal joint is casted into maximum possible extension, the proximal interphalangeal joint is flexed and casted into maximum possible flexion with the cast extending over the casted distal interphalangeal joint.

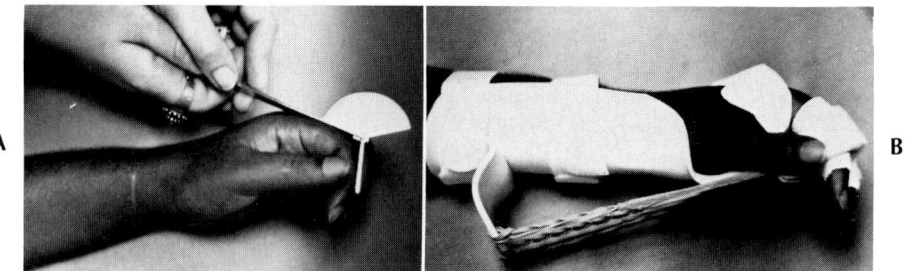

Fig. 91-11 **A,** Maximum extension of interphalangeal joints and maximum flexion of metacarpophalangeal joints after reflex sympathetic dystrophy. **B,** Same patient as progressively casted into extension of the interphalangeal joints and as placed into flexion traction at the metacarpophalangeal joints.

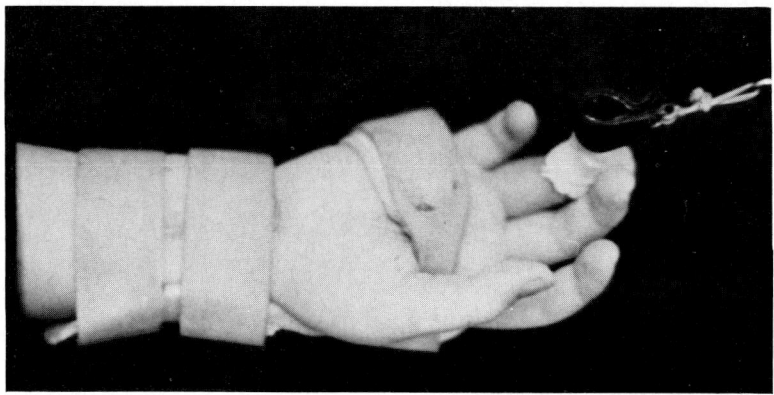

Fig. 91-12 Casting to increase extension of the distal interphalangeal joint and traction to increase extension of the proximal interphalangeal joint in a patient with residual flexion contracture 8 weeks after second-stage flexor tendon graft.

7. Once joint correction is achieved, the final cast can be worn as a retainer at night until after that period of time when joint contracture tends to recur.

8. The cast can be made to last an indefinite period of time by being coated with lacquer or fingernail polish once the plaster is dry.

ADAPTIVE CASTING
Two planes of movement

The use of the plaster casts can be coordinated with other conventional forms of therapy and splinting. The casting is particularly helpful in the treatment of fingers that require correction in two planes of movement, such as fingers with swan-neck deformities (Fig. 91-10) and contracted fingers as seen in nerve injuries and RSD (Fig. 91-11).

Transfer of moment

Casting of individual joints can also be used to block or transfer power of movement to other joints in the same plane of movement.[1] After silicone rubber implants of the MP joints, the patient will often begin early movement of the fingers by undesired flexion at the interphalangeal joints. By casting the interphalangeal joints one restricts the power of flexion at the interphalangeal joints and transfers it to the MP joints, until the patient is able to accomplish active flexion of the MP joints.

In other words, a static splint is not always "static" in function. It can "dynamically" function to transfer an additional force on joint movement of another joint or joints when the hand is moved.

When the PIP joint of the finger is casted, the DIP joint is often included in the cast. It can be left out intentionally, for exercise, for instance, if flexor tendon adhesions are present.

By casting a boutonnière deformity of the finger into extension at the interphalangeal joint, the lateral bands become slightly relaxed, and the power of flexion can be concentrated to flex the DIP joint. Casting of the DIP joint can be done to increase traction at the PIP joint (Fig. 91-12). For a stiff PIP joint, casting of the DIP joint will transfer the full power of the flexor digitorum profundus to the PIP joint (Fig. 91-13).

OTHER JOINTS AND TENDONS

The technique of plaster casting for remodeling can be used on other joints and muscle-tendon unit contractures.

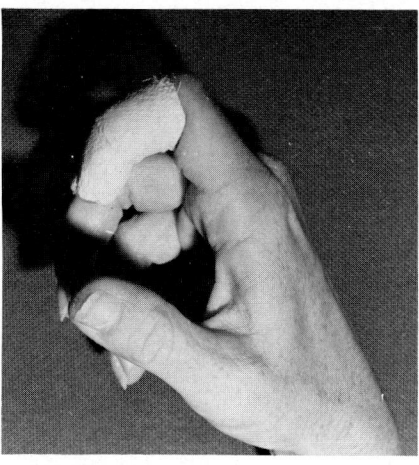

Fig. 91-13 Casting of distal interphalangeal joint to transfer power of the profundus flexion to the stiff proximal interphalangeal joint.

While the method has most often been applied to interphalangeal joint contractures, contractures of the wrist, thumb web space, and elbow have been treated successfully. Muscle-tendon unit contractures usually require slab casting. The technique for casting other parts is based on the same principles as casting for finger interphalangeal joint contractures.

REFERENCES

1. Bell JA: Plaster casting in the remodeling of soft tissue. In Fess E and Philips C: Hand splinting: principles and methods, ed 2, St. Louis, 1987, The CV Mosby Co.
2. Brand PW: The reconstruction of the hand in leprosy, Ann R Coll Surg Engl 11:350, 1952.
3. Flowers KR and Pheasant SD: The use of torque angle curves in the assessment of digital joint stiffness, J Hand Ther 1:69, 1988.
4. Kolumban SL: The use of dynamic and static splints in straightening contracted proximal interphalangeal joints in leprosy patients: a comparative study. Paper read at the forty-seventh annual conference of the American Physical Therapy Association, Washington, DC, 1960.
5. Kolumban SL: Master's thesis, New York University, 1967.
6. Kolumban SL: The role of static and dynamic splints, physiotherapy techniques and time in straightening contractures of the interphalangeal joints, Leprosy in India, p 323-328, Oct 1969.

92

Dynamic pronation-supination splint

Kay Colello-Abraham

This chapter discusses principles of splinting applied to the distal radioulnar joint and presents a dynamic splint designed to achieve pronation/supination of the forearm. The splint consists of two portions. The proximal, or upper, portion is a humoral cuff with two lateral bars that run parallel to the forearm. The lateral bars act as a point of attachment for the dynamic forces. The distal, or lower, portion is a cock-up splint to which the dynamic forces are applied, pulling the forearm in a rotational direction (Fig. 92-1).

SPLINTING PRINCIPLES APPLIED TO THE DISTAL RADIOULNAR JOINT

It is necessary to understand the anatomy and dynamics of the distal radioulnar (RU) joint to be able to properly construct a dynamic splint. The anatomy and dynamics of this joint are not particularly difficult; however, they are different from the other joints of the upper extremity in terms of splinting. Because the motion of the forearm is circular, the direction of the dynamic force must also be circular. The mechanical principles of dynamic splinting as discussed by Fess[3] still apply, although they must be applied to a circular motion rather than an angular one. Some differences in application are as follows:

1. Most joints have a very short axis of rotation, usually the width of the joint (Fig. 92-2). In the forearm, motion takes place equally in both the upper and lower RU joints. Thus the axis of rotation is the length of the forearm (Fig. 92-3). This allows for placement of multiple force arms (Fig. 92-4). In this splint the levers attached to the cock-up splint are considered the force arms, which is the perpendicular distance between the axis of rotation and the force line of action or the dynamic force. Use of multiple force arms will increase the mechanical advantage in two ways: (1) The force will be distributed throughout the multiple force arms, increasing the area of force application. This will increase the amount of force tolerated as the area of pressure distribution is enlarged. (2) Using equal force throughout the length of the axis of rotation will result in equal movement at both the distal and proximal RU joints. Applying force at only the distal RU joint possibly may result in greater movement at the distal end than the proximal end.

2. Fess[3] describes the use of optimum rotational force in terms of rectangular components as applied to hinge joints. Optimum rotational force is the term used to define a dynamic force that is applied at a 90-degree angle to the segment being mobilized, resulting in the full magnitude of the force being applied in a rotational direction. Obtaining optimum rotational force in the forearm requires the use of rectangular components

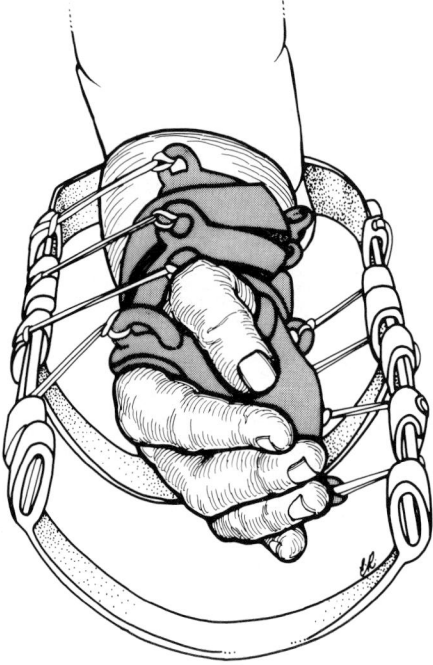

Fig. 92-1   Completed dynamic pronation-supination splint.

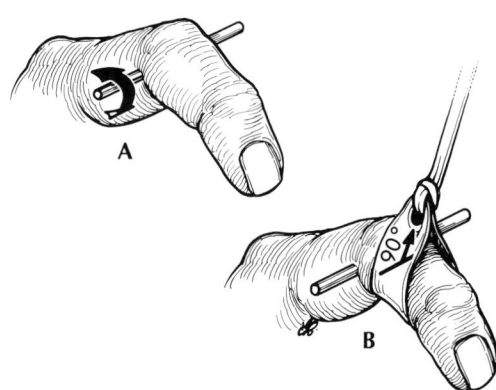

Fig. 92-2   **A,** Axis of rotation of proximal interphalangeal joint is very narrow. **B,** Narrow axis of the proximal interphalangeal allows room for only one force arm.

1134

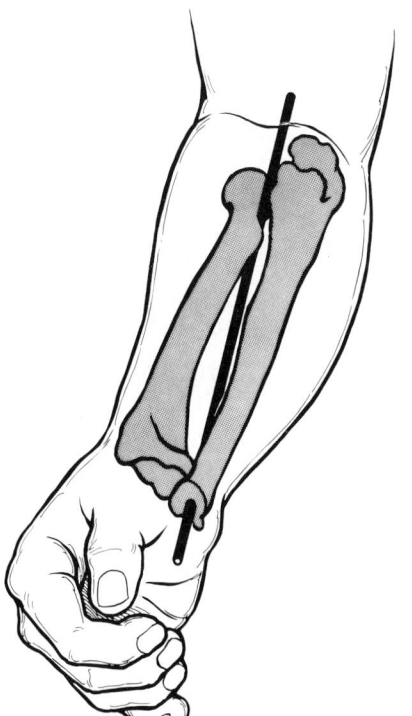

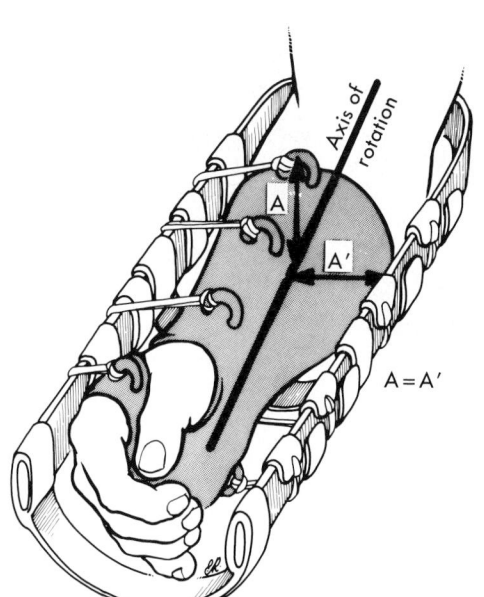

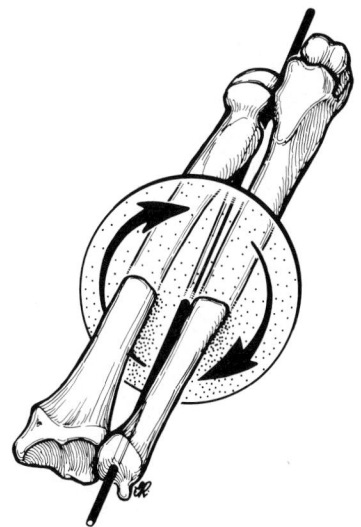

Fig. 92-3 The axis of rotation of the radioulnar joint is the length of the forearm.

Fig. 92-4 The long axis of rotation allows for multiple force arms. The small lever arm increases the length of the force arm, resulting in increased torque. Distances *A* and *A'* should be equal to achieve a circular motion.

Fig. 92-5 Dynamic traction is applied at a 90-degree angle to the axis, but should approximate a 360-degree curve.

and one circular component. One still must apply the dynamic traction at a 90-degree angle to the axis of rotation; however, the motion itself is circular rather than angular (Fig. 92-5). If the dynamic traction does not approximate a 360-degree curve, translational forces will result. Translational forces are forces produced by the dynamic traction that are nonrotary or, in other words, do not move the joint in the desired direction. The placement of the lateral bars will determine the direction of force. If the bars are placed dorsal or volar to the midline of the forearm, a translational force will result in elbow flexion or extension. If the bars are placed too far from the forearm, a lateral pull to the ulnar bar will work against the lateral pull to the radial bar, eliminating or decreasing the rotational forces.

3. Fess also states that torque is equal to the amount of pull from the dynamic assist times the length of the force arm. The force arm is the distance between the joint axis and the point of attachment of the dynamic assist. To increase torque one must increase the length of the force arm or increase the force of the dynamic assist. With a digit the force arm is lengthened by placing the dynamic assist more distally from the joint axis. This is not possible in the forearm. In the forearm the length of the force arm is relatively short, being the distance from the axis of rotation to the radial or ulnar surface (approximately half the width of the forearm). To lengthen the force arm, the dynamic

assist needs to be placed beyond the surface of the forearm. This is done by attaching small lever arms to the cock-up splint (see Fig. 92-4). In other words, when the motion is circular as with the forearm, torque is increased by enlarging the arc of motion.

4. Theoretically, a splint designed to rotate the forearm does not need to extend into the palm. The palm has been included in this design for several reasons. Since forearm rotation influences carpal alignment, rotation, and positioning, and vice versa,[4] the wrist has been included and positioned in neutral. By extending the cock-up splint to the distal palmar crease, one is essentially eliminating all wrist motion except rotation. The axis of rotation is then lengthened to the point of the distal palmar crease, thus providing for additional application of force and increased mechanical advantage. Also, the thenar eminence will help prevent the splint from sliding around the forearm once the dynamic forces are applied. Not including the wrist and hand would tend to leave the hand "hanging" over the distal edge of the volar forearm splint, creating the possibility of compression at the volar wrist crease.

HISTORY

A review of the literature shows Sterling Bunnell was the first to discuss a dynamic pronation-supination device. In 1944 he stated, "Encase the arm in a right angle elbow splint. The hand and wrist are encased in plaster or the wrist is grasped with a broad oval ring. Two extension rods from

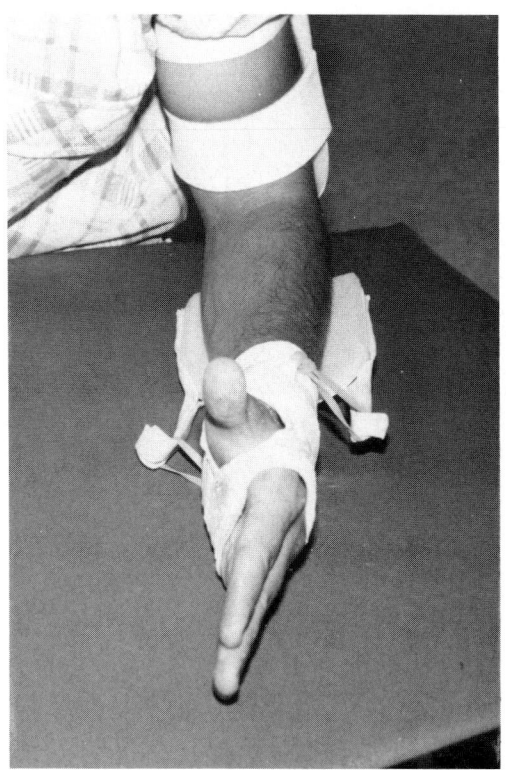

Fig. 92-6 Dynamic forearm device described by Bunnell in 1944.

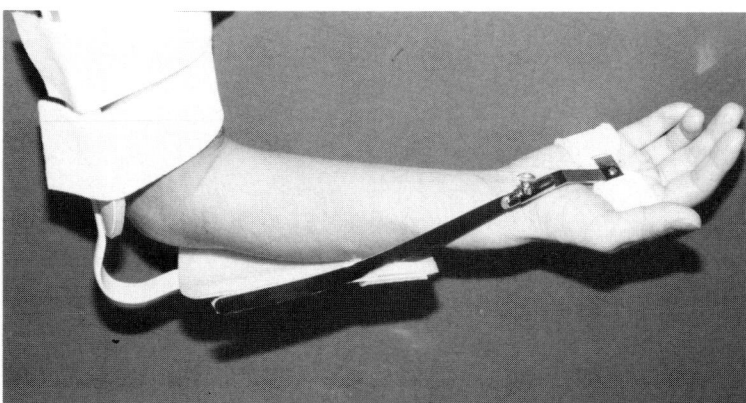

Fig. 92-7 Forearm torsion bar by Bunnell, commercially available today.

the forearm piece of the elbow splint are used as attachments to draw by a rubber band from each rod, the hand-wrist member in rotation."[2] Refer to Fig. 92-6 for a device constructed following these directions. This is essentially using the same design principle as the splint described in this chapter. The differences are a result of our increased knowledge of mechanical and dynamic principles as they relate to splinting. The elbow splint, described by Bunnell, extends distally on the forearm, thus creating friction between the skin and the splint as the forearm is pulled into rotation. The friction will also undermine the strength of the dynamic assist. The splint is composed of only one force arm each on the radial and ulnar sides, which minimizes the mechanical advantage and increases the application of force to a very small area. As stated before, the forearm moves equally at the proximal and distal RU joints, so it is important to apply the dynamic force equally throughout the length of the forearm.

In 1954 Bunnell[1] also wrote an article describing a spring splint designed to pronate or supinate the forearm. This

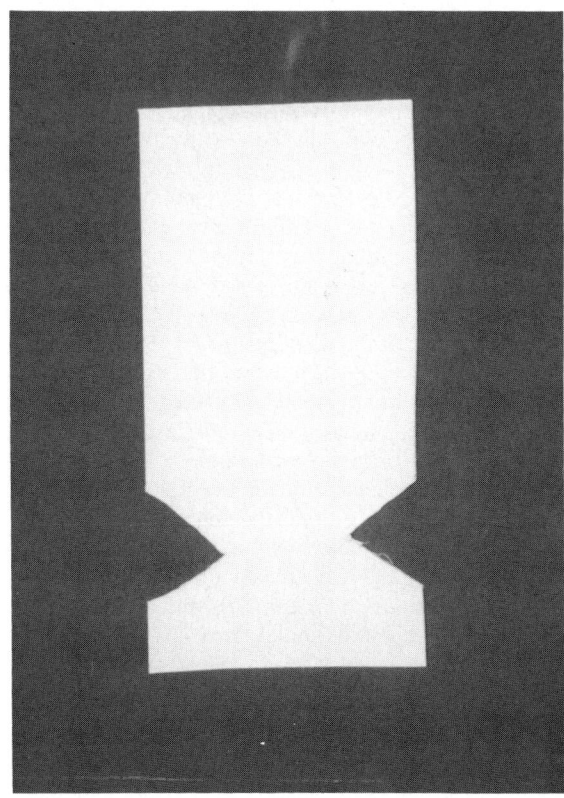

Fig. 92-8 Upper-arm splint pattern.

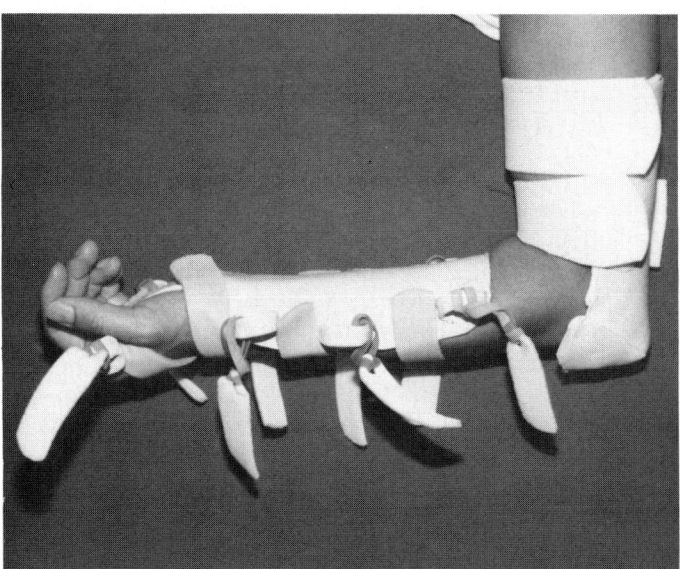

Fig. 92-9 Upper-arm and lower-arm splints.

splint is still commercially available today (Fig. 92-7). This is not a dynamic forearm splint so much as an adjustable forearm positioner. Once the splint is in place, there are no dynamic or movable parts.

CONSTRUCTION OF SPLINT
Step 1, upper portion

Begin with a rectangular piece of low-temperature thermoplastic, approximately 7 to 9 inches by 6 to 7 inches. After heating, cut out triangular sections on both sides, approximately 1 to 2 inches from the distal border (Fig. 92-8). Mold the plastic to the posterior surface of the upper arm, placing the cutout portions at the medial and lateral epicondyles. The splint should be formed with the elbow in 90 degrees of flexion, and care should be taken to avoid pressure points around the bony prominences of the elbow. Mold the splint loosely enough around the elbow to provide room for a thick padding material. The distal edge of the splint should end approximately 1 inch distal to the elbow. Extending more distally on the forearm will interfere with forearm rotation.

Next, line the upper splint with a comfortable padding. A padding thicker than moleskin is preferable, since it

will provide more protection to the bony prominences of the elbow. Attach two straps proximal to the elbow (Fig. 92-9).

Step 2, lower portion

Form a cock-up splint out of a low-temperature thermoplastic. The splint should extend two-thirds the length of the forearm for better purchase and greater distribution of pressures. The distal end should extend only to the distal palmar crease so as not to limit finger flexion. Be sure to construct the thumb web space wide enough to accommodate a strap and the attachment of a lever arm (Fig. 92-10). It is important that the cock-up splint is trimmed so that it comes only to the midline of the forearm on the radial and ulnar sides. If the splint extends beyond the midline, the straps will not hug the forearm and the cock-up splint will tend to rotate.

Next, line the splint with a soft padding that will "grip" the arm rather than slide around the arm. Then attach Velcro straps, leaving room in between the straps for the attachment of lever arms (Fig 92-11).

Construct each lever arm using a strip of thermoplastic ¼-inch wide by 2 inches long. You will need 8 to 10 of these lever arms. While the plastic is warm, form a circle and press it onto the cock-up splint (Fig. 92-12). Use the heat gun to strengthen the attachment. Place four to five lever arms on both the radial and ulnar sides of the cock-up splint—one at the distal palmar crease on each side, one

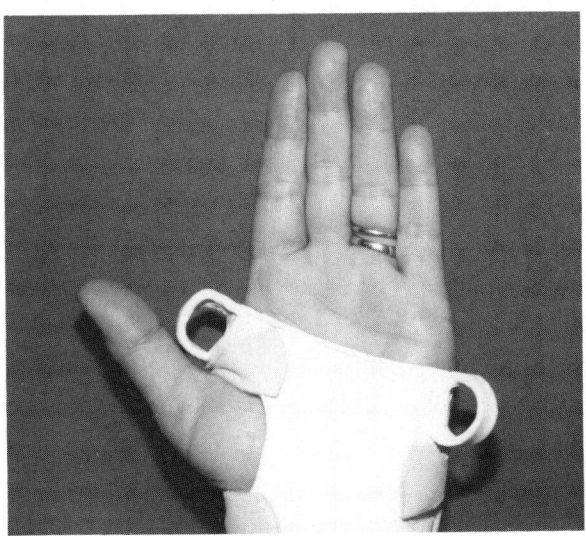

Fig. 92-10 Thumb web space should be wide enough to accommodate a strap and a lever arm.

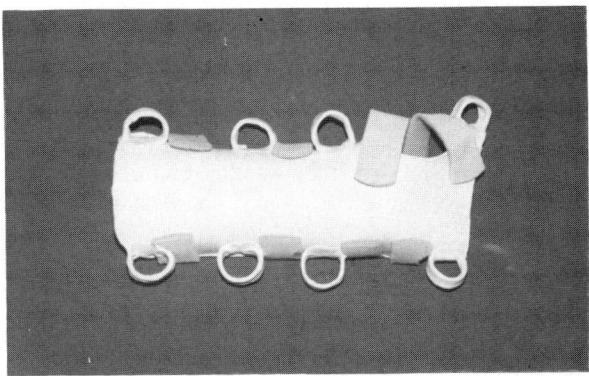

Fig. 92-11 Space straps, leaving room for attachment of the lever arms.

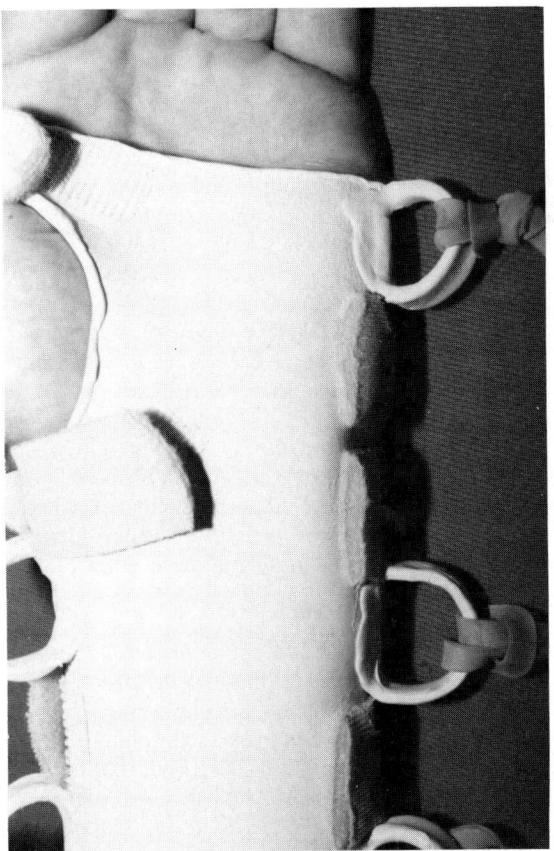

Fig. 92-12 Small piece of plastic is used to form lever arm.

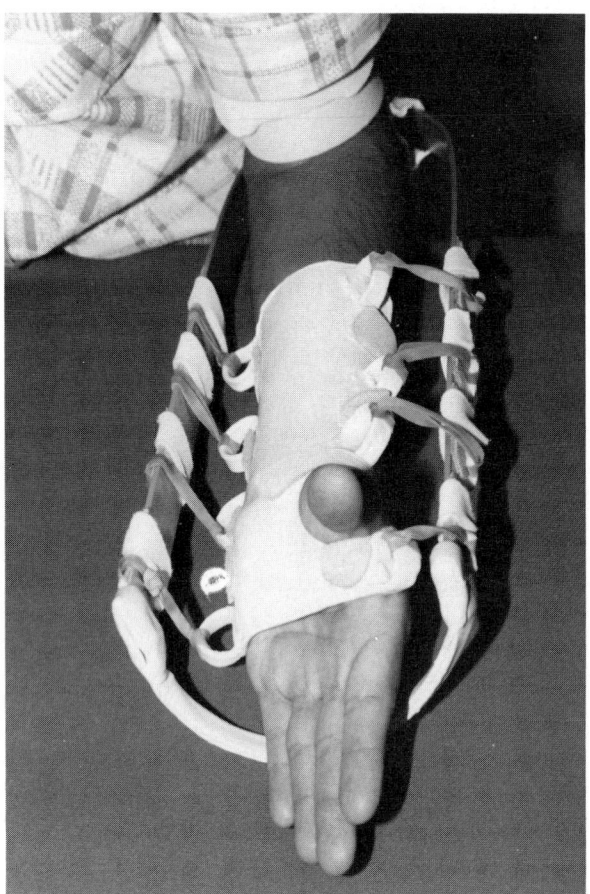

Fig. 92-13 Completed splint with dynamic traction applied.

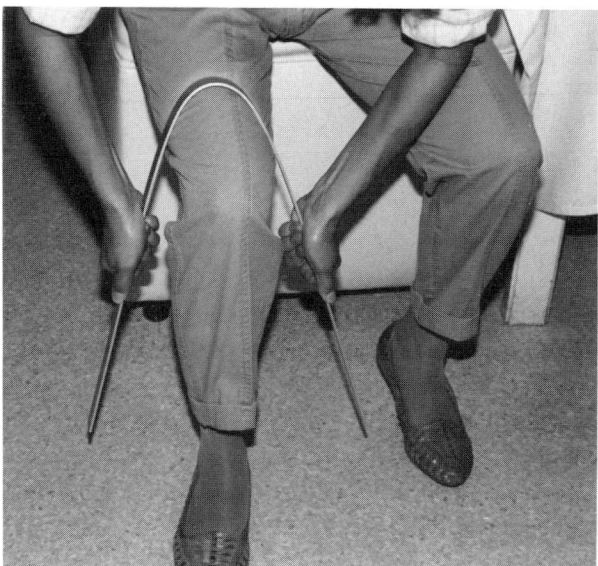

Fig. 92-14 Bend the bar to approximate the curve of the upper arm.

at the proximal end on each side, and two to three in between (Fig. 92-11).

Next, make 8 to 10 tabs out of Velcro pile, and punch a hole in one end of each. The tabs should be approximately ¼ inch wide by 3 to 4 inches long. Attach a rubber band to each tab. Attach the other ends of the rubber bands to the lever arms of the cock-up splint (Fig. 92-13). The length of the rubber bands will depend upon the severity of loss of range of motion. With a very severe loss of range of motion, the rubber bands may need to span a distance of 7 inches to reach the lateral bar. As forearm rotation improves, the lever arms on the cock-up splint move closer to the lateral bars, so the rubber bands may need to span only a 2-inch distance. Obviously, shorter rubber bands would then be required. Because there are multiple force arms, total force is determined by adding them all together.

Step 3, lateral bars

The lateral bars are made from an andonized aluminum flat bar. These bars can be purchased at hardware stores and measure 1 inch by ⅛ inch by 72 inches. Have the bar cut in two pieces, each 36 inches long. Each splint requires one bar 1 inch by ⅛ inch by 36 inches. Bend the bar around your knee or other rounded object that approximates the upper arm in diameter (Fig. 92-14). Adjust the bar until both sides are parallel to the forearm at both the proximal and distal ends (Fig. 92-15). The bar should extend distally to the distal palmar crease. Some therapists prefer to con-

struct the bars out of thermoplastic material. For these bars, forming one at a time, use a piece of plastic 15 to 17 inches long by 2 inches wide. Fold the heated plastic in half. Then mold the proximal portion around the posterior of the upper-arm splint and the remaining portion parallel to the midline of the forearm on the radial or ulnar side. As with the metal bars, attach the plastic bars first with Velcro, and then reinforce them with plastic. (Refer to the following paragraph.)

Put the upper-arm and lower-arm splints on the patient. Hold the bar in place, and determine the attachment position. With the elbow in 90 degrees flexion, the bars should run parallel with the midline of the forearm on both the radial and ulnar sides. The lateral bars should be as close to the forearm as possible, leaving just enough clearance for the cock-up splint to rotate. If the bars are spaced wider than necessary, the circular forces will be decreased and the horizontal forces increased. Fig. 92-4 shows the distance from the axis of rotation to the top of the lever arm being equal to the distance from the axis of rotation to the lateral bars. Now refer to Fig. 92-5. Imagine the lever arm at the 12 o'clock position on this circle and the lateral bar at the 3 o'clock position. When the rubber-band traction is applied, it will pull the forearm in a circular motion. If the lateral bars are spaced wider apart, they will not fall within this arc of motion. The rubber-band traction would have to pull horizontally to reach out to the bar. Next, attach a piece of hook Velcro to the posterior of the upper-arm splint, and loop the Velcro to the inside curve portion of the bar. Attach the bar to the splint. You may want to reinforce this with a piece of thermoplastic. For a more secure attachment you may prefer to use Sabre Grip, Poly-Lock, or a molded-plastic hook Velcro.

Then place 1½- to 2-inch–long pieces of sticky-backed Velcro hook onto the outer sides of the bars. These pieces are placed at intervals corresponding to the levers on the cock-up splint.

To prevent the lateral bars from bending towards the cock-up splint once the dynamic forces are applied, it is necessary

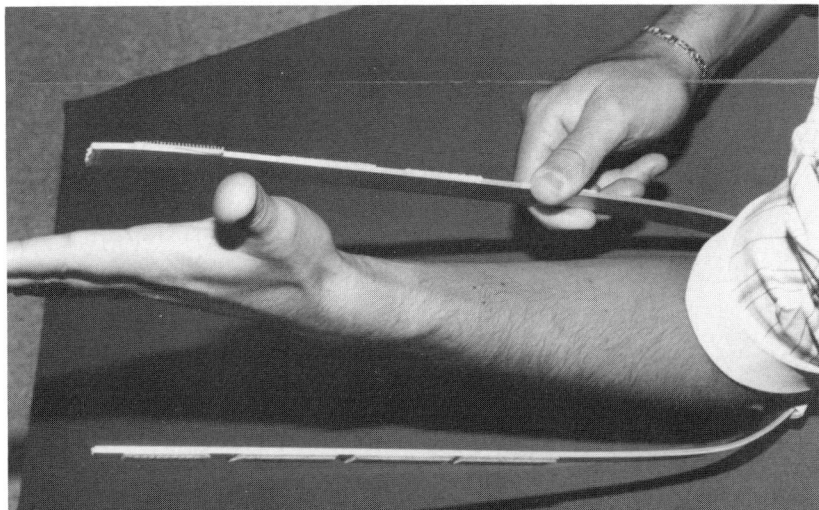

Fig. 92-15   Both sides should be parallel to the forearm at the proximal and distal ends.

to add cross struts. The cross struts are made of thermoplastic (double thickness). Wrap the plastic around the metal bar, and adhere it to itself; then do the same on the opposite bar. Place one cross strut on the distal end and one midway up the forearm. It is preferable to place the cross struts on the volar surface, so when the patient rests the forearm on a table the cross struts will prevent interference with the dynamic traction. The distally placed cross strut should cover the sharp edges of the metal flat bar. Be sure to allow for clearance of the cock-up splint (Fig. 92-16).

Step 4, application and wearing time

Pull the Velcro pile tabs to the lateral bar. Pull each tab around the inside of the bar and attach them to the Velcro hooks. Adjust the tension as necessary. The patient may want to begin by attaching only three tabs on each side and increasing the number as tolerance improves. The tension can be increased by wrapping the tab around the bar twice.

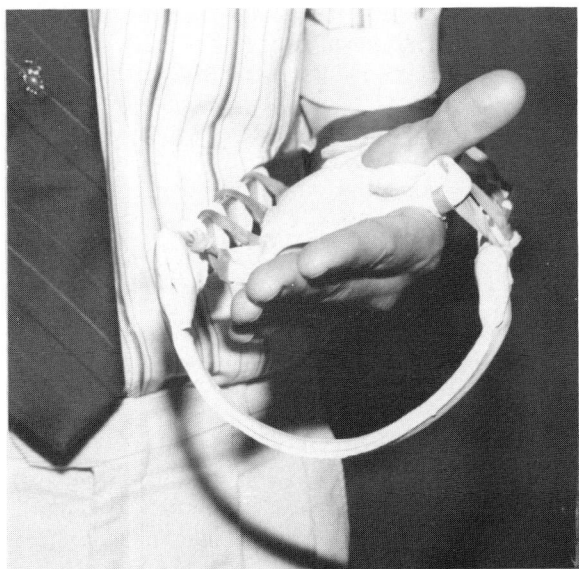

Fig. 92-16   Cross struts should be curved to allow for clearance of the rotating cock-up splint.

The splint is usually worn 15 to 30 minutes every 2 hours. The short wearing time is often a matter of necessity, since many of the patients also have an involved exercise program and possibly other splints to wear frequently during the day. If forearm rotation is the only or most severe problem, the splint can be worn at a lower tension for longer periods, which is more ideal.

Require the patient to apply and remove the splint independently. Also give the patient instruction in how to apply the proper amount of force. The force can vary greatly depending on how far each tab is stretched around the bar, so proper use depends on the patient's knowledge.

INDICATIONS FOR USE

This dynamic splint is appropriate for any patient lacking full passive pronation and/or supination. Possible diagnoses include Colles' fractures, Smith's fractures, proximal radial-head fractures, proximal radial head prostheses, Lowenstein's procedure, Darrach's procedure, radial-lunate fusion, and other partial fusions of the carpus. Normally this splint is applied after sufficient bone healing and removal of pins and after the physician has given approval for passive stretching. The timing varies greatly from patient to patient and thus should be discussed with the physician before application.

REFERENCES

1. Bunnell S: Splint spring to supinate or pronate the hand, J Bone Joint Surg 31A:664, 1949.
2. Bunnell S: Surgery of the hand, ed 3, Philadelphia, 1956, JB Lippincott.
3. Fess E and Philips C: Hand splinting: principles and methods, ed 2, St Louis, 1987, The CV Mosby Co.
4. Green: Operative hand surgery, vol 2, New York, 1982, Churchill Livingstone Inc.

ADDITIONAL READINGS

Frykman G: Fracture of the distal radius including sequelae, Acta Orthop Scand 108:95, 1967.
Hunter JM, Schneider LH, Mackin EJ, and Callahan AD, editors: Rehabilitation of the Hand, ed 2, St Louis, 1984, The CV Mosby Co.
Palmer AK, Werner FW: Biomechanics of the distal radio-ulnar joint, Clin Orthop 187:26, 1984.
Pequignot JP: Distal radio-ulnar involvement in trauma of the wrist, Ann Chir Main 4:273, 1985.

93

Continuous passive motion for the upper extremity

Mary P. Dimick

The development of continuous passive motion (CPM) devices for the upper extremity has added a new dimension to hand therapy. CPM can augment most therapy efforts, which are directed at preventing complications and correcting existing deformities, but it potentially serves a more critical role in recovery—by enhancing healing and ensuring connective tissue homeostasis.

CPM is continual, reciprocal passive joint motion performed by a mechanical device. Most CPM devices consist of a motor, controls that determine the range, rate, and force of movement, and a carriage that moves the anatomic part through a predetermined arc. Ideally, a CPM device can be adjusted to fit the anatomy and move the joint consistently through a controlled and tolerable range of motion (ROM) (Fig. 93-1).

The benefits of CPM are well-documented in the animal model, but clinical data based on CPM results are very limited. Empirical use has met with success and clinical use is increasing. The therapist who chooses to incorporate it should do so cautiously and on an individual basis. The practitioner should be familiar with the theoretical framework on which CPM is based, guidelines for performing passive motion, and specific precautions and expectations for the condition being treated. Clinical use must include careful monitoring of device parameters and objective measurement of patient response. Critical review of results will help to determine the benefits of CPM in the individual case and the efficacy of its overall use in hand therapy.

THEORETICAL FRAMEWORK FOR CPM

The conceptual framework for the use of CPM in hand therapy is based on the effects of motion on connective tissue. It is known that stress deprivation has serious deleterious effects on connective tissue homeostasis, whereas mobilization serves to enhance it.[1-6,11] To understand why this phenomenon occurs, one must have a basic understanding of the properties of dense ordinary periarticular connective tissue, which forms tendons, ligaments, synovial membranes, fascia, and fibrous joint capsules.

Connective tissue is composed of collagen fibers and a ground substance. The mechanical properties of dense connective tissue are determined by the arrangement of the collagen fibers and by bonds of adjacent collagen molecules. Ligaments and tendons, which receive primarily unidirectional stress, are organized mainly in parallel arrays, whereas joint capsules, synovium, sheaths, and aponeuroses, which accommodate stress in many directions, are in a mesh pattern.[2] Collagen is held together by intramolecular and intermolecular bonds known as cross-links. The cross-

links bridge immature collagen with preexisting fibers during collagen synthesis.[2] The extensibility of all connective tissue is determined by the ability of collagen fibers to glide. The ground substance, which consists mainly of water and glycosaminoglycans, serves as a spacer and the lubricant that allows the individual fibrils to glide freely past one another at intercept points.[2] (Fig. 93-2).

Experiments with animals have produced a number of studies on the effects of immobilization and motion on synovial joints.* It was found that immobilization causes profound alterations in joint mechanics leading to restricted mobility. Fibrofatty tissue proliferates within the joint and joint recesses causing intraarticular adhesions, which mature into scar tissue and result in joint stiffness. The lack of movement causes a reduction in ground substance, and it perpetuates random orientation of newly synthesized collagen. This leads to irregular cross-link formation, thereby limiting the extensibility of the tissue[2] (Fig. 93-3).

Early mobilization of these joints was shown to prevent abnormal cross-link formation by assuring the orderly deposition of new collagen fibrils and maintaining the lubrication and critical fiber distance within the cellular matrix.[3,4,22] During healing mobilized tissues showed significant increases over immobilized tissues in cellularity, cell products, strength, and mobility.[7,12,15,16]

The concept of using continuous motion as a possible means to stimulate healing and regeneration of articular tissues and to either prevent or overcome joint stiffness was originated in 1970 by R.B. Salter.[44] He hypothesized that since intermittent motion is better for joints than immobilization, continuous motion should be even better. Passive motion was selected instead of active motion because of the fatigability of skeletal muscle. He studied the effects of CPM on the knee joints of rabbits.[26-28,31,32,34-43] His research found CPM to be significantly more effective than intermittent active motion or immobilization in stimulating the healing and regeneration of articular tissues, as well as preventing joint stiffness. Conclusions drawn from Salter's research are that CPM is well-tolerated, has a healing effect on cartilage, tendons, and ligaments, prevents adhesions and joint stiffness, and does not interfere with the healing of incisions over a moving joint.[44]

THE CLINICAL USE OF CPM

The success of CPM in Salter's animal models has led to experimentation with patients. Currently, the clinical use of CPM is not well-represented in the literature; however,

---

*References 1-6, 12, 14-17, 20-23, 27, 28, 30-43, 47, 48.

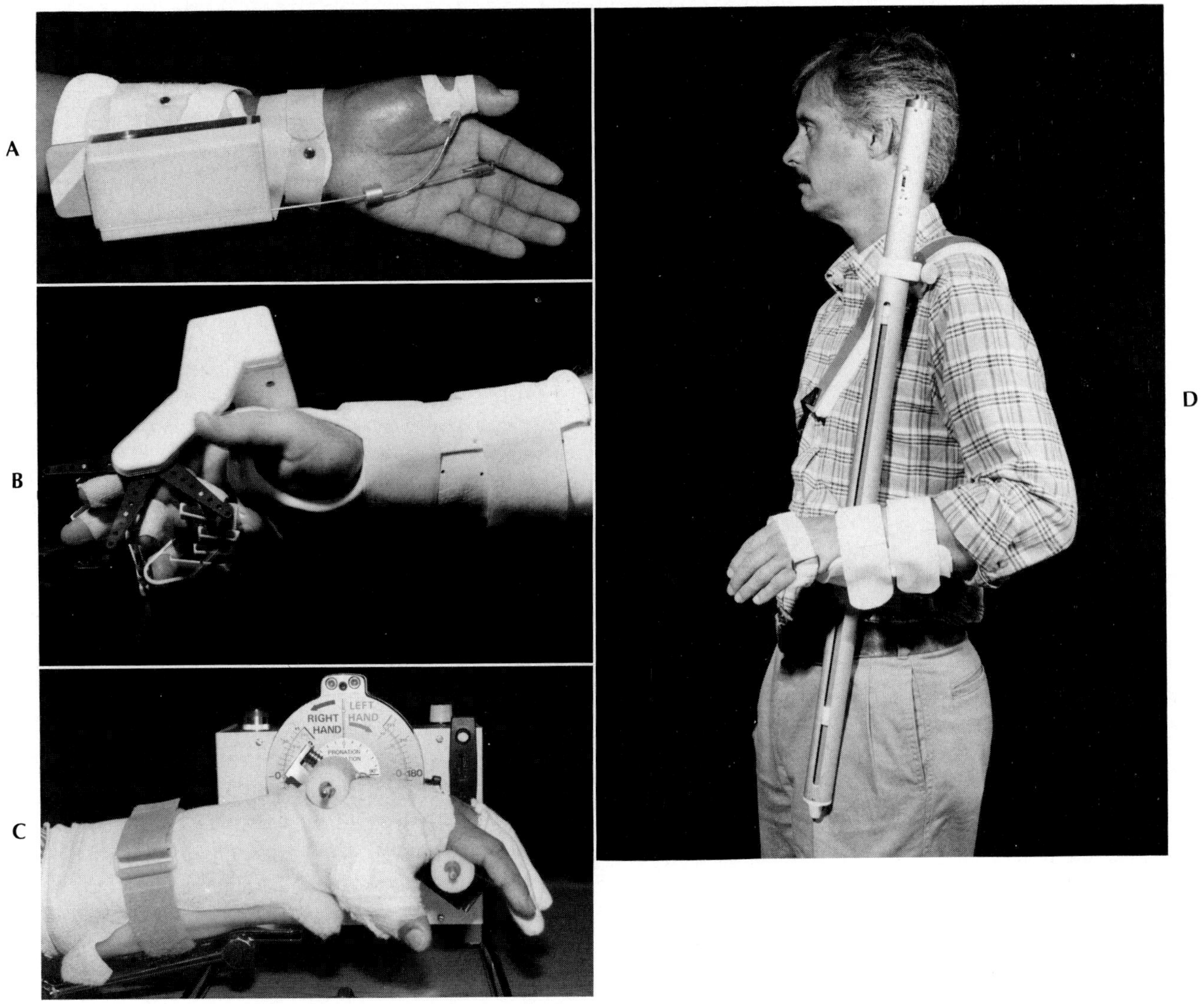

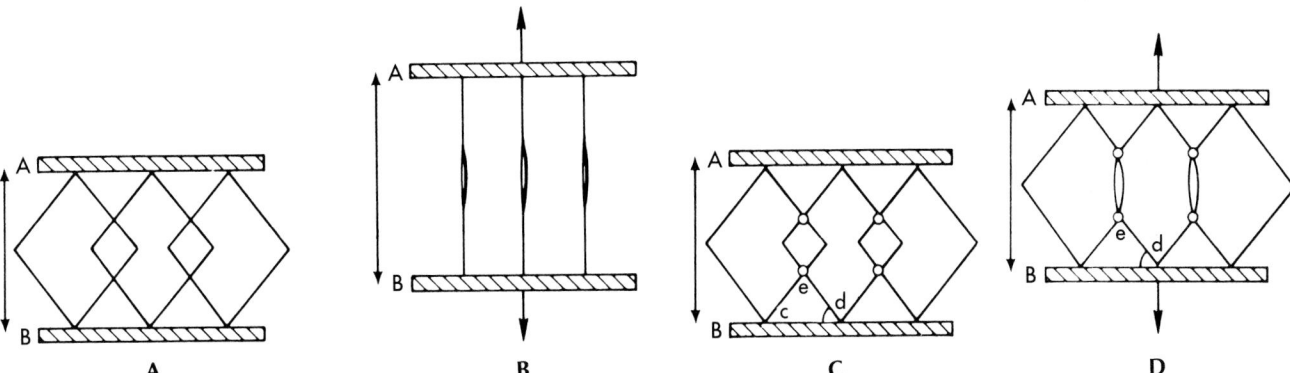

Fig. 93-1   Continuous passive motion (CPM) devices are composed of a motor, limb carriage, and a control unit. Adjustability, reliability, portability, and ease of operation are desirable features in an upper-extremity CPM device. A sample of the various designs available include **A,** the Danniger Mobilimb Hand CPM for the thumb; **B,** the Sutter CPM 5000 for the fingers; **C,** the Kinetec Hand and Wrist CPM Machine for the wrist; and **D,** the Danniger Mobilimb Upper Limb CPM for the elbow.

Fig. 93-2   A diagram showing the idealized weave pattern of collagen fibers. It can be demonstrated that fixed contact at strategic sites (e.g., points d and e) can severely restrict the extensibility of the collagen weave.[1] **A,** Collagen fiber arrangement. **B,** Normal extensibility. **C,** Fixed contact at nodal points. **D,** Restricted extensibility. (Reprinted with permission from Biorheology 17, Akeson WH, Amiel D, and Woo SL-Y: Immobility effects on synovial joints: the pathomechanics of joint contracture, 1980, Pergamon Press, Inc.)

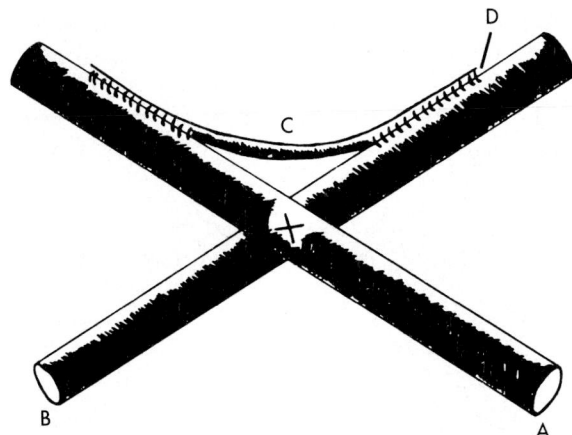

Fig. 93-3 Mechanism of contracture formation at the tissue level. Collagen fibrils, **A** and **B,** come into close contact at point *X* because of loss of spacing-ground substance. New collagen fibrils, **C,** become fixed by cross-linking **D** to inhibit normal gliding. (Reprinted with permission from Biorheology 17, Akeson WH, Amiel D, and Woo SL-Y: Immobility effects on synovial joints: the pathomechanics of joint contracture, 1980, Pergamon Press, Inc.)

many have reported empiric success with its use. R.D. Coutts published the first clinical study on CPM in 1984.[8] He compared the use of CPM following total knee replacement with the standard postoperative treatment protocol. He reported that the use of CPM resulted in a more rapid recovery of range of motion, improved patient comfort, improved wound healing, improved venous dynamics, and a decreased length of hospitalization.

Despite a lack of research that unequivocally supports the use of CPM, its use in the upper extremity is rapidly increasing. Case studies[9,44,45] and research in progress at many centers have suggested using CPM for a wide variety of upper extremity disorders. Currently, it has been used for the postoperative management of synovectomy, open reduction and internal fixation of intraarticular fractures, capsulotomy, tendon repair, tenolysis, implant arthroplasty, Dupuytren's contracture release, drainage of acute septic arthritis, and skin grafts. Nonsurgical upper extremity conditions in which CPM is being used include crush injuries in which there is no bone or tendon involvement, burns, reflex sympathetic dystrophy, and conditions such as stroke that benefit from neuromuscular reeducation.

INDICATIONS FOR CPM USE

Currently specific indications and guidelines have not been established for the clinical application of CPM. Empiric success and the apparent lack of complications[8,44] has led to the assumption by some that CPM is safe[44,45] as long as the parameters of motion are carefully controlled and monitored. Commonly cited reasons for using CPM are to enhance healing and prevent complications, to correct joint contractures, to control pain, to facilitate neuromuscular reeducation, and to augment therapy sessions. It is important that the practitioner understand the rationale behind each of these indications so that CPM can be used to its full potential and the maximum benefit can be attained.

Enhancement of healing and prevention of complications

The early application of CPM after injury or surgery is done to prevent the complications of healing inhibition, joint contracture, and neuromuscular degeneration. Research regarding the effects of immobilization and mobilization on collagen synthesis and connective tissue extensibility support the argument for early, controlled use of CPM. Studies by Gelberman[13-17] and others[48] show that early passive motion actually enhances the mechanism and quality of connective tissue healing.

The optimal timing of CPM initiation and the exact parameters of movement that will not disrupt healing are not known. However, the wound-healing process suggests that the earlier motion is begun, the better it is, as long as it is not excessive.[7] Research has demonstrated that stress applied to healing wounds influences tissue flexibility. New collagen appears in healing wounds as early as 2 days after injury and is deposited in and about the wound at a rate higher than normal connective tissue.[8,10] This process occurs in a random fashion, which limits gliding unless influenced by passive motion.[10] Newly synthesized collagen fibrils are very weak in the early stage.[10] Therefore the early application of CPM must be carefully controlled and monitored, so that it will serve to enhance healing, not disrupt it, thereby causing complications. When CPM is used in conditions of intraarticular fracture, tendon repair, synovectomy, and capsulotomy, the primary purposes are to enhance healing and to prevent complications.

Correction of joint contracture

CPM has potential application in the correction of joint restrictions. Methods such as splinting, active range of motion (AROM) and mobilization may be more appropriate than CPM in the treatment of contracture, but there are some situations in which CPM may be beneficial. These include joint contractures of short duration; joint restrictions in more than one direction that would require alternation of flexion and extension dynamic splints; and patients who either because of pain, an inability to relax, or noncompliance, respond better to the rhythm of CPM than to regular passive motion.

Success will depend on the duration and severity of the joint contracture. Arem and Madden have shown that scar elongation is not possible after 14 weeks of scar maturation; but at 3 weeks scar can be significantly lengthened when subjected to tension.[7] "Stretching" or an increase in length of the scar is a result of straightening or reorientation of collagen fibers without a change in their dimensions. This can occur only with a restored gliding mechanism.[10,19] Peacock hypothesized that the "mechanism" by which scar length is increased becomes critical for restoration of the gliding mechanism.[24,25] This offers support for the administration of carefully controlled motion such as CPM.

Pain control

CPM can be used to control pain. A review of the literature on CPM reveals almost unanimous reports of relief or reduction of pain with CPM use. This may result from both psychologic and physiologic influences. The rhythmic joint movement in CPM is similar to a relaxation technique that has been shown to retard the pain-spasm reflex.[46] Another explanation for the pain relief phenomenon in CPM is the "gate control theory" of pain as proposed by Melzack.[18] It is possible that the continuous generation of proprioceptive impulses from the moving joint and their transmission to the spinal cord or brain may "block" the transmission of pain impulses to the brain.[8,44] This pain relief benefit of CPM may be particularly helpful in conditions such as Dupuytren's contracture, tenolysis, and reflex sympathetic dystrophy, in which active motion is a vital component of early rehabilitation. The patient may be more willing to fully participate with active motion if he is pain-free and convinced that motion will not be painful.

Neuromuscular reeducation

The use of CPM to facilitate neuromuscular reeducation in conditions of stroke and neuroparesis is a fairly new concept. It is known that passive motion increases tension in muscles and provides proprioceptive and sensory feedback to the central nervous system.[12] CPM can be used to maintain this feedback during recovery and the period of restricted active motion, perhaps negating the need for retraining.

Augmentation of therapy

The use of CPM devices as treatment modalities during therapy sessions can help the clinician achieve therapy goals. This is indicated when optimal therapy time is limited by the therapist/patient ratio; the nature, extent, and criticality of other injuries; infrequent or short therapy sessions; or poor compliance by the patient with independent exercise. The use of these devices for passive range of motion (PROM) can allow individual therapy time to be more productive because the therapist can focus on the critical areas which need expert intervention.

LIMITATIONS OF CPM

A review of CPM would not be complete without mention of its shortcomings. The practitioner must take these into account when planning the CPM treatment regimen. The limitations of CPM relate to the lack of specific guidelines for use, the inability of a single modality to do all things, and the problems with being "device dependent." CPM will be optimally used only if these limitations are considered and direct measures are undertaken to compensate for them.

The lack of specificity regarding when and how to institute CPM should challenge the therapist to carefully monitor the the dose-response curve of CPM treatment. Parameters such as time of application, duration, force, speed, and range should be documented and compared to the effects on the joint being moved. It will be only through repeated CPM use and review of results that the type and dose of CPM for a particular joint can be applied with confidence and consistency.

Another deficiency of CPM is that is cannot take the place of active motion. Active motion is often preferred over passive motion in rehabilitation. However, there are some instances, such as when stressing newly healing tissues, that movement must be carefully controlled and repetitive. The lack of external controls over active movement and the fatigability of skeletal muscle during active movement make passive motion the better choice in these cases.

There are often problems with the fit of CPM devices. The current upper extremity CPM devices are designed to be used bilaterally, to move more than one joint, and for extremities of all shapes and sizes. The CPM device must be carefully adjusted, and often straps and splints must be added to ensure that the joints are moved properly. Frequently, the device can not achieve the extremes of joint motion. If the goal is to achieve normal range of motion, other measures such as active range of motion, joint mobilization, or splints must also be used.

Another problem with the use of CPM is a tendency for patients to become overly reliant on the CPM device at the exclusion of all other modalities. This is often reinforced by the enthusiasm of the physician, nurses, and others over the novelty of the device. It should be standard procedure that CPM is introduced only after the patient is completely educated about the importance of his active participation in his entire rehabilitation program.

The last area of concern is related to the cost of CPM. Currently, most units are obtained on a rental basis. At first glance, the cost of this rental and the amount of therapy time needed to initiate CPM treatment may look excessive. However, if this is weighed against other factors, such as the number of subsequent therapy sessions required, the frequency of complications, and the final results, the use of CPM may be found to be cost-effective. It is important that the therapist gather both quantitative and qualitative data to determine the cost benefits of CPM.

SELECTION OF CPM DEVICES

The selection of a CPM device should be based on the critical needs of the individual case. Factors to be considered in the selection process include the joint or joints to be moved, as well as those that must be stabilized; the criticality of the injury or surgery; postoperative or postinjury precautions, especially those related to the allowable arc of motion; the goals of treatment; the length of time CPM will be used; the duration of each CPM session; the skill of the therapist in splint design and fabrication; and the availability and cost of the device. A general rule is that the greater the criticality of the postinjury precautions, the greater the need is for a sophisticated device and a skilled therapist.

Several CPM devices are available for use in the upper extremity. The cost of the device often depends on the sophistication of its features. Adjustability, reliability, portability, and easily-operated controls are desirable features in an upper extremity CPM device.

Adjustability

The ability to isolate the joints to be moved and stabilize surrounding joints is critical. It is also important that the device can be applied to correlate with proper anatomic motion, i.e., the rotational movement must follow the anatomic axis of the joint (Fig. 93-4). It is necessary that parameters, especially those related to the arc of motion, can be changed to progress the patient.

Reliability

The CPM devices are subjected to stresses, which eventually work to fatigue the components and affect the reliability of the device. These stresses include the "continuous"

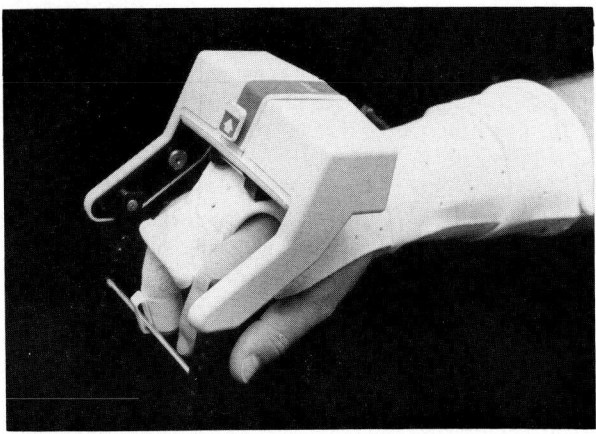

Fig. 93-4 An intraarticular fracture is stabilized within a custom splint. The Sutter CPM 5000 is positioned to correlate with the axis of rotation of the proximal interphalangeal joint, thus providing proper anatomic motion.

nature of motion, the weight of the anatomic part, and changes in direction of movement. The mechanical components, as well as the operating controls, must be dependable and easily checked to prevent machine breakdown while in use.

Portability

The portability of the CPM device will influence patient satisfaction and compliance. The weight of the device is a significant factor in determining portability. The patients with upper extremity injuries have only one arm free to safely lift and move the device. The devices that fit directly on the limb must be very light. External supports are often necessary to properly position the extremity and prevent fatigue of proximal muscles; e.g., foam cushions are used to support the extremity when patients are sitting.

Patient controls

CPM is a passive modality. Any active participation by the patient in this aspect of his rehabilitation should help to ensure compliance. Controls should be clear, easily operated by one hand, and foolproof. It is critical that an emergency "stop" switch be easily accessible in case of machine malfunction. A locking switch on the parameters is beneficial to prevent interference either inadvertently or by an unreliable patient.

APPLICATION OF CPM
CPM planning

Not enough emphasis can be placed on the advisability of CPM planning. This is particularly helpful if the CPM is to be used after surgery. It is often the actual logistics of obtaining the device, setting it up, dealing with the postoperative dressing and splints, and instructing the patient, that preclude the early use of CPM. This is unfortunate because, if goal of use is to enhance healing and prevent complications, every attempt should be made to initiate CPM as early as possible. Planning with the physician, CPM supplier, and patient and preoperative evaluation, splint fabrication, and patient education will do much to enlist patient

cooperation with the CPM protocol and ensure the optimal results of CPM treatment.

Referral

The lack of established protocols for CPM makes it necessary to plan and discuss the CPM regimen directly with the physician. It is important to know the purpose for which CPM is being ordered and the goals and expectations of the physician. The therapist should be familiar with the injury, planned surgical procedures related to the area to be moved, and injuries and surgical procedures to adjacent areas. It is also helpful to know the planned location for incisions and fixation devices such as Kirshner (K) wires and the type and size of the postoperative dressing. It is at this time that potential conflicts, which could preclude the use of CPM, can be resolved. The physician may be willing to try other available options for incision sites or wound dressings if he knows that the ones planned may interfere with the application of CPM. This is the time to outline the general parameters of CPM, but they must be "fine tuned" at the time of surgery.

Obtaining the CPM device

Procuring a CPM device can be time consuming and therefore should be attempted well in advance. Many distributors of CPM devices will screen the patient's insurance policy, set up the rental agreement, make the CPM delivery, and ensure that the device is in good working order.

Preoperative evaluation

The purposes of the preoperative evaluation are to assess the patient's potential for compliance with the protocol and to determine realistic goals for treatment. Critical areas to be assessed include the patient's motivation, his ability to follow instructions, and his living situation. The preoperative evaluation should include objective measurements of joint range of motion, edema, strength, pain, and function. These measurements are imperative because of the lack of clinical studies on the efficacy of CPM. It may be necessary to use these for justification of treatment, and they are critical in both prospective and retrospective studies.

Splint fabrication

Most of the hand CPM devices require a splint component to stabilize the wrist and mount the device. Although prefabricated splints are available with some devices, it is often better to fabricate a custom splint for the patient. This is especially true when the restrictions on the arc of joint motion are critical and the surrounding joints require stability.

Anyone who has ever made a splint in the operating room or at bedside can appreciate the advocacy of prefabricating the splint on the patient. A mock dressing is applied to the patient, the splint is loosely fabricated, and all component parts are prepared. Major adjustments to the device, such as setting it for the right or left extremity, are also done at this time. This preplanning leaves only the final adjustments and assembly to be done at the time of CPM initiation.

Patient education

Patient education is the most important aspect of CPM planning. It is critical in enlisting the patient's cooperation and in influencing a favorable experience with CPM. This education should be done before surgery because after surgery there are innumerable factors (medication, pain, bleeding, drowsiness, anxiety) that conflict with the patient's ability to attend to the education. It is very helpful to have written instructions that include the CPM protocol, device operations and care, a home program, and a backup plan in case of machine breakdown. The device operation, home program, and backup plan should be practiced by the patient until he demonstrates the ability to perform each accurately.

INITIAL CPM SESSION

The above-mentioned preparations must be completed at the time of the initial CPM session if they were not done previously. The remainder of the session usually consists of a brief evaluation of joint range of motion, edema, and pain; application of the CPM device; setting CPM parameters; and review of the home program. Proposed guidelines for applying and adjusting the CPM follow.

1. If necessary and allowable, adjust postoperative dressings to conform with the splint or CPM device.
2. Make necessary splint adjustments and apply splint as indicated.
3. Position the patient and extremity properly for optimum CPM use.
4. Make all necessary adjustments in the CPM device to ensure proper fit. Position the extremity, then fit the CPM device to the extremity.
5. Remove the CPM device.
6. Determine the parameters for the arc of motion by moving the joint within the patient's pain tolerance through the *allowable* arc of motion as prescribed by the physician. Measure this arc.
7. Set device parameters for an arc of motion slightly less than measurement in #6.
8. Set the speed of the device at the slowest point.
9. Set the force at a mild to moderate setting.
10. Run the device to ensure that the parameters are properly set.
11. Position the device at a point in the arc that corresponds to the resting position of the joint.
12. Apply the CPM device to the extremity.
13. Turn on the device and proceed at these settings for 10 minutes.
14. After the 10 minutes are over, the rest of the treatment session is spent gradually increasing the parameters until the patient is at his maximum comfortable or allowable limits.

The dosage of CPM, that is, the length of each session should be determined by the physician. Typically, CPM sessions range from 8 to 24 hours a day with patients being allowed out of the device for eating, hygiene, and in some cases, for sleeping.

FOLLOW-UP THERAPY SESSIONS

The frequency and content of follow-up therapy sessions depend on a number of factors. The initial follow-up session should be scheduled soon after the initiation of CPM to check the extremity and adjust the program. The frequency of subsequent appointments will depend on the patient's progress and compliance with the CPM program, the nature of his injury, and the need for other aspects of therapy.

Often, especially when CPM is applied soon after injury, the frequency of therapy sessions is less during the acute phase than later when active motion, strengthening, and functional activities are instituted. Objective measurements of joint range of motion and edema and subjective measurements of pain and patient tolerance must be taken at each therapy session because they provide the guidelines for CPM use. Progress must be monitored to determine the optimal dose and duration of CPM and the need to augment CPM with other treatment modalities. If CPM is not maintaining the passive range of motion, the dose may need to be increased or other measures such as splints or joint mobilization may have to be instituted. The patient should be taught how to progress himself by changing device parameters as soon as it is considered safe to do so. The tendency for the patient to become dependent on the device can be discouraged by instituting early performance of functional activities and active motion.

DISCONTINUANCE OF CPM TREATMENT

The duration of CPM treatment usually depends on the purpose for which it was instituted and the progress that has been made.[44] The literature suggests that it should last at least 1 week.[44] Durations beyond 6 weeks are unusual. The decision about when to discontinue CPM should be made on a case-by-case basis. Factors to be considered in this decision include completion of a preexisting treatment protocol, removal of restrictions on motion, a plateau in progress, active motion that is as effective as passive motion in maintaining or increasing joint range of motion, or the situation in which CPM is the only thing maintaining joint motion despite attempts at augmenting it with other modalities. In this latter case the long-term goals of treatment should be reassessed because indefinite use of CPM to maintain joint motion is neither advisable nor cost-effective.

The discontinuance of CPM represents a significant decrease in daily exercise. Unless this is replaced by an increase in active and passive motion, functional activities, or splinting, there is apt to be a loss in joint motion and perhaps an increase in edema. The patient should be gradually weaned from CPM whenever possible. This process takes about 1 week. The extremity should be monitored frequently during this period to determine the optimal balance of exercise, splinting, and activity to continue progress toward improved function.

SUMMARY

CPM is being used with increased frequency in upper extremity rehabilitation despite the lack of clinical research and established protocols for its use. The practitioner who chooses to incorporate it into the therapy regimen must rely on guidelines recommended for performing passive joint motion and the available knowledge on the effects of motion on wound healing and connective tissue homeostasis. The appropriate selection of a CPM device can be achieved only if the patient's needs are thoroughly assessed and specific goals are established for CPM treatment. The CPM protocol should be tailored for each case by frequent monitoring of results. Comparison of these results with those of "matched controls" will be necessary to determine the benefits of CPM in an individual case and the overall efficacy of CPM in upper extremity rehabilitation.

REFERENCES

1. Akeson WH, Amiel D, and La Violette D: The connective tissue response to immobility: an accelerated aging response? Exp Gerontol 3:289, 1986.
2. Akeson WH, Amiel D, and Woo SL-Y: Immobility effects on synovial joints. The pathomechanics of joint contracture, Biorheology 17:95, 1980.
3. Akeson, WH and others: The connective tissue response to immobility: biochemical changes in periarticular connective tissue of the immobilized rabbit knee, Clin Orthop 93:356, 1973.
4. Akeson, WH and others: Collagen crosslinking alterations in joint contractures: changes in reducible crosslinks in periarticular connective tissue collagen after nine weeks of immobilization, Connect Tissue Res 5:5, 1977.
5. Amiel, D and others: The effect of immobilization on collagen turnover in connective tissue: a biochemical-biomechanical correlation, Acta Orthop Scand 53:425, 1982.
6. Amiel, D and others: Stress deprivation effect on metabolic turnover of the medial collateral ligament collagen—a comparison between nine and 12 week immobilization, Clin Orthop 172:265, 1983.
7. Arem AJ and Madden JW: Effects of stress on healing wounds. I. Intermittent noncyclical tension, J Surg Res 29:93, 1976.
8. Coutts RD, Toth C, and Kaita J: The role of continuous passive motion in the rehabilitation of the total knee patient. In Hungerford D, editor: Total knee arthroplasty—a comprehensive approach, Baltimore, 1984, Williams & Wilkins.
9. Dimick MP: The use of continuous passive motion in the upper extremity: a preliminary report. Proceedings of the eighth annual meeting of the American Society of Hand Therapists, J Hand Surg 10A(4):584, 1985 (abstract).
10. Donatelli R: Physical therapy of the shoulder, New York, 1987, Churchill Livingstone, Inc.
11. Donatelli R and Owens-Burkhart H: Effects of immobilization on the extensibility of periarticular connective tissue, J Ortho Sports Phys Ther 3(2):67, 1981.
12. Frank, C and others: Physiology and therapeutic value of passive joint motion, Clin Orthop 185:113, 1984.
13. Gelberman RH and Manske PR: Effects of early motion on the tendon healing process: experimental studies in Hunter, J and others, editors: Tendon surgery in the hand, St Louis, 1987, The CV Mosby Co.
14. Gelberman, RH and others: The effects of mobilization on the vascularization of healing flexor tendons in dogs, Clin Orthop 153:283, 1980.
15. Gelberman, RH and others: The influence of protected passive mobilization on the healing of flexor tendons: a biochemical and microangiographic study, Hand 13:120, 1981.
16. Gelberman, RH and others: Effects of early intermittent passive mobilization on healing canine flexor tendons, J Hand Surg 7:170, 1982.
17. Gelberman, RH and others: Flexor tendon healing and restoration of the gliding surface, J Bone Joint Surg 65A:70, 1983.
18. Harris FA: Facilitation techniques. In Basmajian JV, editor: therapeutic exercise, Baltimore, 1978, Williams & Wilkins.
19. Madden JW: Wound healing: the biological basis of hand surgery, Clin Plast Surg 3(1):3, 1976.
20. O'Driscoll SW, Kumar A, and Salter RB: The effect of continuous passive motion on the clearance of a hemarthrosis from a synovial joint, Clin Orthop Rel Res 176:305, 1983.
21. O'Driscoll SW, Kumar A, and Salter RB: The effect of volume of effusion, joint position and continuous passive motion on intraarticular pressure in the rabbit knee, J Rheumatol 10:3, 1983.
22. O'Driscoll SW and Salter RB: The induction of neochrondrogenesis in free periosteal autografts under the influence of continuous passive motion, Proc Orthop Res Soc 8:167, 1983 (abstract).
23. O'Driscoll SW and Salter RB: The influence of neochrondrogenesis in free periosteal autografts under the influence of continuous passive motion. Orthop Trans, 1983. J Bone Joint Surg 7(2):310, 1983.
24. Peacock EE: Collagen metabolism during healing of long tendons. In Hunter, JM and others: tendon surgery in the hand, St Louis, 1987, The CV Mosby Co.
25. Peacock EE, Madden JW, and Trier WC: Postoperative recovery of flexor tendon function, Am J Surg 44A:49, 1962.
26. Salter RB: The healing of bone and cartilage in intraarticular fractures with continuous passive motion. Transactions of the twenty-fourth annual meeting of the Orthopaedic Research Society, vol 3, Feb. 1978 (abstract). Also Orthop Trans, J Bone Joint Surg 2(1):77, 1978.
27. Salter RB: The effect of motion on regeneration of cartilage. Proceedings of International Workshop on Rehabilitation of Articular Joints by Biological Resurfacing, Nov. 15-17, 1979, Dallas, Texas.
28. Salter RB: The prevention of arthritis through the preservation of cartilage. Royal College Lecture, J Can Assoc Radiol 32:5, 1981.
29. Salter RB: Motion vs. rest: why immobilize joints? Presidential address, Canadian Orthopaedic Association, Halifax, June 1981. J Bone Joint Surg 64B(2):251, 1982.
30. Salter RB: Regeneration of articular cartilage through continuous passive motion past, present and future. In Straub R and Wilson PD, editors: Clinical trends in orthopaedics, New York, 1982, Thieme-Stratton Inc.
31. Salter RB and Bell RS: The effect of continuous passive motion in the healing of partial thickness lacerations of the patellar tendon of the rabbit. Ann Royal Coll Phys Surg Can 14(3):209, 1981 (abstract).
32. Salter RB, Bell RS, and Keeley F: The protective effect of continuous passive motion on living articular cartilage in acute septic arthritis: an experimental investigation in the rabbit, Clin Orthop Rel Res 159:223, 1981.
33. Salter RB and Field P: The effects of continuous compression on living articular cartilage, J Bone Joint Surg 42A:31, 1960.
34. Salter RB, Harris DJ, and Bogoch E: Further studies in continuous passive motion. Orthop Trans 212, 1978 (abstract).
35. Salter RB and Harris DJ: The healing of intraarticular fractures with continuous passive motion. American Academy of Orthopaedic Surgeons, Instructional course lectures 28:102, St Louis, 1979, The CV Mosby Co.
36. Salter RB and Minster RR: The effects of continuous passive motion on a semitendinosus tenodesis in the rabbit knee, Proc Orthop Res Soc 7:225, 1982 (abstract).
37. Salter RB and Minster RR: The effects of continuous passive motion on a semi-tendinosus tenodesis in the rabbit knee, Orthop Trans (Orthop Res Soc), 6(2):292, 1983.
38. Salter RB and O'Driscoll SW: The effects of continuous passive motion on repair of full thickness defects in a joint surface with autogenous osteoperiosteal grafts, Ann Royal Coll Phys Surg Can 16(4):360, 1983 (abstract).
39. Salter RB, Wong DA, and Keeley FW: Collagen typing of early repair tissue in healing articular cartilage: an experimental study in the rabbit, Orthop Trans 4(3):397, 1980.
40. Salter, RB and others: The biological effect of continuous passive motion in the healing of full thickness defects in articular cartilage, J Bone Joint Surg 62A:1232, 1980.
41. Salter, RB and others: The effect of continuous passive motion on the healing of full thickness defects in articular cartilage: an experimental investigation in the rabbit, J Bone Joint Surg 62A(8):1232, 1980.
42. Salter, RB and others: Continuous passive motion and the repair of full thickness defects—a one-year follow-up, Orthop Trans (Orthop Res Soc) 6(2):266, 1982.
43. Salter, RB and others: The healing of articular tissues through continuous passive motion: essence of the first ten years of personal experimental investigations, Orthop Trans 6(3):470, 1982. Also J Bone Joint Surg 64-B(5):640, 1982.
44. Salter, RB and others: Clinical application of basic research on continuous passive motion for disorders and injuries of synovial joints: a preliminary report of a feasibility study, Orthop Res 1(3):325, 1984.
45. Skirven T, Osterman A, and Lee FW: The use of continuous passive motion in hand rehabilitation. Presentation at fortieth annual meeting of ASSH at San Antonio, Texas, Sept. 1987.
46. Sullivan PE, Markos PD, and Minor MA: An integrated approach to therapeutic exercise: theory and clinical application, Reston, 1982, Reston Publishing Company, Inc.
47. Woo, S and others: Connective tissue response to immobility: correlative study of biomechanical and biochemical measurements of normal and immobilized rabbit knees, Arthritis Rheum 18:257, 1975.
48. Woo, SL-Y and others: The importance of controlled passive mobilization on flexor tendon healing. A biomechanical study, Acta Orthop Scand 52:615, 1981.

94

Splinting the hand of a child

Patricia M. Byron

Management of the child who has sustained an injury or undergone surgery to the upper extremity poses a unique challenge to the surgeon-therapist-patient team. Most upper extremity surgery and reconstruction require a high degree of cooperation and participation on the part of the patient to achieve optimal results. The child is unable to participate on this level. Parents are asked to participate for and with the child. Together the treatment team is challenged to new limits of creativity to accomplish the desired result with the child. Splinting is often a large part of the management of a child's hand problem because of the difficulty in cooperation.

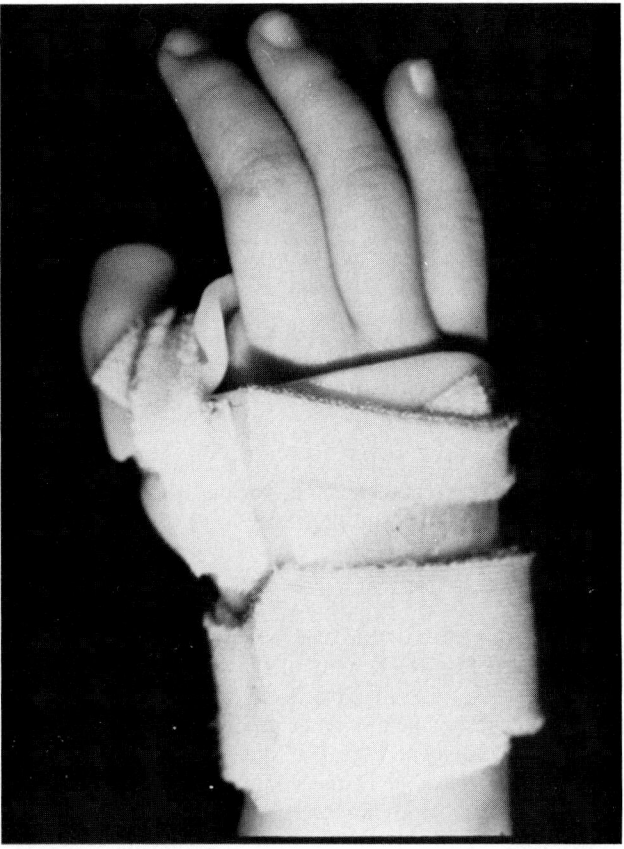

Fig. 94-1 The hand of this 3-year-old girl is shown postcentralization and opponensplasty. Her original diagnosis was radial club hand with absence of the thumb. She is using a static positioning splint for her wrist during the day, with the addition of a thumb web stretcher at night to maintain thumb abduction.

The upper extremity child population is composed of three groups: infants with congenital or birth injuries that require splinting to prevent development of deformity or correct existing deformities,[1,2] children with congenital defects who have undergone corrective surgery, and those who require treatment secondary to trauma.[6,10]

Splinting may be designed to prevent development of deformity, correct an existing problem, position for function, or protect an injured or repaired structure. Within these groups either static (Fig. 94-1), serial static (Figs. 94-2 and 94-3), or dynamic splinting (Fig. 94-4) options may be used.

The specific problems associated with splinting a child vary considerably with the age and developmental level of the individual. The infant cannot actively cooperate. The young child who is aware of his environment and has begun interacting with it but cannot yet be reasoned with poses the greatest challenge.

PARENTAL INVOLVEMENT

The ability or inability of the child to cooperate with splint fabrication is the key and is related to the age and specific abilities of the child and to the parent's ability to work with the child. Communication with parents or caregivers is important before, during, and after splint application. The parent often communicates so much anxiety to the child nonverbally that the child can do nothing but become fearful or anxious himself. Parents often have more difficulty dealing with an injury or disability than the child because of underlying guilt or other unknown factors. It is helpful to begin by establishing a working relationship with the parent.

Reassure the parents as much as possible. Show them a sample of the type of splint their child will be receiving. Inform them about the fabrication process. They may feel that they have to remember every bit of information from the session; let them know ahead of time that written instructions will be provided.

SPLINTING MATERIALS

In the past, it was necessary to thin splint materials by rolling them to obtain a thickness that could be molded accurately to the contour of tiny arms. Recently, several manufacturers have introduced a $\frac{1}{16}$ inch thickness of their materials that is more appropriate for use in children. These materials are also available in perforated form. When nonperforated material is used it is sometimes necessary to introduce a limited number of strategically placed perforations into the splints following fabrication to prevent maceration and increase comfort.

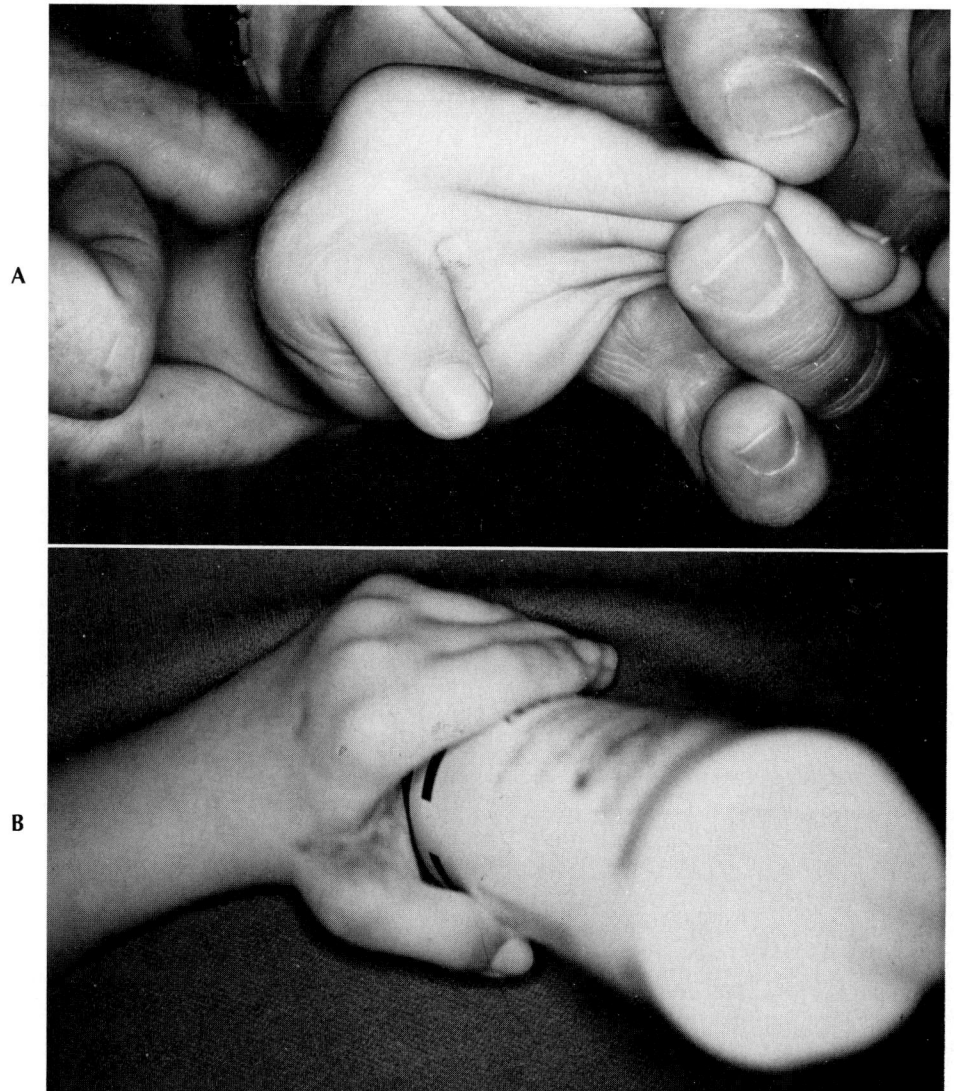

Fig. 94-2 **A,** In preparation for surgery, this 3-year-old boy with arthrogryposis wore a thumb web stretcher with deviation components to correct the severe ulnar drift of his digits. **B,** After web space deepening and grafting, this child's functional ability is significantly improved.

For long arm splints standard thickness material is usually acceptable (Fig. 94-5). Good conformation is still important, and a material with this quality must be chosen.

Plaster of paris is often used for splints and casts for children. The disadvantages of this material are its weight, difficulty in cleaning, and the inability to make changes in the design or contour without redoing the splint.

In some cases, unorthodox materials serve the child's need better than any of the splinting materials in general use.[4] The therapist must be alert to the advent of new materials and be creative in their use.

SPLINT DESIGN

Fortunately, stiffness is an infrequent complication of immobilization and splinting in children.[8] Maintaining splint position is a frequent problem. To increase splint stability and maintain a desired position, splints for children may need to include joints that would not be included for the adult. For example, following flexor tendon repair in a child, in addition to flexing the metacarpophalangeal (MP) and wrist joints to protect the healing tendons, the elbow is also included in the splint and flexed to 90 degrees to improve splint stability.[3,7,9]

GETTING STARTED

If the splint to be fabricated is a functional splint, the therapist should observe the child using his hands (Figs. 94-6 and 94-7). The therapist must be aware of developmental prehension patterns and tasks that are appropriate for each developmental level.[5,11] Age-appropriate toys and games should be kept in the clinic or be brought to the treatment session from home.

The child who is aware of what is going on should be involved in the splint fabrication process. Application of a splint to a favorite toy or to a parent can help allay the child's fear. Later when splint wear is intermittent the splint can be applied to the toy when the child is required to wear his splint.

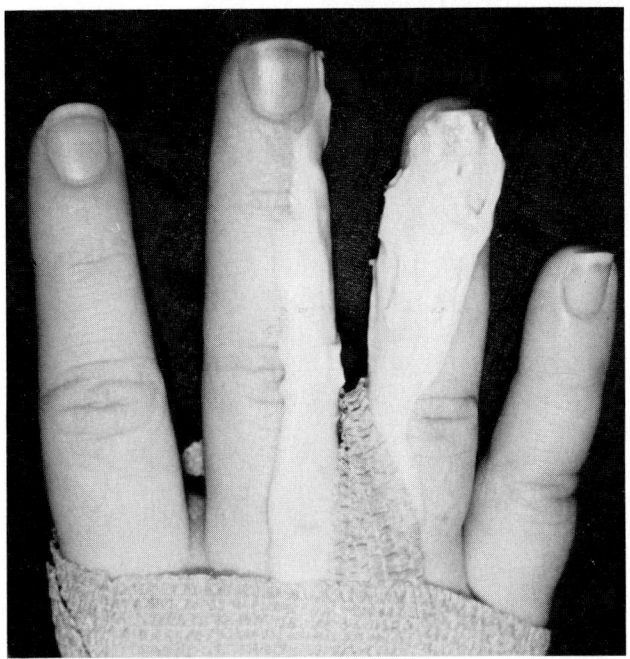

Fig. 94-3 After dyctalization Elastomer inserts secured with Coban were used to maintain the digital web space. Inserts were not used until the skin was healed well. Before this point, bulky dressing was used to maintain the space.

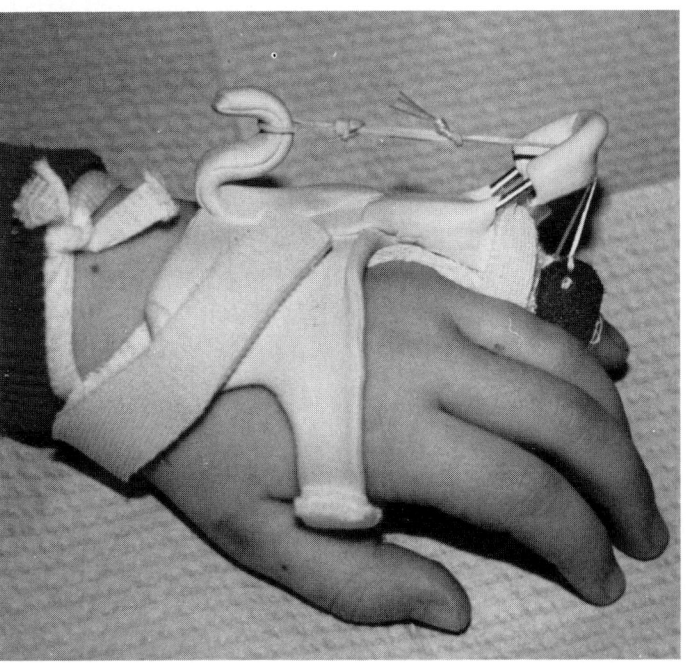

Fig. 94-4 This hand-based dynamic extension splint was fabricated for a 7-year-old child after proximal interphalangeal joint reconstruction. The splint was worn on a full-time basis. The child cooperated fully with the splinting program.

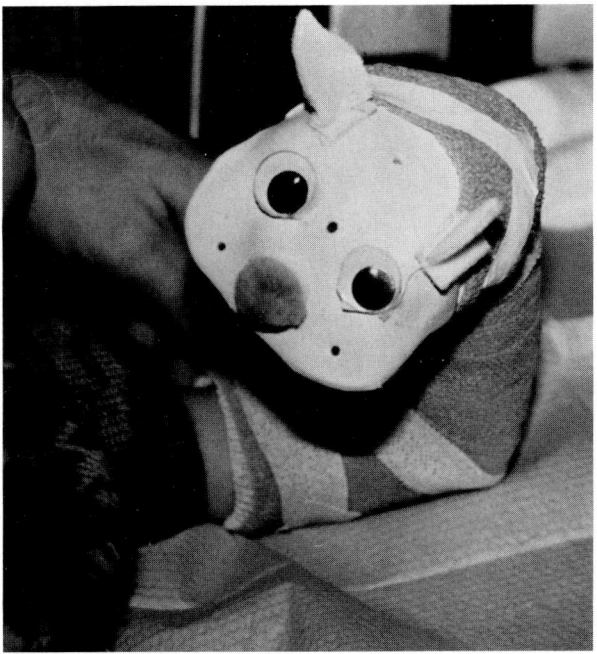

Fig. 94-5 A 3-year-old child was placed in a long arm thermoplastic splint after flexor tenolysis and insertion of a Hunter passive rod. The patient was maintained in the splint full time between therapy sessions. The home exercise program was performed with the splint in place. The splint was secured with a Coban wrap. The addition of the "puppy" face decreased resistance to splint wear considerably.

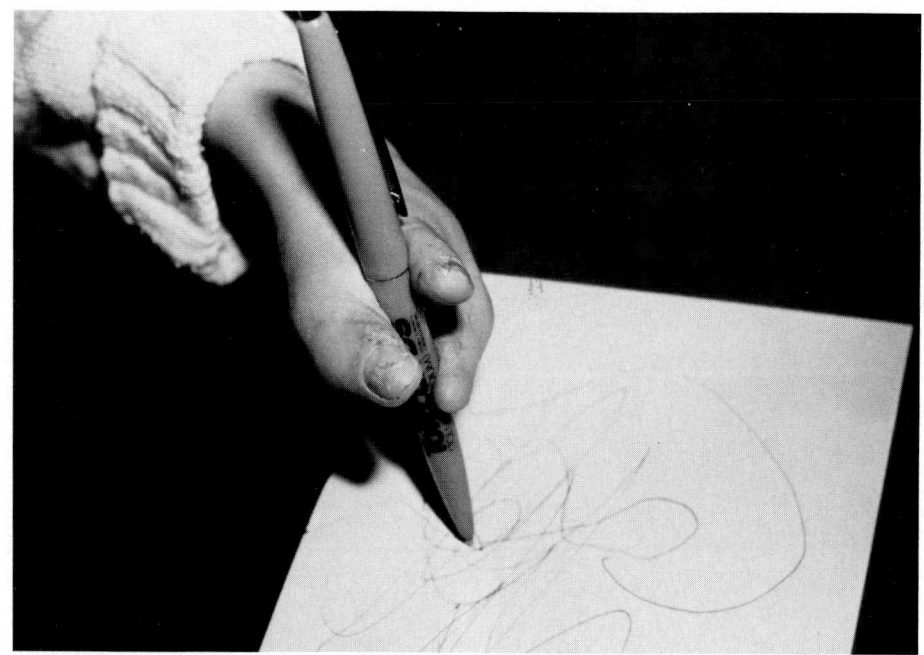

Fig. 94-6   Despite significant absence of digits, this 4-year-old child displayed good fine coordination.

When thermoplastic splint materials are used, it is helpful to seat the child away from the splint pan—just seeing the steam coming from the pan can cause the child to be afraid of being burned especially if the child has ever been burned.

SPLINT FABRICATION

Trace the child's hand on a paper towel to make a pattern. After the child's surgery or when a specific hand position must be maintained, the uninvolved extremity is used. This activity is familiar to many young children through nursery school or kindergarten. Keep a variety of colored markers available so that a second tracing can become a turkey or a special gift for mom.

The splint pattern is traced and cut out as for any splint. Scraps of material may be given to the child or parent to play with while the splint is being prepared.

The child's arm should be protected by a layer of stockinette because the young child's skin is more sensitive to heat than that of an older child or adult. When the skin is very fair a second layer of stockinette may be necessary. One inch tubular cotton stockinette or wide finger stockinette works well.

Bony prominences are padded well. This is especially important because prominences may be used to maintain splint position. This can be done without causing discomfort or pressure areas by maintaining even distribution of pressure over the entire area. After the splint has been formed, any padding that was used is transferred into the splint.

SECURING THE SPLINT

When the purpose of the splint is immobilization, the splint can be secured in therapy and left in place until the next visit. Coban with additional elastic or adhesive tape strips at palm, wrist, and elbow levels maintain good splint position (see Fig. 94-5). Care must be taken in application

of Coban to lay the wrap on lightly from distal to proximal in a graded figure-eight fashion. The wrap must not be applied circumferentially and must not be pulled tightly. This type of application secures the splint well and prevents pooling of edema between straps that have been applied too tightly.[2]

When the splint is to be removed at home for dressing changes or exercise, complications can increase (Fig. 94-8). Velcro straps work very well, but there is the danger that the splint will be removed by the child when he is unsupervised. Stockinette applied over the entire splint and then taped lightly at the proximal ends helps to keep the splint in place in many cases.

When the splint can be removed for exercise or hygiene and there is no danger of injuring the involved area, straps may be color-coded to allow the young child to participate in donning and doffing the splint. (This helps parents feel more comfortable as well.) The hook and loop areas of the Velcro that belong together are given the same color. Shapes or letters may be used in place of color depending on the age of the child.

HOME PROGRAM

Parents should feel comfortable caring for their child and the new splint by the end of the treatment session. They must be provided with written instructions regarding care of the splint, wearing schedule, what problems may occur and how to handle them. Potential problems include change in color of the involved extremity, increase in swelling, and increase in pain or temperature. Every problem should be checked as soon as possible especially because of the increased incidence of Volkmann ischemia in children.[8]

If the splint is to be removed at home, the parent must practice application and removal of the splint several times before leaving the clinic. The splint must be worn for 15

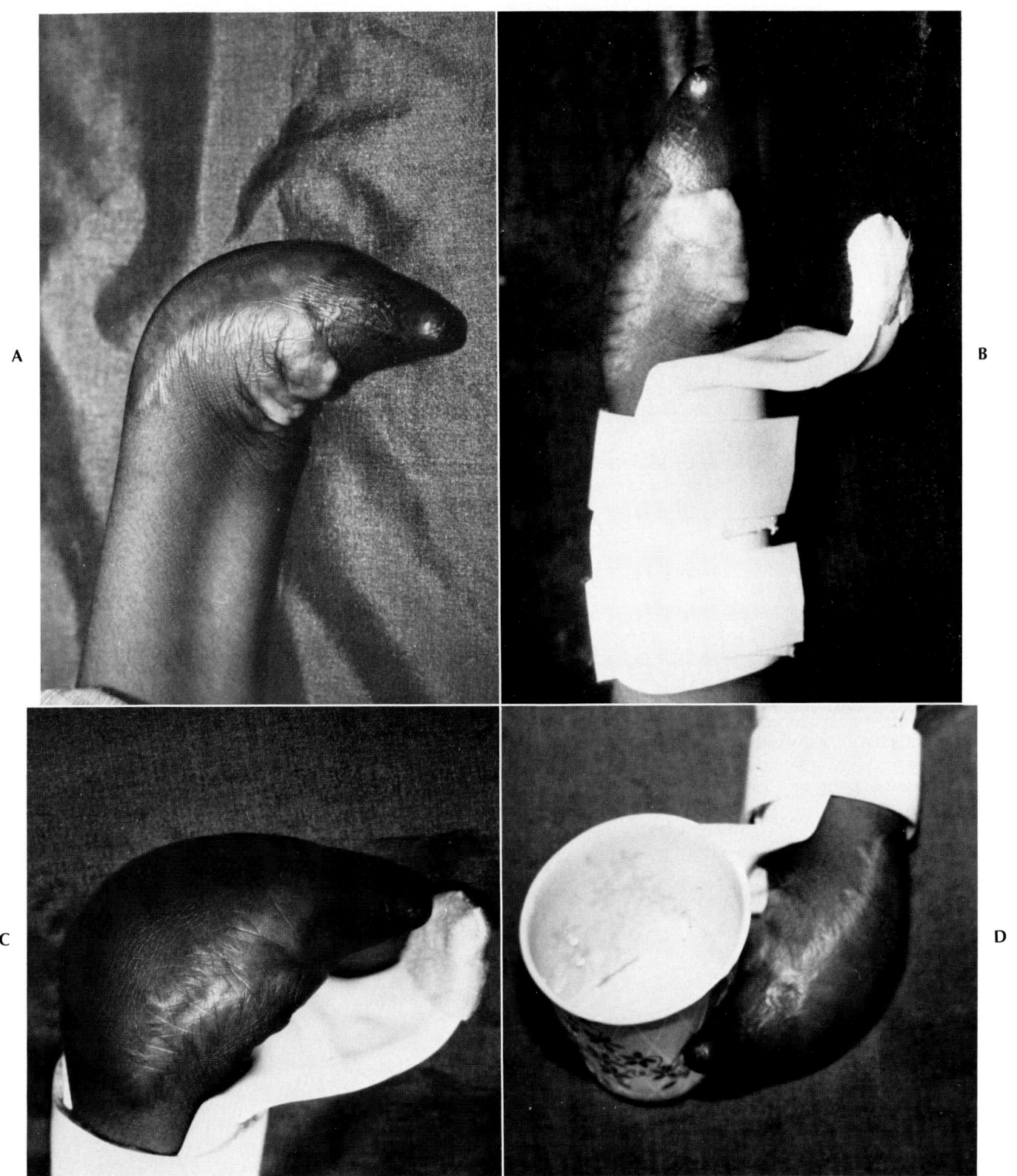

Fig. 94-7   A, This 8-year-old child lost all but one ray in a blast injury. Functional motion of the remnant was minimal; however, good wrist motion remained. **B,** An opposition post was fabricated for the child. **C,** The post allowed prehension of small objects by tip to post contact. **D,** Larger objects could also be grasped because of the range of motion available at the wrist.

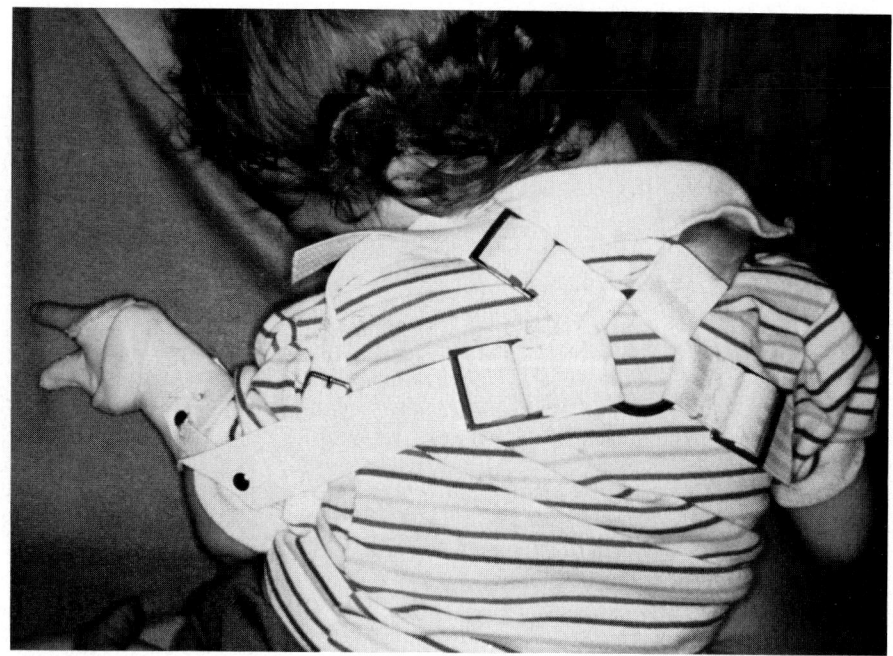

Fig. 94-8 Occasionally extraordinary means are required to secure a splint until the child learns its functional advantages. A figure-eight harness was used to secure an opposition post for this 2-year-old child. As the child adapted to and accepted the splint, the strapping necessary to keep it in place was gradually reduced.

minutes and then removed and the skin checked for signs of pressure before leaving the office.

Parents are given extra copies of home program instructions for other caregivers. The importance of follow-through throughout the child's day is stressed.

SUMMARY

After surgery or trauma, splinting may be a necessary part of a child's hand treatment program. The success of this program is related to the effectiveness of communication between members of the treatment team and caregivers, as well as to the quality of the splint that is fabricated.

REFERENCES

1. Anderson LJ, Anderson JM, and Cohen BS: Principles and techniques of orthotic design and fabrication for hand dysfunction in the neonate and very young infant. Poster presentation, American Academy of Physical Medicine and Rehabilitation, 1985.
2. Anderson LJ and Anderson JM: Hand splinting for infants in the intensive care and special care nurseries, Am J Occup Ther 42(4):222, 1988.
3. Bora FW: The pediatric upper extremity: diagnosis and management, Philadelphia, 1986, WB Saunders Co.
4. Casey CA and Kratz EJ: Soft splinting with neoprene: the thumb abduction supinator splint, Am J Occup Ther 42(6):395, 1988.
5. Erhardt RP: Developmental hand dysfunction, Maryland, 1982, Ramsco Publishing Co.
6. Forsyth-Brown E: The slot-through splint, Physiotherapy 69(2):43, 1983.
7. Herndon JH: Treatment of tendon injuries in children, Orthop Clin North Am 7(3):717, 1976.
8. Herndon JH: Hand injuries—special considerations in children, Emergency Med Clin North Am 3(2):405, 1985.
9. Lindsay WK: Hand injuries in children, Clin Plastic Surg 3(1):65, 1976.
10. Merrell SW and others: Full-thickness skin grafting for contact burns of the palm in children, JBCR 7(6):501, 1986.
11. Skerik SK, Weiss MW, and Flatt AE: Functional evaluation of congenital hand anomalies, Am J Occup Ther 25(2):98, 1971.

XVI

THE WORKER AND PERFORMER IN A HAND REHABILITATION SETTING

95

Work therapy program of the Hand Rehabilitation Center in Philadelphia

Patricia L. Baxter-Petralia, Laura A. Bruening, and Susan M. Blackmore

Work therapy is a program that includes therapeutic activities and progressive resistive exercises to achieve short- and long-term goals. Other terms that are interchangeable with work therapy are *work hardening* and *work tolerance*. Each patient's program is designed to facilitate the maximum recovery of functional use of his injured extremity. The purpose of the work therapy program includes promoting active use, minimizing physical complications from disuse, and most important, increasing the patient's strength, endurance, and coordination, which facilitates his adjustment to his injury and his return to work and normal functional activities.

Work therapy is an integral part of the treatment program at the Hand Rehabilitation Center in Philadelphia. There are two main services provided in the hand therapy program. In primary care, therapists provide preoperative and early postoperative management, splinting, sensibility evaluations, and instruction in active and passive exercise programs. In work therapy, the therapist provides resistive exercises, therapeutic activities, physical capacity evaluations, functional evaluations, on-site visits, and industrial consultations.

The staff of the work therapy program consists of five occupational therapists, a woodworking instructor, a ceramics instructor, a woodcarving instructor, and two therapy aides. The therapist evaluates each patient and plans the treatment. The patient receives instruction initially by the

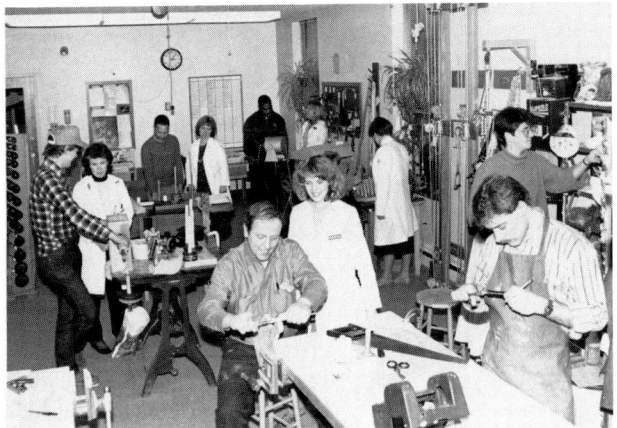

Fig. 95-1 Patients in work therapy under supervision of therapists.

therapist on each therapeutic exercise and activity to be performed. The aides and instructors implement treatment techniques as instructed by the therapist. Participation is monitored in a group setting (Fig. 95-1).

A patient is referred directly to work therapy by a hand surgeon. Other referring sources include insurance companies, rehabilitation companies, and other physicians. The patient's surgeon communicates to the therapist the amount of stress or resistance the patient's injured structures can tolerate considering the extent of the injury. Wound healing, fracture stability, the surgical procedure, and the length of time since the injury or surgery are considerd before the patient begins the work tolerance program.

Each patient is assigned therapeutic activities and exercises according to his condition. The patient may be referred initially to the work tolerance program based on the following schedule:

Diagnosis	Initiation of work therapy
Tendon repair	5½ to 8 weeks after injury
Crush injury	3 to 6 weeks after injury
Partial amputation of digit	3 weeks after injury
Replantation	6 to 8 weeks after injury
Amputation of hand	4 to 6 weeks after injury
Fracture	4 to 6 weeks after injury
Nerve compression releases	3 weeks after surgery
Burn	3 to 6 weeks after injury
Tendon transfers	4 to 8 weeks after surgery
Reflex sympathetic dystrophy	3 to 6 weeks after injury
Soft tissue laceration	2 weeks after injury
Muscle/ligament injuries	4 to 6 weeks after injury
Nerve injury	6 to 8 weeks after injury
Joint fusion	8 to 12 weeks after surgery
Dupuytren's release	4 to 6 weeks after surgery
Frostbite	3 to 4 weeks after injury

Work tolerance activities and exercises are divided into five levels of resistance, that is, the number of pounds the patient can grasp or lift safely. When the patient is referred to work therapy, he starts in a specific level of resistance rather than a certain activity or exercise (Table 95-1).

Level I resistance includes activities and exercises of no greater than **1 pound** of resistance. This level promotes early purposeful hand motion. Prehension activities are performed in elevation to reduce posttrauma or postoperative edema (Fig. 95-2).

A level II program provides resistance of **1 to 3 pounds;** improves prehension and coordination skills and initiates strengthening.

A level III program provides resistance of **3 to 30 pounds.**

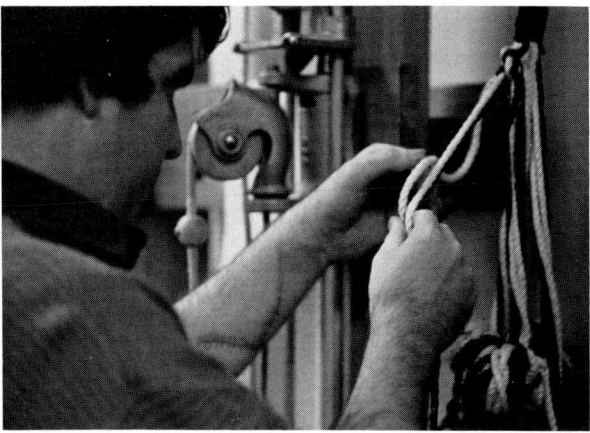

Fig. 95-2 Macramé is a low-resistive activity that allows the incorporation of elevation for edema reduction.

Table 95-1 Levels of resistance

Level	Resistance (pounds)
I	0-1
II	1-3
III	3-30
IV	30-60
V	60-100

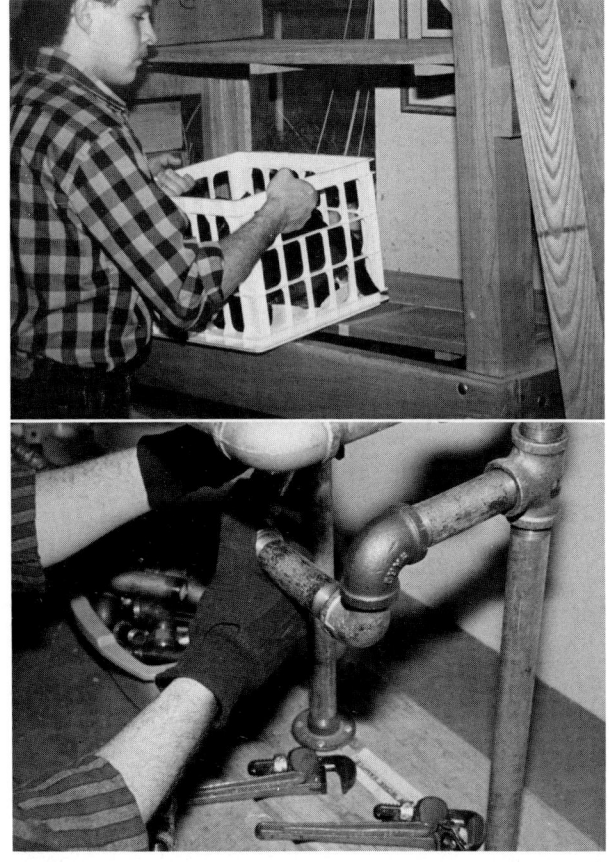

Fig. 95-3 **A** and **B,** Job simulation requires the patient to perform the physical demands of his job such as lifting and tool handling on the pipe assembly.

This level increases strength and endurance through the execution of moderately resistive activities.

A level IV program provides resistance of **30 to 60 pounds.** Moderate to heavy resistive exercises encourage maximum strengthening and improve the patient's endurance.

A level V resistive program provides activities and exercises with resistance of **60 to 100 pounds.** This level promotes heavy resistive exercise that simulates the physical demands of a patient's job to prepare him to return to work (Fig. 95-3).

EVALUATION

The work therapy evaluation includes an occupational interview to determine the physical demands of each person's job. Also, measurements of range of motion, strength, edema, pain, sensibility, coordination, and functional ability are recorded.

Occupational interview

During the occupational interview, the therapist asks the patient to describe the physical demands of his work. The amount of weight the patient lifts, carries, pushes, and pulls during the work day is recorded. Tools that are frequently used are documented. Repetition and frequency of all the tasks are estimated. The length of time the patient assumes or maintains sitting, standing, crouching, crawling, kneeling, or climbing is reviewed (see Chapter 7).

Range of motion

Range of motion is measured with a goniometer.[6] All upper extremity joints are assessed, and limitations in range of motion are noted. Specific joint measurements may be deferred if a primary care therapist has recorded them in the acute phase of treatment and continues to follow the patient.

Strength

A variety of methods are used to evaluate muscle strength in a work tolerance program. The most precise method is to test the strength of individual muscles through a manual muscle test.[9] The comprehensive manual muscle test is where one muscle is isolated and stabilized. The examiner provides resistance to grade the strength from a 0-to-5 scale or from poor to normal.[9] This test should be performed by the same evaluator with each reexamination, because of the subjective component involved. The validity of the manual muscle test depends on the consistency of the procedure, accurate palpation, correct positioning, and the experience of the examiner.[14] Manual muscle testing is often performed when the patient has sustained a nerve laceration or is to undergo tendon transfers. This test is not used when the patient displays spasticity caused by an upper motor neuron disorder.

Grip strength measurements recorded with the Jamar Dynamometer,* assess the group muscle strength of the finger flexors. Grip measurements are taken alternately on all five levels of the dynamometer with each hand. Strokes reported that when a patient exerts his maximum effort on the dynamometer, the scores when plotted will fall into a bell

*Jamar Dynamometer, Asimow Engineering Co, Santa Monica, Calif.

curve.[16] That is, the highest scores will fall on levels II, III, or IV, and the lowest scores on levels I and V. When the dynamometer is used, the patient's elbow should be at 90 degrees of flexion, the forearm in neutral rotation, and the wrist at 0 to 10 degrees of extension.[6] The dynamometer should not rest on the table.[11]

Pinch strength is measured with a Pinch Gauge.* Tip pinch is measured alternately for each digit of both hands. Lateral pinch and three-point pinch measurements are recorded for each hand. The upper extremity is positioned as described for the grip test.

Finally, the strength of muscles can be assessed during a functional muscle test. The patient is instructed to perform ordinary activities of daily living. The therapist notes the patient's ability to complete the self-maintenance or mobility task and documents the patient's subjective report of fatigue after performance.

Endurance

Endurance is the ability of muscles to sustain effort over time.[18] General body endurance or endurance of one muscle or a muscle group may be impaired. Trombly and Scott recommend using a lightly resistive activity that requires approximately 15% to 40% of maximum effort and measuring the number of repetitions or time spent with the activity before fatigue is noted (that is, when the complete motion involved in the activity can no longer be performed).[18]

The BTE Work Simulator† can evaluate endurance. During the initial evaluation, the patient performs repetitive motion on five individual tools until he fatigues (Fig. 95-4). The baseline measurements for each hand are compared with sequential tests weekly. A percentage of increased endurance (force times distance divided by time) is calculated for each tool.

Endurance can also be measured by the length of time the patient can maintain a position. Electromyogram (EMG) biofeedback can be used to evaluate endurance. The electrodes can be placed over the muscles that maintain the

---

*Pinch Gauge, B & L Engineering, Santa Fe Springs, Calif.
†BTE Work Simulator, Baltimore.

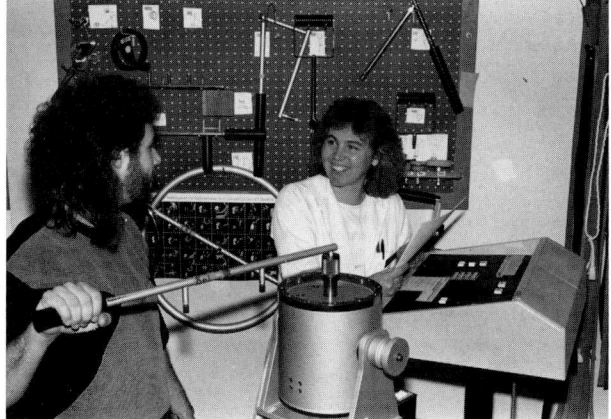

Fig. 95-4 Weekly evaluation on the work simulator determines if endurance has improved.

upper extremity in a specific position. The activity of the muscles will be displayed on the biofeedback monitor and will indicate fatigue by a decrease in the motor unit activity (see Chapter 79).

Edema

Edema is measured circumferentially with a tape measure if there are open wounds or if the extremity cannot be submerged in water. For consistency of measurements, a bone landmark or skin creases should be used when measuring the circumference. The Volumeter* is used to measure edema when wounds are closed, becasue it provides accurate serial measurements. The amount of water displaced by the hand when immersed in the Volumeter is documented. Specific guidelines are outlined for use of the Volumeter.[20]

Pain

Pain is assessed using a pain analog scale. A patient indicates on a 10 cm horizontal line the level of his pain (Fig. 95-5). The right side of the line indicates the worst pain, and the left indicates no pain. Also, a patient may illustrate his areas of pain on a drawing of a body. This technique enables the therapist to understand the patient's perception of the location and intensity of the pain. The pain assessment is usually completed at the beginning and end of each therapy visit.

Functional ability

Functional abilities and limitations are reviewed with an activities-of-daily-living checklist. The patient is asked specific questions regarding his abilities, limitations, or roles in home-care activities, self-care activities, and leisure interests. Demonstration of some of these skills may be included in the evaluation.

Sensibility

Sensibility is assessed with the Semmes-Weinstein Pressure Aesthesiometer† (see Chapter 43) for light touch/deep pressure perception, the Boley gauge for moving and static two-point discrimination, and the Moberg Pickup Test for speed of prehension with vision occluded. Touch localization, using the Semmes-Weinstein Pressure Aesthesiometer, may be added if sensory reeducation is necessary as part of treatment. Also the therapist may ask the patient to locate the specific area that is stimulated by moving touch or constant touch with a blunt instrument.[5]

Light touch/deep pressure, two-point discrimination, and coordination speed are usually tested at 3-month intervals. Moving touch, constant touch, and area localization can be tested weekly or monthly as part of the sensory reeducation program.

---

*Volumeters Unlimited, Idyllwild, Calif.
†Semmes-Weinstein Pressure Aesthesiometer, North Coast Medical, Inc., Campbell, Calif.

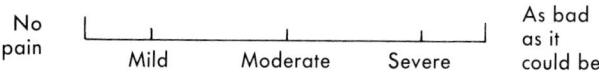

Fig. 95-5 Pain analog scale. (Modified from Phipps WJ, Long BC, and Woods NF, editors: Medical surgical nursing: concepts and clinical practice, ed 3, St Louis, 1987, The CV Mosby Co.)

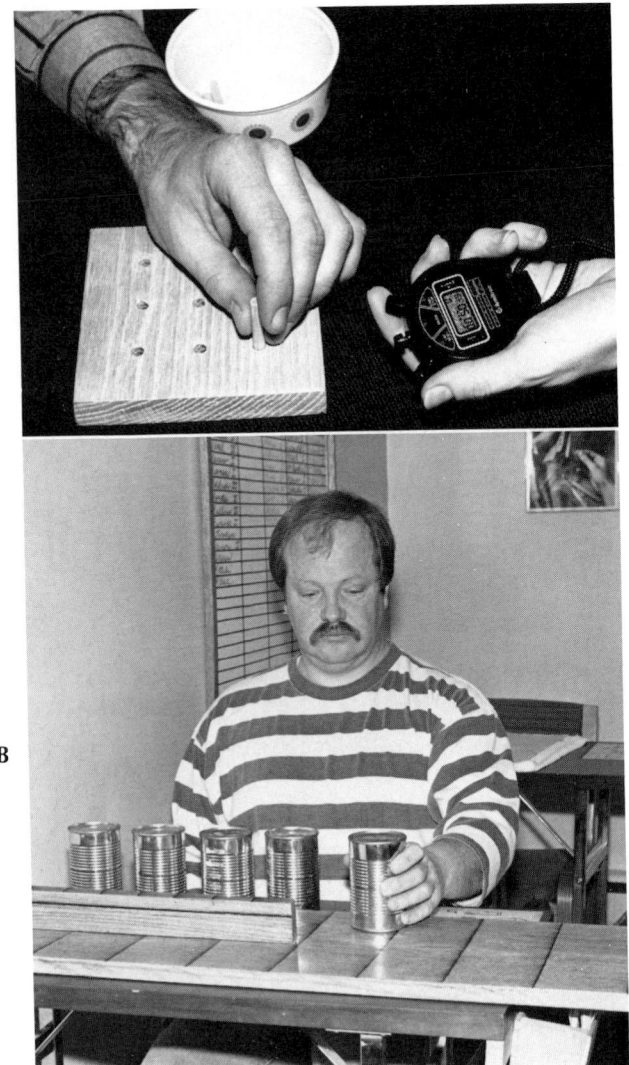

Fig. 95-6 Coordination can be evaluated quickly by using **A,** the Nine Hole Pegboard and **B,** the Jebson Hand Function Evaluation. Normative data are available for each test.

Coordination

Coordination is assessed through standardized evaluations (see Chapter 7). The Nine Hole Peg Test[12] and the Jebson-Taylor hand function evaluation[8] can be quickly administered (Fig. 95-6). They are inexpensive and effective measurements of dexterity. The Minnesota Rate of Manipulation Test,[1] Purdue Pegboard Test,[17] and various Valpar Work Samples[19] are frequently used to measure coordination.

A comprehensive evaluation is vital to ensure an appropriate treatment plan to achieve functional goals. The full battery of evaluations is not assessed on the patient's first visit to the work tolerance program. The evaluation is ongoing, and during the course of the patient's treatment, other problems may be identified and assessed.

GENERAL PROGRAM

Most patients attend work therapy 3 days each week. Each patient is monitored closely throughout his time in work therapy, and the length of each session increases as work tolerance improves. The length of therapy is determined by the patient's progress and physical endurance. He must perform progressive resistive exercises and activities that are increased as he improves.

Therapeutic modalities are used in the work tolerance program both before and after treatment. Heat is applied by hot packs, paraffin, and fluidotherapy, or more directly to a small area by ultrasound applied by a physical therapist. These modalities can provide pain relief, decrease muscle spasms, decrease joint stiffness, and increase connective tissue extensibility. Cold packs are applied to decrease edema, reduce acute tissue inflammation, decrease muscle guarding spasms, and relieve pain. A contrast bath (the patient alternates placing his hand in cool then warm water) is used to facilitate vasodilation and vasoconstriction, which stimulates an increase in local circulation.[13] The choice of modality will depend on therapeutic goals and the patient's tolerance.

Each patient is educated to adhere to specific precautions for his injury. A patient with a peripheral nerve laceration is instructed to inspect his skin frequently and to avoid injuries, such as abrasions and burns, on the insensate part of his hand. A patient with a painful neuroma may learn to increase the use of his injured hand by using appropriate padding over the painful area. Each patient is provided with a written home program that includes specific precautions.

The purpose of the work tolerance program is to help each patient regain strength, coordination, endurance, ability to work, and ability to engage in leisure activities. The resistance in each patient's program is upgraded based on the patient's tolerance. If a patient's hand swells, the resistance must be decreased in the program. If a patient tolerates the resistive program without pain or swelling, resistance is increased.

Communication among the patient, surgeon, and therapist is an essential component of a successful program. The patient is encouraged to ask questions regarding his program. During the patient's rehabilitation program, the work therapy staff maintains ongoing communication between the patient, the primary care therapist, and the surgeon. The work therapist also communicates with the patient's insurance carrier, rehabilitation specialist, and employer to coordinate the patient's reentry into his work environment.

TREATMENT PLANNING
Therapeutic activities and therapeutic exercises

The referral form for work therapy divides the exercises and activities into five levels, from zero to 100 pounds of resistance. This ensures that the surgeon communicates with the therapist about the maximum resistance the patient can tolerate safely. Level I and level II activities are designed to promote active hand use, facilitate coordination, and initiate strengthening. Beasley stated that "the patient must be an active participant in his therapy if it is to be of lasting benefit."[4] The patient cannot drop off his hand for therapy and collect it an hour later. This attitude by some patients must be prevented or corrected early through patient education, evaluation, and close supervision as therapeutic tasks are performed. Levels III to V exercises are used to improve the patient's strength and endurance.

Level I. Prehension tasks, such as manipulation of blocks on dowels, are used (Fig. 95-7). Games are used to en-

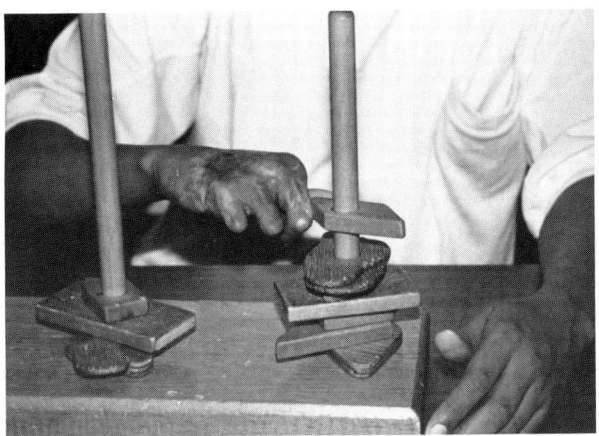

Fig. 95-7 Blocks on dowels require the patient to use a variety of prehension patterns.

courage active motion. For example, in air soccer the patient propels a lightweight ball down the "court" by grasping and squeezing an ear syringe (pediatric size). Alternately, the patient can move the ball with a paddle that requires intrinsic-plus pinch. The game Hi-Q can be modified so that the patient picks up hex nuts with tweezers. Hi-Q can also be played on a large frame with padded dowels. The patient squeezes each dowel together with forceful flexion of the digits to remove it from the board. An extension ball roll game requires the patient to move the ball up an incline with isolated or group finger extension (Fig. 95-8).

EMG biofeedback is initiated in the patient's work tolerance program when active motion is allowed. Some of the indications include isolated training of tendon transfers during the 4 to 6 weeks after surgery and active motion of extrinsic muscles 5 weeks after tendon repairs. EMG biofeedback is used to encourage the use of specific muscle groups while performing therapeutic activity programs (see Chapter 79).

Level II. Macramé is used to encourage active motion, reduce edema, and promote bilateral use of the patient's upper extremities. Macramé is taught to a patient while he is in the acute stage of wound healing. A patient can work on a macramé project in elevation to reduce edema. It is an appropriate activity to train a patient to use a prosthesis. This activity can be graded by reducing the size of cord. It is frequently an integral part of a patient's home program. Patient projects include plant hangers, place mats, and wall hangings.

Leatherwork is used when the surgeon authorizes level II activities. The size of the project and the selection of lacing, stamping, or carving determine its level of difficulty. Generally, lacing increases elbow range of motion and digital flexion, stamping encourages bilateral digit flexion, and carving encourages three-point pinch. Leatherwork is a good project for desensitization, prosthetic training, and strengthening. Patient projects include personal items, such as belts and wallets.

Ceramics is frequently prescribed to increase upper extremity range of motion and strength. It is versatile and easily graded. Patients use hand-molding techniques of coiling, pinching pots, or rolling slabs in ceramics. Coil projects promote digital extension. Pinch-pot projects encourage digital flexion and thumb opposition. Slab projects encourage digital flexion and elbow range of motion through the use of a rolling pin.

Throwing clay on a potter's wheel is more resistive than hand molding. This activity requires bilateral coordination, wrist extension, and digital extension and opposition. Potter's wheel projects can be adapted to a specific patient's needs, whether to gain flexion or extension. The importance of the improved self-esteem of the patients who finish a ceramic project cannot be overestimated (see Chapter 96).

Wax sculpture is less resistive than ceramics and is acceptable to patients who have tactile sensitivity to clay. Foundry wax is made pliable by submersion in warm water (98° to 100° F). The patient works the warm wax and returns it to the water to maintain its softness. Wax sculpture promotes gross grasp, pinch strength, and digit flexion and opposition. Patients with arthritis or reflex sympathetic dystrophy frequently use wax sculpture in their treatment program (Fig. 95-9).

Desensitization of scar or other hypersensitive areas is initiated during the patient's first therapy session. Hypersensitivity can cause limitation of functional use of an affected hand, resulting in weakness, stiffness, and a longer

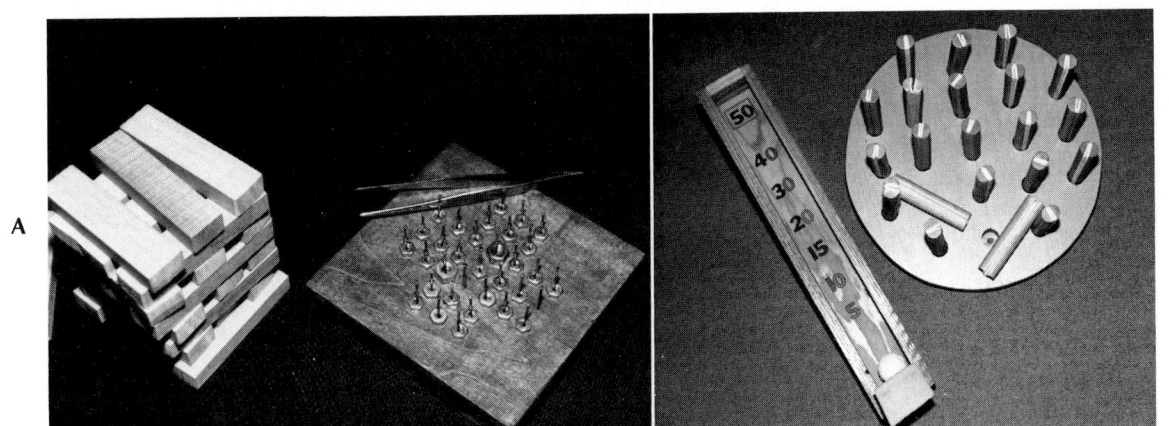

Fig. 95-8 **A,** Active prehension is obtained with block stacking and the Hi-Q game. **B,** Finger extension is required to push the ball up the inclined board. Dowel Squeeze strengthens finger flexion.

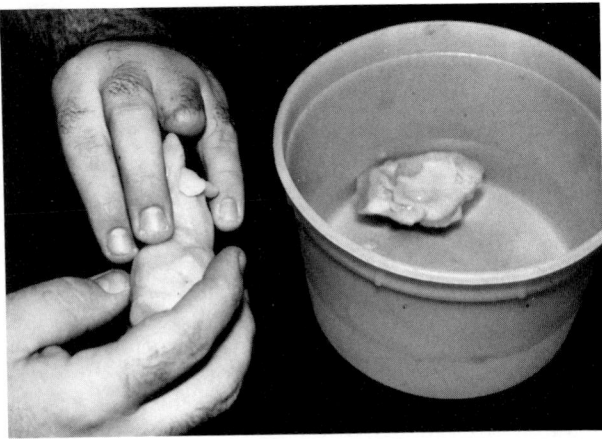

Fig. 95-9 Wax sculpture is less resistive than clay; it promotes gross grasp, prehension, and digital flexion.

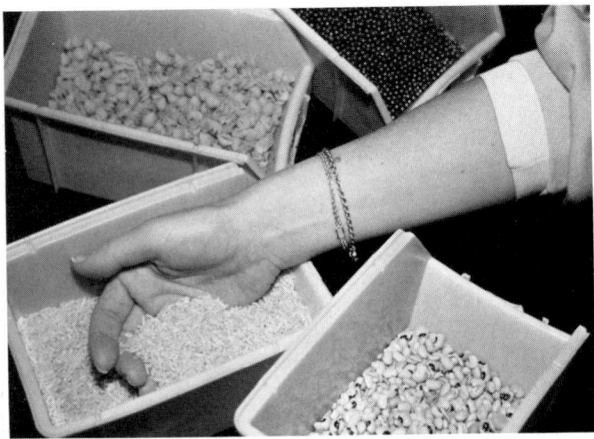

Fig. 95-10 A variety of textures are used to desensitize hypersensitive digital nerves.

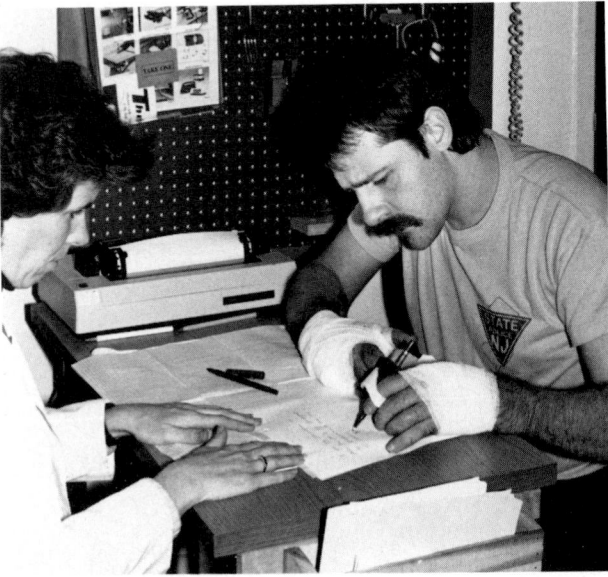

Fig. 95-11 Adaptive writing devices enable a patient to write with his dominant injured hand.

recovery. Patients are instructed to rub the sensitive area 2 minutes each waking hour with textures such as fur, yarn, rice, Styrofoam, or BBs. Each patient is instructed to continue this process at home with textures such as terrycloth towels, clothing, dry beans, or rice or to tap on soft and hard surfaces.[3] (Fig. 95-10).

A peripheral nerve injury can result in cold intolerance. Polyfill or down mittens and thermal liners for gloves are provided to protect patient's hands when outdoors or during job tasks that require exposure to cold.

Coordination training may be necessary to help the patient recover functional use of his injured hand. Activities, such as buttoning, tying, and manipulating various form boards, can increase the patient's gross coordination abilities. Specific tasks, such as writing, should not focus on accuracy, but rather on endurance with submaximal contraction of the muscle groups. As the patient's endurance improves, writing sessions focus on the patient's accuracy and speed.

Patients who have difficulties with activities of daily living are instructed in adaptive techniques or in the use of adaptive equipment. Postoperative patients usually need instructions in one-handed techniques; however, patients with injuries such as amputations may need adaptive equipment. Special adaptive equipment is ordered as necessary from medical supply sources. Rocker knives and buttonhooks are frequently ordered for patients with amputation. Supplies to build up tools and utensil handles include black foam tubing, foam hair rollers, or Styrofoam cylinders (Fig. 95-11).

An arthritic patient is referred by his surgeon for joint-protection instructions and energy conservation techniques. A joint-protection booklet published by the American Occupational Therapy Association is used.[2] The patient is instructed to incorporate joint-protection techniques as he is observed performing activities, such as macramé, foundry-wax sculpture and clay sculpture. It is vital to encourage each patient to make joint-protection techniques a habit.

For all activities within levels I and II, prehension and functional use are emphasized. Photographs of completed projects are available as reference for other patient projects.

Levels III to V. Levels III to V of the work therapy program provide progressive resistive exercises and activities to facilitate the return of a patient's strength and endurance. Trombley and Scott state that muscle strength is related to the maximum tension that can be produced by a muscle during voluntary contraction.[18] The principle to increase muscle strength is to require maximum or near-maximum contractions of weak muscles. This implies use of resistance. As resistance increases, more motor units are recruited, thereby increasing the strength of the contraction of the muscle.

Strengthening exercises include isometric, isotonic, and isokinetic exercises. The benefits and contraindications of the various strengthening exercises are considered for each patient.

An isometric contraction (Gr. *isos* equal and *metron* measure) is a static or holding contraction.[10] The tension in the muscle changes, but the length of the muscle remains the same. There is no change in the joint angle. Isometric exercise involves performance of a static contraction of muscle by either pushing or pulling against an immovable object or by sustaining muscle tension as the patient holds a weight.

This exercise is prescribed for patients who require strengthening early after injury, when their injured structures cannot tolerate resistance throughout full range of joint motion. Patients who experience pain with other strengthening exercises are instructed in isometric exercises. Isometric exercise causes an increase in systolic and diastolic blood pressure; therefore, patients with high blood pressure should not perform isometrics.[15]

Isotonic exercises can facilitate either concentric (a shortening contraction) or eccentric (a lengthening contraction) of the muscles. Isotonic exercise involves physically moving an object to a set point and then returning it to its original position. Rapid improvement in muscle strength is possible if the patient can tolerate frequent increases in the resistance. The Delorme technique has been used in many rehabilitation settings.[18] However, hand-injured patients appear to fatigue less with the modified Oxford technique of regressive resistive exercises[21] (Fig. 95-12).

There are two considerations in selecting weight resistance with isotonic exercises. First, the maximum weight the patient can tolerate is limited to the maximum weight he can move at the weakest angle throughout his range of motion. This may limit the patient's ability to increase the maximum weight and may slow his progress. Isotonic exercise may cause muscle soreness. This is attributed to the patient's performance of concentric and eccentric muscle contractions in the isotonic exercise. Muscle soreness is not a contraindication for this type of activity; however, the patient should be educated to expect it.[18]

An isokinetic contraction (Gr. *isos* equal and *kinetos* moving) occurs when the rate of movement is constant.[10] The resistance accommodates the external force at the skeletal lever so that the muscle maintains maximum output throughout the full range of motion.[7] Isokinetic exercises are performed on the Mini-Gym.* The patient exerts the forces, and the speed of exercises are controlled by the Mini-Gym. The Mini-Gym has a pulley mechanism that provides resistance equal to the force the patient exerts throughout the full range of exercise (Fig. 95-13). Various handles are available for this equipment. The patient performs exercises pulling as hard as possible throughout his full range of joint motion. If the patient has pain in one point of his range of motion, he will not exert as much force and the resistance is decreased automatically. As the painful point is passed, the patient can continue exercising, applying maximum resistance throughout the remaining range of motion. There is one precaution when considering isokinetic exercise. People with cardiovascular dysfuction should not perform isokinetic exercise, because this exercise increases systolic and diastolic blood pressure.[15]

Endurance training is an integral part of the work tolerance program. The principles include (1) grading the activity to involve moderate resistance and (2) requiring perfor-

*Mini-Gym Health and Fitness Systems, Independence, Mo.

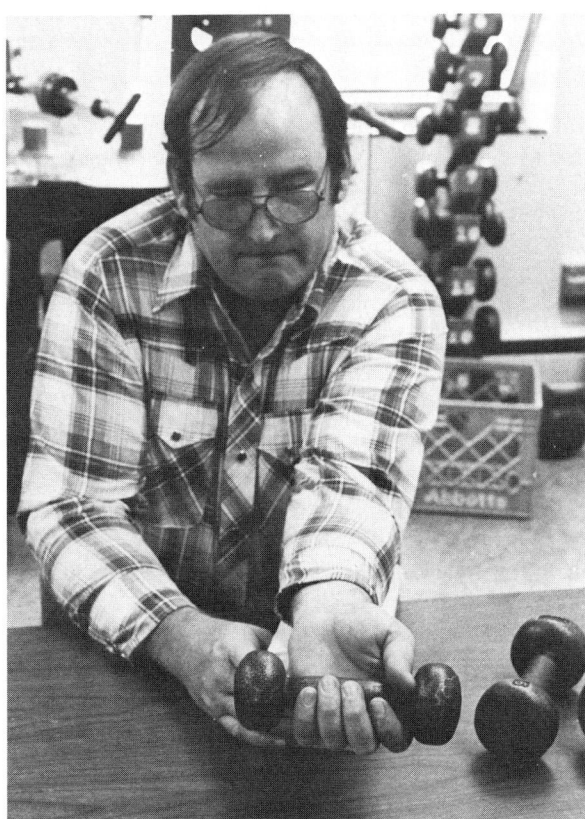

Fig. 95-12 The patient lifts three weights, progressing from the heaviest to the lightest, using the modified Oxford technique.

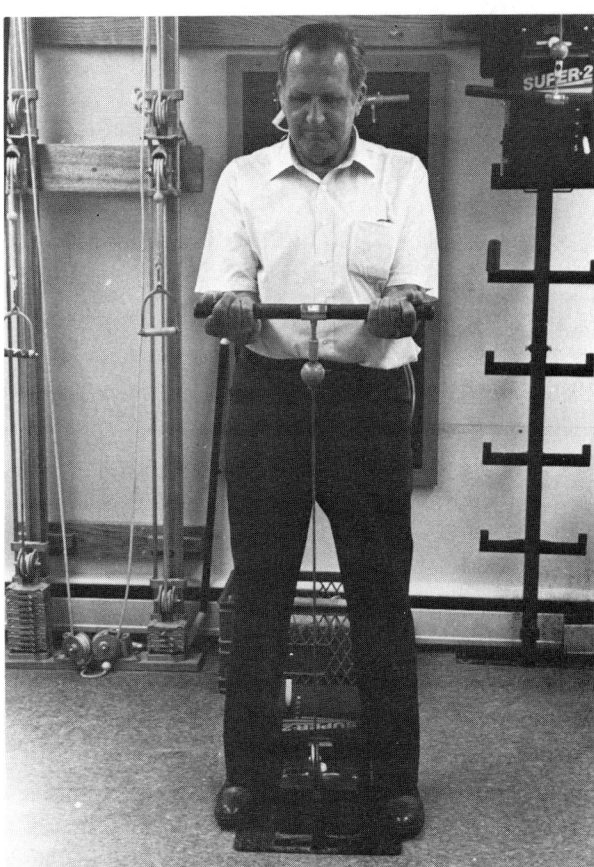

Fig. 95-13 The Mini-Gym pulley mechanism supplies resistance equal to the force applied by the patient during performance of each exercise.

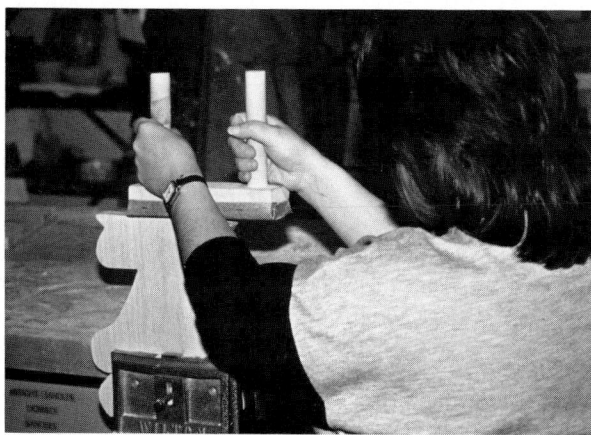

Fig. 95-14   Edema reduction is achieved as the patient performs woodworking with hands elevated above the heart level.

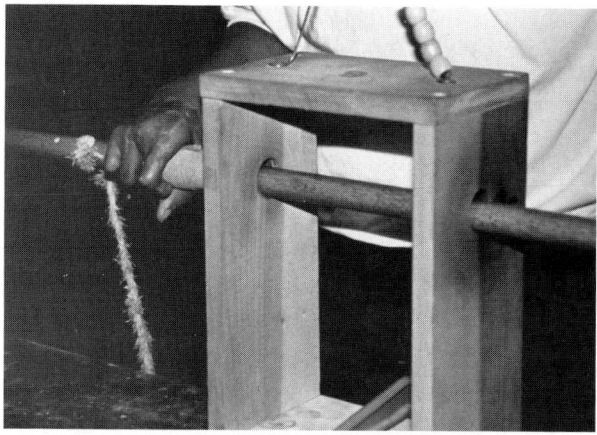

Fig. 95-15   The use of the weight well improves grip strength.

mance of a greater number of repetitions. Strengthening gains will also occur if the activity is repeated to the point of fatigue. The most frequently used activities to increase strength and endurance are those that require a combination of sustained grip and repetitive elbow and shoulder movements.[18]

Woodworking is an excellent therapeutic activity to increase strength and endurance. If the patient performs sustained grip of tool handles, such as a handsander, his muscle strength improves without requiring excessive stress on injured structures, such as tendons. The activity can be initiated earlier than weight lifting. Patients with edema can work in an elevated position to encourage edema reduction (Fig. 95-14). Woodworking is a versatile activity in that it is easily graded and adapted.

Several ways of grading woodworking are possible, including (1) the use of soft and hard wood for projects, (2) the selection of tools (a handsander requires the patient to use less force than a file rasp or handsaw) and (3) the patient's use of tools with either one hand or both. Sanders are fabricated to adapt to the patient's particular problem. Handles that require sustained digital flexion are used most commonly; they can be either unilateral or bilateral. There are sanders that require digital extension, wrist pronation, or wrist extension during use. A common adaptation for a woodworking tool is a larger foam handle. The adapted handle should provide total finger surface contact to encourage individual tendon excursion. Therapists can modify tool handles with adhesive-backed foam or Styrofoam cylinders.

Woodcarving facilitates increased endurance, because it is more resistive than woodworking. A patient may be given a woodcarving project when he has adequate grip strength (approximately 40 pounds) to hold the tools. Woodcarving requires the patient to hold a chisel in his nondominant hand and a mallet in his dominant hand. The patient carves a log by hammering, chiseling, rasping, filing, and sanding.

Repetitive resistive exercisers are used to improve strength and endurance. The weight well* (Fig. 95-15), circumferential weight well, supination/pronation exer-

ciser, and Bioflex wrist exerciser* are frequently used by each patient. The amount of weight and the number of repetitions are increased with patient tolerance. These exercisers can be fabricated or purchased through commercial vendors.

Another form of endurance training is the performance of job-simulated tasks. The goal of the work tolerance program is to prepare each injured worker to return to his job or modified employment. The patient must regain strength and endurance to meet the physical demands of the job. The job demands are the physical movements that are required to perform each task. For example, if a patient is a waiter and his job requires lifting as much as 40 pounds on a tray, he is instructed to lift progressively more weight in therapy. If the patient's job is plumbing, job simulation may include pipe assembly and disassembly, repetitive lifting of weight as it is required on the job, and working in various body postures (see Fig. 95-3, *A*; see also Chapter 7).

The BTE Work Simulator also provides appropriate job simulation. The work simulator (see Chapter 100) is a therapeutic instrument that provides resistance to the patient as he performs physical movements that simulate job tasks. The tool attachments are used to simulate actual tools used on several different jobs. The patient works against progressively more resistance on the work simulator increasingly longer to improve his strength and endurance. The patient performs job simulation on the work simulator at an exercise level that is challenging but comfortable. The patient's performance on each job-simulated task is documented, and the work and power output are compared on sequential tests each week. A percentage of the patient's improvement is documented for each tool used.

HOME PROGRAM

Because a few hours of intensive therapy does not provide sufficient exercise to achieve maximum hand function, each patient is given a home program. Patients from a five-state area are seen at the Hand Rehabilitatioan Center in Philadelphia. Some patients live beyond commuting distance and can attend therapy only once a week for evaluation and

---

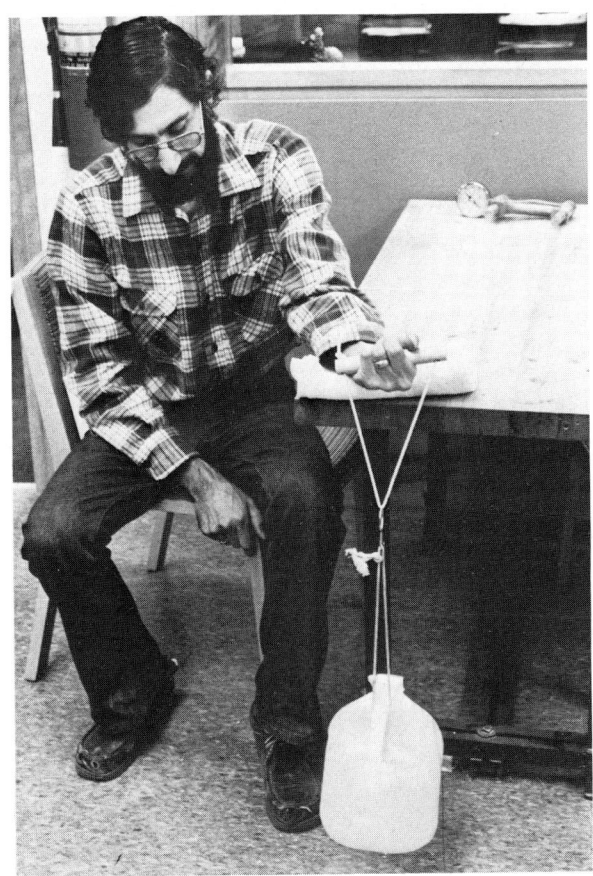

Fig. 95-16 Home exercise device for weight lifting. The patient fills the container with water equal to the amount of weight lifted in therapy.

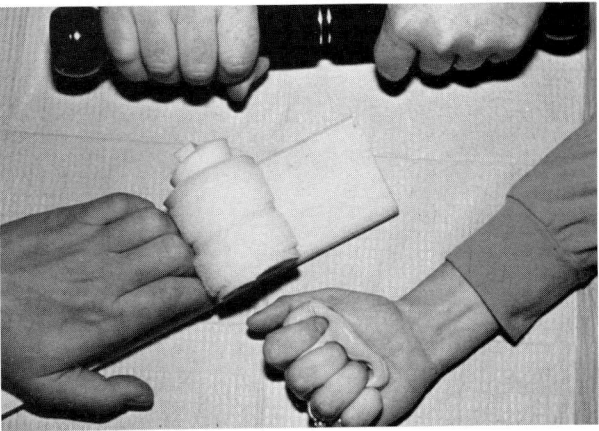

Fig. 95-17 Exer-stick and Velcro. The Velcro extension roll is one of several devices frequently provided for home exercise.

follow-up instructions. Most patients drive an average of 2 hours to attend therapy 3 days each week. Each patient must perform activities and exercises several times each day at home to obtain optimum function when they are not attending therapy. Full instructions are given to each patient, and his ability to carry out the program must be reinforced by verbal, written, and graphic instructions. The patient is requested to demonstrate segments of his home program at each therapy visit.

Written home programs have been developed for weight lifting, desensitization, range of motion exercises, tendon gliding, and blocking exercises for the digits. An individualized home program is given to the patient. Therapeutic activities also are provided for patients to perform at home. Materials and tools for the activities can be loaned to the patient. Each patient is give instructions for the amount of repetitions or time spent on each therapeutic activity at home. Woodworking and macramé are frequently given to patients in addition to job-simulation tasks and weight-lifting.

Isometric and isotonic exercises with weights are prescribed for home use. Because dumbbells are not usually available at home, patients are instructed to use a 1-gallon plastic container that is attached to a wooden dowel by a rope and a shower curtain hook (Fig. 95-16). Additional exercise devices may be provided, such as the extension roll, Hand Helper, and the Exerstick (Fig. 95-17). In the final stages of the therapy program, tool-handling and other job-simulated tasks are included in the patient's home program to prepare him to return to work.

To conclude, the Work Tolerance Program at the Hand Rehabilitation Center in Philadelphia provides comprehensive treatment of the hand-injured patient. The focus for intervention actively involves the patient during goal-setting and planning. The process advances the patient from light active hand use to strengthening and endurance training. The patient continues in the program until he can perform necessary home care tasks and can complete the physical demands of the workplace. If full functional recovery is not achieved, treatment emphasizes maximizing the patient's remaining abilities. This may involve adaptations for the home and workplace.

ACKNOWLEDGMENT

The authors acknowledge the editorial contributions of Patricia Totten and Veronica Keirans.

REFERENCES

1. American Guidance Service, Minnesota Rate of Manipulation Test: examiner's manual, Circles, Minn.
2. American Occupational Therapy Association: A workbook for consumers with rheumatoid arthritis, 1383 Piccard Dr, Rockville, Md 20805.
3. Barber L: Treatment of patients with shoulder-hand-finger syndrome. In Hunter JM and others, editors: Rehabilitation of the hand, St Louis, 1978, The CV Mosby Co.
4. Beasley R: Hand injuries, Philadelphia, 1981, WB Saunders Co.
5. Callahan A: Sensibility testing: clincal methods, In Hunter JM and others, editors: Rehabilitation of the hand, ed 2, St Louis, 1984, The CV Mosby Co.
6. American Society for Surgery of the Hand: The hand examination and diagnosis, ed 2, New York, 1983, Churchill Livingstone Inc.
7. Hislop HJ and Perrine JJ: The isokinetic concept of exercise, Phys Ther 47:114, 1967.
8. Jebsen RH and others: An objective and standardized test of hand function, Arch Phys Med Rehabil 50:311, 1969.
9. Kendall H, Kendall F, and Wadsworth G, : Muscle testing and function, ed 2, Baltimore, 1971, Williams & Wilkins.
10. Lehmkuhl LD and Smith LK: Brunnstrom's clinical kinesiology, ed 4, Philadelphia, 1983, FA Davis Co.
11. Mathiowetz V and others: Grip and pinch strength: normative data for adults, Arch Phys Med Rehabil 66:69, 1984.
12. Mathiowetz V and others: Adult norms for the nine hole peg test of finger dexterity, Occup Ther J Res 5:(1):25, 1984.

13. Michlovitz S and Wolf S, editors: Thermal agents in rehabilitation, Philadelphia, 1986, FA Davis Co.
14. Pedritti LW: Occupational therapy: practice skills for physical dysfunction, ed 2, St Louis, 1985, The CV Mosby Co.
15. Sharkey B: Physiology of fitness, Champion, Ill, 1979, Human Kinetics Publishers, Inc.
16. Strokes M: The seriously uninjured hand: weakness of grip, J Occup Med 25:683, 1983.
17. Tifflin J: Purdue Pegboard examiner manual, Chicago, 1968, Science Research Associates, Inc.
18. Trombly C and Scott S: Occupational therapy for physical dysfunction, Baltimore, 1977, Williams & Wilkins.
19. Valpar Component Work Samples Series, 3801 E 34th Street, Suite 105, Tucson, Ariz.
20. Wood H: Hand Volumeter instruction sheet, US Public Health Service Hospital, Carville, La.
21. Zinovieff AN: Heavy resistance exercise: the Oxford technique, Phys Med 14:129, 1951.

96

Woodcarving and ceramics as therapeutic activities

Adolph Dioda and Kimberly Hunter

WOODCARVING

The human by nature is an activity-oriented person who takes great pleasure in the exercise of creativity.[2] Working in different creative activities has long been used in the healing of the disabled.[1] By participating in creative activity, the patient improves many things—his or her strength, coordination, self-esteem, and well-being. At the Hand Rehabilitation Center in Philadelphia woodcarving and ceramics are two activities that the hand-injured patient engages in to explore his or her creativity while achieving a therapeutic goal.

Woodcarving is a greatly beneficial form of therapy for patients recovering from hand surgery. The patient is prepared for his venture into woodcarving by the hand therapist. Generally, patients for whom woodcarving is prescribed as a therapeutic activity have already been engaged in lighter woodworking and have learned to work with such basic tools as hammers, saws, hand drills, and screwdrivers. Carving, however, allows for more control and a more varied manipulation of tools without strain. The total carving process takes considerable time, and the progression from cutting to rasping to sanding affords the hand a wide range of strengthening exercises.

Practice in carving develops the knack for working with the devious grain in wood while strengthening the long flexors of both forearms. In using the mallet and chisel (Fig. 96-1), the patient can rapidly recover both joint function and muscle power. This is also an excellent means of strengthening the chisel-holding, or nondominant, hand. At the beginning, the voluntary motion is tedious and requires complete concentration.

Not only does the exercise benefit the patient physically, it also gives the patient a feeling of accomplishment that contributes to his general sense of well-being. Woodcarving, in contrast to more traditional modes of therapy, excites the patient's interest. Because accomplishment is immediately visible, the patient's self-competence is promoted. Praise and encouragement by the hand therapy personnel and interaction among patients, with their mutual assistance and advice, help sustain this feeling.

Work area

The recommended height of the work bench is 28 inches. This allows the carver to work down on his piece with far less effort than is required at more conventional bench heights (Fig. 96-2). An 8-foot long work bench accommodates three patients. Three rope slings are used to secure work in progress (Fig. 96-3). The slings are simple loops of half inch ropes that issue from a pair of ¾ inch holes, 12 inches apart on the far side of the table. The ends of the rope have been secured by being knotted below the bench top. When a log is placed on the bench, the loop is easily

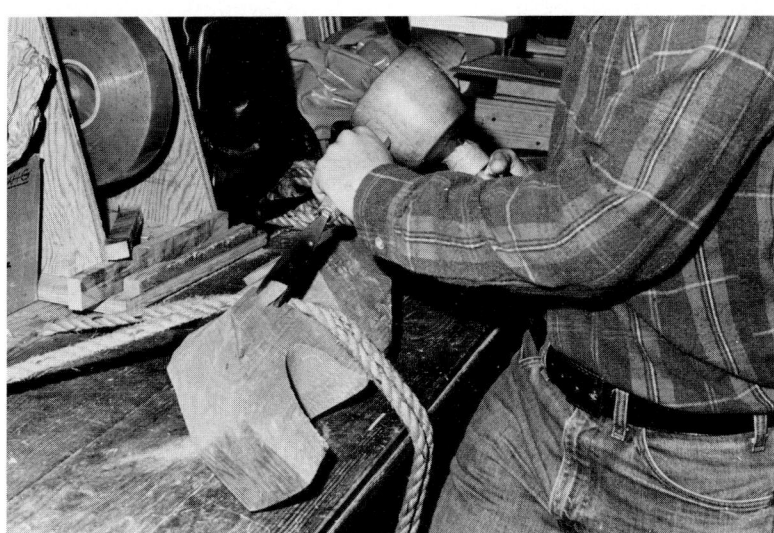

Fig. 96-1   Patient using mallet and chisel. Woodcarving is an excellent activity to strengthen nondominant hand holding chisel.

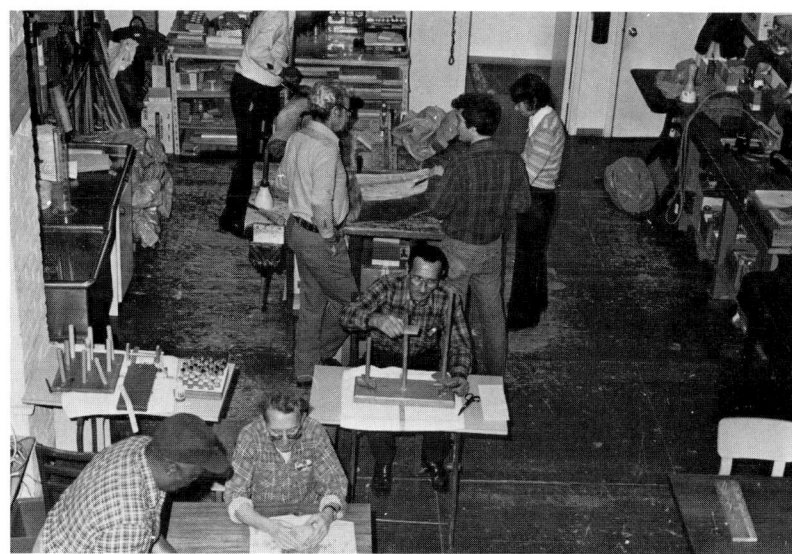

Fig. 96-2   Workbench is 28 inches high, permitting carver to work down on his piece with far less effort than that required at more conventional bench heights.

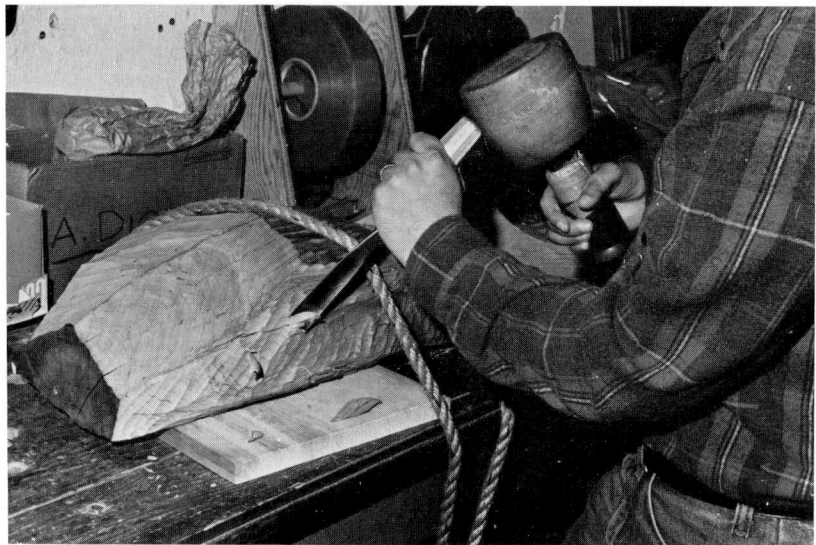

Fig. 96-3   Three foot-controlled rope slings along the bench's 8-foot length are used to secure the work in progress.

raised, passed over the log, and dropped over the side of the table. The loop of the sling should rest a few inches above the floor when the log is in position for carving. A foot placed in the loop and knee pressure on the rope controls rope tension. Wedges may then be placed under the log for additional stabilization.

Procedure and wood selection

Because wood of high moisture content can be carved with comparative ease, lessening impact to the patient's sensitive hand, it is imperative that patients begin carving on freshly cut logs. In a wet state, almost any wood is suitable for carving. Once cut, however, all wood is subject to drying. The less compacted or soft woods such as poplar,

willow, aspen, and tulip carve well, becoming difficult as they dry out and surface fibers tend to tear. In contrast, cherry, walnut, elm, apple, and other hard woods can be worked very satisfactorily because their greater density slows evaporation and deters cracking.

To retain moisture and prevent checking, logs are stored in closed plastic bags. Periodically, they are unbagged to permit the evaporation of surface moisture and are then rebagged. This exposure allows the logs' outer surface to absorb internal moisture gradually, permitting a more uniform shrinkage of the entire log.

Size and shape, too, are important considerations when selecting pieces for carving. To facilitate handling and storage, the ideal unit size should measure 18 to 24 inches in

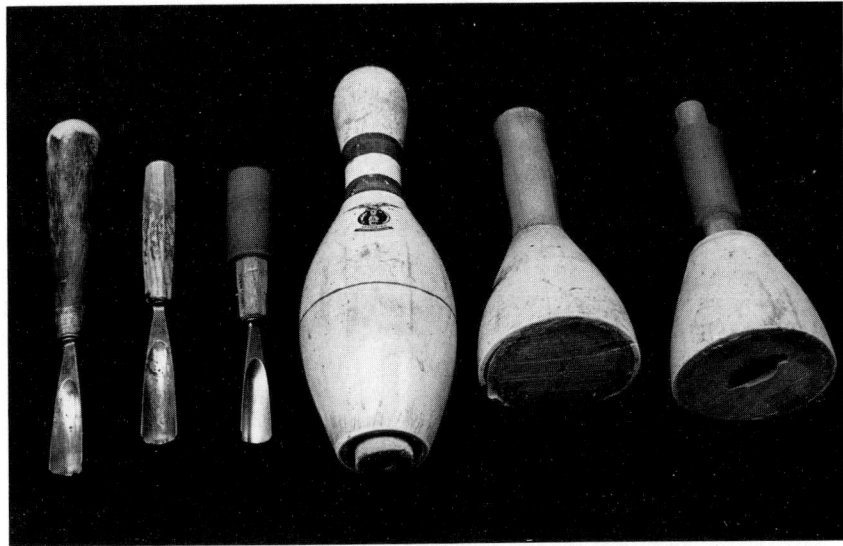

Fig. 96-4   Few tools and relatively simple equipment are needed for woodcarving.

length and 8 to 12 inches in diameter. Shapes may range from the more readily available cylindrical to the more conceptionally stimulating assymetrical, where a confluence of limbs, a knobby projection, or an unexpected twist can suggest a subject, and, at the same time, offer the patient a visible contour to develop in any direction he may choose.

Tools and supplies

Few tools and relatively simple equipment are needed for carving (Fig. 96-4). The chisels we use include a 1 inch deep veiner, a half-inch deep veiner, and a 1 inch, half-round gouge. Cutting edges on the tools used for carving soft and grain woods should have a long bevel on the underside of the blade for a thin, tapering edge. Such a blade produces clean cuts and will not tear the wood. Steel used in woodcarving is very brittle. For hard wood, a blunt edge is required. Thin edges tend to break when forced into a more resistant material.

Mallets are made of discarded bowling pins, two from each pin. Centering the pin in a lathe, one reshapes the neck to form a slight bulge in the center of the handle to fit the contour of the hand. Sizes may vary from 1¼ inches to 1¾ inches at the handle's fullest diameter. This range in size permits the patient to choose the size that most comfortably fits his or her hand. A hole 2 inches deep and 1 inch in diameter is drilled in the center of the remaining pin half. A dowel, 8 inches long and with a diameter to match the hole, is glued and forced into the drilled hole, thus completing the second mallet. Sections of foam rubber tubing can be slipped over these handles to cushion them. The bowling pin's plastic cover is retained; it will serve to protect the mallet head. A Surform rasp with a half-round blade attached is an indispensable tool. Cabinetmaker's rasps are equally valuable, and an ample supply c⁻ sandpaper of various grits is very useful.

Carving

Patients selected for woodcarving sessions are shown photographs of contemporary carvings in which elimination of details and simplicity of form are stressed, an approach that makes the activity of carving attractive. The initial piece is often a nonobjective free form where movement and wood grain are prominent. This approach encourages graduation to more complex projects, usually abstract representations that maintain the intrinsic nature of the wood.

With mallet and chisel, the patient begins his project by first stripping the bark from the selected log (Fig. 96-5). The time involved depends on the physical condition of the disabled hand. The first session is usually short. Sessions that follow are lengthened by degrees as manual strength and flexibility increase. After stripping is done, the log's shape, knobs, protuberances, and so on are noted for possible inclusion in the final carved form. The bottom of the log is then cut so that the log stands in balance. Next, front and side contours are blocked (Fig. 96-6). With the silhouette defined from all visual angles, the process of determining the change of direction of surface planes follows. As work progresses, changes are made to accommodate the unexpected defect. The surface at this stage is rasped and reduced to its final form (Fig. 96-7). The final surface is accomplished in stages as one works from coarse to medium to fine sandpapers (Fig. 96-8). Drying out and cutting away have reduced moisture and bulk, but the sanded piece may require even more time in its plastic bag to insure absolutely thorough drying. It is imperative that the plastic bag be examined periodically for holes. The presence of these may cause too rapid a loss of moisture from the log. When cracks, or checks, develop, insertion of long wedges of the same wood into the opening remedies the condition. These wedges are cut to the length of the opening, dipped in a solution of two parts water and one part white glue and forced into the check. On the following day, any wedge portion projecting above the sculpture's surface can be shaved away and then sanded.

Patients are encouraged to visit Philadelphia's fine museums and art galleries, where exposure to great collections of contemporary, ancient, and primitive sculpture often serves to intensify budding interest. Involved in the creation of sculpture themselves, they find they are better able to relate to the vision of other artists in a totally new and unique way, often engendering a very special insight that may alter for all time the way each relates to every new experience (Figs. 96-9 and 96-10).

CERAMICS

Ceramics is a beneficial therapeutic activity that enhances prehension and coordination and increases strength. Ceramics may be started relatively early in the patient's rehabilitative program; however, wounds must be healed and pins and sutures removed.

Ceramics is initiated by the therapist as part of the patient's work hardening program but can be carried out under the supervision of an aide knowledgeable in ceramics or an

art instructor. The therapist should give the instructor information about the injury, precautions, and therapeutic goals for the patient. The therapist determines which molding technique is most beneficial for that particular patient's goals.

Three basic hand molding techniques are used: pinch, coil, and slab. As the patient advances, the potter's wheel can be used.

Preparing clay

Before any form of activity is begun, the clay must be prepared properly. This process, called wedging, helps deter the cracking of air-dried items and the exploding of products in the kiln resulting from moisture trapped in air pockets. A determined amount of clay is gathered into a ball shape

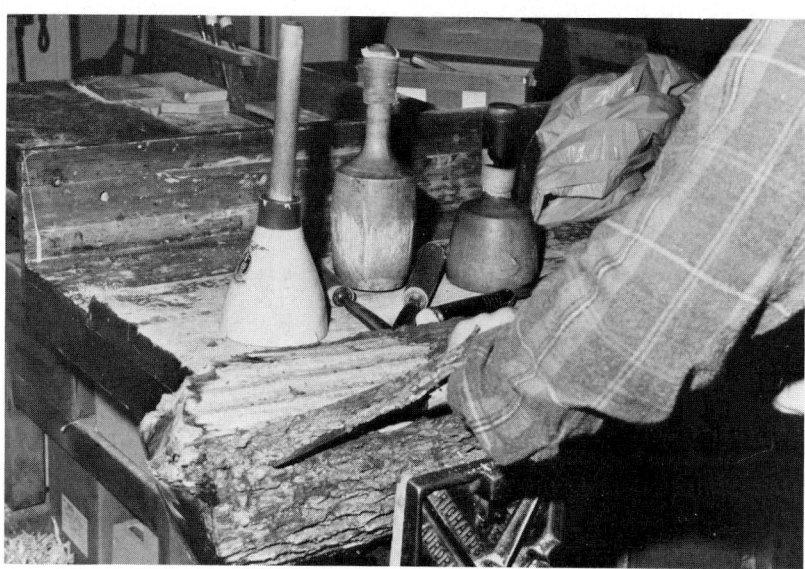

Fig. 96-5 Carving is started on freshly cut logs.

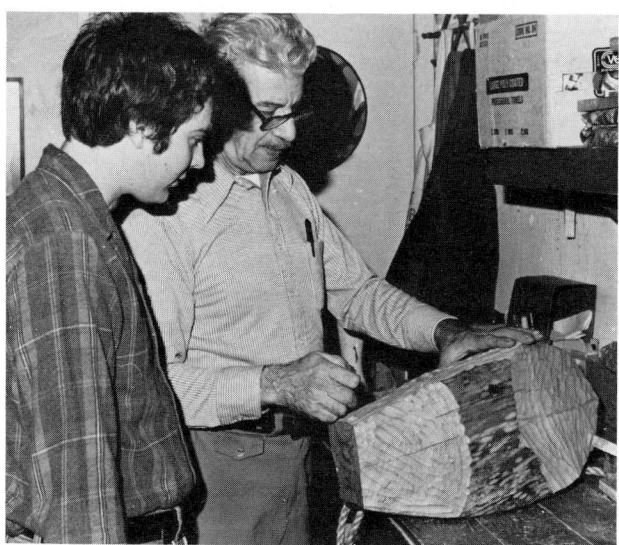

Fig. 96-6 Front and side contours are blocked.

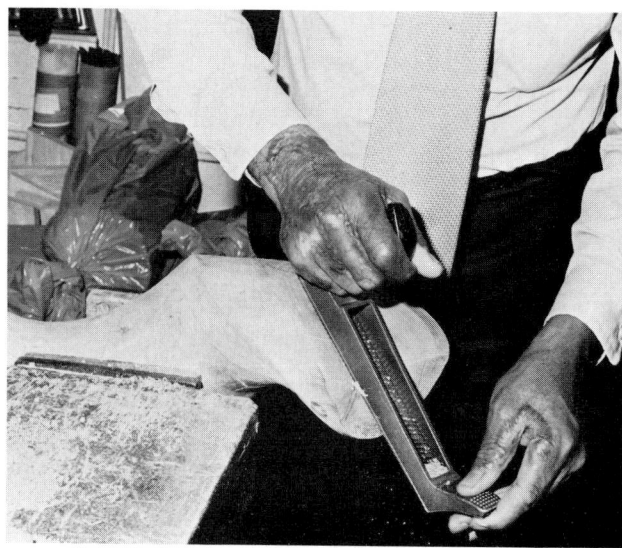

Fig. 96-7 Surface of wood is rasped and reduced to its final form.

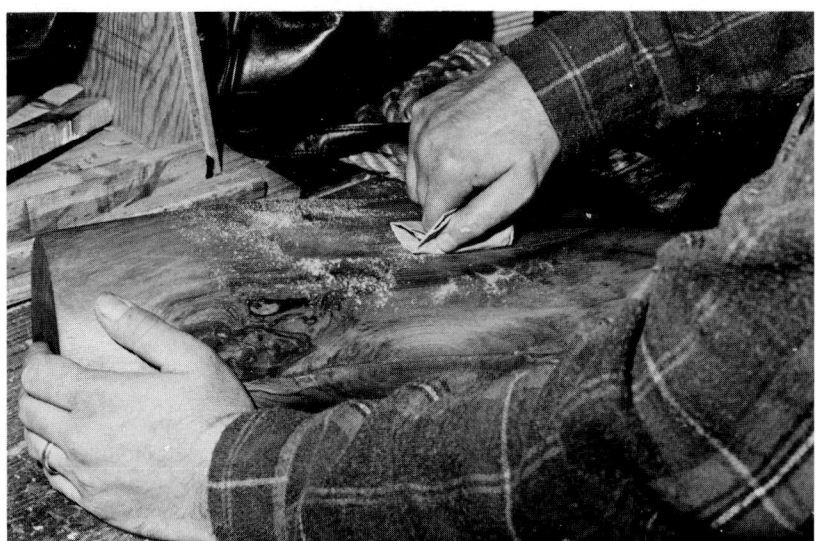

Fig. 96-8   Surface refinement is accomplished in stages working with coarse to medium to fine sandpaper.

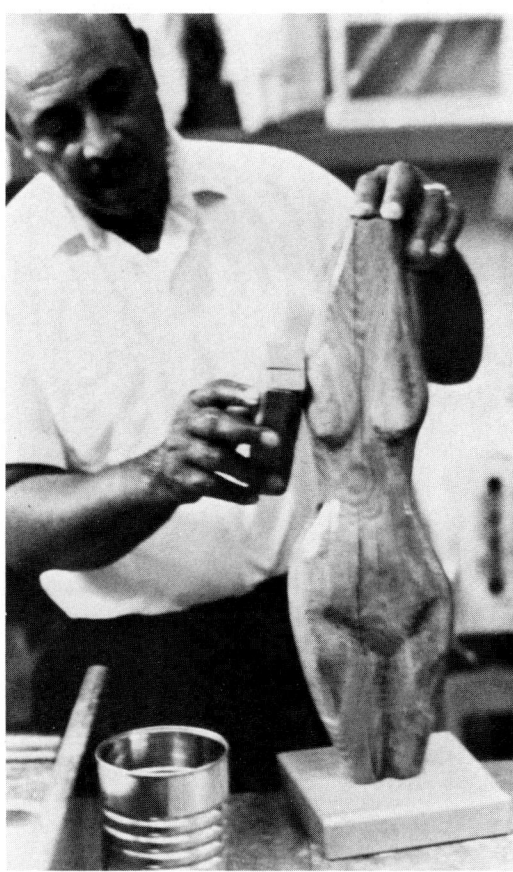

Fig. 96-9   Final sanding of sculpture by patient.

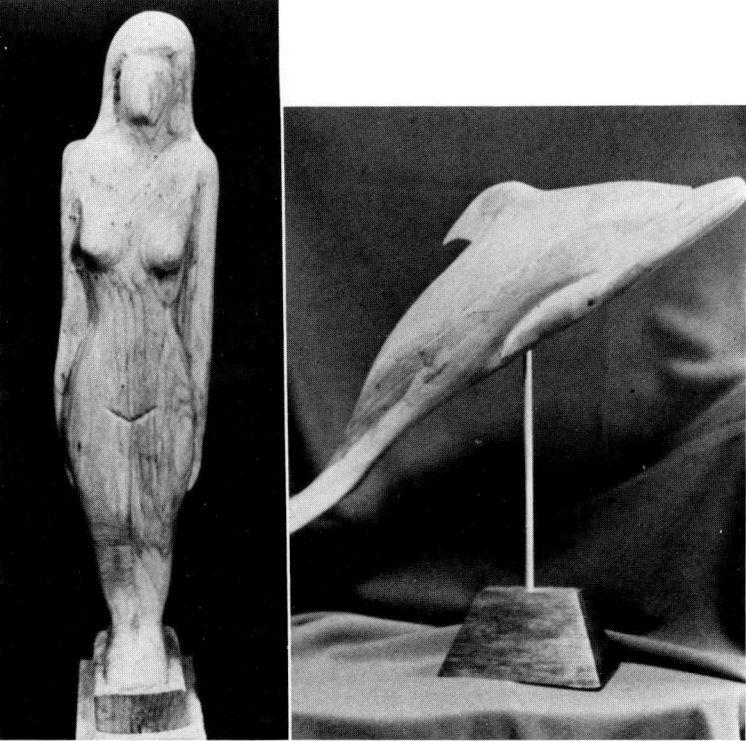

Fig. 96-10   Two pieces of sculpture completed by patients.

and set on the work surface. With the weight of the body, the heels of the patient's hands are pressed into the clay. The clay is then rocked up toward the body and given a clockwise quarter turn. This process is repeated in a rhythmic repetitive motion. The clay is cut into slices with a toggle wire and inspected for air holes. If the clay is wedged properly, it will have a smooth and regular consistency. After the wedging process is completed, hand molding is initiated.

Hand molding methods

Pinch molding. The pinch molding technique (Fig. 96-11) is used for desensitization and for strengthening of extrinsic finger flexors and intrinsic thenar and hypothenar muscles. Most patients start with a basic pinch pot bowl or other simple project. The bowl is beautiful in its simplicity, although desired decorations can be added. Simple patterns carved in or painted on the surface when the pot is in the leather hard stage can form nice textures and make the pot more interesting. The clay is leather hard when it can be cut or carved cleanly.

Lidded forms such as small round jars can be made from hollow forms. The hollow form is made by making two pinch pots having an opening of the same diameter. These two pots should be left to stiffen or dry to leather hard. At this stage the rims of both pots are painted with slip (clay and water mixed to a mayonnaise-like consistency). Both sides are then scored and carefully fitted together (Fig. 96-12). The seam is worked gently and carefully with the fingers so as not to dent the surface now that the form is closed. To smooth and round out the pot a wooden spoon is used. The patient paddles the pot with the spoon in one hand while slowly and evenly turning the pot with the other hand. This is done until the desired shape is reached. When the shape is attained, a knob is added and a lid is cut.

The knob allows further creativity and personalization of the pot. One idea is to trace around a favorite cookie cutter or stencil. This drawing can then be reduced to knob size on a xerographic machine. The patient then traces the outline into the clay and cuts out the shape. The edges are smoothed and detail added if necessary. Because a knob is functional, it is important that it be able to be easily grasped. When the patient can cut into the surface and not have the clay depressed, the lid can be cut. The most effective way to have a clean edge on the finished pot is to gently pull the sharp edge of the knife through the clay. Short, even pulls, rather than sawing, will achieve a cleaner cut.

The process of making a lidded form has several therapeutic advantages. Tracing with a small tool facilitates sustained grip on the tool and is a job simulation activity for patients who use small tools at work. The tool can be built up with foam for patients who lack opposition of the thumb to index finger. Such patients can make a mobile or build a pot and then carve designs into its surface. The carving or cutting out of the pieces facilitates the use of small tools.

The pinch method of building can also be used to make larger forms. Sections can be pinched into flat, square pieces. The pieces are then used to build projects. They can be secured by overlapping and smoothing together if the clay is soft, or by slipping and scoring if the clay is stiff. With either method, the pieces should thoroughly adhere together on the inside. The outside walls in this process of building will have their own texture, which can be left as is or smoothed with the fingertips or by paddling. A decorative touch may then be added to finish the pot.

Coil molding method. Coils are pieces of clay rolled with the palms of the hands. With the thumbs together, the hands move rhythmically from one end of the coil to the other, until the coil is the desired length and width. The process of rolling coils works well for desensitizing sensitive scars in the palm and fingers and for strengthening finger extensors.

Coiling can be taken in many directions. The patient starts with a flat slab base about ¼ to ½ inches thick. The coils

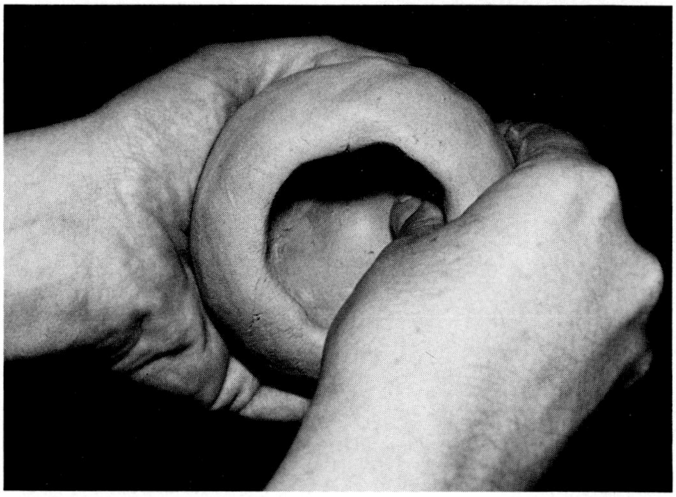

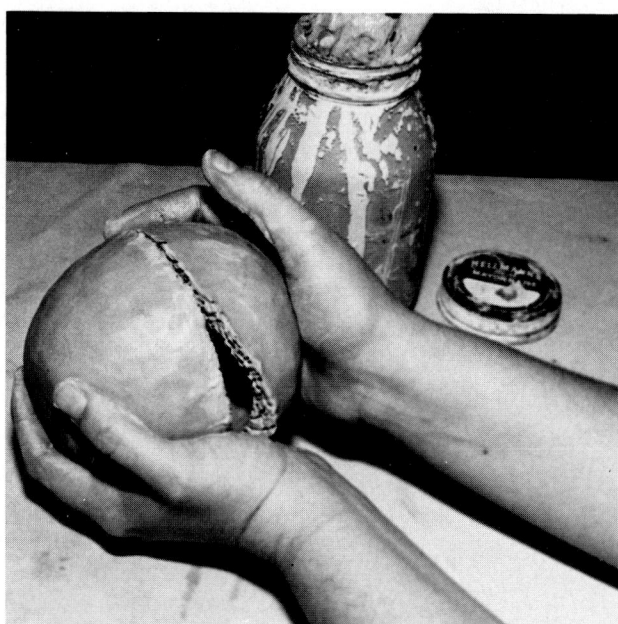

Fig. 96-11   Pinch molding is used for desensitization, strengthening of extrinsic finger flexors, intrinsics, and thenar muscles.

Fig. 96-12   The rims of both pots are slipped and scored and carefully fit together.

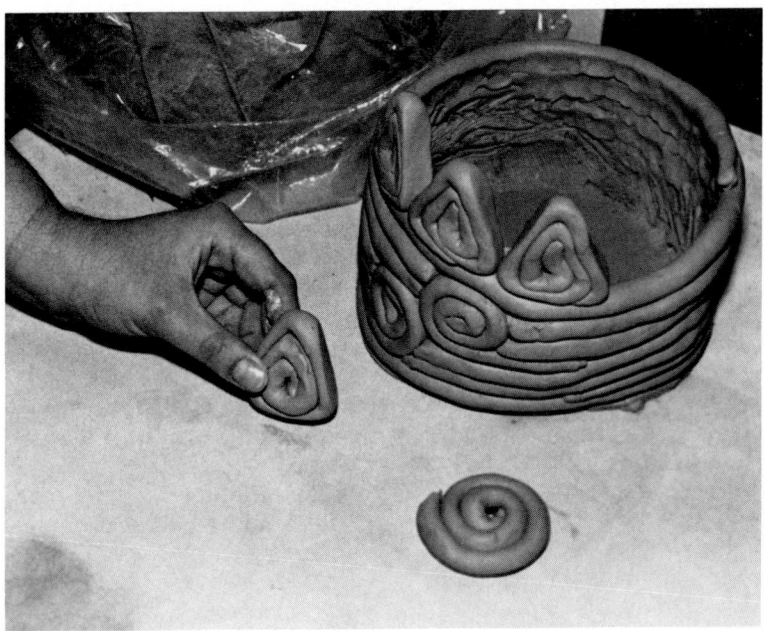

Fig. 96-13   The rolled coil can be left in a spiral or can be tapped on its sides to form squares or triangles.

of clay are then layered one on top of another. If the injury is such that the patient cannot roll even coils, then thicker ones may be slightly flattened and applied on their sides. As the coils are being layered, it is necessary to adhere them well from the inside to prevent leaking and cracking.

The shape of the pot can be changed during the process of building with coils. To enlarge the opening, the coil added should be placed on the outer half of the preceding coil. To decrease the opening the coil added is placed on the inner half of the preceding coil. This process can be repeated on the same pot for interesting and shapely effects. When building with clay it is important to remember that each coil should have adequate support. If the clay is sagging, it needs to be allowed to harden before more clay can be added. The moisture level of clay is controlled by the material in which it is wrapped. If the patient will not return for a few days, the project should be well wrapped in plastic. Plastic garment covers supplied by drycleaners work well. Even an hour in the air can make the clay almost unworkable.

One relatively simple way of adding a pattern to the coil pot is to make a coil and roll it into a spiral. These rolled coils can be left in a circle, or they can be tapped on their sides to form squares or triangles (Fig. 96-13) and added as a band of design or placed sporadically for an interesting effect. The backs of these pieces should be thoroughly sealed together by pulling a flat tool across the cracks, filling them with clay. If a patient can benefit from the therapeutic value of rolling coils but does not enjoy the coiled projects, the coils can be smoothed by using the fingers, wooden rib, or scraper. After the surface has been smoothed, a pattern or design can be added.

Slab technique. The third hand molding method is the slab technique. The patient grips the rolling pin while flexing and extending his elbows and shoulders to roll the clay into a slab. Once rolled, the slab pieces can be used in a variety

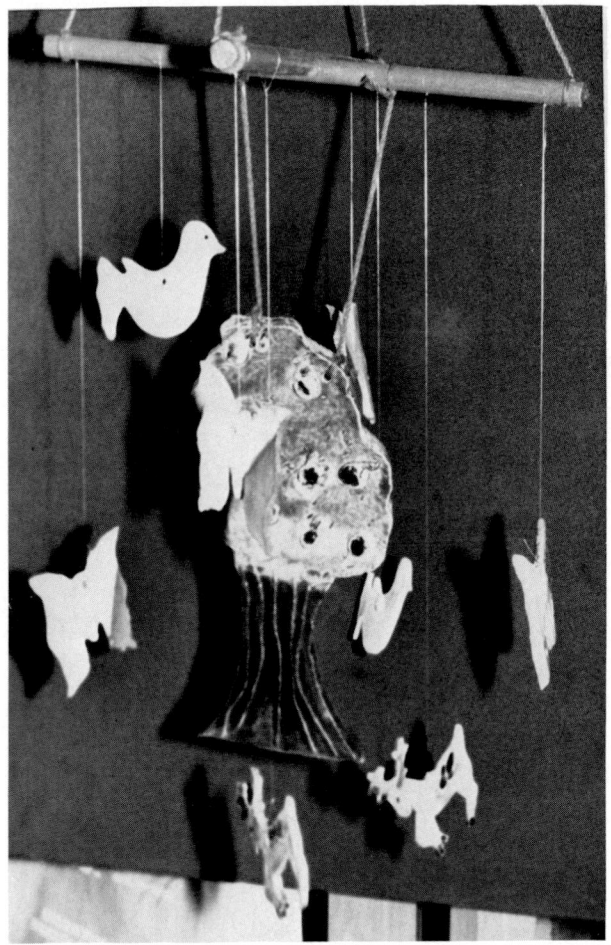

Fig. 96-14   Some of the simpler projects include wind chimes and mobiles, which can take on any theme.

of ways. The simpler projects include wind chimes and mobiles, which can take on any theme. A cookie cutter or a stencil can help vary ideas such as bears and balloons, chickens and cows, cats, boats and fish (Fig. 96-14). These projects are fun and less complicated and can produce quicker gratification. An excellent knot for tying mobiles and chimes is a modification of the midshipman's knot used by fisherman to hold hooks, because it is small and strong (Fig. 96-15). This knot is also used by therapists when making outrigger splints.

Slab boxes and cylindrical forms are somewhat more advanced. Boxes are made from measured and cut leather hard pieces of clay. A patient may roll and measure the slabs, then leave it to stiffen while he does the rest of his exercises (an electric fan on low can be used to quicken slab drying). After a period of ½ hour to 1 hour when the clay is leather hard, the pieces may be assembled. When the slab project is assembled, the edges are cut on angles, then slipped and scored. A reinforcing coil can then be pressed on the inside of each seam to ensure strength. If the box is closed on all sides, the lid can be cut out as described earlier for the pinch closed form. A lid that fits flat requires a flange to hold the lid in place. The flange can be on the inside or added as a decoration on the outside.

Slab cylinders can be molded around a cylindrical object with no undercut. Soda cans with their sharp holes covered with heavy duct tape may be used. A single can works well for a glass or a mug. Two cans taped end to end with the opening at the top is a good size for a vase. To begin the process, thin material or paper towels should be wrapped around the can and taped to it to prevent the wet clay from sticking. The well-taped can opening should be exposed and the paper should be able to slide freely from the can. The exposed opening is used to pull the can free of the clay.

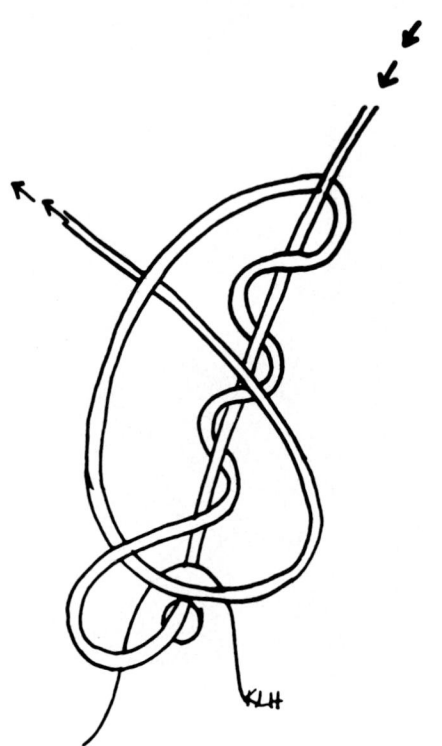

Fig. 96-15 A modified "midshipman's" knot is used to tie mobile pieces.

The slab is rolled, measured, cut, and then wrapped around the can. Care should be taken not to press the clay into any indentations in the can's surface. After the clay is laid in place, the seam is slipped and scored. The bottom is then measured, cut, and applied. It can be difficult to have seams well sealed and still attractive, but with practice it will get easier. The cans should stay in only long enough for the clay to become slightly firm, not leather hard. The clay will shrink and crack. In approximately ½ hour the clay and paper should be removed from the can and be allowed to dry. The finger is hooked into the well-taped opening, and with gentle assistance the clay should slide from the can.

The potter's wheel

Seeing clay thrown on the potter's wheel seems like magic to a beginner, and this can be very motivating. The process of throwing can be deceiving; it seems very simple, but achievement of any amount of skill takes patience and practice.

Many kinds of potter's wheels are available. To choose one suitable for a facility, consider how many patients will be using the wheel and the facility's electrical ability. We have chosen the Brent* Model A wheel designed for a junior or senior high school setting. This wheel requires 110 volts and needs a grounded three-prong outlet. This size wheel is light and easily transported, yet heavy enough to be stable while centering.

Centering the clay is the first step when working on the potter's wheel. To center the clay, a well-wedged piece of clay (approximately 4 inches in diameter) is thrown firmly into the center of the wheel head. A bucket of water and a sponge are placed within easy reach. When the clay is firmly on the wheel, the wheel is started at a high speed. Water is very important when working on the wheel. Without enough water, the clay will not flow smoothly through the hands. One has to guard against too much water, which will cause the clay to become saturated and lose support. The worker will learn this compromise with practice. Usually, for a right hand dominant person, the heel of the right hand does most of the work and vice versa for the left hand dominant person. The hand-injured patient may have to adapt this, but the end result should be the same—a nicely centered lump of clay.

The hands are dipped in water, and the arms are positioned firmly against the rib cage or thighs. While the wheel is turning rapidly the palms are held firmly against the clay, with the thumbs riding on top. The clay is forced into a cone and is then pushed down from the top of the cone to form a low, round hump. This process is repeated several times to center the clay on the wheel. Clay responds to what the hands are doing; therefore this step may require much practice and can be an excellent strengthening activity. During this process the hands and clay may become dry and cause dragging. When this occurs water must again be introduced.

The clay is opened after the ball is centered. The potter's wheel is set at moderate to fast speed. The dominant, or strong, thumb is gradually and evenly drawn into the center of the clay until there is a thickness of ½ to ¼ inch of clay on the wheel head. The beginner should check this thickness with a needle tool. Both hands should work together, each

---

*Robert Brent Corp., Healdsburg, Calif.

responding to the other's actions. Once at the bottom, the thumb guides the clay and pulls it over to the right with an even, steady movement. As the wall of clay comes over, the bottom should be left flat, with right-angle corners. The goal is to shape a low, thick-walled cylinder.

To increase the height of the form, the patient pulls the clay up into a taller cylinder. For this stage the wheel should be at moderate to slow speed. Just enough water should be applied to provide a friction-free surface. Friction could weaken or rip the pot. To apply water while the wheel is moving, squeeze a sponge above the edge of the pot. As the wheel turns, the clay will become evenly lubricated. The left hand is placed in the pot and the index or long and middle fingers ride against the inside right wall. The fingertips of the right hand are placed parallel to the left fingers inside the pot. Both hands apply even pressure and rise together up the side of the pot while pulling up even and straight. The fingers should follow through and rise at the same even, steady speed up and off the pot. Quick movements will make the pot lopsided. The cylinder is the first form to master on the wheel. Once this is achieved, then other shapes can be investigated.

When the pot is finished, slow the wheel to barely turning and run toggle wire under the clay. A puddle of water is splashed on the wheel head and pulled under the form with the wire. The piece is allowed to dry until the surface is not tacky and is then lifted off the wheel. A piece of plastic should be draped over the top to dry the pot more slowly. Clay drying too quickly or unevenly can crack or warp.

When the pot is close to leather hard, the excess clay can be trimmed away by "trimming" the pot. To do this the pot is turned upside down and centered on the wheel. To center the pot hold a pencil in one hand and steady it. Turn the wheel on very low speed and bring the pencil just in contact with the surface of the pot. The pencil should touch smoothly around the pot. When the pot can be felt pushing against the pencil, stop the wheel and tap the pot over just a fraction. Repeat this process until the pencil rides smoothly on the surface. When the pot is centered it is then held down by three evenly placed lumps of soft clay. These lumps of clay are just to hold the pot still. Be careful not to crack or dent the pot when pressing the soft clay in place. The wheel is turned to moderate speed and a loop tool starting in the center trims the pot to the desired shape. Trimming adds to the finished form.

Psychological motivators

Working with clay can be exciting; however, patients may initially focus on their pain, inability to work, or family problems. Any number of things may keep injured people from being motivated. Participating in a craft such as ceramics may be intrinsically motivating and help the injured person become an active participant in his treatment. All the methods of building can be combined together for interesting effects. A rounded pinch pot with coils added or a slab and coil project encourages patients to try different combinations.

Clay is very pliable and takes impressions well. The imprints of bolts, washers, and rubber stamps can make nice designs (Fig. 96-16). Textured fabric such as lace or burlap can also be paddled in; the fabric is then removed. Any one or a combination can make a pot more pleasing.

Many glazes are available. Having a selection of colors available encourages a patient to try more than one. Samples of fired glazes on display proves to be helpful to patients who must select colors for their projects.

A depressed person may become encouraged after seeing his finished project glazed and fired. Many patients benefit by working in a group setting where interaction is a motivator. They enjoy conversation and get their mind off their problems. During these sessions the staff can observe each patient to see how he or she can be best motivated. Some patients need to know exactly what to do for each step of the process of building with clay, whereas others need the freedom to change and experiment as they please.

Equipment

White low-fire clay is suitable for hand building and the potter's wheel; this clay matures at cone 06. Cones are an increment of measurement and range from 018 to 01, then from 1 to 10; 018 is the lowest and 10 is the highest. Choose the cone that melts at the maturing temperature of the clay being used. Many companies offer clay, pyrometric cones, tools, air dry clay, and acrylic or poster paint for the air dry clay. Some company catalogs have extensive lists of supplies and descriptions. A large selection of glazes and many colors

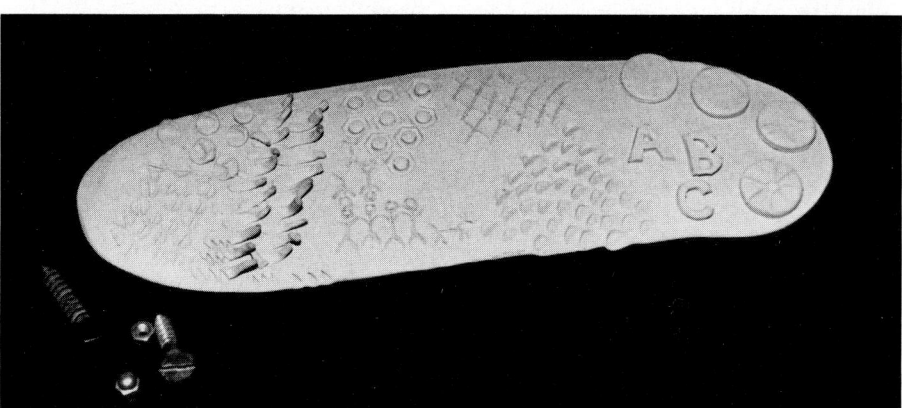

Fig. 96-16 Clay is pliable and adheres well to itself. Decorative effects can be achieved by making impressions with objects such as bolts, screws, or washers or by adding more clay pieces.

are available. Leading catalogs have pictures of the glazes after firing and helpful information. Well-known brands of potter's wheels, kilns, and ceramic equipment are usually available in these catalogs.

Equipment

Suggested equipment includes the following items:

1. A work area approximately 12 square feet, or 2 square feet per patient; this work area should be clean of foreign objects like staples, woodchips, or any foreign body that could get into the clay
2. A sturdy work table about 33 to 36 inches high
3. Slip (clay and water in the consistency of mayonnaise) is used to adhere clay to clay
4. Two or three 24 inch square boards covered with canvas; canvas prevents the clay from sticking
5. Scrap pieces of wood to set projects on while working and moving them (covered with thick plastic so the wood does not warp)
6. Shelves for storage of projects
7. Plastic to wrap projects; laundry plastic works well
8. Wood or plastic modeling tools with various flat surfaces or with angular edges
9. Toggle wire to cut clay during wedging and to cut pots off the wheel (different sized dials can be attached to the ends for comfort while pulling the wire)
10. Fettling knife and a couple of tools with short, sharp blades
11. Sponges
12. Various sized paint or ceramic brushes (for slip, decorating, and glazing)
13. Spray bottle to moisten projects
14. Two turntables about 6 inches in diameter to aid in decorating and general working
15. Rolling pin
16. Wooden spoon for paddling of surface
17. Tight clothing bucket for clay storage

Kilns

One can choose from many types of kilns. Our kiln is 22 inches in height and 25 inches in width. It is octagonal and is top loading. It is equipped with an automatic kiln sitter. The electric kiln is best for clinic use because it is much safer and easier to operate. The kiln sitter enables the staff to insert a pyrometric cone that melts at a specific temperature, signaling the kiln to shut off.

In considering a kiln, the following guidelines should be met:

1. The kiln should be 6 to 8 inches above a cement or stone floor and be situated 1 foot away from the wall.
2. Ventilation must be provided if people will be in the room during firing. A ceiling or exhaust fan is recommended. The exhaust fan pulls air to the outside and can be mounted in a window or a ceiling. There are also vents made specifically to fit above kilns.
3. The electrical system must be adequate for the kiln. The voltages run from 210 amps to 240 amps.
4. The outlet and circuit breaker must be wired to accommodate the power of the kiln.
5. When fired, kilns should be free standing. Combustible objects must not be placed on or near the surface.

Firing the kiln. The amount of time that the kiln is on will vary depending on the type of clay or glaze being fired. Neither should be turned to high too quickly. If the kiln is heated too quickly, the projects may crack or even explode. The safe practice is to turn on one switch an hour. The first firing is called bisque firing. The wares should be completely dry before they are set in the kiln; they should not feel cool to the touch. Clay can be deceiving; it can look dry and still be quite damp. If unsure of dryness, turn the bottom switch on and leave the kiln door propped open for a couple of hours, then close the lid and proceed as described above.

In all firings the top switch is turned on for an hour, which forces the heat down. The bottom switch is turned on next; in an hour another switch is turned on and so on. For earthenware clay fired from 08 to 05 the kiln should be allowed to cool for 24 hours. When ware is taken out it can be warm but not hot. If the lid is open while the pots are still hot, they risk cracking.

In a therapy department that does not have the electrical capacity for a kiln, air dry clay can be used. This clay can be used for all of the projects mentioned for earthen ware clay, but air dry clay will not have the permanence of fired clay. The air dry projects can be painted with tempora or acrylic paint, then coated with polyurethane or some other plastic medium. It must be noted that air dry clay, whether coated or just painted, is unsuitable for food or drink.

Supplies for the kiln

1. Kiln shelves
2. Shelf supports of various sizes
3. Pyrometric cones from 08 to 05
4. Stilts to hold pieces in the glaze firing
5. Glaze
6. Kiln wash; this is painted on the kiln shelf to prevent drips from glaze or glazed pots from sticking to the shelf
7. An automatic shut-off mechanism

SUMMARY

Woodcarving and ceramics are beneficial, versatile therapeutic activities. Woodcarving improves a patient's strength and endurance, and improves his ability to manipulate tools. Ceramics is a versatile activity appropriate for improving hand coordination and muscle strength. Group interaction in therapeutic activities such as woodcarving and ceramics enhances each individual's motivation and determination to regain functional use of his or her injured hand.

REFERENCES

1. Department of the Army: Craft techniques in occupational therapy, St Louis, 1971, US Army AG Publications Center.
2. Wilkinson VC and Heater SL: Therapeutic media and techniques of application, New York, 1979, Van Nostrand Reinhold Co.

BIBLIOGRAPHY

Baxter PL and Fried SL: The Work Tolerance Program of the Hand Rehabilitation Center of Philadelphia. In Hunter JM and others, editors: Rehabilitation of the hand, ed 2, St Louis, 1984, The CV Mosby Co.

Berensohn P: Finding one's way with clay, New York, 1968, Simon & Schuster.

Clark K: The potter's manual, Secaucus, NJ, 1983, Chartwell Books, Inc.

Kempin LS: Psychological motivation in successful hand therapy. In Hunter JM and others, editors: Rehabilitation of the hand, ed 2, St Louis, 1984, The CV Mosby Co.

Nelson GC: Ceramics, New York, 1960, Holt, Rinehart & Winston, Inc.

Woody ES: Hand building ceramic forms, New York, 1982, Farrar Straus Giroux.

97

Ergonomics and cumulative trauma disorders of the hand and wrist*

Thomas J. Armstrong

This chapter is concerned with ergonomics and cumulative trauma disorders of the hand and wrist. Ergonomics has been defined as the process of fitting the task to the person[41]; it is concerned with the design of work equipment, methods, and environments so that workers can achieve maximum productivity without excessive risk of injury or illness. The medical literature contains numerous accounts of workers who have experienced carpal tunnel syndrome, tendinitis, and epicondylitis because of failure to adequately deal with these design issues. This chapter will review some of the history and morbidity patterns of cumulative trauma disorders and will discuss job analysis and design.

CUMULATIVE TRAUMA DISORDERS

Although he did not use the terms ergonomics or cumulative trauma, Ramazinni (1713) did describe the concepts well over two hundred years ago:

Various and manifold is the harvest of diseases reaped by certain workers from the crafts and trades that they pursue. All the profit that they get is fatal injury to their health, mostly from two causes. The first and most potent is the harmful character of the materials they handle. The second, I ascribe to certain violent and irregular motions and unnatural postures of the body, by reason of which, the natural structure of the vital machine is so impaired that serious diseases gradually develop therefrom.[89]

The concept of a "harvest of diseases" is an aptly suited term because the modern literature shows that numerous nerve and tendon problems are associated with repeated or sustained exertions with certain postures. The term "unnatural posture" suggests that these are postures workers do not voluntarily assume and maintain, unless it is the only way a job can be performed. As a result, the afflictions of these postures are given the name of the job in which they arise. Ramazinni went on to describe how bakers, weavers, lathe workers, and writers were affected by their occupations. Gray[42] talked about "washer woman's sprain," which is known as DeQuervain's disease. Rosen and Ronchese compiled an extensive list of occupations and corresponding upper limb lesions or "marks."[94,95] Later investigators talked about gamekeepers thumb[21], drummer's palsy, flute player's hand, pizza cutter's palsy, pipetter's thumb,[73] reed-maker's elbow,[27] tobacco-primer's wrist,[83] wall washer's thumb.[112] These conditions may also occur in sport and recreational activities, e.g., tennis elbow[40], bowler's thumb,[29,49,55,74]

cuber's thumb,[120] space-invaders wrist,[70,91] slot-machine tendinitis,[79] and racket ball wrist.[97]

Cumulative trauma disorders are disorders of the soft tissues caused by repeated exertions and movements of the body. Although they can occur in nearly all tissues, the nerves, tendons, tendon sheaths, and muscles of the upper extremity are the most frequently reported sites. Other commonly used terms include the following:

Repetitive trauma disorders[50,82]
Cumulative trauma disorders[4,45]
Repetitive strain injuries[14,19,33,34,71]
Occupational cervicobrachial disorders[68,118]
Overuse syndrome[38,52,61,105]
Regional musculoskeletal disorders[43]
Work-related disorders[125]

There is no unanimous agreement about which of these terms is best, and arguments can be made for all of them. Some of the common characteristics ascribed to these disorders follow:

1. They are related to the intensity of work.
2. They involve both biomechanical and physiologic mechanisms.
3. They may occur after weeks, months, or years on the jobs.
4. They may require weeks, months, and years for recovery.
5. Their symptoms often are poorly localized and nonspecific.
6. They may have both occupational and nonoccupational causes.

Because there often is a long time between beginning work and the onset of cumulative trauma disorders, because they are not immediately life threatening and may go unreported, and because workers change jobs and employers, it is difficult to determine the exact morbidity patterns. Epidemiologic methods usually are required to isolate jobs, tools, areas, plants, or industries with excessive risk.

MORBIDITY

The overall incidence rate and prevalence of cumulative trauma disorders is not known; however, reports from insurance companies, clinics, and work sites suggest that they approach epidemic proportions and are a major cause of lost work in some settings. Studies[26,127] as early as 1927 by Zollinger and 1930 by Conn suggested that tendinitis was a major cause of lost work and insurance claims. In studies of medical clinic records for two separate military groups

---

*Adapted from Hand Clinics, Philadelphia, 1988, WB Saunders.

assigned to manual agricultural work in Great Britain, approximately 30% were found to have developed tendonitis within several months[36,86] Reed and Harcot[90] reported that 70 cases of tenosynovitis accounted for 0.54% of all visits at a U.S. industrial clinic located in the Midwest. Thompson and Plewes[111] reported that 466 of 544 peritendinitis and tenosynovitis cases seen from 1941 to 1950 at a British hospital and outpatient service were manual workers and agricultural workers.

Hymovich and Lyndholm[50] reported 62 cumulative trauma disorders during 6 years in an electronics firm with an average work force of 160 people. This amounted to an incidence rate of 6.6 cases per 200,000 work hours and resulted in a severity of 410 lost work days per 200,000 hours. Two of the disorders were classified as permanent disabilities.

In a NIOSH Health Hazard Investigation of a film manufacturing and packaging plant with 3300 workers, 104 OSHA-reportable cumulative trauma disorders—including 84 cases of tendinitis, 10 ganglionic cysts, 2 cases of epicondylitis, 4 cases of bursitis, 1 case of myositis, 2 cases of carpal tunnel syndrome, and 1 case of thoracic outlet syndrome—were reported.[1,124] Eighty-four percent of the cases came from two departments that employed 250 people, resulting in an average incidence rate of 7.0 cases per 200,000 work hours.

In a retrospective study of personal and occupational factors of carpal tunnel syndrome, Cannon, Bernacki, and Walter[22] discovered 30 cases from June 1977 to July 1978 in a work population of 20,000 workers. Sixteen of these cases were identified from worker compensation claims; although the remainder were known to medical department personnel, worker compensation claims had not been initiated.

In a study by Armstrong and others,[8] the incidence of cumulative trauma disorders reported to the medical department of a poultry processing plant was 12.8 cases per 200,000 hours.[10] For one job, thigh skinning, the rate was 129.6, or an average of 1.3 cases per worker per year.

In a study of 1979 worker's compensation claims for wrist injuries from 26 states, Jensen and others[51] discovered that more than 6% (3027 cases) were related to inflammation or irritation of the joint, tendons, or muscles or diseases of the nerves or peripheral ganglia. These injuries were all related to repetitive pressure, voluntary motions, overexertion: lifting, pulling, or throwing. The average cost per claim was $618 in medical payments and $1026 in indemnity compensation. In a study by Fine and associates[35] of two automobile plants, it was found that from 7 to 31 more cumulative trauma disorders were reported through personal medical records than through worker's compensation reports.

Worker interviews and physical examinations may provide the most sensitive measures of cumulative trauma disorders. Margolis and colleagues[69] used a mail survey to determine that 62% of female supermarket checkers between 18 and 49 years of age had symptoms of carpal tunnel syndrome. Silverstein and others[101] reported prevalences of 0.6% to 5.6% among 652 male and female industrial workers, depending on the repetitiveness and forcefulness of their jobs; these data were based on interviews and physical examinations. Armstrong and others[12] reported prevalences of 0.6% to 10.8% for hand and wrist tendinitis in the same population. Nathan and associates[78] reported sensory slowing of the median nerve in 39% of 471 industrial employees from 27 occupations in 4 industries. These studies suggest that the prevalence of carpal tunnel syndrome and hand and wrist tendinitis is much higher than indicated by medical visits and compensation claims.

It can be concluded that cumulative trauma disorders are a major health problem in some work settings. The remainder of this paper will elaborate on the character, causes, and prevention of some of the most common work-related disorders.

OCCUPATIONAL FACTORS

Most of the papers published on cumulative trauma disorders during the past 100 years deal mainly with their diagnosis or treatment. Within these papers are numerous references to occupational factors. A few papers describe studies of pathomechanics; a few, epidemiologic studies; and a few, prevention through the design of work equipment and methods. Repetitiveness, forcefulness, mechanical stress, posture, vibration, low temperatures, and unaccustomed work activities are consistently implicated as factors of cumulative trauma disorders of the hand and wrist. Because these factors arise in the performance of work or the interaction of the worker and work equipment, these risk factors are referred to here as "ergonomic factors." Although ergonomic factors are commonly cited, the data are insufficient to predict the effect of changing any one of them. The ability to predict is further complicated by the occurrence of more than one factor in a given work situation. For example, a job may be repetitive and forceful and involve occasional postural stresses and exposure to vibration. While reducing any one of these stresses should reduce risk of cumulative trauma disorders, the amount of risk and its significance is difficult to predict. For these reasons it is essential that any work changes to control cumulative trauma disorders be evaluated. Several iterations may be required to achieve the desired level of control. This section will discuss each of the risk factors, how they are evaluated, and some of the ways in which they can be controlled.

JOB DOCUMENTATION

Before ergonomic stresses can be identified, it is necessary to document what the worker does. This entails:
1. The work objective
2. The work standard
3. The work method
4. Workplace layout
5. Work equipment
6. Materials

The work objective

The work objective is the reason the job is performed, for example, putting wheels on cars, entering data into the computer, and removing fat from hams. Often the job title will reflect the objective.

The work standard

The work standard is an expression of the quantity and quality of work expected in a given period. Manufacturing work standards usually are expressed in numbers of assemblies or parts.[15,81] In office settings, they may be expressed in terms of key strokes, numbers of documents, transactions, or other tasks. Standards are based on the concept of a fair day's work and should be within the work capacity of 95% of the work force.[15,81] In addition to the base standard, there may be incentives or bonuses by which workers can earn additional income for working above the standard. In some cases these are based on individual performance and in others on group performance. Work incentives also should be documented.

The work method

The work method is the procedure used to accomplish the work objective and is described as a sequence of steps or elements. Generally, there are many ways by which a given job can be performed; however, the work standard is based on the assumption of a "standard method."[15,81] The work standard should include a description of the standard method on which it is based. As a practical matter, the method employed by the worker may, in fact, be significantly different from the standard method. These differences should be documented.

Workplace layout

The workplace layout describes how the work equipment is arranged in the workplace. This description may be verbal, such as "worker seated at work bench," or the description may be graphic, such as a blueprint.

Work equipment

Work equipment is any device used to accomplish or facilitate accomplishing the work objective. Examples include presses, jigs, hoists, hand tools, document holders, and seating. In some cases equipment is commercially available, so it may be only necessary to look in a catalogue to determine exact sizes, weights, and capacities. In other cases the equipment may be unique to that job and require complete on-the-job documentation. In some cases the equipment may be improvised by the worker and provide insight into ways of reducing ergonomic stresses.

Materials

The materials include objects that go into the product. In assembly operations these might include parts, lubricants, coatings, and packing materials; in clerical work, documents and information; in meat processing, pieces of meat and bags of additives.

Sources of information

Sources of information include:
1. Industrial engineering
2. Personnel departments
3. Engineering drawing and equipment manuals and catalogues
4. On-site inspection
5. Supervisor interviews
6. Worker interviews

Engineering, personnel, drawings. Work standards, methods, process data, and plant layouts often can be obtained from industrial, manufacturing, product, facility, and plant engineering departments. Depending on the sophistication of these data, it may be possible to complete much

of the job analysis off-site. Formal job descriptions often can be obtained from personnel departments; however, these descriptions tend to emphasize worker qualifications in terms of worker attributes such as education or strength and dexterity, rather than in terms of job attributes such as reach distances, forces, and work rates.

On-site inspection. An on-site inspection should always be performed to verify information obtained in job descriptions and drawings and to collect other information needed for the analysis. The on-site visit will also afford an opportunity to interview supervisors and workers. Differences between the published method and layout and the actual method and layout are not uncommon. Workers often find ways of arranging their work and performing the motions that are faster and easier than those designed by engineers. Also, there may be difficulties with certain pieces of work equipment that cause workers to abandon them in favor of manual methods. Similarly, there may be differences from worker to worker owing to differences in body size, strength, and skill or to differences in work equipment. In a recent visit to a work site in which all workers were using the same kind of equipment to do the same job, the author found that some people spent most of their time watching the machines run while others spent most of their time working on them. Further investigation revealed that machines were assigned according to seniority and that low seniority people inevitably got the old machines, which frequently jammed. The old machines required much more work to achieve the production standard than the new ones. These differences often provide insight into how the job can be simplified to reduce ergonomic stresses on the worker. Consequently, in the example just cited, a progressive maintenance program to reduce machine jams was recommended.

Supervisor and worker interviews. Worker and supervisor interviews require care not to suggest responses. For example, when a person of authority asks a worker, "Doesn't that tool hurt your hand?" it suggests that there is something wrong with the tool. Whenever possible, questions should be asked in ways that provide choices. For example, ask "what do you like best about the tool?" followed by "what do you like the least?" Follow-up questions can be used to provide additional information. It is desirable to complete the job documentation before proceeding with the ergonomic assessment, although additional detail can be added as specific ergonomic factors are considered.

REPETITIVENESS

Repetitiveness of work is one of the most commonly cited risk factors of cumulative trauma disorders.* As early as 1927 Obolenskaja and Glojanitzki[57] talked about hand motions per minute and per shift as factors of tendinitis. In 1934 Hammer[44] expressed repetitiveness in terms of the manipulations per hour. Later in 1979 Kuorinka and Koskinen[56] expressed repetitiveness in terms of the number of parts handled per year. Armstrong and colleagues[8] and Silverstein and colleagues[101] expressed repetitiveness in terms of fundamental cycles to relate physiologic measures to work measures.

These concepts are illustrated in the job shown in the box on p. 1178. In this job the worker gets a wheel from the

---

*References 8, 44, 50, 76, 101, 111, 113, 114, 121, 123.

JOB DOCUMENTATION FOR "PUT WHEELS ON CAR"

Objective

Install wheels on front and rear of car

Standard

60 cars per hour

Method

With both hands:
1. Reach for wheel with both hands
2. Grasp wheel
3. Move wheel to car
4. Position wheel on car
5. Release wheel

With right hand:	With left hand:	
6. Reach for screwgun	6. Reach for lugbolt	
7. Grasp screwgun	7. Grasp bolt	
8. Move screwgun near wheel	8. Move bolt to wheel	
9. Hold screwgun	9. Position bolt in wheel	×5
10. Move screwgun to wheel	10. Idle	
11. Position screwgun	11. Idle	
12. Use screwgun	12. Idle	
13. Move screwgun to belt	13. Idle	
14. Release screwgun		

Work equipment

Nut runner

Materials

Wheels
Lug bolts
Automobile

Work layout

Rack with wheels (center of wheels 36 inches high)
Assembly line (center of wheels 30 inches high)

---

rack, carries it to the front of a car passing on the assembly line, and drives five stud-bolts. The process is then repeated for the rear wheel. The line speed is 60 cars per hour.

Steps 6 through 12 are repeated five times for both the front and the rear wheel. To compare with other jobs, repetitiveness of the wheel install job could be expressed as 60 cars per hour, 120 wheels per hour, 600 bolts per hour, or 720 exertions per hour.

The detail can be varied to suit the purpose of the analysis. For example, "get part" may be sufficient to describe a situation where parts are taken at random from a fixed location, whereas "reach," "grasp," "inspect," and "move" may be required to describe a situation where extra movements are required for inspection. In the above example it is sufficient to say "get" the wheel. Work methods analyses can be performed by observing a worker do the job, by observing films or videotapes or from workplace drawings.

Many companies keep files of methods as part of their work standards program.

In addition to counting the number of exertions, it is necessary to look at the part of the body performing the exertion. For example, the exertions required to put wheels on cars are different from those required to enter data on a keyboard or to trim meat. This information should be taken into consideration in the placement of restricted workers and in the selecton of work regimens that minimize loading on any one part of the body.

Cumulative trauma

Although safe limits of repetitiveness are not yet known, it has been shown that risk of cumulative trauma disorders such as tendinitis and carpal tunnel syndrome increase with increasing repetitiveness and force. Studies by Silverstein and others[101] showed that the risk of carpal tunnel syndrome was 5.5 times greater in persons performing highly repetitive jobs where the same motions were repeated at less than 30-second cycles for more than 50% of the work shift, than in persons performing low repetitive jobs where the motions were repeated at more than 30-second cycles or for less than 50% of the work shift. The risk in persons performing highly repetitive jobs combined with high forces was 15.5 times greater than those performing low force and low repetitive jobs. Similar findings were reported by Armstrong and others[8] for hand and wrist tendinitis and by Feldman and others[32] for upper extremity pain and numbness in an electronics plant.

Reducing repetitiveness

It suffices to say that if a cumulative trauma problem exists and it cannot be controlled by regulation of other factors, then the repetitiveness should be reduced. This may be done by doing the following:
1. Changing the work standard
2. Using mechanical aids
3. Rotating workers
4. Enlarging the work content

Changing the work standard. From a technical standpoint, changing work standards is perhaps the simplest measure; but from a practical standpoint, it may be difficult to implement. Management may be concerned about lost work; labor may be concerned about lost incentives or bonuses. I have heard patients admit reluctance to report problems because they were afraid of being put on a restriction where they would not earn a bonus, or they were afraid of being placed in a lower paying job. Management and labor have to be convinced to take a long-term view of the situation. Profits are not a simple function of the revenue from parts produced. They are related to the revenue from parts produced and the human costs. The human costs resulting from cumulative trauma disorders is becoming a major profit factor in many work situations. Similarly, workers need to realize that they have to assume a pace and a pay scale that they can maintain for their working lifetime. It may be difficult for a worker who is well-adapted to high work pace to accept the work pace and pay scale of the person next to him, who may not be well-adapted. The treating physician or rehabilitation professional has an important job educating management and labor about these issues.

Using mechanical aids. Mechanical aids include jigs and

fixtures for holding parts, feeders for loading hand tools and machines, ejectors for unloading machines, and power tools. In the above "wheel install" example, it may be possible to use a multiple spindle nut runner to drive all five studs at once and thus eliminate four movements per wheel. The advantages of mechanical aids may be offset if there is a corresponding increase in production standards.

Worker rotation. Worker rotations entail moving workers among different jobs to reduce the loading on any one part of the body. Rotation is a relatively simple concept, but often it is hard to implement. First, a detailed methods analysis is required. It probably will not do any good to rotate workers among jobs that require the same pattern of exertions. Also, desirable rotation patterns may conflict with seniority schedules, labor contracts, and worker preferences. Rotation requires workers to be qualified on multiple jobs, which requires training time. If these obstacles can be overcome, there are some advantages in flexibility in dealing with changes in production schedules and absenteeism. Rotations may be facilitated by employee involvement programs in which workers participate in the designing of rotation patterns and schedules.

Work enlargement. Work enlargement entails combining jobs of different motion patterns. The concepts and problems are similar to those of worker rotations. In addition, work enlargement may require redesign of the production line and will require resetting of production standards. For example, a production process may be changed from a moving line to a bench assembly operation. This may be a good opportunity to implement mechanical aids that cannot be used on a moving line.

FORCEFUL EXERTIONS

Virtually all hand activities involve the exertion of force to propel or stabilize the fingers and wrist against gravity, inertia, and external loads. These forces are produced by the contractile proteins in muscles and transmitted through myofacial sheaths, tendons, bones, and ligaments. These forces require the expenditure of energy and result in elastic and viscous deformation of tissues. Some investigators have observed that the risk of cumulative trauma disorders increases with the force of exertion.* There is not yet agreement about what constitutes excessive force, and the effect of reducing force cannot be predicted. It should be safe to assume that reducing force probably will have a greater effect if it is exerted throughout the work cycles than if it is exerted only occasionally. Steps for reducing force should be considered if cumulative trauma disorders have been reported for a given job.

Identification of forceful elements

The forceful elements of a job can be identified from the work methods analysis performed in the job documentation. Exertions are required to move objects, to lift, lower, or slide, or to hold objects against gravity or reaction forces. For example, in the wheel install job shown in the box on p. 1178, exertions are required to lift and hold the wheel while it is carried and to hold the screwgun against the force of gravity and its own reaction forces. In many cases, information about the tools and materials can be used to es-

timate the minimum force requirements or at least to rank order tasks and tools in terms of their force requirements. For example, it will probably require more force to hold a 5 kg tool than a 2 kg tool. Similarly, all things being the same, it will require more force to tighten bolts to 100 newton-meters than to 50 newton-meters.

Estimation of task force requirements

In some cases it is possible to actually estimate the task force requirements. The amount of finger force required to hold an object as shown in Fig. 97-1 is proportional to the force causing it to slip out of the hand and inversely proportional to the coefficient of friction.[20,25] Coefficients of friction for various materials in contact with skin are shown in Table 97-1. Some materials such as paper and suede are sensitive to the moistness of the skin. This can be seen by estimating the minimum force required to hold a 2 kg (20 n) book. The minimum force requirements of tasks such as those shown in Fig. 97-1 can be computed. For example, to calculate the pinch force required to hold a 5-pound book as shown above (see Table 97-1):

$$\text{Moist skin: } F_p = 20/(2 \times 0.42) = 24.0 \text{ newtons}$$
$$\text{Dry skin: } F_p = 20/(2 \times 0.27) = 37.0 \text{ newtons}$$

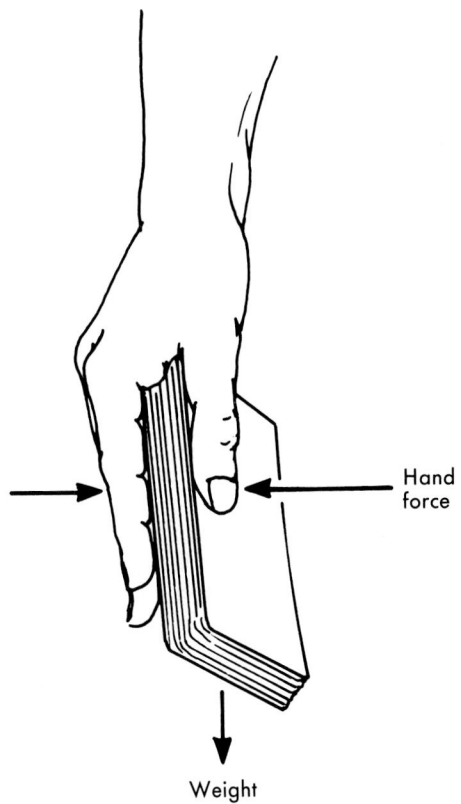

$$\text{Hand force} = \frac{\text{Weight}}{2 \times \text{coefficient of friction}}$$

Fig. 97-1 Hand force is proportional to the force causing the object to slip out of the hand and inversely proportional to its slipperiness (coefficient of friction). (From Armstrong TJ: Hand Clin 2:553, 1986.)

---

*References 6, 7, 8, 76, 101, 111, 113, 114, 123.

Table 97-1 Coefficients of friction for human palmer skin against various materials, n = 7 subjects

Material	Dry (n = 42)	Moist (n = 42)	Combined (n = 84)
Sand paper (#320)	—	—	0.61 + 0.10
Smooth vinyl	—	—	0.53 + 0.18
Textured vinyl	—	—	0.50 + 0.11
Adhesive tape	0.41 + 0.10	0.66 + 0.14	—
Suede	0.39 + 0.06	0.66 + 0.11	—
Aluminum	—	—	0.38 + 0.13
Paper	0.27 + 0.09	0.42 + 0.07	—

Approximately 53% more force is required to hold the tool when the skin is dry than is required to hold it when the skin is moist. The moisture content of the skin will be affected by the objects that are being handled. If the objects are dry and absorbent, the skin can be expected to lose moisture and the force requirements to increase.

These are minimum strength requirements. Most people will exert more than the minimum required and some will exert considerably more.[20,88]

Evaluation of work pace, use of gloves, and hand posture

Other important factors affecting force include work pace, use of gloves, and hand posture. The effect of pace on force has been studied using surface electromyography.[13,60,65,66,110] Arndt[13] reported that the magnitude of the integrated surface electromyogram was nearly twice as great in a fast-paced materials handling task as in a correspondingly slow-paced task. Thus increasing the work standard may increase task force requirements, as well as repetitiveness.

Gloves may increase or decrease the force requirements depending on how the task is performed. Hertzberg[46] showed that 25% to 30% of the hand strength may be required to overcome the stiffness and bulk of Air Force pilot gloves. Thus gloves can significantly increase the strength requirements unless great care is exercised in their selection. Gloves may also decrease the force required to hold objects by altering friction. Studies by Riley[92] and others (1985) have shown that use of certain gloves may decrease the strength requirements by increasing friction. It can be anticipated that in other cases where it is desirable that objects slide through the hand, use of certain gloves would reduce friction. The friction and force requirements of a given brand of gloves must be determined empirically as described by Hertzburg,[46] Riley[92] or Buchholz[20].

The load and physiologic cost of an exertion of the hand also is affected by hand posture. Studies by Swansen and associates[107] show that from 15% to 20% of the amount of force can be exerted in pinch grip as in power grip.[59,63,77] Studies by Chao and others[23] and Armstrong[2] show that approximately three times as much muscle force is required to exert the same force levels in "pinch" as in "power grip." The tasks that must be performed with a pinch grip will carry a higher physiologic cost than those that can be performed with a power grip.

Reduction of force requirements

Safe force levels for repetitive work have not yet been determined. Common sense dictates that the force require-

ments of a task be minimized wherever possible, particularly if experience shows there has been a problem with cumulative trauma disorders. Steps for reducing the load include the following:

1. Friction enhancement
2. Picking up fewer objects at a time
3. Changing the weight of tools
4. Balancing tools
5. Use of torque control devices
6. Use of hoists or articulating arms
7. Use of conveyors, nonpowered or powered
8. Use of work surfaces to facilitate materials handling
9. Use of gravity to facilitate materials handling
10. Use of jigs and fixtures to hold parts
11. Use of handles that can be gripped
12. Selection of gloves
13. Maintenance
14. Quality control

Friction enhancement may entail increasing friction to reduce the force to hold objects or decreasing friction to make it easier for them to slide through the hands. Friction can be changed through the use of surface treatments using Table 97-1 as a guide. For example, covering an aluminum handle with textured rubber will enhance its friction. In other cases where it is not possible to alter the material's friction characteristics, it may be possible to enhance friction using gloves. The information in Table 97-1 may be used to provide insight into how glove materials might affect friction, but testing should be performed to identify the best glove for a given task.

Picking up fewer objects at a time may need to be considered against the need for additional movements that may increase repetitiveness and force. Handling fewer objects at a time should not result in difficulty achieving the work standard.

Reducing the weight of a tool, either through selection or redesign, will reduce the force required to support it against gravity; but reducing the weight of some tools may increase the force required to use them. The decision to decrease or increase weight should be based on how the tool is used. For example, if a power tool is used to drive screws in a horizontal surface as shown in Fig. 97-2, then increasing the weight will reduce the force required to hold it in place, but increase the force to hold it in between tasks (Fig. 97-2). If the tool is used to drive screws in a vertical surface, then reducing the force will reduce the effort to hold the tool but will not increase the effort to keep it engaged in the screw (Fig. 97-2).

The balance of a tool is related to the magnitude of the gravity and reaction forces acting on the tool and their distance from the center of the tool. An unbalanced tool will have a tendency to twist out of the hand and will require more force than a balanced tool. For example, a cut that is performed with the tip of a long knife blade will require more grip force than one that is performed with the tip of a short blade knife (see Fig. 97-3). Tools can be balanced by changing their shape or by adding, removing, or rearranging weight. For example, an in-line powered screwdriver may be balanced by rearranging its airline attachment as shown in Fig. 97-4. A task analysis is required to determine the best solution for a given tool and situation.

The tendency for a tool to twist in the hand may also be caused by its torquing action on turn-to-tighten fasteners.

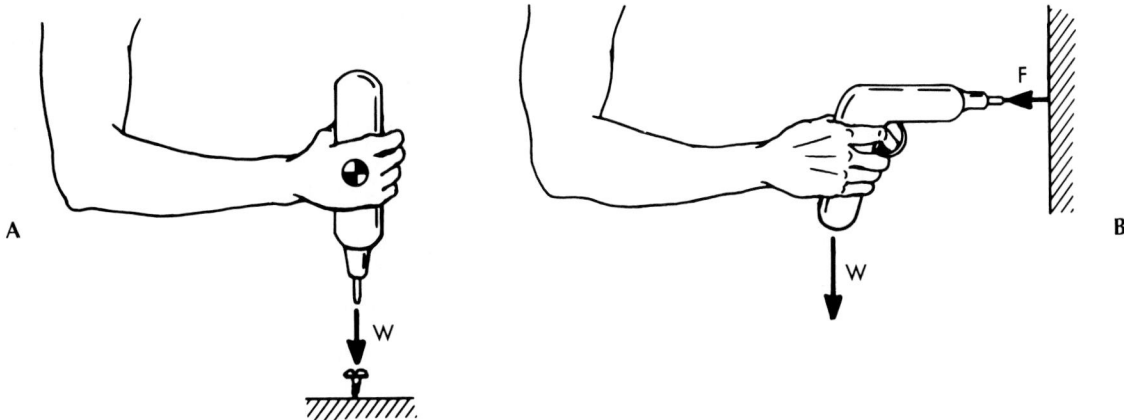

Fig. 97-2   **A,** Increasing weight helps to keep the bit engaged on the horizontal surface, but will make the tool heavier to lift. **B,** Increasing weight only will increase task strength requirements on the vertical surface.

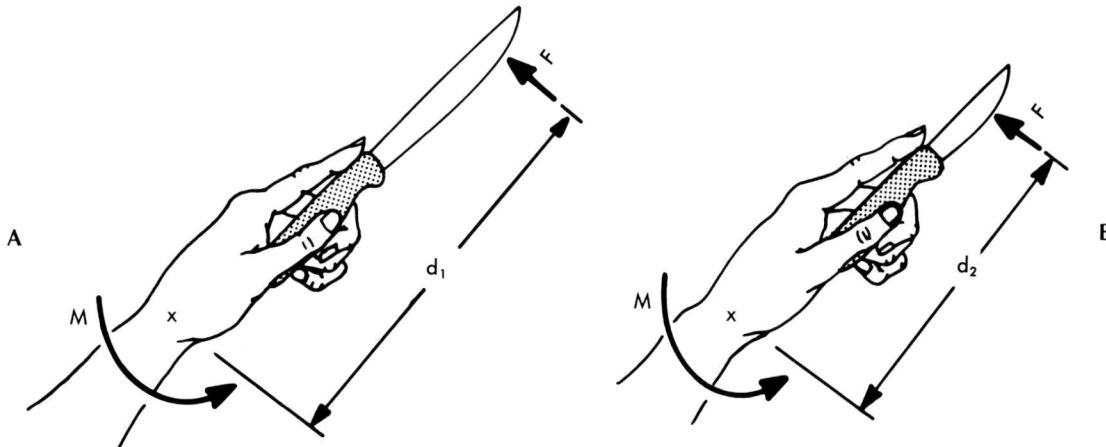

Fig. 97-3   **A,** Cutting with the tip of the blade tends to twist the knife out of the worker's hand. **B,** Using a shorter blade will reduce the twisting moment and the task force requirements.

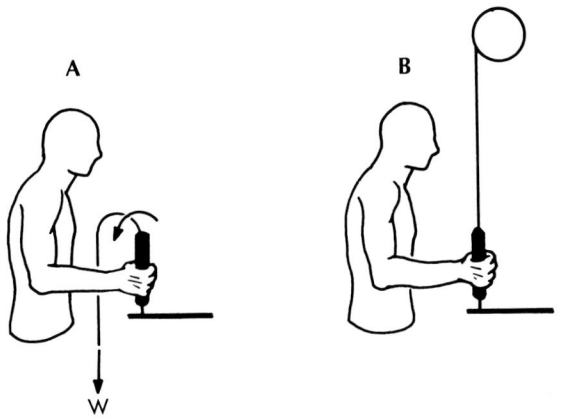

Fig. 97-4   The strength required to keep the tool from twisting out of the hand, **A,** can be eliminated by using an overhead airline attachment, **B.** (From Armstrong TJ: Hand Clin 2:553, 1986.)

These reaction forces may be reduced by reducing the speed or torque setting of the tool, lengthening the handle of the tool, or by the use of a torque reaction bar (Fig. 97-5). A task analysis is required to determine the best solution for a given tool and situation.

Hoists and articulating arms often can be used to support the weight of tools. These devices are particularly useful where it is not possible to change the tool or the number of parts handled at a time. In fact, such devices may even make possible the use of larger tools and handling of more parts at a time while at the same time decreasing force and repetitiveness. Articulating arms may be advantageous over hoists because they can be used to reach in and around workplace obstructions. They can be mounted at a fixed location or on a track to follow a production line, and they can be used to control torque forces transmitted to the worker as shown in Fig. 97-6.[117]

It often is possible to design the work surface, jigs, or fixtures to support materials and assemblies. This may reduce or eliminate a force exertion, as well as free one or both hands. It is important that the materials and assemblies

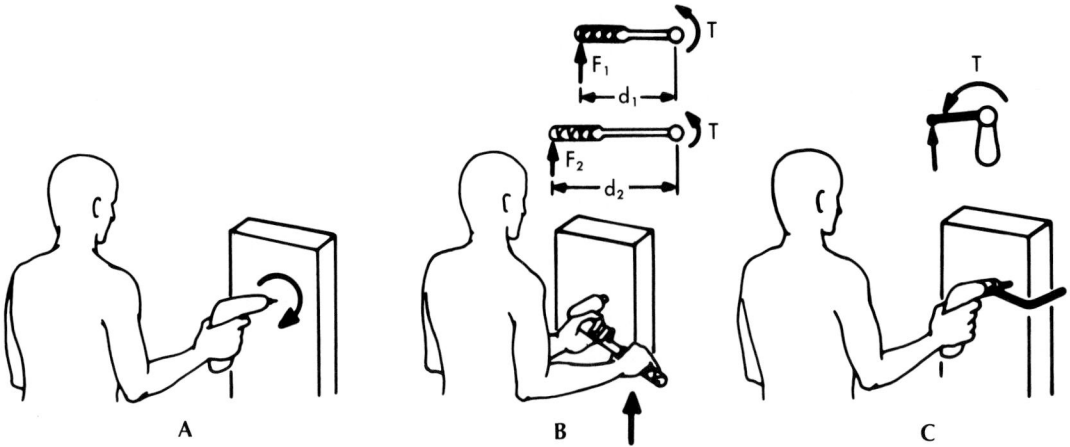

Fig. 97-5 **A,** The hand force required to hold a power screwgun is related to the tightness of the fastener and torque setting of the tool. **B,** Hand force often can be reduced by using a longer tool, or, **C,** by using a reaction bar.

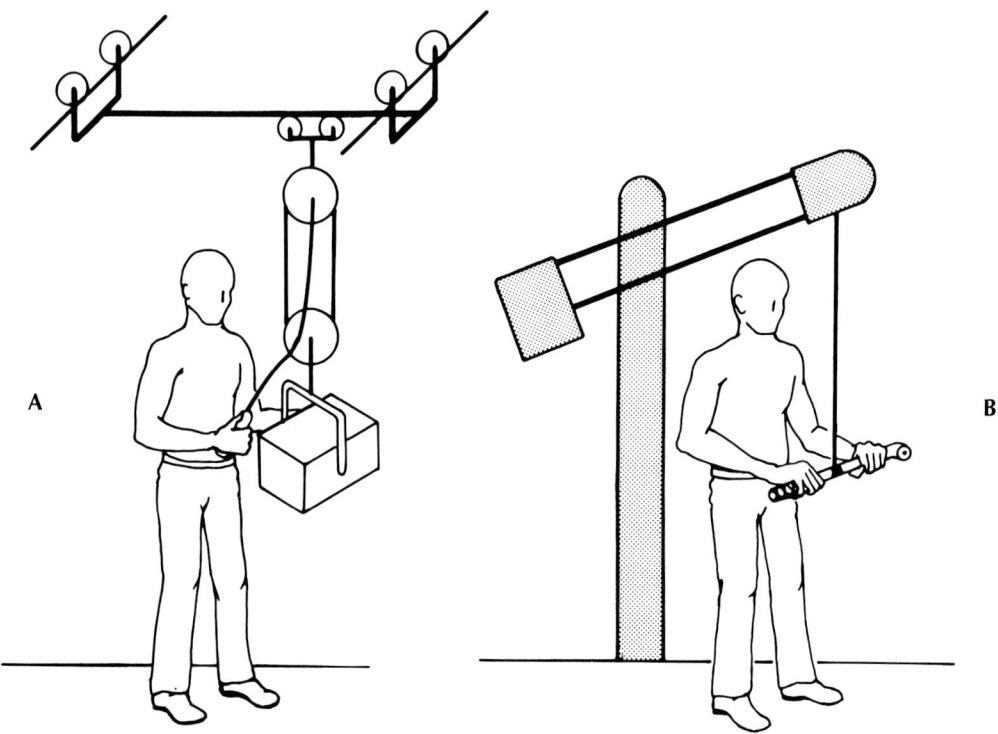

Fig. 97-6 **A,** Hoists can be used to reduce the force requirements of manual materials-handling tasks. **B,** Articulating arms also can be used to reduce the force requirements caused by tool weight and torque.

be supported at a location and orientation at which the task can be performed conveniently without undue postural stress (Fig. 97-7).

It may be possible to slope the work surface so that gravity can be used to propel the part or assembly to the next step in the production process or into a container (Fig. 97-7). It also may be possible to use nonpowered roller conveyors or powered belt conveyors.

Where possible, objects that are to be held in the hands should have handles that can be held using a power grip.

Cartons and tote pans should have cutouts as shown in Fig. 97-8.

The force requirements may also be affected by quality control. Poor quality control may result in size differences among parts, which requires extra effort to put together. Examples of this often are seen in mechanical assembly and upholstery operations.

Poor quality control may be the result of poor maintenance. Examples of this often are seen in molding operations. The dimensions of parts may change as the dies of

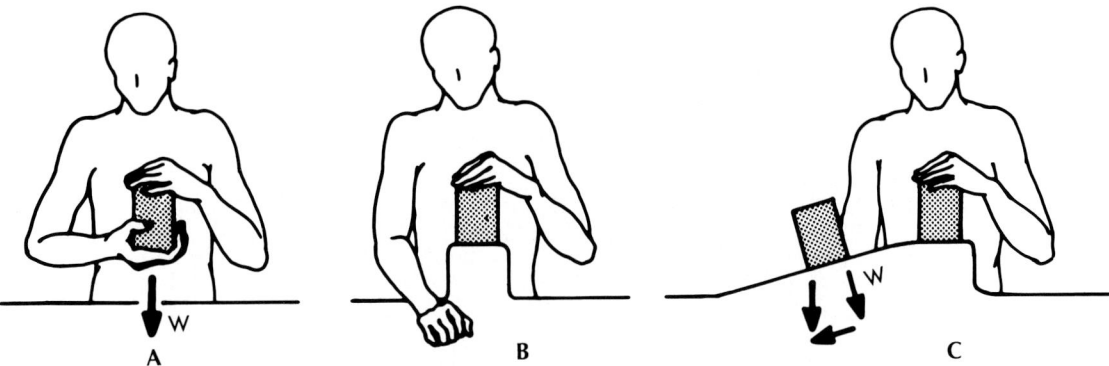

Fig. 97-7 The force required to hold parts, **A,** can be reduced by providing an elevated work surface or fixture, **B.** Gravity can be used to facilitate moving the part to the next location, **C.**

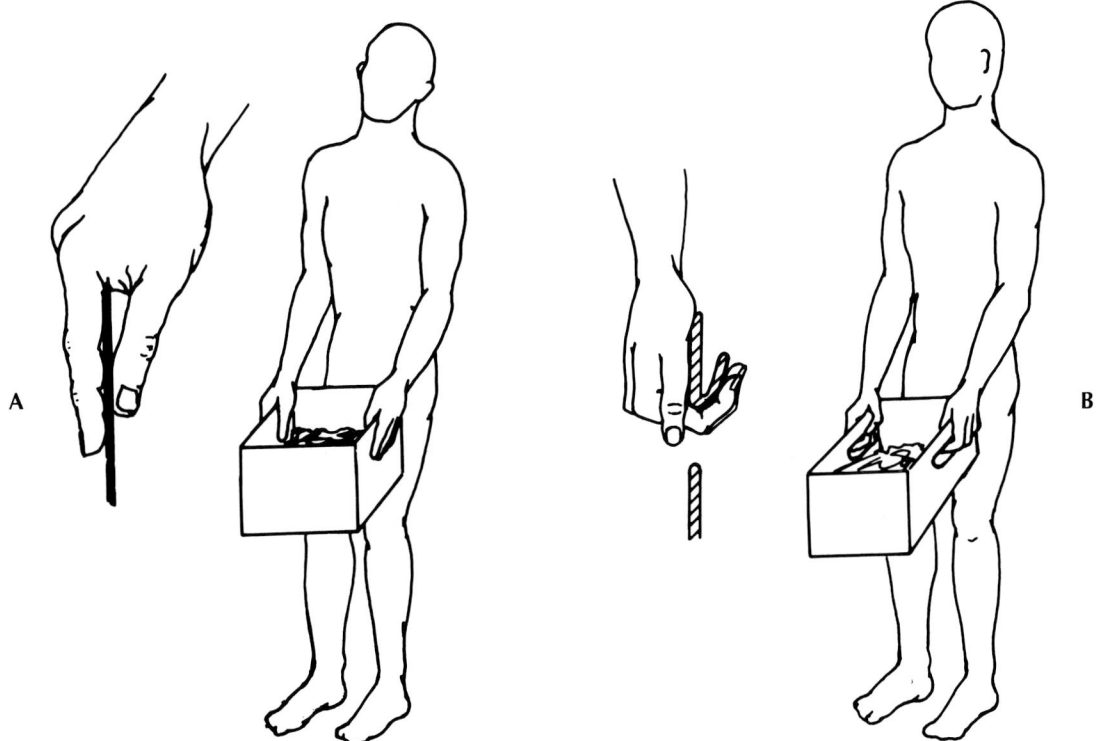

Fig. 97-8 More effort is required to hold cartons and tote pans by pinching, **A,** than gripping, **B.** Cutouts can be used to facilitate gripping. (Modified from Armstrong TJ: Hand Clin 2:553, 1986.)

the press change. Maintenance may also affect the force required to use cutting and finishing tools such as knives, scissors, and sanders, and screwdrivers.[80]

The use of gloves should be reviewed to be sure that they fit well to minimize the strength required for a given job. In some cases, where only palm protection is required, it may be possible to remove the fingers from the gloves. In other cases, where only finger protection is required, it may be possible to protect the fingers with tape. Tests should be performed to determine the best gloves for a given task. Tests might entail hand strength measurements or subjective ratings while performing the job or laboratory simulations.

There is not yet agreement on a safe force level for re-petitive work. It is hard to rationalize anything greater than what is technically feasible, particularly for jobs where workers have had cumulative trauma disorders.

MECHANICAL STRESSES

Mechanical stresses are produced when the soft tissues are squeezed between bone and external objects, such as tools, parts, and the work station. Fig. 97-9 illustrates how the skin is deformed and the stresses are concentrated on the underlying bone when squeezing a clothespin. The magnitude of these stresses is related to the contact force and the area of contact. The contact force can be very high. An average male can exert 540 to 640 newtons of hand force,

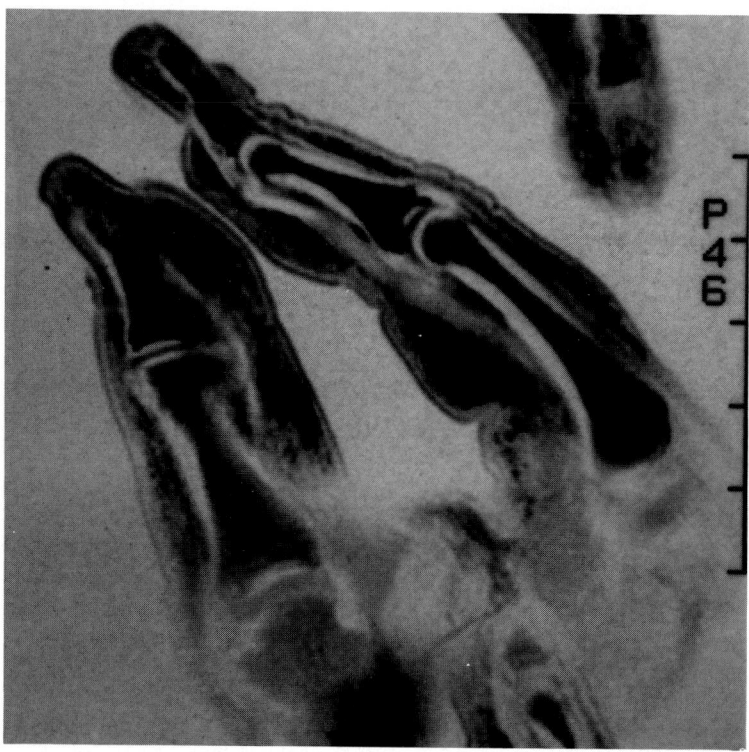

Fig. 97-9 Nuclear magnetic resonance (NMR) scan of hand pinching clothespin shows skin deformation and stress concentration on underlying bone.

and an average female can exert 290 to 340 newtons.[99,107] Even higher forces may be produced when the hand is used for pounding. Exertion of this force results in reaction forces that are transmitted through the skin of the hand to the underlying tendons. The finger flexor tendons are a common site of stenosing-tenosynovitis-crepitans or "trigger fingers."[87,104] Trigger finger may be associated with tools that have hard or sharp handles as shown in Fig. 97-10, *A*.

Another cumulative trauma disorder attributable to mechanical stress involves the digital nerves in the fingers.[29,55]

Compression of the digital nerves is produced by tools such as scissors that rub on the sides of the fingers (Fig. 97-11, *A*).

Tools and parts that are supported over the base of the palm as shown in Fig. 97-12, *A* can cause pressure on the median nerve and thus contribute to carpal tunnel syndrome.* Percussion over the median nerve (Tinel's test) often is used to diagnose a median nerve compression injury inside the wrist.

---

*References 48, 54, 84, 108, 113, 114.

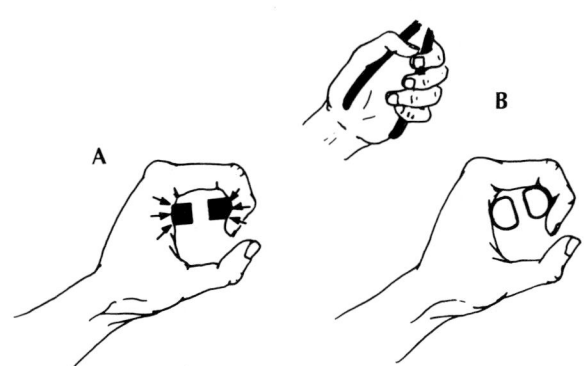

Fig. 97-10 **A,** Gripping objects with hard sharp edges produces stress concentrations on the skin and underlying tendons. **B,** Objects that are held in the hand should be made from compliant materials and have well-rounded corners. (From Armstrong TJ: Hand Clin 2:553, 1986.)

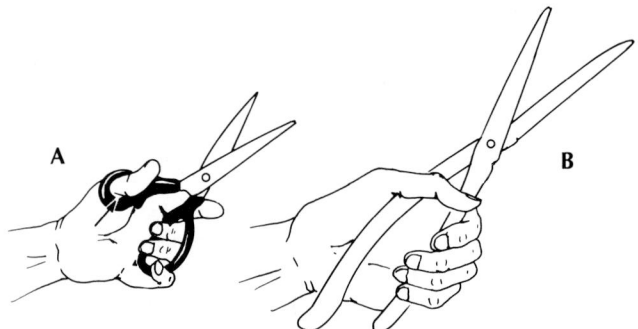

Fig. 97-11 **A,** Scissors produce stress concentrated over the sides of fingers. **B,** Handles should be designed to distribute forces only on the palmar surfaces of the fingers. (From Armstrong TJ: Hand Clin 2:553, 1986.)

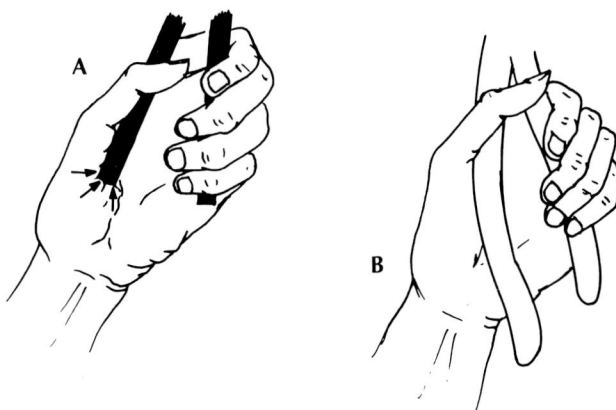

Fig. 97-12 A, Handles supported over the base of the palm produce pressure on the median nerve. **B,** Handles should be as large as possible so that forces are distributed uniformly over the thenar eminences. (From Armstrong TJ: Hand Clin 2:553, 1986.)

Identification of mechanical stresses

Mechanical stresses are identified from inspection of the work elements. Any element that entails the exertion of force involves the risk of a mechanical stress. Mechanical stresses may also result from bumping or resting on objects in the work place.

Control measures

Control measures for mechanical stresses include these:
1. Enlarging handles
2. Rounding edges of handles and benches
3. Use of compliant handle materials
4. Use of tools for pounding
5. Padding the hand.

As a general rule, handles should be as large as possible for a given task, have well-rounded corners, and be covered with compliant rubber or plastic (Figs. 97-10, *B,* and 97-11, *B*). Handles should be long enough to distribute the forces over the muscular eminences at the base of the thumb and little finger as shown in Fig. 97-12, *B*.[3,113,114]

Stresses on the sides, as well as the backs, of the fingers can be controlled by using straight, plastic-coated handles with a spring-opening device (Fig. 97-10, *B*).

In some cases, hammers or other percussive tools can be used to eliminate mechanical stresses produced by pounding with the hand. In other cases, pads may be used to cushion these stresses, but care should be exercised not to interfere with grasping.

POSTURE

Movements of the wrist, flexion-extension, and radial-ulnar deviation cause the tendons to be displaced past and against adjacent anatomic surfaces. For example, flexion and extension of the wrist are associated with tenosynovitis of the flexor and extensor tendons in the wrist and with carpal tunnel syndrome.* Nerves also may be stretched and compressed by exertions in certain postures. Flexing the wrist causes the median nerve to be compressed between

the finger flexor tendons and the flexor retinaculum, whereas extending the wrist causes the nerve to be stretched around the tendons. Phalen[84,85] recognized this and proposed what has become known as the "wrist flexion," or "Phalen's test" for carpal tunnel syndrome in which the forearms are held vertically and the wrists are flexed under the weight of the hands for 1 minute. Precipitation of numbness and tingling in the median innervated areas of the hand is considered a positive sign of carpal tunnel syndrome. Smith and others[103] suggested that this test could be accelerated if subjects pinched at the same time. Phalen went on to suggest, "Occupations that require active finger flexion with the wrist flexed should certainly predispose to carpal tunnel syndrome. . ."[84] Examples of this posture often are seen in materials handling, use of hand tools and keyboards, and in assembly operations.

Ulnar and radial deviation of the wrist are associated with tenosynovitis at the base of the thumb, or DeQuervain's disease†. Examples of these postures often are seen in the use of hand tools and in assembly and packing operations. Jobs should be designed so that the wrist is maintained in a neutral position that is not flexed, hyperextended, or deviated side-to-side. This posture can be demonstrated by letting the arm hang relaxed at the side of the body.

Identification of stressful postures

Stressful postures can be identified by watching workers perform the job. The postural analysis can be facilitated by films or videotapes that can be replayed in slow motion.[10]

Control measures

Stressful postures can be controlled through:
1. Work location
2. Work orientation
3. Tool design
4. Consideration of worker size

Tool design. Tichauer[113] showed that an outbreak of DeQuervain's disease and related cumulative trauma disorders at an electronics manufacturing plant was associated with the use of needle-nose pliers that required workers to deviate their wrists (Fig. 97-13, *A*). The problem was solved by redesigning the handles of the pliers to reduce wrist deviation (Fig. 97-13, *B*).

In another study, Armstrong and others[10] found that ulnar wrist deviation and flexion were required by poultry cutters to hold and use a knife for boning thighs (Fig. 97-14, *A*). A pistol-shaped knife was proposed to reduce this deviation (Fig. 97-14, *B*). The efficacy of this proposal was evaluated by laboratory and field testing of a prototype.[5]

The concept of bent-handled tools is not new.[102,115,119] Some examples of nineteenth century tools are shown in Fig. 97-15. One of the greatest differences between modern tools and tools of the past is that tools of the past usually were made or purchased by the person who used them. Consequently, much attention was given to the size and shape. Today, tools usually are specified by an engineer, ordered by a purchasing agent, and supplied by a tool room attendant; the users may be completely left out of the selection process.

Work location and orientation and worker size. An

---

*References 2, 6, 9, 17, 84, 93, 109, 113.

*References 47, 53, 58, 76, 106, 111, 113, 114, 126.

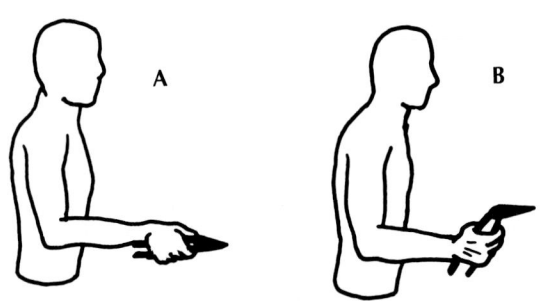

Fig. 97-13   **A,** Ulnar wrist deviation is required to hold needle-nose pliers for bench assembly work. **B,** Wrist posture can be controlled by bending the handles of the pliers with respect to the chuck. (From Armstrong TJ: Hand Clin 2:553, 1986.)

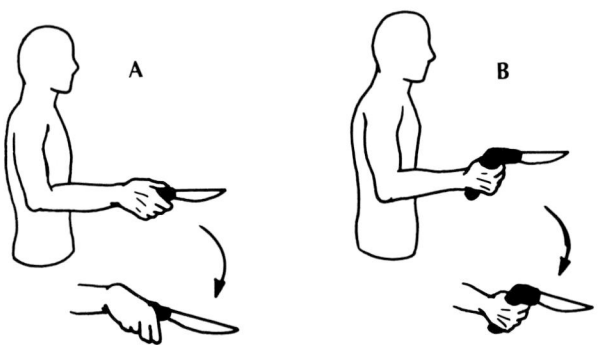

Fig. 97-14   **A,** Ulnar wrist deviation is required to hold the knife for boning turkey thighs. **B,** Wrist posture can be controlled by using a pistol-shaped handle. (From Armstrong TJ: Hand Clin 2:553, 1986.)

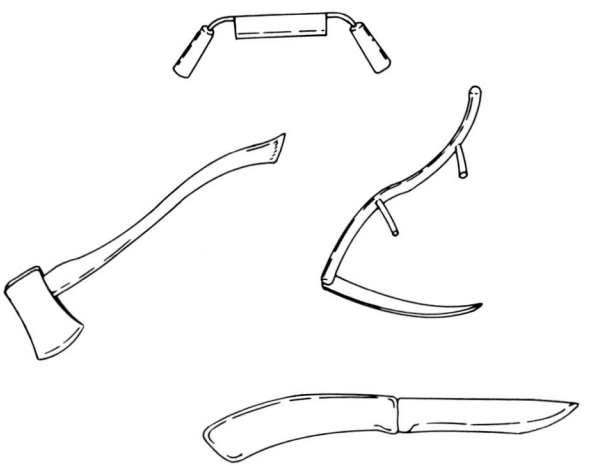

Fig. 97-15   Early tool designs often had bent handles to facilitate use. (From Armstrong TJ: Hand Clin 2:553, 1986.)

example of an automobile assembly job in which the wrist must be flexed to use a pistol-shaped screwgun on a horizontal surface is shown in Fig. 97-16, *A*. In some cases it may be possible to use an in-line screwgun as shown in Fig. 97-16, *B* to control wrist posture. In other cases requiring high torque levels, in-line drivers may not be feasible. In these cases it may be possible to reorient or relocate the work as shown in Fig. 97-16, *C*. The ideal work location and orientation also depends on the size of the worker. The height that is ideal for a tall worker may require the short worker to deviate his wrist or abduct his shoulder. The relationship between worker size, work location, and orientation, tool design, and posture for a given task can be shown graphically with stick figure representations of the human body as shown in Fig. 97-17.

A typical stick figure based on the work of Drillis and Contini[29a] in which the length of each segment is expressed as a fraction of total stature is shown in Fig. 97-18. Average segment lengths for a given stature are estimated by multiplying the segment fraction by the stature. Most stick figure analyses are for individuals of known size or one of the population extremes. The extremes used most frequently are first and ninety-ninth or fifth and ninety-fifth percentiles. According to the USDHEW,[116] the fifth percentile female is 151.1 cm tall, and the ninety-fifth percentile male is 186.9 cm tall. A postural analysis based on these population extremes should be applicable to most people. Ideally, stick figure analyses should be performed in three dimensions; however, two-dimensional analyses are much easier and, in most cases, provide a reasonable approximation of posture. Two-dimensional figures can be dressed up or made to look more lifelike by using silhouettes of each segment. Silhouettes proposed by Dempster[28] in 1955 for a drawing board template of an average male are shown in Fig. 97-18, *B*. These silhouettes can be scaled to fit other percentiles for the sake of appearance.

Stick figures and templates can be used to estimate the best work location for a person of given stature performing a given task. For example, to keep the wrist straight while using a pistol-shaped screwgun on a vertical surface, the work should be located at a height equal to the height of the elbow plus the height of the tool. Simulations of this posture for persons with fifth-percentile female and a ninety-fifth percentile male statures and average proportions are shown in Fig. 97-19. The ideal work location varies from 105.4 cm for the small female to 128.0 cm for the large male. Additional adjustments should be made for shoe height, floor mats, and work platforms.

Fig. 97-20 shows how a stick figure or template can be used to evaluate a keyboard data entry work station for postural stresses. It can be seen that a small female with her feet on the floor and elbows at the side of the body will have to reach over the edge of 76 cm high table and keyboard. This work station will be likely to flex her wrist while resting them on the sharp edge of the table. The situation may be controlled by adjusting the elevation or orientation of the keyboard as shown in Fig. 97-21.

Although stick figure and template manipulations can be performed on drawings of workplaces and equipment using standard drafting techniques, they are more easily performed using computer-aided drafting (CAD) systems.[11] CAD systems provide the ability to create engineering drawings that

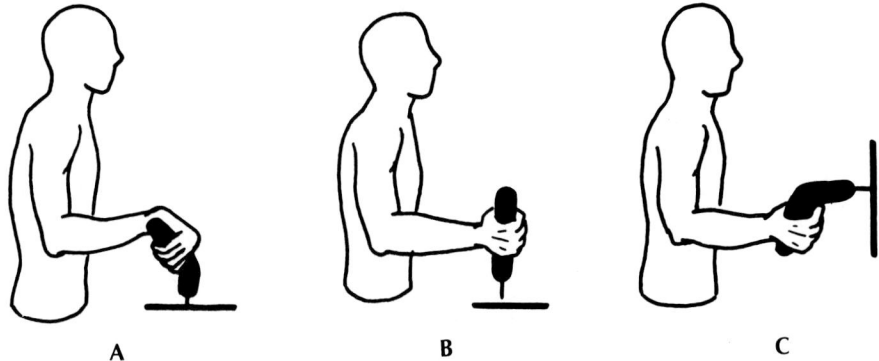

Fig. 97-16   **A,** Wrist flexion is required to use the pistol-shaped screwgun on a horizontal surface at midtorso height. **B,** Wrist posture can be controlled by using an in-line handle or, **C,** by tilting the work surface toward the worker. (From Armstrong TJ: Hand Clin 2:553, 1986.)

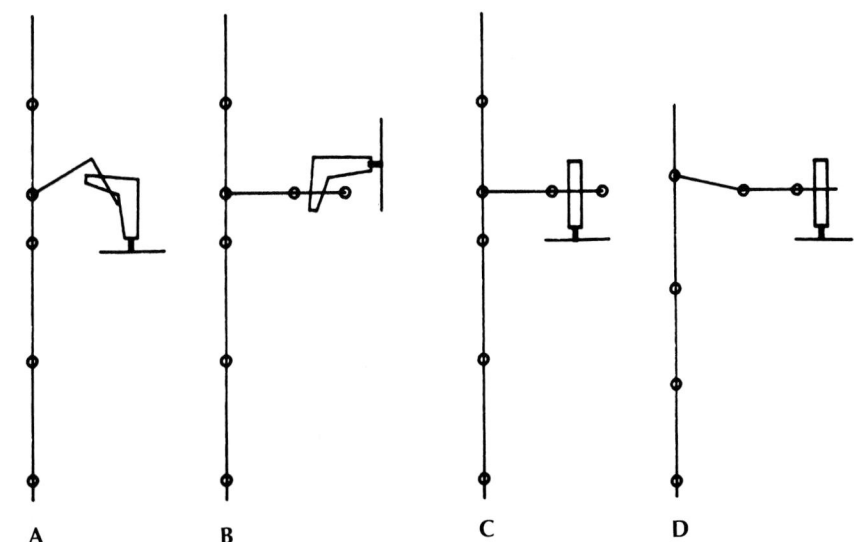

Fig. 97-17   Stick-figure representations of workers can be used to evaluate the effect of work orientation, **A** and **B,** tool shape, **B** and **C,** and stature, **C** and **D,** on posture. (From Armstrong TJ: Hand Clin 2:553, 1986.)

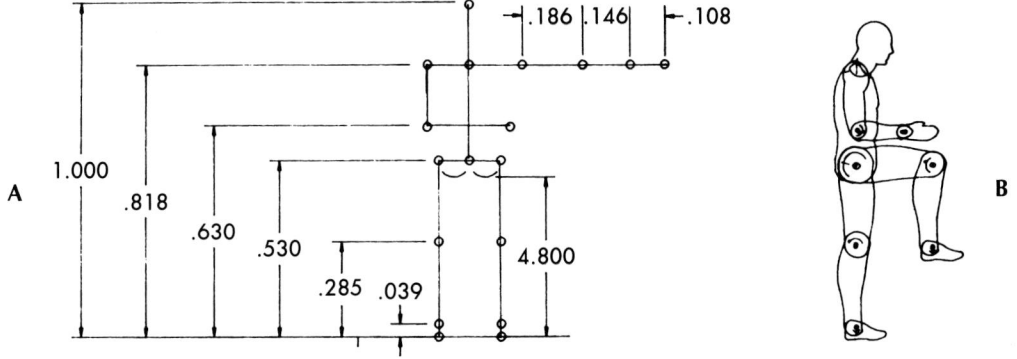

Fig. 97-18   **A,** Average link-length proportions from Drillis and Continni (1966) can be used to evaluate work station design and posture. **B,** Stick figures can be made to look realistic by using silhouettes from Dempster.[28] (From Armstrong TJ: Hand Clin 2:553, 1986.)

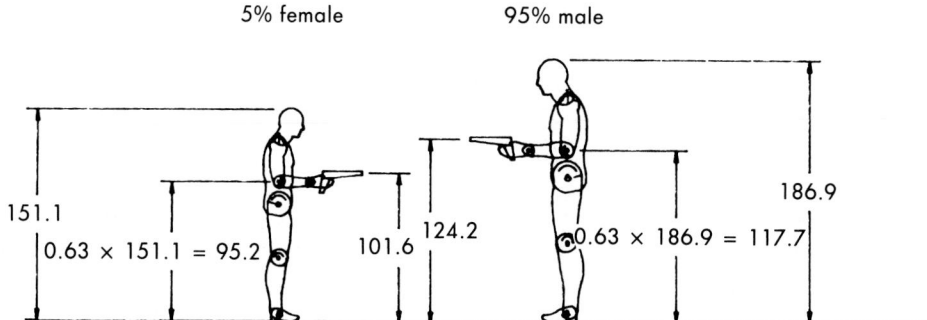

5% female   95% male

Fig. 97-19 Drawing board templates[28] can be used to estimate the best work location for the use of pistol-shaped screwguns. Statures are based on USDHEW[116] and link lengths are based on Drillis and Continni (1966). (From Armstrong TJ: Hand Clin 2:553, 1986.)

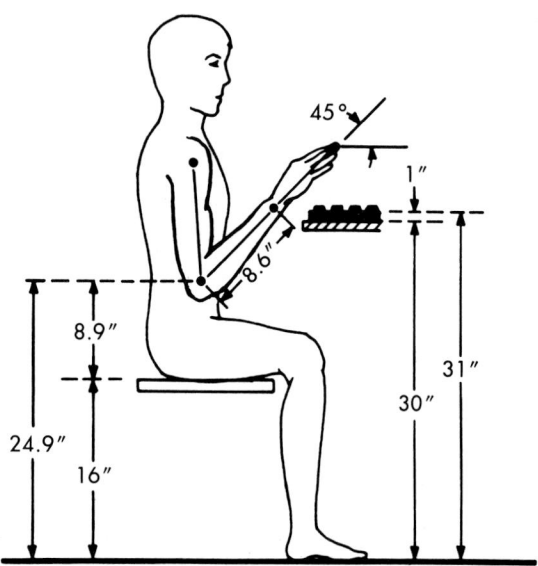

Fig. 97-20 Analysis with a stick figure or mannequin shows that a small woman will have to reach over the edge of the work surface to operate the keyboard.

can be stored on disk or tape and can be recalled for later editing or plotting. Recent advances in microcomputer hardware and software have resulted in widespread availability of inexpensive systems that do not require extensive computer experience.

There is no single best location, orientation, or tool. All of the above-mentioned factors must be considered in the context of a given operation. For example, it may not be possible to reorient an automobile body as it travels down a conveyor line. In this case it may be necessary to focus on the shape of the tool. The ideal work location also is dependent on the size of the worker.

VIBRATION

Another frequently reported factor of cumulative trauma disorders that deserves final mention is vibration.[9,22,64,88,96] Causes of vibration include holding a part in contact with a power or impact tool, holding a power tool, holding a control, and pounding. Unless vibration is of high intensity or exposure is continuous, it may be of secondary importance after repetitiveness, forcefulness, mechanical stress, posture, and low temperature. The job analysis should serve to put these factors into proper perspective. A discussion of engineering vibration control is beyond the scope of this chapter; it suffices to say that where problems exist, exposure should be minimized.[18]

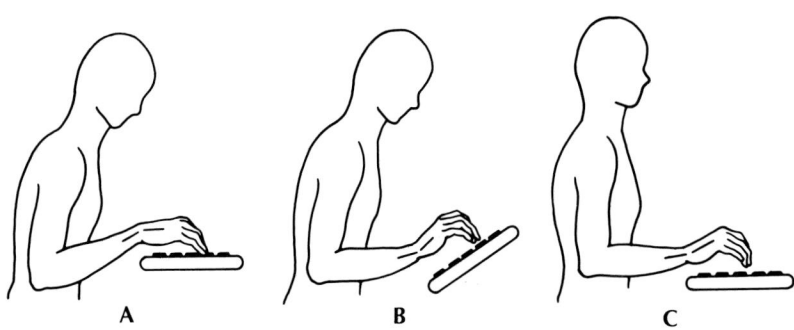

Fig. 97-21 The posture required to use the keyboard, **A**, can be controlled by tilting the keyboard, **B**, or lowering it, **C**. (From Armstrong TJ and Silverstein BA: Upper-extremity pain in the workplace-role of usage in causality. In Clinical concepts in regional musculoskeletal illness, Philadelphia, 1987, WB Saunders Co.)

TEMPERATURE

Tenosynovitis without dermal necrosis has been reported as a result of hand exposure to freezing conditions.[39] In addition, substantial data document the sensory, motor, and circulatory impairments caused by exposure to low temperatures between 0° C and 20° C.* These impairments have two effects: one, to reduce manual dexterity, and, two, to accentuate the symptoms of a nerve impairment. The fingers may be cooled as a result of low environmental temperatures, handling cold materials, or exposure to cold exhaust from an air-powered tool. There are no standards for finger temperatures, but it is recommended that they be kept above 25° C to prevent effects on dexterity. Finger temperature often can be increased by use of gloves, constructing handles from materials with low thermal conductivity, directing exhaust air away from the worker, and wearing additional garments on the torso.

EVALUATION

As stated, there are no absolute standards for repetitiveness, forcefulness, mechanical stresses, postures, temperatures, and vibration. Most cumulative trauma problems are identified after the fact. A job analysis can be performed to identify the major stresses so that interventions can be designed. It is essential that these interventions be evaluated to ascertain their effectiveness. It is not always possible to predict all of the effects of a given intervention. It is possible that an intervention may not have any effect or that it may actually make the job worse. Ideally, epidemiologic studies should be used to evaluate all interventions; however, this usually is not possible and, in fact, may not be desirable. Formal epidemiologic studies require large numbers of workers to perform the same job for months and years.[100] Seldom are work populations and settings this stable. Furthermore, it is desirable to identify problems with interventions before injuries and diseases occur.

Job analysis

The first step in evaluating interventions is the job analysis. This may be performed on the drawing board, on mock-ups, and on prototypes.

User feedback

The second step is obtaining user feedback. Both new and experienced workers should be asked to try the new design. In both cases the workers should be trained how to adjust and operate the new equipment. Workers should be observed and interviewed. A formal interview should be administered to obtain feedback about each design feature. The job analysis may be used to develop an interview checklist for each job. Where possible, workers should be asked to give relative ratings, e.g., "Is the work too high, too low, or just right?" or "Demonstrate the most comfortable work height for you." It is important that the workers studied include a full range of critical anthropometric extremes, e.g., tall males to short women.

Implementation of new equipment

The third step is the implementation of new equipment. All new users should be trained how to adjust and operate the equipment. They should then be observed and interviewed. The interviews should be repeated at frequent intervals initially and at longer intervals later to detect the development of chronic muscle, tendon, or nerve disorders.

Medical surveillance

Finally, there should be ongoing medical surveillance to determine if there has been a change in the incidence rates of injuries and illnesses on the jobs under study versus other jobs in the plant. Control of cumulative trauma disorders requires an ongoing effort and may require several attempts to determine effective interventions.

SUMMARY

Cumulative trauma disorders are a major cause of lost time in many hand-intensive industries. Reported occupational risk factors include repetitive exertions, forceful exertions, mechanical stress, certain postures, vibration, and low temperatures. Although there are no standards for what constitutes excessively repetitive or forceful work, common sense dictates that such factors should be minimized to the extent possible, especially in situations where cumulative trauma disorders have been reported. Mechanical stresses can be produced by holding tools with hard and sharp corners that press on the palm, sides of the fingers, or base of the palm. They also can be produced by pounding with the hand. Tools should be selected that distribute grip forces over as large an area as possible and that avoid delicate nerve tissues. The most frequently reported postural stresses are work with a deviated wrist, a flexed wrist, or a hyperextended wrist. It is recommended that jobs be designed so that the forearm and wrist are in the position that is assumed when the arm hangs relaxed at the side of the body. Processes and tools should be selected to minimize vibration exposure. The hand should be kept above 25° C. All interventions should be evaluated to verify their effectiveness.

REFERENCES

1. Armstrong TJ: Carpal tunnel syndrome and the female worker. Transactions of the forty-third annual meeting of the American Conference of the Governmental Industrial Hygienist, Portland, Ore, May 24-29, 1981, 1982.
2. Armstrong TJ: Development of a biomechanical hand model for study of manual activities. In Easterby R and Kroemer KHE, editors: Anthropometry and biomechanics: theory and application, New York, 1982, Plenum Publishing Corp.
3. Armstrong TJ: An ergonomics guide to carpal tunnel syndrome, American Industral Hygiene Association, 1983.
4. Armstrong T: Ergonomics and cumulative trauma disorders, Hand Clinics 2:553, 1986a.
5. Armstrong T: Upper-extremity posture: definition, measurement and control. In Corlett N, Wilson J, and Manenica I, editors: The ergonomics of working postures, London, 1986b, Taylor & Francis.
6. Armstrong TJ and others: Some histological changes in carpal tunnel contents and their biomechanical implications, J Occup Med 26:197, 1984.
7. Armstrong T and Chaffin D: Carpal tunnel syndrome and selected personal attributes, J Occup Med 21:481, 1979.
8. Armstrong TJ and others: Ergonomics considerations in hand and wrist tendinitis, J Hand Surg 12A(5)(Part 2):830, 1987.
9. Armstrong TJ and others: Ergonomics and the effects of vibration in hand-intensive work, Scand J Work Environ Health 13:286, 1987.
10. Armstrong TJ and others: An investigation of cumulative trauma disorders in a poultry processing plant, Am Ind Hyg Assoc J 43:103, 1982.
11. Armstrong T and others: Repetitive trauma disorders: job evaluation and design, Hum Factors 28:325, 1986.
12. Armstrong TJ and Silverstein BA: Upper-extremity pain in the work-

*References 24, 30, 37, 62, 67, 75, 98, 122.

place—role of usage in causality. In Hadler N, editor: Clinical concepts in regional musculoskeletal illness, New York, 1987, Grune & Stratton, Inc.

13. Arndt R: Work pace, stress, and cumulative trauma disorders, J Hand Surg 12A(5)(Part 2):866, 1987.
14. Australian National Occupations Health and Safety Commission. Interim Report of the RSI Committee. Canberra, 1985, Canberra Publishing and Printing.
15. Barnes R: Motion and time study, design and measurement of work, New York, 1968, John Wiley & Sons.
16. Bennahum DA and Williams W: Waiter's shoulder, N Engl J Med 288:799, 1973.
17. Brain W, Wright A, and Wilkinson M: Spontaneous compression of both median nerves in the carpal tunnel, Lancet 1:277, 1947.
18. Brammer AJ and Talor W, editors: Vibration effects on the hand and arm in industry, New York, 1982, John Wiley & Sons.
19. Browne C, Nolan B, and Faithfull D: Occupational repetitive strain injuries: guidelines for diagnosis and treatment, Med J Aust 17:329, 1984.
20. Buchholz B, Frederick L, and Armstron T: An investigation of human palmer skin friction and the effects of materials, pinch force, and moisture, Ergonomics 31:317, 1988.
21. Campbell CS: Gamekeeper's thumb, J Bone Joint Surg 37B(1):148, 1955.
22. Cannon L, Bernacki E, and Walter S: Personal and occupational factors associated with carpal tunnel syndrome, J Occup Med 23:255, 1981.
23. Chao E, Opgrande J, and Axmear F: Three-dimensional force analysis of finger joints in selected isometric hand functions, J Biomech 9:387, 1976.
24. Clark R: The limiting hand skin temperature unaffected manual performance in the cold, J Appl Psychol 45:193, 1961.
25. Comaish S and Bottoms E: The skin and friction: deviations from Amonton's laws and effect of hydration and lubrication, Br J Derm 84:37, 1971.
26. Conn HR: Tenosynovitis, Ohio State Med J 27:713, 1931.
27. Dawson WJ: Reed-maker's elbow, Medical Problems of Performing Artists.
28. Dempster W: Space requirements of the seated operator; geometrical, kinematic and mechanical aspects of the body with special reference to the limbs, WADC Tech Rep No. 55-159, 1955.
29. Dobyns JH and others: Bowler's thumb: diagnosis and treatment, J Bone Joint Surg 54A(4):751, 1972.
29a. Drillis R and Contini R: Body segment parameters, rep No 1166-03 (Office of Vocational Rehabilitation, Department of Health, Education and Welfare). New York, 1966, New York University School of Engineering and Science.
30. Dusek R: Effect of temperature on manual performance. In Fisher R, editor: Production and functioning of the hands in cold climates, Washington, DC, 1957, National Academy of Sciences, National Research Council.
31. Feldman R, Goldman R, and Keyserling W: Peripheral nerve entrapment syndromes and ergonomic factors, Am J Ind Med 4:661, 1983.
32. Feldman, RG and others; Risk assessment in electronic assembly workers: carpal tunnel syndrome, J Hand Surg 12A(5)(Part 2):849, 1987.
33. Ferguson D: An Australian study of telegraphists' cramp, Br J Ind Med 28:280, 1971.
34. Ferguson D: A study of neurosis and occupation, Br J Ind Med 30:187, 1973.
35. Fine L and others: An alternative way of detecting cumulative trauma disorders of the upper extremities in the workplace, Toronto, May 1984. Proceedings of the International Conference of Occupational Ergonomics,
36. Flowerdew RE and Bode OB: Tenosynovitis in untrained farm-workers, Br Med J II(4264):367, 1942.
37. Fox W: Human performance in the cold, Hum Factors 9:203, 1967.
38. Fry HJH: Incidence of overuse syndrome in the symphony orchestra, Med Prob Perf Arts 51, 1986.
39. Georgitis J: Extensor tenosynovitis of the hand from cold exposure, J Maine Med Assoc 69:129, 1978.
40. Goldie I: Epicondylitis lateralis humeri (epicodylalgia or tennis elbow): a pathogenetical study, Acta Chir Scan (Suppl 339):1, 1964.
41. Grandjean E: Fitting the task to the man: an ergonomic approach, London, 1980, Tayor & Francis Ltd.
42. Gray H: Anatomy, descriptive and surgical, ed 13, Philadelphia, 1983, Lea Bros & Co.
43. Hadler N: Medical management of the regional musculoskeletal diseases, New York, 1984, Grune & Stratton.
44. Hammer A: Tenosynovitis, Med Rec 140:353, 1934.
45. Hershenson A: Cumulative injury: a national problem, J Occup Med 21(10):674, 1979.
46. Hertzberg T: Some contributions of applied physical anthropometry to human engineering, Ann Acad Sci 63(4):616, 1955.
47. Hoffman G: Tendinitis and bursitis, Am Fam Pract 23:103, 1981.
48. Hoffman J and Hoffman PL: Staple gun carpal tunnel syndrome, J Occup Med 27(11):848, 1985.
49. Howell AE and Leach RE: Bowler's thumb: perineural fibrosis of the digital nerve, J Bone Joint Surg 52A(2):379, 1970.
50. Hymovich L and Lindholm M: Hand, wrist, and forearm injuries: the result of repetitive motion, J Occup Med 8(11):573, 1966.
51. Jensen R, Klein B, and Sanderson L: Motion-related wrist disorders traced to industries, occupational groups, Monthly Labor Review, p 13, Sept 1983.
52. Johnson J, Sim F, and Scott S: Musculoskeletal injuries in competitive swimmers, Mayo Clinic Proc 62:289, 1987.
53. Kelly A and Jacobson H: Hand disability due to tenosynovitis, Ind Med Surg 33:570, 1964.
54. Kendall D: Aetiology, diagnosis and treatment of paraesthesiae in hands, Br Med J 2:1633, 1960.
55. Kisner W: Thumb neuroma: a hazard of ten pin bowling, Br J Plast Surg 29:225, 1976.
56. Kuorinka I and Koskinen P: Occupational rheumatic diseases and upper limb strain in manual jobs in a light mechanical industry, Scand J Work Environ Health (Suppl 3) 5:39, 1979.
57. Kurppa K, Warris P, and Kokkanen P: Tennis elbow, Scand J Work Environ Health (Suppl 3) 5:15, 1979.
58. Lamphier T, Crooker C, and Crooker J: DeQuervain's disease, Ind Med Surg 34:847, 1965.
59. Landsmeer JMF: Power grip and precision handling, Ann Rheum Dis 21:164, 1962.
60. Laville A: Cadence de travail et posture, Le Travail Humain 31:1, 1968.
61. Lederman RJ and Calabrese LH: Overuse syndromes in instrumentalists, Med Prob Perf Arts 7, 1986.
62. Lockhart J and Kiess H: Auxiliary heating of the hands during cold exposure and manual performance, Hum Factors 13:457, 1971.
63. Long D and others: Intrinsic and extrinsic muscle control of the hand in power grip and precision handling, J Bone Joint Surg 52:853, 1970.
64. Lucas E: Lesion of the peripheral nervous system due to vibration, Work Environ Health 7:67, 1970.
65. Lundervold A: Electromyographic investigations of position and manner of typewriting, Acta Physiol Scand 24(suppl 84), pp 1-171, 1951.
66. Lundervold A: Electromyographic investigations during typewriting, Ergonomics 1:226, 1958.
67. Mackworth N: Cold acclimatization and finger numbness, Proc Royal Soc 143:392, 1955.
68. Maeda K: Expansion of the occupations which induce neck-shoulder-arm disorders and some problems in taking measures against the disorders—from experience in labor hygiene consultation activities, Sumitomo Sangyo Eisei 10:135, 1974.
69. Margolis W and Kraus JF: The prevalence of carpal tunnel syndrome symptoms in female supermarket checkers, J Occup Med 28(12):953, 1987.
70. McCowan TC: Space-invaders wrist, N Engl J Med 304:1368, 1981.
71. McPhee B: Deficiencies in the ergonomic design of keyboard work and upper limb and neck disorders in operators, J Hum Ergol 11:31, 1982.
72. Melville ID: The differential diagnosis of nerve compression syndromes in the arms and hand, Hand 4(2):114, 1972.
73. Minuk GY and others: Pipetter's thumb, N Engl J Med 306(12):751, 1982.
74. Moidel RA: Bowler's thumb, Arthritis Rheum 24(7):972, 1981.
75. Morton R and Provins K: Finger numbness after acute local exposure to cold, J Appl Physiol 15:149, 1960.
76. Muckart R: Stenosing tendovaginitis of abductor pollicis longus and extensor pollicis brevis at the radial styloid (DeQuervains's disease), Clin Orthop 33:201, 1964.

77. Napier JR: The prehensile movement of the human hand, J Bone Joint Surg 38B:902, 1956.
78. Nathan PA, Meadows KD, and Doyle, LS: Occupation as a risk factor for impaired sensory conduction of the median nerve at the carpal tunnel, J Hand Surg 13-B(2):167, 1988.
79. Neiman R and Ushiroda S: Slot-machine tendinitis, N Engl J Med 304:1368, 1981.
80. Nenzen B: Worn tools: another cause of injury, Work Environ 22, 1987.
81. Niebel B: Motion and time study, Homewood, Ill, 1982, Richard D Irwin, Inc.
82. OSHA: Recordkeeping requirements under the Occupational Safety and Health Act of 1970, OSHA No 200, US Dept of Labor, Occupational Safety and Health Administration, 1978.
83. Parsons JS: Tobacco-primer's wrist, N Engl J Med 305(13):768, 1981.
84. Phalen G: The carpal-tunnel syndrome, J Bone Joint Surg 48A:211, 1966.
85. Phalen G: The carpal-tunnel syndrome: clinical evaluation of 598 hands, Clin Orthop 83:29, 1972.
86. Pozner H: A report on a series of causes of simple acute tenosynovitis, J Roy Army Corps 78:142, 1942.
87. Quinnell R: Conservative management of trigger finger, Practitioner 224:187, 1980.
88. Radwin RG, Armstrong TJ, and Chaffin DB: Power hand tool vibration effects on grip exertions, Ergonomics 30:833, 1987.
89. Ramazzini B: Treatise on the diseases of workers (1713) New York, 1964, Hafner Publ Co. (Translated by WC Wright, 1940).
90. Reed JV and Harcourt AK: Tenosynovitis* An industrial disability, Am J Surg 62(3):392, 1983.
91. Reinstein L: DeQuervain's stenosing tenosynovitis in a video games player, Arch Phys Med Rehabil 64:434, 1983.
92. Riley MW, Cochran DJ, and Schanbacher CA: Force capability differences due to gloves, Ergonomics 28:441, 1983.
93. Robbins H: Anatomical study of the median nerve in the carpal tunnel and etiologies of the carpal-tunnel syndrome, J Bone Joint Surg 45A:953, 1963.
94. Ronchese F: Occupation marks, Practitioner 210:507, 1973.
95. Rosen G: The workers hand, Ciba Found Symp 4:1307, 1942.
96. Rothfleisch S and Sherman D: Carpal tunnel syndrome, biomechanical aspects of occupational occurrence and implications regarding surgical management, Orthop Rev 7:777, 1978.
97. Sandler SA: Racquetball wrist, N Engl J Med 299:494, 1978.
98. Schiefer R and others: Finger skin temperature and manual dexterity—some inter-group differences, Appl Ergonomics 15:135, 1984.
99. Schmidt R and Toews J: Grip strength as measured by the jamar dynamometer, Arch Phys Med Rehabil 51:321, 1970.
100. Silverstein BA: Evaluation of interventions for control of cumulative trauma disorders. In Ergonomic interventions to prevent musculoskeletal injuries in industry, ACGIH, Chelsea, Mich, 1987, Lewis Publishers, Inc.
101. Silverstein BA, Fine LJ, and Armstrong TJ: Occupational factors and carpal tunnel syndrome, Am J Ind Med 11:343, 1987.
102. Sloane E: A museum of early American tools, New York, 1973, Ballantine Books.
103. Smith E, Sonstegard D, and Anderson W: Contribution of flexor tendons to the carpal tunnel syndrome, Arch Phys Med Rehabil 58:379, 1977.
104. Sperling W: Snapping finger, roentgen treatment and experimental producton, Acta Radiol 37:74, 1951.
105. Stanish WD: Overuse injuries in athletes: a perspective, Med Sci Sports Exerc 16:1, 1984.
106. Stein A, Ramsey R, and Key J: Stenosing tendovaginitis at the radial styloid process (DeQuervain's disease), Arch Surg 63:216, 1951.
107. Swanson A, Matev I, and Groot G: The strength of the hand, Bull Pros Res, 10(14):145, 1970.
108. Szabo RM and Gelberman RH: The pathophysiology of nerve entrapment syndromes, J Hand Surg 12A(5)(part 2):880, 1987.
109. Tanzer R: The carpal tunnel syndrome, J Bone Joint Surg 41A:626, 1959.
110. Teiger C: Regulation of activity: an analytical tool for studying workload in perceptual motor tasks. Ergonomics 21:203, 1978.
111. Thompson A, Plewes L, and Shaw E: Peritendinitis crepitans and simple tenosynovitis: a clinical study of 544 cases in industry, Br J Ind Med 8:150, 1951.
112. Thurn JR: Wall washer's thumb, Ann Internal Med 99(3):412, 1983.
113. Tichauer E: Some aspects of stress on forearm and hand in industry, J Occup Med 8:63, 1966.
114. Tichauer E: Biomechanics sustains occupational safety and health, Ind Engin 8:45, 1976.
115. Underhill R: The wood wright's companion: exploring traditional woodcraft, Chapel Hill, 1983, University of North Carolina Press.
116. USDHEW: Weight and height of adults 18–74 years of age: United States 1971-74. Vital and Health Statistics Series Number 211, US Dept HEW PHS, Office of Health Research, Statistics, and Technology. National Center for Health Statistics, Hyattsville, Md, 1979.
117. VanBergeijk E: Selection of power tools and mechanical assists for control of occupational hand and wrist injuries. In Ergonomic interventions to prevent musculoskeletal injuries in industry, ACGIH, Chelsea, Mich, 1987, Lewis Publishers.
118. Waris P, Kuorinka I, and Kurppa K: Epidemiologic screening of occupational neck and upper limb disorders, Scand J Work Environ Health 5(suppl 3):25, 1979.
119. Warner K: The practice of knives, New York, 1976, Winchester Press.
120. Waugh D: Cuber's thumb, N Engl J Med 305:768, 1981.
121. Welch R: The causes of tenosynovitis in industry, Ind Med 41:16, 1972.
122. Williamson D, Chrenko F, and Hamley E: A study of exposure to cold in cold stores, Appl Ergonomics 15:25, 1984.
123. Wilson R and Wilson S: Tenosynovitis in industry, Practitioner 178:612, 1957.
124. Wisseman C and Badger D: Hazard evaluation and technical assistance, Rep #TA 76-93, DHEW, CDC, NIOSH, Cincinnati, Oh, 1970.
125. WHO: Identification and control of work-related diseases, Report of a WHO Expert Committee, WHO Technical Report Series 714, Geneva, 1985, WHO.
126. Younghusband O and Black J: DeQuervain's disease: stenosing tenovaginitis at the radial styloid process, Can Med Assoc 89:508, 1963.
127. Zellinger F: Einige Bemerkungen zur Frage der tuberkulosen Tendovaginitis und Bursitis nach Unfall. Archiv Fur Orthopadischf und Unfall-Chirugic 24:456, 1927.

98

The return to work phase
for the patient with cumulative trauma

Laura A. Bruening and Debra Beaulieu

Cumulative trauma disease (CTD) is an inflammation of soft tissue associated with repetitive activity, stress or overexertion. Other terms that are synonomous with cumulative trauma are repetitive motion disease, repetitive strain injuries, overuse syndrome, and repetitive motion syndrome.[3] Diagnoses commonly associated with CTD are carpal tunnel syndrome, lateral epicondylitis, de Quervain's syndrome, Raynaud's disease, trigger finger, and thoracic outlet syndrome.

The current focus on CTD by industry may seem to imply that it is a new condition. However, Bernardino Ramazzi clearly described in the work-related injuries in the seventeenth century.[3] The National Safety Council reports that hand and arm injuries are second only to the back injuries that occur in the United States.[8] It has been only recently that the incidence of cumulative trauma has been looked at as a separate issue with regard to work-related injuries. The placement of workers on assembly lines, the establishment of production quotas, and incentive programs have increased speed, repetition, and abnormal postures. All of these factors contribute to the development of CTD.

Over 400,000 hand and arm injuries occur each year, accounting for 16 million lost days annually.[8] Workers' compensation costs resulting from hand injuries are 1.3 billion dollars annually, which include hospital, medical, and wage compensation.[8] The Bureau of Labor Statistics reported 34,700 new cases of occupational illnesses associated with repetitive trauma in 1984.[4]

The purpose of this chapter is to describe the return-to-work phase for the patient with CTD. The role of the rehabilitation specialist in the rehabilitation process will be outlined. Several of the functions of the rehabilitation specialist can be completed by the therapist, depending on the nature of the therapist's practice and the involvement of a rehabilitation specialist in the particular patient's case. Particular emphasis will be placed on the job analysis, tool modification, warm-up and stretches, work station modification, and job rotation.

THE RETURN TO WORK PHASE

An important part of the rehabilitation of individuals with cumulative trauma disorders is to address the work environment itself. The worker's ability to return to the work place must be established. This is an issue whether the patient has been managed conservatively or through surgical intervention.

The fields of ergonomics and occupational medicine have made major contributions in identifying the relationship between certain types of work and the development of cumulative trauma conditions. The physical demands of the worker's position need to be evaluated. Communication with the employee and the employer should be established early. Requirements for full return to work might include job change or job modification.

THE ROLE OF THE REHABILITATION SPECIALIST

Workmen's compensation law requires that medical care, rehabilitation, and lost wages be covered when an individual is injured on the job. These costs are incurred by insurance companies who support the concept that timely and quality rehabilitation is cost effective. Insurance companies often employ or consult with rehabilitation specialists to manage the medical and rehabilitation needs of the injured worker. Rehabilitation specialists often are professionals such as registered nurses, occupational or physical therapists, or vocational rehabilitation counselors. Their role is to ensure that the individual is receiving proper medical and rehabilitation services, which may include vocational rehabilitation if the injured worker is unable to return to the original employer. Rehabilitation specialists act as liaisons among physicians, therapists, employers, the insurance carrier, and the injured worker. Vocational rehabilitation is often covered by the insurance carrier because successful placement can resolve the compensation claim.

COMMUNICATION WITH THE INJURED WORKER

The involvement of the rehabilitation specialist is usually initiated by the employer's insurance carrier. The rehabilitation specialist begins the process by meeting with the injured worker. To obtain information about the individual's understanding of his diagnosis and prognosis, the worker's medical care is reviewed with him. His educational and vocational history are discussed, and he is asked to describe his current job and attitudes about the employer and type of work. The rehabilitation specialist also evaluates the individual's social and family roles and financial situation. This initial evaluation is important to begin establishing rapport with the injured worker. The rehabilitation specialist should explain his role as an advocate and resource to assist the individual through the often complex and confusing compensation system. It is essential that a positive supportive relationship be developed; however, the individual should realize that the rehabilitation specialist's final goal is to assist the injured worker in the transition back to appropriate, productive work.

COMMUNICATION WITH THE PHYSICIAN AND HEALTH CARE PROVIDERS

The rehabilitation specialist should also establish contact with the injured worker's treating physician, therapist, and other health care providers to clarify the injured worker's diagnosis, prognosis, and treatment plan. It is important to review with the physician information gathered in the job analysis so that he has a better understanding of the individual's job. The physician is responsible for offering an opinion regarding the injured worker's ability to return to work and any appropriate physical restrictions.

COMMUNICATION WITH THE EMPLOYER

Initiating communication with the patient's employer as early as possible in the rehabilitation process is wise when considering the vocational prognosis of the individual with cumulative trauma. This communication aids in understanding the type and physical demands of the individual's job, the general atmosphere of the work environment, and the employer's concerns.

When making initial contact with employers, the rehabilitation specialist or therapist should be sensitive to the attitudes and concerns of the employer. Most employers are not receptive to the enthusiastic therapist or rehabilitation specialist who makes suggestions for major changes or modifications for the entire plant. It is better to deal with one particular case at first before attempting to launch a complete industrial consultation program. Listen to the employer's remarks about his feelings about the worker's performance, light duty work, and work-related injuries in general. Dobyns states that many attempts to return to work fail because of disbelieving, harassing, and provocative attitudes of employers and coworkers.[4]

In the case of cumulative trauma disorders, the rehabilitation specialist can educate the employer about the nature of the condition, the relationship between the type of work and the development of the condition, and the patient's prognosis for return to work. Some employers are skeptical of the term *overuse syndrome*. They may resist consideration of any modifications or light duty work if they do not thoroughly understand the etiology of the condition. The employer may not realize the need to practice preventive measures to avoid recurrence or development of these conditions among other employees. Many employers are not anxious to consider light duty placement because of the negative effect on other employees. It is helpful to learn how many employees are on workmen's compensation because of direct trauma or cumulative trauma. The employer may doubt the validity of the cumulative trauma condition if numerous workers developed the problem at the same time or if the condition developed concurrently with an imminent layoff. The rehabilitation specialist or therapist must respect and understand the employer's position but still encourage him to consider options that will enhance a successful return to work. If the therapist or rehabilitation specialist is successful in resolving the return-to-work issues of one case, the employer will be more receptive to suggestions regarding the overall impact of the work environment in the development of cumulative trauma disorders.

COMMUNICATION WITH THE INSURANCE CARRIER

The rehabilitation specialist is also responsible for updating the insurance carrier on the initial contacts made with the injured worker, physician, and employer. It is important for the insurance carrier to have a clear understanding of the diagnosis, estimated time for rehabilitation, and prognosis for return to work at the original employer. The rehabilitation specialist can also discuss the injured worker's possible needs for special splints, orthotic devices, or ergonomic tools that may assist the individual with cumulative trauma disorder in resuming productive employment.

The insurance carrier can also be very helpful in the process of convincing an employer to consider job modifications, light duty, or alternate placement by providing financial information to the employer about the potential cost of maintaining the individual on workmen's compensation or providing vocational rehabilitation services. Finding appropriate alternative employment can be a detailed process during which time the individual continues, in some states, to receive compensation benefits for wage loss. The alternate position obtained may not pay the same salary as the worker's original job, and in many states, workmen's compensation laws require payment of a differential wage loss benefit for a period of time. All of these costs indirectly affect the employer in premium rates and can have an impact on his attitude regarding light duty options.

JOB ANALYSIS

Another objective of establishing early contact with the patient's employer is to complete a detailed job analysis of the patient's position. This information should be shared with the treating physician and therapist if the rehabilitation specialist is completing the analysis. It is helpful if the therapist can observe and analyze the patient's job, but often time does not allow the therapist to leave the clinic and evaluate each patient's job. Some companies are now using videotape as a method of job analysis. This information can help the therapist design an appropriate work tolerance program through job simulation and exercise. This information also helps in evaluating whether the patient has the capacity to return to the job. The physician can have a better understanding of the patient's job by reviewing the job analysis.

If able to perform an on-site visit, the therapist should obtain approval from the insurance carrier before the visit so he or she is assured reimbursement for his or her time. If the therapist is not able to perform the on-site visit and a rehabilitation specialist is not involved with the case, information regarding the individual's job can be obtained directly from the injured worker and/or employer.

The job analysis should be completed by the therapist or rehabilitation specialist during an on-site visit. It is helpful if the individual performing the job analysis has an understanding of factors related to cumulative trauma disorders, including anatomy, kinesiology, and ergonomics, so that a biomechanical framework can be used. Various forms can be used to make data collection easier, but an additional narrative description of the injured worker's job is usually helpful.

General information that should be included in the job analysis follows:
1. Length of work shift
2. Schedule of breaks
3. Possibilities for job rotation
4. Possibility for part-time return to work (initially)
5. Employer's attitude and experience with job modification.

It is also important to understand the policies of the union, if one is present, because union rules may limit the options for job rotation, part-time work, and job transfers. Generally, a tour of the work environment is allowed. The rehabilitation specialist or therapist should note overall trends or specific job positions that may be appropriate for the injured worker. If the employer indicates that certain jobs are light duty positions, they must be thoroughly evaluated because they may not be appropriate for an individual with a cumulative trauma condition. For example, the employer may consider a position to be light duty, because the amount of weight lifted is 1 to 2 pounds. However, the frequency of lifting may be excessive, or the tools used may require stressful positioning of the injured extremity. Often, time does not allow for the complete analysis of all the available jobs. However, thorough evaluation of the physical demands of the injured worker's position is necessary.

The physical demands to be evaluated include:
1. Lifting—amount, frequency, and range through which objects are lifted, bilateral versus unilateral
2. Carrying—amount, frequency, bilateral versus unilateral, position of extremity, grasp pattern
3. Reaching—range, frequency
4. Pushing-Pulling—position, frequency, unilateral versus bilateral
5. Grasping—the grasp-prehension patterns required

General requirements of standing, walking, and climbing should be noted. The repetitive nature of the physical demands and the position of the extremity are perhaps the most important factors to evaluate in the injured worker with cumulative trauma. Along with wrist position, the position

of the entire arm is to be considered. The evaluator should note tasks that require working with the elbows raised or the arms outstretched above shoulder height. The evaluator should also note job tasks or tools that subject the worker to prolonged vibration. Exposure to vibration has been associated with the development of cumulative trauma and Raynaud's phenomenon.[6]

TOOL DESIGN AND MODIFICATION

Tools are extensions of the human hand. They allow humans to complete tasks that require more force, grip, or prehension than the hand is able to complete. The correct tool fit in the hand is vital for proper tool usage. Historically, tools were made to fit the hand of the designer. Very little concern was placed on how the tool fit the user's hand. The field of ergonomic engineering has researched the importance of tool and machine interaction with the worker. Proper tool size will contribute to efficient work and conservation of energy. The tool circumference should be approximately 4 to 5 inches. As a rough guideline, placement of the tool in the hand should be similar to that of a tennis racket. The fingertips should not touch the palm.[2]

Handle surfaces were designed with edges for traction. This can be seen in most screwdriver handles. However, with prolonged use, the edges can create pressure areas. This is especially evident in the palm, where the flexor tendons pass close to the skin. A smooth surface allows for gripping without pressure. A nonslip covering can be applied[7]; it will provide traction without edges (Fig. 98-1).

Handles that have grooves for finger placement, i.e., bicycle handlebars or saws, can also cause pressure. All hands will not fit into the finger spaces perfectly, causing pressure buildup on the volar surface of the hand. A handle that is free of finger grooves will provide a more comfortable fit. The tool may then be used by hands of all sizes.[2]

Workers who must use scissors for extended periods of

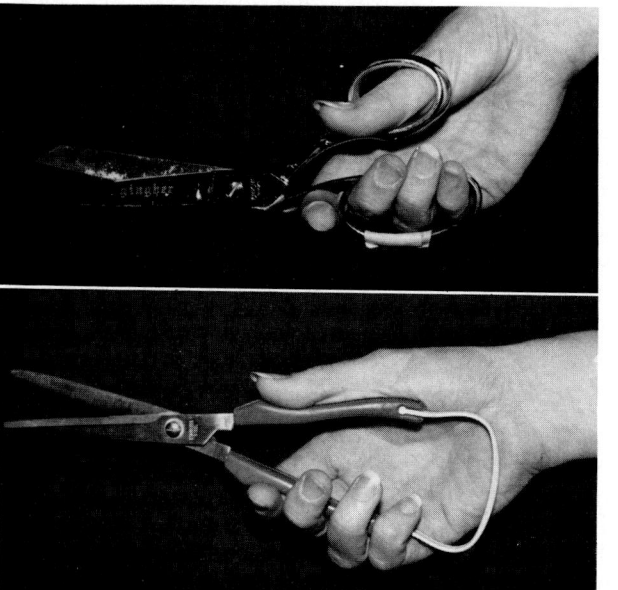

A

B

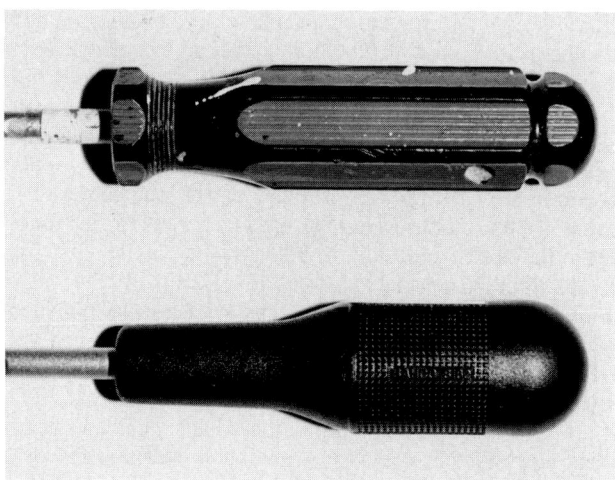

Fig. 98-1 The handle on the top has edges that can cause pressure areas. The bottom handle has traction without edges.

Fig. 98-2 **A,** These scissors apply pressure over the dorsal aspect of the thumb and fingers. **B,** The spring-loaded scissors eliminate the pressure areas on the dorsum; they are able to spring open.

time report fatigue and pain. The pain is usually located on the dorsal surface of the hand where the finger loops rest on the hand. Spring-loaded scissors are available. They require finger flexion to close, but the spring assists in opening. This design eliminates pressure on the dorsum of the hand[2] (Fig. 98-2).

Pressure should be distributed to parts of the hand that are well padded. A longer handle would allow the pressure to be equally distributed in the hand. The pressure then is concentrated in the hypothenar emminence. Handles that end in the palm apply pressure to an area where the flexor tendons lie close to the skin[2] (Fig. 98-3).

McKenzie and colleagues[6] outlined several tool modifications that contributed to a decrease in the incidence of CTD in a telecommunications manufacturing facility. These included use of sleeve guards to reduce the physical stress involved in gripping air-powered screwdrivers and the application of an antitorque radial arm to screwdrivers to reduce torque and vibration. Wire wrap guns were adapted with pneumatic triggers to decrease the amount of force needed to activate the trigger.

Goel and Sim found that Poron and Sorbothane padded gloves reduced the vibration levels transmitted to the hand in simulation of pneumatic chipping. These findings suggest that virbation-isolating gloves should be used by workers exposed to vibration.[5]

WORK STATION MODIFICATION

To modify a work station that requires abnormal posture, a simple solution is always preferred to a complicated one. A solution for a work station that is too high may be to build an elevated platform for the employee. If the work station is too low, providing a seat for the employee may obtain the proper position. Careful attention should be addressed to table and chair height with employees who work at a computer terminal or typewriter for extended periods. A terminal that is low may require long periods of wrist flexion. Modification should be made so that the wrists are maintained in a straight or neutral position if possible (Fig. 98-4, *A* & *B*). This can be accomplished by elevating the desk or by using supports or arm rests. This will eliminate prolonged positioning of an unsupported extremity. Repositioning may be accomplished by using vices or clamps or by tilting the work.

JOB ROTATION

An effective method of reducing prolonged repetition, postures, or tool use is job rotation. Employees are rotated throughout the day to a variety of jobs. An important factor in successful job rotation is jobs that do not require similar movements.

WARM UP AND STRETCHES

The Japanese were among the first to recognize that total body wellness is essential for good work habits. Japanese companies begin the work day with an exercise program. Their philosophy is that exercise prepares the worker for his job, physically and mentally. American companies have begun to provide exercise programs as a benefit, either on the industrial site or at a participating health club. Warm up and stretching are important factors in a fitness program and can be incorporated into a work program. Employees who work in one position for extended periods should stretch before work and periodically throughout the day.

SUMMARY

Individuals with CTD will not have visual trauma to their extremities, such as amputations or lacerations. Although these individuals look healthy, their condition will cause increased pain, resulting in an inability to complete their jobs, hobbies, or normal routines.

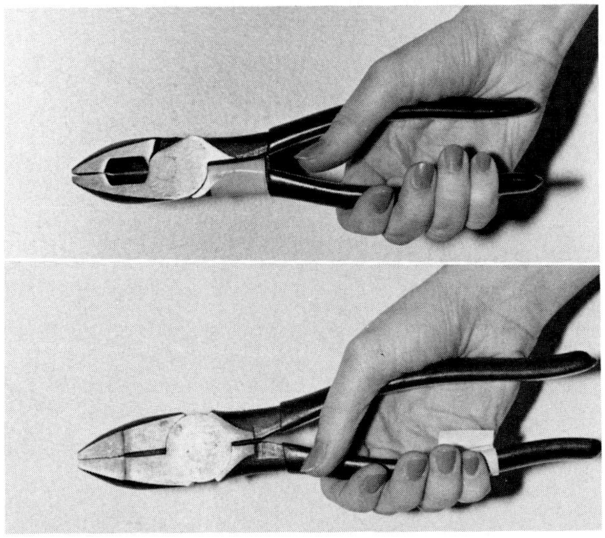

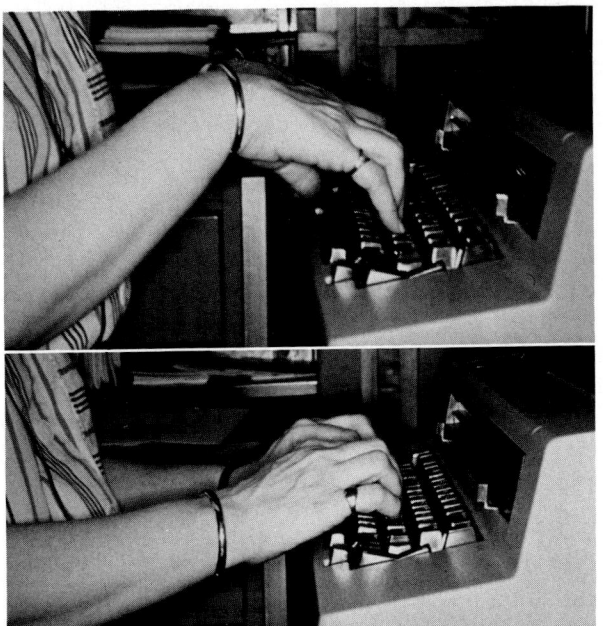

Fig. 98-3 **A,** This tool concentrates pressure in the palm. **B,** With the extended handle, the pressure is primarily in the hypothenar aspect.

Fig. 98-4 **A,** A typewriter setting at an incorrect height can cause poor wrist position. **B,** Proper typewriter height will provide stability and a biomechanical advantage.

Carpal tunnel syndrome, de Quervain disease, and lateral epicondylitis are just a few of the conditions considered in the category of CTD. Thoracic outlet syndrome, radial tunnel syndrome, trigger finger, and pronator syndrome are also related to repetitive trauma disease.

General education regarding CTD is necessary. Employees need to learn how to control their symptoms and modify work postures. Employers need to understand that cumulative trauma is as devastating as blunt trauma. Light duty, job modifications, and job changes may be necessary to reduce the lost time at work. Insurance companies need to be educated by the medical team regarding diagnosis, prognosis, and treatment plan.

Progress has been made in identifying occupational factors that affect a worker's performance and health. The focus now must be on increasing accuracy in reporting cases, so that trends can be identified. Also, evaluation of the treatment of CTD and the functional and vocational outcome need to be addressed.

Therefore open communication and follow-up are necessary among the team members involved in the rehabilitation of the individual with cumulative trauma disorders. Once the patient has returned to work, a follow-up visit is recommended to assure that the worker is practicing warm-up stretches, tendon protection concepts, and appropriate body positions.[1]

REFERENCES

1. Carlton RS: The effects of body mechanics instruction on work performance, Am J Occup Ther 41(1):16, 1987.
2. Chaffin D and Anderson G: Occupational biomechanics, New York, 1984, John Wiley & Sons.
3. Dean L: Cumulative trauma disorders, J Hand Surg 12A(5) (Part 2):823, 1987.
4. Dobyns J: Role of the physician in workers' compensation injuries, J Hand Surg 12A(2) Part 2):826, 1987.
5. Goel V and Sim K: Role of gloves in reducing vibration: an analysis for pneumatic chipping hammer, Am Ind Hyg Assoc J 48(1):9, 1987.
6. McKenzie F and others: A program for control of repetitive trauma disorders associated with hand tool operations in a telecommunications manufacturing facility, Am Ind Hyg Assoc J 46(11):262, 1985.
7. Meagher S: Tool design for prevention of hand and wrist injuries, J Hand Surg 12A(5) (Part 2): 1987.
8. National Safety Council: Accident facts, Chicago, 1981 ed.

BIBLIOGRAGHY

Benner C, Schilling A, and Klein L: Coordinated teamwork in California industrial rehabilitation, J Hand Surg 12A:936, 1987.

Blair S, McCormick E, and Bear-Lehman J: Industrial hand injuries: prevention and rehabilitation. In Hunter JM and others, editors: Rehabilitation of the hand, ed 2, St Louis, 1984, The CV Mosby Co.

Bleecker M: Medical surveillance for carpal tunnel syndrome in workers, J Hand Surg 12A:845, 1987.

Blumenthal S: Vocational rehabilitation with the industrially injured worker, J hand Surg 12A:926, 1987.

Buckle P: Musculoskeletal disorders of the upper extremities: the use of epidemiologic approaches in industrial settings, J Hand Surg 12A:885, 1987.

Cannon L, Bernacki E, and Walter S: Personal and occupational factors associated with carpal tunnel syndrome, J Occup Med 23(4):255, 1981.

Feldman RG, Goldman R, and Keyserling Wm: Classical syndromes in occupational medicine: peripheral nerve entrapment syndrome and ergonomic factors, Am J Ind Med 4(5):66, 1983.

Ferguson D: Repetition injuries in process workers, Med J Aust 408, 1971.

Hadler N: Industrial Rheumatology, Arthritis and Rheumatism 20(4), 1019, 1977.

Hymovich L and Lindholm M: Hand, wrist and forearm injuries, the result of repetitive motions, J Occup Med 8(11):573, 1966.

Lutz G and Hansford T: Cumulative trauma disorder controls: the ergonomics program in Ethicon, Inc., J Hand Surg 12A:863, 1987.

Mattila MK: Job load and hazard analysis—a method for the analysis of workplace conditions for occupational health care, Br J Ind Med 42:656, 1985.

Peterson R: Prevention! A new approach to tendinitis, Occup Health Nurs 1977.

Silverstein B and others: Hand-wrist disorders among investment casting plant workers, J Hand Surg 12A(5) (part 2):838, 1987.

Szabo R and Gelberman H: The pathophysiology of nerve entrapment syndromes, J Hand Surg 12A(5) (part 2):880, 1987.

Taylor W: Vibration white finger in the workplace, J Soc Occup Med 32:159, 1982.

Truskowsky M: The insurance rehabilitation nurse as a team member. In Hunter JM and others, editors: Rehabilitation of the hand, ed 2, St Louis, 1984, The CV Mosby Co.

US Department of Labor: Work-related hand injuries and upper extremity amputations, Bulletin 2160, Washington, DC, December 1982, US Government Printing Office.

99

The upper extremity difficulties of musicians

Fred H. Hochberg

The amateur and professional musician are unique athletes prone to specialized difficulties of the arms and hands. These afflictions create symptoms that alter musical performance or instrumental technique. Not uncommonly, the performer seeks medical aid only after rejecting alternative therapies including alterations or substitution of their instrument, refingering of particular passages, changes in practice habits, and the benefits of lotions, manipulations, and relaxation techniques. This chapter provides a basis for the understanding of the complaints of the instrumental musician.

HISTORY

The appearance of pain, infacility, weakness, or slowness of movement creates for the musician a strong link to the historical difficulties of Robert Schumann. As a performer, Schumann noted infacility during rapid movements of the fourth finger of his right hand. Despite self-designed remedies, his symptoms progressed and became associated with emotional difficulties. Similar poignant stories of medical difficulties are associated with the lives of Haydn, Beethoven, Schubert, Ravel, and Paganini, in addition to modern virtuoso performers.[6] Well known to physicians of the late nineteenth and early twentieth centuries, these difficulties were often called occupational neuroses. Early neurologists described "scrivener's palsy" and writer's cramp (Sir Charles Bell) and similar hand difficulties of telegraphers, typists, and musicians (W.R. Gowers). During the past 5 years, our understanding of these difficulties among musicians has benefitted from the establishment of musical-medicine clinics in 12 locations, the creation of the Internation Arts Medicine Association, and the publication of the *Journal of Medical Problems of Performing Artists*.

To understand the origin of arm and hand difficulties among musicians, the observer is aided by a brief review of the origin of modern instruments. The best studied of these is the piano. The modern piano represents a beautiful but vexing instrument—one that allows the passage of hundreds of percussive movements each minute. Each movement may require down-pressures of all five fingers. Pressures required are measured in the gram-to-kilogram range. It is not uncommon for a musician in practice to devote 5 to 7 hours per day during a career that often spans four decades. The piano before the midnineteenth century was vastly different. It was played with the second, third, and fourth fingers and possessed little capacity for hammer return or counterpulsion (introduced in 1823). Its sound, a product of iron wire and a wooden frame, improved dramatically with the introduction of a cast-iron frame, which allowed the use of high tensile strength steel wire. By the 1850s both the piano and its performer had changed. The latter, formerly both composer and performer, soon gave way to virtuoso performers performing intricate pieces in large salons. Not uncommonly, these performers explored technical devices and surgical procedures to improve their technique. Devices such as the "Chiroplast," "Dactylion," and Schumann's "cigar box" offered the hope of increasing the agility and strength of the right fourth finger, as did operations performed to liberate the communal linkage between the extensor tendons of the third, fourth, and fifth fingers.

The concerned physician, first evaluating a musician, is often faced with arm and hand difficulties expressed in musical terms. The performer, faced with alterations in a well-established, often virtuoso, technique or with the appearance of subtle symptoms affecting the arm or hand, does not complain of these difficulties in medical terms. He provides a history replete with details concerning his teacher's pedagogic techniques, pieces played, practice habits, and the intricate relationship between his technical ability, desire, and the demands of performance. Although these details are

Text continued on p. 1202.

THE APPROACH TO THE MUSICIAN WITH ARM AND HAND COMPLAINTS

History (see Questionnaire, pp. 1198-1201)

Length of study
Current demands of practice and performance
Instrument(s) played
Additional hand use: typing, mechanical trade, shifting car, bicycling
Prior trauma
Instrumental technique: perceived deficiencies, current goals of practice sessions
Occurence of arm or hand fatigue

Examination at instrument (often without shirt)

Careful attention to joint laxity at shoulder, elbow, phalanges; limitation of range of movement, especially shoulder; scapula winging
Videotape analysis

Examination away from instrument

Neurophysiologic studies

Serologic studies

NAME _____ DATE _____
       Last   First   Middle

ADDRESS _____ SEX _____

             _____ AGE _____

Instrument _____ right or left handed _____

Glove size for nonpianists _____

Pianists, please indicate stretch on the keyboard. _____

Describe your general physical condition. _____

- I HAVE NEVER HAD INSTRUMENT-RELATED DIFFICULTIES.   ☐
  Please answer music-related questions only.

- I HAVE HAD INSTRUMENT-RELATED DIFFICULTIES AND HAVE RESOLVED THEM.   ☐
  Please answer questions A through D and all music-related questions.

- I AM CURRENTLY EXPERIENCING INSTRUMENT-RELATED DIFFICULTIES.   ☐
  Please begin with question D and answer all medical and music-related questions. The music-related questions should be answered with a pre-difficulty perspective.

  A. What do you believe was the cause of your difficulties? _____

     _____

  B. How did you resolve them? _____

     _____

  C. Please indicate all successful therapies, drugs used, and medical procedures performed. _____

     _____

  D. Please indicate on the figures below the precise location of the problem:

           Left   Right

  E. What do you believe is the cause of your present difficulty? _____

     _____

     _____

music section

The following questions should be answered by all instrumentalists.

Do you precede repertoire work with purely technical study? Yes ☐ No ☐

List the titles of most used exercises. _____

_____

Does your technical practice focus on any of the following?

Scales ☐   Octaves ☐
Arpeggios ☐   3rds and 6ths ☐
Trills ☐   Other _____

Describe your manner of practicing for speed and volume. _____

_____

Length and frequency of practice session: _____

Do you break up these sessions, and if so, how? _____

When practicing repertoire, do you

Practice predominantly slowly ☐   Practice at normal speed ☐
Practice at normal volume ☐   Practice for endurance ☐
Practice in small segments ☐   If so, how? _____
Play through the piece ☐   Other _____

Is your approach to your instrument reflective of a particular school or method? If so, please specify. _____

_____

_____

Do you favor a certain repertoire? If so, please specify. _____

_____

_____

Please describe as best you can the manner in which you were taught to play your instrument. _____

_____

_____

List any technical advice that was strongly implanted in you during your formative years of study. _____

_____

_____

If your approach to your instrument has changed over the years, please detail the nature of the change. _____

_____

Continued.

surgical procedures

Exploration of nerve entrapment ☐

   Median ☐

   Posterior interosseous nerve ☐

Other _____

_____

_____

Could you or did you try to alleviate your problem through:

Increased practice time ☐
Refingering ☐
Change of technique ☐

Decreased practice time ☐
Change of repertoire ☐
Other _____

At the onset of difficulties what specific repertoire were you studying?

_____

_____

How did your current problem initially manifest itself?

_____

_____

Which of the following areas presented significant difficulty?

Scales ☐
Arpeggios ☐
Octaves ☐
Speed ☐
Other _____

Trills ☐
Staccato playing ☐
Volume ☐
Control ☐

Length of time between onset of difficulties and seeking of medical help:

Less than a month ☐
More than a year ☐
Other _____

Less than a year ☐
More than 2 years ☐

Has this problem ever been induced by:

Typing ☐
Lifting or carrying ☐
Use of toothbrush ☐
Other _____

Writing ☐
Use of eating utensils ☐
Shaking hands ☐

Additional comments, suggestions, observations:

_____

_____

_____

_____

_____

medical section

Physical sensations associated with complaint:

Pain ☐
Fatigue ☐
Swelling ☐
Redness ☐
Stiffness ☐
Pins and needles ☐

Weakness ☐
Tightening ☐
Cramping ☐
Loss of control ☐
Curling/drooping ☐
Other _____

Have you ever suffered from:

Stroke ☐
Seizure ☐
Paralysis ☐

Arm/hand injury ☐
Tumor ☐

Were you ever diagnosed as having:

Tendinitis ☐
Nerve entrapment syndrome ☐
Posterior interosseous nerve syndrome ☐
Cervical spondylosis ☐
Parkinsonism ☐

Inflammatory arthritis ☐
Carpal tunnel syndrome ☐
Thoracic outlet syndrome ☐
Dystonia ☐
Stretched tendons ☐

Rheumatologic history

HUMAN LEUKOCYTE ANTIGEN FEATURES
Neck ☐
Back pain ☐
Psoriasis ☐
Iritis ☐
Urethritis ☐

EXTRAARTICULAR FEATURES
Rheumatoid arthritis ☐
Lupus ☐
Alopecia ☐
Raynaud's sun sensitivity ☐

Prior therapy

MEDICAL
Nonsteroidal anti-inflammatory drugs ☐
Per os (oral) steroids ☐
Local steroid injection ☐
ALTERNATIVE THERAPY
Acupuncture ☐
Chiropractics ☐
Acupressure ☐
Myotherapy ☐
Other _____

PHYSIOTHERAPY
Biofeedback ☐
Splinting ☐
Muscle reeducating ☐
Transcutaneous nerve stimulation ☐
Ultrasound ☐
Traction ☐ Collar ☐
PSYCHOLOGIC
Anti-depressants ☐
Hypnotherapy ☐
Psychotherapy ☐

The following questions should be answered only by keyboard players.

Do you sit either especially high or low at the keyboard? _____
Do you employ a high, vigorous finger action, or do you maintain contact with the key surface?
      High ☐   Close ☐   In between ☐
Do you concentrate on one hand during technical work, and if so, which?
      Right ☐   Left ☐   Equal attention ☐
Do you concentrate particularly on the fourth or fifth fingers of either or both hands?
      Yes ☐   No ☐
What are your favorite right hand trill fingers? _____
What are your favorite left hand trill fingers? _____
Are your physical motions at the keyboard basically
An attempt to isolate activity in the fingers ☐
An attempt to blend the use of upper arm, forearm, wrist, and fingers ☐
Other _____
Is your octave and repeated chord playing
From the wrist exclusively ☐
A combination of wrist and forearm ☐

From the forearm exclusively ☐
Other _____

The following questions should be answered by all touring musicians.

Describe your practice habits while on tour: _____

_____

Please indicate the frequency of public appearances:
10-25 concerts per year ☐
50-75 concerts per year ☐

25-50 concerts per year ☐
75-100 concerts per year ☐

If you are a keyboard player, do you consciously adapt to the instrument at hand or is your approach uniform?
      Adapt ☐   Uniform ☐
Do you believe that a certain degree of pain is acceptable when attempting to overcome technical difficulties?
      Yes ☐   No ☐
Have you continued practicing while experiencing pain?
      Yes ☐   No ☐

THE COMMON SOURCES OF ARM OR HAND DIFFICULTIES AMONG MUSICIANS

Changes in instrument

Increasing size (violin, cello), playing of two instruments, increased weight (electric guitar), altered sound (amplified versus nonamplified percussion, guitar), dead versus live piano

Altered instrument

Summer versus winter bridge (cello, viola), altered angle of instrument (cello pin height), chin rest (violin, viola), drum height, string tension (violin, viola, guitar), drumstick weight, thumb rest position (wind instrument)

Altered repertoire

Percussive versus nonpercussive pieces, pieces requiring large hand stretches for octaves

Altered schedule

Master classes, performance demands versus practice demands, competitions

Altered technique

Emphasis on individualized finger movements (piano or string instrument trills), technical drills used (Hannon, Czerny), new teacher, attempt to change "sound" produced

Intercurrent difficulties

Hand or arm trauma, second instrument, job requirements

---

not to be taken lightly, the medical personnel need not have a musical background to understand the information being provided. If the performer is examined at his instrument, the muscular, skeletal, or neurologic nature of difficulties soon are apparent. Musicians make skilled, highly accurate historians. Most are driven to perform but lack significant psychopathology.

Historical details emerge from a self-administered questionnaire provided to all patients (see questionnaire, pp. 1198-1201). Often multiple symptomatic sites are identified. Commonly, the musician separates difficulties into those associated with practice or playing (e.g., infacility or slowness of movement) and those noted after playing.

Key information is provided concerning previous medical conditions, familial neurologic, rheumatologic, and technical difficulties. Often symptoms emerge from changes in instrument, performance technique, stage position, or demands (see box, p. 1202).

EXAMINATION AT THE INSTRUMENT

Much can be learned by watching the performer, often shirtless, at his instrument. Careful attention should be paid to the position and angulation of the head, the extent of shoulder stability and scapula winging, as well as supination and pronation of the arm. Most musicians chose instruments keeping in mind only sound production. The skilled clinician can provide useful ways of shaping the instrument to the anatomy of the performer.

EXAMINATION AWAY FROM THE INSTRUMENT

Rarely do systemic disorders first present themselves during performance. Our clinical files contain descriptions of virtuoso performers with newly diagnosed multiple sclerosis, primary or secondary malignancies within the brain or spinal axis, disorders of the thyroid and parathyroid glands, diabetes mellitus, and soft tissue involvement by lupus erythematosus, rheumatoid arthritis, and Lyme disease.

The evaluation of musicians is easily performed by the orthopod. The vast majority of patients have well-defined, localized difficulties reflecting shoulder instability or restricted movement, the vascular components of thoracic outlet syndrome, joint laxity at the elbow or metacarpophalangeal (MP) joints, or localized pain reflecting inflammation of synovia or joint or tendon. These overuse syndromes represent the single most common source of pain in musicians. Disorders of movement, focal dystonia, represent a rarer but intriguing form of motor control difficulty in musicians.

PRESENTING DIFFICULTIES OF MUSICIANS

Although many instruments are represented in most clinics, medical disorders of musicians fall into four basic groups[8]:

1. The overuse syndromes—localized pain and inflammation in joints and tendons[16]
2. The consequences of thoracic outlet compression
3. Localized entrapment of a single peripheral nerve
4. Motor control difficulties (box, p. 1203)

Overuse syndrome

Reference to a clinical syndrome related to overuse can be found as far back as the early eighteenth century in the work of Bernardina Ramazzini, who described in his treatise, "Diseases of workers," pain and fatigue in the upper limb of scribes.[20] Even then, repetitive movement, unnatural or constrained postures, and psychologic factors were recognized as contributing to the development of these disorders. Since that time, painful upper limb disorders have been variously identified in the multitude of occupational and recreational settings. Among the most commonly used terms, other than *overuse*, are *regional musculoskeletal pain disorders, cumulative trauma disorders, occupational cervicobrachial disorder* (OCD), and *repetition strain injury* (RSI). More specific terms such as *tendonitis, tenosynovitis,* and *peritendinitis crepitans* have been used generically to refer to focal pain syndromes, as well as to relatively specific localized inflammatory conditions. Uncertain is the relationship of these localized musculotendinous pain disorders to the myofascial pain syndromes and to the more generalized muscle pain syndromes with multifocal tenderness, including fibromyalgia/fibrositis. For the musician, overuse syndrome includes symptoms and signs resulting from stress that exceeds the anatomic or physiologic limits of a particular tissue.

Few pathologic studies of overuse are available. Howard[10] and Thompson and associates[23] have both reported biopsies in manual workers diagnosed as having inflammatory muscle-tendon disorders. Microscopic examination has shown variable and often unimpressive changes of localized edema, increased vascularization, thrombosis of small

PRIMARY PRESENTING DIFFICULTIES OF
MUSICIANS SEEN AT THE MUSICAL MEDICINE
CLINIC AT THE MASSACHUSETTS
GENERAL HOSPITAL
N = 1000

Overuse—local pain and inflammation		*33%*
Tendonitis, tenosynovitis	30%	
Systemic collagen-vascular	3%	
Neurologic		*32%*
Motor control (dystonia)		14%
Peripheral nerve entrapped		11%
Median nerve	4%	
Ulnar nerve	4%	
Posterior interosseus	<1%	
Anterior interosseus	<1%	
Polyneuritis	<1%	
Thoracic outlet syndrome		7%
Structural (joint, bone)		*21%*
Laxity, deformity limited range	9%	
Posttraumatic deformity	5%	
"Gamekeeper's thumb"	4%	
Cervical spondylosis	1%	
Shoulder (sublux or scapular winging)	1%	
Neuroma	1%	
Sympathetic dystrophy	<1%	
Back pain	<1%	
Muscular		*9%*
Cocontraction	6%	
Weakness	3%	
Muscle hypertrophy	<1%	
Miscellaneous		*5%*
Psychiatric	4%	
Technical	<1%	
Brain or systemic cancer	<1%	
Postmastectomy	<1%	
Total		*100%*

veins, and scattered collections of inflammatory cells in the soft tissues and in muscle itself. Muscle biopsies in patients with both myofascial pain syndromes and fibromyalgia have similarly revealed changes that can only be considered nonspecific and of questionable importance. Dennett and Fry[3] recently reported muscle biopsy findings in 29 women with painful overuse involving the first dorsal interosseous of the hand. The most consistent observations included changes in fiber count and type distribution, mitochondrial abnormalities, and ultrastructural changes.

The epidemiology of painful overuse disorders in musicians has been looked at in various ways. Caldron and others[1] surveyed a group of 380 instrumental muscians in northeast Ohio; 58% were students and nearly all the others were professional performers or teachers. Of 250 nonwind instrumentalists, 59% reported musculoskeletal problems related to instrument playing. The most extensive surveys of musicians are those of Fry,[4] who interviewed and carried out local examination of 485 symphony orchestra musicians. Fully 64% had some evidence of painful overuse, and 206, or 42%, of the total group had multifocal pain associated with instrument playing.

Fry's data suggested that these patterns were established early in the musician's career. In a survey of instrumentalists belonging to orchestras in the International Conference of Symphony and Orchestra Musicians (ICSOM)[15] among the 2212 respondents, 67% reported having musculoskeletal symptoms and 58% characterized these as severe. A restricted study of incidence of overuse in a group of amateur instrumentalists at high risk indicated that 72% developed overuse symptoms during a week of intensive instrumental playing.[18]

Studies of study populations include those of Fry[5] in Australia and Manchester[13] in the United States. A prevalence rate of painful overuse of about 9% was found in the Australian music school setting, comparable to conservatory or college-aged students in the United States.[5] The large majority of these involved the upper extremity. Manchester[13] studied the incidence of overuse in a university-level music school and identified an average rate of 8.5 upper extremity episodes per 100 instrumentalists per year.

Virtually all prevalence and incidence studies have suggested that women are more frequently affected than men. In addition to gender differences, the instrument played also accounts for substantial variability in both incidence and prevalence of musculoskeletal problems. In general, keyboard instrumentalists are more likely to have problems with the right arm, whereas string players are afflicted on the left.

Many tissues are subject to overuse.[12] Changes may be identified in bones (stress fractures, molding, and hypertrophy), joints (degenerative arthritis), ligaments (sprain), bursae (bursitis), and nerves (entrapment and inflammation). The major tissue involved remains the muscle tendon unit.

The clinical syndrome is characterized primarily by pain and tenderness. The pain is usually localized and characterized as aching and dull or as sharp, burning, and squeezing. Tightness, stiffness, cramping, and fatigue are also frequently noted. Swelling is often a complaint but is rarely apparent on examination. Patients often note numbness and tingling and a "catch" or a "click." Findings are infrequent except in actual nerve entrapment syndromes along with impaired dexterity, speed, or control. Most performers diminish or cease playing at the onset of symptoms. One quarter, however, assume the problem can be cured by refingering, altering their repertoire, or increasing the intensity of practice.

Tenderness is present in all but the most mild cases and may be unifocal or multifocal. The line between "normal" sensitivity to palpation and pathologic tenderness may not be easy to define. Discomfort can often be produced by provocative maneuvers such as placing the limb in a specific position of stress or activating affected muscle groups against resistance. Muscle weakness is commonly difficult to evaluate in the presence of pain. Reflex abnormalities are not to be expected.

Most reports on the clinical pattern of involvement have emphasized the frequency of symptoms in the hand, wrists, and forearms, although shoulder, upper trunk, and neck are

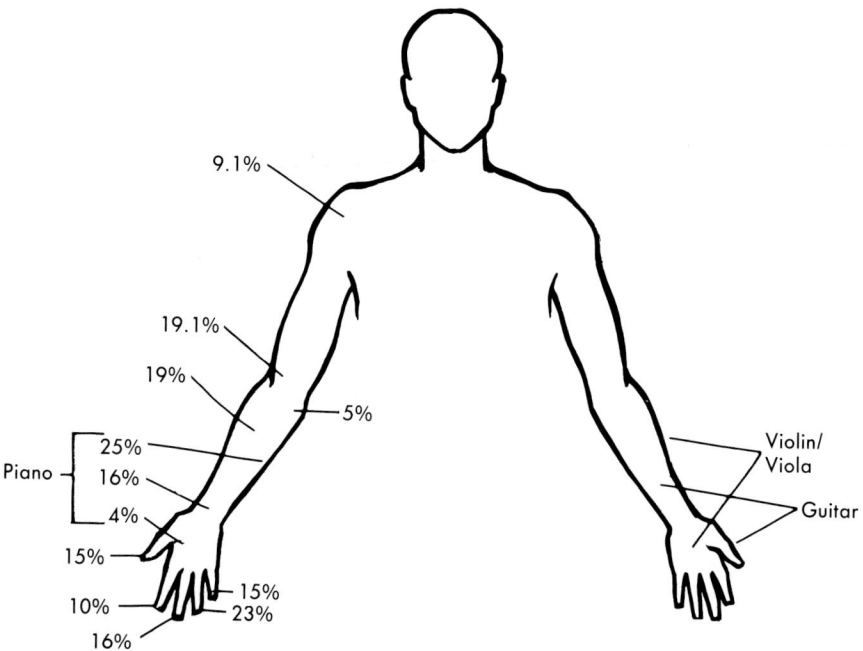

Fig. 99-1 Site of occurrence of playing-related pain.

not infrequently affected as well (Fig. 99-1). The location of pain reflects the instrument played. Pianists are prone to involvement of the lateral portions of the right arm and the flexors of the fourth and fifth fingers of the right hand (reflecting the strength necessary to play the thinner treble strings on the more demanding technique required for the right hand). Most commonly affected among string players is the shoulder of the right bow arm and the left finger flexors and extensors and the wrist extensors. Wind players are prone to pain in the right hand (usually thumb), which supports the weight of the instrument.

A number of factors predispose the musician to the development of these painful disorders. As in other occupational groups, symptoms reflect the frequency of repetitive movement, the degree of resistance to be overcome by movement, and the effects of muscular cocontraction. Contributory causes may be characterized as intrinsic and extrinsic. Among the former are body habitus and local abnormalities (including joint laxity at the shoulder and MP joints, as well as the collateral ligaments of the fingers). Strength, flexibility, and level of conditioning may be considered important. Personality and mood may well play a prominent role. Of the *extrinsic* factors, technique, practice habits, and the instrument itself may be contributory. Technical faults, however subtle, may through repetition and over time cause intolerable stress to muscle and other tissues. Both duration and intensity of playing appear to be important. Many students and young professionals first develop arm problems while preparing for auditions or recitals; an addition to the instrumentalist's repertoire may require hundreds or even thousands of repetitions of a particular passage. A larger viola or a gold flute may offer distinct advantages in sound production or appearance but may be disastrous in terms of ergonomic requirements to hold or play the instrument. No one should underestimate the effects of emotion and stress on these disorders. A feared or disliked

conductor or teacher, a sense of competition and the need to excel, the proximity of an orchestra seat to the next performer or the stage edge, a perceived impression of being "drowned out" by other performers combine with economic pressures in the development of overuse symptoms and signs. The view that these painful muscle-tendon disorders are largely, if not entirely, psychogenic is not uncommon. In our series fewer than 5% of musicians have a functional, nonanatomic disorder.

The diagnosis of muscle/tendon overuse is largely a clinical one. The musician-patient complains of pain only after playing, but as the disorder progresses, pain accompanies any attempt to play and alters the technique. In later states, the discomfort is constant and interferes with all functions. Initially, pain is localized to one area but soon spreads to become multifocal or diffuse.

Attempting to make a diagnosis of a playing-related problem without directly observing the musician playing his instrument would be as egregious an omission as failing to perform ECG monitoring during exercise in a patient who complains of crushing chest pain while walking uphill. Although the examining physician cannot be expected to be an expert in the technique of playing any one instrument, let alone all those he or she may encounter, he or she can be expected to recognize ergonomically unsound technique, which may produce intolerable biomechanical stresses.

Ancillary studies are of relatively little help. However, blood studies may identify systemic predisposing factors, such as a rheumatologic diathesis; radiologic studies may reveal a congenital bony anomaly or degenerative changes; and physiologic studies, such as nerve conduction and needle electromyography, may help identify nerve entrapments. The role or other techniques such as dolorimetry and thermography is debated.

Management of the patient with muscle-tendon overuse may be divided into acute and rehabilitative phases.[12] The cornerstone of acute treatment remains rest, which may be absolute or relative depending on the severity of the disorder. Some reduction in playing and some modification of other activities is almost always indicated. This may be supplemented by splinting, medication such as nonsteroidal anti-inflammatory drugs or analgesics, and other modalities including cold, heat, massage, and ultrasound. Topical salicylates may also be helpful.[9] Surgical intervention other than for nerve entrapment and an occasional skeletal disorder is rarely indicated.

Physical therapy centers on stabilizing the shoulder girdle and hand. The playing of most instruments *appears* to require only finger or wrist stability, and most overuse symptoms are noted in the fingers or wrists. It is our experience that these distal overuse pains often have a more proximal cause. Performers lacking shoulder stability often unconsciously rely on excessive cocontraction of extrinsic hand muscles to stabilize the "platform" from which fine finger movements emerge. Thus a violinist who is unable to support his instrument between chin and shoulder, uses thumb and finger opposition to both stabilize the instrument and create notes. Several rules govern the therapy of these performers:

1. Shoulder instability or hypomobility must be treated during any therapy designed to improve distal overuse difficulties.
2. Patients invariably lack adequate strength in interossei and lumbricals. Musical performance is never adequate exercise for these muscles.
3. The patient with overuse is best treated with a graded set of exercises, initially isometric, then nonresistive, and then resistive in increasing increments of one-third pound.
4. Exercises for endurance are of greatest value.

Musicians need to recruit the serratus anterior and inferior trapezius muscles to stabilize the scapula. In addition, most suffer from hypomobility of the glenohumeral joint and require slow therapeutic stretching. The same requirements for stability exist at the wrist and metacarpal bones. This is especially true for pianists whose interosseus and lumbrical muscles stabilize the metacarpals and allow the finger flexors and extensors to move over long periods of time. Strengthening of atrophied intrinsic hand muscles is a primary goal of physical and occupational therapists providing care for musicians with overuse syndromes. Therapy makes use of training for muscle endurance by emphasizing low-resistance repetitions. Secondary concerns of therapy often involve correction of hypermobility or hypomobility about the shoulder, wrist, and thumb. We use repetitive isometric contractions of supporting muscles to correct hypermobility in patients with overuse, bearing in mind that musicians often view this laxity as a "professional advantage."

The performer should be made aware that 90% of patients with overuse syndrome return to function within 3 months. With subsidence of pain comes the critical rehabilitation phase. It begins with assessment of the technique and the instrument, and here a skilled teacher or performer may be of immense assistance. Technical faults and idiosyncrasies need to be corrected before playing is resumed. Certain faults are predictable and may be easily corrected (see box). Practice habits are reviewed and playing time is sensibly allocated because performers, left unguided, often opt to

---

THE ANATOMIC BASIS OF COMMON TECHNICAL FAULTS THAT PREDISPOSE TO OVERUSE

Neck

Piano—excessive lordosis with right strap muscles
Violin/viola—poorly fit chin rest (instrument not held firmly)
Guitar—improper neck strap

Shoulder

Piano—tight intrinsic muscles diminish "reach" ascending arpeggios and octaves engage thoracic outlet
Violin/viola—bowing limited by limited flexion and internal rotation
　　　　　—bowing limited by thoracic outlet
　　　　　—bowing limited by scapula winging
Cello/bass—high bow arm engages rotator cuff or thoracic outlet
Guitar—finger picking limited by TOS
Percussion—high cymbals engage TOS

Elbow

Piano—limited pronation limits right fourth and fifth finger trills
String—bowing compresses ulnar nerve

Hand

Piano—weak interossei and lumbricales diminish trills and reach
　　　—weak thumb adductor limits arpeggio
　　　—playing in ulnar deviation limits fourth and fifth finger extension
Violin—weakness of left fourth and fifth intrinsics limits vibrato and trills
　　　—lax proximal interphalangeal (PIP) and distal interphalangeal (DIP) joints during vibrato encourage overuse
　　　—left ulnar deviation weakens double stops
Guitar—weak thumb (left adductor limits octaves)
Percussion—"match grip" triggers abductor and extensor pollices overuse
　　　　　—"gamekeeper's thumb" worsened by conga drum
Wind—lax MP joint overused in supporting instrument on thumb rest

---

accept higher levels of pain in exchange for increased practice. Emotional factors may need to be identified. Changes may be made in the instrument. Easily obtained are various shoulder supports and chin rests for a violin or viola, changes of the thumb rest on an oboe or clarinet, support devices for bass clarinet (Fig. 99-2). String players with short fingers benefit from reduction of the distance between the string and the finger board.

Prevention will clearly prove a more effective approach to these problems. Education of teachers, students, and performers should include the following:

1. Identification of the physical and emotional stresses associated with instrumental playing.

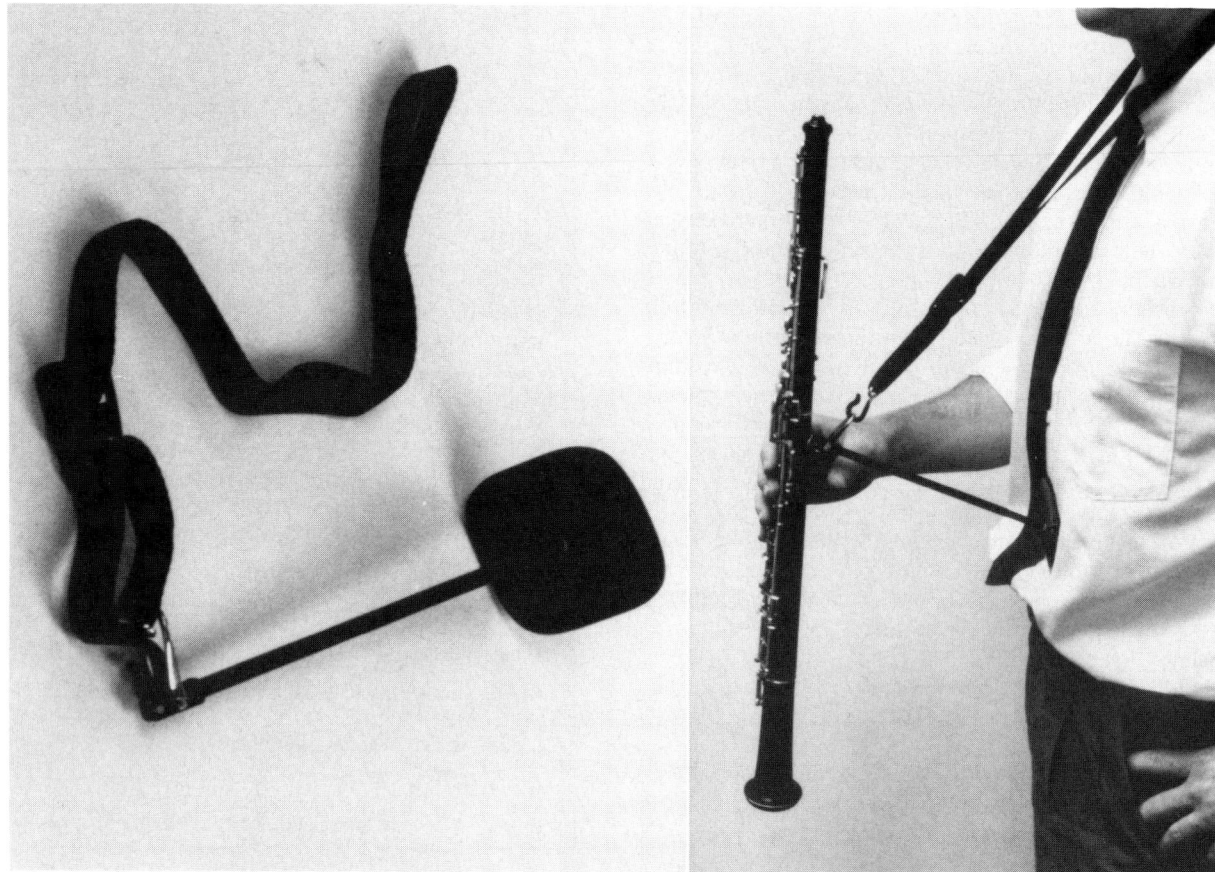

Fig. 99-2 Support post and strap for oboe. (Courtesy Reger, SI, Department of Musculoskeletal Research, Cleveland Clinic Foundation.)

2. Recognition of the role of shoulder and hand anatomy and ergonomy in performance.
3. Realization that pain as distinguished from fatigue is not a necessary part of musicianship.
4. Early identification of technical errors in playing and assiduous attempts to reduce the physical and emotional stresses on the young music student.
5. Recognition that the instrument, the repertoire, the instrumental technique, as well as the teaching method, must be geared to the individual student.
6. Early realization by music students that the body is not indestructible and that strategies for coping involve alterations in the environment, musical obligations, and stresses *not* in the body.

Thoracic outlet syndrome[11]

There are few entities in medicine that provoke as vigorous a dialogue as the thoracic outlet syndrome (TOS). Doubts have been expressed about the very existence of the disorder, let alone finding agreement about terminology, causative factors, methods of diagnosis, and methods of treatment.

Both vascular and neurogenic forms of TOS appear to exist. In clinical practice, the latter are much more common but among musicians "vascular TOS" is a major underappreciated source of difficulty. "True" neurogenic TOS is associated with a cervical rib or elongated transverse cervical process; it is generally acknowledged to be rare.[7] This form is characterized by limb pain and typical pattern of weakness, atrophy, sensory loss, consistent electrodiagnostic changes, and response to surgical decompression. To our knowledge there has not been a single report of such a case in an instrumental musician, although this is likely a reflection only of the low frequency of this disorder, in the range of 1 per 1,000,000, according to Gilliatt.[7]

A much larger group of patients, including a substantial number of instrumental musicians, have limb pain, mostly in the forearm and hand but less commonly in the upper arm, shoulder, and periscapular region, accompanied by paresthesias, primarily along the medial or ulnar aspect of the forearm and hand into the little and ring fingers. Other complaints that mimic a variety of overuse syndromes or are heralded by them include disorders of the muscle-tendon unit and other types of nerve entrapment.[17] Characteristically, symptoms are position-related, often being provoked specifically by playing of the instrument. Verifiable weakness, atrophy, and sensory loss are minimal or nonexistent. This clinical complex has been called the "symptomatic" form of TOS by one of us (RJL) and the "disputed" type by Wilbourn.[11,25]

The role of various provocative positions in diagnosing TOS is also controversial. These maneuvers, including hy-

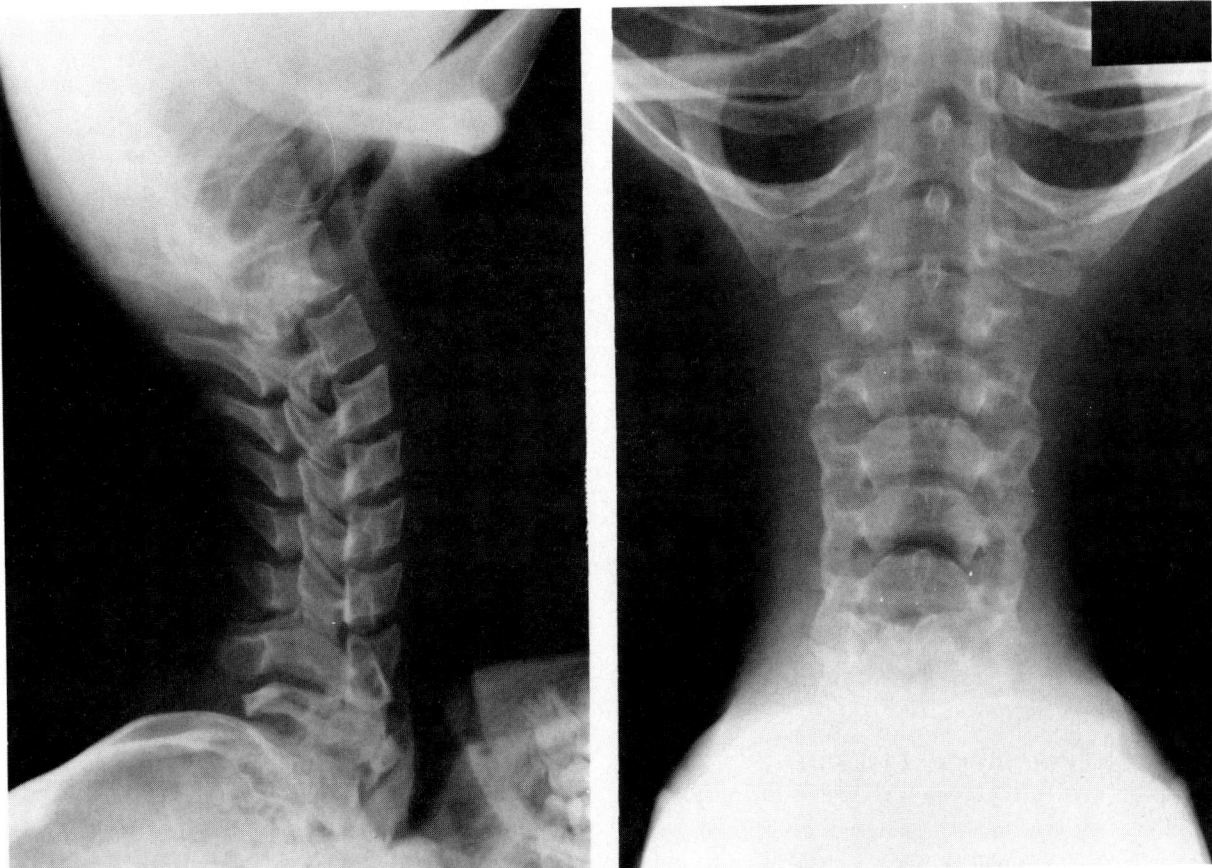

Fig. 99-3   Cervical spine films, frontal *(left)* and lateral *(right)* views in patient with "droopy shoulders." Horizontally placed clavicles are apparent on the frontal view *(curved arrow)*; on the lateral view, the arrow points to the upper border of the T$_3$ vertebral body. (From Lederman RJ: Med Probl Perform Art 2:90, 1987.)

perabduction, the Adson maneuver, the costoclavicular maneuver, and downward arm traction with internal rotation of the shoulder and the elevated arm stress test (EAST) of Roos,[21] are unfortunately nonspecific and not infrequently have positive results in asymptomatic patients or in the uninvolved limb of the symptomatic musician. However, in musicians, the application of these maneuvers may faithfully reproduce symptoms noted during performance. Conversely, the inability to provoke symptoms by one or another of these maneuvers should lead to some skepticism about the diagnosis.

Electrodiagnostic studies are similarly problematic. Abundant evidence now exists that the "classic" ulnar nerve conduction test for TOS is unreliable at best. Nonetheless, nerve conduction studies and needle electromyography are often helpful in excluding other nerve entrapments such as median neuropathy at the wrist, ulnar neuropathy at the elbow, or cervical radiculopathy. The role of somatosensory-evoked potentials is also controversial; our collective experience is that these studies are not helpful, even when performed in provocative positions. Arteriography is useful only for the diagnosis of the vascular forms. The role of magnetic resonance imaging (MRI) remains untested. The clinician must rely on a high index of suspicion, a careful assessment by history and examination to identify a compatible clinical picture, and a thorough search for alternate and more readily diagnosed mechanisms. A substantial subset of TOS patients has either "droopy shoulder" configuration, or a "dead arm" caused by shoulder laxity. Droopy shoulder (Fig. 99-3) is characterized by a long curved neck, sloping shoulder, and concave trunk posture. A characteristic finding on x-ray examination is the presence of horizontally placed clavicles, rather than the more normal angulation upward from medial to lateral, and the ability to visualize on lateral cervical spine films the second or even third thoracic vertebrae, which is normally obscured by the shoulder tissues. While this configuration is not infrequently seen in asymptomatic individuals, it does seem to predispose to brachial plexus or subclavian artery compression in some.

The therapeutic approach to the "symptomatic" form of neurogenic TOS is also controversial. A trial of physical therapy is invariably indicated. At the Massachusetts General Hospital, one physical therapist, David Roberts, instructs the musicians about the correct postural alignment of the head, neck, dorsal spine, and shoulder girdle, as well as scapula positioning. Most commonly, performers play in a position in which their head is held forward and the scapula is protracted. Postural exercises start with mildly extending the middorsal spine. This allows (1) the head and neck to balance on the trunk without over-recruitment of the scaleni muscles and (2) the scapula to "set" on the ribs to reduce protraction.

Musicians are taught to use the correct scapula muscles to control the shoulder blade. This is achieved by a balance between the serratus anterior and the lower trapezius. Left to their own devices, musicians overuse the upper trapezius, rhomboid, and levator scapula muscles to elevate the scapula. These unfortunately increase scapular protraction. Musicians are taught to elevate the scapula by holding it against the posterior rib cage with the serratus anterior muscles. Often weeks of activity are required until the patient can identify and learn the proper movement. This movement is then integrated with playing skills at the instrument.

Clinicians differ with regard to their threshold for advocating surgical intervention. It has been stated that the droopy shoulder syndrome is not generally amenable to such an exercise program but may respond to specific forms of bracing.[22] Surgical intervention is suggested for exercise program failures. In our combined series, fewer than 10% are subjected to surgery. For these, the axillary approach to first rib resection has been the most popular since its initial description. We have not seen a surgical failure to this date among our instrumental musicians, but the numbers are small, particularly in comparison to the enormous surgical series that are reported.

MOTOR CONTROL DIFFICULTIES OF MUSICIANS—FOCAL DYSTONIC MOVEMENTS

Disorders of movement are the cause of difficulty in one quarter of musicians whom we have examined[17] (see box at right). The over-representation of this population reflects awareness of similar difficulties afflicting the right fourth finger of Robert Schumann, as well as the modern pianists Gary Graffman and Leon Fleisher.[14] Characteristic and stereotyped syndromes have involved, in addition to pianists (the right fourth and fifth finger in flexion), guitarists (the right third finger in flexion), cellists and violinists (the right thumb and wrist), wind instrument players (right fourth finger in flexion), and harpists (right second finger in flexion) (Table 99-1). These spontaneous occupation-triggered movements fall into a class of disorders that also afflicts writers (thumb and wrist), telegraphers (first or index finger), typists and legal stenographers (right third and fourth fingers), and may approximate embouchure difficulties of brass players and spasmodic laryngeal difficulties of vocalists. Although initial symptoms are often ascribed to "tension," "cramping," "stress," or the "battle fatigue" of the

---

MOTOR CONTROL DIFFICULTIES OF MUSICIANS—FOCAL DYSTONIC MOVEMENTS

Painless
Usually one extremity
Slow evolution (weeks to months)
No sensory difficulties
Initially single movement (e.g., flexion) may become complex (e.g., flexion and pronation)
Unremarkable x-ray and electrophysiologic studies
No evidence of features of Parkinson's disease, multiple sclerosis, intracranial or spinal mass, familial dystonic disorder
No evidence of posterior interosseus or median neuropathy

---

concert performer, these initial trivial symptoms soon become sources of painless frustration whenever the instrument is approached. Nonmusical activities are seldom initially involved. The right hand difficulties are never mirrored in the left, although the latter may be the sole site of involvement.

Most often, a performer of extended experience or professional caliber, regarded for a style emphasizing highly individual forte finger movements, has slight involuntary flexion of the affected digit. This may follow a trivial painful overuse inflammation of the flexor sheath. Over months, progression of the difficulty results in refingering of chords, and broken octaves and arpeggios at the piano. As the curling worsens, the third finger held in extension is used as a prop. As pain, weakness, or altered sensation are not apparent, the performer assumes the problem is one of "technique." After medical consultation, an erroneous diagnosis is reached of Parkinson disease, multiple sclerosis, an inherited disorder of the basal ganglia, or a mass lesion within the brain or spinal cord. Neuroradiologic, neurophysiologic, and endocrinologic studies add little to the confusing picture. However, examination at the instrument with coincident electromyographic sampling from forearm muscles reveals spontaneous and uncontrolled contraction of flexor muscles with corresponding inhibition of activity in anatagonist extensor groups. Denervation potentials are not seen, nor is there evidence of nerve entrapment, fasciculation, or decremental response to trains of stimuli.

Table 99-1 Motor difficulties of musicians—focal dystonic movements

Instrument played	Hand	Finger	Uncontrolled motion	Compensation
Piano	Right	4,5	Flexion	Extension right 3
Guitar	Right	3	Flexion	Extension right 2
Violin	Left	1,2	Flexion	
	Right	1	Opponens	Flexion wrist
Recorder, oboe	Right	4	Flexion	
Harp	Right	2,3	Flexion	

The origin of these movement disorders has defied evaluation. Neurologists of the early twentieth century viewed these movements as "occupational neuroses," implying a functional component. Equally untested are the contributions of the musician's hand or arm structure, subclinical overuse syndromes and pain, hypoxia within the forearm resulting from localized "compartment syndromes," or the physiologic consequences of rapid finger movement necessary for virtuosity. In fact, little is known of the physiology of the performer's hand. The last major works on the physiology of piano playing were published before the availability of modern electrophysiologic measurement and computer-assisted movement analysis.[19]

Therapy consists of exercises designed to strengthen weakened muscles, along with reeducation techniques (biofeedback) designed to limit the involuntary contractions. Both the spontaneous movement and rare associated tremor may respond to the use of trihexyphenidyl (Artane), low doses of the beta-adrenergic blocker propranolol (Inderal), or the judicious use of medications commonly used for the therapy of Parkinson's disease (such as dopamine agonists). Patients failing these therapies are now treated with the experimental intramuscular injection of Type A botulinum toxin. This agent has been remarkably successful in controlling analogous dystonic movement of the face (blepharospasm and Meige's disease), larynx (spastic dysphonia), and neck (spasmodic torticollis).[24] Injections of the agent produce chemical denervation of afflicted neuromuscular endplates without producing systemic evidence of botulism. Fully three quarters of the approximately 40 patients treated have had some degree of improvement.[2]

REFERENCES

1. Caldron PH and others: A survey of musculoskeletal problems encountered in high-level musicians, Med Probl Perform Art 1:136, 1986.
2. Cohen LG and others: Treatment of focal dystonias of the hand with botulinum toxin, J Neurol Neurosurg Psychiatry, 1988 (in press).
3. Dennett X and Fry HGH: Overuse syndrome: a muscle biopsy study, Lancet 1:905, 1988.
4. Fry HGH: Incidence of overuse syndrome in the symphony orchestra, Med Probl Perform Art 1:51, 1986.
5. Fry HGH: Prevalence of overuse (injury) syndrome In Australian music schools, Br J Ind Med 44:35, 1987.
6. Gerig R: Famous pianists and their techniques, Washington, 1974, Robert B. Luce.
7. Gilliatt RW: Thoracic outlet syndrome. In Dyck PJ and others, editors: Peripheral neuropathy, Philadelphia, 1984, WB Saunders.
8. Hochberg FH and others: Hand difficulties among musicians, JAMA 249:1869, 1983.
9. Hochberg FH and others: Topical therapy of localized inflammation in musicians: a clinical evaluation of Aspercreme versus placebo, Med Probl Perform Art 3:9, 1988.
10. Howard NJ: Peritendinitis crepitans: a muscle-effort syndrome, J Bone Joint Surg 19:447, 1937.
11. Lederman RJ: Thoracic outlet syndrome: review of the controversies and a report of 17 instrumental musicians, Med Probl Perform Art 2:87, 1986.
12. Lederman RJ and Calabrese LH: Overuse syndrome in instrumentalists, Med Probl Perform Art 1:7, 1986.
13. Manchester RA: The incidence of hand problems in music studies, Med Probl Perform Art 3:15, 1988.
14. Merriman L and others: A focal movement disorder of the hand in six patients, Med Probl Perform Art 1:17, 1986.
15. Middlestadt SE and Fishbein M: The prevalence of severe musculoskeletal problems among male and female symphony orchestra string players. Presented at the sixth annual Symposium on Medical Problems of Musicians and Dancers, Aspen, Colo, July 29, 1988.
16. Newmark J and Hochberg FH: Doctor, it hurts when I play: painful disorders among instrumental musicians, Med Probl Perform Art 2:93, 1987.
17. Newmark J and Hochberg FH: Isolated painless manual incoordination in 57 musicians, J Neuro Neurosurg Psychiatry 50:291, 1987.
18. Newmark J and Lederman RJ: Practice doesn't necessarily make perfect: incidence of overuse syndromes in amateur instrumentalists, Med Probl Perform Art 2:142, 1987.
19. Ortmann O: The physiologic mechanics of piano technique, London, 1929, Kegan Paul, Trench, Trubner and Co.
20. Diseases of workers, Chicago, 1940, University of Chicago (originally published in 1713; revised and translated by WC Wright).
21. Roos DB: Thoracic outlet syndromes: symptoms, diagnosis, anatomy and surgical treatment, Med Probl Perform Art 1:90, 1986.
22. Swift TR and Nichols FT: The droopy shoulder syndrome, Neurology (NY) 34:212, 1984.
23. Thompson AR, Plewes LW and Shaw EG: Peritendinitis crepitans and simpled tenosynovitis: a clinical study of 544 cases in industry, Br J Ind Med 8:150, 1951.
24. Tsui JK and others: Double blind study of botulinum toxin in spasmodic torticollis, Lancet 2:245, 1986.
25. Wilbourn AJ: Thoracic outlet syndrome. In course syllabus: Controversies in entrapment neuropathies, Rochester, Minn, 1984, American Association of Electromyography and Electrodiagnosis.

100

The BTE Work Simulator

Katrina Jones Pendergraft, Jonathan K. Cooper, and Gaylord L. Clark

Traditional measures of upper extremity strength and function following trauma typically include use of the grip dynamometer, pinch gauge, and the goniometer for joint range of motion. These testing devices provide objective information and are more often used to gauge progress in recovery from trauma. As medical recovery nears completion, additional questions are commonly asked of physicians and therapists regarding work function and ability to return to full active employment. The traditional measures mentioned above do not provide all the information needed to determine return-to-work status or regarding hand function in relation to job tasks. In the hand rehabilitation setting it is not always feasible or space efficient to have many different machines or tools from industry available. These machines and tools usually have specific functions and do not provide cost-effective treatment alternatives or measurable performance information. The BTE Work Simulator can bridge this information gap and assist in providing the information needed to make determinations regarding progress in therapy and return-to-work status.

The BTE (Baltimore Therapeutic Equipment Company) Work Simulator was invented in 1979 by John Engalitcheff, Jr., in collaboration with Dr. Raymond M. Curtis, at The Union Memorial Hospital, Baltimore, Maryland. The initial goal was to develop a space efficient machine that could provide physical rehabilitation through exercise of the upper extremity and simulation of a wide variety of job tasks.[3] Since 1979 the BTE Work Simulator has undergone many changes and is used internationally for rehabilitation and evaluation of upper extremity function.

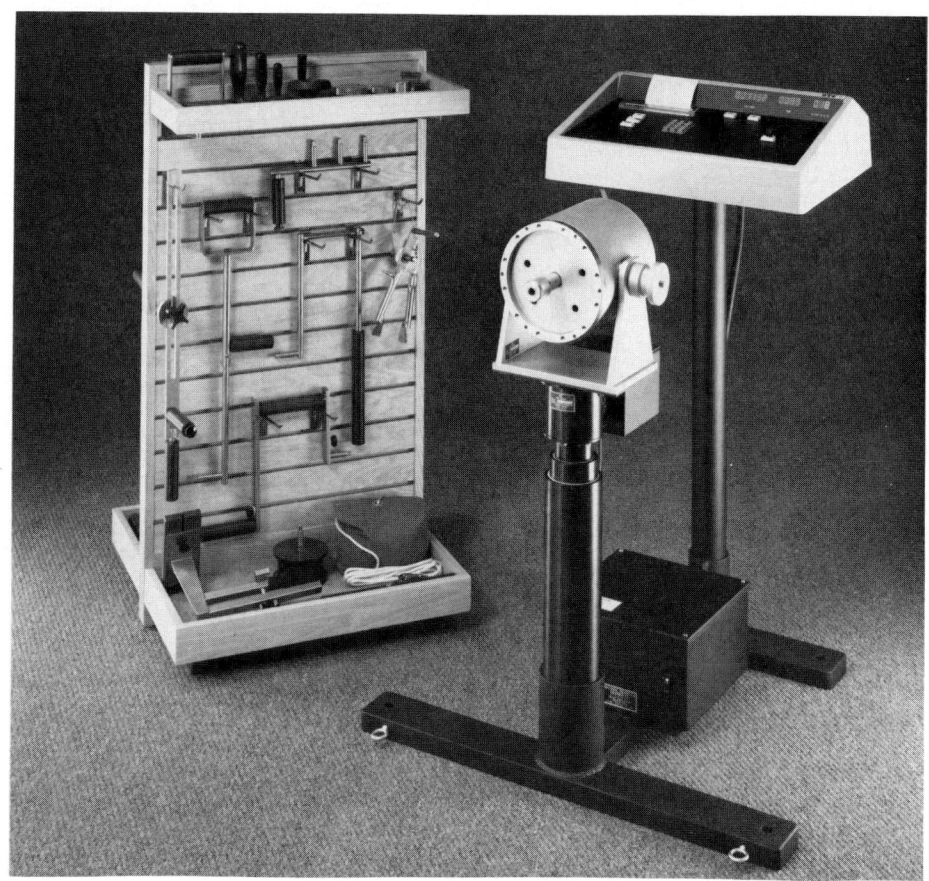

Fig. 100-1　BTE model WS10 with numerous attachments.

GENERAL DESCRIPTION

The BTE Work Simulator can be described as having three major components: (1) the computer console, (2) the exercise head, and (3) various attachments (Fig. 100-1).

The computer console is the control panel for the work simulator. User feedback is provided by displaying resistance level, distance of shaft rotation, and time. The console can provide a printout of these three variables, as well as calculations for dynamic power output, records of patient identification, date of documentation, and attachment number.

The exercise head is an electrical braking system that delivers a controlled amount of resistance to an axial shaft. The height of the exercise head is adjustable with a range of 13 to 66 inches. It swivels to one of seven different positions for increased variability of exercises. The individual exercise attachments lock into the exercise head for operation (Fig. 100-2).

Nineteen attachments for exercise and simulation of specific job tasks are included with the machine. Specifically, these tools include three different-sized knobs, a key, a lathe crank, three different-sized screwdriver handles, and a U-shaped handle. A small three-position crank handle, a large variable-position crank handle, a linear motion articulating tool, a rotational ergometer, two steering wheels, a grip and pinch device, a linear motion golf club, a rotational ladder and a lifting simulator are also included. Each attachment is identified by a number that is universally used with the BTE Work Simulator. Modification of these tools or development of new tools is encouraged based on individual patient need and therapist expertise.

These tools and attachments are used to simulate a wide variety of job tasks including making machine adjustments, rotating small valves, and hand drilling, as well as operating lathe cranks, screwdrivers, and other small hand tools. Gross upper extremity functions such as lifting, pushing, pulling, sawing, driving, shoveling, troweling, hammering, and climbing can be simulated with the larger attachments. Activities of daily living such as ironing, sweeping, vacuuming, opening jar lids, key turning, and pencil sharpening can also be simulated.

Specific exercise use of the work simulator can include pinch and grip strengthening, supination and pronation, radial and ulnar wrist deviation, wrist flexion and extension, palmar and fingertip desensitization, finger flexion and extension, elbow flexion and extension, internal and external shoulder rotation, and shoulder flexion and extension. Total upper extremity range of motion, upper torso motion, upper body conditioning, and bilateral range of motion are also exercise possibilities using the BTE Work Simulator. Each tool can be used creatively to meet the rehabilitation and vocational needs of the patient. Variations in height, shaft angle, and patient position create a wide range of possible uses for each attachment.

The BTE Work Simulator may be used in three modes of operation: automatic, manual-dynamic, and manual-static. In the automatic mode the console will "talk" the user through the exercise program, providing step-by-step instruction for machine setup and operation. The user is also given a computer printout at the end of the exercise. This printout documents strength and power output by recording the resistance level, distance, and time involved with the

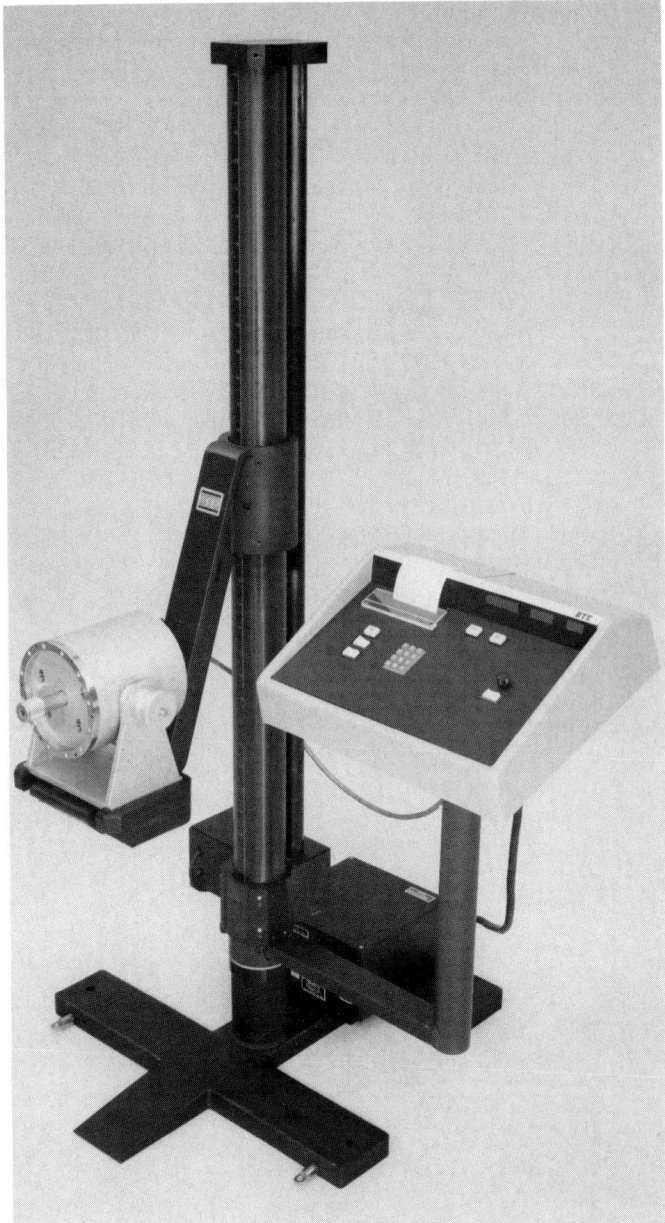

Fig. 100-2 BTE model WS20 has a height range of 13 to 66 inches.

exercise prescribed. The automatic mode is used when accurate assessment of exercise time and power output is desired. The manual-dynamic mode does not automatically provide a printout when the exercise is completed. This mode is most frequently used when power output is not needed, as in routine exercise. The manual-static mode is used for isometric strength testing.

DOCUMENTATION AND CALCULATIONS

The BTE Work Simulator documents information based on three elements of power output. These principles are load, distance, and time. In relation to the work simulator, these variables translate to resistance (inch-pounds), distance (degrees of shaft rotation), and time (seconds), respectively. Static testing generates maximum isometric force exhibited in terms of inch-pounds. This type of testing is usually used to determine maximum strength effort and is similar to the Jaymar dynamometer in testing concept. Dynamic power and endurance test calculations are based on the equation for horsepower. Because the power generated by the human hand cannot be easily measured in horsepower, a smaller unit of measure has been devised by Engalitcheff. This unit has been termed an "engal" (378,000 engals = 1 horsepower). The formula reads as follows:

$$\text{Power} = \frac{\text{Resistance} \times \text{Distance}}{\text{Time}}$$

Documentation of work output is often used to determine patient performance. In a treatment setting, evaluation of daily exercise records can provide information regarding treatment progress and strength and endurance changes. Periodic static strength and dynamic testing can also provide valuable information. Typically, these data are used to compare strength and endurance differences between the injured and uninjured extremity. Repeat testing can also determine improvement percentages as treatment continues. These data are valuable not only to the treating therapist and physician,

but also to the patient. The use of objective feedback during the treatment program allows the patient the opportunity to assess personal progress and formulate realistic goals regarding physical capabilities, limitations, and return to work. The BTE Work Simulator is becoming increasingly popular as an evaluative tool as well. When information regarding functional differences between an injured and an uninjured extremity is needed, static and dynamic strength testing can be used effectively. Some normative data are available for general population comparisons.

A software program called "Quest" and necessary hardware are available for use with the BTE Work Simulator (Fig. 100-3). The computer connects directly to the work simulator console for interaction between the work simulator and "Quest." The program provides a format for storing patient history and daily treatment results. It also performs data calculations and comparisons. Written or graphic exercise and evaluation results for both static and dynamic testing is provided. The program is also capable of graphically comparing test-retest results. In addition, "Quest" generates evaluation reports, converts inch-pounds to

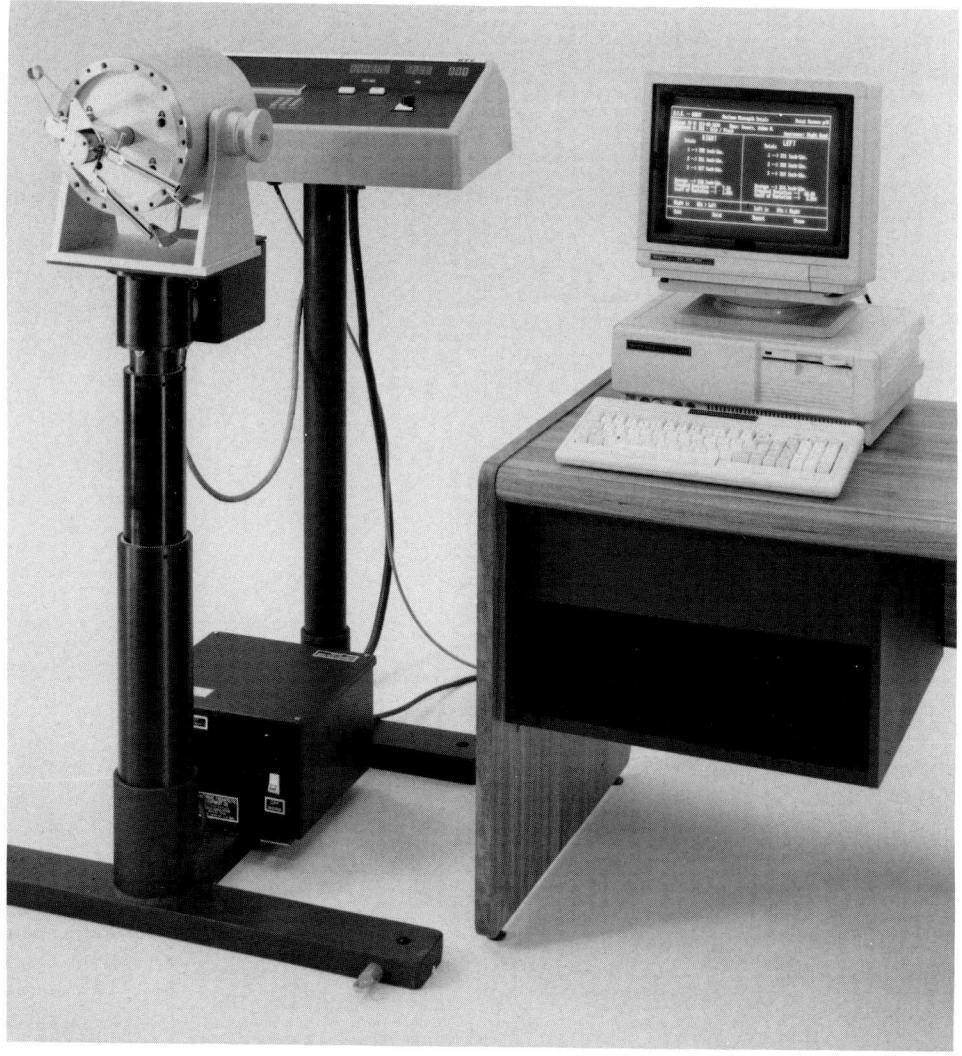

Fig. 100-3 BTE model WS10 and QUEST.

pounds for most attachments, and prints this information in a standardized report format.[4]

Because the BTE Work Simulator has become more widely used as an evaluation instrument, increased questions regarding machine reliability have been addressed. A recent study has been completed revealing reliability coefficients for grip and wrist flexion norms for healthy male subjects. A test-retest design was incorporated to measure intrainstrument reliability. Grip strength reliability coefficients were reported at 0.979. Wrist flexion reliability coefficients were reported at 0.913.[5] To date, intermachine reliability testing has not been statistically measured or reported.

The initial research study performed using the BTE Work Simulator was completed by Berlin and Vermette.[2] Normative data for static and dynamic grip and static and dynamic wrist flexion were developed. A healthy but numerically limited subject population was used for this study. Several other studies, however, have been designed to develop more complete normative data.[1,8,9]

CASE STUDY

J.C. is a 35-year-old male bricklayer who sustained a work-related injury, rupturing the scapholunate ligament of the right, dominant hand. Six weeks after injury this patient underwent a surgical repair of the ligament. Following approximately 8 weeks of physical therapy, J.C. was referred to The Union Memorial Hospital for participation in the work hardening program at the Raymond M. Curtis Hand Center. The patient had normal sensation but had range-of-motion (ROM) deficits of the right wrist. The referring physician's goals for the work hardening program were for the patient to increase strength, endurance, and functional use of the injured right hand in preparation for return to work.

To successfully perform the job duties of a bricklayer, bilateral strength, endurance, and coordination are required. Sample job tasks required of a bricklayer[7] include the ability to lay out brick and cinder blocks using blueprints, level and marking tools; mix mortar; spread mortar using a trowel; and position bricks in mortar. Bricklayers are also required to use a trowel and a level to align bricks and allow for specified thicknesses of mortar. This often requires tapping and measuring activity. The trowel is also used to remove excess mortar from the face of the bricks. All trowel work is performed with the dominant hand. Other job duties include climbing scaffolding and using various hand tools. This occupation requires lifting of up to 50 pounds on occasion and frequent lifting of 25 pounds or less. Climbing, balancing, stooping, kneeling, reaching, and handling are extensively required.[6]

J.C.'s initial physical limitations regarding his work as a bricklayer included ROM deficits, strength and endurance deficits, and a decreased ability to perform tasks requiring bilateral coordination. A work hardening program was individually designed to reduce these physical limitations. Components of this patient's work hardening program included (a) small part assembly-disassembly activity for fine coordination improvements (b) woodworking for improving gross bilateral coordination, overall strength, endurance, and function, (c) work simulation to improve job task performance (mortar mixing, troweling, climbing, lifting, hammering, and bricklaying), (d) periodic BTE Work Simulator evaluations to determine treatment progress, and (e) BTE Work Simulator exercise for strengthening, endurance, and ROM improvements.

Fourteen daily exercises were prescribed. After 9 weeks of participation in the work hardening program, J.C. had increased BTE Work Simulator resistance levels by 33% and distance levels by 53%. Three separate BTE Work Simulator evaluations were performed throughout the duration of the work hardening program. J.C. exhibited right hand strength improvements throughout the program. These improvements are summarized below:

Isometric grip strength—56% increase
Dynamic grip strength—48% increase
Isometric wrist flexion—53% increase
Dynamic wrist flexion—65% increase

Improvements in left hand strength and endurance were also noted during participation in the work hardening program.

After 9 weeks of consistent participation in the work hardening program, this patient was released to return to work as a bricklayer by his treating physician.

SUMMARY

The BTE Work Simulator has widespread use in the hand rehabilitation setting. It is a space efficient machine capable of simulating many job tasks and upper body functions. It can be used in treatment setting where strength and endurance improvements are necessary. It can be used as an evaluation tool to determine treatment progress, return-to-work status, and strength differences between injured and injured extremities. The BTE Work Simulator is also capable of documenting the work output of machine users for accurate record keeping. The BTE Work Simulator has proved to be a valuable tool to the physicians and therapists providing upper extremity rehabilitation services.

ACKNOWLEDGMENT

A special thank you to Janna Jacobs, RPT, of the Baltimore Therapeutic Equipment Company for her assistance in the preparation of this article.

REFERENCES

1. Beck H and Sigmon G: The use of regressive analysis to evaluate static and dynamic performance on tool no. 162 of the BTE Work Simulator. In Issues Papers: Fourth National Forum on Issues in Vocational Assessment, Menomonie, Wis, MDC (in press).
2. Berlin S and Vermette J: An exploratory study of work simulator norms for grip and wrist flexion, Vocational Evaluation and Work Adjustment Bulletin 18(2):61, 1985.
3. BTE Work Simulator operation manual, Baltimore, Md, Baltimore Therapeutic Equipment Co.
4. BTE Newsletter, Fall 1987, Baltimore, Md, Baltimore Therapeutic Equipment Co.
5. BTE Newsletter, Jan 15, 1988, Baltimore, Md, Baltimore Therapeutic Equipment Co.
6. Classification of jobs according to worker trait factors (addendum to dictionary of occupational titles, ed 4), Athens, Ga, 1984, VDARE Service Bureau, Inc.
7. Dictionary of occupational titles, ed 4, US Dep of Labor, Employment and Training Administration, Washington DC, 1977, US Government Printing Office.
8. Lowery D, Beck H, and Sigmon G: The relationship of endurance to static and dynamic performance as measured by the BTE Work Simulator. In Issues Papers: Fourth National Forum on Issues in Vocational Assessment, Menomonie, Wis, MDC (in press).
9. Youngblood K and others: A comparison of static and dynamic strength as measured by BTE and West 4. In Issues Papers: Fourth National Forum on Issues in Vocational Assessment, Menomonie, Wis, MDC (in press).

101

On-site evaluation of the industrial worker

Stanley Berlin

A comprehensive upper extremity rehabilitation program should include work adjustment services designed to help the patient return to work. A preliminary assessment of job readiness serves to decide which services are most appropriate for each patient. The first, and perhaps the most critical, step in this assessment is to obtain reliable information about the physical demands of employment. The most accurate method of gathering this data is to go to the job site to perform an on-site evaluation. The information gathered can then be used to analyze which job tasks may present a problem in terms of performance.

On-site evaluation benefits all parties involved in the rehabilitation process. It benefits the employer by opening and maintaining lines of communication with the medical community. Most employers are genuinely interested in the well-being and recovery of their employees. However, they may feel confused about understanding medical jargon and frustrated about finding out what effect the injury has had on the employee's ability to perform work. The health care professional who makes contact with the employer during the on-site evaluation is in an ideal position to explain the treatment program and how it relates to returning the employee to work as soon as possible.

The employee benefits from the on-site evaluation by maintaining contact with fellow workers. The stability and support provided by these relationships is invaluable, especially during the initial period of returning to work. In addition, the evaluation provides an opportunity for the employer to give support and encouragement.

The insurance company benefits from the on-site evaluation because it results in an accurate assessment of job readiness and serves as the foundation for the most effective and expedient vocational planning.

On-site evaluation benefits the health care provider by serving as the source for the most accurate information regarding the physical demands of employment. It is not uncommon to discover important changes in the nature of the tools, processes, or materials used since the time of injury. For instance, the weight of packages that must be transported on a daily basis may be reduced or the shape of the container may be redesigned to incorporate side handles. These changes can have a dramatic effect on the level of recovery and function needed to resume employment. The on-site evaluation frequently results in the patient being able to return to work sooner than previously expected.

The personal contact made during the on-site evaluation can also provide an opportunity to explore the availability of alternate work if the patient is unable to perform in his or her previous position. Many employers will go to great lengths to provide adaptive equipment or modify the work station to fit the physical capabilities of the injured worker.

Because of the considerable amount of time and money required to perform an on-site evaluation, it is rare that a facility will be able to allocate the resources needed to carry out this process for every patient. When resources are limited, discretion must be used in determining who is best able to benefit from the process. The following situations may indicate that an on-site visit is appropriate:

1. The patient expresses extreme anxiety about returning to work. These feelings may be related to returning to work operating a machine on which the injury occurred or performing a job task that the patient perceives to be hazardous. Some degree of apprehension related to returning to work is normal. Performing an on-site visit can help ascertain why the injury occurred and assess the probability of reinjury. The rehabilitation team should include a health care professional trained to provide psychologic assessment and support. This will ensure that these issues are addressed just as the physical barriers to return to work are confronted.

2. The patient exhibits overconfidence in the ability to return to work. In occupations that require above-average physical strength, some individuals may have difficulty accepting the idea that they may no longer be capable of performing this work. Sometimes there is a family tradition of working in a specific industry. The health care provider has a responsibility to verify the physical demands of employment to make a realistic assessment of the patient's ability to return to their preinjury occupation. This will reduce the risk of the patient returning to a job where the possibility of reinjury is high because of overconfidence.

3. The patient or employer appears to be either exaggerating or minimizing the physical demands of employment. The Workers' Compensation and legal system in some states provide financial incentives for the injured worker to remain in the rehabilitation system for an extended period of time. Alternatively, the employer may be eager to regain the services of a key employee, which could lead to a tendency to minimize the physical demands of employment. An on-site evaluation can resolve many of the questions that must be answered to make an informed decision about the feasibility of return to work.

PREPARATION FOR AN ON-SITE EVALUATION

Before arranging the on-site evaluation, it is important to gather as much information as possible about the position. Sources for this information include a job description from the patient, a written or verbal job description from the employer, and the *Dictionary Of Occupational Titles*[3]. The *Dictionary Of Occupational Titles* provides a written job description for nearly every occupation in the United States economy. However, a study by the National Academy of Sciences[2] has revealed serious deficiencies in the quality of the information as well as the methods used to gather and classify data in the *Dictionary Of Occupational Titles*. Consequently, this book should be used only for general descriptions, not for definitive occupational information.

Every effort should be made to determine if a rehabilitation nurse or rehabilitation specialist has been employed by the insurance company to manage the patient's medical and vocational rehabilitation. Early contact and frequent communication with this professional can help to secure the full cooperation of the employer and claims adjuster in arranging an on-site evaluation and vocational planning. Occasionally, this professional can carry out the on-site evaluation and send a detailed report to the health care provider.

The employer should be contacted in advance to arrange the on-site evaluation. It is prudent to make this initial contact by telephone since waiting for response to a letter may cause unnecessary delay in obtaining approval. The patient can usually provide the name of the appropriate person to contact. If not, it is advisable to contact the personnel department, medical department, or plant manager.

When contacting the employer, it is prudent to keep the conversation short and to the point. Explain that you are the health care professional working with his or her employee. Emphasize that you are interested in helping the employee return to work as soon as possible and that an on-site evaluation would be helpful in understanding the physical stress associated with the position. It is not advisable to make references to any type of safety evaluation or inspection. Also, assure the employer that the on-site evaluation will not interrupt production or work flow.

Before contacting the employer, it is advisable to have several time slots in mind to focus on the most active segments of the work cycle. If the occupational information you have gathered indicates a time of day when the most critical job tasks are performed, then this would be the best time to carry out the on-site evaluation. The ideal method for gathering accurate information during the evaluation is to observe an employee actually performing the job tasks that must be performed by the patient. It is nonproductive to arrive at the job site and receive a tour of the facility to view equipment and materials when the process is not in operation.

When the employer agrees to the on-site evaluation, it is advantageous to ask if the patient can accompany you during the visit. The patient can frequently point out aspects of job task performance that may be overlooked or unfamiliar to the person giving the tour.

The initial contact with the employer is also an appropriate time to request permission to take pictures. Some larger companies require that this request be processed through corporate headquarters. The rationale for taking photographs is that it will give the other members of the rehabilitation team, including the physician, a chance to better understand the physical demands of employment. In addition, it also serves as a foundation for setting up work simulation activities for work hardening or work capacity testing if these services are contemplated.

EQUIPMENT

A variety of equipment should be on hand when performing an on-site evaluation. Safety gear should receive the highest priority. This includes hard hat, safety glasses,

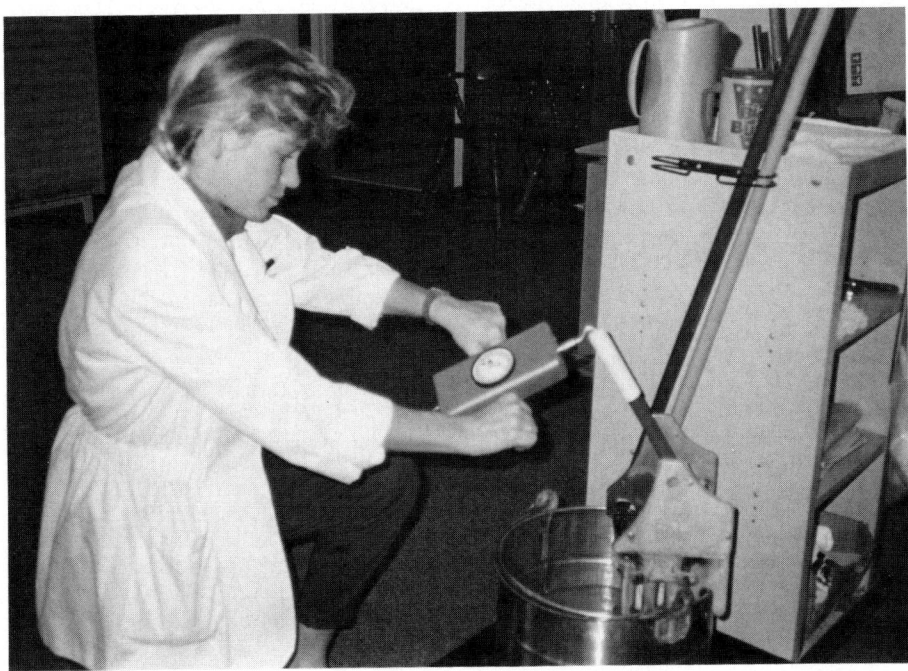

Fig. 101-1 The Chatillon gauge can be used to measure the amount of force required to push and pull during the performance of job tasks.

ear plugs, and safety shoes (with steel reinforced toes). The safety equipment required for each evaluation can be determined at the time the initial telephone contact is made with the employer. Additional equipment that should be used routinely includes a Chatillon push/pull gauge model DPPH 150 (Fig. 101-1), stopwatch, pedometer, tape measure, heavy duty scale, goniometer, indoor/outdoor thermometer, 35 mm camera, and video camera.

DOCUMENTATION OF PHYSICAL DEMANDS

There are many methods and formats for collecting data during an on-site evaluation. An excellent source of information is *A Guide To Job Analysis*.[1] Since documentation time is very limited during the evaluation, it is important to experiment to find the most efficient format. One example is illustrated in Fig. 101-2.

When arriving at the job site, it is helpful to ask some general questions about the nature of the work and the work flow. It is also important to determine the length of the work shift and the number and duration of meal and rest breaks. When time is limited, it is prudent to steer the conversation toward the physical demands of employment as soon as possible.

During the on-site evaluation, it is advisable not to speak to any employee without first asking for permission from the supervisor. Stay alert at all times and stay close to the guide. Always ask questions when more information is needed.

The success of the on-site evaluation depends on being able to record fundamental characteristics about the work being observed. Listing the job tasks that make up a position is an efficient way to group physical activities. A job task is one or more actions carried out to achieve one objective in the performance of work. Each job task can be separated into different elements, or separate actions, necessary to complete the task. Each element can be further separated into separate subelements, or actions required to complete an element.

For example, the job tasks required of a delicatessen clerk include waiting on customers, cleaning the meat case, baking hams and chickens, stocking the meat case, and cleaning the meat slicers.

The single job task of waiting on customers can be separated into the following elements:

greet the customer	wrap the meat
take the customer's order	mark price on package
cut the meat	give package to customer
weigh the meat	

The single element of *cutting the meat* can be separated into the following subelements (a notation is made after each subelement to signify which hand is used to perform the activity):

grasp the handle of meat case door—right
slide door to open the case—right or left
lift package of meat—right and left
carry meat to slicer—right or both
place meat on slicer carriage—right or both
set thickness dial for proper setting—right or left
switch machine on—left or right
place wax paper on base of slicer—left
grasp carriage handle - push and pull—right
place meat slices on wax paper—left
place meat on scale to check weight—right or both
add or take meat off package to reach proper weight—left or right
carry meat to wrapping table—left
unroll wrapping paper from dispenser—right
place meat on wrapping paper—left
wrap meat—left and right
place tape on package—right
write price on package—right

It is extremely time consuming to record all of this information for each job task during the on-site visit. That is why it is desirable to use a video camera to record the job tasks. The videotape can then be played back and viewed at the health care facility during a convenient time. With the proper equipment, the hand and upper extremity movements can be examined more closely by playing the tape in slow motion. When analyzing job tasks performed by a patient with a hand injury, it is almost always necessary to review the subelements associated with selected areas of work performance.

If a video camera is not available, discrimination must be used to decide which aspects of job task performance deserve the most attention. This can be accomplished by analyzing the patient's medical file before making the on-site visit. This enables one to focus on potential problem areas and screen out unnecessary information.

For example, if the patient has had an injury that limits full finger flexion of all fingers of the right hand, we would isolate the following subelements of the job task previously outlined:

grasp handle of meat case door
grasp carriage handle—push and pull
write price on package

Task	Elements	Task criticality	Frequency of performance

Key
Task criticality: 1 2 3 4 5, Low — High
Frequency of performance: 1 2 3 4 5, Low — High

Fig. 101-2 On-site evaluation form.

These subelements all require finger flexion of the right hand and thereby warrant further examination. Subelements requiring finger flexion of the right hand (setting the thickness dial, for instance) have been omitted because they can also be accomplished using the noninjured hand.

Using this technique, we can learn to examine only those areas of job task performance that may be affected by the injury. It takes extensive practice to become proficient at isolating the work activities that may be affected by the patient's injury. Each on-site evaluation should be a learning experience.

The on-site evaluation equipment previously mentioned is used to record characteristics and measurements of the environment and work station. In the previous example, for instance, it was determined that grasping the handle of the meat case door could pose a problem for the patient. The tape measure should be used to determine the diameter of the handle, height of the door, length of the handle, clearance between the handle and door, and the distance over which the door travels from an open to closed position. The goniometer can be used to measure the angle of the door handle. The Chatillon gauge should be used to measure the push/pull force required to open and close the door. The stopwatch can be used to determine how many times the door must be opened and closed within a given time period. The frequency with which a job task is performed is an important factor in determining job readiness and should be ascertained during the on-site evaluation.

It is often helpful to make a sketch of the work area for future reference. This can be invaluable when setting up a simulation of the work station. Every effort should be made to record as much information as possible about those areas of job task performance that may pose a problem when returning to work.

The on-site visit should also be used to determine the criticality of each job task. Although the patient may not be able to perform a given job task, it may be of such minor importance that the employer is willing to overlook the problem or assign the task to another employee. It is important to identify the job tasks that are highly critical and must be performed to retain the position.

It is a good practice to follow up the job site visit with a letter of thanks to the employer. This also provides an opportunity to invite the employer to visit the health care facility to see the work adjustment program in action.

ASSESSING EMPLOYABILITY

Using the information gathered during the on-site evaluation, it is possible to assess the ability of the patient to return to work. This can be accomplished by administering a work capacity evaluation. This evaluation is a comprehensive process designed to determine if the patient is capable of returning to one specific position.

The work capacity evaluation is a four-step process consisting of an interview to document employment history and to explain the purpose of the evaluation, a medical assessment to identify special precautions, testing that includes appropriate measures of function, and a written report with vocational recommendations.

The information gathered at the job site can be used to devise appropriate work simulations and tests. It is frequently possible to borrow material from the employer to test the patient's ability to manipulate and transport the product in the work adjustment area of the rehabilitation center. The measurements taken at the job site should be used to ensure that the work simulation is realistic.

The BTE Work Simulator is a variable resistance device used to simulate aspects of job task performance. It has 19 attachments that can be inserted into the machine to test isometric and dynamic strength. It is particularly useful for simulating upper extremity movements used during the performance of work. By selecting the appropriate attachments and correct positioning, it is possible to test the patient's ability to carry out many job task elements and subelements.

If the work capacity evaluation reveals that the patient is not ready to return to work, participation in the work hardening program may be recommended. Work hardening is a structured program of graded work simulation and conditioning activities designed to improve the patients' ability to perform job tasks.

Work conditioning may include any activity not directly job related, but it is designed to improve overall upper extremity strength, endurance, and function. This includes using exercise machines, lifting weights, or working on a project-oriented activity such as woodworking or metalworking.

Work simulation activities include using the BTE Work Simulator with attachments selected to simulate areas of job task performance. Work simulation activities also include performing critical job tasks at simulated work stations. The information obtained during the on-site evaluation is used as a foundation for planning the work stations. Examples of simulated work stations include:

1. A warehouse worker lifts a set of three boxes without handles onto adjustable shelving. The shelving is set to the heights encountered at work. The weight in the boxes is gradually increased to the weight lifted on the job. Boxes with side handles are not used because they are not used at work.
2. A carpenter hammers nails into a piece of 4 × 4 inch pressure-treated lumber. The 8 foot long section of lumber is bolted vertically to a wall so that the patient can work at a variety of heights from ground level to overhead.
3. An electrician uses wire cutters, pliers, and screwdrivers to wire a series of receptacles and switches on a 4 × 4 foot piece of drywall.

SUMMARY

The advent of precise and portable measuring tools and improved work simulation techniques has made the on-site evaluation a valuable rehabilitation tool. The on-site evaluation also results in documentation of the physical demands of employment. This information serves as the basis for the most accurate assessment of employability through work capacity evaluation and work hardening.

REFERENCES

1. Materials Development Center: A guide to job analysis, Menominee, Wis, 1982, Stout Vocational Rehabilitation Institute.
2. National Research Council Committee On Occupational Classification And Analysis: Work, jobs, and occupations: a critical review of the dictionary titles, Washington DC, 1980, National Acadamy Press.
3. US Department of Labor: Dictionary of occupational titles, Washington DC, 1977, Superintendent of Documents.

102

Industrial hand injuries: prevention and rehabilitation

Sidney J. Blair, Jane Bear-Lehman, and Eva McCormick

The purposes of this chapter are to present the statistics of industrial hand injuries, to discuss the more common injuries, and to present the role of the hand surgeon and the hand therapist in dealing with and searching for solutions. The role of ergonomics and hand therapy in prevention and rehabilitation will also be addressed.

INCIDENCE

There are a tremendous number of industrial upper extremity injuries. These accidents not only severely affect the lives of the patient and the members of his family, but also increase the costs to the community. According to state labor department reports, trunk injuries occurred most frequently, followed by injuries to the thumb and finger.[1]

The National Safety Council's *Accident Facts*[1] reported the following statistics regarding the number of disabling work injuries:

	Arm injuries	Hand injuries	Finger injuries
1979	2,300,000	210,000	160,000	234,000
1984	2,100,000	190,000	150,000	320,000
1986	1,800,000	160,000	90,000	250,000

Hand injuries account for a larger number of days lost from work because of disability than any other kind of occupational injury. The National Institute for Occupational Safety and Health in collaboration with the Consumer Product Safety Commission reported that in 1982 there were 1,129,392 occupational hand and finger injuries treated in hospital emergency rooms (35% of total injuries).[24] Total arm, hand, and finger injuries constituted 20% of the compensation costs of all injuries. The cost of all accidents in 1980, including motor vehicle, work, home, and public, came to 83 billion dollars. Work accidents cost 30 billion dollars, with 20% of them involving the upper extremity.

How accidents occur has been tabulated by the U.S. Department of Labor,[31] the U.S. Consumer Products Safety Commission,[26] and other organizations. Insurance carriers tabulate lists of occurrences. According to one survey, 22% of the emergency room patients with finger amputations gave up their original jobs.

The Occupational Safety and Health Administration (OSHA), part of the U.S. Department of Labor, was created by the Occupational Safety and Health Act of 1970. The purpose of the act is to encourage employers and employees to reduce hazards in the work place. Most employers are covered under this act. OSHA often conducts work-place inspections without advance notice. OSHA has brought about a decrease in the occurrence of accidents, although they are still prevalent.

There are many tools with which a worker can injure his hands. Furthermore, safeguarding is a problem. Safety standards have been established, and organizations make safety equipment and conduct education programs, yet accidents, especially those involving power presses, still occur. For example, an investigation from February to July of 1979 conducted by the Office of Standards Development reported 50 amputations. They occurred in heavily industrial areas, mainly in the northeastern United States.[16]

Data for 1980 indicate that there are about 151,000 mechanical press operators in the United States. About 10%, or 2000, per year of all amputations, which were about 20,000 per year, occur among power press operators. It was noted that 49% of the total injuries on mechanical power presses result in amputation. NIOSH, the National Institute of Occupational Health and Safety, found that young men under the age of 31 were more commonly injured because of their greater hand speed and their ability to move their hands into the presses. Other causes included inadvertent activation of the machine with foot controls and inadequate guards.[23]

Education of supervisors and redesigning of equipment are essential to the reduction of accidents. The medical community, represented by hand surgeons and others, can help to reduce injuries by contacting local safety groups and industries and by developing committees to investigate injuries.

In a study on injuries caused by woodworking equipment, Justis and colleagues[18] found 720,000 injuries per year causing severe psychological and functional impairment. In a survey carried out on 1000 injured woodworkers, the most significant causal factor reported was failure to use properly installed guards, but personal factors such as fatigue and postprandial somnolence was also implicated.

COMMON INDUSTRIAL HAND INJURIES
Ring injuries

Many industrial accidents involve a worker catching his ring on an object and then falling from a height. A fall from a height greater than 5 feet often produces an avulsion of all of the soft tissues of the ring finger. A ring can strip back the soft tissues of the wearer's finger, constrict circulation of bone and joint, and disrupt the skin flap. Amputation is the common result. Dr. William Frackelton of Columbia Hospital, Department of Surgery, Milwaukee, Wisconsin, developed modifications to make a ring safer for its wearer. This simple, inexpensive method slots the ring in three quadrants, thereby protecting the wearer in case of an accident. Caught on a projection, the ring spreads

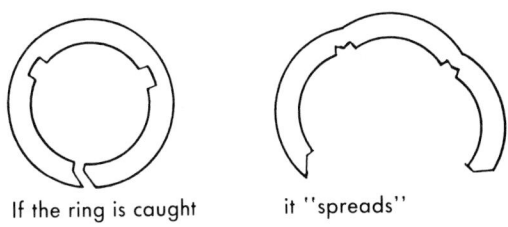

If the ring is caught   it "spreads"

Fig. 102-1   Safety ring designed by William H. Frankelton, Milwaukee, Wisconsin.

open, and the finger is spared (Fig. 102-1). If one were to send out this diagram to jewelers so that they could implement the design, ring avulsion injuries could be effectively reduced.

Grain auger injuries

There is a high prevalence of injuries among agricultural workers. In 1974 the Bureau of Labor Statistics reported that one in 10 farm workers suffered an occupational injury. Although power takeoff and grain auger injuries account for 50% of all farm machinery deaths, little is written about the grain auger. The National Safety Council report of 1979 stated that 22% of farm machinery injuries involved a grain auger and that 18% involved a corn picker. The augers are fitted with protective devices, yet 50% of the injured farm workers admitted removing or altering them for efficiency purposes. Most sustained upper extremity injuries, and about 50% suffered significant permanent disability and could not return to work. The grain auger is now being used in factories producing ground coal and plastic beads. Unfortunately, grain auger–related injuries are now prevalent among both farm and factory workers. In an effort to reduce grain auger injuries in southern Illinois, a media blitz focusing on increased awareness of the hazards of grain auger misuse was initiated in 1980. The report brought a significant reduction in injuries.[7]

Occupational nerve entrapments

The National Institute for Occupational Safety and Health (NIOSH) reports that more than 23,000 manual laborers from manufacturing or similar industries, including production, garment, assembly, upholstery, meat cutting, and letter sorting, are annually afflicted with carpal tunnel syndrome.[27] It is suspected that the actual incidence may significantly exceed the reported occurrences. Many injuries may be related to an overuse syndrome that results in a tenosynovitis in the hand, including the carpal canal. Entrapment of the ulnar nerve may also occur, because of repetitive elbow motion.

Cumulative trauma disorders

There has been an increased incidence of cumulative trauma disorders of the upper extremity reported in the United States. Synonyms for this disorder include repetitive motion disease, repetition strain injuries, upper limb syndrome, shoulder-arm syndrome, and overuse syndrome. The increase in these problems has been confirmed by the United States Bureau of Labor Statistics. They listed new occupational injuries associated with repetitive trauma as fol-

lows: in 1980, 23,000; in 1983, 26,000; in 1984, 34,700.[8]

There have been many studies in the last hundred years that implicate the tendinous structures of the upper extremity to be at risk in hand intensive work. There is a 29 times greater risk of tendonitis in persons who perform highly repetitive forceful jobs than in workers who perform jobs that are low in repetition and force.[3]

The successful program for management of cumulative trauma disorders is based on a multidisciplinary approach through an ergonomic task force, which maintains an ongoing interaction among medical, health and safety, engineering, and managerial departments.[20]

Raynaud's phenomenon

Exposure to vibration may be an etiologic factor in Raynaud's phenomenon.[32] In vibration-induced Raynaud's phenomenon, commonly referred to as "vibration-induced white finger (VWF)," the symptoms are initially mild. Symptoms usually begin with the experience of frequent episodes of cold-induced numbness and blanching of the fingers. A decrease in blood supply causes fingers to become white and numb because of a spasm of the small vessels. The tip of one finger becomes white and numb when the hand is exposed to extreme cold. As the condition progresses, the symptoms occur more frequently and additional fingers become involved. The disease may occur in workers who repeatedly use air hammers, grinding tools, and chain saws, because the operation of vibrating hand tools has been shown to increase the risk of developing Raynaud's phenomenon. More than 500 studies in the medical literature have reported increased incidences of these symptoms in workers using these tools. Studies conducted among British and Scandinavian foundry chippers, grinders, and loggers who use chain saws show Raynaud's phenomenon ranging from 20% to 90%, depending on work force, length of employment, and daily severity of vibration exposure.

PREVENTION AND REHABILITATION
Ergonomics[19]

Ergonomics experts have joined the fight to reduce industrially related injuries. The field of ergonomics originated in Poland over a hundred years ago, and not until 1950 was it introduced into England. The term was coined from the Greek words *ergon*, meaning "work," and *nomos*, meaning "law" or "custom." Ergonomics is a branch of industrial engineering that aims to humanize jobs by fitting the work to the worker by studying man and his relationship to machines. It is an interdisciplinary approach composed of engineering, physiology, and psychology, with philosophical ideas also included in the general theory. Ergonomics revolves around a simple idea: adapt the man-made world to man, instead of the other way around. Ergonomics blends human characteristics with the living and working environment.

Ergonomics experts apply their knowledge to the design and use of hand tools, making the following recommendations:

1. The tool should be designed for operation with a straight wrist; the tool should be bent, not the wrist.
2. Workers should use power tools whenever feasible.
3. Tools should be light, and heavy tools should be suspended or otherwise counterbalanced.

4. Tools should be balanced with handles that are aligned at the center of the mass, so that no rotational moments of torque act on the hand.
5. Tools should be usable with either hand.
6. The grip span of a one-hand tool is best at about 2 inches and should not exceed 4 inches.
7. Handles of tongs and pliers should be designed so that the user will not pinch hands or fingers.
8. The handle surfaces should be so shaped as to contact the largest possible surface of the inner hand and fingers, thereby distributing forces evenly to resist creation of pressure points.

One improvement in hand tools was originated by John Bennett, of Peoria, Illinois. He studied the handle and noticed that with a closed hand an ellipse is formed by the bottom of the hand and the knuckles of the closed fingers. From that he created a 19-degree angle for most tools, which, according to Bennett, contours the hand properly (Fig. 102-2).

Ergonomics experts have begun to investigate industries and have successfully achieved reductions in repetitive trauma disorders, including strains, tendonitis, irritation, ganglions, and carpal tunnel syndrome.[2] Methods of reduction include a task force for direction, training for education, engineering for prevention, and medical prevention and treatment. The engineering controls have led to changes being made in tools. Training consists in explanations of pertinent disorders and exploration of methods of alternative upper extremity postures and movements for work services, elevations, and orientations. Medical personnel have kept careful records to pinpoint sections of departments that have problems. By proper medical management, work restrictions, education of employee and section chiefs regarding the basic mechanics of the repetitive trauma process, and involvement of the product and biomechanical engineers to alter work positions and tool design, repetitive motion disorders have been decreased. Ergonomics engineers have also found that women have a greater risk of developing carpal tunnel syndrome and related tendon disorders than men do. Further research, however, has suggested that the gender variable is less important than work patterns, segmental vibrations, and hand stress.

Workmen's compensation

Workmen's compensation laws were enacted in the United States in 1911. They require employers to assume

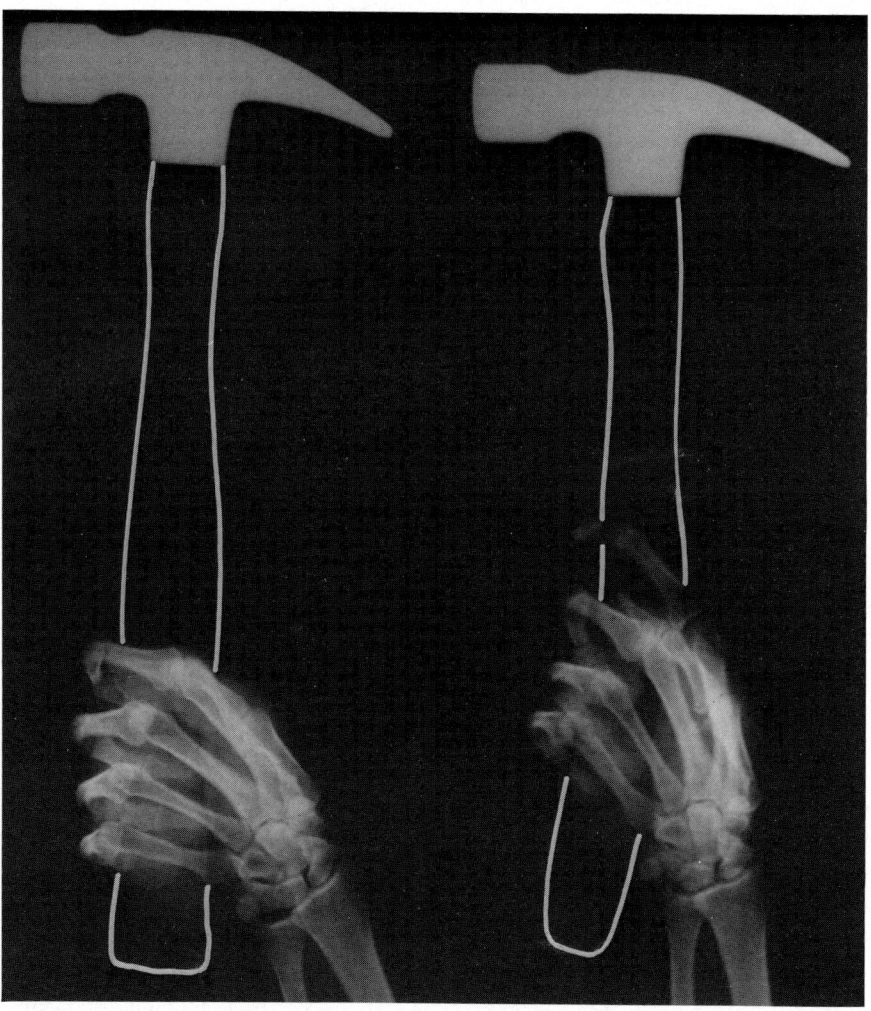

Fig. 102-2 Hammer with 19-degree angle, created by John Bennett of Peoria, Illinois.

the cost of occupational disability. Financial losses resulting from worker disability are part of the cost of production. The basic purposes of the workmen's compensation law are as follows:

1. To encourage safety and effective delivery of benefits
2. To provide medical and rehabilitative services
3. To cover work-related injuries and protect income

While most people conclude that workman's compensation is essential in an industrialized society, some believe that the amount and length of workmen's compensation sometimes influences a patient's response to treatment and the degree of residual disability. According to this point of view, compensated patients get more treatment and have greater residual disability than noncompensated patients. Disability is learned behavior. Since disability is what determines compensation, compensation is based on learned behavior.

In many ways financial compensation does not help the patient or the employer. It can discourage the patient from returning to work. The appeals process can increase the duration of disability. The open claim can inhibit a return to work; thus recovering patients are often unable to return to work. How can ineffective therapy be terminated and claims closed so that recovery is maximized and the patient can return to work? To encourage and facilitate the return, rehabilitation centers have been developed in the United States. Rehabilitation experts act as a liaison between the worker and the company. The problems of trying to locate appropriate jobs and getting a worker back to his previous employment present no easy solution.

Role of the hand therapist

ASHT Committee on Safety and Prevention. An American Society of Hand Therapists (ASHT) committee was formed in 1981 to study the relevance of hand therapy to the issues of safety and prevention for the injured industrial worker. The committee consisted of ASHT members who either work in industry or who have direct relationships with industries in their communities for the purpose of returning injured employees to work. Initial goals included identifying the present state of practice with regard to safety and prevention, establishing both evaluation and treatment goals for the incorporation of safety and prevention into a treatment regimen, increasing awareness, and demonstrating how safety and prevention are part of the hand therapist's domain. The task force became a standing committee in 1986, thereby confirming the importance the American Society of Hand Therapists places on this area of hand rehabilitation.

Evaluation and treatment. In addition to the acute care management of the hand-injured worker, the hand therapist provides evaluation and treatment directed toward return to work. The work of Baxter,[4,5] Matheson,[21] and Smith[30] has broadened our attention so that we are concerned not only with acute care hand therapy but also with the development of physical capacity evaluation, on-site evaluation, and the use of work therapy or work hardening.[21,22] Implicit in such hand therapy programs during the rehabilitation phase is the concept of safe work. In regard to safe work, the following questions are asked.[15] Does the patient employ proper body mechanics? Does he use his hand appropriately? Does he have an adequate number of rest periods? Does he know

when he has done too much? These programs promote the rehearsal of work and worklike behaviors to minimize reinjury.

Primary prevention. The role of hand therapy in safety is not limited to minimizing the risk of repeated injury. Much effort recently has been devoted to primary prevention, that is, preventing an injury from occurring.[6] To do this, therapists and surgeons have begun to trace the symptoms and the injuries to their beginnings.[6,9] Resultant documentation demonstrates the correlation between industrial events and hand problems. For example, tenosynovitis and carpal tunnel syndrome have been linked to the use of crimpers in microassembly and electronics industries. This evidence has provided the foundation for the start of many industry-based prevention programs using education and exercise to diminish the overall incidence of injuries as reported by Lutz[20] and Smith.[29]

Up to now, lack of documentation had meant that industrial prevention programs have been on a limited individual basis. It is of growing concern to attend to the symptoms that develop from repeated mechanical forces before the pain and the disability affects productivity and safety.[14] Documentation facilitates interaction with ergonomics experts, exercise physiologists, and industrial engineers in developing programs.

Screening of employees. Certain anatomic sites and certain job tasks when matched over a prolonged period of time may invite a risk to muscle-tendon units or facilitate an unwanted peripheral nerve entrapment in a worker.[14] Research and surveillance studies[9,11,29] have begun using the latest techniques and a team approach to identify those job tasks that may be at risk. These surveillance studies evaluate the work station and the worker in the work station. It generally begins with the walk-around phase so that the workers can first be observed as they perform their job tasks without intrusion. Those job tasks and work stations that are identified as being at risk are then further scrutinized on an individual basis. The work stations that have a high incidence of physical complaints from the workers, of absenteeism, or of reported injuries are videotaped to obtain scientific biomechanical analysis of the job and its tasks. When the risk is evident, the next step is evaluation. The biomechanical and neurologic body effects are then observed and recorded over time. Should it be determined that the interface between the work station and the worker is a problem, the resulting information can lead to remediation by either work station modification or by changing the way the worker performs the job or a combination of the two.

The majority of these screening tools and surveillance studies recently described in the medical literature have attended to those workers already in their jobs and the jobs that have been perceived to be at risk. However, some industries have shown both an awareness and an interest in screening workers at the time of employment. To be effective and lawful, this form of assessment not only must focus on creating a better match between the physical capacities of the applicant and the physical demands of the job, but also must be in compliance with nondiscriminatory hiring procedures and practices required by law.

Secondary prevention. Historically, therapists have worked as primary treatment agents to facilitate rehabilitation, but the secondary level of prevention is now receiving close attention as therapists attempt to qualitatively identify the achieved level of the patient and determine whether this status is adequate for the resumption of work.[6]

These objective findings from combined evaluations and clinical observations provide valuable information for predicting the ability to return to work safely and for minimizing the chances of repeated injury. Review of the total clinic populations in hand therapy centers could suggest trends in occupational injury that may contribute to the achievement of prevention. Continued education in the principles of ergonomics, including emphasis on preparing an injured worker for a safe return to work, facilitates communication between the medical and industrial communities.

To face the challenges successfully, we must begin to gather informaton about our patients' work in the beginning stages of treatment. Our evaluation tools provide us with information about the patient's functional status and his job requirements. The *Dictionary of Occupational Titles*[12] confirms the physical demands of the job. The information needs to be gathered early and communicated to the medical team, the insurance carrier, and the employer to form a coordinated plan for successful return to work. This type of communication is appreciated by insurance companies who are interested in efficient and cost-effective procedures.

The therapist at this point must decide whether his or her role is to facilitate the return to work through other professionals, with the therapist remaining in the acute care arena, or whether he or she feels comfortable providing the direct care through the longer rehabilitation phase.[10] A therapist should ask himself or herself the following questions:

Do I have knowledge of industries in the local area and their specific job requirements?

Have I made the necessary assessments and performed the tests necessary to determine the patient's readiness to return to work?

Do I understand the therapist's expanding role that includes the industrial sector, the legal process, and all the rules and regulations that apply?

With continued interest and investment in this phase of the rehabilitation perhaps therapists can further the concept of work as therapy and transfer it from hand rehabilitation centers to the work place. The use of modified work setups through supervision may minimize the confusion caused in the blanket referral of "return to work—light duty."

Although much has been accomplished in reducing the number of hand injuries in the United States, there is much to be done, and therapists need to develop epidemiologic information about acute injuries, true number of repetitive injuries, and true incidence of carpal tunnel syndrome. With safety engineers, ergonomists, labor leaders, employers, therapists, and surgeons working as a team, great strides can be made.

REFERENCES

1. Accident facts. Chicago, 1987, National Safety Council.
2. Armstrong TJ and others: Investigation of cumulative trauma disorders in a poultry processing plant, Am Ind Hyg Assoc J 43(2):103, 1982.
3. Armstrong TJ and others: Ergonomics considerations in hand and wrist tendinitis, J Hand Surg 12A(5)(part 2):830, 1987.
4. Baxter P: A focus on work, therapy, and vocational direction. In Hunter JM and others, editors: Rehabilitation of the hand, St Louis, 1978, The CV Mosby Co.
5. Baxter P and McEntee PM: Physical capacity evaluation. In Hunter JM and others, editors: Rehabilitation of the hand, St Louis, 1984, The CV Mosby Co.
6. Bear-Lehman J and McCormick E: The expanding role of occupational therapy in the treatment of industrial hand injuries, Occup Ther Health Care 2:79, 1985.
7. Beatty ME and others: Grain auger injuries: the replacement of the corn picker injury? Plast Reconstr J 69(1):96, 1982.
8. Blair SJ and Bear-Lehman J: Editorial comment: occupational disorders of the upper extremity, J Hand Surg 12(A)(5)(part 2):821, 1987.
9. Bleecker ML: Medical surveillance for carpal tunnel syndrome in workers, J Hand Surg 12A(part 2):845, 1987.
10. Cantor SG: Occupational therapy and occupational medicine—a merger, Am J Occup Ther 33(10):631, 1979.
11. Chaffin DB: Biomechanics of manual materials handling and low back pain. In Lenz C, editor: Occupational medicine principles and practical applications, Chicago, 1988,
12. Dictionary of occupational titles, US Department of Labor, Washington, DC 1977, US Government Printing Office.
13. Douglas, J: Personal communication, Chicago, 1982.
14. Feldman RG and others: Risk assessment in electronic assembly workers: carpal tunnel syndrome, J Hand Surg 12A(2):849, 1987.
15. Holmes D: The role of the occupational therapist–work evaluator, Am J Occup Ther 39:308, 1985.
16. Investigation and analysis of fifty reports of injury to operators of mechanical power presses. Office of Standard Development, final report, Washington, DC, Nov 1975, US Department of Labor (OSHA).
17. Barbara Johnson: Personal communication, United Hospitals of St Paul, St Paul, Minn, 1982.
18. Justis EJ, Moore SV, and LaVelle DG: Woodworking injuries: an epidemiologic survey of injuries sustained using woodworking machinery and hand tools, J Hand Surg 12A(2):890, 1987.
19. Leamon TB: The introduction of ergonomics: a problem of industrial practice, Appl Ergonomics 11(3):161, 1980.
20. Lutz G and Hansford T: Cumulative trauma disorder controls: the ergonomics program at Ethicon, Inc, J Hand Surg 12A(5)(part 2):863, 1987.
21. Matheson LN: Work capacity evaluation, Trabuco Canyon, Calif, 1982, Rehabilitation Institute of Southern California.
22. Matheson LN and others: Work hardening: occupational therapy in industrial rehabilitation, Amer J Occup Ther 39:314, 1985.
23. NIOSH current intelligence bulletin #49, NIOSH Pub No 87-107, Washington, DC, 1987, US Department of Health and Human Services, Public Health Service, Centers for Disease Control, National Institute for Occupational Safety and Health.
24. Occupational finger injuries—United States, 1982. Morbid Mortal Week Rep 32(45):589, 1983.
25. Rehm R: Personal communication, San Jose, Calif, 1982.
26. Report of the US Consumer Products Safety Commission, Washington, DC 1980, US Government Printing Office.
27. Sager M: Hazards in the workplace, The Washington Post, p D1, Feb 22, 1982.
28. Slack DA: Occupational therapy in industrial rheumatology. Presented at American Occupational Therapists Association meeting, 1982.
29. Smith BL: An inside look: hand injury-prevention program, J Hand Surg 12A(part 2):940, 1987.
30. Smith SL: Physical capacity evaluation. In Hopkins HL and Smith HD, editors: Willard and Spackman's occupational therapy, Philadelphia, 1978, JB Lippincott Co.
31. US Department of Labor, Bureau of Labor Statistics, 1974, Washington, DC.
32. Vibration white finger disease in U.S. workers using pneumatic chipping and grinding hand tools. Section I. Epidemiology. Section II. Engineering Testing (NIOSH), US Department of Health and Human Services, Washington, DC, 1981, 1982, US Government Printing Office.

XVII

DEVELOPMENT OF HAND CENTERS

103

Hand therapy as an integral part of the surgical office

Mary C. Kasch and Richard L. Petzoldt

INTRODUCTION TO THE THIRD EDITION

When this chapter was prepared for the first edition of *Rehabilitation of the Hand*, there were very few hand centers or even specialized clinics in hospitals or out-patient facilities. Hand therapy as a specialty area of occupational and physical therapy was a new concept, and the primary sources of learning for therapists were through working closely with hand surgeons and independent study. As the third edition of *Rehabilitation of the Hand* is being prepared, major changes have been made in the provision of hand therapy services. Legal, professional, and economic factors have mitigated against the "physician-owned practice." National and state professional therapy associations have encouraged their members to become independent of their referring physicians and some states are considering legislation that would limit referral to a physician-owned practice. Therefore hand therapists are more frequently found in independent private practice, as employees of free-standing hand centers or in contractual arrangements with physicians. In addition, more literature is available, more continuing education courses and more opportunities for professional interaction with other hand therapists are available; therefore there is, perhaps, less dependence on surgeons for training.

Despite these changes, this chapter reflects the early history of hand rehabilitation in which a surgeon who was concerned about his patients reaching their maximal level of function sought out therapists who were eager to participate in this new and exciting specialty. Many surgeons and therapists in the late 1960s and early 1970s shared small offices and provided the best care possible, based on the overall treatment goals and rendered in a very individualized and personal way. The surgeons and therapists learned together and forged a new profession called hand therapy out of this common concern. Today, many surgeons may not want to administrate a "hand center" in their office, and therapists may feel the need to be more independent while maintaining the goal of working together to achieve the integrated treatment approach described in this chapter. For those surgeons just leaving residency and therapists new to hand therapy, the ideas contained in this chapter may be helpful in guiding them. No matter how a practice is established, the principle of surgeon, therapist, and patient working together as a team is as meaningful today as it was 15 years ago.

INTRODUCTION TO THE FIRST EDITION

It is our strong belief that hand therapy plays a significant and important part in the success of hand surgery. Typically, the surgeon may assume this responsibility himself, send the patient off to a therapist, or simply leave the patient to his own devices. If the surgeon attempts to play the dual role, he soon finds that he must spend an inordinate amount of time with the patient, explaining the nature of the problem and the necessity and techniques of therapy and attempting to supervise the patient's progress. From the standpoint of the therapist working in a separate clinic, there may be a lack of communication with the surgeon regarding the initial trauma or surgery involved and the treatment goals and timetables. This may result in inadequate or inappropriate treatment for the patient. Further, if the patient does not receive proper and specific instructions for therapy, he feels uncertain about his responsibilities and participation postoperatively and fails to obtain the full potential benefit of both the surgery and the therapy.

We believed that a much better and more satisfying relationship could exist if the surgeon, the therapist, and the patient all worked together in the same setting. With this concept (Fig. 103-1), we established therapy as an integral part of our office.

PROBLEMS

Our office is small. Our staff consists of one hand surgeon, one hand therapist, and two medical assistants who do both front and back office work. In addition to the usual reception, clerical, and private consultation areas, we have three examination rooms with a total office area of 840 square feet. The problems of time and space are apparent. We solved the time problem by dovetailing our schedules during the week: the surgeon sees patients in the office full days on Tuesdays and Thursdays, and the therapist works with patients in the office on Mondays, Wednesdays, and Fridays. The space problem is solved by use of a common examination and therapy table in each of the examination rooms (Fig. 103-2).

Ideally, an office would have sufficient space for separate but concurrent use by the surgeon and the therapist. However, we have found that it is possible and practical to use common space in the manner described.

COMMUNICATION

Communication is the key to success of the concept of a three-way interchange between the surgeon, the therapist, and the patient. A direct relationship is established and continued between surgeon and patient and between therapist and patient during respective visits. Communication between the surgeon and the therapist includes regular meetings to discuss new patients to be referred for therapy and periodic follow-up reviews on all therapy patients (Fig. 103-3).

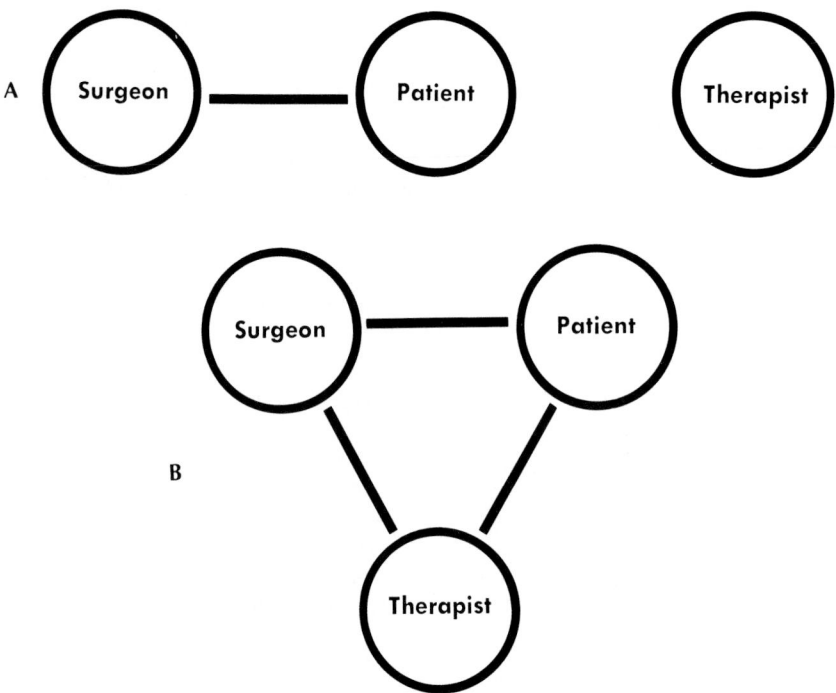

Fig. 103-1 **A,** Typical and often indefinite relationship between surgeon, patient, and therapist. **B,** Relationship that exists when therapy is made an integral part of the office.

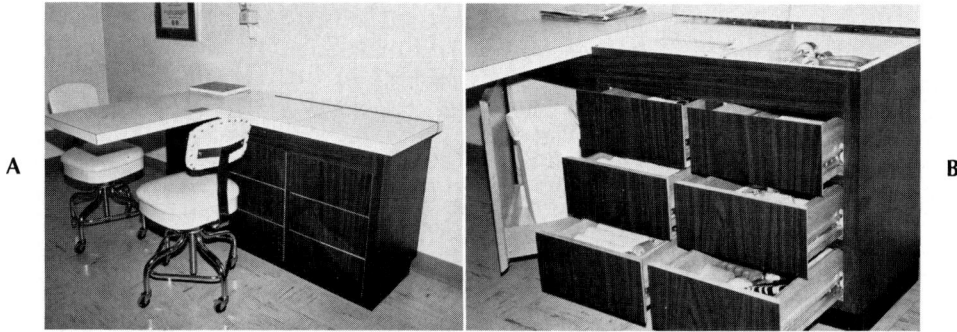

Fig. 103-2 **A,** Hand table used by both surgeon and therapist. (Design modified after others.) **B,** Each table is equipped identically with diagnostic tools, dressing supplies, therapy equipment in hinged-top compartments, and sliding drawers.

The most important form of communication is the patient's chart. This contains the history and physical examination, impressions, problems, treatment goals and plans, roentgenograms, operative reports, and other relevant material (Fig. 103-4). A problem-oriented approach is used. Specific problems, as well as treatment goals and methods, are defined. Dates of initiation and termination of treatment can be entered on the patient's chart. This establishes a clear progression of treatment goals and results. Progress notes are made individually by the surgeon and therapist on separate color-coded sheets, which permit a continuing means of written exchange.

To further simplify communication and to assure optimal progress and integration of efforts, standard protocols are used for all major and common operative procedures. These are developed together by the surgeon and therapist and include the specific techniques and timetables that may be employed for each problem. In this way, there is complete understanding of the treatment goals, and the therapist can still alter the methods and pace as necessary for the best progress of any one patient toward those goals.

It is very important that the patient has some understanding of the nature of his problem. He must also have sufficient motivation to actively participate in his rehabilitation program for optimal results. To help in both these respects, we use a detailed plastic model of the hand as a teaching device to point out and describe in layman's terms the significant structures and relationships and the importance of the patient's own therapy efforts (Fig. 103-5). Simple line drawings are often used for the same purpose.

In addition to the verbal and visual communication, the patient receives printed copies of his individualized home

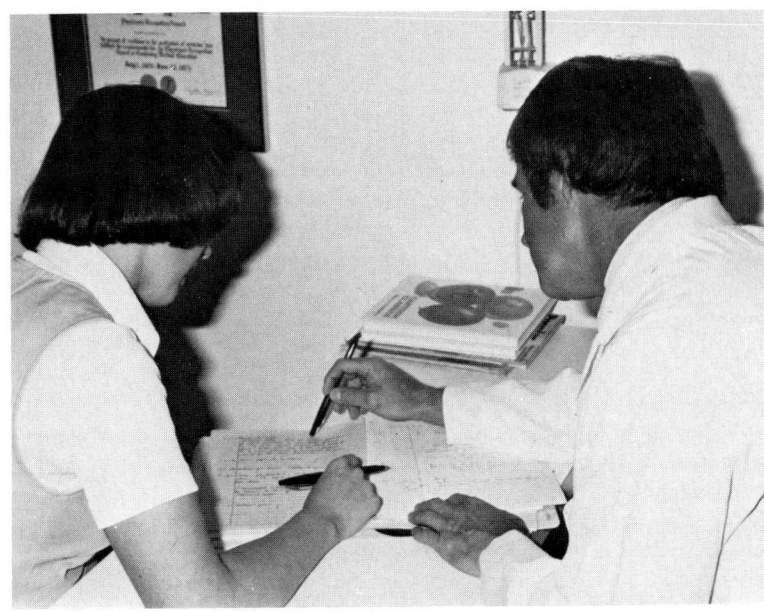

Fig. 103-3 Surgeon and therapist discuss treatment goals and timetables for each therapy patient.

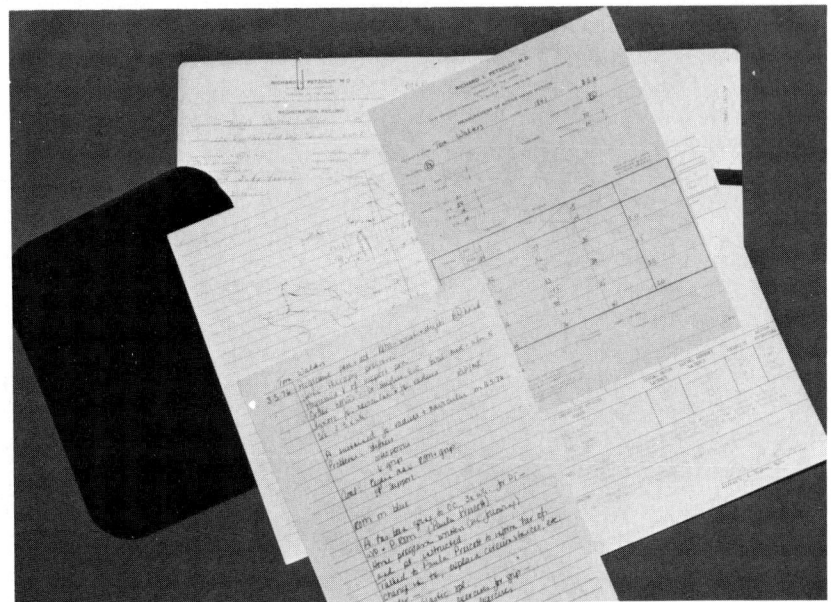

Fig. 103-4 Patient's chart provides a common means of communication, coordination, and documentation for the surgeon and therapist.

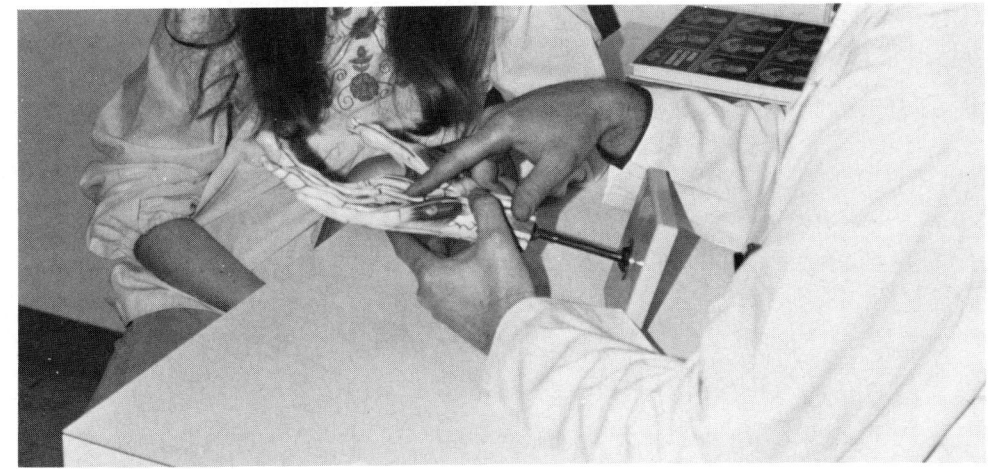

Fig. 103-5 Hand model is useful to help explain the fundamental problem to the patient, which increases the patient's interest and cooperation.

care program and some of the standard procedures. For example, before hospitalization for an elective procedure, the patient is given a printed instruction form to reinforce verbal instructions regarding his postoperative responsibilities for elevation and dressing care.

The patient also communicates with us. An injury to the hand affects the patient psychologically, as well as physically. We find that by providing a supportive atmosphere in which the patient is given a structured program and responsibility for his own rehabilitation and in which he is free to verbalize his feelings, negative attitudes are minimized and more positive efforts are achieved.

REHABILITATION

Not all hand surgery patients require special hand therapy treatment. We reserve participation of the therapist to those cases where such therapy and rehabilitation are considered or become necessary for an improved postinjury or postoperative course or for conservative management.

For those patients referred for therapy, the therapist becomes involved at an early stage. For elective surgery cases he frequently does evaluations preoperatively and then works with the patient closely postoperatively for active continuation of rehabilitation. For elective and trauma cases, he sees the patient as soon as the initial dressings are removed. He reviews the chart and the treatment goals with the surgeon and then initiates a rehabilitation program designed specifically for the patient.

The frequency of patient appointments varies according to individual requirements. Some therapy patients require only one or two visits to receive supplemental instructions, supervision for simpler problems, and splints. More complex or resistant problems of stiffness or weakness require more frequent appointments, which are then decreased as improvement is obtained. The therapist assumes the responsibility for determining the frequency of appointments based on the patient's treatment goals and progress.

Therapy sessions may provide a variety of evaluations and treatment techniques to meet each person's requirements. These may include a selective combination of heat, cryotherapy, vibration, and other facilitation techniques. In addition, the patient's program may include splinting, edema-control techniques, muscle reeducation and strengthening, reeducation of sensibility, desensitization, functional and prevocational activities, activities of daily living, and work hardening.

At appropriate intervals, the therapist remeasures ranges of joint motion, individual muscle and grip strengths, sensory status, and hand volume. Patterns of hand use are observed and recorded. Objective data are recorded and reviewed with the patient, consecutive figures are compared, and red ink is used to record gains, providing a vivid indication to the patient of his progress (Fig. 103-6). Range-of-motion flow sheets and graphs of range of motion and grip strength are used to demonstrate relative progress to help motivate the patient. In addition, the surgeon has available a ready record of the patient's progress without having to repeat all the measurements at each visit.

The fabrication, fitting, and adjustment of splints are also accomplished during therapy sessions. These may include

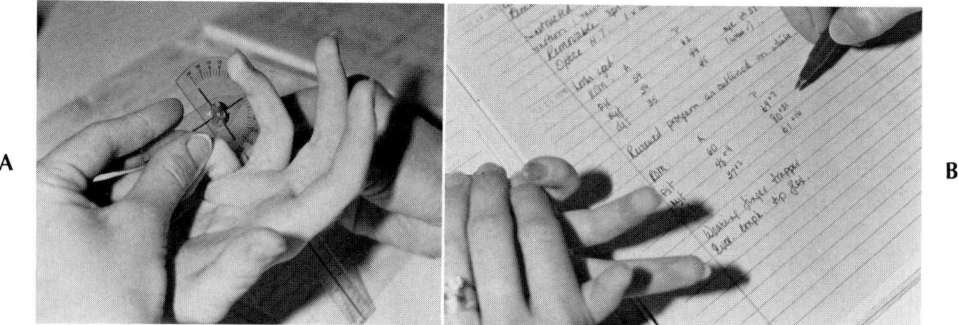

Fig. 103-6 **A,** Therapist periodically measures and records ranges of motion. **B,** Respective gains or losses are reviewed with the patient, which provides a stimulus for continued effort.

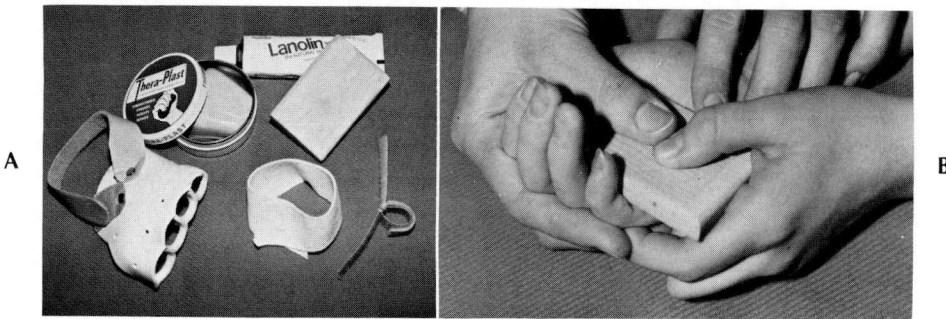

Fig. 103-7 **A,** Equipment for home therapy varies according to patient's needs but is always kept simple. **B,** Patient receives full instructions for the use of any specific device and must demonstrate an understanding of the procedure.

custom-made splints of lightweight plastic material with adjustable straps and dynamic outriggers, webbing straps to improve passive motion, traction gloves, and finger trappers made of Tubigauze or Velcro. Commercial splints may be provided after careful evaluation, and adjustments are made.

The patient's home therapy program is considered the most important aspect of therapy, and the goal is to train the patient sufficiently so that he may continue on his own at home on a daily basis. This is done with the oral, visual, and written techniques mentioned previously. The patient is thoroughly instructed in the use of each piece of equipment he is given as well as the proper positioning, extent of exercising, and danger signals (Fig. 103-7). His program is reviewed by the therapist frequently to assure proper techniques and progress and to make any necessary adjustments.

As part of rehabilitation, the therapist evaluates the patient's hand use in relation to his work and devises exercises and activities to simulate those needs. A patient who is unable to return to his former job may be assigned to a vocational rehabilitation counselor. We assist these counselors by recommending job limitations and by analyzing work requirements in terms of hand use.

Approximately 70% of the therapy patients are industrial compensation cases, and most of the rest are insured privately. Therapy is a financially self-sustaining function of the office. The billing is done through the office, and the therapist is salaried as an employee of the surgeon. With the availability of therapy in our own office, it is possible to offer it to those patients who need it but cannot pay and who otherwise would not have the benefit of it.

ADVANTAGES

As a result of this concept and working relationship, certain advantages for the surgeon, the therapist, and the patient have become apparent. For the surgeon, the biggest single advantage is the amount of time saved in activities that do not require his specific expertise. Basic and initial instruction for therapy is still given personally to the patient by the surgeon, but the more detailed and follow-up visits can be spaced alternately with the therapist and surgeon, thus decreasing the total number of visits with the surgeon. The longer and more tedious evaluations and the making of splints can also be done by the therapist, decreasing the total time of any one visit with the surgeon.

There are also multiple advantages for the therapist. Since many postoperative regimens are standardized in our office, treatment goals and timetables are clearly established. However, the therapist retains the flexibility to adapt modalities and treatment to the individual patient. Time is more efficiently used for the therapist and patient because of limited paperwork and decreased patient waiting time. The patient places a greater value on the importance of therapy because of the surgeon's positive attitude toward it. As a result, his attendance is more regular, he follows through on his home program more diligently, and he cooperates more fully with the therapist.

The patient derives advantages from the continuity of care. When he goes from the surgeon to the therapist in the same office, he recognizes the team approach and the existence of a common effort in his behalf. The patient also feels that everything possible is being done to help him on his road to recovery. With the continued reinforcement from both the surgeon and the therapist, the patient progresses at an optimal rate and to an optimal level.

CONCLUSION

The goal of the hand surgeon is to obtain the best result possible for the patient. The therapist has the same goal but has not always had the opportunity to contribute the full potential of his or her abilities. By combining the two disciplines in the same office we believe we have come closer to achieving this common goal.

ACKNOWLEDGMENT

This chapter is dedicated in fond memory to R. L. Petzoldt, M.D., teacher, mentor, and friend. Dr. Petzoldt was an early supporter of hand therapy and of the American Society of Hand Therapists. His vision of what hand therapy could become served as inspiration to many therapists who worked with him. I am grateful for the opportunities Dr. Petzoldt provided for professional growth in a career that has been personally enriching. He was a fine surgeon who is missed by his colleagues and patients.

104

Hand rehabilitation unit in a hospital setting

Rodney W. Schlegel and Gaylord L. Clark

The formation of a center for management of upper extremity and hand problems goes beyond the traditional surgical approach to disease or injury. As our collective knowledge increases and our technical capability grows, we find most often that it is impossible for one person to render optimum care to the complex hand cases. It is this realization that stimulated us to create the Raymond M. Curtis Hand Center at The Union Memorial Hospital in Baltimore, Maryland. The Center is designed to care for patients with upper limb problems efficiently by means of the expertise of specialists interested in the field (Fig. 104-1).

SURGICAL TEAM

The hand surgeon is the major catalyst in crystallizing the formation of a center. We believe that a team of surgeons is necessary, and their surgical backgrounds should be varied. A general surgeon, an orthopedic surgeon, and a plastic surgeon constitute the ideal team. Each member of this team should be highly skilled in his own right but should be able to call freely for help from any other team member should he believe there is a need for it. The members of the surgical team should be capable of working interchangeably with each other either in or out of the operating theater.

THERAPY TEAM

Closely allied with the surgical team in establishing a hand center and in planning and implementing treatment for the care of the patient with hand injuries are the physical therapists and occupational therapists on the hand team. Their knowledge of the function and dynamics of the hand has increased concurrently with the surgical team. These therapists should have a flexible attitude regarding their identification with physical or occupational therapy so that they may freely exchange certain skills and concepts. This therapy team is fully included in the activities of the hand center. It is recognized that members of these two professional groups have overlapping treatment and teaching responsibilities, regardless of their backgrounds. The specific functions of these therapists must be guided by the scope of practice authorized in their state and in concert with the logistical demands of the specific hand center in which they practice. This allows for the maximum use of individual talent and encourages cooperation in areas of mutual interests.

The center needs to have a nucleus of hand therapists who not only have a high level of clinical expertise, but also have the ability to teach hand rehabilitation concepts

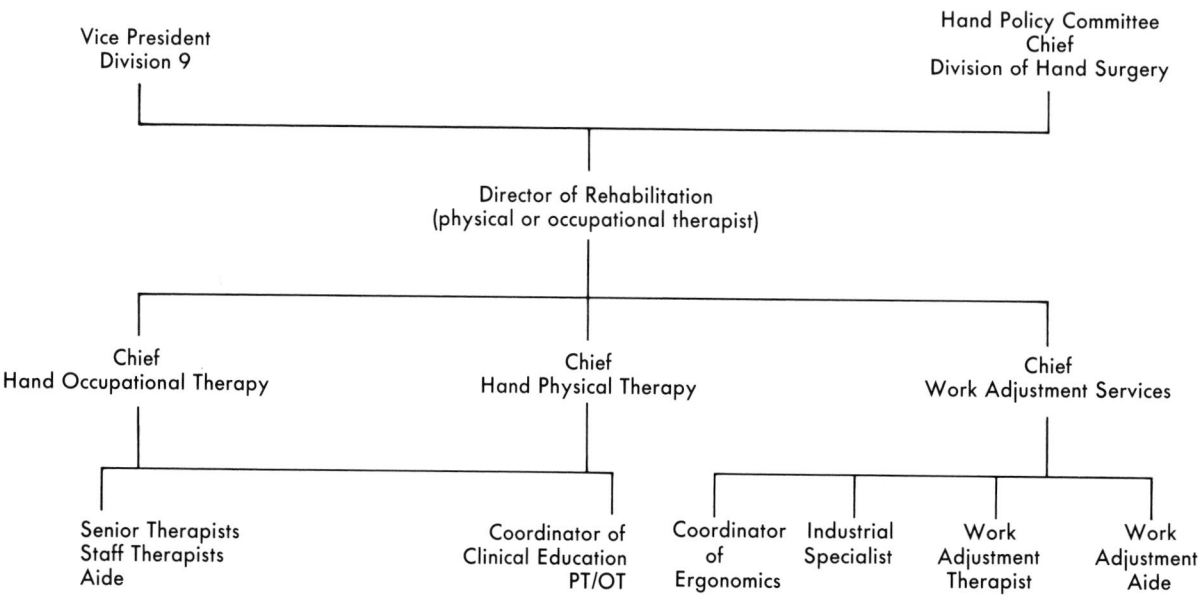

Fig. 104-1 Organizational structure of the Union Memorial Hospital Raymond C. Curtis Hand Rehabilitation Center.

to other practitioners. All therapy members should be able to conduct patient evaluations in a competent manner, including goniometry, manual muscle testing, limited noninvasive vascular testing, electrophysiologic evaluation, sensory evaluation, prevocational assessments, and functional activity testing. All therapists need to demonstrate competence in the application of physical agents, pain management, edema management, and specific exercise systems to enhance the patient's recovery. Members of the staff should be well versed in patient education techniques including directions for activities of daily living, work simplification, joint protection techniques, sensory reeducation, and home exercise programs. Splinting plays a major role in the hand center, and all therapists should attain expertise in the techniques of evaluating patients' conditions for fabrication and application of appropriate splints.

WORK ADJUSTMENT SERVICES

The work adjustment services is staffed by industrial specialists, who have added a special dimension to hand rehabilitation services. The work adjustment services department offers services that act as the final realistic link between therapy and return to work. Members of the work adjustment services department, whom we refer to in our setting as "industrial specialists," may be industrial scientists, vocational evaluators, or vocational rehabilitation therapists. The industrial specialists, in cooperation with the hand therapy staff, are responsible for prevocational testing, job and task analysis, identification of transferrable job skills, work capacity, and work tolerance, along with job site visits. Treatment is oriented to actual work simulation and physical activities having a direct relationship to the patient's employment or specific functional hand needs. The hand center workshops and work simulation programs are the primary responsibility of the industrial specialist.

An exciting program associated with our work adjustment services department is the Center for Industrial Ergonomics. The ergonomics program is responsible for intervention in the industrial community to assist in the prevention or reduction of cumulative trauma disorders. The ergonomics department is staffed as a cooperative effort between an industrial specialist and a hand therapist. The program has been successful in returning patients to previous employment through the modification of job tasks or tools or the industrial environment (Figs. 104-2 and 104-3).

CLINICAL SOCIAL WORK SERVICES

The availability of a clinical social worker is of paramount importance to the well-being of those patients being served by the hand center. We recognize that recovery from a physical injury is dependent not only on the physical rehabilitation of a patient, but also on recognizing the psychosocial concerns of the patient and assisting the patient in resolving those concerns. These psychosocial factors may be presented in a variety of forms such as loss of body parts, self-identity, changes in economic status of self and family, changing social and familial roles and obligations, and loss of normal sexual performance.

The social worker in our setting has been very effective in directing patients through the medical-legal-economic issues they face as a result of an injury. The clinical social worker also serves the patient in matters related to substance abuse and psychic depression.

OTHER HEALTH PROFESSIONALS

Various other medical personnel play important roles, particularly, the physician interested in infectious diseases. It is with this physician's knowledge of the sophisticated use of antibiotic therapy for unusual cases of infection, or potential infection, that the patient can be best cared for. A rheumatologist is important to the center to give advice concerning the care of patients having systemic arthritic conditions. Additionally, it is important to have available to the hand therapy staff other therapists trained in the specialty areas of pediatrics and sports therapy.

HAND POLICY COMMITTEE

A governing committee is important. The chairman is the director of the center. In addition, other hand surgeons and the therapist director are included. It is responsible for the hand rehabilitation unit and acts as the coordinating body to facilitate use of the center by the attending hand surgical staff. It administers quality assurance policies and initiates and approves research projects. The committee serves as a liaison to insurance carriers, industrial nurses, and other persons or agencies interested in the work of the hand center.

OVERNIGHT FACILITY

If the rehabilitation unit draws from a large geographic area, a number of low-cost, overnight, nonmedical beds are needed for patients living at a distance and requiring daily therapy treatments. Ideally, an overnight facility is located immediately adjacent to the unit. When this is not possible, it is recommended that a nearby facility be contracted to house appropriate patients. The number of beds required will vary with each center's patient needs.

LOCATION OF CENTER

A hospital with a concentration of hand and upper limb problems is the ideal place to establish a hand center. In addition to being able to provide established hand rehabilitation programs, the hospital offers an advantage of being able to respond to hand trauma and comprehensive reconstruction services. For a hand center to maintain its effectiveness there must be strong administrative support that understands the necessity of a fiscally sound program that provides excellence in health care.

SOURCES OF PATIENTS

The state of Maryland has an emergency medical system that refers many varied trauma cases from a wide geographic area to a single hand center for acute care. Many of these patients from the same geographic region are then referred for hand rehabilitation. Individual referrals are also accepted from the local medical community. We believe that it is important for the referring physician to be able to refer directly to the hand rehabilitation unit without necessarily being on the hospital staff unless a specific consultation is requested. The referring physician must provide all pertinent information regarding the patient's medical-surgical-accident history along with a written request for treatment so that appropriate care may be provided.

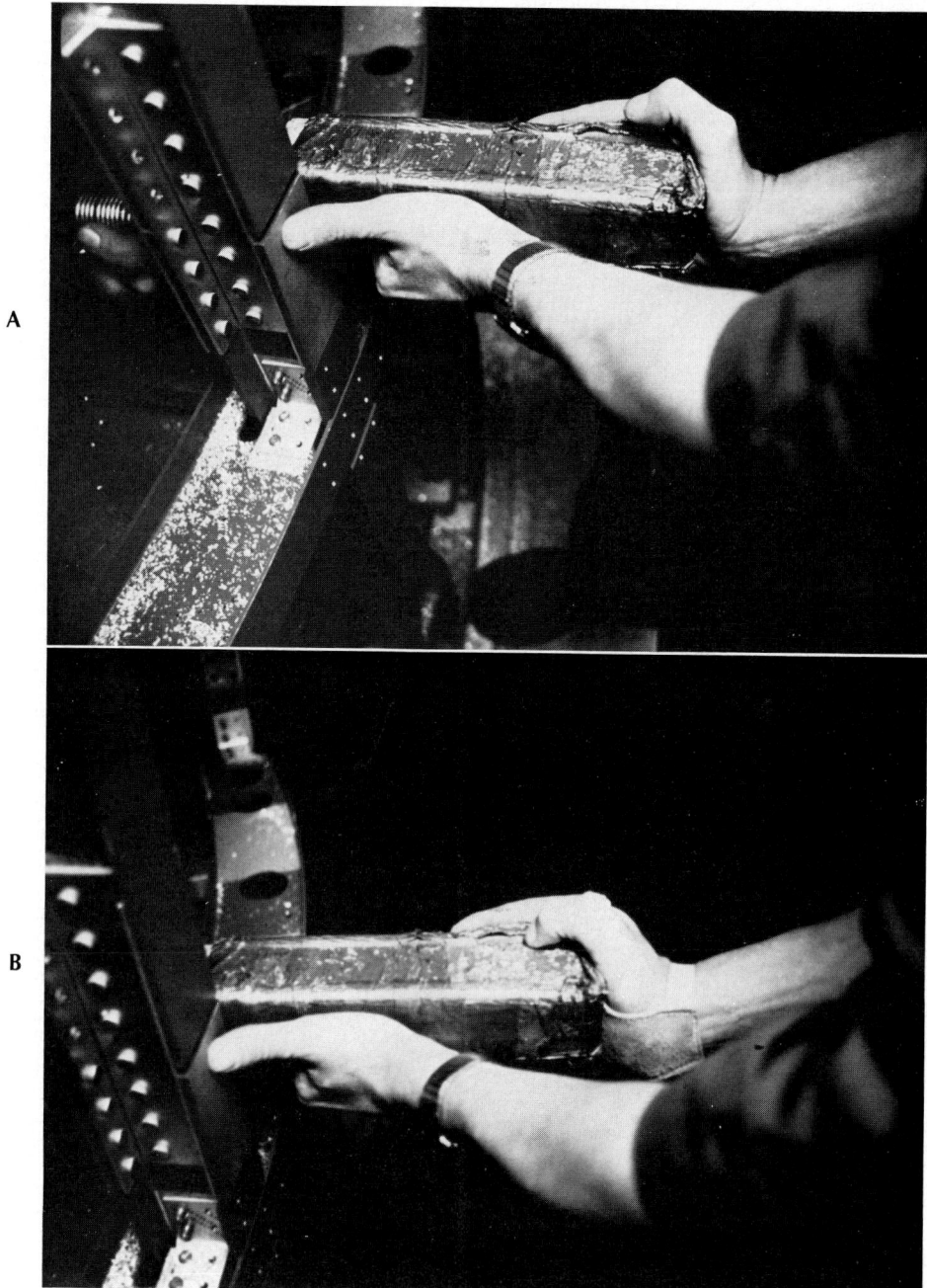

Fig. 104-2   Tool modification to prevent trauma resulting from direct mechanical force. This employee "buckles" rivets for up to 10 hours per day. His job involves holding a metal bar against the surface being secured with rivets. The usual technique is to hold the bar with the carpal tunnel surface against the bar. A partner shoots the rivets through the metal into the bar. **A,** The direct, repetitive pressure on the carpal tunnel increases the potential for carpal tunnel syndrome. **B,** Cushioning the hand with thick gel covered with leather reduces the intensity of the force.

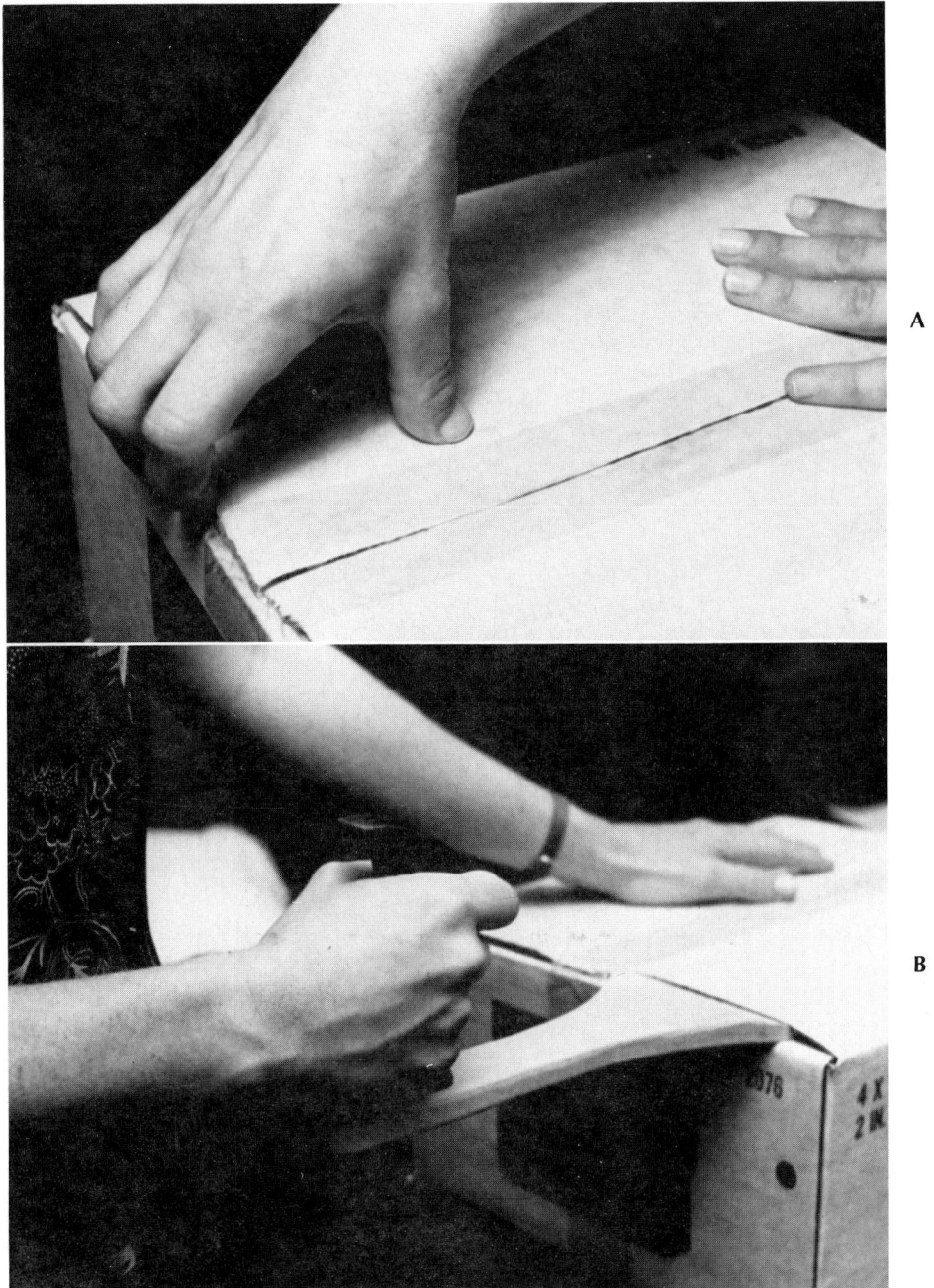

Fig. 104-3 Box opener designed to prevent cumulative trauma. This employee repeatedly opens boxes to check the quality of the contents. **A,** Opening the box tops using the extrinsic flexor muscles. Repeatedly flexing against resistance can potentially irritate the tendons in the carpal canal and the muscles themselves. **B,** The tool transfers the force proximally to the larger muscles of the shoulder. These muscles are less likely to be stressed than the smaller muscles of the forearm.

SUPPORT STAFF

The entire operation of a hand center is greatly dependent on the effectiveness of the supporting office clerical staff. We have found it advantageous to have an office manager directly responsible to the hand surgical and fellowship staff. The office manager is responsible for the coordination of all clerical aspects of the department, including medical secretaries, registrars, and the computer operations of the center. These individuals are usually the first line of communication between the center and those using it.

SPACE AND EQUIPMENT

Space and equipment requirements will vary depending on the needs, demands, and constraints of the institution. Besides the acute care facility, consideration should be given to rehabilitation, microsurgery laboratory, and an inexpensive overnight suite. The equipment will differ from center to center and should reflect the specific needs of that particular center, as well as the ingenuity of those involved.

TRAINING PROGRAMS

Training programs should be incorporated into the center's activities. A residency or fellowship in hand surgery is important if feasible. The hand therapy and work adjustment services will provide internships for students from accredited academic institutions. Where there is teaching, there is excellence of care.

SUMMARY

The hand center is a relatively new and needed phenomenon in the sphere of medicine. It includes the treatment of acute and reconstructive problems while offering the best services for rehabilitation that can be assembled. Quality of care that cannot otherwise be achieved is the goal. It is probable that smaller versions of what has been described can be established. It must be understood that with today's sophisticated knowledge, no one person can offer total care to all of his or her patients.

ACKNOWLEDGMENT

The authors acknowledge with appreciation the assistance of Stanley Berlin, Chief of Work Adjustment Services, and Arlynne Pack, Physical Therapy Coordinator, Center for Industrial Ergonomics, Raymond M. Curtis Hand Center.

Index

Osteophyte, 889
Osteoplastic reconstruction
  radial hemiamputation and, 230
  thumb and, 1028-1030
Osteoporosis
  reflex sympathetic dystrophy and, 764-765
  Sudeck's, 11
Osteotomy
  angulatory, 1001
  elective amputation of digit and, 235
Otto-Beck Greifer, 1079, 1080
Output display for electrographic feedback,
  981
Outrigger
  extension, 947-948
  mechanical properties of, 151
  thumb, 921
Overexertion
  de Quervain's syndrome and, 304-308
  musician and, 1202-1206
  mutilated hand and, 249, 251
Overnight facility, 1231
Overstretching
  nerve injury and, 647
  tendon transfer and, 665-666
Overuse syndrome
  de Quervain's syndrome and, 304-308
  musician and, 1202-1206
Oxybenzamine, 759

P

Pack
  cold
    edema and, 194
    technique of, 208
  hot, 197-198
Packing, wound, 177
Pad
  doughnut, 142
  volar thumb, 1019-1020
Pain
  brachial plexus injury and, 628, 634, 636-
    637
  capsulectomy and, 364
  carpal tunnel syndrome and, 641
  continuous passive motion and, 1142-1143
  cryotherapy and, 206
  de Quervain's syndrome and, 310
  heat and, 196-197
  high-voltage galvanic stimulation and, 215-
    216
  impairment evaluation and, 117-118
  mutilated hand and, 248-249
  myofascial, 731-756
    case studies and, 738-743, 750-755
    evaluation and, 733-738
    historical review and, 731-733
    treatment and, 743-750
  nerve injury and, 9
  nocturnal, 640
  personality and, 757
  referred; see Pain, myofascial
  reflex sympathetic dystrophy and, 764-765,
    780, 788-789
  replantation and, 813
  rheumatoid arthritis and, 905
    thumb and, 898
  transcutaneous electrical nerve stimulation
    and, 793-799
  treatment of, 757-760
  ultrasound and, 205
  work therapy and, 1157
Paint-injection injury, 168
Paleospinothalamic tract, 518
Pallor, 764

Palm
  gunshot wound and, 222
  laceration and, 381, 382
  tendon graft and, 415
Palmar abduction of thumb, 354
  median nerve injury and, 706-707
Palmar bar, 346
Palmar branch of median nerve, 767
Palmar crease, 83
Palmar fascia
  anatomy and, 15
  reflex sympathetic dystrophy and, 765
Palmar flexion in Barton's fracture, 272
Palmar ligament, 322
Palmar pan splint, 879
Palmar plate, rupture of, 484
Palmar sensation, 120
Palmaris longus
  palmar fascia and, 15
  tendon transfer for radial nerve injury and,
    703
Palpation
  rheumatoid arthritis and, 903
  trigger points and, 741
Palsy
  birth, 1003
  brachial plexus and
    elbow and, 626
    postanesthetic, 623
  median and ulnar nerve, 361-362
  posterior interosseous, 656
  radial nerve and
    Saturday night palsy and, 696
    splinting, 653-657
  ulnar nerve and
    electromyography and, 716-718
    splinting and, 649-651
Paper tape, Coban elasticized, 246
Paraffin
  burned hand and, 854
  edema and, 192-194
  heat and, 198-199, 200
  implant arthroplasty and, 926-927
Paralysis
  brachial plexus injury and, 627
  prosthetic devices for, 1015
  tendon graft and, 416
  tendon transfer and, 1008; see also Tendon
    transfer
  radial nerve injury and, 696-704
Paresthesia
  de Quervain's syndrome, 315
  myofascial pain and, 753
  transcutaneous electrical nerve stimulation
    and, 796
Paronychia, self-inflicted, 11
Partial amputation
  finger and, 797
  prosthesis and, 1009-1015
  reconstruction and, 998-1001
  thumb and, 8
    phalanx and, 1018-1020
Partial laceration of flexor tendon, 389, 394-
  395
Partial longitudinal sensory loss, 121
Partial tear of retinacular ligament, 470-471
Partial transverse sensory loss, 120-121
Particles, contact, 723, 726
Passive cosmetic effect, 117
Passive exercise
  brachial plexus injury and, 635-636
  passive tendon implant and, 450
  stiffness and, 321
Passive fist-making, 422
Passive gliding program, 429

Passive motion
  burned hand and, 849
  continuous, 1140-1146
    tendon healing and, 375
  extensor tendon injury and, 498-499, 505-
    509
  fingers and, 87-90
  flexor tendon laceration and, 410-413
  measurement of, 83, 85
  total
    definition of, 65
    measurement techniques for, 83
Passive range of motion
  assessment of, 64-65
  burned hand and, 846-847
  capsulectomy and, 365-366
  chronic stiffness and, 335-336
  Dupuytren's contracture, 876-877, 881
  evaluation for splinting and, 347-347
  measurements of, 153
  median nerve injury and, 707
  muscle flap and, 262
  mutilated hand and, 247
  replantation and, 814, 824, 826
  stiffness and, 329-330
  tendon transfer for median nerve injury and,
    711-712
Passive stretch for mutilated hand, 247
Passive tendon implant
  postoperative therapy and, 445-450, 446-450
  stage I surgery and, 435-441
  stage II surgery and, 441-446
  technique of, 435-450
Patient education, 242-243
Pectoral transfer, 627
Pectoralis major muscle, 976
Pedicled flap, 258-259
Pegs, allograft intramedullary bone, 808
PEMF; see Pulsed electromagnetic field
Percussion
  median nerve and, 46, 48
  neuroma and, 758
Percutaneous injection of neuroma, 758
Perfusion, 381-383
Perilunate dislocation, 275, 276
Perineural infusion, periodic, 775
Perineurium, 525
Periodic perineural infusion, 775
Peripheral nerve; see also Nerve; Nerve injury
  electromyography and, 718
  injury and
    repair and, 515-522
    work therapy and, 1160
  pain and, 758
  replantation and, 822
  testing of, 577
  wound healing and, 242
Peripheral nociceptive stimulus, 758
Peritendinitis crepitans, 304
Peritendinous fascia, 462
Peritendinous fibrosis, Sudeck's, 11
Peritendinous tissue, 665
Permeability
  electrotherapeutic current and, 210
  ultrasound and, 202
Personality and pain, 757, 760
Phagocytic cell
  rheumatoid arthritis and, 885-886
  scar formation and, 181
Phalangization
  metacarpal and, 999
  metacarpophalangeal joint and, 1025
  thumb cleft and, 1005
Phalanx
  aesthetic prosthesis and, 1043